MW01258460

NEWMAN AND CARRANZA'S

CLINICAL PERIODONTOLOGY AND IMPLANTOLOGY

NEWMAN AND CARRANZA'S

CLINICAL PERIODONTOLOGY AND IMPLANTOLOGY

14TH EDITION

MICHAEL G. NEWMAN, DDS, FACD
Professor Emeritus
Periodontics
University of California, Los Angeles School of Dentistry
Los Angeles, California;
Editor-in-Chief
PracticeUpdate Clinical Dentistry
American Dental Association
Chicago, Illinois;
Past President
American Academy of Periodontology
Chicago, Illinois

PERRY R. KLOKKEVOLD, DDS, MS, FACD
Professor of Clinical Dentistry Emeritus
Section of Periodontics
University of California, Los Angeles School of Dentistry
Los Angeles, California;
Private Practice
PermaDent
Torrance, California

SATHEESH ELANGOVAN, BDS, DSc, DMSc
Professor Emeritus
Department of Periodontics
The University of Iowa College of Dentistry and Dental Clinics
Iowa City, Iowa;
Adjunct Professor
Department of Periodontics and Dental Hygiene
University of Texas Health Science Center at Houston School of Dentistry
Houston, Texas

YVONNE L. HERNANDEZ-KAPILA, DDS, PhD
Felix and Mildred Yip Endowed Chair in Dentistry
Professor and Associate Dean for Research
Periodontics, Biosystems and Function
University of California, Los Angeles School of Dentistry
Los Angeles, California

Editors Emeriti

FERMIN A. CARRANZA, DR. ODONT, FACD
Professor Emeritus
Periodontics
University of California, Los Angeles School of Dentistry
Los Angeles, California

HENRY H. TAKEI, DDS, MS
Distinguished Clinical Professor Emeritus
Section of Periodontics
University of California, Los Angeles School of Dentistry;
Consultant
Periodontics
Veterans Administration Hospital Los Angeles
Los Angeles, California

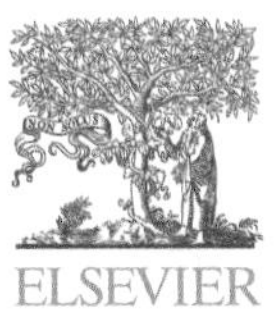

Elsevier
3251 Riverport Lane
St. Louis, Missouri 63043

NEWMAN AND CARRANZA'S CLINICAL PERIODONTOLOGY AND IMPLANTOLOGY, FOURTEENTH EDITION
ISBN: 978-0-323-87887-6

Content Strategist: Lauren Boyle
Director, Content Development: Ellen Wurm-Cutter
Publishing Services Manager: Julie Eddy
Senior Project Manager: Rachel E. McMullen
Design Direction: Brian Salisbury

Printed in Canada

Last digit is the print number: 9 8 7 6 5 4 3 2 1

ABOUT THE AUTHORS

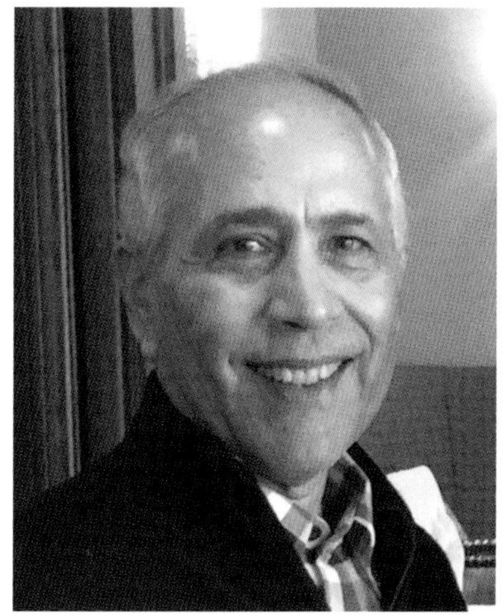

Michael G. Newman, DDS, FACD

Dr. Newman is the Editor in Chief of Elsevier and the American Dental Association PracticeUpdate Clinical Dentistry Channel and he is the Editor in Chief of the following two first edition textbooks: *Newman and Carranza's Clinical Periodontology for Dental Hygienists* and *Newman and Carranza's Essentials of Clinical Periodontology—An Integrated Study Companion*.

Dr. Newman graduated from the University of California, Los Angeles (UCLA), College of Letters and Sciences with a degree in psychology. He completed his dental training at the UCLA School of Dentistry in 1972. He received a Certificate in Periodontics and Oral Medicine at the Harvard School of Dental Medicine and a Certificate in Oral Microbiology from the Forsyth Dental Institute under the mentorship of Dr. Sigmund Socransky. He is a Diplomate of the American Board of Periodontology and Professor Emeritus at the UCLA School of Dentistry. He is a fellow and Past President of the American Academy of Periodontology. In 1975, he won the Balint Orban Memorial Prize from the American Academy of Periodontology. He has been in private practice of periodontics for more than 25 years. In 2007, he received the Gold Medal, the highest honor bestowed by the American Academy of Periodontology. He has published more than 260 abstracts, journal articles, and book chapters and has co-edited nine textbooks. He has served as an ad-hoc reviewer for the National Institute of Dental and Craniofacial Research, was a consultant to the Council on Scientific Affairs of the American Dental Association and is a reviewer for numerous scientific and professional journals and governmental research organizations. He was a founding Board Member of the McGuire Institute in Houston, Texas.

Professor Newman has lectured throughout the world to both dentists' and dental hygienists' audiences. Topics include: microbiology, antimicrobials, evidence-based methodology, risk factors, diagnostic strategies for periodontal disease, clinical outcomes assessments, real world evidence, and big data analytics. He has a strong interest in applied science and the transfer of new technology for practical use. He is a co-author of the first online digital app simulation on a periodontal procedure at Medtronic Touch Surgery. Dr. Newman is a consultant to major dental and pharmaceutical companies throughout the world. He is the Founding Editor-in-Chief Emeritus of the *Journal of Evidence-Based Dental Practice* (JEBDP) and was the Associate Editor of the *International Journal of Oral and Maxillofacial Implants*.

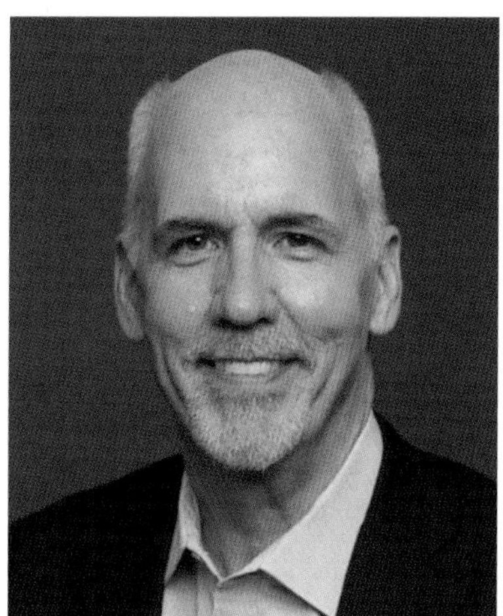

Perry R. Klokkevold, DDS, MS, FACD

Dr. Perry R. Klokkevold attended the University of California, Los Angeles (UCLA), College of Letters and Sciences majoring in Mathematics/Computer Science and Microbiology. He completed his dental education and training at the University of California, San Francisco (UCSF) School of Dentistry where he received his Bachelor of Science and Doctor of Dental Surgery degrees in 1986. He completed multiple postgraduate clinical training and postdoctoral education programs at UCLA School of Dentistry including the Hospital Dentistry General Practice Residency in 1987, the Postgraduate Periodontics Residency in 1994, the Surgical Implant Fellowship in 1995, and the Oral Biology Master of Science degree in 1995.

Dr. Klokkevold is a Diplomate of the American Board of Periodontology and a Fellow of the American College of Dentists. He is Professor of Clinical Dentistry Emeritus in the Division of Regenerative and Reconstructive Sciences, Section of Periodontics, at the UCLA School of Dentistry and served as Clinical Director (1995–2002) and Program Director (2002–2022) for the UCLA Postgraduate Periodontics and Implant Surgery Residency program. He previously served as Clinical Director (1987–1990) and Program Director (1990–1992) for the UCLA Hospital Dentistry General Practice Residency program. He practiced all aspects of general dentistry while in Hospital Dentistry (1987–1992). Since completing his advanced clinical training in 1995, his practice has been limited to the specialty of periodontics and dental implant surgery. He served as President of the California Society of Periodontists for two terms in 2021 and 2022.

Dr. Klokkevold has published more than 70 articles for international peer-reviewed journals and has written more than 125 book chapters for 14 textbooks including five editions of *Clinical Periodontology* on topics ranging from periodontal medicine, influence of systemic disease, and risk factors on periodontitis to bone regeneration and dental implants. He has served as a reviewer for several journals, including the *Journal of Periodontology* and the *International Journal of Oral and Maxillofacial Implants*. He has lectured nationally and internationally on many periodontal and implant-related topics. He has been invited to serve as an expert consultant and reviewer for five major International Conferences organized by the American Academy of Periodontology and the Academy of Osseointegration on topics ranging from Implant Therapy, Bone Augmentation, and Implant Site Development to Periodontal Regeneration and Lasers in Periodontal Therapy.

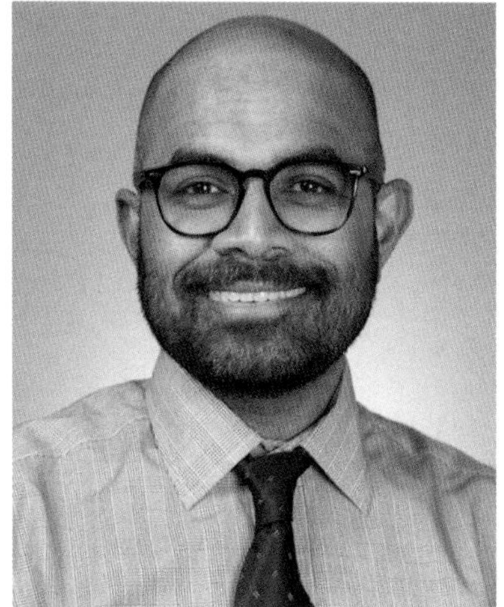

Satheesh Elangovan, BDS, DSc, DMSc

Dr. Satheesh Elangovan completed his dental training from Tamil Nadu Dr. MGR Medical University, India. He subsequently received a Doctor of Science degree from Boston University and combined Doctor of Medical Science degree in Oral Biology and a certificate in Periodontology from Harvard University. He is a Diplomate of the American Board of Periodontology and is a fellow of the International College of Dentists and the American College of Dentists. He is currently Professor Emeritus in the Department of Periodontics at the University of Iowa College of Dentistry and Dental Clinics. In addition, he serves as an Adjunct Professor in the Department of Periodontics and Dental Hygiene at the UT Health Houston School of Dentistry. His research focuses on biomaterials and bone tissue engineering, and evidence-based dentistry. He has published or presented more than 150 articles, abstracts, multimedia contributions, and book chapters. He has received several national honors and awards in the past, for his teaching and research efforts. He has served on the Editorial Board of the *Journal of Dental Education* and served as an Associate Editor for the 13th Edition of this textbook, for which he also served as an Online Editor. In addition, he is an Editor of the following two first edition textbooks: *Newman and Carranza's Clinical Periodontology for Dental Hygienists* and *Newman and Carranza's Essentials of Clinical Periodontology—An Integrated Study Companion*. He is currently an Associate Editor of the American Dental Association's PracticeUpdate Clinical Dentistry channel.

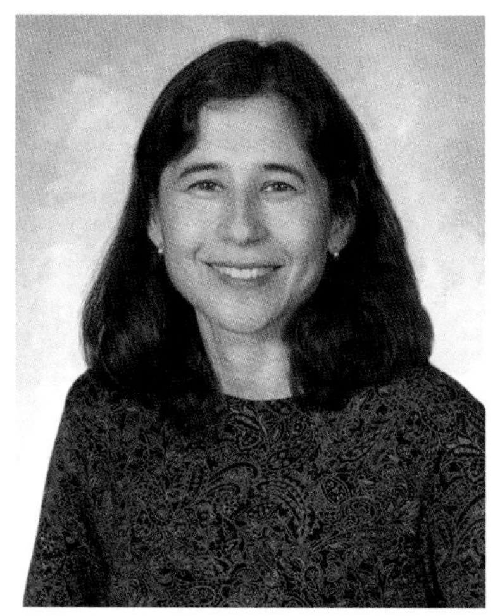

Yvonne L. Hernandez-Kapila, DDS, PhD

Dr. Yvonne L. Hernandez-Kapila graduated from Stanford University with a bachelor's degree in Human Biology. She then completed her dental and graduate training at the University of California San Francisco (UCSF) where she received a Bachelor of Science, Doctor of Dental Surgery, Certificate in Periodontology, Doctor of Philosophy, and Post-Doctoral training. She is a Diplomate of the American Board of Periodontology, a fellow of the American College of Dentists, a fellow of the International College of Dentists, and an ELAM (Executive Leadership in Academic Medicine) Fellow.

She has served as a full-time Professor in academia for 25 years at UCSF, University of Michigan, and currently at UCLA. She has held several leadership positions, including the Inaugural Director of Global Initiatives at the University of Michigan School of Dentistry and leadership roles in the American Academy of Periodontology, including the Chair of the Research Submissions Committee. She has served as Chair of Periodontology at UCSF where she concurrently held the R. Earl Robinson Distinguished Professor of Periodontology. She is currently the Associate Dean for Research at the UCLA School of Dentistry.

She is an internationally recognized expert on periodontal disease pathogenesis, oral cancer carcinogenesis, perio-systemic disease relationships with a special focus on oral cancer, host-microbe interactions, the oral microbiome, oral biofilm biology, and antimicrobial-based therapeutics. She has authored over 140 peer-reviewed publications in such journals as *Biochimica et Biophysica Acta Cancer Reviews, Cell Death and Differentiation, Cancer, Molecular Biology of the Cell, Journal of Proteome Research, Journal of Biological Chemistry, Genes and Cancer, PLOS Pathogens, NPJ Biofilms and Microbiomes,* and *Journal of Controlled Release*. She has been continuously funded by the National Institutes of Health (NIH) for over 25 years. She serves on the Editorial Board of the journal *Scientific Reports* and *International Journal of Oral Science*, and as Editor to a Volume of *Periodontology 2000* on Special Populations in 2021.

Her innovative research studies have been recognized with several major research awards: In 1997, she was awarded the prestigious American Association for Dental Research (AADR) Edward H. Hatton Award and the American Academy of Periodontology (AAP) Balint Orban Award; The International Association for Dental Research (IADR) GSK Innovation in Oral Care

Award in 2014, the UCSF Chancellor's Mid-Career Faculty Award in 2016, the AAP Sunstar Innovation Research Award in 2017, and the AAP Distinguished Scientist Award in 2019. She was selected to give the Annual Research Lecture for the UCSF School of Dentistry Research and Clinical Excellence Day in 2019. In 2021, she received the UCSF Alumni Discovery Award and in 2022 the UCSF Alumni Medal of Honor.

Over the course of her career, she has mentored over 100 PhD, DDS, DDS/PhD, MD, Masters, and undergraduate students with a focus on diversity and inclusion. She was recognized several times at the University of Michigan at the campus-wide level with mentoring awards and she received national recognition for her mentoring contributions, including receiving the prestigious national American Association for Dental Research Irwin D. Mandel Distinguished Mentoring Award in 2019.

She serves her local and national community in several capacities. Nationally, she served on the NIH Oral Dental and Craniofacial Sciences (ODCS) study section for many years, the National Institute of Dental and Craniofacial Research (NIDCR) council as a standing member, and currently she serves on the National Cancer Institute (NCI) and NIDCR on special emphasis panels.

PREFACE

To view the following videos, please visit the companion website at eBooks.Health.Elsevier.com.
Overview of the 14th Edition: Perry R. Klokkevold
Introduction to *Clinical Periodontology and Implantology:* Henry H. Takei

With the help of Elsevier's advanced technology and high standards of quality, a recognized team of editors, contributors, and production staff have developed the most comprehensive periodontal resource ever created. This body of work represents the fundamental knowledge base of the profession providing readers an important digitally accessible information resource.

Since publication of the first edition of the parent *Clinical Periodontology* book in 1953, periodontology has made tremendous advancements. Scientific analysis of periodontal tissues and the elucidation of mechanisms and causes of disease have extended far beyond histology and physiology into the realm of cellular and molecular biologic understanding.

Importantly, oral health, especially periodontal health, is now an integral part of overall systemic health. Precision medicine explicitly incorporates periodontal health considerations and the bidirectional influence of periodontal and systemic health.

The patient is the focus of prevention and therapeutic goals and recent advances in patient reported outcomes allows the clinician to assess the patients' feelings and how their functions improve from the rendered treatment. *Newman and Carranza's Clinical Periodontology and Implantology,* 14th edition, is the first textbook in the field that includes background on this important aspect of integrated health care.

Implant dentistry has become a major component of periodontology, and this book offers a wide coverage of important treatment modalities that are relevant to the practice of dentistry. Digital technology is now an integral part of implant treatment, and this edition provides coverage of many essential topics and techniques. Basic and advanced topics are covered with informative illustrations, videos, and insights from leading clinicians.

This new edition is rich with images, animations and videos (marked with ▶ throughout the text), question sets, case reports, PowerPoint slides, audio slides, a virtual microscope, multidisciplinary case scenarios, and more. No other resource offers such a comprehensive approach to providing high-quality content for dental students and clinicians alike. The addition of images and video from PerioPixel company throughout the resource has been an important contribution to learning. With the interactive glossary, the readers can learn terminologies and definitions as they go through the text.

New therapeutic goals and clinical techniques, based on an improved understanding of disease and healing, have facilitated better outcomes and brought us closer to achieving the ultimate goal of optimal periodontal health and function. Today, reconstruction and regeneration of lost periodontal structures, replacement of compromised teeth with implants, and creation of esthetic results are integral parts of clinical practice.

The multifaceted, complex task of producing a major resource required the collaboration of numerous experts from various fields, and their contributions are invaluable. We know that this edition will be an essential part of the continuous progress of our profession.

ABOUT THE ONLINE RESOURCES

Newman and Carranza's Clinical Periodontology and Implantology, 14th edition, is the most definitive and advanced global reference text and information portal in periodontics. No other resource offers such a comprehensive approach to providing high-quality content ranging from foundational knowledge to advanced clinical procedures in periodontics. Implant dentistry is a major component of periodontology, and this book offers a wide coverage of important implant treatment modalities.

This edition has:

- a unifying view of the basic information related to the science and technology of modern periodontics
- essential core information of periodontology and state-of-the-art methods in both the science and clinical knowledge base
- seamless integration of basic science and the clinical management of periodontal diseases and conditions
- a much-improved online resource, including better speed, quality, functionality, access, and connectivity
- more high-quality and realistic animations, videos, and case reports
- one of the most comprehensive image libraries on periodontal pathology ever assembled
- new case scenarios that offer readers the opportunity to challenge their knowledge of integrated information for better learning and exam preparation
- a print book and companion website that is rich with images, animations, question sets, PowerPoint slides, audio slides, virtual microscope and more.

This integrated learning and information resource has always emphasized science as the cornerstone of good treatment. Since publication of the first edition of this book in 1953, periodontology has made tremendous advancements. Scientific analysis of periodontal tissues and the elucidation of mechanisms and etiology of disease have transcended far beyond histology and physiology into the realm of understanding processes at the cellular and molecular level.

Learning a clinical discipline involves many components that have to come together in order to deliver optimal clinical care. Conceptual knowledge, facts, data, terminology, and evidence are required so that problem solving, clinical decision-making, and clinical reasoning can be accomplished. These elements provide the foundation for the development of good diagnostic and procedural skills (Fig. 1). Knowing why, when, and what to do is as important as the physical performance of the procedure. Understanding when a procedure is not indicated is equally important.

Terminology is a critical part of learning, communication, and keeping up to date. This edition expands the complete and updated Glossary and makes it more usable. To enhance reader experience, many terms within the text of each chapter are connected to the glossary and will appear as pop-ups to provide readers with instant access to information and definitions.

Modern periodontology embraces scientific advancement and more rapid technology transfer is emerging whereby artificial intelligence systems will become an important part of clinical practice. The electronic dental record is the central hub of practice, integrating all aspects of the patient's overall health and current status. Precision medicine and dentistry will soon be incorporated into routine care. It is also the place where technology is accessed and used to improve communications with the patient via teledentistry and patient management tools. In this edition, we are introducing these novel concepts and will be an underlying thread in several chapters, making it a unique resource in dentistry.

The 14th edition is truly transformational. It fully utilizes the current information technology tools to effectively engage the learner, while maintaining and refining its decades of educational excellence.

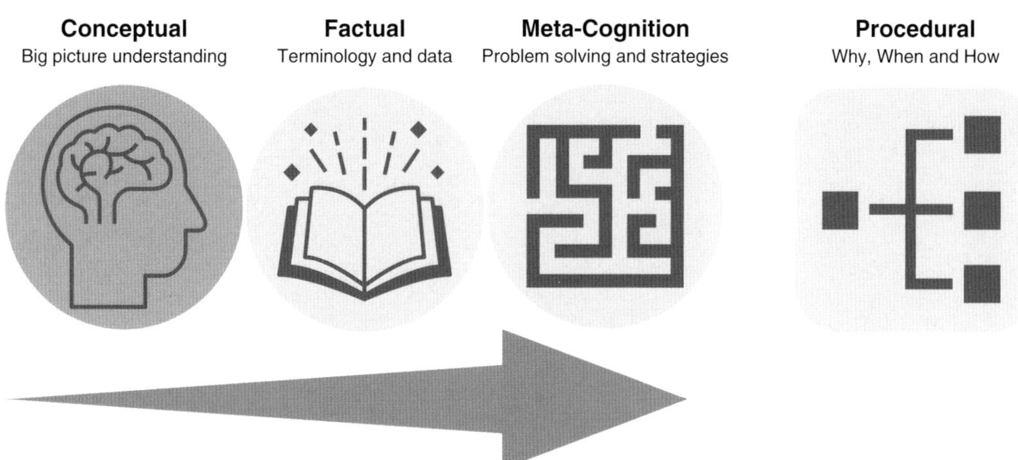

Fig. 1 Elements of learning a clinical discipline. Starting on the left with understanding the goals of treatment (conceptual and factual) to using the acquired information to solve clinical problems (meta-cognition). Once the supporting information is obtained, clinical reasoning can be acquired. Finally, on the right, the actual physical procedure can be learned, practiced, and mastered.

ACKNOWLEDGMENTS

We express our deep gratitude to all those contributors whose expertise, ideas, and efforts built the original book/resource over the years. Many scientists and clinicians have shared their wisdom and expertise in previous editions as associate editors, section editors, and contributors, though some of their names no longer appear.

Special mention of thanks goes to Dr. Ion Zabalegui and PerioPixel company for their extensive effort to provide rich and beautiful illustrations and videos throughout the resource.

Our appreciation goes to Elsevier and particularly to Joslyn Dumas, Lauren Boyle, and Beth LoGiudice. Their expertise and detailed attention to every word and every concept contributed greatly to producing a quality book and a resourceful online component.

CONTRIBUTORS

Alfredo Aguirre, DDS, MS
Professor
Oral Diagnostic Sciences
School of Dental Medicine, University at Buffalo
The State University of New York
Buffalo, New York

Edward P. Allen, DD, PhD
Private Practice
Dallas, Texas

Rana Alshagroud, DS, MS
Assistant Professor
Oral Medicine and Diagnostic Science
King Saud University
Riyadh, Saudi Arabia

Gustavo Avila-Ortiz, DDS, PhD, MS
Private Practice
Atelier Dental Madrid
Madrid, Spain;
Visiting Professor
Department of Oral Medicine, Infection, and Immunity
Harvard School of Dental Medicine
Boston, Massachusetts

Robert R. Azzi, DDS
Department of Periodontology
University of Paris, VII
Paris, France

Adam Barsoum, BDS, DMD, Certificate Periodontics and Oral Implantology
Adjunct Clinical Assistant Professor
Ashman Department of Periodontics and Implant Dentistry
New York University College of Dentistry
New York, New York

Christopher A. Barwacz, DDS, FACD, FAGD
Associate Professor and Department Chair (DEO)
Department of Family Dentistry
The University of Iowa
Iowa City, Iowa

Seyed Hossein Bassir, DDS, DMSc
Private Practice
Los Angeles, California

Marco Bergamini, DDS
Ashman Department of Periodontology and Implant Dentistry
New York University College of Dentistry
New York, New York

Beatriz Bezerra, DDS, PhD
Assistant Clinical Professor
Section of Periodontics
University of California, Los Angeles School of Dentistry
Los Angeles, California

Lucy Bickett, BA, MJur
Program Manager
Dental Informatics
Indiana University School of Dentistry
Indianapolis, Indiana

Mitchell J. Bloom, DMD
Clinical Associate Professor
Ashman Department of Periodontology and Implant Dentistry
New York University College of Dentistry;
Private Practice
Periodontology and Implant Dentistry
New York, New York

Paulo M. Camargo, DDS, MS, MBA, FACD
Professor of Periodontics
Section of Periodontics
University of California, Los Angeles School of Dentistry
Los Angeles, California

Fermin A. Carranza, Dr. Odont, FACD
Professor Emeritus
Section of Periodontics
University of California, Los Angeles School of Dentistry
Los Angeles, California

Frank Celenza, DDS, Cert Periodontology, Cert Orthodontics
Associate Clinical Professor
Post Graduate Orthodontics and Periodontics
Rutgers University School of Dental Medicine
Newark, New Jersey;
Private Practice
New York, New York

Leandro Chambrone, DDS, MSc, PhD
Associate Professor
Evidence-Based Hub
Centro de Investigação Interdisciplinar Egas Moniz
Egas Moniz-Cooperativa de Ensino Superior
Caparica, Almada, Portugal

Ting-Ling Chang, DDS
Clinical Professor
Division of Regenerative and Reconstructive Sciences
University of California, Los Angeles School of Dentistry
Los Angeles, California

Yu-Cheng Chang, DDS, MS, DMD
Assistant Professor
Periodontics
University of Pennsylvania
Philadelphia, Pennsylvania

Denny Chao, DMD
Assistant Clinical Professor
Division of Regenerative and Reconstructive Sciences
University of California, Los Angeles School of Dentistry
Los Angeles, California

Sang Choon Cho, DDS
Clinical Associate Professor
Director, International Programs of Implant Dentistry
New York University
New York, New York

Yong-Hee Patricia Chun, DDS, Med Dent, MS, PhD, Dr
Associate Professor
Periodontics
University of Texas Health Science Center at San Antonio
San Antonio, Texas

Evelyn Chung, DDS
Clinical Professor
Division of Advanced Prosthodontics
University of California, Los Angeles School of Dentistry
Los Angeles, California

Daniel R. Clark, DDS, MS, PhD
Assistant Professor
Department of Periodontics and Preventive Dentistry
University of Pittsburgh School of Dental Medicine
Pittsburgh, Pennsylvania

Charles M. Cobb, DDS, MS, PhD
Professor Emeritus
Periodontics
University of Missouri-Kansas City
Kansas City, Missouri

David L. Cochran, DDS, PhD, MMSci
Professor and Chair
Periodontics
School of Dentistry
University of Texas Health Science Center at San Antonio
San Antonio, Texas

Joseph P. Cooney, BDS, MS
Clinical Professor Emeritus
Restorative Dentistry
University of California, Los Angeles
Los Angeles, California

Russell J. Crocket, DMD
Assistant Professor of Prosthodontics
Arizona School of Dentistry & Oral Health
A.T. Still University
Mesa, Arizona

J. David Cross, DDS
Private Practice of Microsurgical Periodontics and Dental Implants
Springfield, Illinois

Jesica Dadamio, PhD, MSc
Doctor in Biomedical Sciences
Oral Health Sciences, Periodontology Section
Katholieke Universiteit Leuven
Leuven, Belgium

Ann Decker, DMD, PhD
Assistant Professor
Periodontics and Oral Medicine
University of Michigan School of Dentistry
Ann Arbor, Michigan

Christel Dekeyser, DDS, MSc
Clinical Head of Periodontology Section
Oral Health Sciences, Periodontology Section
Katholieke Universiteit Leuven
Leuven, Belgium

Scott R. Diehl, BS, PhD
Professor
Department of Oral Biology
Rutgers School of Dental Medicine;
Professor
Department of Health Informatics
Rutgers School of Health Professions
Newark, New Jersey

Kimon Divaris, DDS, PhD
Associate Professor
Pediatric Dentistry
School of Dentistry
University of North Carolina-Chapel Hill;
Associate Professor
Epidemiology
Gillings School of Global Public Health
University of North Carolina-Chapel Hill
Chapel Hill, North Carolina

Jonathan H. Do, DDS
Assistant Clinical Professor
Section of Periodontics
University of California, Los Angeles School of Dentistry
Los Angeles, California;
Private Practice
San Diego, California

Henrik Dommisch, DDS, PhD
Professor and Chairman
Periodontology, Oral Medicine and Oral Surgery
Charité—Universitätsmedizin Berlin
Berlin, Germany;
Affiliate Professor
Periodontology
University of Washington
Seattle, Washington

Irina F. Dragan, DDS, DMD, MS
Associate Professor
Periodontology
Tufts University
Boston, Massachusetts;
Periodontist
Brookline Periodontal Associates
Brookline, Massachusetts

Satheesh Elangovan, BDS, DSc, DMSc
Professor Emeritus
Department of Periodontics
The University of Iowa College of Dentistry and Dental Clinics
Iowa City, Iowa;
Adjunct Professor
Department of Periodontics and Dental Hygiene
University of Texas Health Science Center at Houston School of Dentistry
Houston, Texas

Grace Gomez Felix Gomez, BDS, MPH, PhD
Postdoctoral Researcher
Dental Informatics
Indiana University School of Dentistry
Indianapolis, Indiana

Magda Feres, DDS, MSc, DMSc
Department of Oral Medicine, Infection and Immunity
Harvard School of Dental Medicine
Boston, Massachusetts

Richard D. Finkelman, DDS, PhD
Senior Medical Director, Clinical Sciences
Rare Genetics & Hematology Therapeutic Area
Takeda Development Center Americas, Inc.
Cambridge, Massachusetts

Joseph P. Fiorellini, DMD, DMSc
Professor
Periodontics
Penn Dental Medicine
Philadelphia, Pennsylvania

Jane L. Forrest, BSDH, MS, EdD
Professor Emerita of Clinical Dentistry
Dental Public Health & Pediatric Dentistry
University of Southern California;
Director
National Center for Dental Hygiene Research & Practice, Inc.
Los Angeles, California

Marcelo Freire, DDS, PhD, DMedSc
Associate Professor
Genomic Medicine, Infectious Diseases
J. Craig Venter Institute
University California, San Diego
La Jolla, California

Scott H. Froum, DDS
Clinical Assistant Professor
Periodontology
SUNY Stony Brook School of Dental Medicine
Stony Brook, New York

Stuart J. Froum, DDS
Clinical Adjunct Professor and Director of Clinical Research
Ashman Department of Periodontology and Implant Dentistry
New York University College of Dentistry
New York, New York

Sukirth M. Ganesan, BDS, PhD
Assistant Professor and Graduate Program Director
Department of Periodontics
The University of Iowa College of Dentistry and Dental Clinics
Iowa City, Iowa

Mark David Gidley, BSc (Hons), PhD, BDS (Hons)
Clinical Lecturer
School of Dental Sciences
Newcastle University
Newcastle upon Tyne, United Kingdom

Ying Gu, DDS, PhD
Professor and Chair
General Dentistry
SUNY Stony Brook School of Dental Medicine
Stony Brook, New York

George Hajishengallis, DDS, PhD
Thomas W. Evans Centennial Professor
Basic and Translational Sciences
University of Pennsylvania
Philadelphia, Pennsylvania

Thomas J. Han, DDS, MS, FACD
Clinical Professor
Periodontics
Herman Ostrow School of Dentistry
University of Southern California
Los Angeles, California

M. Cenk Haytac, PhD
Professor
Periodontology
Cukurova University
Adana, Turkey

James E. Hinrichs, DDS, MS
Professor in Periodontology
Developmental and Surgical Sciences
University of Minnesota School of Dentistry
Minneapolis, Minnesota

Richard Holliday, BDS, M Perio RCSEd, FDS (Rest Dent) RCSEd, PhD
Senior Lecturer and Honorary Consultant in Restorative Dentistry
School of Dental Sciences
Faculty of Medical Sciences
Newcastle University
Newcastle upon Tyne, United Kingdom

Philippe P. Hujoel, DDS, MS, MSD, PhD
Professor
Oral Health Sciences & Epidemiology
University of Washington
Seattle, Washington

Mohammed Husain, DDS
Associate Clinical Professor and Residency Program Director
Section of Oral and Maxillofacial Radiology
University of California, Los Angeles School of Dentistry
Los Angeles, California

Carol A. Jahn, RDH, MS
Director Professional Relations & Educator
Marketing
Water Pik, Inc.
Fort Collins, Colorado

Nicholas S. Jakubovics, BSc, PhD
Senior Lecturer in Oral Microbiology
Centre for Oral Health Research, School of Dental Sciences
Newcastle University
Newcastle upon Tyne, United Kingdom

Stephen John, DDS
Private Practice
San Mateo, California

Mo K. Kang, DDS, PhD
Professor and Chair
Endodontics
University of California, Los Angeles School of Dentistry
Los Angeles, California

Alpdogan Kantarci, DDS, PhD, CAGS
Senior Member of Staff/Professor
Applied Oral Sciences
Forsyth Institute
Cambridge, Massachusetts

Richard T. Kao, DDS, PhD
Clinical Professor
Department of Orofacial Sciences
University of California, San Francisco
San Francisco, California

Yvonne L. Hernandez-Kapila, DDS, PhD
Felix and Mildred Yip Endowed Chair in Dentistry
Professor and Associate Dean for Research
Periodontics, Biosystems and Function
University of California, Los Angeles School of Dentistry
Los Angeles, California

Moritz Kebschull, Dr. Med Dent, Dr. Med Dent Habil. MBA
Chair of Restorative Dentistry
University of Birmingham School of Dentistry
Birmingham, United Kingdom

David M. Kim, DDS, DMSc
Associate Professor
Oral Medicine, Infection and Immunity
Harvard School of Dental Medicine
Boston, Massachusetts

Keith L. Kirkwood, DDS, PhD
Professor and Senior Associate Dean for Research
Oral Biology
School of Dental Medicine
The University at Buffalo, State University of New York
Buffalo, New York

Perry R. Klokkevold, DDS, MS, FACD
Professor of Clinical Dentistry Emeritus
Section of Periodontics
University of California, Los Angeles School of Dentistry
Los Angeles, California;
Private Practice
PermaDent
Torrance, California

Vincent G. Kokich, DDS, MSD†
Department of Orthodontics
School of Dentistry
University of Washington
Seattle, Washington

Olga A. Korczeniewska, PhD
Assistant Professor
Department of Diagnostic Sciences
Rutgers School of Dental Medicine
Newark, New Jersey

Georgios A. Kotsakis, DDS, MS
Associate Professor of Periodontics & Roland Meffert Endowed Scholar
University of Texas Health Science Center at San Antonio
San Antonio, Texas;
Affiliate Associate Professor
Global Health
University of Washington
Seattle, Washington

Jill Marie Kramer, DDS, PhD
Associate Professor
Oral Biology
The University at Buffalo, The State University of New York
Buffalo, New York

Purnima S. Kumar, DDS, PhD
Najjar Professor of Dentistry and Chair
Department of Periodontics and Oral Medicine
University of Michigan School of Dentistry
Ann Arbor, Michigan

Chun-Teh Lee, DDS, MS, DMSc
Associate Professor
Periodontics and Dental Hygiene
The University of Texas Health Science Center at Houston School of Dentistry
Houston, Texas

†Deceased.

Shuning Li, PhD
Assistant Research Scientist
Department of Cardiology, Operative Dentistry & Dental Public Health
Indiana University School of Dentistry
Indianapolis, Indiana

Guo-Hao Lin, DDS, MS
Associate Professor
Department of Orofacial Sciences
University of California, San Francisco
San Francisco, California

Kevin W. Luan, BDS, MS, MEd
Chief of Periodontics
Northwestern Dental Center;
Clinical Associate Professor
Department of Periodontics
University of Illinois at Chicago College of Dentistry.;
Private Practice
Chicago, Illinois

Yasmin Mair, BDS, MS
Assistant Professor
Oral Diagnostic Sciences
Faculty of Dentistry
King Abdulaziz University
Jeddah, Saudi Arabia

Sanjay M. Mallya, BDS, MDS, PhD
Professor and Chair
Section of Oral & Maxillofacial Radiology
University of California, Los Angeles School of Dentistry
Los Angeles, California

Deborah Mancinelli-Lyle, RDH, BS, MS
CEO
Research & Strategy
Scientific Dental Consulting, LLC
Morris Plains, New Jersey

Julie Teresa Marchesan, DDS, PhD
Assistant Professor
Adams School of Dentistry, Comprehensive Health
University of North Carolina at Chapel Hill
Chapel Hill, North Carolina

Angelo Mariotti, BS, DDS, PhD
Professor and Chair
Periodontology
The Ohio State University
Columbus, Ohio

Conchita Martín, DDS, PhD
Professor
Orthodontics
Faculty of Odontology
Complutense University of Madrid
Madrid, Spain

April Guadalupe Martinez, BS
Periodontology Resident
Periodontology Department
University of California, San Francisco
San Francisco, California

Michael J. McDevitt, DDS
Visiting Faculty
Periodontics
Dental College of Georgia
Augusta, Georgia;
Visiting Faculty
L.D. Pankey Institute
Key Biscayne, Florida;
Contributing Faculty
Online Learning
Spear
Scottsdale, Arizona;
Private Practice (Periodontics)
Atlanta, Georgia

Adriana McGregor, DDS
Private Practice of Microsurgical Periodontics and Dental Implants
Thousand Oaks, California

Brian L. Mealey, DDS, MS
Clinical Professor
Department of Periodontics
University of Texas Health Science Center at San Antonio
San Antonio, Texas

Philip R. Melnick, DMD, FACD
Continuing Lecturer
Section of Periodontics and Implant Surgery
University of California, Los Angeles School of Dentistry
Los Angeles, California

Robert L. Merin, DDS, MS
Lecturer, Retired
University of California, Los Angeles School of Dentistry
Los Angeles, California;
Past President
California Society of Periodontists;
Board Director
California Dental Society of Anesthesia
Calabasas, California

Shebli Mehrazarin, DDS, PhD
Private Practice
Chicago, Illinois

Greg W. Miller, DDS
Private Practice
General Dentistry
Deer Park, Washington

Joseph M. Miller, PhD
Division of Integrative Anatomy
Department of Pathology and Laboratory Medicine
University of California, Los Angeles David Geffen School of Medicine
Los Angeles, California

Syrene A. Miller, MSW
Project Manager
National Center for Dental Hygiene Research
Cave Creek, Arizona

Reeva Mincer, DDS
Lecturer
Division of Regenerative and Reconstructive Sciences
University of California, Los Angeles School of Dentistry
Los Angeles, California

Julie Mitchell, DDS, MS
Private Practice
Boston, Massachusetts

Srinivas Myneni, BDS, MS, PhD
Assistant Professor
Periodontology;
Director of Periodontal Research
Periodontology;
SUNY Stony Brook School of Dental Medicine
Stony Brook, New York

Radhakrishnan Nagarajan, PhD
Director
Center for Oral and Systemic Health
Marshfield Clinic Research Institute
Marshfield Clinic Health System
Marshfield, Wisconsin

Ian Needleman, BDS, MSc, PhD, MRDRCS(Eng), FDSRCS(Eng), FFPH, FHEA
Professor of Periodontology and Evidence-Informed Healthcare
Periodontology
UCL Eastman Dental Institute
London, United Kingdom

Michael G. Newman, DDS, FACD
Professor Emeritus
Periodontics
University of California, Los Angeles School of Dentistry
Los Angeles, California;
Editor-in-Chief
PracticeUpdate Clinical Dentistry
American Dental Association
Chicago, Illinois;
Past President
American Academy of Periodontology
Chicago, Illinois

Karen F. Novak, DDS, MS, PhD
Clinical Professor
Department of Periodontics and Dental Hygiene;
Special Assistant to the Dean
School of Dentistry
University of Texas Health Science Center at Houston
Houston, Texas

Joan Otomo-Corgel, DDS, MPH
Clinical Professor
Periodontics
University of California, Los Angeles School of Dentistry;
Faculty
Greater Los Angeles VA Healthcare System—Dental Service
Veterans Administration Medical Center;
Partner
Perio Implant Health Professionals
Los Angeles, California

Kwang-Bum Park
CEO
MegaGen
Daegu, Republic of Korea

Anna M. Pattison, BS, MS
Co-Director
Pattison Institute;
Former Associate Professor and Chair
Dental Hygiene
Herman Ostrow School of Dentistry
University of Southern California
Los Angeles, California

Gordon L. Pattison, DDS
Former Assistant Professor
Periodontology
University of California, Los Angeles School of Dentistry
Los Angeles, California

Flavia Q. Pirih, PhD. DDD
Tarrson Family Endowed Chair in Periodontics
Professor
Periodontics
University of California, Los Angeles School of Dentistry
Los Angeles, California

Alan M. Polson, DDS, MS
Professor Emeritus
Department of Periodontics
School of Dental Medicine
University of Pennsylvania
Philadelphia, Pennsylvania

Philip M. Preshaw, BDS, FDS RCSEd, FDS (Rest Dent) RCSEd, PhD
Professor of Periodontology and Dean of Dentistry
School of Dentistry
University of Dundee
Dundee, United Kingdom

Marc Quirynen, DDS, PhD
Professor Emeritus
Oral Health Sciences, Periodontology Section
Katholieke Universiteit Leuven
Leuven, Belgium

Anushri Singh Rajapuri, BDS, MS
Research Specialist
Regenstrief Institute, Inc.
Indiana University School of Dentistry
Indianapolis, Indiana

Natacha Reis, DDS, MFDRCSI, DICOI
Ashman Department of Periodontology and Implant Dentistry
New York University College of Dentistry
New York, New York

Jits Robben, DDS
Clinical Resident in Dentistry
Oral Health Sciences, Periodontology Section
Katholieke Universiteit Leuven
Leuven, Belgium

Carlos Rossa Jr., DDS, MSc, PhD
Associate Professor
Diagnosis and Surgery
State University of São Paulo (UNESP) School of Dentistry
Araraquara, Brazil

Maria Emanuel Ryan, DDS, PhD
VP and Chief Clinical Officer
Global Research and Development
Colgate Palmolive Company
Piscataway, New Jersey

Hector L. Sarmiento, DMD, MSc
Assistant Clinical Professor
Department of Periodontics
University of Pennsylvania
Philadelphia, Pennsylvania;
Private Practice
New York, New York

E. Todd Scheyer, DDS, MS
Private Practice, Periodontist
Perio Health Professionals;
Associate Professor
University of Texas School of Dentistry at Houston
Houston, Texas

Titus Schleyer, DMD, PhD
Research Scientist
Center for Biomedical Informatics
Regenstrief Institute;
Professor of Biomedical Informatics
Department of Medicine
Indiana University
Indianapolis, Indiana

Todd R. Schoenbaum, DDS, MS, FACD
Professor
Restorative Sciences
Dental College of Georgia
Augusta, Georgia

Dennis A. Shanelec, DDS†
Private Practice, Microsurgical Periodontics and Dental Implants
Santa Barbara, California

Kitetsu Shin, DDS, PhD
Professor
Periodontology
Meikai University School of Dentistry
Sakado, Saitama, Japan

Daniela Rodrigues P. Silva, DDS, MS
Chair & Residency Program Director
Pediatric Dentistry
University of California, Los Angeles School of Dentistry
Los Angeles, California

Dennis Sourvanos, BSDH, DDS
Resident, Advanced Graduate Education Student
Periodontics
School of Dental Medicine;
TL-1 Scholar TL1TR001880
Institute Translational Medicine and Therapeutics (ITMAT)
Perelman School of Medicine;
T-90 Postdoctoral Fellow & Scholar T90DE030854;
Center for Innovation and Precision Dentistry (CiPD)
School of Dental Medicine & Engineering
University of Pennsylvania
Philadelphia, Pennsylvania

Frank M. Spear, DDS, MSD
Founder and Director
Spear Education
Scottsdale, Arizona

Claudio Stacchi, DDS, MSc
Adjunct Professor
Department of Medical, Surgical, and Health Sciences
University of Trieste
Trieste, Italy

Corey Stein, DMD, MS
Private Practice
Brooklyn, New York

Henry H. Takei, DDS, MS, FACD
Distinguished Clinical Professor Emeritus
Section of Periodontics
University of California, Los Angeles School of Dentistry;
Consultant
Periodontics
Veterans Administration Hospital Los Angeles
Los Angeles, California

Kai Soo Tan, BSc (Hons), PhD
Associate Professor
Faculty of Dentistry
National University of Singapore
Singapore

†Deceased.

Dennis P. Tarnow, DDS
Clinical Professor of Dental Medicine
Division of Periodontics, Section of Oral & Diagnostics Service
Columbia University College of Dental Medicine;
Director of Implant Education
Columbia University College of Dental Medicine
New York, New York

Sotirios Tetradis, DDS, PhD
Professor and Senior Associate Dean
Oral and Maxillofacial Radiology
University of California, Los Angeles School of Dentistry
Los Angeles, California

Wim Teughels, DDS, PhD
Professor Doctor
Oral Health Sciences, Periodontology Section
Katholieke Universiteit Leuven
Leuven, Belgium

Vivek Thumbigere-Math, BDS, PhD
Assistant Professor
Division of Periodontics
University of Maryland School of Dentistry
Baltimore, Maryland

Thankam P. Thyvalikakath, DMD, MDS, PhD
Professor & Director of Dental Informatics
Cariology, Operative Dentistry & Dental Public Health
Indiana University School of Dentistry;
Research Scientist
Center for Biomedical Informatics
Regenstrief Institute
Indianapolis, Indiana

Leonard S. Tibbetts, DDS, MSD
Private Practice, Microsurgical Periodontics and Dental Implants
Arlington, Texas

Kenneth C. Trabert, DDS, MEd
Emeritus Club Professor
Endodontics
University of California, Los Angeles School of Dentistry
Los Angeles, California

Onur Ucak Turer, PhD
Professor
Department of Periodontology
Cukurova University
Adana, Turkey

Istvan A. Urban, DMD, MD, PhD
Adjunct Associate Professor
Periodontics
University of Michigan
Ann Arbor, Michigan;
Private Practice
Urban Regeneration Institute
Budapest, Hungary

Jose Luis Tapia Vazquez, DDS, MS
Clinical Associate Professor
Oral Diagnostic Sciences
School of Dental Medicine
The University at Buffalo, The State University of New York
Buffalo, New York

Giuseppe Vercellotti, PhD
Adjunct Assistant Professor
Division of Health Sciences
The Ohio State University
Columbus, Ohio

Tomaso Vercellotti, MD, DDS
Honorary Professor
Periodontology
UCL Eastman Dental Institute of London
London, United Kingdom

Keisuke Wada, DDS, PhD, DMS, DMD
Director
Periodontology/Implantology
i-Smile Dental Clinic Tokyo
Tokyo, Japan

Michael Whang, DDS, FACD
Lecturer
Section of Periodontics
University of California, Los Angeles School of Dentistry
Los Angeles, California

Joel M. White, DDS, MS
Professor
Preventive and Restorative Dental Sciences
University of California, San Francisco School of Dentistry
San Francisco, California

Megumi A. Williamson, DDS, MS, PhD
Assistant Professor
Department of Periodontics
University of Iowa
Iowa City, Iowa

Wichaya Wisitrasameewong, DDS, MSc, DMSc
Lecturer and Clinical Instructor
Periodontology
Faculty of Dentistry
Chulalongkorn University
Bangkok, Thailand

Carilynne Yarascavitch, DDS, MSc
Assistant Professor
Faculty of Dentistry, University of Toronto;
Courtesy Staff
Department of Dental and Maxillofacial Sciences
Sunnybrook Health Sciences Centre
Toronto, Ontario, Canada

Adrian Karl Zacher, MBA
Chief Executive Officer
Executive
British Society of Pharmacy Sleep Services;
Managing Director
Snorer.com
Oxford, United Kingdom

CONTENTS

PART 1 FUNDAMENTALS OF PERIODONTOLOGY

SECTION I FUNDAMENTALS AND ESSENTIAL EVIDENCE, 1

SECTION II ETIOLOGY AND PATHOGENESIS, 91

SECTION III GINGIVAL PATHOLOGY, 196

SECTION IV PERIODONTAL PATHOLOGY, 295

†Deceased.

†Deceased.

†Deceased.

VIDEO CONTENTS

CHAPTER 1

Clinical Periodontology and Implantology in the Era of Precision Medicine

Satheesh Elangovan | Chun-Teh Lee | Georgios A. Kotsakis | Irina F. Dragan | Michael G. Newman

CHAPTER OUTLINE

Periodontology and Its Contemporary Practice

Periodontology is a field of dentistry that focuses on the prevention, diagnosis, and treatment of periodontal diseases (and conditions) and on the placement of dental implants to treat edentulism. In this chapter, we will present some of the recent developments and concepts that will change the way periodontics will be practiced in the near future. Periodontal diseases and conditions are pathologic processes affecting the tooth-supporting apparatus called "periodontium" (see Chapter 5). Of these diseases and conditions, gingivitis and periodontitis are highly prevalent across the globe, with gingivitis being the inflammation of gingiva without loss of periodontal attachment, whereas in periodontitis, there will be loss of periodontal attachment, making the latter condition irreversible.

Periodontitis is one of the most prevalent diseases in the world, with an estimated 538 million people affected by its severe form.[19,29] Periodontitis is initiated by specific bacteria in the dental biofilm, but the signs and symptoms of the disease are a result of the host immune response (inflammation) to the bacteria and its by-products (Fig. 1.1). When uncontrolled, the inflammatory mediators that are supposed to be protective attack the host tissues of the periodontium, leading to its loss (see Chapter 8). There is emerging evidence that inflammation can also drive the microbial shift from a nonpathogenic to a pathogenic dental biofilm (see Chapters 8 and 10). The clinical signs of periodontitis include pocket formation and increase in tooth mobility. The typical symptoms patients with periodontitis present with include pain or discomfort, bad breath, bleeding while brushing, or a mobile tooth or teeth. It is important to remember that periodontitis is a noncommunicable chronic condition (NCCC) that shares several of the social and other risk factors of other NCCCs that will be discussed later.[69] There is also a large body of evidence to suggest associations between periodontitis and systemic conditions such as diabetes or cardiovascular conditions, with inflammation being the bridge between the two disease entities.

As mentioned earlier, placement and maintenance of dental implants are an integral part of periodontology, and it is an understatement to say that implants revolutionized the way dentistry is currently practiced and that it has positively impacted countless patients by improving their quality of life (Fig. 1.2). Dental implants, like natural dentition, are prone to pathologic conditions, with periimplant mucositis and periimplantitis being the implant counterpart of gingivitis and periodontitis of natural dentition, respectively. Periodontists, specialists in periodontology and implant dentistry, have extensive additional training beyond dental school and often partner with referring dentists to maximize the overall treatment of the patient. The subsequent chapters of this book will go in depth into all aspects of periodontology and oral implantology.

Fig. 1.3 provides an overview of the currently used workflow in the management of patients with periodontal diseases and conditions. Currently, when patients present to clinic for a periodontal evaluation, most of the time, they already have periodontal or periimplant disease or conditions, with or without symptoms. Often these patients are self-referred or referred by another oral health care provider for treatment. Clinicians with conventional training perform the clinical exam, which is composed of extraoral and intraoral examinations. Clinical periodontal examination involves both visual and tactile examination in the form of periodontal probing to assess probing depths, clinical attachment levels, and several other measures (see Chapter 38). Radiographic examination then follows, which typically involves interpretation of radiographic images of the dentition or implant and its relationship to the alveolar bone. Findings from both the clinical and radiographic assessments are then taken into account to come up with a diagnosis. Then prognosis

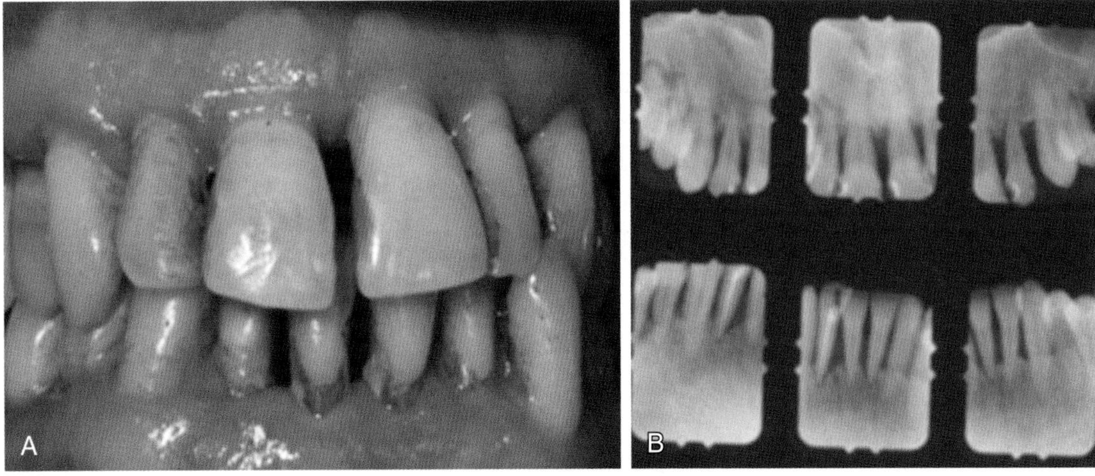

Fig. 1.1 Clinical (A) and radiographic (B) images of a patient suffering from periodontitis showing the classical clinical signs of the disease. The clinical signs include signs of inflammation of the gingiva, deepening of periodontal sulcus (becoming a pocket), and the presence of deposits. Radiographically, bone loss is characteristic of periodontitis, and in the example shown (B) there is bone loss all the way up to the apical third of the root of the anterior dentition.

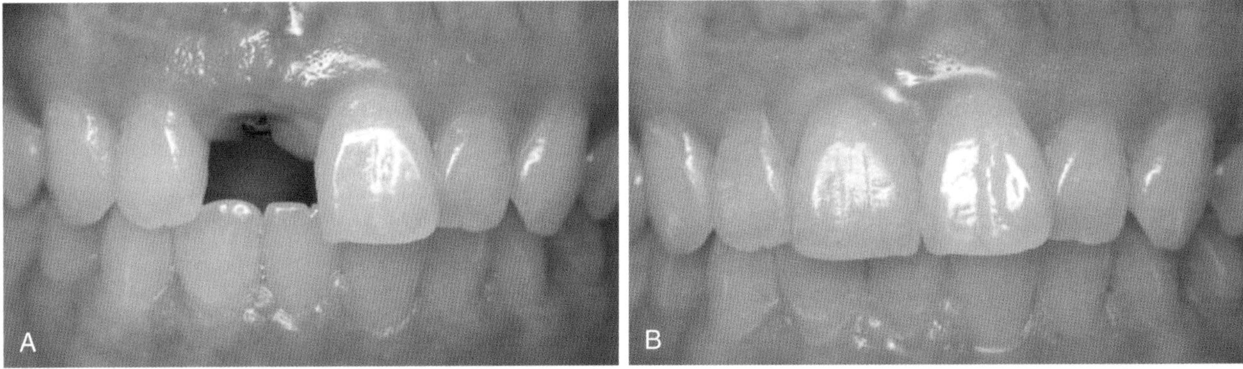

Fig. 1.2 Restoration of an edentulous site (#8) (A) with an implant supported single crown (B). Note the significant improvement in esthetics for this patient following an implant-based fixed restorative solution.

will be assigned for each tooth or implant and for the overall dentition, and subsequently, a treatment plan is devised.

Using the treatment plan as a roadmap, patients typically start with nonsurgical therapy (NST) (see Chapter 51), which will be followed by periodontal reevaluation, to assess outcomes of NST (see Fig. 1.3). Depending on the clinical presentation at the time of reevaluation, the need for additional therapy such as surgery will be assessed. If a patient does not require additional therapy or is not a candidate for surgical therapy, the patient will be placed on a maintenance program (or supportive periodontal therapy) that involves periodic exams and professional cleanings (see Chapter 70).

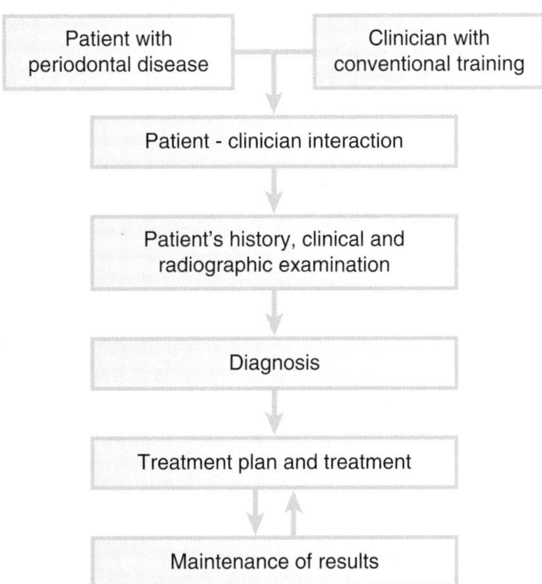

Fig. 1.3 Flowchart depicting the current clinical workflow in the management of patients with periodontal diseases and conditions. To an extent this is a one-size-fits-all approach, and it is more of a reactive approach to disease that already exists than preventative.

Contemporary Practice of Medicine

Currently there is a greater emphasis given to patients' well-being and how *they* feel and function, versus the mere presence or absence of disease that can be detected and measured using clinical tests and other diagnostic tools. Yet, still, health care primarily focuses on the physical signs or surrogate measures of disease and addresses those using interventions, giving less regard to the patient's mental and social well-being and how they perceive the disease. In addition, the outcomes used to assess the effectiveness of those interventions both in clinical studies and in practice often does not correlate with patients' perception or well-being.[72] Moreover, the health care system traditionally has been very good at being reactive to an already existing disease rather than being preventive.[70] With the advancements in systems medicine—big-data and digital technologies including machine learning (ML)—modern medicine is going through a rapid transformation.

The aforementioned advances allow for a more thorough risk assessment that takes several factors into consideration, that were not available or accessible earlier. These will also facilitate the provision of preventive care and a treatment that is highly customized to the patient rather than taking a "one-size-fits-all" approach. The problem with the latter approach is that it works with the assumption that all the patients will respond to a particular intervention in a similar manner, which is not the case. A good example is the way an individual patient metabolizes a given pharmacologic agent. Using genetics to guide drug prescribing decisions ("pharmacogenetics") now allows the clinician to select a drug based on the genetic makeup of the patient to maximize its safety and efficacy (see Chapter 9). This is a good example of what precision medicine can offer.

Precision Health Care

Clinicians must always strive to come up with the best possible treatment available for a given clinical situation. In precision medicine, the treatment plan generated will be customized to the patient, based on personal history, medical history, and clinical factors, supplemented with environmental factors and biologic information. Therefore the aim of precision treatment is to tailor health care for individuals using their own unique characteristics to enhance treatment outcomes and minimize adverse effects.

Although the terms precision medicine and personalized medicine are used interchangeably, it is important to note that there is a distinction between the two. Precision medicine encompasses personalized medicine, and it harnesses clinical and biologic information to stratify patients and to guide clinical decision-making.

With the assistance of advanced and novel technology, information derived from biologic specimens such as blood or saliva can now be effectively and rapidly analyzed by computers through informatics. In addition, artificial intelligence (AI) has improved the accuracy of diagnostic interpretation of clinical and radiographic images, and the patient's behavioral information can be collected through wearable electronic devices. The other major advancement is the widespread use of electronic health records (EHRs) in clinics, which is an ideal platform to connect and integrate all of the aforementioned advancements to aid the clinician chairside in developing a personalized treatment plan that incorporates all of the aforementioned factors.

Emerging Practice Model in Periodontology

The contemporary clinical protocol that uses just surrogate outcomes of periodontitis such as probing depths is geared toward detecting periodontal diseases that have already occurred and therefore does not offer any guidance for *preventive* strategies. The current workflow (see Fig. 1.3) also lacks the ability to *predict* the degree of responsiveness to a proposed therapy. In addition, the existing workflow is set up in a way that is not conducive for patients to *participate* and be engaged in their health management process.

The alternative model of care shown in Fig. 1.4 allows the care to be *predictive, preventive, personalized,* and *participatory* (the cornerstones of "precision health care" and often referred to as the 4Ps).[73] With this approach, the expectation is that the patients will see the health care provider before the initiation of disease *(preventive),* and this is feasible by knowing the patient's risk profile (for the disease), based on the biologic makeup of the individual. When information, such as a patient's biologic makeup, is routinely integrated into the clinical assessment and with effective amalgamation of digital innovations such as AI and ML in the EHRs, clinicians will be able to assemble a more accurate diagnosis and prognosis. This allows for the development of a more personalized treatment plan *(personalized)* for the patient that is far more predictable *(predictive).* Oral hygiene aids such as brushes or intraoral appliances, when fitted with biosensors, can detect plaque levels or biomarker analytes in saliva and can provide real time notifications to patients regarding their oral and systemic health *(participatory).*[2,31] Equally important to provide personalized care is the availability and application of scientific evidence with dental patient-reported outcome (dPRO) measures in the clinical decision-making process.[54]

Components of Precision Periodontics

This section is focused on introducing some of the key components associated with precision and patient-centered periodontics (see Fig. 1.4).

Biologic Information

Microbiologic and Host Response Information

Maintaining the host-microorganism balance and homeostasis is a prerequisite for maintaining periodontal health. Comprehensively deciphering the host response and microbiome, at the patient level, will be critical to stratify patients for precise diagnosis and effective treatment. Periodontitis is an inflammatory disease initiated by microorganisms, primarily bacteria (see Fig. 1.1). However, tissue damage in periodontitis is primarily mediated by the host response, with a smaller contribution by bacteria. In other words, the presence of periodontal pathogens is required but not sufficient for disease initiation. Therefore understanding the host response in periodontitis patients is critical to assess patients' periodontal conditions and risk for future progression. Analysis of genetic polymorphisms, evaluating cytokine levels in saliva, gingival crevicular fluid (GCF) or serum, and measuring blood immune cell counts are some of the ways clinicians can assess the patient's host response.

Historically, several bacterial species, such as *Aggregatibacter actinomycetemcomitans*, *Porphyromonas gingivalis*, *Treponema denticola*, and *Tanerella forsythia* were known to be the major periodontal pathogens. Keystone pathogens, such as *P. gingivalis*, with a relatively low abundance in dental plaque, can cause dysbiosis, which can instigate periodontal inflammation[38] (see Chapter 10). Recently, more and more bacterial species and other members of the microbial world, such as viruses, bacteriophages, and fungi are being identified (through novel technologies, such as 16S sequencing, shotgun sequencing, and metagenomics) to be associated with periodontitis. In general, excessive putative and opportunistic pathogens induce inflammation, but specific bacterial species are more important for pathogenesis than others. Analyzing oral plaque samples can provide information on microbial composition and abundance that may help clinicians to assess periodontal disease risk at the individual patient level. For detailed information on periodontal microbiology and the role of host response in the pathogenesis of periodontal diseases, refer to Chapters 10 and 11.

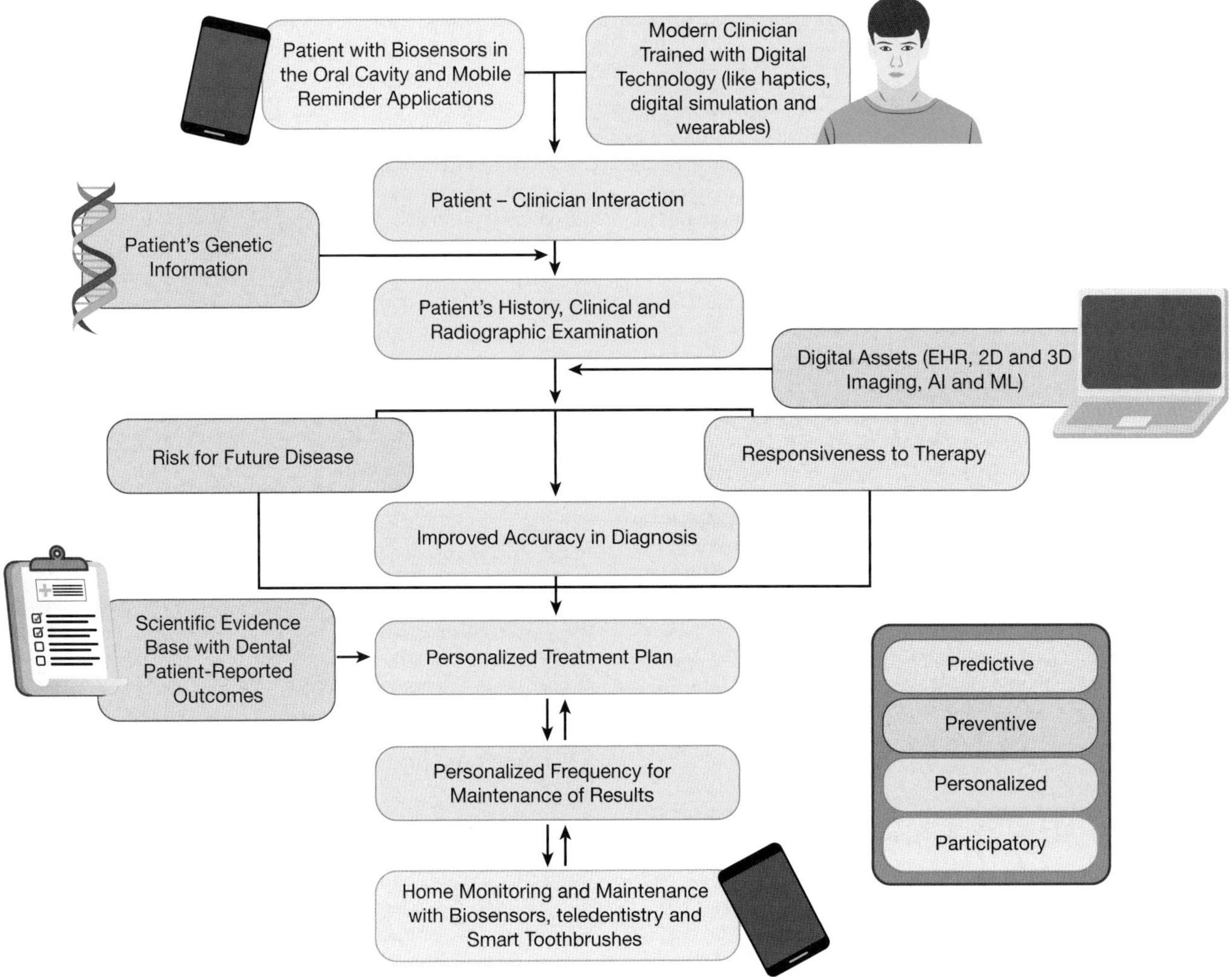

Fig. 1.4 Periodontology and implant dentistry as an integral part of overall connected health and personalized care. At the center is the digital home that maintains the electronic dental record and information from other dentists, practice guidelines, physicians, family, patient-reported outcomes, medication history, pharmacy, and more. Artificial intelligence, virtual reality, teledentistry, sensors, connected devices, and wearables are linked to provide clinical decision support, training, and remote connectivity between the provider and the patient. Biological information such as the microbiome, genetic, environmental, immune status and other info in one central location where algorithms assist the dental professional to provide optimum treatment and prevention guidance. (*Figure by Dr. Ryutaro Kuraji.*)

Genetic Information

It is well known that specific genetic mutations are associated with disorders and diseases (see Chapter 9). Due to the complexity of associations and interactions between a large number of genes and disorders, the single gene–single disorder ("candidate gene") approach to study the impact of genetic factors on diseases is no longer effective. By using advanced informatics technology, a conceptual framework can now be developed to systematically link all genetic disorders (disease phenome) with all of the disease-associated genes (disease genome), resulting in a global view or "diseasome" that comprises of comprehensive known disorder/disease gene associations.[20]

Biomarkers in Periodontitis

A biomarker, or "biologic marker," is defined as a characteristic that is objectively measured and evaluated as an indicator of normal biologic processes, pathogenic processes, or responses to a therapeutic intervention or a hazard.[6,74] This section is focused on providing a brief overview of biomarkers (molecules) that can be measured in biologic samples that correlate with the severity and progression of periodontal inflammation.

GCF is a physiologic fluid and an inflammatory exudate originating from the gingival vascular plexus and exists in the gingival sulcus.[5] GCF is composed of a mixture of molecules that originate from the blood, host tissues, and bacteria, including, electrolytes, metabolites, cytokines, antibodies, bacterial antigens, and enzymes. GCF can be easily collected from both healthy and diseased sites using special paper strips (Fig. 1.5) or micropipette, and its volume increases when periodontal tissues are inflamed. The concentration of specific molecules (biomarkers) from GCF can be assessed by techniques such as enzyme-linked immunosorbent assay (ELISA), proteomics, or metabolomics, depending on the purpose and characteristics of the molecules of interest.

Omics Technologies

Omics technologies help analyze the characteristics of a large number of biologic molecules in samples in a cost-effective and high-throughput fashion. Depending on the type of biologic molecules analyzed, these technologies have been named by appending the suffix "-omics." For example, genomics is focused on studying genes and their function, and transcriptomics is focused on studying the organism's transcriptome (the sum of all RNA transcripts). Proteomics, lipidomics, and metabolomics are focused on quantifying and studying the structure and functions of proteins, lipids, and cellular metabolites, respectively. With the assistance of newly developed equipment and analytical tools, advances in "omics" technologies contribute to innovative breakthroughs in science with far-reaching clinical applications. A good example of such a technologic advancement is Next-Generation Sequencing (NGS), which enables the completion of genomics or transcriptomics analyses in hours. Having access to the results of such analyses will assist the clinician to understand the inherent differences in host response and plaque microbial composition in periodontitis patients at a much deeper level and plan treatments accordingly.[10,15]

Biosensor

A biosensor is an analytic device that detects analytes with specific biologic activities. A typical biosensor has two fundamental units: a "bioreceptor," such as an enzyme, an antibody, or DNA, responsible for selective recognition of the target analyte, and a "physicochemical transducer," which can be a(n) electrochemical, optical, or mechanical transducer, converting the detected activity into a signal.[32] Then, the signal is exported and transformed into clinically meaningful results. Some biosensors were designed to detect specific biologic events in the oral cavity. For example, a highly sensitive peptide-graphene nanosensor can be placed on tooth enamel to detect salivary bacteria at single-cell levels (Fig. 1.6).[44] A biosensor[38] which has antibodies coated on a small chip can detect and quantify salivary matrix metalloproteinase-8 (MMP-8), a biomarker associated with periodontitis. These biosensors can offer either real time biologic data collection or can be used for point-of-care testing.

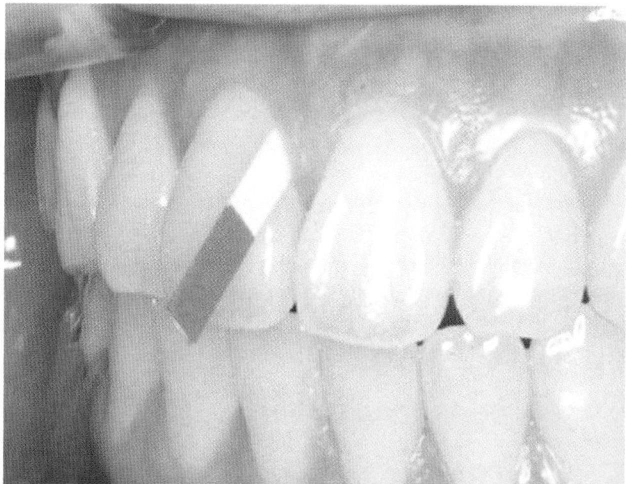

Fig. 1.5 Gingival crevicular fluid collection using a special filter paper that is inserted into the gingival crevice. (*From Papagerakis P, Zheng L, Kim D, et al. Saliva and gingival crevicular fluid (GCF) collection for biomarker screening.* Methods Mol Biol. *2019;1922:549–562. doi: 10.1007/978-1-4939-9012-2_41. PMID: 30838599.*)

Electronic Health Record Capabilities

An EHR is a digital version of the traditional patient paper chart. As compared with the paper chart, an EHR can save much more information and provide standardization of patient records. In addition, the EHR system has the capability to provide reminders, deliver warning messages about medical conditions, including drug allergies, and can help to perform risk assessment for oral and systemic diseases. *In the United States, the "Health Information Technology for Economic and Clinical Health (HITECH) Act" was enacted in 2009. The HITECH Act listed the "meaningful use" of interoperable EHRs throughout the US health care delivery system as a critical national goal. "Meaningful Use" was defined as the use of certified EHR technology in a meaningful manner, ensuring effective electronic exchange of health information to improve the quality of care. The Consortium for Oral Health Research and Informatics (COHRI) was convened in February 2007 by several dental schools that use the same EHR platform as its members. COHRI aims to facilitate the advancement of education, research, and patient care outcomes through collaborative development and by promoting the use of standardized tools and processes in EHR data. BigMouth is an oral health database[71] developed from partially deidentified EHR data contributed by COHRI member institutions for clinical and research purposes.*

The following is an example of how EHRs can be used for precision periodontics. Diabetes is a well-known risk factor for periodontitis (Fig. 1.7). Cross sectional studies have shown that certain clinical thresholds such as the presence of 26% or greater teeth with deep pockets (≥5 mm) or four or more missing teeth could accurately identify greater than 70% of patients with prediabetes

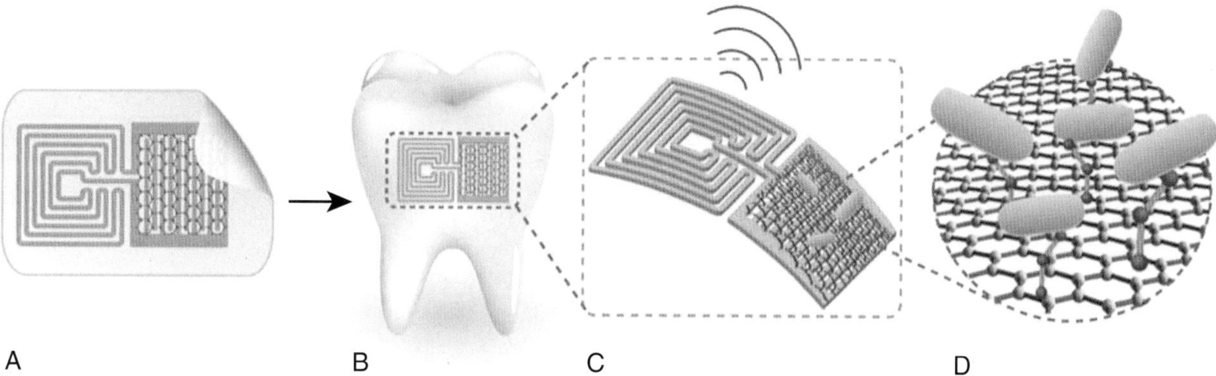

Fig. 1.6 Illustration showing graphene wireless nanosensor that can be attached to tooth enamel for remote monitoring of pathogenic bacteria. Graphene printed onto bioresorbable silk (A) and attached onto tooth surface (B). Magnified schematic of the sensing element is shown in part C, while part D shows how the pathogenic bacteria binds to the nano transducer. (*From Mannoor MS, Tao H, Clayton JD, et al. Graphene-based wireless bacteria detection on tooth enamel.* Nat Commun. *2012 Mar 27;3:763. doi: 10.1038/ncomms1767. Erratum in:* Nat Commun. *2013;4:1900. PMID: 22453836.*)

or diabetes presenting with at least one of the risk factors associated with hyperglycemia.[35,36] By setting up these thresholds in the EHR system, a clinician can be notified of the potential risk of the patient for diabetes, based on the findings from dental examination and personal information. Once these potential diabetic patients are identified, dentists can refer the patients to physicians for further testing and management.[37] In addition, several risk-assessment tools, such as Periodontal Risk Assessment (PRA),[39] and Periodontal Management by Risk Assessment (PEMBRA),[49,53] that are available to assess the risk for periodontal disease progression can be integrated into the EHR (see Chapter 40). This allows for chairside risk determination that can be used for treatment planning and patient education purposes.

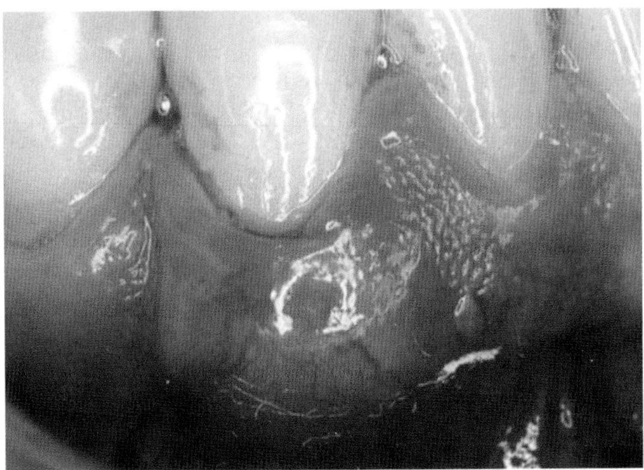

Fig. 1.7 Localized periodontal abscess of a mandibular right canine in a poorly controlled diabetic patient. Diabetes, when uncontrolled, predisposes a patient to periodontal abscess formation.

Artificial Intelligence–Assisted Clinical Data and Radiographic Image Analyses

Artificial intelligence refers to the ability to build machines with the capability of performing tasks that are performed normally by humans.[60] The utilization of AI to assist and supplement clinicians to improve the overall accuracy of diagnosis is called augmented intelligence.[61] In contrast, ML is a subset of AI applications that refers to the ability of self-learning by the machine itself with the capability to detect patterns and make predictions.[25,60] Deep learning (DL) is a subset of ML applications that teaches itself to perform a specific task with increasingly greater accuracy as compared with ML.[25] (ML or DL models have been extensively applied to perform complex data analysis, to identify anatomic structures and pathologic findings on radiographs, and for disease detection; Fig. 1.8.) A research group using ML, recently demonstrated that a well-designed combination of salivary bacteria can distinguish periodontally healthy from the disease group.[30] In separate studies, a DL-based computer-aided diagnosis (CAD) tool was shown to assist in making periodontal diagnosis by measuring alveolar bone levels on oral radiographic images.[8,34] *Very recently, authors applied ML algorithms to a large national database and identified predictors of tooth loss.*[16]

Wearable/Portable Electronic Devices

Many wearable or portable electronic devices, such as a smart phone and a smart watch, that are used in day to day lives can collect and transfer data effectively. These devices are developed based on the concept called the "Internet of Things" (IoT), which is about connecting and exchanging data between a variety of devices and systems over the Internet. The Internet of Medical Things (IoMT) is a cloud network–based advanced technology which is basically IoT that is applied to the medical field. It allows for collection and active monitoring of patients' health status information for disease prevention (Fig. 1.9). The same concept can be applied in dentistry

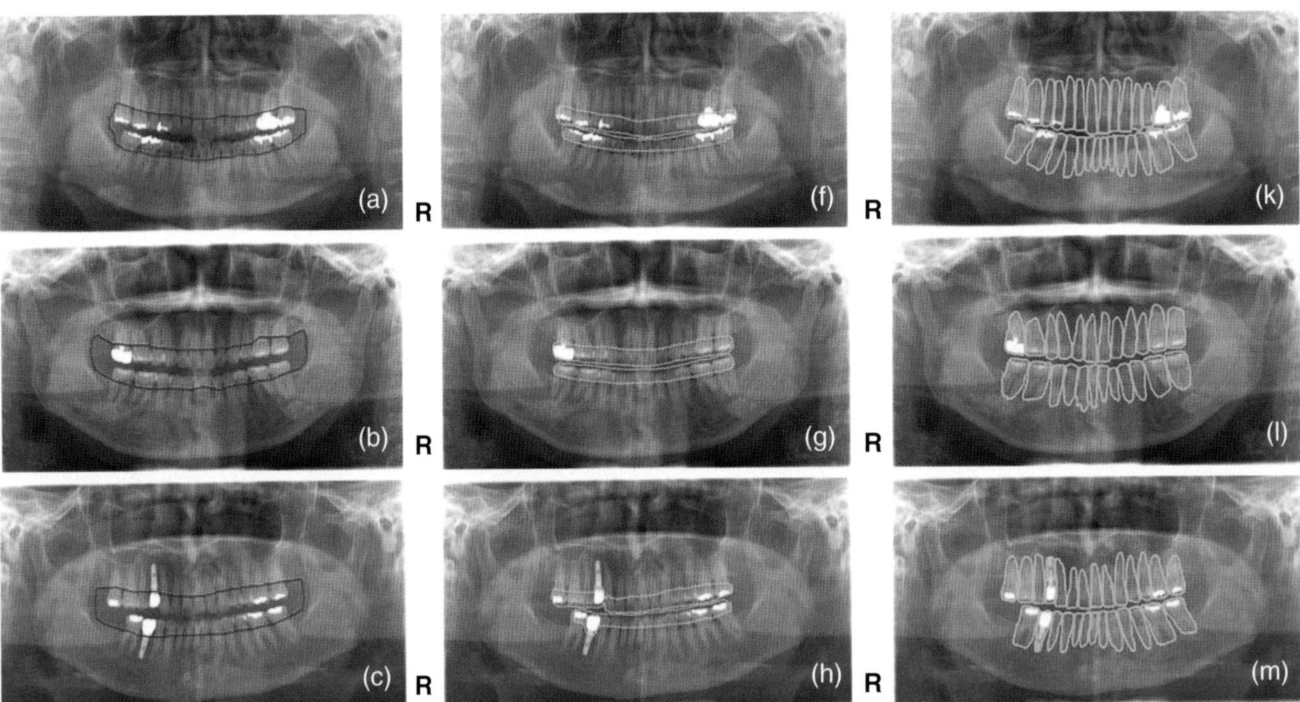

Fig. 1.8 Use of deep learning (DL) program to diagnose periodontal disease. DL program was used to detect bone levels (a, b, and c), cementoenamel junctions (f, g, and h), and tooth/implant morphology (k, l, and m) in three different patients. (*From Chang HJ, Lee SJ, Yong TH, et al. Deep learning hybrid method to automatically diagnose periodontal bone loss and stage periodontitis.* Sci Rep. *2020 May 5;10[1]:7531. doi: 10.1038/s41598-020-64509-z. PMID: 32372049; PMCID: PMC7200807.*)

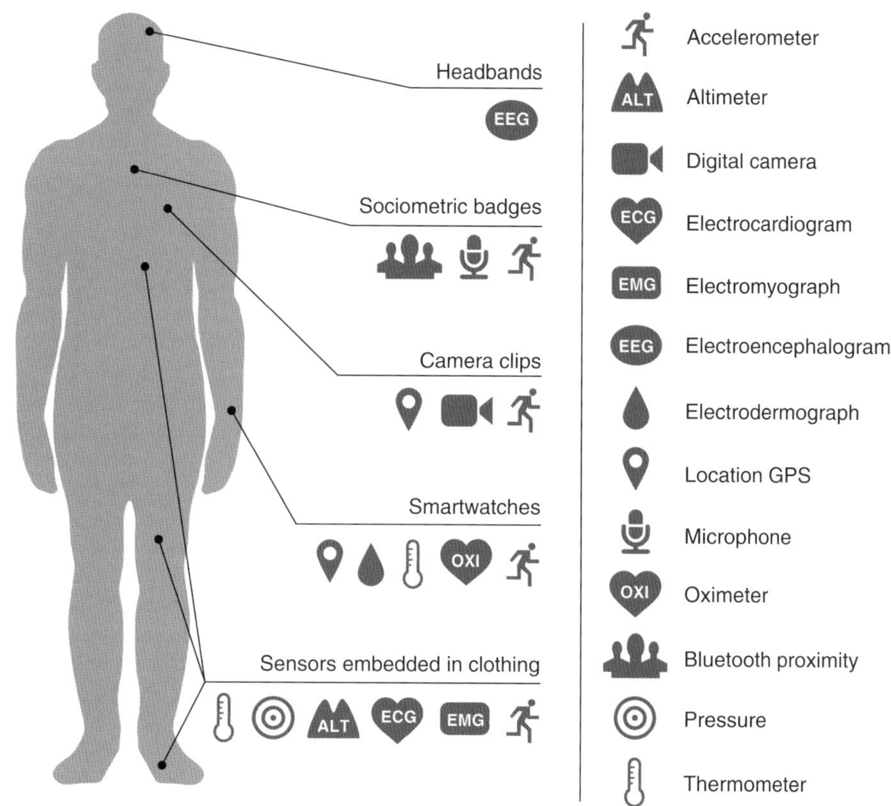

Fig. 1.9 Examples of consumer wearables to monitor health. (*From Piwek L, Ellis DA, Andrews S, et al. The rise of consumer health wearables: promises and barriers.* PLoS Med. *2016 Feb 2;13[2]:e1001953. doi: 10.1371/journal.pmed.1001953. PMID: 26836780; PMCID: PMC4737495.*)

as the Internet of Dental Things (IoDT).[59] For example, a Bluetooth-incorporated smart toothbrush can detect dental plaque, monitor real-time brushing location, sense brushing pressure, and document brushing behavior. These connected devices can then transfer this information to the dental EHR to aid clinicians in improving their patient's home care by customized behavioral modifications.

Teledentistry

Teledentistry is an effective way to remotely interact with patients by videoconferencing to provide dental consultations and instructions. With the increased availability and access to broadband internet services, teledentistry is gaining popularity. It can be a good medium to reach patients who would otherwise not have access to dental care (e.g., in rural areas, patients in nursing facilities, or during a pandemic). Although a large majority of dental treatments can be only provided in person, teledentistry offers an alternative approach to screen for oral diseases and potentially help patients to manage oral diseases when immediate dental care is unavailable. The coronavirus disease 2019 (COVID-19) pandemic has brought to light the importance and usefulness of teledentistry, which would potentially pave way for its regular future use even in nonpandemic situations.[66]

Patient-Reported Outcomes and Clinical Research

Periodontal practice has made tremendous progress toward evidence-based treatment over the past decade, but in some aspects, it is still trailing behind medical practice. This important progress can be further accelerated with the availability of patient-perceived outcomes of periodontal and implant interventions. One critical aspect of personalized medicine is that each person perceives disease burden differently.[51] Disease-related morbidity has an experiential component that cannot be captured by clinical disease measures. In periodontal practice, treatment effects are routinely based on clinician measured surrogate outcomes, such as probing depth and attachment levels, which are not easily communicated to or perceived by dental patients. The fact that in most cases these physical measures are not readily perceived by patients generates a communication gap in the dentist-patient relationship that ultimately affects care. For instance, a clinician would be concerned with a 6-mm probing depth on an anterior central incisor, whereas this would mean very little to a patient without a dental background. Therefore proper diagnosis and communication is key to devising tailored treatment plans that meets patient preferences and expectations.

Tailored treatment plans go beyond precision dentistry, which considers individual host inflammatory characteristics, to encompass behavioral characteristics and individually perceived treatment needs. A periodontal patient who strongly prioritizes function and pain over esthetics or over social interactions and appearance may not be necessarily amenable to undergoing a surgical procedure to retain a tooth and maintain esthetics. To address the communication gap and to include patient-specific quality of life considerations in treatment planning, dPROs, which are true outcomes of disease, have gained significant momentum in dental and medical research to better capture disease burden and treatment effects.[54]

KEY FACT

Examples of dental patient-reported outcome measures (PROMs) include how a patient feels and functions and the overall *patient-reported* satisfaction, phonetics, chewing comfort, stability, cleanability, and esthetics.[50] PROMs must be reported directly by the patient without interpretation by anyone else, including the dentist.

As dPROs gain momentum in dental practice, our understanding of the true outcome of dental therapies will vastly increase. One key question that the utilization of dPROs is poised to address is, "To what extent does periodontal disease contribute to an individual's burden of disease?" *As mentioned earlier, the Global Burden of Diseases study has consistently revealed that periodontitis is one of the most prevalent noncommunicable diseases in adults worldwide.*[29] *The global epidemiology of population health has fundamentally changed during the past decades. Since 2000, the burden of NCCC has become the leading cause affecting population health worldwide, with communicable diseases negatively impacting population health, only in limited developing regions, or areas affected by war.*[15] *Therefore new health metrics are being developed, such as years lived with disability and proportion of years spent in ill health, to capture the extent of diseases on nonfatal health loss. Nonetheless, although periodontitis is highly prevalent, its contribution to nonfatal yet negative impact on health is consistently underappreciated, in comparison with medical conditions, such as diabetes mellitus, because the patient-perceived burden of periodontitis is not adequately captured in dental practice and research settings.*[29] *Despite the understanding that periodontal diseases affect a person's well-being and oral health–related quality of life (OHRQoL), in most cases, physical measures of diseases are solely captured to track an individual's oral health status.* [54]

In clinic, treatment interventions seem to lead to varying levels of patient-perceived improvements; however, these effects are not routinely captured by clinicians. As a result, the individual patient perspective is not adequately influencing clinical decisions. To implement a real world change in the practice of periodontics and implantology by centering clinical practice on dPROs and complementing them with disease-relevant clinically measured outcomes, a clinically relevant and valid instrument for assessing OHRQoL becomes necessary. *Previous efforts to incorporate psychosocial measures in clinical practice have focused on the assessment of OHRQoL. The most frequently used OHRQoL instruments have been modeled after a seven-dimensional theoretical model of OHRQoL, based on Locker's conceptual model of oral health,*[41] *leading to the development of lengthy instruments that may be too burdensome to be used in real life situations. For example, the most commonly used measuring instrument for OHRQoL in dental research has been the Oral Health Impact Profile (OHIP), which in its original version included seven self-report items for each of the seven dimensions of OHRQoL.*[64] *Therefore the OHIP-49 requires considerable time and dedication by dental patients to complete, making it impractical for routine use at each dental visit. The use of lengthy measurement instruments and the practical limitations that they impose in clinical care settings and in large-scale research studies have remained the main impediment in the incorporation of the assessment of OHRQoL as a standard outcome in periodontology and implant dentistry.*[26]

Future Clinical Trials

In addition to the inclusion of dPROs in clinical trials, it is extremely important to rethink the way clinical trials are conducted. Due to inherent variations between patients, there will be responders and nonresponders to any given treatment intervention. Based on the response to prior intervention and patient characteristics at any given point in therapy, the next decision in treatment sequence is made, and this is the principle behind the concept of dynamic treatment regimens (DTRs). Traditional clinical trials in periodontics will not allow researchers to identify DTRs or validate interventions that have to be adapted based on patient responses called "adaptive interventions." Sequential Multiple Assignment Randomized Trial (SMART) clinical trials with the help of advanced statistical techniques will allow researchers to identify DTRs and adaptive treatment interventions in a given patient population.[3,40] *Multiple nodes of key clinical decision-making steps along with specific outcomes embedded within the SMART designs make it an ideal design to identify and validate DTRs. Therefore, in the near future, clinical trials embedded with SMART design will have an important place in the development of dynamic treatment protocols in periodontics.*

Periodontal Education to Support Future Clinical Practice

With the forthcoming changes in the landscape of clinical practice, educators will be required to adapt and update the curriculum accordingly to prepare clinicians for the future. The Commission on Dental Accreditation, the accreditation body of dental education in the United States, requires academic institutions to integrate technologies in a meaningful way in the training offered for both dental students and postgraduate residents.[9] Significant efforts have been made by different institutions to offer consistent programs able to inform faculty members on the best pedagogic practices in their teaching activities.[27] Framing these activities using validated educational models can positively impact not only the students (Logic Model) but also the patients (Kirkpatrick Model).[17] The release of the new Integrated National Board Dental Examination in the United States in August 2020, with a focus on case-based assessment, is consistent with the ongoing shift in clinical practice to a more person-centered approach.[28] Most chapters in this book will have a case-based learning exercise. Students are now required to apply fundamentals in basic and clinical sciences in a specific clinical scenario.[14] *To expand on the scope of the American Academy of Periodontology's In-Service examination offered to all postgraduate residents in the United States, a case-based component has been piloted in 2021. This initiative might be able to leverage on the benefits of case-based assessment for different clinical scenarios, testing key concepts in diagnosis, etiology, prognosis, treatment plan options, and maintenance.*

Surgical Education

Multiple studies in various health care professions have shown the key role of simulators in surgical education, but there is only sparse evidence in the field of dentistry.[67] The pedagogic principles that support this type of technology are cognitive task analysis (CTA) and constructivism.[68,69] Applying the CTA framework, clinicians will be able to divide a complex task into its cognitive phases, enabling their decision-making process.[68] When applying such a process into the teaching activity, an educator can assess whether the students were able to comprehend a complex task step by step (Fig. 1.10). Furthermore, one can modify the complex procedure by adding intraoperative complications and assess the situational awareness of the student.

Virtual reality (VR) is an advanced computer-generated technology that offers realistic experience by three-dimensional visual rendering of the background or surroundings. The students or clinicians can wear a special electronic device (e.g., VR headset) to interact with virtual patients or perform virtual procedures to gain experience and practice clinical procedures in a simulated environment. These VR devices can also help patients as a tool to reduce their dental anxiety.[45] VR is becoming an important part of medical education, and dental education is not too far from this.[57] With more and more dental schools investing in virtual simulators in the fields of operative dentistry, prosthodontics, and endodontics, the use of VR will soon be a standard in periodontal education as well.[13] As these technologies make their way into clinical education, it is prudent to evaluate their impact not only on the students' attitudes, behaviors, and learning but also on other key stakeholders (faculty, staff, and patients).[47]

Augmented reality (AR) is simulation of the real world environment, where the real objects are enhanced by computer-generated perceptual information to provide interactive experience (Fig. 1.11). By

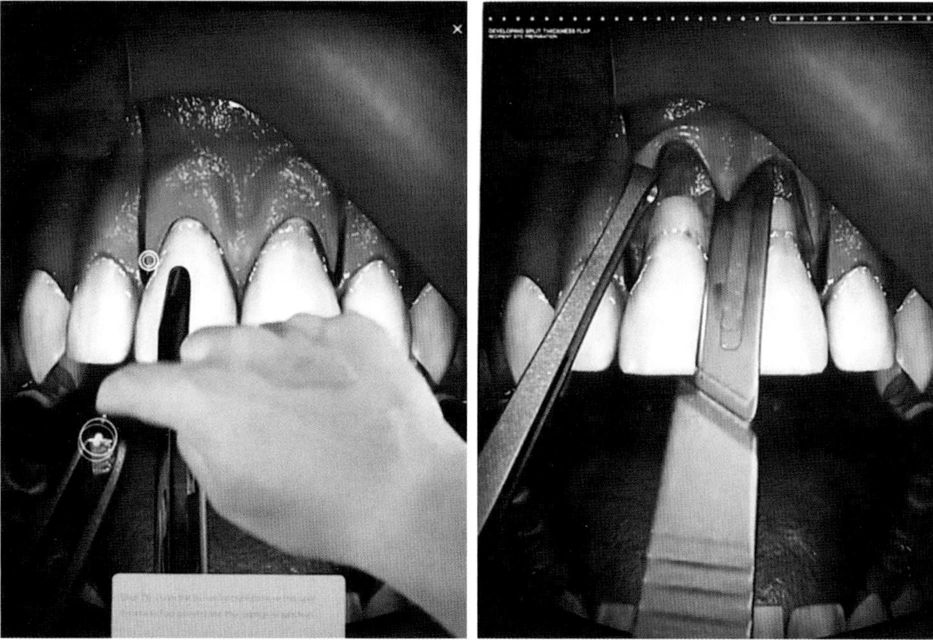

Fig. 1.10 Screenshots showing an interactive learning experience using a surgical simulation program (*Touch Surgery, Medtronic* https://www.youtube.com/watch?v=pL-amyBgu6Q)

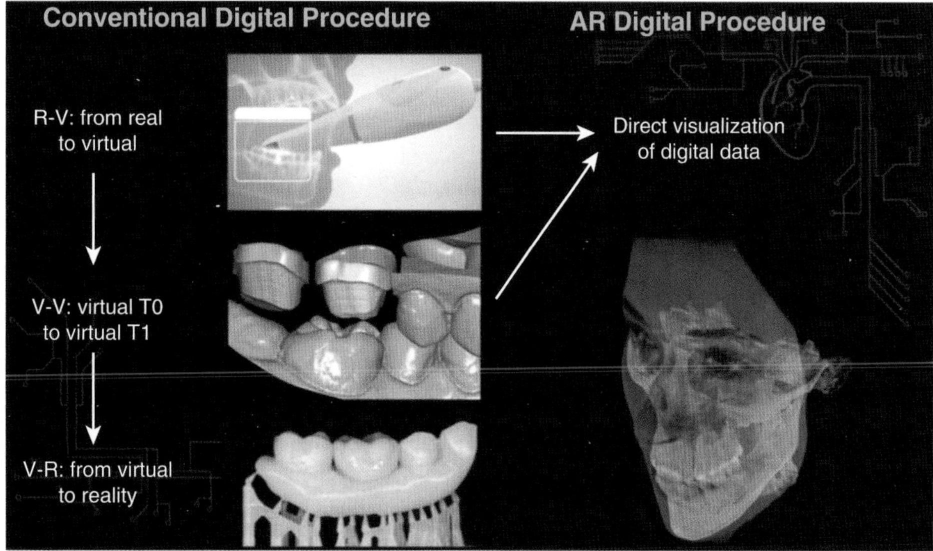

Fig. 1.11 Illustration showing how augmented reality can enhance the current digital dentistry workflow. *(From Farronato M, Maspero C, Lanteri V, et al. Current state of the art in the use of augmented reality in dentistry: a systematic review of the literature.* BMC Oral Health. *2019 Jul 8;19[1]:135. doi: 10.1186/s12903-019-0808-3. PMID: 31286904; PMCID: PMC6613250.)*

wearing a specific device (e.g., AR glasses), the user can see virtual objects seamlessly integrated with the real environment. The key difference between VR and AR is that VR attempts to create an artificial environment in which the user interacts through the senses, whereas AR also provides an interactive experience by supplementing the real environment rather than creating a new artificial environment.[48] In addition to their potential uses in dental education, emerging evidence points to the application of AR-based technologies in the clinics.[48] An example would be an AR-based implant navigation system developed to increase the accuracy of implant placement.[56]

Conclusion

Recent biologic and technologic innovations are rapidly changing the health care landscape, and dentistry is no exception. Periodontists, despite tailoring treatment based on patient needs, still follows a one-size-fits-all approach when it comes to providing periodontal care. Now with the availability of biologic information from innovative technologies, continuously monitorable real world data from biosensors, all well integrated into an EHR that is powered by AI and ML, periodontics now enters into a precision care model that allows the treatment to be predictive, preventive, personalized, and participatory. These changes in clinical care should be supplemented by changes in the dental education curriculum to adequately prepare clinicians for this model and by rethinking how clinical trials should be conducted and by giving greater emphasis to dPROs in those trials.

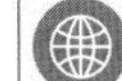

References for this chapter are found on the companion website eBooks.Health.Elsevier.com.

CHAPTER 2

Evidence-Based Decision Making

Satheesh Elangovan | Jane L. Forrest | Syrene A. Miller | Greg W. Miller | Michael G. Newman

CHAPTER OUTLINE

Dental care professionals make decisions about clinical care on a daily basis. It is important that these decisions incorporate the best available scientific evidence to maximize the potential for successful patient care outcomes. It is also important for readers of this book to have the background and skills necessary to evaluate information they read and hear about. These evaluative skills are as important as learning facts and clinical procedures. *The ability to find, discriminate, evaluate, and use information is the most important skill that can be learned as a professional and lifelong learner.* Honing this skill will provide a rewarding and fulfilling professional career.

Background and Definition

Using evidence from the medical literature to answer questions, direct clinical action, and guide practice was pioneered at McMaster University, Ontario, Canada, in the 1980s. As clinical research and the publication of findings increased, so did the need to use the medical literature to guide practice. The traditional clinical problem-solving model based on individual experience or the use of information gained by consulting authorities (colleagues or textbooks) gave way to a new methodology for practice and restructured the way in which more effective clinical problem solving should be conducted. This new methodology was termed *evidence-based medicine* (EBM).[14]

KEY DEFINITIONS

Evidence: Evidence is considered the synthesis of all valid research that answers a specific question and that, in most cases, distinguishes it from a single research study.[2]

Evidence-based medicine: The integration of the best research evidence with our clinical expertise and our patient's unique values and circumstances.[36]

Evidence-based dentistry: An approach to oral health care that requires the judicious integration of systematic assessments of clinically relevant scientific evidence, relating to the patient's oral and medical condition and history, with the dentist's clinical expertise and the patient's treatment needs and preferences.[4]

The use of evidence to help guide clinical decisions is not new. However, the following aspects of EBM are relatively new:

- The methods of generating high-quality evidence, such as **randomized controlled trials** (RCTs) and other well-designed methods
- The statistical tools for synthesizing and analyzing the evidence (**systematic reviews** [SRs] and **meta-analysis** [MA])
- The ways for accessing the evidence (electronic databases) and applying it (**evidence-based decision making** [EBDM] and practice guidelines)[11,12]

These changes have evolved along with the understanding of what constitutes the evidence and how to minimize sources of bias, quantify the magnitude of benefits and risks, and incorporate patient values.[9,15] "In other words, evidence-based practice is not just a new term for an old concept and as a result of advances, practitioners need (1) more efficient and effective online searching skills to find relevant evidence and (2) critical appraisal skills to rapidly evaluate and sort out what is valid and useful and what is not."[33]

EBDM is the formalized process and structure for learning and using the skills for identifying, searching for, and interpreting the results of the best scientific evidence, which is considered in conjunction with the clinician's experience and judgment, the patient's preferences and values, and the clinical and patient circumstances when making patient care decisions. Translating the EBDM process into action is based on the abilities and skills identified in Box 2.1.[36]

Principles of Evidence-Based Decision Making

The use of current best evidence does not replace clinical expertise or input from the patient but rather provides another dimension to the decision-making process,[13,19,22] which is also placed in context with the patient's clinical circumstances (Fig. 2.1). It is this decision-making process that we refer to as "evidence-based decision making" and is not unique to medicine or any specific health discipline; it represents a concise way of referring to the application of evidence to clinical decision making.

BOX 2.1 Skills and Abilities Needed to Apply an Evidence-Based Decision-Making Process

1. Convert information needs and problems into clinical questions so that they can be answered.
2. Conduct a computerized search with maximum efficiency for finding the best external evidence with which to answer the question.
3. Critically appraise the evidence for its validity and usefulness (clinical applicability).
4. Apply the results of the appraisal, or evidence, in clinical practice.
5. Evaluate the process and your performance.

National Library of Medicine: MEDLINE, PubMed, and PMC (PubMed Central). How are they different? https://www.nlm.nih.gov/bsd/difference.html.

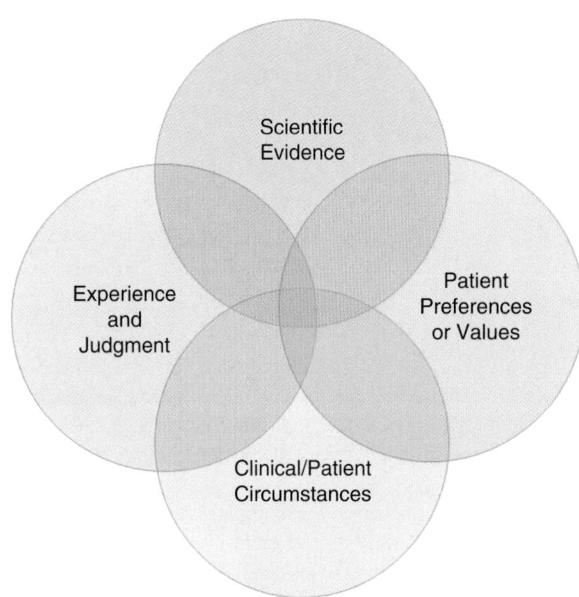

Fig. 2.1 Evidence-based decision making. *(Adapted from Image Copyright Jane L. Forrest, reprinted with permission.)*

EBDM focuses on solving clinical problems and involves two fundamental principles, as follows[15]:

1. Evidence alone is never sufficient to make a clinical decision.
2. Hierarchies of quality and applicability of evidence exist to guide clinical decision making.

EBDM is a structured process that incorporates a formal set of rules for interpreting the results of clinical research and places a lower value on authority or custom. In contrast to EBDM, traditional decision making relies more on intuition, unsystematic clinical experience, and pathophysiologic (biologic) rationale.[15]

Evidence-Based Dentistry

Since the 1990s, the evidence-based movement has continued to advance and is widely accepted among the health care professions, with some refining the definition to make it more specific to their area of health care. The American Dental Association (ADA) has defined evidence-based dentistry (EBD) as "an approach to oral health care that requires the judicious integration of systematic assessments of clinically relevant scientific evidence, relating to the patient's oral and medical condition and history, with the dentist's clinical expertise and the patient's treatment needs and preferences."[4] They have also established the ADA Center for Evidence-Based Dentistry (ebd.ada.org) to facilitate the integration of EBD into clinical practice.

The ADA's definition is now incorporated in the Accreditation Standards for Dental Education Programs.[3] Dental schools are expected to develop specific core competencies that focus on the need for graduates to become critical thinkers, problem solvers, and consumers of current research findings to enable them to become lifelong learners. The accreditation standards require learning EBDM skills so that graduates are competent in being able to find, evaluate, and incorporate current evidence into their decision making.[3]

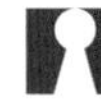

KEY FACT

PICO

The first step in evidence-based decision making is asking the right question. The key is to frame a question that is simple and at the same time highly specific to the clinical scenario. Dissecting the question you want to ask into its components—problem or population (P), intervention (I), comparison group (C), and outcomes (O)—and then combining them will facilitate a thorough and precise evidence search.[36] In some cases, the time duration that it takes to demonstrate a measurable clinical outcome or the observation period (T) is also included in the research question.

Evidence-Based Decision-Making Process and Skills

The growth of evidence-based practice has been made possible through the development of online scientific databases, such as MEDLINE (PubMed) and internet-based software, along with the use of computers and mobile devices (e.g., smartphones) that enable users to quickly access relevant clinical evidence from almost anywhere. This combination of *technology* and *good evidence* allows health care professionals to readily apply the benefits from clinical research to patient care.[34] EBDM recognizes that clinicians can never be completely current with all conditions, medications, materials, or available products, and it provides a mechanism for assimilating current research findings into everyday practice to answer questions and to stay current with innovations in dentistry. A critical thinking skillset is an important prerequisite in EBDM. Fig. 2.2 depicts the traits that overlap between critical thinking and EBDM processes and how they are interconnected to tackle everyday clinical problems. Translating the EBDM process into action is based on the abilities and skills identified in Box 2.1.[36] This is illustrated clearly in a real patient case scenario (management of a patient with trauma-related avulsion and luxation of teeth) that is introduced in Case Scenario 2.1 (Figs. 2.3 and 2.4) and used throughout the chapter.

Asking Good Questions: The PICO Process

Converting information needs and problems into clinical questions is a difficult skill to learn, but it is fundamental to evidence-based practice. The EBDM process almost always begins with a patient question or problem. A "well-built" question should include four parts that identify the patient problem or population *(P)*, intervention *(I)*, comparison *(C)*, and outcome(s) *(O)*, referred to as PICO.[36] Once these four components are clearly and succinctly identified, the following format can be used to structure the question:

"For a patient with _____ (P), will _____ (I) as compared with _____ (C) increase/decrease/provide better/in doing _____ (O)?"

The formality of using PICO to frame the question serves two key purposes, as follows:

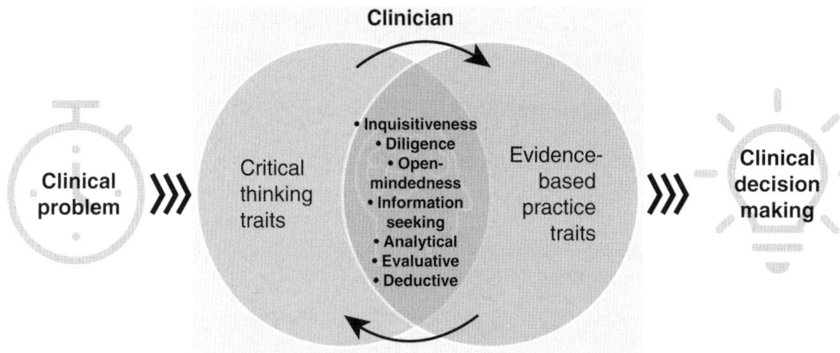

Fig. 2.2 Schematic illustrating traits that overlap critical thinking and evidence-based practice that serve the clinician to tackle day-to-day time-sensitive clinical problems and aid in clinical decision making. Critical thinking is important in evidence-based practice, and the systematic approach in evidence-based clinical practice bolsters critical thinking ability.

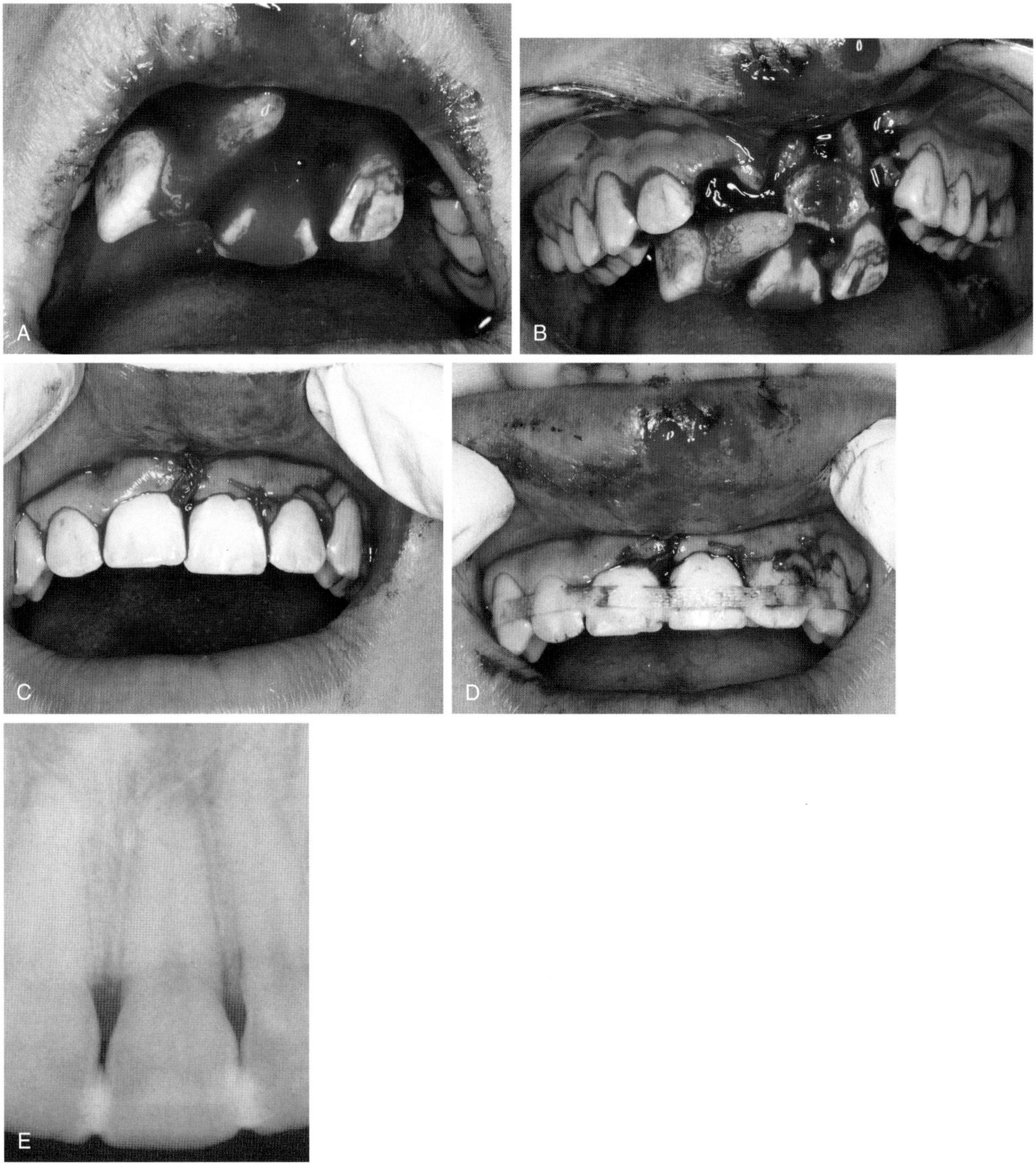

Fig. 2.3 (A) Initial examination of the patient. (B) Trauma site following irrigation. (C) Replantation of avulsed and luxated teeth. (D) Replanted and splinted teeth. (E) Radiograph after placement of the splint. (*Copyright Greg W. Miller, DDS, reprinted with permission.*)

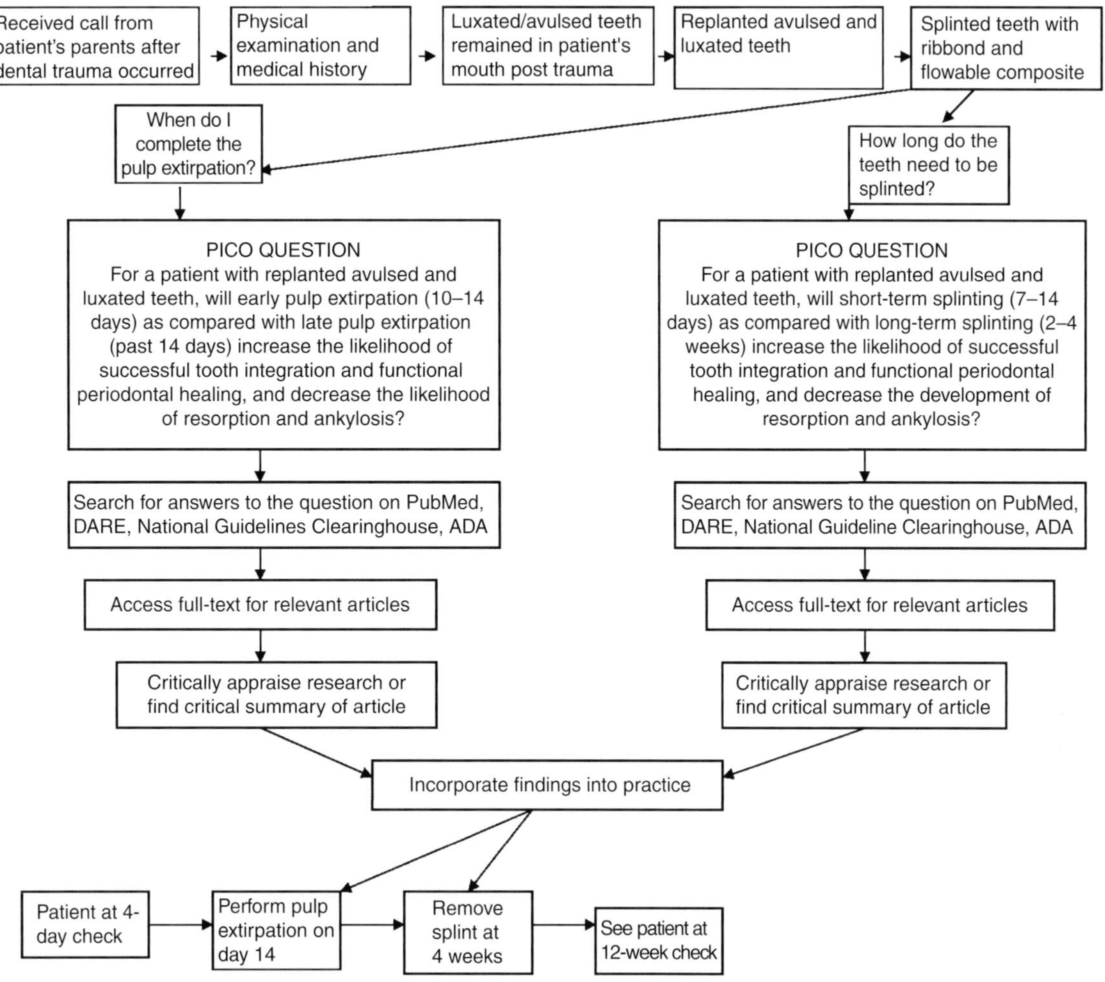

Fig. 2.4 Decision-making pathway from telephone call to resolution. *ADA,* American Dental Association; *DARE,* Database of Abstracts of Review of Effectiveness; *PICO,* patient problem or population, intervention, comparison, and outcome(s). (*Copyright Greg W. Miller, DDS, reprinted with permission.*)

1. PICO forces the clinician to focus on what he or she and the patient believe to be the most important single issue and outcome.
2. PICO facilitates the next step in the process, the computerized search, by identifying key terms that will be used in the search.[36]

The conversion of information needs into a clinical question is demonstrated using Case Scenario 2.1. Two separate PICO questions were written as follows:

1. For a patient with replanted **avulsed and luxated teeth** (P), will early pulp extirpation (10 to 14 days) (I) as compared with late pulp extirpation (past 14 days) (C) increase the likelihood of successful tooth integration and functional periodontal healing and decrease the likelihood of resorption and ankylosis (O)?
2. For a patient with replanted avulsed and luxated teeth (P), will short-term splinting (7 to 14 days) (I) as compared with long-term splinting (2 to 4 weeks) (C) increase the likelihood of successful tooth integration and functional periodontal healing and decrease the development of resorption and ankylosis (O)?

PICO directs the clinician to identify clearly the problem, the results, and the outcomes related to the specific care provided to that patient. This, in turn, helps identify the search terms that should be used to conduct an efficient search. It also allows identification of the type of evidence and information required to solve the problem, as well as considerations for measuring the effectiveness of the intervention and the application of the EBDM process. Thus EBDM supports continuous quality improvements through measuring outcomes of care and self-reflection.

Before conducting a computerized search, it is important to have an understanding of the types of research study methodologies and the appropriate methodology that relates to different types of clinical questions. The methodology, in turn, relates to the levels of evidence. Table 2.1 shows these relationships.

Becoming a Competent Consumer of the Evidence

Evidence typically comes from studies related to questions about treatment and prevention, diagnosis, etiology and harm, and prognosis of disease, as well as from questions about the quality and economics of care. Evidence is considered the synthesis of all valid research that answers a specific question and that, in most cases, distinguishes it from a single research study.[18] Once synthesized, evidence can help inform decisions about whether a method of diagnosis or a treatment is effective relative to other methods of diagnoses or to other treatments and under what circumstances. The challenge in using EBDM arises when only one research study is available on a particular topic. In these cases, individuals should be cautious in relying on the study, because it can be contradicted by another study and it may test only efficacy and not effectiveness. This underscores the importance of staying current with the scientific literature because the body of evidence evolves over time as more research is conducted. Another challenge in using EBDM occurs when the limited research available is weak in quality or poorly conducted. In these cases, one may rely more heavily on clinical experience and patients' preferences and values than the scientific evidence (see Fig. 2.1).

TABLE 2.1 Type of Question Related to Type of Methodology and Levels of Evidence

Type of Question	Methodology of Choice[32]	Question Focus[25]
Therapy, prevention	MA or SR of randomized controlled trials SR of cohort studies	Study effect of therapy or test on real patients; allows for comparison between intervention and control groups; largest volume of evidence-based literature
Diagnosis	MA or SR of controlled trials (prospective cohort study) *Controlled trial* (Prospective: compare tests with a reference or "gold standard" test)	Measures reliability of a particular diagnostic measure for a disease against the "gold standard" diagnostic measure for the same disease
Etiology, causation, harm	MA or SR of cohort studies *Cohort study* (Prospective data collection with formal control group)	Compares a group exposed to a particular agent with an unexposed group; important for understanding prevention and control of disease
Prognosis	MA or SR of inception cohort studies *Inception cohort study* (All have disease but free of the outcome of interest) *Retrospective cohort*	Follows progression of a group with a particular disease and compares with a group without the disease

MA, Meta-analysis; *SR*, systematic review.

Sources of Evidence

The two types of evidence-based sources are primary and secondary, as follows:

- *Primary sources* are original research studies and publications that have not been filtered or synthesized, such as an RCT or a cohort study.
- *Secondary sources* are synthesized studies and publications of the already conducted primary research. These include **clinical practice guidelines** (CPGs), SRs, MAs, and evidence-based article reviews and protocols. This terminology is often confusing to individuals new to the EBDM approach because, although SRs are *secondary* sources of evidence, they are considered a higher level of evidence than a *primary* source, such as an individual RCT.

Both primary and secondary sources can be found by conducting a search using such biomedical databases as MEDLINE (accessed through PubMed), Embase, and Database of Abstracts of Review of Effectiveness (DARE). Other sources of secondary evidence, such as CPGs, clinical recommendations, parameters of care, position papers, academy statements, and critical summaries related to dental practice, can be found on the websites of professional organizations and journals, as listed in Table 2.2. Additional EBDM resources for clinicians are available online in eTable 2.1.

Levels of Evidence

As previously mentioned, one principle of EBDM is that hierarchies of evidence exist to guide decision making. At the top of the hierarchy for therapy are CPGs (Fig. 2.5). These are systematically developed statements to assist clinicians and patients about appropriate health care for specific clinical circumstances.[10] CPGs should be based on the best available scientific evidence, typically from MAs and SRs, which put together all that is known about a topic in an objective manner. The level and quality of the evidence are then analyzed by a panel of experts who formulate the CPGs. Thus guidelines are intended to translate the research into practical application.

Guidelines also will change over time as the evidence evolves, thereby underscoring the importance of keeping current with the scientific literature. One example of this is the change in the American Heart Association guidelines for the prevention of infective endocarditis related to the need for premedication before dental and dental hygiene procedures.[5] Before the 2007 guidelines, the last update was in 1997, and before then, eight updates were added to the primary regimens for dental procedures since the original guideline was first published in 1955. In the 2007 update, the rationale for revising the 1997 document was provided, notably that the prior guidelines were largely based on expert opinion and a few case-controlled studies. With more research conducted, the ability now existed to synthesize those findings to provide a more objective body of evidence on which to base recommendations.[5]

If a CPG does not exist, other sources of preappraised evidence (critical summaries, critically appraised topics [CATs], SRs, MAs, or reviews of individual research studies) are available to help stay current. MAs and SRs have strict protocols to reduce bias and the synthesis of research from more than one study. These reviews provide a summary of multiple research studies that have investigated the same specific question. SRs use explicit criteria for retrieval, assessment, and synthesis of evidence from individual RCTs and other well-controlled methods. SRs facilitate decision making by providing a clear summary of the current state of the existing evidence on a specific topic. SRs provide a way of managing large quantities of information,[28] thus making it easier to keep current with new research.

MA is a statistical process used when the data from the individual studies in the SR can be combined into one analysis. When data from these studies are pooled, the sample size and power usually increase. As a result, the combined effect can increase the precision of estimates of treatment effects and exposure risks.[28]

SRs and MAs are followed respectively by individual RCT studies, cohort studies, case-control studies, and then studies not involving human subjects.[32] In the absence of scientific evidence, the consensus opinion of experts in appropriate fields of research and clinical practice is used (see Fig. 2.5). This hierarchy of evidence is based on the concept of causation and the need to control bias.[24,25] Although each level may contribute to the total body of knowledge, "not all levels are equally useful for making patient care decisions."[25] In progressing up the hierarchy, the number of studies and, correspondingly, the amount of available literature decrease, while at the same time their relevance to answering clinical questions increases.

Evidence is judged on its rigor of methodology, and the level of evidence is directly related to the type of question asked, such as those derived from issues of therapy or prevention, diagnosis, etiology, and prognosis (see Table 2.1). For example, the highest level of evidence associated with questions about therapy or prevention is from CPGs based on MAs and/or SRs of RCT studies. However, the highest level of evidence associated with questions about prognosis

TABLE 2.2 Sources of Secondary Evidence

Sources	Websites
American Academy of Pediatric Dentistry (AAPD): 2017–2018 definitions, oral health policies, and clinical practice guidelines	http://www.aapd.org/policies
American Academy of Periodontology (AAP): Clinical and scientific papers[1]	https://www.perio.org/resources-products/clinical-scientific-papers.html
American Dental Association (ADA), Center for Evidence-Based Dentistry	http://ebd.ada.org
American Heart Association (AHA): Prevention of bacterial endocarditis, recommendations	http://circ.ahajournals.org/content/116/15/1736.full.pdf+html?sid=ada268bd-1f10-4496-bae4-b91806aaf341
Centers for Disease Control and Prevention (CDC): Guidelines and recommendations	http://www.cdc.gov/OralHealth/guidelines.htm
Cochrane Collaboration: A nonprofit organization dedicated to producing systematic reviews as a reliable and relevant source of evidence about the effects of health care for making informed decisions.[9]	http://www.cochrane.org Cochrane Oral Health Group: http://ohg.cochrane.org
Journal: *Evidence-Based Dentistry*	http://www.nature.com/ebd/index.html
Journal: *Journal of Evidence-Based Dental Practice*	http://www.jebdp.com

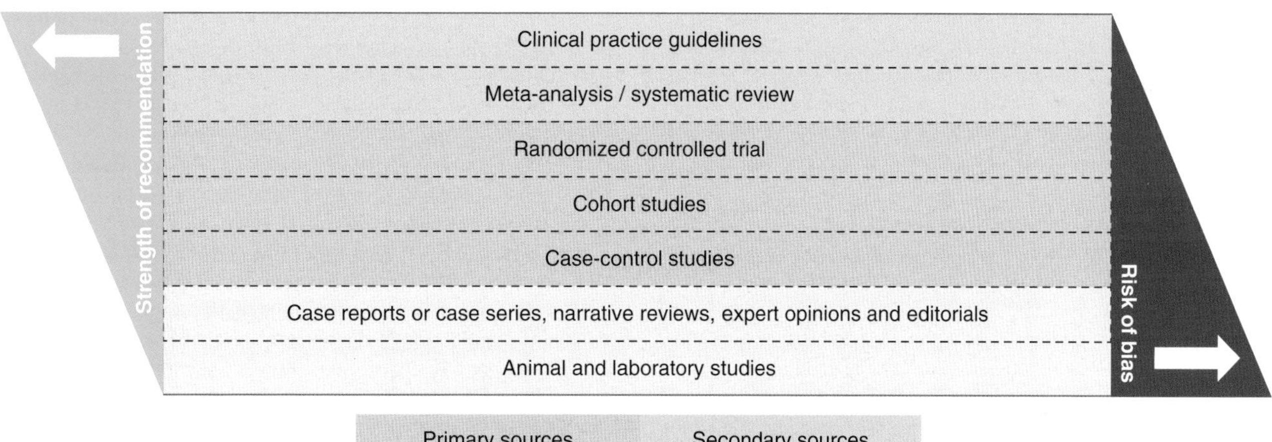

Fig. 2.5 Hierarchy of research and levels of clinical evidence. (*Adapted from an Image Copyright 2012 JL Forrest, SA Miller: National Center for Dental Hygiene Research & Practice.*)

is from CPGs based on MAs and/or SRs of inception cohort studies.[32] Because the two case scenario questions are related to prognosis, the highest level of evidence for them is a CPG based on MAs and/or SRs of inception cohort studies. If no CPG is found, then the next highest level would be a critical summary of an MA or SR of cohort studies. In the event that a critical summary is not found, MAs or SRs of cohort studies followed by individual cohort studies provide the next highest levels of evidence.

Knowing what constitutes the highest levels of evidence and knowing how to apply evidence-based filters are necessary skills to search the literature with maximum efficiency.[25] By using filters, one can refine the search to limit the citations to publication types such as practice guidelines, MAs, SRs, RCTs, and clinical trials, the highest levels of evidence.

Having talked about the hierarchy of evidence, it important to know that, although SRs or MAs occupy the highest echelon in the hierarchy of evidence, they are as good as the studies they encompass. If there were inherent deficiencies in the design and conduction of RCTs and therefore have a high risk of bias, then an SR that includes those trials, even if well conducted, will carry over those deficiencies. On the contrary, an SR or MA of observational studies with low risk of bias will have better quality of evidence and strength of recommendation, in comparison to the previous situation. Therefore it is important to note that not all SRs and MAs can be treated the same with respect to evidence quality and strength of recommendation. For this reason, some authors proposed changing the horizontal lines that separate the categories in the hierarchy to wavy lines and to separate SRs and MAs from the top of the hierarchy ladder and to make it into a lens through which other study designs are viewed.[29]

Searching for and Acquiring the Evidence

PubMed is designed to provide access to both primary and secondary research from the biomedical literature. PubMed provides free access to MEDLINE, the National Library of Medicine's premier bibliographic database covering the fields of medicine, nursing, dentistry, veterinary medicine, the health care system, and the preclinical sciences. MEDLINE contains bibliographic citations and author abstracts from more than 5200 biomedical journals published in the United States and 80 other countries. The database contains more than 26 million citations dating back to 1946.[31]

It is often helpful to identify the appropriate terminology when searching PubMed. This is done by using the Medical Subject Heading (MeSH) database. It provides the definition of terms and illustrates how the terms are indexed in MEDLINE. The PICO terms from the question can be typed into the MeSH database to

TABLE 2.3 Search Terms for Each PICO Question

PICO Question 1 Search Terms		PICO Question 2 Search Terms
Tooth avulsion (MeSH)[26] OR Tooth replantation (MeSH)[26]	P	Tooth avulsion (MeSH)[26] OR Tooth replantation (MeSH)[26]
Pulp extirpation OR Root canal therapy (MeSH)[26]	I	Splints (MeSH)[26]
(Same intervention as above; however, timing is the real comparison so that is the factor in the final article selection.)	C	(Same intervention as above; however, timing is the real comparison so that is the factor in the final article selection.)
Tooth integration OR Functional periodontal healing OR Root resorption (MeSH)[26] OR Tooth ankylosis (MeSH)[26]	O These terms were used as inclusion criteria and were not used when searching PubMed because only a few systematic reviews and guidelines were found using just the P, I, and C terms	Tooth integration OR Functional periodontal healing OR Root resorption (MeSH)[26] OR Tooth ankylosis (MeSH)[26]

MeSH, Medical Subject Heading (database); *PICO,* patient problem or population, intervention, comparison, and outcome(s).

maximize searching efficiency. For example, by typing "avulsed tooth" into the MeSH database, a term from the case scenario, it is learned that the MeSH term is "tooth avulsion." It is defined as partial or complete displacement of a tooth from its alveolar support. It is commonly the result of trauma. It is also learned that "tooth luxation" links to the MeSH term "tooth avulsion." This informs the searcher that "tooth avulsion" is the best term to use for the search because it encompasses both avulsed and luxated teeth.[26]

Using PubMed's Clinical Queries feature, one can quickly pinpoint a set of citations that will potentially provide an answer to the question being posed. Although online databases provide quicker access to the literature, knowing how databases filter information and having an understanding of how to use search terms and database features allow a more efficient search to be conducted.

Because two focused clinical (PICO) questions were generated from the clinical case, two separate searches were conducted, one for each PICO question. In addition to PubMed, several other databases were used to find high levels of evidence. These included the Database of Abstracts of Reviews of Effects (https://www.crd.york.ac.uk/CRDWeb/), Scopus (https://www.scopus.com/), Web of Science (https://apps.webofknowledge.com/), the National Guideline Clearinghouse (http://www.guideline.gov), the ADA Center for Evidence-Based Dentistry website (http://ebd.ada.org), the American Academy of Pediatric Dentistry website (www.aapd.org), and the American Association of Endodontists (www.aae.org), resulting in several relevant references. In addition, clinicians can subscribe to portals such as PracticeUpdate-Clinical Dentistry channel (https://www.practiceupdate.com/explore/channel/clinical-dentistry/sp23) that allow them to stay updated on recent advances in clinical dentistry. The subscribers of this ADA-Elsevier joint initiative receive daily updates of recently published relevant articles with brief take-home messages with or without additional expert commentaries.

When searching for evidence, the PICO question guides the search (Table 2.3).[4,6] By using key terms identified in the PICO question and combining them using the Boolean operators "OR" and "AND," relevant articles can be narrowed to a manageable number.

The first search used the terms "(tooth avulsion OR tooth replantation) AND (pulp extirpation OR root canal therapy)." This resulted in 590 papers. Studies were limited to practice guidelines, MAs, and SRs by using each of these three filters separately so that each of these types of studies could be identified. The findings included four practice guidelines, including those of the American Association of Endodontists and the International Association of Dental Traumatology, one critical summary of an SR, and one SR. The second search used the terms "(tooth avulsion OR tooth replantation) AND splints." This resulted in 340 papers. Again, studies were limited to practice guidelines, MAs, and SRs by using the filter for each publication type separately. Relevant results included four practice guidelines from the International Association of Dental Traumatology and Pediatric Dentistry, one MA, and one SR. Fig. 2.3 provides a detailed review of the decision-making steps in this case and the outcomes.[27]

The articles that were selected as relevant research included each aspect of the PICO question. Inclusion criteria were the following: The patient population studied had to have replanted avulsed or luxated teeth; the research studied the intervention for each of the two PICO questions, pulp extirpation and splint duration, respectively; and the research measured at least one of the outcomes of tooth integration, functional periodontal healing, or the levels of resorption or ankylosis. To reduce the requirement of critical appraisal, the search also looked for critical summaries of the SRs that were found.

Critical Summary

A critical summary is a brief article that effectively summarizes and critically appraises an already published systematic review (SR). Because it includes a critical appraisal component, it makes it easier for clinicians to apply the results to a given clinical situation without having to read the entire SR. Several critical summaries can be found at the ADA Center for Evidence-Based Dentistry website (https://ebd.ada.org/en/evidence).

Appraising the Evidence

After identifying the evidence gathered to answer a question, it is important to have the skills to understand the evidence found. In all cases, it is necessary to review the evidence, whether it is a CPG, an MA, an SR, or an original study, to determine whether the methods were conducted rigorously and appropriately. International evidence-based groups have made this easier by developing appraisal forms and checklists that guide the user through a structured series of "YES/NO" questions to determine the validity of the individual study or SR. Table 2.4 provides the names and websites of three different guides that can be used for critical analysis.

TABLE 2.4 Examples of Critical Analysis Guides

Guide	Purpose
CONSORT (Consolidated Standards of Reporting Trials) statement[3] http://www.consort-statement.org	To improve the reporting and review of RCTs
PRISMA (Preferred Reporting Items for Systematic Reviews and Meta-analyses) http://www.prisma-statement.org	To improve the reporting and review of SRs
CASP (Critical Appraisal Skills Program)[11] http://www.casp-uk.net	To review RCTs, SRs, and several other types of studies

RCTs, Randomized controlled trials; *SRs*, systematic reviews.

Common Ways Used to Report Results

Once the results are determined to be valid, the next step is to determine whether the results and potential benefits (or harms) are important. Straus and colleagues[36] identified the clinically useful measures for each type of study. For example, in determining the magnitude of therapy results, we would expect articles to report the control event rate (CER), the experimental event rate (EER), the absolute and relative risk reduction (ARR or RRR), and number needed to treat (NNT). The NNT provides the number of patients (e.g., surfaces, periodontal pockets) who would need to be treated with the experimental treatment or intervention to achieve one additional patient (surfaces, periodontal pockets) who has a favorable response. Another way of assessing evidence is presented in Chapter 3, which introduces 12 tools that may be useful in assessing causality in clinical sciences.

In appraising the evidence found for the case scenario, the first research study retrieved that answered the first PICO question was a well-conducted SR published in *Dental Traumatology* in 2009.[20] Results indicated an association between pulp extirpations performed after 14 days following replantation and the development of inflammatory resorption. A corresponding critical summary was also found.[35] This evidence was consistent with the 2007 clinical guidelines from the International Association of Dental Traumatology for pulp extirpation within 10 to 14 days of replantation.[16]

The Practice Guideline on the Management of Acute Dental Trauma from the American Academy of Pediatric Dentistry answered the second PICO question. It recommended a "flexible splint for 1 week" for avulsed teeth. However, for lateral luxation, an additional 2 to 4 weeks may be needed when there is breakdown of marginal bone.[2] In addition, a well-conducted SR about splinting duration reported inconclusive evidence of an association between short-term splinting and an increased likelihood of functional periodontal healing, acceptable healing, or decreased development of replacement resorption.[21] The study found no evidence to contraindicate the current guidelines and suggested that the likelihood of successful periodontal healing after replantation was unaffected by splinting duration. Although this SR excluded studies of luxated teeth, this SR is still applicable to the patient. It concluded that dentists should continue to use the currently recommended splinting periods when replanting avulsed permanent teeth, pending future research to the contrary.[21] Consistent with previous reviews, another SR on splinting luxated, avulsed, and root-fractured teeth reported that "the types of splint and the fixation period are generally not significant variables when related to healing outcomes."[23] These two SRs were appraised using the Critical Appraisal Skills Program (CASP) form for appraising reviews (see Table 2.4).

Applying the Evidence: Evidence-Based Dentistry in Action

Throughout this chapter, the EBDM process has illustrated the application of evidence in clinical decision making. The clinician used the EBDM process to answer two clinical questions. Several relevant resources were incorporated into the decision-making process and the treatment of the patient. The clinician performed pulp extirpations on the avulsed and luxated teeth within the recommended time period of 10 to 14 days (Fig. 2.6A). Healing at 2 weeks post trauma is seen in Fig. 2.6B. The clinician also removed the splint within the recommended time frame for luxated teeth of 2 to 4 weeks. The evidence, in combination with clinical experience, helped provide care for this patient that resulted in the best possible prognosis given the extent of the patient's dental trauma. It also allowed the patient to keep her own teeth, which incorporated the patient preferences aspect of the EBDM process. Fig. 2.6C shows the healing at 4 weeks post trauma; Fig. 2.6D shows the healing at 12 weeks; and Fig. 2.6E shows the patient 2 years post trauma.

Evaluating the Outcomes

The final steps in the EBDM process are to evaluate the effectiveness of the intervention and clinical outcomes and to determine how effectively the EBDM process was applied. For example, one question to ask in evaluating the effectiveness of the intervention is, "Did the selected intervention or treatment achieve the desired result?" In this specific case, the answer is yes.

EBDM is a valuable tool that guides practice decisions to achieve optimal results. In the case of tooth avulsion, the key PICO questions were established to identify research that studied the outcomes of reducing the risk of root resorption and tooth ankylosis and increasing periodontal healing. In using the EBDM process, providers can be confident that they have the most current and relevant evidence available on which to base treatment decisions to provide the best treatment to improve the possibility of a successful outcome.

Using an EBDM approach requires understanding new concepts and developing new skills. In addition to evaluating patient care outcomes, another aspect of evaluation is in using the EBDM process. Questions that parallel each step in the EBDM process can be asked in evaluating self-performance. For example, "How well was the search conducted to find appropriate and relevant evidence to answer the question?" As with most learning, time and practice are essential to mastering new techniques.

Real World Clinical Evidence

It is important to note that RCTs are typically conducted in a well-controlled environment so that the investigators are able to clearly discern the true effects of the intervention. The study participants in RCTs are typically selected based on a predetermined set of inclusion and exclusion criteria. This means that certain patients with uncontrolled diabetes or current smokers at the time of study recruitment were potentially excluded from the trial. Therefore it is important for the clinician reading the published RCTs to know the differences between the characteristics of study participants and the patients they would typically encounter in their clinical practice. It is equally important to be cognizant of the differences between the clinical expertise of the authors conducting the trial and the clinician consuming the evidence. Being aware of these differences while reading RCTs will allow the clinician to accurately extrapolate the results of the study and apply the findings to their patient situations in a judicious manner to get predictable treatment outcomes. To improve the translatability of clinical research findings and to overcome some of the aforementioned barriers, the National Dental Practice-Based Research Network

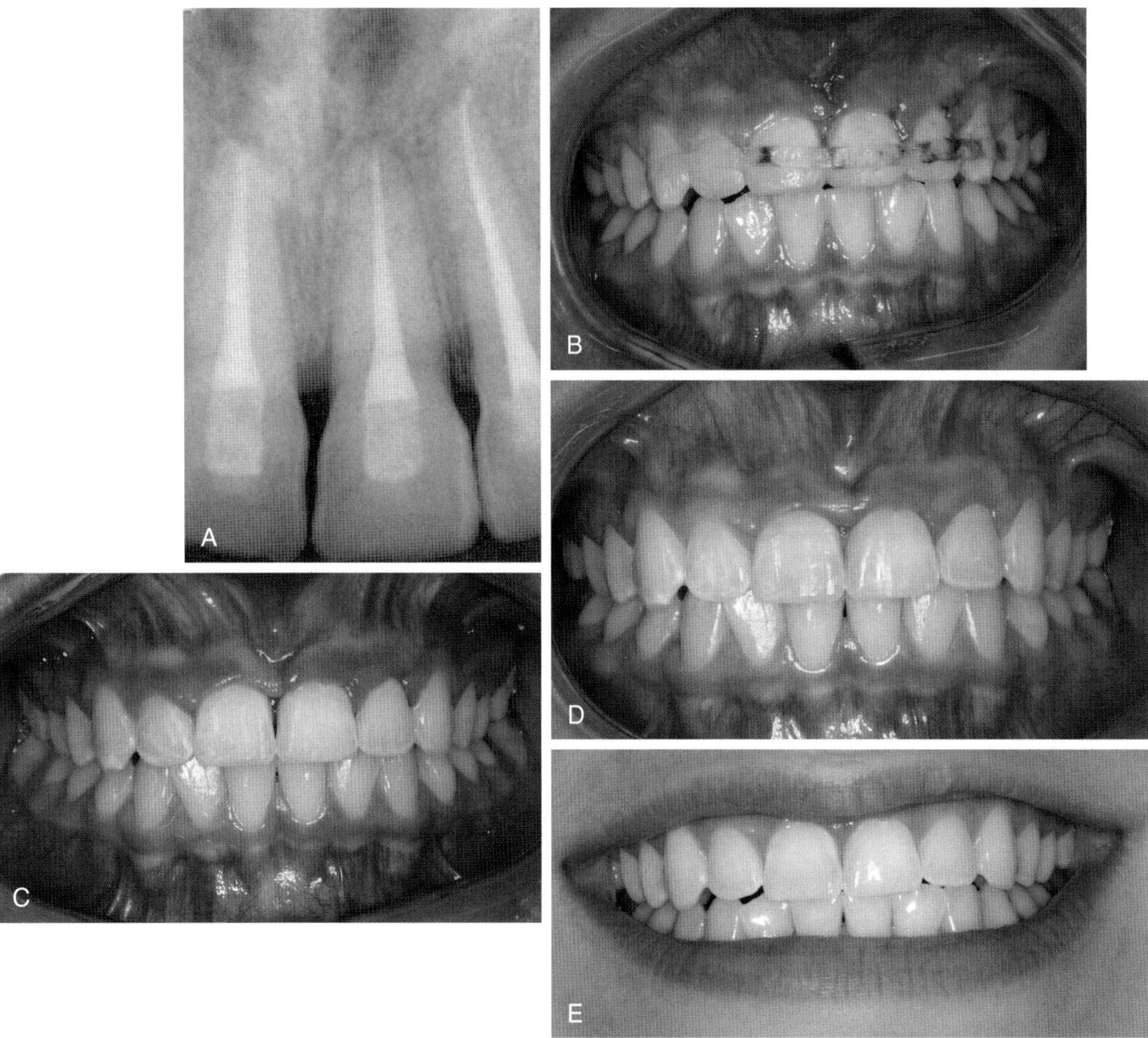

Fig. 2.6 (A) Periapical radiograph following pulp extirpations. (B) Healing at 2 weeks post trauma. (C) Healing at 4 weeks post trauma. (D) Healing at 12 weeks post trauma. (E) Patient 2 years post trauma (*Copyright Greg W. Miller, DDS, reprinted with permission.*)

was created with funding from the National Institutes of Health.[30] The network is a consortium of dental practices across the United States that allows the research to be conducted in the real world of clinical practice by clinicians with varying levels of clinical experience. This effort has led to several publications addressing important clinically applicable questions.[30]

Clinical Decision Support System

Computerized clinical decision support systems (CDSSs), either integrated within the electronic health records (EHR) or as stand-alone systems, are being developed to provide point-of-care patient-specific alerts and guidance to clinicians to aid in informed clinical decision making, be it for prevention, diagnosis, or treatment.[17] A good example is drug interactions alerts provided by CDSSs, prior to prescribing a medication or suggestion alerts for diagnosis based on all the available information. The primary goals of CDSSs are to reduce harm for the patients, improve clinical outcomes, and minimize cost. The available scientific evidence on several health conditions and medications is constantly being fed as data source into CDSSs to keep the system as updated and relevant as it can be. CDSSs are broadly classified into two types: knowledge based and non–knowledge based. In the knowledge-based CDSSs, specific algorithms (IF-THEN) are created (from available scientific evidence) within the system that for a given clinical situation provide an output or actionable item. In the non–knowledge-based CDSSs, data source is still required but the system harnesses the power of artificial intelligence and machine learning to provide patient-specific alerts and clinical recommendations for a given clinical situation.[37] Therefore it is clear that CDSSs have the potential to aid in point-of-care EBDM and SRs confirm their clinical utility and effectiveness.[7,8]

CHAPTER HIGHLIGHTS

- Evidence-based decision making (EB[illegible] [illegible]es clinicians the skills t[illegible] find, efficiently filter, interpret, and apply research findings so that what is known is reflected in the care provided.
- EBDM takes time and practice to learn to use.
- When mastered, EBDM is an efficient way for clinicians to stay current, and it maximizes the potential for successful patient care outcomes

Conclusion

An EBDM approach closes the gap between clinical research and the realities of practice by providing dental practitioners with the skills to find, efficiently filter, interpret, and apply research findings so that what is known is reflected in the care provided. This approach assists clinicians in keeping current with conditions that a patient may have by providing a mechanism for addressing gaps in knowledge to provide the best care possible.

As EBDM becomes standard practice, individuals must be knowledgeable about what constitutes the evidence and how it is reported. Understanding evidence-based methodology and distinctions among different types of articles allows the clinician to better judge the validity and relevance of reported findings. To assist practitioners with this endeavor, SRs and MAs are being conducted to answer specific clinical questions and to support the development of CPGs. Journals devoted to evidence-based practice are published to alert readers about important advances in a concise and user-friendly manner. By integrating good science with clinical judgment and patient preferences, clinicians can enhance their decision-making ability and maximize the potential for successful patient care outcomes.

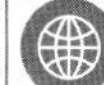

References for this chapter are found on the companion website eBooks.Health.Elsevier.com.

CHAPTER 3

Critical Thinking: Assessing Evidence

Philippe P. Hujoel

CHAPTER OUTLINE

Between 1950 and 2020, 2772 scientific articles were published that have the terms "periodontal diseases" and "antibacterial agents" as Medical Subject Headings. Which of these articles provide information that is clinically relevant? Are those articles that are clinically relevant selected and accurately summarized in educational courses, textbooks, or systematic reviews? Relying completely on authority to ensure that this happens can be dangerous.

Einstein purportedly said that "his own major scientific talent was his ability to look at an enormous number of experiments and journal articles, select the very few that were both correct and important, ignore the rest, and build a theory on the right ones."[6] Most evidence-based clinicians aspire to the same goal when evaluating clinical evidence. In this search for good evidence, a "baloney detection kit"[73] can be helpful to separate salesmanship from science and suggestive hints from unequivocal evidence. This chapter introduces 12 tools that may be useful in assessing causality in clinical sciences.

Twelve Tools for Assessing Evidence

Be Skeptical

Of all machines, ours is the most complicated and inexplicable.

—Thomas Jefferson

By 1990, it was concluded that "available data thus strongly support the hypothesis that dietary carotenoids reduce the risk of lung cancer."[87] Beta-carotene (β-carotene) was hypothesized to interfere passively with oxidative damage to deoxyribonucleic acid (DNA) and lipoproteins,[40] and these beliefs in part translated into $210 million sales of β-carotene in 1997 in the United States. Was this convincing evidence, or should it be evaluated skeptically? Two large randomized controlled trials (RCTs) were initiated, and both were stopped prematurely because β-carotene increased lung cancer risk, cardiovascular disease risk, and overall mortality risk.[62,81] In 2005, the primary investigator of one of the trials reported that "beta-carotene should be regulated as a human carcinogen."[61] In 2015, mechanistic studies started to demonstrate how antioxidants, such as β-carotene, accelerate the growth and invasiveness of tumors.[45,64] Similar dramatic turnarounds are in process on the topic of the "heart-healthy" effects of vegetable oils,[68] dietary salt restriction,[2] or high-carbohydrate diets.[79]

Evidence on how to cure, manage, or prevent chronic diseases is notoriously contradictory, inconsistent, and unreliable. Mark Twain reminded people to be careful when reading health books because one may die of a misprint.[72] Powerful forces conspire to deliver a preponderance of misleading results:

1. Identifying a successful treatment for chronic diseases can be challenging. It has been estimated that less than 0.1% of all investigated treatments are effective. Because the odds of identifying successful interventions for chronic diseases are so small, most so-called effective treatments identified in small clinical trials turn out to be ineffective or harmful when they are evaluated in rigorously conducted pivotal trials.
2. Chronic diseases can be complex and include both environmental and genetic causes. The "obvious" causes of disease, such as tobacco and sugars for periodontitis, are often ignored.[49] As a result of such biased epidemiologic research, incomplete and mistaken understandings of chronic disease etiology can lead to a cascade of wrong turns in the exploration of possible diagnosis, prognosis, and treatment.
3. Poor scientific methodology is a common problem permeating most of the evidence that surrounds us. Popular press headlines tell it all: "Lies, Damned Lies and Medical Statistics,"[71] "Undermined by an Error of Significance: A Widespread Misconception Among Scientists Casts Doubt on the Reliability of a Huge Amount of Research,"[55] "Sloppy Stats Shame Science,"[74] or "How Science Goes Wrong."[28]

4. Finally, the possibility needs to be considered that no magic bullets exist against certain noxious aspects of civilized lifestyles. It was a popular idea in the 20th century that the harmful effects of smoking could be prevented by prescription (e.g., vitamin A), and not proscription (e.g., quit smoking). The experiences so far with finding prescriptions as protection against harmful lifestyles have been largely disastrous.

These factors may all be at play in periodontics, thus suggesting that skepticism is required in the evaluation of scientific evidence. First, the large number of "effective" periodontal treatments may be a telltale sign of a challenging chronic disease. Before 1917, hundreds of pneumonia treatments were available, none of which worked. Before the advent of antibiotics in the 1940s, the wealth of available tuberculosis treatments was misleading in the sense that none really worked. The current "therapeutic wealth" for periodontal diseases may well mean poverty—an indication of the absence of truly effective treatments—and a suggestion that we are dealing with a challenging chronic disease. Second, many no longer regard periodontal diseases as the simple, plaque-related diseases they were thought to be in the mid-20th century but, rather, as complex diseases. Complex diseases are challenging to diagnose, treat, and investigate. Third, the scientific quality of periodontal studies has been rated as low.[4] Major landmark trials were analyzed using wrong statistics,[36,48] most randomized studies were not properly randomized,[55] and the primary drivers of the periodontitis epidemic may have been misunderstood because of the definition of periodontal diseases as an infectious disease without properly controlled epidemiologic studies.[30,31,49] The chance that periodontal research somehow managed to escape the scientific challenges and hurdles that were present in research in medicine appears slim. The opposite appears more likely.

Do Not Trust Biologic Plausibility

Born but to die, and reasoning but to err.

—Alexander Pope

If an irregular heartbeat increases mortality risk, and if encainide can turn an irregular heartbeat into a normal heartbeat, then encainide should improve survival.[66] If high serum lipid levels increase myocardial infarction risk, and if clofibrate can successfully decrease lipid levels, clofibrate should improve survival.[69] If *Streptococcus mutans* causes dental decay, and if chlorhexidine can eradicate *S. mutans,* then chlorhexidine can wipe out dental decay. Such "causal chain thinking" (A causes B, B causes C, and, therefore, A causes C) is common and dangerous. These examples of treatment rationales, although seemingly reasonable and biologically plausible, turned out not to help but to harm patients. Causal chain thinking is sometimes referred to as "deductive inference," "deductive reasoning," or a "logical system."

In mathematics, "once the Greeks had developed the deductive method, they were correct in what they did, correct for all time."[5] In medicine or dentistry, decisions based on deductive reasoning have not been "correct for all time" and are certainly not universal. Because of an incomplete understanding of biology, the use of deductive reasoning for clinical decisions may be dangerous. For thousands of years, deductive reasoning largely failed to lead to medical breakthroughs. In evidence-based medicine, evidence that is based on deductive inference is classified as level 5, which is the lowest level of evidence available.

CLINICAL CORRELATION

The Dietary Guidelines for Americans dropped their recommendation to floss because of the lack of scientific evidence. Dental floss has been recommended by oral hygiene companies and the dental profession based on the following biologic plausibility argument: dental plaque causes dental caries; floss removes dental plaque. Therefore, flossing will lower the risk of dental caries. Such reasoning is no longer accepted as evidence for effectiveness in the 21st century.

Unfortunately, much of our knowledge on how to prevent, manage, and treat periodontitis depends largely on deductive reasoning. Small, short-term changes in pocket depth or attachment levels have been assumed to translate into tangible, long-term benefits to patients, but minimal evidence to support this deductive inference leap is available. In one small study without statistical hypothesis testing, dental plaque was related to the transition from an unnatural, inflammation-free condition referred to as "Aarhus superhealthy gingiva" to experimental gingivitis (which is different from clinical gingivitis).[50] Such studies do not offer proof that dental plaque bacteria cause destructive periodontal disease. It is even unclear whether experimental gingivitis and plaque are correlated at a site-specific level above and beyond what would be expected by chance alone. One subsequent study at the same university, using a similar population, and using a similar experimental design, failed to identify an association between plaque and gingivitis.[50] Evidence that personal plaque control affects the most common forms of periodontal diseases is still weak and largely based on "biologic plausibility" arguments.[33] A move toward a higher level of evidence (higher than biologic plausibility) is needed to put periodontics on a firmer scientific footing.

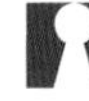

KEY FACT

Biologic plausibility will increasingly become an unacceptable rationale to recommend dental treatments.

What Level of Controlled Evidence Is Available?

Development of Western science is based on two great achievements: the invention of a formal logical system (in Euclidean geometry) by the Greek philosophers, and the discovery of the possibility to find out causal relationships by systematic experiment (during the Renaissance).

—Albert Einstein

Rational thought requires reliance on either deductive reasoning (biologic plausibility) or systematic experiments (sometimes referred to as inductive reasoning). Galileo is typically credited with the start of systematic experimentation in physics. Puzzlingly, it took until the latter half of the 20th century before systematic experiments became part of clinical research. Three systematic experiments are now routine in clinical research: the case-control study, the cohort study, and the RCT. In the following brief descriptions of these three systematic experimental designs, the term *exposure* refers to a suspected etiologic factor or an intervention, such as a treatment or a diagnostic test, and the term *endpoint* refers to the outcome of disease, quality-of-life measures, or any type of condition that may be of interest in clinical studies.

1. *RCT.* Individuals or clusters of individuals are randomly assigned to different exposures and monitored longitudinally for the endpoint of interest. An association between the exposure and the endpoint is present when frequency of the endpoint occurrence differs among the exposure groups. The RCT is the "gold standard" design in clinical research. In evidence-based medicine, RCTs, when properly executed, are referred to as level 1 evidence and the highest (best) level of evidence available.
2. *Cohort study.* Exposed individuals are compared with nonexposed individuals and monitored longitudinally for the occurrence of the primary endpoint of interest. An association between the exposure and endpoint is present when the frequency of endpoint occurrences differs between exposed and nonexposed individuals. A cohort study is often considered the optimal study design in nonexperimental clinical research (i.e., for those study designs where randomization may not be feasible). In evidence-based medicine, cohort studies, when properly executed, are referred to as level 2 evidence.
3. *Case-control study.* Cases (individuals with the endpoint of interest) are compared with controls (individuals without the endpoint of interest) with respect to the prevalence of the exposure. If the prevalence of exposure differs between cases and controls, an association between the exposure and the endpoint is present. In a case-control study, it is challenging to select cases and controls in an unbiased manner and to obtain reliable information on possible causes of disease that occurred in the past. The case-control study is the most challenging study design to use for obtaining reliable evidence. As a result, in evidence-based medicine, case-control studies, when properly executed, are considered the lowest level of evidence.

All three study designs permit us to study the association between the exposure and the endpoint. This association can be represented schematically as follows:

$$\text{Exposure} \rightarrow \text{Endpoint}$$

An important challenge in the assessment of controlled evidence is determining whether the association identified (→) is causal. Criteria used to assess causality include factors, such as the assessment of temporality, the presence of a pretrial hypothesis, and the size or strength of the reported association. Unlike deductive reasoning, in which associations are either true or false, such absolute truths cannot be achieved with systematic experiments. Conclusions based on controlled study designs are always surrounded by a degree of uncertainty, a frustrating limitation to real-world clinicians who have to make yes/no decisions.

Did the Cause Precede the Effect?

You can't change the laws of physics, Captain.

—"Scotty" in Star Trek

In 2001, a study published in the *British Medical Journal* suggested that retroactive prayer shortened hospital stays in patients with bloodstream infection.[47] The only problem was that patients were already dismissed from the hospital when the nonspecified prayer to the nonspecified deity was made. To most scientists, findings in which the effect (shorter hospital stay) precedes the cause (the prayer) are impossible, and this provides an unequivocal example of a violation of correct temporality; the effect preceded the hypothesized cause. In chronic disease research, it is often challenging to disentangle temporality, and fundamental questions regarding temporality often remain disputed. For example, in Alzheimer disease research the amyloid in the senile plaques in the brain is often considered to be the cause of Alzheimer disease, but some researchers suggested that amyloid may be the result, rather than the cause, of Alzheimer disease and that the amyloid may be protective.[46] Or, it is widely believed that obesity is caused by overeating and insufficient physical activity. Yet, increasing evidence points to the opposite—that obesity is a disease induced by carbohydrates that leads to internal starvation and consequent overeating and physical inactivity.[78] Vigorous investigation of temporality is a key aspect in scientific investigation.

Temporality is the only criterion that needs to be satisfied for claiming causality; the cause needs to precede the effect. In periodontal research, almost all studies relating plaque or specific infections to periodontal diseases suffer from unclear temporality.[49] Are observed microbial profiles the result or the cause of periodontitis? No cohort studies in adults have established that an infectious cause precedes the onset of periodontitis.[49] Unequivocal establishment of temporality is an essential element of causality and can be surprisingly difficult to establish for chronic diseases, including periodontal diseases.

No Betting on the Horse After the Race Is Over

Predictions are difficult, especially about the future.

—Niels Bohr

One of the most pervasive cancers in clinical research is the inability of researchers to stick to a hypothesis. Science is about formulating a specific hypothesis, testing it in a clinical experiment, and accepting the findings for what they are. Not only does this rarely happen, but also powerful forces sometimes actively try to prevent regulations that would enforce such scientific behavior.

An acquired immunodeficiency syndrome (AIDS) researcher at an international AIDS conference was jeered when she claimed that AIDS therapy provided a significant benefit for a subgroup of trial participants.[60] A study published in the *New England Journal of Medicine*[51] was taken as a textbook example of poor science[20] when it claimed that coffee drinking was responsible for more than 50% of the pancreatic cancers in the United States. Results of a large collaborative study demonstrating that aspirin use after myocardial infarction increased mortality risk in patients born under Gemini or Libra provided a comical example of an important scientific principle: data-generated ideas are unreliable.

An essential characteristic of science is that hypotheses or ideas predict observations, not that hypotheses or ideas can be fitted to observations. This essential characteristic of scientific enterprise—prediction—is often lost in medical and dental research when poorly defined prestudy hypotheses result in convoluted data-generated ideas or hypotheses that fit the observed data. It has been reported that, even for well-organized studies with carefully written protocols, investigators often do not remember which hypotheses were defined in advance, which hypotheses were data derived, which hypotheses were "a priori" considered plausible, and which were unlikely.[89] A wealth of data-generated ideas can be created by exploring patient subgroups, exposures, and endpoints, as shown by the following:

1. Modifying study sample definition. A commonly observed post-trial modification of a hypothesis is to evaluate improper or proper subgroups of the original study sample. Improper subgroups are based on patients' characteristics that may have been influenced by the exposure. For example, one may evaluate tumor size only in those patients who survived or pocket depths only in those teeth that were not lost during maintenance. Results of improper

subgroup analyses are almost always meaningless when establishing causality. Proper subgroups are based on patients' characteristics that cannot be influenced by the exposure, such as sex, race, or age. A review of trials in the area of cardiovascular disease suggested that even the results of proper subgroup analyses turn out to be misleading in a majority of cases.[89] In the human immunodeficiency virus (HIV) area, one proper subgroup analysis (based on racial characteristics) drew an investor lawsuit on the basis that company officials "deceived" investors with a "fraudulent scheme."[15]

2. Modifying exposure definition. After or during the conduct of a study, the exposure definition can be changed, or the number of exposures under study can be modified. In a controversial trial on the use of antibiotics for middle ear infections, the placebo treatment was replaced with a boutique antibiotic, thus causing a potentially misleading perception of the antibiotics' effectiveness.[16,17,52] In another example of "betting on the horse after the race was over," a negative finding for cigarette smoking (the primary exposure) as a cause of pancreatic cancer reportedly led to the data-generated hypothesis that coffee drinking increased pancreatic cancer risk.[51] When this study was repeated in the same hospital, using the same protocol, but now with the pretrial hypothesis to evaluate coffee drinking, the results of the prior study could not be duplicated.
3. Modifying endpoint definition. Almost all pivotal trials specify one primary endpoint in the pretrial hypothesis. In periodontal research the absence of a specific pretrial defined endpoint is common and permits effortless changing of the endpoint definition. The typical periodontal trial has six endpoints and does not specify which endpoint is primary, and it is not always clear what is a good or a bad outcome.[20] Similarly, the definition of adverse pregnancy outcomes is flexible and susceptible to post hoc manipulations to squeeze out statistical significance. Statistical trickery to reach desired conclusions under such circumstances may be child's play. These problems have remained rampant in clinical research, despite all efforts at preventing them. Two surveys of RCTs published in 2015 reported that 18% to 31% of the trials still changed primary endpoints, and 64% of the trials still changed secondary endpoints.[22,41]

Deviating from the pretrial hypothesis is often compared to data torturing.[56] Detecting the presence of data torturing in a published article is often challenging; just as the talented torturer leaves no scars on the victim's body, the talented data torturer leaves no marks on the published study. Long-term efforts at registering all trials (e.g., see www.alltrials.net) have still not solved this problem.[11] Opportunistic data torturing refers to exploring data without the goal of "proving" a particular point of view. Opportunistic data torturing is an essential aspect of scientific activity and hypothesis generation. Procrustean data torturing refers to exploring data with the goal of proving a particular point of view. Just as the Greek mortal Procrustes fitted guests perfectly to his guest bed either through bodily stretching or through chopping of the legs to ensure correspondence between body height and bed length, so can data be fitted to the pretrial hypothesis by Procrustean means.

What Is a Clinically Relevant Pretrial Hypothesis?

Clinically relevant questions are designed to have an impact on improving patients' outcomes. Usually, clinically relevant questions share four important characteristics of the pretrial hypothesis: (1) a clinically relevant endpoint (referred to as the Outcome in the PICO question), (2) relevant exposure comparisons (referred to as the Intervention and the Control in the PICO question), (3) a study sample representative of real-world clinical patients (should be representative of the patient defined in the PICO question), and (4) small error rates.

Clinically Relevant Endpoint

An endpoint is a measurement related to a disease process or a condition and is used to assess the exposure effect. Two different types of endpoints are recognized. True endpoints are tangible outcomes that directly measure how a patient feels, functions, or survives[80]; examples include tooth loss, death, and pain. Surrogate endpoints are intangible outcomes used as a substitute for true endpoints[23]; examples include blood pressure and probing depths of periodontal pockets. Treatment effects on surrogates do not necessarily translate into real clinical benefit (Table 3.1). Reliance on surrogate endpoints in clinical trials has led to widespread use of deadly medications, and such disasters have prompted minor changes in the drug approval process.[67] Most major causes of human disease (e.g., cigarette smoking) were identified through studies using true endpoints. A first requirement for a clinically relevant study is the pretrial specification of a true endpoint.

Common and Relevant Comparisons

The more prevalent a studied exposure is, the more relevant is the clinical question. A clinically relevant comparison implies the absence of comparator bias, which is defined as the presence of contrived or unethical control groups.[53] Providing the control subjects with less than the standard dose of the standard treatment and providing a control therapy that avoids the real clinical questions are examples of clinically irrelevant research. Similarly, the presence of a placebo treatment, instead of "no" treatment, in clinical trials can be critical given the large therapeutic effects that can be obtained by proper attention and care in medical settings. For instance, the absence of placebo controls in fluoride varnish trials for primary teeth raises serious doubts whether or not fluoride varnish has an effect above and beyond what would be observed with only a placebo. In case-control or cohort studies, the measurement and characterization of exposures (e.g., mercury, fluoride, chewing tobacco) can be difficult and imprecise, thus making answers to the questions almost unavoidably imprecise.

Representative Study Sample

The larger the discrepancy between the typical subjects enrolled in clinical studies and the patient you seek to treat, the more questionable the applicability of the study's conclusions becomes. When cholesterol-lowering drugs provided a small benefit in middle-aged men with abnormally high cholesterol levels, it was concluded that those benefits "could and should be extended" to other age groups and women with "more modest elevations" of cholesterol levels.[82] Findings on blood lipids and heart disease that were derived mostly from Polish immigrants in the Framingham Study were generalized to a much more diverse population. An antidepressant that was approved for use in adults was widely prescribed for children, with unexpected, serious consequences.[1]

Ideally, clinical trials should use simple entry criteria in which the enrolled patients reflect the real-world clinical practice situation as closely as possible. Legislation has been enacted to reach this goal. In 1993, US policy ensured the recruitment of women and minority groups in clinical trials.[10] A US policy for the inclusion of children in clinical studies was then set into law in 1998. Experiments with long lists of inclusion and exclusion criteria can be expensive recipes for failure because they can lead to study subjects who are unrepresentative of most real-world clinical patients.

TABLE 3.1 Examples of Potentially Misleading Surrogates[a]

Disease or Condition	Experimental Treatment	Control Treatment	Effect on Surrogate Endpoint	Effect on True Endpoint	Misleading Conclusion	Reference
AIDS	Immediate zidovudine	Delayed zidovudine	Significant increase of 30–35 CD4 cells/mm^3	No change in incidence of AIDS, AIDS-related complex, or survival	False-positive	82
Osteoporosis	Fluoride	Placebo	Significant increase of 16% in bone mineral density of lumbar spine	Nonvertebral fracture rates increased by 85%	False-positive	
Lung cancer	ZD1839 (Iressa)	Placebo	Dramatic tumor shrinkage in 10% of patients	No effect	False-positive	84
Aphthous ulcers	Thalidomide	Placebo	Although thalidomide expected to decrease TNF-α production, significant increase of 4.4 pg/mL in TNF-α production occurred, suggesting harm	Pain diminished and ability to eat improved	False-negative	34
Edentulism dentures	Implant-supported	Conventional dentures	No impact on chewing cycles	Improved oral health–related quality of life	False-negative	5
Prostate cancer	Radical prostatectomy	Watchful waiting	Substantial elimination of tumor mass	No effect on overall mortality risk	False-positive	80
Advanced colorectal cancer	5-FU + LV	5-FU	23% of patients had 50% or greater reduction in tumor volume	No effect on overall survival	False-positive	38
Periodontitis	Surgery	Scaling	Mean pocket depth reduced by 0.5 mm	Effect on tooth loss or quality of life unknown	?	32

[a]For some examples, the experimental treatment led to improvements in surrogate endpoints, whereas the true endpoint was either unaffected or worsened (a false-positive conclusion). For other examples, the experimental treatment had no impact or worsened the surrogate endpoint, whereas the true endpoint improved (a false-negative conclusion).
AIDS, Acquired immunodeficiency syndrome; *5-FU,* 5-fluorouracil; *LV,* leucovorin; *TNF-α,* tumor necrosis factor-alpha.

Small Type I and Type II Error Rates

The type I error rate is the likelihood of concluding that an effect exists when, in truth, no effect exists. The type I error rate is set by the investigator, and common values are 1% or 5%. The type II error rate is the likelihood of concluding that no effect exists when, in truth, an effect does exist. The type II error rate is typically set by the investigator at 10% or 20%. The complement of the type II error rate (i.e., 1—type II error rate) is referred to as the power of the study. The likelihood of a false-positive or false-negative result depends, in addition to the type I and II error rates, on the likelihood that the treatment under investigation is truly effective. This last component is obviously not under the investigator's control, and yet it determines the likelihood of making correct conclusions. For chronic diseases, in which the likelihood of identifying effective treatments or true causes is low, the false-positive rate can be high, even when the type I error rate is low. Clinically relevant studies require small type I and type II error rates to minimize false-positive and false-negative conclusions.[38]

Size Does Matter

Chronic hepatitis B infection increased the chances for liver cancer by more than 23,000%.[7] Proximity to electromagnetic radiation increased the chance for leukemia in children by 49%.[86] Periodontitis in populations with smokers increased the chance for coronary heart disease by 12%.[34] No one doubts the causality of the association between chronic hepatitis B infection and liver cancer, but the role of periodontitis in coronary heart disease or electromagnetic radiation in childhood leukemia remain controversial. Why? To a large extent, the size of the association drives the interpretation of causality.

The larger an association, the less likely it is to be caused by bias, and the more likely it is causal. One simple way to calculate the size of the association is to calculate an odds ratio. The odds of an event represent the probability that an event happens divided by the probability that an event does not happen. An odds ratio is a ratio of odds. To calculate an odds ratio, a two-by-two (2 × 2) table is constructed in which the outcome is cross-tabulated with the exposure (Table 3.2). Odds ratios can be calculated for data from RCTs, cohort studies, and case-control studies.

The odds ratio is the ratio of the cross-products (ad/bc). The odds ratio associated with penciclovir use for oral lesion healing is (376 × 757) / (526 × 878) = 0.62 (Table 3.3). The odds ratio associated with periodontitis (previously called "chronic periodontitis") for a fatal myocardial infarction is (2 × 1241) / (8 × 257) = 1.21 (Table 3.4). The 95% confidence interval can be approximated by exp[ln(odds ratio) ± 1.96 √ (1/a + 1/b + 1/c + 1/d)]. The 95% confidence intervals of the odds ratio for lesion healing and fatal myocardial infarction are, respectively, exp(−0.48 ± 1.96 √ 0.007), or 0.52 to 0.73, and exp(0.18 ± 1.96 √ 0.63), or 0.25 to 5.72.

TABLE 3.2 Two-by-Two Table Cross-Classifying Exposure and Endpoint[a]

		ENDPOINT	
		Failure	**Success**
Exposure	Experimental	A	B
	Control	C	D

[a]Note that the top left cell, by convention, tallies the number of failures for the experimental group.

TABLE 3.3 Two-by-Two Table on Association Between Penciclovir and Oral Lesion Healing

		ENDPOINT	
		No Lesion Healing by Day 6	**Lesion Healing by Day 6**
Exposure	1% Penciclovir	376	878
	Placebo	526	757

TABLE 3.4 Two-by-Two Table on Association between Periodontitis (Previously Called "Chronic Periodontitis") and Fatal Myocardial Infarction

		ENDPOINT	
		Fatal MI	**No Fatal MI**
Exposure	CP	2	257
	No gingivitis or CP	8	1241

CP, Chronic periodontitis; *MI,* myocardial infarction.

The size of the odds ratio ranges between 0 and infinity. An odds ratio of 1 indicates the absence of an association, and, if the two-by-two table is set up with the reference cell (poor outcome exposure of interest) in the left-hand side of the top data row, an odds ratio larger than 1 means a harmful effect (e.g., periodontitis increases the odds of a fatal myocardial infarction by 20%), and an odds ratio smaller than 1 means a protective effect (e.g., penciclovir decreases the odds of failed lesion healing by day 6 by 38%).

The confidence interval is the range of numbers between the upper confidence limit and the lower confidence limit. The confidence interval contains the true odds ratio with a certain predetermined probability (e.g., 95%). In a properly executed randomized trial, a conclusion of causality is typically made if the 95% confidence interval does not include the possibility of "no association" (e.g., odds ratio = 1). For example, because the 95% confidence interval for the odds ratio associated with penciclovir use is 0.52 to 0.73 and does not include 1, the effect can be referred to as "statistically significant." For the periodontitis (previously called "chronic periodontitis")–myocardial infarction example, the 95% confidence interval ranges from 0.25 to 5.72, includes 1, and is, therefore, referred to as "statistically insignificant."

In epidemiology, where no randomization of individuals to exposures occurs, the interpretation of a confidence interval is challenging because no probabilistic basis (in the form of randomization) exists for making causal inference. A pessimist will claim that, because no randomization was present, no statistical interpretations are allowed.[25] The emphasis should be on visual display of the identified associations and on sensitivity analyses where the results are interpreted under "what if" assumptions. An optimist will argue that the absence of randomization does not preclude the making of statistical inferences, and that one always starts from the assumption that "assignments were random" (even when they were not).[90]

When individuals are randomly assigned to exposures, very small associations (i.e., associations very close to 1, such as 1.1) can reliably be identified. When individuals are not randomly assigned to exposures, as is the case in cohort studies and case-control studies, the size of the reported association (e.g., the odds ratio) becomes key in the interpretation of the findings. Because of the inherent biases in epidemiologic research, small odds ratios cannot be reliably identified. Yet, what is small? Leading epidemiologists provide some guidelines on how to interpret the size of an association with respect to possible causality. Richard Doll, one of the founders of epidemiology, said, "No single epidemiological study is persuasive by itself unless the lower limit of its 95% confidence level falls above a threefold (200%) increased risk." Dimitrios Trichopoulos, past chairperson of the Department of Epidemiology at Harvard University, opted "for a fourfold (300%) increase at the lower limit (of the 95% confidence interval)." Marcia Angell, former editor of the *New England Journal of Medicine,* reported: "As a general rule of thumb we are looking for an odds ratio of 3 or more (≥200% increased odds) [before accepting a paper for publication]." Robert Temple, Director of the Food and Drug Administration, stated: "My basic rule is if the odds ratio isn't at least 3 or 4 (a 200% or 300% increased risk), forget it."[77] Textbooks on evidence-based medicine report an odds ratio of 3 for cohort studies and 4 for case-control studies as a reflection of a reliable result.[76] These opinions provide some guidelines on what size of odds ratio to look for when determining causality.

CLINICAL CORRELATION

Periodontitis during pregnancy was reported to increase the risk for preterm low birth weight eightfold.[21]

Is a Better Alternative Explanation Available?

No amount of experimentation can ever prove me right; a single experiment can prove me wrong.

—Albert Einstein

When you have eliminated the impossible, whatever remains, however improbable, must be the truth.

—Sir Arthur Conan Doyle

Dozens of epidemiologic studies appeared to support the hypothesis that β-carotene intake lowered lung cancer risk. However, RCTs provided unequivocal evidence to the contrary. What went wrong? Different explanations that worked as well or better may have been inadequately explored. Possibly, smoking was not adequately considered as an alternative explanation and led to a misunderstanding of the health effects of β-carotene.[21,75] Similarly, a systematic review of epidemiologic studies appeared to support the hypothesis that periodontitis (previously called "chronic periodontitis") caused low birth weight.[84] In contrast, however, a systematic review of RCTs suggested that the periodontitis–low birth weight theory may be dead.[85] Why was epidemiology misleading? Again, different explanations may have been inadequately

Association present? (not necessarily causal)
Confounding variable
Causal association
Exposure
Endpoint
Investigated causal association

Fig. 3.1 Schematic representation of the two necessary criteria for a variable to induce spurious associations (i.e., to be a confounding variable). The confounding variable has to be associated with the exposure and causally linked to the outcome. When both criteria are satisfied, confounding is said to be present.

explored. More efforts may have been expended toward proving associations by ignoring common causal factors, rather than disproving associations. The highest goal of a scientist is the attempt to refute, disprove, and vigorously explore factors and alternative hypotheses that may "explain away" the observed association.[12] The efforts at refuting smoking and nutrition as potential confounders in periodontics have been minimal and may have led to a significant waste of clinical research resources.

Epidemiologic studies are by nature unreliable. It has been estimated that 80% of the epidemiologic studies report false-positive findings. Two large pivotal trials on periodontal treatments and adverse pregnancy outcomes funded by the National Institutes of Health,[21,75] as well as subsequent epidemiologic studies,[88] failed to confirm the dramatic claims of previously published epidemiologic studies.

For a factor (i.e., a potential confounder) to explain away an observed association, two criteria need to be fulfilled. First, the factor must be related to the exposure, but not necessarily in a causal way. Second, the factor must be causally related to the outcome and must not be in the causal pathway. If both criteria are satisfied, the factor is referred to as a confounder, and confounding is said to be present. For example, smoking satisfied the criteria for a confounder in the β-carotene–lung cancer association because (1) cigarette smokers consumed less β-carotene than nonsmokers, and (2) smoking caused lung cancer. Confounding is often represented schematically (Fig. 3.1).

In randomized studies, confounding is typically not an issue because randomization balances known and unknown confounders across the compared groups with a high degree of certainty. In epidemiologic studies, in which no randomization is present, three questions related to confounding need to be considered in the assessment of the causality, as addressed next.

First, were all important confounders identified? Complex diseases have multiple risk factors, which may act as confounders in the reported association. The multiple confounders need to be included in the statistical analyses. An association unadjusted for any potential confounders is sometimes referred to as the *crude association*. When this crude association is adjusted for potential confounders, it is referred to as an *adjusted association*. Typically, crude and adjusted odds ratios are both presented so that readers can evaluate the direction of the bias.

KEY FACT

Single epidemiologic studies reporting large odds ratios are unreliable.

Second, how accurately were confounders measured? Some potential confounders, such as age, sex, and race, can be measured relatively accurately. Other potential confounders, such as smoking or lifestyle factors, such as nutrition, are notoriously more difficult to measure. A discrepancy between what is measured and what is the truth will result in the incomplete removal of bias and lead to spurious associations. The remaining bias is sometimes referred to as *residual confounding*. Residual confounding is common in epidemiology and is one of the reasons that case-control and cohort studies are less effective research tools than randomized trials in identifying small effects. For instance, an accurate summary of smoking history over a person's lifetime may be impossible.

Third, was the statistical modeling of the confounders appropriate? Any mis-specification of the functional relationships causes bias. For example, assuming a linear relationship between a confounder and an endpoint, whereas, in truth, the relationship is quadratic, causes bias.

Evaluating the impact of confounding can be a challenge. The goal of an epidemiologist is to come up with the best possible defense for why an identified association is spurious. All possible efforts should be spent identifying known confounders, obtaining accurate measurements of the confounders, and exploring different analytic approaches to refute the observed association. Smoking, a potential confounder in many studies, has been found to be such a strong confounder that several leading epidemiologists have suggested that restriction to those who have never been smokers is required to eliminate the potential for residual confounding by smoking. Control for confounding is the major methodologic challenge in epidemiology, and randomization is the only tool available to eliminate confounding reliably.

CLINICAL CORRELATION

Epidemiologic evidence has suggested that periodontal patients who comply with periodontal maintenance procedures lose fewer teeth.[35]

Was the Study Properly Randomized?

It is often taken for granted that randomization is properly performed in RCTs. This is, unfortunately, not the case. Attempts by physicians to circumvent randomization are not isolated events; they used to be part of an endemic problem stemming from ignorance.[60]

Randomization can be a counterintuitive process because it (1) creates heterogeneity, (2) takes control over treatment assignment away from the physician, and (3) leads to apparently illogical situations in which patients randomly assigned to a treatment but refusing compliance still are analyzed as if they received the treatment. Although randomization was a radical innovation introduced for agriculture, some have suggested that it is doubtful whether it would have ever been widely introduced into medicine (and subsequently dentistry) if not for a confluence of factors surrounding the end of World War II in Great Britain. Because of the revolutionary nature of randomization, fundamental misunderstandings of this process remained prevalent until recently. In 1994, about one-third of the clinical trials published in elite medical journals apparently did not ensure that patients are assigned to different treatments by chance.[60] The majority of reported periodontal trials failed to convince reviewers that (1) the studies were properly randomized, (2) randomization was concealed, or (3) randomized patients were accounted for.[57] Tampering with the delicate process of randomization can quickly, according to Ronald Fisher, a statistician and geneticist, turn an experiment into an experience.

KEY FACT

Patients who comply with medical or dental recommendations are typically healthier. As a result, interventions that increase mortality risk in randomized trials will spuriously appear to decrease mortality in epidemiologic studies. The reason for this discrepancy is healthy user bias. A Canadian study[18] demonstrated that patients compliant with taking statins are less likely to have accidents (e.g., burns), more likely to undergo medical screening (e.g., eye examination), less likely to have dental problems, and less likely to have other serious medical problems, such as deep vein thrombosis. Such effects are typically interpreted as examples of healthy user bias. The effectiveness of periodontal treatments in providing tangible patient benefits cannot reliably be estimated in epidemiologic studies due to the healthy user bias.

Several studies have shown how an inadequate randomization process will bias study findings. In one review study, the ability to reject patients from the study after random treatment assignment tripled the likelihood of finding significant results and doubled the likelihood that confounders were unequally distributed among the compared groups.[13] Trials where clinicians can break the randomization code reported treatment effects that averaged 30% larger than effects in trials where the randomization could not be broken.[13] The common desire to eliminate noncompliant patients can similarly lead to biases, as shown by the following two examples. First, in one cardiovascular disease trial, patients compliant with a placebo pill had a 10% reduction in mortality risk compared with patients who were noncompliant with the placebo.[69] Second, in a caries trial, adolescents compliant with a placebo varnish had, on average, 2.2 fewer new caries lesions than adolescents noncompliant with a placebo varnish.[24] Such findings suggest that factors related to compliance and unrelated to the treatments under investigation have a powerful influence on the outcome measured. Deleting such noncompliant patients may lead to biases.

Proper randomization ideally includes the following elements. First, subjects are enrolled into a study before randomization: important baseline disease characteristics are recorded and provided to an independent person or organization. This step ensures that baseline information is available for every patient who will be randomized. Without this step, randomized patients can be "lost," thus leading to biases. Subsequently, an independent person or organization randomly assigns subjects to treatments and informs the clinician regarding the treatment assignment. This randomization process needs to be auditable, a requirement that makes pseudorandom processes, such as coin tosses, unacceptable. The concealment of the randomization process ensures that clinicians cannot crack the code and that they will enroll only those patients they think are suited for the treatment that will be assigned. Finally, the outcome in the subject is evaluated, regardless of follow-up time or compliance and according to the treatment assigned, not the treatment received. Imputation is used in sensitivity analyses to determine the extent that subjects with missing information can bias the conclusions. The whole process of randomization is complex and often deviated from, thereby leading to unreliable results.

When to Rely on Nonrandomized Evidence

Randomize the first patient.

—**Thomas Chalmers**

To tell the truth, all of the discussion today about the patient's informed consent still strikes me as absolute rubbish.

—**Sir Austin Bradford Hill**

Scores of epidemiologic studies reported evidence that hormone replacement therapy provided benefits to postmenopausal women. Despite this "strong" evidence from "leading" researchers, and despite the opposition on ethical grounds to begin a placebo-controlled trial, the Women's Health Initiative trial was initiated. The "miracle" of hormone replacement therapy was shown to lead to increased breast cancer risk, dementia, myocardial infarction, and stroke. This example illustrates the need for randomized studies and for questioning well-established and widely accepted beliefs based on numerous epidemiologic studies. Nonetheless, the initiation of randomized trials can become difficult because of ethical considerations and expensively large sample sizes.

Ethical principles dictate that proposed interventions do more good than harm, that the populations in whom the study will be conducted will benefit from the findings, that informed consent is obtained from enrolled subjects, and that a genuine uncertainty exists with respect to treatment efficacy. The interpretation of these ethical principles is largely determined by culture and era. Ethical principles also play an important role in determining which clinical questions are sufficiently important to warrant the conduct of an RCT.

Sample size requirements represent another consideration that may prevent the conduct of RCTs. The smaller the rate at which endpoints occur in an RCT, the larger the required sample size will be. For rare events, such as bacterial endocarditis subsequent to a dental procedure or HIV conversion after exposure to an HIV-contaminated dental needle, RCTs may never be possible because the required sample sizes are in the 100,000s or millions of subjects.

In addition to both ethical and practical reasons, powerful political issues can surround the decision to initiate clinical trials. It has been pointed out that specialists are unlikely to support clinical trials that evaluate their main source of income.[65] This observation for medical specialties may also hold for periodontics. Although dental professional organizations commonly claim that periodontal disease is a major cause of tooth loss, evidence indicates that standard periodontal therapy is not effective at reducing tooth loss. Hopefully, well-designed and well-conducted studies in the future will allow us to compare different treatments effectively. Unequivocal evidence requires the conduct of rigorously designed and executed RCTs. The absence of RCT evidence for important and answerable clinical questions can be frustrating to those who seek reliable, evidence-based practice guidelines.

Did the Investigators Take Into Account the Placebo or Nocebo Effects?

I never knew any advantage from electricity in (the treatment of) palsies that was permanent. And how far the apparent temporary advantage might arise from the exercise in the patient's journey, and coming daily to my house, or from the spirits given by the hope of success, enabling them to exert more strength in moving their limbs, I will not pretend to say.

—**Benjamin Franklin**[84]

Sham or mock surgical procedures have been used to evaluate whether implanting human fetal tissue in the brain decreases symptoms of Parkinson disease, whether surgical lavage and debridement decrease pain in arthritic knee joints,[58] whether mammary artery ligation improves heart disease outcomes,[14] and whether alveolar trephination relieves the pain of acute apical periodontitis.[27,59]

What motivates clinical investigators to subject patients to surgical risks and yet knowingly provide no hypothesized benefits to these patients? A partial answer to this question lies in a phenomenon known as placebo or nocebo effects: the beneficial or harmful effects patients may experience by participating in a study, by patient–physician interaction, by the patient's anticipation for improvement, or by the patient's desire to please the physician. One group of researchers suspects that the placebo or nocebo effect may be related to the balance of the parasympathetic and sympathetic nervous system, which could explain both placebo and nocebo effects.[43] Without mock surgical procedures it would be impossible to tell whether the improvements observed in clinical trials are caused by the placebo effects associated with the surgical procedures or by the hypothesized active ingredient of the surgery itself.

Two studies have quantified the placebo effect. In the first study, the magnitude of the placebo effect was estimated by evaluating patients' responses to ineffective treatments.[70] Five treatments were identified as ineffective (all these treatments had been abandoned by the medical profession and, in at least one controlled study, confirmed its ineffectiveness). With these ineffective treatments, good to excellent treatment responses were observed in 45% to 90% of the patients, a powerful placebo effect indeed. In the second study, placebo interventions (pharmacologic placebo, physical, or psychological interventions) were compared with true "no-treatment" interventions.[29] A significant placebo effect was observed for pain, the condition that was evaluated in the largest number of trials and that had the largest number of evaluated participants.

Placebo effects can reliably be estimated only when clinical trials randomly assign patients to a placebo treatment and no treatment. Such studies are rare. Some systematic reviews may provide a hint at the magnitude of placebo effects. One systematic review of 133 studies reported that the fluoride effect on caries was significantly larger when a no-treatment control group was used versus a placebo control group.[54] One possible interpretation for these differences is a placebo effect: the placebo lowered caries rates possible through re-equilibrating of parasympathetic and sympathetic nervous activity, which may influence factors, such as improved saliva flow. Other explanations, such as the scientific quality of the studies, may, of course, also be responsible for such observed differences, especially for pain. Overall, sufficient evidence is available to suggest that placebo effects can be real and measurable, and that the magnitude of the placebo effect may depend on the treatment under study and the type of outcome evaluated.

Was Protection in Place Against Conflict of Interest?

In evidence-based medicine, the data from clinical research remain largely esoteric and of no real-world significance if the evidence fails to be translated into clinical practice. Spinal fusion, vertebroplasty, and arthroscopic surgery for knee pain have all shown ineffectiveness in clinical trials, yet these trials had no impact on clinical practice. In some instances, the use of surgical procedures actually increased after a demonstration of ineffectiveness.[39,44] Such discrepancies between clinical practice and science have been in part attributed to "perverse financial incentives."[39]

Can one trust clinical recommendations regarding a novel, noninvasive cardiac bypass operation by a physician who has a $100 million stake in the procedure he or she is recommending? Is it possible that financial stakes are preventing physicians from disclosing a 10-fold increased mortality risk? Can one trust guidelines establishing sharply lowered lipid levels while knowing that eight of the nine panel experts have financial connections to the manufacturers of lipid-lowering drugs? Is it possible that panelists are picked for ideology?[8] Can one trust clinical guidelines published by professional dental organizations? The answers to these questions are not straightforward and, in general, are discussed under the heading of "conflicts of interest."

Conflict of interest has been defined as "a set of conditions in which professional judgment concerning a primary interest (such as patient's welfare or validity of research) tends to be unduly influenced by a secondary interest."[3] A common secondary interest is financial but can include others, such as religious or scientific beliefs, ideological or political beliefs, or academic interests (e.g., promotion). Some examples of how conflicts of interests can bias evidence are the following:

1. Evidence can be suppressed by lawsuits. For example, a company initiated a multimillion-dollar legal action[15] against the investigator who reported that the company's HIV vaccine was ineffective.[42] Companies can attempt to suppress submitted scientific articles that they perceive as incorrect.
2. Negative evidence can disappear into a "black hole."[26] One can expect that 2 of 40 trials of an ineffective treatment will provide positive results by chance if the experiments are run with a type I error rate of 5%. If the 38 negative trial reports go into a file drawer, and if the 2 positive reports lead to drug approval and are published in leading journals, a misleading perception of the drug's effectiveness will be given to the practicing community. Although a Food and Drug Administration official indicated that such situations have never happened,[19] reports on nondisclosed negative trials of an antidepressant drug suggests the contrary.[83] Although registries of clinical trials should succeed at eliminating the problem of disappearing trial results, and although many leading journals request a priori trial registration as a prerequisite for publishing, the problem of disappearing trial results remains with us today.
3. Conflicts of interest can lead to distortion of study designs and analyses to provide the desired results. Such distortions can range from data fabrication and data falsification to design and analysis "tweaks," such as contrived control groups, unplanned subgroup analyses, and only showing that time point in the analysis where the differences favor the investigated drug.
4. Conflicts of interests related to loss of patents or orphan drugs can shunt available research resources to the conduct of clinical trials that are not necessarily in the best interest of public health. The potential for conflict of interest appears to be ever increasing. The prevalence of industry-funded trials is increasing, and more and more universities hold stock in start-up companies that support clinical trials within those institutions. Such connections can be viewed with a skeptical eye. It has been confirmed over and over again that industry-sponsored studies are more likely to have proindustry conclusions than are non-industry-sponsored studies.[9]

Protection against potential conflict of interest is an important aspect of clinical research. Mandatory registration of clinical trials helps. The appointment of independent data and safety monitoring boards for trial monitoring provides protection against biases. Policy regulations established by journals, academic institutions, and governments can further decrease the impact of perceived conflicts of interests. For instance, all the work that has been done toward establishing registries of RCTs helps in decreasing biases.

Conflict of interest issues may be just as prevalent in dental research as in other medical areas dealing with chronic disease. In 2002, an article published in a leading dental journal ended up on the cover of the *New York Times*.[63] In part, the reason was a perceived conflict of interest; the article did not disclose that funding for the study came from an advertising company. Disclosure of conflict of interest is often poorly enforced, and some dental journals do not have regulations in place to reveal potential conflicts of interest of authors. Such situations (1) make it challenging for clinicians to recognize the potential for conflicts of interest, (2) may reduce trust in dental journals, and (3) may affect the scientific integrity of dental research.

Conclusion

Lessons learned from other chronic disease areas do apply to the evaluation of evidence in the periodontal disease research arena. Randomization and confounding are as important in periodontal research as they are in cancer research. Work remains to be done to integrate evidence-based thinking into clinical practice. One challenging task is to lessen the excessive reliance on biologic plausibility in determining both research priorities and patient management and to transition to clinical thinking that is based on controlled clinical observations. Perhaps, however, the most challenging task for the dental profession to eliminate this bias will be to comply with the Institute of Medicine guideline largely to exclude experts from writing clinical guidelines.[37] Although the 12 discussed tools for assessing evidence do not cover all necessary tools, or maybe even the most important tools, it is hoped that they provide a useful starting point for the further exploration of the issues and principles involved in the conduct of systematic experiments in periodontal disease research.

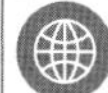
References for this chapter are found on the companion website eBooks.Health.Elsevier.com.

CHAPTER 4

Anatomy, Structure, and Function of the Periodontium

Joseph P. Fiorellini | David M. Kim | Yong-Hee Patricia Chun | Yu-Cheng Chang

For online-only content on the gingival epithelium, the alveolar process, and the attachment apparatus, please visit the companion website at eBooks.Health.Elsevier.com.

CHAPTER OUTLINE

The normal periodontium provides the support necessary to maintain teeth in function. It consists of four principal components: gingiva, periodontal ligament (PDL), cementum, and alveolar bone. Each of these periodontal components is distinct in its location, tissue architecture, biochemical composition, and chemical composition, but all of these components function together as a single unit. Healthy periodontium is usually defined by the absence of inflammation or disease progression. Despite this, there are limited reports that define periodontal health. Research has revealed that the extracellular matrix components of one periodontal compartment can influence the cellular activities of adjacent structures. Therefore, the pathologic changes that occur in one periodontal component may have significant ramifications for the maintenance, repair, or regeneration of other components of the periodontium.[19]

This chapter first discusses the structural components of the normal periodontium; it then describes their development, vascularization, innervation, and functions.

Periodontal Phenotype

The term periodontal biotype was first defined by Seibert in 1989 to categorize periodontium into "thin-scalloped" and "thick-flat" and "thick-scalloped" biotypes (Fig. 4.1).[249] Other terms such as, "gingival biotype," "periodontal morphotype," "gingival morphotype," and "gingival phenotype" were also widely used to refer to the clinical variations in the gingival thickness, the amount of the keratinized tissue width, bone morphotypes, the shape of the tooth, and other morphological characteristics of the gingiva and the periodontium.

The 2017 World Workshop on the Classification of Periodontal and Peri-Implant Diseases and Conditions recommended the adoption of the term "periodontal phenotype" to describe the combination of gingival phenotype (three-dimensional gingival volume and the width of the keratinized tissue) and bone morphotype. This classification system categorizes periodontal phenotype into "thin-scalloped," "thick-scalloped," and "thick-flat." Periodontal phenotype is considered as the combination of the gingival phenotype and bone morphotype.[55,135,144]

Phenotype is influenced by a combination of genetic traits and environmental factors. It is important to know that the periodontal phenotype changes over time due to environmental factors or by phenotype modification therapy. The periodontal phenotype may play an important role in disease progression such as gingival recession and bone resorption. However, further studies are needed to evaluate the correlation between the periodontal phenotype and the therapy outcome.

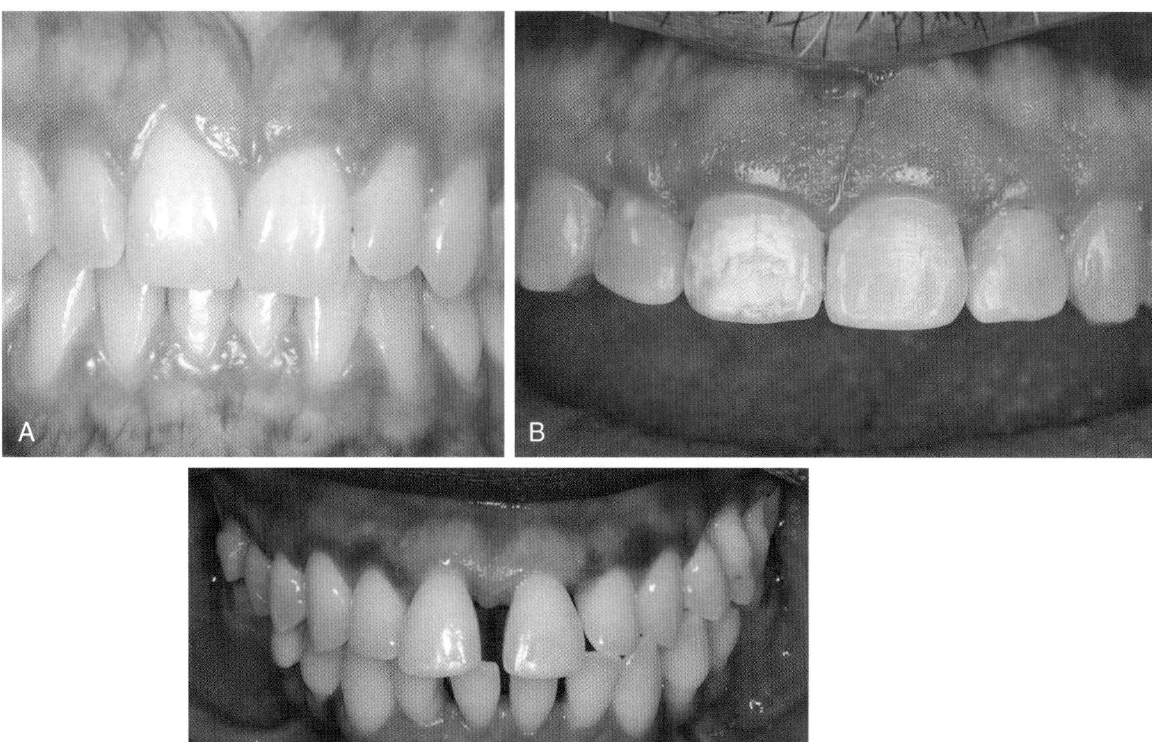

Fig. 4.1 (A) Thin-scalloped biotype. (B) Thick-flat biotype. (C) Thick-scalloped biotype. (Courtesy Dr. Wael Isleem and Dr. Vicky Choi.)

Oral Mucosa

The *oral mucosa* consists of the following three zones:

1. The gingiva and the covering of the hard palate, termed the *masticatory mucosa* (the *gingiva* is the part of the oral mucosa that covers the alveolar processes of the jaws and surrounds the necks of the teeth)
2. The dorsum of the tongue, covered by *specialized mucosa*
3. The oral mucous membrane lining the remainder of the oral cavity

Gingiva

Clinical Features

In an adult, normal gingiva covers the alveolar bone and tooth root to a level just coronal to the cementoenamel junction. The gingiva is divided anatomically into *marginal, attached,* and *interdental areas.* Although each type of gingiva exhibits considerable variation in differentiation, histology, and thickness according to its functional demands, all types are specifically structured to function appropriately against mechanical and microbial damage.[7] In other words, the specific structure of different types of gingiva reflects each one's effectiveness as a barrier to the penetration by microbes and noxious agents into the deeper tissue. The periodontal phenotype may serve as a critical component in disease progression and in treatment outcomes.

Marginal Gingiva

The marginal or unattached or free gingiva is the terminal edge or border of the gingiva that surrounds the teeth in a collar-like fashion (Figs. 4.2 and 4.3).[6] In about 50% of cases, it is demarcated from the adjacent attached gingiva by a shallow linear depression called the *free gingival groove.*[6] The marginal gingiva is usually about 1 mm wide, and it forms the soft-tissue wall of the gingival sulcus. It may be separated from the tooth surface with a periodontal probe. The most apical point of the marginal gingival scallop is called the *gingival zenith.* Its apicocoronal and mesiodistal dimensions vary between 0.06 and 0.96 mm.[175]

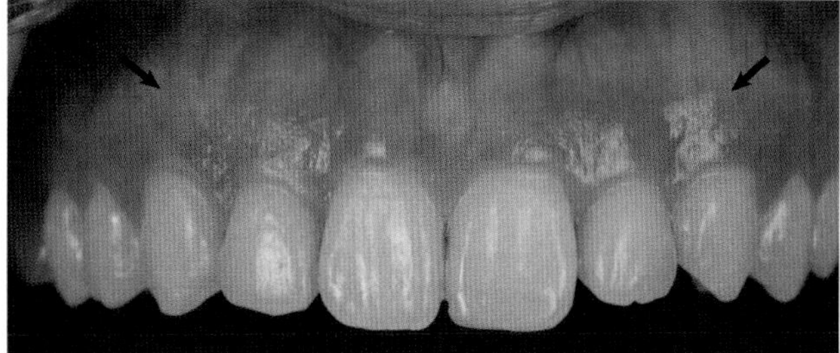

Fig. 4.2 Normal gingiva in a young adult. Note the demarcation (mucogingival line) *(arrows)* between the attached gingiva and the alveolar mucosa. (Courtesy Dr. Tun Juan Wang.)

Gingival Sulcus

The gingival sulcus is the shallow crevice or space around the tooth bounded by the surface of the tooth on one side and the epithelium lining the free margin of the gingiva on the other side. It is V-shaped and barely permits the entrance of a periodontal probe. The clinical determination of the depth of the gingival sulcus is an important diagnostic parameter. Under absolutely normal or ideal conditions, the depth of the gingival sulcus is 0 mm or close to 0 mm.[105] These strict conditions of normalcy can be produced experimentally only in germ-free animals or after intense and prolonged plaque control.[13,49]

In clinically healthy human gingiva, a sulcus of some depth can be found. The depth of this sulcus, as determined in histologic sections, has been reported as 1.8 mm, with variations from 0 to 6 mm[206]; other studies have reported 1.5 mm[289] and 0.69 mm.[93] The clinical evaluation used to determine the depth of the sulcus involves the introduction of a metallic instrument (i.e., the periodontal probe) and the estimation of the distance it penetrates (i.e., the probing depth). The histologic depth of a sulcus does not need to be exactly equal to the depth of penetration of the probe. The penetration of the probe depends on several factors, such as probe diameter, probing force, and level of inflammation.[91] Consequently, the probing depth is not necessarily exactly equal to the histologic depth of the sulcus. The so-called probing depth of a clinically normal gingival sulcus in humans is 2 to 3 mm (see Chapter 38). The visibility of the periodontal probe through the gingiva during probing is also commonly used as a technique to measure gingiva thickness. If the periodontal probe is visible through the gingiva after being inserted in the sulcus, the periodontal phenotype is considered as thin. On the other hand, it is considered as thick when the probe is not visible (Fig. 4.4).[88]

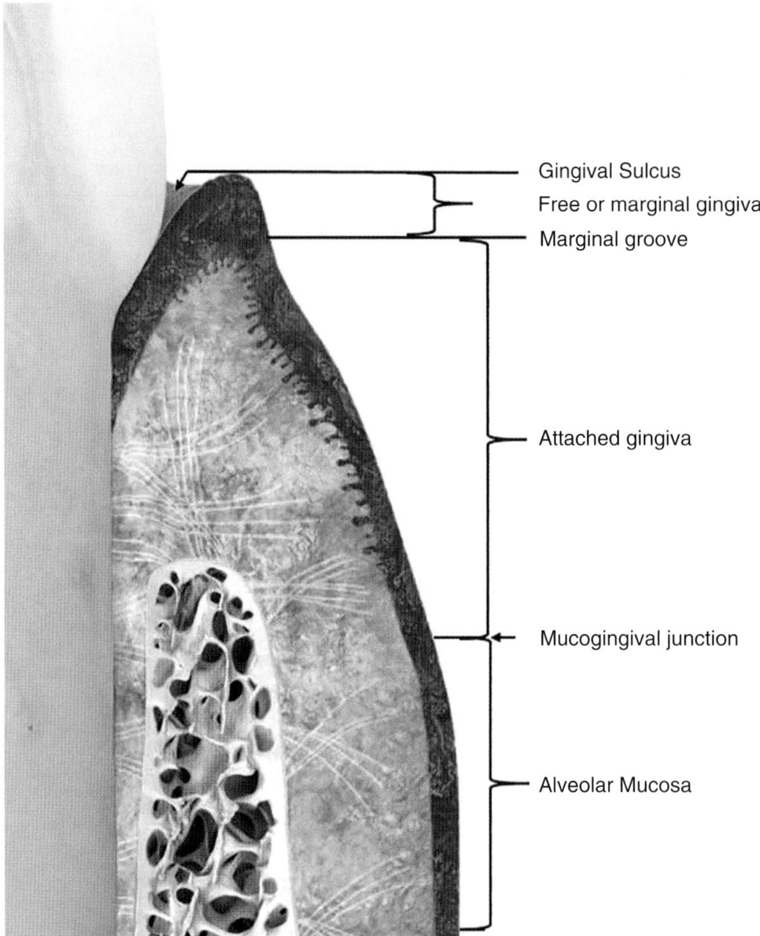

Fig. 4.3 Diagram showing the anatomic landmarks of the gingiva. (© Periopixel.)

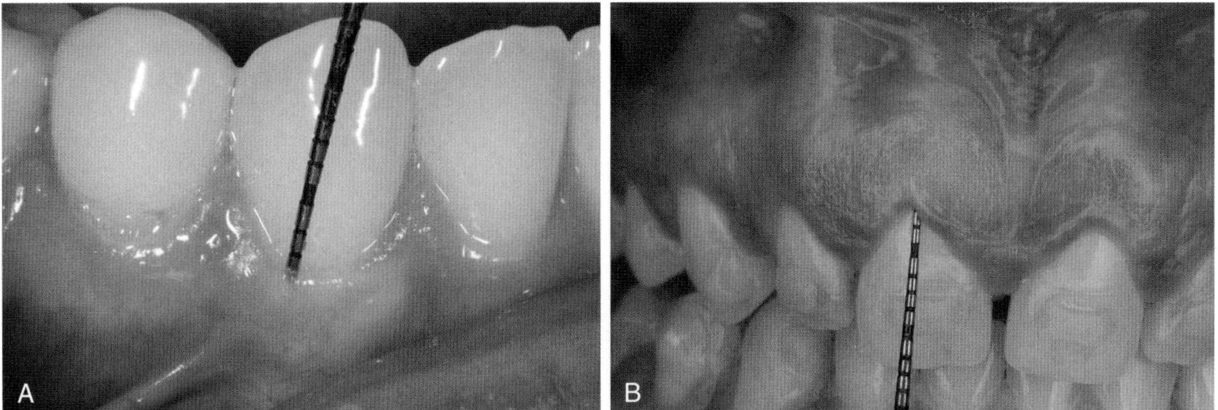

Fig. 4.4 (A) Thin Periodontal phenotype: The periodontal probe visible through the gingival sulcus. (B) Thick Periodontal phenotype: The Perio probe is not visible through the gingival sulcus.

Attached Gingiva

The attached gingiva is continuous with the marginal gingiva. It is firm, resilient, and tightly bound to the underlying periosteum of the alveolar bone. The facial aspect of the attached gingiva extends to the relatively loose and movable alveolar mucosa; it is demarcated by the mucogingival junction (see Fig. 4.3).

The *width of the attached gingiva* is another important clinical parameter.[7] It is the distance between the mucogingival junction and the projection on the external surface of the bottom of the gingival sulcus or the periodontal pocket. It should not be confused with the *width of the keratinized gingiva,* although this also includes the marginal gingiva (see Fig. 4.3).

The width of the attached gingiva on the facial aspect differs in different areas of the mouth.[40] It is generally greatest in the incisor region (i.e., 3.5 to 4.5 mm in the maxilla, 3.3 to 3.9 mm in the mandible) and narrower in the posterior segments (i.e., 1.9 mm in the maxillary first premolars and 1.8 mm in the mandibular first premolars)[6] (Fig. 4.5). Additional considerations with respect to the measurement of attached gingiva is presented in Box 4.1.[270]

Because the mucogingival junction remains stationary throughout adult life,[4] changes in the width of the attached gingiva are caused by modifications in the position of its coronal portion. The width of the attached gingiva increases by the age of 4 years and in supraerupted teeth.[5] On the lingual aspect of the mandible, the attached gingiva terminates at the junction of the lingual alveolar mucosa, which is continuous with the mucous membrane that lines the floor of the mouth. The palatal surface of the attached gingiva in the maxilla blends imperceptibly with the equally firm and resilient palatal mucosa.

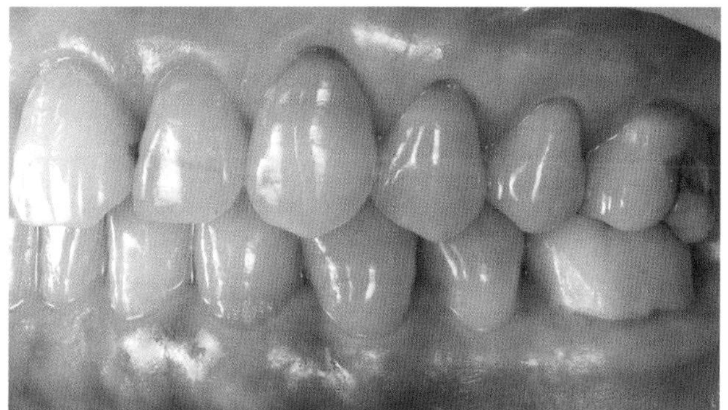

Fig. 4.5 Mean width of the attached gingiva in the human permanent dentition. (Courtesy Dr. Tun Juan Wang.)

Interdental Gingiva

The interdental gingiva occupies the gingival embrasure, which is the interproximal space beneath the area of tooth contact. The interdental gingiva can be pyramidal, or it can have a "col" shape. In the former, the tip of one papilla is located immediately beneath the contact point; the latter presents a valley-like depression that connects a facial and lingual papilla and that conforms to the shape of the interproximal contact (Figs. 4.6 and 4.7).[63] The shape of the gingiva in a given interdental space depends on the presence or absence of a contact point between the adjacent teeth, the distance between the contact point and the osseous crest,[271] and the presence or absence of some degree of recession. Fig. 4.8 depicts the variations in normal interdental gingiva.

The facial and lingual surfaces are tapered toward the interproximal contact area, whereas the mesial and distal surfaces are slightly concave. The lateral borders and tips of the interdental papillae are formed by the marginal gingiva of the adjoining teeth. The intervening portion consists of attached gingiva (Fig. 4.9). If a diastema is present, the gingiva is firmly bound over the interdental bone to form a smooth, rounded surface without interdental papillae (Fig. 4.10).

Microscopic Features

Microscopic examination reveals that gingiva is composed of the overlying stratified squamous epithelium and the underlying central core of connective tissue. Although the epithelium is predominantly cellular in nature, the connective tissue is less cellular and composed primarily of collagen fibers and ground substance. These two tissues are considered separately. (A detailed description of gingival

BOX 4.1 Measurement of Attached Gingiva—Additional Considerations

When measuring the attached gingiva (AG), the supracrestal tissue attachment in healthy and diseased periodontium should be considered. In a healthy periodontium with supracrestal tissue attachment that is bound to tooth and bone (Fig. A) or tooth only, AG is measured from the base of the sulcus to the mucogingival junction. In a periodontally involved site with an infrabony defect on the facial aspect, the AG may only be attached to the alveolar bone (Fig. B) or may be absent (Fig. C). In such periodontally involved sites, AG is measured from the bone crest (instead of sulcus) to the mucogingival junction.

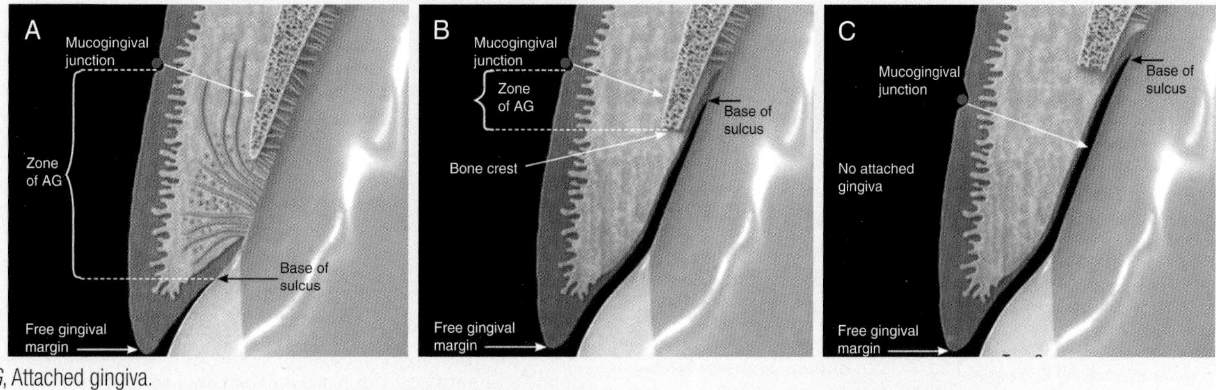

AG, Attached gingiva.

Printed with permission from Tarnow D, Hochman M, Chu S, Fletcher P. A new definition of attached gingiva around teeth and implants in healthy and diseased sites. *Int J Periodontics Restorative Dent.* 2021 Jan–Feb;41(1):43–49.

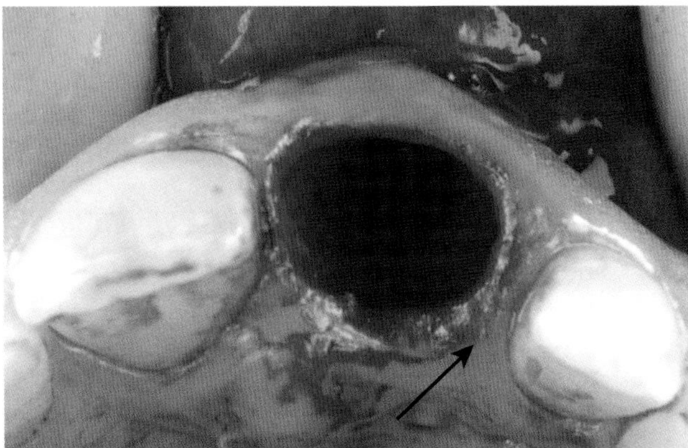

Fig. 4.6 Site of extraction showing the facial and palatal interdental papillae and the intervening col *(arrow)*.

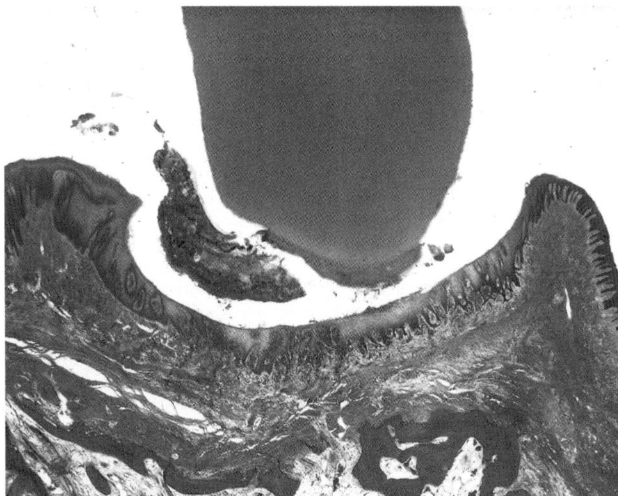

Fig. 4.7 Faciolingual section of a monkey showing the col between the facial and lingual interdental papillae. The col is covered with nonkeratinized stratified squamous epithelium.

histology can be found in Schroeder HE. *The Periodontium*. New York: Springer-Verlag; 1986; and in Biological structure of the normal and diseased periodontium, *Periodontol 2000*. 1997;13:1.)

Gingival Epithelium

General Aspects of Gingival Epithelium Biology

Historically, the epithelial compartment was thought to provide only a physical barrier to infection and the underlying gingival attachment. However, we now believe that epithelial cells play an active role in innate host defense by responding to bacteria in an interactive manner,[68] which means that the epithelium participates actively in responding to infection, in signaling further host reactions, and in integrating innate and acquired immune responses. For example, epithelial cells may respond to bacteria by increased proliferation, the alteration of cell-signaling events, changes in differentiation and cell death, and, ultimately, the alteration of tissue homeostasis.[68] To understand this new perspective of the epithelial innate defense responses and the role of the epithelium in gingival health and disease, it is important to understand its basic structure and function (Box 4.2).

The gingival epithelium consists of a continuous lining of stratified squamous epithelium. There are three different areas that can be defined from the morphologic and functional points of view: the oral or outer epithelium, the sulcular epithelium, and the junctional epithelium.

The principal cell type of the gingival epithelium—as well as of other stratified squamous epithelia—is the *keratinocyte.* Other cells found in the epithelium are the clear cells or nonkeratinocytes, which include the Langerhans cells, the Merkel cells, and the melanocytes.

The main function of the gingival epithelium is to protect the deep structures while allowing for a selective interchange with the oral environment. This is achieved via the proliferation and differentiation of the keratinocytes. The *proliferation* of keratinocytes takes place by mitosis in the basal layer and less frequently in the suprabasal layers, in which a small proportion of cells remain as a proliferative compartment while a larger number begin to migrate to the surface.

Differentiation involves the process of keratinization, which consists of progressions of biochemical and morphologic events that occur in the cell as they migrate from the basal layer to the keratinized layer (Fig. 4.11). The main morphologic changes include the following: (1) the progressive flattening of the cell with an increasing prevalence of tonofilaments ("bundled cytokeratin"); (2) the coupling of intercellular junctions (desmosomes) with the production of keratohyalin granules in the granulous layer; (3) the disappearance of the nucleus and cell organelles in the keratinized layer; and (4) the accumulation and assembly of keratins (consisting of cross-linked cytokeratin, filaggrin, loricrin, and involucrin) and lipids in the plasma membrane, forming the cell envelope. (See Nanci[195] for further details.)

A complete keratinization process leads to the production of an *orthokeratinized* superficial horny layer similar to that of the skin, with no nuclei in the stratum corneum and a well-defined stratum granulosum provided by the keratohyalin granules (Fig. 4.12). When the lipid content of the keratohyalin granules merges with the plasma membrane of the cell in the keratinized layer, the granules are no longer present intracellularly.

Only some areas of the outer gingival epithelium are orthokeratinized; the other gingival areas are covered by parakeratinized or nonkeratinized epithelium[46] and are considered to be at intermediate stages of keratinization. These areas can progress to maturity or dedifferentiate under different physiologic or pathologic conditions.

In *parakeratinized epithelia,* the stratum corneum retains pyknotic nuclei, and the keratohyalin granules are dispersed rather than giving rise to a stratum granulosum. The *nonkeratinized epithelium* (although cytokeratins are the major component, as in all epithelia) has neither granulosum nor corneum strata, whereas superficial cells have viable nuclei.

Nonkeratinocyte cells are present in the gingival epithelium as in other non-keratinizing epithelia. *Melanocytes* are cells with dendritic processes and are located in the basal and spinous layers of the gingival epithelium between keratinocytes. They store melanin in organelles called *premelanosomes* or *melanosomes* (Fig. 4.13).[62,238,263] The color pigmentation of the oral mucosa presents a wide range of shades. While the melanocyte number is similar, the differences lie in the rate of production and breakdown of melanin.[117]

Langerhans cells are dendritic cells that contain elongated granules (Birbeck granules) and are located among keratinocytes at all suprabasal levels (Fig. 4.14). They belong to the mononuclear phagocyte system (reticuloendothelial system) as modified monocytes derived from the bone marrow and present antigens to lymphocytes.[73]

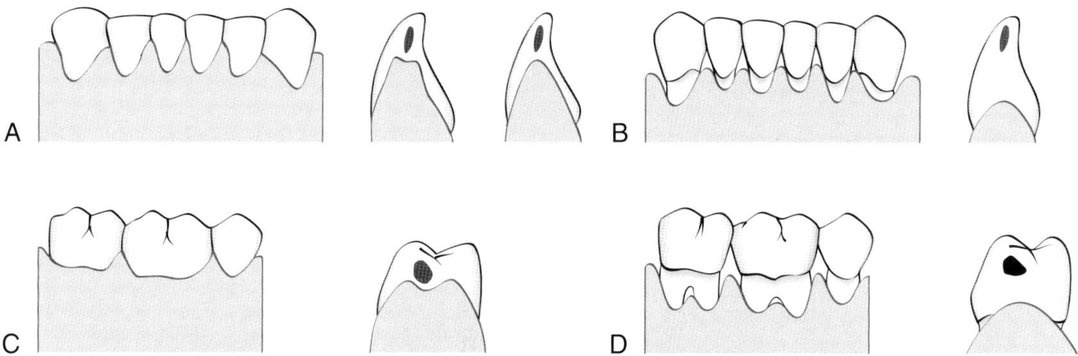

Fig. 4.8 A diagram that compares anatomic variations of the interdental col in the normal gingiva *(left side)* and after gingival recession *(right side)*. (A and B) Mandibular anterior segment, facial and buccolingual views, respectively. (C and D) Mandibular posterior region, facial and buccolingual views, respectively. Tooth contact points are shown with black marks in the lower individual teeth.

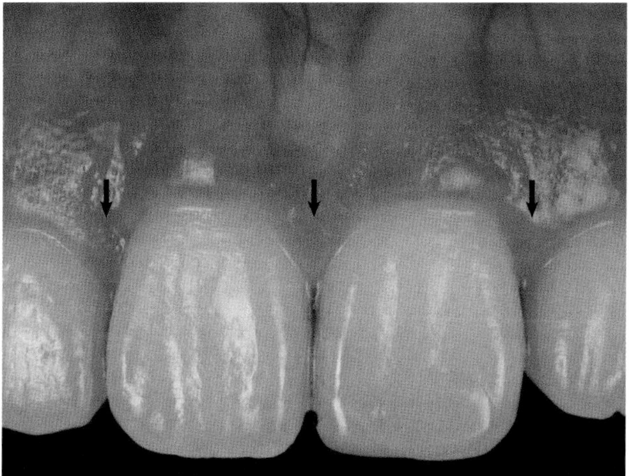

Fig. 4.9 Interdental papillae *(arrows)* with a central portion formed by the attached gingiva. The shape of the papillae varies according to the dimension of the gingival embrasure.

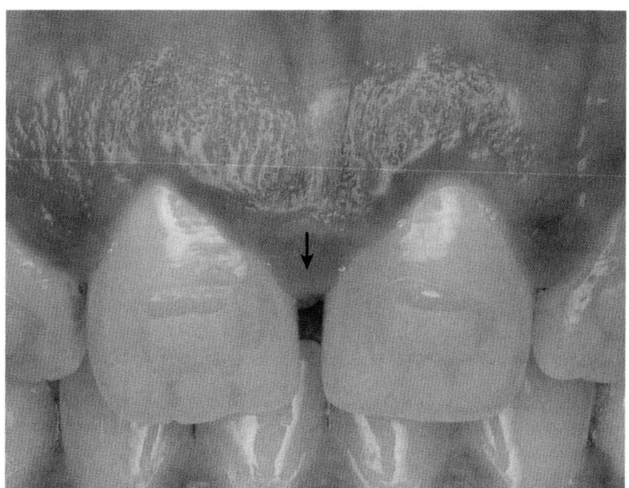

Fig. 4.10 An absence of interdental papillae and col where the proximal tooth contact is missing. (Courtesy Dr. Osvaldo Costa.)

BOX 4.2 Functions and Features of Gingival Epithelium

Functions
Mechanical, chemical, water, and microbial barrier
Signaling functions

Architectural Integrity
Cell-cell attachments
Cell-basal lamina attachments
Basal lamina
Keratin cytoskeleton

Major Cell Type
Keratinocyte

Other Cell Types
Langerhans cells
Melanocytes
Merkel cells

Constant Renewal
Replacement of damaged cells

Cell–Cell Attachments
Desmosomes
Adherens junctions
Tight junctions
Gap junctions

Cell–Basal Lamina
Synthesis of basal lamina components
Hemidesmosome

Modified from Dale BA. Periodontal epithelium: a newly recognized role in health and disease. *Periodontol 2000.* 2002;30:71.

Langerhans cells are found in the oral epithelium of normal gingiva and in fewer numbers in the sulcular epithelium; they are probably absent from the junctional epithelium of normal gingiva.

Merkel cells are located in the deeper layers of the epithelium; they harbor nerve endings, and they are connected to adjacent cells by desmosomes. They have been identified as tactile preceptors.[197]

The epithelium is joined to the underlying connective tissue by a *basal lamina* 300 to 400 Å thick and lying approximately 400 Å beneath the epithelial basal layer.[151,245,265] The terms "basal lamina" and "basement membrane" refer to the same structure. "Basal lamina" is used in conjunction with electron microscopy and "basement membrane" with light microscopy. The functions of this sheet-like structure are to connect tissues that would be separated otherwise and to control the exchange of molecules between tissues. The basal lamina consists of lamina lucida and lamina densa. The lamina lucida is the zone where integrin $\alpha4\beta6$ interacts with the glycoprotein, laminin-332 (formerly laminin-5).[210] Hemidesmosomes are electron-dense structures inserted into the plasma membrane of epithelial cells adjacent to the extracellular matrix. Their function is

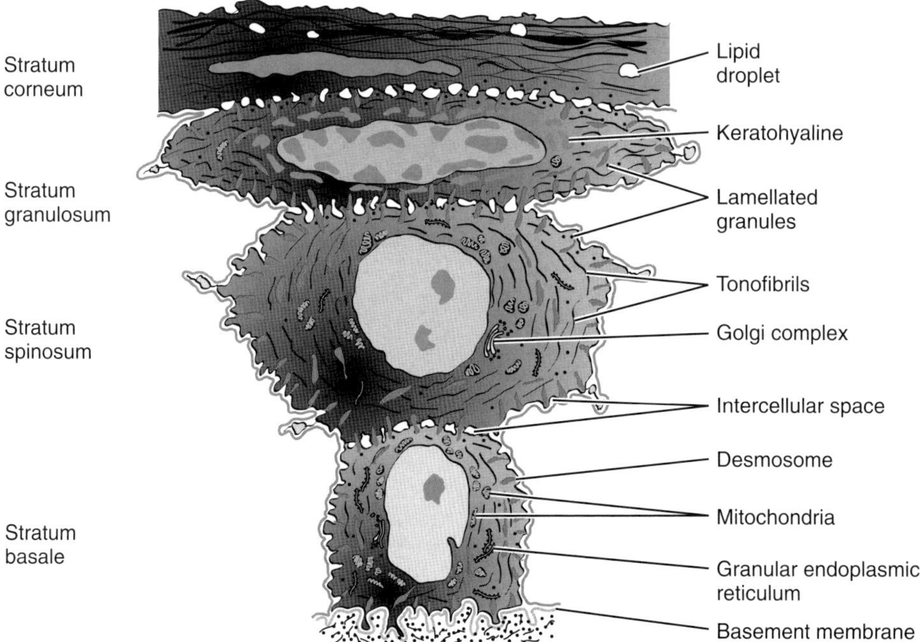

Fig. 4.11 Diagram showing representative cells from the various layers of stratified squamous epithelium as seen by electron microscopy. (Modified from Weinstock A. In: Ham AW, ed. *Histology*. 7th ed. Philadelphia: Lippincott; 1974.)

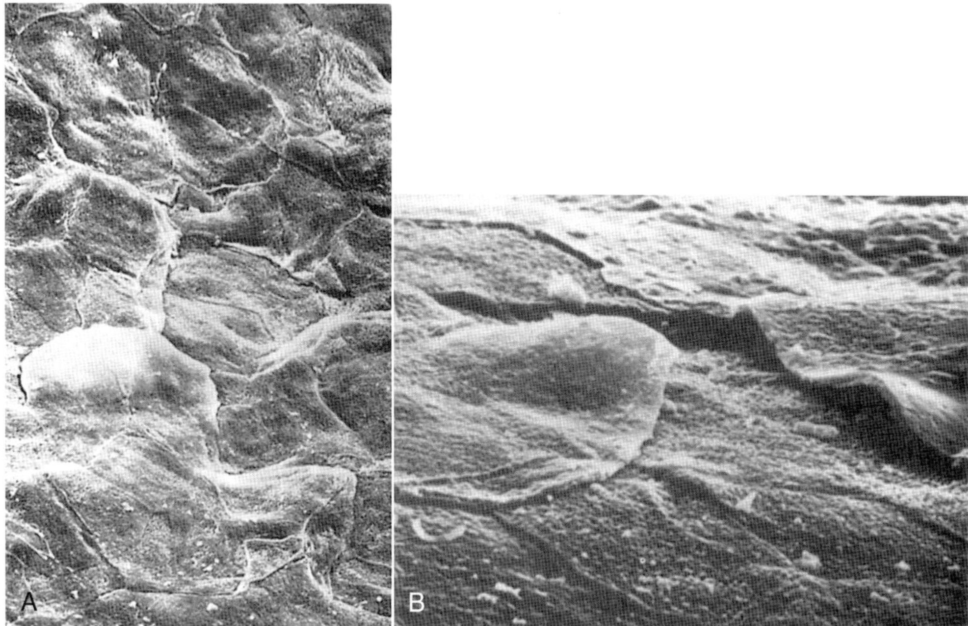

Fig. 4.12 (A) Scanning electron micrograph of keratinized gingiva showing the flattened keratinocytes and their boundaries on the surface of the gingiva (×1000). (B) Scanning electron micrograph of the gingival margin at the edge of the gingival sulcus showing several keratinocytes about to be exfoliated (×3000). (From Kaplan GB, Pameijer CH, Ruben MP. Scanning electron microscopy of sulcular and junctional epithelia correlated with histology (part 1). *J Periodontol.* 1977;48:446.)

to attach the epithelial cells to the basal lamina and to send signals from the matrix to the cell.

Structural and Metabolic Characteristics of Different Areas of Gingival Epithelium

The epithelial component of the gingiva shows regional morphologic variations that reflect tissue adaptation to the tooth and alveolar bone.[241] These variations include the oral epithelium, the sulcular epithelium, and the junctional epithelium. Whereas the oral epithelium and the sulcular epithelium are largely protective in function, the junctional epithelium serves many more roles and is of considerable importance in the regulation of tissue health.[19] It is now recognized that epithelial cells are not passive bystanders in the gingival tissues; rather, they are metabolically active and capable of reacting to external stimuli by synthesizing a number of cytokines, adhesion molecules, growth factors, and enzymes.[19]

The degree of gingival keratinization diminishes with age and the onset of menopause,[211] but it is not necessarily related to the

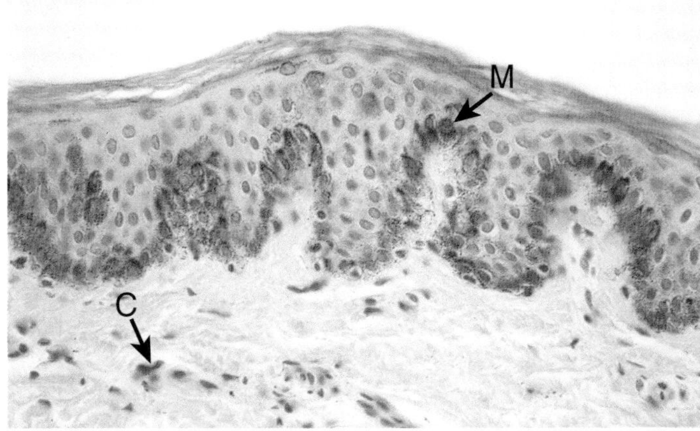

Fig. 4.13 Pigmented gingiva of dog showing melanocytes *(M)* in the basal epithelial layer and melanophores *(C)* in the connective tissue (Glucksman technique.)

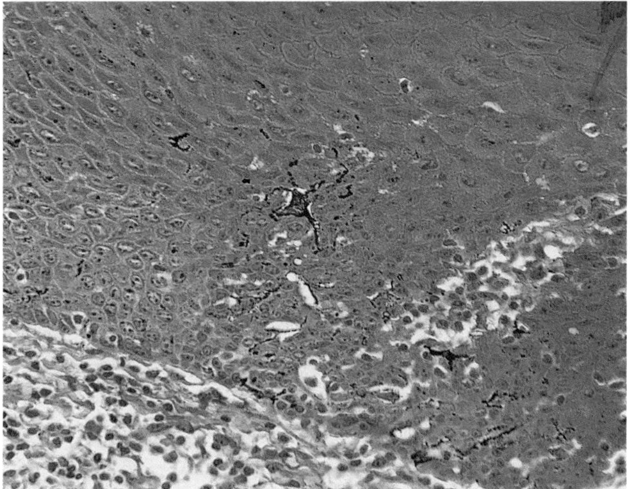

Fig. 4.14 Human gingival epithelium, oral aspect. Immunoperoxidase technique showing Langerhans cells.

different phases of the menstrual cycle.[134] Keratinization of the oral mucosa varies in different areas in the following order: palate (most keratinized), gingiva, ventral aspect of the tongue, and cheek (least keratinized).[185]

Oral (Outer) Epithelium

The oral or outer epithelium covers the crest and outer surface of the marginal gingiva and the surface of the attached gingiva. It is composed of four layers: stratum basale (basal layer), stratum spinosum (prickle cell layer), stratum granulosum (granular layer), and stratum corneum (cornified layer). On average, the oral epithelium is 0.2 to 0.3 mm in thickness. It is keratinized or parakeratinized, or it may present various combinations of these conditions (Fig. 4.15). The prevalent surface, however, is parakeratinized.[46,295]

Sulcular Epithelium

The sulcular epithelium lines the gingival sulcus (Fig. 4.16). It is a thin, nonkeratinized stratified squamous epithelium without rete pegs, and it extends from the coronal limit of the junctional epithelium to the crest of the gingival margin (Fig. 4.17). It usually shows many cells with hydropic degeneration.

Despite these morphologic and chemical characteristics, the sulcular epithelium has the potential to keratinize if it is reflected and exposed to the oral cavity[44,48] or if the bacterial flora of the sulcus is totally eliminated.[50] Conversely, the outer epithelium loses its keratinization when it is placed in contact with the tooth.[50] These findings suggest that the local irritation of the sulcus prevents sulcular keratinization.

The sulcular epithelium is extremely important; it may act as a semipermeable membrane through which injurious bacterial products pass into the gingiva and through which tissue fluid from the gingiva seeps into the sulcus.[277] Unlike the junctional epithelium, however, the sulcular epithelium is not heavily infiltrated by polymorphonuclear neutrophil leukocytes, and it appears to be less permeable.[19]

Junctional Epithelium

The junctional epithelium consists of a collar-like band of stratified squamous nonkeratinizing epithelium. It is three to four layers thick in early life, but that number increases with age to 10 or even 20 layers. In addition, the junctional epithelium tapers from its coronal end, which may be 10 to 29 cells wide to one or two cells wide at its apical termination, which is located at the cementoenamel junction in healthy tissue. These cells can be grouped into two strata: the basal layer that faces the connective tissue and the suprabasal layer that extends to the tooth surface. The length of the junctional epithelium ranges from 0.97 to 1.14 mm (Fig. 4.18).[93,285]

The junctional epithelium is formed by the confluence of the oral epithelium and the reduced enamel epithelium (REE) during tooth eruption. However, the REE is not essential for its formation; in fact, the junctional epithelium is completely restored after pocket instrumentation or surgery, and it forms around an implant.[243]

The junctional epithelium is attached to the tooth surface (epithelial attachment) by means of an internal basal lamina. It is attached to the gingival connective tissue by an external basal lamina that has the same structure as other epithelial–connective tissue attachments elsewhere in the body.[158,164]

The internal basal lamina consists of a lamina densa (adjacent to the enamel) and a lamina lucida to which hemidesmosomes are attached. Hemidesmosomes are integrated into the plasma membrane of epithelial cells facing the internal basal lamina and attach the junctional epithelium to the internal basal lamina on the tooth surface.[123] Hemidesmosomes recognize signals from the basal lamina and relay them to the cell for the regulation of gene expression, cell proliferation, and cell differentiation.[138] Hemidesmosomes contain integrin $\alpha 4\beta 6$ receptors that span the membrane as heterodimers and bind laminin-332 with the $\beta 6$ domain. The hemidesmosome connects to keratin filaments through plectin, BP230, and

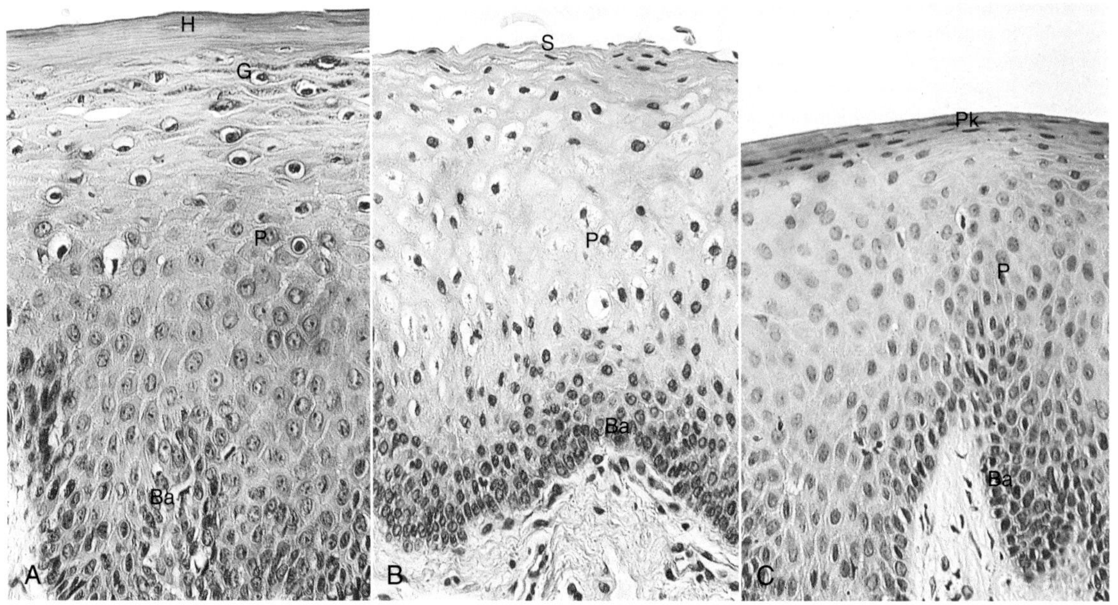

Fig. 4.15 Variations in the gingival epithelium. (A) Keratinized. (B) Nonkeratinized. (C) Parakeratinized. *Ba*, Basal cell layer; *G*, granular layer; *H*, Horny layer; *P*, prickle cell layer; *Pk*, parakeratotic layer; *S*, flattened surface cells.

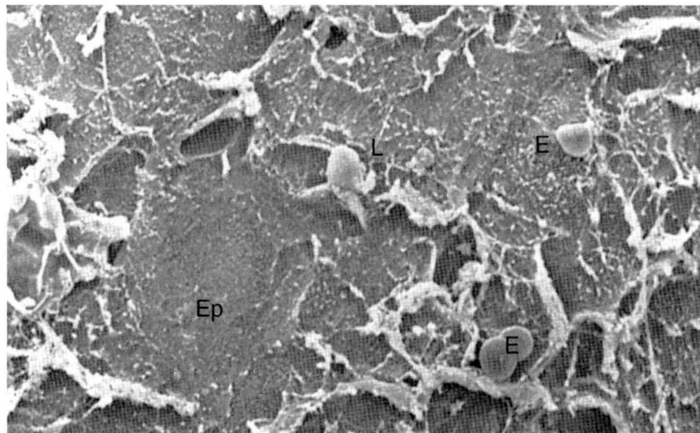

Fig. 4.16 Scanning electron microscopic view of the epithelial surface facing the tooth in a normal human gingival sulcus. The epithelium *(Ep)* shows desquamating cells, some scattered erythrocytes *(E)*, and a few emerging leukocytes *(L)*. (×1000.)

collagen type XVII. The lamina densa of the internal basal lamina lacks type IV collagen.[123,124] Recently, basement membrane proteins of the secreted calcium-binding phosphoproteins were identified to attach to the junctional epithelium.[146,187,188] The secreted calcium-binding phosphoproteins are a cluster of genes on human chromosome 4 that arose through multiple gene duplication. In the developing tooth, ODAM (odontogenic ameloblast-associated), and amelotin are expressed in maturation stage ameloblasts and form the basement membrane for the maturing enamel (Fig. 4.19). After tooth eruption, the REE contributes to the junctional epithelium, and the secretion of basement membrane proteins continues, now serving as the internal basal lamina for the junctional epithelium. ODAM, amelotin, and SCPPPQ1 form a network and create an attachment, specific for interfacing the tooth at the internal basal lamina.[86] The epithelial attachment is mediated by the combination of hemidesmosomes and internal basal lamina. The basal lamina is permeable to fluids, but it acts as a barrier to particulate matter. The external basal lamina is clearly distinguishable at the ultrastructural level and at the optical level as periodic acid–Schiff–positive and by argyrophilic lines (Fig. 4.20).[246,268] The main difference between the internal basal lamina and lamina densa is in the composition of

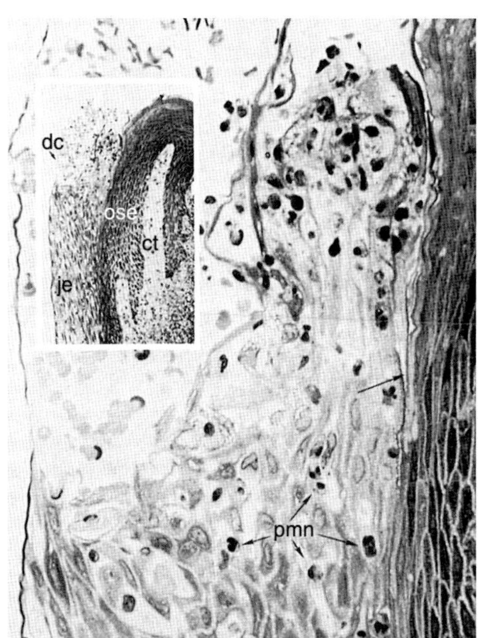

Fig. 4.17 Epon-embedded human biopsy specimen showing a relatively normal gingival sulcus. The soft-tissue wall of the gingival sulcus is made up of the oral sulcular epithelium *(ose)* and its underlying connective tissue *(ct)*, whereas the base of the gingival sulcus is formed by the sloughing surface of the junctional epithelium *(je)*. The enamel space is delineated by a dense cuticular structure *(dc)*. A relatively sharp line of demarcation exists between the junctional epithelium and the oral sulcular epithelium *(arrow)*, and several polymorphonuclear leukocytes *(pmn)* can be seen traversing the junctional epithelium. The sulcus contains red blood cells that resulted from the hemorrhage that occurred at the time of biopsy. (×391; *inset* ×55.) (From Schluger S, Youdelis R, Page RC. *Periodontal Disease.* 2nd ed. Philadelphia: Lea & Febiger; 1990.)

proteins. Collagen type IV forms a network from tetramers resembling chicken wire. Nidogen and perlecan bind to this network, as well as to laminin-332, to interconnect lamina lucida and lamina densa.[14,202] The lamina reticularis underneath the lamina densa contains anchoring fibrils (collagen type VII). Anchoring fibrils have

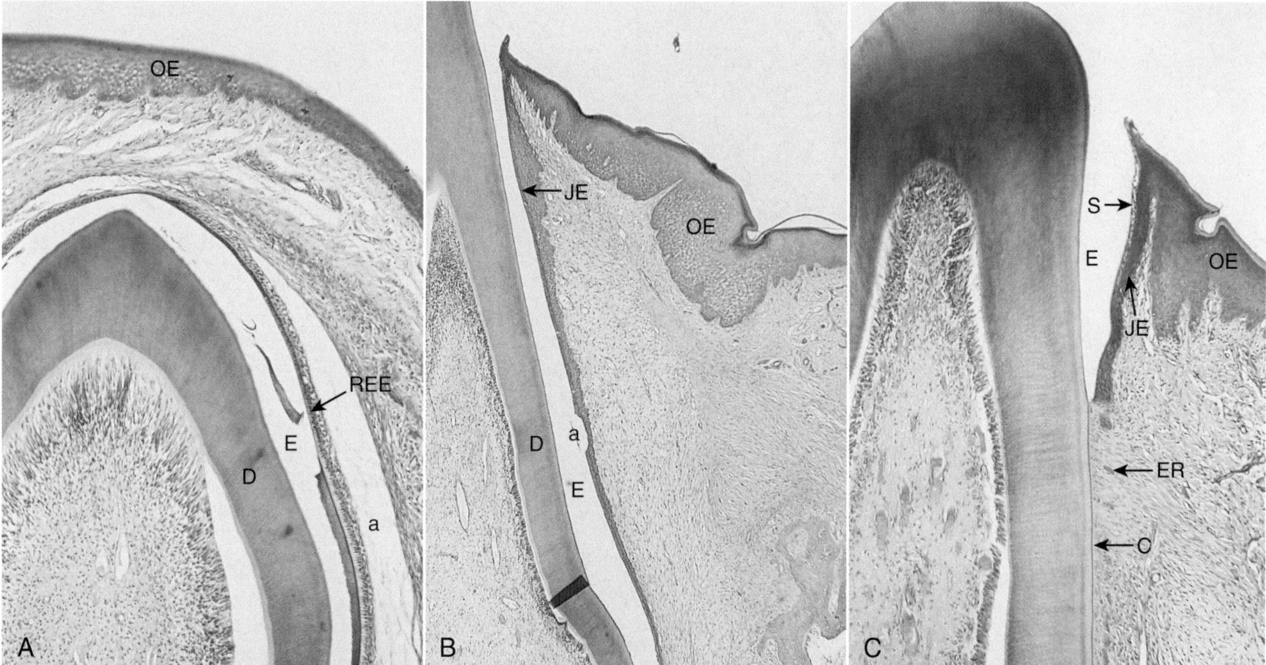

Fig. 4.18 Eruption process in cat's tooth. (A) Unerupted tooth. Dentin *(D)*, remnants of enamel matrix *(E)*, reduced enamel epithelium *(REE)*, oral epithelium *(OE)*, and artifact *(a)*. (B) Erupting tooth forming junctional epithelium *(JE)*. (C) Completely erupted tooth. Sulcus with epithelial debris *(S)*, cementum *(C)*, and epithelial rests *(ER)*.

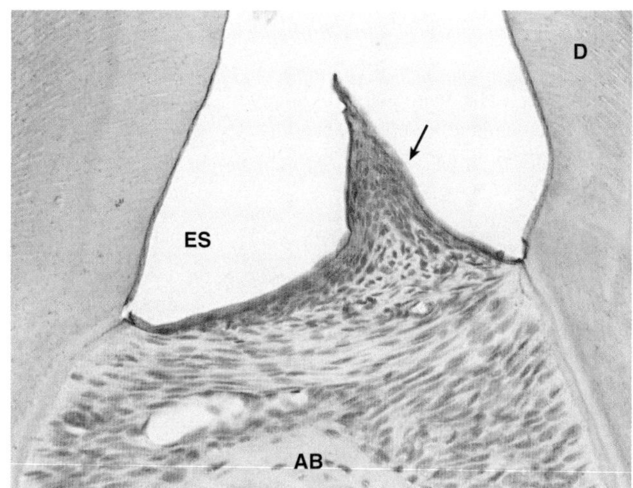

Fig. 4.19 Immunohistochemistry of anti-ODAM (odontogenic ameloblast-associated) of the interdental region of mouse mandibular molars. The junctional epithelium displays strong ODAM localization to the internal basal lamina and cells close to the tooth surface *(arrow)*. *AB*, Alveolar bone; *D*, dentin; *ES*, enamel space. (Courtesy Y.P. Chun and D.N. Dullnig.)

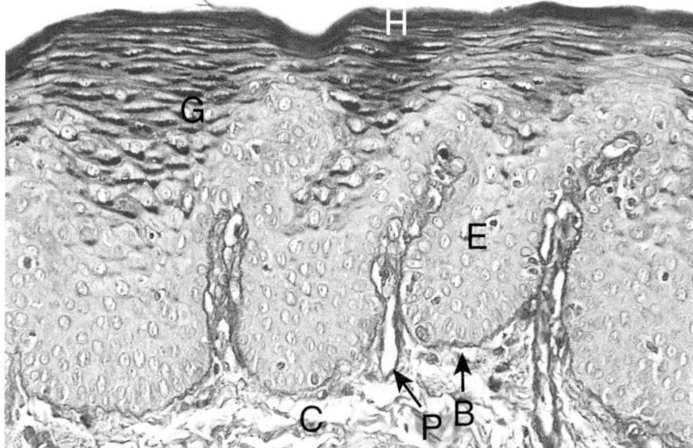

Fig. 4.20 Normal human gingiva stained with the periodic acid–Schiff histochemical method. The basement membrane *(B)* is seen between the epithelium *(E)* and the underlying connective tissue *(C)*. In the epithelium, glycoprotein material occurs in cells and cell membranes of the superficial hornified *(H)* and underlying granular layers *(G)*. The connective tissue presents a diffuse, amorphous ground substance and collagen fibers. The blood vessel walls stand out clearly in the papillary projections of the connective tissue *(P)*.

been measured to be 750 nm in length from their epithelial end to their connective tissue end, where they appear to form loops around collagen fibers (type I and III) by interacting with type IV collagen.[289] The proteins of the internal and external basal lamina interact within the lamina lucida, lamina densa, lamina reticularis, and the tooth surface to create attachment across different tissues.

The attachment of the junctional epithelium to the tooth is reinforced by the gingival fibers, which brace the marginal gingiva against the tooth surface (Fig. 4.21). For this reason, the junctional epithelium and the gingival fibers are considered together as a functional unit referred to as the *dentogingival unit*.[161] In conclusion, it is usually accepted that the junctional epithelium exhibits several unique structural and functional features that contribute to preventing pathogenic bacterial flora from colonizing the subgingival tooth surface.[217] First, junctional epithelium is firmly attached to the tooth surface, thereby forming an epithelial barrier against plaque bacteria. Second, it allows access of gingival fluid, inflammatory cells, and components of the immunologic host defense to the gingival margin. Third, junctional epithelial cells exhibit rapid turnover, which contributes to the host-parasite equilibrium and the rapid repair of damaged tissue.

Development of Gingival Sulcus

After enamel formation is complete, the enamel is covered with *REE*, which is attached to the tooth by a basal lamina and hemidesmosomes.[159,266] When the tooth penetrates the oral mucosa, the REE unites with the oral epithelium and transforms into the junctional

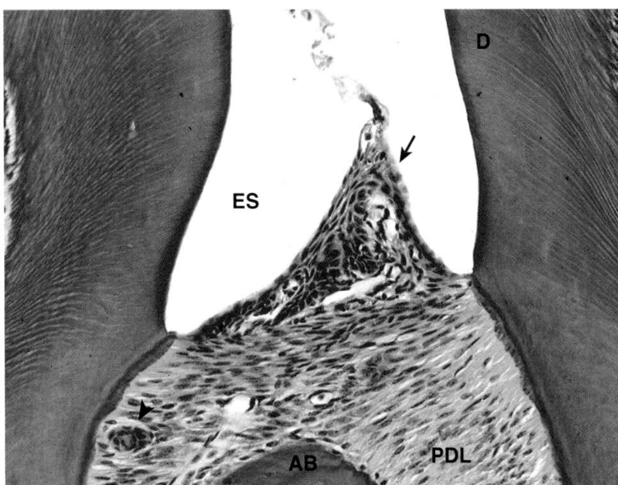

Fig. 4.21 Periodic acid-Schiff staining of the interdental region of mouse mandibular molars. The junctional epithelium is directly adjacent to the tooth surface *(arrow)*. Epithelial rests of Malassez. *AB*, Alveolar bone; *D*, dentin; *ES*, enamel space; *PDL*, periodontal ligament. (Courtesy Y.P. Chun and D.N. Dullnig.)

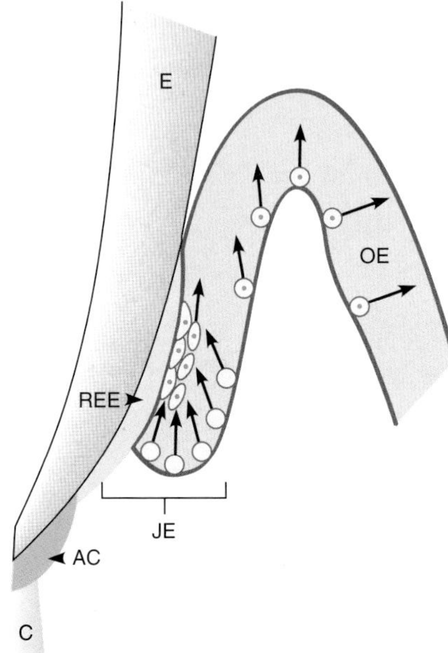

Fig. 4.22 Junctional epithelium on an erupting tooth. The junctional epithelium *(JE)* is formed by the joining of the oral epithelium *(OE)* and the reduced enamel epithelium *(REE)*. Afibrillar cementum *(AC)* is sometimes formed on enamel after the degeneration of the REE. The *arrows* indicate the coronal movement of the regenerating epithelial cells, which multiply more rapidly in the JE than in the OE. *C*, Root cementum; *E*, Enamel. A similar cell turnover pattern exists in the fully erupted tooth. (Modified from Listgarten MA. Changing concepts about the dento-gingival junction. *J Can Dent Assoc*. 1970;36:70.)

epithelium. As the tooth erupts, this united epithelium condenses along the crown, and the ameloblasts, which form the inner layer of the REE (see Fig. 4.18), gradually become squamous epithelial cells. The transformation of the REE into a junctional epithelium proceeds in an apical direction without interrupting the attachment to the tooth. According to Schroeder and Listgarten,[243] this process takes between 1 and 2 years.

The junctional epithelium is a continually self-renewing structure, with mitotic activity occurring in all cell layers.[159,266] The regenerating epithelial cells move toward the tooth surface and along it in a coronal direction to the gingival sulcus, where they are shed (Fig. 4.22).[24] The migrating daughter cells provide a continuous attachment to the tooth surface. The strength of the epithelial attachment to the tooth has not been measured.

The gingival sulcus is formed when the tooth erupts into the oral cavity. At that time, the junctional epithelium and the REE form a broad band that is attached to the tooth surface from near the tip of the crown to the cementoenamel junction. The gingival sulcus is the shallow, V-shaped space or groove between the tooth and the gingiva that encircles the newly erupted tip of the crown. In the fully erupted tooth, only the junctional epithelium persists. *The sulcus consists of the shallow space that is coronal to the attachment of the junctional epithelium and bounded by the tooth on one side and the sulcular epithelium on the other. The coronal extent of the gingival sulcus is the gingival margin.*

Renewal of Gingival Epithelium

The oral epithelium undergoes continuous renewal that relies on the proliferation and stemness of basal cells. Its thickness is maintained by a balance between new cell formation in the basal and spinous layers and the shedding of old cells at the surface. The mitotic activity exhibits a 24-hour periodicity, with the highest and lowest rates occurring in the morning and evening, respectively.[267] The mitotic rate is higher in nonkeratinized areas and increased in gingivitis, without significant gender differences. Opinions differ with regard to whether the mitotic rate is increased[163,164,183] or decreased[16] with age.

With regard to junctional epithelium, the epithelial cells facing the external basal lamina form the basal layer and divide rapidly and progress towards the internal basal lamina.[231,232] The rapid adding of cells effectively removes bacteria that adhere to the epithelial cells and therefore is an important part of the antimicrobial defense mechanisms at the dentogingival junction.[217] In addition to the role of epithelial cells in microbial shedding, the gingiva produces and secretes small antimicrobial peptides, known as defensins to maintain bacterial homeostasis.[294]

Gingival Fluid (Sulcular Fluid)

The value of the gingival fluid is that it can be represented as either a transudate or an exudate. The gingival fluid contains a vast array of biochemical factors, thereby offering its potential use as a diagnostic or prognostic biomarker of the biologic state of the periodontium in health and disease (see Chapter 14).[79] It is derived from blood and also contains components of connective tissue, epithelium, inflammatory cells, serum, and microbial flora that inhabit the gingival margin or the sulcus (pocket).[78]

In the healthy sulcus, the amount of gingival fluid is very small. During inflammation, however, the gingival fluid flow increases, and its composition resembles that of an inflammatory exudate.[60] The main route of the gingival fluid diffusion is through the endothelium, connective tissue, external basal lamina, wide intercellular spaces of the junctional epithelium, internal basal lamina, and then into the sulcus.[217] The gingival fluid contributes to the host defense by (1) cleansing particles from the sulcus; (2) containing antimicrobial peptides; and (3) exerting antibody activity to defend the gingiva.

Gingival Connective Tissue

The major components of the gingival connective tissue are the extracellular matrix consisting of collagen fibers (about 60% by volume), other proteins of the extracellular matrix (about 35%), fibroblasts (5%), vessels, and nerves. The connective tissue of the gingiva is known as the *lamina propria,* and it consists of two layers: (1) a *papillary layer* subjacent to the epithelium that consists of papillary projections between the epithelial rete pegs or epithelial ridges and (2) a *reticular layer* that is contiguous with the periosteum of the alveolar bone.

Connective tissue has a cellular compartment and an extracellular compartment composed of fibers and ground substance. Thus, the gingival connective tissue is largely a fibrous connective tissue that has elements that originate directly from the oral mucosal connective tissue as well as some fibers (dentogingival) that originate from the developing dental follicle.[19]

The *ground substance* fills the space between fibers and cells; it is amorphous, and it has a high water content. It is composed of proteoglycans (mainly hyaluronic acid and chondroitin sulfate) and glycoproteins (mainly fibronectin). Glycoproteins account for the faint periodic acid–Schiff–positive reaction of the ground substance.[80] Fibronectin binds fibroblasts to the fibers and many other components of the intercellular matrix, thereby helping to mediate cell adhesion and migration. Laminin-332, which is another glycoprotein found in the basal lamina, serves to attach it to epithelial cells.

The three types of connective tissue fibers are collagen, reticular, and elastic. Collagen type I forms the bulk of the lamina propria and provides the tensile strength to the gingival tissue. Type IV collagen (argyrophilic reticulum fiber) branches between the collagen type I bundles, and it is continuous with fibers of the basement membrane and the blood vessel walls.[164]

The elastic fiber system is composed of oxytalan, elaunin, and elastin fibers distributed among collagen fibers.[57] Therefore, densely packed collagen bundles that are anchored into the acellular extrinsic fiber cementum just below the terminal point of the junctional epithelium form the connective tissue attachment. The stability of this attachment is a key factor in the limitation of the migration of junctional epithelium.[58]

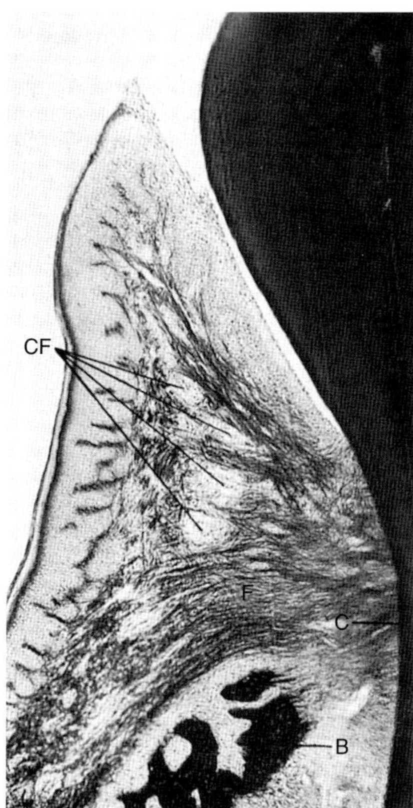

Fig. 4.23 Faciolingual section of marginal gingiva showing gingival fibers *(F)* that extend from the cementum *(C)* to the crest of the gingiva, to the outer gingival surface, and external to the periosteum of the bone *(B)*. Circular fibers *(CF)* are shown in crosssection between the other groups. (Courtesy Sol Bernick.)

Gingival Fibers

The connective tissue of the marginal gingiva is densely collagenous, and it contains a prominent system of collagen fiber bundles called the *gingival fibers*. These fibers consist of type I collagen.[225] The gingival fibers have the following functions:

1. To brace the marginal gingiva firmly against the tooth
2. To provide the rigidity necessary to withstand the forces of mastication without being deflected away from the tooth surface
3. To unite the free marginal gingiva with the cementum of the root and the adjacent attached gingiva

The gingival fibers are arranged in three groups: gingivodental, circular, and transseptal.[150]

The *gingivodental fibers* are those on the facial, lingual, and interproximal surfaces. They are embedded in the cementum just beneath the epithelium at the base of the gingival sulcus and junctional epithelium. On the facial and lingual surfaces, they project from the cementum in a fanlike conformation toward the crest and outer surface of the marginal gingiva, where they terminate short of the epithelium (Figs. 4.23 and 4.24). They also extend externally to the periosteum of the facial and lingual alveolar bones, terminating in the attached gingiva or blending with the periosteum of the alveolar bone. Interproximally, the gingivodental fibers extend toward the crest of the interdental gingiva.

The *circular fibers* course through the connective tissue of the marginal and interdental gingivae and encircle the tooth in a ringlike fashion.

The *transseptal fibers,* which are located interproximally, form horizontal bundles that extend between the cementum of the approximating teeth into which they are embedded. They lie in the area between the epithelium at the base of the gingival sulcus and the crest of the interdental bone, and they are sometimes classified with the principal fibers of the PDL.

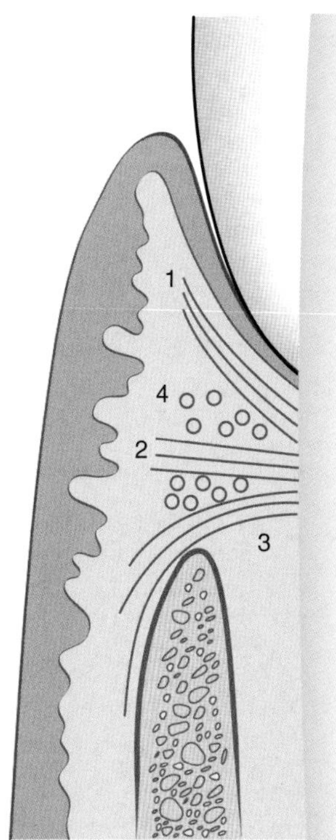

Fig. 4.24 Diagram of the gingivodental fibers that extend from the cementum *(1)* to the crest of the gingiva, *(2)* to the outer surface, and *(3)* external to the periosteum of the labial plate. Circular fibers *(4)* are shown in crosssection.

Page and colleagues[209] described a group of *semicircular fibers* that attach at the proximal surface of a tooth immediately below the cementoenamel junction, go around the facial or lingual marginal gingiva of the tooth, and attach on the other proximal surface of the same tooth; they also discussed a group of *transgingival fibers* that attach in the proximal surface of one tooth, traverse the interdental space diagonally, go around the facial or lingual surface of the adjacent tooth, again traverse the interdental space diagonally, and then attach in the proximal surface of the next tooth.

Altogether, the fibers of the connective tissue form a dense network to provide shape to the gingiva and attachment to individual teeth, between adjacent teeth, and to the alveolar bone.

Cellular Elements

The preponderant cellular element in the gingival connective tissue is the *fibroblast.* Numerous fibroblasts are found between the fiber bundles. Fibroblasts are of mesenchymal origin and play a major role in the development, maintenance, and repair of gingival connective tissue. As with connective tissue elsewhere in the body, fibroblasts synthesize collagen and elastic fibers as well as the glycoproteins and glycosaminoglycans of the amorphous intercellular substance. Fibroblasts also regulate collagen degradation through phagocytosis and the secretion of collagenases.

Fibroblast heterogeneity is a well-established feature of fibroblasts in the periodontium.[236] Although the biologic and clinical significance of such heterogeneity is not yet clear, it seems that this is necessary for the normal functioning of tissues in health, disease, and repair.[19]

Mast cells, which are distributed throughout the body, are numerous in the connective tissue of the oral mucosa and the gingiva.[52,254,255,297] *Fixed* macrophages and *histiocytes* are present in the gingival connective tissue as components of the mononuclear phagocyte system (reticuloendothelial system) and are derived from blood monocytes. *Adipose cells* and *eosinophils,* although scarce, are also present in the lamina propria.

In clinically normal gingiva, small foci of plasma cells and lymphocytes are found in the connective tissue near the base of the sulcus (Fig. 4.25). Neutrophils can be seen in relatively high numbers in both the gingival connective tissue and the sulcus. These inflammatory cells are usually present in small amounts in clinically normal gingiva.

Repair of Gingival Connective Tissue

Because of the high turnover rate, the connective tissue of the gingiva has remarkable healing and regenerative capacity. Indeed, it may be one of the fastest healing tissues in the body, and it generally shows little evidence of scarring after surgical procedures.

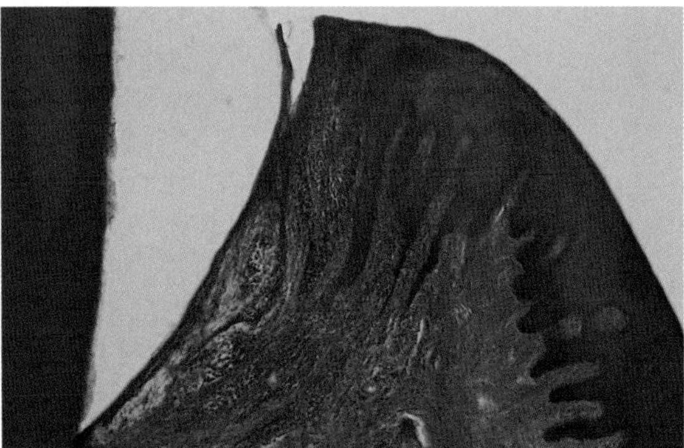

Fig. 4.25 Section of clinically normal gingiva showing some degree of inflammation, which is almost always present near the base of the sulcus.

This is likely facilitated by the rapid synthesis and reconstruction of the fibrous architecture of the tissues.[182] However, it is important to know the regenerative capacity is better in the PDL than the connective tissue.

Blood Supply, Lymphatics, and Nerves

Microcirculatory tracts, blood vessels, and lymphatic vessels play an important role in the drainage of tissue fluid and in the spread of inflammation. In individuals with gingivitis and periodontitis, the microcirculation and vascular formation change greatly in the vascular network directly under the gingival sulcular epithelium and the junctional epithelium.[174]

Three sources of blood supply to the gingiva are as follows (Figs. 4.26 and 4.27):

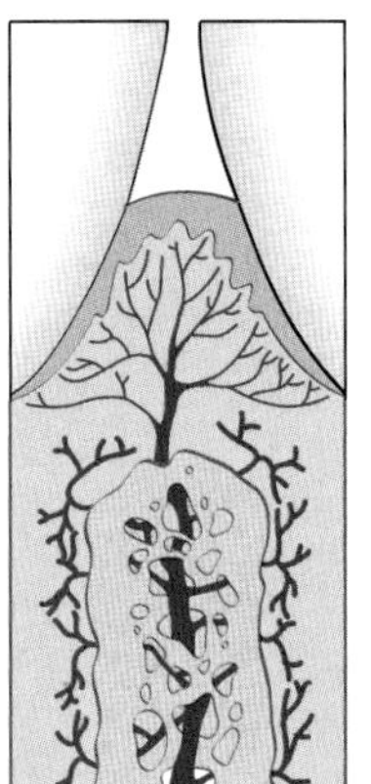

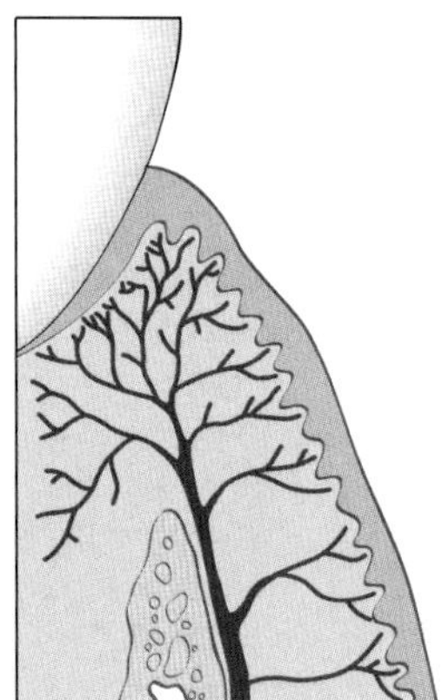

Fig. 4.26 Diagram of an arteriole penetrating the interdental alveolar bone to supply the interdental tissues *(left)* and a supraperiosteal arteriole overlying the facial alveolar bone, sending branches to the surrounding tissue *(right).*

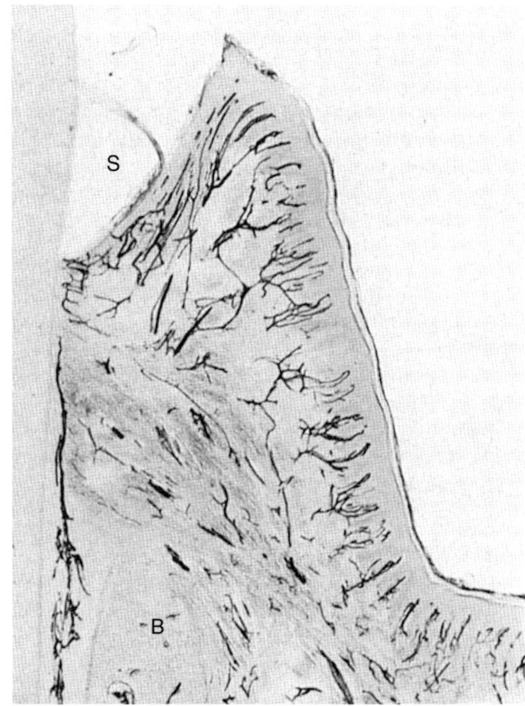

Fig. 4.27 Blood supply and peripheral circulation of the gingiva. Tissues perfused with India ink. Note the capillary plexus parallel to the sulcus *(S)* and the capillary loops in the outer papillary layer. Note also the supraperiosteal vessels external to the bone *(B)*, which supply the gingiva, and a periodontal ligament vessel anastomosing with the sulcus plexus. (Courtesy Sol Bernick.)

1. *Supraperiosteal arterioles* along the facial and lingual surfaces of the alveolar bone from which capillaries extend along the sulcular epithelium and between the rete pegs of the external gingival surface.[8,75,113] Occasional branches of the arterioles pass through the alveolar bone to the periodontal ligament or run over the crest of the alveolar bone.
2. *Vessels of the periodontal ligament,* which extend from the root apices into the gingiva and anastomose with capillaries in the sulcus area.
3. *Arterioles,* which emerge from the crest of the interdental alveolar bone[83] and extend parallel to the crest of the bone to anastomose with vessels of the periodontal ligament, with capillaries in the gingival crevicular areas and supraperiosteal arterioles.

Beneath the epithelium on the outer gingival surface, capillaries of the supraperiosteal arterioles extend into the papillary connective tissue between the epithelial rete pegs in the form of terminal hairpin loops with efferent and afferent branches, spirals, and varices (Fig. 4.28; also see Fig. 4.27).[54,113] The loops are sometimes linked by cross-communications,[85] and flattened capillaries serve as reserve vessels when the circulation is increased in response to irritation.[99]

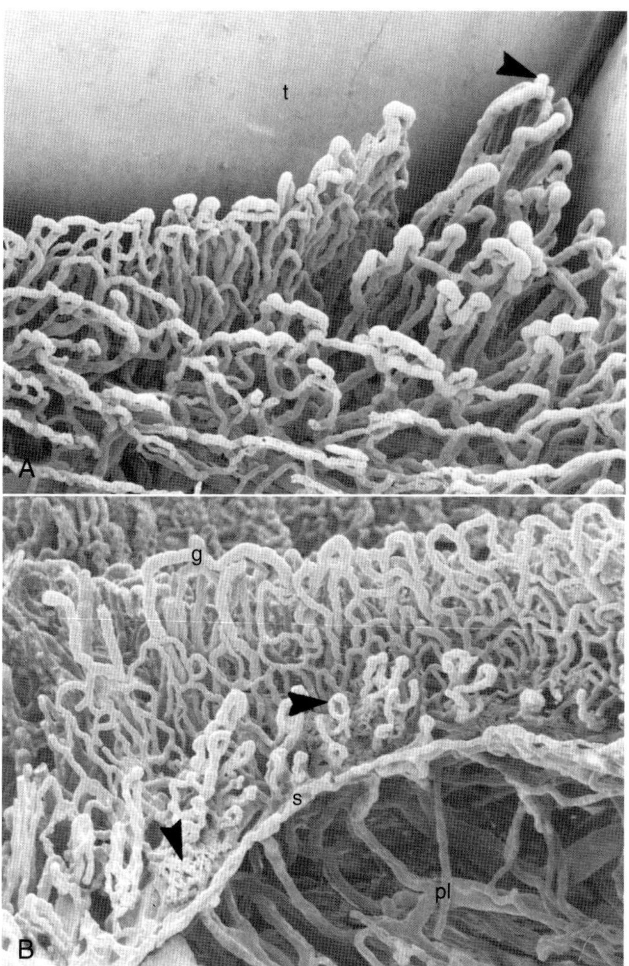

Fig. 4.28 Scanning electron microscopic view of the gingival tissues of rat molar palatal gingiva after the vascular perfusion of plastic and the corrosion of soft tissue. (A) Oral view of gingival capillaries: *t*, tooth; interdental papilla *(arrowhead)* (×180). (B) View from the tooth side. Note the vessels of the plexus next to the sulcular and junctional epithelium. The *arrowheads* point to vessels in the sulcus area with mild inflammatory changes. *g*, Crest of the marginal gingiva; *pl*, periodontal ligament vessels; *s*, bottom of the gingival sulcus. (×150.) (Courtesy N.J. Selliseth and K. Selvig, University of Bergen, Norway.)

Along the sulcular epithelium, capillaries are arranged in a flat, anastomosing plexus that extends parallel to the tooth surface from the base of the sulcus to the gingival margin.[54] In the col area, a mixed pattern of anastomosing capillaries and loops occurs.

As mentioned previously, anatomic and histologic changes have been shown to occur in the gingival microcirculation of individuals with gingivitis. Studies of the gingival vasculature in animals have demonstrated that, in the absence of inflammation, the vascular network is arranged in a regular, repetitive, and layered pattern.[54] In contrast, the inflamed gingival vasculature exhibits an irregular vascular plexus pattern, with looped, dilated, and convoluted.[200]

Microvessels

The lymphatic system in removing excess fluids, cellular and protein debris, microorganisms, and other elements is important for controlling diffusion and the resolution of inflammatory processes.[172] The *lymphatic drainage of the gingiva* collects the lymphatics of the connective tissue papillae.[247] It progresses into the collecting network external to the periosteum of the alveolar process and then moves to the regional lymph nodes, particularly the submaxillary group. In addition, lymphatics just beneath the junctional epithelium extend into the periodontal ligament and accompany the blood vessels.

Neural elements are extensively distributed throughout the gingival tissues. Within the gingival connective tissues, most nerve fibers are myelinated and closely associated with the blood vessels.[165] *Gingival innervation* is derived from fibers that arise from nerves in the periodontal ligament and from the labial, buccal, and palatal nerves.[45] The following nerve structures are present in the connective tissue: a meshwork of terminal fibers, some of which extend into the epithelium; Meissner-type tactile corpuscles; Krause-type end bulbs, which are temperature receptors; and encapsulated spindles.[15,186]

Correlation of Clinical and Microscopic Features

An understanding of the normal clinical features of the gingiva requires the ability to interpret them in terms of the microscopic structures that they represent.

Color

The color of the attached and marginal gingiva displays a range from brown, orange to pink; it results from the colors of the vascular supply, the thickness and degree of keratinization of the epithelium, and the pigment-containing cells. The color varies among different persons and correlates with the cutaneous pigmentation (Fig. 4.29).

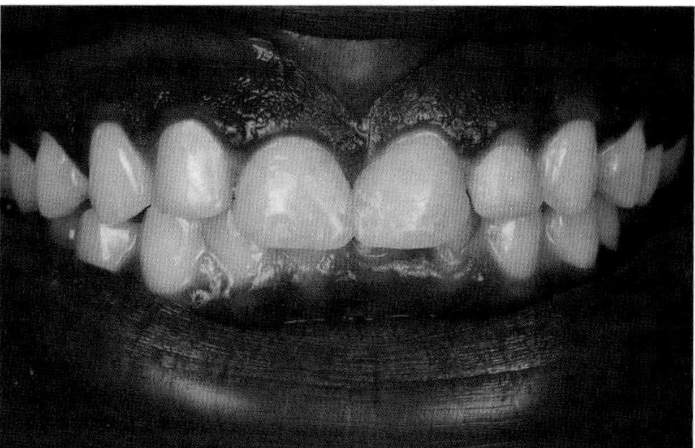

Fig. 4.29 Heavily pigmented (melanotic) gingiva in a middle-aged adult. (Courtesy Dr. Howard Yen.)

The attached gingiva is demarcated from the adjacent alveolar mucosa on the buccal and lingual aspects by a clearly defined mucogingival line. The alveolar mucosa is red, smooth, and shiny. A comparison of the microscopic structure of the attached gingiva with that of the alveolar mucosa provides an explanation for the difference in appearance. The epithelium of the alveolar mucosa is thinner and nonkeratinized, and it contains no rete pegs (Fig. 4.30). The connective tissue of the alveolar mucosa is loosely arranged, and the blood vessels are more numerous.

Physiologic Pigmentation (Melanin)

Melanin is a non–hemoglobin-derived brown pigment with the following characteristics:

- It is located in the intercellular vesicles of melanosomes.
- It is responsible for the pigmentation of the skin, the gingiva, and the remainder of the oral mucous membrane.
- It is present in all individuals (often not in sufficient quantities to be detected clinically), but it is absent or severely diminished in individuals with genetic pigmentation disorders.

Color variations relate to the quantity of melanin synthesized and degraded.

- Ascorbic acid directly downregulates melanin pigmentation in gingival tissues.[256]

Size

The size of the gingiva corresponds with the sum total of the bulk of cellular and intercellular elements and their vascular supply. Alteration in size is a common feature of gingival disease.

Contour

The contour or shape of the gingiva varies considerably and depends on the shape of the teeth and their alignment in the arch, the location and size of the area of proximal contact, and the dimensions of the facial and lingual gingival embrasures.

The marginal gingiva envelops the teeth in a collar-like fashion and follows a scalloped outline on the facial and lingual surfaces. It forms a straight line along teeth with relatively flat surfaces. On teeth with pronounced mesiodistal convexity (e.g., maxillary canines) or teeth in labial version, the normal arcuate contour is accentuated, and the gingiva is located farther apically. On teeth in lingual version, the gingiva is horizontal and thickened (Fig. 4.31). In addition, the gingival tissue phenotype varies significantly. A thin and clear gingiva is found in one-third of the population and primarily in females with slender teeth with a narrow zone of keratinized tissue, whereas a clear, thick gingiva with a broad zone of keratinized tissue is present in two-thirds of the population and primarily in males.[72]

Shape

The shape of the interdental gingiva is governed by the contour of the proximal tooth surfaces and the location and shape of the gingival embrasures.

When the proximal surfaces of the crowns are relatively flat faciolingually, the roots are close together, the interdental bone is thin mesiodistally, and the gingival embrasures and interdental gingiva are narrow mesiodistally. Conversely, with proximal surfaces that flare away from the area of contact, the mesiodistal diameter of the interdental gingiva is broad (Fig. 4.32). The height of the interdental gingiva varies with the location of the proximal contact. Thus, in the anterior region of the dentition, the interdental papilla is pyramidal in form, whereas the papilla is more flattened in a buccolingual direction in the molar region.

Consistency

The gingiva is firm and resilient and, with the exception of the movable free margin, tightly bound to the underlying bone. The collagenous nature of the lamina propria and its contiguity with the mucoperiosteum of the alveolar bone determine the firmness of the attached gingiva. The gingival fibers contribute to the firmness of the gingival margin.

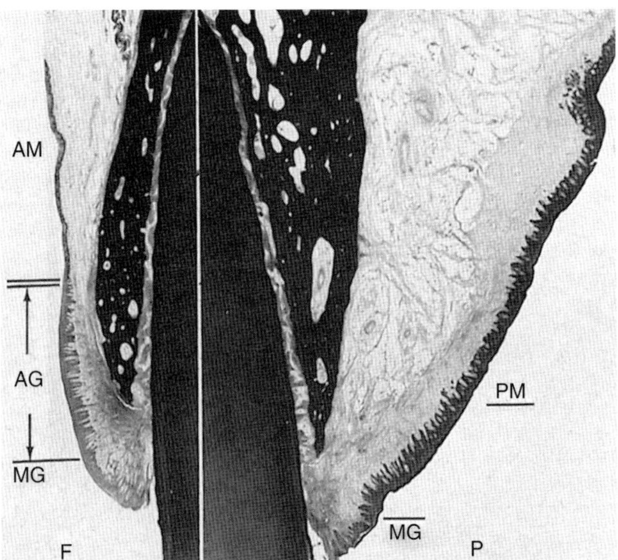

Fig. 4.30 Oral mucosa, facial and palatal surfaces. The facial surface *(F)* shows the marginal gingiva *(MG)*, the attached gingiva *(AG)*, and the alveolar mucosa *(AM)*. The double line marks the mucogingival junction. Note the differences in the epithelium and the connective tissue in the attached gingiva and the alveolar mucosa. The palatal surface *(P)* shows the marginal gingiva *(MG)* and the thick, keratinized palatal mucosa *(PM)*.

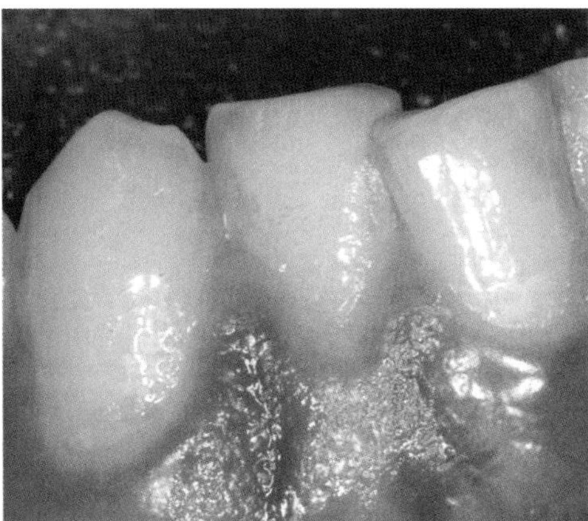

Fig. 4.31 A thickened, shelflike contour of gingiva on a tooth in lingual version aggravated by local irritation caused by plaque accumulation.

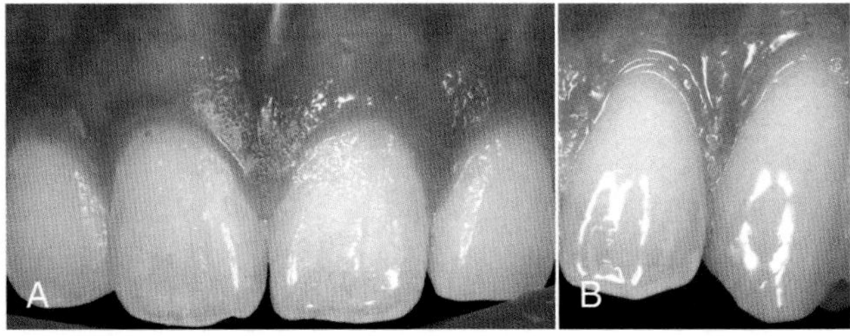

Fig. 4.32 Shape of the interdental gingival papillae correlated with the shape of the teeth and the embrasures. (A) Broad interdental papillae. (B) Narrow interdental papillae.

Surface Texture

The gingiva presents a textured surface similar to that of an orange peel and is referred to as *stippled* (see Fig. 4.29). Stippling is best viewed by drying the gingiva. *The attached gingiva is stippled; the marginal gingiva is not.* The central portion of the interdental papillae is usually stippled, but the marginal borders are smooth. The pattern and extent of stippling vary among individuals and among different areas of the same mouth.[108,227] Stippling is less prominent on lingual than facial surfaces and may be absent in some persons.

Stippling varies with age. It is absent during infancy, it appears in some children at about 5 years of age, it increases until adulthood, and it frequently begins to disappear during old age.

Microscopically, stippling is produced by alternate rounded protuberances and depressions in the gingival surface. The papillary layer of the connective tissue projects into the elevations, and the elevated and depressed areas are covered by stratified squamous epithelium (Fig. 4.33). The degree of keratinization and the prominence of stippling appear to be related.

Scanning electron microscopy has shown considerable variation in shape but a relatively constant depth of stippling. At low magnification, a rippled surface is seen, and this is interrupted by irregular depressions that are 50 μm in diameter. At higher magnification, cell micropits are seen.[62]

Stippling is a form of adaptive specialization or reinforcement for function. It is a feature of healthy gingiva, and the reduction or loss of stippling is a common sign of gingival disease due to edema in the gingiva. When the gingiva is restored to health after treatment, the stippled appearance returns.

The surface texture of the gingiva is also related to the presence and degree of epithelial keratinization. Keratinization is considered a protective adaptation to function. It increases when the gingiva is stimulated by toothbrushing. However, research on free gingival grafts (see Chapter 65) has shown that when connective tissue is transplanted from a keratinized area to a nonkeratinized area, it becomes covered by a keratinized epithelium.[145] This finding suggests a connective-tissue–based genetic determination of the type of epithelial surface.

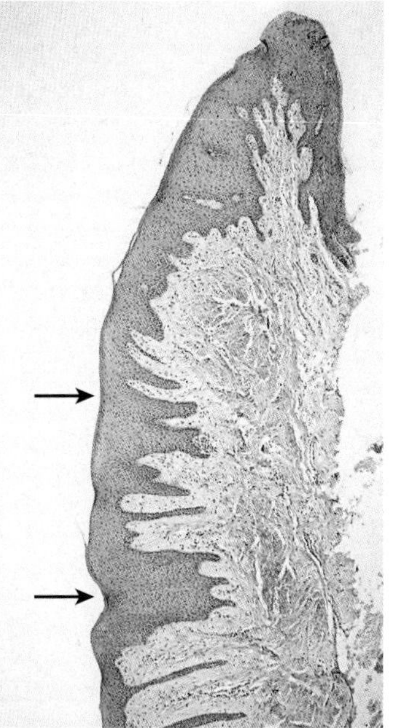

Fig. 4.33 Gingival biopsy of the patient shown in Fig. 4.9 demonstrating alternate elevations and depressions *(arrows)* in the attached gingiva that are responsible for the stippled appearance.

Position

The *position* of the gingiva is the level at which the gingival margin is attached to the tooth. When the tooth erupts into the oral cavity, the margin and sulcus are at the tip of the crown; as eruption progresses, they are seen closer to the root. During this eruption process, as described previously, the junctional epithelium, the oral epithelium, and the REE undergo extensive alterations and remodeling while maintaining the shallow physiologic depth of the sulcus. Without this remodeling of the epithelia, an abnormal anatomic relationship between the gingiva and the tooth would result.

Continuous Tooth Eruption

According to the concept of continuous eruption,[105] eruption does not cease when the teeth meet their functional antagonists; rather, it continues throughout life. Eruption consists of an active phase and a passive phase. *Active eruption* is the movement of the teeth in the direction of the occlusal plane, whereas *passive eruption* is the exposure of the teeth via apical migration of the gingiva.

This concept distinguishes between the anatomic crown (i.e., the portion of the tooth covered by enamel) and the anatomic root (i.e., the portion of the tooth covered by cementum) and between the clinical crown (i.e., the part of the tooth that has been denuded of its gingiva and projects into the oral cavity) and the clinical root (i.e., the portion of the tooth covered by periodontal tissues). When the teeth reach their functional antagonists, the gingival sulcus and the junctional epithelium are still on the enamel, and the clinical crown is approximately two-thirds of the anatomic crown.

Gottlieb and Orban[105] believed that active and passive eruption proceed together. Active eruption is coordinated with attrition; the teeth erupt to compensate for tooth substance that has been worn away by attrition. Attrition reduces the clinical crown and prevents it from becoming disproportionately long in relation to the clinical root, thus avoiding excessive leverage on the periodontal tissues. Ideally, the rate of active eruption keeps pace with tooth wear, thereby preserving the vertical dimension of the dentition.

As teeth erupt, cementum is deposited at the apices and furcations of the roots, and bone is formed along the fundus of the alveolus and at the crest of the alveolar bone. As a result, part of the tooth substance lost by attrition is replaced by the lengthening of the root, and the socket depth is maintained to support the root.

Passive eruption is divided into the following four stages (Fig. 4.34):

Stage 1: The teeth reach the line of occlusion. The junctional epithelium and the base of the gingival sulcus are on the enamel.

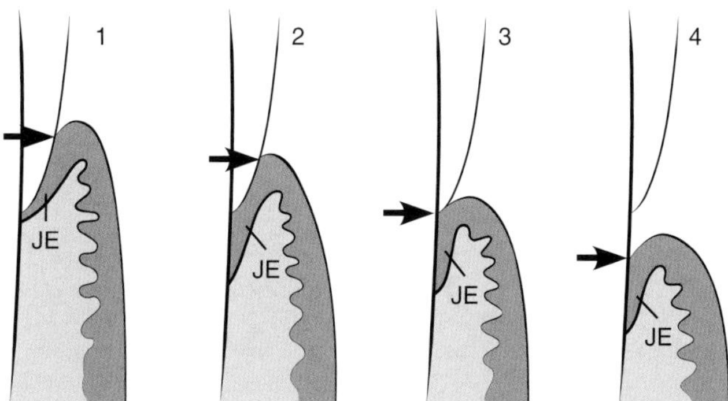

Fig. 4.34 Diagrammatic representation of the four steps of passive eruption according to Gottlieb and Orban.[105] *1,* The base of the gingival sulcus *(arrow)* and the junctional epithelium *(JE)* are on the enamel. *2,* The base of the gingival sulcus *(arrow)* is on the enamel, and part of the junctional epithelium is on the root. *3,* The base of the gingival sulcus *(arrow)* is at the cementoenamel line, and the entire junctional epithelium is on the root. *4,* The base of the gingival sulcus *(arrow)* and the junctional epithelium are on the root.

Stage 2: The junctional epithelium proliferates so that part is on the cementum and part is on the enamel. The base of the sulcus is still on the enamel.

Stage 3: The entire junctional epithelium is on the cementum, and the base of the sulcus is at the cementoenamel junction. As the junctional epithelium proliferates from the crown onto the root, it does not remain at the cementoenamel junction any longer than at any other area of the tooth.

Stage 4: The junctional epithelium has proliferated farther on the cementum. The base of the sulcus is on the cementum, a portion of which is exposed. Proliferation of the junctional epithelium onto the root is accompanied by degeneration of the gingival and periodontal ligament fibers and their detachment from the tooth. The cause of this degeneration is not understood. At present, it is believed to be the result of chronic inflammation and therefore a pathologic process.

As noted, apposition of bone accompanies active eruption. The distance between the apical end of the junctional epithelium and the crest of the alveolus remains constant throughout continuous tooth eruption (i.e., 1.07 mm).[93]

Exposure of the tooth via the apical migration of the gingiva is called *gingival recession* or *atrophy*. According to the concept of continuous eruption, the gingival sulcus may be located on the crown, the cementoenamel junction, or the root, depending on the age of the patient and the stage of eruption. Therefore, some root exposure with age would be considered normal and referred to as *physiologic recession*. Again, this concept is not accepted at present. Excessive exposure is termed *pathologic recession* (see Chapter 22).

Periodontal Ligament

The periodontal ligament is composed of a complex vascular and highly cellular connective tissue that surrounds the tooth root and connects it to the inner wall of the alveolar bone.[179] It is continuous with the connective tissue of the gingiva, and it communicates with the marrow spaces through vascular channels in the bone. Although the average width of the periodontal ligament space is about 0.2 mm, considerable variation exists. The periodontal space is diminished around teeth that are not in function and in unerupted teeth, but it is increased in teeth that have been subjected to hyperfunction.

Periodontal Fibers

The most important elements of the periodontal ligament are the *principal fibers,* which are collagenous and arranged in bundles and which follow a wavy course when viewed in a longitudinal section (Fig. 4.35). The terminal portions of the principal fibers that are inserted into cementum and bone are termed *Sharpey fibers* (Fig. 4.36). The principal fiber bundles consist of individual fibers that form a continuous anastomosing network between tooth and bone.[26,59] Once embedded in the wall of the alveolus or in the tooth, Sharpey fibers calcify to a significant degree. They are associated with abundant noncollagenous proteins that are typically found in bone, and they have also been identified in tooth cementum.[33,137,179] Notable among these proteins are osteopontin and bone sialoprotein.[167,262] These proteins are thought to contribute to the regulation of mineralization and to tissue cohesion at sites of increased biomechanical strain.[179,196]

Type I collagen is a protein that is composed of three chains twisted into a triple helix. The amino acid sequence contains characteristic repeats of Gly-X-Y, with proline occupying the X or Y position, and hydroxylysine and hydroxyproline in the Y position.[51] The amount of collagen in a tissue can be determined by its hydroxyproline content. Collagen is responsible for the maintenance of the periodontal framework and the tone of tissue. There are at least 19 recognized collagen types encoded by at least 25 separate genes dispersed among 12 chromosomes.[18,79]

Collagen biosynthesis occurs inside the fibroblasts to form tropocollagen molecules. These aggregate into microfibrils that are packed together to form fibrils. Collagen fibrils have a transverse striation with a characteristic periodicity of 64 μm; this striation is caused by the overlapping arrangement of the tropocollagen molecules. In collagen types I and III, these fibrils associate to form fibers; in collagen type I, the fibers associate to form bundles (Fig. 4.37).

Collagen is synthesized by fibroblasts, chondroblasts, osteoblasts, odontoblasts, and other cells. The several types of collagen are all distinguishable by their chemical composition, distribution, function, and morphology.[142] The principal fibers are composed

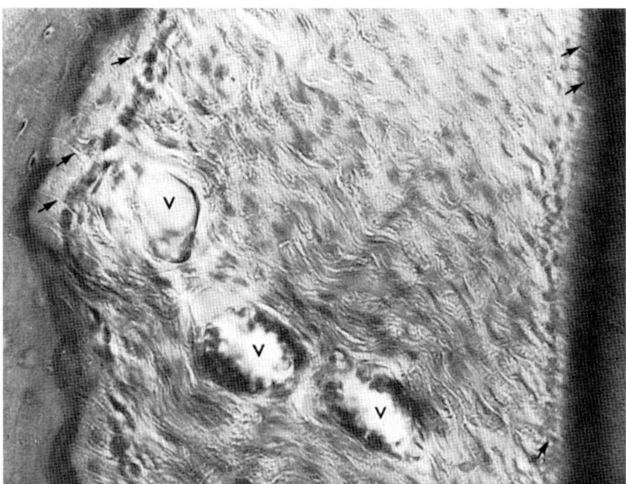

Fig. 4.35 Principal fibers of the periodontal ligament follow a wavy course when sectioned longitudinally. The formative function of the periodontal ligament is illustrated by the newly formed osteoid and osteoblasts along a previously resorbed bone surface *(left)* and the cementoid and cementoblasts *(right)*. Note the fibers embedded in the forming calcified tissues *(arrows)*. *V*, Vascular channels.

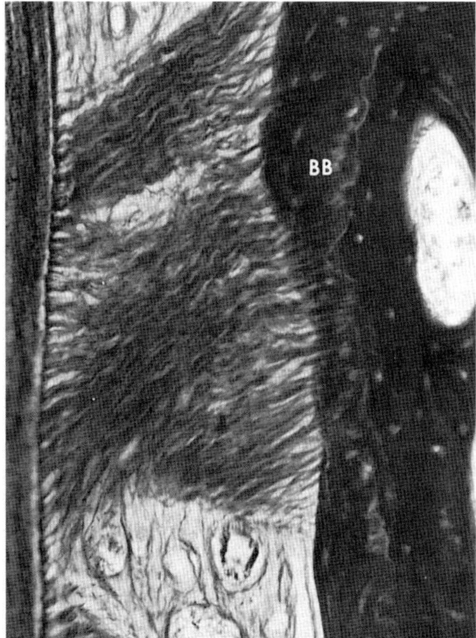

Fig. 4.36 Collagen fibers embedded in the cementum *(left)* and the bone *(right)* (silver stain). Note the Sharpey fibers within the bundle bone *(BB)* overlying the lamellar bone.

mainly of collagen type I,[223] whereas reticular fibers are composed of collagen type III. Collagen type IV is found in the basal lamina.[224] The expression of type XII collagen during tooth development is timed with the alignment and organization of periodontal fibers and is limited in tooth development to cells within the periodontal ligament.[168] Type VI collagen has also been immunolocalized in the periodontal ligament and the gingiva.[81]

The molecular configuration of collagen fibers provides them with a tensile strength that is greater than that of steel. Consequently, collagen imparts a unique combination of flexibility and strength to the tissues.[142]

The principal fibers of the periodontal ligament are arranged in six groups that develop sequentially in the developing root: the transseptal, alveolar crest, horizontal, oblique, apical, and interradicular fibers (Fig. 4.38).

Transseptal fibers extend interproximally over the alveolar bone crest and are embedded in the cementum of adjacent teeth (Fig. 4.39). They are reconstructed even after the destruction of the alveolar bone that results from periodontal disease. These fibers may be considered as belonging to the gingiva because they do not have osseous attachment.

Alveolar crest fibers extend obliquely from the cementum just beneath the junctional epithelium to the alveolar crest (Fig. 4.40). Fibers also run from the cementum over the alveolar crest and to the fibrous layer of the periosteum that covers the alveolar bone. The alveolar crest fibers prevent the extrusion of the tooth[53] and resist lateral tooth movements. The incision of these fibers during periodontal surgery does not increase tooth mobility unless significant attachment loss has occurred.[97]

Horizontal fibers extend at right angles to the long axis of the tooth from the cementum to the alveolar bone.

Oblique fibers, which constitute the largest group in the periodontal ligament, extend from the cementum in a coronal direction obliquely to the bone (see Fig. 4.38). They bear the brunt of vertical masticatory stresses and transform such stresses into tension on the alveolar bone.

The *apical fibers* radiate in a rather irregular manner from the cementum to the bone at the apical region of the socket. They do not occur on incompletely formed roots.

The *interradicular fibers* fan out from the cementum to the tooth in the furcation areas of multirooted teeth.

Other well-formed fiber bundles interdigitate at right angles or splay around and between regularly arranged fiber bundles. Less regularly arranged collagen fibers are found in the interstitial

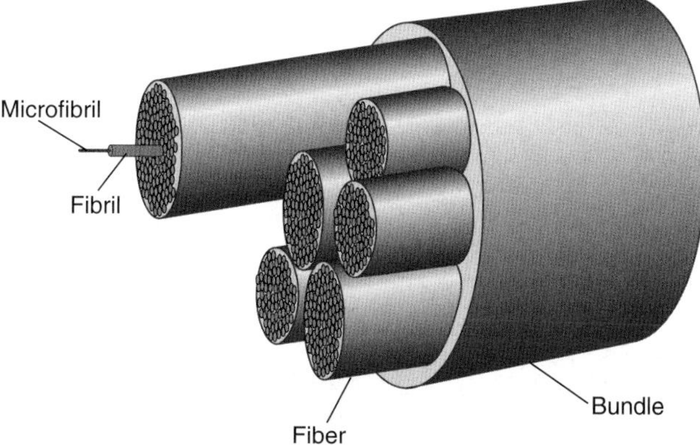

Fig. 4.37 Collagen microfibrils, fibrils, fibers, and bundles.

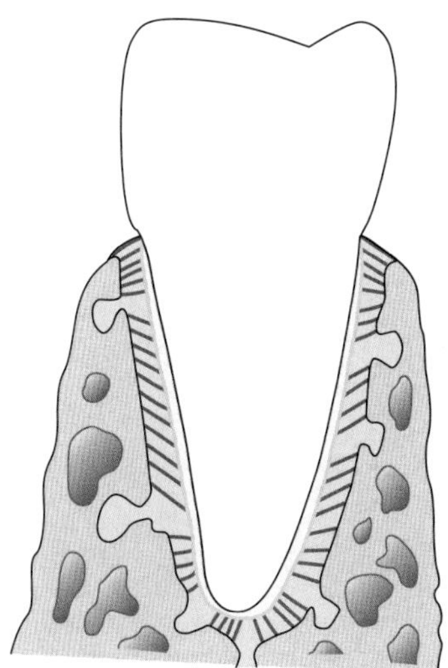
Fig. 4.38 Diagram of the principal fiber groups.

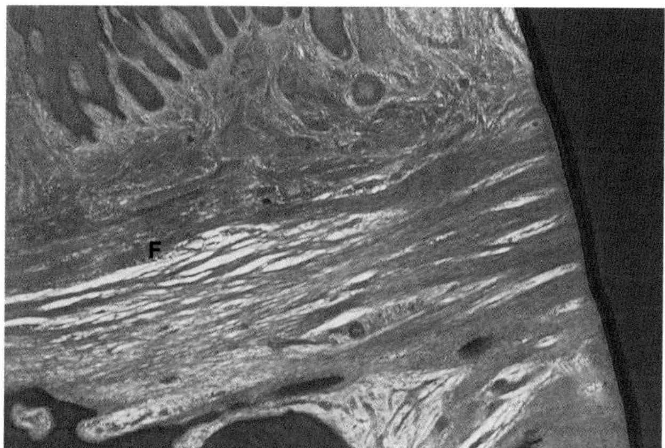

Fig. 4.39 Transseptal fibers *(F)* at the crest of the interdental bone.

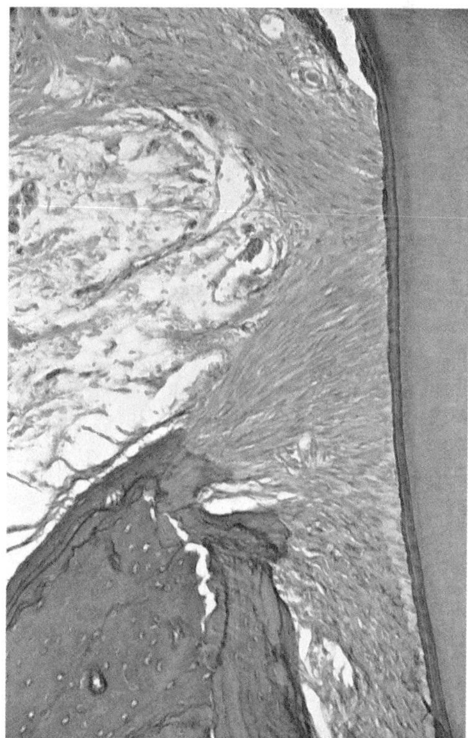
Fig. 4.40 Rat molar section showing alveolar crest fibers radiating coronally.

connective tissue between the principal fiber groups; this tissue contains the blood vessels, lymphatics, and nerves.

Although the periodontal ligament does not contain mature elastin, two immature forms are expressed by fibroblasts: oxytalan and elaunin. An elastic meshwork has been described in the periodontal ligament[137] as being composed of many elastin lamellae with peripheral oxytalan fibers and elaunin fibers. The so-called oxytalan fibers[89,103] run parallel to the root surface in a vertical direction and bend to attach to the cementum[89] in the cervical third of the root. They are thought to regulate vascular flow.[87] Oxytalan fibers have been shown to develop de novo in the regenerated periodontal ligament.[230] Oxytalan fibers consist of the glycoproteins fibrillin-1 and fibrillin-2, forming microfibrils. When microfibrils assemble with an elastin core, they are called elaunin (immature form) and elastin (mature form).

The principal fibers are remodeled by the periodontal ligament cells to adapt to physiologic needs[275,304] and in response to different stimuli.[284] In addition to these fiber types, small collagen fibers associated with the larger principal collagen fibers have been described. These fibers run in all directions and form a plexus called the *indifferent fiber plexus.*[253]

Cellular Elements

Four types of cells have been identified in the periodontal ligament: connective tissue cells, epithelial rest cells, immune system cells, and cells associated with neurovascular elements.[27,28]

Connective tissue cells include fibroblasts, cementoblasts, and osteoblasts. Fibroblasts are the most common cells in the periodontal ligament; they appear as ovoid or elongated cells oriented along the principal fibers, and they exhibit pseudopodia-like processes.[222] These cells synthesize collagen and possess the capacity to phagocytose "old" collagen fibers and degrade them via enzyme hydrolysis.[275] Thus, collagen turnover appears to be regulated by fibroblasts in a process of intracellular degradation of collagen that does not involve the action of collagenase.[25]

Phenotypically distinct and functionally different subpopulations of fibroblasts exist in the adult periodontal ligament. They appear to be identical at both the light and electron microscopic levels,[115] but they may have different functions, such as the secretion of different collagen types and the production of collagenase.

Osteoblasts, cementoblasts, osteoclasts, and odontoclasts are also seen in the cemental and osseous surfaces of the periodontal ligament.

The *epithelial rests of Malassez* form a latticework in the periodontal ligament and appear as either isolated clusters of cells or interlacing strands (Fig. 4.41), depending on the plane in which the microscopic section is cut. Continuity with the junctional epithelium has been suggested in experimental animals.[106] The epithelial rests are considered remnants of the Hertwig root sheath, which disintegrates during root development (see Fig. 4.41A).

Epithelial rests are distributed close to the cementum throughout the periodontal ligament of most teeth; they are most numerous in the apical area[219] and the cervical area.[287,288] They diminish in number with age[258] by degenerating and disappearing or by undergoing calcification to become cementicles. The cells are surrounded by a distinct basal lamina, they are interconnected by hemidesmosomes, and they contain tonofilaments.[25]

Although their functional properties are still considered to be unclear,[269] the epithelial rests are reported to contain keratinocyte growth factors, and they have been shown to be positive for tyrosine kinase A neurotrophin receptor.[92,290,300] In addition, epithelial rests proliferate when stimulated,[272,276,283] and they participate in the formation of periapical cysts and lateral root cysts.

The *defense cells* in the periodontal ligament include neutrophils, lymphocytes, macrophages, mast cells, and eosinophils. These cells, as well as those associated with neurovascular elements, are similar to the cells found in other connective tissues.

Ground Substance

The periodontal ligament also contains a large proportion of ground substance that fills the spaces between fibers and cells. This substance consists of two main components: *glycosaminoglycans,* such as hyaluronic acid and proteoglycans, and *glycoproteins,* such as fibronectin and laminin-332. It also has a high water content (i.e., 70%).

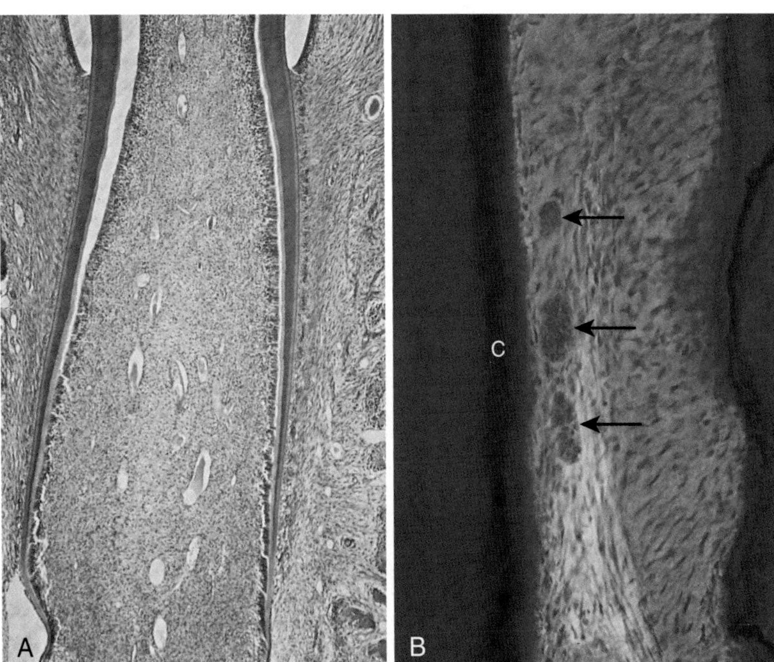

Fig. 4.41 Epithelial rests of Malassez. (A) Erupting tooth in a cat. Note the fragmentation of the Hertwig epithelial root sheath giving rise to epithelial rests located along and close to the root surface. (B) Human periodontal ligament with rosette-shaped epithelial rests *(arrows)* lying close to the cementum *(C).*

The cell surface proteoglycans participate in several biologic functions, including cell adhesion, cell-cell and cell-matrix interactions, binding to various growth factors as co-receptors, and cell repair.[301] For example, fibromodulin (a small proteoglycan rich in keratan sulfate and leucine) has been identified in the bovine periodontal ligament.[292] The most comprehensive study of the proteoglycans in periodontal ligament was performed with the use of fibroblast cultures of human ligament.[153]

The periodontal ligament may also contain calcified masses called *cementicles,* which are adherent to or detached from the root surfaces (Fig. 4.42).

Cementicles may develop from calcified epithelial rests; around small spicules of cementum or alveolar bone traumatically displaced into the periodontal ligament; from calcified Sharpey fibers; and from calcified, thrombosed vessels within the periodontal ligament.[184]

Functions of Periodontal Ligament

The functions of the periodontal ligament are categorized as physical, formative and remodeling, nutritional, and sensory.

Physical Functions

The physical functions of the periodontal ligament entail the following:

1. Provision of a soft-tissue "casing" to protect the vessels and nerves from injury by mechanical forces.
2. Transmission of occlusal forces to the bone.
3. Attachment of the teeth to the bone.
4. Maintenance of the gingival tissues in their proper relationship to the teeth.
5. Resistance to the impact of occlusal forces (i.e., shock absorption).

Resistance to Impact of Occlusal Forces (Shock Absorption)

Two theories pertaining to the mechanism of tooth support have been considered: the tensional theory and the viscoelastic system theory.

The tensional theory of tooth support states that the principal fibers of the periodontal ligament are the major factor in supporting the tooth and transmitting forces to the bone. When a force is applied to the crown, the principal fibers first unfold and straighten, and they then transmit forces to the alveolar bone, thereby causing an elastic deformation of the bony socket. Finally, when the alveolar bone has reached its limit, the load is transmitted to the basal bone. Many investigators find this theory insufficient to explain available experimental evidence.

The viscoelastic system theory states that the displacement of the tooth is largely controlled by fluid movements, with fibers having only a secondary role.[32,43] When forces are transmitted to the tooth, the extracellular fluid passes from the periodontal ligament into the marrow spaces of the bone through the foramina in the cribriform plate. These perforations of the cribriform plate link the periodontal ligament with the cancellous portion of the alveolar bone; they are more abundant in the cervical third than in the middle and apical thirds (Fig. 4.43).

After the depletion of tissue fluids, the fiber bundles absorb the slack and tighten. This leads to a blood vessel stenosis. Arterial back pressure causes ballooning of the vessels and passage of the blood ultrafiltrates into the tissues, thereby replenishing the tissue fluids.[32]

Transmission of Occlusal Forces to Bone

The arrangement of the principal fibers is similar to that of a suspension bridge or a hammock. When an axial force is applied to a tooth, a tendency toward a displacement of the root into the alveolus occurs. The oblique fibers alter their wavy, untensed pattern, assume their full length, and sustain the major part of the axial force. When a horizontal or tipping force is applied, two phases of tooth movement occur. The first is within the confines of the periodontal ligament, and the second produces a displacement of the facial and lingual bony plates.[71] The tooth rotates about an axis that may change as the force is increased.

The apical portion of the root moves in a direction that is opposite to the coronal portion. In areas of tension, the principal fiber bundles are taut rather than wavy. In areas of pressure, the fibers are compressed, the tooth is displaced, and a corresponding distortion of bone exists in the direction of root movement.[215]

In single-rooted teeth, the axis of rotation is located in the area between the apical third and the middle third of the root (Fig. 4.44). The root apex[191] and the coronal half of the clinical root have been suggested as other locations of the axis of rotation. The periodontal ligament, which has an hourglass shape, is narrowest in the region of the axis of rotation (Table 4.1).[66,149] In multirooted teeth, the axis of rotation is located in the bone between the roots (Fig. 4.45). In compliance with the physiologic mesial migration of the teeth, the periodontal ligament is thinner on the mesial root surface than on the distal surface.

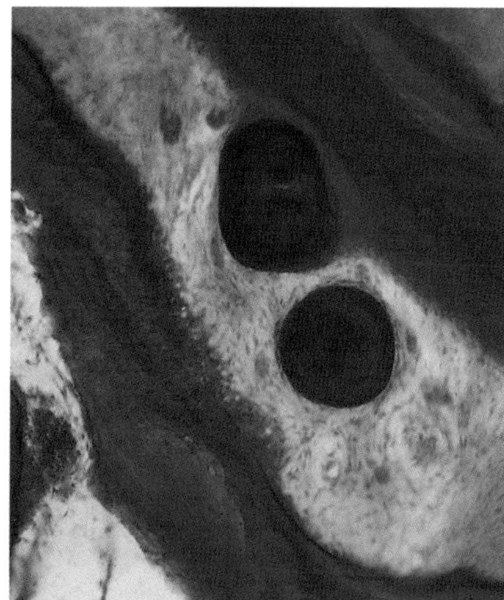

Fig. 4.42 Cementicles in the periodontal ligament. One is lying free and the other is adherent to the tooth surface.

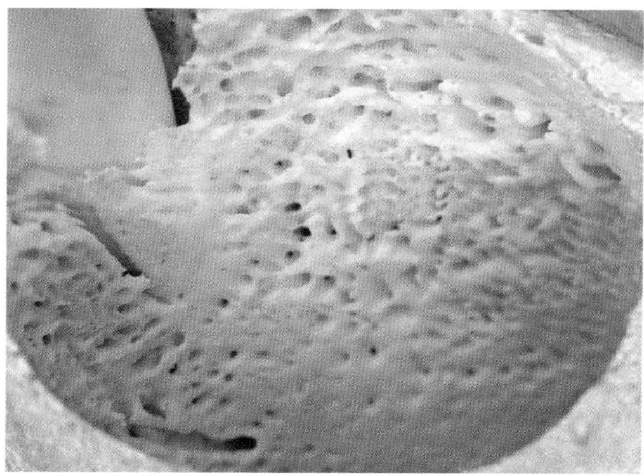

Fig. 4.43 Foramina perforating the lamina dura of a dog jaw.

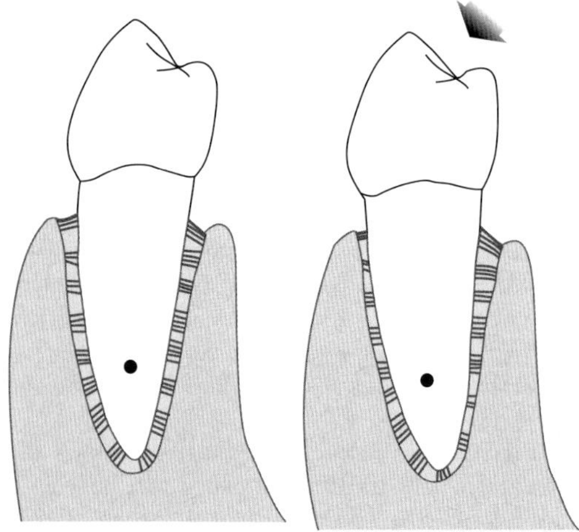

Fig. 4.44 *Left,* Diagram of a mandibular premolar in a resting state. *Right,* When a force is exerted on the tooth—in this case, in faciolingual direction *(arrow)*—the tooth rotates around the fulcrum or axis of rotation *(black circle on root).* The periodontal ligament is compressed in areas of pressure and distended in areas of tension.

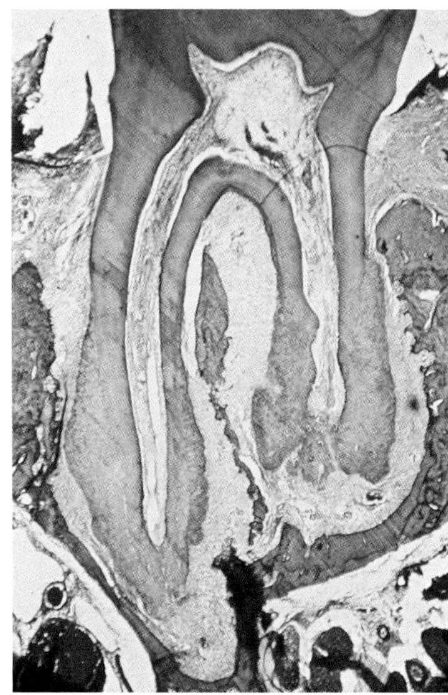

Fig. 4.45 Microscopic view of a rat molar subjected to occlusohorizontal forces. Note the alternating widened and narrowed areas of the periodontal ligament as the tooth rotates around its axis of rotation. The axis of rotation is in the interradicular space.

TABLE 4.1 Thickness of the Periodontal Ligaments of 172 Teeth From 15 Human Subjects

	Average of Alveolar Crest (mm)	Average of Midroot (mm)	Average of Apex (mm)	Average of Tooth (mm)
Ages 11 through 16 years	0.23	0.17	0.24	0.21
83 teeth from 4 jaws				
Ages 32 through 50 years	0.20	0.14	0.19	0.18
36 teeth from 5 jaws				
Ages 51 through 67 years	0.17	0.12	0.16	0.15
35 teeth from 5 jaws				
Age 24 years (1 case)	0.16	0.09	0.15	0.13
18 teeth from 1 jaw				

Modified from Coolidge ED. The thickness of the human periodontal membrane. *J Am Dent Assoc.* 1937;24:1260.

Formative and Remodeling Function

Periodontal ligament and alveolar bone cells are exposed to physical forces in response to mastication, parafunction, speech, and orthodontic tooth movement.[177] Cells of the periodontal ligament participate in the formation and resorption of cementum and bone, which occur during physiologic tooth movement, during the accommodation of the periodontium to occlusal forces, and during the repair of injuries.

Variations in cellular enzyme activity are correlated with the remodeling process.[94–96] Although applied loads may induce vascular and inflammatory reactive changes in periodontal ligament cells, current evidence suggests that these cells have a mechanism to respond directly to mechanical forces via the activation of various mechanosensory signaling systems, including adenylate cyclase, stretch-activated ion channels, and via changes in cytoskeletal organization.[177]

Cartilage formation in the periodontal ligament, although unusual, may represent a metaplastic phenomenon in the repair of this ligament after injury.[21]

The periodontal ligament is constantly undergoing remodeling. Old cells and fibers are broken down and replaced by new ones, and mitotic activity can be observed in the fibroblasts and the endothelial cells.[192] Fibroblasts form the collagen fibers, and the residual mesenchymal cells develop into osteoblasts and cementoblasts. Therefore, the rate of formation and the differentiation of osteoblasts, cementoblasts, and fibroblasts affect the rate of formation of collagen, cementum, and bone.

Radioautographic studies with radioactive thymidine, proline, and glycine indicate a high turnover rate of collagen in the periodontal ligament. The rate of collagen synthesis is twice as fast as that in the gingiva and four times as fast as that in the skin, as established in the rat molar.[260] A rapid turnover of sulfated glycosaminoglycans in the cells and amorphous ground substance of the periodontal ligament also occurs.[22] It should be noted that most of these studies have been performed in rodents and that information about primates and humans is scarce.[242]

Nutritional and Sensory Functions

The periodontal ligament supplies nutrients to the cementum, bone, and gingiva by way of the blood vessels, and it also provides lymphatic drainage as discussed later in this chapter. In relation to other ligaments and tendons, the periodontal ligament is highly vascularized tissue; almost 10% of its volume in the rodent molar is blood vessels.[35,178] This relatively high blood vessel content may provide hydrodynamic damping to applied forces as well as high perfusion rates to the periodontal ligament.[177]

The periodontal ligament is abundantly supplied with sensory nerve fibers that are capable of transmitting tactile, pressure, and pain sensations via the trigeminal pathways.[15,31] Nerve bundles pass into the periodontal ligament from the periapical area and through channels from the alveolar bone that follow the course of the blood vessels. The bundles divide into single myelinated fibers, which ultimately lose their myelin sheaths and end in one of four types of neural termination: (1) free endings, which have a treelike configuration and carry pain sensation; (2) Ruffini-like mechanoreceptors, which are located primarily in the apical area; (3) coiled Meissner corpuscles and mechanoreceptors, which are found mainly in the midroot region; and (4) spindle-like pressure and vibration endings, which are surrounded by a fibrous capsule and located mainly in the apex.[87,170]

Regulation of Periodontal Ligament Width

Some of the most interesting features of the periodontal ligament in animals are its adaptability to rapidly changing applied force and its capacity to maintain its width at constant dimensions throughout its lifetime.[178] These are important measures of periodontal ligament homeostasis that provide insight into the function of the biologic mechanisms that tightly regulate the metabolism and spatial locations of the cell populations involved in the formation of bone, cementum, and periodontal ligament fibers. In addition, the ability of periodontal ligament cells to synthesize and secrete a wide range of regulatory molecules is an essential component of tissue remodeling and periodontal ligament homeostasis.[177]

Cementum

Cementum is the calcified, avascular mesenchymal tissue that forms the outer covering of the anatomic root. The two main types of cementum are acellular *(primary)* and cellular *(secondary)* cementum.[104] Both consist of a calcified interfibrillar matrix and collagen fibrils.

The two main sources of collagen fibers in cementum are Sharpey fibers *(extrinsic)*, which are the embedded portion of the principal fibers of the periodontal ligament and which are formed by the fibroblasts, and fibers that belong to the cementum matrix *(intrinsic)*, which are produced by the cementoblasts.[250] Cementoblasts also form the noncollagenous components of the interfibrillar ground substance, such as proteoglycans, glycoproteins, and phosphoproteins. Proteoglycans are most likely to play a role in regulating cell-cell and cell-matrix interactions, both during normal development and during the regeneration of the cementum.[18] In addition, immunohistochemical studies have shown that the distribution of proteoglycans is closely associated with the cementoblasts and the cementocytes.[1,2]

The major proportion of the organic matrix of cementum is composed of type I (90%) and type III (about 5%) collagens. Sharpey fibers, which constitute a considerable proportion of the bulk of cementum, are composed of mainly type I collagen.[218] Type III collagen appears to coat the type I collagen of the Sharpey fibers.[17]

Acellular cementum is the first cementum formed; it covers approximately the cervical third or half of the root, and it does not contain cells (Fig. 4.46). This cementum is formed before the tooth reaches the occlusal plane, and its thickness ranges from 30 to 230 µm.[258] Sharpey fibers make up most of the structure of acellular cementum, which has a principal role in supporting the tooth. Most fibers are inserted at approximately right angles into the root surface and penetrate deep into the cementum, but others enter from several different directions. Their size, number, and distribution increase with function.[126] Sharpey fibers are completely calcified, with the mineral crystals oriented parallel to the fibrils as in dentin and bone, except in a 10- to 50-µm–wide zone near the cementodentinal junction, where they are only partially calcified. The peripheral portions of Sharpey fibers in actively mineralizing cementum tend to be more calcified than the interior regions, according to evidence obtained by scanning electron microscopy.[141] Acellular cementum also contains intrinsic collagen fibrils that are calcified and irregularly arranged or parallel to the surface.[242]

Cellular cementum, which is formed after the tooth reaches the occlusal plane, is more irregular and contains cells (cementocytes) in individual spaces (lacunae) that communicate with each other through a system of anastomosing canaliculi (Fig. 4.47). Cellular cementum is less calcified than the acellular type.[127] Sharpey fibers occupy a smaller portion of cellular cementum and are separated by other

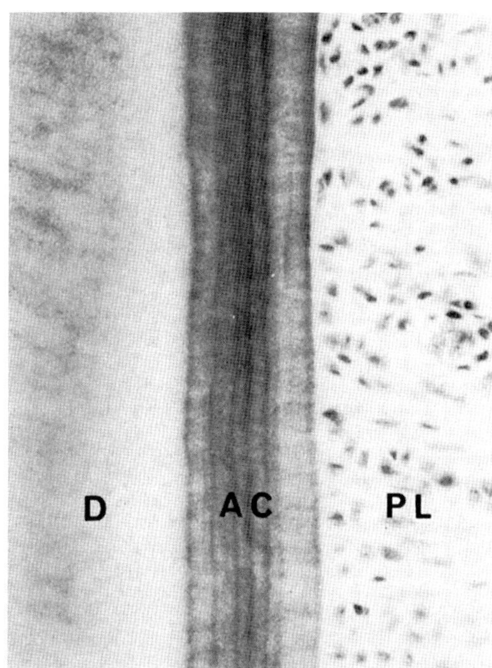

Fig. 4.46 Acellular cementum *(AC)* showing incremental lines running parallel to the long axis of the tooth. These lines represent the appositional growth of cementum. Note the thin, light lines running into the cementum perpendicular to the surface; these represent the Sharpey fibers of the periodontal ligament *(PL)*. *D*, Dentin. (×300.)

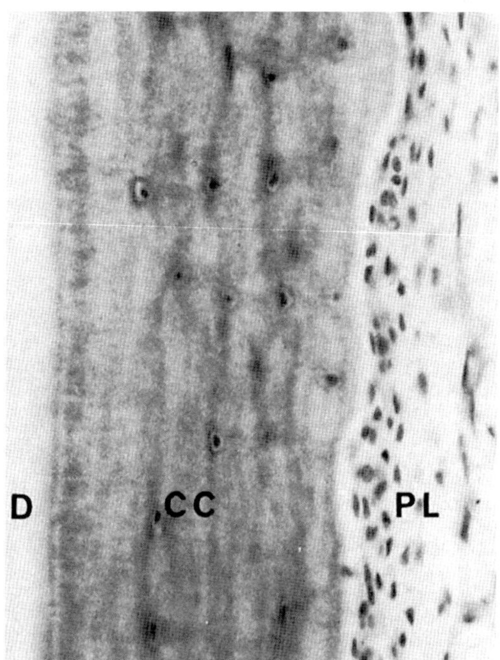

Fig. 4.47 Cellular cementum *(CC)* showing cementocytes lying within the lacunae. Cellular cementum is thicker than acellular cementum. The evidence of incremental lines also exists, but they are less distinct than in the acellular cementum. The cells adjacent to the surface of the cementum in the periodontal ligament *(PL)* space are cementoblasts. *D*, Dentin. (×300.)

fibers that are arranged either parallel to the root surface or at random. Sharpey fibers may be completely or partially calcified, or they may have a central, uncalcified core surrounded by a calcified border.[139,250]

Both acellular cementum and cellular cementum are arranged in lamellae separated by incremental lines parallel to the long axis of the root (see Figs. 4.46 and 4.47). These lines represent "rest periods" in cementum formation, and they are more mineralized than the adjacent cementum.[226] In addition, the loss of the cervical part of the REE at the time of tooth eruption may place portions of mature enamel in contact with the connective tissue, which then will deposit an acellular and afibrillar type of cementum over the enamel.[160]

On the basis of these findings, Schroeder[137,138] has classified cementum as follows:

- Acellular afibrillar cementum contains neither cells nor extrinsic or intrinsic collagen fibers, except for a mineralized ground substance. Acellular afibrillar cementum is a product of cementoblasts and is found as coronal cementum in humans, with a thickness of 1 to 15 μm.
- Acellular extrinsic fiber cementum is composed almost entirely of densely packed bundles of Sharpey fibers and lacks cells. Acellular extrinsic fiber cementum is a product of fibroblasts and cementoblasts. It is found in the cervical third of roots in humans, but it may extend farther apically. Its thickness is between 30 and 230 μm.
- Cellular mixed stratified cementum is composed of extrinsic (Sharpey) and intrinsic fibers, and it may contain cells. Cellular mixed stratified cementum is a co-product of fibroblasts and cementoblasts. In humans, it appears primarily in the apical third of the roots and apices and in furcation areas. Its thickness ranges from 100 to 1000 μm.
- Cellular intrinsic fiber cementum contains cells but no extrinsic collagen fibers. Cellular intrinsic fiber cementum is formed by cementoblasts, and, in humans, it fills the resorption lacunae.

Intermediate cementum is a poorly defined zone near the cementodentinal junction of certain teeth that appears to contain cellular remnants of the Hertwig epithelial sheath embedded in a calcified ground substance.[76,156]

Inorganic content of cementum (hydroxyapatite; $Ca_{10}[PO_4]_6[OH]_2$) is 45% to 50%, which is less than that of bone (65%), enamel (97%), or dentin (70%).[308] Opinions differ with regard to whether the microhardness increases[198] or decreases with age,[291] and no relationship has been established between aging and the mineral content of cementum.

Permeability of Cementum

In very young animals, acellular cementum and cellular cementum are very permeable and permit the diffusion of dyes from the pulp and the external root surface. In cellular cementum, the canaliculi in some areas are contiguous with the dentinal tubuli. The permeability of cementum diminishes with age.[36]

Cementoenamel Junction

The cementum at and immediately subjacent to the *cementoenamel junction* is of particular clinical importance in root-scaling procedures. Three types of relationships involving the cementum may exist at the cementoenamel junction.[199] In about 60% to 65% of cases, cementum overlaps the enamel (Fig. 4.48); in about 30%, an edge-to-edge butt joint exists; and in 5% to 10%, the cementum and enamel fail to meet. In the last case, gingival recession may result in accentuated sensitivity as a result of exposed dentin.

Cementodentinal Junction

The terminal apical area of the cementum where it joins the internal root canal dentin is known as the *cementodentinal junction.* When root canal treatment is performed, the obturating material should be at the cementodentinal junction. There appears to be no increase or decrease in the width of the cementodentinal junction with age; its width appears to remain relatively stable.[264] Scanning electron microscopy of the human teeth reveals that the cementodentinal junction is 2 to 3 μm wide. The fibril-poor layer contains a significant amount of proteoglycans, and fibrils intermingle between the cementum and the dentin.[302,303]

Thickness of Cementum

Cementum deposition is a continuous process that proceeds at varying rates throughout life. Cementum formation is most rapid in the apical regions, where it compensates for tooth eruption, which itself compensates for attrition.

The thickness of cementum on the coronal half of the root varies from 16 to 60 μm, which is about the thickness of a hair. It attains its greatest thickness (≤150 to 200 μm) in the apical third and in the furcation areas. It is thicker in distal surfaces than in mesial surfaces, probably because of functional stimulation from mesial drift over time.[70] Between the ages of 11 and 70 years, the average thickness of the cementum increases threefold, with the greatest increase seen in the apical region. Average thicknesses of 95 μm at the age of 20 years and of 215 μm at the age of 60 years have been reported.[307]

Abnormalities in the thickness of cementum may range from an absence or paucity of cellular cementum (i.e., cemental aplasia or hypoplasia) to an excessive deposition of cementum (i.e., cemental hyperplasia or hypercementosis).[155]

The term *hypercementosis* refers to a prominent thickening of the cementum. It is largely an age-related phenomenon, and it may be localized to one tooth or affect the entire dentition. As a result of considerable physiologic variation in the thickness of cementum among different teeth in the same person and also among different persons, distinguishing between hypercementosis and the physiologic thickening of cementum is sometimes difficult. Nevertheless, the excessive proliferation of cementum may occur with a broad spectrum of neoplastic and non-neoplastic conditions, including benign cementoblastoma, cementifying fibroma, periapical cemental dysplasia, florid cemento-osseous dysplasia, and other benign fibro-osseous lesions.[155]

Hypercementosis itself does not require treatment. It could pose a problem if an affected tooth requires extraction. In a multirooted tooth, sectioning of the tooth may be required before extraction.[20]

Cementum Resorption and Repair

Permanent teeth do not undergo physiologic resorption as primary teeth do. However, the cementum of erupted (as well as unerupted) teeth is subject to resorptive changes that may be of microscopic proportion or sufficiently extensive to present a radiographically detectable alteration in the root contour.

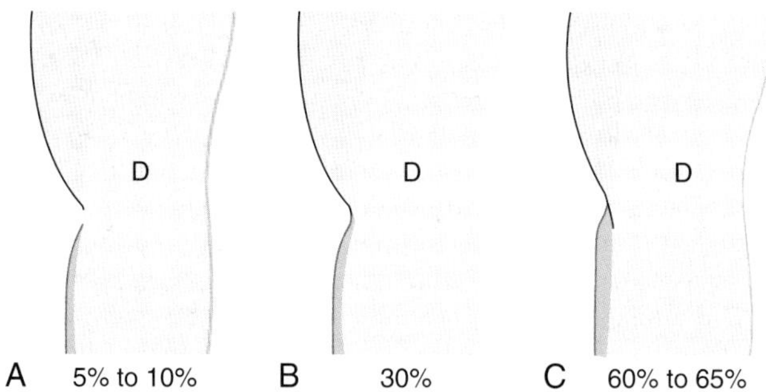

Fig. 4.48 Normal variations in tooth morphology at the cementoenamel junction. (A) Space between the enamel and the cementum with the dentin *(D)* exposed. (B) End-to-end relationship of enamel and cementum. (C) Cementum overlapping the enamel.

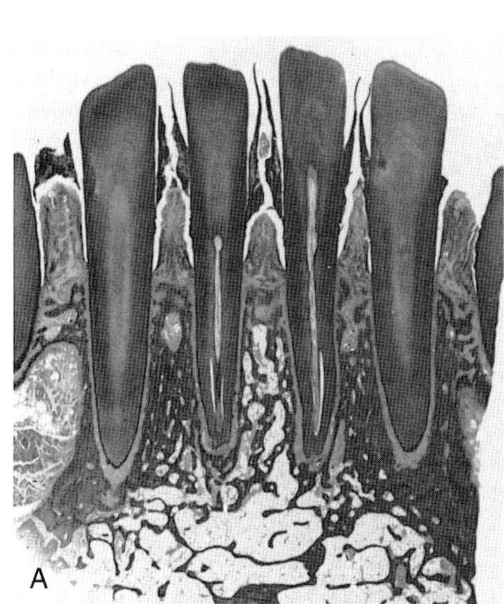

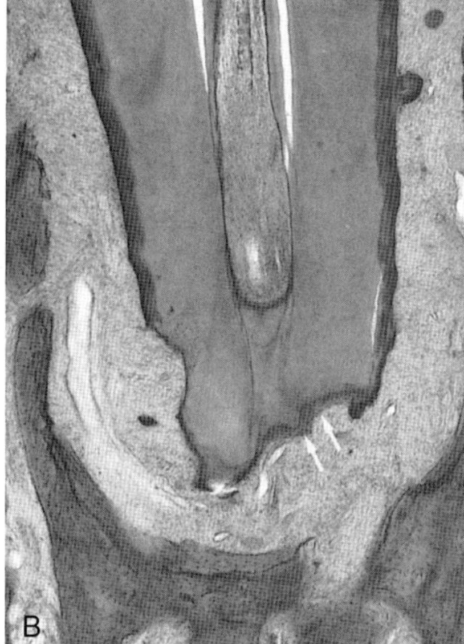

Fig. 4.49 Cemental resorption associated with excessive occlusal forces. (A) Low-power histologic section of the mandibular anterior teeth. (B) High-power micrograph of the apex of the left central incisor shortened by the resorption of cementum and dentin. Note the partial repair of the eroded areas *(arrows)* and the cementicle at the upper right.

Microscopic cementum resorption is extremely common; in one study, it occurred in 236 of 261 teeth (90.5%).[120] The average number of resorption areas per tooth was 3.5. Of the 922 areas of resorption, 708 (76.8%) were located in the apical third of the root, 177 (19.2%) in the middle third, and 37 (4.0%) in the gingival third. Approximately 70% of all resorption areas were confined to the cementum without involving the dentin.

Cementum resorption may be caused by local or systemic factors, or it may occur without apparent etiology (i.e., idiopathic). Local conditions that cause cementum resorption include trauma from occlusion (Fig. 4.49)[205]; orthodontic movement[119,204,228]; pressure from malaligned erupting teeth, cysts, and tumors[148]; teeth without functional antagonists; embedded teeth; replanted and transplanted teeth[3,139]; periapical disease; and periodontal disease. Systemic conditions that are cited as predisposing an individual to or inducing cemental resorption include calcium deficiency,[140] hypothyroidism,[24] hereditary fibrous osteodystrophy,[279] and Paget disease.[229]

Cementum resorption appears microscopically as baylike concavities in the root surface (Fig. 4.50). Multinucleated giant cells and large mononuclear macrophages are generally found adjacent to cementum that is undergoing active resorption (Fig. 4.51). Several sites of resorption may coalesce to form a large area of destruction. The resorptive process may extend into the underlying dentin and even into the pulp, but it is usually painless. Cementum resorption is not necessarily continuous and may alternate with periods of repair and the deposition of new cementum. The newly formed cementum is demarcated from the root by a deeply staining irregular line termed a *reversal line,* which delineates the border of the previous resorption. One study showed that the reversal lines of human teeth contain a few collagen fibrils and highly accumulated proteoglycans with mucopolysaccharides (glycosaminoglycans) and that fibril intermingling occurs only in some places between reparative cementum and resorbed dentin or cementum.[302,303] Embedded fibers of the periodontal ligament reestablish a functional relationship in the new cementum.

Cementum repair requires the presence of viable connective tissue. If epithelium proliferates into an area of resorption, repair will not take place. Cementum repair can occur in devitalized as well as in vital teeth.

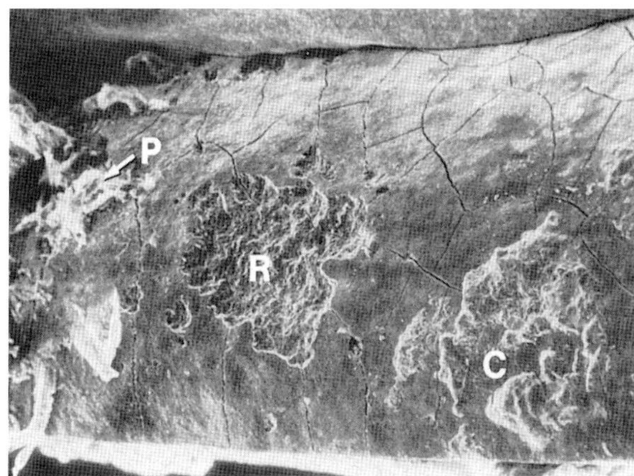

Fig. 4.50 Scanning electron micrograph of a root exposed by periodontal disease showing a large resorption bay *(R)*. Remnants of the periodontal ligament *(P)* and **calculus** *(C)* are visible. Cracking of the tooth surface occurs as a result of the preparation technique. (×160.). (Courtesy Dr. John Sottosanti, La Jolla, California.)

Histologic evidence demonstrates that cementum formation is critical for the appropriate maturation of the periodontium, both during development and during the regeneration of lost periodontal tissues.[235] In other words, a variety of macromolecules present in the extracellular matrix of the periodontium are likely to play a regulatory role in cementogenesis.[173]

The regeneration of cementum requires cementoblasts, but the origin of the cementoblasts and the molecular factors that regulate their recruitment and differentiation are not fully understood. However, research provides a better understanding; for example, the epithelial cell rests of Malassez are the only odontogenic epithelial cells that remain in the periodontal ligament after the eruption of teeth, and they may have some function in cementum repair and regeneration under specific conditions.[114] The rests of Malassez may be related to cementum repair by activating their potential to secrete matrix proteins

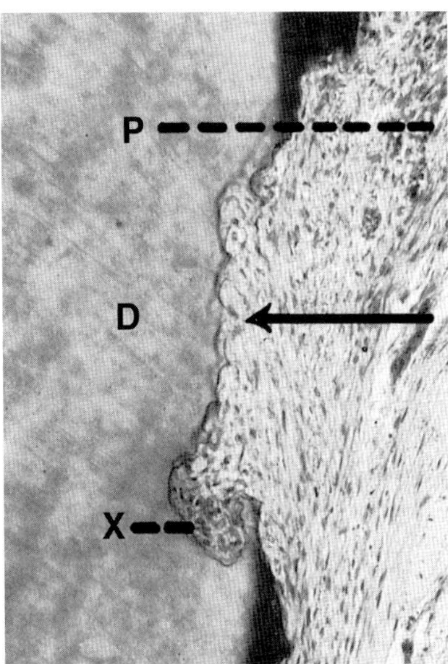

Fig. 4.51 Resorption of cementum and dentin. A multinuclear osteoclast in seen *(X)*. The direction of resorption is indicated by the arrow. Note the scalloped resorption front in the dentin *(D)*. The cementum is the darkly stained band at the upper and lower right. *P*, Periodontal ligament.

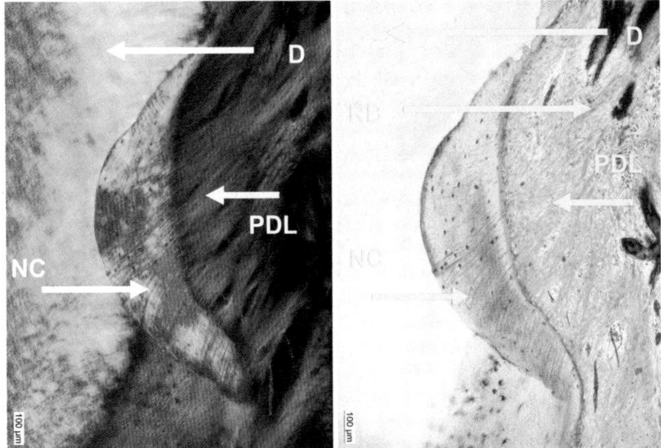

Fig. 4.52 A clinical human histology shows that new cementum and new periodontal ligament fiber formed at a previous periodontal defect treated with recombinant human platelet-derived growth factor-BB with β-tricalcium phosphate. (Courtesy Dr. Daniel W.K. Kao, Philadelphia, Pennsylvania.)

that have been expressed in enamel formation, such as amelogenins, enamelins, and ameloblastins.[189] Several growth factors have been shown to be effective in cementum regeneration, including members of the transforming growth factor superfamily (i.e., bone morphogenetic proteins), platelet-derived growth factor, insulin-like growth factor, and enamel matrix derivatives (Fig. 4.52).[235]

Ankylosis

Fusion of the cementum and the alveolar bone with obliteration of the periodontal ligament is termed *ankylosis*. Ankylosis occurs in teeth with cemental resorption, which suggests that it may represent a form of abnormal repair. Ankylosis may also develop after chronic periapical inflammation, tooth replantation, and occlusal trauma and around embedded teeth. This condition is relatively uncommon, and it occurs most frequently in the primary dentition.[180]

Exposure of Cementum to the Oral Environment

Cementum becomes exposed to the oral environment in cases of gingival recession and as a result of the loss of attachment in pocket formation. The cementum is sufficiently permeable to be penetrated in these cases by organic substances, inorganic ions, and bacteria. Bacterial invasion of the cementum occurs frequently in individuals with periodontal disease, and cementum caries can develop (see Chapter 22).

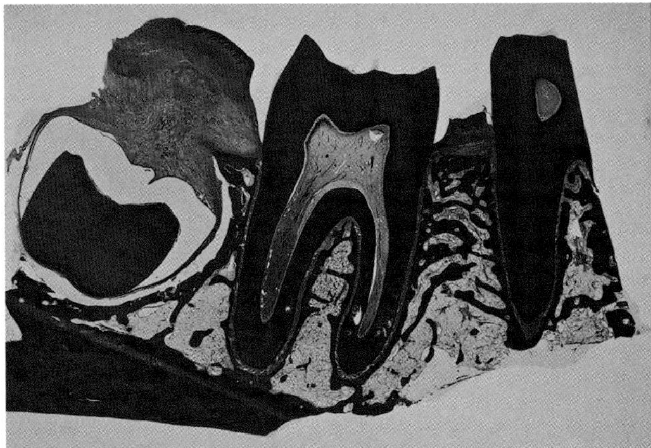

Fig. 4.53 Mesiodistal section through the mandibular molars of a 17-year-old girl obtained at autopsy. Note the interdental bony septa between the first and second molars. The dense cortical bony plates represent the alveolar bone proper (i.e., the cribriform plates) and are supported by cancellous bony trabeculae. The third molar is still in the early stages of root formation and eruption.

Alveolar Process

The alveolar process is the portion of the maxilla and mandible that forms and supports the tooth sockets (alveoli). It forms when the tooth erupts to provide the osseous attachment to the forming periodontal ligament; it disappears gradually after the tooth is lost.

Because the alveolar processes develop and undergo remodeling with tooth formation and eruption, they are tooth-dependent bony structures.[237] Therefore, the size, shape, location, and function of the teeth determine their morphology. Interestingly, although the growth and development of the bones of the jaw determine the position of the teeth, a certain degree of repositioning of the teeth can be accomplished through occlusal forces and in response to orthodontic procedures that rely on the adaptability of the alveolar bone and the associated periodontal tissues.[261]

The alveolar process consists of the following:

1. An external plate of cortical bone is formed by haversian bone and compacted bone lamellae.
2. The inner socket wall of thin, compact bone called the *alveolar bone proper* is seen as the lamina dura in radiographs. Histologically, it contains a series of openings (i.e., the *cribriform plate*) through which neurovascular bundles link the periodontal ligament with the central component of the alveolar bone: the cancellous bone.
3. Cancellous trabeculae between these two compact layers act as supporting alveolar bone. The *interdental septum* consists of cancellous supporting bone enclosed within a compact border (Fig. 4.53).

In addition, the bones of the jaw include the basal bone, which is the portion of the jaw located apically but unrelated to the teeth (Fig. 4.54).

The alveolar process is divisible into separate areas on an anatomic basis, but it functions as a unit, with all parts interrelated in the support of the teeth. Figs. 4.55 and 4.56 show the relative proportions of cancellous bone and compact bone that form the alveolar process. Most of the facial and lingual portions of the sockets

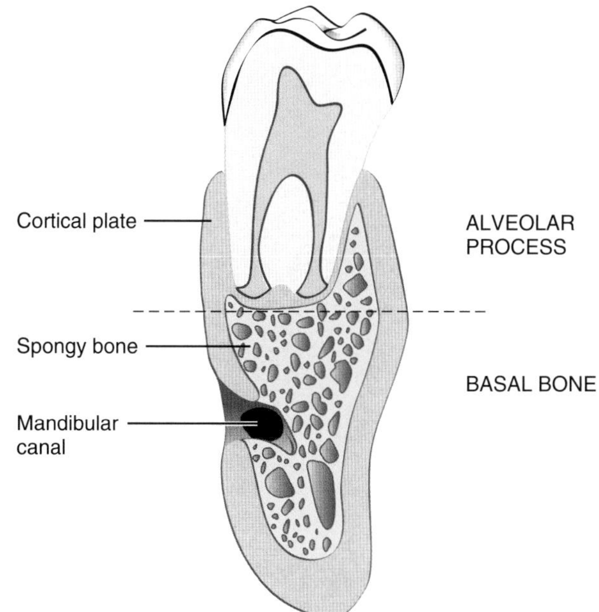

Fig. 4.54 Section through a human jaw with a tooth in situ. The dotted line indicates the separation between the basal bone and the alveolar bone. (Redrawn from Ten Cate AR. *Oral Histology: Development, Structure, and Function.* 4th ed. St Louis: Mosby; 1994.)

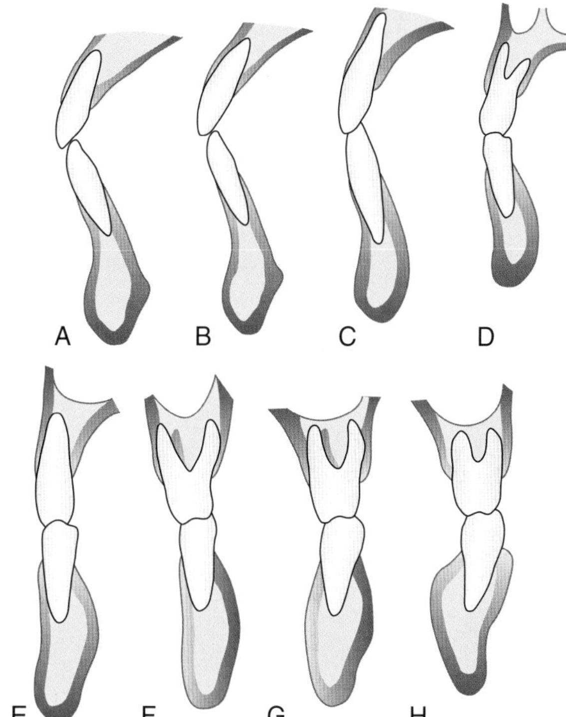

Fig. 4.55 Relative proportions of cancellous bone and compact bone in a longitudinal faciolingual section of (A) central incisors, (B) lateral incisors, (C) canines, (D) first premolars, (E) second premolars, (F) first molars, (G) second molars, and (H) third molars.

are formed by compact bone alone; cancellous bone surrounds the lamina dura in apical, apicolingual, and interradicular areas.

Bone consists of two-thirds inorganic matter and one-third organic matrix. The inorganic matter is composed principally of the hydroxyapatite minerals composed of calcium and phosphate, along with hydroxyl, carbonate, citrate, and trace amounts of other ions[101,102] such as sodium, magnesium, and fluorine.

The organic matrix[74] consists mainly of collagen type I (90%),[192] with small amounts of noncollagenous proteins such as osteocalcin, osteonectin, bone morphogenetic protein, phosphoproteins, and proteoglycans.[221] Osteopontin and bone sialoprotein are cell-adhesion proteins that appear to be important for the adhesion of both osteoclasts and osteoblasts.[166] In addition, paracrine factors, including cytokines, chemokines, and growth factors, have been implicated in the local control of mesenchymal condensations that occur at the onset of organogenesis. These factors probably play a prominent role in the development of the alveolar processes.[261]

Although the alveolar bone tissue is constantly changing its internal organization, it retains approximately the same form from childhood through adult life. Bone deposition by osteoblasts is balanced by resorption by osteoclasts during tissue remodeling and renewal. It is well known that the number of osteoblasts decreases with aging; however, no remarkable change in the number of osteoclasts has ever been reported.[201]

Remodeling is the major pathway of bony changes in shape, resistance to forces, repair of wounds, and calcium and phosphate homeostasis in the body. Indeed, the coupling of bone resorption with bone formation constitutes one of the fundamental principles by which bone is necessarily remodeled throughout its life. Bone remodeling involves the coordination of activities of cells from two distinct lineages, the osteoblasts, and the osteoclasts, which form and resorb the mineralized connective tissues of bone.[261]

The bone matrix that is laid down by osteoblasts is nonmineralized osteoid. While new osteoid is being deposited, the older osteoid located below the surface becomes mineralized as the mineralization front advances.

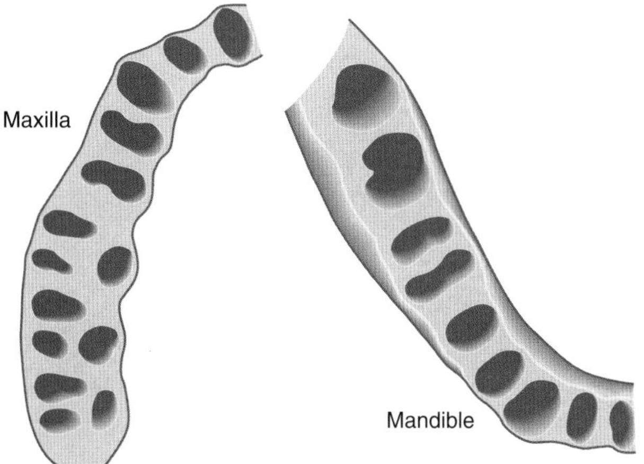

Fig. 4.56 The shape of the roots and the surrounding bone distribution in a transverse section of maxilla and mandible at the midroot level.

Bone resorption is a complex process that is morphologically related to the appearance of eroded bone surfaces (i.e., Howship lacunae) and large, multinucleated cells (osteoclasts) (Fig. 4.57). Osteoclasts originate from hematopoietic tissue[56,110,208] and are formed by the fusion of mononuclear cells of asynchronous populations.[147,195,213] When osteoclasts are active rather than resting, they possess an elaborately developed ruffled border from which hydrolytic enzymes are thought to be secreted.[286] These enzymes digest the organic portion of bone. The activity of osteoclasts and the morphology of the ruffled border can be modified and regulated by hormones such as parathyroid hormone (indirectly) and calcitonin, which has receptors on the osteoclast membrane.

Another mechanism of bone resorption involves the creation of an acidic environment on the bone surface, thereby leading to the

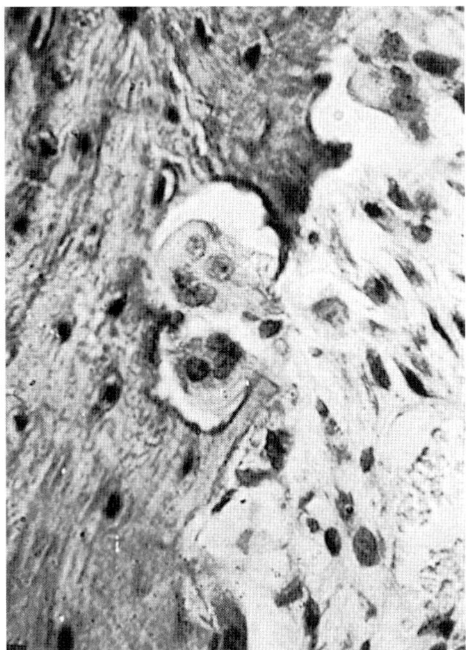

Fig. 4.57 Rat alveolar bone. This histologic view shows two multinucleated osteoclasts in the Howship lacuna.

dissolution of the mineral component of bone. This event can be produced by different conditions, including a proton pump through the cell membrane of the osteoclast,[34] bone tumors, and local pressure[208] translated through the secretory activity of the osteoclast.

Ten Cate[195] described the sequence of events in the resorptive process as follows:

1. Attachment of osteoclasts to the mineralized surface of bone
2. Creation of a sealed acidic environment through the action of the proton pump, which demineralizes bone and exposes the organic matrix
3. Degradation of the exposed organic matrix to its constituent amino acids via the action of released enzymes (e.g., acid phosphatase, cathepsin K)
4. Sequestering of mineral ions and amino acids within the osteoclast

Notably, the cellular and molecular events involved in bone remodeling have a strong similarity to many aspects of inflammation and repair. The relationships among matrix molecules (e.g., osteopontin, bone sialoprotein, SPARC [secreted protein, acidic, rich in cysteine], osteocalcin), blood clotting, and wound healing are clearly evident.[261]

Cells and Intercellular Matrix

Osteoblasts, which are the cells that produce the organic matrix of bone, are differentiated from pluripotent follicle cells. Alveolar bone is formed during fetal growth by intramembranous ossification, and it consists of a calcified matrix with osteocytes enclosed within spaces called *lacunae.* The osteocytes extend processes into *canaliculi* that radiate from the lacunae. The canaliculi form an anastomosing system through the intercellular matrix of the bone, which brings oxygen and nutrients to the osteocytes through the blood and removes metabolic waste products. Blood vessels branch extensively and travel through the periosteum. The endosteum lies adjacent to the marrow vasculature. Bone growth occurs via the apposition of an organic matrix that is deposited by osteoblasts. Haversian systems (i.e., *osteons*) are the internal mechanisms that bring a vascular supply to bones that are too thick to be supplied only by surface vessels. These are found primarily in the outer cortical plates and the alveolar bone proper.

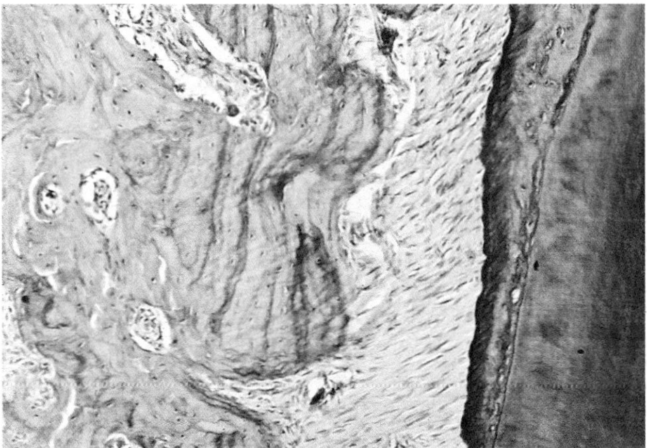

Fig. 4.58 Deep penetration of Sharpey fibers into bundle bone of a rat molar.

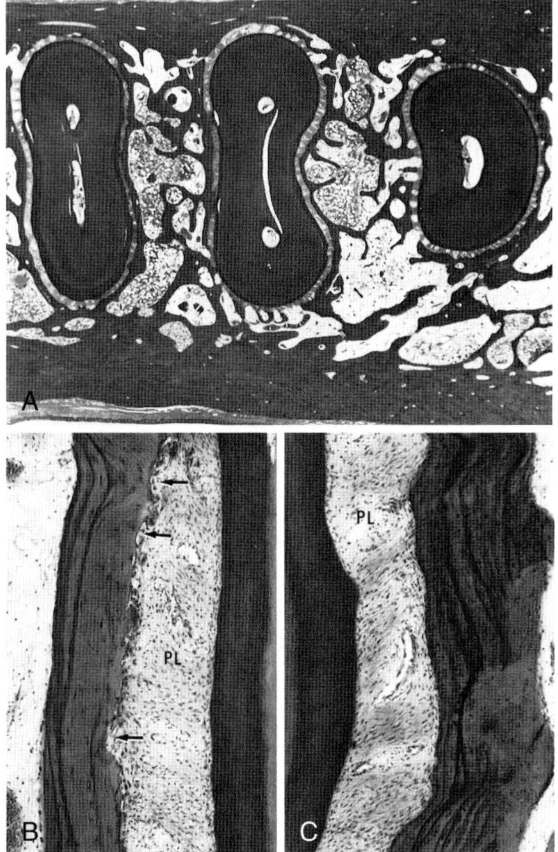

Fig. 4.59 Bundle bone associated with the physiologic mesial migration of the teeth. (A) Horizontal section through the molar roots during the process of mesial migration (*left,* mesial; *right,* distal). (B) Mesial root surface showing osteoclasis of bone *(arrows).* (C) Distal root surface showing bundle bone that has been partially replaced with dense bone on the marrow side. *PL,* Periodontal ligament.

Socket Wall

The socket wall consists of dense, lamellated bone, some of which is arranged in haversian systems and bundle bone. *Bundle bone* is the term given to bone adjacent to the periodontal ligament that contains a great number of Sharpey fibers (Fig. 4.58).[296] It is characterized by thin lamellae arranged in layers parallel to the root, with intervening appositional lines (Fig. 4.59). Bundle bone is localized within the alveolar bone proper. Some Sharpey fibers are completely calcified, but most contain an uncalcified central core within a calcified outer layer.[250] Bundle bone is not unique to the jaws; it occurs throughout the skeletal system wherever ligaments and muscles are attached.

The cancellous portion of the alveolar bone consists of trabeculae that enclose irregularly shaped marrow spaces lined with a layer of thin, flattened endosteal cells. Wide variation occurs in the trabecular pattern of cancellous bone,[212] which is affected by occlusal forces. The matrix of the cancellous trabeculae consists of irregularly arranged lamellae separated by deeply staining incremental and resorption lines indicative of previous bone activity, with an occasional haversian system.

Cancellous bone is found predominantly in the interradicular and interdental spaces and in limited amounts facially or lingually, except in the palate. In the adult human, more cancellous bone exists in the maxilla than in the mandible.

Bone Marrow

In the embryo and the newborn, the cavities of all bones are occupied by red hematopoietic marrow. The red marrow gradually undergoes a physiologic change to the fatty or yellow inactive type of marrow. In the adult, the marrow of the jaw is normally of the latter type, and red marrow is found only in the ribs, sternum, vertebrae, skull, and humerus. However, foci of the red bone marrow are occasionally seen in the jaws, often accompanied by the resorption of bony trabeculae.[41] Common locations are the maxillary tuberosity, the maxillary and mandibular molar and premolar areas, and the mandibular symphysis and ramus angle, which may be visible radiographically as zones of radiolucency.

Periosteum and Endosteum

Layers of differentiated osteogenic connective tissue cover all of the bone surfaces. The tissue that covers the outer surface of bone is termed *periosteum,* whereas the tissue that lines the internal bone cavities is called *endosteum.*

The periosteum consists of an *inner layer* composed of osteoblasts surrounded by osteoprogenitor cells, which have the potential to differentiate into osteoblasts, and an *outer layer* rich in blood vessels and nerves and composed of collagen fibers and fibroblasts. Bundles of periosteal collagen fibers penetrate the bone, thereby binding the periosteum to the bone. The endosteum is composed of a single layer of osteoblasts and sometimes a small amount of connective tissue. The inner layer is the osteogenic layer, and the outer layer is the fibrous layer.

Cellular events at the periosteum modulate bone size throughout an individual's life span, and a change in bone size is probably the result of the balance between periosteal osteoblastic and osteoclastic activities. Little is currently known about the control of periosteal osteoblastic activity or the clinical importance of variations in periosteal bone formation.[207] Moreover, the nature and impact of periosteal bone resorption are virtually unexplored.

Interdental Septum

The interdental septum consists of cancellous bone that is bordered by the socket wall cribriform plates (i.e., lamina dura or alveolar bone proper) of approximating teeth and the facial and lingual cortical plates (Fig. 4.60). If the interdental space is narrow, the septum may consist of only the cribriform plate. In one study, for example, the space between the mandibular second premolars and first molars consisted of cribriform plate and cancellous bone in 85% of the cases and of only cribriform plate in the remaining 15%.[118] If the roots are too close together, an irregular "window" can appear in the bone between adjacent roots (Fig. 4.61). Between maxillary molars, the septum consisted of cribriform plate and cancellous bone in 66.6% of cases; it was composed of only cribriform plate in 20.8%, and it had a fenestration in 12.5%.[118]

Determining root proximity radiographically is important (see Chapters 39 and 41). The mesiodistal angulation of the crest of the interdental septum usually parallels a line drawn between the cementoenamel junctions of the approximating teeth.[198] The distance between the crest of the alveolar bone and the cementoenamel junction in young adults varies between 0.75 and 1.49 mm (average, 1.08 mm). This distance increases with age to an average of 2.81 mm.[93] However, this phenomenon may not be as much a function of age as of a periodontal disease.

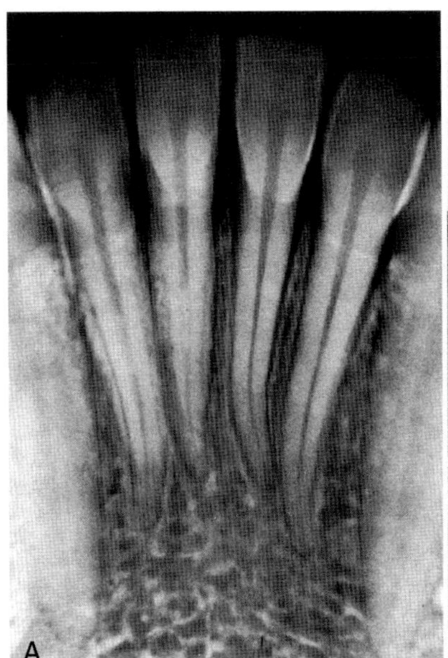

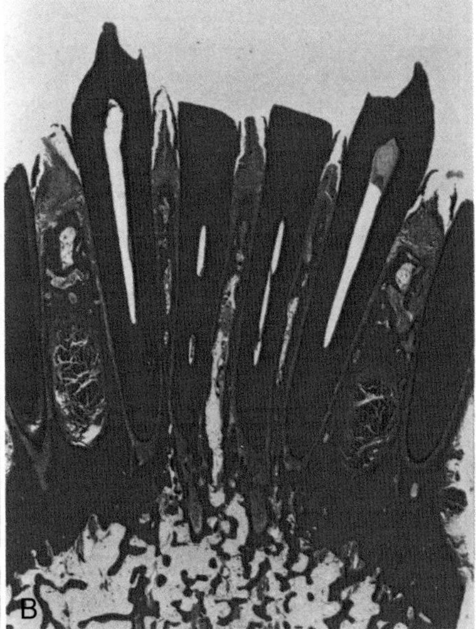

Fig. 4.60 Interdental septa. (A) Radiograph of the mandibular incisor area. Note the prominent lamina dura. (B) Interdental septa between the mandibular anterior teeth shown in A. There is a slight reduction in bone height with widening of the periodontal ligament in the coronal areas. The central cancellous portion is bordered by the dense bony cribriform plates of the socket, which form the lamina dura around the teeth in the radiograph. Attachments for the mentalis muscle are seen between the canine and lateral incisors. (From Glickman I, Smulow J. *Periodontal Disease: Clinical, Radiographic, and Histopathologic Features.* Philadelphia: Saunders; 1974.)

The mesiodistal and faciolingual dimensions and shape of the interdental septum are governed by the size and convexity of the crowns of the two approximating teeth as well as by the position of the teeth in the jaw and their degree of eruption.[221]

Osseous Topography

The bone contour normally conforms to the prominence of the roots, with intervening vertical depressions that taper toward the margin (Fig. 4.62). Alveolar bone anatomy varies among patients and has important clinical implications. The height and thickness of the facial and lingual bony plates are affected by the alignment of the teeth, the angulation of the root to the bone, and occlusal forces.

On teeth in labial version, the margin of the labial bone is located farther apically than it is on teeth that are in proper alignment. The bone margin is thinned to a knife edge, and it presents an accentuated arc in the direction of the apex. On teeth in lingual version, the facial bony plate is thicker than normal. The margin is blunt, rounded, and horizontal rather than arcuate. The effect of the root-to-bone angulation on the height of alveolar bone is most noticeable on the palatal roots of the maxillary molars. The bone margin is located farther apically on the roots, and it forms relatively acute angles with the palatal bone.[122] The cervical portion of the alveolar plate is sometimes considerably thickened on the facial surface, apparently as reinforcement against occlusal forces (Fig. 4.63).

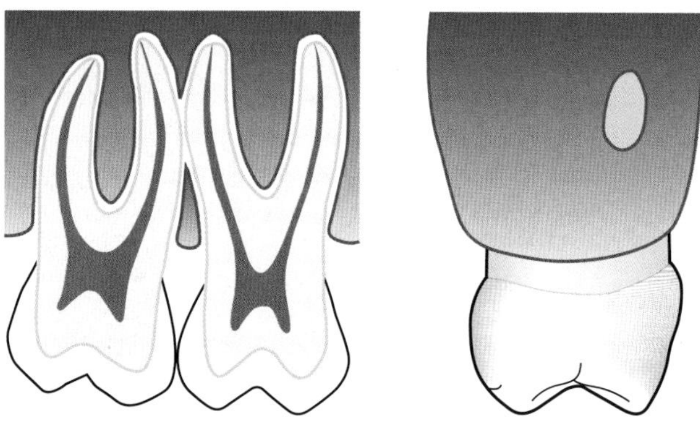

Fig. 4.61 Boneless "window" between adjoining close roots of molars.

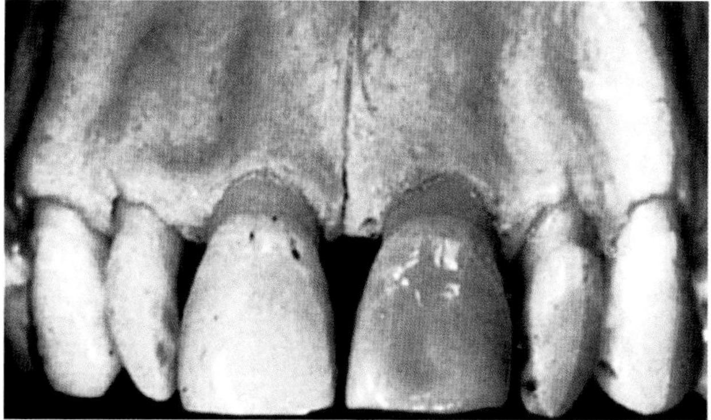

Fig. 4.62 Normal that the bone contour conforms to the prominence of the roots.

Fenestration and Dehiscence

Isolated areas in which the root is denuded of bone and the root surface is covered only by periosteum and overlying gingiva are termed *fenestrations*. In these areas, the marginal bone is intact. When the denuded areas extend through the marginal bone, the defect is called a *dehiscence* (Fig. 4.64).

Such defects occur on approximately 20% of the teeth; they occur more often on the facial bone than on the lingual bone, they are more common on anterior teeth than on posterior teeth, and they are frequently bilateral. Microscopic evidence of lacunar resorption may be present at the margins. The cause of these defects is not clear. Prominent root contours, malposition, and labial protrusion of the root in combination with a thin bony plate are predisposing factors.[77] Fenestration and dehiscence are important because they may complicate the outcome of periodontal surgery.

Remodeling of Alveolar Bone

In contrast with its apparent rigidity, alveolar bone is the least stable of the periodontal tissues, because its structure is in a constant state of flux. A considerable amount of internal remodeling takes place by means of resorption and formation, and this is regulated by local and systemic influences. Local influences include functional requirements on the tooth and age-related changes in bone cells. Systemic influences are hormonal and nutritional (e.g., parathyroid hormone, calcitonin, vitamin D_3).

The remodeling of the alveolar bone affects its height, contour, and density and is manifested in the following three areas: adjacent to the periodontal ligament, in relation to the periosteum of the facial and lingual plates, and along the endosteal surface of the marrow spaces.

Development of the Attachment Apparatus

After the crown has formed, the stratum intermedium and the stellate reticulum of the enamel organ disappear. The outer and inner epithelia of the enamel organ merge into the REE. The apical portion of epithelial double layer loops and constitutes the Hertwig epithelial root sheath, which will continue to grow apically and determines the shape of the root. Before the beginning of root formation, the root

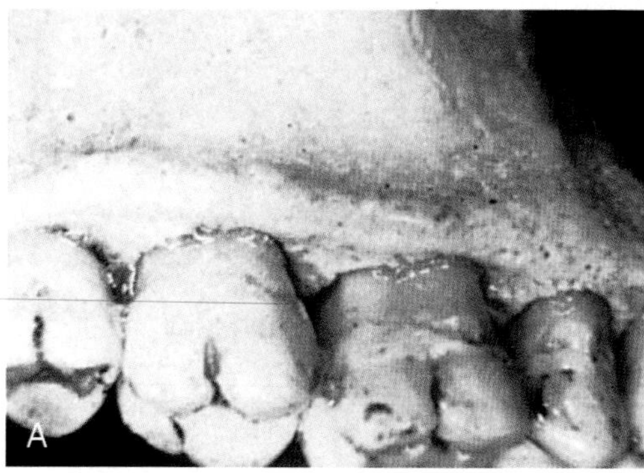

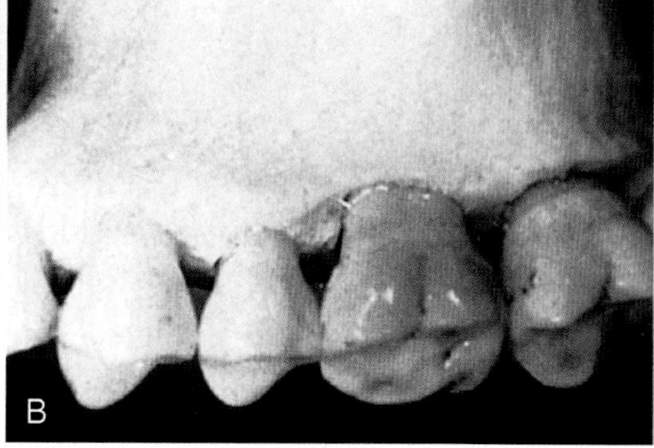

Fig. 4.63 Variations in the cervical portion of the buccal alveolar plate. (A) Shelflike conformation. (B) Comparatively thin buccal plate.

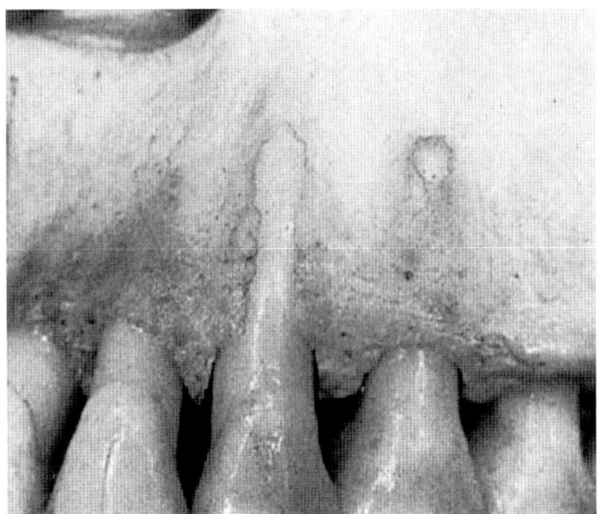

Fig. 4.64 Dehiscence on the canine and fenestration of the first premolar.

sheath bends horizontally at the future cementoenamel junction, thereby narrowing the cervical opening and forming the epithelial diaphragm. The epithelial diaphragm separates the dental follicle from the dental papilla.

After root dentin formation begins, the Hertwig root sheath breaks up as the root grows in an apical direction; the remaining cells form the epithelial clusters or strands known as the *epithelial rests of Malassez* (see Fig. 4.41A). In multirooted teeth, the epithelial diaphragm grows in such a way that tongue-like extensions develop horizontally, thereby leaving spaces for each of the future roots to form.

The role of the Hertwig epithelial root sheath in root development, especially as it relates to the initiation of cementogenesis, includes the expression and secretion of bone sialoprotein, osteopontin, and ameloblastin by the cells of the Hertwig epithelial root sheath.[38,84,281] In addition, research shows that growth and differentiation factors may play roles in the development of the attachment apparatus of periodontal tissues. Pluripotent dental follicle cells have been shown to differentiate into osteoblasts, cementoblasts, and periodontal fibroblasts.[251]

Cementum

The rupture of the Hertwig epithelial root sheath allows the mesenchymal cells of the dental follicle to contact the dentin, where they start forming a continuous layer of cementoblasts. On the basis of immunochemical and ultrastructural studies, Thomas[280] and others[35,169] have speculated that cementoblasts can be of epithelial origin (i.e., the Hertwig's epithelial root sheath), having undergone an epithelial mesenchymal transformation.

Cementum formation begins with the deposition of a meshwork of irregularly arranged collagen fibrils sparsely distributed in a ground substance or matrix called *precementum* or *cementoid.* This is followed by a phase of matrix maturation, which subsequently mineralizes to form cementum. Cementoblasts, which are initially separated from the cementum by uncalcified cementoid, sometimes become enclosed within the matrix and are trapped. After they are enclosed, they are referred to as *cementocytes,* and they will remain viable in a manner similar to that of osteocytes.

A layer of connective tissue known as the *dental sac* surrounds the enamel organ and includes the epithelial root sheath as it develops. The zone that is immediately in contact with the dental organ and continuous with the ectomesenchyme of the dental papilla is called the *dental follicle,*[273,274,276] and it consists of undifferentiated, pluripotent fibroblasts.

Periodontal Ligament

As the crown approaches the oral mucosa during tooth eruption, the fibroblasts of the dental follicle become active and start producing collagen fibrils. They initially lack orientation, but they soon acquire an orientation that is oblique to the tooth. The first collagen bundles then appear in the region immediately apical to the cementoenamel junction and give rise to the gingivodental fiber groups. As tooth eruption progresses, additional oblique fibers appear and become attached to the newly formed cementum and bone. The transseptal and alveolar crest fibers develop when the tooth merges into the oral cavity. Alveolar bone deposition occurs simultaneously with periodontal ligament organization.[260]

The developing periodontal ligament and the mature periodontal ligament contain undifferentiated stem cells that retain the potential to differentiate into osteoblasts, cementoblasts, and fibroblasts.[176]

Alveolar Bone

Just before mineralization, osteoblasts start producing matrix vesicles. These vesicles contain enzymes (e.g., alkaline phosphatase) that help to jump-start the nucleation of hydroxyapatite crystals. As these crystals grow and develop, they form coalescing bone nodules, which, with fast-growing nonoriented collagen fibers, are the substructure of woven bone and the first bone formed in the alveolus. Later, through bone deposition, remodeling, and the secretion of oriented collagen fibers in sheets, mature lamellar bone is formed.[29,30]

The hydroxyapatite crystals are generally aligned with their long axes parallel to the collagen fibers, and they appear to be deposited on and within the collagen fibers in mature lamellar bone. In this way, bone matrix is able to withstand the heavy mechanical stresses applied to it during function.

The alveolar bone develops around each tooth follicle during odontogenesis. When a deciduous tooth is shed, its alveolar bone is resorbed. The succedaneous permanent tooth moves into place and develops its own alveolar bone from its own dental follicle. As the tooth root forms and the surrounding tissues develop and mature, alveolar bone merges with the separately developing basal bone, and the two become one continuous structure. Although alveolar bone and basal bone have different intermediate origins, both are ultimately derived from neural crest ectomesenchyme.

Mandibular basal bone begins mineralization at the exit of the mental nerve from the mental foramen, whereas the maxillary basal bone begins at the exit of the infraorbital nerve from the infraorbital foramen.

Physiologic Migration of the Teeth

Tooth movement does not end when active eruption is completed and the tooth is in functional occlusion. With time and wear, the proximal contact areas of the teeth are flattened, and the teeth tend to move mesially. This is referred to as *physiologic mesial migration.* By the age of 40 years, this process results in a reduction of about 0.5 cm in the length of the dental arch from the midline to the third molars. Alveolar bone is reconstructed in compliance with the physiologic mesial migration of the teeth. Bone resorption is increased in areas of pressure along the mesial surfaces of the teeth, and new layers of bundle bone are formed in areas of tension on the distal surfaces (see Fig. 4.59).

External Forces and the Periodontium

The periodontium exists for the purpose of supporting teeth during function, and it depends on the stimulation that it receives from function for the preservation of its structure. Therefore a constant and sensitive balance is present between external forces and the periodontal structures.

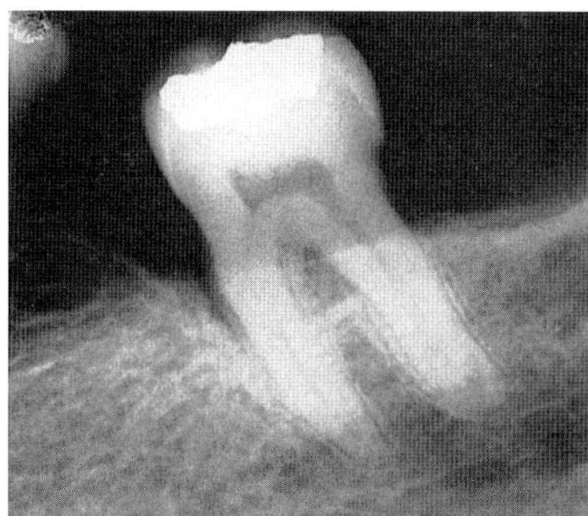

Fig. 4.65 Bony trabeculae realigned perpendicular to the mesial root of a tilted molar.

TABLE 4.2 Comparison of Periodontal Width of Functioning and Functionless Teeth in a 38-Year-Old Man

	AVERAGE WIDTH OF PERIODONTAL SPACE		
	Entrance of Alveolus (mm)	**Middle of Alveolus (mm)**	**Fundus of Alveolus (mm)**
Heavy Function	0.35	0.28	0.30
Left upper second bicuspid			
Light Function	0.14	0.10	0.12
Left lower first bicuspid			
Functionless	0.10	0.06	0.06
Left upper third molar			

Modified from Kronfeld R. Histologic study of the influence of function on the human periodontal membrane. *J Am Dent Assoc.* 1931;18:1242 and Tarnow D, Hochman M, Chu S, Fletcher P. A new definition of attached gingiva around teeth and implants in healthy and diseased sites. *Int J Periodontics Restorative Dent.* 2021 Jan–Feb;41(1):43–49.

Alveolar bone undergoes constant physiologic remodeling in response to external forces, particularly occlusal forces. Bone is removed from areas where it is no longer needed and added to areas where it is presently needed.

The socket wall reflects the responsiveness of the alveolar bone to external forces. Osteoblasts and newly formed osteoid line the socket in areas of tension; osteoclasts and bone resorption occur in areas of pressure. Forces exerted on the tooth also influence the number, density, and alignment of cancellous trabeculae. The bony trabeculae are aligned in the path of the tensile and compressive stresses to provide maximal resistance to the occlusal force with a minimum of bone substance (Fig. 4.65).[100,257] When forces are increased, the cancellous bony trabeculae increase in number and thickness, and bone may be added to the external surface of the labial and lingual plates.

A study has shown that the presence of antagonists of occlusal force and the severity of periodontal disease increase the extension of periodontal tissue resorption.[67]

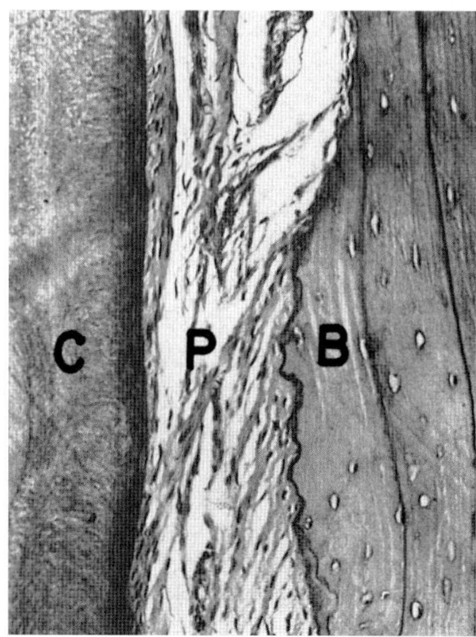

Fig. 4.66 Atrophic periodontal ligament *(P)* of a tooth devoid of function. Note the scalloped edge of the alveolar bone *(B)*, which indicates that resorption has occurred. *C*, Cementum.

The periodontal ligament also depends on the stimulation provided by function to preserve its structure. Within physiologic limits, the periodontal ligament can accommodate increased function with an increase in width (Table 4.2), a thickening of its fiber bundles, and an increase in the diameter and number of Sharpey fibers. Forces that exceed the adaptive capacity of the periodontium produce injury called *trauma from occlusion.* Because trauma from occlusion can only be confirmed histologically, the clinician is challenged to use clinical and radiographic surrogate indicators in an attempt to facilitate and assist with its diagnosis (see Chapter 34).[111]

When occlusal forces are reduced, the number and thickness of the trabeculae are reduced.[65] The periodontal ligament also atrophies and appears thinned; the fibers are reduced in number and density, disoriented,[11,220] and ultimately arranged parallel to the root surface (Fig. 4.66). This phenomenon is termed *disuse atrophy* or *afunctional atrophy.* With this condition, the cementum is either unaffected[65] or thickened, and the distance from the cementoenamel junction to the alveolar crest is increased.[216]

Decreased occlusal function causes changes in the periodontal microvasculature, such as the occlusion of blood vessels and a decrease in the number of blood vessels.[125] For example, Murrell and colleagues[194] reported that the application and removal of orthodontic force produced significant changes in blood vessel number and density; however, no evidence-based explanation exists for why the force stimulated such changes in the number of blood vessels.

Orthodontic tooth movement is thought to result from site-specific bone remodeling in the absence of inflammation. It is well recognized that tensional forces will stimulate the formation and activity of osteoblastic cells, whereas compressive forces promote osteoclastic activity.[261]

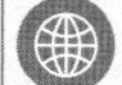
References for this chapter are found on the companion website eBooks.Health.Elsevier.com.

CHAPTER 5

Classification of Diseases and Conditions Affecting the Periodontium

Georgios A. Kotsakis | Chun-Teh Lee | James E. Hinrichs 

CHAPTER OUTLINE

Diagnosis Calculator

Readers will be able to access an interactive periodontal disease diagnosis calculator in the online version (expertconsult.inkling.com) of this chapter. This calculator is only for educational purposes and is intended to act as an interactive guide to arrive at a periodontal diagnosis. Clinicians should take into consideration the available clinical and radiographic findings along with presenting risk factors before finalizing the diagnosis on a case-by-case basis.

Introduction

Our understanding of the causes and pathogenesis of oral diseases and conditions changes continually with increased scientific knowledge. In light of this fact, the new classification scheme of periodontal and peri-implant diseases and conditions is primarily defined by the differences in the clinical and radiographic manifestations of disease, as well as risk factors and potential for disease progression; they are clinically consistent and require little, if any, clarification by laboratory testing. As new diagnostic strategies and therapeutic approaches are developed, so do the options for characterizing and classifying diseases. In 1999, a classification system for diseases and conditions that affect the periodontium was introduced by the International Workshop for a Classification of Periodontal Diseases and Conditions, which has served our profession well for close to two decades.[4] The 1999 classification of periodontal diseases was based on their extent (generalized versus localized); severity (slight, moderate, or severe); rate of progression (aggressive versus chronic); and localization (i.e., contained within the gingiva, as in gingivitis, or further involving alveolar bone, as in periodontitis) that are briefly mentioned for historical purposes and continuity. Since then, periodontology has seen major advances over the last two decades. Therefore, in 2017, the American Academy of Periodontology (AAP) and the European Federation of Periodontology (EFP) convened periodontal experts from around the world to develop updated definitions for periodontal health, gingival disease, periodontitis, periodontal manifestations of systemic diseases, and peri-implant diseases.[8] These redefined classifications, especially for periodontitis, are intended to provide a more precise diagnosis characterized by a multidimensional staging and grading system while still being user-friendly to clinicians.[57] In this new classification, staging is predominately determined by the severity of the disease at time of presentation, as well as complexity of disease management:

- Stages I through IV are assigned according to the degree of clinical attachment loss, amount of bone loss, tooth loss due to periodontitis, probing depth, presence of vertical bone loss, furcation involvement, tooth mobility, and other complexity factors (e.g., ridge deficiency, masticatory dysfunction).
- Grades A through C are designated according to the risk of progressive periodontitis associated with systemic disease status, exposure to smoking, level of metabolic control of diabetes, historic rate of progression and other individualized risk predictors. One major addition to the periodontal classification system is the introduction of a new category for peri-implant conditions that are stratified as peri-implant health, peri-implant mucositis, or peri-implantitis.

Peri-implant health is clinically characterized by the absence of visual signs of inflammation and lack of bleeding on probing (BOP). In contrast, peri-implant mucositis exhibits visual signs of inflammation and/or BOP but without loss of supportive or marginal bone. Peri-implantitis is a pathological condition with inflammation and/or BOP accompanied by progressive loss of supportive bone. In addition, there is ample evidence now that points to several factors that contribute to hard and soft tissue deficiencies at implant sites and these conditions are now categorized separately under peri-implant diseases and conditions.[18]

The existing definitions encompass the best available way to define a spectrum of diseases affecting the periodontal tissues and to guide therapeutic approaches. The new periodontal classification establishes a definition for a widely accepted but not previously defined state; that of periodontal health. This is a major improvement from earlier classifications since periodontal health is much more than the mere absence of disease.[8] On a molecular level, periodontal health is consistent with well-regulated immune surveillance and maintenance of homeostasis. Clinically, periodontal health is determined by the absence of signs of inflammation but also necessitates the absence of patient-perceived symptoms of disease. For instance, a periodontium with no evidence of attachment loss or BOP cannot be defined as healthy, if the person in the dental chair complains of halitosis and gingival swelling. It cannot be overstated that, as clinicians, we best serve a person by treating them as a whole entity and not as the findings of a metal probe.

The current definition of periodontal health further provides specific criteria for defining what was previously empirically referred to as a "reduced periodontium," i.e., a periodontium with previous loss of structural alveolar support and clinical findings of attachment loss. For instance, a patient diagnosed with existing periodontitis who undergoes successful periodontal therapy may be classified as a case of gingival health in a reduced periodontium in a successfully treated stable periodontitis patient with slight, moderate, or severe attachment loss once the disease is well controlled and stable. Subsequently, if the same individual presents with gingival inflammation without signs of further attachment loss at a future appointment, the appropriate diagnosis would be "gingivitis on a reduced periodontium in a patient with a history of periodontitis." Depending on their future compliance with home care and maintenance visits, patients may have a recurrence of periodontitis or maintain a healthy but reduced periodontium. The case example highlights the importance of conceptualizing the dynamic nature of inflammatory diseases that affect the periodontium, while appreciating the importance of commonly accepted definitions for periodontal diseases.

The classification presented in this chapter is based on the most recent internationally accepted consensus on the diseases and conditions that affect the tissues of the periodontium.[8] More recent views on the Classification of Periodontal Diseases and Conditions are also discussed. Each disease or condition is briefly discussed, and the reader is referred to pertinent chapters within this book that discuss the topics in more detail.

A new classification system, which has already been implemented in clinical practice in most regions globally, was introduced in the 2018 proceedings of a joint workshop by the American Academy of Periodontology (AAP) and the European Federation of Periodontology (EFP). This chapter provides an overview of this AAP/EFP 2018 classification system and examples of its implementation in practice.

Periodontal Health

Periodontal health is defined as a state free from inflammatory periodontal disease such as gingivitis, periodontitis, and other periodontal conditions. In addition to the patients without a history of periodontal diseases, periodontal health can be applied to patients who had a history of successfully treated periodontal diseases and are able to maintain periodontal tissues without clinical inflammation. Clinically, there are two categories of periodontal health diagnosis: (1) clinical health on an intact periodontium; (2) clinical gingival health on a reduced periodontium in a stable periodontitis patient or non-periodontitis patient.[9] The classification system recognizes a difference between the spectrum of health on a site basis as compared to a case basis. A patient with a healthy periodontium may exhibit a few sites with signs of inflammation, such as BOP. On a case basis, clinical health on an intact periodontium is defined as less than 10% sites with BOP, all sites with probing depths ≤ 3 mm and absence of clinical attachment loss and bone loss (intact periodontium). Clinical gingival health on a reduced periodontium in a non-periodontitis patient is also defined as less than 10% sites with BOP, all sites with probing depths ≤ 3 mm but a presence of attachment loss and bone loss (reduced periodontium) due to non-periodontitis reason (e.g., crown lengthening surgery). A diagnosis of clinical gingival health on a reduced periodontium in a stable periodontitis is given to a patient with less than 10% sites with BOP, all sites with probing depths ≤ 4 mm and presence of attachment loss and bone loss due to periodontitis. In these successfully treated periodontitis patients diagnosed with clinical gingival health, the sites with probing depths of 4mm should have no BOP. Clinically, it is important to distinguish a case of clinical gingival health on a reduced periodontium in a stable periodontitis patient from a case of clinical gingival health on a reduced periodontium in a non-periodontitis patient, as the patient with a history of periodontitis has a higher risk for periodontal disease progression than the patient without the history. Less than 10% of BOP sites is used to define clinical health because it is not common to identify an adult who has no BOP during the periodontal examination. See Table 5.1 for different scenarios of periodontal health.

Gingival Diseases

Dental Biofilm-Induced Gingivitis

Gingivitis that is associated with retained dental biofilm (plaque) is the most common form of gingival disease (Fig. 5.1). As compared to periodontal health, patients with gingivitis present with signs of inflammation such as swelling, bleeding, and/or redness in the gingiva. The gingivitis patients may feel pain or soreness from the inflamed gingiva. Gingivitis can be categorized as localized or generalized based on the percentage of BOP sites. Localized gingivitis is defined as 10% to 30% BOP sites and generalized gingivitis is defined as greater than 30% BOP sites.[9] So far, there is not strong evidence to classify the severity of gingivitis. However, to facilitate communications, clinicians may use terms like mild, moderate or severe gingivitis based on percentages of sites with BOP (mild = <10%; moderate = 10% to 30%; severe = >30%).

Gingivitis may occur on an intact periodontium or on a reduced periodontium (Fig. 5.2) in the successfully treated periodontitis patient or non-periodontitis patient. For all gingivitis patients, the probing depth of all sites should be ≤3 mm. The epidemiology of periodontal diseases is reviewed in Chapter 6. What separates gingivitis from periodontitis is the containment of the inflammatory lesion within the gingiva in the former. As such, gingivitis is generally not associated with progressive attachment loss. However, it should be noted that a successfully treated periodontitis patient diagnosed with gingivitis on a reduced periodontium still has the increased risk of periodontitis progression if the disease is not well controlled. A patient diagnosed with gingivitis on an intact periodontium is not associated with the risk of progressive attachment loss or bone loss.

TABLE 5.1 Different Scenarios

Parameters	Intact Periodontium	Reduced Periodontium Non-Periodontitis Patient (example: toothbrush trauma induced generalized gingival recession)	Successfully Treated Stable Periodontitis Patient (example: patient with a past history of 4 quadrants of osseous surgery)
Probing attachment loss	No	Yes	Yes
Probing pocket depths (assuming no pseudopockets	≤3 mm	≤3 mm	≤4 mm (no site 4 mm or greater with BOP)
Bleeding on probing (BOP) %	<10	<10	<10
Radiographic bone loss	No	Possible	Yes

BOP, Bleeding on probing.
Adapted from Chapple ILC, Mealey BL, Van Dyke TE, et al. Periodontal health and gingival diseases and conditions on an intact and a reduced periodontium: consensus report of workgroup 1 of the 2017 World Workshop on the Classification of Periodontal and Peri-Implant Diseases and Conditions. *J Periodontol.* 2018;89(Suppl 1):S74–S84, with permission.

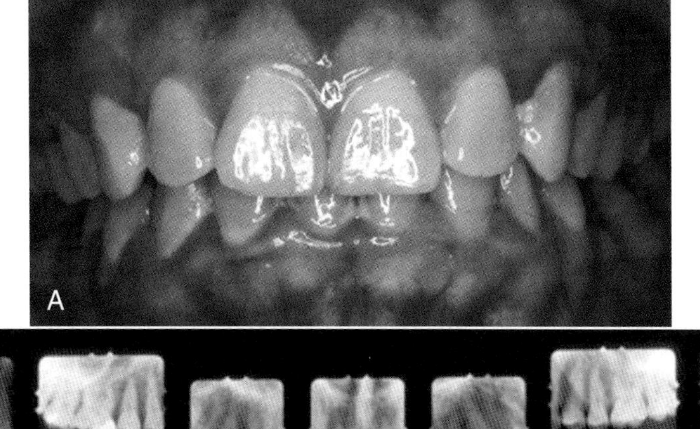

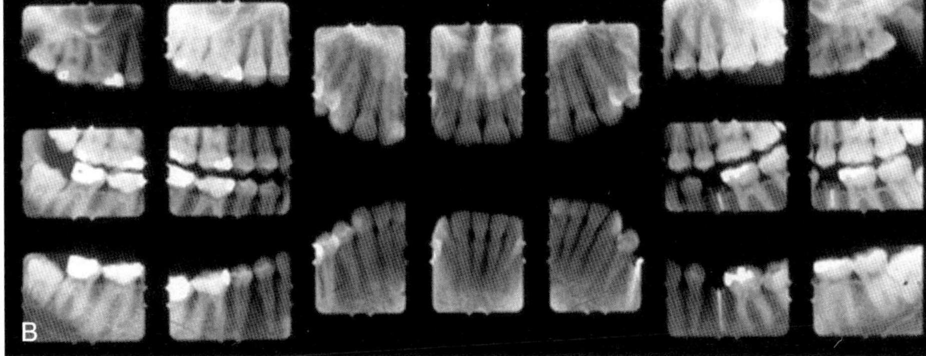

Fig. 5.1 (A) Dental biofilm-induced gingivitis depicts marginal and papillary inflammation, with 1- to 4-mm probing depths and generalized zero clinical attachment loss, except recession in tooth #28. (B) Radiographic images of the patient.

KEY FACT

Gingivitis may be the diagnosis for inflamed gingival tissues, associated with a tooth without previous attachment loss or with a tooth that has previously undergone attachment and bone loss (i.e., with reduced periodontal support) but exhibits probing depths ≤3 mm and is not currently losing attachment, even though gingival inflammation is present. In the latter case, the appropriate definition would be "gingivitis on a reduced periodontium."

Dental Biofilm-Induced Gingivitis Associated With Biofilm Alone

Biofilm-induced gingival disease is the result of an interaction between the microorganisms found in the dental biofilm and the inflammatory host response. A cause-and-effect relationship between microbial plaque and gingivitis has been elegantly demonstrated by a classic experiment demonstrating that the cessation of oral hygiene consistently leads to the manifestation of gingivitis within 2 to 3 weeks in healthy adults.[5,33] Gingivitis is histologically characterized by a dense infiltrate of lymphocytes and other mononuclear cells, fibroblast alterations, increased vascular permeability, and continuing loss of collagen in response to the microbial challenge. However, the alveolar bone is not affected. Microbial biofilm is thus considered the primary etiologic factor for gingivitis. The extent, severity, and duration of the inflammatory response interaction can be altered by the local (see Chapter 24) or systemic factors (see Chapters 23 and 25). Gingivitis is fully reversible in otherwise healthy persons shortly following the removal of local factors and reduction of the microbial load around the teeth. As noted earlier, gingivitis is rapidly established in cases of inefficient plaque removal. Therefore, it is crucial that patients are instructed in oral hygiene to maintain long-term gingival health.

Gingival Diseases Mediated by Systemic Factors

Several systemic risk factors (i.e., modifying factors) may contribute to gingivitis by exacerbating the gingival inflammatory response

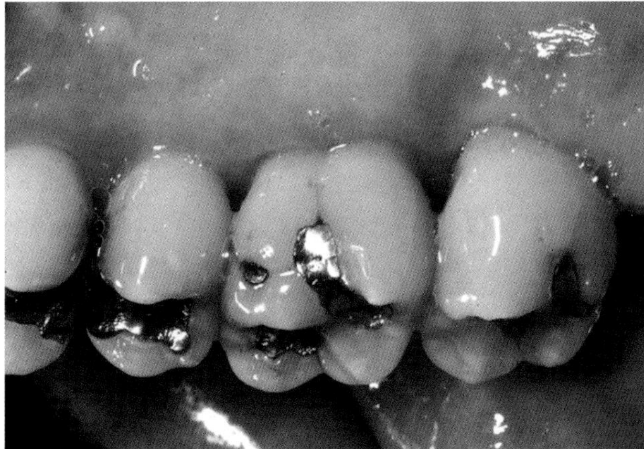

Fig. 5.2 Maxillary second molar exhibits mild inflammation at mesial-palatal surface. However, the clinical attachment loss has been stable for 15 years after apical positioned flap and periodontal maintenance, which is consistent with remission. The appropriate diagnosis is dental biofilm-induced gingivitis on a reduced periodontium.

to dental biofilm.[28,49] This altered response appears to result from the effects of systemic conditions on the host's cellular and immunologic functions, but microbial biofilm is still the primary etiologic factor. These systemic factors include: (a) smoking; (b) hyperglycemia; (c) nutritional factors; (d) pharmacological agents (prescription, non-prescription, and recreational); (e) sex steroid hormones (puberty [Fig. 5.3], menstrual cycle, pregnancy [Fig. 5.4], oral contraceptives); (f) hematological conditions.[9,40]

Smoking is a major risk factor for both gingivitis and periodontitis. The chemical components of cigarette can affect systemic immune response and induce microvascular vasoconstriction as well as fibrosis in gingiva (see Chapter 23). The vasoconstriction may reduce BOP which influences clinical diagnosis of gingivitis.

Gingival diseases modified by malnutrition have received attention because of clinical descriptions of bright red, swollen, and bleeding gingiva associated with severe ascorbic acid (vitamin C) deficiency or scurvy.[34,40,44] Various nutrients, such as long-chain omega-3 fatty acids, have been found to have immunomodulatory properties, whereas others act to ameliorate the destructive effects of reactive oxygen species (ROS) functioning as ROS scavengers. Nonetheless, the available evidence to support a clinically impactful role for mild nutritional deficiencies in the development or severity of gingival inflammation in humans is limited.

Elevations in sex steroid hormones may mediate inflammatory response in gingiva. One example is apparent during pregnancy when the incidence and severity of gingival inflammation may increase even in the presence of low levels of dental biofilm.

In blood dyscrasias (e.g., leukemia), the reduced number of immunocompetent lymphocytes in the periodontal tissues is associated with increased edema, erythema, and bleeding of the gingiva. Gingival enlargement caused by the excessive infiltration of malignant blood cells is often associated with the swollen and spongy gingival tissues (Fig. 5.5).

Gingival Diseases Mediated by Local Factors

Local risk factors (i.e., predisposing factors), including dental plaque biofilm retention factors and oral dryness, can increase plaque accumulation by inhibiting plaque removal from daily oral care or providing an environment conducive to plaque development. Poorly contoured subgingival restorations are associated with increased gingival inflammation and progressive attachment loss.[30,54] Oral dryness caused by medications, Sjögren's syndrome, radiation therapy for cancer, and other medical conditions result in increased plaque accumulation. These patients with oral dryness can have an increased percentage of BOP.[37]

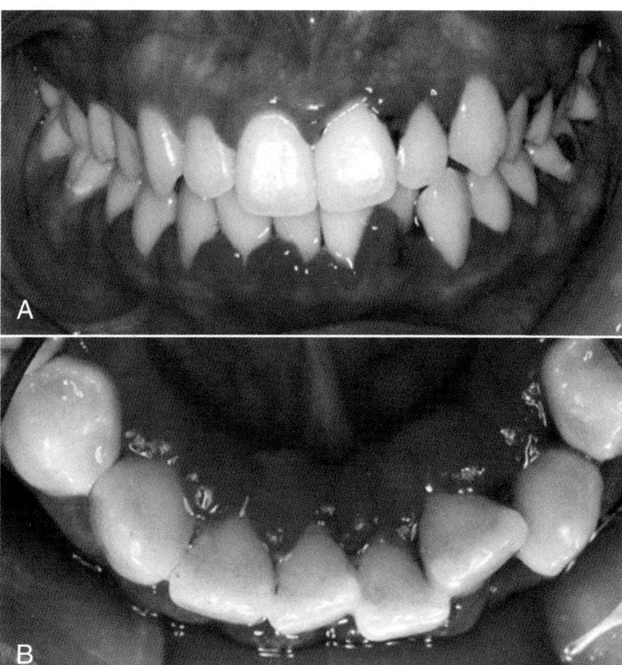

Fig. 5.3 A 13-year-old female with hormone-exaggerated marginal and papillary inflammation, with 1- to 4-mm probing depths yet minimal clinical attachment loss. (A) Facial view. (B) Lingual view.

Drug Influenced Gingival Enlargement

Gingival diseases that are modified by medications include gingival overgrowth due to anticonvulsant drugs such as phenytoin, immunosuppressive drugs such as cyclosporine (Fig. 5.6), and calcium channel blockers such as nifedipine (Fig. 5.7), verapamil, diltiazem, and sodium valproate.[17,34,40,49] The development and severity of gingival enlargement in response to medications is patient specific and is influenced by uncontrolled plaque accumulation.

Non–Dental Biofilm-Induced Gingival Diseases

Oral manifestations of systemic conditions that produce lesions in the tissues of the periodontium are less common than biofilm-induced gingivitis. Non-dental biofilm-induced gingival diseases encompass a variety of conditions including: (a) genetic/developmental disorders (hereditary gingival fibromatosis); (b) specific infections (bacterial, viral, or fungal origin); (c) inflammatory and immune conditions (hypersensitivity reactions, autoimmune diseases of skin and mucous membranes, granulomatous inflammatory lesions); (d) reactive processes (epulides); (e) neoplasms; (f) endocrine disorders, nutritional (vitamin C deficiency) and metabolic diseases; (g) traumatic lesions; and (h) gingival pigmentations.[9,22] These gingival conditions will not be fully resolved by removal of dental biofilm alone. However, uncontrolled plaque accumulation can worsen these conditions. Some of these conditions are further discussed below.

Genetic/Developmental Disorders

Gingival diseases of genetic origin may involve the tissues of the periodontium and have been described in detail.[47] One of the most clinically evident conditions is *hereditary gingival fibromatosis,* which exhibits autosomal-dominant or (rarely) autosomal-recessive modes of inheritance. The gingival enlargement may completely

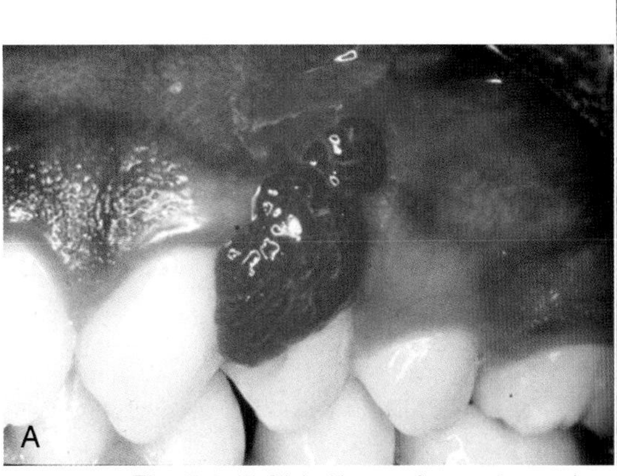
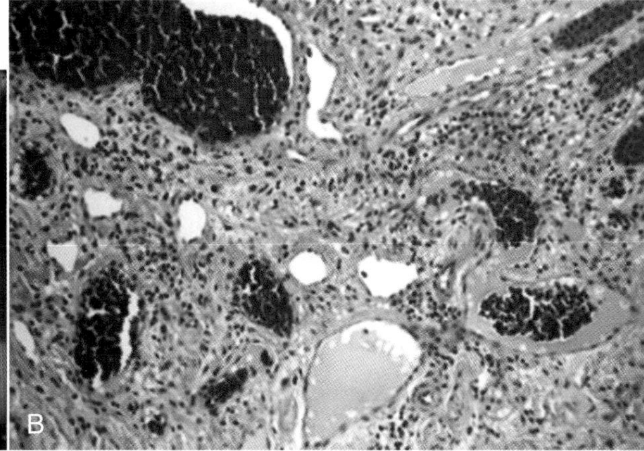

Fig. 5.4 (A) Clinical image of pyogenic granuloma in a 27-year-old pregnant female. (B) Histologic image depicts dense inflammatory infiltrate and prominent vessels.

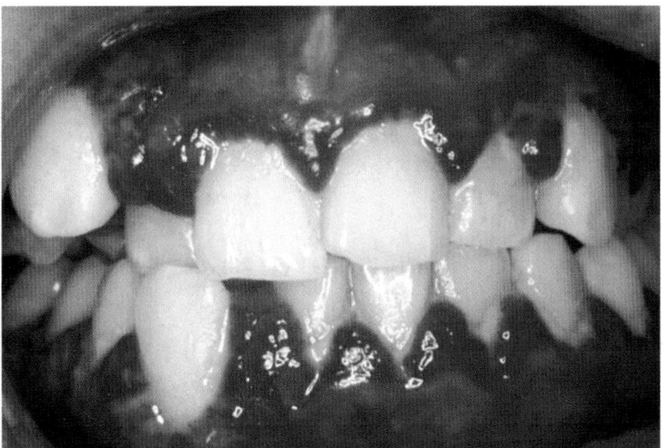

Fig. 5.5 A 12-year-old female with a primary medical diagnosis of leukemia that exhibits swollen/spongy gingiva.

cover the teeth, delay eruption, and present as an isolated finding; alternatively, it may be associated with several more generalized syndromes.

Specific Infections

Infections from three types of microorganisms, bacteria, fungi, or viruses can cause gingival diseases. Two bacterial species, *Neisseria gonorrhoeae* and *Treponema pallidum,* which can be transferred as a result of sexually transmitted diseases such as gonorrhea and syphilis, respectively, cause characteristic lesions in the gingiva.[6,50] Streptococcal gingivitis or gingivostomatitis is a rare entity that may present as an acute condition with fever, malaise, and pain associated with acutely inflamed, diffuse, red, and swollen gingiva with increased bleeding and occasional gingival abscess formation. The gingival infections are usually preceded by tonsillitis. Necrotizing gingival disease is an infectious disease affecting gingiva that is discussed later in this chapter.

Gingival diseases of viral origin may be caused by a variety of deoxyribonucleic acid (DNA) and ribonucleic acid (RNA) viruses, with the most common being the herpesviruses. A case example of herpetic stomatitis is demonstrated in Fig. 5.8A and B. Herpetic lesions are not uncommon and develop as intraoral blisters, usually grouped together, that quickly burst, leaving minuscule ulcerations. Lesions are frequently related to the reactivation of latent viruses, especially as a result of reduced immune function. The oral manifestations of viral infection have been comprehensively reviewed.[6] Viral gingival diseases are treated with topical or systemic antiviral drugs (see Fig. 5.8C and D).

CLINICAL CORRELATION

Unlike other herpetic recurrences, varicella zoster virus (VZV) usually manifests with a prodrome of tingling, itching, burning, or a unilateral numbness (shingles) at the affected dermatome. These symptoms are followed by moderate to severe pain shortly after initiation and are very important for differential diagnosis.

Gingival diseases of fungal origin are relatively uncommon in immunocompetent individuals, but they occur more frequently in immunocompromised individuals and in those with disturbed microbiota from the long-term use of broad-spectrum antibiotics.[55,56] The most common oral fungal infection is candidiasis (*Candida albicans* is often implicated). Candidiasis can also be seen under prosthetic devices, in individuals using topical steroids, and in individuals with decreased salivary flow, increased salivary glucose, or decreased salivary pH. A generalized candidal infection may manifest as white patches on the gingiva, tongue, or oral mucous membrane that can potentially be removed with gauze and leave a red, bleeding surface. In human immunodeficiency virus (HIV) seropositive persons, candidal infection may present as continuous erythematous stripe of the attached gingiva; this has been referred to as *linear gingival erythema* or *HIV-associated gingivitis* (see Chapter 27). The diagnosis of candidal infection can be made by culture, smear, or biopsy. Less common fungal infections have also been described.[55,56]

Inflammatory and Immune Conditions

Gingival manifestations of altered inflammatory and immune conditions may appear as desquamative lesions, ulcerations of the gingiva, or both.[23,32,48,55] Mucous membrane pemphigoid is a systemic autoimmune disease that affects mucous membranes and sometimes the skin. Oral and ocular mucosal tissues are most frequently affected. It is characterized by sloughing gingival tissues that leave painful ulcerations of the gingiva (Fig. 5.9). Autoantibodies are targeted at the basement membrane, and histologically the destruction resembles a subepithelial blister (see Fig. 5.9C and D). Case Scenario 5.2 depicts gingival recession accompanied by a mucosal lesion located on the gingiva manifesting with a white lacy pattern with characteristic striations.

Allergic reactions that manifest with gingival changes are uncommon but have been observed in association with several restorative

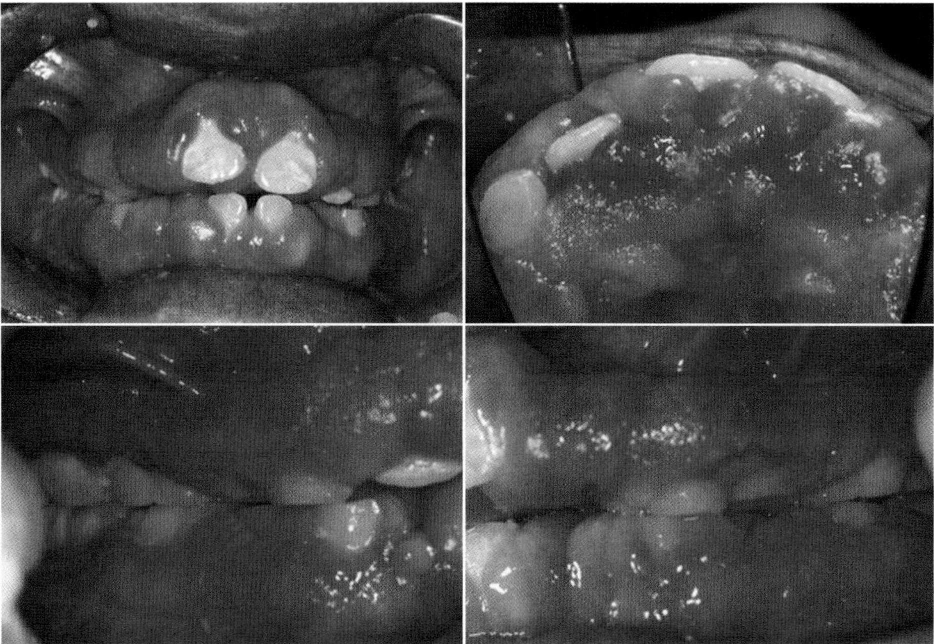

Fig. 5.6 Clinical images of a 9-year-old male with severe gingival enlargement secondary to heart transplant and cyclosporine therapy.

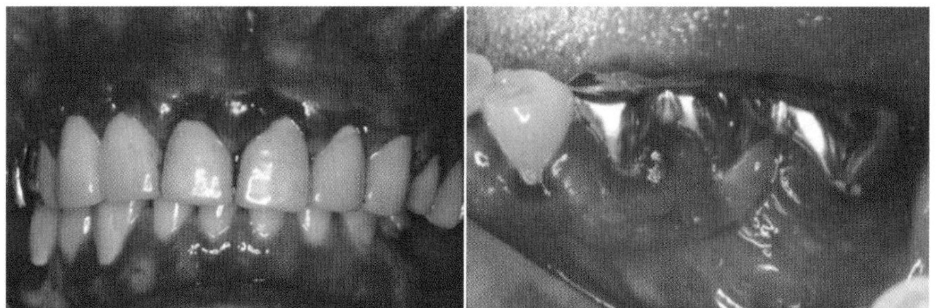

Fig. 5.7 Clinical images of gingival enlargement following use a of calcium channel blocker to control hypertension.

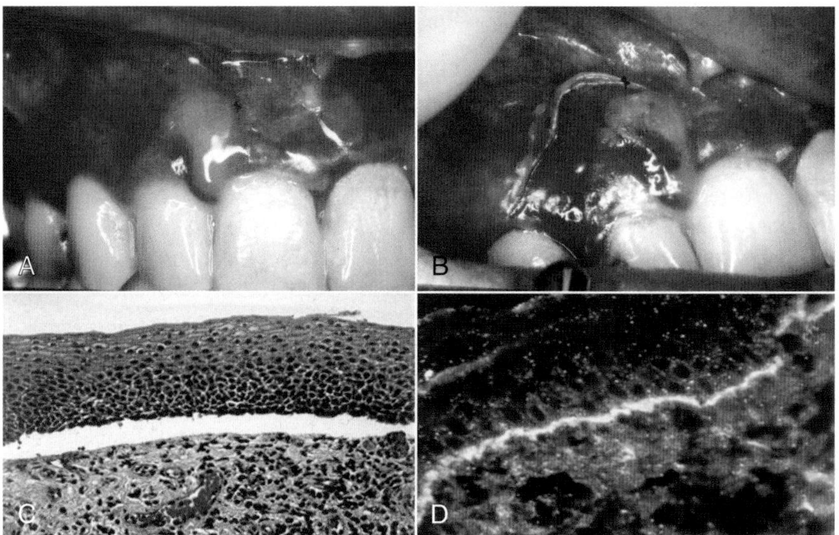

Fig. 5.8 (A and B) A 29-year-old male with primary herpetic infection and severe gingival inflammation. (C and D) Six weeks post systemic acyclovir.

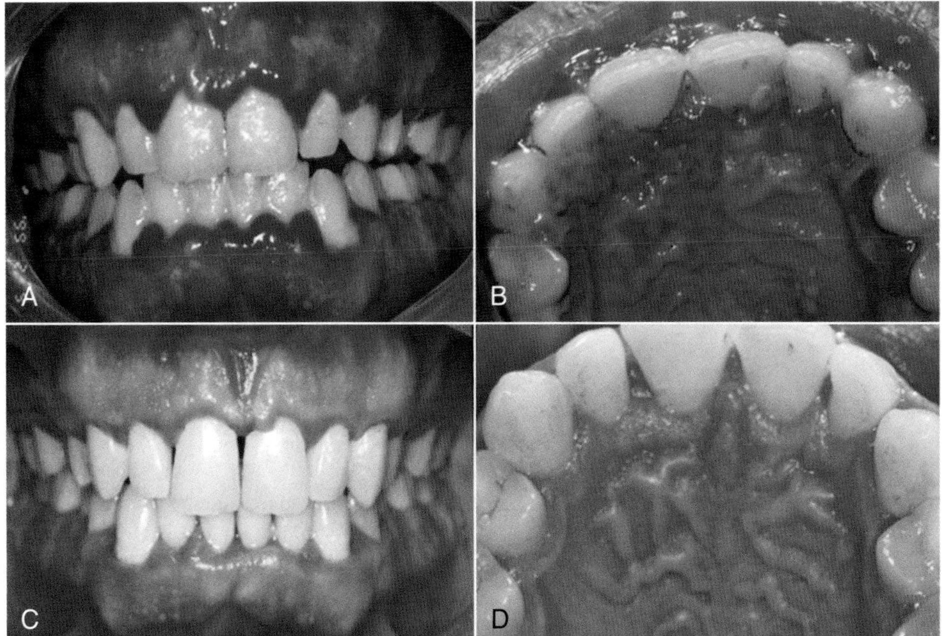

Fig. 5.9 A 62-year-old female with benign mucous membrane pemphigoid. (A and B) Clinical image with sloughing epithelial surface. (C) Hematoxylin and eosin (H&E) stain depicting separation of epithelium from connective tissue. (D) Immunofluorescent-labeled antibodies to basement membrane.

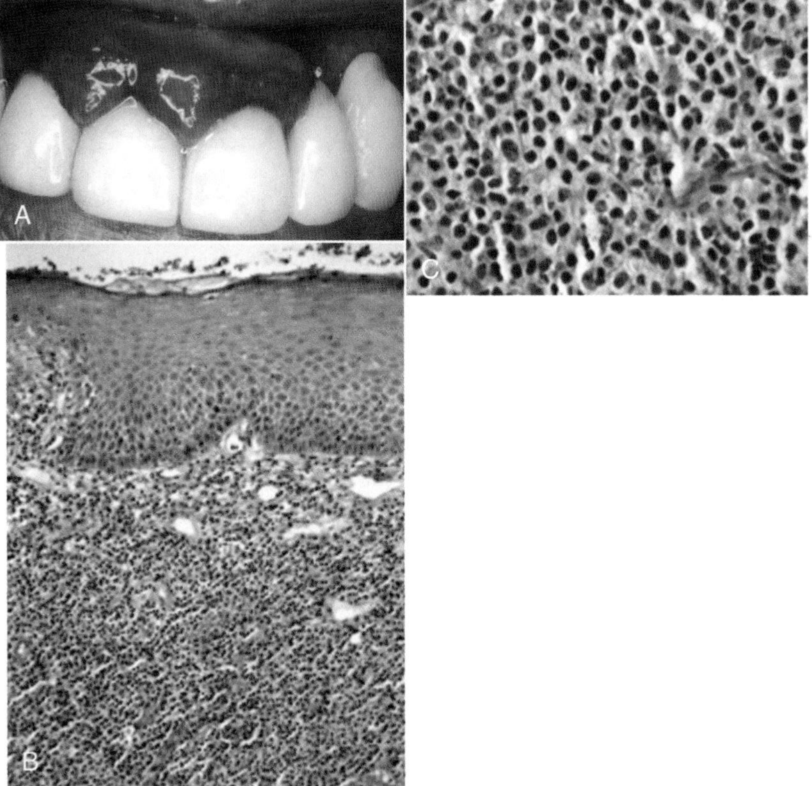

Fig. 5.10 (A) Localized pronounced gingival inflammation secondary to nickel allergy. (B and C) Biopsy depicts dense infiltrate of plasma cells.

materials (Fig. 5.10A), dentifrices, mouthwashes, chewing gums (Fig. 5.11), and foods. The diagnosis of these conditions may prove difficult and may require an extensive history and the selective elimination of potential causes. Conjoint assessment with an allergy specialist is indicated, and percutaneous tests are often recommended. Histologic traits of biopsies from gingival allergic reactions include a dense infiltrate of eosinophilic cells (see Fig. 5.10B and C).

Traumatic Lesions

Traumatic lesions may be self-inflicted and *factitious* in origin, which means that they are intentionally or unintentionally produced by artificial means (Fig. 5.12). Other examples of traumatic lesions include toothbrush trauma that results in gingival ulceration, recession, or both.

CLINICAL CORRELATION

Individuals who perform aggressive horizontal brushing are often found to have gingival recession or cervical abrasion on the teeth quadrants contralateral to their dominant hand.

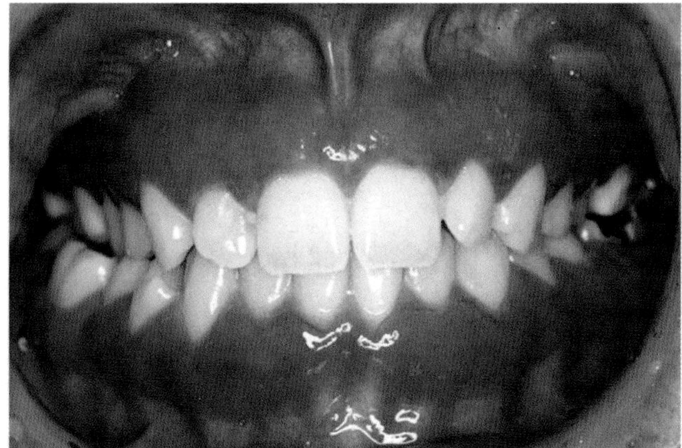

Fig. 5.11 Generalized severe allergic response of gingiva as a result of additive in chewing gum.

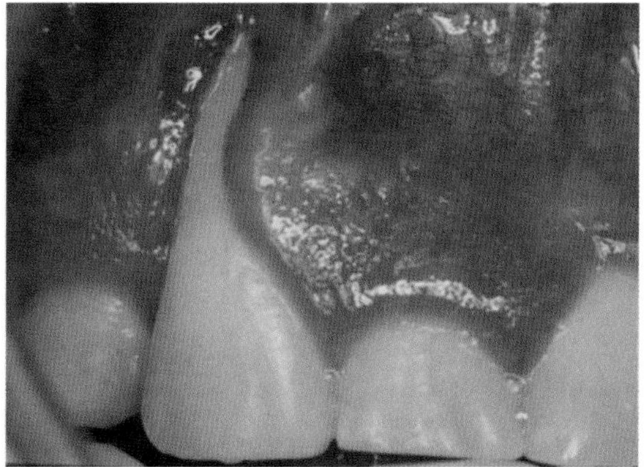

Fig. 5.12 Self-inflicted gingival dehiscence induced via patient's fingernail.

Iatrogenic trauma (i.e., induced by the dentist or health professional) to the gingiva may also lead to a gingival lesion. Such trauma may be caused directly (i.e., via use of dental instruments) or by the induction of cement or preventive or restorative materials. Peripheral ossifying fibroma may develop in response to the embedment of a foreign body (Fig. 5.13). Self-inflicted *accidental damage* to the gingiva may also occur as a result of minor burns from hot foods and drinks.[23]

Periodontiti

Periodontitis is defined as "an inflammatory disease of the supporting tissues of the teeth caused by specific microorganisms or groups of specific microorganisms, resulting in progressive destruction of the periodontal ligament and alveolar bone, with increased probing depth formation, recession, or both."[60] The clinical feature that distinguishes periodontitis from gingivitis is the presence of a clinically detectable attachment loss as a result of inflammatory destruction of the periodontal ligament and alveolar bone. This loss is often accompanied by periodontal pocket formation and changes in the density and height of the subjacent alveolar bone. In some cases, recession of the marginal gingiva may accompany attachment loss, thereby masking ongoing disease progression only if probing depth measurements are taken without measurements of **clinical attachment levels**.

For a definitive diagnosis of periodontitis, it is required that the patient present with detectable interdental clinical attachment loss in at least two non-adjacent teeth, or buccal or lingual clinical attachment loss (≥3 mm) jointly with probing depths (>3 mm) on two or more teeth. It is important to ensure that tissue destruction (clinical attachment loss) took place due to periodontal diseases and not due to other conditions such as: (a) trauma-induced gingival recession, (b) dental caries extending subgingivally, (c) clinical attachment loss on the distal aspect of the second molar (associated with malposition or extraction of the third molar), (d) endodontic pathology draining through periodontium, and (e) vertical root fracture.[59] Depending on the percentage of teeth at the stage defining severity level, the extent can be categorized into localized (<30% of teeth involved), generalized (≥30% of the teeth involved), or to present with the distinct molar-incisor pattern of disease involvement.[59]

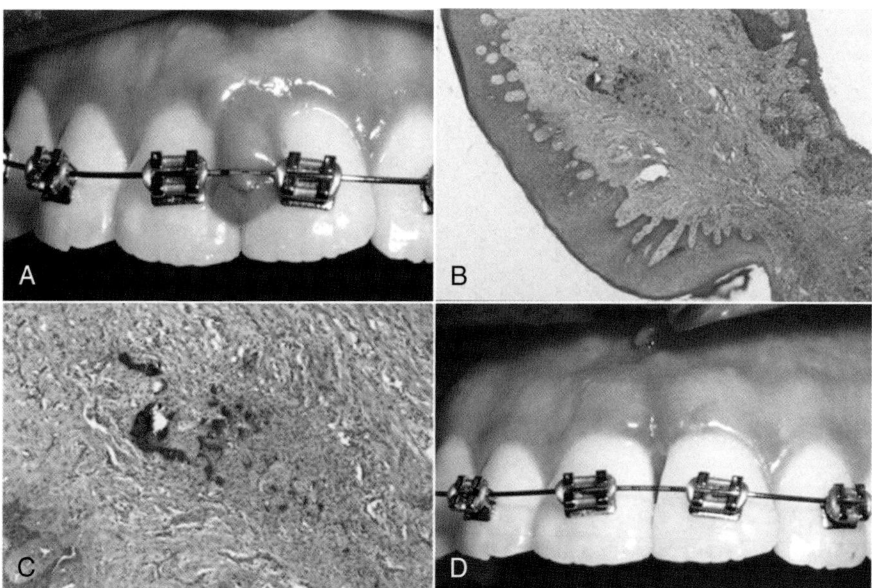

Fig. 5.13 (A) Proliferative gingival overgrowth secondary to impaction of foreign body. (B) Histology of peripheral ossifying fibroma. (C) Higher magnification of image in part B. (D) Four weeks post excisional biopsy.

TABLE 5.2 Key Periodontitis Staging Elements

	Periodontitis	Stage I	Stage II	Stage III	Stage IV
Severity	Clinical attachment loss	1–2 mm	3–4 mm	≥5 mm	≥5 mm
	Radiographic bone loss	Coronal third of the root (<15%)	Coronal third of the root (15%–33%)	Middle or apical third of the root	Middle or apical third of the root
	Tooth loss due to periodontitis	No tooth loss		≤4 teeth	≥5 teeth
Complexity		• PD ≤4 mm • Mostly horizontal bone loss	• PD ≤5 mm • Mostly horizontal bone loss	In addition to Stage II: • PD ≥6 mm • Vertical bone loss ≥3 mm • Class II or III furcation involvement • Moderate ridge defects	In addition to Stage III: • Need for complex rehabilitation due to masticatory dysfunction, tooth mobility, bite collapse, pathologic migration, <20 remaining teeth
Extent and distribution		• Localized (<30% of the teeth involved) • Generalized (≥30% of the teeth involved) • Molar-incisor pattern			

Adapted from Tonetti MS, Greenwell H, Kornman KS. Staging and grading of periodontitis: framework and proposal of a new classification and case definition. *J Periodontol.* 2018;89(Suppl 1):S159–S172, with permission.

KEY FACT

Probing depth measurement alone is inadequate for an assessment of periodontitis. Clinical attachment loss is usually assessed by adding the extent of gingival recession to the probing depth measurement to estimate the total extent of tissue loss from the cementoenamel junction (CEJ) of the tooth. However, when recession is not visible, it is essential that the height of the marginal gingiva coronal to the CEJ be determined, and that the measurement is subtracted from the probing depth to establish the extent of clinical attachment loss. The measurement of clinical attachment around a tooth provides insights on the history and extent of periodontal destruction around the tooth. One common pitfall of clinical periodontal examination is the direct translation of probing depths as clinical attachment levels when the gingival margin lies above the cementoenamel junction, leading to an overestimation of attachment levels.

Clinical signs of inflammation—such as changes in color, contour, and consistency as well as BOP—may not always be positive indicators of ongoing attachment loss, but the absence of bleeding is a good indicator of periodontal stability. The attachment loss associated with periodontitis may occur in a cyclic fashion, with attachment loss progressing either continuously or in episodic bursts of disease activity. However, the available clinical instruments for detecting disease are not sensitive enough to capture the cycles of attachment loss and repair that occur during disease activity and remission, respectively (i.e., the periodontal probe is graded in 1-mm increments).

KEY FACT

In the AAP/EFP 2018 classification of periodontal diseases, a multidimensional staging and grading system was introduced to subclassify periodontitis disease entities. The severity of periodontal disease at the time of presentation and the complexity of disease management dictate the staging, while grading offers additional information, including the rate of past progression of the disease and the risk for future progression. A periodontal calculator, provided for educational purposes, has been devised exclusively for the readers of this book.

Many classifications of periodontitis have been presented since the late 1980s; these considered the rate of disease progression and classified disease into distinct phenotypes, such as adult periodontitis, refractory periodontitis, and the various different forms of early-onset periodontitis. In the 2018 classification, these have been unified into the overarching "Periodontitis" category using stage and grade of disease to capture the phenotypic variations across age groups and levels of host susceptibility. The classification discussed in this chapter will focus on the currently accepted 2018 classification with references to the 1999 classification in parentheses when appropriate.

The 1999 classification established three descriptors for periodontitis that have been widely used in the literature for the past two decades: extent, severity, and rate of progression (chronic vs. aggressive). Chronic periodontitis was previously considered the most common form of periodontitis[16]; as mentioned above, in the 2018 classification "chronic" and "aggressive," the two descriptors of rate of progression of periodontitis were combined into one category of "periodontitis." Consequently, the remaining descriptors where "extent" and "severity." While "extent" remained as a descriptor of periodontitis (generalized, localized, or molar-incisor pattern), the severity and progression of disease were replaced by two new dimensions, "staging" and "grading," respectively.

Staging

Staging describes the severity and complexity of each case and incorporates the following elements:

- Severity of the disease and tooth loss due to periodontitis.
- Management complexity of the patient's periodontal condition and overall oral rehabilitation needs.

Staging is based on a full-mouth diagnosis and is not subdivided into different severity levels for different parts of the mouth (Table 5.2). Staging is designed to give information about the whole mouth, relative to the severity and complexity of the patient's periodontal status. The stage will also inform the clinician of the initial difficulty and complexity of required treatment. Although staging is not equivalent to severity, based on the determinants of each periodontitis stage, it is expected that the majority of cases of mild to moderate periodontitis will typically be either Stage I or Stage II,

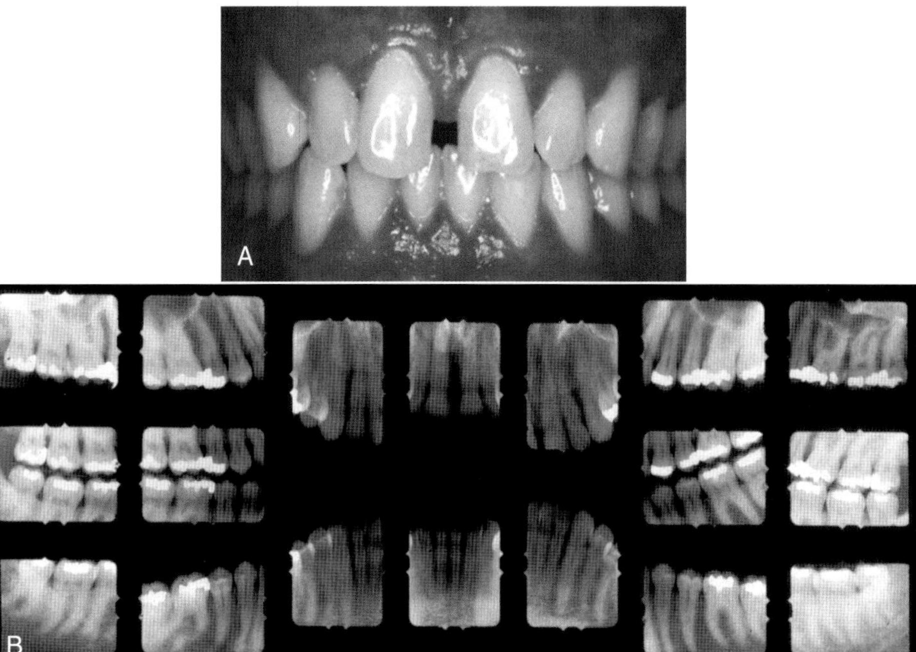

Fig. 5.14 (A) Clinical image of Generalized Stage I Grade B periodontitis with 1- to 2-mm clinical attachment loss in a 40-year-old female. (B) Radiographic images of the patient.

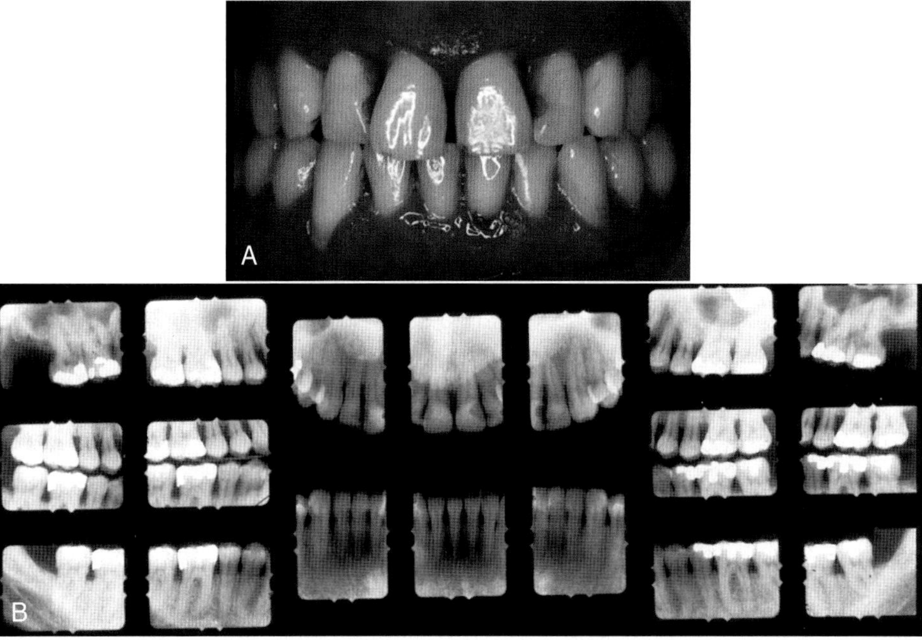

Fig. 5.15 (A) Clinical image of Generalized Stage II Grade B periodontitis with 3- to 4-mm clinical attachment loss in a 53-year-old male smoker. (B) Radiographic images of the patient.

while severe periodontitis will typically be either Stage III or Stage IV (Figs. 5.14–5.17). The staging system is designed to highlight the patient's most severe areas of destruction and it considers the sites with the maximum attachment loss or bone loss as one of its determinants. Determining the tooth loss number should include teeth that have been identified for extraction, due to periodontitis, as part of active therapy. See Table 5.2 and Box 5.1 for elements that make up periodontitis staging system and the characteristics of different stages. Assessment of extent describes the percentage of teeth at the stage-defining severity level based on a 30% threshold.[29,53] Localized periodontitis is defined as periodontitis affecting less than 30% of teeth, while periodontitis affecting ≥30% of teeth is considered generalized. Although, some complexity factors (e.g., deep probing depth) might be controlled or eliminated after treatment, the Stage generally should not retrogress to a lower level. It is because the existing disease severity (based on clinical attachment loss and bone loss) and previous complexity factors are associated with potential future disease progression. However, if significant bone gain was achieved following successful regenerative therapy, the Stage could potentially be retrograded, this being the only exception.

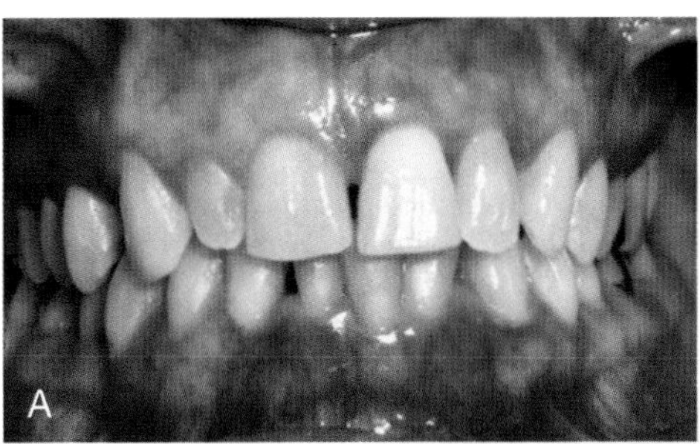

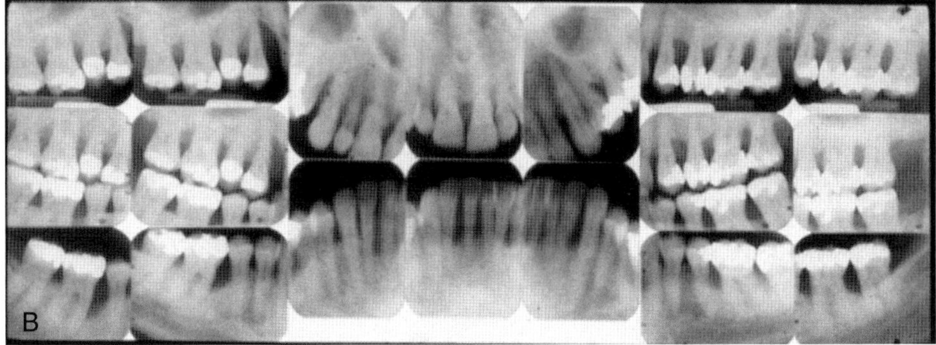

Fig. 5.16 (A) Clinical image of Generalized Stage III Grade C periodontitis with ≥5 mm clinical attachment loss in a 47-year-old female. (B) Radiographic images of the patient.

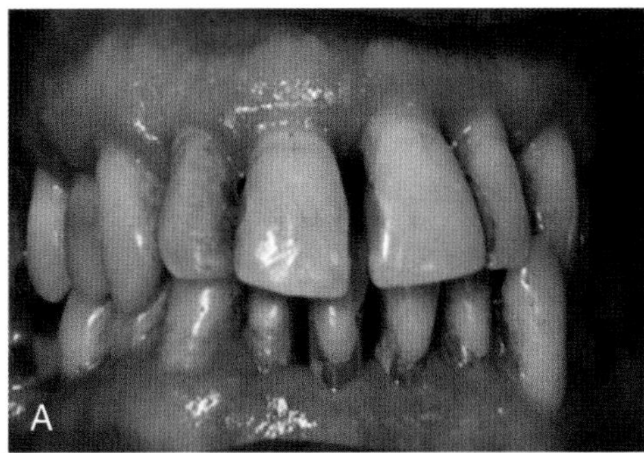

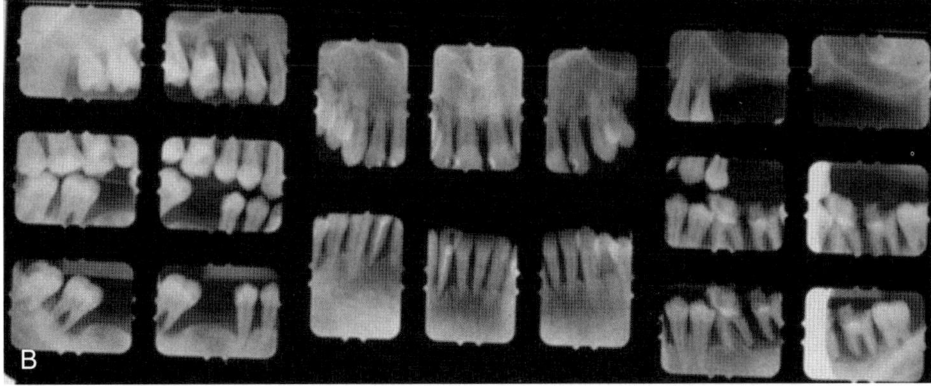

Fig. 5.17 (A) Clinical image of what we used to diagnose as aggressive periodontitis with 3- to 13-mm periodontal diseases and 7- to 15-mm clinical attachment loss in a 32-year-old male. Following the 2018 American Academy of Periodontology/European Federation of Periodontology classification system, this patient is diagnosed with Generalized Stage IV Grade C periodontitis. (B) Radiographic images of the patient.

KEY FACT

In the 1999 classification of periodontal diseases, a separate category of "aggressive periodontitis" was employed to define rampant progression of disease in certain individuals, oftentimes associated with young age or lack of local factor. In the 2018 classification, both chronic and aggressive periodontitis disease entities are grouped together and simply called *periodontitis. The rate of progression and risk for future progression are now captured by the multidimensional grading system.*

Grading

As discussed previously, in the 1999 classification the term "aggressive periodontitis" characterized a disease that differed from the chronic form primarily by the rapid rate of disease progression seen in an otherwise healthy individual (see Fig. 5.17). In the new classification, the rate of progression of disease is captured within the grading domain.

Grading provides the likelihood of post-treatment disease progression, and it can change along the way because it depends on the state of the patient at the time of examination. In essence, grading

BOX 5.1 Periodontitis Staging

Stage I Periodontitis (Mild Disease) (Fig. 5.14)

- Probing depths ≤4 mm
- Interdental CAL ≤1–2 mm
- Horizontal bone loss (<15%)
- Will require nonsurgical treatment
- No posttreatment tooth loss expected

Stage II Periodontitis (Moderate Disease) (Fig. 5.15)

- Probing depths ≤5 mm
- Interdental CAL ≤3–4 mm
- Primarily horizontal bone loss (15%–33%)
- Will require nonsurgical *and* maybe surgical treatment
- No posttreatment tooth loss is expected

Stage III Periodontitis (Severe Disease) (Fig. 5.16)

- Probing depths ≥6 mm
- Interdental CAL ≥5 mm
- Bone loss extending to middle third of root and beyond; may have vertical bone loss and/or furcation involvement of Class II or III
- Will require initial nonsurgical treatment followed, most probably, by surgical treatments
- Loss of four or fewer teeth due to periodontitis
- Higher risk of tooth loss due to periodontitis
- Moderate ridge defects
- Complexity of implant and/or restorative treatment is increased and may require multispecialty treatment

Stage IV Periodontitis (Very Severe Disease) (Fig. 5.17)

- Probing depths ≥6 mm
- Interdental CAL ≥5 mm
- Bone loss extending to middle third of root and beyond; may have vertical bone loss and/or furcation involvement of class II or III
- Loss of five or more teeth due to periodontitis; less than 20 teeth may be present
- Higher risk for tooth loss due to periodontitis; patients will require initial nonsurgical treatment likely followed by advanced surgical treatment and/or regenerative therapy, including augmentation treatment to facilitate implant therapy
- Severe ridge defects
- Very complex implant and/or restorative treatment may be needed usually requiring multispecialty treatment

CAL, Clinical attachment loss.

is this dimension of the new classification enables clinicians to incorporate individual characteristics into the diagnosis and related treatment plans. These include history-based and/or anticipated rate of periodontitis progression, presence and control of risk factors, and general health modifiers (Table 5.3). See Table 5.3 and Box 5.2 for elements that make up periodontitis grading scheme and their characteristics.

Incorporating grading in clinical practice will likely require some modifications as compared to the previously established 1999 classification scheme. For example, the rate of radiographic bone loss/clinical attachment loss (primary criteria determining the grade) can be directly assessed via longitudinal radiographic evaluation or review of clinical measurements from successive examinations. This is indeed the gold standard approach for grading periodontitis but not always feasible due to the lack of prior documentation or multiple providers. As a result, the 2018 classification recommends that the percentage of bone loss with respect to the patient's age be considered. Staging of periodontitis determines the case's severity and complexity, while grading is used to incorporate a temporal characterization of the disease progress that takes into account risk factors like smoking and diabetes, in order to assess risk for disease progression. Based on the changes in disease progression rate or in risk factors, the grade will be modified accordingly.

In the case presented in Fig. 5.16, the Stage is III based on the interdental clinical attachment loss exceeding 5 mm at the most involved site, the severity of bone loss and the loss of fewer than four teeth due to periodontitis. However, determining grading requires consideration of the rate of progression of disease as well as consideration of the underlying risk factors. For educational purposes, let us consider that the patient presented in Fig. 5.16 is self-referred and there is no access to previous examination or radiographic records. The person's age is 47 years and the bone loss of the tooth with the most periodontal tissue destruction is approximately 80%. A simple calculation of % bone loss/age equals to 1.7, which puts her at grade C rate of progression. Modifiable risk factors, such as smoking and glycemic control also have to be considered in all cases and could modify the rate of progression, which highlights the need for careful medical history review and frequent updates.

Periodontal Manifestations of Systemic Diseases

Several hematologic and genetic disorders have been associated with the development of periodontitis in affected individuals.[2,26,27]

TABLE 5.3 Key Periodontitis Grading Elements

Progression			Grade A: Slow Rate	Grade B: Moderate Rate	Grade C: Rapid Rate
Primary criteria (Direct evidence should be used when available)	Direct evidence of progression	Radiographic bone loss or CAL	No loss over 5 years	<2 mm over 5 years	≥2 mm over 5 years
	Indirect evidence of progression	% bone loss/age	<0.25	0.25–1	>1
		Case phenotype	Heavy biofilm with low levels of destruction	Destruction commensurate with biofilm deposits	Destruction inconsistent with biofilm deposits; clinical patterns suggestive of periods of rapid progression and/or early onset
Grade modifiers	Risk factors	Smoking	Nonsmoker	<10 cigarettes/day	≥10 cigarettes/day
		Diabetes	Nondiabetic	Diabetic with HbA1c <7%	Diabetic with HbA1c ≥7%

CAL, Clinical attachment loss.

Adapted from Tonetti MS, Greenwell H, Kornman KS. Staging and grading of periodontitis: framework and proposal of a new classification and case definition. *J Periodontol.* 2018;89(Suppl 1): S159–S172, with permission.

The majority of existing publications are case reports, whereas only a few research studies have investigated the exact nature of the effect of the specific condition on the tissues of the periodontium primarily because of the rare occurrence of many of these diseases. It is speculated that the major effect of these disorders is through alterations in immune response, such as in the case of interleukin-17 overexpression in leukocyte adhesion deficiency[38] or due to tissue metabolic disorders, such as in some forms of Ehlers–Danlos syndrome.[3] The clinical manifestation of many of these disorders appears at an early age and may be confused with aggressive forms of periodontitis, depicting rapid attachment loss and the potential for early tooth loss. This was one of the drivers of the use of the term *early-onset periodontitis* in the past. In reality, periodontitis occurs as a manifestation of these systemic diseases when the underlying disease is the major predisposing factor and the local factors (e.g., large quantities of plaque and calculus) are not clearly evident or their presence alone does not justify the severity or progression of disease. This definition is reserved for a specific group of diseases and syndromes that have been documented to have a profound destructive effect on the periodontium. The removal of local factors as part of conventional periodontal therapy in such cases is often inadequate to arrest the periodontal destruction due to the systemic effect (Figs. 5.18 and 5.19).[24]

Papillon–Lefèvre syndrome (PLS) is one example of a condition that causes severe periodontitis as one of its manifestations. PLS is an autosomal-recessive disorder caused by mutations in the cathepsin C gene located on chromosome 11q14.[20] The clinical manifestations of the syndrome include severe periodontitis with rapid destruction and diffuse keratoderma on the palms, soles, knees, or all three (Figs. 5.20 and 5.21).[19] The consanguinity of the parents is a common finding in approximately one-third of the cases.[39]

BOX 5.2 Periodontitis Grading

- A, slow or no progression risk
- B, moderate progression risk
- C, rapid progression risk

CLINICAL CORRELATION

When monogenic diseases are encountered, consanguinity can be a common finding, particularly in certain ethnic cultures. Appropriate genetic counseling is advisable. In addition, when the diagnosis for the proband (the first offspring for whom disease is noted) is established, it is crucial that the siblings are carefully examined for prompt diagnosis of additional cases.

Impaired neutrophil function is considered to be the primary cause of PLS and eventually results in the deregulation of the polymorphonuclear leukocyte response to microbial infection.[36] Although the subgingival microbiota associated with PLS is diverse, opportunistic periodontal pathogens such as *Aggregatibacter actinomycetemcomitans* (Aa), *Porphyromonas gingivalis, Tannerella forsythia, Fusobacterium nucleatum,* and *Prevotella intermedia* are frequently identified among plaque samples from PLS patients.[1,58] Serum immunoglobulin G titers against Aa are typically elevated in individuals with PLS, thereby implicating Aa as a significant causative factor.[58] Individuals with PLS are often initially screened by a dermatologist or a pediatrician, and the phenotype of the syndrome may be mistaken for atopic dermatitis (eczema) or palmoplantar keratoderma.[43] The case presented in Figs. 5.20 and 5.21 was treated for several years by a dermatologist as atopic dermatitis with occasional cauterization of misdiagnosed "plantar warts." The diagnosis of PLS was established in a periodontal office. A multidisciplinary treatment approach for these patients including referral to a periodontist cannot be overemphasized. After a diagnosis of PLS has been established, it is important to collect a complete family history and to construct a pedigree to help identify undiagnosed or misdiagnosed siblings (Fig. 5.22). In 1979, Haneke proposed palmoplantar

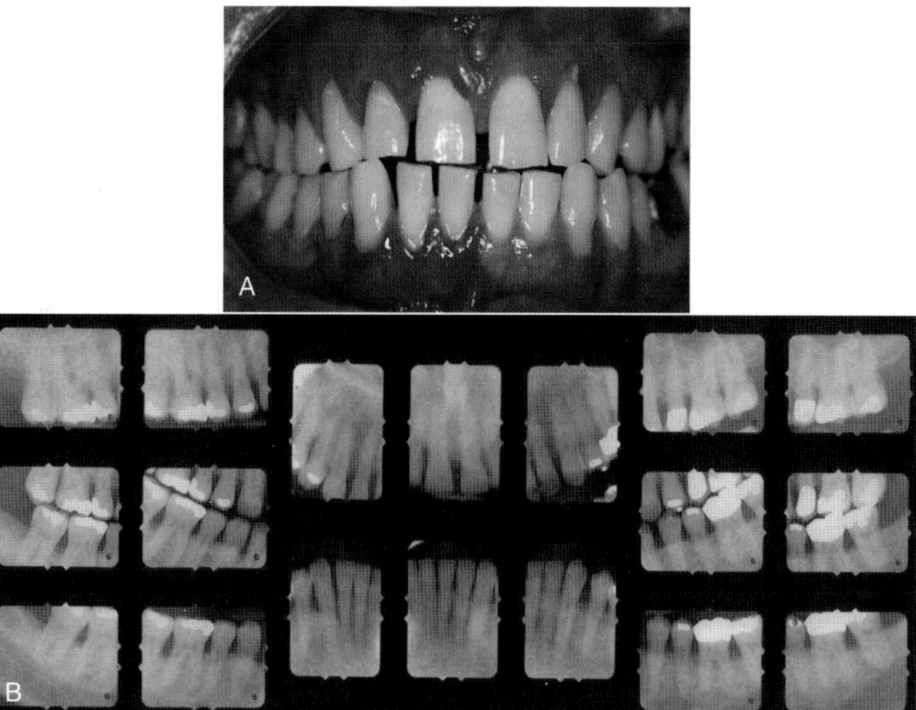

Fig. 5.18 (A) Clinical image of severe periodontitis (localized Stage III Grade C periodontitis) in a 53-year-old male smoker with diabetes and hemoglobin A_{1c} (HbA_{1c}) = 10.7. (B) Radiographic images of the patient.

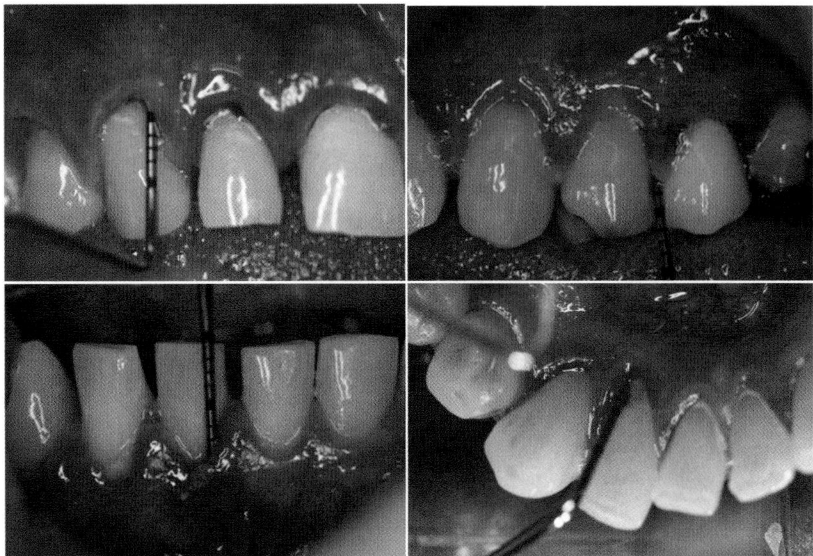

Fig. 5.19 Selective probing depths of the same 53-year-old diabetic patient shown in Fig. 5.18 with severe periodontitis.

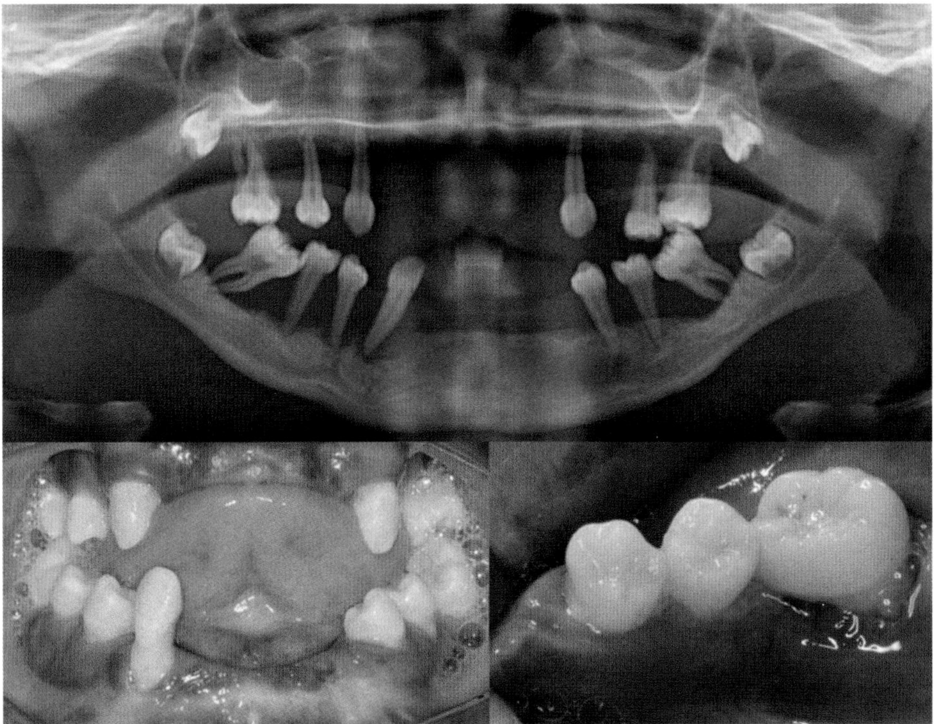

Fig. 5.20 Panoramic radiograph and clinical photos of a 13-year-old female with Papillon–Lefèvre syndrome (PLS). PLS is an autosomal recessive disorder caused by mutations in the cathepsin C gene located on chromosome 11q14. The clinical manifestations of the syndrome are severe periodontitis as well as diffuse keratoderma on the palms, soles, or knees. In PLS patients, by the age of 4 to 5 years, the primary teeth have typically exfoliated or been extracted due to severe periodontal destruction. Subsequently, an edentulous phase occurs during which a reduction in the oral microbial load is noted and gingival health is restored. Following eruption of the permanent dentition, a similar cycle of severe periodontal inflammation is repeated that generally does not respond to conventional periodontal therapy. An increase in tooth mobility and periodontal abscesses is frequently observed shortly after the eruption of permanent teeth. (*Courtesy Dr. Georgios Kotsakis, San Antonio, Texas.*)

hyperkeratosis, the loss of primary and permanent teeth, and an autosomal-recessive pattern of inheritance as being essential criteria to verify a diagnosis of PLS.[19] Secondary manifestations of PLS may include ectopic intracranial calcifications and increased susceptibility to infections, including pyogenic liver abscesses that can be fatal.[10]

Sarcoidosis is a chronic disease that is expressed as a cell-mediated, delayed-type hypersensitivity that primarily affects the lungs, lymph nodes, skin, eyes, liver, spleen, and small bones of the hands and feet.[45] Sarcoidosis rarely affects the oral cavity, with incidence of occurrence in descending order noted in the lymph nodes, lips, soft palate, buccal mucosa, gingiva, tongue, and bone.[45] Fig. 5.23

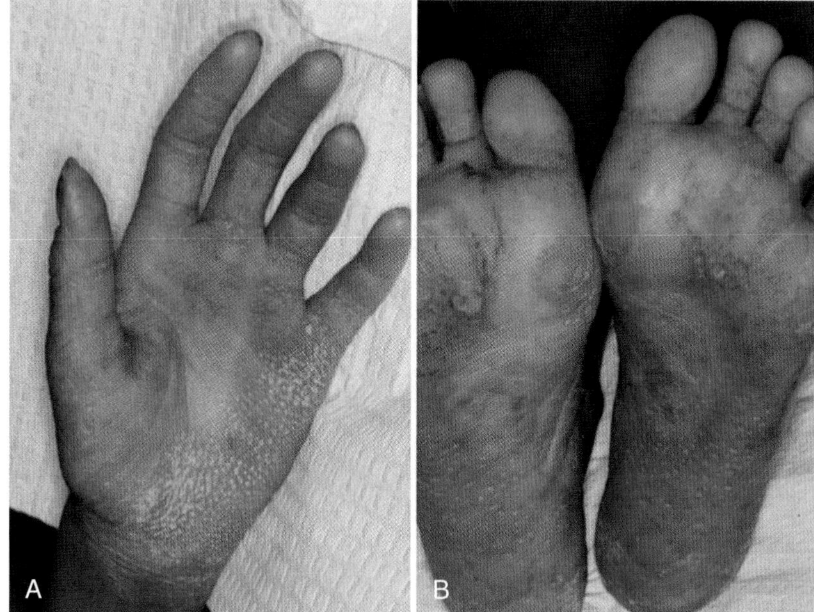

Fig. 5.21 Patient with Papillon-Lefèvre (PLS) syndrome exhibiting hyperkeratosis on palms of the hand (A) and soles of the feet (B). PLS clinically affects both the primary and permanent dentition. Signs of palmoplantar keratoderma usually appear simultaneously with the eruption of the first primary teeth (5 to 6 months) but may appear as early as 1 month of age. (*Courtesy Dr. Georgios Kotsakis, San Antonio, Texas.*)

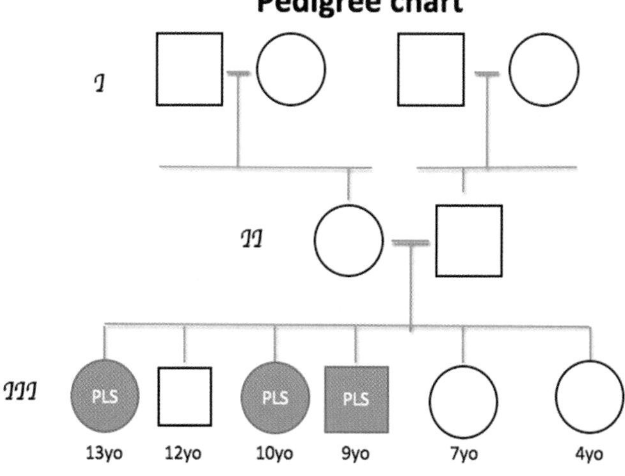

Fig. 5.22 No history of consanguinity was reported in this case. However, approximately one-third of the diagnosed Papillon-Lefèvre (PLS) cases descend from same ancestor. Offsprings III1, III3, and III4 display a PLS phenotype. A periodontist should thoroughly examine all siblings once a case of PLS has been diagnosed.

depicts the pretreatment pattern of bone loss and recession associated with sarcoidosis, with pulmonary parenchymal fibrous infiltrate noted in the lungs, as depicted by a white lacy pattern on a chest radiograph (see Fig. 5.23C). Histologic features of sarcoidosis include the presence of an intense chronic inflammatory infiltrate with focal areas of noncaseating granulomas and a positive Kveim test (Fig. 5.24C). The remineralization of alveolar bone is noted on radiographs obtained 1 year after the systemic administration of steroids (e.g., prednisone) (see Fig. 5.24A).

In the same category of manifestations of systemic diseases in the periodontium the subcategory of systemic disorders that can result in loss of periodontal tissue independent of periodontitis was introduced in 2018. This subcategory includes neoplasms, such as oral squamous cell carcinoma, and other disorders, such as Langerhans cell histiocytosis that can lead to periodontal bone loss, independent of local factors as described in Table 5.4.

Necrotizing Periodontal Diseases

The clinical characteristics of necrotizing periodontal diseases (NPD) may include (but are not limited to) ulcerated and necrotic papillary and marginal gingiva that is covered by a yellowish white or grayish slough or pseudomembrane, blunting and cratering of the papillae, bleeding on provocation or spontaneous bleeding, pain, and fetid breath. Similar to periodontal abscess, NPD also belong to acute periodontal lesions. NPDs may be accompanied by fever, malaise, and lymphadenopathy, although these characteristics are not consistent. NPDs are microbial, infectious conditions but a compromised host immune response can make the condition worse. Three forms of NPD have been described: *necrotizing gingivitis (NG)* (Fig. 5.25), *necrotizing periodontitis (NP)* (Fig. 5.26), and *necrotizing stomatitis (NS)*. With the presence of necrosis/ulcer of the interdental papillae, gingival bleeding and pain, the major difference between NG and NP is that there is no rapid bone loss in NG. In general populations, the prevalence of NG ranges from 0.51% to 3.3% and occurrence is higher in immunocompromised patients.[21]

The clinical and causative characteristics of NG[51] are described in detail in Chapter 17. The defining characteristics of NG are its bacterial cause, necrotic lesion, and predisposing factors, such as psychological stress, smoking, and immunosuppression. In addition, malnutrition may be a contributing factor in developing countries. NG is usually seen as an acute lesion that responds well to antimicrobial therapy in combination with professional plaque and calculus removal as well as improved oral hygiene.

NP differs from NG in that in NP, the loss of clinical attachment and alveolar bone is a consistent feature originating from the proximal region.[21] The characteristics of NP are described in detail in Chapter 30. NP is often observed in HIV seropositive individuals with low CD4 counts. Clinical manifestations include local

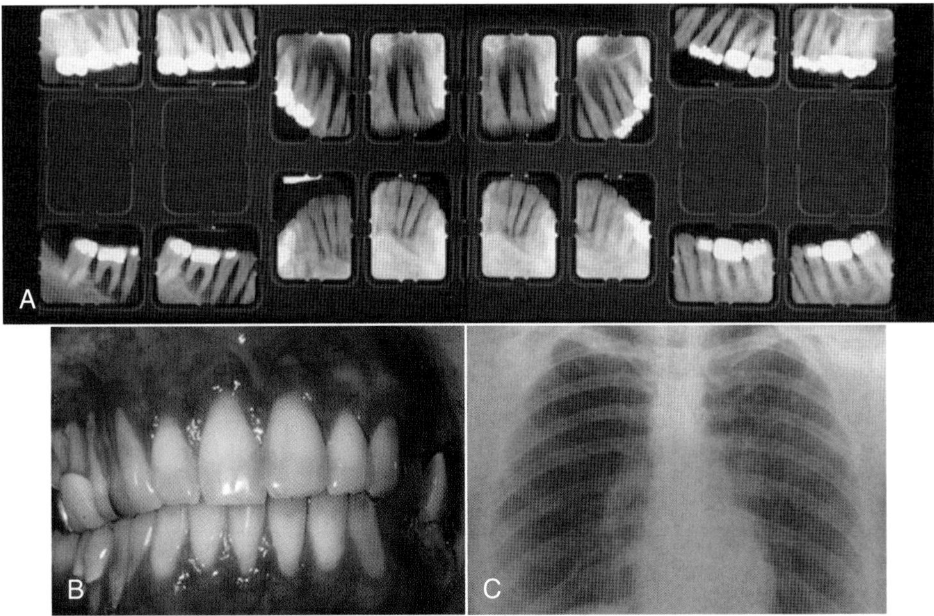

Fig. 5.23 Sarcoidosis pretreatment. (A) Intraoral x-rays depict extensive bone loss for anterior teeth. (B) Extensive recession plus clinical attachment loss. (C) Pulmonary parenchymal fibrous infiltrate.

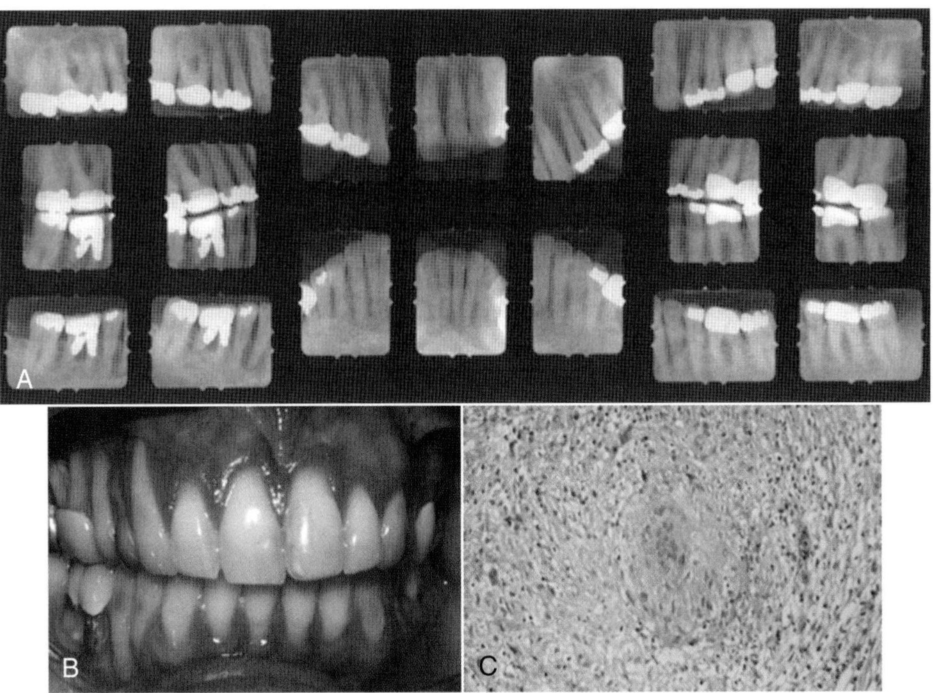

Fig. 5.24 Sarcoidosis after treatment with prednisone. (A) Intraoral x-rays depict remineralization of bone. (B) Reduction in gingival inflammation while extensive recession and clinical attachment loss persist. (C) Pretreatment biopsy.

ulceration and the necrosis of gingival tissue with the exposure and rapid destruction of underlying bone, as well as spontaneous bleeding and severe pain. Like NG, NP has also been associated with severe malnutrition in developing countries. NS is a more severe form of NPDs with soft tissue necrosis extending beyond the gingiva and bone denudation occurring in the area of alveolar mucosa, with potential bony sequestrum formation or osteitis. It usually occurs in patients with significant systemic co-morbidities.

KEY FACT

Necrotizing stomatitis is a serious inflammatory condition that develops in systemically compromised individuals and is characterized by soft tissue necrosis that extends beyond the gingiva, with potential bony sequestrum formation.

TABLE 5.4 Systemic Disorders That Can Result in Loss of Periodontal Tissue Independent of Periodontitis

1. Neoplasms
a. Oral squamous cell carcinoma
b. Odontogenic tumors
c. Other primary neoplasms
d. Secondary metastatic neoplasms
2. Other disorders
a. Granulomatosis with polyangiitis
b. Langerhans cell histiocytosis
c. Giant cell granulomas
d. Hyperparathyroidism
e. Systemic sclerosis (scleroderma)
f. Vanishing bone disease (Gorham-Stout syndrome)

Adapted from Albandar JM, Susin C, Hughes FJ. Manifestations of systemic diseases and conditions that affect the periodontal attachment apparatus: case definitions and diagnostic considerations. *J Clin Periodontol.* 2018;45(Suppl 20):S171–S189.

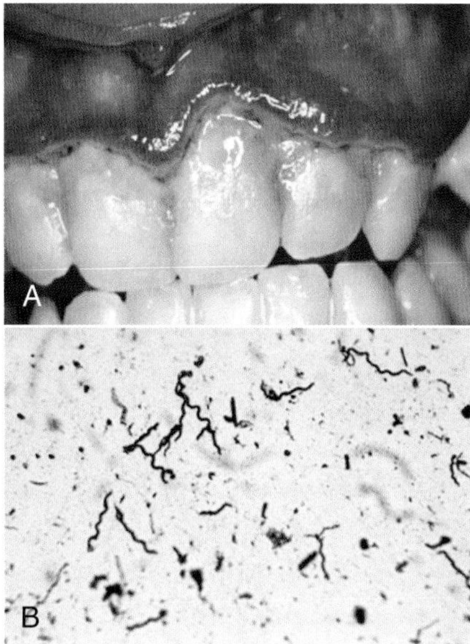

Fig. 5.25 (A) Necrotizing gingivitis illustrating sloughing of marginal gingiva. (B) Phase-contrast microscopy reveals spirochetes in subgingival plaque sample.

Other Periodontal Conditions: Periodontal Abscesses

A periodontal abscess is a localized acute and purulent infection within the gingival wall of the periodontal pocket. The tissue destruction is rapid, and the infection is associated with risk of systemic dissemination.[42] Periodontal abscesses are common infections in the oral cavity that require immediate management. These abscesses should be classified according to the etiological factors, including pre-existing deep periodontal pockets, foreign body reactions, overgrowth of opportunistic bacteria, or inadequate orthodontic forces. Identifying these etiologic factors can help clinical management. The clinical, microbiologic, immunologic, and predisposing characteristics are discussed in Chapters 10, 11, and 24.

Other Periodontal Conditions: Endodontic–Periodontal Lesions

Endodontic-periodontal lesions (EPLs) are clinical conditions present in a tooth with a pathological communication between the pulpal and periodontal tissues and can manifest in acute or chronic forms.[21,42] The primary etiological factors include: (1) endodontic and/or periodontal infections; (2) trauma and/or iatrogenic factors (e.g., root fracture or cracking, root/pulp chamber/furcation perforation, external root resorption or pulp necrosis). The endodontic and periodontal infections may happen in sequence or simultaneously: EPLs might be triggered by pulp infection first that then affect the periodontium (Figs. 5.27 and 5.28); triggered by periodontal destruction first which then affect pulp tissues; or triggered by both pulp and periodontal infections concomitantly. It is somewhat uncommon for periodontal infection to lead to endodontic infection than vice versa.

The most common signs and symptoms of EPLs are deep periodontal pockets reaching or close to the root apex with negative or altered response to pulp vitality tests. Spontaneous pain, pain on percussion, presence of sinus tract, suppuration, gingival inflammation, tooth mobility, and bone loss in the periapical or furcation region are commonly reported. The symptoms might be less evident when the lesion is primarily induced by periodontal infection. EPLs are classified by signs and symptoms that have direct impact on tooth prognosis and treatment options.[21] Two major classifications are (1) EPL with root damage, and (2) EPL without root damage. When the EPL has root damage, the lesion can be further categorized based on the etiological factors: (i) root fracture or cracking, (ii) root canal or pulp chamber perforation, or (iii) external root resorption. When there is no root damage associated with EPL, the lesion can be further categorized into (i) EPL in periodontitis patients or (ii) EPL in non-periodontitis patients. Then a grade can be assigned to EPLs according to the extent of periodontal destruction: Grade 1: narrow deep periodontal pocket in one tooth surface; Grade 2: wide deep periodontal pocket in one tooth surface; Grade 3: deep periodontal pockets in greater than one tooth surface. Generally, a tooth with EPL caused by root fracture, perforation, or severe periodontal destruction has the worst prognosis.

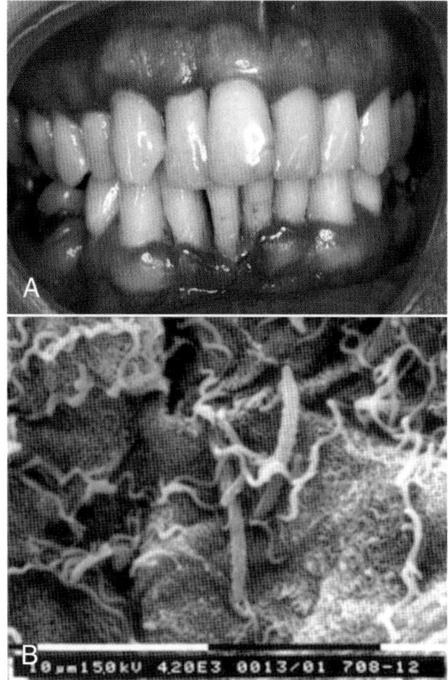

Fig. 5.26 (A) Necrotizing periodontitis with severe clinical attachment loss in a 28-year-old male infected with human immunodeficiency virus. (B) Spirochetes noted on surface of sloughed epithelial cells.

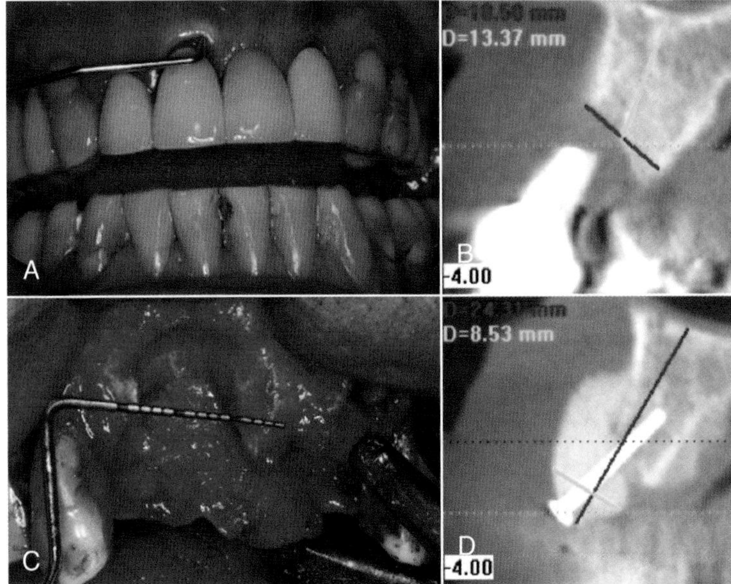

Fig. 5.27 (A) and (C) Clinical images of extensive loss of alveolar ridge secondary to periapical endodontic lesion. (B) CT scan depicts alveolar bone loss. (D) CT image of regenerated ridge via allogenic bone graft, tenting screw, and membrane.

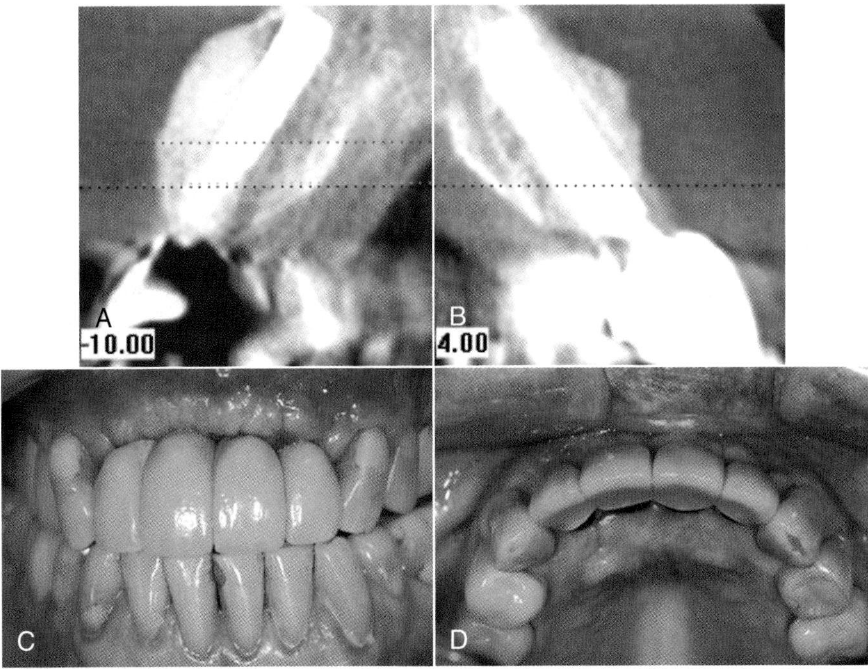

Fig. 5.28 Same patient depicted in Fig. 5.27. (A and B) CT scans of regenerated ridge with implants placed in areas 7, 9, and 10. (C and D) Clinical images of implant-supported bridge.

CLINICAL CORRELATION

If endodontic infection is the primary factor, root canal therapy may be the only treatment necessary to restore the periodontal apparatus of the tooth with endodontic-periodontal lesions.

Other Periodontal Conditions: Mucogingival Deformities and Conditions

Mucogingival deformity is a generic term used to describe the mucogingival junction and its relationship to the gingiva (Fig. 5.29), the alveolar mucosa, and frenula muscle attachments. A mucogingival deformity is a significant departure from the normal shape of the gingiva and the alveolar mucosa, and it may involve the underlying alveolar bone. Mucogingival surgery and periodontal plastic and aesthetic surgery correct defects in the morphology, position, or amount of gingiva. This subject is described in detail in Chapter 65. The surgical correction of mucogingival deformities may be performed for aesthetic reasons, to enhance function, or to facilitate oral hygiene.[46]

Other Periodontal Conditions: Occlusal Trauma and Traumatic Occlusal Forces

Traumatic occlusal force is defined as any occlusal force, which may exceed the adaptive capacity of the individual person or site, resulting in injury of the teeth and/or the periodontal attachment

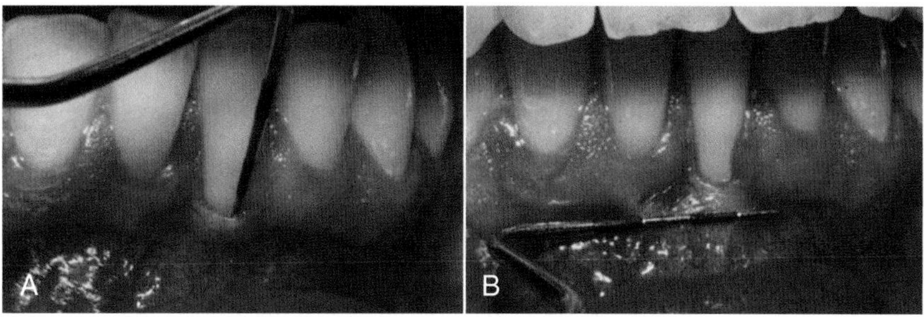

Fig. 5.29 (A) Mucogingival defect depicted by recession. (B) Defects extend into alveolar mucosa and lack keratinized tissue.

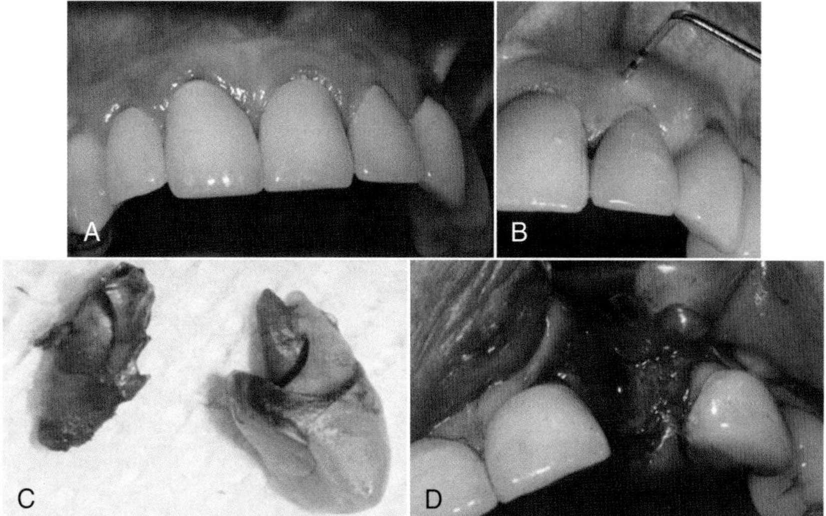

Fig. 5.30 (A and B) Clinical images of fistula tract. (C) Root fracture. (D) Resultant alveolar ridge defect.

apparatus.[24] The signs and symptoms of traumatic occlusal forces include fremitus, tooth mobility, tooth migration, excessive occlusal wear, thermal sensitivity, discomfort/pain on chewing, fractured teeth, radiographically widened periodontal ligament space, root resorption, and hypercementosis. Occlusal trauma is a histologic term describing the injury to the periodontal attachment apparatus. Traumatic occlusal forces can be classified into primary occlusal trauma (injury resulting in tissue changes at a tooth or teeth with normal periodontal support); secondary occlusal trauma (injury resulting in tissue changes at a tooth or teeth with reduced support); or orthodontic forces. So far, there is no strong clinical evidence that traumatic occlusal forces result in periodontal attachment loss, non-carious cervical lesions, or gingival recessions.[15,24] The causes of traumatic occlusal forces and the effect of this trauma on the periodontium[15] are discussed in detail in Chapters 34 and 35.

Other Periodontal Conditions: Prostheses and Tooth-Related Factors That Modify or Predispose to Plaque-Induced Gingival Diseases/Periodontitis

Several conditions, associated with prostheses and teeth, may predispose to plaque accumulation resulting in periodontal diseases. Localized tooth related factors include tooth anatomic factors, root fractures, cervical root resorption, cemental tears, root proximity and altered passive eruption.[14] Tooth anatomic factors are associated with malformations of tooth development or tooth location. Anatomic factors (e.g., cervical enamel projections, palatal grooves, enamel pearls) have been associated with clinical attachment loss, especially in furcation areas. Cervical enamel projections are found on 15% to 24% of mandibular molars and on 9% to 25% of maxillary molars, and strongly associated with furcation involvement.[35]

Palatogingival grooves, which are found primarily on maxillary incisors, are observed in 1% to 8.5% of the population and are associated with increased plaque accumulation and clinical attachment, as well as bone loss.[59] Proximal root grooves on incisors and maxillary premolars also predispose individuals to plaque accumulation, inflammation, and the loss of clinical attachment and bone. Tooth location is considered important for the initiation and development of disease. Misaligned teeth predispose individuals to plaque accumulation with resultant inflammation in children, and they may predispose adults to clinical attachment loss, especially when they are associated with poor oral hygiene habits. Open interproximal contacts that contribute to food impaction have been associated with an increased loss of attachment.[25]

Root fractures may be associated with endodontic or restorative procedures, as well as traumatic forces (Fig. 5.30A–C) and may lead to periodontal involvement through the apical migration of plaque along the fracture line (see Fig. 5.30D). Invasive cervical root resorption (ICR) (as noted on the cone-beam computed tomography scans shown in Fig. 5.31A and B) and cemental tears may lead to periodontal destruction when the lesion communicates with the oral cavity and allows bacteria to migrate subgingivally. The atraumatic removal of teeth with extensive cervical resorption lesions and the reconstruction of resultant ridge defects with bone grafts, dental implants, and prostheses are viable solutions for such defects (Fig. 5.32). Avulsed teeth that are reimplanted frequently develop ankylosis and cervical root resorption many years after reimplantation.

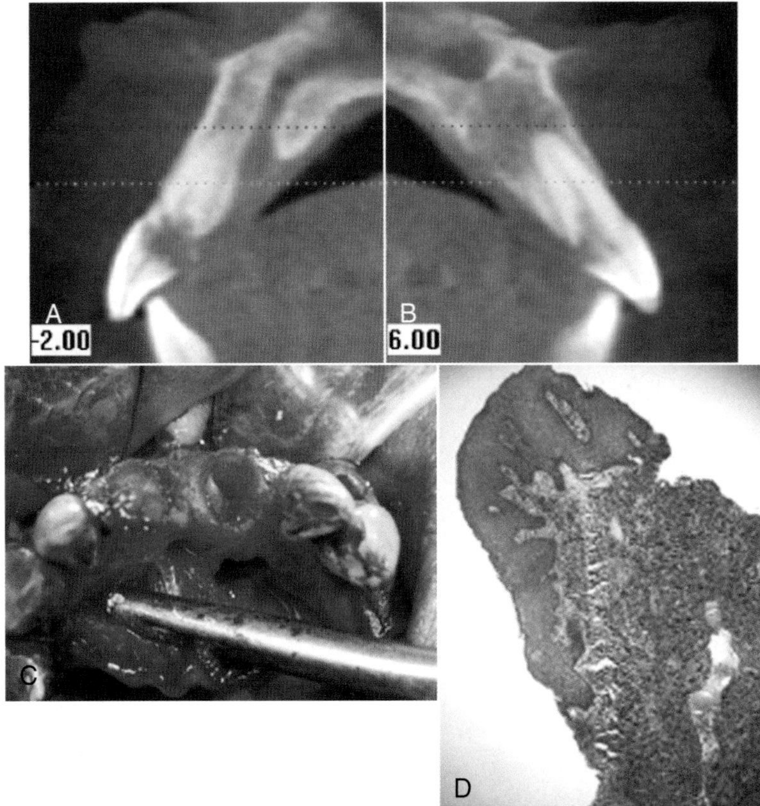

Fig. 5.31 (A and B) CT scans reveal severe cervical root resorption of maxillary central incisors and periapical abscess. (C) Crowns fractured because of resorption. (D) Biopsy of soft tissue from resorption.

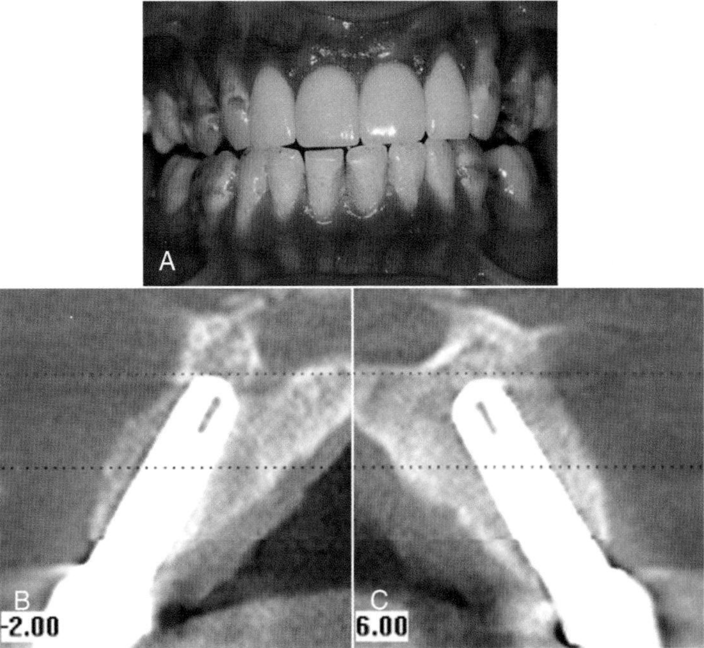

Fig. 5.32 (A) Posttreatment clinical image of same patient depicted in Fig. 5.31 with implant-supported crowns and veneers on laterals. (B and C) CT scans of bone grafts and implants replacing central incisors lost as the result of severe cervical root resorption.

If the patient is still in the phase of skeletal growth, decoronation may be the treatment of choice for ridge preservation. In adults with completed skeletal growth, atraumatic removal of such ankylosed teeth, followed by ridge reconstruction and placement of implants and prosthesis, is a viable treatment option (see Fig. 5.32).

Localized dental prosthesis related factors include restoration margins placed within the supracrestal attached tissues (previous biologic width), clinical procedures related to the fabrication of indirect restorations, and hypersensitivity/toxicity reactions to dental materials.

Dental restorations or appliances are frequently associated with the development of gingival inflammation. Restorations placed deep in the sulcus or within the junctional epithelium may impinge on the supracresal tissue attachment (previous biologic width) resulting in inflammation and the loss of clinical attachment and bone. Contour of a complete crown restoration can affect plaque retention, with flat surfaces being more hygienic as compared to convex restorations exhibiting increased bulk of material at the cervical region. Optimal restoration margins located within the gingival sulcus may not cause gingival inflammation if patients are compliant with oral care and professional cleaning. Detailed information on the interactions between restorative factors and periodontium can be found in Chapter 45.

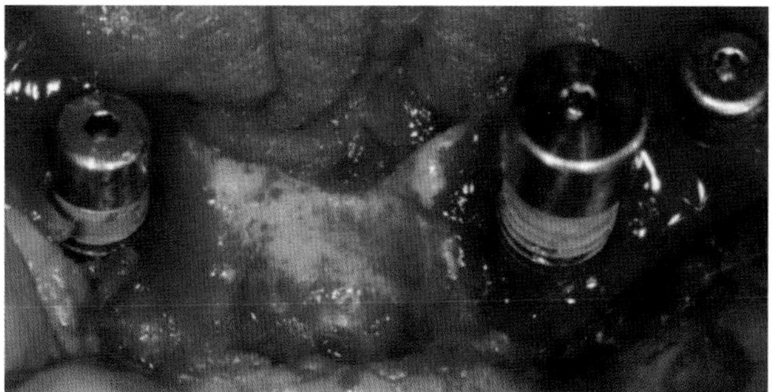

Fig. 5.34 A case of peri-implantitis. (Note the exposed threads of the two implants that are denuded of bone. Also note the bony socket following explantation of the implant.)

Peri-Implant Diseases and Conditions

One major addition to the periodontal classification system is the introduction of a new category for peri-implant conditions (Box 5.3).[7]

Peri-implant health is clinically characterized by the absence of visual signs of inflammation and lack of BOP. In contrast, peri-implant mucositis exhibits visual signs of inflammation and/or BOP but without loss of supportive or marginal bone. Peri-implantitis is a pathological condition with inflammation and/or BOP accompanied by progressive loss of supportive bone (Figs. 5.33 and 5.34). If longitudinal data are unavailable to determine bone level changes over time, peri-implantitis can be diagnosed by the presence of BOP and/or suppuration, probing depths ≥6 mm and bone levels (≥3 mm) apical to the most coronal portion of the intraosseous part of the implant. Further, based on ample evidence that hard and soft tissue ridge profiles are diminished following tooth loss these peri-implant hard and soft tissue deficiencies are now included in the classification under the category of Peri-implant Soft and Hard Tissue Deficiencies. Detailed description of these conditions and their management can be found in Chapter 86.

Endodontic-Peri-Implant Lesions

Recently, it was reported that endodontic lesions may affect peri-implant tissues in addition to periodontal tissues. Previously, it was known that residual endodontic bacteria can cause a condition referred to as "retrograde peri-implantitis," which is radiographically defined as a radiolucent lesion surrounding the apex of an implant. These lesions are generally non-progressive and do not compromise implant functional stability. However, a new disease entity was described in 2020 and referred to as Endodontic-Peri-implant (aka Endo-implant) defects. In the description of this entity, two cases were reported, in which peri-implant bone loss occurred in the coronal half of the implant adjacent to a tooth with an EPL. In both cases the defects were resolved by dental treatment either via endodontic therapy or tooth extraction.[11] This entity was first described following the world workshop for classification of periodontal and peri-implant diseases. Further studies are needed to determine the prevalence of such lesions and to confirm whether endodontic treatment results in resolution of peri-implant bone loss.

BOX 5.3 Peri-Implant Diseases and Conditions (Fig. 5.33)

- Peri-implant health
- Peri-implant mucositis
- Peri-implantitis
- Peri-implant soft and hard tissue deficiencies

Acknowledgment

The authors would like to thank Dr. Georgia K. Johnson (the University of Iowa) for her thorough review of this chapter.

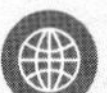

Case Scenarios are found on the companion website eBooks.Health.Elsevier.com.

References for this chapter are found on the companion website eBooks.Health.Elsevier.com.

Fig 5.33 Schematic showing peri-implant health, peri-implant mucositis, and peri-implantitis. (Note the bone loss noted in peri-implantitis.) (From Pirih FQ, Galvan M, Ishii M. Core concepts: Introduction to peri-implant health, mucositis and peri-implantitis. In Newman MG, et al. *Newman and Carranza's clinical periodontology*, ebook, 13th edition. Elsevier; 2019.)

CHAPTER 6

Fundamentals in the Methods of Periodontal Disease Epidemiology

Philippe P. Hujoel | Georgios A. Kotsakis

CHAPTER OUTLINE

The Need for Epidemiology

The World Health Organization (WHO) defines epidemiology as "the study of the distribution and determinants of health-related states or events (including disease), and the application of this study to the control of diseases and other health problems." Distinct study designs are employed to examine the distribution of periodontal diseases in populations and determine their etiology and association with other diseases; the ultimate goal is to determine evidence-driven preventive and therapeutic strategies. "Periodontal [gum] diseases, including gingivitis and destructive periodontal disease, are serious infections."[75] This 2009 statement from a professional dental organization reflected the dominating belief accepted since the 1960s that bacteria cause periodontal conditions.[19] This bacterial dogma had several consequences. Clinical management and research became largely focused on vaccines, microbial diagnosis, antimicrobials, antibiotics, dental plaque, and immunology. Clinical diagnoses that did not fit the infection paradigm (e.g., periodontal atrophy) were eliminated from some periodontal disease classifications, and it was hypothesized that periodontal infections caused systemic diseases.

However, are periodontal diseases infectious? A reliable answer to this question requires epidemiologic evidence. This chapter focuses on the role of epidemiology in the study of human diseases. ***Case-control studies*** and ***cohort studies*** are two epidemiologic study designs that identify common causes of chronic diseases (e.g., smoking, ionizing radiation, hepatitis B, and high blood pressure). *Randomized controlled trials* are study designs that assess the diagnosis, management, and prognosis of chronic diseases and that either confirm or refute the suspected causes of disease identified in case-control or cohort studies. Prostate surface antigen screening, polio vaccination, and hormone replacement therapy are examples of diagnoses and treatments for chronic diseases that were evaluated by means of randomized controlled trials.

> **Study Designs**
>
> Epidemiologic study designs fall within two broad categories: observational and interventional studies. As the terms imply, assigning a study to one of these categories depends on if the investigators assess the efficacy of an intervention (interventional) or if the intervention is not under control of the investigators (observational). Examples of interventional studies in oral health research are randomized clinical trials and nonrandomized clinical trials. Examples of observational studies are cross-sectional studies, cohort studies, and case-control studies.

Some essential characteristics of epidemiologic studies are that they are conducted in humans, a control or a comparison group, and clinically relevant endpoints are evaluated. Such studies are available to support the direct effects that oral bacteria have on reversible gingival inflammation.[76] However, studies commonly cited in support of the periodontal infection hypothesis often lack these elements. For instance, is a "burst" of bone loss[21] subsequent to the implantation of *Bacteroides gingivalis* (now *Porphyromonas gingivalis*) in an animal model, proof that "this microorganism [is] of great importance to the control of destructive periodontal disease"? Opponents of this hypothesis could argue that in similar animal models nicotine injections alone have a direct effect on periodontal bone loss, thus satisfying the biologic plausibility criterion for causality.[56] Nevertheless, in contemporary practice, the strength of scientific evidence is formally ranked based on the study design. One widely used level of evidence classification by the Oxford Center for Evidence-Based Medicine (http://www.cebm.net/wp-content/uploads/2014/06/CEBM-Levels-of-Evidence-2.1.pdf) generally considers animal studies (i.e., mechanism-based reasoning) as having the lowest level of evidence to impact clinical thinking. In contrast, systematic reviews of randomized controlled trials generally are considered the highest available level of evidence.

Systematic Review Versus Expert Opinion

A systematic review is considered a form of secondary research that aims to screen the entire breadth of information on a selected topic, identify relevant research studies, and summarize their findings. The critical difference between an expert opinion review and a systematic review is that the latter is more objective than the former. It intends to summarize the available body of literature inclusively and not based on the author's opinion on which studies are noteworthy or impactful. Systematic reviews are considered high level and are often used to guide clinical decision-making, but the clinicians should be aware that their conclusions suffer from the shortcomings of the included studies.

Epidemiologic studies, which are at a higher level than case reports and animal studies, have had a powerful impact on reducing the incidence of some chronic diseases by reliably identifying their primary causes. Reliable evidence on what causes disease allows laboratory research to focus on elucidating the causal pathways of disease, which can then lead to clinical trials. "Medical science continually passes the baton of discovery from [epidemiologic] observation to laboratory studies to human clinical trials."[42] For example, epidemiologic observations identified hepatitis B as the leading cause of liver carcinoma, one of the most common cancers globally.[3] Subsequently, the baton of discovery was passed to basic science, with which a recombinant engineered vaccine for hepatitis B was developed. The baton of discovery then passed to clinical trialists, who assessed the effectiveness of vaccinations and documented dramatic declines in mortality rates from liver cancer.[41] Similar success stories in managing chronic diseases in which epidemiology played a critical role include coronary heart disease and blood pressure medication, dental caries and fluoride, and lung cancer and smoking intervention programs.

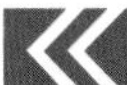

FLASH BACK

Recall that well-designed interventional studies generally are higher level than observational studies.

The emerging epidemiologic evidence regarding the cause of periodontal diseases suggests that factors such as cigarette smoking, sugar, cereals, and chronic diseases such as diabetes could be primary causes of periodontal disease.[5,22,67] Notably, the 2004 US Surgeon General report concluded that the evidence was sufficient to infer a causal relationship between smoking and periodontitis.[77] Organizations such as the WHO suggest that periodontal disease prevention be made an integral part of programs that focus on tobacco control, diet, and physical activity, which are also shared risk factors with other prevalent chronic diseases such as cardiovascular diseases.[58] Regardless of an individual's personal beliefs concerning the causes of periodontal disease, becoming familiar with the epidemiologic methodology may be necessary to judge this emerging evidence independently and critically.

Measuring the Occurrence of Conditions or Diseases

The fundamental tools of epidemiology are simple sums and divisions that reflect how many individuals or sites have or will develop a particular condition or disease.

The ***prevalence*** is the sum of all examined individuals or sites that exhibit the condition or disease of interest divided by the sum of the number of individuals or sites examined. The prevalence can range from 0% (no one has the condition or disease of interest) to 100% (everyone has the condition or disease of interest).

As an example of prevalence, the Centers for Disease Control and Prevention reported about the prevalence of individuals with at least one periodontal pocket depth of 4 mm or deeper. From 1988 to 1994, slightly more than 1 in 5 Americans had such a condition, for a prevalence of approximately 20%; from 1999 to 2004, only 1 in 10 Americans fell into this category,[15] for a prevalence of approximately 10%. These findings suggest greater than a 50% decline in the prevalence of pocket depths greater than or equal to 4 mm for adults between the ages of 20 and 64 years, which occurred over approximately a decade. These epidemiologic data confirm another report of declining destructive periodontal disease prevalence in the United States.[7] Such information regarding prevalence measures of periodontal conditions may have implications for human resource needs in the United States and may provide clues concerning the causative factors that drive such changes. Unfortunately, many countries do not have prevalence surveillance systems,[58] making it difficult to determine whether these trends observed in the United States are isolated events or part of a more general trend.

The *risk* is the probability that an individual or a site will develop a particular condition or disease during follow-up. The risk for a condition or a disease is a number that ranges between 0% and 100%. The simplest way to estimate risk is to have a fixed number of persons or sites at risk at some defining moment (i.e., time zero [t_0]). Individuals or sites within individuals are followed up over time after this defining moment. After a follow-up period (i.e., from t_0 to t_n), the risk can be calculated as the proportion of persons or sites in which the clinical outcome of interest develops during the follow-up period. Because the risk is estimated as a proportion, it is without dimension, and it ranges between 0 and 1. When a risk is reported, it should be accompanied by a specific time period to which it is applied. For example, a 5% risk for death may be considered small when it refers to a 20-year period but significant when it refers to a 3-month period.

For example, consider concerns regarding occupational human immunodeficiency virus (HIV) infection among dentists. It has been reported that the risk for developing an HIV infection within 1 year of an accidental needlestick with HIV-contaminated blood is 0.3%. Such a statistic has an intuitive appeal and can be related to patients or colleagues. For example, a risk of 0.003 (0.3%) indicates that for every 1000 individuals who have an accidental HIV-contaminated needlestick, 3 are expected to develop an HIV infection within 1 year of the event.

The *odds* for an event is the probability that an event occurred divided by the probability that an event did not occur. Whereas probability is a value that ranges between 0 and 1, odds values range from 0 to infinity. If the probability for observing an event is small, then the odds and the probability are almost identical. For example, if the probability for a vertical root fracture after an endodontic procedure is 0.001, then the odds are 0.001/0.999 or 0.001001. Odds are commonly reported in studies because they are often easier to estimate with statistical models than probabilities. For example, the odds for developing an HIV infection after an accidental needlestick with HIV-contaminated blood are 0.003 (0.003/0.997).

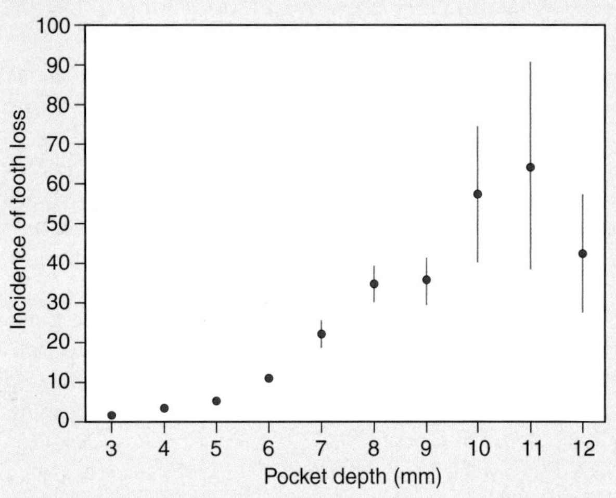

Fig. 6.1 Rate of tooth loss per 1000 tooth-years as a function of maximum probing depth per tooth in a cohort of 1021 patients between the ages of 40 and 65 years under periodontal specialist care for destructive form of periodontal disease. (Data from Hujoel PP, Cunha-Cruz J, Selipsky H, et al. Abnormal pocket depth and gingival recession as distinct phenotypes. *Periodontol 2000*. 2005;39:22–29.)

***Incidence** rates* are an alternative measure to describe disease occurrence. One example of an incidence rate is the speedometer in a car that displays at any given time the number of kilometers being traveled per hour. In clinical trials or epidemiology, the rate reflects the number of disease occurrences per person-time or site-time. The *disease rate* is a ratio in which the numerator is the number of subjects or sites diagnosed with the disease of interest and the denominator is the sum of the time at risk over all subjects or sites in the population.

Incidence Versus Prevalence

Recall that prevalence is the proportion of a population found to have a condition at a given point in time (e.g., 9% of the US population had severe periodontitis in the 2009–10 NHANES survey), while incidence is the probability that a disease will occur in a previously healthy population over a period of time (e.g., the incidence of peri-implantitis for patients with mandibular over-dentures is 17% after 5 years).

Incidence rates—as opposed to the previously introduced measures of disease occurrence—imply an element of time. The denominator in the incidence rate has time as the dimension. Thus, the dimension of incidence rate is 1/time. This dimension is often referred to as "person-time" or "site-time" to distinguish the time summation from ordinary clock-time. The magnitude of the incidence rate can vary between 0 and infinity. When there are no new disease onsets during the study period, the incidence rate is 0. When every person observed dies instantaneously at the start of the study (thus, the sum of the periods is 0), the incidence rate is infinity.

An example of the application of rates in which the number of teeth lost per 1000 tooth-years is plotted as a function of the maximum probing depth at the start of follow-up is provided in Fig. 6.1. The plot suggests a nonlinear relationship between maximum pocket depth and tooth loss, with a substantial increase in tooth loss rate for teeth with 7 mm or deeper periodontal pockets.

For the study of risk, the population studied is usually limited to those individuals at risk for the outcome of interest. Thus, if the outcome of interest is a disease, the following subjects are excluded from the cohort: persons who already have the disease, persons who have immunity to the disease, and persons who are biologically incapable of developing the disease.

Periodontal Measures Typically Recorded Clinically

A periodontal examination can measure various characteristics of the periodontium. Dental records of periodontal patients typically contain information regarding the teeth that are present, missing, or impacted, and measurable information about the periodontal status of those teeth. Information such as clinical probing depth, bleeding on probing (BOP), gingival recession, mobility of teeth, and the presence of furcation involvements can be charted. In addition, some clinicians may collect information about the presence of gingivitis by evaluating the color and form of the gingival tissues. These measures can be complemented with radiographic examinations that may provide information about marginal bone levels.

In research settings or in some selected private practices, additional periodontal measures may be collected, such as clinical attachment levels, microbiologic measures, gingival crevicular fluid volume, biomarkers in the crevicular fluid, and indices that measure the amount of gingival inflammation or dental plaque or debris accumulation.

Two standard measures of gingival inflammation are the Gingival Index (GI) and BOP.[25] The GI was proposed in 1963 as a method for assessing the severity and quantity of gingival inflammation.[46,47] With this particular index, only gingival tissues are assessed. Each of the four gingival areas of the tooth (i.e., facial, mesial, distal, and lingual) are assessed for inflammation and rated as normal gingiva (a score of 0) to severely inflamed gingiva with a tendency to bleed spontaneously (a score of 3). Gingiva that is mildly inflamed but without BOP is given a score of 1, whereas moderately inflamed gingiva with bleeding is given a score of 2. The scores can be averaged for each patient to provide patient means. Alternatively, site-specific analyses can relate local and patient-specific factors to the GI that is measured at individual sites.[13]

Bleeding on Probing Versus Gingival Index

In clinical settings, the term *gingival index* is often misused in lieu of bleeding on probing (BOP). According to the existing nomenclature, gingival index is a categorical index that assesses the severity of gingival inflammation on a scale from 0 to 3. Conversely, BOP is a binary index (i.e., Yes/No) that determines whether or not a site is BOP. The two must not be confused.

BOP is another measure of periodontal inflammation. The specific approach to obtaining a bleeding measure can vary from one study to the next and from one clinician to another. For example, in the third National Health and Nutrition Examination Survey (NHANES III),[54] bleeding measures were obtained. First, the facial and mesiofacial sites of teeth in two randomly selected quadrants—one maxillary and one mandibular—were selected. A special probe known as the *National Institute of Dental Research probe* was used in these assessments. This color-coded probe is marked at 2, 4, 6, 8, 10, and 12 mm. Next, the examiner dried a quadrant of teeth with air to begin the assessment.

Then, starting with the most posterior tooth in the quadrant (excluding the third molar), the examiner placed a periodontal probe 2 mm into the gingival sulcus at the facial site and carefully swept the probe from the mesiofacial to the mesial interproximal area. After probing the sites in the quadrant, the examiner assessed the presence or absence of bleeding at each probed site. The same procedure was repeated for the remaining quadrant.

Commonly used measures of periodontal tissue destruction include mean probing depth, mean attachment loss, and mean recession level.[32] The clinical protocols regarding how such mean values are collected and calculated can vary considerably. One example of how such values can be ascertained clinically is described in the National Institute of Dental and Craniofacial Research "periodontal destruction" examination.[54] This examination includes an assessment of periodontal attachment loss[65] as the distance in millimeters from the cemento-enamel junction to the bottom of the gingival sulcus. This distance was measured at the facial and mesiofacial sites of teeth in a randomly selected maxillary and mandibular quadrant with the use of the indirect measurement method developed by Ramfjord.[65]

Sensitivity Versus Specificity

Sensitivity is defined as the number of diseased patients who are correctly identified as having disease—that is, the diagnostic marker leads to a minimum number of false negative diagnoses. *Specificity* is defined as the number of healthy persons who are correctly determined to not have the disease—that is, the diagnostic marker leads to a minimum number of false positive diagnoses.

Translating Periodontal Measures Into Traditional Epidemiologic Measures of Disease Occurrence

Applying the traditional epidemiologic methods of risk, prevalence, and rate was challenging, because medical epidemiologists typically deal with patients. Dental epidemiologists deal with as many as 188 sites per patient. These periodontal sites within patients are correlated with many host-related factors. For example, gingival bleeding is suppressed in smokers.[6] Therefore BOP in periodontal sites in smokers tends to be more alike than BOP in periodontal sites among nonsmokers. Sites within patients are not statistically independent. The statistical methodology that is used to deal with correlated observations can be complex, and for most of the 20th century it was challenging to calculate the confidence intervals for site-specific risks or prevalence.[34] As a result, clinicians could not obtain reliable information regarding whether a periodontal site colonized with a particular microbiologic species was at an increased risk for periodontal attachment loss. These challenges may have hampered progress in building causal models of periodontal disease.

A common approach to dealing with this challenge of correlated observations was to summarize site-specific periodontal data at the patient level. These summaries could be calculated in a variety of ways. For example, the information about the presence of bleeding in up to 188 periodontal sites in a patient could be summarized as the presence of at least 1 bleeding site, the presence of at least 5 bleeding sites, or a patient mean value.

The advent of modern statistical techniques to deal with the problem of correlated data made it possible to avoid summarizing site-specific information at a patient level.[13,14,28,33,34] These methods allow for the exploration of the role of patient- and site-specific factors in local site-specific events. For example, this can be used to determine whether the 3-mm loss of attachment at a site is related to site-specific factors (e.g., microflora present at that site), host factors (e.g., serum cotinine levels), or an interaction between a site-specific factor and a host factor.

True and Surrogate Measures of the Periodontal Condition

The epidemiology of true and surrogate endpoints of periodontal disease do not necessarily coincide. *True endpoints* are tangible outcomes that directly measure how a patient feels, functions, or survives.[17] True endpoints include oral health-related quality-of-life measurements[40,48,71] and self-reported problems, such as a positive answer to the following question: "When you brush or floss your teeth, do you notice bleeding that is both regular and that involves spitting blood-stained saliva?" Dental patient reported outcome measures (PROMs) include how patients feel and function and their overall patient-reported satisfaction, phonetics, chewing comfort, stability, cleanability, and aesthetics.[53] PROMs must be reported directly by the patient without interpretation by anyone else, including the dentist. (See Chapter 1 for more information about PROMs.)

Surrogate endpoints are intangible to the patient.[74] Surrogate endpoints in periodontal research include anatomic measures (e.g., probing depth), measures of inflammation (e.g., bleeding), microbiologic measures, and immunologic measures.[13] Surrogate endpoints are often objective because they can be measured by the clinician (rather than relying on self-report by patients) or by laboratory methods.

Surrogate endpoints can be misleading when the goal is to provide reliable information about clinical decisions related to diagnosis, etiology, treatment, or prognosis. An overview of situations in clinical research in which surrogate endpoints have led to misleading conclusions is provided in Table 3.1 on the Expert Consult website. One periodontal example is the use of systemic antibiotics that may have a beneficial impact on attachment gain[19] but a potential increased risk for tooth loss.[11]

Periodontal Endpoints: Examples

True endpoints: Tooth loss, patient's quality of life, and oral function
Surrogate endpoints: Probing depths, BOP, microbial measures

Challenges of Obtaining Epidemiologic Measures of Periodontal Conditions and Diseases

Among the challenges that periodontal epidemiologists face are the continuous changes in the type of surrogate data collected, the paucity of information about whether surrogate information provides reliable information regarding outcomes of tangible patient benefit (i.e., outcomes that the patient cares about), and the lack of diagnostic codes for the reasons for tooth loss. Accruing evidence points in the direction of commonly used surrogate measures being poor predictors of periodontal status.[52]

The diversity of measures used to assess periodontal condition or disease is staggering. One survey of periodontal clinical trials conducted over a mere 4-year period indicated that 153 distinct surrogate endpoints were defined and that more than 80% of these endpoints were used in fewer than 5 of the 82 trials.[25] Another survey similarly identified the diversity of methodologies and definitions as a challenging issue when systematically reviewing evidence.[62] This continuous creation of "new and improved" surrogate outcomes in periodontal research is likely an essential driver of false-positive conclusions.[27]

The types of periodontal measures that are favored also depend on the era. Russell developed the Periodontal Index,[66] which scored the supporting tissues for each tooth in the mouth according to a progressive scale that gives little weight to gingival inflammation and relatively great weight to advanced periodontal disease. Although the Periodontal Index was used in the first National Health and Nutrition Examination Survey (NHANES), thereby gaining national prominence in the United States, it was never used again in any of the subsequent NHANES versions. Since then, most periodontal surveys in the United States have employed different examination protocols. The survey methodology has been changed yet again, leading to significant variations in disease estimates.[16] Studies of decreases in the use of scaling and root planing procedures in the state of Washington and at a national level,[8,64] long-term trends in decreasing edentulism, and decreasing periodontitis prevalence estimates in national surveys with consistent methodology[15] suggest that periodontitis prevalence in the United States is dropping rapidly (Tables 6.1 and 6.2).

A second challenge when interpreting periodontal statistics is the common lack of information about measures that matter to patients (e.g., tooth loss, quality-of-life issues related to oral health). This situation creates challenges when interpreting evidence. For example, it is similar to tracking prostate cancer by measuring inflammation or swelling of the prostate gland without knowing how this information relates to prostate cancer mortality. This challenge is further compounded by the absence of diagnostic codes for tooth loss, which has largely prevented the obtaining of reliable information about how many teeth are lost as a result of periodontal disease as opposed to dental caries.

Finally, the attempt to track a disease by only collecting a surrogate outcome measure such as probing depth from the teeth that are present leads to a type of bias that is typically referred to as *survival bias*. Most periodontal clinical trials performed during the 20th century evaluated the effect of periodontal therapies on those teeth that survived the treatment. The more teeth that are lost, the more meaningless such data become. The imputation of data can provide an understanding of the extent to which such biases may alter the conclusions of studies.

In summary, the fundamental tool of periodontal epidemiology is a measure of the occurrence of periodontal conditions. These measures include epidemiologic statistics (e.g., prevalence, risk, rate) and focus on either patient- or site-specific markers (e.g., oral health-related quality of life, tooth loss, anatomic measures, and measures of gingival inflammation). This wealth of possibilities when defining periodontal conditions in combination with statistical challenges when handling correlated data has made it difficult to answer even a simple question such as whether a hidden periodontal disease epidemic occurred during the 20th century.[29]

TABLE 6.1 Periodontal Status of the US Population Among Adults Age 20 to 64 Years

Status	1988–1994	1999–2004
Number of teeth present	24	25
Edentulism	6%	4%
Periodontal disease (i.e., one site with ≥3-mm attachment loss and ≥4-mm pocket depth)	15%	9%
Periodontal disease among the poor	28%	14%
Dental visits	66%	6%
Mean pocket depth	1.47 mm	1.02 mm
Mean loss of attachment	1.07 mm	0.72 mm
≥2-mm recession in at least one site	32%	21%
≥4-mm pocket depth in at least one site	23%	10%
≥4-mm attachment loss in at least one site	25%	17%

TABLE 6.2 Periodontal Status of the US Population Among Adults Aged 65 Years and Older

Status	1988–1994	1999–2004
Number of teeth present	18	19
Edentulism	34.0%	27.0%
Periodontal disease (one site with ≥3-mm attachment loss and ≥4-mm pocket depth)	19.5%	10.5%
Periodontal disease among the poor	26.3%	16.6%
Dental visits	54.0%	55.0%
Mean pocket depth	1.47 mm	1.07 mm
Mean loss of attachment	2.04 mm	1.55 mm
≥2-mm recession in at least one site	73.0%	48.0%
≥4-mm pocket depth in at least one site	22.0%	12.0%
≥4-mm attachment loss in at least one site	59.0%	50.0%

Epidemiologic Study Designs

The essence of epidemiology and clinical epidemiology is to relate measures of disease occurrence to suspected causes or interventions. For example, can the dramatic drop in destructive periodontal disease prevalence in the United States be attributed to a change in smoking prevalence? Can the presence of particular microbiologic species around a tooth be related to the risk of future tooth loss? Can the rate of tooth loss in a sample of elderly patients be related to using an antimicrobial rinse? These questions can be most reliably answered by three epidemiologic study designs with an evidence-based approach. As mentioned earlier in this chapter and briefly introduced in Chapter 2, these study designs (in order of decreasing reliability) are the randomized controlled trial, the cohort study, and the case-control study.

Randomized Controlled Trials

Randomized controlled trials in periodontics typically assign patients or some teeth within a patient randomly to a treatment. Patients are then monitored, and subsequent outcomes are assessed. Table 6.3 provides two examples of randomized controlled trials.

The randomized controlled trial is the only study design that can provide a probabilistic basis for making a causal inference between an intervention and an outcome. Reliable inference regarding the causality of associations can be obtained if the delicate machinery of clinical trial design and analysis is strictly respected. For example, there needs to be a pretrial hypothesis that specifies the endpoint, the treatments to be compared, the patient population, and the degree of required precision. Other important factors for obtaining reliable answers include a secure randomization process, the masking of patients and clinicians, the presence of an independent data and safety monitoring board, and strict adherence to the pretrial hypothesis, which must include an intent-to-treat analysis. Trials with exquisite attention to detail are referred to as *definitive trials,* and they are rare in any field, including periodontal research. Definitive trials are required to provide reliable answers about treatment efficacy. Most of the trials published in the literature are in the category of exploratory trials. These trials typically do not report a pretrial hypothesis, and they conclude that the intervention was successful when compared to the control.[26] These are almost always false-positive conclusions.[27]

TABLE 6.3 Examples of Periodontal Randomized Controlled Trials

Periodontal Treatment	Outcome	Sample Size
Scaling and root planing for pregnant women[51]	Infants with low birth weights	823
Biphasic calcium phosphate ceramic[55]	Clinical attachment level	137

TABLE 6.4 Examples of Periodontal Cohort Studies

Periodontal Exposure	Outcome	Sample Size
Periodontal disease and tooth loss[35]	Coronary heart disease	51,529
Gingivitis[9]	Tooth loss	>500

Cohort Studies

Cohort studies can also be referred to as *exposure-based study designs.* Subjects who are free of the disease of interest are classified with respect to exposure (e.g., cigarette smoking, diabetes) and followed longitudinally to assess periodontal outcomes. Table 6.4 provides two examples of cohort studies.

Cohorts can be defined by a geographic area, records, exposure status, or a combination of different criteria. For example, in one study of the causal factors of edentulism, the population of interest was defined as the inhabitants of the town of Tecumseh, Michigan. Persons within this community were examined in 1959 as part of a community-wide health study. Twenty-eight years later, a subset of these patients was reexamined to study the risk factors for edentulism.[54] Some natural disease history studies of destructive periodontal disease have been conducted based on geographic location (e.g., Norwegian Longitudinal Study[1]; Veterans Administration Longitudinal Study[39]; Sri Lanka Study[2]). A cohort can be defined by records (e.g., schools, health insurance plans, unions, industries, professional organizations). Many cohort studies of periodontal disease outcomes are performed in patients who belong to a particular dental insurance company[12] or to a professional group.[36] Finally, cohorts can be defined based on a specific exposure. For example, different levels of fluoride concentrations in the water supply have been used for the definition of cohorts.

Case-Control Studies

Case-control studies typically are referred to as *outcome-based study designs.* Persons with a condition or outcome of interest (i.e., cases) are compared with persons without a condition of interest (i.e., controls) with respect to the history of the suspected causal factors. Many people intuitively think along the lines of a case-control study when evaluating disease causes. For example, if an individual suffers from food poisoning after a party, he or she is likely to compare past food intake with those individuals who did *not* experience food poisoning. Similarly, if one is diagnosed with a serious illness, a common reaction is to ask, "Why me?" This is usually followed by a comparison of one's history of exposures with those of other individuals who did *not* develop the serious illness. The primary goal of a case-control study is to find out what *past* exposures or factors are different between patients with a disease versus those without the disease. Table 6.5 provides two examples of case-control studies.

TABLE 6.5 Examples of Periodontal Case-Control Studies

Case-Control Criteria	Investigated Risk Factors	Sample Size
Destructive periodontal disease[48]	Smoking	177
Acute myocardial infarction[62]	Dental health	202

The case-control study is a challenging type of study to conduct. Trying to minimize the role of bias in case-control studies requires careful planning, conduct, and analysis. Even when everything is done perfectly, one can come to the wrong conclusions in case-control studies. A review of the quality of periodontal case-control studies suggested that they are frequently inadequately conducted and reported.[45]

Two critical elements of the case-control study design are the definitions of the terms *case* and *control.* A *case* is a person in the population or study group who has been identified as having a particular disease, health disorder, or condition.[10] The case definition should be rigorous to minimize bias and misclassification; it can be based on symptoms, signs, or the results of diagnostic tests. For example, the case definition for a myocardial infarction in a case-control study of the relationship between dental health and acute myocardial infarction was as follows[2]:

1. Symptoms start within 36 hours before the admission
2. No prior myocardial infarction
3. Residing in Helsinki or an immediate neighborhood
4. Younger than 60 years for men and younger than 65 years for women
5. Blood samples available at admission and at 4 weeks

In a case-control study, the *controls* should be at risk for developing the investigated disease and come from the same population that generated the cases. For example, if the investigated disease is root caries, the controls should be at risk for developing root caries (i.e., have exposed root surfaces) and originate from the same population that generated the cases that have root caries.

Causes

Human chronic diseases such as cancer, diabetes, and destructive periodontal disease have complex causes. The terms *necessary cause, component cause,* and *sufficient cause* help define the challenges of determining the cause of a disease and of verbalizing the complexity of chronic disease causes.[65]

The set of causes that initiate a chronic disease is referred to as a *sufficient cause.* Each sufficient cause consists of multiple component causes. Consider the hypothetical example in which four sufficient causes exist for noniatrogenic destructive periodontal disease (Fig. 6.2). The first sufficient cause in this example includes the following component causes: smoking, delayed neutrophil apoptosis, an interleukin-1 gene defect, dental plaque, a tooth, and an unspecified gene defect. These different elements of a sufficient cause are referred to as *component causes.* All component causes of a sufficient cause must be present for the disease process to be initiated. Multiple sufficient causes may be responsible for a given disease. For example, two sufficient causes exist for destructive periodontal diseases that do not include smoking.

A component cause—an element of all the sufficient causes for a given disease—is referred to as a *necessary cause.* For example, fermentable carbohydrates are a necessary cause for dental caries. However, there are very few examples of necessary causes:

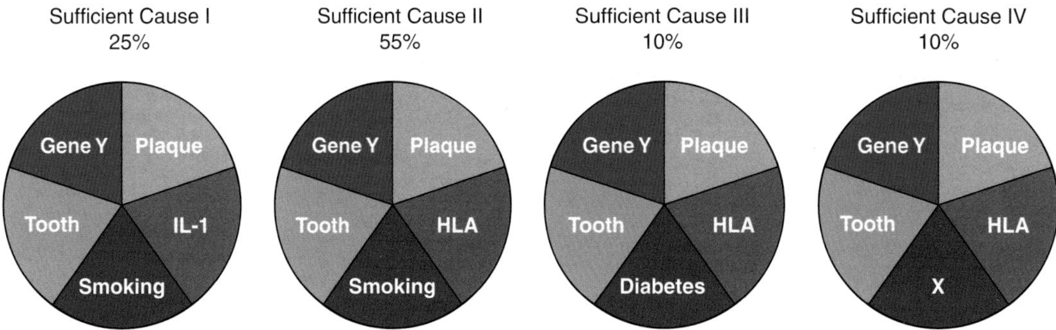

Fig. 6.2 Causes of noniatrogenic periodontitis. *IL-1*, Interleukin-1; *HLA*, human leukocyte antigen. (Data from Rothman KJ. Causes. 1976. *Am J Epidemiol.* 1995;141:90–95.)

smoking is not a necessary cause of lung cancer or destructive periodontal disease, hepatitis B infection is not a necessary cause of liver cancer, and *Streptococcus viridans* is not a necessary cause of bacterial endocarditis. The search for necessary causes of disease is important, because the elimination of such causes could eradicate a disease.

The proportion of disease that results from different component causes is greater than 100%. The component cause "smoking" is responsible for 80% of destructive periodontal disease cases; plaque is responsible for 100%; and diabetes is responsible for 10%.

The complex causal web that leads to the initiation and progression of chronic disease makes the reliable identification of causal components difficult. Since the 1960s, epidemiology has succeeded in reliably identifying some of the causes of human chronic diseases. Now that component causes responsible for a large proportion of cases for particular diseases (e.g., smoking for lung cancer) have been identified, the search for new causes is becoming significantly more challenging. For example, the hope existed that the Human Genome Project would lead to quick advances, but these hopes have not yet been fulfilled. Chronic diseases are typically caused not by one gene but rather by a set of many different genes, with each one responsible for only a small proportion of cases and acting in a variety of synergistic mechanisms for disease initiation.

Suspected Modifiable Causative Factors for Periodontal Disease

Tobacco Smoking

Several organizations recognize tobacco smoking as one of the primary drivers of periodontal disease epidemiology.[5] Many criteria for causality have been satisfied,[18] and smoking cessation has been shown to slow the progression of periodontal disease.[38,39,59] The strong impact of tobacco smoking on periodontal disease has the potential to induce spurious causal associations in other suspected risk factors for periodontal disease. For example, smoking is a risk factor for both type 2 diabetes[78] and periodontal disease, thereby making associations between type 2 diabetes and periodontal disease susceptible to biases. To obtain reliable inferences about causal factors other than smoking, studies of periodontal disease epidemiology may need to be restricted to those who have never smoked.

Nutrition

Several studies have demonstrated relationships between periodontal disease and a variety of medical conditions that center on carbohydrate metabolism, including intake of dietary carbohydrates, exercise, obesity, prediabetes, and diabetes. A systematic review of randomized controlled trials involving carbohydrates suggested that the increased intake of fermentable carbohydrates may cause an increase in gingivitis.[26] Two systematic reviews suggested that diabetes was a risk factor for destructive periodontal disease.[67,70]

Dental Plaque

Several systematic reviews have shown that chemotherapeutic and mechanical plaque control will reduce gingival inflammation. Essential oils[4] and cetylpyridinium-chloride-containing mouthrinses[20] may reduce gingival inflammation. Interdental brushes may reduce dental plaque, bleeding, and probing pocket depth.[72] Power-driven toothbrushes may be more effective than manual toothbrushes for removing plaque and reducing inflammation.[69] Self-performed dental flossing may not be effective for reducing plaque and gingival inflammation.[4] Although these systematic reviews provide evidence about the role of dental plaque in gingival inflammation, they do not necessarily suggest that dental plaque is the primary cause of gingival inflammation.[24] Stomach acids may cause heartburn, and antacids may be effective at eliminating heartburn symptoms. However, this evidence does not make stomach acids a primary cause of heartburn. The primary cause of heartburn may, for instance, be a gluten allergy, and thus the cure of the heartburn requires the elimination of gluten from the diet. Antacids can be considered a palliative that is needed as long as the primary cause has not been identified.

Neither is there reliable evidence that gingival inflammation precedes destructive periodontal disease. There is no reliable randomized controlled trial evidence that oral hygiene has a beneficial impact on the prevention of periodontal destruction.[27,30]

The Cause of Periodontal Disease for the Patient Sitting in Your Chair

In clinical epidemiology, in a court of law, and in modern-day clinical practice, uncertainty regarding the "cause" is an important consideration when discussing causality. The term *attributable risk percentage* is used to express the probability that a suspected causative agent causes a disease. For example, in a smoker with lung cancer, there may be a 20% probability that the lung cancer was caused by a factor other than smoking (e.g., radon). In an obese person with diabetes, there may be a 10% chance that obesity played no role in the onset of diabetes. For a worker with leukemia in the nuclear industry, there may be an 80% chance that the leukemia was not caused by the low-level protracted radiation exposures. One can rarely determine with certainty what caused a particular condition or disease to appear in a patient; all one can do is assign probabilities to the likelihood that a particular causal factor was responsible for the disease diagnosed in the patient. Destructive periodontal disease and periodontal inflammation are no exception to this general rule of uncertainty for determining a disease's cause. As a result, diagnostic names (e.g., plaque-induced gingival disease, non-plaque-induced inflammatory gingival lesions[43]) can be considered misnomers because such names imply diagnostic certainty that leads to circular reasoning.[2] The principle of diagnostic uncertainty is also essential when it comes to diagnosing periodontal conditions.

Diagnosis

Periodontal Conditions Versus Periodontal Diseases

Disease is defined as an attribute or a characteristic of a person, and *diagnosis* is the clinician's belief that the person has the attribute.[73] The WHO defined disease as those adverse health consequences that include physical or psychological impairment, activity restrictions, and role limitations.[73] Certain periodontal conditions have been associated with such adverse consequences, and thus certain periodontal conditions qualify as diseases according to the WHO definition. In one study, about one in five patients who presented to a periodontal specialist reported that their teeth, gums, or dentures had an impact fairly often or very often on either eating; relaxing; avoiding going out; or feeling self-conscious, pain, or discomfort. In this same study, 4 out of 10 patients rated their oral health as fair or poor.[11] Other studies have shown that gingival conditions (e.g., necrotizing ulcerative gingivitis, attachment loss in high school students) are similarly related to oral health-related quality of life.[44]

An important thing to consider during periodontal diagnosis is to determine which periodontal conditions can be diagnosed as "diseased." Can a patient with a couple of sites with 1 or 2 mm of attachment loss be classified in this way? What about a patient with such subtle gingival inflammation that the majority of clinicians would not notice the inflammation and that even highly trained clinical examiners agree poorly about the presence of gingivitis? Disagreement regarding such questions is one of the reasons that the prevalence of gingivitis and destructive periodontal disease can range widely, depending on which reference levels are considered to be the cutoff for normal as compared with diseased.

Diagnostic Tests Available to Assess Periodontal Conditions

Diagnostic tests for periodontal disease can include anatomic measures of tissue destruction (e.g., probing pocket depth, clinical attachment loss); measures of gingival inflammation (e.g., redness, suppuration, bleeding, BOP, elevated gingival temperature, gingival crevicular fluid markers); radiographic measures of bone destruction and tooth mobility; and microbiologic measures. These test results—in combination with factors such as age, dental history, and systemic conditions—can be translated into a distinct set of periodontal diagnoses.

Translating Periodontal Diagnostic Test Results Into Periodontal Disease Diagnosis

Three different methods can be distinguished to translate clinical conditions into diseases: (1) normative or arbitrary values, (2) risk-based reference values, and (3) treatment-based reference values.[32]

Normative or Arbitrary Values to Diagnose Periodontal Disease

Diseases can be defined based on normative or arbitrary reference values. If the normal periodontium is assumed to have no pockets deeper than 3 mm, then one could define destructive periodontal disease as being present in a patient with any pocket equal to or deeper than 4 mm, or a patient with three pockets equal to or deeper than 5 mm could be classified as having destructive periodontal disease.

Alternatively, normative values could be based on parametric or nonparametric percentage cutoff values as derived from national surveys. For instance, the 97.5th percentile of the age-specific number of pockets deeper than 5 mm could be used to define destructive periodontal disease. Based on NHANES III data, a 28-year-old individual with two pockets deeper than 5 mm could be diagnosed as having destructive periodontal disease, whereas five periodontal pockets deeper than 5 mm would be required in a 58-year-old individual.[31]

Diagnoses that are based on normative or arbitrary cutoffs result in normative or arbitrary disease prevalence levels, regardless of the distribution of underlying risk factors. Whether 5% or 95% of the population smoked two packs a day for 40 years, the prevalence of destructive periodontal disease would remain equal to the selected cutoff value. If all human chronic diseases were defined based on an arbitrary 10th percentile cutoff value, the prevalence of all chronic disease would be equal to 5% (e.g., 5% of the population would have blood pressure that is too high, 5% would have a blood glucose level that is too high).

Risk-Based Reference Values to Diagnose Periodontal Disease

The diagnosis of disease can be set at the point on the diagnostic marker at which a steep increased risk for adverse health outcomes is present. The cutoff is still somewhat arbitrary, but it is connected to clinical realities in terms of the risk of adverse health outcomes. There is a tradeoff between the dangers of missed diagnoses when the cutoff is made too high (i.e., more specific) and the dangers of false-positive diagnoses when the cutoff is too low (i.e., more sensitive).

A risk-based diagnosis of destructive periodontal disease requires the conducting of longitudinal studies in which pocket depth at baseline is related to the risk of subsequent adverse outcomes (e.g., tooth loss). Fig. 6.1 represents such a plot and suggests that a pocket depth of 6 mm could be a diagnostic marker for destructive periodontal disease because a distinctive increased risk for tooth loss is associated with pocket depth values of 6 mm or deeper.

The risk-based diagnosis of chronic diseases, much like the use of normative or arbitrary values, can do more harm than good. A diagnosis of obesity that is based on a body mass index of 28 may do more harm than good if weight loss treatments increase mortality risk.[37] A diagnosis of high blood pressure[61] or diabetes[50] may cause more harm than good if the prescribed treatment further increases the mortality risk. Similarly, a diagnosis of destructive periodontal disease that is based on the presence of periodontal pockets 6 mm or deeper may cause more harm than good if the suggested periodontal treatments increase periodontal morbidity.

Therapeutic Reference Values to Diagnose Periodontal Disease

A more attractive definition of disease is the therapeutic or treatment-based diagnosis. With this definition, a person is defined as diseased only if the diagnosis of disease leads to tangible benefits. Most commonly, it is best to avoid diagnosing disease unless it can be shown that the diagnosis and the subsequent treatment actually provide tangible patient outcomes. With such an approach to diagnoses, periodontal disease should only be diagnosed if it leads to less morbidity.

Periodontal Disease Diagnoses

The Medical Subject Heading (MeSH) term headings for periodontal disease, the classification systems for periodontal diseases developed by professional organizations, and a sampling of

English-language periodontal textbooks indicate that periodontal disease diagnoses come and go at a fast rate. On PubMed, seven different entry terms are currently listed under the MeSH heading of *Periodontitis,* which reflects some of the distinct periodontal diagnoses that have been used in the literature since 1965. However, a conference consensus[35] concluded that five of the seven terms listed were obsolete. The American Academy of Periodontology reported 10 different classification systems in 20 years.[2] Periodontal textbooks have similarly reported different sets of periodontal diagnoses every decade.

Periodontal dystrophies provide one example on the apparent arbitrariness by which periodontal diagnoses come and go. Periodontal dystrophies were commonly reported from the 18th century until the 1960s. However, this diagnosis was subsequently decided to be obsolete,[58] because it did not appear to fit the infection paradigm. Periodontal textbooks no longer referred to the diagnosis of "periodontosis." However, an argument was made that this diagnosis should be resurrected.[57]

This example illustrates how profoundly the belief that periodontal disease is infectious has influenced all aspects of clinical periodontics, including the system for classifying periodontal conditions. Periodontal diagnoses in some circles are based on the premise that periodontal diseases "follow an infection/host paradigm in which it is held that noxious materials from dental plaque bacteria induce an inflammatory response in the adjacent periodontal tissue.... Central to this paradigm is the notion that the destruction of periodontal tissues is accompanied by an inflammatory response."[1]

The diagnostic classification of periodontal diseases should not be based on the infection paradigm or on any other assumed cause for two reasons. First, high-level evidence from epidemiologic studies is required to determine that periodontal disease is indeed an infection. Such evidence remains largely missing.[23] Smoking and diabetes appear to be associated with destructive periodontal disease independent of microbial colonization. Second, for chronic diseases with multiple causes, it is not possible to determine the cause of the disease; therefore, it is of little clinical value to name the disease after a suspected cause. For example, periodontal disease in a diabetic patient cannot be referred to as "diabetic periodontitis." The clinician can only say that there is a certain probability that the periodontal disease in a diabetic patient is attributable to the diabetic condition.

From a clinical perspective, the ever-changing diagnostic classification systems that result from consensus conferences may be irrelevant because no reliable evidence exists that the clinical use of such diagnostic systems improves patient outcomes. Simple diagnostic systems of periodontal disease can have several advantages for patient care because they provide useful information about both the severity of the disease and its prognosis. See Chapter 5 for an in-depth discussion of periodontitis classification systems.

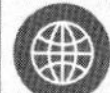

References for this chapter are found on the companion website eBooks.Health.Elsevier.com.

CHAPTER 7

Atlas of Periodontal Diseases

M. Cenk Haytac | Onur Ucak Turer

CHAPTER OUTLINE

This chapter provides additional illustrations for many chapters in this book. All illustrations are from the Archives of the Department of Periodontology, School of Dentistry, Cukurova University, Adana, Turkey (Box 7.1).

BOX 7.1 Gingival Diseases

Plaque-Induced Gingival Diseases

I. Gingivitis associated with dental plaque only
   A. Without local contributing factors
   B. With local contributing factors (eFigs. 7.1–7.32)
II. Gingival diseases modified by systemic factors
   A. Associated with endocrine system
      1. Puberty-associated gingivitis (eFig. 7.33)
      2. Menstrual cycle–associated gingivitis (eFig. 7.34)
      3. Pregnancy-associated gingivitis (eFigs. 7.35–7.37)
         a. Gingivitis
         b. Pyogenic granuloma
      4. Diabetes mellitus–associated gingivitis
   B. Associated with blood dyscrasias
      1. Leukemia-associated gingivitis (eFigs. 7.38–7.40)
      2. Other (eFigs. 7.41–7.46)
III. Gingival diseases modified by medications
   A. Drug-induced gingival diseases
      1. Drug-influenced gingival enlargement (eFigs. 7.47–7.51)
      2. Drug-influenced gingivitis
         a. Oral contraceptive–associated gingivitis
         b. Other
IV. Gingival diseases modified by malnutrition
   A. Ascorbic acid–deficiency gingivitis
   B. Other

Non–Plaque-Induced Gingival Lesions

I. Gingival diseases of specific bacterial origin
   A. *Neisseria gonorrhoeae*
   B. *Treponema pallidum*
   C. *Streptococcus* species (eFig. 7.52)
   D. Other
II. Gingival diseases of viral origin
   A. Herpesvirus infection (eFig. 7.53)
      1. Primary herpetic gingivostomatitis
      2. Recurrent oral herpesvirus infection
      3. Varicella zoster
   B. Other (eFig. 7.54)
III. Gingival diseases of fungal origin
   A. *Candida* species infections: generalized gingival candidiasis (eFigs. 7.55 and 7.56)
   B. Linear gingival erythema
   C. Histoplasmosis
   D. Other (eFigs. 7.57 and 7.58)

Continued

BOX 7.1 Gingival Diseases—cont'd

IV. Gingival lesions of genetic origin
    A. Hereditary gingival fibromatosis (eFigs. 7.59–7.61)
    B. Other
V. Gingival manifestations of systemic conditions
    A. Mucocutaneous lesions
        1. Lichen planus (eFigs. 7.62–7.65)
        2. Pemphigoid
        3. Pemphigus vulgaris (eFig. 7.66)
        4. Erythema multiforme
        5. Lupus erythematosus
        6. Drug induced
        7. Other (eFigs. 7.67–7.73)
    B. Allergic reactions
        1. Dental restorative materials
            a. Mercury
            b. Nickel
            c. Acrylic
            d. Other
        2. Reactions attributable to the following
            a. Toothpastes or dentifrices
            b. Mouthrinses or mouthwashes
            c. Chewing gum additives
            d. Foods and additives (eFig. 7.74)
        3. Other
VI. Traumatic lesions: factitious, iatrogenic, or accidental (eFigs. 7.75–7.92)
    A. Chemical injury
    B. Physical injury
    C. Thermal injury
VII. Foreign body reactions
VIII. Not otherwise specified
    A. Cysts and tumors (eFigs. 7.93–7.102)

Periodontitis (eFigs. 7.103–7.108)

I. Localized
II. Generalized
III. Periodontitis modified by systemic disorders
    A. Diabetes mellitus (eFigs. 7.109–7.113)

Periodontitis (eFigs. 7.114–7.119)

I. Localized
II. Generalized

Periodontitis as a Manifestation of Systemic Diseases

I. Hematologic disorders
    A. Acquired neutropenia
    B. Leukemias (see eFigs. 7.120–7.122)
    C. Other
II. Genetic disorders
    A. Familial and cyclic neutropenia (eFig. 7.123)
    B. Down syndrome
    C. Leukocyte adhesion deficiency syndromes (eFigs. 7.124 and 7.125)
    D. Papillon-Lefèvre syndrome (eFigs. 7.126 and 7.127)
    E. Chediak-Higashi syndrome
    F. Histiocytosis syndromes
    G. Glycogen storage disease
    H. Infantile genetic agranulocytosis
    I. Cohen syndrome
    J. Ehlers-Danlos syndrome (types 4 and 8)
    K. Hypophosphatasia (eFig. 7.128)
    L. Other
III. Not otherwise specified

Necrotizing Periodontal Diseases

I. Necrotizing ulcerative gingivitis (NUG) (eFigs. 7.129–7.131)
II. Necrotizing ulcerative periodontitis (NUP) (eFig. 7.132)
III. Bisphosphonate-related osteonecrosis (eFigs. 7.133 and 7.134)

Abscesses of the Periodontium

I. Gingival abscess
II. Periodontal abscess (eFigs. 7.135 to 7.137)
III. Pericoronal abscess (eFig. 7.138)

Periodontitis Associated With Endodontic Lesions

I. Endodontic-periodontal lesions (eFigs. 7.139 and 7.140)
II. Periodontal-endodontic lesions
III. Combined lesions

Developmental or Acquired Deformities and Conditions

I. Localized tooth-related factors
II. Mucogingival deformities around teeth
III. Mucogingival deformities on edentulous ridges
IV. Occlusal trauma

CHAPTER 8

Periodontal Disease Pathogenesis

Philip M. Preshaw | Kai Soo Tan

For online-only content on interleukin-1 family cytokines, bacterial invasion of epithelial tissues, terminology, and CD4+ T-cell subsets, please visit the companion website at eBooks.Health.Elsevier.com.

CHAPTER OUTLINE

Understanding periodontal pathogenesis is key to improving management strategies for this common yet complex disease. The term *pathogenesis,* according to *Merriam Webster's Collegiate Dictionary*, is defined as "the origination and development of a disease." Essentially, this refers to the step-by-step processes that lead to the development of a disease and that result in a series of changes in the structure and function of, in this case, the periodontium. In broad terms, the pathogenesis of a disease is the mechanism by which a causative factor (or factors) causes the disease. The word itself is derived from the Greek roots *pathos* (meaning "suffering") and *genesis* (meaning "generation or creation").

Our knowledge of periodontal pathogenesis has evolved over the years. It is important to be aware of this because treatment philosophies have changed in parallel with our improving understanding of the disease processes and will likely continue to change as our knowledge improves. During the late 1800s, Willoughby D. Miller[96] (an eminent dental researcher who established the important causal role of oral bacteria for dental caries) asserted that "during the last few years the conviction has grown continually stronger, among physicians as well as dentists, that the human mouth, as a gathering-place and incubator of diverse pathogenic germs, performs a significant role in the production of varied disorders of the body, and that if many diseases whose origin is enveloped in mystery could be traced to their source, they would be found to have originated in the oral cavity." This statement marked the beginning of an era of dental treatment strategies that aimed to treat systemic diseases by eliminating the so-called "foci of infection" in the mouth. As a result, many patients underwent unnecessary dental clearances to manage their systemic diseases.

By the 1930s, such approaches were beginning to be questioned. In an analysis of 200 patients with rheumatoid arthritis, of whom 92 had their tonsils removed as treatment for the arthritis (even though only about 15% gave any history of tonsillitis or sore throat) and of whom 52 had some or all of their teeth removed, no improvements in the rheumatoid arthritis symptoms were noted in any of the patients.[21] These authors wrote that "focal infection is a splendid example of a plausible medical theory which is in danger of being converted by its too enthusiastic supporters into the status of an accepted fact."[21] The end of the focal infection era was signaled by an editorial in the *Journal of the American Medical Association* in 1952, which stated that "many patients with diseases presumably caused by foci of infection have not been relieved of their symptoms by removal of the foci, many patients with these same systemic diseases have no evident focus of infection, foci of infection are as common in apparently healthy persons as in those with disease."[141]

In more recent times, advances in the management of periodontitis have been driven by improved knowledge of the epidemiology, causation, and pathogenesis of the disease.[160] During the 1970s, the role of plaque as the sole causative factor for periodontitis was unquestioned. In those days, nonsurgical treatment was in its infancy, and many treatment options involved surgery (e.g., gingivectomy for elimination of pockets). When looking back, it becomes clear that the treatment strategies used during a given time period depend entirely on the prevailing understanding of pathogenesis at that particular point in time. It is, therefore, very likely that the management options that we take for granted now will change again in the future. This is to be welcomed because a progressive clinical discipline, such as periodontology, which is well founded in science and with patient benefit as its primary value, should strive to improve therapeutic strategies in parallel with continued discovery.

CLINICIAN'S CORNER

Why is studying periodontal pathogenesis important?

Pathogenesis refers to the processes that cause disease. In periodontitis, bacteria in the biofilm stimulate an immune–inflammatory response that causes the tissue damage that we recognize clinically as periodontitis. Understanding the disease processes is important because it may lead to the development of improved treatment strategies.

Periodontitis results from a complex interplay between the subgingival biofilm and the host immune–inflammatory events that develop in the gingival and periodontal tissues in response to the challenge presented by the bacteria. The tissue damage that results from the immune–inflammatory response is recognized clinically as periodontitis. Gingivitis precedes periodontitis, but it is clear that not all cases of gingivitis progress to periodontitis. In gingivitis, the inflammatory lesion is confined to the gingiva; however, with periodontitis, the inflammatory processes extend to affect the periodontal ligament and alveolar bone. The net result of these inflammatory changes is the breakdown of the fibers of the periodontal ligament, resulting in clinical attachment loss, together with resorption of the alveolar bone.

During the 1970s and 1980s, bacterial plaque was generally considered to be preeminent as the cause of periodontitis. It was clear (as it is now) that poor oral hygiene results in increased plaque accumulation, and it was accepted that this, in turn, resulted in periodontal disease. However, this model failed to take into account observations, such as the finding that there are many individuals with poor oral hygiene who do not develop advanced periodontitis, and, conversely, some individuals, despite good oral hygiene and compliance with periodontal treatment protocols, present with advanced and progressing periodontitis. These findings were confirmed by the work of Löe and colleagues,[89] who studied Sri Lankan tea laborers who had no access to dental care and who could be divided into three main categories: (1) individuals (≈8% of the population studied) who had rapid progression of periodontitis, (2) those (≈81%) who had moderate progression, and (3) those (≈11%) who demonstrated no progression of periodontal disease beyond gingivitis. All individuals in this population displayed abundant plaque and calculus deposits, so clearly susceptibility to disease is influenced by more than just presence of dental biofilm. The causative role of bacteria in the biofilm is clear in that the bacteria initiate and perpetuate the inflammatory responses that develop in the gingival tissues. However, the main determinant of susceptibility to disease is the nature of the immune–inflammatory response. It is somewhat paradoxical that these defensive processes, which are protective by intent (i.e., to prevent the ingress of the bacteria and their products into the tissues), result in the majority of tissue damage that leads to the clinical manifestations of disease.

Periodontal disease is, therefore, a unique clinical entity. It is not an infection in the classic sense of the word. With many infections, a single infective organism causes the disease (e.g., human immunodeficiency virus, syphilis, tuberculosis), and the identification of that organism can provide the basis for the diagnosis. However, it is impossible to conclude that a single species, or even a group of species, causes periodontal disease. Many of the species that are considered important in periodontal pathogenesis may predominate in deep pockets because this is a favorable environment in which they can survive (i.e., it is warm, moist, and anaerobic, with a ready supply of nutrients). Many of the unique features of periodontitis result from the anatomy of the periodontium, in which a hard, nonshedding surface (the tooth) is partly embedded within the body (within connective tissue), crosses an epithelial surface, and is partly exposed to the outside world (within the confines of the mouth). The bacteria that colonize this surface are effectively outside of the body (although they are in the gingival crevice or pocket), yet the inflammatory response that develops is located within the body (i.e., within the tissues). These factors add complexity to our understanding of the role of the biofilm and the immune–inflammatory responses in the progression of periodontal tissue breakdown.

Histopathology of Periodontal Disease

To understand periodontal pathogenesis better, it is important to have an appreciation of the histology of clinically healthy tissues, as well as of inflamed gingival and periodontal tissues. Even healthy gingival tissues that clinically would be considered to be noninflamed always have evidence of inflammatory responses occurring at the microscopic level. This is normal given the chronic low-grade challenge presented by the subgingival biofilm. The low-grade inflammatory response that results is not detectable macroscopically at the clinical level but is an essential protective mechanism for combating the microbial challenge and for preventing bacteria and their products from infiltrating tissues and causing tissue damage. Our current understanding of susceptibility to periodontitis suggests that individuals who are susceptible to disease mount an excessive or dysregulated immune–inflammatory response for a given bacterial challenge that leads to increased tissue breakdown as compared with those individuals who have a more normal inflammatory response.

Clinically Healthy Gingival Tissues

Clinically healthy gingival tissues appear pink, are not swollen or inflamed, and are firmly attached to the underlying tooth and bone, with minimal bleeding on probing. The dentogingival junction is a unique anatomic feature that functions to attach the gingiva to the tooth. It has an epithelial portion and a connective tissue portion, both of which are of fundamental importance for periodontal pathogenesis. The epithelial portion can be divided into three distinct epithelial structures: the gingival epithelium, the sulcular epithelium, and the junctional epithelium (Fig. 8.1). These epithelial structures are in continuity with each other, but they have distinct structures and functions, as indicated in Box 8.1.

The junctional epithelium is a unique epithelial structure because the surface cells are specialized for the purpose of attachment to the tooth.[10] Therefore, unlike other epithelial tissues elsewhere in the body, no opportunity exists for the sloughing of cells from the surface. Instead, cells at the basal layer continually divide and move to within two or three cell layers of the tooth surface and then migrate coronally and parallel to the tooth surface to reach the floor of the sulcus and then be sloughed off into the gingival crevice. The spaces between cells of the junctional epithelium are also greater than those seen in other epithelial tissues, with the intercellular spaces comprising approximately 18% of the volume of the epithelium. This configuration is a result of a lower density of desmosomes in the junctional epithelium as compared with the gingival epithelium; the junctional epithelium is, therefore, intrinsically "leaky." This situation has great relevance for periodontal pathogenesis because the widened intercellular spaces in the junctional epithelium permit the migration of neutrophils (polymorphonuclear leukocytes); they also allow macrophages from the gingival connective tissues to enter the sulcus to phagocytose bacteria, and the ingress of bacterial products and antigens occurs, as well.

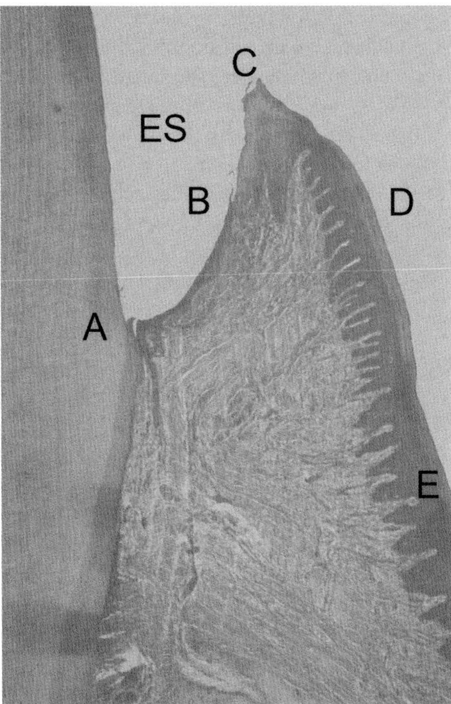

Fig. 8.1 Histologic appearance of healthy gingiva. A photomicrograph of a demineralized tooth with the gingival tissues in situ (hematoxylin and eosin staining, low magnification). Cementoenamel junction *(A)*. Enamel space *(ES)*. Gingival health is characterized by the organization of the epithelium into distinct zones: junctional epithelium *(A–B)*, sulcular epithelium *(B–C)*, free gingiva *(C–D)*, and attached gingiva *(D–E)*. The gingival connective tissue is composed of densely packed, organized, and interlacing collagen bundles. A few scattered inflammatory cells are present but no significant inflammatory cell infiltrate.

The connective tissue component of the dentogingival unit contains densely packed collagen fiber bundles (a mixture of type I and III collagen fibers) that are arranged in distinct patterns that maintain the functional integrity of the tissues and the tight adaptation of the soft tissues to the teeth (see Chapter 4).

Even in clinically healthy gingiva, the gingival connective tissue contains at least some inflammatory cells, particularly neutrophils. Neutrophils continually migrate through the connective tissues and pass through the junctional epithelium to enter the sulcus or pocket. These findings were reported in the classic investigations of the histology of periodontal disease reported by Page and Schroeder in 1976.[111] This low-grade inflammation occurs in response to the continued presence of bacteria and their products in the gingival crevice. There is a continuous exudate of fluid from the gingival tissues that enters the crevice and flows out as gingival crevicular fluid (GCF). In addition to the continuous migration of neutrophils through the gingival tissues, lymphocytes and macrophages also accumulate. The presence of leukocytes in the gingival connective tissues results from the chemotactic stimulus created by the subgingival biofilm and bacterial products, as well as from the chemoattractant factors produced by the host.

In clinically healthy tissues, this steady-state equilibrium between low-grade inflammation in the tissues and the continual presence of the bacterial biofilm may persist for many years or, indeed, for the lifetime of the individual. Overt clinical signs of gingivitis (i.e., redness, swelling, bleeding) may not develop because of several innate and structural defense mechanisms, including:

- Maintenance of an intact epithelial barrier (the junctional and sulcular epithelia).
- Outflow of GCF from the sulcus (dilution effect and flushing action).
- Sloughing of surface epithelial cells of the junctional and sulcular epithelia.
- Presence of neutrophils and macrophages in the sulcus to phagocytose bacteria.
- Presence of antibodies in the GCF.

However, if plaque accumulation increases, then inflammation and the classic clinical signs of gingivitis may develop. Although the development of gingivitis in response to the accumulation of plaque biofilm is fairly predictable, research has identified that a spectrum of responses may be observed, with some individuals developing more pronounced gingival inflammation for a given plaque challenge and others developing minimal gingival inflammation.[4] These observations highlight the importance of the host response in determining susceptibility to disease. For example, some individuals may never develop periodontitis, despite having widespread gingivitis. The immune–inflammatory response is fundamental for determining which individuals may progress to developing periodontitis, and it is likely that inflammatory responses vary between individuals who develop periodontitis as compared with those who never progress beyond gingivitis. The challenge that this presents clinically is that we do not yet know enough about susceptibility to periodontitis to identify these individuals before they actually develop signs of disease.

BOX 8.1 Characteristics of the Epithelial Component of the Dentogingival Unit

Gingival Epithelium

- Stratified squamous keratinized and parakeratinized epithelium
- Continuous with the sulcular epithelium at the gingival crest/gingival margin
- Covers the gingiva and forms the clinically visible gingival tissues
- Covers both the free and attached gingival tissues

Sulcular Epithelium

- Stratified squamous epithelium
- Nonkeratinized
- Faces the tooth surface but is not attached to it
- Forms the soft tissue lining of the gingival sulcus or the periodontal pocket

Junctional Epithelium

- Forms the epithelial attachment between the gingiva and the tooth
- Nonkeratinized
- Forms the floor of the sulcus/pocket
- Wraps around the tooth like a collar in health following the morphology of the cementoenamel junction
- Wider at the floor of the sulcus (i.e., 15–30 cells thick) and tapers apically to 3–4 cells thick
- Composed of layers of flattened squamous cells oriented parallel to the tooth surface
- Surface cells attach to the tooth surface through hemidesmosomes
- Basal lamina differs from other basal laminae that oppose connective tissue in that type IV collagen is absent

Histopathology of Gingivitis and Periodontitis

The development of gingivitis can be clearly observed clinically. In addition, the changes that occur within the tissues are obvious when examined under a microscope. In broad terms, infiltration of the connective tissues by numerous defense cells, particularly neutrophils, macrophages, plasma cells, and lymphocytes is seen. As a result of

BOX 8.2 Key Features of the Histologic Stages of Gingivitis and Periodontitis

Initial Lesion (Corresponds With Clinically Healthy Gingival Tissues)

- Slightly elevated vascular permeability and vasodilation
- Gingival crevicular fluid flows out of the sulcus
- Migration of leukocytes, primarily neutrophils, in relatively small numbers through the gingival connective tissue, across the junctional epithelium, and into the sulcus

Early Lesion (Corresponds With Early Gingivitis That Is Evident Clinically)

- Increased vascular permeability, vasodilation, and gingival crevicular fluid flow
- Large numbers of infiltrating leukocytes (mainly neutrophils and lymphocytes)
- Degeneration of fibroblasts
- Collagen destruction that results in collagen-depleted areas of the connective tissue
- Proliferation of the junctional and sulcular epithelia into collagen-depleted areas

Established Lesion (Corresponds With Established Gingivitis)

- Dense inflammatory cell infiltrate (i.e., plasma cells, lymphocytes, and neutrophils)
- Accumulation of inflammatory cells in the connective tissues
- Elevated release of matrix metalloproteinases and lysosomal contents from neutrophils
- Significant collagen depletion and proliferation of epithelium
- Formation of pocket epithelium that contains large numbers of neutrophils

Advanced Lesion (Marks the Transition From Gingivitis to Periodontitis)

- Predominance of neutrophils in the pocket epithelium and in the pocket
- Dense inflammatory cell infiltrate in the connective tissues (primarily plasma cells)
- Apical migration of junctional epithelium to preserve an intact epithelial barrier
- Continued collagen breakdown that results in large areas of collagen-depleted connective tissue
- Osteoclastic resorption of alveolar bone

Note: These classic descriptions are primarily based on findings in experimental animals, and the correlation with the clinical situation in humans is approximate.

Adapted from Page RC, Schroeder HE. Pathogenesis of inflammatory periodontal disease: a summary of current work. *Lab Invest.* 1976;34(3):235–249.

the accumulation of these defense cells and the extracellular release of their destructive enzymes, disruption of the normal anatomy of the connective tissues occurs and causes collagen depletion and subsequent proliferation of the junctional epithelium. Vasodilation and increased vascular permeability lead to increased leakage of fluid out of the vessels and facilitate the passage of defense cells from the vasculature into the tissues, thus resulting in enlargement of the tissues, which appear erythematous and edematous (i.e., the clinical appearance of gingivitis). These changes are all reversible if the bacterial challenge is substantially reduced by improved oral hygiene.

In their landmark study, Page and Schroeder[111] described the histologic changes that occur in the gingival tissues as the *initial*, *early*, *established*, and *advanced* gingival lesions (Box 8.2). In broad terms, the initial lesion corresponds with clinically healthy tissues (but, nonetheless, with transmigrating defense cells, such as neutrophils, which can be observed histologically), the early lesion corresponds with the early stages of (clinically evident) gingivitis, the established lesion corresponds with established gingivitis, and the advanced lesion marks the transition to periodontitis, with attachment loss and bone resorption. These are *histologic descriptions only*, and they should not form part of a clinical diagnosis. Moreover, these classic descriptions are primarily based on findings in experimental animals. The histologic appearances of gingivitis and periodontitis are shown in Figs. 8.2 and 8.3, respectively.

The Initial Lesion

The initial lesion was reported to develop within 2 to 4 days of the accumulation of plaque at a site that was otherwise free of plaque and at which no inflammation was evident microscopically. However, this situation is probably never encountered in reality, and, as already described, the gingival tissues usually have characteristics of a low-grade chronic inflammatory response (as observed histologically) as a result of the presence of the subgingival biofilm. In other words, the initial lesion corresponds to the histologic picture that is evident in clinically healthy gingival tissues. This low-grade inflammation is characterized by dilation of the vascular network and increased vascular permeability, thus permitting the neutrophils and monocytes from the gingival vasculature to migrate through the connective tissues toward the source of the chemotactic stimulus: the bacterial products in the gingival sulcus. The up-regulation of adhesion molecules, such as intercellular adhesion molecule-1 (ICAM-1) and E-selectin in the gingival vasculature, facilitates the migration of neutrophils from the capillaries into the connective tissues. The increased leakage of fluid from the vessels increases the hydrostatic pressure in the local microcirculation, and, as a result, GCF flow increases. Increased GCF flow has the effect of diluting bacterial products, and it also potentially has a flushing action to remove bacteria and their products from the crevice. However, given the nature of the bacterial biofilm, it is likely that mainly only planktonic (free-floating) bacteria are removed in this way.

The Early Lesion

The early lesion was said to develop after about 1 week of continued plaque accumulation and corresponds to the early clinical signs of gingivitis. The gingiva is erythematous in appearance as a result of the proliferation of capillaries, the opening up of microvascular beds, and continued vasodilation.[87] Increasing vascular permeability leads to increased GCF flow, and transmigrating neutrophils increase significantly in number. The predominant infiltrating cell types are neutrophils and lymphocytes (primarily thymic lymphocytes [T cells]),[113] and the neutrophils migrate through the tissues to the sulcus and phagocytose bacteria. Fibroblasts degenerate, primarily by apoptosis (programmed cell death), which increases the space available for infiltrating leukocytes. Collagen destruction occurs, which results in collagen depletion in the areas apical and lateral to the junctional and sulcular epithelium. The basal cells of these epithelial structures begin to proliferate to maintain an intact barrier against the bacteria and their products, and the epithelium can then be seen proliferating into the collagen-depleted areas of the connective tissues (see Fig. 8.2).[129] As a result of edema of the gingival tissues, the gingiva may appear slightly swollen, and, accordingly, the gingival sulcus becomes slightly deeper. The subgingival biofilm exploits this ecologic niche and proliferates apically (thereby rendering effective plaque control more difficult). The early gingival lesion may persist indefinitely, or resolve (e.g., with improved oral hygiene), or it may progress further.

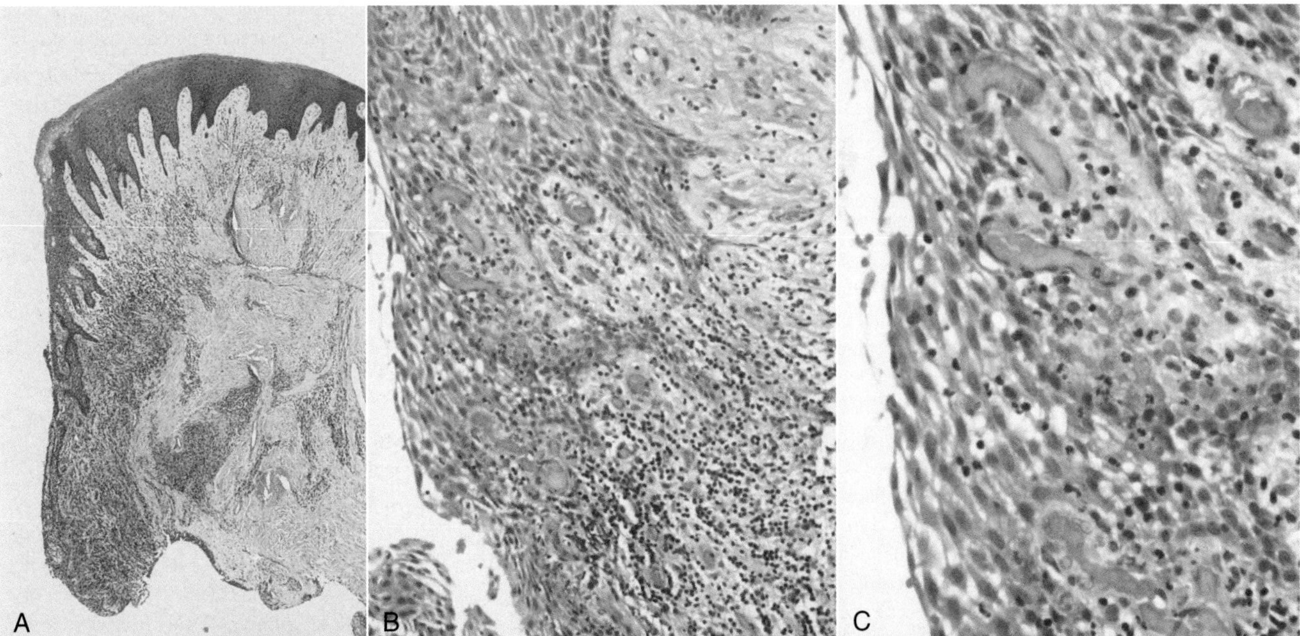

Fig. 8.2 A series of photomicrographs illustrating the histologic appearance of gingivitis (hematoxylin and eosin staining). In all cases, the tooth is to the left side of the image. (A) Low magnification of the gingiva demonstrates hyperplastic junctional and sulcular epithelia with a dense inflammatory cell infiltrate in the adjacent connective tissue. (B) Medium magnification of the epithelial–connective tissue interface shows numerous intraepithelial inflammatory cells along with intercellular edema. The connective tissue contains dilated capillaries (hyperemia), and a dense inflammatory cell infiltrate is noted. (C) High magnification shows neutrophils and small lymphocytes transiting the sulcular epithelium.

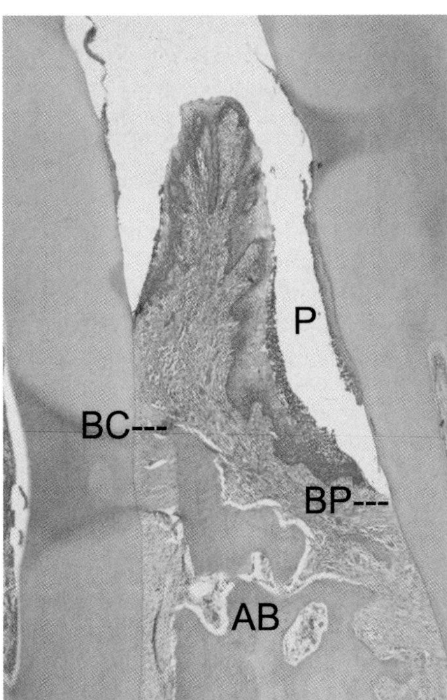

Fig. 8.3 Histologic appearance of periodontitis. A photomicrograph of adjacent demineralized teeth with the interproximal gingiva and periodontium in situ (hematoxylin and eosin staining, low magnification). The root of the tooth on the *right* is coated with a layer of dental biofilm or calculus, and attachment loss is noted with the formation of a periodontal pocket *(P)*. The periodontium is densely inflamed, and alveolar bone *(AB)* loss produces a triangular defect in addition to vertical bone loss. The base of the pocket *(BP)* is apical to the alveolar bone crest *(BC)*; this is called an *infrabony periodontal pocket*. (*From Soames JV, Southam JC.* Oral Pathology. *4th ed. Oxford, UK: Oxford University Press; 2005.*)

The Established Lesion

The established lesion roughly corresponds to what clinicians might describe as an established case of gingivitis. The progression from the early lesion to the established lesion depends on many factors, including the bacterial challenge (the composition and quantity of the biofilm), host susceptibility factors, and risk factors (both local and systemic). In the initial work by Page and Schroeder,[111] the established lesion was defined as being dominated by plasma cells, and the significant inflammatory cell infiltrate that occurs occupies a considerable volume of the inflamed connective tissues. Large numbers of infiltrating cells can be identified adjacent and lateral to the junctional and sulcular epithelia, around blood vessels, and between collagen fiber bundles.[18] Collagen depletion continues, with further proliferation of the epithelium into the connective tissue spaces. Neutrophils accumulate in the tissues and release their lysosomal contents extracellularly (in an attempt to kill bacteria that are not phagocytosed), thereby resulting in further tissue destruction. Neutrophils are also a major source of matrix metalloproteinase-8 (MMP-8; also called neutrophil collagenase) and MMP-9 (also called gelatinase B), and these enzymes are produced in large quantities in the inflamed gingival tissues as the neutrophils migrate through the densely packed collagen fiber bundles to enter the sulcus. The junctional and sulcular epithelia form a pocket epithelium that is not firmly attached to the tooth surface, that contains large numbers of neutrophils, and that is more permeable to the passage of substances into or out of the underlying connective tissue. The pocket epithelium may be ulcerated and less able to resist penetration by a periodontal probe, so bleeding upon probing is a common feature in gingivitis. These inflammatory changes are still completely reversible if effective plaque control is reinstituted.

The Advanced Lesion

The advanced lesion, as described by Page and Schroeder,[111] marks the transition from gingivitis to periodontitis. This transition is determined by many factors, the relative importance of which is currently unknown but which includes the bacterial challenge (both the composition and the quantity of the biofilm), the host inflammatory response, and susceptibility factors, including environmental (e.g., smoking) and genetic risk factors. Histologic examination reveals continued evidence of collagen destruction that extends into the periodontal ligament and the alveolar bone. Neutrophils predominate in the pocket epithelium and the periodontal pocket, and plasma cells dominate in the connective tissues. The junctional epithelium migrates apically along the root surface into the collagen-depleted areas to maintain an intact epithelial barrier. Osteoclastic bone resorption commences, and the bone retreats from the advancing inflammatory front as a defense mechanism to prevent the spread of bacteria into the bone (see Fig. 8.3). As the pocket deepens, bacteria proliferate apically into this niche, which is very favorable for many of the species that are regarded as periodontal pathogens. The pocket presents a protected, warm, moist, and anaerobic environment with a ready nutrient supply, and, because the bacteria are effectively outside of the body (even though they are in the periodontal pocket), they are not easily eliminated by the inflammatory response. Thus, a cycle develops in which chronic inflammation and associated tissue damage continue. The tissue damage is mainly caused by the inflammatory response, yet the initiating factor—the biofilm—is not eliminated. The destruction of collagen fibers in the periodontal ligament continues, bone resorption progresses, the junctional epithelium migrates apically to maintain an intact barrier, and, as a result, the pocket deepens fractionally. This makes it even more difficult to remove the bacteria and to disrupt the biofilm through oral hygiene techniques, and, thus, the cycle is perpetuated.

Inflammatory Responses in the Periodontium

The molecules that play a role in the pathogenesis of periodontitis can be broadly divided into two main groups: those derived from the subgingival bacteria (i.e., microbial virulence factors) and those derived from the host immune–inflammatory response. In terms of the relative importance of each, it is clear that most of the tissue breakdown results from the host inflammatory processes.

Microbial Virulence Factors

The subgingival biofilm initiates and perpetuates inflammatory responses in the gingival and periodontal tissues. The subgingival bacteria also contribute directly to tissue damage by the release of noxious substances, but their primary importance in periodontal pathogenesis is that of activating immune–inflammatory responses.

Lipopolysaccharide

Lipopolysaccharides (LPSs) are large molecules composed of a lipid component (lipid A) and a polysaccharide component. They are the major component of the outer membrane of gram-negative bacteria. LPS is frequently referred to as *endotoxin* and it elicits strong immune responses in animals. LPSs are highly conserved in gram-negative bacterial species, a finding that reflects their importance in maintaining the structural integrity of the bacterial cells. LPS is an example of *microbe-associated molecular patterns* (MAMPs), which are recognized by cells of the innate immune systems through Toll-like receptors (TLRs). TLRs, a family of transmembrane proteins are highly conserved in animal species ranging from *Drosophila* (a genus of fruit flies) to humans, thereby reflecting their importance in innate immune responses.[1] At least 10 TLRs (TLR-1 to TLR-10) have been discovered in humans. Specifically, TLR-4 recognizes LPS from gram-negative bacteria and functions as part of a complex of cell surface molecules, including CD14 and MD-2 (also known as lymphocyte antigen 96). The interaction of this CD14/TLR-4/MD-2 complex with LPS increases production of inflammatory mediators (most notably cytokines) and the differentiation of immune cells (e.g., dendritic cells) for the development of effective immune responses against the pathogens. LPS is of key importance for initiating and sustaining inflammatory responses in the gingival and periodontal tissues. *Porphyromonas gingivalis*, a gram-negative anaerobic black-pigmented bacterium that is associated with periodontitis, has an atypical form of LPS that is recognized by both TLR-2 and TLR-4.[31]

Biologic Properties of Lipopolysaccharide

- Located in the outer membrane of gram-negative bacteria.
- Fundamental for maintaining structural integrity of the bacteria.
- Elicits a strong immune response in animals.
- Interacts with the CD14/TLR-4/MD-2 receptor complex on immune cells, such as macrophages, monocytes, dendritic cells, and B cells, with resulting release of proinflammatory mediators, such as cytokines, from these cells.

TLR, Toll-like receptors.

Lipoteichoic Acid

Lipoteichoic acid (LTA), a major component of cell walls of gram-positive bacteria, also stimulates immune responses, although less potently than LPS. LTA signals through TLR-2. Both LPS and LTA are released from the bacteria present in the biofilm and stimulate inflammatory responses in the tissues, thereby resulting in increased vasodilation and vascular permeability, the recruitment of inflammatory cells by chemotaxis, and the release of proinflammatory mediators by the leukocytes that are recruited to the area.

Exotoxins

Exotoxins are heat-labile proteins secreted by both gram-positive and gram-negative bacteria. In periodontitis, exotoxins produced by bacteria primarily cause cell/tissue destruction or cause dysregulation of host inflammatory immune responses, facilitating the survival of bacteria. Plaque bacteria produce proteases, which are capable of breaking down structural proteins of the periodontium, such as collagen, elastin, and fibronectin. Bacteria produce these proteases to digest proteins and, thereby, provide peptides for bacterial nutrition. Bacterial proteases disrupt host responses, compromise tissue integrity, and facilitate the microbial invasion of the tissues. *P. gingivalis* produces two classes of cysteine proteases that have been implicated in periodontal pathogenesis. These are known as *gingipains,* and they include the lysine-specific gingipain Kgp and the arginine-specific gingipains RgpA and RgpB. The gingipains can modulate the immune system and disrupt immune–inflammatory responses, thus potentially leading to increased tissue breakdown.[115]

Aggregatibacter actinomycetemcomitans, a gram-negative capnophilic bacterium associated with rapidly progressing forms of periodontitis, produces two exotoxins, namely leukotoxin (Ltx) and cytolethal-distending toxin (Cdt). Ltx specifically targets leukocytes due to its binding affinity to LFA-1 which is specifically expressed on the surface of white blood cells. At the cellular level, Ltx triggers the rapid degranulation of lysosomal enzymes of neutrophils,[63] causes apoptosis of T-cells,[90] and stimulates the activation and secretion of the pro-inflammatory cytokines IL-1β and IL-18 from monocytes/macrophages.[68] The *A. actinomycetemcomitans*

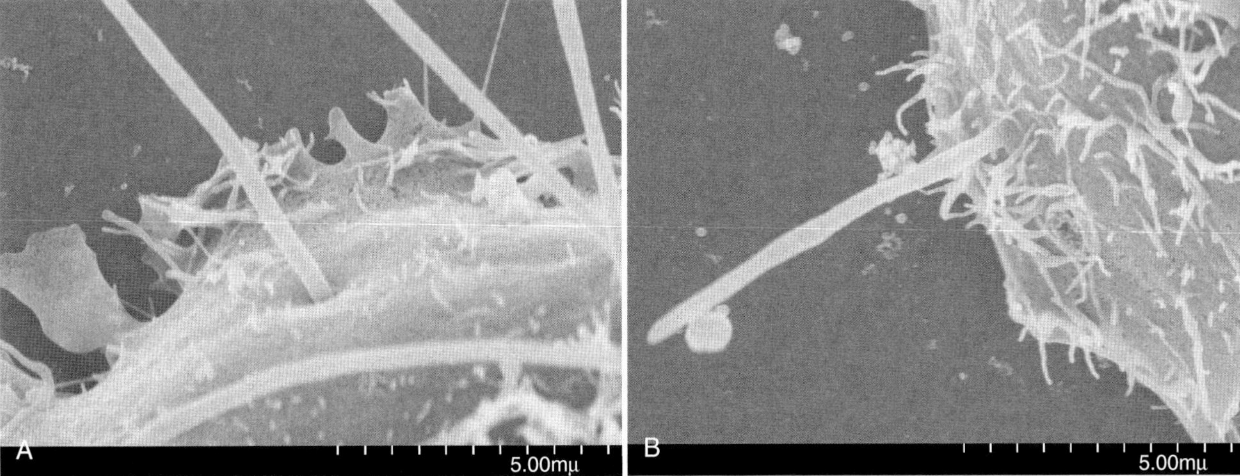

Fig. 8.4 Invasion of epithelial cells by *Fusobacterium nucleatum*. In both images, a single epithelial cell is shown being penetrated by invading *F. nucleatum* bacteria; four bacteria are evident in (A), and one bacterium is evident in (B). (A) The ruffled surface of the epithelial cells (multiple small fingerlike projections that are much smaller than the *F. nucleatum* bacteria) is likely to be an artifact. (B) *F. nucleatum* may facilitate the colonization of epithelial cells by bacteria that are unable to adhere or invade directly as evidenced by the single coccoid bacterium *(Streptococcus cristatus)* that has coaggregated with the *F. nucleatum* bacterium as it penetrates the epithelial cell. *(A and B, Courtesy Dr. A. E. Edwards, Imperial College, London, UK; Dr. J. D. Rudney, Bath University, Bath, UK; and Dr. T. J. Grossman, the University of Minnesota, Minneapolis, Minn.)*

Cdt consists of three subunit proteins, A, B, and C. CdtA and C facilitate the binding and entry of the toxin to the target cells,[30] while CdtB, the enzymatic components of the toxin, possesses nuclease and phosphatidylinositol 3,4,5-trisphosphate phosphatase activities.[138] Cdt causes deoxyribonucleic acid (DNA) damage, thereby triggering cell cycle arrest, and cell death by apoptosis.[139]

Noxious By-Products

Plaque bacteria produce several metabolic waste products that contribute directly to tissue damage. These include noxious agents, such as ammonia (NH_3) and hydrogen sulfide (H_2S), as well as short-chain carboxylic acids, such as butyric acid and propionic acid. These acids are detectable in GCF and are found in increasing concentrations as the severity of periodontal disease increases. These substances have profound effects on host cells (e.g., butyric acid induces apoptosis in T cells, B cells, fibroblasts, and gingival epithelial cells).[79,80] The short-chain fatty acids may aid *P. gingivalis* infection through tissue destruction, and they may also create a nutrient supply for the organism by increasing bleeding into the periodontal pocket. The short-chain fatty acids also influence cytokine secretion by immune cells, and they may potentiate inflammatory responses after exposure to proinflammatory stimuli, such as LPS, interleukin-1β (IL-1β), and tumor necrosis factor alpha (TNF-α).[102]

Microbial Invasion

Microbial invasion of the periodontal tissues has long been a contentious topic.[9] In histologic specimens, bacteria (including cocci, filaments, and rods) have been identified in the intercellular spaces of the epithelium.[40] Periodontal pathogens, such as *P. gingivalis* and *A. actinomycetemcomitans*, have been reported to invade the gingival tissues,[24,124] including the connective tissues.[125] *Fusobacterium nucleatum* can invade oral epithelial cells, and bacteria that routinely invade host cells may facilitate the entry of noninvasive bacteria by coaggregating with them (Fig. 8.4).[37] It has also been shown that *A. actinomycetemcomitans* can invade epithelial cells and persist intracellularly.[39] The clinical relevance of these various findings is unclear, however, and more recent studies have reported that, although species, such as *P. gingivalis*, can be found located within the tissues, they are mainly within the epithelium, and it is unusual for the bacteria to reach the connective tissue until extensive tissue destruction has occurred, and even then it is as a result of inflammation, rather than "invading" bacteria.[9]

CLINICAL CORRELATION

Is bacterial invasion of the tissues a valid concept, and does it have implications for therapy?

Good evidence indicates that certain species of subgingival bacteria are able to invade epithelial cells, thereby providing a shelter from the host defenses (and also highlighting the important role of epithelium in host defenses by release of cytokines to activate inflammatory responses). However, invasion of the deeper connective tissues by live bacteria, such as *Porphyromonas gingivalis*, seems to occur (if it occurs at all) at a much later stage in advanced disease, probably as a result of inflammation and resultant tissue destruction. Reports of bacteria present in the tissues (described as a "reservoir of infection") have sometimes been used to justify the use of antibiotics for treatment of periodontitis as a means to try to eliminate those organisms that are located in the tissues and that are, therefore, "protected" from mechanical disruption by root debridement. However, until the clinical relevance of the presence of bacteria in the tissues is better defined, it is inappropriate to make clinical treatment decisions (e.g., whether to use adjunctive systemic antibiotics) on this premise alone.

Fimbriae

The fimbriae of certain bacterial species, particularly *P. gingivalis*, may also play a role in periodontal pathogenesis. *P. gingivalis* fimbriae stimulate immune responses, such as IL-6 secretion,[81] and the major fimbrial structural component of *P. gingivalis*, FimA, has been shown to stimulate nuclear factor (NF)-κB and IL-8 in a gingival epithelial cell line through TLR-2.[3] Monocytes are also stimulated by *P. gingivalis* FimA, secreting IL-6, IL-8, and TNF-α.[38] *P. gingivalis* fimbriae also interact with complement receptor-3 (CR-3) to activate intracellular signaling pathways that inhibit

IL-12 production mediated by TLR-2 signaling.[51] This may be of clinical relevance because IL-12 is important in the activation of natural killer (NK) cells and $CD8^+$ cytotoxic T cells, which themselves may be important in killing *P. gingivalis*-infected host cells, such as epithelial cells. Indeed, the blockade of the CR-3 receptor promotes IL-12-mediated clearance of *P. gingivalis* and negates its virulence.[51] Bacterial fimbriae are, therefore, important for modifying and stimulating immune responses in the periodontium.

Bacterial Deoxyribonucleic Acid and Extracellular Deoxyribonucleic Acid

Bacterial DNA stimulates immune cells through TLR-9, which recognizes hypomethylated CpG regions of the DNA.[78] (CpG sites are regions of DNA at which a cytosine nucleotide is found next to a guanine nucleotide, separated by a phosphate molecule, which links the C and G nucleotides together; hence, "CpG"). Extracellular DNA (eDNA) is a ubiquitous constituent of all biofilms and of particular interest in biofilms associated with chronic diseases, such as periodontitis.[61] eDNA is derived from the genomic DNA of bacteria in biofilms, and the majority of eDNA is released after bacterial cell lysis.[151] However, evidence also indicates that eDNA secretion may occur from bacterial cells by mechanisms that are independent of cell lysis.[52] The presence of naked pieces of DNA extracellularly may be taken up by competent bacteria in plaque biofilm increasing genetic diversity and facilitate the spread of antibiotic resistance genes.[61] More importantly, it is becoming increasingly clear that eDNA plays a number of important roles in biofilm formation and maintenance of structural integrity of the biofilm slime layer on hard and soft tissues in the oral cavity. These include roles in adhesion and biofilm formation, protection against antimicrobial agents, and nutrient storage, as well as genetic exchange, and it is possible that eDNA may ultimately prove to be an important target for biofilm control.[61]

Host-Derived Inflammatory Mediators

The inflammatory and immune processes that develop in the periodontal tissues in response to the long-term presence of the subgingival biofilm are protective by intent but can result in considerable tissue damage, thereby leading to the clinical signs and symptoms of periodontal disease. It is somewhat paradoxical that the host response is responsible for most of the tissue damage, although this is not unique to periodontal disease. For example, the tissue damage that occurs in the joints in patients with rheumatoid arthritis results from prolonged and excessive inflammatory responses, and this damage is characterized by increased production of many of the cytokines that are also known to be important in periodontal pathogenesis. In the case of rheumatoid arthritis, the initiating factor is an autoimmune response to structural components of the joint; in periodontitis, the initiating factor is the subgingival biofilm. In both cases, the destructive inflammatory events are similar, although the pathogenesis varies as a result of the different anatomy. Key types of mediators that orchestrate the host responses in periodontitis are summarized in the following subsections.

Cytokines

Cytokines play a fundamental role in inflammation, and they are key inflammatory mediators in periodontal disease.[118] They are soluble proteins, and act as messengers to transmit signals from one cell to another. Cytokines bind to specific receptors on target cells and initiate intracellular signaling cascades that result in phenotypic changes in the cell by altered gene regulation.[149] Cytokines are effective in very low concentrations, they are produced transiently in the tissues, and they primarily act locally in the tissues in which they are produced. Cytokines are able to induce their own expression, in either an autocrine or paracrine fashion, and they have pleiotropic effects (i.e., multiple biologic activities) on a large number of cell types. (Autocrine signaling means that the autocrine agent [in this case, cytokines] binds to receptors on the cell that secreted the agent, whereas paracrine signaling affects other nearby cells.) Simply put, cytokines bind to cell surface receptors and trigger a sequence of intracellular events that lead ultimately to the production of protein by the target cell that alters that cell's behavior and could result in, for example, increased secretion of more cytokines in a positive feedback loop.

Cytokines are produced by a large number of cell types, including infiltrating inflammatory cells (e.g., neutrophils, macrophages, lymphocytes), as well as resident cells in the periodontium (e.g., fibroblasts, epithelial cells). Cytokines signal, broadcast, and amplify immune responses, and they are fundamentally important for regulating immune–inflammatory responses and for combating infections. They have profound biologic effects that also lead to tissue damage with chronic inflammation; the prolonged and excessive production of cytokines and other inflammatory mediators in the periodontium leads to the tissue damage that characterizes the clinical signs of disease. For example, cytokines mediate connective tissue and alveolar bone destruction through the induction of fibroblasts and osteoclasts to produce proteolytic enzymes (i.e., MMPs) that break down structural components of these connective tissues.[8]

Significant overlap and redundancy exist in the functions of individual cytokines. Cytokines do not act in isolation; rather, they function in flexible and complex networks that involve both proinflammatory and antiinflammatory effects and that bring together aspects of both innate and acquired immunity.[5] Cytokines play a key role at all stages of the immune response in periodontal diseases.[118]

Prostaglandins

The prostaglandins (PGs) are a group of lipid compounds derived from arachidonic acid, a polyunsaturated fatty acid found in the plasma membrane of most cells. Arachidonic acid is metabolized by cyclooxygenase-1 and -2 (COX-1 and COX-2) to generate a series of related compounds called the prostanoids, which include PGs, thromboxanes, and prostacyclins. PGs are important mediators of inflammation, particularly PG E_2 (PGE_2), which results in vasodilation and induces cytokine production by a variety of cell types. COX-2 is up-regulated by IL-1β, TNF-α, and bacterial LPS, thus resulting in increased production of PGE_2 in inflamed tissues. PGE_2 is produced by various types of cells and, most significantly, in the periodontium by macrophages and fibroblasts. PGE_2 results in the induction of MMPs and osteoclastic bone resorption, and it has a major role in contributing to the tissue damage that characterizes periodontitis.

Matrix Metalloproteinases

Matrix metalloproteinases (MMPs) are a family of proteolytic enzymes that degrade extracellular matrix molecules, such as collagen, gelatin, and elastin. They are produced by a variety of cell types, including neutrophils, macrophages, fibroblasts, epithelial cells, osteoblasts, and osteoclasts. The names and functions of key MMPs are shown in Table 8.1. The nomenclature of MMPs has been based on the perception that each enzyme has its own specific substrate; for example, MMP-8 and MMP-1 are both collagenases (i.e., they break down collagen). However, it is now appreciated that MMPs usually degrade multiple substrates, with significant substrate overlap among individual MMPs.[54] The substrate-based classification is still used, however, and MMPs can be divided into

TABLE 8.1 Classification of Matrix Metalloproteinases

Group	Enzyme	Name
Collagenases	MMP-1	Collagenase 1, fibroblast collagenase
	MMP-8	Collagenase 2, neutrophil collagenase
	MMP-13	Collagenase 3
Gelatinases	MMP-2	Gelatinase A
	MMP-9	Gelatinase B
Stromelysins	MMP-3	Stromelysin 1
	MMP-10	Stromelysin 2
	MMP-11	Stromelysin 3
Matrilysins	MMP-7	Matrilysin 1, pump-1
	MMP-26	Matrilysin 2
Membrane-type MMPs	MMP-14	MT1-MMP
	MMP-15	MT2-MMP
	MMP-16	MT3-MMP
	MMP-17	MT4-MMP
	MMP-24	MT5-MMP
	MMP-25	MT6-MMP
Others	MMP-12	Macrophage elastase
	MMP-19	—
	MMP-20	Enamelysin

MMPs, Matrix metalloproteinases; *MT,* membrane type.
Adapted from Hannas AR, Pereira JC, Granjeiro JM, et al. The role of matrix metalloproteinases in the oral environment. *Acta Odontol Scand.* 2007;65(1):1–13.

collagenases, gelatinases/type IV collagenases, stromelysins, matrilysins, membrane-type metalloproteinases, and others.

MMPs are secreted in a latent form (inactive) and are activated by the proteolytic cleavage of a portion of the latent enzyme. This is achieved by proteases, such as cathepsin G, produced by neutrophils. MMPs are inhibited by proteinase inhibitors, which have antiinflammatory properties. Key inhibitors of MMPs found in the serum include the glycoprotein (gp) α_1-antitrypsin and α_2-macroglobulin, a large plasma protein produced by the liver that is capable of inactivating a wide variety of proteinases. Inhibitors of MMPs that are found in the tissues include the tissue inhibitors of metalloproteinases (TIMPs), which are produced by many cell types; the most important in periodontal disease is TIMP-1.[15]

MMPs are also inhibited by the tetracycline class of antibiotics, which has led to the development of a subantimicrobial formulation of doxycycline as an adjunctive systemic drug treatment for periodontitis. Doxycycline, like all the tetracyclines, possesses the ability to down-regulate MMPs, and this was recognized as representing a potential novel treatment strategy for periodontitis. The subantimicrobial formulation has been shown to inhibit collagenase activity in the gingival tissues and GCF of patients with periodontitis, and clinical trials have investigated the clinical effect of using subantimicrobial dose doxycycline as an adjunct to periodontal therapy (see Chapter 55 for more details).[116]

Properties of Key Types of Inflammatory Mediators in Periodontitis

Cytokines	Proteins that transmit signals from one cell to another. Bind to cell surface receptors to trigger production of protein by the cell. There are proinflammatory and antiinflammatory cytokines. A key proinflammatory cytokine is interleukin-1β, which up-regulates inflammatory responses and is produced by multiple cell types in the periodontium.
Prostaglandins	Lipid compounds derived from arachidonic acid. Prostaglandin E_2 (PGE_2) is a key inflammatory mediator, stimulating production of other inflammatory mediators and cytokine production. PGE_2 also stimulates bone resorption and plays a key role in periodontitis progression.
Matrix metalloproteinases (MMPs)	A group of enzymes that break down structural proteins of the body. MMPs include collagenases, which break down collagen. Key MMPs in periodontitis include MMP-8 and MMP-9, which are produced by neutrophils as they migrate through the periodontal tissues, thus contributing to periodontal tissue breakdown.

Role of Specific Inflammatory Mediators in Periodontal Disease

Interleukin-1 Family Cytokines

The IL-1 family of cytokines comprises at least 11 members, including cytokines with proinflammatory activities (IL-1α, IL-1β, IL-18, IL-33), antiinflammatory properties, and IL-1 receptor antagonist (IL-1Ra).[118]

IL-1α is primarily an intracellular protein that is not normally secreted and that, therefore, is not usually found in the extracellular environment or in the circulation.[34] Unlike IL-1β, biologically active IL-1α is constitutively expressed and likely mediates inflammation only when it is released from necrotic cells, thus acting as an "alarmin" to signal the immune system during cell and tissue damage.[14] The precise role of IL-1α in periodontal pathogenesis is not well defined, although studies have reported elevated IL-1α levels in GCF and gingival tissues in patients with periodontitis.[119] IL-1α is a potent bone-resorbing factor involved in the bone loss that is associated with inflammation.[147] It is possible that the measured level of IL-1α in gingival tissues represents intracellular IL-1α that has been released from damaged or necrotic cells, and it is probable that IL-1α plays a role in periodontal pathogenesis, possibly as a signaling cytokine (signaling tissue damage) and contributing to bone resorptive activity.

IL-1β plays a key role in inflammation and immunity; it is closely linked to the innate immune response, and it induces the synthesis and secretion of other mediators that contribute to inflammatory changes and tissue damage. For example, IL-1β stimulates the synthesis of PGE_2, platelet-activating factor, and nitrous oxide, thereby resulting in vascular changes associated with inflammation and increasing blood flow to the site of infection or tissue injury. IL-1β is mainly produced by monocytes, macrophages, and neutrophils and also by other cell types, such as fibroblasts, keratinocytes, epithelial cells, B cells, and osteocytes.[32] IL-1β increases the expression of ICAM-1 on endothelial cells and stimulates the secretion of the chemokine CXCL8 (IL-8), thereby stimulating and facilitating the infiltration of neutrophils into the affected tissues. IL-1β also synergizes with other proinflammatory cytokines and PGE_2 to induce bone resorption. IL-1β has a role in adaptive immunity; it regulates the development of antigen-presenting cells (APCs) (e.g., dendritic cells), stimulates IL-6 secretion by macrophages (which, in turn, activates B cells), and has been shown to enhance the antigen-mediated stimulation of T cells.[11] GCF concentrations of IL-1β are increased at sites affected by gingivitis[55] and periodontitis,[83] and tissue levels of IL-1β correlate with clinical disease severity.[142] Studies in experimental animals have shown that IL-1β exacerbates inflammation and alveolar bone resorption.[73] It is clear from the multiplicity of studies that have investigated this cytokine that IL-1β plays a fundamental role in the pathogenesis of periodontal disease.[77]

IL-18 is mainly produced by stimulated monocytes and macrophages.[47] Increasing evidence suggests that IL-18 plays a significant role in inflammation and immunity. IL-18 results in proinflammatory responses, including the activation of neutrophils.[85] It is a chemoattractant for T cells,[74] and it interacts with IL-12 and IL-15 to induce interferon gamma (IFN-γ), thereby inducing T-helper (Th1) cells, which activate cell-mediated immunity.[163] Oral epithelial cells secrete IL-18 in response to stimulation with LPS,[122] and a correlation between GCF IL-18 levels and sulcus depth has been reported.[64] IL-18 levels have been reported to be higher than those of IL-1β in patients with periodontitis, thereby suggesting that IL-18—along with IL-1β—is predominant in periodontitis lesions.[108] Because IL-18 has the ability to induce either Th1 or Th2 differentiation, it is likely to play an important role in periodontal disease pathogenesis.[109]

Following microbial challenge and activation of TLRs on cells of the innate immune system, such as monocytes, macrophages, and dendritic cells, upregulation of IL-1β and IL-18 occurs. However, these cytokines are synthesized as immature proteins (termed pro-IL-1β and pro-IL-18), which are biologically inactive. These pro-proteins are then cleaved by the cysteine protease, caspase-1, generating mature IL-1β and IL-18, which are secreted extracellularly, triggering inflammatory responses.[1]

IL-1Ra has structural homology to IL-1β, and it binds to the IL-1 receptor (IL-1R1). However, the binding of IL-1Ra does not result in signal transduction; therefore, IL-1Ra antagonizes the action of IL-1β[33]. IL-1Ra is important for the regulation of inflammatory responses, and it can be considered an antiinflammatory cytokine. IL-1Ra levels have been reported to be elevated in the GCF and tissues of patients with periodontal disease, thereby suggesting that it has a role in immunoregulation in periodontitis.[121]

Tumor Necrosis Factor-α

TNF-α is a key inflammatory mediator in periodontal disease, and it shares many of the cellular actions of IL-1β.[48] It plays a fundamental role in immune responses, it increases neutrophil activity, and it mediates cell and tissue turnover by inducing MMP secretion. TNF-α stimulates the development of osteoclasts and limits tissue repair by the induction of apoptosis in fibroblasts. TNF-α is secreted by activated macrophages, as well as by other cell types, particularly in response to bacterial LPS. The proinflammatory effects of TNF-α include the stimulation of endothelial cells to express selectins that facilitate leukocyte recruitment, the activation of macrophage IL-1β production, and the induction of PGE_2 by macrophages and gingival fibroblasts. TNF-α—although possessing similar activity to IL-1β—has a less potent effect on osteoclasts and is present at lower levels in inflamed gingival tissues than IL-1β.[143] GCF levels of TNF-α increase as gingival inflammation develops, and higher levels are found in individuals with periodontitis.[48,55]

Interleukin-6 and Related Cytokines

The cytokines in this group—which include IL-6, IL-11, leukemia-inhibitory factor (LIF), and oncostatin M—share common signaling pathways through signal transducers; gp 130.[56] IL-6 is the most extensively studied of this group, and it has pleiotropic proinflammatory properties.[71] IL-6 secretion is stimulated by cytokines, such as IL-1β and TNF-α, and it is produced by a range of immune cells (e.g., T cells, B cells, macrophages, dendritic cells), as well as resident cells (e.g., keratinocytes, endothelial cells, fibroblasts). IL-6 is also secreted by osteoblasts, and it stimulates bone resorption and the development of osteoclasts. IL-6 is elevated in the GCF of patients with periodontal disease[86] and may have an influence on monocyte differentiation into osteoclasts and a role in bone resorption in periodontitis.[107] IL-6 also has a key role in regulating the proliferation and differentiation of B cells and T cells, particularly the Th17 subset.[71] IL-6, therefore, has an important role in periodontal disease pathogenesis, although less than that of IL-1β or TNF-α.

IL-6 also has many activities outside of the immune system, such as in the cardiovascular and nervous systems. It has an important role in hematopoiesis and in signaling the production of C-reactive protein (CRP) in the liver. Furthermore, IL-6 stimulates T-cell differentiation and function, and it is important in the regulation of the balance of T-cell subsets, particularly the activation of Th17 cells (a subset of T cells that produce IL-17) and the balance with regulatory T cells (T_{reg} cells).[12]

Prostaglandin E_2

The cells primarily responsible for PGE_2 production in the periodontium are macrophages and fibroblasts. PGE_2 levels are increased in the tissues and in GCF at sites undergoing periodontal attachment loss. PGE_2 induces the secretion of MMPs, as well as osteoclastic bone resorption, and it contributes significantly to the alveolar bone loss seen in periodontitis. PGE_2 release from monocytes in patients with severe periodontitis is greater than that from patients who are periodontally healthy.[43,105] A large body of evidence has demonstrated the importance of PGE_2 in periodontal disease pathogenesis, and, given that PGs are inhibited by nonsteroidal antiinflammatory drugs (NSAIDs), researchers have investigated the use of NSAIDs as potential host–response modulators in the management of periodontal disease.[161] However, daily administration for extended periods is necessary for the periodontal benefits to become apparent, and NSAIDs are associated with significant unwanted side effects, including gastrointestinal problems, hemorrhage (from impaired platelet aggregation resulting from inhibition of thromboxane formation), and renal and hepatic impairment. NSAIDs are therefore not indicated as adjunctive treatments for the management of periodontitis (see Chapter 55).

The PGs, including PGE_2, are derived from the COX pathway of arachidonic acid metabolism. The two main isoforms of the COX enzyme are COX-1 and COX-2. COX-1 is constitutively expressed and has antithrombogenic and cytoprotective functions. COX-2 is induced after stimulation with various cytokines, growth factors, and LPS. The inhibition of COX-1 by nonselective NSAIDs results in the majority of the unwanted side effects associated with NSAID usage, such as gastrointestinal ulceration and impaired hemostasis. The induction of COX-2 results in the production of elevated quantities of PGs (e.g., PGE_2); therefore, the inhibition of COX-2 by NSAIDs that selectively inhibit COX-2 results in a reduction of inflammation without the unwanted effects commonly seen after long-term NSAID use. Preliminary studies in animal models showed that selective COX-2 inhibitors slowed alveolar bone loss,[13,58] and human studies indicated that PG production in the periodontal tissues was modified.[156] However, in an unfortunate development, the selective COX-2 inhibitors were later identified to be associated with significant and life-threatening adverse events, thereby resulting in several of these drugs being withdrawn from the market.[36] The selective COX-2 inhibitors, therefore, cannot be considered as adjunctive treatments for periodontal disease.

Matrix Metalloproteinases

MMPs are a family of zinc-dependent enzymes that are capable of degrading extracellular matrix molecules, including collagens.[15,123] MMPs play a key role in periodontal tissue destruction and are secreted by the majority of cell types in the periodontium, including fibroblasts, keratinocytes, endothelial cells, osteoclasts, neutrophils, and macrophages. In healthy tissues, MMPs are mainly produced by fibroblasts, which produce MMP-1 (also known as *collagenase-1*), and these have a role in the maintenance of the periodontal connective tissues. The transcription of genes coding for MMPs is upregulated by cytokines, such as IL-1β and TNF-α. MMP activity is regulated by specific endogenous TIMPs and serum gps, such as α-macroglobulins, which form complexes with active MMPs and their latent precursors.[120] TIMPs are produced by fibroblasts, macrophages, keratinocytes, and endothelial cells; they are specific inhibitors that bind to MMPs in a 1:1 stoichiometry.[54] MMPs are also produced by some periodontal pathogens, such as *A. actinomycetemcomitans* and *P. gingivalis*, but the relative contribution of these bacterially derived MMPs to periodontal disease pathogenesis is small. Most MMP activity in the periodontal tissues is derived from infiltrating inflammatory cells.

In healthy periodontal tissues, collagen homeostasis is a controlled process that is mediated extracellularly by MMP-1 (expressed by resident cells, primarily fibroblasts) and intracellularly by a variety of lysosomal acid–dependent enzymes. In inflamed periodontal tissues, increased quantities of MMPs are secreted by resident cells and by the large numbers of infiltrating inflammatory cells (particularly neutrophils) as they migrate through the tissues. As a result, the balance between MMPs and their inhibitors is disrupted, resulting in breakdown of the connective tissue matrix[15,150] and leading to the development of collagen-depleted areas within the connective tissues. Neutrophils are key infiltrating cells in periodontitis that accumulate in large numbers in inflamed periodontal tissues (see Fig. 8.2). Neutrophils have evolved to respond rapidly and aggressively to external stimuli, such as bacterial LPS, and they release large quantities of destructive enzymes very rapidly.[101] The predominant MMPs in periodontitis, MMP-8 and MMP-9, are secreted by neutrophils, and they are very effective at degrading type 1 collagen, which is the most abundant collagen type in the periodontal ligament.[91] MMP-8 and MMP-9 levels increase with increasing severity of periodontal disease and decrease after treatment.[69] The prolonged and excessive release of large quantities of MMPs in the periodontium leads to the significant breakdown of structural components of the connective tissues, thereby contributing to the clinical signs of disease.

MMPs play a fundamental role in connective tissue homeostasis, as well as disease pathogenesis, and they possess a wide range of biologic effects that are relevant in periodontitis (Table 8.2). MMPs are important in alveolar bone destruction. They are expressed by osteoclasts, which also express cathepsin K, which is a lysosomal cysteine protease that is mainly expressed in osteoclasts and that plays a key role in bone resorption and remodeling. This enzyme can catabolize collagen, gelatin, and elastin and can, therefore, contribute to the breakdown of bone and cartilage.

TABLE 8.2 Biologic Activities of Selected Matrix Metalloproteinases Relevant to Periodontal Disease

MMP Type	Enzyme	Biologic Activity
Collagenases	All	Degrade interstitial collagens (types I, II, and III)
		Digest ECM and non-ECM molecules
	MMP-1	Keratinocyte migration and re-epithelialization
		Platelet aggregation
	MMP-13	Osteoclast activation
Gelatinases	All	Degrade denatured collagens and gelatin
	MMP-2	Differentiation of mesenchymal cells with inflammatory phenotype
		Epithelial cell migration
		Increased bioavailability of MMP-9
Stromelysins	All	Digest ECM molecules
	MMP-3	Activate pro-MMPs
		Disrupted cell aggregation
		Increased cell invasion
Matrilysins	MMP-7	Disrupted cell aggregation
		Increased cell invasion
Membrane-type MMPs	All	Digest ECM molecules
		Activate pro-MMP-2 (except MT4-MMP)
	MT1-MMP	Epithelial cell migration
		Degrade collagen types I, II, and III

ECM, Extracellular matrix; *MMPs*, matrix metalloproteinases; *MT*, membrane type.
Adapted from Hannas AR, Pereira JC, Granjeiro JM, et al. The role of matrix metalloproteinases in the oral environment. *Acta Odontol Scand.* 2007;65(1):1–13.

MMPs are critical for osteoclast access to the resorption site, particularly for MMP-9 and MMP-14. MMP-14 is located in the ruffled border of osteoclasts, and osteoblasts and osteocytes (but not osteoclasts) express MMP-13, which is present in resorption lacunae and functions to remove collagen remnants left over by osteoclasts.[54] MMPs also contribute to osteoclast recruitment and activity by releasing cytokines and receptor activator of NF-κB ligand (RANKL; see later). MMPs are also important in osteoblastic bone formation, including MMP-2, MMP-9, MMP-13, and MMP-14.

Chemokines

Chemokines are cytokine-like molecules that are characterized by their chemotactic activity.[22] This activity gave rise to the term **chemokine** (i.e., they are chemotactic cytokines). Chemokines orchestrate leukocyte recruitment in physiologic and pathologic conditions,[16] so they are important for periodontal pathogenesis, which results in the chemotactic migration of neutrophils through the periodontal tissues toward the site of the bacterial challenge in the periodontal pocket.[140] Chemokines play a key role in neutrophil recruitment and the recruitment of other adaptive and innate immune cells to the site of immune and inflammatory responses. The chemokines are divided into two subfamilies according to structural similarity: the CC subfamily and the CXC subfamily.[136] The chemokine CXCL8, which is more familiarly known as IL-8, has been demonstrated to be localized in the gingival tissues in areas of plaque accumulation and in the presence of neutrophilic infiltration,[152] and it has also been found in GCF.[92] Interaction between bacteria and keratinocytes results in the up-regulation of IL-8 and ICAM-1 expression in the gingival epithelium and the development of a chemotactic gradient of these molecules in the gingiva, thereby stimulating neutrophil migration into the tissues and the gingival sulcus.[153] Similar chemotactic gradients are also present in the gingiva of periodontally healthy individuals; this suggests a role for this process in the maintenance of periodontal health and supports the findings of infiltrating neutrophils being present even in clinically healthy tissues.[153]

It is becoming clear that chemokines play an important role in leukocyte migration in periodontal disease. CCL2 and CCL5 (also known as *regulated on activation, normal T-cell expressed and secreted* [RANTES]) play a role in macrophage migration, and CCL3 (also known as *macrophage inflammatory protein-1α* [MIP-1α]) and CXCL10 play a role in T-cell migration in inflamed periodontal tissues.[140] Chemokines play important roles in immune responses, repair, and inflammation, and they regulate osteoclast activity by influencing myeloid cell differentiation into osteoclasts, which may be of particular importance in the context of periodontitis.

Antiinflammatory Cytokines

The balance between proinflammatory and antiinflammatory events is crucial for determining disease progression, and it is now clear that individual cytokines do not act in isolation but, rather, as part of complex networks of mediators that have different functional activities. Antiinflammatory cytokines include IL-10, transforming growth factor-beta (TGF-β), and IL-1Ra.

The IL-10 family of cytokines has multiple pleiotropic effects and possesses immunosuppressive properties.[26] IL-10 is produced by T_{reg} cells, monocytes, and B cells, and it suppresses cytokine secretion by Th1 cells, Th2 cells, monocytes, and macrophages. The role of IL-10 in periodontal disease has been minimally studied, but animal models support that IL-10 down-regulates inflammatory responses. For example, IL-10 knockout mice are more susceptible to alveolar bone loss than wild-type mice.[126] IL-10 is also present in GCF and periodontal tissues.[59]

TGF-β is a growth factor that functions as a cytokine and has immunoregulatory roles, such as the regulation of T-cell subsets and the action of T_{reg} cells, and it also plays a role in repair and regeneration.[162] It has multifunctional roles in various cellular functions, including angiogenesis, the synthesis of the extracellular matrix, apoptosis, and the inhibition of cell growth. TGF-β levels are higher in the GCF and periodontal tissues of patients with periodontitis and gingivitis than in patients who are periodontally healthy.[53]

Linking Pathogenesis to Clinical Signs of Disease

Advanced periodontitis is characterized by tooth mobility, tooth loss, and tooth migration. These result from the loss of attachment between the tooth and its supporting tissues after the breakdown of the inserting fibers of the periodontal ligament and resorption of alveolar bone. Having reviewed the histopathology and the inflammatory processes that develop in the periodontal tissues as a result of prolonged accumulation of dental biofilm, it is now necessary to link these changes to the structural damage that occurs in the periodontium, thereby leading to the signs and symptoms of disease.

Even healthy tissues demonstrate signs of inflammation when histologic sections are examined. For example, transmigrating neutrophils are evident in clinically healthy gingival tissues moving toward the sulcus for the purpose of eliminating bacteria. If the inflammation becomes more extensive, vasodilation and increased vascular permeability then lead to edema and erythema of the tissues (i.e., gingival swelling and redness), and a slight deepening of the sulcus that further compromises plaque removal. The increased infiltration of inflammatory cells (particularly neutrophils) and the breakdown of collagen result in the development of collagen-depleted areas below the epithelium; as a result, the epithelium proliferates to maintain tissue integrity.

The epithelium provides a physical barrier to impede the ingress of bacteria and their products; therefore, the disruption of the epithelial barrier can lead to further bacterial invasion and inflammation. Antimicrobial peptides (AMPs), which are also called *defensins*, are expressed by epithelial cells, and gingival epithelial cells express two human β-defensins (hBD-1 and hBD-2). Furthermore, a cathelicidin class AMP, LL-37, which is found in the lysosomes of neutrophils, is also expressed in gingiva. These AMPs are important for determining the outcomes of the host–pathogen interactions at the epithelial barrier.[158] The epithelium is, therefore, more than simply a passive barrier: it also has an active role in innate immunity.[47] Epithelial cells in the junctional and sulcular epithelia are in constant contact with bacterial products and respond to these products by secreting chemokines (e.g., IL-8, CXCL8) to attract neutrophils, which migrate up the chemotactic gradient toward the pocket. Epithelial cells are, therefore, active in responding to infection and signaling further host responses.

If the bacterial challenge persists, the cellular and fluid infiltrate continues to develop, and neutrophils and other inflammatory cells soon occupy a significant volume of the inflamed gingival tissues (see Fig. 8.2). Neutrophils are key components of the innate immune system and play a fundamental role in maintaining periodontal health, despite the constant challenge presented by the plaque biofilm.[124] Neutrophils are protective leukocytes that phagocytose and kill bacteria, and deficiencies in neutrophil functioning result in increased susceptibility to infections in general, as well as periodontal disease.[84] Neutrophils also release large quantities of destructive enzymes (e.g., MMPs) as they migrate through the tissues (particularly MMP-8 and MMP-9), a process that results in the breakdown of structural components of the periodontium and the development of collagen-depleted areas. Neutrophils also release their potent lysosomal enzymes, cytokines, and reactive oxygen species (ROS) extracellularly, thereby causing further collagen depletion and tissue damage. Patients with periodontitis have been reported to have neutrophils that demonstrate enhanced enzymatic activity and that produce increased levels of ROS.[93] At the same time, degeneration of fibroblasts limits opportunities for repair, and the epithelium continues to proliferate apically, thus deepening the pocket further; the pocket is then rapidly colonized by the subgingival bacteria, which further perpetuate the ongoing inflammatory response.

The very first steps in the development of the pocket result from a combination of factors, including the detachment of cells at the coronal aspect of the junctional epithelium, whereas cells at the apical aspect migrate apically into the developing collagen-depleted areas; and intraepithelial cleavage occurs within the junctional epithelium.[88,145] Epithelial tissues do not have their own blood supply and must rely on the diffusion of nutrients from the underlying connective tissues. Thus, as the epithelium proliferates and thickens, necrosis of epithelial cells that are more distant from the connective tissues can lead to intraepithelial clefts and splits, which also contribute to the early stages of pocket formation.

CLINICIAN'S CORNER

How does a pocket develop?

The bacterial biofilm causes inflammation in the gingival tissues, leading to swelling and a slight deepening of the sulcus. The inflammatory response subsequently extends to the deeper tissues and is characterized by infiltration by defense cells and breakdown of collagen in the connective tissues. The junctional epithelium migrates apically to maintain an intact epithelial barrier, and, thus, the sulcus becomes deeper again and is now referred to as a pocket. Bacteria in the biofilm proliferate apically as the pocket deepens, exploiting and perpetuating this environmental niche. The bacteria are not completely eradicated by the host response, and, thus, they continue to provoke an immune–inflammatory response, leading to progressing tissue breakdown, continued apical migration of the junctional epithelium, resorption of alveolar bone, and gradual deepening of the pocket.

A cycle of chronic inflammation is, therefore, established in which the presence of subgingival bacteria drives inflammatory responses in the periodontal tissues; this is characterized by infiltration by leukocytes, the release of inflammatory mediators and destructive enzymes, connective tissue breakdown, and the breakdown and proliferation of the epithelium in an apical direction. The junctional and pocket epithelia become thin and ulcerated and bleed more readily, a condition that results in bleeding on probing. The bacteria in the pocket are not fully eliminated because they are effectively outside the body, but their continued presence drives the destructive inflammatory response in the periodontal tissues. Attempts at effective oral hygiene are rendered more difficult by the deepening of the pocket, and the cycle continues.

Alveolar Bone Resorption

As the advancing inflammatory front approaches the alveolar bone, osteoclastic bone resorption commences.[25] This is a protective mechanism to prevent bacterial invasion of the bone, but it ultimately leads to tooth mobility and even tooth loss. The resorption of alveolar bone occurs simultaneously with the breakdown of the periodontal ligament in the inflamed periodontal tissues. Two factors determine whether bone loss occurs: (1) the concentration of inflammatory mediators in the gingival tissues must be sufficient to activate the pathways that lead to bone resorption; and (2) the inflammatory mediators must penetrate to within a critical distance of the alveolar bone.[48]

Histologic studies have confirmed that the bone resorbs so that a width of noninfiltrated connective tissue of about 0.5 to 1.0 mm overlying the bone is always present.[157] It has also been demonstrated that bone resorption ceases when at least a 2.5-mm distance is present between the bacteria in the pocket and the bone.[112] Osteoclasts are stimulated by proinflammatory cytokines and other inflammatory mediators to resorb the bone, so that the resorbing alveolar bone "retreats" from the advancing inflammatory front. Osteoclasts are multinucleated cells that are formed from osteoclast progenitor cells and macrophages, and osteoclastic bone resorption is activated by a variety of mediators (in particular, IL-1β, TNF-α, IL-6, PGE_2).[99]

Receptor Activator of Nuclear Factor-κB Ligand and Osteoprotegerin

A key system for controlling bone turnover is the receptor activator of NF-κB (RANK)/RANK ligand (RANKL)/osteoprotegerin (OPG) system. RANK is a cell surface receptor expressed by osteoclast progenitor cells, as well as by mature osteoclasts. RANKL is a ligand that binds to RANK and is produced as either a membrane-bound or secreted protein by a range of cells, including fibroblasts, osteoblasts, mesenchymal cells, and T- and B-lymphocytes. OPG is the inhibitor of RANKL and functions as a decoy receptor—that is, it binds to RANKL and prevents it from interacting with RANK. OPG is secreted primarily by osteoblasts, fibroblasts, and bone marrow stromal cells. The binding of RANKL to RANK results in osteoclast differentiation and activation, and, thus, bone resorption. The balance between RANKL and OPG activity (often referred to as the *RANKL:OPG ratio*) can, therefore, determine bone resorption or bone formation.

IL-1β and TNF-α regulate the expression of RANKL and OPG, and T cells express RANKL, which binds directly to RANK on the surfaces of osteoclast progenitors and osteoclasts, thereby resulting in cell activation and differentiation to form mature osteoclasts. In individuals with periodontitis, elevated levels of proinflammatory cytokines (e.g., IL-1β, TNF-α) and increasing numbers of infiltrating T cells result in the activation of osteoclasts by RANK, which results in alveolar bone loss. It has been reported that levels of RANKL are higher and that levels of OPG are lower in sites with active periodontal breakdown as compared with sites with healthy gingiva.[27] In addition, GCF RANKL/OPG ratios are higher in periodontitis than in healthy tissue.[17] It is clear that alterations in the relative levels of these key regulators of osteoclasts play a key role in the bone loss that characterizes periodontal disease.

RANK/RANKL/OPG System

RANK (receptor activator of nuclear factor-κB)	Cell surface receptor on osteoclast progenitor cells
RANKL (RANK ligand)	Cytokine-like molecule that is the ligand for RANK (i.e., binds to RANK) and causes maturation into fully differentiated osteoclasts
OPG (osteoprotegerin)	Cytokine-like molecule that binds to RANKL and inhibits the interaction between RANKL and RANK

The RANK/RANKL/OPG signaling pathway plays a key role in regulating bone resorption. RANKL binds to RANK and stimulates osteoclast differentiation and activation. OPG antagonizes this action by binding to RANKL and preventing it from binding to RANK. The ratio of RANKL to OPG is important, with studies reporting higher levels of RANKL and lower levels of OPG in patients with advanced periodontitis compared with healthy controls.

Resolution of Inflammation

Inflammation is an important defense mechanism to combat the threat of bacterial infection, but inflammation also results in tissue damage associated with the development and progression of most chronic diseases associated with aging, including periodontal disease.[155] It is becoming evident that the resolution of inflammation (i.e., "turning off" inflammation) is an active process that is regulated by specific mechanisms that restore homeostasis (see Chapter 12). It is possible that controlling or augmenting these mechanisms may lead to the development of new treatment strategies for managing chronic diseases, such as periodontitis.[66] The resolution of inflammation is an active process that results in a return to homeostasis, and it is mediated by specific molecules, including a class of endogenous proresolving lipid mediators that includes the lipoxins, resolvins, and protectins.[132] These molecules are actively synthesized during the resolution phases of acute inflammation; they are antiinflammatory and they inhibit neutrophil infiltration. They are also chemoattractants, but they do not cause inflammation. For example, lipoxins stimulate infiltration by monocytes but without stimulating the release of inflammatory cytokines.

Lipoxins

The lipoxins include lipoxin A_4 (LXA_4) and lipoxin B_4 (LXB_4), and the appearance of these molecules signals the resolution of inflammation. Lipoxins are lipoxygenase (LO)-derived eicosanoids that are generated from arachidonic acid. They are highly potent, they possess biologic activity at very low concentrations, and they inhibit neutrophil recruitment, chemotaxis, and adhesion. Lipoxins also signal macrophages to phagocytose the remnants of apoptotic cells at sites of inflammation without generating an inflammatory response. Proinflammatory cytokines (e.g., IL-1β) released during acute inflammation can induce the expression of lipoxins, which promote the resolution of the inflammatory response.[94]

Resolvins and Protectins

Resolvins (i.e., resolution phase interaction products) are derived from the omega-3 fatty acids eicosapentaenoic acid and docosahexaenoic acid; they are classified as E series resolvins (RvE) and D series resolvins (RvD).[133] Resolvins inhibit neutrophil infiltration and transmigration, as well as the production of proinflammatory mediators, and they have potent antiinflammatory and immunoregulatory effects.[131] Resolvins are highly potent and have been shown to reduce neutrophil transmigration by around 50% at concentrations of as low as 10 nm.[144] Protectins are also derived from docosahexaenoic acid, and they reduce cytokine expression and inhibit neutrophil infiltration.[60]

Immune Responses in Periodontal Pathogenesis

The immune system is essential for the maintenance of periodontal health, and it is central to the host response to periodontal pathogens. However, if the immune response is dysregulated, inappropriate, persistent, or excessive in some way, then damaging chronic inflammatory responses, such as those observed in periodontal disease, can ensue. The immune response to biofilm bacteria involves the integration at the molecular, cellular, and organ level of elements that are often categorized as being part of the innate immune system or the adaptive immune system. Previously, host responses in periodontal disease (and many other human diseases) were described as a linear progression from the host's recognition of microbial pathogens, to innate immune responses dominated by the action of phagocytic neutrophils, and culminating in the establishment of adaptive immune responses led by antigen-specific effector functions (e.g., cytotoxic T cells, antibodies). It is now clear, however, that immune responses are complex biologic networks in which pathogen recognition, innate immunity, and adaptive immunity are integrated and mutually dependent.[41] This complex network is flexible and dynamic, with aspects of positive and negative regulation, as well as feedback control; signals are amplified and broadcast, which leads to diverse effector functions. Furthermore, the immune system is integrated with other systems and processes, including the nervous system, hematopoiesis, and hemostasis, as well as elements of tissue repair and regeneration.[100]

Observational studies of periodontal tissues and investigations of animal models and cell and tissue systems have allowed us to identify aspects of the immune response that are relevant to periodontitis.[77] Immune responses, which underpin periodontal disease, have unique facets that must be considered before we can truly rationalize the detailed information that we have about individual immune cell functions and their responses to specific periodontal pathogens. Thus, we need to understand how the polymicrobial biofilm (as opposed to individual species of periodontal pathogens) interacts with host immune defenses. We also need to appreciate specific immunologic properties that relate to the unique anatomy of the periodontium, to understand how immune responses contribute to the dynamic aspects of periodontal disease and its various clinical courses, and to gain a comprehension of how elements of host immunity contribute to tissue destruction, resolution, repair, and regeneration.

Innate Immunity

Defenses against infection include a wide range of mechanical, chemical, and microbiologic barriers that prevent pathogens from invading the cells and tissues of the body. Saliva, GCF, and the epithelial keratinocytes of the oral mucosa all protect the underlying tissues of the oral cavity and the periodontium. The commensal microbiota (e.g., in dental biofilm) may also be important for providing protection against infection by pathogenic microorganisms through effective competition for resources and ecologic niches and also by stimulating protective immune responses. The complex microanatomy of the periodontium, including the diversity of specialized epithelial tissues, presents many interesting challenges for the study of the immunopathogenesis of periodontal disease.

If bacterial products enter the tissues, the cellular and molecular elements of the innate immune response are then activated. The term *innate immunity* refers to the elements of the immune response that are determined by inherited factors (and therefore "innate"), that have limited specificity, and that are "fixed" in that they do not change or improve during an immune response or as a result of previous exposure to a pathogen. The recognition of pathogenic microorganisms and the recruitment of effector cells (e.g., neutrophils) and molecules (e.g., the complement system) are central to effective innate immunity. Innate immune responses are orchestrated by a broad range of cytokines, chemokines, and cell surface receptors, and the stimulation of innate immunity leads to a state of inflammation. If innate immune responses fail to eliminate infection, then the effector cells of adaptive immune responses (lymphocytes) are activated. It is increasingly appreciated that the immune response functions as a network of interacting molecular and cellular elements in which innate immunity and adaptive (antigen-specific) immunity work together toward a common purpose. Aspects of innate immunity that are relevant to periodontal disease are now considered.

Innate Immunity	Adaptive Immunity
Refers to nonspecific defense mechanisms that act as barriers to infection. Components include: • Barriers to infection, such as skin, mucosa, and acid pH in the stomach • Antimicrobial molecules, such as lysozyme, antimicrobial peptides, etc. • Immune system cells, such as neutrophils and macrophages that kill infecting organisms • Receptors (e.g., Toll-like receptors) that recognize pathogen-derived molecules and activate immune–inflammatory responses • Antigen presentation to activate adaptive immune responses	Refers to antigen-specific immune responses. Components include: • Recognition of specific molecules on infecting organisms at the species and strain level • Cellular immune responses focused on defense from intracellular pathogens (e.g., viruses), involving cytokines from T helper cells, macrophages, and natural killer cells • Humoral immune responses focused on defense from extracellular pathogens (e.g., bacteria), involving B cells that differentiate into antibody-producing plasma cells

Innate and adaptive immunity do not function in isolation; close integration exists between the innate and adaptive arms of the immune response.

TABLE 8.3 Constituents of Saliva That Contribute to Innate Immunity

Saliva Constituent	Host Defense Function
Antibodies (e.g., immunoglobulin A)	Inhibit bacterial adherence, promote agglutination
Histatins	Neutralize lipopolysaccharides, inhibit destructive enzymes
Cystatins	Inhibit bacterial growth
Lactoferrin	Inhibits bacterial growth
Lysozyme	Lyses bacterial cell walls
Mucins	Inhibits bacterial adherence, promotes agglutination
Peroxidase	Neutralizes bacterial hydrogen peroxide

TABLE 8.4 Virulence Factors of *Porphyromonas gingivalis* That Interact With the Immune System

Virulence Factor	Effect on Immune System
Proteases (gingipains)	Degradation of signaling molecules (CD14) and cytokines (e.g., interleukin-1β, interleukin-6)
Cell invasion capabilities	Inhibition of interleukin-8 secretion
Lipopolysaccharides	Antagonism of the stimulatory effects of lipopolysaccharides from other species; no up-regulation of E-selectin
Fimbriae	Inhibition of interleukin-12 secretion in macrophages
Cell surface polysaccharides	Resistance to complement
Short-chain fatty acids	Induction of apoptosis in host cells

Saliva

Saliva that is secreted from the three major salivary glands (i.e., parotid, submandibular, and sublingual), as well as from the numerous minor salivary glands, has an important role in the maintenance of oral and dental health. The action of shear forces associated with saliva flow is important for preventing the attachment of bacteria to the dentition and oral mucosal surfaces. Human saliva also contains numerous molecular components that contribute to host defenses against bacterial colonization and periodontal disease (Table 8.3). These components include molecules that non-specifically inhibit the formation of the plaque biofilm by inhibiting adherence to oral surfaces and promoting agglutination (e.g., mucins), those that inhibit specific virulence factors (e.g., histatins that neutralize LPS), and those that inhibit bacterial cell growth (e.g., lactoferrin) and that may induce cell death.[46,82] Saliva also contains specific immunoglobulin A (IgA) antibodies to periodontal pathogens that target specific antigens and that inhibit bacterial adherence.

Epithelial Tissues

The epithelial tissues play a key role in host defense because they are the main site of the initial interactions between plaque bacteria and the host, and they are also the site of the invasion of microbial pathogens. The keratinized epithelium of the sulcular and gingival epithelial tissues provides protection for the underlying periodontal tissue in addition to acting as a barrier against bacteria and their products.[10,130] By contrast, the junctional epithelium has larger intercellular spaces, is not keratinized, and exhibits a higher cellular turnover rate. These properties render the junctional epithelium permeable, thereby allowing the inward movement of microbes and their products and the outward movement of GCF and the cells and molecules of innate immunity. Furthermore, the spaces between the cells of the junctional epithelium widen with inflammation, which results in increased GCF flow.[130]

At the cellular and molecular levels, most in vitro studies of epithelial cell responses to periodontal bacteria have been carried out in primary gingival epithelial cells or various immortalized cell lines derived from oral epithelial tissue; these studies have provided insight into host cell responses to periodontal bacteria.[3,64,67] Epithelial cells also constitutively express AMPs (e.g., hBDs, LL-37), and the synthesis and secretion of these molecules is up-regulated in response to periodontal bacteria. Neutrophils are also a source of AMPs (i.e., α-defensins). AMPs are small, polycationic peptides that disrupt bacterial cell membranes and, thereby, directly kill bacteria with broad specificity.

The different categories of AMPs are defined on the basis of structural homology. The α-defensins (e.g., human neutrophil peptides 1 through 4) are expressed by neutrophils and as such are commonly found in GCF. The human β-defensins (e.g., hBDs 1 through 3) are expressed in the gingival epithelial cells, the salivary glands, and the tongue, as well as in immune cells (e.g., macrophages, dendritic cells); some hBDs are constitutively expressed, and others are expressed only in response to cytokines and bacterial products (e.g., gingipains of *P. gingivalis*).[2,29] A third class of AMPs are the cathelicidins, of which LL-37 is expressed in high levels in the junctional epithelium. Like the hBDs, LL-37 has a widespread expression pattern in the mouth; it is found in the salivary glands, the tongue, and the leukocytes, as well as in the connective tissue. AMPs have more recently assumed greater importance because it has been recognized that they have a wider role in regulating innate and adaptive immune responses to infection. Thus, these molecules have chemokine-like activity in that they stimulate the chemotaxis of a range of leukocytes involved in innate and acquired immunity. AMPs also stimulate mast cell degranulation and cytokine production, and they likely have a role in wound healing through their effect on keratinocyte differentiation.

Epithelial cells that are directly stimulated with bacterial components and cytokines can produce MMPs, which contribute to a loss of connective tissue. Epithelial cells also secrete a range of cytokines in response to periodontal bacteria (e.g., *P. gingivalis*, *A. actinomycetemcomitans*, *F. nucleatum*, *Prevotella intermedia*), which signal immune responses. These include the proinflammatory cytokines IL-1β, TNF-α, and IL-6, as well as the chemokine IL-8 (CXCL8) and the monocyte chemoattractant protein-1 (MCP-1), which serve to signal neutrophil and monocyte migration from the vasculature into the periodontal tissue. In some (but not all) experimental systems, *P. gingivalis* has been shown to inhibit IL-8; it has been suggested that this may result in a temporary local immune suppression in the periodontium and facilitate the accumulation and invasion of pathogenic periodontal bacteria and the initiation of periodontitis.[50] *P. gingivalis* is an example of one periodontal pathogen with a range of virulence factors that affect host immune defenses,[50,81] as indicated in Table 8.4.

Gingival Crevicular Fluid

GCF originates from the postcapillary venules of the gingival plexus. It has a flushing action in the gingival crevice, but it also likely functions to bring the blood components (e.g., neutrophils, antibodies, complement components) of the host defenses into the sulcus.[49] The flow of GCF increases in inflammation, and neutrophils are an especially important component of GCF in periodontal health and disease.[77]

Pathogen Recognition and Activation of Cellular Innate Responses

If plaque bacteria and their products penetrate the periodontal tissues, specialized "sentinel cells" of the immune system recognize their presence and signal protective immune responses. These cells include neutrophils, macrophages, and dendritic cells, which express a range of pattern recognition receptors (PRRs) that interact with MAMPs. Besides these professional immune cells, resident cells of the periodontium, including gingival epithelial cells, gingival fibroblasts, and periodontal fibroblasts, also express PRRs. The activation of PRRs activates innate immune responses to provide immediate protection, and adaptive immunity is also activated with the aim of establishing a sustained antigen-specific defense. Prolonged and dysregulated immune responses lead to chronic inflammation and the concomitant tissue destruction associated with periodontal disease.

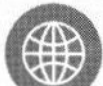
A glossary of terms relevant to periodontal immunobiology is presented in eTable 8.2, which can be accessed on the companion website at eBooks.Health.Elsevier.com.

TLRs are the major PRRs in the recognition of bacterial infections. TLRs are structurally conserved with an extracellular leucine-rich-repeat (LRR) motif, and an intracellular Toll/interleukin-1 receptor (TIR) signaling domain responsible for the initiation of a cascade of intracellular signaling events leading to the initiation of immune responses. TLRs found on the cell surface membrane include TLR-1, TLR-2, TLR-4, TLR-5, and TLR-6, while TLR-3, TLR-7, TLR-8, and TLR-9 are localized in intracellular membranous compartments, such as the endosome or lysosome.[1] TLRs recognize various MAMPs, which are conserved molecular structures located on bacteria. For instance, TLR-1, TLR-2, and TLR-6 recognize bacterial cell wall components, such as lipoproteins and LTA. These TLRs function as heterodimers of TLR-2/TLR-1 or TLR-2/TLR-6, specifically binding tri- or diacylated lipoproteins, respectively.[146] TLR-4 requires the co-receptors, the LPS-binding protein (LBP), CD14, and myeloid differentiation protein-2 (MD-2), to bind to LPS. TLR-5 recognizes flagellin unique to motile bacteria; TLR-3, TLR-7, and TLR-8 recognize viral nucleic acids, while TLR-9 recognizes bacterial DNA via its unmethylated CpG motifs.[1]

The best studied of the signaling systems involved in the recognition of plaque bacteria is the interaction of bacterial LPS with TLRs. *P. gingivalis*, *A. actinomycetemcomitans*, and *F. nucleatum* all possess LPS molecules that interact with TLR-4 to activate myeloid immune cells. While LPS recognition is predominantly mediated by TLR-4, *P. gingivalis* LPS is unique, with heterogeneous chemical structure that differs from enteric bacterium-derived LPS. The ability of *P. gingivalis* LPS to elicit immune response in C3H/HeJ mice,[114] which possess defective TLR-4 signaling, led to a common belief that *P. gingivalis* LPS is a TLR-2 ligand. However, subsequent structural and functional studies revealed that *P. gingivalis* LPS activates cells through TLR-4, and that the TLR-2 activity of *P. gingivalis* LPS may be contributed by lipoprotein contamination in the preparation.[106] To date, the interaction of *P. gingivalis* LPS with TLR-2 or TLR-4 or both remains controversial.[31]

Although the signaling pathways activated by PRRs may be diverse, in general terms, they converge to elicit similar host cell responses in the form of up-regulation of cytokine secretion and, in the case of APCs, such as dendritic cells, cell differentiation that leads to enhanced signaling of the adaptive immune response.

The signaling of cytokine responses by PRRs influences innate immunity (e.g., neutrophil activity), adaptive immunity (e.g., T-cell effector phenotype), and the development of destructive inflammation (e.g., the activation of fibroblasts and osteoclasts). Some cytokines are particularly important to innate immune signaling and clearly have a role in immune responses in periodontitis. The archetypal proinflammatory cytokine is IL-1β, which exerts its action directly by activating other cells that express the IL-1R1 receptor (e.g., endothelial cells) or by stimulating the synthesis and secretion of other, secondary mediators, such as PGE_2. The effect of IL-1β is amplified by synergistic actions with other cytokines, such as TNF-α. The up-regulation of ICAM-1 and E-selectin on endothelial cells is central to the migration of neutrophils into the periodontium, and this is stimulated by IL-1β and TNF-α. IL-1β also stimulates the secretion of the chemokine IL-8, which stimulates neutrophil chemotaxis. IL-1β and TNF-α also activate MMP secretion from fibroblasts and osteoclasts; this facilitates the movement of neutrophils through the connective tissues (and, thus, protective innate responses), but it also contributes to the tissue destruction associated with periodontal disease, along with MMPs from neutrophils.

Other cytokines that are up-regulated as a result of the activation of PRRs include IL-6, which influences the development of a number of immune cells (e.g., B cells, dendritic cells) and stimulates osteoclast differentiation and, thus, bone turnover. Other cytokines provide specific signals that contribute to the development of specific $CD4^+$ Th1 cell subsets (e.g., IL-4, IL-12, IL-18). In addition to cytokines that activate immune responses, other cytokines are up-regulated that have a role in immune regulation by suppressing cytokine activity; these include IL-1Ra, IL-10, and TGF-β. Cytokines from T-cell subsets feedback to and modify innate immune responses; for example, IFN-γ from Th1 cells activates macrophages, IL-17 from Th17 cells synergizes with IL-1β and TNF-α to reinforce inflammatory reactions, and IL-10 and TGF-β suppress immune responses. The action of many cytokines produced in the periodontium is not limited to one aspect of the host immune response; in other words, cytokines are pleiotropic (i.e., they have multiple effects).

Neutrophil Function

Neutrophils are the "professional" phagocytes that are critical to the clearance of bacteria that enter host tissues.[101] Neutrophils are present in clinically healthy gingival tissues, and they migrate through the intercellular spaces of the junctional epithelium into the sulcus.[130] This is part of a "low-grade defense" against plaque bacteria, and it is necessary to prevent infection and periodontal tissue damage. The importance of neutrophils to the maintenance of periodontal health is demonstrated clinically by the observations of severe periodontitis in patients with neutrophil defects.[101]

A small proportion (1% to 2%) of the intercellular spaces in healthy junctional epithelium is occupied by neutrophils (and other leukocytes at various stages of differentiation), but this can increase to 30% with even modest inflammation. In the inflammatory state, changes to the local vasculature occur in the gingiva: high endothelial venules develop from the postcapillary venules of the gingival plexus, which facilitates leukocyte emigration and increases the flow of GCF into the pocket.[130]

Neutrophils migrate from the gingival plexus to the extravascular connective tissue and then into the junctional epithelium through the basement membrane. The presence of a layer of neutrophils in the junctional epithelium forms a host defense barrier between subgingival biofilm and the gingival tissue. At the molecular level, the interaction of adhesion molecules (e.g., ICAM-1) on endothelial and epithelial cells with β2 integrins on neutrophils facilitates neutrophil migration. Indeed, evidence from immunohistochemistry studies indicate the existence of gradients of IL-8 (a "chemotactic gradient"), as well as gradients of ICAM-1, which direct the neutrophils from the vasculature into the tissues and toward the junctional epithelium.[153] The migration of neutrophils contributes to the disruption of the junctional epithelium by the degradation of the basement membrane through protease release and the action of ROS.

An aspect of neutrophil-mediated immunity is the formation of neutrophil extracellular traps (NETs).[159] NETs constitute a highly conserved antimicrobial strategy in which decondensed nuclear DNA and associated histones are extruded from the neutrophil, thus forming web-like strands of DNA in the extracellular environment. These strands, in conjunction with AMPs, facilitate the extracellular killing of microorganisms that become trapped within the NETs. NETs can be released by viable neutrophils, as well as following a form of programmed cell death called NETosis. NETs are produced in response to a wide range of infecting pathogens and likely constitute an important defense strategy, but, due to the concomitant release of cytotoxic molecules, they can also contribute to host tissue damage.

Adaptive Immunity

Adaptive immunity has evolved to provide a focused and intense defense against infections that overwhelm innate immune responses. Adaptive immunity is particularly important as ecologic, social, and demographic changes—which alter susceptibility to existing and emerging infective microorganisms—outpace the natural evolution of biologic systems. Furthermore, the development of effective vaccination is, along with the identification of antibiotics, perhaps one of the greatest triumphs of medical science; this success is based on knowledge of the elements and principles of adaptive immunity.

Adaptive immunity contrasts with innate immunity with regard to the dynamic of the underlying cellular and molecular responses: adaptive immunity is slower and reliant on complex interactions between APCs and T and B lymphocytes. A key element is the antigen specificity of the responses that facilitates the specific targeting of a diverse range of effector elements, including cytotoxic T cells and antibodies. Another facet is the ability of adaptive immune responses to improve during exposure to antigen and on subsequent reinfection events.[20] Our current understanding suggests that the cellular and molecular elements of adaptive immunity are more diverse than those of innate immunity, and, although a role for many of these factors in periodontal disease has been identified, our knowledge is far from complete. The importance of adaptive immune responses in periodontal pathogenesis is endorsed by histologic studies.[77,111] The population of leukocytes in the periodontium in gingivitis (i.e., the early stages of responses to the plaque biofilm) and in stable periodontal lesions (i.e., those in which tissue destruction is apparently not progressing) has been reported to be dominated by T cells, and these cells are clustered mainly around blood vessels. Cell surface marker studies suggest that these cells are activated but not proliferating.[45] In addition, a predominance of the helper T-cell subset (i.e., CD4-expressing T cells) over the cytotoxic T-cell subset (i.e., CD8-expressing T cells) is observed. These T cells are considered to be proactively maintaining tissue homeostasis in the presence of the microbial challenge of the plaque biofilm.[45] By contrast, in active (progressing) periodontitis, B cells and plasma cells predominate and are associated with pocket formation and the progression of disease.

Antigen-Presenting Cells

Central elements of the activation and function of T cells and B cells are the presentation of antigen by specialized APCs to T cells and the development of a specific cytokine milieu that influences the development of T cells with particular effector functions. APCs detect and take up microorganisms and their antigens, after which they may migrate to lymph nodes and interact with T cells to present antigen. The periodontium contains a number of APCs, including B cells, macrophages, and at least two types of dendritic cells (i.e., dermal dendritic cells and Langerhans cells).[28] It is increasingly recognized that the engagement of PRRs (and, in particular, TLRs) by MAMPs from pathogenic microorganisms is not only central to signaling innate immunity in the form of cytokine up-regulation but also a critical element of the activation of APCs and the elaboration of T-cell effector function. Thus, TLR activation increases the expression of costimulatory molecules on APCs, which are critical to the interaction of these cells with T cells. In addition, TLR activation enhances antigen uptake and processing. Different APCs process and present antigens by different pathways and mechanisms, and this variation is one of the factors—along with the presence of specific combinations of cytokines—that influences the phenotype of T-cell effector function produced during specific immune responses.[45]

T Cells

Several different subsets of thymic lymphocytes (i.e., T cells) develop in the bone marrow and thymus and migrate to the peripheral tissues to participate in adaptive immune responses. The expression of the cell surface molecules (CD4 or CD8) or particular T-cell antigen receptors (αβ or γδ) broadly defines functional T-cell subsets that emerge from the thymus. The role of T cells in periodontal disease has been established through immunohistologic studies of diseased tissues.[135] $CD4^+$ helper T cells are the predominant phenotype in the stable periodontal lesion, and it is thought that alterations in the balance of effector T-cell subsets within the $CD4^+$ population may lead to progression toward a destructive, B-cell-dominated lesion.[45] $CD4^+$ T-cell subsets are defined on the basis of their phenotypic characteristics and effector functions. The nature of the APCs, which present antigen to cognate T-cell receptors on T cells, and the presence of specific combinations of cytokines and chemokines locally influence the nature of the $CD4^+$ T-cell effector subset that develops from naive T cells (Fig. 8.5). $CD4^+$ T-cell subsets are defined by the expression of specific transcription factors, and their functional characteristics are associated with their cytokine secretion profile.

The best-defined functional subsets of $CD4^+$ T cells are the Th1 and Th2 cells, and a dynamic interaction between Th1 and Th2 cells may provide, in part, an explanation for fluctuations in disease activity and the progression of periodontal disease (Box 8.3). Th1 cells secrete IFN-γ, which activates cell-mediated immunity (i.e., macrophages, NK cells, and $CD8^+$ cytotoxic T cells) against pathogenic microorganisms. The activation of macrophages promotes phagocytosis and killing of microbial pathogens, whereas NK cells and $CD8^+$ T cells are cytotoxic T cells that kill infected host cells. Conversely, Th2 cells regulate humoral (antibody-mediated) immunity and mast cell activity through the secretion of the cytokines IL-4, IL-5, and IL-13. Thus, the predominance of Th2 cells leads to a B-cell response. The B-cell response may be protective, for example, as a result of the production of specific antibodies that would serve to clear tissue infections through interaction with the complement system and by enhancing neutrophil phagocytosis. However, B cells are also a source of proinflammatory cytokines that contribute to tissue destruction.

T_{reg} cells have an immunosuppressive action that is mediated by the secretion of TGF-β and that is important to the prevention of autoimmune disease. These cells are increased in periodontitis lesions and

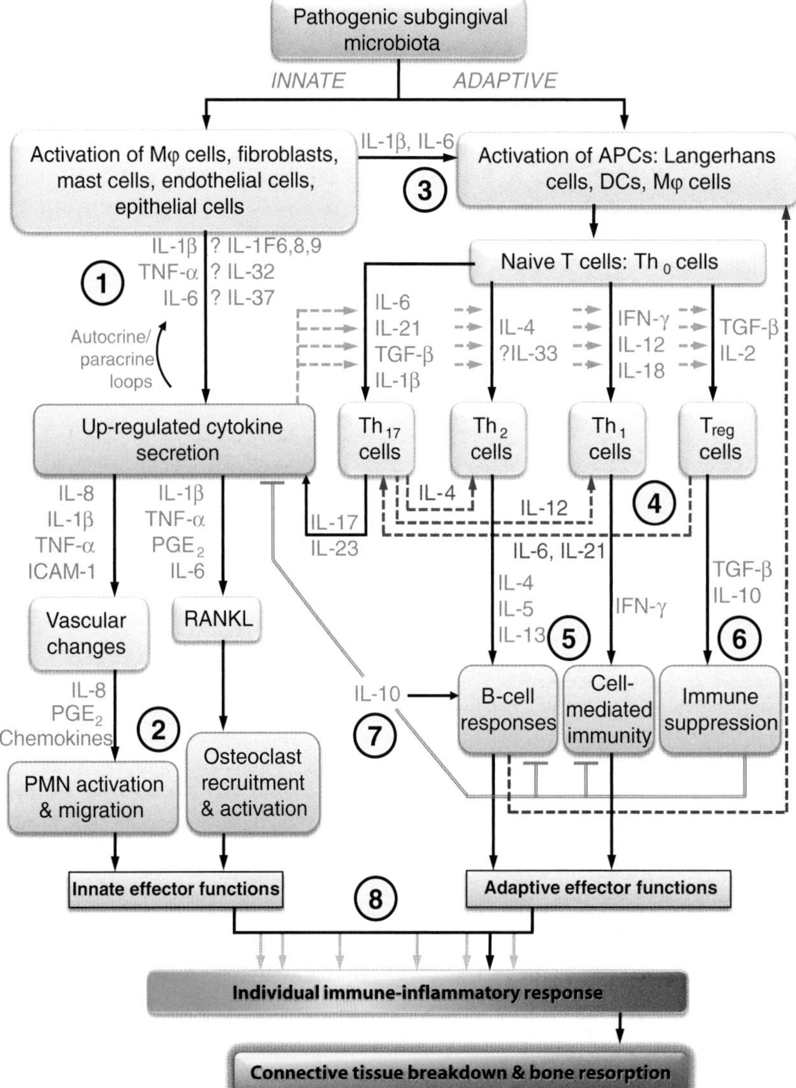

Fig. 8.5 Cytokine networks in periodontal diseases. Schematic to illustrate the multiple interactions between cytokines and cellular functions in periodontal disease. *(1)* Resident and infiltrating cells in the periodontium respond to microbe-associated molecular patterns *(MAMPs)* signaling through pattern-recognition receptors *(PRRs)* by the production of cytokines as an early step in innate immune responses. Cytokine up-regulation is sustained by autocrine and paracrine feedback loops. (Note: *Question marks* indicate more speculative suggestions about the role of specific cytokines in periodontal pathogenesis than are known at present.) *(2)* Up-regulated cytokine activity leads to vascular changes, polymorphonuclear leukocyte *(PMN)* activation and migration, and, ultimately, osteoclastogenesis and osteoclast activation. *(3)* Cytokines produced in innate responses contribute to the activation of antigen-presenting cells *(APCs)*. These present specific antigens to naive CD4+ T cells *(Th_0 cells)*, which differentiate into CD4+ effector T cells (e.g., T-helper cells *[Th_1, Th_2, Th_{17}]*, and T-regulatory *[T_{reg}] cells*) according to the local cytokine milieu (as indicated by the groups of *four parallel horizontal gray dashed arrows*). For example, Th_0 cells differentiate into Th_{17} cells under the influence of interleukin-6 (*IL-6*), IL-21, transforming growth factor beta (*TGF-β*), and IL-1β. (APCs are also activated by B cells, which are themselves activated at a later stage in the cytokine network [indicated by the *brown dashed arrow at the right edge of the figure*]; this is an example of the complexities of sequential feedback loops that develop). *(4)* Th_1 and Th_2 cells have a relatively stable phenotype, but other T-cell subsets can exhibit functional plasticity under the influence of different cytokine environments (indicated by *purple dashed arrows*). For example, Th_{17} cells can develop into Th_1 cells under the influence of IL-12 and into Th_2 cells under the influence of IL-4. *(5)* Different T-cell subsets are associated with various cytokine secretion profiles that regulate different aspects of immune responses and that contribute to up-regulated cytokine activity. For example, Th_1 cells secrete interferon gamma (*IFN-γ*) (which activates cell-mediated immunity), and Th_2 cells regulate antibody-mediated (humoral) immunity through the secretion of cytokines IL-4, IL-5, and IL-13. Cytokines produced by different T-cell subsets increase their further secretion in positive feedback loops and also inhibit the development of other T-cell subsets (e.g., IL-4 from Th_2 cells inhibits Th_1 development, and IFN-γ from Th_1 cells inhibits Th_2 T-cell subsets). *(6)* T_{reg} cells secrete TGF-β and IL-10, which have immunosuppressive functions. For example, IL-10 suppresses Th_1 and Th_2 responses, as well as cells of monocyte/macrophage lineage *(Mф)* and dendritic cell *(DC)* function, and it also down-regulates cytokine production in various cells (i.e., Th_1 cells, Th_2 cells, PMNs, and natural killer *[NK]* cells). (Suppressive effects are indicated by *flat-ended*

green lines.) (7) IL-10 functions as a regulatory mediator, but it can also exhibit other activities (e.g., the activation of B cells). The different aspects of IL-10 biology (i.e., immunosuppressive vs. immunostimulatory) likely depend on the local cytokine environment. These dual roles of IL-10 are indicated by the *green (inhibitory) line* and the *black (stimulatory) arrow. (8)* The sum total of innate and adaptive effector functions results in an immune–inflammatory response, the precise nature of which will vary from person to person (as indicated by the *multiple gray arrows,* with some patients being more susceptible to disease than others), as well as over time within an individual. In this case, the *black arrow* indicates an individual who has a proinflammatory response that leads to connective tissue breakdown and bone resorption. *ICAM-1,* intercellular adhesion molecule-1; *PGE₂,* prostaglandin E_2; *RANKL,* receptor activator of nuclear factor-κB ligand; *TNF-α,* tumor necrosis factor alpha. (*Reproduced with permission from Kinane DF, Preshaw PM, Loos BG. Host-response: understanding the cellular and molecular mechanisms of host-microbial interactions—consensus of the Seventh European Workshop on Periodontology.* J Clin Periodontol. *2011;38[11 Suppl]:44–48.*)

BOX 8.3 The T-Helper 1/T-Helper 2 Concept of Periodontal Disease Progression

A dynamic interaction between T-helper 1 (Th1) and T-helper 2 (Th2) cells represents a possible explanation for aspects of the fluctuations in disease activity and clinical progression seen with periodontal disease. It has been hypothesized that a strong innate response results in interleukin-12 synthesis (e.g., by tissue macrophages) that leads to a Th1 response that provides protective cell-mediated immunity that would be manifested as a "stable" periodontal lesion. Conversely, a poor innate response would lead to reduced interleukin-12, which would permit the development of Th2 responses and lead to the activation of B cells; this, in turn, would mediate a destructive lesion, possibly through enhanced B-cell-derived interleukin-1β.[45,134] However, definitive evidence to support associations of Th1 and Th2 cells with different clinical presentations of periodontal disease has been difficult to obtain. Investigators have suggested that this is a result of variations among experimental studies, which have differed with respect to the material that has been used, the definitions of disease stages, the experimental designs, and analytic methods used.[42,45,134] In addition, in general terms, the Th1/Th2 dichotomy does not explain all aspects of the regulation of adaptive immune responses. Other T-cell subsets have also been identified and defined. For example, regulatory T cells secrete interleukin-10 and transforming growth factor beta and, thereby, suppress immune responses. Th17 cells have a proinflammatory action through the secretion of interleukin-17, a cytokine that synergizes with interleukin-1β and tumor necrosis factor alpha. Therefore, although it is widely accepted that Th1 and Th2 cells are likely to be important in the immunopathogenesis of periodontal disease, it is increasingly recognized that the Th1/Th2 model alone is probably inadequate to explain the role of T cells in this process.

may, therefore, have a role in disease pathogenesis.[98] Certain lines of evidence suggest that the pathogenesis of periodontal disease may involve some elements of autoimmunity.[45] For example, immunologic cross-reactivity occurs between HSP60 expressed on human cells and the GroEL molecule of *P. gingivalis*, and specific serum antibodies and antigen-specific T cells to these molecules have been detected in periodontal disease. Similarly, autoantibodies and specific T cells against other host (i.e., self) molecules, such as type I collagen, have been identified in periodontal disease.

Th17 cells comprise another subset of T cells, and they have a proinflammatory action that is important in immune responses against extracellular infections mediated by the cytokine IL-17. Infections with a diverse range of pathogens have been shown to activate strong Th17 cell responses, and Th17 cells are thought to provide a substantial inflammatory response to clear microorganisms that Th1/Th2 cells have failed to eradicate. IL-17 has a number of activities in common with IL-1β and TNF-α, and it has a synergistic activity with these cytokines, particularly TNF-α. IL-17 induces proinflammatory cytokine expression (including IL-1β and TNF-α) in macrophages, stimulates chemokine expression, and, thereby, activates neutrophil infiltration. Increasing evidence indicates a role of IL-17 and Th17 cells in periodontal disease.[42] IL-17 has been detected in periodontal tissues at sites of advanced disease. IL-17 induces IL-6 and IL-8 secretion by gingival fibroblasts and also up-regulates MMP-1 and MMP-3 in these cells. IL-17 also induces IL-1β and TNF-α secretion from macrophages and gingival epithelial cells.

The complexities of the interactions between cellular and molecular aspects of innate and adaptive immune functioning are presented in Fig. 8.5. It is clear that multiple proinflammatory and antiinflammatory pathways, positive and negative feedback loops, and agonists and antagonists all play a role in determining the nature of the immune–inflammatory response to the bacterial challenge and the degree of tissue damage that is experienced. Furthermore, the nature of the inflammatory response varies among individuals; this could explain why certain people appear to be more susceptible to periodontitis than others.

CLINICIAN'S CORNER

What makes a person susceptible to periodontitis?

We have all seen patients with good oral hygiene yet advanced periodontitis and, conversely, patients with poor oral hygiene who may have gingivitis or mild periodontitis, but who do not develop advanced periodontitis. It is clear that immune functioning and inflammatory responses are highly complex processes that vary from person to person. Our understanding is that the sum total of all the immune–inflammatory events in the periodontal tissues (which are also influenced by environmental factors, such as smoking or diabetes) is the main determinant of how much tissue damage occurs in response to the challenge presented by the bacterial biofilm. This tissue damage is what we recognize clinically as disease. Our challenge for the future is to learn how to identify susceptible patients at a much earlier stage in the disease process, before tissue damage occurs.

Antibodies

Specific antibodies are produced in response to the bacterial challenge in periodontal disease and are the endpoint of B-cell activation. Commensurate with the appearance of antibodies against bacterial antigens is the appearance of differentiated plasma cells. High levels of antibodies appear in GCF (in addition to those in the circulation), and these are produced locally by plasma cells in periodontal tissues.[6] Antibodies to periodontal pathogens are primarily IgG, with few IgM or IgA types produced.

Many species of oral bacteria elicit a polyclonal B-cell response (with the consequent production of specific antibodies against those bacteria). However, these responses augment responses against nonoral bacteria and may lead to the production of autoantibodies (e.g., antibodies against collagen and connective tissue proteins), which may contribute to tissue destruction in periodontal disease.[6,45] The incidence and levels of specific serum and GCF IgG antibodies are raised in periodontitis, a finding suggesting that local and peripheral generation of antibodies may be important in the immune response to periodontal pathogens. Antibodies (i.e., IgA) to periodontal pathogens are also found in saliva.

P. gingivalis molecules (i.e., fimbriae and hemagglutinin) act as antigens for antibodies. Specific antibodies are also generated against serotype-specific carbohydrate antigens (e.g., capsular polysaccharide of *P. gingivalis*, carbohydrate of *A. actinomycetemcomitans* LPS). The distribution of antibodies is influenced by cytokines that are derived from monocytes.[127] For example, IgG_2 production is regulated by IL-1α, IL-1β, and PGE_2 from monocytes, as well as by platelet-activating factor from neutrophils. PGE_2 and platelet-activating factor indirectly induce Th1 responses and, therefore, IFN-γ, which stimulates IgG_2 production.

Some studies have reported an effect of treatment on levels of specific antibodies to periodontal pathogens. For example, plaque removal reduces the titers of antibodies to *P. gingivalis* and *A. actinomycetemcomitans* in serum, GCF, and saliva.[6] Some studies have observed a transient increase in antibody titers after treatment, which may be due to the release of antigens into the tissue and circulation.

The significance of antibodies in periodontitis is not fully clear. It is not known whether these antibodies have a protective function or whether they participate in disease pathogenesis. Although some evidence indicates a correlation between clinical parameters of disease and titers of specific antibodies to periodontal pathogens, other studies report an inverse correlation of antibody levels and avidity with periodontal destruction. In addition, specific antibodies to periodontal pathogens are found in healthy individuals, as well as in persons with periodontal disease.

Concept of Host Susceptibility

The immune and inflammatory processes that result from the challenge presented by the subgingival biofilm are complex and are mediated by a large number of proinflammatory and antiinflammatory cytokines and enzymes that function as a network of mediators with overlapping roles and activity (see Fig. 8.5). Immune responses to the bacterial challenge do not occur in isolation but, rather, take place in the context of other host and environmental factors that influence these responses and, thereby, determine the progression of disease. Certain risk factors increase susceptibility to periodontal disease, particularly smoking[103] and diabetes[117]; these are considered elsewhere in this book.

A feature of human development and evolution has been that quantitative and qualitative differences exist in immune responses among individuals.[57] Indeed, infectious agents (e.g., bacteria) exert evolutionary selection pressures on the species that they infect. This may be relevant in periodontal disease, and some studies have confirmed that immune cells from patients with periodontal disease secrete higher quantities of proinflammatory cytokines than do cells from persons who are periodontally healthy.[149] Cytokine profiles are also different in those individuals with immune-mediated diseases as compared with healthy control subjects.

These observations have led to the concept of the "hyperinflammatory" or "hyperresponsive" trait in which certain individuals possess a hyperinflammatory phenotype that accounts for their increased susceptibility to chronic inflammatory conditions, such as periodontitis.[23] Such a proinflammatory trait may also contribute to shared susceptibility between conditions, such as periodontitis and cardiovascular disease or diabetes. However, at present, it is not

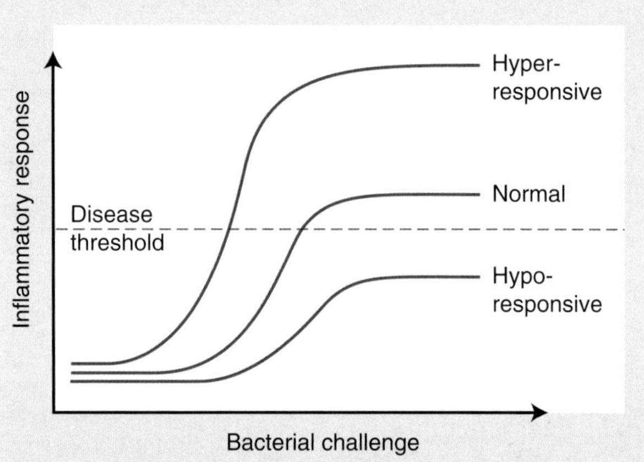

Fig. 8.6 Inflammatory response characteristics in relation to bacterial challenge. A given bacterial challenge results in differing levels of inflammatory response according to the response profile of an individual. Most people are close to normal and produce a certain level of inflammatory mediators for a given challenge. Those who are hyperresponders generate an excessive inflammatory response for the same bacterial challenge and cross the threshold into active disease at an earlier stage. Those who are hyporesponsive produce lower levels of inflammatory mediators and, despite a significant bacterial challenge, may never develop advanced periodontitis. (*Modified from Champagne CM, Buchanan W, Reddy MS, et al. Potential for gingival crevice fluid measures as predictors of risk for periodontal diseases.* Periodontol 2000. *2003;31:167–180.*)

possible to identify with certainty those patients who are hyperresponders. The hyperresponder concept was originally proposed in the context of the responsiveness of monocytes to LPS challenge; this suggests that patients with disease possess an individual hyperresponsive monocytic trait that is characterized by elevated levels of inflammatory mediators released from monocytes in response to bacterial challenge.[105] It is likely that many reasons contribute to disease variations among individuals, such as variations in immune responses, pathogenesis, and the bacterial biofilm; this situation results in an uneven disease experience in the population.

Fig. 8.6 is a schematic illustration of how increasing bacterial challenge can result in differing levels of inflammatory response according to the response profile of an individual patient.[105] Most individuals would be considered normal, and for a given bacterial challenge, would produce a certain level of inflammatory mediators in the periodontal tissues. For those who are hyperresponders, the same bacterial challenge results in a greater inflammatory response, which would result in increased tissue breakdown over time, earlier presentation of the clinical signs of disease, and a clinical interpretation of having increased susceptibility to periodontitis. Those individuals who are hyporesponsive produce lower levels of inflammatory mediators and are, therefore, somewhat resistant to the development of advanced periodontitis, even though plaque may be present and they may have widespread gingivitis and/or mild periodontitis. The nature of the immune–inflammatory response is governed by genetic factors and environmental factors, and it may vary over time within the same individual (e.g., if environmental factors, such as smoking, stress, or systemic disease, should change).[72]

A similar dose–response curve can also be expressed in the context of stable or progressing disease, and, as shown in Fig. 8.7, a certain level of bacterial challenge results in a moderate release of inflammatory cytokines, mediators, and enzymes. These mediators, together with the infiltrating defense cells, have a protective role to eliminate bacteria in the sulcus and do not trigger periodontal disease breakdown. Such a steady-state scenario may persist indefinitely. However, if something changes (e.g., the quantity or

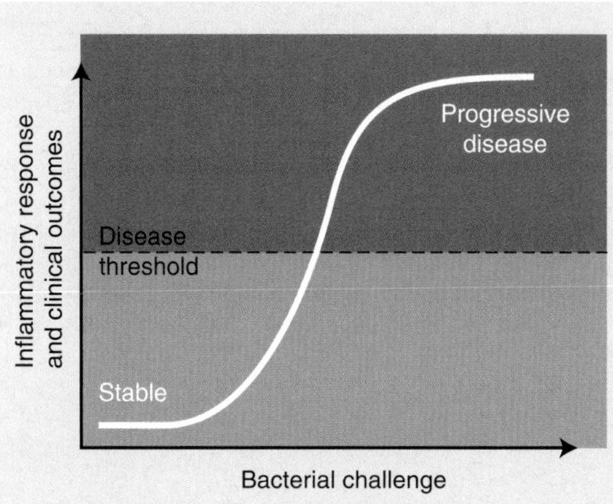

Fig. 8.7 Inflammatory response characteristics in relation to an individual's threshold for periodontitis. A certain level of bacterial challenge results in a moderate inflammatory response, which is protective by intent and may not be sufficient to transition to periodontal disease. This stable condition may persist for many years or even throughout the individual's lifetime. Changes in the bacterial burden (i.e., qualitative, quantitative, or both) or changes in the host response (e.g., as a result of a change in an environmental exposure) could result in an up-regulated inflammatory response characterized by marked cellular infiltrate and the increased secretion of inflammatory mediators leading to tissue damage and a transition from the stable situation to periodontitis. The location of the threshold between stable and active disease varies from person to person. In addition, the dose–response curve for any individual can shift to the left or the right in accordance with environmental changes. A shift to the left would result in an increased inflammatory response to a given bacterial challenge and potentially an exacerbation of disease. A shift to the right would have the opposite effect. (*Modified from Champagne CM, Buchanan W, Reddy MS, et al. Potential for gingival crevice fluid measures as predictors of risk for periodontal diseases.* Periodontol 2000. *2003;31:167–180.*)

quality of the biofilm alters, or the host defenses alter as a result of a change in an environmental exposure), then the secretion of cytokines, prostanoids, MMPs, and other mediators may increase in the tissues, thereby leading to the histopathologic changes described previously and a transition to periodontitis. Thus, a threshold exists between stable and active disease, and this will vary from person to person. The dose–response curve for any individual can shift to the left or the right according to environmental changes. A shift to the left would result in an increase in the quantities of inflammatory mediators produced for a given bacterial challenge and potentially an exacerbation of disease; a shift to the right would have the opposite effect. In all cases, an increase in the bacterial challenge would have the tendency to increase the production of inflammatory mediators, which may tip the balance from stability to a progression of periodontitis.

These are, of course, simplistic models to explain a highly complex phenomenon, and it is clear that cytokines and inflammatory mediators function in complicated networks (see Fig. 8.5).[70,118] Therefore, although increases and decreases in the absolute levels of cytokines have been reported in disease states, it is clear that the dysregulation of cytokine networks and other mediators is the key determinant of disease progression. Thus, the relative proportions of mediators within inflammatory networks are fundamental to determining disease progression, and changes in these proportions are driven by inflammatory challenges and the genetic and environmental factors that govern how the host responds to such challenges.[76,110] Schematic illustrations to explain the pathogenesis of periodontal disease, such as presented in Fig. 8.5, can be useful; however, given the complexity of the disease processes, they are inevitably simplistic. Earlier models were very simplistic indeed, being essentially linear and suggesting that periodontitis resulted directly from the microbial challenge.[76] This concept influenced periodontal treatment over the decades and resulted in treatment strategies that focused primarily on the biofilm. Modern concepts of periodontal pathogenesis describe a host response that transitions from being proportionate and pro-resolving (i.e., in terms of resolving inflammation) to one that is disproportionate and nonresolving and ultimately self-destructive as chronic inflammation develops. These changes occur in parallel with changes in the biofilm, the nature of which is influenced by the development of inflammation in the tissues, as it transitions from being health-promoting to dysbiosis, thus perpetuating the chronic inflammation.[95]

Increasing awareness of the importance of host factors in determining interindividual differences in disease experience has resulted in the realization that, although plaque bacteria initiate and perpetuate the inflammatory response, most of the tissue damage results from the host response, which is influenced by genetic factors, as well as environmental and acquired risk factors. Risk factors, such as smoking, alter the progression of the immune–inflammatory response and shift the balance toward increased periodontal breakdown.[62] This implies that the presence of plaque bacteria does not inevitably lead to advanced tissue destruction, and this concept is supported by a large number of epidemiologic studies, which confirm that more advanced disease (although prevalent) is usually confined to a minority of the population.[67,89]

Our improved understanding of the disease processes in periodontitis has led to the development of a biologic systems model for representing periodontal pathogenesis. This involves bacterial components, environmental factors, specific inflammatory mechanisms, and host–genetic variations that are associated with disease.[76] A biologic systems approach provides a framework for viewing the contributions and relative importance of all the components that contribute to the clinical presentation of disease. Thus, in the context of periodontal disease, such a system would include a person level, a genetic/epigenetic level, the biologic phenotype, and, ultimately, the clinical phenotype (Fig. 8.8).[104] Such systems provide a more comprehensive view of the disease as a complex regulatory network in which aspects of the specific genetic factors, environmental exposures, and other modifying factors that an individual is exposed to determine the development of the disease state.

To summarize, it is clear that the subgingival bacteria initiate and perpetuate the immune–inflammatory responses in the periodontal tissues. These responses are characterized by classic signs of inflammation that are modified as a result of the unique anatomy of the periodontium and the dentogingival apparatus. The inflammatory events that develop in response to the bacterial challenge are protective by intent, but they result in the majority of tissue damage and breakdown that lead to the clinical signs of periodontitis. Individuals vary with regard to their susceptibility to periodontal disease and also in the threshold at which disease progression occurs. Such variations are partly genetically determined and are also influenced by environmental risk factors (e.g., smoking, diabetes), some of which are modifiable and some of which are not. The challenge for the future is to identify susceptible individuals so that disease can be prevented before tissue loss has occurred.

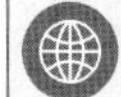
A Case Scenario is found on the companion website at eBooks.Health.Elsevier.com.

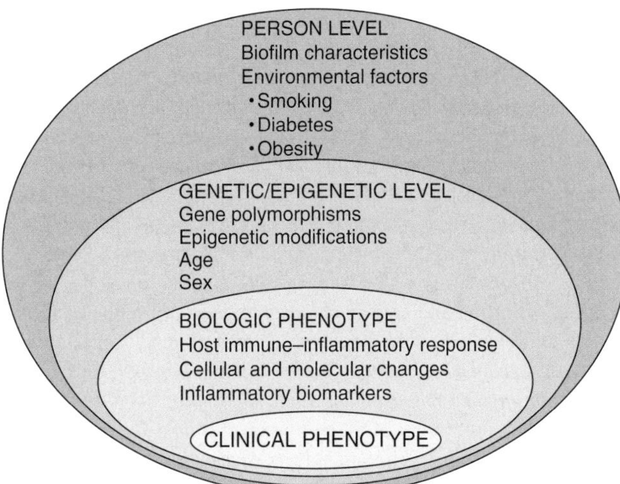

Fig. 8.8 A biologic systems model of periodontitis. The outermost level of this model is the *Person Level*, which represents an individual's unique characteristics as they are related to periodontitis. These include the compositional characteristics of the subgingival biofilm, as well as known risk factors and environmental exposures, such as smoking and diabetes. The *Person Level* characteristics interact with the *Genetic/Epigenetic Level* characteristics, which include nonmodifiable factors, such as age, sex, and genetic composition. Gene polymorphisms are known to be associated with periodontal disease, and epigenetics refers to changes in phenotype (i.e., clinical disease expression) caused by mechanisms other than changes in the underlying deoxyribonucleic acid (DNA) sequence. Epigenetics can be defined as all the meiotically and mitotically inherited changes in gene expression that are not encoded in the DNA sequence itself. Epigenetic modifications are important permissive and suppressive factors for controlling the expressed genome through gene transcription. Two major epigenetic mechanisms are the posttranslational modification of histone proteins in chromatin and the methylation of DNA. The *Genetic/Epigenetic Level* characteristics influence the *Biologic Phenotype*, which is characterized by the specific immune–inflammatory responses (i.e., cellular and molecular events and the production of inflammatory mediators) that are associated with the *Clinical Phenotype* (i.e., the clinical presentation of the disease). This model reflects how different individuals with the same presentation (e.g., periodontitis) may have very different predisposing and risk factors. The model depicts the different biologic factors that underpin the development of periodontal disease in different individuals and that ultimately may be used to classify disease by the contribution provided to the clinical phenotype at each level. (*Modified from Offenbacher S, Barros SP, Beck JD. Rethinking periodontal inflammation.* J Periodontol. *2008;79[8 Suppl]:1577–1584.*)

Suggested Reading

1. Löe H, Anerud A, Boysen H, et al. Natural history of periodontal disease in man. Rapid, moderate and no loss of attachment in Sri Lankan laborers 14 to 46 years of age. *J Clin Periodontol.* 1986;13:431–440.
2. Page RC, Kornman KS. The pathogenesis of human periodontitis: an introduction. *Periodontol 2000.* 1997;14:9–11.
3. Page RC, Schroeder HE. Pathogenesis of inflammatory periodontal disease: a summary of current work. *Lab Invest.* 1976;33:235–249.
4. Preshaw PM, Taylor JJ. How has research into cytokine interactions and their role in driving immune responses impacted our understanding of periodontitis? *J Clin Periodontol.* 2011;38(suppl 11):60–84.
5. Kinane DF, Preshaw PM, Loos BG. Host-response: understanding the cellular and molecular mechanisms of host-microbial interactions—consensus of the Seventh European Workshop on Periodontology. *J Clin Periodontol.* 2011;38(suppl 11):44–48.
6. Meyle J, Chapple I. Molecular aspects of the pathogenesis of periodontitis. *Periodontol 2000.* 2015;69:7–17.
7. Okada H, Murakami S. Cytokine expression in periodontal health and disease. *Crit Rev Oral Biol Med.* 1998;9:248–266.
8. Champagne CM, Buchanan W, Reddy MS, et al. Potential for gingival crevice fluid measures as predictors of risk for periodontal diseases. *Periodontol 2000.* 2003;31:167–180.
9. Offenbacher S, Barros SP, Beck JD. Rethinking periodontal inflammation. *J Periodontol.* 2008;79:1577–1584.
10. Mahanonda R, Pichyangkul S. Toll-like receptors and their role in periodontal health and disease. *Periodontol 2000.* 2007;43:41–55.
11. Dahlen G, Basic A, Bylund J. Importance of virulence factors for the persistence of oral bacteria in the inflamed gingival crevice and in the pathogenesis of periodontal disease. *J Clin Med.* 2019;29:1339.
12. Garlet GP. Destructive and protective roles of cytokines in periodontitis: a re-appraisal from host defense and tissue destruction viewpoints. *J Dent Res.* 2010;89:1349–1363.

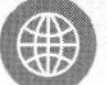
References for this chapter are found on the companion website at eBooks.Health.Elsevier.com.

CHAPTER 9

Precision Dentistry: Genetics and Epigenetics of Periodontitis

Olga A. Korczeniewska | Scott R. Diehl

CHAPTER OUTLINE

It is now widely accepted that differences among individuals who are at risk of the development of most diseases have a substantial inherited component. Factors in the environment (e.g., diet, smoking, preventive care, and exposure to pathogens) interact with each person's genetic predisposition to determine his or her health outcomes. This complex combination of variables determines if and when a disease affects a person, how fast and how severely symptoms of the disease progress, and how the person responds to different treatments in terms of both side effects and the success of alternative therapies. Sometimes—and particularly with diseases such as cystic fibrosis and muscular dystrophy—the genetic component of risk predominates, and differences in environment play only a minor role. With other diseases, factors in the environment are most important, and variation inherited in the person's deoxyribonucleic acid (DNA) has only an infrequent or minor influence on disease susceptibility or progression. Examples of the latter include infectious diseases, such as human immunodeficiency virus/acquired immunodeficiency syndrome (HIV/AIDS) as well as cancers such as mesothelioma, which are strongly associated with asbestos exposure. The majority of human diseases fall about halfway between these two extremes, with genes and the environment both playing important roles.

Most cases of periodontitis appear to fit this complex gene and environment model. With the exception of a handful of rare syndromes caused by mutations of single genes, evidence indicates that inherited variation in DNA has a role roughly equal to that of the environment in determining who remains periodontally healthy versus who is affected by this disease. Beyond this broad generalization, however, and despite more than 800 association studies of periodontitis and genetic polymorphisms reported to date, knowledge of which specific genes are most important remains extremely limited. We know virtually nothing about the role that inherited genetic differences are likely to have in determining how patients respond to alternative treatments. This knowledge is necessary for the development of "personalized" or "individualized" periodontal treatment strategies, an approach that is playing an increasingly important role in improving virtually all other areas of health care today.

This chapter reviews the challenges and barriers that have thus far limited progress in advancing our knowledge of the complex genetics of periodontitis. This requires a basic understanding of not only the architecture of the human genome and the complexity of genetic susceptibility but also of the critical roles that statistical power and sample size play in the process of discovery. These latter issues are important for all areas of research but especially for situations in which a large number of variables need to be evaluated. In genetic studies, about 20,000 genes need to be considered as potential hypotheses or candidates for influencing disease risk. Depending on the gene's size and the frequency of genetic recombination in the gene's chromosomal region, scientists need to evaluate a handful or up to several hundred inherited DNA variants in each gene as potential "biomarkers" of disease risk. Each one of these variants essentially amounts to a test of the hypothesis as to whether the variant is associated with disease risk. Furthermore, many complex diseases have been found to be strongly associated with DNA variation in parts of the human genome where no genes are known to exist but where the genetic material may have important functional effects, nonetheless. Therefore, to fully evaluate the entire human genome, the number of hypotheses that needs to be tested is truly enormous and involves roughly the equivalent of 1 million independent statistical tests. Only since the early 2000s have laboratory and computational tools been available that make this scale of work technically feasible at an affordable cost, and thus far, only a few studies have reported results for a whole genome analysis for periodontitis genetic risk.

Opportunities for advanced study designs and next-generation DNA sequencing and other genomic technologies to improve the understanding of the inherited basis of periodontitis make it likely (although by no means certain) that genetic variation will become an important variable to be routinely considered by practicing dentists within the careers of dental students today, and this is already starting to occur. Therefore, it is essential that dentists learn how to access and interpret the information coded in the human genome, so they can use this wisely to improve periodontal disease prevention, diagnosis, and treatment for their patients. Alternatively, new interdisciplinary teams will need to be established with dentists as key members working closely with experts in bioinformatics, genomics, and genetic counseling so that patients will be able to reap the potentially significant benefits of these scientific advances. However the process evolves, the genomics revolution will surely lead to major changes in both dental education and dental practice in the not-so-distant future.[10,36]

Genomic Advances in the 21st Century

Most health care professionals are aware of the many major advances in genetics accomplished during the decades since the Human Genome Project officially began in 1990.[62] Headlines and announcements of breakthroughs continue to appear regularly in print and television media. All too often, many of these stories seem to promise rapid and significant improvements in health care that are totally unrealistic.[13] Cautious assessments are usually not deemed newsworthy by the media, and understatement is not in the interest of private companies or grant-awarding government agencies supporting basic research and clinical trials. Consequently, the public has too often received overly optimistic pictures of what the future of medical care based on genomic medicine really holds in store for them. Despite this all-too-common overstatement about rapid translation to clinical practice, the actual advances in technical capabilities for genomic data acquisition and the accumulation of knowledge in the field of genetics have been truly enormous. The eventual impact of this explosion of biologic knowledge on all areas of human health, including those concerning the field of dentistry, is certain to be substantial over the longer term.

Unfortunately, for reasons explored further in the next section, genomic advances have thus far contributed little to advance our understanding of the molecular-pathologic causes of periodontitis, nor pointed toward ways to improve treatment through individualized approaches based on patients' inherited genetic variation. Genome-wide association studies (GWAS—pronounced "gee-wahs") and next-generation DNA sequencing techniques are now being used in periodontology research. For these strategies to be successful, however, they must be combined with further improvement in research definitions of periodontal disease and much larger sample sizes than have been used in the majority of previous genetic studies. To provide a refresher on basic concepts and help improve understanding, some of the commonly used terms in genetics are explained in Table 9.1.

TABLE 9.1 Glossary of Terms Relevant to the Genetics of Periodontal Disease

Term	Definition
Allele	One of several possible alternative forms of a gene caused by small or large differences in the DNA sequence within or near the gene. These differences arise by mutation, and some may affect the function of the gene product (i.e., a protein) or its abundance in different kinds of cells.
Autosomal dominant	DNA variation in a gene located on an autosome that has a dominant effect over other forms of variation at this location within the gene. When the dominant DNA sequence is present in combination with some other sequence, the gene's function is entirely or nearly entirely determined by the dominant sequence, whereas the alternative sequence that occurs on the person's other chromosome is essentially silent.
Autosomal recessive	DNA variation in a gene located on an autosome that has an effect on the gene's function only when the person has inherited two copies: one from the mother and the other from the father. For example, if an individual has two copies of an abnormal gene that is autosomal recessive, he or she will be subject to the effects of that gene.
Autosome	A chromosome that is not a sex chromosome.
Chromosome	A nuclear structure that contains genetic information. Humans have 46 chromosomes that are arranged in 23 pairs. There are 22 pairs of autosomes and one pair of sex chromosomes (either XX or XY).
Concordance	The probability that a pair of individuals (e.g., twins) both have a certain characteristic (e.g., periodontal disease), given that one of the pair has the characteristic. Presented as a number from 0 to 1 or as a percentage.
Dizygotic twins	Twins that have resulted from the fertilization of two separate eggs. They are no more similar to each other (from a genetic perspective) than are nontwin siblings. Nonidentical twins.
Epigenetics	Term used to describe the changes in phenotype or gene expression that result from mechanisms other than changes in the underlying DNA sequences (i.e., changes in which the gene is expressed rather than a change in the DNA sequence itself). Nongenetic factors cause the organism's genes to be expressed differently.
Exon	Protein coding regions of DNA.
Frameshift mutation	A mutation that results from the insertion or deletion of one or more nucleotides into a gene, thereby causing the coding regions to be read in the wrong frame and usually causing the protein produced to be defective in function.
Gene	The basic unit of heredity that occupies a specific position (locus) on a chromosome and that has specific effect(s) on the phenotype of the organism. A piece of DNA that is transcribed into a molecule of RNA and then translated into a protein.
Gene expression	The process by which the information in a gene is used via transcription and translation, thereby leading to the production of protein. Differences in gene expression can affect the phenotype of the organism, including the risk of disease.
Genetic code	In RNA and DNA, the consecutive nucleotide triplets (codons) that specify the sequence of amino acids for protein synthesis (translation).
Genome	The entire hereditary information of an organism. This term refers to all of the genes and other nongene portions of DNA carried by an individual cell.

TABLE 9.1 Glossary of Terms Relevant to the Genetics of Periodontal Disease—continued

Genotype	The genetic makeup of an organism or cell as distinct from its expressed features or phenotype.
Haplotype	A contraction of the term *haploid genotype.* This word refers to a combination of alleles at multiple loci, which are usually transmitted together on the same region of a chromosome.
Heredity	The passing of traits to offspring from parents or ancestors. In biology, the study of heredity is referred to as *genetics.* As a result of heredity, variation among individuals allows species to evolve by natural selection in response to changes in their environment or by random change over long periods of time.
Heterozygous	The presence of two different alleles at a specific position in a gene.
Homozygous	The presence of identical alleles at a specific position in a gene.
Intron	A DNA region within a gene that is not translated into protein. These intervening (noncoding) portions of DNA or RNA are removed during RNA processing.
Isoform	Any of several different forms of the same protein. Isoforms may be produced from related genes, or they may arise from the same gene via alternative splicing. Many isoforms are caused by single nucleotide polymorphisms.
Ligand	A molecule that binds to another molecule (usually a cellular receptor molecule).
Linkage	The tendency for certain genes to be transmitted from parent to child together because they are located close to each other on the same chromosome.
Linkage disequilibrium	The occurrence of specific alleles at different locations in the DNA that are relatively close to each other (linked) more often than would be expected by chance alone (disequilibrium).
Locus	The physical location that a gene occupies within a chromosome. (Plural: loci.)
Monozygotic twins	Twins with identical genetic makeup (i.e., identical twins) as a result of the fertilization of a single egg that then splits into two embryos.
Mutation	Changes in the DNA sequence of the genome can result from errors that occur during DNA replication or meiosis and can be caused by radiation, viruses, and mutagenic chemicals. Most mutations have little or no measurable effect on the gene's function; some are harmful, and a rare few may be advantageous.
Nucleotide	Molecules that, when linked, make up the structural units of RNA and DNA. They are composed of a phosphate group; the bases adenine, cytosine, guanine, and thymine; and a pentose sugar. In RNA, the thymine base is replaced by uracil.
Penetrance	The proportion of individuals who have a particular allele/genotype who express an associated trait (phenotype). Genotypes with a high penetrance result in a larger number of individuals in the population with the associated phenotype as compared with genotypes with a low penetrance.
Phenotype	The observable characteristics displayed by an organism (e.g., morphology, development, gender, eye color, physiologic properties, behavior). Phenotype results from the expression of the organism's genes as well as from the influence of environmental factors and interactions between the two.
Polymorphism	Polymorphism exists when two or more different phenotypes exist within different individuals of the same population. In the context of genetics, it refers to a region of the genome that varies between individual members of the population in such proportions that the rarest of them cannot be maintained just by recurrent mutation. Polymorphism may be actively maintained in populations by natural selection and also by random drift.
Sequencing	Determining in the laboratory the linear arrangement of nucleotides (in RNA or DNA) or amino acids (in proteins).
Signal transduction	A cascade of intracellular events that occurs after the binding of an extracellular signal (e.g., a hormone, a cytokine) to a receptor on the cell surface. The intracellular cascade can result in changes in gene expression in the nucleus and hence an altered phenotype of the cell (e.g., as a result of different protein production).
Single nucleotide polymorphism (SNP)	A polymorphism in a gene caused by a change in a single nucleotide in the DNA sequence. A large number of protein isoforms result from SNPs. SNPs occur frequently; approximately every 100 to 1000 base pairs occur as a result of deletions, insertions, and substitutions. There are estimated to be more than 10 million SNPs in the human genome. Many SNPs that occur in genes have no effect on the encoded protein, but some SNPs do influence the function of the protein that the gene produces. An SNP initially arises as a rare mutation, but it is considered to be an SNP if it occurs in at least 1% of the population.
Splicing	The removal of introns from transcribed RNA. The process of removal can vary, and some exons are skipped or excluded from splicing. This causes the production of "splice variants" or "alternatively spliced" protein isoforms, thereby resulting in the formation of different proteins from the same initial RNA.
Transcription	RNA synthesis. The process of creating an RNA copy of an equivalent section of DNA is the first step of gene expression, and it occurs in the nucleus. The RNA copy that is produced is called *messenger RNA* (mRNA).
Translation	The first stage of protein synthesis. mRNA produced during transcription is decoded to produce an amino acid chain that will later fold into an active protein. Translation occurs in the cytoplasm: ribosomes bind to the mRNA and then facilitate decoding via the binding of transfer RNAs (tRNAs) that have complementary anticodon sequences to those of mRNA. The tRNAs carry specific amino acids that are joined to form a polypeptide as the mRNA passes through the ribosome.

DNA, Deoxyribonucleic acid; *RNA,* ribonucleic acid.

Patterns in Populations and Pedigrees

With all of the attention focused on silicon arrays, laser scanners, and the other "glamorous" gadgets of advanced genomic technologies, it is important to consider how much can be learned about the genetic basis of a disease before stepping into a DNA laboratory. In fact, a strong foundation of knowledge about a disease's frequency in different populations and its occurrence among closely and distantly related family members (i.e., pedigrees) is absolutely essential. Without this foundation, endless gigabytes of DNA sequence data will not enable scientist-clinicians to develop a solid understanding of the causes of a disease. The human genome has not evolved in a test tube nor inside a supercomputer; rather, it has existed for millennia in natural populations and been transmitted from generation to generation, from parents to children. Only by carefully studying the genetics of a disease in populations and pedigrees can we hope to begin to unearth the complex interactions between genes and the environment that underlie individual differences in disease susceptibility. This field of research is known as *genetic epidemiology.*

Genetic epidemiologists often first look at whether a disease occurs more often in some human populations than others. These comparisons can include both populations in different geographic areas as well as racial or ethnic groups living in the same region. Does the disease have more severe symptoms, more rapid rates of progression, or an earlier age of onset in some populations? Such findings suggest (but do not prove) that genetic differences that are important for the disease may exist among the populations.

Before the massive human migrations in recent centuries, most human populations existed in semi-isolation from other populations around the globe. As a consequence of natural selection (i.e., differential survival and reproduction), populations sometimes adapted genetically to their local environments. The most famous example of adaptation is the sickle cell hemoglobin variant that protects an individual against the infectious disease malaria. This variant is common among populations that live in areas where this mosquito-borne parasite has long been endemic because it provides strong protection against the severe symptoms of this disease. The variant persists at high frequency in these populations, although persons who inherit two copies of the mutation (i.e., one from the mother and one from the father) are severely affected by the disease sickle cell anemia. A balance between the benefit of malaria resistance in persons who inherit only one copy of the variant versus the disadvantage of sickle cell disease keeps the variant at relatively high frequencies among populations where malaria is present. Another example of population differentiation by natural selection is the ability to digest the milk sugar lactose as an adult that evolved in Europeans in conjunction with the domestication of dairy cattle more than 8000 years ago. In addition to differentiation driven by natural selection, as is seen in these examples, a random process called *genetic drift* also causes populations with little or no migration between them to differentiate genetically over time. Thus one cannot assume that every population difference observed has a functional biologic basis.

Regrettably, the comparison of periodontitis in different populations across the globe is extremely challenging because of the lack of calibrated examiners and standardized disease definitions.[7] One of the most dramatic population differences in which data quality is not an issue is the observation that both localized and generalized forms of early-onset aggressive periodontitis occur about ten times more frequently among African Americans as compared with Caucasians.[45] Human racial and ethnic groups often differ dramatically with regard to the frequency of mutations of genes that have major effects on disease risk. For example, cystic fibrosis is caused exclusively by recessive mutations in the CFTR gene, and it varies in frequency from 1 in 3000 Caucasians to 1 in 15,000 African Americans in the United States, whereas only 1 in 350,000 Japanese individuals is affected.[68] It is possible that the 10-fold higher prevalence of early-onset aggressive periodontitis in African Americans is caused by the elevated frequency of high-risk gene variants in this population. However, additional evidence is needed before such a conclusion can be drawn. Although comparative studies of different populations may provide clues as to possible genetic mechanisms underlying a disease, the environments of the populations may also be dissimilar in important ways. It is possible that variations in diet, exposure to pathogenic oral bacteria, or some unknown and unmeasured environmental factors could entirely explain the observed differences in the frequency of aggressive periodontitis among population groups. Until solid data confirm a genetic basis for population differences, we need to wait before drawing firm conclusions.

The comparison of disease occurrence or severity in identical (monozygotic) versus nonidentical (dizygotic) twins is a powerful method for distinguishing between effects caused by variation in genes versus factors in the environment. This requires us to make what is usually a reasonable assumption that the environments of pairs of identical twins are no more or less similar than the environments shared by pairs of nonidentical twins. If variation among individuals in disease susceptibility or severity is caused entirely by factors in the environment, then we expect pairs of identical twins to be no more similar to each other in terms of disease risk than pairs of nonidentical twins. All twins, whether identical or nonidentical, are expected to be more similar to their co-twins, on average, than to unrelated members of their local population because they were raised in the same family environment with similar diets, microbial exposures, and so on. However, if genetic variation plays an important role in determining a certain trait, then genetically identical twin pairs will be more similar to each other than nonidentical twin pairs. This is because identical twins share 100% of the same genes, whereas nonidentical twin pairs share only 50% of their parents' genes, on average. Genetic epidemiologists calculate a measure called *heritability* that is based on these correlations and that estimates the portion of all variation in the trait attributable to inherited genetic variation. Traits with variation that is determined entirely by differences in environmental exposures have heritabilities of zero, whereas traits with variation attributable solely to inherited genetic differences without any environmental influence have heritabilities of 1.0. Heritabilities are sometimes reported as a percentage that ranges from 0% to 100%.

Most human disease and nondisease traits fall in the middle of this range, with heritability ranging from 0.25 to 0.75. For example, in one study, type 2 diabetes was estimated to have a heritability of 0.26, and abnormal glucose tolerance had a heritability of 0.61.[71] For it to be feasible to use the twin method with adequate statistical power, the disease has to be fairly common so that the researcher can recruit enough twin pairs in which at least one of the twins is affected by the disease. Not surprisingly, with regard to periodontal disease, only chronic periodontitis occurs frequently enough to have been studied using the twin design. Two twin studies of modest size (i.e., 110 and 117 pairs) have been reported, and these estimate the heritability of measures of chronic periodontitis range from 40% to 80%, thereby clearly implicating genetic variation in disease risk.[57,58] Interestingly, a study of bacteria associated with periodontitis found no difference between identical versus nonidentical twins.[59] This suggests (at least for these twins, most of whom did not have severe periodontitis) that inherited variation in risk is not mediated by genes that influence the presence of specific bacteria in subgingival plaque. Another review also failed to find an association between single nucleotide polymorphisms (SNPs, pronounced "snips") at interleukin-1 or other host genes and the presence or counts of subgingival bacteria.[63] These studies were performed before today's high-throughput DNA sequencing technologies were fully available to study the microbiome in depth; however, it remains to be seen whether sharing specific strains of the hundreds of oral microbial species may be related to host genetics.

Another method used by genetic epidemiologists to understand and distinguish different mechanisms of transmission of diseases through families is called *segregation analysis*. This is relatively straightforward for traits in which mutation in a single gene causes the disease to develop with nearly 100% certainty in carriers, whereas persons who do not inherit the mutation are at little or no risk. For example, carriers of a single copy of the Huntington disease gene mutation or carriers of two copies of a cystic fibrosis gene mutation always develop these diseases if they reach the ages at which symptoms of these conditions normally emerge. By tracking the transmission of these diseases in families, it is obvious, for example, that Huntington disease is a dominant single-gene disorder: It is transmitted with 50% probability to offspring of affected individuals, and thus it is often found occurring across many generations of large pedigrees. By contrast, parents of children with cystic fibrosis are rarely affected themselves, and 25% of siblings are affected by cystic fibrosis when the disease is present in a nuclear family. This pattern of transmission is expected if a disease is recessive (i.e., it requires the inheritance of a mutated gene copy from both parents, who themselves have one normal and one mutated copy and so are not affected). For most common complex diseases, however, having a high-risk gene does not automatically lead to development of the disease; this phenomenon is called *reduced penetrance*. Furthermore, several or even dozens or more different genes may influence disease susceptibility; this is known as *oligogenic inheritance* and *genetic heterogeneity*. Environmental exposures are also important modifiers of disease risk. Such highly complex combinations of multiple genetic and environmental risk factors make the challenge of deciphering genetic mechanisms by merely observing transmission patterns in families using the segregation analysis approach unfeasible. The limitations of this approach were illustrated in an analysis that facetiously presented evidence of a recessive gene controlling the trait of attending medical school.[53] "Risk" for this outcome among first-degree relatives of a doctor was elevated 61 times above that of the general population. More recently, a robust quantitative analysis of the family histories of characters in the Harry Potter series suggested that a dominant gene controls the inheritance of magic abilities.[75] Because the etiology of periodontitis is likely to be highly complex, segregation analyses of this disease that have been reported in the literature should be viewed with considerable skepticism. Unfortunately, the simplifying assumptions required for this method make the results unreliable and potentially misleading. For highly complex diseases, such as most cases of periodontitis, assays at the DNA level need to be combined with careful evaluations of clinical measures among related individuals to derive robust conclusions about a disease's genetic architecture. Some of the key features of the different techniques for studying the genetics of periodontal disease are explained in Table 9.2.

Searching for Answers in the DNA

In theory, a *genetic marker* can be any type of biomolecule or assay that allows us to read inherited differences among individuals in their DNA sequences. Blood groups, protein isozymes, and human leukocyte antigens (HLAs) were among the first developed markers, but even simple traits that are controlled by single genes (e.g., eye color) can also serve this purpose. Genomic methods have made these methods obsolete because researchers can now determine a person's inherited variation directly at the DNA level for a much lower cost and with greater speed and accuracy. So-called next-generation DNA sequencing methods are projected to enable researchers and clinicians to obtain nearly the entire 3 billion–DNA base human genetic blueprint for less than $1000.[25,91] At present, most genetic studies use a combination of whole genome arrays that can evaluate up to 1 million variable DNA sites in a single assay in combination with lower-throughput methods that are used for the fine mapping of chromosome regions of special interest.[74] These regions are said to contain *candidate genes* of high priority for further investigation either because of the genes' known biologic functions or because results of previous genome-wide surveys indicate strong statistical chances that disease susceptibility genes are located in certain regions of one or more chromosomes. Types of variation include SNPs in which one DNA base is substituted for another; small insertions and deletions ("in/dels") of one or more DNA bases and larger structural changes in the DNA, such as inversions (in which a piece of DNA of hundreds or thousands of bases in size is cut out and sewn back into the chromosome in the opposite orientation); and copy number changes (in which a given segment of DNA is either missing or occurs in more than the usual two copies inherited as one copy from each parent).

Equipped with these powerful tools for rapidly measuring DNA variation, the next question to address is what kinds of study design are most powerful for identifying the dozen or more variants that influence the risk of disease from among the millions of DNA differences that exist between any two individuals in a typical population. One method that has been highly successful for finding molecular defects related to simple genetic diseases caused by the mutation of a single gene, such as cystic fibrosis and Huntington disease, is *linkage analysis*.[1,9] This gene-mapping strategy requires families with one or more members affected by the disease to be recruited and clinically and molecularly evaluated for a relatively small number of genetic markers. Depending on the type of marker used, as few as 500 markers or up to 10,000 markers distributed evenly across the genome are needed. Investigators usually try to recruit families with two or more close relatives, such as sibling pairs, who are affected by the disease as well as parents and other siblings who may be unaffected. With a *null hypothesis* that suggests that a region of the chromosome does *not* contain genetic variation that influences disease risk, siblings share identical genetic material inherited from their parents an average of 50% of the time. However, if the region of the chromosome being evaluated contains a gene that has a substantial effect on disease risk (i.e., increases the risk by tenfold or more), then pairs of siblings who are both affected by the disease will share the chromosome region that contains the disease gene substantially more often than 50% of the time, and the null hypothesis of 50% sharing will be statistically rejected if the study has an adequately large sample of such families. This simple example illustrates how linkage analysis is performed. In practice, both small and large extended families are studied; this will include the simultaneous evaluation of the sharing of genetic material among both affected and unaffected relatives. Sophisticated mathematical algorithms and computer programs are used to carry out the huge number of calculations required for data analyses.

After achieving many successes with the use of linkage analysis for "simple" diseases caused by the mutation of a single gene, this method was extended to complex diseases caused by combinations of multiple susceptibility genes and environmental risk factors. Unfortunately, these conditions proved to be beyond the reach of linkage analysis in most instances. In numerous studies conducted during the 1990s, either researchers failed to find any genes

TABLE 9.2 Techniques for Studying the Genetics of Periodontal Disease

Candidate gene approach	A gene-mapping approach that tests whether one allele of a gene occurs more often in patients with the disease than in subjects without the disease. These methods are also referred to as *association analyses,* and they aim to identify which genes are associated with the disease. Candidate genes are chosen on the basis of their known or presumed function (i.e., they have some plausible role in the disease process, such as producing a protein that is important in the disease pathogenesis). Conceptually this makes sense, but it requires some knowledge of the candidate gene to look for it.
Case–control studies	Studies in which the genetic makeup is compared between cases (who have the disease in question) and controls (who do not). The populations need to be carefully matched, otherwise apparent observed differences between cases and controls could arise because of ethnic or geographic variation, for example.
Twin studies	Comparisons of traits—including diseases in monozygotic, dizygotic, or usually both types of twins—aimed at determining whether variation in the trait among members of a population is caused by genetic variation in inherited DNA sequences, environmental exposures in the subjects' lives, or some combination of both of these processes. Twin studies often measure the *concordance rates* of twins with regard to a particular trait or disease of interest. Monozygotic (identical) twins are nearly identical in their DNA, whereas dizygotic (nonidentical) twins share an average of half of their DNA as identical sequences inherited from their parents. If a disease has high heritability, identical twins will be more likely to be either both affected or both unaffected (concordant). However, this assumption is complicated in many diseases. A genetic mutation may not have complete *penetrance,* and environmental conditions may contribute to the development of the disease (e.g., one twin may smoke and the other may not). Furthermore, many diseases are polygenic (i.e., caused by alterations in multiple genes).
Familial aggregation and relative risk	Many diseases run in families, and the degree of clustering within the family can be estimated by comparing the number of disease cases in relatives of patients to the risk of disease in the general population. Difficulties with this approach relate to the fact that, in addition to having many genes in common, family members also share many aspects of a common environment (e.g., diet, nutrition, smoking, infectious organisms, shared socioeconomic factors).
Segregation analyses	Statistical analyses of the patterns of transmission of a disease in families in an attempt to determine the relative likelihood that the disease is caused by a single gene with dominant or recessive inheritance, by multiple genes, or entirely by variation in exposure to risk factors. The observed proportions of offspring who have the trait or disease being evaluated (i.e., the phenotype) are compared with the proportions expected to be found in the general population.
Linkage analysis	A technique used to map a gene responsible for a trait to a specific location on a chromosome. These studies are based on the fact that genes that are located close to each other on the chromosome tend to be inherited together as a unit. As such, these genes are said to be "linked." Because linkage analysis initially requires the use of expensive DNA markers, this was originally only considered justified after finding strong evidence of a genetic basis for a trait with the use of segregation analyses or family aggregation studies. One difficulty with linkage analyses is that many diseases are not caused by a single gene of "major" effect but rather by multiple genes of "minor" effect. In the latter situation, multiple genes each contribute a small amount to the phenotype, disease, or trait. The linkage study approach has little power for detection, whereas association analysis methods may still be quite powerful.
Genome-wide analyses	A genome-wide association study (GWAS) investigates genetic variation across the entire genome simultaneously, with the aim of identifying genetic associations related to a trait or disease of interest. The completion of the Human Genome Project in 2003 and the development of microarray technologies capable of assaying more than half a million single nucleotide polymorphisms have made GWASs possible. This method has the potential to identify the genetic contributions to common diseases. Because the entire genome is analyzed, an important advantage of this approach is that the technique permits the genetics of a disease to be investigated in a nonhypothesis-driven way. In other words, it is not necessary to correctly guess which candidate genes are most interesting to evaluate. A GWAS requires that well-characterized cases and controls be identified. A disadvantage of GWASs is that large clinical sample sizes are required to reduce the likelihood of differences between the cases and controls being observed simply by chance as a result of the hundreds of thousands of multiple statistical tests required to search the entire human genome.

or initially positive findings failed to replicate. Linkage studies of large numbers of carefully diagnosed families for complex diseases (e.g., orofacial clefting in which twin studies had firmly established heritability of 70%) identified at most a tiny fraction of this genetic variation. Mathematical analyses have subsequently shown that the linkage analysis gene-mapping strategy has extremely low statistical power for complex diseases in which each individual susceptibility gene has a relatively small effect on risk (i.e., twofold or less) and in which there is extensive heterogeneity among different families that have different combinations of susceptibility genes and environmental exposures.[78] Consequently, it is not surprising that linkage analysis has been successfully applied only to syndromic forms of periodontitis (summarized elsewhere in this book).

Disappointment over this setback in human disease mapping caused by the initially unrecognized limitations of linkage analysis was short lived. An alternative approach called *association analysis* was also available, although this had been relegated to studies of HLA and a few other markers of special interest during the prime time of linkage approaches.[1,9] Mathematical analyses indicated that if we make some reasonable assumptions about the nature of genetic

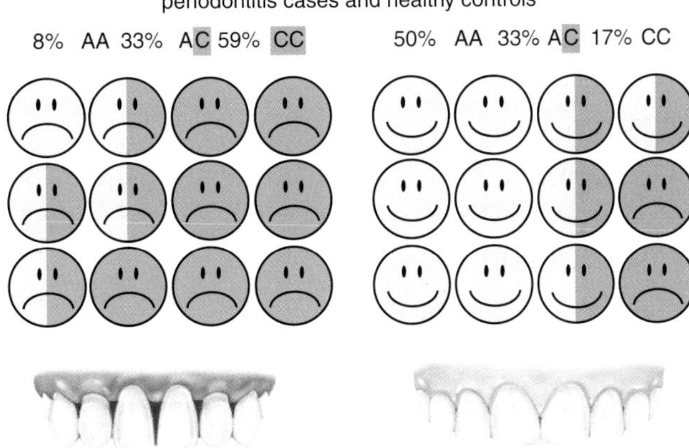

Fig. 9.1 Case–control design for a genetic association study. Periodontitis cases shown on the left have frequencies for a hypothetic genetic marker of 8% AA, 33% AC, and 59% CC, which are substantially different from genotype frequencies found in healthy periodontal controls of 50% AA, 33% AC, and 17% CC. In this example, the CC genotype is associated with increased risk, because it occurs at a much higher frequency in the disease cases; alternatively, the AA allele is protective, because this variant is much more common in the healthy controls.

factors in human disease, this method could provide adequate statistical power for finding genes of small to modest effect on risk while requiring only moderately large sample sizes that would be feasible to recruit.[78] There was, however, one major catch: To search the entire genome using the GWAS method, the number of genetic markers needed was several orders of magnitude greater (i.e., 500,000 to 1 million assays per subject). Fortunately, advances in molecular assay technologies converged in this time period, and several methods of array-based genotyping provided this capability at an acceptable cost.[74]

How association studies are used to find disease susceptibility genes is illustrated for the case–control design in Fig. 9.1. Association analyses are sometimes referred to as *case–control studies,* although this is only one of several sampling methods that can be used (including studies of families). Genotype frequencies of an inherited DNA variant for a group of periodontitis cases are statistically compared with the frequencies of the variant in a matched group of periodontally healthy control subjects. If the genotype frequencies differ so greatly that the results are unlikely to occur by chance, then we conclude that the genotype that is more common in the cases as compared with the controls is associated with increased disease risk. In Fig. 9.1, 59% of the cases have the CC genotype (having inherited a C allele from both of their parents), whereas only 17% of the healthy controls inherited the CC genotype. Therefore, this DNA variant could be used to predict periodontitis risk (but not until after the finding was validated in additional independent studies). Conversely, we can also say that the AA genotype is “protective” against disease because it occurs much more often in the healthy controls (50%) compared with periodontitis cases (8%). Ideally, the cases and healthy controls are matched as closely as possible for race/ethnicity, smoking behavior, age, gender, and so on so that differences in genotype frequency are likely to be caused by real biologic effects on disease development or progression rather than as artifacts of some kind. For example, it is well known that races and ethnic groups sometimes differ dramatically with regard to genotype frequencies as a result of their historic isolation in different geographic regions. Consider, for example, a study that had mostly Swedish cases and mostly Italian controls. We know that there are thousands of DNA variants that differ substantially among these populations because of their geographic isolation throughout human history. Few, if any, of these variants have anything to do with differences in disease risk, but they could falsely appear to be associated because of the failure to carefully match ethnicity in cases and controls. In practice, this is usually not a problem, provided that investigators take reasonable precautions with regard to how cases and controls are selected. It is also now routine practice to use several statistical methods to check for mismatching and then adjust for this during data analysis if it occurs.

The good news is now clearly in: Association studies have been a boon for the discovery of inherited genetic variation important for a wide range of complex diseases, including diabetes, cardiovascular disease, metabolic disorders, obesity, and mental illnesses. Reviews show that dozens of genes have been identified with unquestionable statistical confidence for type 2 diabetes alone, and the list continues to grow.[23,88] Most of these genetic polymorphisms with elevated risk are common in the population (i.e., from 5% up to >50%). Although each variant only increases risk slightly (i.e., twofold or less) because the risk alleles are so common they can account for a nontrivial proportion of the occurrence of disease in the population; this is a measure that epidemiologists call *attributable risk.*

An especially attractive aspect of the GWAS approach is that because the entire human genome is searched, we no longer have to depend on prior hypotheses about the disease’s molecular pathology. In most GWAS studies, about half of the statistically definitive findings point to genes that experts in the field had no suspicion whatsoever were involved in the disease’s etiology. This allows researchers to open up entirely new pathways for investigation that may lead to insights about the disease’s biologic mechanism and suggest novel molecular strategies for pharmaceutical or other therapeutic interventions. In more than a few cases, robust GWAS findings implicate regions of the human genome in which no genes appear to be present, thereby highlighting the limitations of our current knowledge of basic genome functions.

Although great progress has been made toward understanding the etiology of many complex human diseases by using GWAS methods, the approach has nevertheless usually failed to account for most of the heritability known to exist for these conditions.[14,50] One study found that well-established nongenetic diabetes risk factors (e.g., gender, smoking, family history, body mass index, blood lipid and glucose levels) were better predictors of risk than a combination of the top 20 genetic markers for this disease.[89] To improve gene-based risk estimates, the missing heritability needs to be found. The

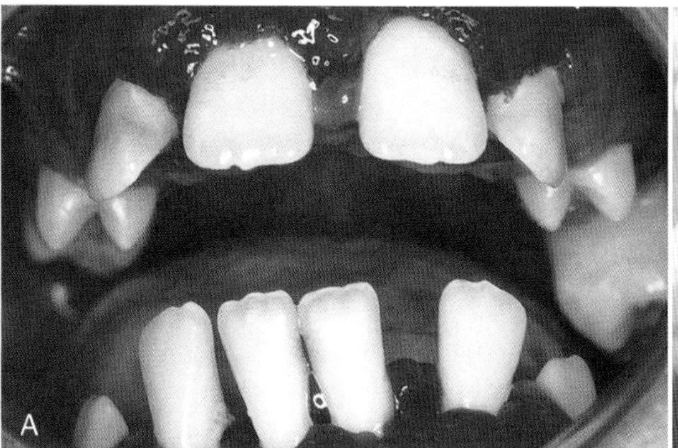

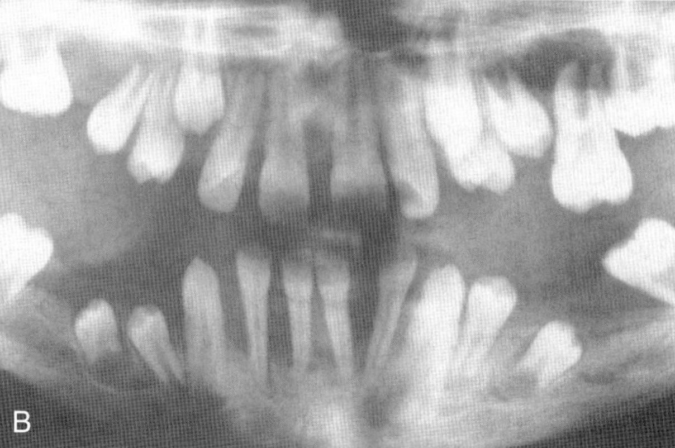

Fig. 9.2 Oral (A) and radiographic (B) appearance of a patient with leukocyte adhesion deficiency. The child was deficient in CD18 (i.e., leukocyte adhesion deficiency type I), which results in absent or severely reduced levels of the β2 integrin molecule. The patient suffered from recurrent infections of the middle ear, the tongue, and the perirectal areas as well as of the periodontium. (B, From Majorana A, Notarangelo LD, Savoldi E, et al. Leukocyte adhesion deficiency in a child with severe oral involvement. *Oral Surg Oral Med Oral Pathol Oral Radiol Endod.* 1999;87:691–694.)

emergence of next-generation DNA-sequencing tools may help advance this search. In theory, data from the entire human genome of more than 3 billion bases may enable researchers to identify the less common (i.e., 1% to 5%) genetic variants that are predicted to have individual gene effects of greater magnitude on disease risk (i.e., greater than twofold but less than tenfold) that cannot readily be found with the use of either GWAS or linkage analysis methods.

Genetic Basis for Individual Differences in Disease Risk

As a result of the appropriate focus on the role of bacterial infections in the disease pathogenesis of periodontitis, inherited human genetic variation is often referred to as *host defense* or, somewhat more broadly, *host response.* However, these terms cover only a small portion of the range of gene functions that may be important for periodontitis risk. Many additional biologic processes that are not directly related to defenses against or responses to infection by microbial pathogens are also likely to play important roles in determining an individual's susceptibility to this disease.

Periodontitis in Genetic Syndromes and Other Diseases

A number of extremely rare conditions consistently include periodontitis among the array of clinical manifestations that define a syndrome. Many genetic syndromes involve mutations of single genes or larger chromosomal regions. However, a number of syndromes, such as fetal alcohol syndrome, are purely environmental in origin. Some of the syndromes that include periodontitis are caused by mutations in specific genes. For example, mutations in the cathepsin C gene have been shown to cause both Papillon–Lefèvre syndrome and Haim–Munk syndrome as well as some forms of nonsyndromic prepubertal periodontitis, and they may also be associated with a risk of aggressive periodontitis.[66] Periodontitis frequently occurs with some subtypes of Ehlers–Danlos syndrome, Kindler syndrome, Down syndrome (trisomy 21), leukocyte adhesion deficiencies (Fig. 9.2), hypophosphatasia, two types of neutropenia, and aplasia of the lacrimal and salivary glands. A large triracial extended family demonstrated evidence of a single gene that caused both early-onset aggressive periodontitis and dentinogenesis imperfecta.

The gene has been mapped with the use of linkage to a chromosomal region that contains a dentin matrix protein gene.[49] Many of these conditions are so rare that few periodontists see even a single case during a lifetime of practice. However, dentists should be aware that these single-gene conditions exist; they need to be prepared to extend clinical evaluations to close relatives and to seek the assistance of or refer to appropriately trained genetic counselors or specialists if a patient's medical history or the presentation of multiple symptoms raises the possibility that he or she may be affected. Clinicians can obtain updated information about these conditions by accessing the publicly available *Online Mendelian Inheritance in Man* database, and typing in "periodontitis OR periodontal disease" as the query term.[2] Further research is necessary to determine whether inherited variation in the genes that cause these rare syndromes may also influence the risk of nonsyndromic forms of aggressive or chronic periodontitis.

Genetic Disorders Associated With Periodontitis

Genetic Syndrome With Periodontitis as an Oral Manifestation	Mutated Gene/ Genes	Functions of Affected Genes
Chédiak–Higashi syndrome	LYST	LYST encodes for lysosomal trafficking regulator that aids in intracellular transport of materials into lysosomes.
Ehlers–Danlos syndrome, periodontal types, 1 and 2; EDSPD1 and EDSPD2 (formerly type VIII)	C1R and C1S	Genes C1r and C1s encode serine proteases that are major constituents of human complement subcomponent C1. Complement is part of the innate immune system and is involved in inflammation.
Papillon–Lefèvre syndrome	CTSC	CTSC encodes for cathepsin C, which is a key activator of serine proteases in immune cells, regulating their function.

Nonsyndromic Aggressive and Chronic Periodontitis

In this section, evidence for the association of inherited genetic variation with aggressive and chronic periodontitis will be considered for cases that present without the co-occurrence of anomalies or disorders of other parts of the body or the affected individual's behavior. Such cases are appropriately classified as *nonsyndromic periodontitis*. This terminology is similar to the way that other human diseases, such as orofacial clefting, have long been recognized as occurring in both syndromic and nonsyndromic forms. The elevated risk of periodontitis that is associated with metabolic conditions (e.g., diabetes, which is addressed elsewhere in this book) is more appropriately considered a comorbidity rather than cause for the designation of a syndrome.

> *A finding of no statistical significance in a well-designed, conceptually sound, adequately powered study testing an important hypothesis is likely to provide more useful information than significance in a study that does not meet these criteria.*[6]

As described previously, twin studies have shown that chronic periodontitis has substantial heritability, and we know that aggressive periodontitis aggregates strongly in families. Because aggressive periodontitis occurs so rarely, it is not feasible to perform a twin study to confirm the heritability of this condition. Neither segregation analyses nor gene-mapping linkage studies are capable of providing reliable information about the genetic etiology of a highly complex disease such as periodontitis. However, large numbers of susceptibility genes have been identified for complex disorders, such as diabetes and cardiovascular disease, using association analysis. It seems reasonable to expect that similar successes could be achieved for periodontitis using this approach. In fact, since the early 2000s, several hundred papers have reported associations of nonsyndromic aggressive and chronic periodontitis with polymorphisms in a number of candidate genes.[8,60,61,85,52] Certain classes of genes (e.g., cytokines) that have long been a focus of attention by immunologists and cell biologists studying pathogenic mechanisms associated with periodontitis have received the most attention. Early reports of relatively weak associations with variation in interleukin-1 (IL-1) genes led to a large number of attempts to replicate and extend these findings.[19] Unfortunately, with few exceptions, association studies of periodontitis have been inadequately powered to detect genetic variation with modest effects on disease risk or progression (i.e., sample sizes that are much too small). In addition, inconsistency with regard to the methods used to classify subjects as periodontal cases versus controls or to quantitatively measure disease severity and extent greatly limit our ability to draw sound conclusions by comparing results reported in different studies.

KEY FACT

Oral Manifestations of Chédiak–Higashi Syndrome

This autosomal recessive condition occurs due to a mutation of the LYST gene that encodes for a lysosomal trafficking regulator protein. The phagocytosis function of immune cells is drastically affected in these patients, making them significantly prone to infections. As a result, severe forms of periodontitis and early exfoliation of both deciduous and permanent teeth are common findings in these patients.

The reason why association studies of periodontitis have largely failed will be challenging to fully address. The first issue is straightforward and simply a matter of numbers. It is noteworthy that the

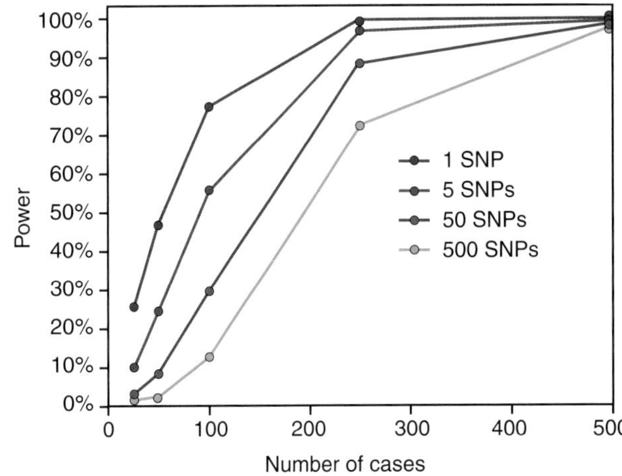

Fig. 9.3 Statistical power estimates are shown for a situation in which we hypothesize that a dominantly transmitted disease susceptibility gene that increases risk twofold and that has an allele frequency in the population of 25% is being mapped by a case–control association study. The lines illustrate the loss of statistical power caused by the requirement to adjust for multiple comparisons when a research study involves the evaluation of not just a single genetic marker but as many as 5, 50, or 500 independent genetic polymorphisms. Although only 100 cases (and 100 controls) may provide sufficient power if only a single marker is being tested, 250 cases and 250 controls are needed if 5 or 50 single nucleotide polymorphisms are assayed; a minimum of 500 cases and 500 controls will be necessary if a study investigates 500 independent genetic markers.

successes achieved for many complex diseases (e.g., diabetes) with the use of the GWAS mapping approach were based on sample sizes involving thousands of cases and controls with multiple replications by *independent* teams of investigators. Statistical theory shows that to detect genes of modest effect, these large sample sizes are absolutely essential. With the use of a statistical power calculator developed for case-control studies,[73] sample sizes required for 80% power are shown in Fig. 9.3 for a study that involves only a single genetic marker as well as for studies that evaluate 5, 50, or 500 independent genetic markers in which the effects of multiple comparisons need to be accommodated. In this example, we assume that the risk gene acts in a dominant manner, with the high-risk allele occurring at a frequency of 25% in the population, and that this allele causes risk among carriers to increase twofold (i.e., a greater effect on risk than observed for many susceptibility alleles found in GWAS studies of other complex diseases).

Many periodontitis association studies reported in the literature involved multiple markers in each publication, and often the same research team reported positive findings for other genes in subsequent papers. Furthermore, because of the difficulties of publishing negative findings (i.e., when no association is found), many research teams working in this area may assay 50 or more genetic markers over the course of their work over several years. Results shown in Fig. 9.3 demonstrate that to obtain 80% power, a study of 50 markers would require more than 200 cases and 200 controls. Even if a research team assays only 5 SNPs, its study would still require 100 cases and 100 controls to achieve adequate power.

Most association findings have been drastically underpowered if periodontitis is assumed to be a complex disease as a majority of association reports for chronic and aggressive periodontitis are based on samples of 100 cases or fewer. As shown in Fig. 9.3, studies of such small sample size have little power to detect a susceptibility gene that increases risk twofold. Given the added concern about publication bias (i.e., that positive findings are more likely to be accepted for publication), we can have little confidence that even the more statistically significant findings are valid and likely to be independently replicated if they are based on such inadequate sample sizes. With only a few exceptions from GWAS, which are noted later in this chapter, publications since 2010 have continued to involve small numbers of cases, and provide marginal statistical support for association.

Aside from important lessons about how *not* to carry out association studies of a complex disease, there are some tentative conclusions that can be drawn from the data available thus far.

CLINICAL CORRELATION

Ehlers–Danlos Syndromes

Ehlers–Danlos syndromes (EDSs) are connective tissue disorders characterized by joint laxity and skin hyperextensibility, scarring, and bruising. Periodontal EDS (EDSPD; previously EDS VIII) is a subtype with autosomal dominant inheritance with severe periodontal inflammation. Children exhibit extensive gingivitis followed by early-onset periodontitis in their teen years, leading to attachment and tooth loss. Serious complications including arterial or gastrointestinal ruptures have also been reported.

For example, when bacteria challenge gingival tissue, CD14 binds to lipopolysaccharide and TLR4 plays a key role in pathogen recognition and the activation of innate immunity.[42] Lactotransferrin (LTF) plays an antimicrobial role as the first line of host defense, and it can also neutralize endotoxin, and inhibit the induction of nuclear factor-κβ (NF-κβ) in monocytes in response to lipopolysaccharides.[37,90] Myeloperoxidase (MPO) is an oxidative enzyme expressed in polymorphonuclear leukocytes. It is involved in the defense against periodontal bacteria and also able to mediate inflammatory tissue destruction in periodontal disease.[54] Glutathione S-transferase mu 1 (GSTM1)[12] and *N*-acetyltransferase 2 (NAT2)[40] genes are responsible for the detoxification of a wide range of chemicals, including tobacco carcinogens. HLA complex genes[87] play a central role in the immune system by presenting extracellular peptides that are important for either self-recognition or initiating immune responses to foreign pathogens. The Fcγ receptor genes (FcγRS) encode receptors for the Fc portion of immunoglobulin G, and they are involved in the removal of antigen-antibody complexes from circulation as well as other antibody-dependent responses.[47] Formyl peptide receptor (FPR1) is a G-protein-coupled receptor of phagocytic cells that interacts with bacterial peptides and mediates chemotaxis, degranulation, and superoxide production involved in inflammation.[27] Cytokines such as the interleukins (IL-1, IL-2, IL-4, IL-6, IL-10), tumor necrosis factor (TNF), and lymphotoxin-alpha (LTA) play a number of important roles in the immunopathology of periodontal disease.[8,65] Prostaglandin-endoperoxide synthase (PTGS2), which is also known as cyclooxygenase-2, is the key enzyme in prostaglandin biosynthesis. It is regulated by specific stimulatory events, which suggests that it is responsible for the prostanoid biosynthesis involved in inflammation.[31] S100 calcium binding protein A8 (S100A8), which is the light subunit of calprotectin, is also associated with inflammatory diseases, including periodontitis.[43] Fibrinogen (FBG) is an acute-phase protein; FBG levels are elevated during inflammation, and the substance has been associated with cardiovascular disease risk.[79] Vitamin D receptor (VDR)[30] and estrogen receptor (ESR1)[92] are hormone receptors involved in skeletal muscle metabolism, including calcium absorption and bone loss. The matrix metalloproteinases (MMPs) are a group of endogenous proteinases that contribute to the degradation of extracellular and basement membrane components.[28] CDKN2B antisense RNA (CDKN2BAS) is a nonprotein coding gene of unknown function that has also been reported to be associated with coronary heart disease.[82] The one GWAS reported for periodontitis, which is described in detail later in this chapter, revealed a strong association of a glycosyltransferase gene (GLT6D1) with aggressive periodontitis,[84] but there is no clear functional relationship of this gene with periodontal disease pathogenesis.

The inconsistency among the reported findings requires a much deeper analysis to understand what may be going on. One possibility is that genetic variation at the candidate gene is *not* associated with periodontitis. When a large number of studies are performed using a multitude of alternative ways of classifying small numbers of cases versus controls, when multiple alternative statistical analyses are run for the same small data sets, and when there may be a bias against the publication of negative results, then a substantial portion of studies should report positive findings, even if no real association exists. Then again, heterogeneity among studies may be real. The negative studies may differ in terms of the racial or ethnic composition of the subjects, and the findings may be valid for some human populations, but not others. Different genetic polymorphisms in the candidate gene may be evaluated in the different studies, and only some of these may actually be associated with disease risk. Different clinical definitions or sources of information (e.g., clinical attachment loss versus bone loss measured from radiographs) may be used to define cases or various quantitative measures may be employed, and these sources of variation may also influence the outcome of association tests. With data limited to mostly small studies, it is not currently possible to definitively determine which of these potential explanations applies to most of the reported findings. To standardize disease definition, the periodontitis classification consensus report has been adopted in which previous "chronic" or "aggressive" periodontitis is classified as periodontitis, and further characterized based on a multidimensional staging and grading system.[70] The new classification raised concerns among researchers who emphasized the importance of distinct phenotypic characteristics of rare localized aggressive periodontitis and the far more common chronic periodontitis affecting older adults.[21,22,69] It is crucial to realize that standardization of the disease phenotype is integral for the discovery of underlying molecular mechanisms of a disease.

CLINICAL CORRELATION

Papillon–Lefèvre Syndrome and Dental Implants

Caused by a mutation in the cathepsin C gene, this syndrome is characterized by advanced periodontitis affecting both deciduous and permanent dentition and palmar plantar hyperkeratosis affecting palms and soles. Patients become edentulous very early in life. Limited scientific evidence in the form of case reports indicates that edentulous patients with this syndrome can be successfully treated with dental implant–supported restorations.

Only a handful of periodontitis association studies have been reported that approach the sample size needed for complex diseases, with more than 400 cases.[20,46,55,56,82,83] This includes the GWAS in which more than 322,825 SNP genetic markers were evaluated for association with the risk of aggressive periodontitis.[84] In the GWAS, statistical testing was performed in sequence for three independent sets of samples with a total of 438 cases and 1320 controls. Interestingly, this relatively powerful analysis failed to yield significant support for the usual suspect candidate genes after adjusting for the large number of hypotheses tested in the analysis. Instead, several novel chromosomal regions and candidate genes were implicated, with among the strongest being a glycosyltransferase gene (GLT6D1),[65] one of several glycosyltransferases in the human genome. This had an unadjusted *P* value of .000000006. However, the *P* value was reduced by three orders of magnitude to .000006 after accounting for the effects of gender, smoking, and diabetes. The adjusted *P* value indicates that we should expect to see a difference in genotype frequency of this magnitude by chance alone about 1 out of 166,666 times under the null hypothesis of no association with disease risk. This may seem to be strong evidence for rejection of the null hypothesis, but this adjusted finding is actually only of marginal statistical significance in the context of a GWAS. In fact, this sometimes occurs by chance alone in the absence of a valid association because this study involved testing more than 300,000 genetic markers. Recently, a sequencing study of five families affected by early onset periodontitis confirmed the presence of deleterious mutations in the GLT6D1 gene. Because there is no obvious functional connection of this gene with what we currently know about the pathogenesis of periodontitis (the protein is thought to play a role in signaling in development), it may be tempting to further downplay the finding's significance. However, experience with GWAS studies of other complex diseases has shown that, quite often, valid gene associations are discovered in pathways that experts in the field did not previously realize were even related to the disease's biology. This makes such discoveries all the more valuable, assuming that they are definitively and independently replicated, because they offer the potential of revealing completely new avenues for further exploration at the cellular and molecular levels and because they potentially may also provide novel targets for therapeutic interventions.

The first genome-wide study that focused on chronic periodontitis included 4504 European Americans, with 43% having moderate chronic periodontitis and 17% having severe chronic periodontitis.[17] No genome-wide significant associations were found in this large sample, with no support whatsoever for the much-studied periodontitis candidate genes IL-1A, IL-1B, IL-1RN, IL-4, IL-6, IL-10, CD14, FCGR2A, MMP1, TLR4, TNF, and VDR. However, intriguing suggestive evidence was found supporting the role of cellular immune response, nervous system, and cytokine signaling pathways. By broadening the phenotype, a subset of these subjects was also analyzed using genome-wide SNP data for periodontal pathogen colonization, but again, only statistically suggestive results were obtained with this smaller sample.[18] A large-scale replication analysis of 23 much-studied candidate genes in 600 aggressive periodontitis cases and 1448 control subjects of German ethnicity found support only for SNPs in IL-10, but this association was not replicated in 1437 chronic periodontitis cases of German ethnicity.[81] Several GWAS of periodontitis have now been completed for moderately large sample sizes, and the results are sobering:[64,80] No statistically strong replicated associations have been found in any of these studies. Furthermore, in two large cohort studies, DNA sequencing of the coding regions of nearly all genes (exome sequencing) also failed to reveal any rare variants with a statistically significant association with chronic periodontitis.[39]

It is clear from these findings that large-scale association studies, possibly involving family-based designs and searches for rare high-risk variants, will be needed to more fully elucidate the role of genetics in periodontal disease. From what we now know, it appears increasingly likely that the high heritability estimated for chronic periodontitis is likely attributable to a large number of inherited DNA variations in more than 100 and possibly 500 or more different genes. This is the genetic architecture that we know underlies other highly heritable traits such as height, and this discovery has important implications, and places limitations on the use of genetic variation for tests to predict risk, as will be addressed later in this chapter.

Challenges and Opportunities for the Future

The classification of disease used for research studies is an especially difficult challenge to be faced if we are to benefit fully from the opportunities offered by the genomics revolution.[72] If we cannot agree which subjects in a study are affected by disease or a particular subtype of disease, how severely they are affected, or how quantitative measures related to disease should be obtained and analyzed, then the chances of making progress will be low, regardless of how advanced our molecular or bioinformatics technologies become. This problem is important for all kinds of research, not only genetics, and the issue of diagnosis is addressed elsewhere in this book. However, genetics may have a unique role to contribute toward solving this dilemma. This may best be illustrated by an example from the early 1980s in which medical geneticists and oncologists could not agree about the classification of the disease neurofibromatosis (NF). "Splitters" argued for up to a dozen different etiologic subtypes, whereas "lumpers" suggested that there may be only a single disease with a lot of variation among individuals as a result of differences in environmental exposures and variation in "genetic background" (a term that encompasses the cumulative influence of all other genes distributed throughout the genome in addition to the "major gene"). It had been discovered in research conducted during earlier decades that NF was transmitted in families as a single dominant gene, but the question remained as to how many different genes were involved (locus heterogeneity). Furthermore, even if only one gene was involved, it was possible that different mutations caused unique patterns of signs and symptoms (allelic heterogeneity). The controversy was largely resolved by the discovery of the NF1[48] and NF2[86] genes. After these genes were identified, DNA testing could distinguish individual patients, and the diagnostic classification controversies were resolved. In hindsight, it became clear that the clustering of signs and symptoms fell into two major categories among different types of families and depended on which NF1 or NF2 mutation was involved and what kind of gene mutation was involved. Although such gene-based clarity is unlikely for a complex multigenic condition, such as periodontitis, the potential exists that subtypes of patients may eventually be classified more effectively by examining their DNA to see what kinds of susceptibility genes they inherited.

To move toward this desired outcome, however, we need to use the best strategies available today to classify research subjects into categories, such as cases versus controls. Alternatively, we can attempt to use quantitative measures of bone loss or attachment loss to classify research subjects along a more continuous gradient that ranges from persons with extremely healthy periodontium and little or no sign of disease to those with tooth loss and high measures of pocket depth and attachment loss in remaining teeth. Family studies have numerous advantages in genetics; for these designs, the use of a quantitative measures approach is especially attractive. When searching for gene associations in unrelated cases and controls, we can decide to select only subjects who are clearly affected as cases, and compare them with control subjects who clearly are periodontally healthy. When studying families, however, one has to assign a disease status to all of the family members to fully make use of all the information in the biologic unit. We may initially recruit the family on the basis of an unambiguous case known as the *proband* (i.e., the subject who makes the family eligible for inclusion in the study), but the handling of parents, siblings, and other close relatives who may be neither clearly periodontally healthy nor clearly diseased is not easy to determine. For example, if we establish a threshold and require that two or more teeth have a minimum of 4 mm of attachment loss for subjects to be classified as affected, then how we handle family members who are borderline becomes the

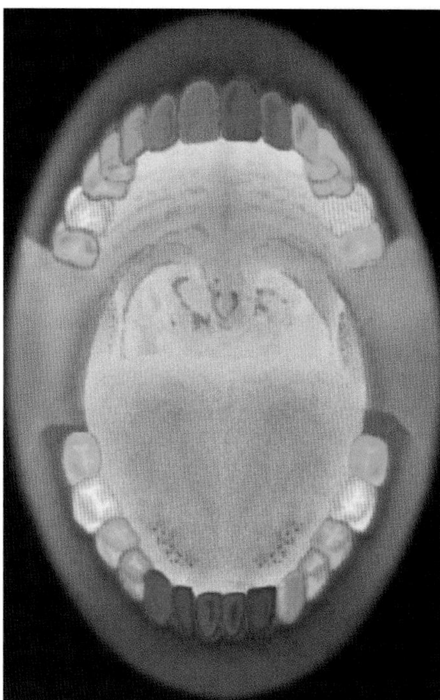

Fig. 9.4 Illustration of the similarities and differences among different kinds of teeth with regard to the frequency and severity of attachment loss observed in early-onset aggressive periodontitis patients and their unaffected family members with the use of the principal components analysis method.[16]

challenge. For example, siblings of the proband may have several teeth with 3 mm of attachment loss in addition to one tooth with 6 mm of loss. Such subjects are close to but not quite over the threshold. They are neither clearly healthy nor clearly diseased, and this makes them problematic for categorical data analyses that require them to be classified as cases versus controls.

One aspect of the diagnosis challenge that is especially poorly understood is how and why different teeth are affected by periodontitis. Dentists have long recognized that incisors and first molars are more likely to be affected during early-onset disease, but it is not straightforward to incorporate this information into threshold disease definitions. One way to begin to address the problem of variation among teeth is to apply multivariate methods, such as principal components analysis, as was done in a study of aggressive periodontitis.[16] This method maximizes the proportion of the total variation in attachment loss among all 28 teeth explained by a limited number of master variables called *principal components.* In this study, three principal components explained 77.8% of the total variance. The results are displayed in Fig. 9.4, with color intensities being used to help visualize the patterns of correlation among different tooth types. Mixtures of red, green, and blue are "painted" onto the teeth, with each color's intensity adjusted according to the tooth's relative "weight" calculated for each of the principal components. This quantitative analysis shows how attachment loss is correlated among different kinds of teeth. First molar teeth are consistently painted yellow by their principal components scores; these teeth are very different from all of the other teeth with regard to their patterns of attachment loss. There is a gradual change in the patterns of attachment loss for the other teeth that extend out from the central incisors (magenta) to the lateral incisors (purple), the cuspids (blue), the premolars (blue-green), and the second molars (green). In addition to generally exploring patterns of periodontal disease dispersed in the geography of the mouth, because these are studies conducted in families, we can also use genetic epidemiologic methods to validate and compare alternative measures of disease.

Specifically, we can calculate heritability for different quantitative variables (e.g., simple mean attachment loss averaged across all teeth or averaged for specific groups of teeth) as well as for more complex variables, like these principal components. In the study of aggressive periodontitis illustrated in Fig. 9.4, the principal component most heavily weighted on the first molars had a heritability of 30%, which was actually slightly higher than the 26% heritability estimated for a simple mean of attachment loss in the first molars. By using heritability and other genetic measures such as association with specific inherited polymorphisms, it may be possible to refine diagnostic and disease classification systems by aligning these according to subgroups of subjects that share homogeneous etiologies. Another example of moving beyond simply classifying subjects as cases versus controls but using principal component analysis to combine multiple measures of disease such as levels of pathogens and inflammatory markers was reported using a GWAS design.[67] The results of this more complex approach to the phenotype pointed to several novel genes of potential interest that now require independent replication.

> *Learning from the experience of other complex diseases, Sir Isaac Newton famously remarked in 1676: "What Descartes did was a good step. You have added much several ways ... If I have seen a little further it is by standing on the shoulders of Giants."*

Although there remains some enthusiasm for further GWAS studies, as noted previously, even the most successful GWAS results (e.g., those that have been obtained for type 2 diabetes) have failed to identify most of the genetic variation responsible for the disease. The discovery of so many gene associations related to risk of type 2 diabetes accounts for a small fraction of the disease's heritability.[14] To track down the missing genetic variation, a great deal of attention is now turning to whole genome DNA and exome sequencing methods[13] that have become available at lower cost in recent years. Sequencing methods also expand the ability to measure gene expression in various tissues. These data, in combination with the ever-increasing availability of proteomic assays, will challenge investigators with huge quantities of information. Aside from generating the many gigabytes of data involved in this technology, the greatest challenges of "systems biology" may lie in developing the bioinformatics tools needed to sift through and identify the key pieces of information that are important for advancing our knowledge from among the vast rising sea of biologic data pouring out of our laboratories.[4]

Strategies for improving our understanding of the genetics of periodontitis as well as for increasing the possibilities for the translation of this knowledge to benefit patients in the clinic are being mapped out today by teams of geneticists, clinicians, and information scientists who are currently focused on major medical conditions. By continuing to learn from the experiences of these early genomic explorers, it is reasonable to hope that dental researchers will be able to avoid some of their mistakes, and follow the quickest path to advances in knowledge about diseases of interest.

Precision Dentistry: Using Genetics for Personalized Treatment

Pharmacogenomics and Individualized Dentistry

If individuals differ in susceptibility to a disease, especially if underlying the superficial signs and symptoms of a disease, there really are etiologically distinct subtypes of disease pathogenesis, and the traditional medical model of "one size fits all" treatment may not

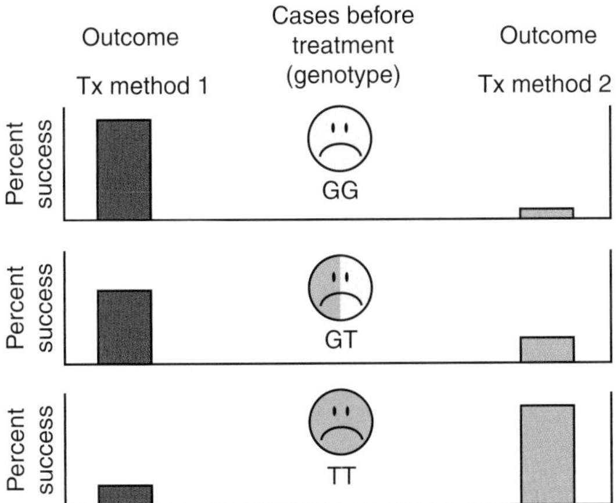

Fig. 9.5 Inherited genetic variation determines treatment success. Individuals who inherited the GG or GT genotypes at a gene involved in a biologic pathway related to either the underlying disease susceptibility mechanisms or to the body's response to the therapy have very good chances for success with treatment method 1 *(Tx method 1)* but poor prognoses with treatment method 2 *(Tx method 2)*, whereas individuals with the TT genotype respond positively to treatment method 2 only.

be optimal. As shown in Fig. 9.5, cases of disease (as illustrated by circles with unhappy faces) may differ with regard to genotype for a gene that determines which treatment works best for each individual. Some cases inherited G alleles from both their mother and their father and thus have a GG genotype, whereas others have a GT or TT genotype.

The gene may distinguish between different subtypes of disease etiology or pathogenesis, or it might code for an enzyme, transporter, or receptor important for the metabolism of a therapeutic drug and have nothing directly to do with disease susceptibility. In the example illustrated in this figure, treatment method 1 *(Tx method 1)* has a high success rate when it is provided to subjects with the GG or GT genotypes, but it usually fails for cases with the TT genotype. TT genotypes experience much better outcomes when provided with treatment method 2 *(Tx method 2)*, but this method often fails for subjects with the GG and GT genotypes. Sometimes concerns about severe side effects that limit the use of a therapy rather than differences in efficacy and risk of side effects can also be genetically determined. If clinicians are not aware of the relationships between these genotypes and treatment success or side effects, it would appear that neither treatment is consistently effective. Clinicians would be forced to use a trial-and-error approach, first trying one method and then switching to another if the first one fails. At best, this causes unnecessary expense and does not provide an optimal quality of care. Furthermore—and especially for deadly diseases such as cancer—precious time may be lost in halting the advance of the disease; by the time the clinician discovers an individual's best treatment, it may be too late. This strategy of individualized medicine is already being practiced for an increasing number of diseases.[11,26]

In dentistry, a test based on inherited genetic variation at the interleukin-1 alpha (IL-1α) and IL-1β cytokine genes was proposed as being able to predict the risk, progression, and severity of periodontitis. The test has been commercialized and gone through multiple versions (PST, PerioPredict, and today's version, ILUSTRA). Although specific numbers are not available, the test does not yet appear to be widely used. A number of reviews of the large number of studies of the IL-1 gene polymorphisms indicate that genetic variation at these loci may be associated with, at most, a modest effect on disease risk.[33,65] In 2007, Huynh-Ba and colleagues concluded that "there is insufficient evidence to establish if a positive IL-1 genotype status contributes to progression of periodontitis or treatment outcomes."[33] A similar lack of supporting evidence for the use of IL-1 genetic testing to predict implant success has also been reported.[3,32] A meta-analysis of the available data suggested that these much-studied IL-1 polymorphisms have a small (odds ratio ≈1.5) but significant effect on periodontitis risk, although only for chronic periodontitis in white populations.[19,38] However, it is essential to emphasize that because heritability for chronic periodontitis is estimated to be 50%,[58] the small effect of the IL-1 polymorphisms makes up at most a tiny fraction of the genetic component of risk for this disease (which remains missing, as discussed previously).

Candidate Genes Possibly Related to Risk of Chronic or Aggressive Periodontitis

- Interleukin (IL)-1 gene cluster (IL-1A, IL-1B, IL-1 receptor antagonist), IL-4, IL-6, and IL-10.
- TNF-alpha
- Leukocyte receptors for the constant (Fc) part of immunoglobulin (FcγR)
- Vitamin D receptor
- Pattern recognition receptor genes (TLRs, cluster of differentiation [CD]-14)
- Matrix metalloproteinase (MMP)-1

As the benefits of individualized or personalized treatments that are optimally matched to the genome of each patient have been demonstrated for cancer and increasing numbers of other human diseases, interest has grown in applying this approach to dentistry.[41,76] The first major study that attempted to develop guidelines for individualized treatment has been reported.[24] This study involved 5117 adults between the ages of 34 and 55 years with no prior diagnosis of early periodontitis who were followed retrospectively for 16 years. The aim was to evaluate whether only a subset of high-risk patients really benefits from two versus only one preventive visit per year to avert tooth loss. The risk factors that were tested were smoking, diabetes, and the IL-1 composite genotype. The authors of the study concluded that all three risk factors predict which patients benefit from two preventive visits. They proposed the use of the IL-1 genetic test[34] to detect the IL-1 composite genotype, which, along with smoking and diabetic status, was looked at as a risk factor for progressive periodontitis. The study claimed that by reducing the preventive dental visits to one per year in so-called low-risk patients, $4.8 billion would be saved annually. However, an independent reanalysis of the findings[15] showed that of the three assessed risk factors, only diabetes and smoking had statistically significant effects on tooth extraction risk. This conclusion was supported by an independent critical commentary by a leading expert in the field of epidemiology.[35] Therefore it is clear that we lack consistent evidence to demonstrate the scientific validity or clinical utility of the IL-1 genetic test that is commercially available as a periodontitis risk prediction tool.[34] This first major attempt to use a genetic test in mainstream dentistry continues to be an area of great controversy, and dentists will need to remain aware of the scientific consensus regarding such tests as these emerge in the future so that they can accurately advise patients on their use and limitations.

As genetic testing becomes widespread, especially if it is marketed through direct-to-consumer models, increasing responsibility will fall on dentists to fully understand and counsel their patients about the implications of test results for their treatment options and their risk of developing various dental diseases in the future. Tests for diseases of the oral cavity may likely combine inherited polymorphisms with oral microbial profiles, and they might also include assays of gene expression or proteomic data measured in saliva or other oral tissues. Few dentists practicing today have been educated to prepare themselves for these future challenges. This major shortfall of knowledge urgently needs to be addressed. This can be done by continually educating today's dental professionals about advances in knowledge of human genetics and the uses and potential misuses of genetic testing, by establishing multidisciplinary teams of health practitioners in which dentists work closely with genetics counselors and medical geneticists, or by combining these approaches.

Epigenetic Control

Epigenetic changes are heritable changes that do not depend on changes in DNA sequence. Epigenetic mechanisms are essential for regulation of transcription and provide a dynamic, reversible, and mechanistic framework that could explain the way in which environmental and behavioral factors interact with the genome to alter disease risk.

Epigenetic modifications include DNA methylation and histone acetylation, both of which are reversible, dynamic changes affecting gene expression. DNA methylation is controlled by DNA methyl transferase enzymes (DNMTs), which add methyl groups to the DNA molecule. When methylation occurs in a gene promoter, it typically suppresses transcription of that gene. Histone acetylation promotes transcription and is controlled by histone acetyltransferases, which add acetyl groups to lysine residues and histone deacetylases, which remove the acetyl groups from lysine residue.

Epigenetics factors play an important role in chronic inflammatory conditions by allowing microbial persistence to play a role in the infectious mechanism, resulting in pathogen interference with the host genome.[5] Thus, periodontal pathogens containing lipopolysaccharides can be a cause of epigenetic modifications affecting expression of inflammatory mediators in periodontal tissue, and low-grade chronic inflammation present in periodontal disease has been shown to promote DNA methylation.[29] Periodontal disease is closely linked with diabetes mellitus complications, which are related to epigenetic changes.[44]

Acknowledgments

We acknowledge the support provided by the National Institutes of Health's National Institute of Dental and Craniofacial Research grants 5R01DE016057 and 5R01DE018635 and the Foundation of the University of Medicine and Dentistry of New Jersey.

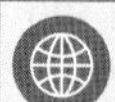
A Case Scenario is found on the companion website eBooks.Health.Elsevier.com.

Suggested Reading

1. Morelli T, Agler CS, Divaris K. Genomics of periodontal disease and tooth morbidity. *Periodontol 2000*. 2020;82(1):143–156.
2. Masumoto R, et al. Identification of genetic risk factors of aggressive periodontitis using genomewide association studies in association with those of chronic periodontitis. *J Periodontal Res*. 2019;54(3):199–206.
3. Richter GM, et al. Exome sequencing of 5 families with severe early-onset periodontitis. *J Dent Res*. 2021:220345211029266.
4. Barros SP, et al. Targeting epigenetic mechanisms in periodontal diseases. *Periodontol 2000*. 2018;78(1):174–184.
5. Hamza SA, et al. Emerging role of epigenetics in explaining relationship of periodontitis and cardiovascular diseases. *Diseases*. 2021;9(3).
6. Li Y, et al. Epigenetic changes caused by diabetes and their potential role in the development of periodontitis. *J Diabetes Investig*. 2021;12(8):1326–1335.

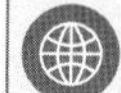
References for this chapter are found on the companion website eBooks.Health.Elsevier.com.

CHAPTER 10

Biofilm and Periodontal Microbiology

Wim Teughels | Magda Feres | Sukirth M. Ganesan | Mark David Gidley | Yvonne L. Hernandez-Kapila | Nicholas S. Jakubovics

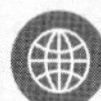 For expanded discussions on microbiology and its relationship to biofilm, please visit the companion website at eBooks.Health.Elsevier.com.

 Videos for this chapter can be viewed on the companion website at eBooks.Health.Elsevier.com.

CHAPTER OUTLINE

Introduction

There is active debate about whether the human fetus inside the uterus is sterile,[549] but there is little question that colonization with microorganisms occurs rapidly during and after birth.[100,139,464] Within 2 weeks, a nearly mature *microbiota* is established in the gut of the newborn baby. After weaning (>2 years), the entire human microbiota is formed and comprises a very complex collection of hundreds of different types of bacteria with approximately 10^{14} microbial cells.[340] From this moment on, our body contains *1.3 to 10 times more bacteria* than human cells.[462] It has been estimated that, for a normal, healthy human being, the bacterial population comprises 2 kg of the total body weight. This is fascinating if one realizes that the average human brain weighs only about 1.4 kg.

Colonization of the oral cavity also starts close to the time of birth, with the types of microorganisms present determined by the mode of delivery.[203] Within hours after birth, the sterile oral cavity is colonized by low numbers of mainly facultative and aerobic bacteria.[502] At that time, the oral microbiota of newborns closely resembles the mother's vaginal microbiota or, for newborns delivered by cesarean section, the mother's skin microbiota.[100] From the second day, anaerobic bacteria can be detected in the infant's edentulous mouth.[112,433] The number of oral bacteria increases gradually as a result of exposure to external environmental microbial sources.[238,276,433]

Because of the paucity of longitudinal studies, relatively little is known about the initial establishment of key microbes found in the oral cavity of children and adults.[264] It is estimated that the oral bacterial microbiome of adults encompasses approximately 700 commonly occurring species,[1] roughly half of which can be present at any time in any individual.[27,367] When one thinks about bacteria, one almost immediately associates them with different pathologic conditions. However, most oral bacteria are harmless commensals under normal circumstances. This means that this microbiota lives in harmony with its host but that, under specific conditions (i.e., increased mass and/or pathogenicity, suppression of commensal or beneficial bacteria, and/or reduced host response), disease can occur. A shift in microbial community leads to an imbalance, or dysbiosis, in the microbiota. This shift in the microbial community can be largely independent of the acquisition of new members of the microbiota and instead reflects changes in the abundance of either individual organisms or consortia of organisms resident within the subgingival biofilm (previously referred to as plaque).[76] The importance of the commensal microbiota is clearly illustrated by the development of *Candida* infections when the normal oral microbiota is reduced, such as after a longer period of systemic antibiotic usage.[548] In addition, it has been shown that severe periodontitis in young adults, previously termed aggressive periodontitis, is associated with a loss of colonization of *S. sanguinis* (see eFig. 10.1D).[507] Conversely, investigators showed in mice that the commensal microbiota is required for *Porphyromonas gingivalis* (see eFig. 10.1H)–induced bone loss.[4,81]

The oral microbiota is extremely complex. Because it both affects and is affected by the host, the oral environment, and the pathogenesis and management of periodontal diseases, a profound knowledge of periodontal microbiology is necessary for dental professionals. This chapter presents the steps and players that drive the microbial colonization of the oral cavity, including a detailed discussion about the interplay between microorganisms and host. Topics such as the interconnection between the oral microbiome and other microbiomes in the body and how the oral microbiota may relate to systemic diseases are also discussed. The composition of the oral biofilm associated with periodontal health and disease is reviewed, from historical to contemporary concepts, as well as the composition of the microbiota associated with different oral conditions, such as necrotizing periodontal diseases, periodontal abscesses, endo-periodontal lesions, and peri-implantitis. Finally, the effects of different periodontal treatments in reverting the dysbiotic biofilm associated with periodontitis are also presented.

The Oral Cavity From a Microbe's Perspective

From an ecologic viewpoint, the oral cavity, which communicates with the pharynx, should be considered an "open growth system" with an uninterrupted ingestion and removal of microorganisms and their nutrients. Any microorganisms that are unable to adhere to a surface within the mouth are washed away in the flow of saliva and swallowed.

KEY FACT

Most micro-organisms can survive in the oropharynx only when they adhere to either the soft tissues or the hard surfaces. Microbes may be removed by:

- Swallowing, mastication, movement of the tongue, or blowing the nose
- Implements used to maintain oral hygiene
- The wash-out effect of the salivary, nasal, and crevicular fluid outflow
- The active motion of the cilia of the nasal and sinus walls

The oral cavity is an extremely varied landscape which forms a dynamic ecosystem with a range of ecological niches that microorganisms are able to colonize. It is an entry point for microbes through dietary intake, direct contact, inhalation, open-mouth breathing, and host-to-host contact. Colonization of the oral cavity is a selective process and not all microbes are well-adapted to thrive in this environment.[316,398,399] The intra-oral environment is subject to significant changes in the prevailing conditions at different times and at different sites within the oral cavity. The composition and diversity of the microbial community is therefore impacted by physical gradients of temperature, humidity, nutrient content, salivary flow, oxygen tension and pH, as well as shear forces due to mastication.[3,399] Frequent exposure to dietary sugars can significantly affect the dynamics of bacterial adhesion and accumulation.[504]

The constant lubrication of the oral cavity by saliva allows microbes to disperse and reach distant sites within the oral cavity, with saliva effectively acting as a transport medium. The three major salivary glands differ in their rates of salivary secretion and salivary composition.[398] There is a dense and expansive network of minor salivary glands associated with the labial, palatal and buccal mucosa, which secrete viscous, proteinaceous saliva with less buffering capacity.[83,398] Although saliva has antimicrobial properties, it has also been reported to promote growth of a health-associated microbiota. This is partly by aiding attachment via selected salivary proteins and glycoproteins that form the acquired enamel pellicle (see later), and also through supplying nutrients such as urea, bicarbonate, lactate, and amino acids released from salivary protein degradation.[56] The proximity to a salivary gland, with fluctuations in salivary flow and salivary composition, could be a source of significant environmental variation[389] and it has been reported that the spatial organization of microbial communities is impacted by salivary flow.[400] In order to persist in the oral cavity, microbes need to adhere to either the soft or hard tissues in order to avoid removal forces such as washing out by the salivary and crevicular flow, swallowing, frictional removal by diet and tongue and masticatory movements, and through oral hygiene regime.[316,521] Surface features of distinct intra-oral habitats providing opportunities for adhesion, therefore, have an impact on microbial colonization and distribution.

Within the oral cavity, there are a diverse range of ecological niches that are colonized by microbial communities (Fig. 10.1). The different ecological niches vary greatly in their physical, chemical, and morphologic characteristics. One of the major distinctions between intra-oral environments colonized by microbes is whether microbial communities are formed on shedding (oral mucosa) or non-shedding surfaces (teeth, dental restorations, dental implants, or dental prostheses[398]). The rapid turnover of oral lining epithelia (shedding three times per day) provides an effective mechanism to reduce bacterial adhesion to the soft tissues;[504] the rapid turnover would allow less time for microbial communities to form. Non-shedding surfaces, such as the enamel surface of teeth, dental implants and dental appliances such as dentures and orthodontic appliances, are potentially susceptible to microbial colonization. Within each ecological niche, a number of physical and chemical factors have a selective effect on microbial communities at any one time, including salivary or gingival crevicular fluid (GCF) flow rates, pH and redox potential, and aspects of the host immune response.[399]

Hard Tissues

In the human body, teeth and nails are the only naturally occurring non-shedding surfaces. Artificial non-shedding surfaces of medical importance include catheters, artificial joints, dental implants, dentures, and heart valves. From a microbiological viewpoint, teeth and implants are unique for two reasons: (1) they provide a hard, non-shedding surface that allows for the development of extensive structured bacterial deposits; and (2) they form a unique ectodermal interruption. A special seal of epithelium (junctional epithelium) and connective tissue is present between the external environment and the internal parts of the body. The accumulation and metabolism

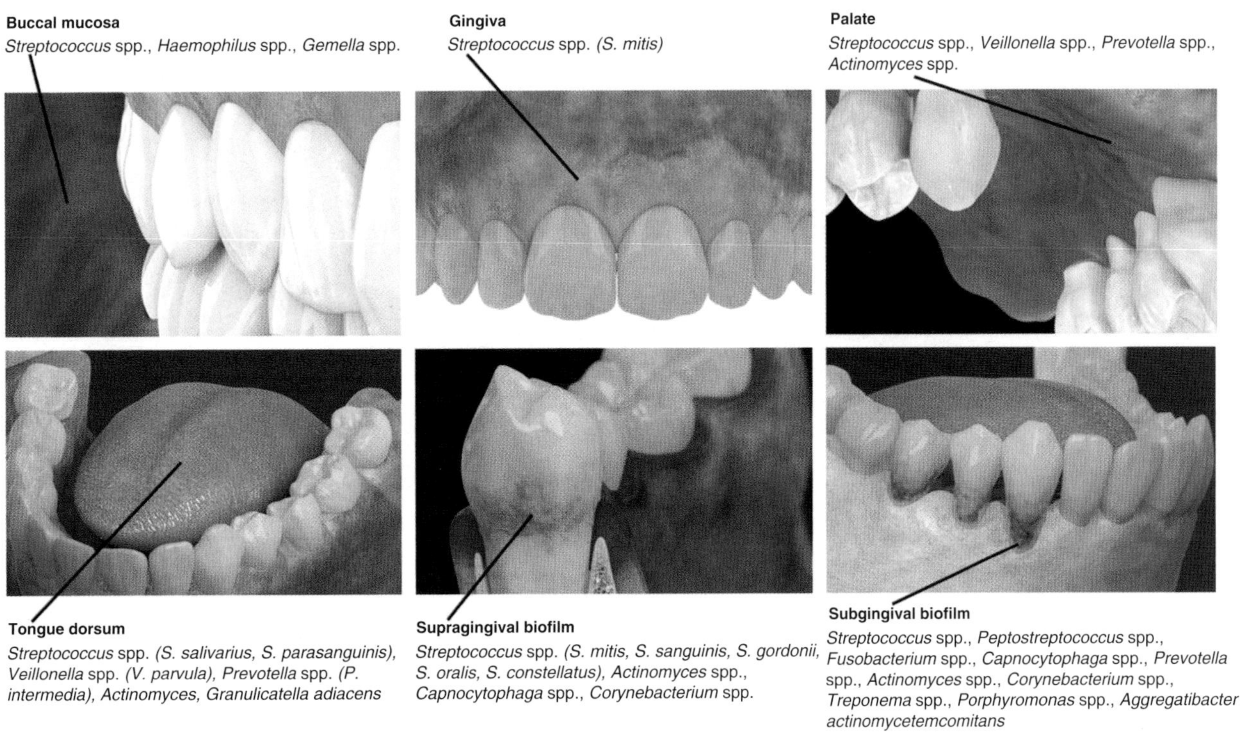

Fig. 10.1 Different intra-oral ecological niches with the most prevalent bacterial species.

of bacteria on these hard surfaces are considered the primary causes of caries, gingivitis, periodontitis, peri-implantitis, and, sometimes, bad breath. The teeth provide hard, smooth, non-shedding surfaces that are accessible to microbial colonization both above the gum line (supragingival) and below the gum line (subgingival) and have been reported to account for approximately 20% of the total surface area of the oral cavity.[307] The teeth are bathed in saliva which enables dispersal of microbes over the surfaces of the teeth. Areas of the teeth such as pits and fissures and proximal surfaces are more protected from salivary flow and also from the activity of the tongue. The rate of saliva flow, therefore, varies over individual tooth surfaces and varies based on tooth position and these variations in saliva flow rate and saliva clearance can directly impact the physiology and ecology of microbial communities.[399] Bacteria do not attach directly to the tooth surface but instead bind to the acquired enamel pellicle, a layer of proteins and glycoproteins that is primarily derived from saliva.

In patients suffering from the onset of periodontitis, the formation of periodontal pockets creates a subgingival ecological niche. Periodontal pocket formation leads to an increase in surface area for microbial colonization on the root surface of teeth leading to the development of a subgingival microbial biofilm. A periodontal pocket has a subgingival tooth surface available for colonization and also the gingival tissue forming one side of the pocket. The increased surface area available for colonization by microorganisms can lead to a significant increase in microbial load between periodontal health and periodontitis.[399] Deeper periodontal pockets lead to the development of low-oxygen microhabitats which favor colonization by anaerobic bacteria. Localized inflammation results from increased microbial colonization of this subgingival environment, leading to increases in temperature and GCF flow rate.[219] The increased flow of GCF provides proteins and glycoproteins that can be used as substrates for bacterial metabolism. In the periodontal pocket, different strategies contribute to bacterial survival, such as adhesion to the pocket epithelium and, when dentine is encountered, the colonization of the dentinal tubules.[405] The crevicular fluid with its constant outflow does not favor the maintenance of unattached bacteria in the periodontal pocket.

The environmental parameters of the subgingival region differ from those of the supragingival region. The gingiva surrounding the teeth provide a keratinized stratified squamous epithelium and the juncture with the teeth creates a nutrient-rich crevice.[316] The gingival crevice or pocket is bathed by the flow of crevicular fluid, which is derived from serum and contains many substances that bacteria may use as nutrients. There can be variations in temperature in the gingival sulcus depending on whether the gingival tissues are in a state of health or disease.[316] Host inflammatory cells and mediators are likely to have considerable influence on the establishment and growth of bacteria in the subgingival region. Both morphologic and microbiologic studies of subgingival biofilm reveal distinctions between the tooth-associated regions and the soft tissue–associated regions of subgingival dental biofilms (Fig 10.2A–C).[282,349] In periodontal pockets, there are high numbers of bacteria attached to pocket epithelial cells in vivo. Areas of gingival inflammation are characterized by an increased number of adhering bacteria.[107,534] These adhering bacteria can also infiltrate the pocket wall in relatively large numbers and reach the underlying stroma (Fig. 10.3).[132,312,441] In general, a positive correlation exists between the adhesion rate of pathogenic bacteria to different epithelia and the susceptibility of the affected patient to certain infections.[360]

Soft Tissues

The dorsal surface of the tongue has a specialized structure of keratinized stratified squamous epithelium with papillae. There are variations within this environment between different types of papillae with a large area of filiform and fungiform papillae and, more posteriorly, large circumvallate and foliate papillae. The densely packed papillae and fissures on the dorsum of the tongue create a rough topography with a high surface area and so the dorsum of the tongue, especially where covered with papillae, creates an environment with crevices with low oxygen tension suitable for anaerobic bacteria.[9,316] A further topographically distinctive location is the

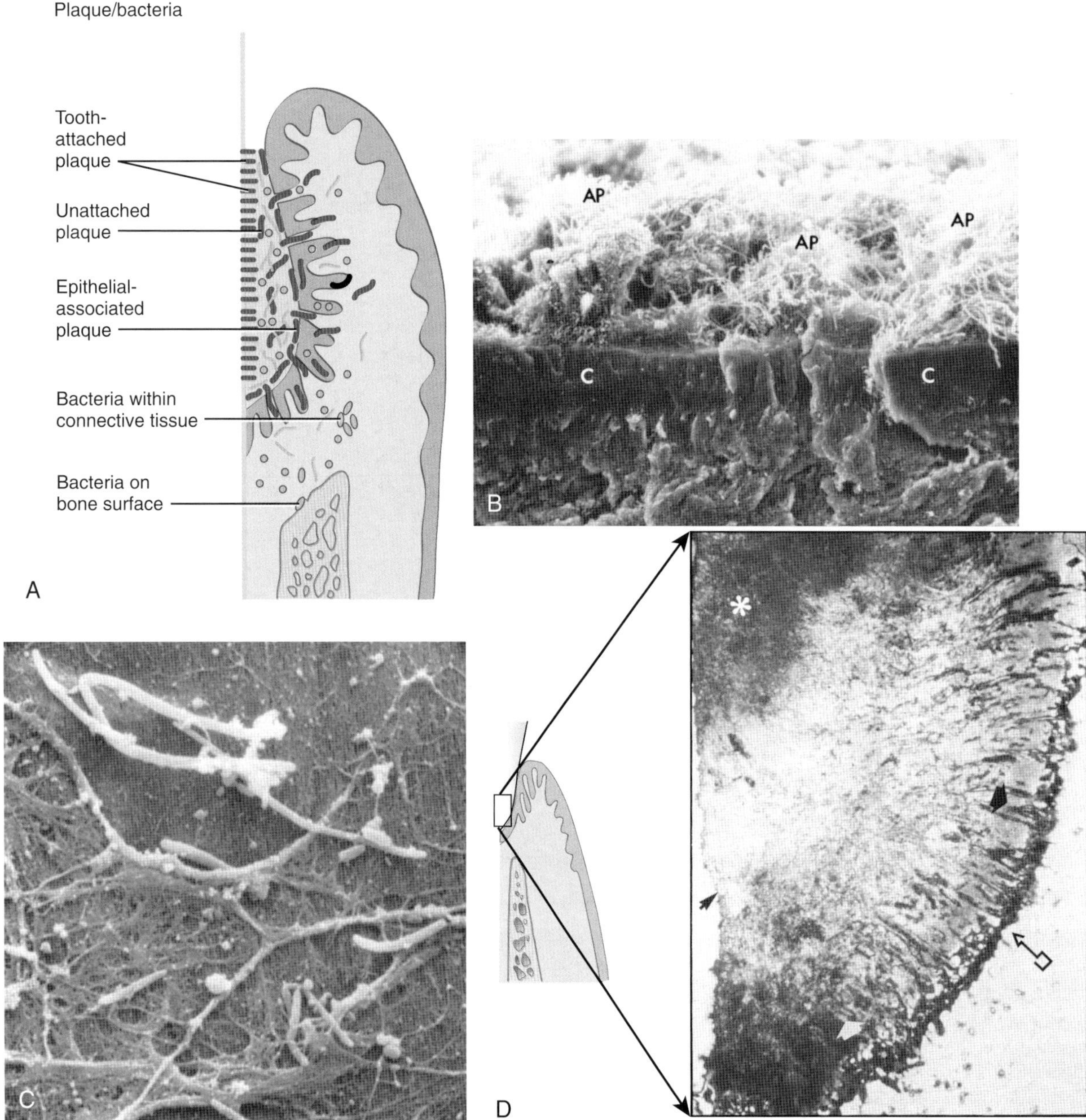

Fig. 10.2 Subgingival plaque. (A) Diagram depicting the plaque–bacteria association between the tooth surface and the periodontal tissues. (B) Scanning electron photomicrograph of a cross-section of cementum *(C)* with attached subgingival plaque *(AP)*. The area shown is within a periodontal pocket. (C) Scanning electron micrograph of cocci and filaments associated with the surface of pocket epithelium in a case of marginal gingivitis. ×3000. (D) *Left,* Diagrammatic representation of the histologic structure of subgingival plaque. *Right,* Histologic section of subgingival plaque. *Arrow with box,* Sulcular epithelium. *White arrow,* Predominantly gram-negative unattached zone. *Black arrow,* Tooth surface. *Asterisk,* Predominantly gram-positive attached zone. (B, Courtesy Dr. J. Sottosanti, La Jolla, California.)

tonsillar crypts which have been reported to have a diverse bacterial microbiota.[1,316] The lateral and ventral surfaces of the tongue are smooth and non-keratinized and lack the characteristic fissures and crevices of the dorsal surface. Consequently, the lateral and ventral surfaces of the tongue differ significantly in surface topography and are also associated with differences in microbial profile.[1,398]

The hard palate comprises a firmer keratinized epithelium.[316] The flexible lining mucosa of the floor of the mouth, buccal mucosa, soft palate, and labial mucosa lacks keratinization. The buccal mucosa is characterized by a high oxygen concentration, lubrication by saliva, and has a high rate of desquamation of epithelial cells.[9] Mucosal surfaces are covered in a pellicle that is distinct from the enamel pellicle. Whilst it is also a subset of salivary proteins, the mucosal pellicle is thought to be composed mainly of large molecular weight glycoproteins such as salivary mucins.[166] Evidence suggests it has a protective role involved in lubrication of the oral epithelia and moisture retention and also protects against excessive bacterial colonization.[166,389]

In health, a core set of microorganisms is almost universally present in these ecosystems. This core microbiome includes members of the phyla Firmicutes (*Streptococcus* spp., *Veillonella* spp., and *Granulicatella* spp.), Proteobacteria (*Neisseria* spp., *Campylobacter* spp., and *Haemophilus* spp.), Actinobacteria (*Corynebacterium* spp., *Rothia* spp., and *Actinomyces* spp. [see eFig. 10.1C],

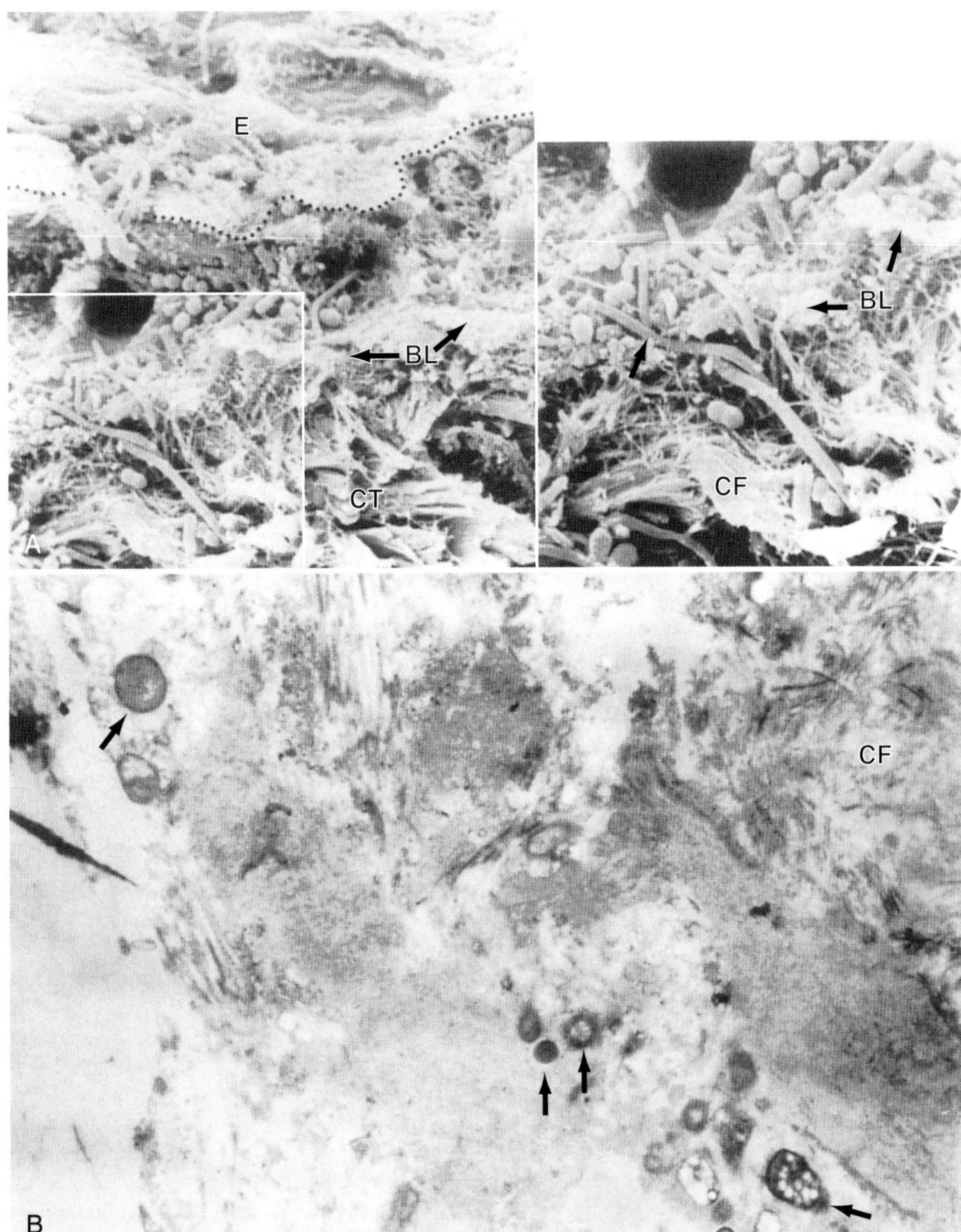

Fig. 10.3 Bacterial penetration into the pocket wall with advanced periodontitis. (A) Penetration through the pocket epithelium *(E)* and the basement lamina *(BL)* into the connective tissue *(CT)* *(arrows)*. *CF*, Collagen fibers. (B) Connective-tissue–associated bacteria *(arrows)* in a patient with advanced periodontitis. ([A] Courtesy Dr. R. Saglie. [A] and [B] From Nissengard RJ, Newman MG. *Oral Microbiology and Immunology*. 2nd ed. Philadelphia: Saunders; 1994.)

Bacteroidetes (*Prevotella* spp., *Capnocytophaga* spp. [see eFig. 10.1Q], *Porphyromonas* spp.), and Fusobacteria (*Fusobacterium* spp.).[190,265,586] Although some species such as *S. mitis* (see eFig. 10.1A) are widely distributed on hard and soft tissues throughout the mouth, other species and strains show marked specificity for particular sites within the oral cavity (see Fig. 10.1).[116] There is evidence that there are significant variations in the microbial population between individuals and across different intra-oral habitats.[111]

A study by Xu and coworkers (2015)[578] reported that the buccal mucosa was associated with lower bacterial diversity and proposed this may be due to challenges associated with colonizing this area, for example, the rapid shedding of the mucosa, exposure to salivary flow rate, increased oxygen tension, masticatory movements, contact with the host innate immune system and generally less protection in comparison with some of the more sheltered intra-oral sites.

As well as site specificity having an impact on microbial colonization of a given niche, there have also been reported variations in surface-associated bacterial communities along an ecological gradient from the anterior to posterior oral cavity irrespective of the type of tissue.[400]

It has been suggested that teeth are the primary habitat for periodontal pathogens because soon after a full-mouth tooth extraction in patients with severe periodontitis, key pathogens such as *Aggregatibacter actinomycetemcomitans* (see eFig. 10.1K) and *P. gingivalis* disappeared from the oral cavity, as determined by bacterial culturing techniques.[80] *Prevotella intermedia* (see eFig. 10.1H) and other black-pigmented *Prevotella* spp. (see eFig. 10.1I) remained, but at lower detection frequencies and numbers. The same applies to edentulous infants and wearers of full dentures in whom significant proportions of periodontal pathogens have

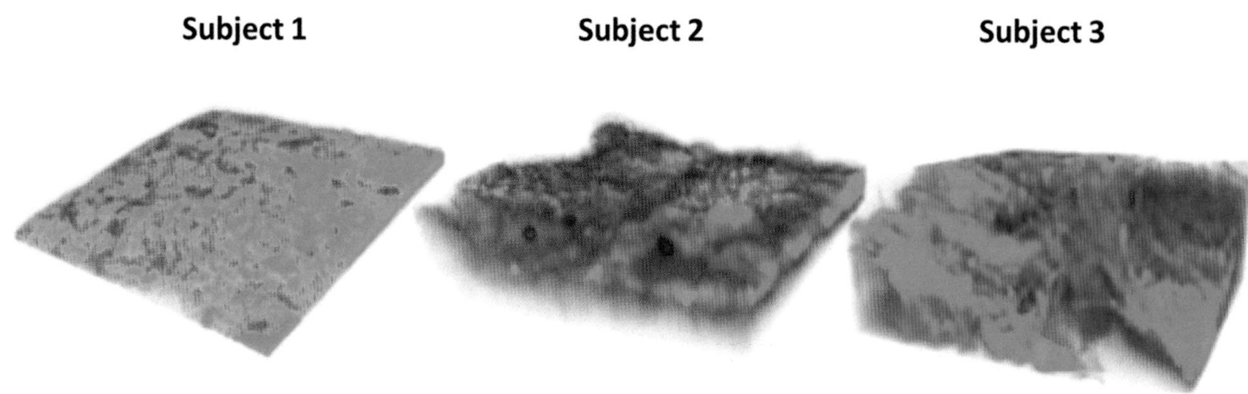

Fig. 10.4 Architecture of oral biofilms formed on enamel discs in situ in three subjects. Biofilms were allowed to develop on the enamel surfaces mounted on healing abutments in the oral cavity for 7 days. The abutments were then removed, stained with BacLight Live/Dead (ThermoFisher Scientific, Waltham, MA) staining, and visualized using confocal laser scanning microscopy. (Adapted from Rabe P, Twetman S, Kinnby B, et al. Effect of fluoride and chlorhexidine digluconate mouthrinses on plaque biofilms. *Open Dent J.* 2015;31:106–111.)

been recorded, with the exception of *A. actinomycetemcomitans* and *P. gingivalis.*[79,238] Therefore, teeth were considered as a "porte d'entrée" for periodontal pathogens. However, studies involving the use of molecular tools to detect and quantify oral bacteria indicate that *A. actinomycetemcomitans* and *P. gingivalis* are not entirely eradicated after full-mouth extraction. They may remain colonizers of the oral cavity, but when teeth are lost, the relative numbers of these bacteria decrease.[410,412]

Bacteria and Their Biofilm Mode of Living—Life in "Slime City"

To many people, the word *microbiologist* conjures images of someone in a laboratory coat swilling a flask of bacterial cells that are growing happily as pure cultures in nutrient-rich broth. In nature, bacteria rarely enjoy such an easy life. The major struggle faced by bacteria lies in obtaining sufficient nutrients to support growth. Competition is rife, and most microbial communities contain many different species, sometimes 100 or more, sharing the same site. Nutrients tend to concentrate at interfaces, and consequently, the densest bacterial populations are located at interfaces of various kinds. In aquatic ecosystems, the major interfaces are the solid-liquid boundaries, such as the surfaces of submerged rocks or soil particles, and the air-water interface that is present in open systems, such as oceans or lakes. Bacteria grow well in the laboratory at the solid-gas interface on the surface of an agar plate. However, desiccation rapidly kills most bacterial cells, and microbial growth at solid–gas interfaces is therefore generally restricted to areas where moisture is available. The human body provides several interfaces that support microbial populations, of which the most important in healthy individuals are the skin, gut, mouth, and female urogenital tract. As mentioned previously, the oral cavity is unusual in this regard because it provides both hard, non-shedding surfaces, as well as shedding surfaces that are accessible for microbial colonization. Microbes need to successfully colonize these surfaces in order to survive in the mouth. The importance of surfaces for microbial growth was recognized as early as the 1920s when a number of workers independently noted that bacteria growing on glass slides submerged in soil were different from bacteria that could be cultured in broth.[263] However, it was not until around 50 years later that sessile microbial populations were considered to be sufficiently different from free-living microorganisms to merit their own name, and the term *biofilms* was coined.[128] Biofilms are composed of microbial cells encased within a matrix of extracellular polymeric substances, such as polysaccharides, proteins, and nucleic acids. Bacteria that grow in multispecies biofilms interact closely with neighboring cells. Sometimes these interactions are mutually beneficial, as is the case when one organism removes another's waste products and uses them as an energy source. In other instances, bacteria compete with their neighbors by secreting antibacterial molecules such as inhibitory peptides (bacteriocins) or hydrogen peroxide (H_2O_2) (Video 10.1). In addition, the biofilm mode of growth facilitates cell-cell signaling and deoxyribonucleic acid (DNA) exchange between bacteria. It is clear that microbial ecology within biofilm communities is highly complex and that, in many cases, knowledge is only emerging at this point.

Biofilms are heterogeneous: variations in structure exist within individual biofilms, between different types of biofilms, and between individuals (Fig. 10.4).[413] However, some structural features that are common to many biofilms have been noted. For example, biofilms frequently contain microcolonies of bacterial cells. Water channels are commonly found in biofilms, and these can form a primitive circulatory system that removes waste products and brings fresh nutrients to the deeper layers of the film. Surface structures, such as fronds, can dissipate the energy of fluid flowing over the biofilm and lead to the rapid blockage of vessels.[103] Mixed-species biofilms often have heterogeneity in the distribution of different species. Steep chemical gradients exist, such as those of oxygen or pH, and these produce distinct microenvironments within the biofilm.

Biofilms are associated with the pathogenesis of a number of chronic human infections and the biofilm mode of living is thought to provide both survival advantages within certain environments and also the potential for enhanced virulence.[372] Parsek and Singh (2003) proposed criteria to define the general characteristics of bacterial biofilm-associated infections.[372] These include association with a surface or association with some substratum, the presence of bacterial cell clusters, or microcolonies, surrounded by an extracellular matrix, the infection is usually within a defined location, and the infection shows elevated resistance to antimicrobials (compared to component microorganisms when in the planktonic state).

Dental Biofilms

Microbial populations on the surfaces of teeth are excellent examples of biofilm communities (Fig. 10.5). The architecture of a dental biofilm has many features in common with other biofilms. It is heterogeneous in structure, with clear evidence of open fluid-filled channels running through the biofilm mass (Fig. 10.6).[72,73,569] Nutrients reach the sessile (attached) microcolonies by diffusion through water channels to microbial microcolonies. The bacteria exist and proliferate within the intercellular matrix through which the channels run. The matrix confers a specialized environment that distinguishes the bacteria that exist within the biofilm from those that are free-floating; this is the so-called planktonic state in solutions such as saliva or crevicular fluid. The biofilm matrix functions as a barrier. Substances produced by bacteria within the biofilm are retained and concentrated, which fosters metabolic interactions among the different bacteria.

The importance of dental biofilms for oral diseases, such as dental caries and periodontitis, together with the relative ease with which tooth surface biofilms can be accessed, has led to dental biofilms becoming some of the most highly studied biofilm systems. It is anticipated that, by understanding the mechanisms involved in the accumulation of dental biofilms and the transition from health to disease, it will be possible to improve our control over these processes and to restrict biofilm-associated oral diseases further.

Formation of the Dental Biofilm

The development of dental biofilms follows a well-established sequence of events where initial colonizers, predominantly streptococci, act as a foundation to establish an environment suitable for later colonization by potentially more pathogenic species (Fig. 10.7).[249] The biofilm develops sequentially with middle and late colonizers joining via processes such as cell-cell coadhesion and coaggregation.[228] Colonization of an intra-oral surface begins immediately after its introduction in the oral cavity. Colonizing bacteria can be detected within 3 minutes after the introduction of sterile enamel into the mouth.[168] The process of dental biofilm formation can be divided into several phases: (1) the formation of the pellicle on the tooth surface, (2) the initial adhesion/attachment of bacteria, and (3) colonization/biofilm maturation (see Fig. 10.7).

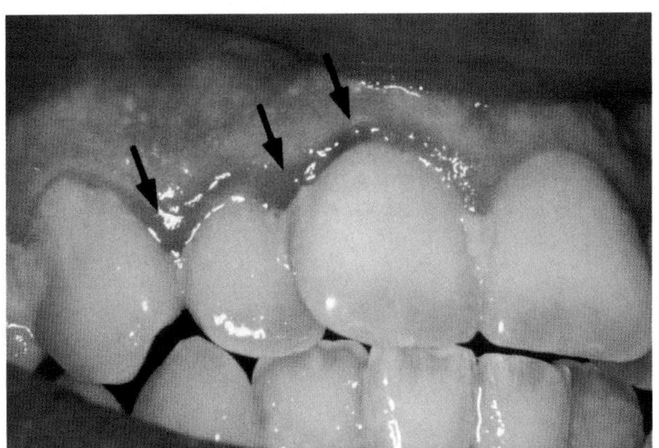

Fig. 10.5 Clinical picture of 10-day-old supragingival plaque. The first signs of gingival inflammation *(arrows)* are becoming visible.

Initial Adhesion/Attachment of Bacteria

The initial steps of transport and interaction with the surface are essentially nonspecific (i.e., they are the same for all bacteria). The proteins and carbohydrates that are exposed on the bacterial cell surface become important when the bacteria are in loose contact with the acquired enamel pellicle. The specific interactions between microbial cell surface "adhesin" molecules and receptors in the salivary pellicle determine whether a bacterial cell will remain associated with the surface. Only a relatively small proportion of oral bacteria possess adhesins that interact with receptors in the host pellicle, and these organisms are generally the most abundant bacteria in biofilms on tooth enamel shortly after cleaning (see Fig. 10.7).

These species are considered the "primary colonizers" of tooth surfaces. The primary colonizers provide new binding sites for adhesion by other oral bacteria. The metabolic activity of the primary colonizers modifies the local microenvironment in ways that can influence the ability of other bacteria to survive in the dental biofilm. For example, by removing oxygen, the primary colonizers provide conditions of low oxygen tension that permit the survival and growth of obligate anaerobes. Initial colonizers such as streptococci produce lactic acid which can be utilized as a carbon and energy source by *Veillonella* species.[597] *Veillonella* spp. are amongst the most prevalent bacterial species in dental biofilms and are thought to have a similar role to oral fusobacteria (such as *Fusobacterium nucleatum* [see eFig. 10.1G]) in that they are able to act as bridging organisms that are able to support the colonization and growth of later colonizers, by their ability to bind to both early and late colonizers.[597,598] The initial steps in the colonization of teeth by bacteria occur in three phases. Phase 1 is transport to the surface, phase 2 is initial reversible adhesion, and phase 3 is strong attachment.

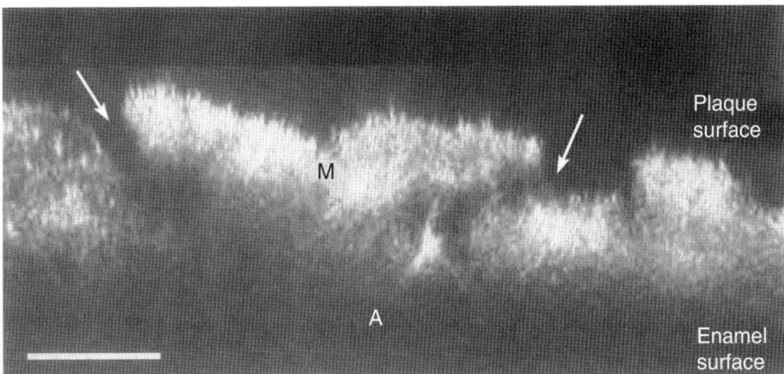

Fig. 10.6 Vertical section through a 4-day human plaque sample. An intraoral device designed for the in vivo generation of plaque biofilms on enamel was used. Confocal microscopy enabled the visualization of the section of plaque without the dehydration steps used in conventional histologic preparations. Notice the open fluid-filled channels *(arrows)* that traverse from the plaque surface through the bacterial mass (*M*; gray-white areas) to the enamel surface. An area in which the bacterial mass appears to attach to the enamel surface *(A)* is indicated. Scale bar = 25 μm. (From Wood SR, Kirkham J, Marsh PD, et al. Architecture of intact natural human plaque biofilms studied by confocal laser scanning microscopy. *J Dent Res.* 2000;79:21.)

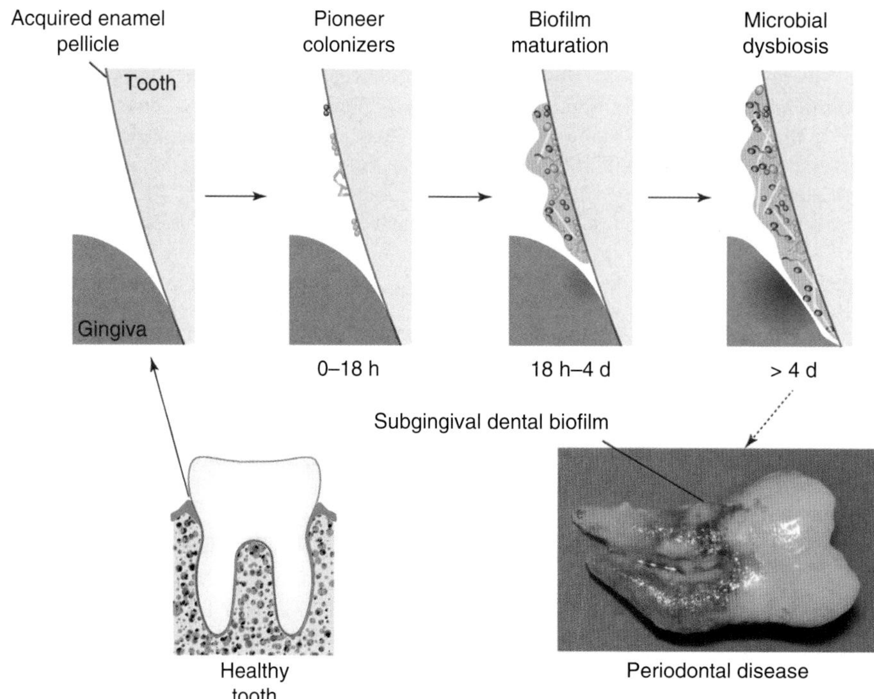

Fig. 10.7 Accumulation of dental biofilm and progression to disease. Good oral hygiene maintains low levels of dental biofilm at the gum margin. The acquired enamel pellicle, a layer of protein and glycoprotein largely derived from saliva, is not removed during tooth cleaning and forms attachment sites for pioneer colonizing bacteria. Initial attachment starts within minutes. Without further oral hygiene, the dental biofilm thickens and an extracellular matrix accumulates ("biofilm maturation") after around 18 h. This mature biofilm reorganizes over the next few days, without dramatically increasing in thickness. Interactions between the biofilm and gingival tissue triggers inflammation, indicated by reddening of the gingiva. Ultimately, this can lead to microbial dysbiosis and the accumulation of significant biofilm below the gingival margin which leads to chronic inflammation and loss of tissue surrounding the tooth. Ultimately, the biofilm-laden tooth becomes mobile and requires extraction. A tooth extracted for periodontal disease is shown.

Colonization and Biofilm Maturation

The primary colonizing bacteria (Table 10.1) adhere to the tooth surface and provide new receptors for attachment by other bacteria as part of a process known as *coadhesion*.[234] Together with the growth of adherent microorganisms, coadhesion leads to the development of microcolonies (Fig. 10.8) and eventually to a mature biofilm.

Cell-cell adhesion between genetically distinct oral bacteria also occurs in the fluid phase (i.e., in saliva). In the laboratory, interactions between genetically distinct cells in suspension result in clumps or coaggregates that are macroscopically visible (Fig. 10.9). Coaggregation is a direct interaction; it is distinct from agglutination, which occurs when cells are stuck together by molecules in solution. At least 18 genera from the oral cavity have shown some form of coaggregation.[232] All oral bacteria possess surface molecules that foster some sort of cell-cell interaction (Fig. 10.10).[233] The initial stages of coaggregation or coadhesion are essentially the same as the first steps involved in bacterial binding to surfaces: bacterial cells come into contact through passive or active transport and bind weakly through nonspecific hydrophobic, electrostatic, and van der Waals forces.[102,130,227,233] These steps can be dramatically accelerated in vitro by vigorously mixing dense suspensions of bacterial cells.[234] Strong cell-cell binding is then determined by the presence of adhesin proteins or carbohydrates on one partner and complementary receptor proteins or carbohydrates on the other. Note that adhesin–receptor interactions are mediated by the fundamental physicochemical forces (i.e., hydrophobic, electrostatic, and van der Waals), but they are highly specific due to complementary conformations of adhesin and receptor that provide a large number of weak bonds and create a strong binding force overall. Different species—or even different strains of a single species—have distinct sets of coaggregation partners (see Fig. 10.10). Fusobacteria coaggregate with all other human oral bacteria, whereas *Veillonella* spp., *Capnocytophaga* spp. (see eFig. 10.1Q), and *Prevotella* spp. bind with streptococci and/or actinomyces.[233,235,559] Each newly accreted cell becomes itself a new surface and therefore may act as a coaggregation bridge to the next potentially accreting cell type that passes by.

Secondary colonizers (see Table 10.1) such as *P. intermedia, P. loescheii, Capnocytophaga* spp., *F. nucleatum,* and *P. gingivalis* do not initially colonize clean tooth surfaces but rather adhere to bacteria that are already in the biofilm mass.[233] The transition from early supragingival dental biofilm to more mature biofilm developing beneath the gingival margin involves a shift in the microbial population from primarily gram-positive organisms to high numbers of gram-negative bacteria. There is an increase in heterogeneity of the biofilm.[176] During the later stages of dental biofilm formation, coaggregation among different gram-negative species is likely to predominate. Examples of these types of interactions are the coaggregation of *F. nucleatum* with *P. gingivalis* or *Treponema denticola* (see eFig. 10.1L).[222,229,235] As the biofilm develops, bacterial cells on the surface utilize oxygen and a hypoxic environment develops beneath the surface.

The continued development of a dental biofilm is dependent on a variety of host and environmental factors but a highly complex structure results as a dental biofilm matures.[504]

TABLE 10.1 Overview of Primary and Secondary Colonizers in Dental Plaque

Primary colonizers	*Streptococcus gordonii* *Streptococcus intermedius* *Streptococcus mitis* *Streptococcus oralis* *Streptococcus sanguinis* *Actinomyces gerencseriae* *Actinomyces israelii* *Actinomyces naeslundii* *Actinomyces oris* *Aggregatibacter actinomycetemcomitans serotype a* *Capnocytophaga gingivalis* *Capnocytophaga ochracea* *Capnocytophaga sputigena* *Eikenella corrodens* *Actinomyces odontolyticus* *Veillonella parvula*
Secondary colonizers	*Campylobacter gracilis* *Campylobacter rectus* *Campylobacter showae* *Eubacterium nodatum* *Aggregatibacter actinomycetemcomitans serotype b* *Fusobacterium nucleatum* spp. *nucleatum* *Fusobacterium nucleatum* spp. *vincentii* *Fusobacterium nucleatum* spp. *polymorphum* *Fusobacterium periodonticum* *Parvimonas micra* *Prevotella intermedia* *Prevotella loescheii* *Prevotella nigrescens* *Streptococcus constellatus* *Tannerella forsythia* *Porphyromonas gingivalis* *Treponema denticola*

Structure of Mature Dental Biofilms

General Aspects of Dental Biofilms

Dental biofilms (see Fig. 10.5) are defined clinically as a structured, resilient, yellow-grayish substance that adheres tenaciously to the intraoral hard surfaces, including removable and fixed restorations.[34] The tough extracellular matrix makes it impossible to remove dental biofilms by rinsing or with the use of sprays and so mechanical biofilm removal via an effective home oral hygiene regime or professional mechanical plaque/biofilm removal (PMPR) is essential to remove the biofilm and maintain oral hygiene.

A dental biofilm is broadly classified as supragingival or subgingival on the basis of its position on the tooth surface toward the gingival margin.

- *Supragingival biofilm* is found at or above the gingival margin; when in direct contact with the gingival margin, it is referred to as *marginal biofilm.*
- *Subgingival biofilm* is found below the gingival margin, between the tooth and the gingival pocket epithelium.

Dental biofilms can be differentiated from other deposits that may be found on the tooth surface, such as materia alba and calculus. *Materia alba* refers to soft accumulations of bacteria, food matter, and tissue cells that lack the organized structure of dental biofilms and that are easily displaced with a water spray. *Calculus* is a hard deposit that forms via the mineralization of dental biofilms and that is generally covered by a layer of unmineralized biofilm (Table 10.2).

A mature dental biofilm is composed primarily of microorganisms. One gram of dental biofilm (wet weight) contains approximately 10^{11} bacteria.[453,499] The number of bacteria in supragingival biofilm on a single tooth surface can exceed 10^9 cells. In a periodontal pocket, counts can range from 10^3 bacteria in a healthy crevice to more than 10^8 bacteria in a deep pocket. With the use of highly sensitive molecular techniques for microbial identification, it has been estimated that more than 750 distinct microbial phylotypes can be present as natural inhabitants of dental biofilms.[2] Any individual may harbor hundreds of different species. Next to bacteria, non-bacterial organisms can also be found in the dental biofilm, including archaea, yeasts, protozoa, and viruses.[69,271]

Supragingival biofilm typically demonstrates the stratified organization of a multilayered accumulation of bacterial morphotypes (Fig. 10.12).[599] Gram-positive cocci and short rods predominate at the tooth surface, whereas gram-negative rods, filaments, and spirochetes predominate on the outer surface of the mature biofilm mass. In general, the subgingival microbiota differs in composition from the supragingival biofilms, primarily because of the local availability of blood products and a low reduction-oxidation (redox) potential, which characterizes the anaerobic environment. Many periodontal pathogens are fastidious strict anaerobes and as such may contribute little to the initiation of disease in shallow gingival pockets. In deep periodontal pockets, however, they find their preferred habitat.

KEY FACT

The specific microbial composition and structure of dental biofilms are highly dependent on the region of the tooth and the local environmental parameters.

The tooth-associated cervical dental biofilm that adheres to the root cementum does not markedly differ from that observed in gingivitis. At this location, filamentous microorganisms dominate, but cocci and rods also occur. This dental biofilm is dominated by gram-positive rods and cocci, including *S. mitis*, *S. sanguinis*, *A. oris*, *Actinomyces naeslundii*, and *Eubacterium* spp. (see eFig. 10.1N). However, in the deeper parts of the pocket, the filamentous organisms become fewer in number; in the apical portion, they seem to be virtually absent. Instead, the microbiota is dominated by smaller organisms without a particular orientation.[282] The apical border of the biofilm mass is separated from the junctional epithelium by a layer of host leukocytes, and the bacterial population of this apical-tooth–associated region shows an increased concentration of gram-negative rods (see Fig. 10.2).

The layers of microorganisms that face the soft tissue lack a definite intermicrobial matrix and contain primarily gram-negative rods and cocci, as well as large numbers of filaments, flagellated rods, and spirochetes. Studies of dental biofilms associated with crevicular epithelial cells indicate a predominance of species such as *S. oralis, S. intermedius*, *Parvimonas*

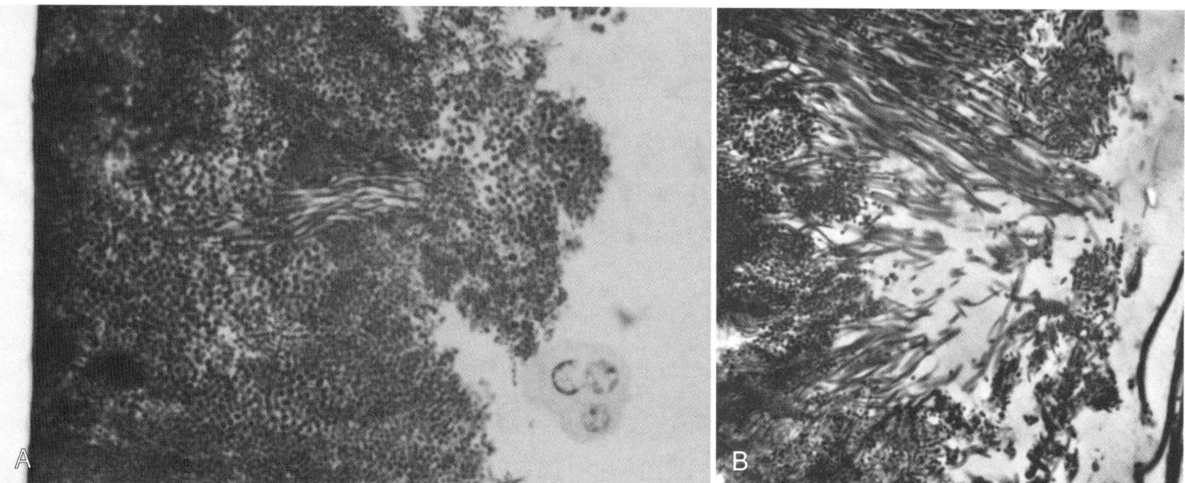

Fig. 10.8 Dental plaque. (A) and (B) When a single microorganism adheres to the tooth surface, it can start to multiply, and it slowly forms a microcolony of daughter cells. These views were taken after plaque formation on a plastic strip (e.g., as shown in Fig. 10.22) glued to a tooth surface.

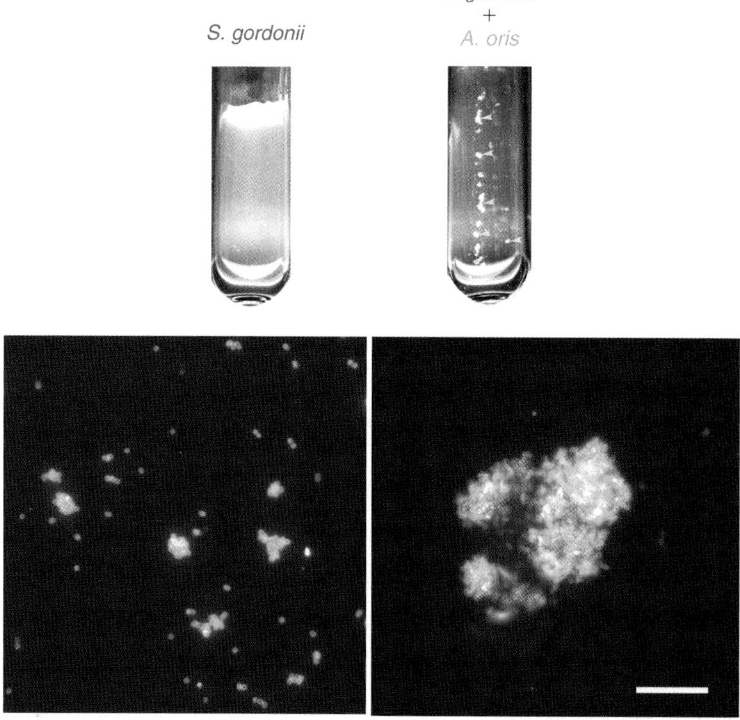

Fig. 10.9 Coaggregation. Coaggregation between *Streptococcus gordonii* DL1 and *Actinomyces oris* MG1 in vitro. A monoculture of *S. gordonii* appears uniformly turbid. Microscopically, cells labeled with specific anti-DL1 antibodies *(green)* are in small chains or clumps. After the addition of *A. oris,* cells clump together to form macroscopic coaggregates *(yellow arrowhead).* Under the microscope, *S. gordonii (green)* are evenly distributed throughout the coaggregates with *A. oris* (*orange*). Bar = 20 μm. (Image reproduced in part from Jakubovics NS, Gill SR, Iobst SE, et al. Regulation of gene expression in a mixed-genus community: stabilized arginine biosynthesis in *Streptococcus gordonii* by coaggregation with *Actinomyces naeslundii. J Bacteriol.* 2008;190:3646.)

micra (formerly *Micromonas micra* and *Peptostreptococcus micros* [see eFig. 10.1J]), *P. gingivalis*, *P. intermedia*, *T. forsythia* (see Fig. 10.12, eFig. 10.10), and *F. nucleatum.*[94,107] Host-tissue cells (e.g., white blood cells, epithelial cells) may also be found in this region (see Fig. 10.12C). Bacteria are also found within the host tissues, such as in the soft tissues (see Fig. 10.3), and within epithelial cells (Fig. 10.13), as well as in the dentinal tubules (Fig. 10.14).[440,441] The composition of the subgingival biofilm depends on the depth of a periodontal pocket. The apical part is more dominated by spirochetes, cocci, and rods, whereas in the coronal part more filaments are observed. The site-specificity of dental biofilms is significantly associated with diseases of the periodontium. Marginal biofilm, for example, is of prime importance during the initiation and development of gingivitis. Supragingival biofilm and tooth-associated subgingival biofilm are critical in calculus formation and root caries, whereas tissue-associated subgingival biofilm is important in the tissue destruction that characterizes

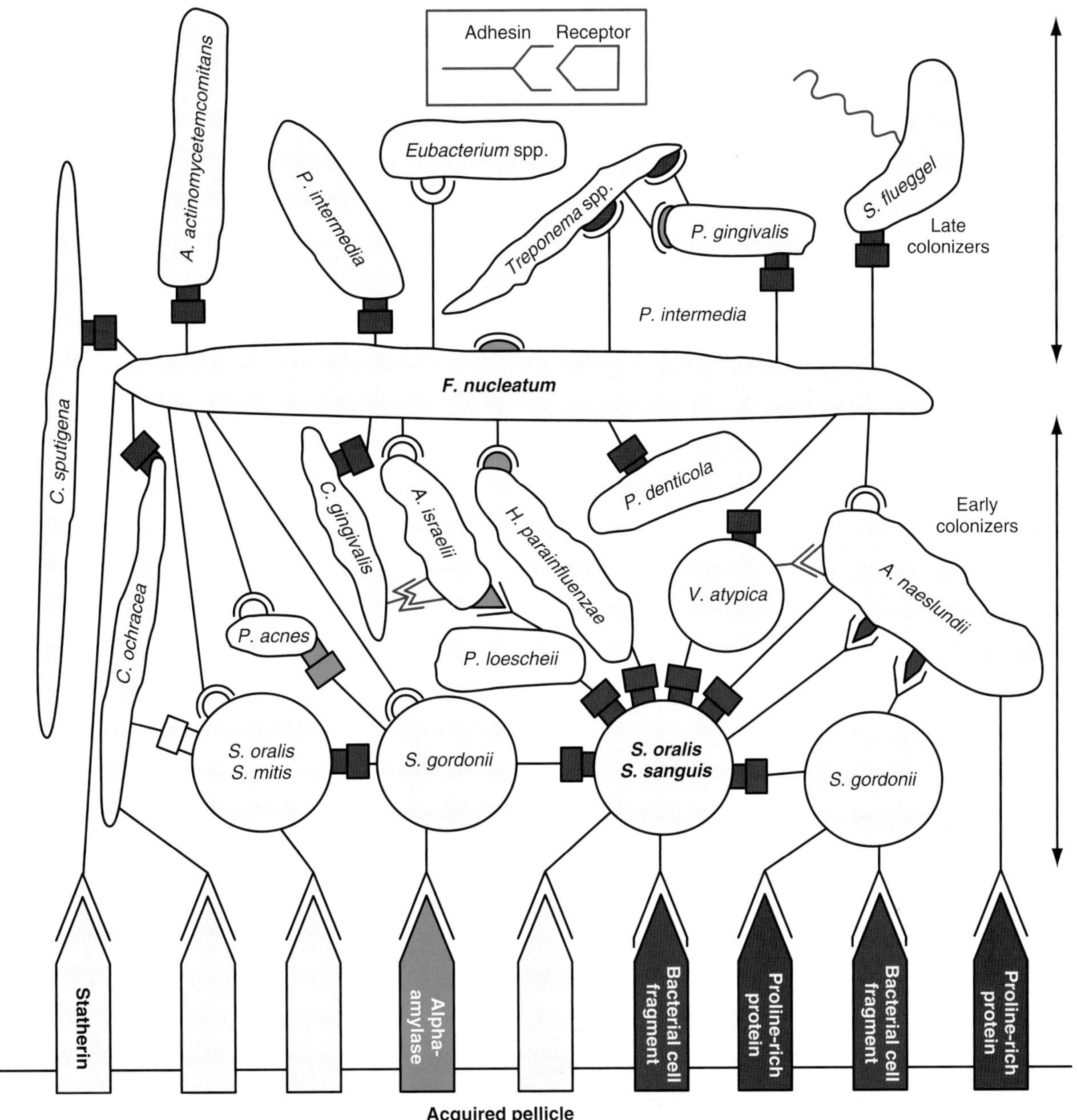

Fig. 10.10 Diagrammatic representation of initial plaque formation. Early colonizers bind to receptors in the pellicle. Each adherent cell becomes in turn the nascent surface and bridge for additional species (secondary colonizers). The complementary sets of adhesin receptor symbols (example in box) represent the various kinds of coaggregations as well as the interactions with molecules in the pellicle. The symbol with a stem (adhesin) represents a cellular component that is heat-inactivated (cell suspension heated to 85°C for 30 minutes) and sensitive to protease treatment. The cell type that exhibits the complementary symbol (receptor) is insensitive to either treatment. The symbols with a rectangular shape represent lactose-inhibitable coaggregations; the others are lactose noninhibitable. *A. actinomycetemcomitans, Aggregatibacter actinomycetemcomitans; A. israelii, Actinomyces israelii; A. naeslundii, Actinomyces naeslundii; C. gingivalis, Capnocytophaga gingivalis; C. ochracea, Capnocytophaga ochracea; C. sputigena, Capnocytophaga sputigena; F. nucleatum, Fusobacterium nucleatum; H. parainfluenzae, Haemophilus parainfluenzae; P. acnes, Propionibacterium acnes; P. denticola, Prevotella denticola; P. gingivalis, Porphyromonas gingivalis; P. loescheii, Prevotella loescheii; S. flueggel, Selenomonas flueggei; S. gordonii, Streptococcus gordonii; S. mitis, Streptococcus mitis; S. oralis, Streptococcus oralis; S. sanguis, Streptococcus sanguis; V. atypica, Veillonella atypica.* (Adapted from Kolenbrander PE, London J. Adhere today, here tomorrow: oral bacterial adherence. *J Bacteriol.* 1993;175:3247.)

different forms of periodontitis. Biofilms also establish on artificial surfaces exposed to the oral environment, such as dental prostheses and implants.

One key aspect of oral biofilms is the extracellular matrix that holds the biofilm together and retains it on the tooth surface.[196] The scaffold of the matrix consists of biological macromolecules such as nucleic acids, proteins, polysaccharides, lipids, and other cell wall fragments. Enzymatic degradation of key macromolecules such as extracellular DNA or polysaccharides inhibits the formation of biofilms.[421,532] Organic and inorganic small molecules including nutrients, waste products, and metal ions are held within this structure and contribute to the homeostasis of the biofilm.

As the mineral content of dental biofilms increases, the biofilm mass becomes calcified to form calculus (Fig. 10.15). Calculus is frequently found in areas of the dentition adjacent to salivary ducts (e.g., the lingual surface of the mandibular incisors and canines, the buccal surface of the maxillary first molars), and this reflects the high concentration of minerals available from saliva in those regions. The inorganic components of subgingival dental biofilms are derived from crevicular fluid (a serum transudate). The

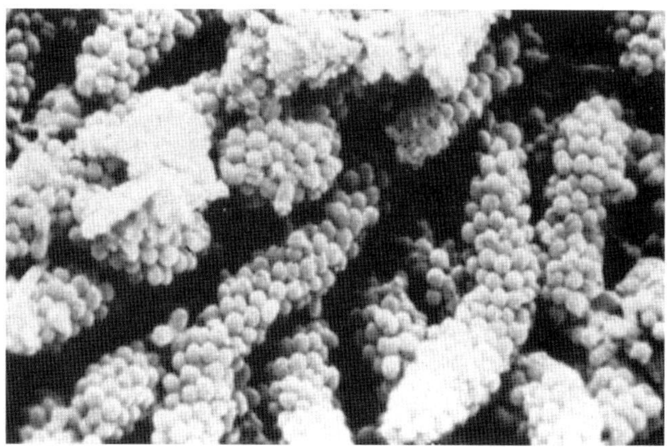

Fig. 10.11 Long-standing supragingival plaque near the gingival margin demonstrating a "corn cob" arrangement. A central gram-negative filamentous core supports the outer coccal cells, which are firmly attached by interbacterial adherence or coaggregation.

TABLE 10.2 Differences Between Tooth Deposits

Materia Alba	Dental Plaque	Calculus
• White, cheeselike accumulation	• Resilient clear to yellow-grayish substance	• Hard deposit that forms via the mineralization of dental plaque
• Soft accumulation of salivary proteins, some bacteria, many desquamated epithelial cells, and occasional disintegrating food debris	• Primarily composed of bacteria in a matrix of salivary glycoproteins and extracellular polysaccharides	• Generally covered by a layer of unmineralized dental plaque
• Lacks an organized structure and is therefore not as complex as dental plaque	• Considered to be a biofilm	
• Easily displaced with a water spray	• Impossible to remove by rinsing or with the use of sprays	

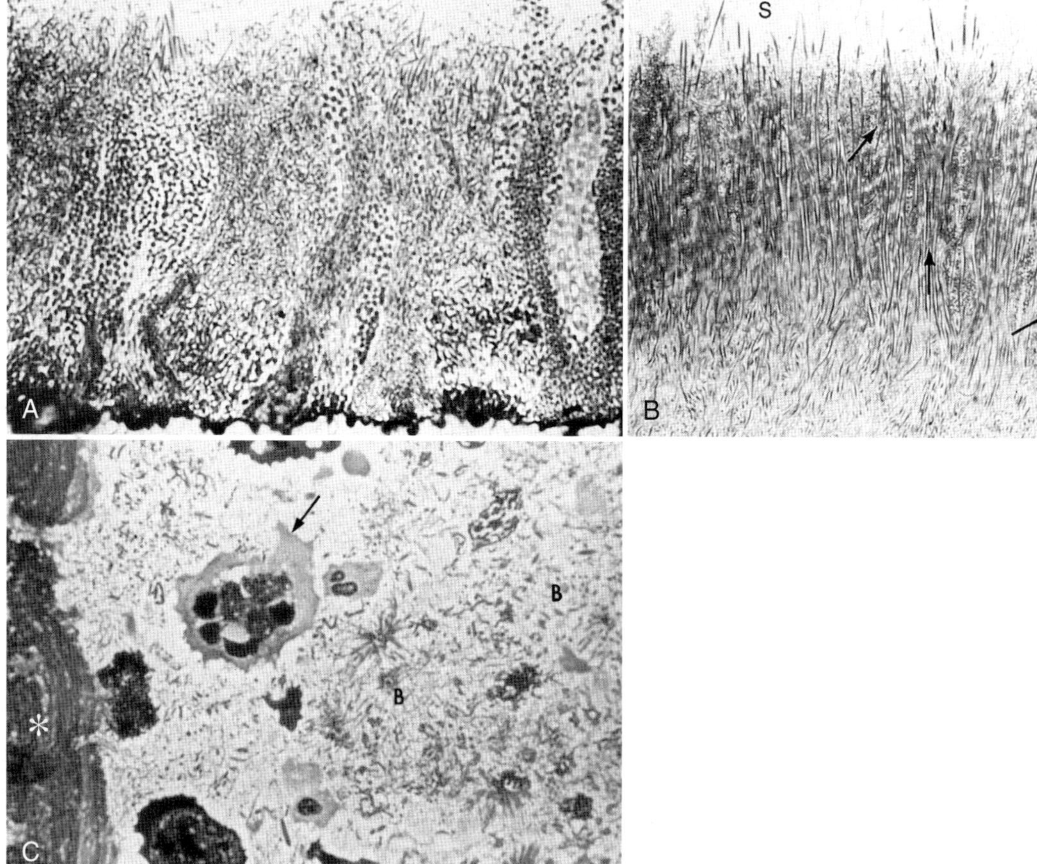

Fig. 10.12 Plaque formation. (A) One-day-old plaque. Microcolonies of plaque bacteria extend perpendicularly away from the tooth surfaces. (B) Developed supragingival plaque showing the overall filamentous nature and the microcolonies *(arrows)* that extend perpendicularly away from the tooth surface. The saliva–plaque interface is shown *(S)*. (C) A histologic section of plaque showing nonbacterial components such as white blood cells *(arrow)* and epithelial cells *(asterisk)* interspersed among bacteria *(B)*. (Courtesy Dr. Max Listgarten, Philadelphia, PA.)

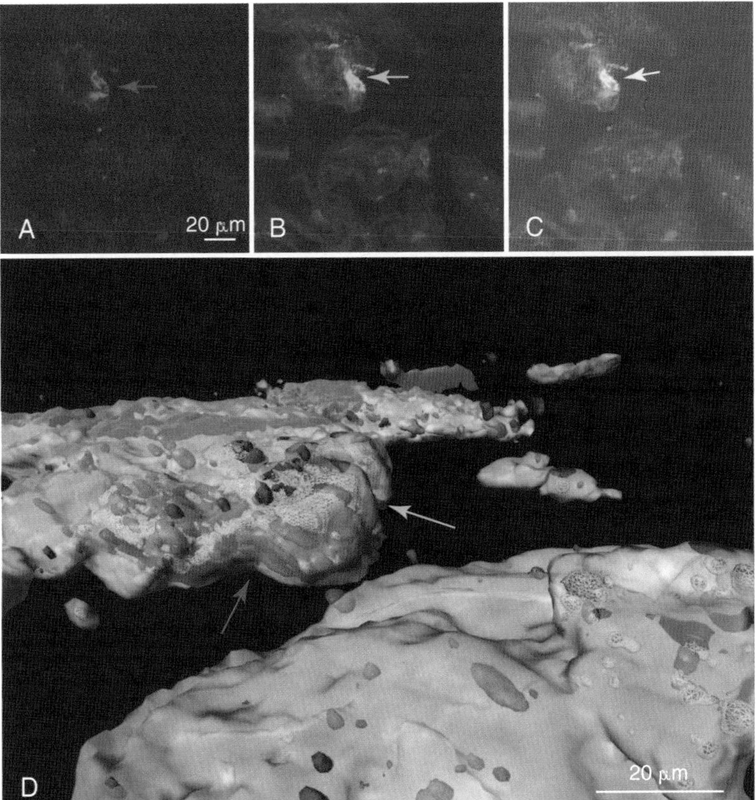

Fig. 10.13 Bacteria in epithelial cells. (A–C) Images of z-section no. 39 from a stack of 74 0.2-μm z-sections (×600; the scale bar in [A] also applies to [B] and [C]). Buccal epithelial cells in this field were double-labeled with (A) the EUB338 universal probe and (B) the *Aggregatibacter actinomycetemcomitans*–specific probe. The cell in the center of (A) contained a large mass of brightly fluorescent intracellular bacteria *(red arrow)*. Other cells in the field contained smaller bacterial masses (not marked). (B) A portion of the large mass labeled with the universal probe also hybridized with the *A. actinomycetemcomitans*–specific probe *(green arrow)*. Images from (A) and (B) were superimposed in (C) to confirm that bacteria labeled with both probes *(yellow arrow)* were adjacent to other bacteria labeled only with the universal probe *(red arrow)*. (D) Three-dimensional reconstruction of the same field. Bacteria recognized only by the universal probe are shown in solid red, whereas the colocalization of the *A. actinomycetemcomitans* and universal probes is depicted by a green wireframe over a red interior. Reconstructed buccal epithelial cell surfaces are presented in blue. The red and green colors are muted when bacterial masses are intracellular and brighter when bacteria appear to project out of the surface. The angle of view was rotated along the z-axis, and the image was zoomed. The large mass that appeared to have a lobular structure in z-section no. 39 was seen to be a cohesive unit that contained *A. actinomycetemcomitans* in direct proximity to other species *(red and green arrows)*. (From Rudney JD, Chen R, Sedgewick GJ. Actinobacillus actinomycetemcomitans, Porphyromonas gingivalis, and Tannerella forsythensis are components of a polymicrobial intracellular flora within human buccal cells. *J Dent Res*. 2005;84:59–63.)

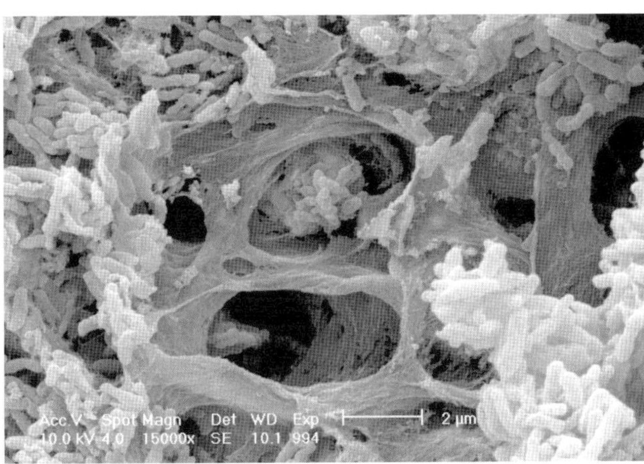

Fig. 10.14 Scanning electron micrograph of bacteria within dentinal tubules.

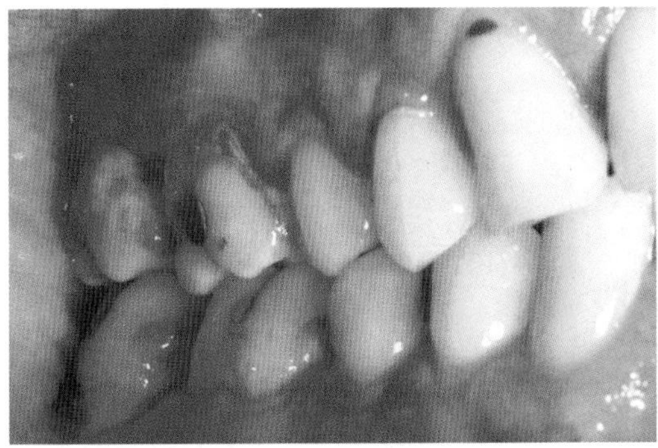

Fig. 10.15 Supragingival calculus is depicted on the buccal surface of the maxillary molars adjacent to the orifice of the parotid duct.

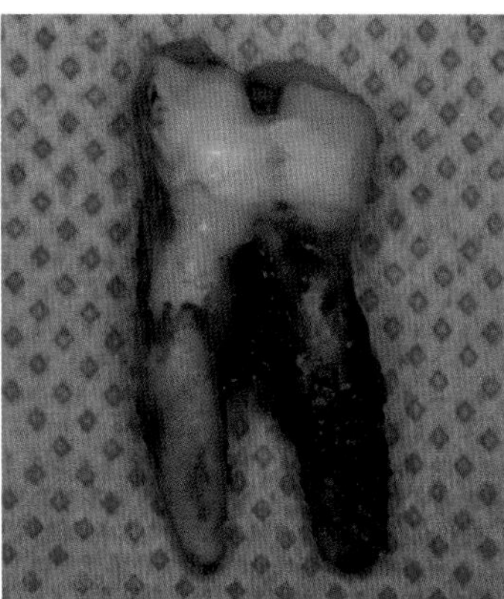

Fig. 10.16 Dark-pigmented deposits of subgingival calculus on the distal root of anextracted lower molar.

calcification of subgingival biofilm also results in calculus formation (Fig. 10.16). Subgingival calculus is typically dark green or dark brown, which probably reflects the presence of blood products that are associated with subgingival hemorrhage.

KEY FACT

Biofilm maturation is a highly specific event that involves a non-random aggregation of different bacteria.

Metabolism of Bacteria in Dental Biofilms

Most nutrients for bacteria within dental biofilms originate from saliva or GCF, although the host diet provides an occasional but nevertheless important food supply. The transition from gram-positive to gram-negative microorganisms observed in the structural development of mature dental biofilms is paralleled by a physiologic transition in the developing biofilm. The early colonizers (e.g., *Streptococcus* and *Actinomyces* spp.) use oxygen and lower the redox potential of the environment, which then favors the growth of anaerobic species.[93,546] Many of the gram-positive early colonizers use sugars as an energy source. The bacteria that predominate in mature dental biofilms are anaerobic and asaccharolytic (i.e., they do not break down sugars), and they use amino acids and small peptides as energy sources.[293] There is a shift towards proteolytic metabolism in a mature dental biofilm within a periodontal pocket.

Laboratory studies have demonstrated many metabolic interactions among the different bacteria found in dental biofilms (Fig. 10.17). For example, lactate and formate are byproducts of the metabolism of streptococci and *Actinomyces* spp.; they may be used in the metabolism of other plaque microorganisms, including *Veillonella* spp. and *A. actinomycetemcomitans*.[43,108] Interestingly, the commensal bacterium *S. gordonii* (see eFig. 10.1F) has also been shown to provide electron acceptors that promote respiratory growth of *A. actinomycetemcomitans* in vivo during abscess formation.[505] The importance of this cross-respiration in dental biofilms is not yet clear. The growth of *P. gingivalis* is also enhanced by metabolic byproducts produced by other microorganisms, such as succinate from *C. ochracea* or *T. denticola* and protoheme from *Campylobacter rectus* (see eFig. 10.1R).[149,150,328] In turn, *P. gingivalis* provides isobutyric acid that stimulates growth of *T. denticola.*[149] Overall, the total microbial population of the dental biofilm is more efficient than any one constituent organism at releasing energy from the available substrates.[560]

Metabolic interactions also occur between the host and microorganisms within the dental biofilm. The bacterial enzymes that

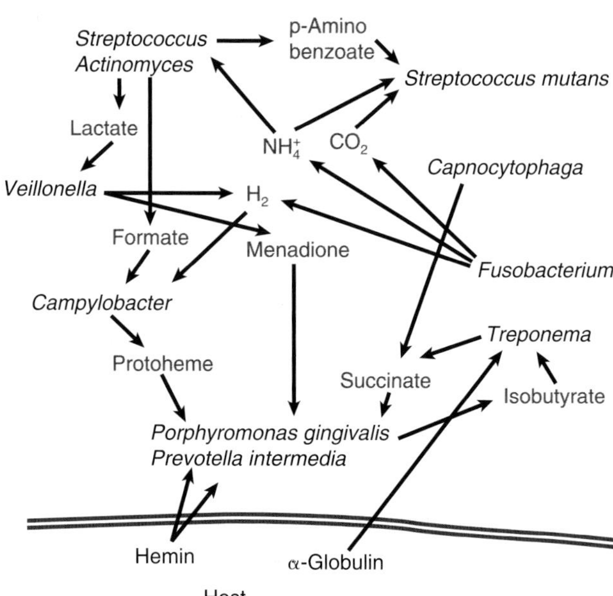

Fig. 10.17 Schematic illustration of metabolic interactions among different bacterial species found in plaque and between the host and the plaque bacteria. These interactions are likely to be important to the survival of bacteria in the periodontal environment. CO_2, Carbon dioxide; H_2, hydrogen; NH^+_4, ammonium. (Data from Carlsson J. Microbiology of plaque associated periodontal disease. In: Lindhe J, ed. *Textbook of Clinical Periodontology.* Munksgaard: Munksgaard International Publishers; 1983; Grenier D. Nutritional interactions between two suspected periodontal pathogens, *Treponema denticola and Porphyromonas gingivalis. Infect Immun.* 1992;60:5298; Loesche WJ. Importance of nutrition in gingival crevice microbial ecology. *Periodontics.* 1968;6:245; and Walden WC, Hentges DJ. Differential effects of oxygen and oxidation–reduction potential on the multiplication of three species of anaerobic intestinal bacteria. *Appl Microbiol.* 1975;30:781.)

degrade host proteins mediate the release of ammonia, which may be used by bacteria as a nitrogen source.[54] Hemin/heme is one of the essential nutrients required by periodontal pathogens such as *P. gingivalis* to grow *in vitro* and, within the oral cavity, this nutrient is thought to be provided by the GCF.[597] As bleeding is clinically associated with periodontitis, subgingival microorganisms residing within periodontal pockets may be frequently exposed to constituents of blood, including erythrocytes.[40] Hemin iron from the breakdown of host hemoglobin may be important in the metabolism of *P. gingivalis.*[38] Increases in steroid hormones are associated with significant increases in the proportions of *P. intermedia* found in subgingival biofilms.[241] Growth of facultatively anaerobic bacteria may be enhanced by host secretion of nitrate in saliva, through the use of nitrate as an electron acceptor for respiration.[317] These nutritional interdependencies are probably critical to the growth and survival of microorganisms in dental biofilms, and they may partly explain the evolution of the highly specific structural interactions observed among bacteria in dental biofilms.

Communication Between Biofilm Bacteria

In a biofilm, bacterial cells have the capacity to communicate with each other. One example of this is quorum sensing, in which bacteria secrete a signaling molecule that accumulates in the local environment and triggers a response such as a change in the expression of specific genes once they reach a critical threshold concentration. The threshold concentration is reached only at a high cell density, and therefore bacteria sense that the population has reached a critical mass or quorum. Some evidence indicates that intercellular communication can occur after cell-cell contact and that, in this case, communication may not involve secreted signaling molecules.[197]

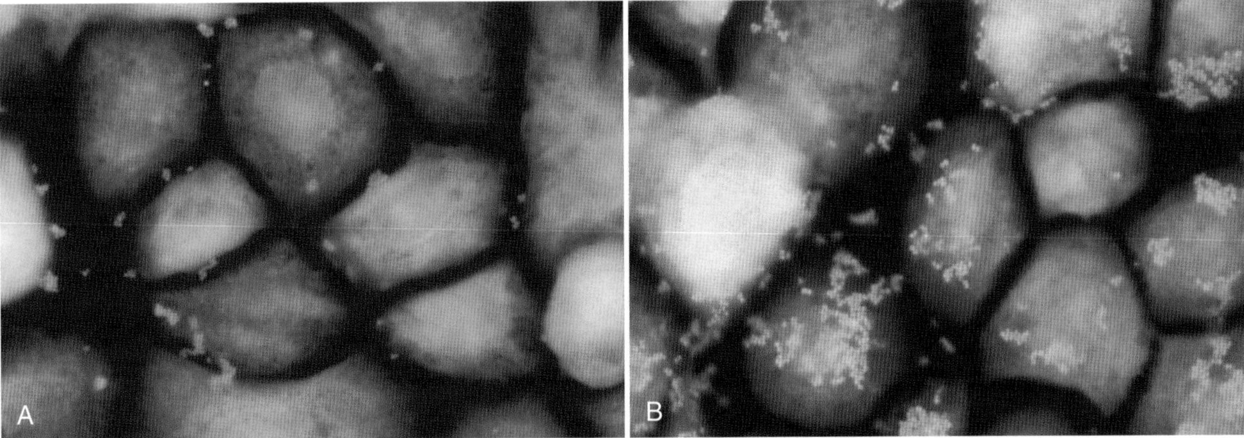

Fig. 10.18 ***Porphyromonas gingivalis*** **adhesion capacity differences. Microscopic confirmation of significant differences in the adhesion capacity of** ***P. gingivalis (small green dots)*** **to epithelial cells from (A) a resistant patient as compared with (B) a patient with severe periodontitis.**

Two types of signaling molecules have been detected from dental biofilm bacteria: peptides released by gram-positive organisms during growth and a "universal" signal molecule called *autoinducer 2* (AI-2).[231] Peptide signals are produced by oral streptococci; they are recognized by cells of the same strain that produced them and possibly also by different species of streptococci.[131] Responses are induced only when a threshold concentration of the peptide is attained, and thus the peptides act as cell density or quorum sensors. Local concentrations of signaling molecules may be enhanced in biofilms if the signals become trapped in the biofilm matrix. The streptococcal peptides are known as *competence-stimulating peptides* because the major response to these signals is the induction of competence, a physiologic state during which cells are primed for DNA uptake and incorporation. In some species, such as *S. mutans* (see eFig. 10.1M), a few of the cells in a population respond to competence-stimulating peptides by lysing.[382] Lysis is considered to be an altruistic behavior that helps to disseminate genetic information throughout the population of *S. mutans* cells.

In contrast to the strain-specific competence-stimulating peptides, AI-2 is produced and detected by many different bacteria. The detection of AI-2 produces wide-ranging changes in gene expression, in some cases affecting up to one-third of the entire genome.[514] Little is known about the specific functions of AI-2 in oral biofilms. However, this molecule has been demonstrated to play a role in mutualistic interactions between *S. oralis* and *A. oris (A. naeslundii)*.[423] Thus, in an in vitro model system, neither *S. oralis* nor *A. oris* formed biofilms in monoculture. When cultured together, these organisms grew abundantly on surfaces to form thick, confluent biofilms. This mutualistic behavior was observed only when AI-2 was present: disrupting the gene for AI-2 in *S. oralis* abrogated mutualistic growth. These data demonstrate that AI-2 is produced and sensed by oral bacteria and suggest that interbacterial communication is important for the development of dental biofilms.

Quorum sensing, therefore, appears to play diverse roles in, for example, modulating the expression of genes for antibiotic resistance, encouraging the growth of beneficial species in the biofilm, and discouraging the growth of competitors.

Interactions Among Dental Biofilm Bacteria

Some evidence from laboratory studies indicates that non-pathogenic organisms in subgingival dental biofilms can modify the behavior of periodontal pathogens. For example, long and short fimbriae of *P. gingivalis* are required for adhesion and biofilm formation. The expression of long fimbriae is down-regulated in the presence of *Streptococcus cristatus,* and short fimbriae are down-regulated by *S. gordonii, S. mitis,* or *S. sanguinis.*[279,370] Changes in bacterial physiology after transitions from monoculture to mixed-species communities may be quite wide-ranging. With the use of a proteomics approach to probe the phenotype of *P. gingivalis*, it has been shown that the expression of almost 500 *P. gingivalis* proteins is changed in model oral microbial communities that contain *S. gordonii* and *F. nucleatum.*[250] At present, it is not clear how these changes affect the interaction between *P. gingivalis* and the host.

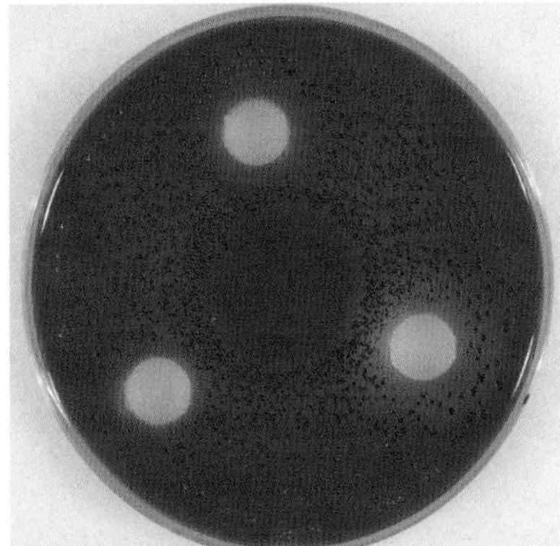

Fig. 10.19 Growth inhibition induced by streptococci. The growth of *Prevotella intermedia (black colonies)* is inhibited by the presence of *Streptococcus mitis, Streptococcus salivarius,* and *Streptococcus sanguinis* (in the *white holes*). This is represented by a zone of no growth (halo) around the white holes. This is a typical example of growth inhibition induced by streptococci.

In multispecies biofilms in which many bacteria are juxtaposed to cells of different species, interactions among genetically distinct microorganisms can be mutually beneficial (Fig. 10.18A). However, many examples of competitive interactions between different bacteria exist (Fig. 10.19). For example, *S. mutans* produces antimicrobial peptides that have broad activity against bacteria in vitro.[244] Other oral streptococci compete with *S. mutans* by excreting the strongly oxidizing molecule H_2O_2.[244] In fact, *Streptococcus oligofermentans* can convert lactic acid produced by *S. mutans* into H_2O_2, which then kills the *S. mutans* cells.[528] In subgingival biofilms, oxygen is scarce, and therefore H_2O_2 production by bacteria is lower. Oxidizing agents may be more important in the interaction between the host and the pathogen because reactive oxygen species are a major component of the neutrophil response to bacteria.

Another example of competitive interaction exists between streptococci and periodontal pathogens. *S. sanguinis*, *S. salivarius*, and *S. mitis* have been shown to inhibit hard and soft tissue coloni-

zation of *A. actinomycetemcomitans* (Video 10.3, *P. gingivalis*, and *P. intermedia* in vitro.[477,522,537]

Interactions between oral bacteria can be strain-specific but have also been reported to be site-specific.[317] A recent review by Mark Welch and coworkers noted that Veillonellae from the tongue bind to streptococci from the tongue while Veillonellae from dental biofilms bind to streptococci from dental biofilms. The authors proposed that if specific interactions between bacterial species in terms of adhesion occur at defined habitats within the oral cavity, then this suggests that spatial positioning within the oral cavity could be important for survival.[317]

Studies have shown that these interactions can also influence the host. Although in a study by Teughels and coworkers[523] no clinical effect was expected, a reduction in bleeding on probing was noted in pockets that received the streptococci. At that time, this observation was explained by the establishment of a more host-compatible microbiota. However, an interaction with the host via the immune system seems to be an additional interesting hypothesis. Oral streptococci have been shown to modulate bacteria–host interactions that involve both *F. nucleatum* and *A. actinomycetemcomitans*. Thus, *S. cristatus* and other oral streptococci attenuate the ability of *F. nucleatum* to stimulate interleukin (IL)-8 production by host oral epithelial cells.[590] Sliepen and coworkers[478] demonstrated similar results for the streptococci that were used in the study by Teughels and coworkers. Another interesting example is the *S. gordonii*–induced increased expression of a complement resistance protein, ApiA, in *A. actinomycetemcomitans,* thereby resulting in a higher resistance to killing by host serum.[419]

Biofilms and Antimicrobial Resistance

Bacteria growing in microbial communities adherent to a surface do not "behave" the same way as bacteria growing suspended in a liquid environment (i.e., in a planktonic or unattached state). For example, the resistance of bacteria to antimicrobial agents is dramatically increased in the biofilm.[8,15,73,181,395] Almost without exception, organisms in a biofilm are 1000 to 1500 times more resistant to antimicrobial agents than their planktonic counterparts.[15,112] The mechanisms of this increased resistance differ from species to species, from antibiotic to antibiotic, and for biofilms growing in different habitats.

It is generally accepted that the resistance of bacteria to antibiotics is affected by their nutritional status, growth rate, temperature, pH, and prior exposure to sub-effective concentrations of antimicrobial agents.[41,42,562] Variations in any of these parameters will lead to a varied response to antibiotics within a biofilm. An important mechanism of resistance appears to be the slower rate of growth of bacterial species in a biofilm, which makes them less susceptible to many but not all antibiotics.[15,39,73,577] The biofilm matrix, although not a significant physical barrier to the diffusion of many antibiotics, does have certain properties that can retard antibiotic penetration. For example, strongly charged or chemically highly reactive agents can fail to reach the deeper zones of the biofilm because the biofilm acts as an ion-exchange resin that removes such molecules from solution.[140,515]

KEY FACT

The bacteria within biofilms are often up to 1000 times more resistant to antimicrobial agents than their planktonic counterparts.

Dental biofilms have been shown to possess increased resistance to antimicrobial agents and elevated virulence compared with planktonic bacteria.[248] The penetration and efficacy of antimicrobials against biofilm bacteria are critical issues for the treatment of periodontal infections. The oral microbiota has been highlighted as a potential reservoir for antimicrobial resistance genes that could be potentially transferred within the bacterial population via horizontal gene transfer,[313] with oral biofilms found to contain numerous antimicrobial resistance determinants that can be transferred within or outside the oral cavity.[221]

Studies on the oral microbiota that have used a metagenomic approach rather than conventional culture techniques have identified several known and novel antibiotic resistance determinants. This suggests that the oral microbiota acts as a reservoir for antimicrobial resistance determinants and it was also proposed that uncultivable bacteria could play a significant role in the acquisition and transfer of antimicrobial resistance.[221,503] A study comparing oral biofilm samples from healthy subjects and periodontitis patients reported increased diversity and abundance in the oral antibiotic resistome in periodontitis patients compared with healthy subjects. The authors proposed that there may be differences in the distribution and diversity of antibiotic resistance in oral biofilms associated with health and disease.[221] When considering the use of antimicrobials in the management of periodontitis (discussed in more detail in the Systemic Antibiotics section in this chapter), global concerns regarding the overuse of antimicrobials and the development of antimicrobial resistance should be considered.[446] Dental professionals should be aware of the issues associated with antimicrobial resistance and embrace the concept of antimicrobial stewardship.[106]

Care is also needed to avoid the overuse of antiseptics since there is evidence that these can promote antimicrobial resistance. Antiseptics are used as part of professional dental care but are also used widely in a range of oral care products, such as mouthwashes or dentifrices.[313] Antiseptics such as chlorhexidine have proven effective in reducing oral biofilm formation[457] and in the disruption and inhibition of dental biofilms.[248] Chlorhexidine is an antiseptic commonly used in dental care settings, as a mouthrinse, a gel, and as a locally delivered antimicrobial therapy. Cetylpyridinium chloride, a quaternary ammonium compound, is another common antiseptic found in oral care products. In periodontitis therapy, adjunctive antiseptics such as chlorhexidine may be considered in specific cases, for a limited period of time, as adjuncts to mechanical instrumentation.[446] It has been reported that adjunctive use of an antiseptic such as chlorhexidine mouthrinse could result in a slightly greater pocket depth reduction than mechanical debridement alone.[77]

Concerns regarding antimicrobial resistance have been publicized more in recent years but the potential issues associated with resistance to antiseptics have been less well covered. It has been proposed that frequent use of cetylpyridinium chloride could result in bacterial resistance[313,437] and the evidence for the potential emergence of phenotypic adaptation or resistance to cetylpyridinium chloride in non-oral bacteria was recently reviewed by Mao and coworkers.[313] Cieplik and coworkers[64] highlighted a growing concern regarding a lack of knowledge about resistance to antiseptics such as chlorhexidine in oral bacteria, in terms of potential resistance mechanisms and the risk of cross-resistance towards antibiotics. The upregulation of microbial efflux pumps can lead to cross-resistance to multiple antibiotics in a manner analogous to the development of resistance to chemotherapeutics by cancer cells.[11] It has been suggested that the widespread use of such antiseptic agents could lead to resistance in oral bacteria[457] and that the use of antiseptic agents should be restricted to cases where there is a clear patient benefit.[210] A recent study using saliva-derived biofilms investigated the antimicrobial efficacy of antiseptics and phenotypic adaptation of bacteria after repeated exposure.[457] Oral bacteria showed phenotypic adaption after repeated exposure to sub-inhibitory concentrations and in mature biofilms, the antiseptics tested showed limited antimicrobial efficacy.[457] It is important for dental professionals to be aware of the potential emergence of resistance to antiseptics commonly used in dentistry and of the potential for cross-resistance to antibiotics.

Factors That Affect Supragingival Dental Biofilm Formation

Clinically, early undisturbed biofilm formation on teeth follows an exponential growth curve when measured planimetrically.[407] During the first 24 hours when starting with a clean tooth surface, biofilm growth is negligible from a clinical viewpoint (i.e., <3% coverage of the vestibular tooth surface, which is an amount nearly undetectable clinically). This "lag time" is a result of the fact that the microbial population must reach a certain size before it can easily be detected visually by a clinician. During the following 3 days, coverage progresses rapidly to the point at which, after 4 days, an average of 30% of the total coronal tooth area will be covered with biofilm (see Video 10.4).

Several reports have shown that the microbial composition of the dental biofilm will change, with a shift toward a more anaerobic and a more gram-negative flora, including an influx of fusobacteria, filaments, spiral forms, and spirochetes (see Fig. 10.7). This was clearly illustrated in experimental gingivitis studies.[511,525] Using next-generation sequencing, the microbiota was shown to shift from baseline to a significantly different community within 1 week of withdrawing oral hygiene measures.[223] With this ecologic shift within the biofilm, a transition occurs from the early aerobic environment, which is characterized by gram-positive facultative species, to a highly oxygen-deprived environment, in which gram-negative anaerobic microorganisms predominate. Bacterial growth in more mature biofilms is much slower than in newly formed dental biofilms, presumably because nutrients become limiting for much of the biomass.[553]

Topography of Supragingival Biofilms

Early biofilm formation on teeth follows a typical topographic pattern (Fig. 10.20), with initial growth along the gingival margin and from the interdental spaces (i.e., the areas protected from shear forces). Later, a further extension in the coronal direction can be observed.[333,409] This pattern may change severely when the tooth surface contains irregularities that offer a favorable growth path (Fig. 10.21). Biofilm formation may also originate from grooves, cracks, perikymata, or pits. Scanning electron microscopy studies clearly revealed that the early colonization of the enamel surface starts from surface irregularities in which bacteria shelter from shear forces, thereby permitting them the time needed to change from reversible to irreversible binding.

KEY FACT

Dental biofilm growth starts at areas that are protected from shear forces such as the gingival margin, the interdental space, and along grooves, cracks, pits, and fissures.

Bacterial cells subsequently multiply and spread out from these starting-up areas as a relatively even monolayer. Surface irregularities are also responsible for the so-called individualized biofilm growth pattern (see Fig. 10.21), which is reproduced in the absence of optimal oral hygiene.[333,334] This phenomenon illustrates the importance of surface roughness in dental biofilm growth and so the surface topography, the 3D characteristics of a surface with peaks and troughs, could highlight the important role of surface roughness in biofilm formation.[174] It is also worth noting that all intraoral surfaces are covered by the salivary pellicle, which can affect the nanotopography and therefore have an impact on the surface roughness.[504]

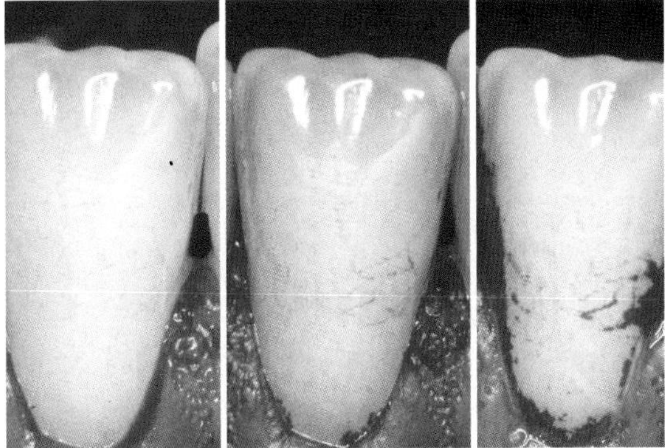

Fig. 10.20 Typical topography of plaque growth. Initial growth starts along the gingival margins and from the interdental spaces (i.e., areas protected from shear forces) to extend farther in a coronal direction. This pattern may fundamentally change, for example, if the tooth surface contains irregularities, such as those evident in Fig. 10.21.

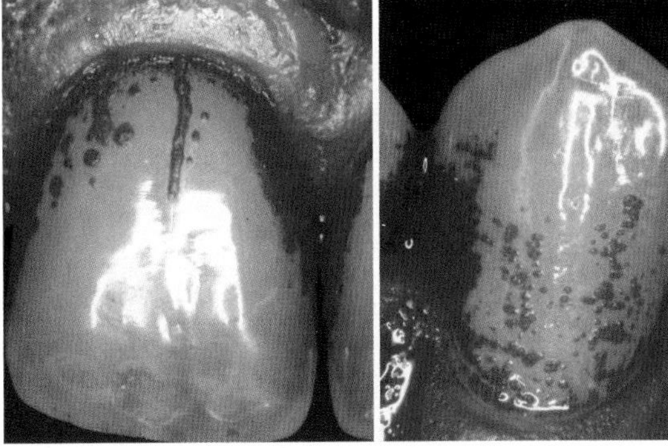

Fig. 10.21 Surface irregularities and plaque growth. Important surface irregularities (i.e., a crack on the central upper incisor, several small pits on the canine) are also responsible for the so-called individualized plaque growth pattern.

Surface Microroughness

Rough intraoral surfaces (e.g., restorations/restoration margins, implant abutments, denture bases) accumulate and retain more biofilm and calculus in terms of thickness, area, and colony-forming units.[404] A more rough intraoral surface provides an increased surface area to promote bacterial attachment as a result of the increased contact area between the surface and bacterial cells[504] and a more rough surface provides protection from shear forces.[521] Accumulation of dental biofilm at these sites results in an increased maturity or pathogenicity of its bacterial components, which is characterized by an increased proportion of motile organisms and spirochetes and/or a denser packing of them (Fig. 10.22). The periodontal tissues adjacent to a rough surface of a tooth, restoration or other intraoral surface are more likely to be inflamed, with a higher bleeding index, increased production of crevicular fluid and/or an increase in inflammatory infiltrate.[521] Smoothing an intraoral surface decreases the rate of biofilm formation. Below a certain surface roughness ($R_a < 0.2$ μm), however, further smoothing does not result

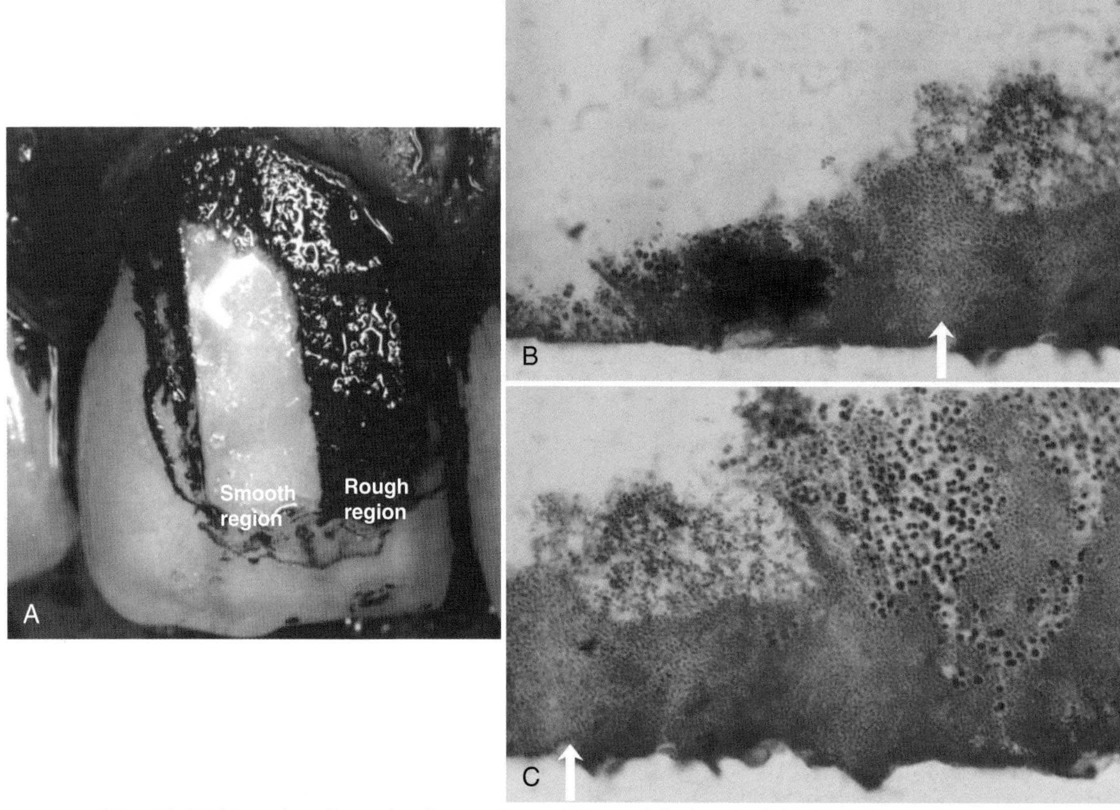

Fig. 10.22 Plaque formation and surface roughness. (A) A small plastic strip, divided in half (a rough region [R_a 2.0 μm] located mesially and a smooth region [R_a 0.1 μm] located distally), had been glued to the central upper incisors of a patient who refrained from oral hygiene for 3 days. (B) and (C) After removal, the strip had been cut into small slices for microscopic evaluation. It is obvious that the rough part (C) contains a thicker plaque layer than the smooth part (B). The *arrow* shows the border between the rough and smooth surfaces. (From Quirynen M, Listgarten MA. Distribution of bacterial morphotypes around natural teeth and titanium implants ad modum Brånemark. *Clin Oral Implants Res.* 1990;1:8.)

in an additional reduction in biofilm formation.[32,405] There seems to be a threshold level for surface roughness ($R_a \approx 0.2$ μm) above which bacterial adhesion will be facilitated.[31]

Dental materials used for restorations in teeth are less likely to be as smooth as enamel and so restorations and restoration margins are therefore potential sites for dental biofilm accumulation.[47] Restoration margins need to be optimized to prevent biofilm accumulation. It has been reported that biofilms on composites and glass-ionomer cements can cause surface deterioration, which in turn enhances biofilm formation.[47]

Dental implants have also been used as a model to study the impact of surface roughness on subgingival biofilm formation.[32,44,153,405,408,424] It was reported that microbial adhesion on titanium-zirconium (TiZr) dental implant abutments is positively correlated with nanoroughness of the surface.[63,497] A study by Bermejo et al. (2019)[24] using an in vitro biofilm model indicated that titanium dental implants with a moderately rough surface accumulated more bacterial biomass and a significantly higher number of pathogenic bacteria (*F. nucleatum* and *A. actinomycetemcomitans*) in comparison to implants with minimally rough surfaces, within a similar biofilm structure. Smooth implant abutments (R_a < 0.2 μm) were found to harbor 25 times fewer bacteria than rough ones, with a slightly higher density of coccoid (i.e., nonpathogenic) cells. The subgingival microbiota was also largely dependent on the remaining presence of teeth and the degree of periodontitis in the remaining natural dentition (for a review, see Persson et al.[383]).

These observations highlight the importance of intraoral bacterial translocation for subgingival biofilms.

Individual Variables That Influence Dental Biofilm Formation

The rate of dental biofilm formation differs significantly among subjects, and these differences may overrule surface characteristics. A distinction is often made between "heavy" (fast) and "light" (slow) dental biofilm formers (Video 10.5).

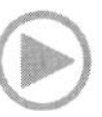

A multiple regression analysis showed that the clinical wettability of the tooth surfaces, the saliva-induced aggregation of oral bacteria, and the relative salivary flow conditions around the sampled teeth explained 90% of the variation. Moreover, the saliva from light biofilm formers reduced the colloidal stability of bacterial suspensions of, for example, *S. san*

CLINICIAN'S CORNER

Do some patients form dental biofilms faster than others?

Yes, so-called heavy and light dental biofilm formers exist. However, in both cases, it takes days before the biofilm is clinically visible. Patients cannot justify poor oral hygiene by being heavy dental biofilm formers.

The intersubject variation in biofilm formation can also be explained by factors such as diet, chewing fibrous food, smoking, the presence of copper amalgam, tongue and palate brushing, the colloid stability of bacteria in the saliva, antimicrobial factors present in the saliva, the chemical composition of the pellicle, and the retention depth of the dentogingival area.

A study by Rosier et al. (2018)[431] looked at the susceptibility of individuals to dental diseases such as periodontal disease and discussed variability within a population whereby some individuals would be more susceptible to disease processes leading to periodontitis than others. Less susceptible individuals possess a higher degree of "resilience" when exposed to disease drivers such as biofilm accumulation and so are less likely to suffer from undesirable changes to their oral microbiome towards a more periopathogenic microbiota. This concept of "resilience" therefore relates to the ability of the oral microbiota to resist pressure to progress to a dysbiotic state that favors disease.[56,431] Resilience could therefore discriminate between susceptible and tolerant individuals when disease drivers were applied and tolerant individuals would have an intrinsic resistance to these stress factors and would have the ability to withstand and recover from any perturbations that are triggered.[431] Health-maintaining mechanisms exist in these more tolerant individuals to maintain resilience and promote resistance to disease drivers. In susceptible individuals, or in previously tolerant individuals, if disease drivers are applied above a certain threshold, then resilience is disrupted and this could then lead to a significant shift in the microbial ecosystem to promote dysbiosis and increase the risk of periodontal breakdown. Further understanding of the markers of microbiome resilience could potentially lead to new strategies to prevent disease.[431]

Variation Within the Dentition

Within a dental arch, large differences in dental biofilm growth rate can be detected. In general, early biofilm formation occurs faster: in the lower jaw (as compared with the upper jaw); in molar areas; on the buccal tooth surfaces (as compared with palatal sites, especially in the upper jaw); and in the interdental regions (as compared with the buccal or lingual surfaces).[262,403]

Impact of Gingival Inflammation and Saliva

Several studies clearly indicate that early in vivo biofilm formation is more rapid on tooth surfaces facing inflamed gingival margins than on those adjacent to healthy gingivae.[406,417,418] These studies suggest that the increase in crevicular fluid production may enhance biofilm formation. Some of the components of this exudate (e.g., minerals, proteins, carbohydrates) favor both the initial adhesion and/or the growth of the early colonizing bacteria. In addition, it is known that, during the night, the biofilm growth rate is reduced by some 50%.[409] This seems surprising because one would expect that reduced biofilm removal and the decreased salivary flow at night would enhance biofilm growth. The fact that the supragingival biofilm obtains its nutrients mainly from the saliva appears to be of greater significance than the antibacterial activity of saliva.[53]

A major role of saliva is to lubricate and protect the oral soft and hard tissues from a microbial challenge.[9] There are a number of factors that can lead to a reduction in saliva flow or hyposalivation, including prescribed medication, conditions such as Sjögren syndrome, and radiation therapy to the head and next region. A reduced salivary flow rate or altered buffering capacity could have an impact on the formation and composition of a dental biofilm. A study investigating the formation of the supragingival dental biofilm in patients with hyposalivation reported that subjects with hyposalivation (due to medicines or of unknown origin) were found to have elevated levels of *S. mutans* and *Lactobacillus* spp., oral bacteria associated with the development of caries, compared with controls.[9] In a study of patients who had undergone radiation therapy, the proportions of the gram-negative anaerobes *P. intermedia/P. nigrescens* and *F. nucleatum* were low in the radiation therapy group and *P. gingivalis* was not detected. The authors of this study inferred that bacteria associated with gingivitis and periodontitis may be suppressed in an oral cavity with a low salivary secretion rate and high proportions of acidogenic bacteria.[9]

Impact of Patient's Age

Although previous studies were contradictory, more recent reports clearly indicate that a subject's age does not influence de novo biofilm formation. In a study by Fransson and colleagues,[133] no differences could be detected in de novo biofilm formation between a group of young (20 to 25 years old) patients and a group of older (65 to 80 years old) subjects who abolished mechanical tooth cleaning measures for 21 days, neither in amount nor in composition.[133] This observation largely confirms data by Holm-Pedersen and colleagues[188] and data by Winkel and coworkers.[565] However, the developed biofilm in the older patient group resulted in more severe gingival inflammation, which seems to indicate an increased susceptibility to gingivitis with aging.

There are various factors that may influence dental biofilm formation in more elderly patients. Various studies have reported that more elderly patients have reduced salivary flow rates and changes in salivary composition. This may be due to the effects of medication, associated with medical conditions, or as a result of age-related physiological changes.[345,601] A reduction in salivary flow bathing the oral tissues may impact on the ability to wash away oral bacteria and food debris and this may affect the formation of supragingival dental biofilms. Elderly patients may also have reduced manual dexterity, which could affect the ability to effectively perform an adequate oral hygiene regime to mechanically disrupt and remove dental biofilms.

De Novo Subgingival Biofilm Formation

It is technically impossible to record the dynamics of subgingival biofilm formation in an established dentition for the simple reason that one cannot sterilize a periodontal pocket. Some early studies involving the use of culturing techniques examined the changes within the subgingival microbiota during the first week after mechanical debridement and reported an only partial reduction of around 3 logs (from 10^8 bacterial cells to 10^5 cells), followed by rapid regrowth toward nearly pretreatment levels (−0.5 log) within 7 days.[148,175,306] A review of the effectiveness of subgingival instrumentation revealed that a high proportion of treated tooth surfaces (5% to 80%) still harbored dental biofilm and/or calculus after instrumentation. These remaining bacteria were considered the primary source for the subgingival recolonization.[385] Some pathogens penetrate the soft tissues or the dentinal tubules and eventually escape instrumentation (see Fig. 10.14).[5,173,435]

The introduction of dental implants, especially of the two-stage type, provided a new experimental setup. When the transmucosal part of the implant (the abutment) is inserted on top of the osseointegrated endosseous part, a new "pristine" surface is created on which the intraoral translocation of bacteria can be investigated.[405] It has been demonstrated that a complex subgingival microbiota, including most periodontal pathogens, is established within 1 week after abutment insertion.[134,411,412]

Relationship Between Oral Microbiome and Other Microbiomes

The human microbiome exists as a complex ecosystem and varies immensely across the body sites and between individuals. Most studied distinct ecological niches in the human body are: (1) oral cavity, (2) gut, (3) skin, (4) respiratory tract, and (5) urogenital tract. These environments demonstrate specific physical and biological conditions and further include microenvironments and sub-niches.[532] These microenvironments have unique properties, including dissimilarities in pH, temperature, oxygen availability, and cellular/tissue properties (e.g., keratinized vs. non-keratinized). For example, within the oral cavity, mucosal surfaces with high cell turnover rates such as buccal mucosa remain close to non-mucosal surfaces such as teeth.[586,587] Thus, there is a high degree of species selectivity and remarkable niche specificity regarding microbial colonization in these microenvironments.

While topographically, the oral cavity is the gateway to the upper respiratory and gastrointestinal tract and is in close proximity to the skin, each of these environments possesses distinct characteristics (Fig. 10.23). Hence the composition and function of the stable resident microbiome native to these environments are distinct among the different niches, as demonstrated by the Human Microbiome Project.[287,532]

Oral-gut Axis

Advances in understanding these microbial niches with the development of new tools and computational biology techniques have led to our latest understanding that although the oral and stool environments share a little taxonomic resemblance, community-type analysis demonstrates that oral bacterial population seed the gut. In particular, the genus *Prevotella* is identified in both the stool and salivary environments with similar frequency and abundances.[98] However, several other bacterial members belonging to the *Streptococcus* and *Bacteroidetes* are also identified in both the oral and the gut environments, with varied relative abundances. For example, *Streptococcus* comprises approximately 20% to 47% of the oral microbiome, while it constitutes only 0.07% of the gut. The relative abundances are reversed for the *Bacteroidetes*.[308,460] In general, the oral microbiome is much more diverse than the gut microbiome.[275] The presence of oral microbial strains that are being discovered now is attributed to the potential translocation of these microbes through swallowing, and those strains that can survive the changes from the oral to the gut environment persist. In disease, global dysbiosis prevails, and a lot more of these translocations are reported.[101,461,529]

Oral-respiratory Tract Axis

The upper respiratory tract is bathed in atmospheric air, inhaled microbes and contaminants, and constantly exposed to changes in humidity and temperature. Therefore, the nasal and the lung environments host a unique microbiome that is dissimilar across these two respiratory tract niches and from that of the oral environment.[253] The nasal microbiome of healthy humans is primarily composed of the phyla Actinobacteria, Bacteroidetes, Firmicutes, and Proteobacteria with representatives of genera *Bifidobacterium, Corneybacterium, Staphylococcus, Streptococcus, Dolosigranulum,* and *Moraxella*. The biomass decreases from the upper to the lower respiratory tracts.[18,510] While most of the lung communities are identified in the oral cavity, specific microbial species belonging to *Enterobacteriaceae, Hemophilus, Methylobacterium, Tropheryma,* and *Ralstonia* were excessively represented in the lungs.[61,95,342]

Oral-skin Axis

The skin is cool, acidic, desiccated with folds, glands, and appendages, and hence select for the distinctive microbiome. Phylum *Actinobacteria*, including genera *Corynebacterium, Propionibacterium, Brevibacterium*, and the genera *Micrococcus* and *Staphylococcus*, are the commensal flora of the skin which is distinct from that of the oral cavity.[151] However, the skin microbiome more closely resembles that of the oral microbiome in disease conditions, such as atopic dermatitis. Unlike the other systemic diseases, the composition and functions of the oral microbiome seem to have an anti-inflammatory role in patients with atopic dermatitis.[277]

Historical and Contemporary Concepts in the Etiology of Periodontitis

The search for the etiologic agents of periodontal diseases started in the 19th century, during the "golden era" of medical bacteriology (1890–1920). Researchers applied the microbiological techniques

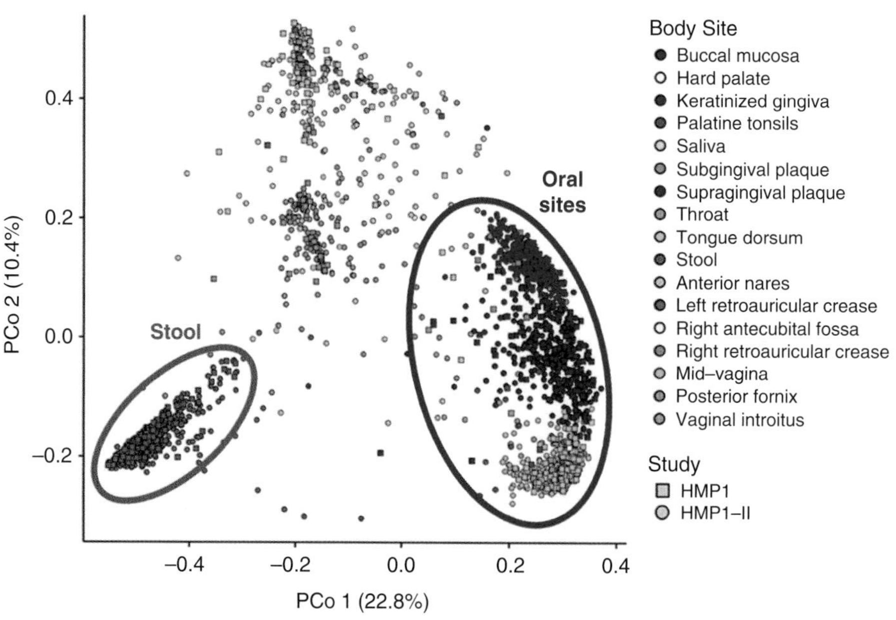

Fig. 10.23 Ordinations show Bray–Curtis principal distances among all microbes at the species-level abundances at each body site. Within-site ecological structure is evident. (Lloyd-Price J, Mahurkar A, Rahnavard G, et al. Strains, functions and dynamics in the expanded Human Microbiome Project. *Nature*. 2017;550:61–66. https://doi.org/10.1038/nature23889.)

available at that time to study the oral microbiota. Unfortunately, these studies were not as successful as those of extraoral diseases, mostly due to the lack of effective diagnostic tests to isolate and characterize the strict anaerobe pathogens colonizing the subgingival environment.[122,495] After the initial attempt to establish the infectious nature of periodontal diseases, this concept was abandoned and rekindled a few times over the course of history. Since then, different hypotheses have been suggested to explain the role of microorganisms in the onset and progression of periodontitis.

Nonspecific Plaque Hypothesis

In the mid-1900s, periodontal diseases were thought to result from an accumulation of biofilm (called plaque at that time) over time, eventually in conjunction with a diminished host response and increased host susceptibility with age. This theory, which was called the *nonspecific plaque hypothesis*, was supported by epidemiologic studies that correlated both age and the amount of biofilm with evidence of periodontitis.[300,438,450] It was thought that periodontitis resulted from the "elaboration of noxious products by the entire biofilm flora."[294] When only small amounts of biofilm are present, the noxious products are neutralized by the host. Similarly, large amounts of biofilm would cause a higher production of noxious products, which would essentially overwhelm the host's defenses. The classic study of "experimental gingivitis" by Löe and coworkers,[289] convincingly demonstrated that biofilm led to gingivitis. This concept was generalized to periodontitis and reinforced the principles of the *nonspecific plaque hypothesis* that periodontal destruction would result from the overall growth of biofilm and that the composition of biofilm was similar from patient to patient and from site to site.

KEY FACT

The classic study of "experimental gingivitis" by Löe and coworkers[289] demonstrated that biofilm leads to gingivitis, confirming the relationship between biofilm accumulation and gingival inflammation.

Inherent in the nonspecific plaque hypothesis was the concept that the control of periodontal disease depended on the reduction of the total amount of biofilm. Thus, in the 1960s and 1970s, periodontal treatment was focused on strict supragingival biofilm control. A group of clinicians and periodontists around the world that supported this protocol were sometimes referred to as the "plaque evangelists."[495]

Several observations contradicted the principles of the nonspecific plaque hypothesis. Newer epidemiological surveys indicated that only certain individuals or sites exhibited attachment loss and that some populations in Sri Lanka[290] and Kenya[16] had a large amount of calculus and biofilm with minimal or no periodontal attachment loss or inflammation. Furthermore, individuals who presented with periodontitis demonstrated considerable site-specificity regarding the pattern of disease. Some sites were unaffected, whereas advanced disease was found in adjacent sites. In the presence of a uniform host response, these findings were inconsistent with the concept that all biofilms were equally pathogenic. These concepts and the results of the first studies recognizing microbiological differences in biofilm at sites of different clinical status (i.e., disease vs. health) (see Video 10.2) led to a renewed search for specific pathogens in periodontal diseases and a conceptual transition from the nonspecific to the specific plaque hypothesis.

Specific Plaque Hypothesis

The specific plaque hypothesis underlines the importance of the qualitative composition of the resident microbiota.[294] The pathogenicity of dental biofilm depends on the presence of or an increase in specific microorganisms.[481] This concept encapsulates that biofilms harboring specific pathogens may provoke periodontal disease because key organisms produce substances that mediate the destruction of host tissues. In the late 1970s and 1980s major advances were made in the techniques used to isolate and identify periodontal microorganisms. These included improvements in procedures to sample subgingival biofilm, in the handling of samples to prevent killing the bacteria, and in the media used to grow the bacteria in the laboratory.[500] The results were a tremendous increase in the ability to isolate periodontal microorganisms and considerable refinement in bacterial taxonomy.[245] Acceptance of the specific plaque hypothesis was spurred by the recognition of *A. actinomycetemcomitans* as a pathogen in localized aggressive periodontitis.[350,483] These advances led to a series of studies focused on identifying specific periodontal pathogens by examining the microbiota associated with states of health and disease in cross-sectional and longitudinal studies.[350,351,481,482]

The introduction of molecular methods for bacterial identification has greatly increased the power of periodontal microbiological studies because these were no longer constrained to analyzing those bacteria that could be cultured (i.e., up to 50% of the total oral microbiota).[497,552,584] Molecular identification techniques such as the checkerboard DNA–DNA hybridization allowed for the first time the identification and enumeration of many different organisms simultaneously and were thus well suited for high-throughput studies (Fig. 10.24).[491] An analysis of more than 13,000 biofilm samples for 40 subgingival microorganisms using a DNA-hybridization methodology defined "complexes" of periodontal microorganisms that tended to occur together in health or disease. The composition of the different complexes was based on the frequency with which different clusters of microorganisms were recovered, and the complexes were color coded for easy conceptualization (see Fig. 10.24).[501] The yellow, purple, and green microbial complexes harbored several species considered to be host-compatible, including *V. parvula* (see eFig. 10.1B), *Schaalia odontolytica* (formerly *Actinomyces odontolyticus*) (see eFig. 10.1D), *Streptococcus* (see eFig. 10.1A, D, F), and *Capnocytophaga* species (see eFig. 10.1Q). Later, a group of four *Actinomyces* species was also pointed out as being important beneficial microorganisms.[493] These species were considered early colonizers of the tooth surface that usually precede the multiplication of the species from the pathogenic orange and red complexes. The orange complex includes microorganisms recognized as pathogens in periodontal and nonperiodontal infections, such as *Fusobacterium, Prevotella,* and *Campylobacter* spp. (see eFig. 10.1R). The red complex consisted of *T. forsythia, P. gingivalis,* and *T. denticola*, three closely related pathogens associated with probing depth and bleeding on probing.[501] The existence of complexes of species in biofilms is an important reflection of bacterial interdependency in the biofilm environment.

These studies convincingly demonstrated the association of certain species with periodontal health or disease. However, they also showed that periodontal destruction could occur even in the absence (or in the presence of very low levels) of defined "pathogens," such as red complex bacteria. Conversely, "pathogens" may be present in the absence of disease. This line of thought supported new theories about the interplay between microorganisms and the immuno-inflammatory host response in the onset and progression of periodontitis.

Ecologic Plaque Hypothesis

During the 1990s, Marsh and coworkers[320] developed the "ecologic plaque hypothesis" as an attempt to unify the existing theories regarding the role of dental biofilms in oral disease (Fig. 10.25). The

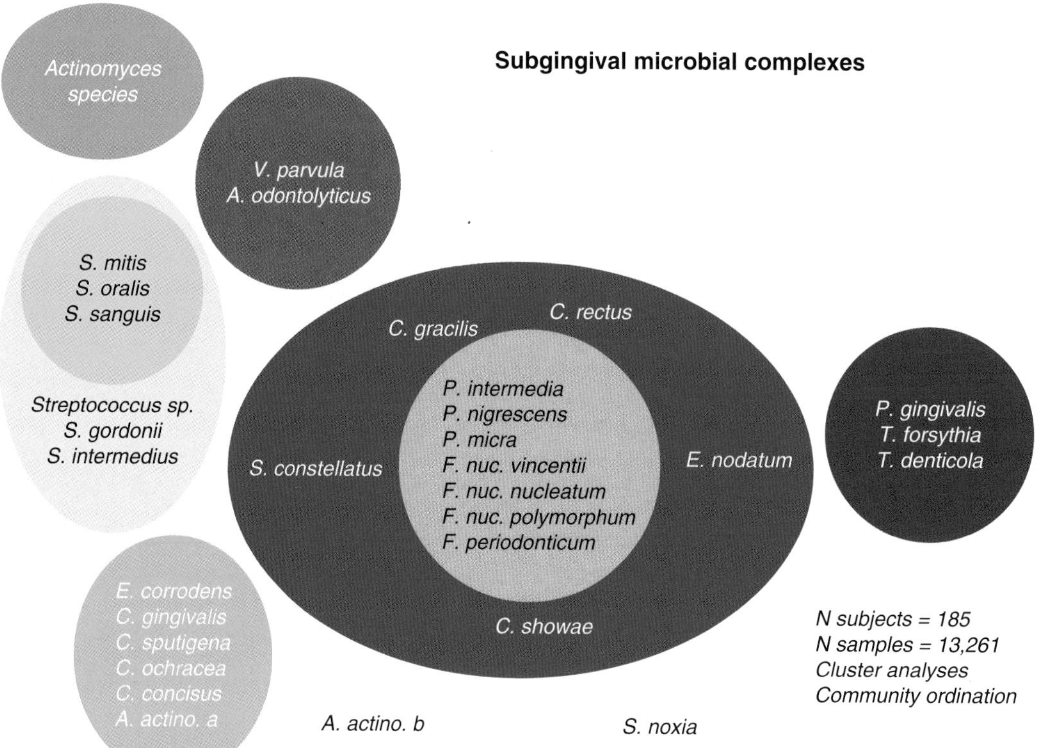

Fig. 10.24 Associations among subgingival species. The data were derived from 13,261 subgingival plaque samples taken from the mesial aspect of each tooth in 185 adult subjects. Each sample was individually analyzed for the presence of 40 subgingival species with the use of checkerboard DNA–DNA hybridization. Associations were sought among species via cluster analysis and community ordination techniques. The complexes to the left consist of species that are thought to colonize the tooth surface and to proliferate at an early stage. The orange complex becomes numerically dominant later; it is thought to bridge the early colonizers and the red complex species, which become numerically more dominant during the later stages of plaque development. *A. actinomycetemcomitans, Aggregatibacter actinomycetemcomitans; A. odontolytica, Actinomyces odontolytica; C. concisus, Campylobacter concisus; C. gingivalis, Capnocytophaga gingivalis; C. gracilis, Campylobacter gracilis; C. ochracea, Capnocytophaga ochracea; C. rectus, Campylobacter rectus; C. showae, Campylobacter showae; C. sputigena, Capnocytophaga sputigena; E. corrodens, Eikenella corrodens; F. nuc., Fusobacterium nucleatum; F. periodonticum, Fusobacterium periodonticum; P. gingivalis, Porphyromonas gingivalis; P. micra, Parvimonas micra; P. nigrescens, Prevotella nigrescens; S. constellatus, Streptococcus constellatus; S. mitis, Streptococcus mitis; S. noxia, Selenomonas noxia; S. oralis, Streptococcus oralis; S. sanguis, Streptococcus sanguis; T. denticola, Treponema denticola; T. forsythia, Tannerella forsythia; V. parvula, Veillonella parvula.* (Adapted from Socransky SS, Haffajee AD, Cugini MA, et al. Microbial complexes in subgingival plaque. *J Clin Periodontol.* 1998;25:134.)

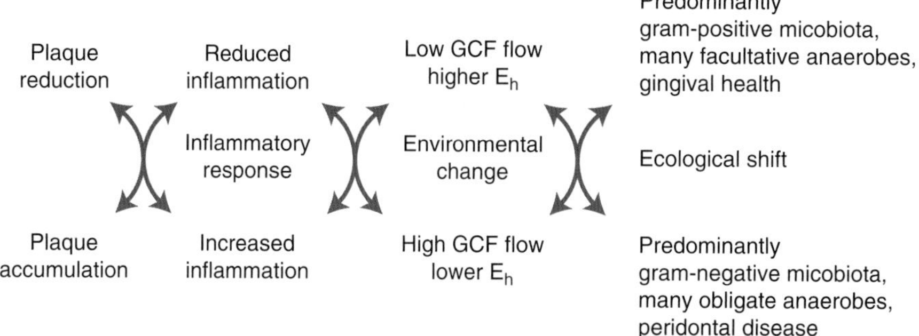

Fig. 10.25 Ecologic plaque hypothesis in relation to periodontal diseases: gingivitis and periodontitis. The accumulation of plaque causes the inflammation of adjacent tissues (gingivitis) and other environmental changes that favor the growth of gram-negative anaerobes and proteolytic species, including periodontal pathogens. The increased proportions of such species result in the destruction of periodontal tissues (i.e., periodontitis). *E_h*, Redox potential; *GCF*, gingival crevicular fluid. (Adapted from Marsh PD. Microbial ecology of dental plaque and its significance in health and disease. *Adv Dent Res.* 1994;8:263.)

principles of this hypothesis are that both the total amount of dental biofilm and the specific microbial composition of biofilms may contribute to the transition from health to disease. The health-associated dental microbiota is considered to be relatively stable over time and in a state of dynamic equilibrium or "microbial homeostasis." The host controls subgingival biofilms to some extent by a tempered immune response and low levels of GCF flow. Perturbations to the host response may be brought about by an excessive accumulation of nonspecific dental biofilm—leading to inflammation, by biofilm-independent host factors (e.g., the onset of an immune disorder, changes in hormonal balance [e.g., during pregnancy]), or by environmental factors (e.g., smoking, diet). Changes in the host status, such as inflammation, tissue degradation, and/or high GCF flow, may lead to a shift in the microbial population in the biofilm. As a result of microenvironmental changes, the number of beneficial species may decrease, whereas the number of potentially pathogenic species increases. This gradual shift in the entire microbial community, known as *dysbiosis*, may result in a chronic disease state such as periodontitis.[21] The ecologic plaque hypothesis is entirely consistent with observations that disease-associated organisms are minor components of the oral microbiota in health; these organisms are kept in check by interspecies competition during microbial homeostasis. Disease is associated with the overgrowth of specific members of the dental biofilm when the local microenvironment changes, but it is not necessarily the same species in each case. An important consideration of the ecologic plaque hypothesis is that therapeutic intervention can be useful on a number of different levels. Eliminating the etiologic stimulus—whether it is microbial, host, or environmental—will help to restore microbial homeostasis. Targeting specific microorganisms may be less effective because the conditions for disease will remain.

The Community as a Pathogen

The community as a pathogen hypothesis emerged in the early 2000s, with newer microbiological studies using next-generation sequencing techniques.[191,373] These studies allowed the evaluation of the whole bacterial community concomitantly, creating a unique opportunity for a deep understanding of the complex periodontal microbiome. The contribution of the studies using next-generation sequencing techniques for our understanding of the periodontal microbiome in health and in disease will be fully covered in the Periodontal Biofilm Composition in Health and Disease section in this chapter. For now, we want to highlight that the results of these investigations combined with the ecological concepts from the previous hypothesis regarding the etiopathogenesis of periodontal diseases led to the idea that periodontitis could be initiated by "a pathogenic microbial community"[21] or by "the community as a pathogen."[420] These theories posit that the periodontal microbial community should be viewed as a meta-organism, and that the united behavior of the community results in disease.[199] An addition to this notion is the theory of "keystone pathogens" which indicates that certain low-abundance microbial pathogens can orchestrate inflammatory disease by remodeling a normally benign microbiota into a dysbiotic one.[162,163] Some evidence indicates that certain pathogens may trigger the disruption of microbial homeostasis, thereby leading to the development of periodontal disease, even when they are present only in low numbers. For example, specific pathogen-free mice exposed to *P. gingivalis* developed periodontal bone loss even when the pathogen was present in less than 0.1% of the total microbiota. Disease did not occur in the absence of other bacteria (i.e., in germ-free mice) or in mice lacking the C3a or C5a complement receptors. These data indicated that *P. gingivalis* subverts the host immune system and changes the microbial composition of dental biofilms, ultimately leading to periodontal bone loss. On this basis, *P. gingivalis* was labeled a "keystone" pathogen; this means that it is an organism that is central to the disease process, even when it is at a relatively low abundance. The keystone pathogen hypothesis has been extended to include the concepts of a disrupted homeostasis in addition to the important roles of keystone pathogens in the "polymicrobial synergy" and "dysbiosis model" of disease.[163] In this model, interspecies communication between keystone pathogens and other members of the community (known as *accessory pathogens*) is considered one important factor that leads to overgrowth of the more pathogenic microbiota and to a dysbiotic microbial community. This model is based on a number of observations of microbial synergy among species that are not considered periodontal pathogens such as the oral streptococci and more pathogenic organisms including *P. gingivalis* and *A. actinomycetemcomitans*.[163] While the theory of "the community as a pathogen" has reasonable biological plausibility, the only keystone pathogen with good supporting evidence so far is *P. gingivalis*—a well-known periodontal pathogen from the red complex. Thus, the idea that other pathogens, or even species associated with health may have a relevant role in dysbiosis is yet to be proved.

Periodontal Biofilm Composition in Health and Disease

The Search for Periodontal Pathogens

During the 1870s, Robert Koch proposed the classic criteria by which a microorganism can be judged to be a causative agent in human infections. These criteria, known as Koch's postulates, stipulated that the causative agent must (i) be routinely isolated from diseased individuals, (ii) be grown in pure culture in the laboratory, (iii) produce a similar disease when inoculated into susceptible laboratory animals, and (iv) be recovered from lesions in a diseased laboratory animal.

Difficulties existed with regard to the application of these criteria to polymicrobial diseases, and the pertinency of Koch's postulates was challenged. In the case of periodontitis, three primary problems exist: (i) the inability to culture all of the organisms that have been associated with disease (e.g., many of the oral spirochetes), (ii) the difficulties inherent in defining and culturing sites of active disease, and (iii) the lack of a good animal model system for the study of periodontitis.[492] In fact, if the ecologic plaque hypothesis proves correct, it must be inherently impossible to fulfill Koch's postulates because no single organism is responsible for all cases of disease. Thus, in 1979, Sigmund Socransky adapted Koch's postulates to fit the periodontal disease model and proposed the following criteria by which periodontal microorganisms may be judged to be potential pathogens[492]:

1. Be associated with disease, as evidenced by increases in the number of organisms at diseased sites (association postulate)
2. Be eliminated or decreased in sites that demonstrate the clinical resolution of disease with treatment (elimination/suppression postulate)
3. Induce a host response in the form of an alteration in the host cellular or humoral immune response
4. Be capable of causing disease in experimental animal models
5. Produce demonstrable virulence factors that are responsible for enabling the microorganism to cause the destruction of the periodontal tissues

Socransky (1979) considered that the most important levels of evidence are provided by association (postulate 1) and elimination (postulate 2) studies. Different groups of investigators have been using these study designs for over a century in an attempt to identify the etiological agents of periodontal diseases.[381,496,518] Regrettably, several technical difficulties such as the need to identify a complex community of microorganisms, many of which are still difficult or impossible to cultivate, have delayed research in this field for many decades.[500] Despite these challenges, a convincing body of evidence of studies using cultivation and molecular techniques such as PCR and checkerboard DNA-DNA hybridization support *A. actinomycetemcomitans*, and the three red complex species (*T. forsythia*, *T. denticola*, and *P. gingivalis*) as key periodontal pathogens. Animal models have recently validated their disease potential as key periodontal pathogens.[136,217,363,390,425] These species have been strongly associated with periodontal disease status, disease progression, and unsuccessful therapy. Those studies also suggested moderate evidence for the role of the following microorganisms as putative periodontal pathogens, at least if their levels pass a certain threshold: *Selenomonas sputigena*, *Eubacterium nodatum* (see eFig. 10.1N), *P. micra*, *Eikenella corrodens* (Fig. 10.26), several *Fusobacteria*, *Prevotella*, and *Campylobacter* species (members of the orange complex), as well as various spirochetes.[13,341,481-483,488,493,500,501,568]

Technologic advancements such as next-generation sequencing techniques and the development of the Human Oral Microbial Database (http://www.homd.org)[110] have enabled the rapid expansion of the list of periodontal microorganisms, including the uncultured segment of the oral microbiota and even the potential involvement of non-bacterial members of this community, including virome and mycobiome members.[90,91,136,302,384,513] It is currently estimated that 30% of the oral microbiota has not yet been cultivated.[539]

A recent publication compiled data from all studies that used next-generation sequencing to compare the composition of subgingival biofilm samples of individuals with periodontitis and periodontal health (association postulate).[120] Overall, the twenty studies selected included 384 volunteers with periodontitis (710 subgingival samples) and 267 with periodontal health (353 subgingival samples). Taken together, the data confirmed the role of classical periodontal pathogens from the red and orange complexes in disease. The species most associated with periodontitis were *P. gingivalis*, *T. denticola*, *T. forsythia* (the three red complex species), and *Filifacor alocis*, a newly identified pathogen.[381] The species *Porphyromonas endodontalis*, *P. intermedia*, *Eubacterium saphenum*, *Phocaeicola abscessus*, *Mycoplasma faucium*, and *Fusobacterium simiae* were pointed out as potential pathogens. Some uncultivated taxa from the genera *Synergistetes*, *Desulfobulbus*, and *Saccharibacteria* (formerly TM7) were also more frequently elevated in periodontitis (Fig. 10.27).

The Role of Beneficial Species

An important notion in periodontal ecology is that not all oral microorganisms are pathogenic. Some of them are host-compatible or even beneficial. While it sounds obvious nowadays, this concept was avant-garde when first proposed in 1989[498,490] and was further consolidated after the publication of the landmark study "Microbial complexes in subgingival plaque" (see the Historical and Contemporary Concepts in the Etiology of Periodontitis section in this chapter).[501] Some theories have been raised over the years to explain the mechanism of protection by these host-compatible

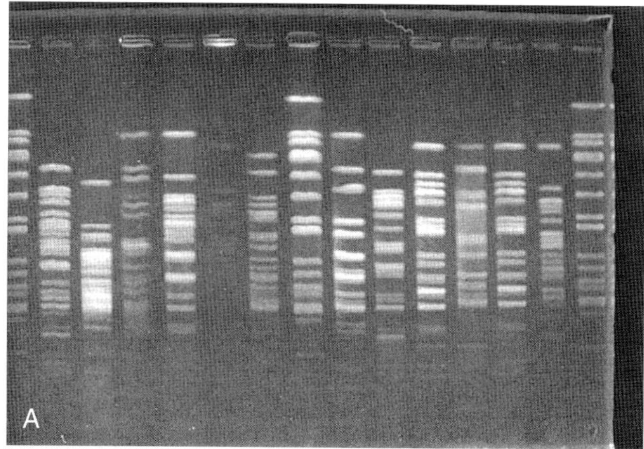

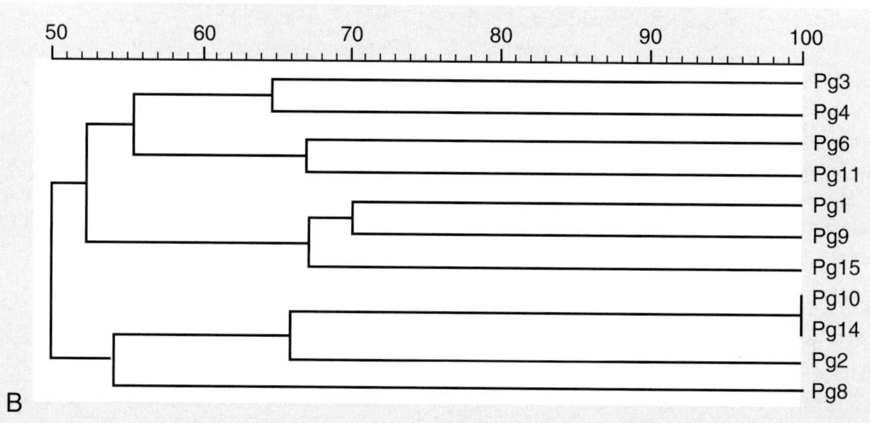

Fig. 10.26 Porphyromonas gingivalis strains. (A) Band pattern of DNA isolated from multiple *Porphyromonas gingivalis* strains after pulsed-field gel electrophoresis. Lanes 1, 8, and 15 contain a reference strain of DNA *(Staphylococcus aureus)* cut with SmaI (a restriction endonuclease) in lanes 2 through 7 and 9 through 14; 12 different *P. gingivalis* strains are compared for their genetic similarity. (B) The genetic similarity is expressed in a dendrogram. Bacteria are considered genetically similar when their band patterns are 80% similar.

microorganisms.[427,500] These bacteria can affect the pathogenic species and host response in different ways and thus modify the disease process as follows: (1) by passively occupying a niche that may otherwise be colonized by pathogens, (2) by actively limiting a pathogen's ability to adhere to appropriate tissue surfaces, (3) by adversely affecting the vitality or growth of a pathogen, (4) by affecting the ability of a pathogen to produce virulence factors, (5) by degrading the virulence factors produced by the pathogen, or (6) by modulating the inflammatory host response. The microorganisms considered host-compatible are those found in higher prevalence, levels, or proportions in health than in disease or in sites that exhibit less active disease and respond better to treatment.[498] Species from the genera *Actinomyces*, *Streptococcus*, *Capnocytophaga* as well as *V. parvula* and *Neisseria mucosa*[397,490,498] are those classically associated with periodontal health. Results from the studies using next-generation sequencing to investigate the periodontal microbiome confirmed these data and advocated that microorganisms from the genus *Rothia, Haemophilus*, *Corynebacterium*, *Leptotrichia*, *Neisseria,* and *Bergeyella* are also closely associated with periodontal health (Fig. 10.28).[120,123]

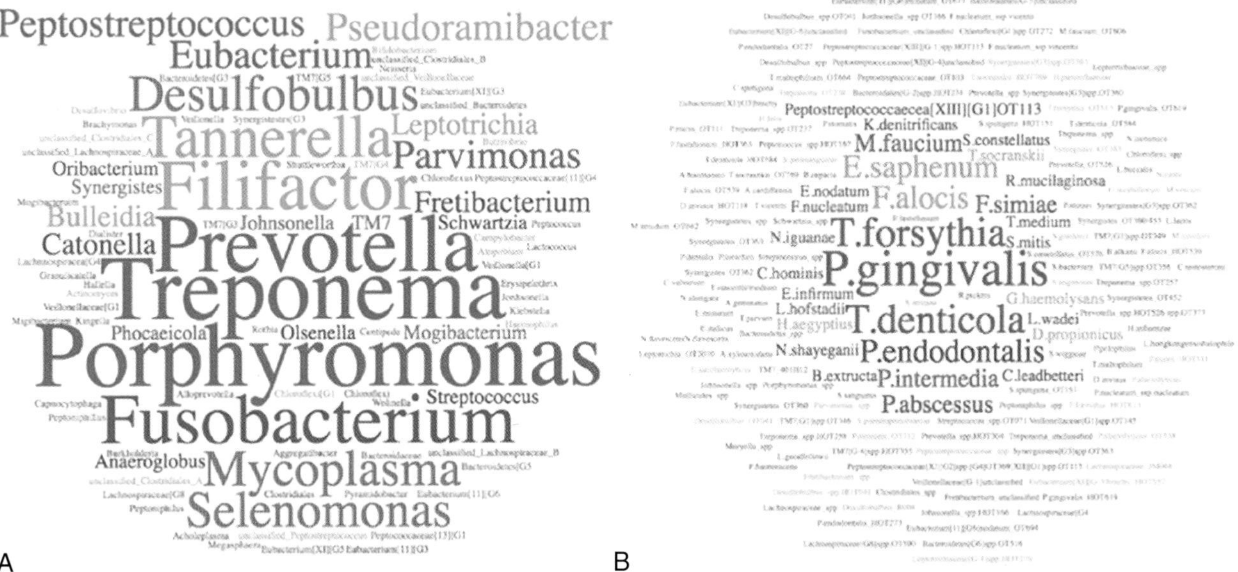

Fig. 10.27 Word clouds of the genera (A) and species (B) increased in periodontitis. Data from the association studies using next-generation sequencing (16S and metagenomic techniques) were combined and the results were used to create the cloud. (Feres M, Retamal-Valdes B, Gonçalves C, et al. Did Omics change periodontal therapy? *Periodontol 2000*. 2021;85[1]:182–209, First published: 23 November 2020. DOI:10.1111/prd.12358.)

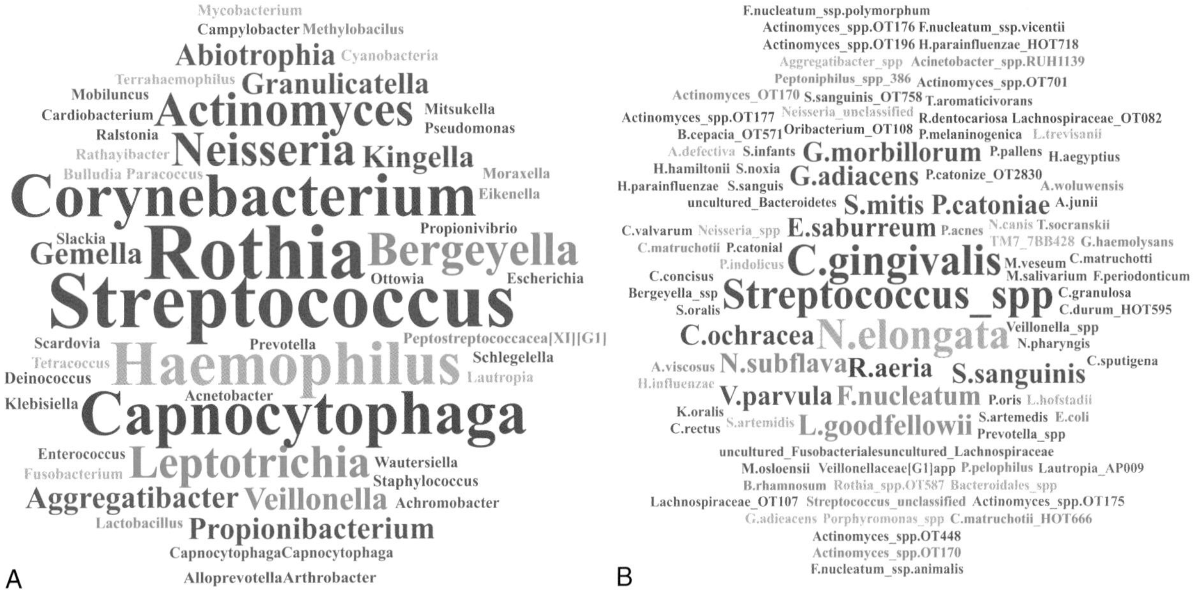

Fig. 10.28 Word clouds of the genera (A) and species (B) increased in periodontal health. Data from the association studies using next-generation sequencing (16S and metagenomic techniques) were combined and the results were used to create the cloud. (Feres M, Retamal-Valdes B, Gonçalves C, et al. Did Omics change periodontal therapy? *Periodontal 2000.* 2021;85[1]:182–209, First published: November 23, 2020. DOI: 10.1111/prd.12358.)

Microbial Profiles

Collectively, the results of the association studies conducted to date, using either target or open-ended diagnostic tests have shown that the subgingival biofilm of patients with periodontitis harbors higher levels/proportions/abundance of several periodontal pathogens and lower levels/proportions/abundance of beneficial species. These studies also extended considerably our knowledge regarding the composition of the microbiota in different oral habitats. For example, deep pockets, especially those ≥5 mm, have a more dysbiotic biofilm than shallower pockets of patients with periodontitis.[380] This was expected, since many periodontal pathogens are strict anaerobes and deep pockets provide an ideal environment for their growth, including reduced oxygen levels. A rather unexpected finding was that healthy sites in periodontally healthy and diseased individuals harbor rather different microbial signatures. The biofilms from shallow healthy sites in periodontitis patients are more dysbiotic and contain more pathogens than the same sites in periodontally healthy individuals.[78,96,307,380] In addition to shallow pockets, strict anaerobe pathogens have also been detected in other aerobic environments in the mouth. This may be explained by the biofilm protection. The biofilm structure may protect colonizing species from the noxious effect of high oxygen levels.[118,119] Anaerobic species, including the three red complex pathogens have been found in supragingival or supramucosal biofilms, tongue, saliva, and oral mucosa.[116,307,467,574,575]

Functional Potential and Metabolic Activity of the Periodontal Microbiome

As previously described in this chapter, the studies using DNA hybridization, and especially those assessing the oral microbiome by the amplification of the 16S rRNA gene have significantly enhanced our understanding of the composition of the biofilm associated with periodontal health and disease. However, it is worth noting that the studies using the 16S sequencing technique can only determine the genera, and at most the species present in the biofilm, but they cannot provide information about different strains, virulence genes, resistance genes, and changes occurring in the biofilm metabolism. The shotgun whole-genome sequencing and metatranscriptomic techniques allow the amplification of all genes in a sample, enabling a comprehensive evaluation of the biofilm composition (including bacteria, viruses, phages, archaea, and fungi), and the functionality of the microorganisms and of the biofilm as a whole. Overall, the studies using these techniques confirmed the findings from 16S (and checkerboard DNA-DNA hybridization) studies, both for periodontal pathogens and host-compatible microorganisms. Species from the genus *Actinomyces* were associated with periodontal health, while those from the genera *Prevotella, Fusobacterium, Treponema, Selenomonas,* and *Porphyromonas* were associated with disease.[78,105,206,512,551] Metatranscriptomics, the analysis of microbial gene expression within the biofilm, has provided important insights into the functionality of the biofilms. Apparently, the microorganisms present in periodontitis—including classical pathogens—encode novel metabolic functions or express more virulence factors, such as motility, enzymes involved in iron metabolism and in antibiotic resistance, in comparison to those found in periodontal health.[105,206,512] Although still embryonic, the results of the functionality and metabolic activity of the microbiome support the notion that pathogenic species and/or the whole biofilm community may have different virulence patterns or metabolic activities in health and in disease, or during disease development. In the future, these findings may open new avenues for the development of therapeutic protocols targeting particular bacterial protein products.

Microbial Profiles of Different Periodontal Phenotypes

Periodontitis has different clinical presentations that may vary substantially according to the patient's age, teeth affected, accumulation of local factors, and severity of the disease. Some patients may have severe periodontal destruction at a relatively young age (i.e., between 20 and 40 years) accompanied by low levels of biofilm and calculus, while others may show heavy accumulation of local factors and less severe disease. Over the years, it has been speculated that these different phenotypes could be associated with specific microbiological profiles or host immune-inflammatory features. Thus, the 1999 classification system of periodontal diseases defined two main clinical categories of disease based on clinical features: aggressive and chronic.[14] The notion that different phenotypes would be associated with different microbial etiologies was greatly influenced by investigations conducted in the 1970s and 1980s showing high prevalence and levels of *A. actinomycetemcomitans* in very young patients with aggressive periodontitis.[154,362,481,487] However, studies conducted for over two decades failed to find specific differences in the pathophysiology of these conditions, either in terms of microbial composition or the immune-inflammatory responses of the affected patients.[12,104,339] In 2009, Faveri et al.[118] and Feres et al.[124] compared the microbial profiles of young subjects with localized aggressive periodontitis, adults with aggressive and chronic periodontitis and periodontally healthy individuals. Although *A. actinomycetemcomitans* was found in significantly higher proportions in subjects with aggressive periodontitis in comparison with those with chronic periodontitis, there were no striking differences in terms of microbial profile among the three groups of diseased patients (Fig. 10.29).[118,124] A recent systematic review integrated data of the 56 studies that compared the composition of subgingival biofilm of patients diagnosed with chronic and aggressive periodontitis and concluded that no species or groups of microorganisms were unique to or could differentiate between these two clinical conditions.[339] These findings suggested little evidence from the literature that aggressive and chronic periodontitis are distinct diseases and supported the development of the new classification scheme for periodontal diseases that grouped aggressive and chronic periodontitis in one single disease named periodontitis.[369,527]

The Transition From Health to Disease

As previously described in this chapter, over the past decades, association, elimination, and animal studies were able to identify several periodontal pathogens. In addition, robust microbiological studies have strengthened the importance of host-compatible microorganisms in maintaining a symbiotic environment between the microbiota and the host in the oral cavity. However, as in the case of most human infections, periodontitis onset and progression are not only dependent on the presence of specific microorganisms or microbial profiles. The mere presence of putative periodontal pathogens in the gingival crevice is not in itself sufficient to initiate or cause periodontal inflammation. An elevation in the relative proportion or number of these pathogens to reach a critical mass seems more crucial to mount an effective tissue-damaging process. Indeed, even in health, periodontal pathogens are or can be present in the gingival crevice, albeit in low numbers, as members of the normal resident microbiota.[298] The oral microbial ecology is dynamic. The presence and numbers of particular microorganisms, even as a part of a community colonizing a niche in a human being, are controlled by the type and quantity of nutrients present (nutritional determinant), their ability to tolerate the specific physicochemical factors

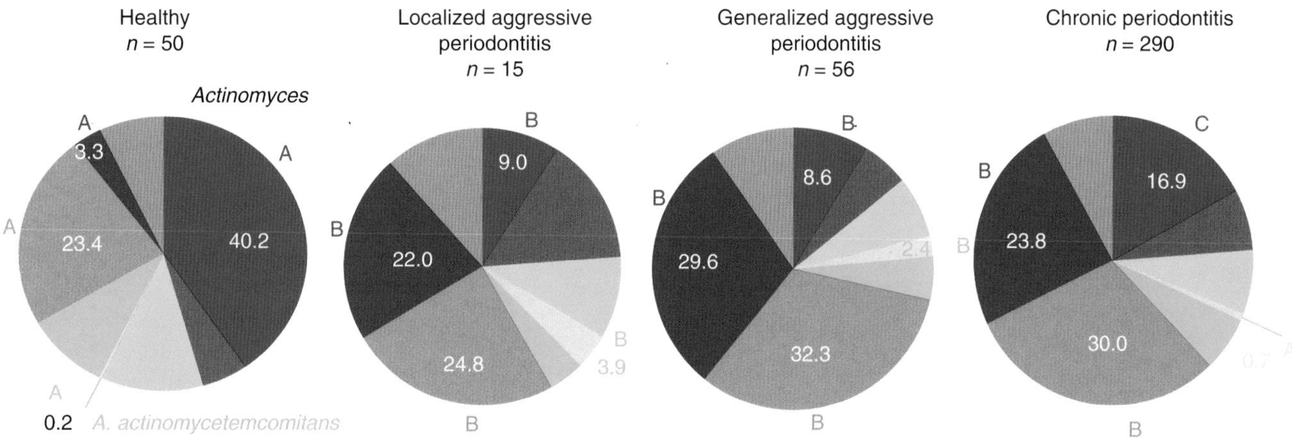

Fig. 10.29 Pie charts describing the mean proportions of microbial complexes in subgingival biofilm samples taken from 50 subjects with periodontal health, 15 subjects with localized aggressive periodontitis, 56 subjects with generalized aggressive periodontitis, and 290 subjects with chronic periodontitis. Nine subgingival biofilm samples were taken from each subject and were analyzed separately to determine their content of 40 species. The percentage of DNA probe counts for each species was determined at each site, then averaged within a subject and then across subjects in each group. The mean proportion of each species was summed in order to determine the proportion of each complex. The colors represent the different complexes described by Socransky et al. *Actinomyces* spp. are represented in blue and *A. actinomycetemcomitans* in light green. The gray color represents species that did not fall into any complex. The significance of differences among groups was determined using analysis of covariance, adjusted for mean age and Tukey's multiple comparison tests (different letters indicate significant differences among groups). (Feres M, Figueiredo LC, Soares GMS, et al. Systemic antibiotics in the treatment of periodontitis. *Periodontol 2000.* 2015; 67[1]:131–186, First published: December 12, 2014. doi:10.1111/prd.12075.)

(physicochemical determinants), and their ability to cope with antimicrobial compounds (biologic determinants) or mechanical removal forces (mechanical determinants). Although these determinants are well defined from a theoretical point of view, in practice they overlap each other, especially in more complex environments (i.e., multispecies environments). Inherent to their biologic nature, bacteria interact with each other, with their environment, and vice versa. Therefore, the microbial ecology will change its composition, or the composition of the microbial ecology will be changed when transitioning from a healthy status to a diseased status or vice versa.

The current concept regarding the etiology of periodontal diseases considers four groups of factors that determine whether active periodontal destruction will occur in a subject: (i) a susceptible host, (ii) the presence of pathogenic species, (iii) the absence or small proportion of so-called beneficial bacteria, and (iv) an altered local environment (e.g., presence of gingival inflammation and deep pockets). The clinical manifestations of periodontal destruction will result from a complex interplay among these etiologic agents. In general, small amounts of bacterial accumulation can be controlled by the body's defense mechanisms without destruction or by the resilience of the biofilm; however, when dysbiosis happens periodontal destruction could occur.[23] The main challenges researchers still have to face while trying to understand the exact events associated with the onset of periodontitis are related to the concepts of "temporality" and "dose". In other words, the *temporal sequence* and the *minimal level of change* in each of these components (i.e., biofilm composition, host susceptibility, and local/systemic inflammation) necessary to initiate disease are yet to be determined.

KEY FACT

Transition from health to disease results from a complex interplay among the host, the local environment, pathogenic bacteria, and commensal bacteria.

The Microbiota of Other Periodontal Conditions

Necrotizing Periodontal Diseases

Necrotizing periodontal diseases (see Case Scenario 10.1; see Chapter 30) are acute lesions characterized by severe inflammation and necrosis of the marginal gingival tissue and the interdental papillae.[182] Clinically, they may be accompanied by malodor and pain and possibly systemic symptoms, including lymphadenopathy, fever, and malaise. These conditions are often associated with stress or HIV infection.[392,454] Microbiologic studies on necrotizing periodontal diseases indicate that they are associated with high levels of spirochetes, fusiform bacteria, and *P. intermedia.* Furthermore, *Treponema, Selenomonas*, and *Fusobacterium* species have been considered "constant flora" in necrotizing periodontal disease lesions.[182,283,284,295] In addition, some specific microorganisms, such as *C. albicans*, herpes viruses, or superinfecting bacterial species, have been identified in patients with necrotizing periodontal disease and systemic conditions like HIV.[182]

Periodontal Abscesses

Periodontal abscesses (see Chapter 30) are acute lesions characterized as a localized purulent inflammation located within the gingival wall of the periodontal pocket and that may result in the very rapid destruction of the periodontal tissues.[182,184,185] They often occur in patients with untreated periodontitis, but they also may be found in patients during maintenance or after the scaling and root planing of deep pockets. Typical clinical symptoms of periodontal abscesses include pain, swelling, suppuration, bleeding on probing, and mobility of the involved tooth. Signs of systemic involvement may be present, including cervical lymphadenopathy and an elevated white blood cell count.[184] The microbial composition of periodontal abscesses is similar to that observed in periodontitis. Classical periodontal pathogens are commonly found in significant numbers/proportion in this lesion, including *P. gingivalis, P. intermedia, P. melaninogenica, F. nucleatum, T. forsythia, Treponema* species, *Campylobacter* species, *Capnocytophaga* species, *A. actinomycetemcomitans* or gram–negative enteric rods.[160,184,369] In addition, the role of viruses has been proposed, but with less evidence.[182]

Endo-periodontal Lesions

Endo-periodontal lesions (see Fig. 85.139; see Chapter 49) are acute or chronic clinical conditions involving both the pulp and periodontal tissues. The two main signs and symptoms associated with a tooth affected by an endo-periodontal lesion are deep periodontal pockets reaching or close to the apex and negative or altered response to pulp tests. In addition, other signs and symptoms have been reported, such as bone resorption, spontaneous pain or pain on palpation and percussion, purulent exudate, tooth mobility, sinus tract, crown, and gingival color alterations.[182] Studies on microbiological composition of endo-periodontal lesions have identified classical periodontal pathogens such as *P. gingivalis*, *T. forsythia*, or *P. micra*, and species from the genera *Fusobacterium*, *Prevotella*, and *Treponema*.[96,182,378,428,436,445,448] In addition, studies using "open–ended" molecular techniques have observed a higher microbial diversity and identified fewer common taxa, such as *F. alocis*, *Enterococcus faecalis*, and species from the genera *Desulfobulbus*, *Dialister*, *Fretibacterium*, or *Rothia*.[144,182,274,571] Overall, no major differences exist between the microorganisms found in the endodontic and periodontal lesions or a specific microbial profile associated with the endo-periodontal lesions.

Peri-implantitis

Peri-implantitis is a pathological condition in tissues around implants, characterized by inflammation in the peri-implant mucosa and progressive loss of supporting bone (see Chapter 86).[261,281,456] As gingivitis often precedes periodontitis, it is accepted that peri-implant mucositis is established before peri-implantitis.[202] Evidence shows that biofilm formation around implants leads to peri-implant inflammation on soft tissues.[391,442,600] A retrospective study evaluating the incidence of peri-implantitis in individuals with pre-existing mucositis observed that the absence of preventive maintenance was associated with a high incidence of peri-implantitis.[71] In animal models, bacterial biofilm formation followed by ligature placement in a submucosal position leads to soft tissue inflammation and bone loss.[7,52,280,455]

Besides the similarities in clinical and histological features with periodontitis, peri-implantitis is also associated with a dysbiotic biofilm.[247,258,379,422] A recent systematic review analyzed the data of eleven association studies comparing microbial data around healthy implants and implants with peri-implantitis.[379] The results suggested moderate evidence supporting the association of the three red complex pathogens, *P. gingivalis*, *T. denticola*, and *T. forsythia*, with the etiology of peri-implantitis. Additionally, there was some evidence supporting the association of *P. intermedia* and *C. rectus* (orange complex species[501]) with peri-implantitis.[379] Another systematic review analyzed studies that compared microbiological data of biofilm samples collected from healthy teeth and implants or teeth with periodontitis and implants with peri-implantitis.[422] The study aimed to determine the weight of the current evidence for the existence of specific differences between these conditions. The authors concluded that there was insufficient evidence to support specific differences between microorganisms colonizing teeth and implants in health or in disease.[422]

Relationship Between Periodontal Microbiome and Systemic Diseases

The oral cavity is the second-largest microbial niche in the human body after the gut. Approximately 2000 bacterial, viral, archaeal, and fungal species that colonize the oral cavity play an active role in maintaining health at the mucosal barrier site by maintaining homeostatic interactions with the host immune response.[89,587] Dysbiosis in this environment is associated with increased inflammation and leads to disease.[260]

The evolution of the human microbiome project, which started in 2008, and the advent of next-generation sequencing approaches have shed light on the distinct characteristics and functions of the microbiome and their dynamic interactions with the host system. These technical advances have ultimately led to identifying the role of the oral microbiome past the local environment into systemic health and disease.[213,287,310,416,459,582]

The oral cavity is an entry point to the alimentary canal that leads to the gut and the respiratory tract. Additionally, the local oral environment is highly vascular, and there is a greater likelihood of disruption of the epithelial barrier (e.g., in periodontal disease or ulcerations), thus increasing the risk of bacteremia. Taken together, all the characteristics mentioned above, the oral environment facilitates the extraoral spread of the oral microbial communities, their toxins, and the metabolite end products to the systemic environment, either through the direct translocation of the bacteria itself to the distant site or via the circulation of the bacterial toxins and end products.

The frequency of bacteremia is the highest (80% to 100%) following dental extractions; however, routine oral hygiene activity such as toothbrushing showed a 28% incidence of bacteremia. Other dental procedures such as endodontic therapy and professional dental cleaning are associated with 20% and 70% incidence rates.[85,178,288,309] In a systemically healthy individual, the bacteremia is only transient, the magnitude and duration are controlled within 40 to 60 minutes, and the bacteria are removed from the circulation effectively.[393] However, in an immunocompromised patient, the bacteremia may persist and lead to extraoral colonization and infection.[252]

The oral microbiome and associated changes in the local and systemic inflammation have been implicated in several non-oral infections, adverse pregnancy outcomes, pneumonia, cardiovascular diseases, inflammatory diseases, gastrointestinal disorders, cancers, stroke, and neurodegenerative diseases.[45,224,252]

Oral Microbiome and Pulmonary Diseases

Several periodontal pathogens, including *P. gingivalis*, *F. nucleatum*, *Prevotella oralis*, *Campylobacter gracilis*, *A. actinomycetemcomitans*, *T. forsythia*, *Rothia* spp., and *T. denticola* have been identified in the bronchial mucosa and lung fluids from patients with pulmonary diseases such as pneumonia and chronic obstructive pulmonary disease (COPD).[25,146,311,439,510] Respiratory pathogens such as *Pseudomonas aeruginosa* and *Chlamydia pneumoniae* were detected in periodontal sulci of patients with bacterial pneumonia and cystic fibrosis.[127,439,449,561] Recently, several bacterial species belonging to the resident oral microbiota, such as *Capnocytophaga* and *Veillonella*, have been identified in the lung fluid of COVID-19 patients.[17,303] The interactions between the oral microbial communities and respiratory infections have been hypothesized to be mediated by (1) inflammatory responses triggered by these pathogenic bacteria, and/or (2) the translocation of the communities between the lung and the oral cavity due to coughing and swallowing.[311]

Oral Microbiome and Cardiovascular Diseases

Several oral bacteria and established periodontal pathogens such as *S. sanguinis*, *S. mutans*, *A. actinomycetemcomitans*, *P. gingivalis*, *P. endodontalis*, *T. denticola*, *T. forsythia*, *P. intermedia*, and *Prevotella nigrescens*, have been commonly found in atherosclerotic plaques.[63,87,463] The burden of many of these periodontal bacteria in subgingival plaque is associated with thickening of the carotid intima-media (carotid intima-media thickness test, measuring the thickness of the inner two layers of the carotid artery is used to diagnose the extent of carotid atherosclerotic vascular disease, even when patients are asymptomatic).[266] In addition to the identification of these bacteria in atherosclerotic plaques, the levels of systemic antibody in response to periodontal pathogens directly correlate to the incidence of coronary artery disease and subclinical atherosclerosis.[19,401] In patients with acute ischemic stroke, oral streptococci and not *P. gingivalis* and *A. actinomycetemcomitans* are identified.[30,375] In addition, by mediating the conversion of dietary nitrates to nitric oxide, the oral microbiome also plays a protective role in cardiovascular health. However, long-term longitudinal studies are required to validate the role of the oral microbiome in maintaining cardiovascular health.[29,99]

Oral Microbiome and Adverse Pregnancy Outcomes

Recently, the oral microbiome has been identified as a significant contributor to the placental microbial colonization.[146] There are proposed associations between periodontal disease, the oral microbiome, and adverse pregnancy outcomes such as preeclampsia and preterm birth, and low-birth-weight birth.[291,361,563,582] However, the evidence remains equivocal. High levels of periodontal pathogens including *T. forsythia, C. rectus, P. intermedia, P. nigrescens*, and *P. gingivalis* in maternal subgingival plaque are associated with low-birth-weight birth.[67,270,371,563] *P. gingivalis* was detected in the subgingival plaque and amniotic fluid in pregnant women with threatened premature labor.[270] Development of an intrauterine proinflammatory environment in response to pathogenic bacteria in the placenta and/or fetal response to the maternal pathogens (such as *F. nucleatum, C. rectus*) are hypothesized to be plausible mechanistic links between the oral microbiome and adverse pregnancy outcomes.[285,305] On the other hand, several clinical studies found that neither the levels of periodontal pathogens nor periodontal therapies were associated with adverse pregnancy outcomes.[254,331,354,355]

Oral Microbiome and Alzheimer Disease

Emerging evidence indicates the existence of the oral-brain axis and the potential role of the oral microbiome in the pathogenesis of Alzheimer disease.[346,426] Investigations in mice with *P. gingivalis* infection exhibit reduced blood-brain barrier (BBB) integrity, as shown by a decrease in the tight junction related proteins and the increased influx of beta-amyloid peptides from the periphery into the brain when compared to the uninfected control group.[471,509,524] In addition to the direct effect, an increase in systemic inflammation via IL-6, tumor necrosis factor-α (TNF-α), and IL-17 pathways due to LPS coupled with *P. gingivalis*, is associated with cognitive decline and Alzheimer disease.[152] Significant increases in levels of *Lactobacillales, Streptococcaceae*, an increased *Firmicutes/Bacteroidetes* ratio, and a significantly decreased number of *Fusobacterium* have also been reported in Alzheimer disease in a recent case-control clinical investigation.[570] Oral *Treponema* spp. have also been implicated in the disease.[426] Periodontal dysbiosis is associated with brain amyloidosis (a preclinical marker for Alzheimer disease) in cognitively normal elderly patients.[209]

Oral Microbiome and Cancers

Since the original reports linking periodontitis and leukemia were published in the 1940s and 1950s,[70,558] the association between periodontal disease, oral microflora, and oral and non-oral cancers have been actively investigated (see Chapter 26).[415] Studies with germ-free mice have shown that there is an increase in size and number of the tumors when the tongue surface is colonized with the microbiome when compared to the negative controls.[386] Mouse models have also validated the specific tumorigenic potential of several periodontal pathogens (*P. gingivalis, T. denticola, F. nucleatum*).[211] Mechanistically, these processes are partly regulated via TLR/MyD88 triggered activation of Integrin/FAK signaling. Furthermore, these studies have discovered the potential to mitigate oral carcinogenesis with a probiotic bacteriocin.[205,211,212,469] These findings highlight an emerging paradigm; namely the ability to mitigate carcinogenesis via the use of antimicrobial therapy. *P. gingivalis*, and *P. intermedia* infection but not *T. forsythia, T. denticola, A. actinomycetemcomitans*, and *F. nucleatum* infection were associated with increased risk for developing oral cancer in a recent meta-analysis.[573] However, due to the heterogeneity of the samples, study design, and the techniques involved, different studies have identified an increase in several of the oral microbial members in oral squamous cell carcinoma (OSCC). Some of the frequently reported alterations in the oral microbiome in OSCC patients include: *Capnocytophaga gingivalis, P. melaninogenica, S. mitis, F. nucleatum, P. aeruginosa, Campylobacter concisus, Prevotella salivae, Prevotella loeschii, Fusobacterium oral taxon 204*, genera *Fusobacterium, Dialister, Peptostreptococcus, Filifactor, Peptococcus, Catonella, Parvimonas, Prevotella oris, Neisseria flava, Neisseria flavescens/subflava, Aggregatibacter segnis*, and *Fusobacterium periodonticum.*[194,257,470,508,573,592] Shifts in microbes from health to primary and metastatic disease have also been reported including a shift toward a high fusobacterial and low streptococcal signature in head and neck cancer.[470]

P. gingivalis and *Fusobacterium* spp. are also associated with an increased risk of developing pancreatic cancer.[332,336] One potential mechanism behind this association is through activation of toll-like receptor 4 (TLR4) followed by a downstream activation of nuclear factor kappa B (NF-κB) through MyD88 dependent and independent pathways. Human pancreatic cancer shows higher expression of TLR4 when compared to a healthy pancreas.[35,359] *F. nucleatum* has been discussed also as a biomarker organism associated with colorectal cancer,[129,434] and identification of *F. nucleatum* has been associated with shorter survival rates in esophageal tissue.[579] Reduction in *F. nucleatum* virulence has also been associated with improved therapeutic outcomes in colorectal cancer.[583] Studies have also reported a predominant association of the genus *Veillonella* with lung cancer.[580,591]

Oral Microbiome and Rheumatoid Arthritis

Oral microbial dysbiosis and periodontal disease have been associated with increased susceptibility and risk for developing rheumatoid arthritis (RA).[216] *P. gingivalis* is frequently identified in RA patients and influences citrullination.[314,557] However, the higher frequency of identification of *P. gingivalis* could be because of the confounding effect with the presence of active periodontal disease in these patients.[26] Higher salivary levels of *Prevotella* and *Veillonella* were identified in early RA and individuals at risk for RA.[62,246] In the absence of periodontal disease, *P. gingivalis* and *A. actinomycetemcomitans* are not differentially detected between the groups (in periodontally healthy patients with RA). *Cryptobacterium curtum*, another organism capable of producing large amounts of citrulline, appears to be a more robust discriminant of the oral microbiome in individuals with RA.[299]

Oral Microbiome and Diabetes Mellitus

Diabetes mellitus (DM) is one of the two established risk factors for periodontal disease, and the bidirectional relationship between the two diseases is well-established.[220,396] The association between oral microbial dysbiosis and diabetes is an active area of investigation.[388,572] Several oral bacteria, including periodontal pathogenic genera such as *Fusobacterium, Parvimonas, Peptostreptococcus, Gemella, Streptococcus, Leptotrichia, Filifactor, Veillonella, Saccharibacteria* (TM7), *Terrahemophilus, Catonella, Bulleidia* have been associated with DM.[135,550,596] Additionally, the oral microbial composition is dependent on the control of the diabetic status and the level of the glycemic index.[135,297,326] For example, adequate control of the glycemic index (HbA1c < 7.8%) is associated with a heterogenous microbiome when compared to poorly controlled DM (HbA1c > 8.0). Fermenting species associated with propionate/succinate production are increased in the subgingival microbiome of poorly controlled diabetics, and those forming butyrate/pyruvate are decreased. In particular, higher abundances of *S. anginosus* group and *Streptococcus agalactiae* are associated with inadequately controlled DM.[59,114,297]

Oral Microbiome and Bacterial Vaginosis

In addition to the above-mentioned systemic diseases, the periodontal pathogen, *F. nucleatum* has been associated with bacterial vaginosis (BV). BV is associated with dysbiosis in the vaginal environment with a reduction of commensal lactobacilli, and an increase in *F. nucleatum,* which further supports the robust outgrowth of *Gardnerella vaginalis,* thus potentiating the development of disease. The metabolite cross-feeding between *F. nucleatum* and *G. vaginalis* thus promoting pathogen colonization is hypothesized to be the underlying mechanism for deciphering the role of *F. nucelatum* in BV.[6,338]

Biofilm and Microbiome Modulation by Different Periodontal Treatments

Although the processes associated with the onset of periodontitis are not yet completely elucidated, it was clear from the concepts and findings presented in this chapter that our knowledge about the composition of the biofilms in health and disease has strikingly evolved in the past decades. We understood that the periodontal microbiota is more diverse than previously thought and that periodontitis is a complex ecological problem associated with an imbalance between beneficial and pathogenic species. The notion that anaerobic pathogens are not restricted to deep pockets but can also be present at high levels even in oxygenated niches of the oral cavity, such as tongue, saliva, supragingival biofilm, and shallow pockets was also crucial for a better understanding of the periodontal ecology. Another important piece of information is the similarity observed among the subgingival microbiological profiles of patients with different phenotypes. As opposed to what was previously thought, most of the severe cases of periodontitis are associated with high levels and proportions of red complex bacteria and other pathogens, and low proportions of *Actinomyces* species and other host-compatible species—independently of the patient's age, amount of local factors, or local inflammation (see Fig. 10.28).

The overall interpretation of these findings was crucial to establish microbiological goals for periodontal treatment. The recognition that the entire oral cavity is in dysbiosis in subjects affected by periodontitis indicates that effective periodontal treatment would require a striking ecological shift in the oral environment. Not only deep pockets, but all oral niches would require anti-infective treatment in order to achieve a new biofilm climax community compatible with periodontal health and, consequently, reestablish homeostasis. Thus, understanding how different periodontal treatments modulate the periodontal biofilm is crucial to guide clinical practice.

As the knowledge about periodontal ecology evolved, it became clearer that in order to determine the effectiveness of periodontal treatments, one would have to track not only the presence or absence of one or a few pathogens before and after treatment but the changes occurring in the entire subgingival microbial profile. In this sense, the checkerboard DNA-DNA hybridization technique provided an essential contribution by allowing the simultaneous enumeration of the 40 bacterial species from the microbial complexes in many biofilm samples. Open-ended next-generation sequencing techniques expanded the list of species found in the periodontal environment, but also confirmed the role of microbial complexes microorganisms as main pathogens (e.g., red complex pathogens) or host-compatible species (e.g., *Actinomyces* and species from yellow and green complexes) (see Figs. 10.28 and 10.29). Thus, the microbial complexes, especially the proportions of red complex and its relation to the proportion of *Actinomyces* species, remain a very good thermometer for identifying states of dysbiosis or homeostasis as well as to monitor treatment. It has been advocated that when red complex pathogens sum 8% or more of the 40 bacterial species of the checkerboard panel,[501] the patient has lower chances to achieve the clinical end point for treatment of "≤4 sites with probing depth ≥5mm" at 1-year post-treatment.[31,121] Thus, most of the information available on the effects of different treatments on the composition of periodontal biofilm (elimination/suppression postulate) has been provided by clinical studies that used checkerboard DNA-DNA hybridization. These studies evaluated the microbial shifts brought by scaling and root planing[57,68,75,126,157-159,193,330,429] treatment with local and systemic antimicrobials[57,115,121,123-125,156,159,189,330,472,494,516,518,530], as well as surgical[46,156,272,494] and laser[49,143,322,402] treatments. Taken together, the results of these studies suggested that clinical benefits and longitudinal clinical stability are associated with a rapid and profound reduction in red and orange complexes pathogens and a concomitant increase in proportions of host-compatible species.

The gold standard scaling and root planing procedure produces a deep beneficial change in the composition of the subgingival microbiota, including a reduction in pathogens and an increase in *Actinomyces* species (Fig. 10.30). The selective reduction of certain pathogens after scaling and root planing—a mechanical treatment that does not target specific bacterial species—is an interesting observation. Most probably, the first colonizers from the yellow, purple and green complexes, as well as *Actinomyces* species recolonize the recently scaled pockets in greater proportions and the pathogens of the red and orange complexes recolonize more slowly—probably because of their fastidious nature—and remain in lower proportions.[124] The final outcome is a healthier biofilm composition. Unfortunately, not all these benefits are sustained over time in patients with severe disease. The data presented in Fig. 10.30 of microbial complexes in subgingival biofilm samples taken from 75 subjects with periodontitis stages III and IV show that red complex pathogens may slowly recolonize the subgingival environment 3 months post-treatment. Thus, apparently nonsurgical mechanical debridement alone is not sufficient to change the climax community of patients with severe disease to a new stable climax community compatible with health. Thus, over the years, researchers have put efforts to search other treatments to be used as adjuncts to subgingival debridement in order to potentiate the effects of this treatment.

Among the adjunctive therapies tested to date, those that reach all the oral environments for a prolonged period of time seem to be the most promising in maintaining a healthy periodontal ecology longitudinally.[446] The clinical and microbiological effects of adjunctive treatment targeting specific oral habitats, such as antimicrobials locally delivered to deep periodontal pockets, were not found to be particularly promising.[124,156,183,494,518] The most consolidated

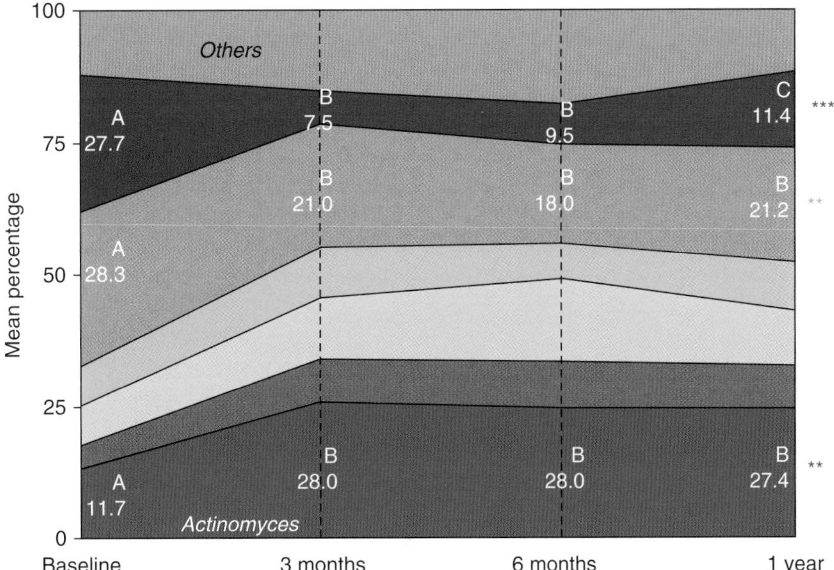

Fig. 10.30 Cumulative mean proportions of microbial complexes in subgingival biofilm samples taken from 75 subjects with advanced periodontitis at baseline, and at 3 months, 6 months, and 1-year post–scaling and root planing. Nine subgingival biofilm samples were taken from each subject at each time point and were analyzed separately to determine their content of 40 species of bacteria. The percentage of DNA probe counts for each species was determined at each site, then averaged within a subject and then across subjects at each time point. The mean proportion of each species was summed in order to determine the proportion of each complex. The colors represent the different complexes described by Socransky et al. The gray color ("Others") represents species that did not fall into any complex, and *Actinomyces* spp. are represented in blue. The significance of differences among time points was determined using repeated–measures analysis of variance (**$P < .01$; ***$P < .001$) and Tukey's multiple comparison test (different letters indicate significant differences between time points). (Feres M, Figueiredo LC, Soares GMS, et al. Systemic antibiotics in the treatment of periodontitis. *Periodontol 2000.* 2015; 67[1]:131–186, First published: December 12, 2014, DOI:10.1111/prd.12075.)

adjunctive treatment to mechanical debridement is systemic antibiotics, followed by probiotics/prebiotics and host-modulators. Although promising, there are still very scarce data from interventional studies on the effects of host-modulators on the composition of the subgingival biofilm,[348] and some evidence for the benefits of probiotics and prebiotics.[204,327,430,517,520,531]

Probiotics

The use of probiotics is a new developing field in oral health care. Probiotics have been defined as living micro-organisms that, when administered in adequate amounts, confer a health benefit to the host.[186] Although the effects of probiotics are considered to be local, studies in which probiotics were given to rats by gavage feeding, so without passing through the mouth, also showed reduced periodontal breakdown in a ligature model for periodontitis.[137,225] This indicates that the effects of probiotics are both local and systemic, presumably by interfering with the host immune system. The clinical benefits of the use of probiotics for oral and periodontal health have been well-documented in several clinical trials. For a detailed discussion of these topics please see two recent reviews.[352,353] For instance, individuals with moderate to severe gingivitis receiving *Lactobacillus reuteri* (now reclassified as *Limosilactobacillus reuteri*) formulations showed decreased biofilm accumulation and less gum bleeding.[243] In another study, the regular consumption of *L. reuteri* lozenges by healthy individuals was shown to significantly improve clinical parameters including bleeding on probing, gingival index, probing attachment level, and probing pocket depth.[451] The benefits of using probiotics as adjuncts to standard periodontal therapies have also been demonstrated in several clinical studies, with improvements in important periodontal clinical parameters such as periodontal pocket depth, clinical attachment loss, gingival index, plaque index, and bleeding on probing.[192,321,352,517,520,543]

In terms of microbiological effects, evidence is more limited, but a few clinical trials also reported beneficial effects on the oral microbial ecology. For instance, the study of Teughels et al. also reported stronger reductions in *P. gingivalis* numbers in saliva, supra- and subgingival samples for the scaling and root planing + probiotic group compared to the scaling and root planing alone group.[520] Patients with chronic periodontitis and treated with a *Bacillus subtilis*-containing mouthrinse showed significantly decreased abundances of the "red complex" periodontal pathogens (*P. gingivalis, T. denticola,* and *T. forsythia*), indirectly measured as changes in the proteolytic activity of these anaerobes, compared to treatment with a classical mouthrinse.[531] In healthy volunteers without severe periodontitis, the oral administration of *Lactobacillus salivarius* (now reclassified as *Ligilactobacillus salivarius*) WB21-containing tablets resulted in a significantly reduced total count of five periodontal pathogens (*A. actinomycetemcomitans, P. gingivalis, P. intermedia, T. forsythia,* and *T. denticola*) in subgingival biofilm samples 4 weeks post-treatment, but not 8 weeks post-treatment.[327] In the study of Tekce et al., reductions in total viable cell counts and proportions of obligate anaerobes were observed at 21, 90, and 180 days post-treatment, but this effect was lost at 360 days post-treatment.[517]

In vitro evidence further highlights the ability of probiotics and their bacteriocins (secreted antimicrobial peptides) to suppress periodontal pathogens in biofilms and in planktonic forms.[208,414,468,536] For example, the probiotic *Lactococcus lactis* and its bacteriocin Nisin both suppressed periodontal pathogens in biofilm structures and planktonic states.[208,468,414] Furthermore, sequencing data has shown that these probiotics and bacteriocins can mediate shifts in oral pathogenic biofilm composition back towards health.[414] These effects can be mediated without negatively affecting human oral cells.[468] Future therapeutic approaches in this area may include the use of nano-sized drug delivery systems to further improve the delivery of bacteriocins, other small antimicrobial peptides, molecules, or prebiotics.[414]

Prebiotics

In light of the continuous search for novel preventive or therapeutic strategies, the modulation of the commensal oral microbiota by means of prebiotics is increasingly gaining attention. Prebiotics are "substrates that are selectively utilized by host microorganisms conferring a health benefit."[138] From this definition, it is evident that the utilization of the prebiotic by the commensal microbiota results in a health benefit to the host. This health benefit can be due to microbiological changes, like stimulation of the growth and abundance of certain species, but also due to metabolic changes, such as the stimulation of certain metabolic activities.[138] The prebiotic concept for oral health was only recently introduced.[479,480] In these in vitro studies, several hundreds of substrates were screened for their ability to selectively stimulate commensal oral bacteria, which consequently results in the inhibition of disease-associated species. Whereas the concept was initially proven at in vitro level for single species and dual-species biofilms,[479] it was quickly expanded to a more complex in vitro 14-species biofilm.[480] In this way, three potential prebiotic substrates for oral health were identified with beneficial effects on microbiological composition (i.e., decreases in periodontal pathogens and increases in commensal species): N-acetyl-D-mannosamine, β-methyl-D-galactoside, and succinic acid. Recently, four other potential prebiotic substrates were shown to beneficially modulate the same in vitro 14-species biofilm model in terms of microbiological composition, metabolism, virulence gene expression, and inflammatory potential towards human oral keratinocytes.[541] Over the past years, several other in vitro and in vivo studies have investigated the potential use of prebiotics for oral health. With increasing knowledge of the pathogenesis of oral diseases, these studies have been focusing on substrates that stimulate bacterial species with inhibitory activities on oral pathogens and/or modify environmental conditions that contribute to disease onset and progression such as environmental pH.[85,585] This has particularly been investigated for dental caries, with several studies proposing arginine, or substrates whose metabolization sets free arginine, as a prebiotic for caries prevention and care.[239,240,595] Arginine is hydrolyzed through the arginine-deiminase system found in several commensal species such as *S. sanguinis*, *S. gordonii*, *S. mitis*, and *Actinomyces* species, which results in the production of ammonia. Subsequently, this contributes to an increase in pH, which counteracts caries-associated environmental and microbiological changes that establish a low pH.[286] The use of toothpastes supplemented with 1.5% or 8% arginine has been shown to stimulate the ADS activity of commensal oral species and to result in beneficial oral microbiota shifts from a caries point of view, both in vitro and in vivo.[239,347,595] Furthermore, arginine has also been shown to destabilize single- or mixed-species oral biofilms and to stimulate H_2O_2 production by *S. gordonii*.[177,195,226] Given the sensitivity of periodontal pathogens to H_2O_2, this suggests that arginine could also be used in the prevention or treatment of periodontal diseases. Recently, nitrate was also suggested as a potential prebiotic substrate for oral health.[204,430] In vitro biofilms derived from salivary samples of healthy individuals grown in the presence of nitrate showed reduced lactate production, elevated ammonium and pH levels, increased abundances of health-associated oral genera and decreased abundances of periodontitis-, caries-, and halitosis-associated oral genera.[430] Another study reported decreased gingival inflammation in individuals following 2 weeks of nitrate-rich lettuce juice consumption.[204] However, the use of potential prebiotics should consider individual factors such as disease susceptibility and the specific composition of the commensal oral microbiota. For instance, individuals with an already highly proteolytic microbiome and elevated oral pH might not benefit from increased ammonium and pH levels caused by arginine or nitrate, as this has been shown to increase the abundance of certain periodontal disease-associated species such as *Porphyromonas* spp., *Prevotella* spp., and *Treponema* spp.[239,595] Altogether, research on prebiotics for oral health is rapidly evolving since this approach counters several of the limitations of the probiotic approach. Through specific modulation of the commensal oral microbiota, the chance of longer-lasting effects is higher with prebiotics. However, it also requires individually tailored strategies, as the commensal oral microbiota can show high inter- and intra-individual variability. Despite their promising potential, further in vitro and in vivo research is required before prebiotics could be widely used in the prevention and treatment of oral diseases.

Systemic Antibiotics

The most well-studied adjunct treatment to mechanical treatment to date is systemic antibiotics. Many studies have assessed the benefits of different antibiotic protocols in periodontal clinical parameters and in their ability to bring about changes in the biofilm composition.[57,115,119,121,123-125,156,330,472,494,516,518,530]

The majority of these studies evaluated patients with severe disease (stages III and IV generalized periodontitis). The few investigations that included patients with less advanced disease[82,155,364,397] did not report clear clinical and microbiological benefits from the adjunctive use of these agents. This is in line with the notion that scaling and root planing/root instrumentation alone is very effective to treat patients with mild to moderate periodontitis.[201] A recent systematic review[519] evaluated the clinical efficacy of all systemic antibiotics tested to date as adjuncts to mechanical periodontal treatment. Consistent clinically relevant and statistically significant benefits were observed for the combination of metronidazole plus amoxicillin, followed by metronidazole alone, and to a lesser extent azithromycin. A convincing body of evidence indicates that the clinical benefits obtained with the adjunctive use of metronidazole and amoxicillin, or with metronidazole are related to the efficacy of these agents in reducing specific periodontal pathogens and in shifting the subgingival microbial profile of periodontitis towards a healthy-associated composition, in systemically healthy adults and in young patients, as well as in subjects with type 2 diabetes and smokers.[57,115,119,121,123-125,156,330,472,494,516,518,530]

Fig. 10.31 depicts the changes occurring in the subgingival biofilm composition before and after mechanical treatment alone and with metronidazole or metronidazole and amoxicillin. An overall reduction in the proportions of pathogens and an increase in host-compatible complexes were observed in all treatment groups. But at 1-year post-treatment, subjects receiving adjunctive antibiotics harbored a more health-compatible biofilm composition. They had lower proportions of pathogens from the red and orange complexes than those receiving mechanical treatment. It is worth noting that subjects taking metronidazole plus amoxicillin had an additional benefit in comparison with the other two groups, including the group taking metronidazole alone which was higher proportions of the host-compatible *Actinomyces* spp. (see Fig. 10.31).

A few clinical studies have used sequencing techniques to assess changes in the microbiome with the use of metronidazole plus amoxicillin.[28,120,139,161,207,259,353] The studies varied substantially in terms of their methods, but in general they showed that treatments

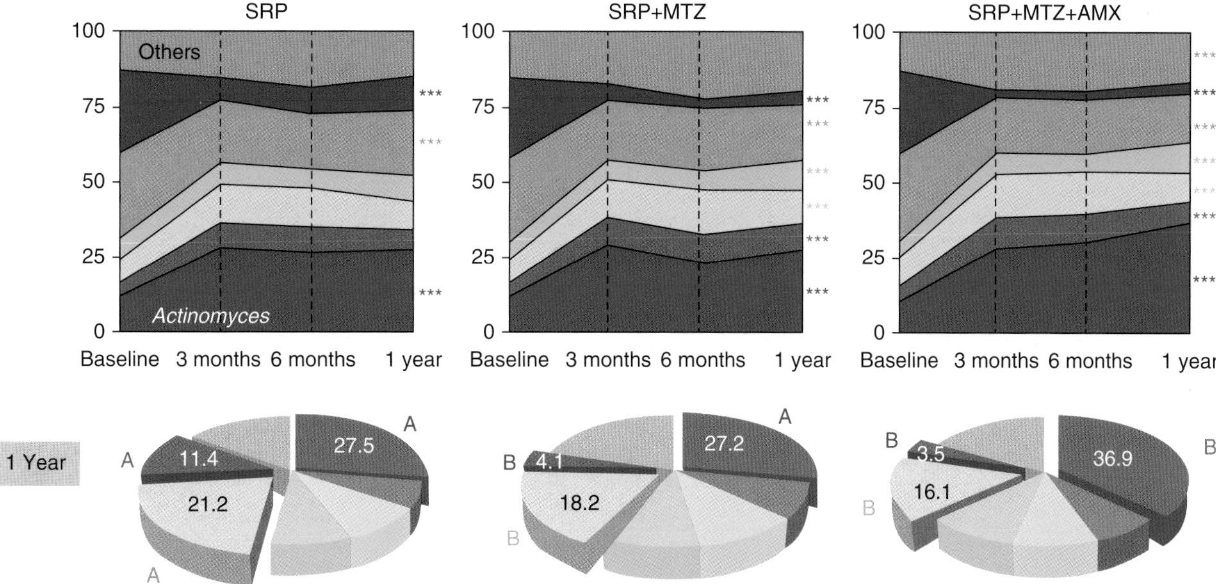

Fig. 10.31 Cumulative mean proportions of microbial complexes, as well as pie charts describing the mean proportion of microbial complexes at 1-year post-treatment in subgingival biofilm samples taken from subjects with advanced periodontitis treated with scaling and root planing (*SRP*), alone ($n = 55$), combined with 400 mg of metronidazole (three times daily for 14 days) *(SRP+MTZ)* ($n = 45$), or combined with 400 mg of metronidazole + 500 mg of amoxicillin (three times daily for 14 days) (*SRP+MTX+AMX*) ($n = 54$), at baseline and at 3 months, 6 months, and 1-year post-treatment. Nine subgingival biofilm samples were taken from each subject at each time point and were analyzed separately to determine their content of the 40 species of bacteria listed in Fig. 10.24. The percentage of DNA probe counts for each species was determined at each site, then averaged within a subject and then across subjects in each group at each time point. The mean proportion of each species was summed in order to determine the proportion of each complex. The colors represent the different complexes described by Socransky et al. (1963). The gray color ("Others") represents species that did not fall into any complex, and *Actinomyces* spp. are represented in blue. The significance of differences among time points was determined using repeated-measures analysis of variance (***$P < .001$). The significance of differences among groups at 1 year post-treatment was determined using one-way analysis of variance and Tukey's multiple comparison tests (different letters indicate significant differences between pairs of groups, $P < .05$). (Feres M, Figueiredo LC, Soares GMS, et al. Systemic antibiotics in the treatment of periodontitis. *Periodontol 2000.* 2015; 67[1]:131–186, First published: December 12, 2014. DOI:10.1111/prd.12075.)

including the adjuncts produced a more beneficial change in the subgingival microbiome.[120] Two randomized clinical trials and one clinical investigation have directly compared mechanical debridement alone or with adjunctive metronidazole plus amoxicillin and showed that several genera containing classical or newly identified pathogens, such as *Porphyromonas, Treponema, Tannerella, Synergistetes*, and *Filifactor*, were more affected by the treatment protocols including antibiotics than by scaling and root planing alone.[161,207,283] Conversely, antibiotics were more effective in fostering host-compatible species from the genera *Veillonella* and *Haemophilus*. These results provide a preliminary view of the effects of treatment in modulating the dysbiotic periodontal microbiome, but future clinical trials evaluating more patients for a longer period of time are necessary.

A series of ecological changes seem to be associated with the benefits in the subgingival microbiome brought about by metronidazole and amoxicillin. These include the effect of the antibiotics in reducing levels of key pathogens such as metronidazole on strict anaerobic pathogens and of metronidazole and amoxicillin on *A. actinomycetemcomitans*.[22,538,564] Antibiotics also benefit the biofilm on other oral surfaces, fluids, and tissues and the broad-spectrum amoxicillin potentiates the effect of scaling and root planing in reducing bacterial load in the subgingival space. These effects would allow the recolonization of recently scaled pockets by a new climax biofilm community more compatible with health. This new microbial community is difficult to disturb and enables the long-term clinical stability of the periodontium.[123,124,161,489,516]

Biofilm Modulation in Peri-implantitis

Treatment of peri-implant diseases is not a simple task and depends on a striking change in the microbial profile around the diseased dental implants, including a reduction in several pathogens associated with periodontitis.[379,467] The nonsurgical treatment of peri-implantitis does not seem very promising in controlling the disease, even in association with other adjunctive treatments.[113] Decontamination of dental implant surfaces by means of mechanical, chemical, and physical methods has been tested in various clinical trials.[526] The main target of all decontamination methods is primarily to decontaminate the implant surface and to remove the inflammatory peri-implant soft tissues.[218]

Because the microbial profile of peri-implantitis presents great similarity to that of periodontitis,[258,379] and adjunctive metronidazole and amoxicillin are very effective in changing the microbial profile of periodontitis towards health, this same effect would be expected in peri-implantitis. Nonetheless, the only two studies that evaluated the effects of these agents adjunctive to nonsurgical debridement did not show similar benefits in the treatment of severe peri-implantitis.[84,466] This lack of effectiveness may be due to mechanical difficulties in decontaminating the implant threads, mainly in deeper pockets. Thus, it could be hypothesized that effective treatment of peri-implantitis would require open flap debridement. Randomized clinical trials testing open flap debridement with other antibiotic protocols such as amoxicillin[51] or azithromycin[164] failed to show important advantages of the use of antibiotics. Although there is some clinical evidence that metronidazole and amoxicillin adjunct to open flap surgery would be an effective protocol to treat peri-implantitis[179] the effects of this treatment in changing the peri-implant biofilm composition have not been determined. Future randomized clinical trials should be designed with the aim of determining the effects of different treatments of peri-implantitis in modulating the submucosal microbiome towards **peri-implant health**.

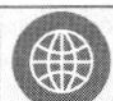
Case Scenarios are found on the companion website eBooks.Health.Elsevier.com.

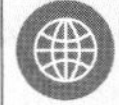
References for this chapter are found on the companion website eBooks.Health.Elsevier.com.

CHAPTER 11

Host-Microbe Interactions and the Inflammatory Response

Keith L. Kirkwood | Carlos Rossa Jr. | George Hajishengallis | Ann Decker | Yvonne L. Hernandez-Kapila

CHAPTER OUTLINE

Chapter Overview

The oral cavity is an important interface with the external environment, and thus is in constant interaction with a great number and variety of microorganisms, mostly organized in plaque biofilms. These microorganisms are required for the most prevalent diseases of the oral cavity: caries and periodontal disease. The periodontium is comprised of dynamic remodeling tissues, that are continuously challenged by bacterial biofilms colonizing proximal odontogenic and mucosal surfaces. Periodontal disease is currently thought to be driven by a dysbiotic microbiome,[87,176,233] in which the nature and dynamic status of host-microbial interactions ultimately dictate the onset and progression of tissue damage observed clinically and radiographically. Preclinical research in gnotobiotic animals demonstrate that microorganisms are fundamental for the occurrence of periodontal disease[201] and clinical observations and experimental studies support the rationale for antimicrobial (mechanical and chemical) therapy for the correction of the dysbiotic status and restoring health.[5,99]

Substantial experimental evidence supports the concept that host immune response is the primary mediator of periodontal tissue destruction.[13,52,129,227] Experimental periodontitis investigations in animal models deficient in specific immune cell subsets,[12,120] receptors,[23,31,108,123,185] and cytokines[4,66,206,250] have contributed to the delineation of the immuno-pathophysiology of periodontal disease. Clinical observations and studies in immunocompromised persons demonstrating increased susceptibility and greater severity of periodontal disease further underscores the significance of the host immune response to the oral bacterial challenge.[61,153]

Thus, comprehension of host-microbial interactions and inflammatory response provides insights into the mechanisms involved in periodontal tissue destruction. This chapter will focus on host aspects of the dysbiotic process associated with periodontal disease by a didactic progression from molecular aspects of early events in host-microbe interactions, the resulting inflammatory response, the cells and endogenous mediators elicited, the evolving dynamics of innate and adaptive immune response, the modulating influences of non-microbial host-associated external factors, and the current therapeutic perspectives derived from this knowledge. Lastly, evidence on the therapeutic potential of immunomodulatory interventions targeting host-microbe molecular interactions and inflammation in periodontitis are explored.

Host-Microbial Interactions

Microbial-Associated Molecular Patterns

The oral microbiome is a highly complex microbial community consisting of over 700 known bacterial species,[44] of which a relatively limited number is associated with periodontal disease. Current understanding of periodontal disease as a dysbiotic condition,[176] defined as a disequilibrium between host immune surveillance mechanisms and the microbial biofilm, supports a prominent role for the host response to the microbial biofilm in disease development. Clinical health is associated with tolerance mechanisms of the host response to microbial biofilm and vigilance mechanisms protecting against the shifts in microbial aggression, such as the increase in the quantity and prevalence of disease-associated microbial species (periodontopathogens). This clinically healthy/homeostatic status is due to the host's capability of discerning among commensal and pathogenic bacteria and proper modulation of the immune response. The prompt and timely direct recognition of microbial-associated molecular patterns (MAMPs) by host pattern-recognition receptors (PRRs) is rapid and critical in homeostasis and dysbiosis.[25,119,224]

MAMPs are evolutionary conserved molecular motifs present in microorganisms, which are not found in higher eukaryotes and that function as ligands having specificity for corresponding PRRs expressed by host cells.[25,119,224] Evidence indicates that periodontal disease is associated with quantitative and qualitative shifts in the microbiota of the oral biofilm that reflect an ecologic adaptation of the microorganisms to microenvironmental conditions,[107,142,150] but individual variability in the onset, rate of progression, and severity of disease-associated tissue destruction in humans has been demonstrated,[11,103,141] verifying the subjective clinical observations of lack of correspondence between microbial load (both in quantity and quality) and occurrence, the severity of periodontal disease, and indicating that there were determinants of disease still unknown. However, preclinical data have more formal evidence where specific antibiotics inhibited bone loss by causing changes in the microbiome without reducing the total microbial mass.[51] While the role of qualitative and quantitative shifts in the dental microbial biofilm in periodontitis remains debated,[39,233] there are distinct microbial signatures associated with periodontal health, gingivitis and periodontitis.[2] Since clinical periodontal health occurs in the presence of a relatively rich and diverse microbial biofilm and of a discrete inflammatory response,[242] this homeostatic condition involves tolerance mechanisms, which are, in part, mediated by MAMPs from commensals or health-associated microorganisms that can modulate the immune response (for a review on this subject, see Ref. 98). Thus, the interaction MAMPs-PRRs can also be involved in the homeostatic status.

Nevertheless, there is extensive literature on the association and role of specific microbial species in periodontal disease, particularly with gram-negative species,[217,231] of which *Porphyromonas gingivalis* is the most intensely studied and best characterized periodontopathogen, considered by some authors as a "keystone pathogen" in periodontitis,[85,88,93] which can elicit unique immune responses and induce a dysbiotic, disease-associated state.[146] To avoid redundancy with information provided in depth in other chapters (see Chapter 10), this subsection will briefly discuss aspects of MAMPs, using *P. gingivalis* as an example, that are important in modulating host-microbial interactions.

Given the predominance of gram-negative microorganisms in periodontitis-associated biofilm, lipopolysaccharide (LPS) is a major MAMP, which is usually only thought of as a Toll-like receptor (TLR) agonist eliciting a protective/inflammatory response. However, the molecular structure of LPS may differ among bacterial species, between serotypes of the same species or even according to microenvironmental conditions.[6] Lipid A (a constituent of bacterial LPS) may have agonistic or antagonistic effects on activation of PRRs.[193] The agonistic effect induces inflammation, which may lead to tissue destruction. The antagonistic effect may allow for evasion of the host immune response enhancing bacterial survival, proliferation, and invasion by dampening the host response. As a component of the bacterial cell wall, LPS may exert its stimulatory/inhibitory effects even after the microorganism is dead, but it may also be secreted by live bacteria in the form of vesicles.[80] Other parts or structural components of bacteria are recognized by different PRRs as MAMPs, including lipoteichoic acid (LTA), lipoprotein, flagellin, fimbriae proteins, peptidoglycans, and nucleic acids.[225] In addition to those MAMPs connected to bacteria, secretory molecules, such as short chain fatty acids, extracellular vesicles, extracellular polysaccharide, and cyclic dinucleotides (CDN) are recognized by distinct PRR.[58,59]

Other bacterial-secreted/expressed virulence factors, including enzymes (proteases and phosphatases) induce immunostimulatory post-translational modifications (e.g., citrullination). These factors directly degrade and inactivate host proteins, including inflammatory mediators,[97] complement factors[104] and T cell surface proteins.[127,143] The reader is referred to other chapters for in-depth information on microbial virulence factors (see Chapter 10).

Pattern-Recognition Receptors

The discovery of PRRs as the cellular sensors of MAMPs is one of the significant discoveries in immunology in the last three decades, which was acknowledged with a Nobel Prize in 2011. Since then, recognition of new PRRs, understanding of their ligand specificity, subcellular localization, signal transduction, and biological relevance has advanced the comprehension of immune response and particularly its role in tissue homeostasis and pathogenic mechanisms, providing insights into therapeutic strategies. As the receptors capable of recognizing MAMPs, PRRs were initially described related to innate immune cells (e.g., macrophages, dendritic cells [DCs]), inducing a cellular response that includes production of inflammatory mediators, such as pro- and anti-inflammatory cytokines, chemokines, and enzymes that catalyze the production of various second messengers and signaling molecules, which ultimately shape and modulate adaptive immunity. Consequently, PRRs were considered the bridge between innate and adaptive immunity.[32,192] Currently, functional PRRs are known to be expressed by "nonprofessional" immune cells (e.g., epithelial cells, fibroblasts, osteoblasts) that have a role in innate immunity, and also by adaptive immune cells (e.g., T and B cells), which blurs the didactic/theoretical boundaries between innate and adaptive immunity.[21,68,96,190,259]

PRRs include cell-associated, both membrane-bound (extracellular and intracellular) and cytosolic, as well as soluble or secreted molecules. TLRs are primarily membrane-bound, nucleotide-binding and oligomerization domain (NOD)-like receptors (from the family of nucleotide-binding domain and leucine-rich repeat containing receptors, NOD-like receptors [NLRs]) and retinoic acid-inducible gene I (RIG-I)-like receptors (RLRs) are primarily cytosolic/intracellular.

In this chapter, we will focus on the PRRs present in the periodontal microenvironment and the evidence for their relevance in host-microbial interactions in this context. There is evidence for an increase in the expression of various PRRs with the onset of periodontal disease,[54] which suggests the mobilization of the host response to the microbial challenge and supports their relevance in host-microbial interactions in periodontitis. RLRs are sensors of RNA and therefore mostly associated with response to RNA viruses. Their possible role in periodontal disease is not known. The two major families of PRRs most extensively studied in the periodontium are the TLRs and the NLRs (Table 11.1).[25,119,224] These are also the families of PRRs conserved from early invertebrates to mammals.[256] In addition to recognizing MAMPs, PRRs also

TABLE 11.1 Host Cell Pattern-Recognition Receptors Present in the Periodontal Microenvironment Cells and Microbial-Associated Molecular Patterns Ligands Present in Oral Biofilm Bacteria

PRRs[a]	Activating MAMPs	Periodontal Bacteria
TLR2	Lipoproteins	*P. gingivalis, T. forsythia, A. viscosus, T. denticola*
	Peptidoglycan	*A. naeslundii*
	Lipoproteins, Lipoteichoic acid, Peptidoglycan	*S. gordonii*
TLR4	LPS	*P. gingivalis, A. actinomycetemcomitans, F. nucleatum*
TLR9	CpG-DNA	*P. gingivalis, T. forsythia*
NOD1	iE-DAP	*P. gingivalis, A. actinomycetemcomitans, F. nucleatum*
NOD2	MDP	
NLRP3	LPS	*P. gingivalis*

[a]Most intensely studied PRRs in the context of periodontal disease. There is evidence for expression of all TLRs, except TLR10, in periodontal tissues.
MAMP, Microbial-associated molecular pattern; *PRR,* pattern-recognition receptor.

recognize immuno-stimulatory by-products derived from damaged host tissues, known as damage-associated molecular patterns (DAMPs).[25,119,224] While PRR recognition of MAMPs and DAMPs are both essential for the host immune defense and normal tissue remodeling, this chapter focuses on MAMPs studied in the context of dental biofilm bacteria.

Toll-Like Receptors

The TLR family currently consists of 10 known functional TLRs in humans,[118,173,137] of which TLR10 is the latest TLR discovered[34] and the only TLR family member that exhibits anti-inflammatory properties, albeit its ligands and biological functions are still not well understood.[100,174] TLR1 through TLR9 have been reported to be expressed in the periodontium, both in health and disease.[15] TLR family members are generally subdivided into two groups according to their localization at the plasma membrane (TLR1, TLR2, TLR4, TLR5, TLR6, TLR10), which sense various types of MAMPs, or at endosomal membranes (TLR3, TLR7, TLR8, TLR9), which sense primarily microbial nucleic acids.[118] Notably, TLR4 is unique in that it has the ability to localize to both the plasma membrane and endosomal membrane.[118,173] Plasma membrane TLR signaling induces the expression of pro-inflammatory cytokines, whereas endosomal TLR signaling predominantly induces the expression of type I interferons.[119,224]

TLRs localized to the plasma membrane recognize extracellular microbial cell wall components (TLR1, TLR2, TLR4, TLR6) or flagellin (TLR5), while TLRs localized to the endolysosomal membrane recognize microbial nucleic acids (TLR3, TLR7, TLR8, TLR9).

This chapter will focus on MAMP ligand recognition at TLR2, TLR4, and TLR9, since these TLR family members have been studied most extensively in the context of sensing periopathogenic bacteria (see Table 11.1). TLR2 and TLR4 will be discussed in the context of recognizing extracellular bacterial cell wall components at the cell surface, and TLR9 will be addressed regarding recognizing bacterial nucleic acids within endosomes (Fig. 11.1).

The TLRs are single-pass transmembrane proteins (see Fig. 11.1) characterized by an N-terminal leucine-rich recognition domain and an intracellular C-terminal Toll/interleukin (IL)-1 receptor signaling domain (TIR). Upon MAMP ligand recognition at the N-terminal domain and subsequent formation of a sustainable homodimer/heterodimer, TIR domains of TLRs act as a scaffold to recruit various TIR domain-containing adaptor proteins, such as myeloid differentiation primary-response protein 88 (MYD88) and MYD88-adaptor-like protein (MAL), or TIR domain-containing adaptor protein inducing IFNβ (TRIF) and TRIF-related adaptor molecule (TRAM).[119,224] With the exception of TLR3, all TLRs engage the MyD88 adaptor protein. TLR3 and endosomal-TLR4 uniquely interact with the TRIF adapter protein.[119,224] Engagement of the adaptor proteins at the TIR domain of TLRs initiates signal transduction (see Fig. 11.1) that involves interactions between the adaptor molecules, IL-1R-associated kinases (IRAKs), and tumor necrosis factor (TNF) receptor-associated factors (TRAFs). In the case of TLR2 and TLR4 localized to the plasma membrane, MyD88-dependent downstream activation of TGF-β-activated kinase 1 (TAK-1) simultaneously induces mitogen-activated protein kinase (MAPK) and nuclear factor-κB (NF-κB) signaling. NF-κB translocates to the nucleus, and MAPK cascades activate activator protein 1 (AP-1), ultimately resulting in the expression of pro-inflammatory cytokine genes. Regarding TLR4 translocated to endosomes, TRIF-dependent signaling leads to the activation of NF-κB and IFN-regulatory factor (IRF)-3, resulting in the expression of pro-inflammatory cytokine and type I IFN genes. Concerning TLR9 localized to the endolysosomal membrane, MyD88-dependent signaling leads to the activation of IRF-7, which upregulates the expression of type I IFN genes.[119,224] The notable crosstalk of the TLR signaling pathways (see Fig. 11.1) highlights the potential for synergy/amplification effects modulating the host immune response.

TLR4—Lipopolysaccharide Recognition

Knowledge of the molecular architecture of gram-positive versus gram-negative bacterial cell walls is central to conceptually understanding MAMP recognition by the host. Oral bacteria interactions with host TLRs are largely dependent on the exposed macromolecules making up the outer membrane of bacterial cell walls. Whereas LPS is unique to the outer membrane of gram-negative bacteria, LTA and peptidoglycan are distinct to the outer membrane of gram-positive bacteria. Importantly, lipoproteins are common constituents of the outer membranes of both gram-negative and gram-positive bacteria.[192]

LPS is the major macromolecule composing the outer surface envelope of gram-negative bacteria, critical to the bacterium for maintaining structural integrity, selective permeability, and proper folding and insertion of outer membrane proteins. LPS is typically made up of three domains (lipid A, a short core oligosaccharide, and an O-antigen), and induces a host immune response through recognition of lipid A.[164,191] Mammalian cells recognize LPS through a TLR4 homodimer protein complex consisting of TLR4, the co-receptor myeloid differentiation factor 2 (MD2), and accessory proteins CD14 and LPS-binding protein (LBP) (see Fig. 11.1). LBP processes and delivers LPS to CD14, which sensitizes cells for LPS binding by the MD2-TLR4 receptor.[118,173]

TLR2—Lipoproteins/Lipoteichoic Acid/Peptidoglycan Recognition

Unlike the TLR4 homodimer protein complex, which is specific for LPS, TLR2 has the capacity to recognize diverse microbial macromolecules due to forming heterodimer protein complexes with other TLR family members (TLR1, TLR6, and TLR10).[118,173] TLR2 ligands highly relevant to oral flora interactions with host cells include lipoproteins, LTA, and peptidoglycan (see Table 11.1).

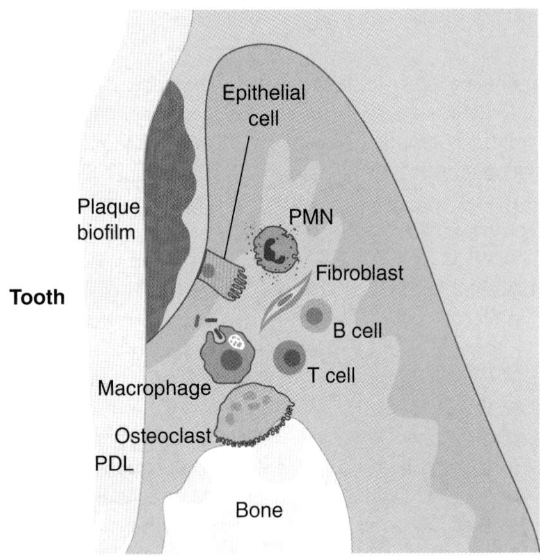

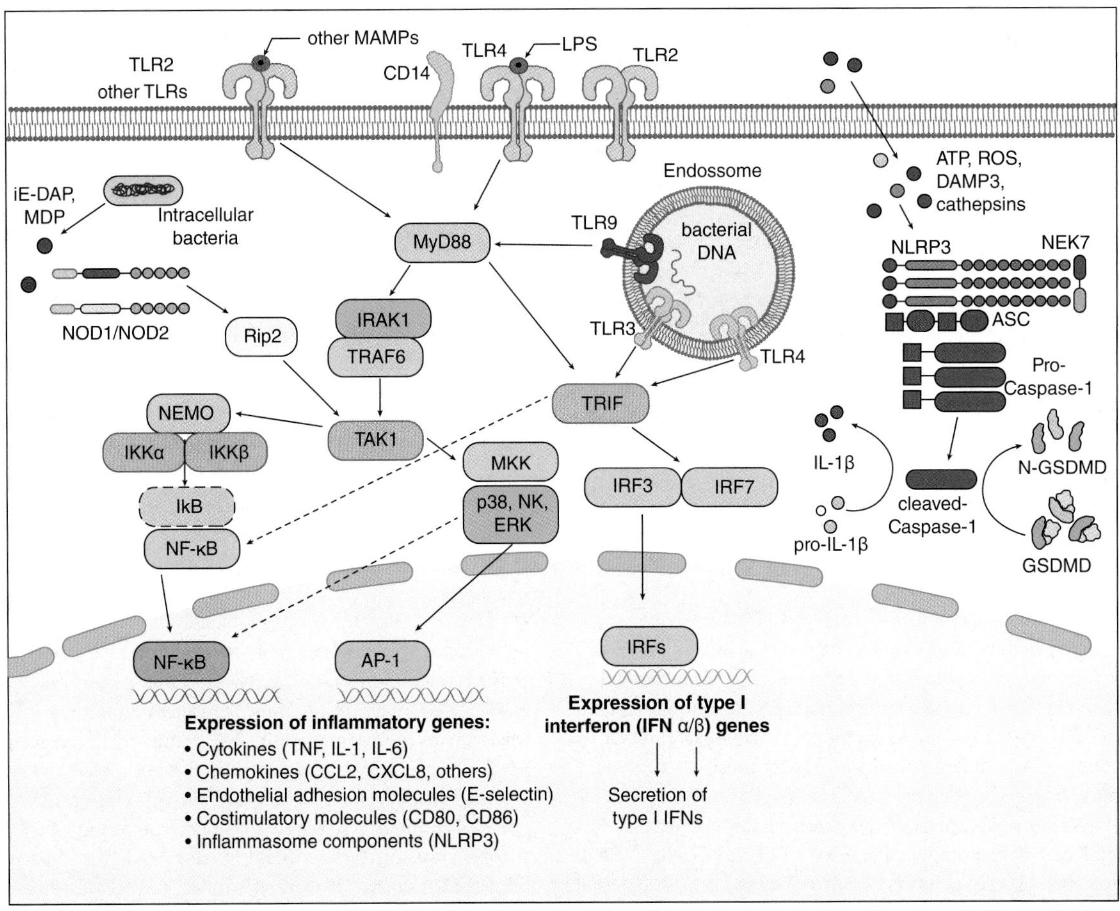

Fig. 11.1 Multiple pattern-recognition receptors *(PRR)* involved in host-microbial interactions in the periodontium. Overview of PRRs involved in recognition and response to microbial-associated molecular patterns *(MAMPs)*. As discussed in the text, these PRRs may be expressed by various cell types, both immune and non-immune resident cells. Membrane-bound Toll-like receptors *(TLRs)* (plasma membrane and endosomes) are sensors of MAMPs and may form homo- and heterodimers. Ligand binding to these PRRs triggers a signal transduction cascade that involves recruitment of various adaptor proteins and kinases. MyD88 is an adaptor protein required for signaling by all TLRs, except TLR3 that signals via TRIF. Intracellular (endosome) TLR4 may also signal in an MyD88-independent manner via TRIF. Downstream of MyD88, common upstream signaling intermediates will be activated (IRAK/TRAF6 and TAK1), which can ultimately activate NF-κβ and MAP kinases inducing expression of pro-inflammatory mediators alongside with expression of inflammasome proteins (first inflammasome-activating signal). TLR9 also signals through MyD88 but activate interferon-regulatory factors, which are the usual downstream effectors of TRIF. NOD1/NOD2 are cytosolic PRRs that recognize peptidoglycan fragments of the bacterial cell wall and can also activate NF-κB and MAPK, signaling via Rip2. NLRP3 inflammasome activation can be induced by various ligands (DAMPs, ROS, ATP) and results in the assembly of a multi-protein complex, including oligomerization of NLRP3, ASC, and pro-Caspase-1 proteins. Autoproteolytic cleavage of oligomerized pro-caspase-1 results in activated (cleaved) caspase-1, which will cleave IL-1β and IL-18 into their biologically active forms and also cleave gasdermin-D, forming pores on the cellular membrane causing death by pyroptosis and allowing the secretion of active IL-1β. *ERK,* Extracellular signal-regulated kinase; *PDL,* periodontal ligament; *PMN,* periodontal ligament; *MDP,* muramyl dipeptide

Lipoproteins, ubiquitously expressed in the outer cell membranes of all bacteria, are anchored to the bacterial cell membrane by lipid chains covalently attached to conserved N-terminal cysteines.[192] Triacylated lipoproteins commonly expressed by gram-negative bacteria are recognized by TLR2/TLR1 heterodimer complexes, whereas diacylated lipoproteins primarily expressed by gram-positive bacteria or mycoplasmas are recognized by TLR2/TLR6 heterodimer complexes.[118,173] Unique to the outer membranes of gram-positive bacteria, LTA and peptidoglycan are recognized by incompletely characterized TLR2/TLR6 heterodimer complexes.[118] Although not as well understood as LPS-TLR4 signaling, differences in extracellular accessory/co-receptor proteins (CD14, CD36) and intracellular adaptor proteins associated with TLR2/TLR1 versus TLR2/TLR6 signal transduction appear to critically regulate TLR2-mediated host immune response mechanisms.[118,173] More recently, there is evidence indicating that TLR2 can form a heterodimer with TLR10 which inhibits pro-inflammatory cytokines[175] by blocking MyD88-dependent and independent signaling, including inhibition of activation of NF-κB, MAPK, and PI3K/Akt signaling.[100,174] This inhibitory heterodimer may be elicited in response to various MAMPs that also activate TLR2 homodimers, TLR2/TLR1 and TLR2/TLR4 heterodimers, such as LPS and diacylated lipopeptides (as well as the synthetic ligand Pam3Cys).[174,236] As TLR10 is expressed in the periodontium and this expression is increased in periodontitis,[15] it may have a role in modulating signaling by TLR2-engaging MAMPs from *P. gingivalis*.

TLR9—CpG DNA Recognition

Whilst TLR2 and TLR4 are localized to the plasma membrane to engage cell surface MAMPs, TLR9 recognizes MAMPs in cytoplasmic endosomes (see Fig. 11.1). TLR9 is the endosomal TLR family member which has been studied most extensively regarding the recognition of intracellular microbial nucleic acids. During infection, microbe-derived nucleic acids are sensed by endosomal TLRs, which facilitates mounting a host immune response to clear the invading microorganisms. While TLR9 recognizes both viral and bacterial CpG-DNA,[119,224] periodontal research has focused on TLR9 due to CpG motifs being abundant in bacterial DNA (see Table 11.1). CpG-DNA localized within lysosomal compartments induces the trafficking of TLR9 from the endoplasmic reticulum to the endosome, which activates TLR9 signal transduction.[119,224]

Role of Toll-Like Receptors in Periodontitis

TLRs are expressed in the periodontium in health, and notably have been reported to be expressed at much higher levels in severe periodontal disease tissues.[15] Both commensal and pathogenic periodontal bacteria stimulate TLR2 signaling,[121,249] which points to the significance of vigilance and tolerance mechanisms in the host immune defense regulation of the colonizing oral microbiota. The fact that lipoproteins derived from gram-positive versus gram-negative bacteria are differentially recognized by TLR2/TLR6 versus TLR2/TLR1 heterodimer complexes,[118,173] highlights the complexity of a single TLR receptor in the modulation of the host immune defense response. Considering that the resident periodontal flora shifts from a predominantly gram-positive microbiota in health, to a predominantly gram-negative microbiota in periodontal disease states, gram-negative periopathogenic bacteria-induced periodontal destruction could be mediated through differential TLR2 signal transduction associated with increased activation of TLR2/TLR1 versus TLR2/TLR6 heterodimer complexes.

Current comprehension of TLR signaling suggests that gram-negative periopathogenic bacterial-induced catabolic actions are due to differential signaling at the TLR2 receptor, as well as the concomitant activation of TLR4 receptor by LPS.[121,171] *P. gingivalis* has been most extensively investigated in its ability to stimulate TLR signal transduction through various MAMPs. Early investigations assessing *P. gingivalis* LPS-induced upregulation of pro-inflammatory cytokine expression in various human and murine cells were controversial as to whether the actions of LPS were mediated through TLR2-versus TLR4-dependent recognition. Understanding that LPS recognition is specific to the lipid A domain, definitive evidence that *P. gingivalis* LPS only activates TLR4 was elucidated through chemically synthesized *P. gingivalis* lipid A analogues which activated TLR4, not TLR2.[130,207,258] Research demonstrating that a *P. gingivalis*-derived lipoprotein that specifically activates TLR2, can be co-isolated with LPS,[171] implies that early contradictory reports concerning *P. gingivalis* LPS recognition at TLR2 versus TLR4 were due to lipoprotein contamination. Highlighting the importance of periopathogenic bacteria-induced activation of concomitant TLR receptors in periodontal tissue destruction, studies employing TLR2 or TLR4 knockout mice have shown that *P. gingivalis* co-activation of TLR2 and TLR4 is critical in stimulating host immune response mechanisms driving alveolar bone loss.[23] Recently, a preclinical study showed that blocking TLR4 with a systemically administered biochemical compound that disrupts interaction of the cytoplasmic portion of TLR4 with adaptor molecules reduced both the production of inflammatory cytokines and alveolar bone resorption-associated experimental periodontitis,[247] supporting the potential for a therapeutic application of TLR modulators.

Relative to TLR2 and TLR4, investigations delineating the role of TLR9 in the pathogenesis of periodontal disease have been scarce to date. Similar to TLR2 and TLR4, TLR9 expression has been reported to be upregulated in clinical periodontitis tissues when compared to gingivitis tissues[114] and healthy gingival biopsies.[199] Notably, an experimental periodontitis investigation assessing *P. gingivalis* challenged TLR9 deficient mice provides evidence indicating that TLR9 contributes to periodontal bone loss.[123] TLR9 knockout versus wild-type mice were resistant to *P. gingivalis*-induced alveolar bone loss, which correlated with lower levels of IL-6, TNF, and receptor activator of nuclear factor kappa B ligand (RANKL) in the gingival tissues of knockout mice. Ex vivo studies performed in the aforementioned report, demonstrating that TLR2 or TLR4 agonist challenge resulted in significantly lower cytokine production in TLR9 knockout versus wild-type cells, highlight the possibility of TLR9 crosstalk with TLR2 and TLR4 signaling in periodontal pathogenesis.[123]

NOD-Like Receptors

There are currently 23 family members which comprise the intracellularly expressed NLRs in humans.[25,43] NLRs are localized to the cytosol and play a critical role in sensing invading microorganisms and prompting the immune response. NLRs are characterized by C-terminal leucine-rich repeats that act as a sensing domain, a central nucleotide-binding and oligomerization domain (i.e., a NOD), and an N-terminal effector domain which mediates downstream signaling.[27,43] This effector N-terminal domain is variable and classifies the subfamilies of NLRs: NLRAs which have an acidic activation domain, NLRBs with a baculovirus inhibitor of apoptosis repeat (BIR)-like domain, NLRCs that feature a caspase activation and recruitment domain (CARD) or a Death domain (DD), and the NLRP subfamily presenting a PYRIN domain.[43,229] The most studied NLRs in the context of periodontal disease are those of the NLRC and NLRP subfamilies.

NOD1/NOD2 (NLRC Subfamily)—Peptidoglycan Recognition

Originally detected in epithelial cells, NOD1 (or NLRC1) is expressed preferentially by mucosal/skin-homing innate immune cells, whereas

NOD2 (or NLRC2) expression is comparable in epithelial, other non-immune and immune cells.[43] NOD1 recognizes g-D-glutamyl-meso-diaminopimelic acid (iE-DAP), a component of peptidoglycan present in most gram-negative and some gram-positive bacteria, whereas NOD2 recognizes muramyl dipeptide (MDP), which is found in peptidoglycan from all gram-negative and gram-positive bacteria.[3,224] As most NLRs, NOD1 and NOD2 remain in an auto-inhibitory state in the cytoplasm and until engagement with their ligands. Peptidoglycan binding to NOD1 and NOD2 receptors cause their binding to early endosomes and oligomerization, which results in recruitment of a serine/threonine kinase adaptor protein, RIP-2/RICK, to a caspase activation and recruitment domain (CARD, one domain in NOD1 and two domains in NOD2) at the effector N-terminal domain. RIP-2/RICK recruitment at the N-terminus activates NF-κB and MAPK dependent upregulation of pro-inflammatory cytokine genes (see Fig. 11.1).[3,224] The outcome of NOD activation may influence both innate and adaptive by inducing the expression of inflammatory mediators (cytokines, chemokines, matrix metalloproteinases [MMPs]), increasing expression of MHC II complexes by antigen-presenting cells, inducing the production of antimicrobial peptides and modulating cellular processes (e.g., migration, chemotaxis) in antigen-presenting cells.[83] More recently, their expression has been detected in T and B cells and there is evidence suggesting a direct role for NOD receptors in these adaptive immune cells.[116,181,213,253]

NLRP3 Inflammasome (NLRP Subfamily)—Activation by MAMPs and DAMPs

Inflammasomes are multi-protein complexes that recognize diverse inflammation-inducing stimuli, including exogenous MAMPs and endogenous DAMPs, to control the production of pro-inflammatory cytokines and regulate pyroptosis (an inflammatory form of cell death).[81,221] NLRP3 is mostly expressed in immune cells, particularly macrophages, but also in epithelial cells. Its activation is a two-step process: a priming signal (which may be an MAMP signaling through other PRRs such as LPS/TLR or MDP/NOD) that induces expression of inflammasome components including NLRP3 itself, and a second activating signal. Diverse molecules have been described as NLRP3 activating signal, including DAMPs and compounds associated with cell perturbation (ATP release, potassium efflux, ROS, cathepsins).[261] Several cytoplasmic PRRs can assemble into an inflammasome complex. The NLR proteins represent the "core" of the multi-protein inflammasome complex, which is named after the central NLR protein. NLRP3, the most extensively investigated inflammasome complex has a critical role in the terminal processing and biological activity of the pro-inflammatory cytokines IL-1β and IL-18.[81,221]

Recognition of cytosolic MAMPs and DAMPs initiates NLRP3 activation, which requires interaction with NEK7 (a serine-threonine kinase) and subsequent conformational change of NLRP3, permitting NACHT domain-mediated oligomerization. This allows recruitment of an adaptor protein (apoptosis-associated speck-like protein containing a CARD—ASC) to the PYRIN domain of NLRP3, and ASC further forms polymers that engages pro-caspase-1 (which has a caspase activation and recruitment domain—CARD), via homotypic binding of CARD domains. Oligomerization of pro-Caspase-1 proteins in the inflammasome leads to their autoproteolytic cleavage into active Caspase-1. Activated Caspase-1 is the biological effector in canonical inflammasome activation, including cleavage of pro-IL-1β and pro-IL-18 into their biologically active forms.[81,221,261]

Role of NLRs in Periodontitis

Clinical investigations of NOD1 and NOD2 receptor expression in oral tissue biopsies and isolated cultured cells have demonstrated that both NOD1 and NOD2 are expressed in human oral epithelium,[223] gingival fibroblast cells,[139,226] and periodontal ligament fibroblast cells.[139,226] Interestingly, there are no reports showing that periodontal disease states alter NOD1 or NOD2 expression levels in the human periodontium.

Experimental periodontitis investigations in NLR-deficient mice have provided limited insight into the critical role of NOD1 and NOD2 in periodontal pathogenesis. While it must be recognized that study methodologies were not consistent across investigations, intriguingly there has been no consistency in reported study outcomes. The initial experimental periodontitis investigation employing the NOD1 and NOD2 knockout mouse models, which induced periodontitis via applying ligatures, found that mice deficient in NOD2 showed comparable levels of alveolar bone resorption, whereas mice deficient in NOD1 demonstrated reduced levels of alveolar bone loss when compared to wild-type control mice.[108] Corresponding with the blunted alveolar bone loss findings, NOD1 knockout mice had fewer osteoclasts and lower pro-inflammatory cytokine expression levels in gingival tissue isolates.[108] A subsequent experimental periodontitis investigation in the NOD1 knockout mouse model, which induced periodontitis via intra-gingival injection of heat-killed gram-negative/-positive bacteria, reported contradictory findings.[31] NOD1 knockout mice had exacerbated alveolar bone loss, increased osteoclast numbers, and upregulated pro-inflammatory cytokine expression levels in cultured bone marrow macrophages.[31] In light of the aforementioned conflicting study outcomes concerning NOD1, other experimental periodontitis reports showing that *P. gingivalis* inoculation induced less alveolar bone loss in NOD2 knockout vs. wild-type mice,[185] a finding confirmed in a gram-negative periopathogenic experimental periodontitis model,[220] but currently the role of NOD1 and NOD2 on periodontal inflammation and alveolar bone loss is unclear.

While ongoing research is indicated to delineate whether NOD1 and NOD2 receptor signaling is required for periodontitis-associated tissue destruction, investigations highlighting the crosstalk between NOD1/2 and TLR receptor signaling provide insight into the role of NOD1/2 in the pathogenesis of periodontitis. Considering the complexity of the oral microbiome and the diversity of MAMPs, simultaneous activation of various TLRs and NOD1/2 commonly converge at the MAPK and NF-κβ signaling pathways, which can result in downstream synergistic or "amplifying" effects that possibly enhance the host response. A seminal report demonstrating NOD1/2 activation has synergistic effects with TLR signaling to enhance the production of pro-inflammatory cytokines in cultured human periodontal ligament fibroblast (IL-1β, IL-6, IL-8)[226] and provides early evidence that periopathogenic biofilms may induce a destructive host immune response via concomitant activation of diverse PRRs.

Considering NLR family inflammasome complexes, studies relative to periodontitis have predominantly focused on NLRP3.[215] Expression of NLRP3 is increased in diseased periodontal tissues,[19,33,177,243] and in vitro gram-negative periopathogens have been shown to induce NLRP3 expression in fibroblasts, monocytes/macrophages, osteoblasts, and epithelial cells.[20,112,124,214,260] There are ambiguous reports regarding the induction or inhibition of NLRP3 by *P. gingivalis* in cells of the periodontal microenvironment, which may be due to differences in experimental conditions such as cell type, microenvironmental conditions (e.g., hypoxia), or presence of other bacterial species/MAMPs.[16,33,248] There is also conflicting information from in vivo preclinical studies using diverse experimental periodontitis models in genetically modified mice lacking the central NLRP3 protein: attenuated inflammation and alveolar bone resorption[244] or no significant difference.[197] Recently, alveolar bone resorption and inflammation was reduced in NLRP3 knockout mice, with these data confirmed using a biochemical inhibitor of NLRP3.[32] The positive correlation between NLRP3 levels with the IL-1β and IL-18 expression levels in periodontally diseased versus healthy tissues and most in vitro and preclinical studies support a role for the NLRP3 inflammasome in the pathogenesis of periodontitis.[135]

Antimicrobial Peptides

Antimicrobial peptides are components of the innate immune response in eukaryotes, providing defense against a wide spectrum of gram-positive and gram-negative bacteria, viruses, and fungi.[216,240,254] In the oral cavity, at least 45 different antimicrobial peptides belonging to different biochemical classes are found in the saliva and the gingival crevicular fluid (GCF).[72,73] The discussion of antimicrobial peptides in this chapter will focus on defensins and the cathelicidin LL-37, in order to highlight another molecular variable impacting PRR signaling and the periodontal host immune response.

Defensins and Cathelicidin LL-37

Defensins and cathelicidin LL-37, the most studied antimicrobial peptides,[79,110] are cationic peptides that bind to negatively charged molecules on the microbial cell surface (e.g., LPS in gram-negative bacteria and LTA in gram-positive bacteria), which ultimately depolarize and permeabilize the cell membrane resulting in bacterial cell death. In addition to their primary antimicrobial function, defensins are modulated by immune response mediators and also present immunomodulatory functions of their own.[128,211]

Defensins can be classified into α-defensins and β-defensins, based on structural distinctions in the connecting patterns of three disulfide bonds and in the spacing of cysteine residues.[110] Six human α-defensins and four human β-defensins have been extensively characterized. α-defensins 1–4, known as human neutrophil peptides due to their expression in neutrophils, are present in the oral cavity, while α-defensins 5–6 are localized to the mucosal Paneth cells of the small intestine. β-defensins 1–4, which are produced by a variety of epithelial cells throughout the body are abundantly produced by epithelial tissues within the oral cavity,[41,42] and found in the GCF and saliva.[41,42,79,203] Cathelicidin LL-37 is another important human defense peptide residing in neutrophils, which can be found in the gingival epithelium.[79]

Role of Antimicrobial Peptides in Periodontitis

In the periodontium the expression of β-defensins 1, 2, and 3 is observed at the mRNA level, both in clinically healthy and diseased tissues; the expression of these epithelium-derived peptides appears to be correlated with periodontal health, thereby suggesting a protective role.[18,22,235] Specific β-defensins are located in different anatomic regions of the periodontal epithelium: β-defensins 1 and 2 are observed in the upper layers of the gingival and sulcular epithelium, adjacent to the microbial biofilm and external environment, which is consistent with the innate immune "barrier" function of the epithelium. Interestingly, neither β-defensin 1 nor 2 are found in the junctional epithelium. Protection in the junctional epithelium may be provided by the higher concentration of α-defensins and LL-37 produced by granulocytes migrating toward the gingival sulcus.[41,42,152]

While the role of defensins and LL-37 in periodontal disease is currently not well understood, the expression of neutrophil-derived α-defensins 1–3 and LL-37 has been reported to be significantly elevated in the GCF of patients with chronic periodontitis.[186,232] The expression of defensins induced by whole periodontal pathogenic bacteria such as *F. nucleatum*, *P. gingivalis*, *A. actinomycetemcomitans*, and *T. denticola* is largely dependent on TLR signaling which reinforces the complexity of host-microbe interactions and the periodontal immune defense.[79,106,182,234]

Inflammatory Response in the Periodontium

Cells and Soluble Mediators of Inflammation

One rare consensus in the periodontal literature is that inflammation is a hallmark of periodontal diseases, with bleeding on gentle probing considered an objective clinical sign of inflammation and disease activity. Inflammation is a process elicited by the immune system. The immune system comprises both cells and soluble molecules that collectively defend the organism from foreign substances of both infectious and non-infectious origin. While innate immune cells were formerly perceived to have been derived solely from the hematopoietic lineage, MAMP-PRR recognition at epithelial cells and other stromal cells revealed that hematopoietic, epithelial, and mesenchymal cells are central to innate immune defense mechanisms regulating colonizing/invading microorganisms. More recently, the realization that MAMPs can be directly recognized by PRRs expressed by adaptive immune cells (i.e., not requiring innate immune cell processing/priming) provided insight demonstrating that the innate and adaptive immune systems act more as a continuum than as separate entities. This is particularly true for chronic inflammatory conditions, such as periodontitis, in which MAMPs are continuously present in the microenvironment alongside with "professional" (myeloid), "non-professional" (mesenchymal, epithelial) innate immune cells, and adaptive (lymphoid) immune cells. Relevant cells participating in the host-microbial interactions in the periodontal microenvironment are listed in Table 11.1. In the complex periodontal microenvironment, there is a multitude of stimuli from both microbial and endogenous origins that may elicit a response from the various cells in an autocrine and paracrine manner. Interestingly endocrine dissemination of these locally produced inflammatory mediators ("metastatic inflammation") is considered one possible biological mechanism for the systemic influences of periodontal disease (see Chapter 26).

Initiation and progression of periodontal tissue destruction (non-mineralized and mineralized) are largely caused by these host-derived inflammatory mediators (Table 11.2).[76] In general, production of these inflammatory mediators is strictly regulated at multiple levels (transcriptional, translational, and post-translational) and by various mechanisms (epigenetic mechanisms, transcriptional activators/repressors, miRNAs, mRNA stability, post-translational processing enzymes). The balance in production of a pro-inflammatory mediator (e.g., IL-1β, MMP, IL-12, RANKL) is usually accompanied by the production of its antagonist/anti-inflammatory counterpart (e.g., IL-1ra, TIMP, IL-10, or OPG). Imbalance in these systems, either by excessive/prolonged production of pro-inflammatory mediators or by reduced production of antagonists/anti-inflammatory mediators, results in autoimmune disease. In periodontitis, the continuous presence of microorganisms (mostly arranged in a biofilm located outside/externally to the periodontal tissues) both overwhelms and stimulates primary local innate immune defenses, generating this periodontal unbalance (Fig. 11.2).

Over the past four decades, multiple studies (in vitro, preclinical, and clinical) have contributed to the understanding of host response and host-microbial interactions in periodontal disease, usually by focusing on the specific relevance/contribution of a single inflammatory (or anti-inflammatory) mediator, PRR or cell type/cell phenotype at a time (for comprehensive reviews, please

TABLE 11.2 Cells Involved in Host-Microbial Interactions in the Periodontal Microenvironment

Cells/Markers	Phenotypes	Inflammatory Mediators[a]	Notes
Epithelial cells E-cadherin+, cytokeratin+	N/A	IL-1β, IL-6, IL-8, G-CSF, GM-CSF, β-defensin-2, MMPs-3/9/13, MIP-1α	First mechanical/biological innate immune barrier in the periodontal tissues, respond to multiple external signals
Dendritic cells CD11c+, CD14+	Activated	IFN-α, IL-1β, IL-6, IL-8, IL-12, IL-23, TNF-α, GM-CSF, CXCL1, NO	There are various subtypes of dendritic cells, myeloid and resident (Langerhans) dendritic cells have the primarily role in antigen-presentation (via MHC-II and cross-presentation via MHC-I) and activation of adaptive immunity in periodontal tissues. May transdifferentiate into osteoclasts.
	Tolerogenic	IL-10, IL-37, VEGF, TGFβ	
Endothelial cells CD31+, CD309 (VEGFR2)+	N/A	IL-6, IL-8, GM-CSF, ICAM-1	These cells have a primary role in angiogenesis and vascular permeability and control immune cell trafficking in inflammation and repair
Gingival fibroblasts FSP1, Col1a1+, fibronectin+	N/A	IL-1β, IL-6, IL-8, TNF-α, PGE_2, MCP-1, MMP-2	Most abundant resident stromal cells in healthy gingival connective tissues, participate in innate recognition of microorganisms Periodontal ligament cells are heterogenous in their stem-like properties, capable of differentiating into mineralized tissue-producing cells
PDL fibroblasts FSP1, Col1a1^{high}, fibronectin^{high}	N/A	IL-1β, IL-6, IL-8, MMP-1/-2/-3/-13, RANKL, TGFβ	
Cementocyte Cementum-derived attachment protein (CAP), cementum protein 1 (CEMP1) ?	N/A	OPN, OCN, RANKL, IL-1β, IL-6	These cells express functional PRRs and produce inflammatory mediators that stimulate other immune cells. Similarly to osteocytes, may support osteoclastic resorption of dental root and alveolar bone
Macrophages CD11b+, CD68+	M1 CD80+, CD86+, MHC-II^{high}	IL-1β, IL-6, IL-12, TNF-α, MMP-1/-9 NO	Highly responsive to external signals, transit between phenotypical extremes and participate in host response to microorganisms by phagocytosing, microbial killing, and antigen presentation via MHC-II
	M2 CD163+, CD206+, MHC-II^{low}	IL-1ra, IL-10, VEGF, TGFβ	
Osteoblasts Osteopontin, RUNX2, Osterix, Osteocalcin	N/A	IL-1β, IL-6, TNF-α, RANKL, PGE_2, NO, MMP-2/-9, OPG	Stromal cells that participate in innate immunity via PRRs and produce inflammatory mediators that stimulate other cells. Can support osteoclastic bone resorption.
Osteocytes Sclerostin, DMP-1, FGF-23	N/A	IL-1β, IL-6, TNF-α, RANKL, OPG, Sclerostin	Most abundant cell type in bone, these cells have an important influence on alveolar bone resorption as a major source of RANKL in the periodontal microenvironment, also produce mediators that regulate osteoblast activity. Recent studies demonstrate that these cells also respond to MAMPs.
Osteoclasts RANK+, TRAP+, Cathepsin K+	N/A	MMP-9, IL-1β, IL-6, TNF-α, IL-10, TGFβ	Derived from erythro-myeloid precursors that also differentiate into monocytes. Directly responsible for bone-resorption, can differentiate in response to the gradient of RANKL/OPG. Can also have activating (antigen-presentation via MHC-II and cross-presentation via MHC-I) and suppressive (efferocytosis, secretion of tolerogenic cytokines) immune functions
Neutrophils CD15+	N1 CD11b+CD16^{bright}CD62L^{bright}	TNF-α, ROS, IL-1β, IL-6, IL-8, NET, LL-37, MMP-8/-9, MPO, RANKL	These are the prototypical innate immune cells, primarily involved in phagocytosing/microbial killing, but may also assume different phenotypes in response to cues from the microenvironment and participate in repair processes
	N2 (tolerogenic/suppressive) CD11b+CD16^{bright}CD62L^{dim}	Arginase, CCL2, CCL5, TGFβ, IL-10, MMP-9, TIMP-1	

TABLE 11.2 Cells Involved in Host-Microbial Interactions in the Periodontal Microenvironment—cont'd

Cells/Markers	Phenotypes	Inflammatory Mediators[a]	Notes
Monocytes $CD11b^+$	Classical $CD14^{bright}CD16^-$	IL-6, IL-8, IL-10, TNF-α, G-CSF, CCL2, CCL5, greater phenotypic plasticity, greater phagocytosing, MPO activity and antibody-mediated cytotoxicity	Monocytes infiltrating the tissues from the circulation differentiate into macrophages. Peripheral blood monocytes exposed in vitro to cells and GCF from periodontitis tissues differentiate into macrophages. Monocytes are phagocytosing, antigen-presenting cells with phenotypic plasticity and important roles in microbial killing and activation of adaptive immunity.
	Non-classical $CD14^+CD16^{bright}$	IL-1β, IL-6, IL-8, TNF-α, better Fc-mediated phagocytosis, patrolling function	
	Intermediate $CD14^{bright}CD16^+$	IL-6, IL-8, TNF-α, greater production of ROS, angiogenic activity, greater MHC-II antigen-presentation, most pro-inflammatory	
B lymphocytes $CD19^+$, $CD20^+$	Follicular $HLA\text{-}DR^+$, $CXCR5^+$	IL-6, IL-12, TNF-α	B cells have a primary role in humoral immunity by producing antibodies, but also can phagocytose, present antigens to T cells and differentiate into osteoclasts
	Breg (B10) $CD1d^{bright}$, $CD40^+$	IL-10, IL-35, TGFβ	
T helper lymphocytes $CD3^+CD4^+$	Th1 T-bet^+, IFN-γ^{high}	IFN-γ, IL-1β, IL-2, IL-6, IL-12, IL-18, TNF-α, RANKL	T helper lymphocytes have phenotypic plasticity in response to cues from the microenvironment, which enable these cells to participate in host defense against microorganisms and repair processes/cessation of inflammation by influencing the chemotaxis and activity/phenotype of other immune cells. It has long been suggested that the prevailing Th subsets and their characteristic inflammatory mediators are associated with the active/progressive or stable/quiescent status of periodontal lesions. Clinical studies associate Th1/Th17 with tissue progressive and Th2/Treg with non-progressive lesions. Preclinical studies support this possibility, particularly for the association between Th17/progression and Treg/stability.
	Th2 GATA-3^+, IL-4^{high}	IL-2, IL-4, IL-5, IL-10, IL-13	
	Th17 ROR γ^+, IL-17 ^{high}	IL-1β, IL-6, IL-12, IL-17, IL-21, CCL20	
	Treg $FOXP3^+CD25^+$	Galectin-1, IL-10, IL-35, TGFβ	
	Th9 PU.1^+, IL-9 ^{high}	IL-9, IL-10, CCL17, CCL22	
	Th22 AHR^+, $IL22^{high}$	IL-22, IL-10, IL-13, CCL7, TNF-α	
Cytotoxic T cells $CD3^+CD8^+$	Based on cytokine expression profiles, may assume different phenotypes, analog to $CD4^+$ Th cells: Tc1, Tc2, Tc9, Tc17, Tc22 Tcreg	IL-4, IL-5, IL-9, IL-10, TGFβ, IFN-γ, IL-17, IL-22	CD8 T cells have MHC-I mediated cytotoxicity and also inflammatory mediator-associated immunoregulatory activities. May also assume different phenotypes depending on external cues, which affect their function/profile of inflammatory mediators secreted. As an example, $CD8^+FOXP3^+$ ($CD8^+$ Tregs) have been shown to attenuate inflammatory bone resorption in preclinical models.
γ/δ T cells $CD44^+$, $CCR6^+$, $CD3^+\alpha\beta TCR^-$ $\gamma\delta TCR^+$	Present functional plasticity associated with the type of inflammatory mediators secreted. IL-17 producing cells are denominated γ/δ17 cells.	IFN-γ, TNF-α, IL-17, amphiregulin	Considered innate immune tissue-resident cells (as opposed to classical αβT cells that enter the tissues from the circulation), these are not limited to MHC- or CD1-presented antigens and may respond to a wide variety of stimuli. They have a role in immune regulation via secreted inflammatory mediators, besides their direct cytotoxic activity. These cells have been detected in periodontal tissues (epithelium and connective tissue, including PDL) but their relevance for periodontal disease is not clearly defined: produce IL-17 that may contribute to tissue destruction; as well as amphiregulin that promote barrier repair and homeostasis.

Continued

TABLE 11.2 Cells Involved in Host-Microbial Interactions in the Periodontal Microenvironment—cont'd

Cells/Markers	Phenotypes	Inflammatory Mediators[a]	Notes
NK T cells $CD3^+CD56^+$	NKT $Th1^-$, $Th2^-$, $Th17^-$, Treg-like	IFN-γ, TNF-α, IL-4, IL-10, IL-13, IL-17, IL-21, IL-22	Recognize antigens via CD1d (CD1d-restricted). Major function is immunoregulatory (pro-inflammatory and suppressive) through production of inflammatory mediators. Predominant secreted mediators characterize different subsets, and these cells may also have cytotoxic activity.
NK cells $CD3^-CD16^+CD56^+$	Considered the founding member of innate lymphoid cells (ILCs) as an ILC1 family member	IFN-γ, TNF-α, GM-CSF, CCL3, CCL4	Have both immunoregulatory ($CD56^{bright}$) and direct cytotoxic functions ($CD56^{dim}$). Can mediate antibody-dependent cell-mediated cytotoxicity via CD16 besides direct cytotoxicity in infected cells with low MHC-I. Have immunoregulatory properties, via activation of other immune cells by secreted cytokines; modulation of B cell activity and stimulation of IgG2.
Innate lymphoid cells (ILCs) $CD3^-CD127^+$	Similar to $CD4^+$ Th cells, subsets of ILCs are characterized by lineage-specific transcription factors and secreted cytokines: ILC1 (tumor/viruses), ILC2 (parasites and allergens), ILC3 (bacteria, fungi)	IFN-γ, TNF-α, IL-4, IL-5, IL-13, IL-17, IL-22, GM-CSF, RANKL	These cells are present in primary and secondary lymphoid organs and also in barrier tissues such as oral mucosa. All subsets have been detected in diseased periodontal tissues (ILC1 was the most prevalent), but their role in periodontal disease is still not demonstrated.

[a]Some selected inflammatory mediators related with inflammation associated with host-microbial interactions in the periodontal microenvironment, common phenotypic markers, some associated inflammatory soluble mediators, and possible role in periodontal disease.

see Refs. 27,45,67,76,140). In the dynamics of immune response in the periodontal microenvironment, the "net balance" of pro- and anti-inflammatory mediators ultimately determines homeostasis or disease. These clinical outcomes are most likely resulting from the prevailing phenotype of immune cells, as the major source of inflammatory mediators.[134] Importantly, there is recent evidence indicating interindividual variability in inflammatory phenotype associated with the onset of biofilm-induced gingival inflammation, which may be related with the microbial (composition, quantity) and/or with the host (genetic/epigenetic makeup, systemic and environmental influences) components.[14]

Macrophages are antigen-presenting cells that are very responsive to microenvironmental cues, assuming a phenotype in a spectrum defined by the opposite M1/classical/pro-inflammatory (e.g., expressing high levels of IL-1β, IL-6, and TNF) and M2/alternative/pro-repair (e.g., expressing high levels of IL-10, TGF-β, specialized pro-resolving mediators). In a diseased state, M1 macrophages predominate,[216,246,252] whereas M2 macrophages are associated with homeostatic and repair states.[154,255,264]

Similar phenotypic plasticity is reported for neutrophils, infiltrating the periodontal tissues in healthy/homeostatic and dysbiotic/diseased states.[28,62,241] DC also may assume different phenotypes in dysbiotic/diseased and homeostatic/healthy states, respectively characterized as "activated" or "tolerogenic" states.[40,50,218,237] These DC phenotypes will determine the phenotype of the adaptive T helper-type response[111,205,222] and, consequently, have a profound influence on the "yin-yang" cytokine balance in the periodontal microenvironment.[101,212,219]

Relevance of B cells is commonly associated with their prevalence in the diseased periodontal microenvironment and in the capacity to secrete immunoglobulins, pro-inflammatory cytokines, and MMPs, but these cells can have other roles including antigen presentation and as osteoclast precursors.[120,265] B cells may also assume distinct phenotypes or activation states associated with the production of various cytokines. $CD25^+$ B and IL-10 secreting B10 cells (or "Bregs") have a suppressive/anti-inflammatory phenotype, associated with production of cytokines such as IL-10, TGF-β, and IL-35, and have been shown to attenuate periodontal tissue destruction in preclinical models.[24,94,239,251] Interestingly, Bregs were induced in vitro by TLR4- and TLR9-activating MAMPs, demonstrating that B cells express functional PRRs.[94] However, the most investigated aspect of the host response in periodontal disease is the T helper-type response. As neutrophils, macrophages and DCs, $CD4^+$ T cells may assume different phenotypes depending on the microenvironmental cues, particularly the balance of soluble inflammatory mediators and membrane-bound co-activating molecules expressed by other immune and stromal cells, as well as a possible direct effect of MAMPs. Current evidence supports a concept that diseased states characterized by increased inflammation and connective tissue destruction are associated with the predominance of Th17 pro-inflammatory phenotype.[51] Conversely, healthy and treated/repair/"quiescent" states are associated with increased prevalence anti-inflammatory Th phenotypes Th2 and Treg (for a comprehensive review, see reference[27]). Of note, there is incipient and conflicting information on the disease-activity or protective roles of more recently described Th9 and Th22 phenotypes in periodontal disease[49,157] and in periapical lesions.[9,49] Regardless, these Th-type phenotypes are characterized by the prevailing cytokines secreted by the $CD4^+$ T cells (see Tables 11.1 and 11.2) and will influence the production of inflammatory mediators by innate immune cells (neutrophils, macrophages, DC, gamma/delta T cells, NK cells, epithelial cells, fibroblasts, mesenchymal stem cells), and adaptive immune

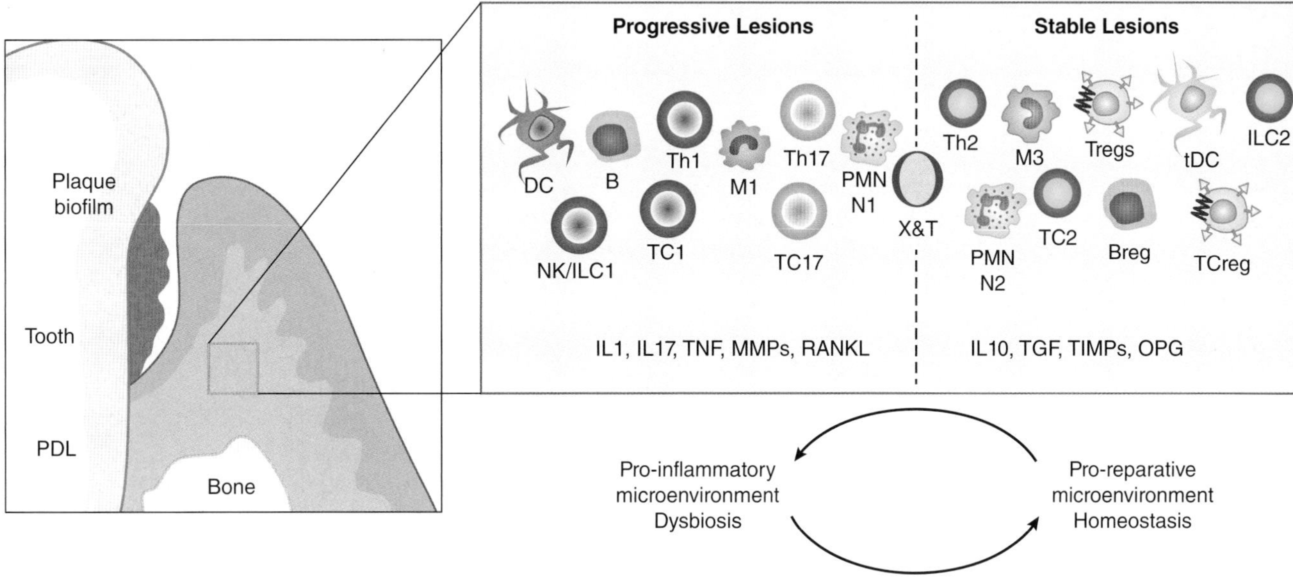

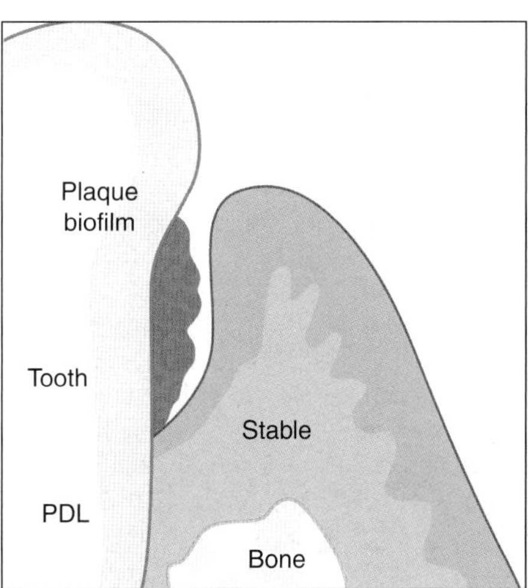

Fig. 11.2 Dynamics of immune/inflammatory response in periodontal disease. The onset and progression of periodontal disease with active destruction of periodontal non-mineralized and mineralized connective tissues detected as clinical attachment loss and/or alveolar bone resorption ultimately result from the immune-inflammatory status. Predominance pro-inflammatory microenvironment, characterized by increased prevalence of immune cells with pro-inflammatory phenotypes that produce higher amounts of pro-inflammatory/catabolic mediators is associated with progressive lesions. The reestablishment of a homeostatic state, either after periodontal treatment or after an adequate host response, occurs in non-progressive/stable lesions and is associated with the predominance of a pro-reparative microenvironment, characterized by the increased prevalence of immune cells with anti-inflammatory/reparative phenotypes, that produce higher amounts of anti-inflammatory/reparative cytokines and growth factors. Limited information indicates that gamma-delta T cells may participate in both "progressive" and "stable" conditions. Note that this is a dynamic process that is not exclusive, and that likely works as a "gradient," with the predominant phenotype and inflammatory mediators that will impart the "pro-inflammatory" or "pro-reparative" character in the microenvironment. This dynamic process may be shifted over time in the same individual/site and that is influenced by microbial factors (quantity and composition of microbial biofilm) and host-associated factors (diseases, medications, genetic variability, smoking, stress). *MMPs,* Matrix metalloproteinases; *OPG,* osteoprotegerin; *PDL,* periodontal ligament; *RANKL,* receptor activator of nuclear factor kappa B ligand; *TIMPs,* tissue inhibitors of metalloproteinases

cells (B cells, NK T cells). This complex interaction network in the periodontal microenvironment cycles back-and-forth between these various cell types in positive- and negative-feedback regulatory loops mediated by MAMPs and soluble inflammatory mediators. This further supports the notion that the didactically categorized innate and adaptive immune responses are in fact a dynamic continuum, as innate immune responses are not "switched off" once adaptive immunity is elicited, as there are reciprocal cross-activating and cross-regulatory effects and both arms of immune response occur simultaneously in the periodontal microenvironment.

The Complement System

Complement has been historically regarded as an antimicrobial enzyme system present in the serum and inflammatory exudates, such as the GCF. In response to microbes, complement can be activated via distinct initiation mechanisms (the classical, lectin, and alternative pathways), involving sequential activation and proteolytic cleavage of a series of proteins, designated C1 through C9 (Fig. 11.3). In addition to the classical components (C1 to C9), the integrated complement system comprises pattern-recognition molecules, convertases and other proteases, regulatory molecules, and receptors for interactions with complement activation fragments and other immune mediators.[195] All three pathways converge at the third component (C3) of complement. C3 is activated by pathway-specific C3 convertases and leads to the generation of effector molecules, which mediate (1) recruitment and activation of inflammatory cells (via the anaphylatoxins C3a and C5a that interact with specific G-protein-coupled receptors on leukocytes); (2) microbial opsonization (through opsonins, such as C3b) to facilitate phagocytosis; and (3) direct lysis of targeted susceptible bacteria (by means of the C5b-9 membrane attack complex) (see Fig. 11.3).

Cross-Talk Interactions of Complement

Advances in the past two decades have established that complement has functions above and beyond the "tagging and elimination" of microbes. It is now well appreciated that the activities of complement involve a network of interactions with other immune or physiological systems, which collectively coordinate the host immune response to infection, tissue injury, and other types of insult.[195] An important cross-talk interaction of complement involves its interplay with TLRs, leading to the amplification of innate immune and inflammatory responses. Upon infection or tissue damage, complement and TLRs are swiftly activated and engage in cross-talk signaling in different myeloid cell types, namely monocytes/macrophages, neutrophils, and DC (see Fig. 11.3).[86] Although these cross-talk interactions can potentially amplify innate immune responses against infection in a beneficial or detrimental manner for the host, they may also contribute to destructive inflammatory responses.

The signaling pathways activated downstream of complement receptors (e.g., C3aR or C5aR1) and TLRs (e.g., TLR2 or TLR4) converge at MAPKs (extracellular signal-regulated kinase-1 and -2 and c-Jun N-terminal kinase), which in turn enhance the activation of activator protein-1 and nuclear factor-κB, key transcription factors involved in the induction of inflammatory cytokines.[257] From an oral perspective, the concomitant activation of C5aR1 and TLR2 in the gingival tissue of mice after local micro-injection of specific ligands (C5a anaphylatoxin and Pam3Cys lipopeptide, respectively) causes the production of significantly higher levels of pro-inflammatory and pro-osteoclastogenic cytokines (interleukin [IL]-1β, IL-6, IL-17, and tumornecrosis factor) in the gingiva than stimulation of either receptor alone.[1] Thus, in principle, co-activation of complement and TLRs might have detrimental effects in the setting of periodontitis.

Complement and Periodontitis: Clinical Observations

The GCF in the gingival crevice contains a functional complement system.[93] Therefore, the subgingival bacteria likely constantly encounter complement and the generated complement-dependent host defense mechanisms may contribute to host-microbe homeostasis in the healthy periodontium. This notion is consistent with the concept that complement, in general, plays a crucial role in mediating immune surveillance and maintaining overall health. However, when dysregulated or overactivated, complement switches from a homeostatic to a pathological effector, as evidenced by its involvement in several inflammatory disorders.[196] Similarly, at least in principle, complement may contribute to inflammatory tissue destruction in the setting of chronic periodontitis, a perception that has been proven by a combination of clinical and experimental studies.

Clinical observational studies have associated periodontitis with increased complement activation in gingival biopsies and GCF collected from patients as compared to healthy control samples.[38,162,165,178,208] An experimental human gingivitis study correlated progressive elevation of complement cleavage (activation) products with increased clinical periodontal inflammation.[178] Conversely, albeit consistently, successful treatment of periodontitis leading to inflammation resolution resulted in decreased activation of C3 in the GCF.[163] A recent study has suggested that the complement activation product C3c may be a potential salivary biomarker for periodontitis.[75]

Complement and Periodontitis: Animal Model-Based Studies

Cause-and-effect studies in preclinical models of periodontitis have conclusively implicated complement in the pathogenesis of this oral disease. Indeed, mice genetically deficient in C3, C3aR, or C5aR1 are all protected from developing gingival inflammation and alveolar bone loss, as compared to wild-type littermate control mice.[89,136,144] In particular, the protective effect of C3 deficiency was confirmed in three distinct disease models, namely, ligature-induced periodontitis, *P. gingivalis*-induced periodontitis, and naturally occurring periodontitis.[146] The protective effect of C3 deficiency was associated with decreased production of pro-inflammatory and pro-osteoclastogenic cytokines, such as IL-23 and IL-17,[146] which are derived mainly from antigen-presenting cells[5] and $CD4^+$ T helper 17 (Th17) cells,[51] respectively. This observation is consistent with the notion that complement can cross-talk with and regulate both the innate and adaptive immune response.[195]

Studies in a more relevant model of periodontitis, specifically in non-human primates (NHP), were undertaken to determine whether inhibition of complement C3 can restrain periodontitis and pave the way to clinical trials for the treatment of the human disease (see *Immunomodulatory Therapies* section). The C3 inhibitor used in these studies was Cp40 (a.k.a. AMY-101), a third-generation analog of the compstatin family of cyclic peptidic inhibitors with specificity for NHP and human C3.[151,189] In the first study, young adult cynomolgus monkeys were subjected to ligature-induced periodontitis under a split-mouth experimental design.[146] Sites that were locally treated with intragingival injections of Cp40 showed significantly less radiographic bone loss than sites treated with a sequence-scrambled control peptide.[146] Moreover, Cp40 significantly inhibited gingival inflammation and clinical attachment loss. These clinical effects were associated with lower concentrations of pro-inflammatory and pro-osteoclastogenic cytokines (e.g., IL-17 and RANKL) in the GCF.[146]

Cp40 was additionally used in a therapeutic, rather than preventive, setting. In other words, this C3 inhibitor was tested for its ability to inhibit preexisting, naturally occurring periodontitis in aged cynomolgus monkeys.[145] The experimental design of this study involved a 6-week treatment regimen with injections of Cp40 in the interdental papillae (0.1 mg/site) followed by a 6-week monitoring period without further treatment. Regardless of the frequency of drug administration (once or three times weekly), Cp40 caused significant reduction of clinical indices related to inflammation, pocket formation and tissue destruction. These beneficial clinical effects were associated with significant reduction of pro-inflammatory cytokines and complement activation fragments (C3a and C5a) in the GCF, as well as with decreased numbers of osteoclasts in bone biopsies. The therapeutic effects of Cp40 persisted for at least 6 weeks after treatment completion.

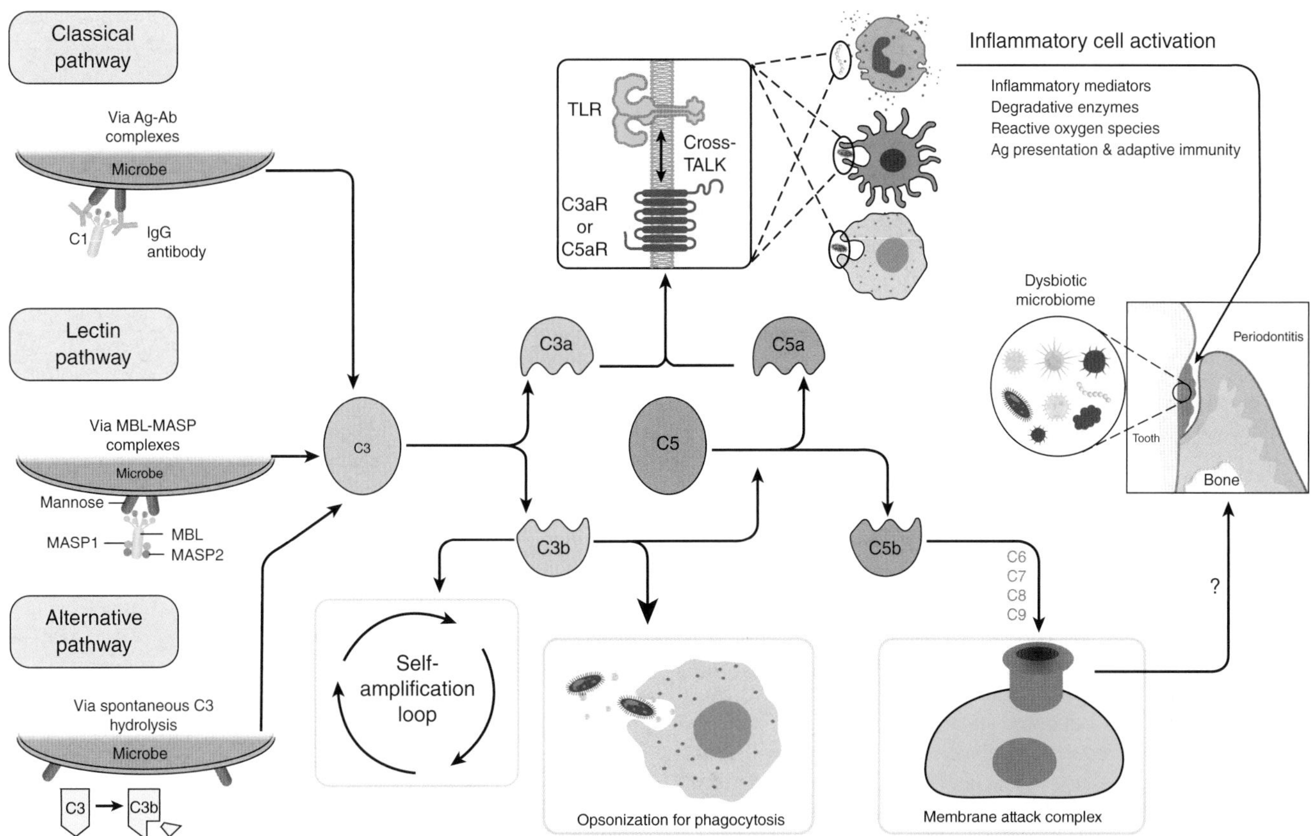

Fig. 11.3 Complement activation and periodontal disease. The complement system can be activated by distinct initiation mechanisms: The classical pathway is triggered by antigen-antibody complex-mediated activation of the C1 complex. The lectin pathway is initiated when complexes of mannose-binding lectin *(MBL)* and MBL-associated serine proteases *(MASPs)* recognize and adhere to microbial surfaces. The alternative pathway is triggered by a "tick-over" mechanism that involves spontaneous C3 hydrolysis, which occurs in the absence of complement regulatory molecules (as is typically the case with foreign surfaces such as microbial cells). In the so-called alternative pathway-amplification loop, additional C3 is cleaved into even more C3b which further fuels the loop, thereby amplifying complement activation irrespective of the initiating mechanism. All three mechanisms of complement initiation and amplification converge at C3. The downstream effects of C3 activation include the generation of effectors that promote inflammation *(C3a and C5a)*, opsonization for phagocytosis (C3b) and the generation C5b-C9 membrane attack complex (MAC). MAC can lyse susceptible targeted bacteria but has also been implicated in destructive inflammation. Whereas the role of MAC in periodontitis is uncertain, C3a and C5a activate specific G-protein-coupled receptors *(C3aR and C5aR1)*, which cross-talk with Toll-like receptors *(TLRs)*. This cross-talk interaction between complement and TLRs activates synergistically inflammatory leukocytes, which directly or indirectly mediate destructive inflammation that leads to periodontal tissue breakdown and alveolar bone loss in periodontitis.

Taken together, the preclinical studies in mice and NHPs have conclusively shown that complement is involved in the pathogenesis of periodontitis (see Fig. 11.3) and provided proof-of-concept for a complement-targeted host-modulation therapy in periodontitis.

Complement and Periodontal Pathogens

A potential concern is whether complement inhibition could undermine the competency of antimicrobial mechanisms in the periodontium. On the basis of available evidence, local blockade of complement is unlikely to cause uncontrolled growth of periodontal pathogens in periodontitis. In this regard, complement is exploited by periodontal pathogens to subvert the host immune response and promote the persistence of a dysbiotic microbial community.[146] Moreover, many periodontal pathogens have developed mechanisms to protect themselves from the antimicrobial effects of complement. For instance, *P. gingivalis* and *Prevotella intermedia* can capture and co-opt a soluble inhibitor of complement activation, namely the C4b-binding protein.[149,184] In this manner, these bacteria prevent complement activation on their cell surface, which could otherwise lead to their opsonization by C3b and phagocytic uptake. Moreover, *Treponema denticola* expresses a virulence protein that binds and exploits complement factor H, another major soluble inhibitor of complement activation.[155] Periodontal pathogens may not only hijack soluble negative regulators of complement for their own protection, but can also degrade host cell-associated regulatory molecules to potentially instigate complement attack against host cells. For example, *P. gingivalis* causes the shedding from oral epithelial cells of membrane-anchored CD46 (a.k.a. membrane cofactor protein), an action that might render the host cells susceptible to the destructive effects of complement activation.[147]

Therefore, in the context of periodontal disease, complement activation is unlikely to restrain periodontal pathogens, thus its inhibition should not entail a risk. Consistently, C3-deficient mice subjected to experimental periodontitis exhibit decreased periodontal bacterial load relative to wild-type littermate controls.[144] The diminished periodontal inflammation seen in C3 deficiency may also contribute to the reduced microbial burden. In this respect, inflammation is a major ecological factor that drives the selective expansion of pathogenic species in periodontitis, presumably by generating a nutritionally favorable environment through accumulation of tissue breakdown products that are used as nutrients by the bacteria.[122,133]

Dynamics of Host Response/Interactions and Intersections Between Innate and Adaptive Responses

The immune system is classically defined into two components: innate and adaptive. The innate immune system components include myeloid lineage derivatives including macrophages, neutrophils, natural killer cells, and DC. In addition, innate immune system components also include non-hematopoietic derivatives including complement proteins and oral epithelial cell barriers. The adaptive immune system arm includes B cells and T lymphocytes and their derivatives.[82] There is an important connection between these two arms of the immune system through antigen presentation modalities and cytokine secretion.[204]

Cells of the Adaptive Immune System: Lymphocytes

Once innate immune modalities are activated, adaptive immune system components—lymphocytes—are recruited by local cytokine gradients and activated through antigen presentation systems. Lymphocytes then produce clonally distributed receptors that are specific to diverse antigens. Lymphocytes include two large subtypes: B cells and T cells. These cells are identified based on surface proteins, CD (cluster of differentiation).

Cell types can also be described by surface proteins that characterize their interaction. An essential modality of communication between antigen-presenting cells and adaptive immune cells includes the specialized peptide display molecules called major histocompatibility complex (MHC). These proteins were discovered in the field of organ transplant compatibility and these studies delineated the important role in MHC proteins binding antigen (either self or pathogens) for recognition by the appropriate T-lymphocytes.[105]

B Lymphocytes

B lymphocytes recognize antigen and differentiate into plasma cells that produce antibodies specific to that presented antigen. B lymphocytes are the only cells capable of producing antibodies. They are characterized by CD19, CD23, and their receptors exhibit a class II MHC. They are activated when membrane-bound antibodies (serving in this capacity as receptors) recognize antigens either soluble, on the surface of microbes, or on the surface of host cells trying to present antigen to the B cells. This results in proliferation and differentiation of the antigen-specific B cells that secrete soluble forms of antibodies with the same antigen specificity as the membrane receptors.

T Lymphocytes

T lymphocytes are a subset of adaptive immune cells activated in response to protein antigens that are presented while bound to MHC molecules of antigen-presenting cells. T cells can be characterized by the T-cell receptor (TCR) on their surface. The majority of circulating T cells have two glycoprotein chains called alpha (α) and beta (β) TCR chains, whereas a small subset of T cells that specifically reside in the mucosal tissues express one gamma (γ) and one delta (δ) chain.[194] The α/β T cells are further classified by their CD surface proteins and MHC recognition capacity described below and in Table 11.3:

CD4⁺ helper T lymphocytes are called helper T cells because they help B lymphocytes produce antibodies and also help phagocytes destroy ingested microbes. They recognize antigens on class II MHC complexes. Their surface protein profile is characterized as $CD3^+$, $CD4^+$, and $CD8^-$. $CD4^+$ subsets can be further divided into Th1, Th17, Th2.[63,158] Th1 T lymphocytes have broad implications in terms of cell-mediated immunity, because they secrete IFNγ (activating macrophages, NK cells, and $CD8^+$ T cells) in addition to influencing B cells to secrete opsonizing antibody isotypes that further enhance antigen uptake and presentation to T cells.[170] In response to bacterial lipopeptides, Th17 cells produce IL-17, TNFα, and GM-CSF 102. In contrast, Th2 cells mediate production of IgE and activate mast cells in humoral immunity responses and allergy-type responses.[245]

$CD8^+$ cytotoxic T lymphocytes are called cytotoxic T cells because they are responsible for killing cells that are infected with intracellular microbes. They recognize antigens on class I MHC complexes. Their surface protein profile is characterized as $CD3^+$, $CD4^-$, $CD8^+$.

Regulatory T lymphocytes function to regulate the response of the immune system and maintain self-tolerance. These cells often suppress other T cells to achieve these goals. They recognize antigen presented on class II MHC complexes and are specific for self (and minimal amounts of foreign) antigens. They are characterized by the surface protein profile of $CD3^+$, $CD4^+$, $CD25^+$, $FoxP3^+$.

Inflammatory Mechanisms Lead to Bone Loss in Periodontitis

As the microbiota at the gingival crevice shift to a dysbiotic state, neutrophils are initially recruited to the localized gingival connective tissue, junctional epithelium, and the periodontal pocket (Fig. 11.4).[169] In response to neutrophil recognition of microbial antigens, neutrophils release MMPs and express membrane bound RANKL that potentially initiate matrix (soft and hard tissue) destruction.[29] In addition, neutrophils also secrete CCL2 and CCL20, which are cytokines that are released to recruit adaptive counterparts to the gingival spaces to exacerbate the immune response to the localized microbial dysbiosis and invasion.[179]

Dysbiotic microbiota also activate antigen-presenting cells including macrophages, DC, and γ/δ T cells. These specialized cells "sound the alarm" within the localized context and both secrete cytokines (TNF, IL-16, IL-17) that recruit the adaptive immune defense (B, Th1, Th17 cells) and directly present antigen to the adaptive immune cells.[65,93] These adaptive immune cells have a positive feedback to innate immune cells, resulting in a more robust innate population to the localized gingival area perpetuating the inflammatory cycle. In addition, adaptive immune cells both express and secrete large quantities of RANKL,[115,156] supporting osteoclastic differentiation and subsequent periodontal bone loss observed in periodontal disease diagnosis.

Systemic Modulators of Immune Responses

In the above sections, we have reviewed the complex role of dysbiotic oral bacterial communities that elicit an exacerbated, chronic, and pathogenic host response involving all components of the immune defense system, which ultimately result in the clinical features of inflammation and alveolar bone loss. Susceptibility to periodontitis and other inflammatory diseases appears to change in response to genetic, environmental, and stochastic factors throughout the life span of our patients. Many of these modifiable risk factors have effects on the innate and adaptive immune cells and thus alter susceptibility of the patient to periodontal disease; therefore,

TABLE 11.3 Compilation of Risk Factors in Periodontal Disease Progression and Their Impact on Immune System Dysregulation and Oral Clinical Manifestations

Risk Factors	Immune Response Modifications	Clinical Outcomes	References
Smoking	Increased macrophage percentage Macrophage phagocytosis altered Increased NK cell secretion of IL-17A Increased Th1, Th17 cells Decreased Th2 cells by nicotine Decreased B cells and Treg	Exacerbated osteoclastogenesis and bone loss	Nociti et al. 2015[166] Qiu et al. 2017[188]
Diabetes	Increased M1 macrophages and secretion of TNFα Increased Th1, Th17, CD8 T cells Increased secretion of IFNγ, TNFα, and IL-17 from CD8 T cells Decreased neutrophils, eosinophils, NK cells, M2 macrophages, Th2 cells, Treg	Elevated inflammation Susceptibility to infection Delayed wound healing Increased osteoclastogenesis, bone loss, attachment loss	Zhou et al. 2018[262] Graves et al. 2020[77]
Obesity and metabolic syndrome	Insulin resistance Increased chronic systemic inflammation and cytokines Impaired immune response to *P. gingivalis*	Delayed wound healing Increased clinical inflammatory features Increased osteoclastogenesis	Amar et al. 2007[7] Falagas et al. 2006[60]
Aging	Increased immunosenescence Increased myelopoiesis Increased chronic systemic inflammation and cytokines Low-level state of immune activation	Delayed and impaired wound healing Increased clinical inflammatory features Increased osteoclastogenesis Increased bone fragility	Ebersole et al. 2016[53] Kirkwood et al. 2018[126] Clark et al. 2021[35]
Stress	Increased Th1, Th17, B cells Increased production of IL-1β, IL-17 Decreased leukocyte mobilization Decreased Treg cells	Susceptibility to infection Delayed wound healing	Genco et al. 1999[69] Schmidt et al. 2010[210] Decker et al. 2020[46] Decker et al. 2021[48]
Genetic Disorders (including leukocyte adhesion deficiency, cyclic neutropenia)	Decreased neutrophil recruitment to the gingiva Overproduction of IL-17	Microbial overgrowth and bacteria-driven inflammation Increased osteoclastogenesis	Hajishengallis et al. 2016a[91] Hajishengallis et al. 2016b[90] Moutsopoulos et al. 2017[160]
Rheumatoid arthritis	T cells and B cells presented antigen by dendritic cells and macrophages Fibroblasts produce RANKL CD4+ T cells produce IL-17 and TNF Anti-citrullinated protein antibodies produced by B cells	Elevated inflammation systemically and in the periodontium Increased C-reactive protein, IL-1β in the periodontium Increased osteoclastogenesis, bone loss, attachment loss	Kaur et al., 2013[117] Bingham III et al. 2013[17] Walsh et al. 2018[238]

understanding of these modifiable risk factors and how they modulate the immune response/alveolar bone resorption is essential for clinical practice (see Fig. 11.4).

Tobacco Use

Clinical notations of the caustic effects that smoking induces on the periodontal tissues is long standing.[183] More recently, epidemiological studies presenting adequate methodologies and statistical analyses (capable of controlling for confounding factors) have clearly demonstrated a strong association between tobacco use and periodontal diseases in a diverse population.[55,230] Furthermore, we have recent biological and microbiological studies that delineate more precisely the mechanisms by which tobacco use can alter the immune system to cause periodontal tissue destruction and periodontal disease progression.[167,187] Tobacco smoking can alter the innate immune response through increased macrophage percentages and altered phagocytosis capacity, as well as increase NK cell production of IL-17. These altered innate immune responses subsequently recruit adaptive counterparts Th1 and Th17 cells to the gingival tissues. In addition, decreased numbers of Th2, B cells, and Tregs are observed with tobacco use. These immune response modifications can result in exacerbated osteoclastogenesis and alveolar bone loss observed in periodontal disease progression.

Diabetes Mellitus

Studies investigating the effects of diabetes on all organ systems is a growing area of interest and concern with the global rise in prevalence of the disease.[172] The systemic effects of diabetes are abundant, in part, due to modulation of the inflammatory and immunological dysregulation.[84] In this disease process, increased M1 macrophages are observed along with additive secretion of TNFα. In the adaptive response, increased Th1, Th17, and CD8 T cells are observed along with additive secretion of IFNγ, TNFα, and IL-17 from CD8 T cells. Conversely, decreased neutrophils, eosinophils, NK cells,

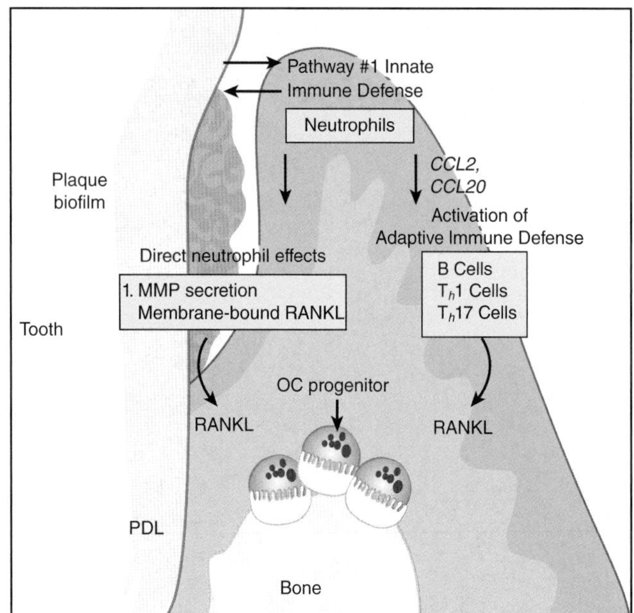

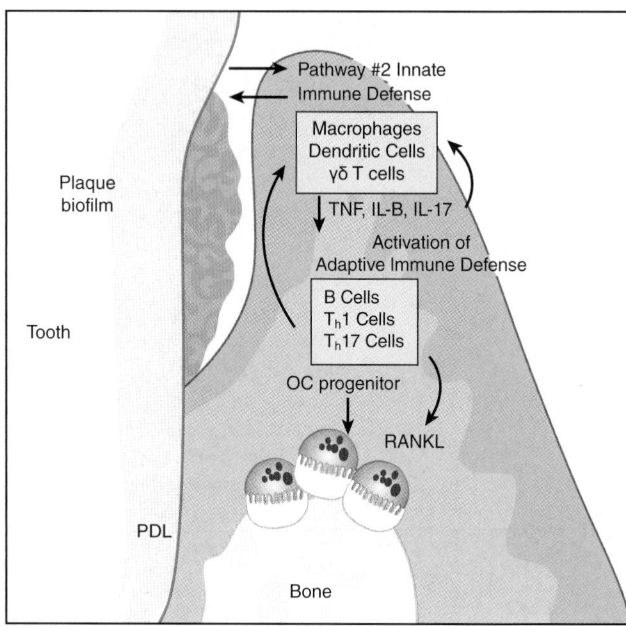

Fig. 11.4 Dynamics of host response in periodontal disease. Dysbiotic bacteria and their biofilm secretory products can infiltrate the oral epithelium and activate the innate immune defenses including neutrophils *(Pathway #1)*, macrophages, dendritic cells, and γδ T cells *(Pathway #2)*. Neutrophils can both activate the adaptive immune defense cells via secretion of CCL2 and CCL20, as well as affect extracellular matrix integrity through the secretion of enzymes (i.e., matrix metalloproteinases *[MMPs]*) and in a limited sense increase osteoclastogenesis with membrane-bound receptor activator of nuclear factor kappa B ligand *(RANKL)*. Macrophages, dendritic cells, and γδ T cells can activate the adaptive immune defense as well through secretion of tumor necrosis factor *(TNF)*, interleukin *(IL)*-6, IL-17, which in turn promote osteoblastic secretion of RANKL and subsequent bone resorption by osteoclastogenesis. In addition, there is a notable autocrine and paracrine positive feedback loop among innate and adaptive players that amplify osteoclastogenesis phenotypes. *PDL,* Periodontal ligament.

M2 macrophages, Th2 cells, and Treg cells are observed.[78,263] This immunological dysregulation results in the characteristic of elevated inflammation, heightened susceptibility to infection, delayed wound healing, and increased osteoclastogenesis/bone loss/attachment loss observed in uncontrolled diabetic patients that have periodontal tissue comorbidities.[77]

Obesity and Metabolic Syndrome

Obesity and metabolic syndrome are emerging public health problems in modern society. Overweight/obesity designations are measures of body mass index, waist to hip ratio, waist circumference, and body weight changes.[71] Obesity and metabolic disorders can have general effects on health and local effects on the periodontium, including insulin resistance, chronic systemic inflammation, and impaired immune response to periodontal pathogens including *P. gingivalis*.[7,60]

Aging

Increased prevalence and severity of periodontal disease have long been associated with aging.[56] However, recent studies have illuminated that the immune system undergoes quantitative and qualitative modifications with aging.[53] With aging, increased "immunosenescence" is observed, whereby modifications of the immune system leads to greater susceptibility to infection, neoplasia, and autoimmunity.[53] This global reduction in immune response efficacy is notably coupled with a progressive increase in the general, non-specified pro-inflammatory status of an aged individual, referred to as "inflammaging."[126] This expression of inflammaging and low-level state of immune activation can also have direct and damaging implications on bone density, volume, and phenotype, including that of the periodontium, through increased levels of osteoclastogenesis.[126] Readers are referred to a recent review on the basic biological aspects on aging and periodontal disease.[36]

Stress

Effects of chronic psychosocial stress on systemic organ and tissue systems is an increasing area of relevance.[138,209] Psychobiological connections between chronic psychosocial stress and periodontal disease progression specifically have grown with more evidence from both epidemiological studies and biological mechanistic studies combined.[47,70,132,209] These observations of periodontal severity and exacerbated progression with chronic psychosocial stress appear as a result between alterations in behavior and altered immune response mechanisms. Modifications of the immunological profile include increased levels of Th1, Th17, and B cells with concomitant increases in IL-1β and IL-17 production. In addition, there is a decrease of leukocyte mobility and a decreased number of Treg cells. The combination of these immunological effects in the presence of a dysbiotic microbial profile results in the clinical results of increased gingival inflammation and subsequent bone loss observed in processing periodontal disease.

Neutrophil Dysfunction Disorders: Leukocyte Adhesion Deficiency and Neutropenia

Neutrophil dysfunction is a feature in several diseases, including, but not limited to, leukocyte adhesion deficiency and neutropenia, that directly affect periodontal tissues.[57,74] Importantly, gingival presentation of oral mucosal inflammation or periodontal tissue destruction noted by a dentist can be one of the first flags for these systemic disorders or relapse of a previously treated systemic disorder.[37,180] Mechanistic biological insights into how neutrophil dysfunction can produce these oral phenotypes have been recently elucidated in the context of subsequent immunological dysregulation within the gingival substructures.[86,91,159,160] For instance, in periodontitis associated with leukocyte adhesion deficiency, there is a decreased neutrophil recruitment to the gingiva (due to genetic mutations in β2 integrins, i.e., adhesive molecules required for the transmigration of neutrophils). The paucity of neutrophils in the gingival tissue leads to overproduction of IL-17 (owing to alterations in local factors, such as microbial dysbiosis and diminished efferocytosis due to lack of apoptotic neutrophils) by T cells which thereby mediate local periodontal tissue destruction. This destruction perpetuates microbial overgrowth fueled by breakdown products of the gingival tissues and increased osteoclastogenesis.

Rheumatoid Arthritis

Growing evidence in both dental and rheumatology fields of study suggest a dynamic cross-reactive relationship between rheumatoid arthritis and periodontal disease progression to tooth loss.[17,117] The rheumatoid arthritic autoimmune response is induced by inflammation, whereby T cells and B cells are activated by antigen presenting cells, including macrophages and DC.[238] Local to the joint at a rheumatoid site, synovial fibroblasts produce RANKL, while CD4+ T cells produce osteoclastogenic cytokines IL-17 and TNF.[238] Anti-citrullinated protein antibodies are produced by B cells, which also promote osteoclastogenesis and osteoclast activity.[238] Local to the periodontium, rheumatoid patients exhibit erythrocyte sedimentation rates, clinical attachment loss, and elevated pro-inflammatory conditions, including raised C-reactive protein and IL-1β levels.[117] In addition, some evidence for a positive outcome of periodontal treatment on the clinical features of rheumatoid arthritis was also noted.[117]

An etiopathic mechanism involving rheumatoid arthritis onset and periodontopathogen, *P. gingivalis,* which uniquely possesses a prokaryotic citrullinating enzyme and could potentially give rise to cross-reactive antibodies, is currently a matter of debate.[200] However, these hypotheses are still being generated and tested with no clear consensus at this time.[148,161]

Immunomodulatory Therapies

A variety of treatment strategies have been developed to target the host response to LPS-mediated tissue destruction. MMP inhibitors (e.g., low-dose formulations of doxycycline) have been used in combination with scaling and root planing[26] or surgical therapy.[64] In addition, high-risk patient populations (e.g., diabetic patients, patients with refractory periodontal disease) have benefited from the systemic administration of MMP inhibitors.[30,168,202] Encouraging results have been shown with the use of soluble antagonists of TNF-α and IL-1β delivered locally to periodontal tissues in nonhuman primates.[10] Other therapeutic strategies that are being explored are aimed at inhibiting the signal transduction pathways involved in inflammation. Pharmacological inhibitors of NF-κβ and p38 MAPK pathways are actively being developed to manage rheumatoid arthritis and inflammatory bone diseases,[10,109,131] and they have been applied in periodontal disease models with noteworthy accomplishments.[125,198] With the use of this novel strategy, inflammatory mediators including pro-inflammatory cytokines (e.g., IL-1, TNF, IL-6), MMPs, and others would be inhibited at the level of the cell-signaling pathways required for the transcription factor activation necessary for inflammatory gene expression or mRNA stability. Indeed, the targeting of RNA-binding proteins that mediate the effects of inflammatory cytokines does have therapeutic value in small animal models of periodontal disease progression.[198] These therapies may provide the next wave of adjuvant chemotherapeutics that may be used to manage chronic periodontitis.

The antimicrobial and immunomodulatory roles of defensins also have obvious attractiveness for therapeutic applications. However, the biochemical purification process is cost-inefficient and the synthesis process is complicated by the size and tridimensional structure of the peptides. Recently, novel analogs of defensins have shown even higher antibacterial activity than the endogenous β-defensins 1 and 3, without any cytotoxic effects on host cells,[241] thus indicating the promise of this approach.

Following complement-targeted host-modulation therapy in periodontitis success as host-modulation therapeutic in preclinical models of periodontitis,[113,145,146] Cp40 was clinically developed for human use as AMY-101, which completed a phase 1 safety trial in 2017.[151] A randomized, placebo-controlled, double-blind phase 2a clinical trial assessed the safety and efficacy of AMY-101 in 40 patients with existing periodontal inflammation. Clinical and laboratory assessments of safety showed that the drug was safe and well-tolerated in all study participants. Consistent with the NHP proof-of-concept studies of C3 inhibition,[145,146] a once-per-week intragingival injection of AMY-101 for 3 weeks resulted in a pronounced and sustainable resolution of gingival inflammation in human subjects, which was evident even 3 months after treatment initiation. In particular, the clinical efficacy of AMY-101 was reflected by statistically significant reductions in two key periodontal indices measuring gingival inflammation.[8] AMY-101 will be further tested in a pivotal Phase 3 study as an adjunctive therapeutic in patients with periodontitis.[8] In the studies performed to date, AMY-101 was applied as a stand-alone treatment. Eventually, this C3-targeted drug is intended for use as an adjunctive therapy to the standard periodontal treatment.

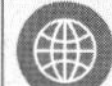
References for this chapter are found on the companion website eBooks.Health.Elsevier.com.

CHAPTER 12

Resolution of Inflammation

Marcelo Freire | Julie Teresa Marchesan | George Hajishengallis

 For additional content on systemic links, including type 2 diabetes, cardiovascular diseases, cancer, and pregnancy outcomes, please visit the companion website at eBooks.Health.Elsevier.com.

CHAPTER OUTLINE

Inflammation has protective functions that are regulated by multiple endogenous interactions with host cells, microbiome, and external antigens. Acute inflammation is temporally and spatially regulated to maintain homeostasis. There are signals that control activation and termination of inflammation. The signals activating inflammation are well known, and the repertoire of cells and signals controlling resolution (termination) are emerging. Four specialized lipid mediator (SLM) families activate resolution signals (lipoxins, resolvins, protectins, and maresins). There are cellular actions, such as phagocytosis and efferocytosis, that are key in activating these signals. Understanding the crosstalk between cells and signals that mediate resolution in the tissue response to injury has the potential to prevent and treat chronic diseases. The therapeutic applications of inflammation resolution include prevention, maintenance, and regeneration of periodontal tissues. This chapter presents fundamental concepts of resolution as an active biochemical mechanism regulated by endogenous/therapeutic lipid mediators (LMs). Novel concepts of resolution mediators in tissue regeneration and potential therapeutic applications are also discussed.

Inflammation

Inflammation is an essential biologic response observed across species with particular importance to human health and disease. The first description of a localized response to injury and infection that resembled signs of inflammation was recorded by the ancient Egyptian and Greek cultures. Four cardinal signs describing inflammation were identified: *rubor et tumor cum calore et dolore* (redness and swelling with heat and pain).[115] In 1958, Virchow's investigations led to the understanding of the cellular basis of inflammation as a pathologic condition, and his observations led to the addition of a new cardinal sign, *functio laesa* (loss of organ/tissue function).[115]

More recently, advanced cellular and molecular mechanisms governing the fate of inflammation have been identified. The initiation of an acute response is accepted to be a physiologic response occurring in vascularized tissues to defend the host and maintain homeostasis. Inflammation, or "set on fire," is an active cellular and molecular response that aims to control challenge.[79] When activated, inflammation is protective to host tissues against stimuli such as pathobionts, foreign bodies, toxic chemicals, and trauma.

Innate immunity, characterized by the local inflammatory response, is the early response to identifying and eliminating infectious agents or damaged tissues. As an initial and protective response to challenges presented by host tissues, inflammation is characterized by increased blood flow, vascular dilation, increased vascular permeability, and cellular recruitment. This response requires four biologic components: inflammation inducers, detecting sensors, downstream mediators, and target tissues. The type and degree of an inflammatory response are dependent on the underlying biology of the host itself, the nature of the trigger (e.g., bacterial, viral, parasitic, or chemical), and its duration.[78] With specific cellular and molecular cues, inducers will be detected by the first line of response and activate a cascade of events that are tightly regulated.

The major sensors for the inflammatory response are epithelial and innate immune cells that migrate to the injured site and resident stromal cells. Polymorphonuclear leukocytes (PMNs) or neutrophils (named for their staining characteristics with hematoxylin and eosin) constitute the cellular arm of the first line of defense of the innate immune system. PMNs are phagocytes with potent oxidative and nonoxidative killing mechanisms that combat bacteria.[13] PMN infiltration is followed by the entry of mononuclear cells, monocytes, and activated macrophages into the inflammatory site that clears cellular debris, bacteria, and apoptotic PMNs by efferocytosis without prolonging inflammation. Together, innate cells trigger production of mediators that modulate the fate of inflammation. Neutrophils, macrophages, dendritic cells, and mast cells produce low-molecular-weight proteins called cytokines that control initiation, maintenance, and regulation of the amplitude and duration of the inflammatory response.

In response to bacteria, conserved receptors expressed in innate immune cells, namely Toll-like receptors (TLRs), sense molecules expressed on pathogens, such as pathogen-associated molecular patterns (PAMPs). Binding of TLRs to specific pathogen molecules induces a signal that activates downstream events. As a consequence, the production of communicating molecules, such as inflammatory cytokines, interleukins (ILs), chemokines (CXCs), and inflammatory LMs, is key to signaling an effective response.[17,18] The inflammatory mediators are communicators establishing the "language" responsible to signal bacterial clearance. A didactic and functional classification of mediators categorized the inflammatory molecules according to their functions in the context of activation (pro) or inhibition (anti) of inflammation. It is important to note that the binary terminologies of proinflammatory and antiinflammatory are more dynamic than first described. This complex relationship is controlled by the molecule concentration, the interaction with its receptors and other interactants, and finally the time of production and activity. The binary view of a molecule's activity is still the convention and the accepted terminology, but it is crucial to contextualize these concepts as part of a dynamic system where multiple markers and cells are overlapping continuously to respond to injury. For example, proinflammatory mediators are produced locally in the tissues or systemically in the bloodstream (e.g., IL-1β, IL-6, tumor necrosis factor-α [TNF-α], and prostaglandin E2 [PGE2]). In response to the direct challenge or the production of proinflammatory molecules, antiinflammatory cytokines control the response and maintain the reaction in check (e.g., IL-10, IL-13, transforming growth factor-β [TGF-β], IL-1RA).[101]

The regulation leading to transcription of proinflammatory cytokine genes, their translation, and secretion from a variety of cells is dependent on nuclear factor kappa-light-chain-enhancer of activated B cells (NF-κB). NF-κB gene clusters and proteins function as dimeric transcription factors that regulate a broad range of biologic processes, including innate and adaptive immunity, inflammation, stress responses, B-cell development, lymphoid organogenesis, and cytokine production. Cytokines are low-molecular-weight proteins that modulate inflammation positively or negatively. Cytokines are released by local cells, such as epithelial cells and fibroblasts, and phagocytes in the acute inflammation phase, and by immune cells in adaptive immunity. *(Please refer to Chapter 11 for more details on inflammation.)* Phagocytes are known to initiate clearance and present antigens. In addition, we discuss efferocytosis (i.e., the phagocytic clearance of apoptotic cells) and host heterogeneity in the context of inflammation and tissue response to infection and injury.

Although the inflammatory response is protective, unresolved, continuous inflammation is detrimental to tissue function, promoting dysbiosis. Failure to resolve inflammation leads to chronic diseases, including inflammatory bowel syndrome, type 2 diabetes, cardiovascular diseases (CVDs), Alzheimer disease, cancer, and periodontal diseases. Resolution of inflammation is an active biochemical mechanism regulated by mediators that switch gene expression, protein functions, and cells to return to homeostasis. Among the mediators that regulate this process, SPMs activate cells to start resolution. Thus beneficial acute inflammation is spatially and temporally regulated by SPMs.[12,24,87,94,107]

KEY FACT

Proresolution Versus Antiinflammation

Proresolution lipid mediators are fatty acids that are expressed endogenously to activate cells and tissues to control inflammation. Initiation of inflammation requires external and internal cellular signals that in turn activate proresolution enzymes to produce lipid ligand signals. Upon interaction with a cellular receptor, agonist lipid ligands activate cells to produce proresolution or antiinflammation signals. The stereospecificity guides the cell function to either suppress and/or proresolve. In antiinflammation, blocking and suppressing pathways that activate inflammation are the usual mechanism. In proresolution, specific lipids are able to activate cell switching from proinflammation to proresolution, and phagocytosis and efferocytosis are stimulated, while antiinflammation is inhibited. For example, the endogenous mediators are able to enhance deficient phagocytosis seen in type 2 diabetes, increase chemotaxis in localized aggressive periodontitis (LAP), and prevent gingivitis. Thus stimulating resolution either endogenously or exogenously/therapeutically activates protective signals that prevent collateral damage and limit acute or continuous inflammation.

Acute Inflammation Is Self-Limited

To maintain homeostasis, a class switch activity of enzymes from proinflammation to proresolution controls temporal regulation of acute inflammation.[34,39] For many years, our understanding of inflammation was mostly on initiation as an active process, whereas termination (a.k.a. resolution) was thought to be a passive process with decay of inflammation, (Fig. 12.1) until basic and translational studies from Drs. Charles Serhan and Thomas Van Dyke came to light that proved otherwise. Contrary to old belief, they showed that resolution is an active process that can be initiated only when enzymes produce bioactive proresolution lipids.[40,97,111]

In the context of acute inflammation initiation, locally produced LMs, such as prostaglandins, prostacyclin, leukotrienes (LTs), and thromboxanes (TXAs), regulate major processes and act as autacoids (short-lived molecules that act at the site of synthesis). These LMs are synthesized in a sequence of enzymatic activations when arachidonic acid (AA) is released from the cell membrane due to trauma or via cell-cell communication. Structurally, most of the lipids of inflammation are eicosanoids (20-carbon chains) and act as endogenous precursors for biosynthesis of a chain of several molecules. In fact, the enzyme phospholipase A2 releases AA from the phospholipid membrane. This release constitutes the rate-determining step in the generation of eicosanoids produced by most phagocytic and immune cells.[70] AA is rapidly converted into various potent LMs with specific functions in a cell-specific manner by cyclooxygenases (COXs), lipoxygenases (LOs), or epoxygenases to yield prostaglandins, LTs, and endoperoxides, respectively.

AAs are metabolized mostly by two major enzyme pathways: COXs and LOs. COX-1 (constitutively expressed COX) is responsible for basal levels of prostaglandin synthesis, whereas COX-2 (inducible COX) catalyzes the conversion of AA to LMs during inflammation. Prostaglandins comprise 10 subclasses, of which, D, E, F G, H, and I are the most important in inflammation. Specifically, PGE2 is generated via PGE synthase in leukocytes, whereas PGI2 is generated by prostacyclin synthase in endothelial cells and TXAs are generated via TXA synthase in platelets.[20,40]

LOs catalyze the formation of hydroxyeicosatetraenoic acids (HETEs) from AA, leading to the formation of LTs and other

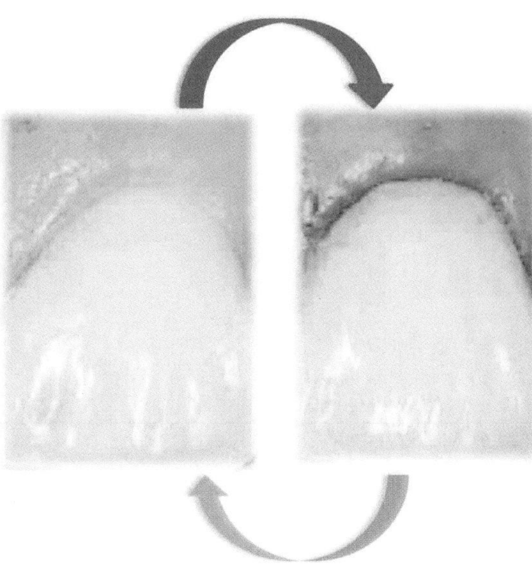

Fig. 12.1 Acute inflammation is self-limited. In clinical scenarios of health, resident cells, molecular mediators, and tissues respond to injury effectively and return to homeostasis. If acute inflammation is unresolved, chronic inflammation and disease will establish. Tissue healing is effective when a class switch from proinflammation to proresolution is activated. *CXC motif,* Chemokine; *IL,* interleukin; *NF-κB,* nuclear factor-κB; *TGF,* transforming growth factor; *TNF-α,* tumor necrosis factor-α.

biologically active compounds.[116] LTs are predominantly produced by inflammatory cells, including PMNs, macrophages, and mast cells. There are three distinct LOs that are cell specific: 5-LO in myeloid cells, 12-LO in platelets, and 15-LO in epithelial/endothelial cells. Cellular activation by pathogens and immune complexes results in activation of a sequential enzymatic reaction that includes cPLA2 and 5-LO. 5-LO converts released AA to the epoxide LTA4, which undergoes transformation by distinct pathways—one to generate LTB4, which is a potent regulator of neutrophil chemotaxis and leukocyte adhesion to endothelial cells.[40] The end products of 12- and 15-LO are 12- and 15-HETE, which are further metabolized. Excessive production of inflammatory mediators, such as prostaglandins and LTs, with an exacerbated sensing response to inflammatory triggers is correlated with progression from acute inflammation to chronic inflammation in many diseases. Favorable inflammatory processes are self-limiting, which implies the existence of termination signals that regulate acute inflammation. Endogenous proresolution lipids are produced by enzymatic pathways that switch inflammation to resolution.[95] In addition to proinflammatory mediators that turn on inflammation, there is a separate set of LMs that act as endogenous agonists to activate termination of inflammation by stimulating resolution.[92] The following sections provide a more detailed look at SLMs in the resolution of acute inflammation.

Specialized Lipid Mediators

Proresolution signals are activated mostly by resolvins, lipoxins, maresins, and protectins. LM class-switches biosynthesize proresolution LMs, such as lipoxin A4, eicosapentaenoic acid (EPA)-derived resolvins (i.e., RvE1, RvE2), and docosahexaenoic acid (DHA)-derived LMs including D-series resolvins, protectins, and maresins (Fig. 12.2).[114] More details on the key proresolution mediators are given next.

Lipoxins

Derived from AA, lipoxins are natural proresolving molecules produced from endogenous fatty acids. Lipoxins have strong dual antiinflammatory and proresolution actions. Lipoxins A4 and B4 were first isolated and identified as inhibitors of PMN infiltration and stimulators of nonphlogistic (nonfever) recruitment of macrophages.[35,45,91] Three main pathways of lipoxin synthesis have been identified. In humans, sequential oxygenation of AA-derived lipids by 15-LO and 5-LO, followed by enzymatic hydrolysis, leads to LXA4, and LXB4 occurs in the mucosal tissues, including the oral cavity, gastrointestinal tract, and airways, while in blood vessels, 5-LO biosynthesizes LXA4, and 12-LO in platelets produces LXB4. Lipoxin receptors are ubiquitously expressed by many cells, including neutrophils and monocytes. Aspirin triggers a third synthetic pathway. Aspirin promotes acetylation of COX-2, leading to a change in COX-2 activity and the chirality of the products, which are termed *aspirin-triggered lipoxins* (ATLs).[43] Cells that express COX-2 include vascular endothelial cells, epithelial cells, macrophages, and neutrophils.[100] In addition to the synthesis of lipoxin, aspirin also blocks prostaglandin synthesis by acetylation of COX-2, inhibiting inflammation.[85]

Resolvins

Resolvins are endogenous LMs induced during the resolution phase of inflammation. These LMs are biosynthesized from the essential ω-3 polyunsaturated fatty acids (PUFAs) (EPA and DHA) derived from the diet. The two primary groups of the resolvin family have distinct chemical structures: E-series, obtained from EPA,

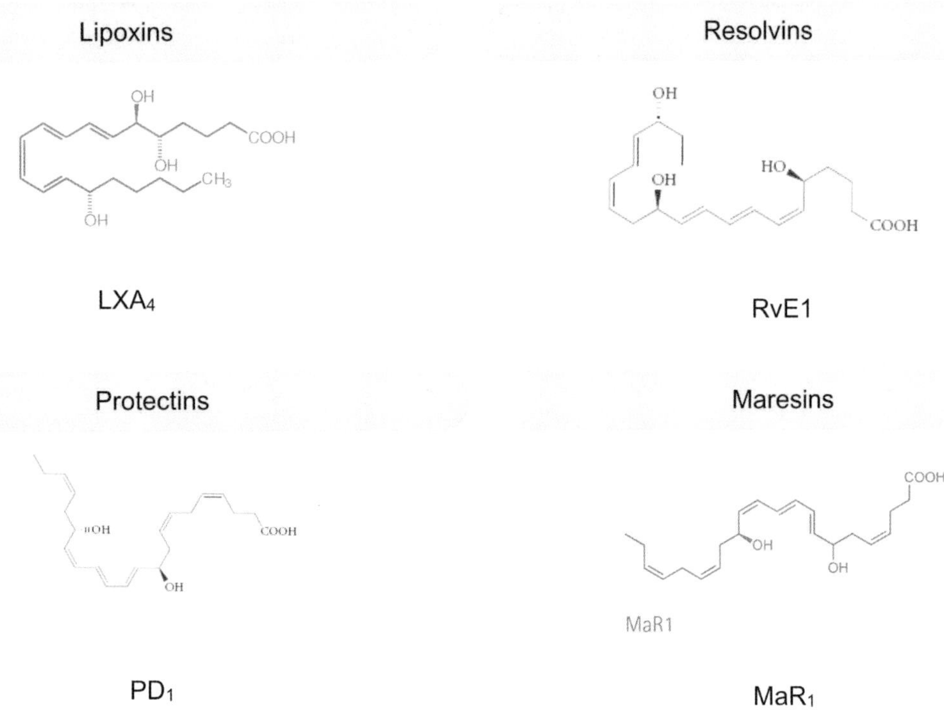

Fig. 12.2 Chemical structure of proresolution lipid mediators. Lipid mediator class switches yield lipoxins, eicosapentaenoic acid–derived E-series resolvins, and docosahexaenoic-acid derived D series resolvins, protectins, and maresins. *LXA_4*, Lipoxin A4; *MaR_1*, maresin 1; *PD_1*, protectin D1; *RvE_1*, resolvin E1.

and D-series, derived from DHA. Vascular endothelium produces E-series resolvins via aspirin-modified COX-2 that converts EPA to 18R-hydroperoxyeicoapentaenoic acid (18R-HPEPE) and 18S-HPEPE. Neutrophils are rapidly taken up by human monocytes and metabolized to RvE1 and RvE2 by 5-LO. Resolvin E1 production increases in plasma of individuals taking aspirin or EPA, resulting in amelioration of clinical signs of inflammation.[74] Similarly, DHA-derived D-series resolvins have been shown to reduce inflammation by decreasing platelet-leukocyte adhesion, and aspirin-triggered DHA conversion produces molecules with dual antiinflammatory and proresolution function.[98]

The interaction between resolvins and specific receptors modulates the fate of innate immune cells and counterregulates active inflammation. Selective target sites for resolvins are G protein–coupled receptors (GPCRs).[99] The ERV1 receptor (also known as ChemR23 or CMKLR1) is a GPCR expressed on monocytes and dendritic cells. BLT1, an LT receptor, is the resolvin E1 receptor on neutrophils. Upon selective binding to the receptors, RvE1 attenuates NF-κB signaling and production of proinflammatory cytokines including TNF-α.[16,83] D-series resolvins target GPR32 and ALX receptors[119] expressed on platelets and PMNs. Activation of CB2 leads to inhibition of P-selectin expression, decreasing PMN chemotaxis. Resolvins induce hallmark functions of resolution of inflammation, including decreasing neutrophil migration, phagocytosis of apoptotic cells, and increasing clearance of infection to activate tissue healing.[99]

Protectins

Protectins are also biosynthesized via an LO-mediated pathway. The pathway converts DHA into a 17S-hydroxyperoxide–containing intermediate that is taken up by leukocytes and converted into 10,17-diH-DHA, known as protectin D1 or neuroprotectin.[15] The name accounts for the protective actions observed in neural tissues and within the immune system. Human peripheral blood lymphocytes produce protectin D1 with a T helper 2 (Th2) phenotype, thereby reducing TNF-α and interferon-γ secretion, blocking T-cell migration, and promoting T-cell apoptosis.[77] A novel protectin synthesis pathway was found that uses aspirin-triggered COX-2 to synthesize epimeric 17R-hydroxyperoxide from DHA, called AT-PD1, and has shown a positive interaction with CB2 and peroxisome proliferator-activated receptor (PPAR) family receptors. Protectins reduce PMN transmigration through endothelial cells and enhance clearance (efferocytosis) of apoptotic PMN by human macrophages.[64]

Maresins

Macrophage mediators in resolving inflammation (maresins or MaR) have been identified as primordial molecules produced by macrophages with homeostatic functions. Metabololipidomic approaches in peritonitis models led to the identification of a novel pathway of DHA metabolism.[1] Macrophage phagocytosis of apoptotic cells triggers biosynthesis of RvE1, PD1, LXA4, and MaR1. Conversion of DHA into 14-hydroxy diHA was identified via the 14-LO cascade. MaR1 effectively stimulates efferocytosis of human cells and also has regenerative functions.[25]

In sum, the local LMs constitute a new genus of proresolving endogenous compounds with potent actions in treating immune-metabolic human diseases. Lipoxin A4/ATL and resolvin E1 have been shown to inhibit neutrophil recruitment, attenuate proinflammatory gene expression, and reduce the severity of colitis in a murine model. PMN infiltration and lymphatic removal of phagocytes were observed when resolvin E1, D2, protectin D1, lipoxin, and maresin were used to ameliorate colitis.[5,58]

Efferocytosis and Resolution

In addition to lipid and cytokine mediator signaling, cell death controls tissue response to inflammation. Apoptosis is a major mechanism of programmed cell death seen in inflamed tissues. The majority of apoptotic cells in inflamed gingival tissue are the neutrophils.[41] Apoptotic cells need to be cleared by macrophages, and their phagocytosis is designated efferocytosis (from *effere;* Latin for take to the grave, bury).

Efferocytosis is mediated by distinct receptors on macrophages, such as the T-cell immunoglobulin- and mucin domain–containing molecule-4 (TIMD-4), c-Mer tyrosine kinase receptor (MerTK), and the integrins αvβ3 and αvβ5.[86] Phosphatidylserine residues on the outer membrane surface of apoptotic cells serve as "eat-me" signals and thereby promote efferocytosis by interacting, either directly or indirectly, with efferocytic receptors on macrophages.[86] An example of the direct interaction involves TIMD-4, which can bind directly to phosphatidylserine on apoptotic cells.[35] The indirect mechanism involves the participation of opsonins, or "bridging molecules," such as the secreted protein developmental endothelial locus-1 (DEL-1) and the structurally related milk-fat-globule epidermal growth factor 8 (MFG-E8). Both DEL-1 and MFG-E8 facilitate efferocytosis by each binding to integrin αvβ3 via an RGD (Arg-Gly-Asp) motif present on their *N*-terminal segment that contains epidermal growth factor (EGF)-like repeats. At the same time, DEL-1 and MFG-E8 engage apoptotic cell-associated phosphatidylserine via their discoidin-I like domains in their *C*-terminal segments.[50,51,67] This structure-function relationship is depicted for DEL-1 in Fig. 12.3.

Efferocytosis Pathways and Resolution

The clearance of apoptotic cells through the process of efferocytosis prevents secondary necrosis and inflammation. However, efferocytosis acts above and beyond a "waste disposal" function, as it rewires the transcriptional profile of the macrophage, switching its phenotype from a proinflammatory to a proresolving macrophage (see Fig. 12.3). Indeed, during efferocytosis, macrophages are reprogrammed to downregulate the expression of proinflammatory cytokines and upregulate the expression of antiinflammatory cytokines such as TGF-β and IL-10.[67,68,84,105] Ligand-activated transcription factors of the nuclear receptor superfamily, such as liver X receptors (LXRs), play critical roles in efferocytosis and downstream signaling events that promote the resolution of inflammation.

LXRs occur in two isoforms (LXRα and LXRβ) that are triggered by oxidized derivatives of cholesterol. The uptake of apoptotic cells activates LXR signaling in the efferocytic macrophage, presumably in response to sterol lipids of the apoptotic plasma membrane. LXR signaling in turn upregulates the expression of efferocytic receptors (e.g., MerTK), thereby promoting further clearance of apoptotic cells, as well as the expression of molecules that contribute to inflammation resolution and tissue repair.[3,66] Such molecules include TGF-β, IL-1 receptor antagonist, and arachidonate 15-LO (ALOX15), an enzyme involved in the biosynthesis of precursor lipids required for the generation of SPMs. Moreover, LXR activation during efferocytosis blocks the expression of proinflammatory cytokines.[3,55,67,104,106]

It is important to note that not all efferocytic receptors are expressed by a given phagocyte and that the associated clearance mechanisms may operate in a tissue-specific manner. In a similar context involving efferocytic opsonins, although DEL-1 and MFG-E8 have an overall 50% identity at the amino acid sequence level and share several functions, they are typically expressed by different cell subsets and are regulated by distinct transcription factors.[48] We will next focus on DEL-1, which has been shown to promote resolution of periodontal inflammation.

Developmental Endothelial Locus-1–Mediated Efferocytosis and Resolution of Periodontitis

In the context of periodontitis, DEL-1 was originally shown to regulate the initiation of gingival inflammation by restraining the β_2 integrin–dependent recruitment of neutrophils.[31] In particular, endothelial cell–derived DEL-1 binds the αLβ2 integrin (a.k.a. lymphocyte function–associated antigen-1 [LFA-1]) on circulating neutrophils and prevents the interaction of this integrin with the

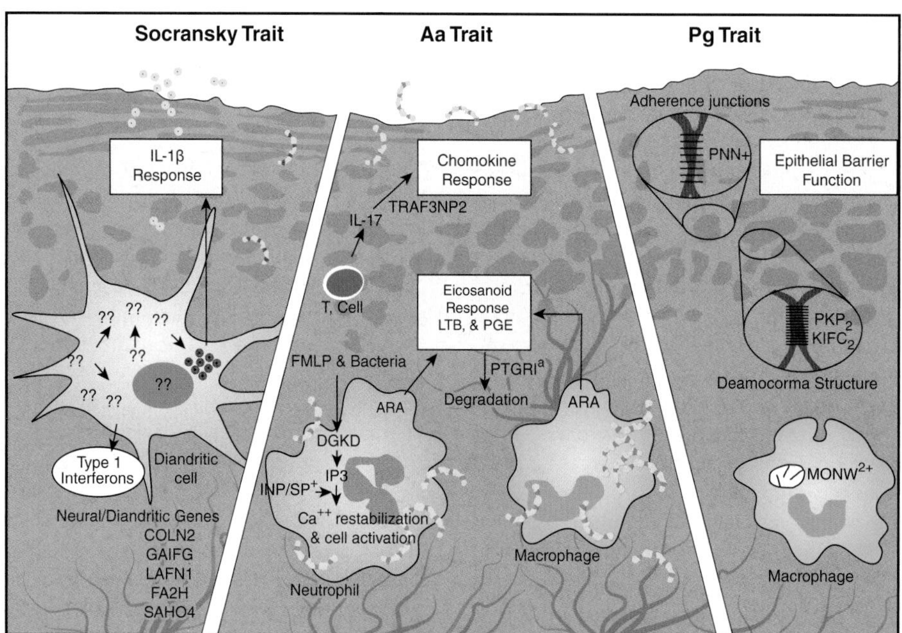

Fig. 12.3 Developmental endothelial locus-1 *(DEL-1)* promotes efferocytosis and the resolution of inflammation. DEL-1 binds, via its discoidin-I–like domains, to the "eat-me" signal phosphatidylserine (PS) on apoptotic neutrophils and, via its RGD site in the second EGF-like repeat, to the αvβ3 integrin on macrophages, thereby acting as an efferocytic "bridge" that promotes efferocytosis. In this manner, DEL-1 enhances liver X receptor *(LXR)*-dependent reprogramming of the efferocytic macrophage to adopt a proresolving phenotype. The release of factors, such as transforming growth factor-β *(TGF-β)* and resolvins, contributes to the resolution of periodontal inflammation. *EGF,* Epidermal growth factor.

intercellular adhesion molecule-1 (ICAM-1) on the vascular endothelium.[21] Since the αLβ2 integrin–ICAM-1 interaction is required for firm neutrophil adhesion on the endothelium and subsequent transendothelial migration, the interception of this adhesive interaction by DEL-1 attenuates neutrophil infiltration of the gingiva.[31] However, the levels of DEL-1 are relatively low during periodontitis, which contributes to increased neutrophil infiltration of the periodontium.

Interestingly, DEL-1 production is markedly upregulated during periodontal inflammation resolution in both mice and humans; importantly moreover, DEL-1 proactively contributes to the resolution of periodontal inflammation.[67] The proresolving function of DEL-1 was linked to its capacity to promote efferocytosis of apoptotic neutrophils by macrophages, which are thereby rewired to adopt a proresolving state. This reprogramming requires LXR-dependent signaling and leads to the upregulation of proresolving factors such as TGF-β and resolvins (see Fig. 12.3).[67] The anti–neutrophil-recruitment action is associated with endothelial cell–derived DEL-1, whereas the efferocytic/pro-resolving action is attributed to macrophage-derived DEL-1.[67]

DEL-1–deficient mice are unable to resolve periodontal inflammation and regenerate alveolar bone lost due to periodontitis, unless they are treated locally with recombinant DEL-1.[67,120] Furthermore, during inflammation resolution, DEL-1 enhances the stability and repressive function of T regulatory (Treg) cells, which restrain the expansion and effector functions of Th17 cells[71] that are pathogenic in periodontitis in both mice and humans.[27]

Intriguingly, resolvins contribute to the rising levels of DEL-1 during resolution.[67,73] This finding together with the observation that DEL-1–mediated efferocytosis increases the levels of resolvins (at least of RVD1 and RvE1) suggests a feedforward loop linking DEL-1 to resolvins and presumably reinforcing the resolution of inflammation. DEL-1 could thus be therapeutically exploited not only to inhibit the initiation of destructive inflammation but also to enhance resolution of inflammation and reconstitution of tissue integrity in the context of periodontal disease treatment.

Host Response Heterogeneity

The concept of a host response heterogeneity in periodontal disease pathogenesis is best exemplified by the "hyperinflammatory," unresolved response presented by some patients that leads to uncontrolled destruction of the periodontium. Currently, this exaggerated response has most often been attributed to the IL-1 genotype.[63] However, progress in the oral health domain to better understand disease underlying biology has illuminated previously unrecognized aspects of host susceptibility.[2,8,12] Recently, new periodontal disease taxonomies were developed to incorporate biologic information into the traditional clinical and radiographic parameters of periodontitis. This includes indirect measurements that are known to affect the oral microbiome and host response (risk factors diabetes and smoking)[108] and direct measurements derived from the oral cavity (levels of IL-1β and levels of periodontal pathogens).[26,82] The creation of these multidimensional traits aims to address disease heterogeneity, thereby improving the identification of periodontal disease subphenotypes and allowing patient care based on the biologic etiologic component.

Genetic studies have enlightened our understanding on periodontal host susceptibility and disease heterogeneity. Supplementation of clinical data with levels of eight periodontal pathogens and IL-1β identified six periodontal complex traits. Constructing biologically informed phenotypes has led to the identification of subgroups of periodontal disease with distinct "genetic signatures" but overlapping clinical presentations, each presenting distinct molecular pathways of inflammation (some never investigated in the context of

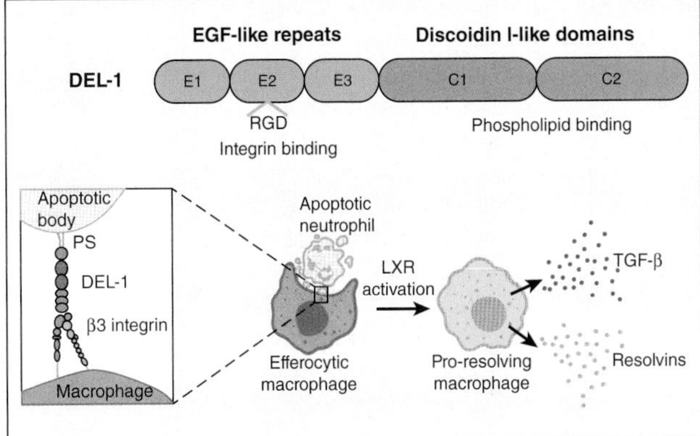

Fig. 12.4 Model of genetic and microbial patterns of periodontal disease defined by supplementing clinical data with biologic intermediates of microbial burden (levels of eight classic periodontal pathogens) and local inflammatory response (gingival crevicular fluid–interleukin [IL]-1b). (Figure derived from Zhang S, Divaris K, Moss K, et al. The novel ASIC2 locus is associated with severe gingival inflammation. *JDR Clin Trans Res.* 2016;1:163–170.)

periodontitis).[2,26,75,76,82,122] These genetic variants associated with immune responses and the epithelial barrier function, including the regulation of IL-1β activation (inflammasome sensors IFI16 and AIM2), prostanoid and LT metabolism (prostaglandin reductase 1), mucosal surface integrity (IL-17R adaptor protein gene TRAF3IP2), epithelial cell-cell adhesion function (desmosome structural protein PKP2 and tight junctions), phagocytosis (phagosome protein of macrophages MORN2), and nervous system–signaling proteins (BEGAIN and DLK1)[81]; see Fig. 12.4. These findings reveal a host heterogeneity that may be closer to the biologic and physiologic parameters that reflect the disease process. The dissection of these distinct molecular pathways may assist with the identification of druggable pathways and further development of tailored care, which is distinct from the current one-size-fits-all health care approach.[90] For example, proresolvin mediators may offer significant therapeutic advantages for the periodontal trait characterized by high *A. actinomycetemcomitans* levels and impaired neutrophilic phagocytosis (Aa trait shown in Fig. 12.4). However, adjuvant therapies for patients with the "Socransky trait" may be centered on inflammasome modulation.[128,130] We have initiated an exciting journey ahead of us that requires testing and validation of whether these genetic variants lead to distinct periodontitis-associated inflammatory networks that can be used to control periodontitis development and improve response to care.

KEY FACT

- Resolution of inflammation is an active biochemical process regulated by a class switch of enzymes and lipid mediators.
- A novel class of lipid mediators is known to modulate the resolution of inflammation; it consists of lipoxins, resolvins, maresins, and protectins.
- Efferocytosis is a process that promotes the clearance of apoptotic cells, thereby promoting inflammation resolution and tissue homeostasis.
- Host modifiers and variability, including genetic, behavioral, anatomic, metabolic, and environmental, modulate the magnitude of the disease and response to periodontal care.

Unresolved Chronic Inflammation in Periodontal Diseases

The oral host-microbial interactome modulates oral and systemic immune development, and a physiologic interaction maintains the homeostatic response. Periodontal diseases are chronic inflammatory diseases initiated by dybiosis and microbial biofilms.[21] In the case of gingivitis, acute inflammation is self-limited and reversible. When the etiologic factor and modifiers are "removed," the host returns to health. When stimuli persist, unresolved inflammation causes chronic lesions, loss of attachment, disease progression, and tissue loss. The host immune response functions as a protective mechanism, but continuous or exacerbated response risks the tissue integrity.[80]

The presence of plaque bacteria is highly prevalent in humans; in fact, 90% of the adult dentate population presents with some form of gingivitis.[27] Through coevolution, host-microbiota interactions result in host benefits including, nutrient utilization, colonization resistance, and immune development.[21,45]

Although plaque is an evident etiologic factor in gingivitis, in periodontitis the specificity or number of the pathogens has not explained the variability in individual host response. Despite abundant microbial deposits in most people, the prevalence of moderate periodontitis is only around 40% of the population.[64] It is therefore possible that bacteria are not the primary factor of gingivitis-periodontitis transition. Although "plaque" is a traditional concept in etiology, the host presents multiple variations that provide increased susceptibility to changing taxonomic composition of the plaque and metabolomic functions.[112] Resolution failure is a plausible explanation of this health-pathologic transition.

Host modifiers and variability, including genetic, behavioral, anatomic, metabolic, and environmental, modulate the magnitude of the disease. These factors influence the disease severity, progression, and response to therapy. Classic studies in the 1980s showed that intake of antiinflammatory medications prevented the progression of periodontal disease.[57] Although this was promising, it is now clear that inflammation is an important biologic process, and complete suppression of its cascade influences the host entirely. Instead of suppressing the system, resolution aims to enhance "good" inflammation to terminate the disease process.[65,88] In fact, deficient phagocytosis is seen in aggressive forms of periodontitis and is reversed by resolution mediators.[37,48] Thus host-derived etiology is now well accepted and is a target for future therapies.

In a clinical trial of patients with moderate to severe periodontitis, the actions of dietary supplementation of ω-3 PUFA and aspirin were evaluated. In patients taking the preceding supplements, in addition to scaling and root planing (SRP), significant improvements were noted in pocket depth reduction and clinical attachment level gain, with lower levels of inflammatory mediators in saliva compared with patients who underwent SRP alone.[29] LMs are considered excellent candidates for the prevention and treatment of periodontal diseases.

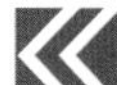

FLASH BACK

Bacteria have been recognized for years as the main etiologic factor for periodontal diseases. With advances in molecular immunology and genetics, inflammation and resolution pathways have shown to play an integral part in the multifactorial pathogenesis of periodontal diseases.

Therapeutic Actions of Resolution Mediators

Periodontal diseases, including gingivitis and periodontitis, are leukocyte-driven inflammatory conditions characterized by soft-tissue and osteoclast-mediated bone loss.[64,80,102] Resolution mediators are needed to control and treat periodontal diseases. In animal models, restoration of tissue health by resolution lipids is initiated after acute response generates classic eicosanoids, prostanoids, and prostacyclins and LTs. The synthesis of immune-resolvents by key enzymes that induce a class switch is partially known.[93] Thus return to homoeostasis is highly regulated by resolution pathways (Table 12.1).

Evidence from animal studies demonstrated that overexpression of 15-LO type I in rabbits increased endogenous levels of LXA4, protecting the host from developing periodontal disease. Although no animal model is a perfect fit for humans, as proof-of principle, these concepts could be translated. In addition, RvE1 when topically applied to the tissues ameliorates signs of disease activity, decreasing bone loss by 95% and significantly reducing the number of tissue neutrophils. Leukocyte infiltration was also reduced when RvE1 was applied in a murine dorsal air pouch model.[59] Similarly, in human cells obtained from LAP, RvE1 and LXA4 treatment decreased neutrophil superoxide production in response to TNF-α and the bacterial surrogate peptide marker N-formyl-methionyl-leucyl-phenylalanine by 80%.[37,109,121]

The potential for treatment of periodontal diseases with one or a combination of SLMs is clear and requires further investigation clinically. In one trial, SRP with dietary supplementation of ω-3 PUFA and lower dose of aspirin reduced pocket depths and increased clinical attachment levels significantly when compared with SRP alone.[30] The clinical benefits were accompanied by lower levels of inflammatory mediators in saliva compared with SRP alone.[29]

Failure to remove pathobions and inefficient clearance of the innate immune cells (mainly dead neutrophils) characterize the progression to chronic pathologic lesion. In susceptible individuals, periodontal inflammation fails to resolve, and chronic inflammation becomes periodontal pathology. In periodontitis, primed neutrophils can mediate destruction and feedforward destruction of the extracellular matrix, bone, scarring, and loss of periodontal tissue function.[21] In an inflammatory model, resolvin D1 has been associated with the regulation of miRNAs and target genes and the reduction of LTB4, PGD2, TXA2, PGF2α, and TXA2 in peritoneal exudates.

CLINICAL CORRELATION

- Inflammation is a biologic protective mechanism against injury.
- Acute inflammation seen in gingivitis is reversible and self-limited.
- Chronic inflammation in periodontitis has a failure of signals that activate resolution and return to homeostasis.
- Inflammation and resolution are connecting links with systemic conditions (e.g., type 2 diabetes, cancer, autoimmune and cardiovascular diseases) and periodontal diseases.

Tissue regeneration has also been a target of specialized resolution mediators. Treatment with maresin 1 has been demonstrated to stimulate tissue regeneration in system models, including planaria models.[97] Consistently in periodontal disease models, lipoxin A4/ATL prevented connective tissue and bone loss. Treatment of experimental periodontitis with LMs completely resolved inflammation and rescued tissue loss with the regeneration of periodontal tissues.[111,113] It has been suggested that defective endogenous resolution of inflammation underlies the inflammatory phenotype presented in chronic diseases and that exogenous therapeutic molecules rescue this phenotype. Proresolution LMs play a role as natural molecules in the maintenance of homeostasis with promising potential as therapeutic agents in human diseases.[36,39]

TABLE 12.1 Therapeutic Actions of Proresolution Lipid Mediators

Disease Models	Lipid Mediator Therapeutic Actions	References
Periodontitis	**Lipoxin A4/ATL**	
	Rescues attachment loss	Van Dyke et al. (2008)
	Enhances tissue healing	Serhan et al. (2003)
	Promotes periodontal regeneration	Van Dyke et al. (2015)
	Ceases infiltration of neutrophils	Van Dyke et al. (2015)
	Resolvin E1	
	Decreases bone loss	Hasturk et al. (2005)
	Lowers number of osteoclasts	Hasturk et al. (2007)
Type 2 diabetes	**Resolvin E1**	
	Increases cell counts	Herrera et al. (2015)
	Increases chemotaxis	Tang et al. (2013)
	Rescues phagocytosis	Freire et al. (2017)
	Resolvin D1	
	Increases monocyte recruitment	Spite et al. (2014)
	Decreases inflammation in adipocytes	Spite et al. (2014)
Colitis	**Lipoxin A4/ATL**	
	Decreases severe colitis	Aliberti et al. (2002)
	Proinflammatory gene expression is	Gewirtz et al. (2002)
	downexpressed	Gewirtz et al. (2002)
	Reduces immune dysregulation	Wallace et al. (2003)
	Resolvin E1	
	Improves animal survival rate	Arita et al. (2005)
	Reduces weight loss	Arita et al. (2005)
	Activates LPS detoxification	Campbell et al. (2010)
	Inhibits neutrophil recruitment	Ishida et al. (2010)
	AT-Resolvin D1	
	Reduces diseases activity index	Bento et al. (2011)
	Attenuates proinflammatory mediators' gene expression	Bento et al. (2011)
	Attenuates neutrophil recruitment	Bento et al. (2011)
	Resolvin D-2	
	Ameliorates disease activity index	Bento et al. (2011)
	Reduces colonic polymorphonuclear leukocyte infiltration	Bento et al. (2011)
Retinopathy	**Protectin D1**	
	Protects against neovascularization	Connor et al. (2007)
Calvaria defects	**Resolvin E1**	
	Promotes bone regeneration in calvaria defects	Gao et al. (2012)

ATL, Aspirin-triggered lipoxins; *LPS*, lipopolysaccharide.

Final Remarks

The role of acute inflammation is protection of the host and development of tissue integrity. The fate of this process is determined by the balance and magnitude of how cells and mediators amplify the inflammatory process or control the restoration to normal health. It is now evident that the resolution of inflammation is modulated by protective mediators, such as AA-derived lipoxins and ATLs, ω-3 EPA–derived resolvins of the E-series, DHA-derived resolvins of the D series, protectins, and maresins. The selective interaction of the LMs with GPCR receptors of innate immune cells induces the cessation of leukocyte infiltration; the return to normal levels of vascular permeability/edema; PMN death (mostly via apoptosis); and nonphlogistic infiltration of monocyte/macrophages. Macrophage removal of apoptotic PMN via efferocytosis, foreign agents (bacteria), and necrotic debris from the site via phagocytosis initiates clearance. Macrophages and other phagocytes migrate to lymphatics. These cellular events lead to resolution with a return

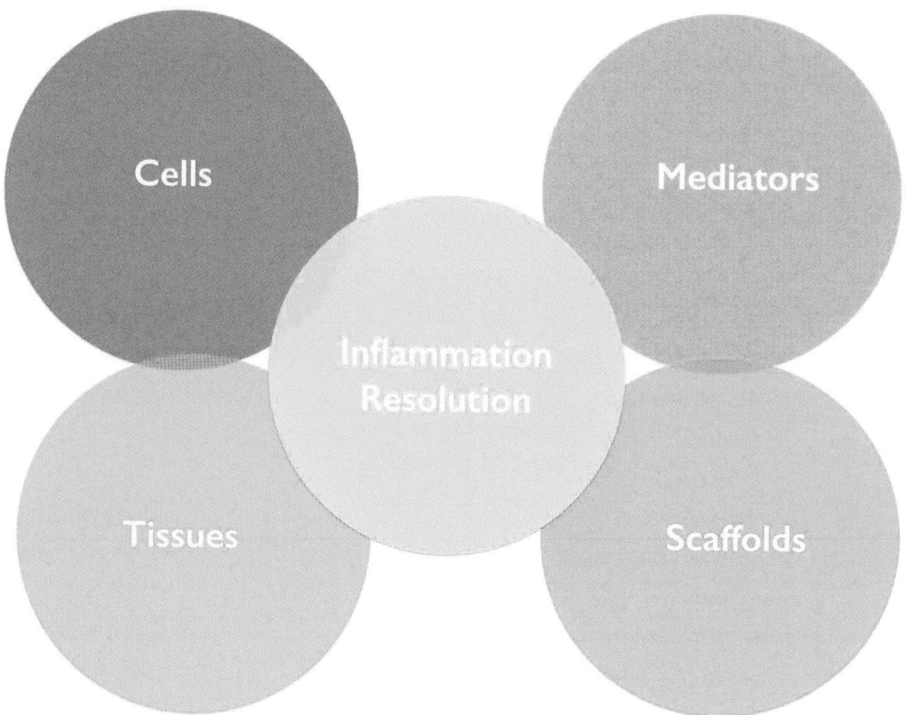

Fig. 12.5 Inflammation resolution is a key component of tissue healing and regeneration. Upon antigenic challenge, cells, tissue, vasculature, and mediators have to synchronize the host response to adequately remove triggers and protect the host prior to regeneration. Resolution of inflammation has main functions in the activation of cells to promote clearance, return to homeostasis, and together with the factors described promote tissue regeneration.

to predisease homeostasis. Unresolved inflammation is a hallmark of various human diseases including diabetes, ulcerative colitis, rheumatoid arthritis, cancer, CVDs, and periodontitis. The fate of acute inflammation determines the restoration to homeostasis versus disease establishment. Diseases associated with uncontrolled acute inflammation are characterized by a continuous release of histotoxic substances that results in local tissue damage, prolonged inflammatory response, and loss of function. In contrast, in health, the fate of inflammation is influenced by endogenous mediators, cells, tissue, and scaffolds to resolve the acute process and reestablish homeostasis, thereby promoting tissue healing and regeneration (Fig. 12.5).[7]

A localized inflammatory response to an injury or infection is a spatially defined and temporally regulated process that ideally should be self-limited as previously described. If the lesion does not resolve and becomes chronic, the acquired immune system is stimulated, including broad activation of lymphocytic pathways as well as cell-mediated and humoral immunity. The chronicity of the lesion alters molecular, cellular, and overall tissue responses in remote regions of the body having a transient or permanent impact on overall health.

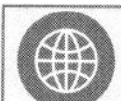 A Case Scenario is found on the companion website eBooks.Health.Elsevier.com.

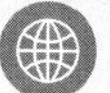 References for this chapter are found on the companion website eBooks.Health.Elsevier.com.

CHAPTER 13

Aging and the Periodontium

Ian Needleman | Daniel R. Clark

CHAPTER OUTLINE

Changing Patterns of Periodontal Health in Older People

Increased health awareness and improvements in preventive dentistry have led to decreasing tooth loss for all age groups, although the prevalence of periodontitis in older populations remains high.[18] In some populations, it is predicted that by 2030, one-third of older adults will have no tooth loss[32] with a 27% increase in the number of teeth requiring periodontal treatment.[70] The effects of this shift in tooth retention need to be considered carefully. Clearly, there will be an increased public health need for periodontal care in older individuals and an increase in demand might also be anticipated. However, policy recommendations from the European Geriatric Medicine Society and European College of Gerodontology have identified that poor oral health including periodontitis is prevalent in the elderly and largely undiagnosed because those who are frail (or thought to be so) do not receive routine dental care due to a number of barriers and misconceptions.[35] It has also been reported that older age is associated with a greater simultaneous occurrence of both caries and periodontitis, highlighting an increased need for health management.[53] Current research is also identifying important and wider implications for health in older people. Poor periodontal health is associated with increased medical costs of dementia[67] as well as increased levels of disability and poor physical function.[36] Perhaps unsurprisingly, decreased oral function, for which periodontitis-associated tooth loss is a major contributor, is a risk for poorer nutrition and sarcopenia (progressive loss of skeletal muscle mass and strength), introducing a concept of "oral frailty."[80] Therefore an understanding of the impact of aging on the periodontium is critical to contribute to overall management of health. This chapter will first review the literature concerning the fundamental aspects of aging on the periodontal tissues; broader aspects of aging will then be examined and their possible effects on treatment outcomes discussed. The chapter has been updated following a detailed search of new research published since 2016.

The evidence base is not without problems, many of which make it difficult to draw conclusions about the effects of aging. Some of these problems include inconsistency with regard to the definition of a true "older" group, the inadequate exclusion of adults with systemic diseases that can modify study findings, and attempts to extrapolate results from animal research. For the purposes of this chapter, the effects of aging will be limited to a narrow review of possible biologic and microbiologic changes. For further reading about the effects of aging on the dental and periodontal patient, the reader should consult Holm-Pedersen, Walls & Ship: Textbook of Geriatric Dentistry, Wiley-Blackwell, 2015, Oxford 3rd edition.[30] The reader should be fully aware that this excludes many important age-associated phenomena, including reductions in an individual's cognitive or motor function skills, which may have a direct impact on periodontal management. These will be discussed more fully in Chapter 29.[65]

CLINICAL CORRELATION

For a full understanding of aging and managing periodontal health, in addition to this chapter on biology, readers should understand aging more broadly including cognitive and motor function effects that might affect oral hygiene for instance.

Since first writing this chapter more than 20 years ago, the volume of new research into aging and the periodontium has increased slowly. This is particularly the case in relation to human clinical studies. Despite the limited data directly related to periodontal health, much effort and many resources have been employed to research questions at least partially related to this topic. These include the effect of periodontal infection on general health (see Chapter 26) and the impact of osteoporosis on periodontal status (see Chapter 25).

Effects of Aging on the Periodontium

Gingival Epithelium

Thinning and decreased keratinization of the gingival epithelium have been reported with age.[72] The significance of these findings

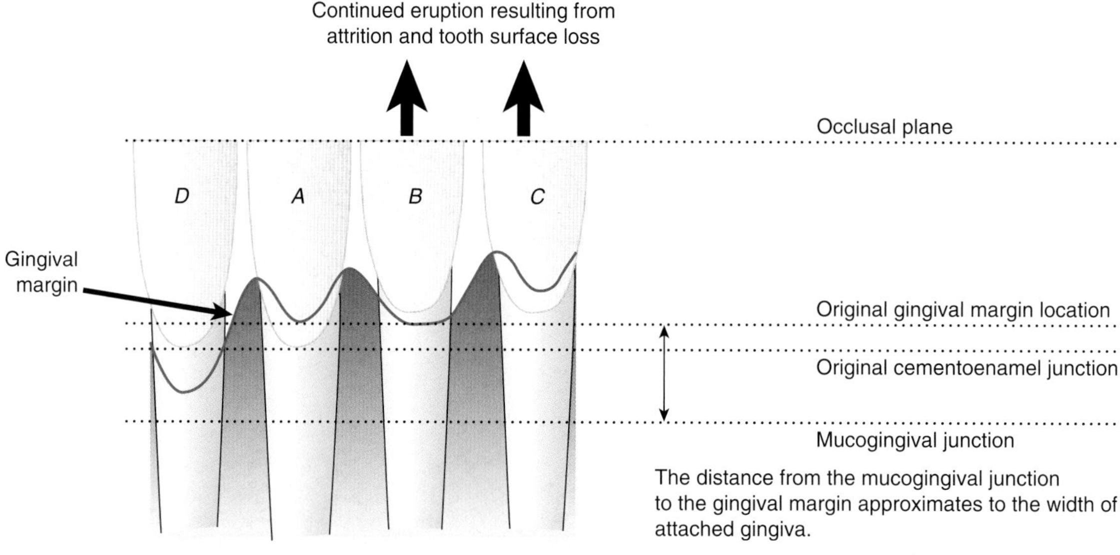

Fig. 13.1 Diagram showing the relationship of the gingival margin with the crown and root surface. (A) Normal relationship with the gingival margin 1 to 2 mm above the cementoenamel junction. (B) Wear of the incisal edge and continued tooth eruption. The gingival margin remains in the same position as shown in (A). Therefore the root surface is exposed, and clinical recession is evident. The width of the attached gingiva has not changed. (C) Wear of the incisal edge and continued tooth eruption. The gingival margin has moved with the tooth; therefore the entire dentogingival complex has moved coronally, with a resulting increase in the width of the attached gingiva. (D) No wear of incisal edge is evident. The gingiva has moved apically, and clinical recession is evident. The width of attached gingiva is reduced.

could mean an increase in epithelial permeability to bacterial antigens, a decreased resistance to functional trauma, or both. If so, such changes may influence long-term periodontal outcomes. However, other studies have found no age-related differences in the gingival epithelium of humans or dogs.[11,33] Other reported changes with aging include the flattening of rete pegs and altered cell density. Conflicting data regarding the surgical regeneration times for gingival epithelium have been ascribed to problems with research methodology.[79]

The effect of aging on the location of the junctional epithelium has been the subject of much speculation. Some reports show migration of the junctional epithelium from its position in healthy individuals (i.e., on the enamel) to a more apical position on the root surface with accompanying gingival recession.[11] However, in other animal studies, no apical migration has been noted.[40] With continuing gingival recession, the width of the attached gingiva would be expected to decrease with age, but the opposite appears to be true.[2,3] Alternatively, the migration of the junctional epithelium to the root surface could be caused by the tooth erupting through the gingiva in an attempt to maintain occlusal contact with its opposing tooth (i.e., passive eruption) as a result of tooth surface loss from attrition (Fig. 13.1). The consensus is that gingival recession is not an inevitable physiologic process of aging, but rather that it can be explained by the cumulative effects of inflammation or trauma on the periodontium (Fig. 13.2)[8,11]; this is discussed in more detail later in this chapter. Changes in the apoptotic gene expression of gingival tissue with age have recently been reported in nonhuman primates.[26] This finding requires further research to understand its potential impact on gingival homeostasis and the pathogenesis of periodontal diseases.

KEY FACT

Gingival recession is not an inevitable consequence of aging but is the cumulative result of trauma or periodontitis.

Gingival Connective Tissue

Increasing age results in coarser and denser gingival connective tissues.[83] Qualitative and quantitative changes to collagen have been reported. These include an increased rate of conversion of soluble to insoluble collagen, increased mechanical strength, and increased denaturing temperature. These results indicate increased collagen stabilization caused by changes in the macromolecular conformation.[66] Not surprisingly, an increased collagen content has been found in the gingivae of older animals, despite a lower rate of collagen synthesis decreasing with age.[11,79]

Periodontal Ligament

Changes in the periodontal ligament that have been reported with aging include decreased numbers of fibroblasts and a more irregular structure, thus paralleling the changes seen in the gingival connective tissues.[11,66,79] Other findings include decreased organic matrix production, epithelial cell rests, and increased amounts of elastic fiber.[79] Conflicting results have been reported for changes in the width of the periodontal ligament in human and animal models. Although true variation may exist, this finding probably reflects the functional status of the teeth in the studies: the width of the space will decrease if the tooth is unopposed (i.e., hypofunction) or increase with excessive occlusal loading.[79] Both scenarios can be anticipated as a result of tooth loss in this population. These effects may also explain the variability in studies that have reported qualitative changes within the periodontal ligament.

Recognition that the periodontal ligament has an important role in alveolar bone metabolism has led to an increased interest in investigating this role in relation to the maintenance of periodontal health and the pathogenesis of periodontitis. One approach to investigating this role is to examine mediators of bone homeostasis, such as receptor activator of nuclear factor-κB ligand (RANKL) and osteoprotegerin (OPG). RANKL is widely recognized for its role in activating osteoclasts, whereas OPG antagonizes RANKL binding, thus helping to maintain balance. The interplay of cytokines—and,

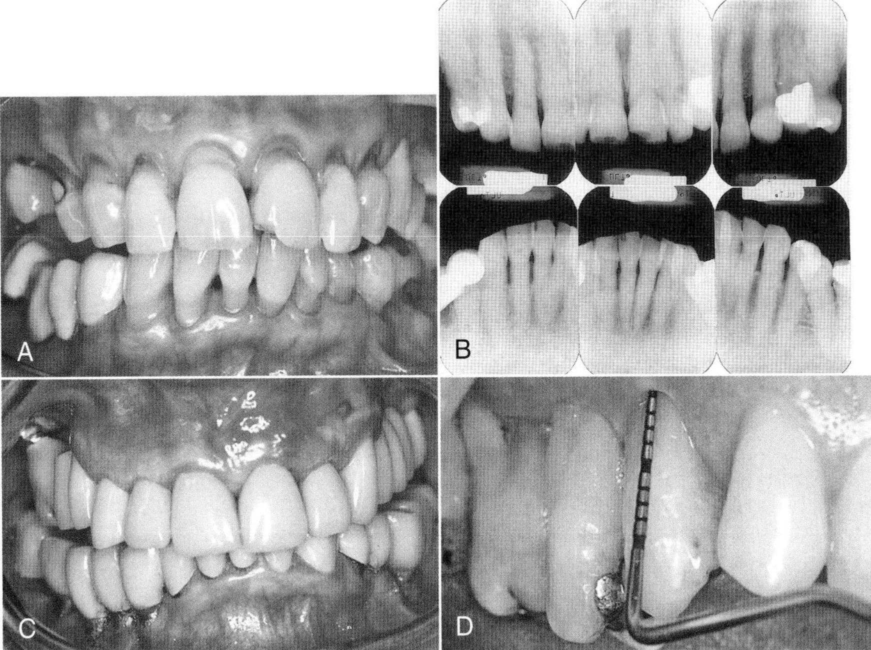

Fig. 13.2 Three scenarios illustrating the variation of the position of the gingival margin with age. (A) Overeruption with recession in an older individual (i.e., a 68-year-old woman) with generalized recession and a history of previously treated periodontitis. Note some overeruption of the lower anterior teeth and wear of teeth related to oral hygiene measures. (B) Radiographs of the patient shown in (A). (C) Overeruption without recession in an older individual (i.e., a 72-year-old woman) with no periodontitis but marked lower incisor tooth wear and overeruption. Note how the gingival margin has migrated coronally with the erupting teeth. (D) Extensive recession in a younger individual (i.e., a 32-year-old man) with marked recession and no history of periodontitis. The recession has resulted from a combination of anatomically thin tissues and toothbrush-related trauma.

in particular, the interleukin family—has also been extensively researched in periodontal disease pathogenesis. Some of the interleukins are potent mediators of inflammation (e.g., IL-1), whereas others have been shown to downregulate this process (e.g., IL-4, IL-10). Therefore evaluating the balance between these homeostatic processes would seem to be of great merit when evaluating possible negative changes in the periodontium. Such a strategy appears to be predictive of hard-tissue destruction among individuals with rheumatoid arthritis.[24] Recent findings comparing periodontal ligament cells in older individuals (i.e., >60 years old) with those of younger individuals (i.e., 15 to 20 years old) have suggested greater gene expression for pro-inflammatory cytokines.[10] This has been reported more widely as an age-associated change, although it is unclear whether it is a cause or an effect.[57] However, in addition to increased IL-1 and IL-6 expression, OPG was also increased, which suggests that increased OPG may be a homeostatic response to the upregulation of inflammation.[10] If this homeostatic mechanism was effective, it may explain why an increase in inflammation did not result in greater tissue damage with age. Periodontal ligament cell proliferation was decreased with age, thereby suggesting an impairment of repair potential, although such an impact does not appear to be manifested clinically.[82] Further research investigating periodontal ligament cells from individuals diagnosed with periodontitis will be important to understand the potentially important relationship between aging and periodontal ligament cells.

Cementum

Some consensus regarding the effect of aging on cementum exists. An increase in cemental width is a common finding; this increase may be 5 to 10 times with increasing age.[11] This finding is not surprising, because deposition continues after tooth eruption. The increase in width is greater apically and lingually.[79] Although cementum has limited capacity for remodeling, an accumulation of resorption bays explains the finding of increasing surface irregularity.[27]

Alveolar Bone

Reports of morphologic changes in alveolar bone mirror age-related changes in other bony sites. Specific to the periodontium are findings of a more irregular periodontal surface of bone and the less-regular insertion of collagen fibers.[79] Although age is a risk factor for the bone mass reductions in individuals with osteoporosis, it is not causative and therefore should be distinguished from physiologic aging processes.[31] Overriding the diverse observations of bony changes with age is the important finding that the healing rate of bone in extraction sockets appears to be unaffected by increasing age.[4] Indeed, the success of osseointegrated dental implants, which relies on intact bone healing responses, does not appear to be age related.[12] However, balancing this view is the observation that bone graft preparations (i.e., decalcified freeze-dried bone) from donors who were more than 50 years old possessed significantly less osteogenic potential than graft material from younger donors.[69] The possible significance of this phenomenon for normal healing responses needs to be investigated.

Bacterial Plaque

In a classic experimental gingivitis study, participants were rendered free of plaque and inflammation through frequent professional cleaning. After this was achieved, they abstained from oral hygiene measures for periods of 3 weeks to allow gingivitis to develop.[44] In this experimental model, a comparison of developing gingivitis between younger and older individuals demonstrated a greater inflammatory response in older participants, in both humans and dogs.[11,21,22,29] In the older age group (i.e., 65 to 80 years), the findings included a greater amount of infiltrated connective tissue, increased gingival crevicular fluid flow, and an increased gingival index.[21,22] The increased severity of gingivitis in the older group may be explained by age-related changes to the microbial plaque or age-related changes to the host inflammatory response. Our understanding of how the oral microbiome and the host inflammatory response change with age is discussed later. Dentogingival plaque accumulation has been suggested to increase with age.[29] This might be explained by the increase in hard-tissue surface area as a result of gingival recession and the surface characteristics of the exposed root surface as a substrate for plaque formation as compared with enamel. Other studies have shown no difference in plaque quantity with age. This contradiction might reflect the different age ranges of experimental groups as variable degrees of gingival recession and root surface exposure. For supragingival plaque, no real qualitative differences have been shown for plaque composition.[29] With regard to subgingival plaque, one study has shown subgingival flora to be similar to normal flora, whereas another study reported increased numbers of enteric rods and pseudomonads in older adults.[52,75] Recent advances in high-throughput 16S ribosomal RNA gene sequencing have enhanced our understanding of the complexity of the oral microbiome in health and disease. Research using the sequencing technologies has largely supported the earlier findings that the subgingival microbiome is largely unaffected by age in healthy human subjects, with no significant changes in the quantity or proportions of the bacterial species reported.[19,38] The most significant age-related change in the subgingival microbiota of healthy older individuals compared to young was an increase in *Actinomyces* species.[19] Similar age-related changes have previously been demonstrated by others using culture-dependent techniques.[61] The significance of the increased *Actinomyces* species in older adults has yet to be determined and may be a function of age-related changes in ecologic determinants for periodontal bacteria, such as increased presence of protheses or increased exposed root surfaces.[9] In addition, periodontitis results in a significant shift in the composition of the subgingival microbiome and this change in microbial species was similar within old and young age groups.[19]

Another approach to investigating the microbiological aspects is to conduct intervention studies and to examine their impact on the microflora. Among individuals who were 60 to 75 years old, the prevalence of *Porphyromonas gingivalis, Treponema forsythia, Treponema denticola, Aggregatibacter actinomycetemcomitans,* and *Prevotella intermedia* was high and not clearly related to probing depth.[62] The finding of high levels of the organisms could have been related to the sample of individuals: the participants were mostly those with low incomes and with no recent dental care. Long-term use (i.e., 5 years) of a 0.12% chlorhexidine mouthrinse did not promote reductions in the proportions of the organisms in individuals experiencing alveolar bone loss as compared with the placebo mouthrinse, possibly as a result of the mouthrinse routine being less frequent than daily.[62]

KEY FACT

There is no clear evidence that aging affects the microbiology of dental plaque.

Immune and Inflammatory Responses

Increased age does not appear to result in an obvious shift toward a more pathogenic microbial population. Therefore, it is reasonable to consider that age-related changes to the host response may contribute to the increased periodontitis experience in older populations.

The study of the biology of aging has demonstrated many pathophysiological changes that occur with aging including a chronically elevated and dysregulated inflammatory response that has been termed inflamm-aging.[20] Examples of inflamm-aging have been demonstrated systemically with studies measuring increased levels of circulating IL-6, tumor necrosis factor-α (TNF-α), and C-reactive protein (CRP) in older adults compared with young adults even after all systemic disease and conditions are controlled for.[50] Inflamm-aging has been proposed to contribute to the increased prevalence of many age-related diseases. As proper inflammatory regulation is critical to maintaining periodontal health, inflamm-aging may, in part, drive the increased prevalence of periodontitis in older adults.

Immune cells, including neutrophils, macrophages, and T cells, which are critical for host defense and inflammatory regulation to maintain periodontal health, have demonstrated age-related changes that may contribute to the increased prevalence of disease in older populations (Fig. 13.3). Neutrophils, the first line of defense

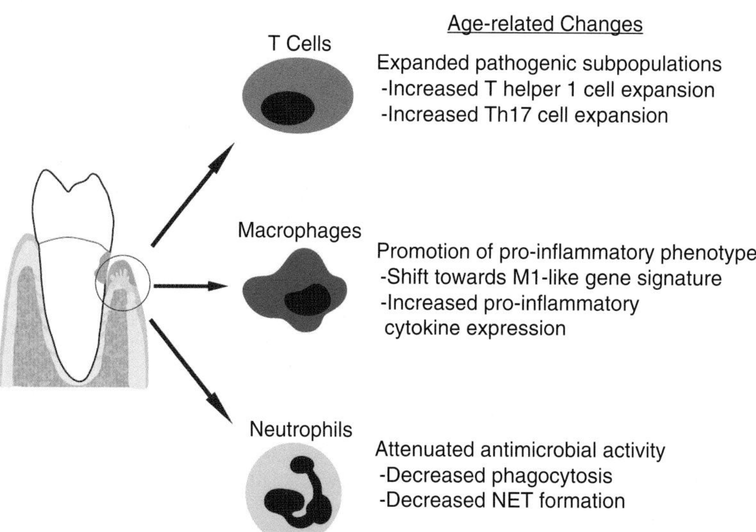

Fig. 13.3 Age-related changes to immune cells may promote periodontal diseases in aging populations. Immune cells, including T cells, macrophages, and neutrophils, are critical host defense mechanisms within the periodontium. These cells are also implicated in the pathogenesis of periodontal diseases. Age-related changes in these immune cells have been observed and may enhance their pathogenicity in periodontal diseases. The pathogenic changes that have been observed with increased age are described.

to bacteria in relation to periodontal diseases, show decreased antimicrobial activity with increasing age. Bacterial phagocytosis by neutrophils is decreased with age.[81] Similarly, formation of neutrophil extracellular traps, a mechanism for trapping and killing bacterial extracellularly, is decreased with increasing age.[28] Additionally, macrophages are key regulators of inflammation in periodontal diseases that respond early during infection to propagate inflammation and are also present later to actively resolve inflammation. Intrinsic age-related changes appear to shift the macrophage toward a more pro-inflammatory (M1-type) phenotype.[14] In addition, increased inflammatory cytokines produced by M1-type macrophages were present in the gingiva of old mice compared with young.[39] In a mouse model, therapeutically depleting the macrophages resulted in improved resolution of periodontitis in old mice while having no effect in young mice, further suggesting the pathogenic contribution of macrophages in old populations.[15]

Subsets of T cells are implicated in the pathogenesis of periodontitis. With increased age, T-cell differentiation is promoted toward T helper 1 (Th1) cells.[86] Th1 cells demonstrate pro-inflammatory cytokine expression and are associated with increased bone resorption.[77] Another pathogenic subset of T cells involved in periodontitis is the Th17 cell. Th17 cells produce the pro-inflammatory cytokine IL-17, and inhibition of Th17 expansion was shown to decrease periodontitis severity in animal models.[17] Increased expansion of Th17 cells was demonstrated in circulating blood samples of older humans compared with young, and increased quantities of Th17 cells were also shown in the periodontium of old humans and mice compared with young.[16,68] The age-related changes to innate and adaptive immune cells involved in the pathogenesis of periodontitis further demonstrate the potential impact of aging on periodontal health.

In relation to systematic inflammatory responses, CRP is an acute phase protein that is widely regarded as a marker of inflammatory burden and response to bacterial infection.[73] When investigating serum CRP levels among individuals who are 60 to 75 years old and comparing individuals having progressive periodontitis with those with stable disease, CRP levels were increased in those with progressive periodontitis and no other systemic conditions.[76] This may indicate that inflammatory burden can be investigated with the use of CRP, although there is growing evidence that CRP alone may not be as reliable a marker in older people.[63]

A further modulator of the immune and inflammatory responses is nutrition. Interest in this field is increasing rapidly as part of both medicine and periodontology.[13] Nutrition has been studied extensively in geriatric medicine as a result of the nutritional intake changes that occur with age. The impact of this as a potential risk factor for periodontal diseases and their progression is therefore of interest. Data have started to appear that suggest a negative association of serum folate with periodontitis. After controlling for major known confounders, lower serum folate levels in dentate adults who are more than 60 years old are associated with greater levels of periodontitis.[85] These cross-sectional data cannot demonstrate causality alone, but the recognized relationship between folate protection for chronic inflammatory diseases (e.g., cardiovascular disease[48]) offers biologic plausibility to a potential relationship that merits further investigation with prospective studies.

Although many contradictions exist, a survey of the literature demonstrates that some age-related changes are evident in the periodontium and the host response. Whether these changes are significant in the alteration of the progression of periodontal diseases or the response of an older adult to periodontal treatment will be examined next.

KEY FACT

Cellular mediators of the host inflammatory response demonstrate age-related changes that may contribute to the pathogenesis of periodontitis.

Effects of Aging on the Progression of Periodontal Diseases

In a classic experimental gingivitis study, subjects were rendered free of plaque and inflammation through frequent professional cleaning. After this was achieved, the subjects abstained from oral hygiene measures for periods of 3 weeks to allow gingivitis to develop.[45] In this experimental model, a comparison of developing gingivitis between younger and older individuals demonstrated a greater inflammatory response in older subjects, in both humans and dogs.[11,21,22,29] In the older age group (i.e., 65 to 80 years), the findings included a greater amount of infiltrated connective tissue, increased gingival crevicular fluid flow, and an increased gingival index.[21,22] Other studies have not demonstrated differences between subjects; this may be related to smaller differences between the ages of the younger and older experimental groups.[84] Intriguingly, even at the baseline level of excellent gingival health before the commencement of plaque accumulation, differences may exist between groups, with older individuals demonstrating more inflammation.[21,22] However, older individuals reporting regular floss use had better periodontal health, highlighting the benefits of preventive health behaviors.[46]

The phrase *getting long in the tooth* expresses a widespread belief that age is inevitably associated with an increased loss of connective tissue attachment. However, this observation may equally well reflect cumulative exposure to a number of potentially destructive processes. These exposures may include plaque-associated periodontitis, chronic mechanical trauma from toothbrushing, and iatrogenic damage from unfavorable restorative dentistry or repeated scaling and root planing. The effects of these exposures act in one direction only (i.e., an increased loss of attachment).

In an attempt to differentiate the effects of age from these other processes, several studies have been designed to eliminate confounding issues and to address more clearly the question of age as a risk factor for periodontitis. A ***risk factor*** is defined as "any characteristic, behavior, or exposure with an association to a particular disease." The relationship is not necessarily causal in nature. Some risk factors, if causal, can be modified to reduce one's risk of initiation or progression of disease, such as smoking or improved oral hygiene … while other factors cannot be modified, such as genetic factors.[23] The conclusions from these studies are strikingly consistent and show that the effect of age either is nonexistent or provides a small and clinically insignificant increased risk of loss of periodontal support.[43,49,54,58,59] Indeed, in comparison with the odds ratio of 20.52 for poor oral hygiene status and periodontitis, the odds ratio for age was only 1.24,[1] and smoking was much more influential than age.[54] Therefore age has been suggested to be not a true risk factor but rather a background or associated factor for periodontitis.[58] In addition, the clarification of a genetic basis for susceptibility to severe forms of periodontitis underlines the overriding importance of plaque, smoking, and susceptibility in explaining most of the variations in periodontal disease severity among individuals.[34] Nevertheless, a longitudinal study of essentially untreated periodontitis in an elderly (≥70 years old) Japanese population indicated that 296 of 394 individuals (75%) had a least one site with 3 mm or more loss of attachment over a 2-year period.[55] Smoking and a baseline attachment level of 6 mm or more were significantly associated with disease progression. A more recent study modeling the transition of periodontal health states over a 2-year period estimated that the risk of transiting from health to gingivitis was overall reduced by 3% with age.[47] Each year of age increase was associated with a 2% decreased risk of such a transition. Furthermore, increased age was not statistically associated with an increased risk of transiting from health or gingivitis to periodontitis.

Nevertheless, recent work has demonstrated the potential to reduce the severity of periodontitis with increasing age by targeting the basic biological changes that occur with aging. A large body of work in the aging biology field has been focused on the mammalian target of the rapamycin (mTOR) signaling pathway. mTOR is a protein kinase involved in multiple cellular processes across most eukaryotic cells, including cytokine production, autophagy, and cellular metabolism.[37] Interestingly, inhibition of mTOR activity, through genetic or pharmacologic means, has been well demonstrated to increase the lifespan and health span in experimental animal models, suggesting mTOR to be a key pathway in the aging process.[42] Interestingly animal models have shown the potential of therapeutically targeting mTOR for the management of periodontitis. In one experiment, mice were treated with rapamycin, a pharmacologic inhibitor of mTOR, for their entire adult life. Upon reaching old age (35 months), the mice that were treated with rapamycin demonstrated significantly less alveolar bone loss compared with the non-treated controls.[6] In another study, old mice were treated with a short course (2 months) of rapamycin. The short course of treatment resulted in significantly less alveolar bone loss, decreased pro-inflammatory cytokine signaling, and evidence of new alveolar bone formation compared with non-treated old mice.[5] These studies suggest aging as a contributor to periodontitis, as targeting mTOR activity, a well-demonstrated pathway that contributes to aging, was beneficial at reducing disease severity.

KEY FACT

Aging does not appear to be a true risk factor of developing periodontitis.

Aging and the Response to Treatment of the Periodontium

The successful treatment of periodontitis requires both meticulous home plaque control by the patient and meticulous supragingival and subgingival instrumentation by the therapist.[51] Unfortunately, only a few studies have directly compared such an approach among patients of different age groups. The few studies that have done so clearly demonstrate that, despite the histologic changes in the periodontium with aging, no differences in response to nonsurgical or surgical treatment have been shown for periodontitis.[7,82,41] However, if plaque control is not ideal, the continued loss of attachment is inevitable. Furthermore, without effective periodontal therapy, the progression of disease may be faster with increasing age.[60] Attempts to increase plaque control by chemical means have also been reported.[74]

A purely biologic or physiologic review indicates that aging has some impact on the structure and function of the periodontium as well as on the immune response and the nature of either supragingival or subgingival plaque. However, these changes have a negligible impact on an individual's responsiveness to treatment. Aging may affect other aspects of the management of periodontal health (e.g., the risk of root caries[64]; see Chapter 29), and the resulting difficulties should not be underestimated. Interestingly, a recent study has identified greater compliance with supportive maintenance among older individuals as compared with younger patients.[56]

Conclusions

Periodontal health should be a goal for all ages. In older individuals, it is clear that periodontal diseases can be prevented and treated. This is important for life quality and to prevent physical decline and dependency. Improving periodontal health in older people will be facilitated by a contemporary understanding of the limited effects of aging on the periodontium, planning care based on individual patient assessment rather than chronological age, and health policies that promote access for care.[35,78]

KEY FACT

The biologic effects of aging have either no or a minimal impact on an individual's response to periodontal treatment. However, other factors may have a profound impact including cognitive and motor skills as well as medical history.

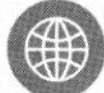

A Case Scenario is found on the companion website eBooks.Health.Elsevier.com.

Suggested Readings

An JY, Kerns KA, Ouellette A, et al. Rapamycin rejuvenates oral health in aging mice. *eLife*. 2020;9:e54318.

Baker DL, Seymour GJ. The possible pathogenesis of gingival recession. *J Clin Periodontol*. 1976;3(4):208–219.

Belibasakis GN. Microbiological changes of the ageing oral cavity. *Arch Oral Biol*. 2018;96:230–232.

Berglundh T, Lindhe J, Sterrett JD. Clinical and structural characteristics of periodontal tissues in young and old dogs. *J Clin Periodontol*. 1991;18(8):616–623.

Chapple ILC. Potential mechanisms underpinning the nutritional modulation of periodontal inflammation. *J Am Dent Assoc*. 2009;140(2):178–184.

Clark D, Brazina S, Yang F, et al. Age-related changes to macrophages are detrimental to fracture healing in mice. *Aging Cell*. 2020;19(3):e13112.

Clark D, Halpern B, Miclau T, Nakamura M, Kapila Y, Marcucio R. The contribution of macrophages in old mice to periodontal disease. *J Dent Res*. 2021;0(0):00220345211009463.

Eke PI, Wei L, Borgnakke WS, et al. Periodontitis prevalence in adults ≥ 65 years of age, in the USA. *Periodontol 2000*. 2016;72(1):76–95.

Feres M, Teles F, Teles R, Figueiredo LC, Faveri M. Th subgingival periodontal microbiota of the aging mouth. *Periodontol 2000*. 2016;72(1):30–53.

Franceschi C, Bonafè M, Valensin S, et al. Inflamm-aging. An evolutionary perspective on immunosenescence. *Ann N Y Acad Sci*. 2000;908:244–254.

Fransson C, Mooney J, Kinane DF, Berglundh T. Differences in the inflammatory response in young and old human subjects during the course of experimental gingivitis. *J Clin Periodontol*. 1999;26(7):453–460.

Holm-Pedersen P, Walls AWG, Ship JA. *Textbook of Geriatric Dentistry*, 3rd ed. Oxford: Wiley-Backwell; 2015.

Kossioni AE, Hajto-Bryk J, Maggi S, et al. An Expert Opinion from the European College of Gerodontology and the European Geriatric Medicine Society: European Policy Recommendations on Oral Health in Older Adults. *J Am Geriatr Soc*. 2018;66(3):609–613.

Lindhe J, Socransky S, Nyman S, Westfelt E, Haffajee A. Effect of age on healing following periodontal therapy. *J Clin Periodontol*. 1985;12(9):774–787.

Liu GY, Sabatini DM. mTOR at the nexus of nutrition, growth, ageing and disease. *Nat Rev Mol Cell Biol*. 2020;21(4):183–203.

Marchesan JT, Byrd KM, Moss K, et al. Flossing is associated with improved oral health in older adults. *J Dent Res*. 2020;99(9):1047–1053.

Needleman I, Nibali L, Di Iorio A. Professional mechanical plaque removal for prevention of periodontal diseases in adults – systematic review update. *J Clin Periodontol.* 2015;42:S12–S35.

Russell SL, Ship JS. Normal oral mucosal, dental, periodontal and alveolar bone changes associated with aging. In: Lamster IB, Northridge ME, eds. *Improving Oral Health for the Elderly: An Interdisciplinary Approach.* New York: Springer; 2008:233–246.

Scannapieco FA, Cantos A. Oral inflammation and infection, and chronic medical diseases: implications for the elderly. *Periodontol 2000.* 2016;72(1):153–175.

Tonetti MS, Bottenberg P, Conrads G, et al. Dental caries and periodontal diseases in the ageing population: call to action to protect and enhance oral health and well-being as an essential component of healthy ageing – Consensus report of group 4 of the joint EFP/ORCA workshop on the boundaries between caries and periodontal diseases. *J Clin Periodontol.* 2017;44(suppl 18):S135–S144.

Wennström JL. Treatment of periodontal disease in older adults. *Periodontol 2000.* 1998;16(1):106–112.

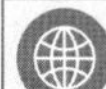
References for this chapter are found on the companion website eBooks.Health.Elsevier.com.

CHAPTER 14

Defense Mechanisms of the Gingiva

Marcelo Freire | Wichaya Wisitrasameewong | Fermin A. Carranza

CHAPTER OUTLINE

The mouth is part of the mucosal immune system, and it plays a role as a protective and constitutive tissue of the human mucosal tissues. The gingival tissue host and immune responses are in constant interaction with the complex oral environment that is exposed to microorganisms, external antigens, and chemicals. The establishment of a healthy mucosal system is characterized by a commensal microbiome with a continuous immune response that keeps the challenge in check and maintains the integrity of the tissue. When the challenge is continuous, cellular and molecular modifications characterize the host response. A sequential immune response will build, and clinical manifestations of the cellular outcomes become more evident. The initial lesion is characterized by inflammatory activation with subclinical changes. Upon bacterial metabolism and persistence, the early lesion appears clinically as early gingivitis. As this process progresses, periodontal tissue loss occurs and reversible disease ends, while the advanced lesion phase begins. Gingival tissue integrity is key in maintaining the barrier intact for protecting against microorganisms, while the junctional epithelium (JE) allows for a more dynamic interaction between the host and the microbiome.

The Junctional Epithelium

The JE is structurally and functionally unique. It has several specific features that differ from those of other oral epithelium. A crucial role of the JE in maintaining periodontal homeostasis is due to its strategic location as a frontline barrier against bacterial infection. The JE is located at the interface between the gingival sulcus and the underlying soft and mineralized connective tissues of the periodontium, and therefore, is constantly exposed to environmental stimuli, particularly, microbial invasion.

Anatomical and Structural Aspects

The JE is classified as non-keratinized stratified squamous epithelium that is made up of two strata only, namely a basal layer (the stratum basale) and a suprabasal layer (the stratum suprabasale). It consists of 15 to 30 cell layers coronally and tapers off in the apical direction to only 1 to 3 cell layers at its apical termination.[17] The coronal termination of the JE is a free surface and forms the bottom of the gingival sulcus. At its apical and lateral aspects, the JE is bordered by soft connective tissue.[117] The cell layer toward the tooth surface provides an attachment to the gingiva to the tooth surface by means of a structural complex called the *epithelial attachment*. This complex consists of a basal lamina-like structure that is adherent to the tooth surface and to which the superficial cell layer is attached by hemidesmosomes.[87] This provides physical attachment between the gingiva and the tooth via hemidesmosomes. By simply providing an attachment to the tooth surface, the JE has a significant role in host-microbial interactions, as it actively engages in the defense mechanism of gingiva with its unique functional features.

Junctional Epithelium as a First-Line Defense of Periodontal Tissues Against Microbial Challenge

The cellular turnover rate of the JE is extremely high when compared to other epithelium types.[121] All cells at the JE are in continual coronal migration and then exfoliate into the gingival sulcus. The regenerating epithelial cells then reestablish their hemidesmosome and immediately and continuously attach to the tooth surface.[117,120] With its rapid shedding of junctional epithelial cells, bacteria and their products, adhering to the epithelial cells are effectively removed. Thus, shedding of the JE is one of the important antimicrobial defense mechanisms at the dentogingival junction.

The JE is remarkably permeable, and this is due to intercellular junctions formed in the JE that are relatively loose and contain only a small number of desmosomes and gap junctions.[51] This provides a pathway for tissue exudate and transmigrating inflammatory cells from the connective tissue underneath toward the gingival sulcus. In the physiological state, roughly 30,000 polymorphonuclear cells (PMNs) per minute migrate through the JE of all teeth into the oral cavity, implying that modest inflammation occurs histologically even when the clinical signs of inflammation are absent.[17,116,124] These intracellular spaces are normally occupied by both, transmigrating PMNs (also called neutrophils) and infiltrating mononuclear cells, such as macrophages and lymphocytes, in various phases of activation. All such cells occupy about 12% of these spaces under noninflammatory states, but with inflammation, when the defense system is activated, that percentage can increase to 30% or more.[118] Antigen-presenting cells, as well as Langerhans and other dendritic cells, can also be found.[17] Neutrophils which are amongst the most abundant leukocytes within the periodontal tissues,[52] are retained near the sulcus bottom as a result of a high IL-8 gradient concentration synthesized by the JE.[124] Therefore neutrophils play an important role in defending the gingiva from bacterial invasion.[119] Together with junctional epithelial cells, they stand ready to phagocytose any pathogens that attempt to invade the JE.[74]

Finally, the JE expresses defensive factors by producing natural antimicrobial peptides and proteins in response to the bacterial challenge, such as β-defensins, cathelicidin LL-37, and calprotectin (Table 14.1).[17,26] Furthermore, the JE constitutively expresses numerous cell adhesion molecules (CAMs) and produces chemokines and cytokines, such as IL-8 and IL-1β. Integrins, cadherins, intercellular adhesion molecule-1 (ICAM-1) and lymphocyte function antigen-3 (LFA-3) are among the CAMs expressed by cells of the junctional epithelia. The latter two play key roles in directing PMNs toward the sulcus bottom and controlling leukocyte migration to inflammatory sites.[17,87] These findings demonstrate the active role of the JE in the innate host defense.

Sulcular Fluid

Sulcular fluid, or *gingival crevicular fluid (GCF)*, contains an array of biologic mediators, cells, and bacteria. Recognized since the 19th century, its possible role in oral defense was first elucidated by the pioneering work of Waerhaug[125] and Brill and Krasse[15] during the 1950s. The latter investigators applied filter paper to the gingival sulci of dogs that had previously been injected intramuscularly with fluorescein; within 3 minutes, the fluorescent material was recovered on the paper strips. This indicated the passage of fluid from the bloodstream through the tissues and the exiting of fluid via the gingival sulcus.

In subsequent studies, Brill[12,14] confirmed the presence of GCF in humans and considered it as "transudate." However, others[73,126] demonstrated that GCF is an inflammatory exudate rather than a continuous transudate. In strictly normal gingiva, little or no fluid can be collected.

More recently, interest in the development of tests for the detection or prediction of periodontal disease has resulted in numerous research papers about the components, origin, and function of GCF.[21] Potential markers from crevicular fluid are now used as diagnostic tools for the activity of periodontal diseases and a return to homeostasis, with potential for the evaluation of systemic markers.

Methods of Collection

The most difficult hurdle to overcome when collecting GCF is the scarcity of material that can be obtained from the sulcus. Many collection methods have been tried.[11,13,61,64,76,78,103] These methods include the use of absorbing paper strips, the placement of twisted threads around and into the sulcus, and techniques involving micropipettes and intracrevicular washings. There are limitations to the techniques, including fluid collection, collection time, flow rate, contamination, and reproducibility.

The absorbing paper strips are placed within the sulcus (intrasulcular method) or at its entrance (extrasulcular method) (Fig. 14.1). Placement of the filter paper strip in relation to the sulcus or pocket is important. The Brill technique involves inserting it into the pocket until resistance is encountered (see Fig. 14.1A). This method produces some degree of irritation of the sulcular epithelium that by itself can trigger the flow of fluid.

To minimize this irritation, Löe and Holm-Pedersen[73] placed the filter paper strip just at or over the pocket entrance (see Fig. 14.1B and C). In this way, fluid that seeps out is picked up by the strip, but the sulcular epithelium is not in contact with the paper.

Weinstein and colleagues[126] used preweighed twisted threads. The threads were placed in the gingival crevice around the tooth, and the amount of fluid collected was estimated by weighing the sample thread.

The use of micropipettes permits the collection of fluid by capillarity. Capillary tubes of standardized length and diameter are placed in the pocket, and their contents are later centrifuged and analyzed.[11–13]

Crevicular washings can be used to study GCF from clinically normal gingiva. One method involves the use of an appliance that consists of a hard acrylic plate that covers the maxilla, with soft borders and a groove that follows the gingival margins; it is connected to four collection tubes. Washings are obtained by rinsing the crevicular areas from one side to the other with the use of a peristaltic pump.[22]

A modification of the previous method involves the use of two injection needles that have been fitted one within the other so that, during sampling, the inside (ejection) needle is at the bottom of the pocket and the outside (collecting) needle is at the gingival margin. The collection needle is drained into a sample tube via continuous suction.[103]

Permeability of Junctional and Sulcular Epithelia

The initial studies by Brill and Krasse[15] involving the use of fluorescein were later confirmed with substances such as India ink[97] and saccharated iron oxide.[22] Substances that have been shown to penetrate the sulcular epithelium include albumin,[96] endotoxin,[95,100] thymidine,[49] histamine,[28] phenytoin,[113] and horseradish peroxidase.[80] These findings indicate permeability to substances with a molecular weight of up to 1000 kD.

Squier and Johnson[112] reviewed the mechanisms of penetration through an intact epithelium. The intercellular movement of molecules and ions along intercellular spaces appears to be a possible mechanism. Substances that take this route do not traverse the cell membranes.

Amount

The amount of GCF collected on a paper strip can be studied in multiple ways. The wetted area can be made more visible by staining with Ninhydrin; it is then measured planimetrically on an enlarged photograph or with a magnifying glass or a microscope.

An electronic method has been devised for measuring the fluid collected on a "blotter" (Periopaper) with the use of an electronic transducer (Periotron, Harco Electronics, Winnipeg, Manitoba, Canada) (Fig. 14.2). The wetness of the paper strip affects the flow of an electric current and provides a digital readout. A comparison between the Ninhydrin-staining method and the electronic method performed in vitro revealed no significant differences between the two techniques.[115]

The amount of GCF collected is extremely small. Measurements performed by Cimasoni[22] showed that a strip of paper 1.5-mm wide and inserted 1 mm within the gingival sulcus of a slightly inflamed gingiva absorbs about 0.1 mg of GCF in 3 minutes. Challacombe[20] used an isotope dilution method to measure the amount of GCF

TABLE 14.1 Locations and Functions of Molecular Factors Associated with the Junctional Epithelium

Molecular Factors	Locations and Functions the Junctional Epithelium	Suggested Functions	References
Cell Adhesion Molecules (CAMs)			
Integrins	Cell membrane of junctional epithelial cells	Mediate cell–matrix and cell–cell interactions	Hormia et al. (1992, 2001) Del castillo et al. (1996) Thorup et al. (1997) Gures et al. (1999)
Epithelial cadherin (E-cadherin)	Epithelial intercellular junctions	Critical in intercellular adhesion and thus crucial for maintaining structural integrity	Ye et al. (2000)
Carcino-embryonic Ag-related cell adhesion molecule 1 (CEACAM1)	Cell membranes of leukocytes and junctional epithelial cells	Adhesion between epithelial cells; contributes to the guidance of PMNs through the junctional epithelium; participates in the regulation of cell proliferation, stimulation, and co-regulation of activated T-cells; cell receptor for certain bacteria	Odin et al. (1988) Öbrink (1997) Hauck et al. (1998) Kammerer et al. (1998) Singer et al. (2000)
Intercelluar adhesion moleule-1 (ICAM-1 or CD54)	Cell membranes of junctional epithelial cells	Mediates cell–cell interactions in inflammatory reactions; guiding PMNs toward the sulcus bottom	Heymann et al. (2001) Crawford and Hopp (1990) Crawford (1992)
Lymphocyte function antigen-3 (LFA-3)	Cell membranes of junctional epithelial cells	Mediates cell–cell interactions in inflammatory reactions; controls leukocyte migration to inflammatory sites	Gao and Mackenzie (1992) Tonetti (1997) Tonetti et al. (1998) Crawford (1992)
Cytokines/Chemokines			
Interleukin-8 (Il-8)	In junctional epithelial cells near the sulcus bottom	Chemotaxis; guiding PMNs toward the sulcus bottom	Tonetti et al. (1994, 1998)
Interleukin-1α (Il-1α) Interleukin-1β (Il-1β) Tumor necrosis factor-α (TNF-α)	In junctional epithelial cells and macrophages in the coronal portion of the junctional epithelium	Pro-inflammatory cytokines that contribute to the innate immune defense	Miyauchi et al. (2001)
Cell-membrane-associated Blood-group-specific Carbohydrates			
N-acetyllactosamine	Cell membrane of junctional epithelial cells	Indicates a low level of cell differentiation	Steffensen et al. (1987)
Growth Factors and Corresponding Receptors			
Epidermal growth factor (EGF)	In junctional epithelial cells	Mitogen that participates in epithelial growth, differentiation, and wound healing	Tajima (1992)
Epidermal growth factor receptor (EGFR)	Cell membrane of junctional epithelial cells	Signal transduction	Nordlund et al. (1991)
Proteases			
Tissue plasminogen activator (t-PA)	In junctional epithelial cells	Serine protease that converts plasminogen into plasmin, which in turn degrades extracellular matrix proteins and activates matrix metalloproteinases	Schmid et al. (1991)
Matrix metalloproteinase-7 (MMP-7 or matrilysin)	In suprabasal junctional epithelial cells	Proteolytic degradation of the extracellular matrix	Uitto et al. (2002)
Natural Antimicrobial Peptides and Proteins			
α-defensins	In PMNs and gingival crevicular fluid	PMNs-produced antimicrobial substances that contribute to the innate immune defense	Dale (2002)
Human β-defensin-1 (hBD-1) Human β-defensin-2 (hBD-2)	Weak expression in junctional epithelial cells	Epithelially produced antimicrobial substances that contribute to innate host defense	Dale (2002)
Cathelicidin LL-37	In junctional epithelial and inflammatory cells	Antimicrobial and chemotactic substance produced by both PMNs and epithelial cells; contributes to the regulation of the innate immune defense	Dale (2002)

From Bosshardt DD, Lang NP. The junctional epithelium: from health to disease. *J Dent Res.* 2005;84(1):9–20.

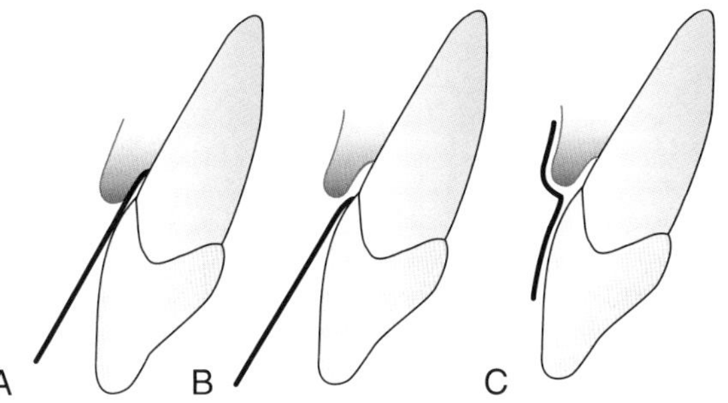

Fig. 14.1 Placement of a filter strip in the gingival sulcus for the collection of fluid. (A) Intrasulcular method. (B and C) Extrasulcular methods.

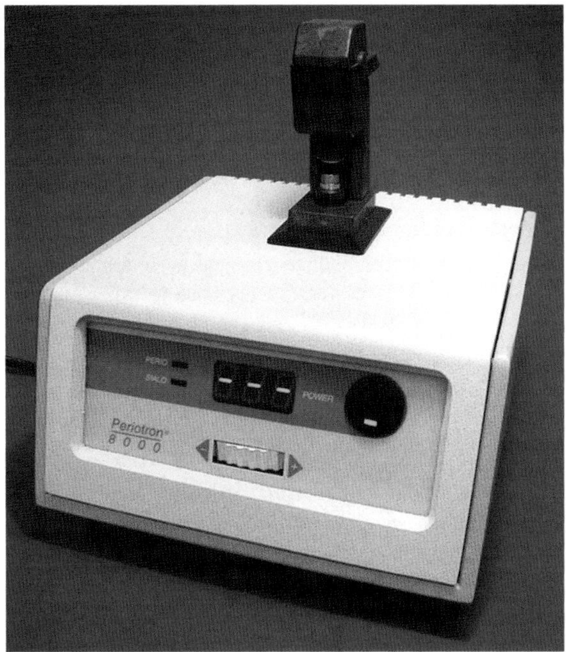

Fig. 14.2 Electronic device for measuring the amount of fluid collected on filter paper.

present in a particular space at any given time. His calculations for human volunteers with mean gingival indices of less than 1 showed that the mean GCF volume in the proximal spaces from the molar teeth ranged from 0.43 to 1.56 μL.

Composition

The components of GCF are characterized by individual proteins, metabolites,[73,86,104] specific antibodies, antigens,[36,94] and enzymes of several specificities.[16] The GCF also contains cellular elements from both host and microbes, and tissue breakdown porducts.[7,28,31,50,128]

Multiple research efforts have attempted to use GCF components to detect or diagnose an active disease or to predict which patients are at risk for periodontal disease (see Table 14.1).[3] So far, more than 40 compounds found in GCF have been analyzed,[91] but their origin is not known with certainty. These compounds can be derived from the host or produced by bacteria in the gingival crevice, but their source can be difficult to elucidate; examples include β-glucuronidase, which is a lysosomal enzyme, and lactic acid dehydrogenase, which is a cytoplasmic enzyme. The sources of collagenases may be fibroblasts or polymorphonuclear leukocytes (PMNs [neutrophils]),[5,89] or collagenases may be secreted by bacteria.[36] Phospholipases are lysosomal and cytoplasmic enzymes, but they are also produced by microorganisms.[16] The majority of GCF elements detected thus far have been enzymes, but there are nonenzymatic substances as well.

Cellular Elements

Cellular elements found in GCF include bacteria, desquamated epithelial cells, and leukocytes (i.e., PMNs, lymphocytes, and monocytes/macrophages), which migrate through the sulcular epithelium.[28,31]

Electrolytes

Potassium, sodium, and calcium have been studied in the GCF. Most studies have demonstrated a positive correlation of calcium and sodium concentrations with the sodium/potassium ratio seen with inflammation.[58–60] (For more information, see references.[58,59])

Organic Compounds

Both carbohydrates and proteins have been investigated. Glucose hexosamine and hexuronic acid are two compounds that are found in GCF.[47] Blood glucose levels do not correlate with GCF glucose levels; glucose concentration in GCF is three to four times greater than that in serum.[47] This is interpreted not only as a result of the metabolic activity of adjacent tissues but also as a function of the local microbial flora.

The total protein content of GCF is much less than that of serum.[13,15] No significant correlations have been found between the concentration of proteins in GCF and the severity of gingivitis, pocket depth, or extent of bone loss.[9] Metabolic and bacterial products identified in GCF include lactic acid,[48] urea,[42] hydroxyproline,[93] endotoxins,[109] cytotoxic substances, hydrogen sulfide,[111] and antibacterial factors.[27] Many enzymes have also been identified.

The methodology used to analyze GCF components is as varied as the diversity of those components. Examples include fluorometry to detect metalloproteinases,[28] enzyme-linked immunosorbent assays to detect enzyme levels and interleukin-1β (IL-1β),[71] radioimmunoassays to detect cyclooxygenase derivatives[88] and procollagen III,[122] high-pressure liquid chromatography to detect tinidazole,[68] and direct and indirect immunodot tests to detect acute-phase proteins.[108]

Cellular and Humoral Activity in Gingival Crevicular Fluid

Monitoring periodontal disease is a complicated task because few noninvasive procedures can follow the initiation and progress of the disease. Analyzing GCF constituents in health and disease may be extremely useful as a result of GCF's simplicity and because GCF can be obtained with noninvasive methods.

The analysis of GCF has identified cell and humoral responses in both healthy individuals and those with periodontal disease.[66] The cellular immune response includes the appearance of cytokines in GCF, but there is no clear evidence of a relationship between cytokines and disease. However, IL-1α and IL-1β are known to increase the binding of PMNs and monocytes/macrophages to endothelial cells, to stimulate the production of prostaglandin E_2 and the release of lysosomal enzymes, and to stimulate bone resorption.[69] Preliminary evidence also indicates the presence of interferon-α in GCF,[66] which may have a protective role in periodontal disease because of its ability to inhibit the bone resorption activity of IL-1β.[44]

Because the amount of fluid recoverable from gingival crevices is small, only the use of very sensitive immunoassays permits the analysis of the specificity of antibodies.[27,29,30] A study that compared antibodies in different crevices with serum antibodies directed at specific microorganisms did not provide any conclusive evidence regarding the significance of the presence of antibodies in GCF among individuals with periodontal disease.[66]

Although the role of antibodies in the gingival defense mechanisms is difficult to ascertain, the consensus is that in a patient with periodontal disease, a reduction in antibody response is detrimental, and an antibody response plays a protective role.[65]

TABLE 14.2 Gingival Crevicular Fluid Diagnostic Tests

Test Name	Target	References
Periocheck	Proteinases	Page RC. Host response tests designed for diagnosing periodontal disease. *J Periodontol.* 1992;63(4 Suppl):356–366.
Prognostik	Elastase	Oswal S, Dwarakanath CD. Relevance of gingival crevice fluid components in assessment of periodontal disease–A critical analysis. *J Indian Soc Periodontol* 2010;14(4):282–286.
Biolise	Elastase	Oswal S, Dwarakanath CD. Relevance of gingival crevice fluid components in assessment of periodontal disease–A critical analysis. *J Indian Soc Periodontol* 2010;14(4):282–286.
MMP dipstick	MMPs	Mäntylä P, Stenman M, Kinane DF, Tikanoja S, Luoto H, Salo T, Sorsa T. Gingival crevicular fluid collagenase-2 (MMP-8) test stick for chair-side monitoring of periodontitis. *J Periodontal Res.* 2003;38(4):436–439.
TOPAS	Bacterial toxins and proteases	Oswal S, Dwarakanath CD. Relevance of gingival crevice fluid components in assessment of periodontal disease–A critical analysis. *J Indian Soc Periodontol* 2010;14(4):282–286.
Pocket watch	AST	Mäntylä P, Stenman M, Kinane DF, Tikanoja S, Luoto H, Salo T, Sorsa T. Gingival crevicular fluid collagenase-2 (MMP-8) test stick for chair-side monitoring of periodontitis. *J Periodontal Res.* 2003;38:436–439.

MMP, Mucous membrane pemphigoid.

Clinical Significance

As an exudate, GCF is a biologic fluid that has potential in diagnostics and disease management.[73] Its presence in clinically normal sulci can be explained because gingiva that appears clinically normal invariably exhibits inflammation when it is examined microscopically. Commercially available kits for diagnosis are now available (Table 14.2).

CLINICAL CORRELATION

- Novel diagnostics tools allow evaluations of biomarkers from tissue and oral biofluids.
- Drug delivery targeting oral tissues has optimal absorption and bioavailability.
- Gingival fluid and saliva are biologic fluids that can provide information on human genomics and metagenomics (microbiome, transcriptome, metabolome, and proteome).
- Oral immunity is activated through rapid response from innate immune components (fluids, mucosal surfaces, epithelium, cell mediators, molecules, host-bacterial interactions).

The amount of GCF is greater when inflammation is present,[35,106] and it is sometimes proportional to the severity of inflammation.[90] GCF production is not increased by trauma from occlusion,[79] but it is increased by the mastication of coarse foods, toothbrushing and gingival massage, ovulation,[71] hormonal contraceptives,[72] prosthetic appliances,[84] and smoking.[81] Other factors that influence the amount of GCF are circadian periodicity and periodontal therapy.

Circadian Periodicity

There is a gradual increase in the amount of GCF from 6 a.m. to 10 p.m. and a decrease thereafter.[10]

Sex Hormones

Female sex hormones increase GCF flow, probably because they enhance vascular permeability.[69] Pregnancy, ovulation,[68] and hormonal contraceptives[70] all increase GCF production.

Mechanical Stimulation

Chewing[12] and vigorous gingival brushing stimulate the flow of GCF. Even minor stimuli represented by intrasulcular placement of paper strips increases the production of fluid.

Smoking

Smoking produces an immediate transient but marked increase in GCF flow but, in the long term, a decrease in salivary and GCF flow.[81]

Periodontal Therapy

There is an increase in GCF production during the healing period after periodontal surgery.[4]

Drugs in Gingival Crevicular Fluid

Drugs that are excreted through the GCF may be used advantageously in periodontal therapy. Bader and Goldhaber[8] demonstrated in dogs that tetracyclines are excreted through the GCF; this finding triggered extensive research that showed a concentration of tetracyclines in GCF as compared with serum.[43] Metronidazole is another antibiotic that has been detected in human GCF (see Chapter 53).[32]

Leukocytes in the Dentogingival Area

Leukocytes have been found in clinically healthy gingival sulci in humans and experimental animals. The leukocytes found are predominantly PMNs. They appear in small numbers extravascularly in the connective tissue adjacent to the apical portion of the sulcus; from there, they travel across the epithelium[19,45] to the gingival sulcus, where they are expelled. These cells then migrate to saliva and execute *in situ* biological responses (Figs. 14.3 and 14.4).

Leukocytes are present in sulci even when histologic sections of adjacent tissue are free of inflammatory infiltrate.[98] Differential counts of leukocytes from clinically healthy human gingival sulci have shown 91.2% to 91.5% PMNs and 8.5% to 8.8% mononuclear cells.[110,128]

Mononuclear cells were identified as 58% B lymphocytes, 24% T lymphocytes, and 18% mononuclear phagocytes. The ratio of T lymphocytes to B lymphocytes was found to be reversed from the normal ratio of about 3:1 found in peripheral blood to about 1:3 in GCF.[128]

Leukocytes are attracted by different plaque bacteria,[56,127] but they can also be found in the dentogingival region of germ-free adult animals.[75,102] Leukocytes were reported in the gingival sulcus in nonmechanically irritated (resting) healthy gingiva, thereby indicating that their migration may be independent of an increase in vascular permeability.[6] The majority of these cells are viable and have phagocytic and killing capacity.[63,92,99] Therefore leukocytes

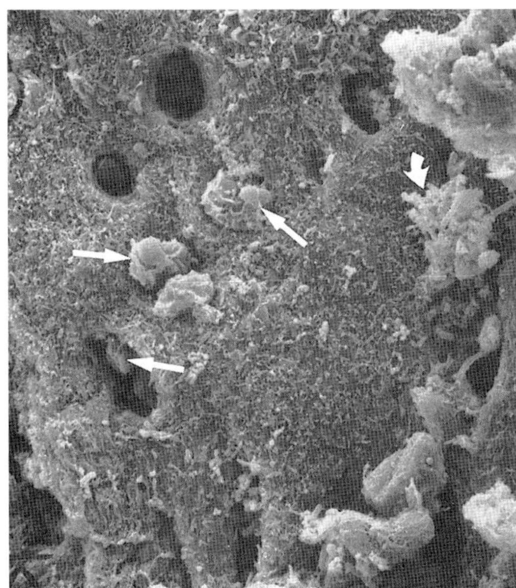

Fig. 14.3 Scanning electron microscope view of the periodontal pocket wall. Several leukocytes are emerging *(straight arrows)*, some of which are partially covered by bacteria *(curved arrow)*. Empty holes correspond to tunnels through which leukocytes have emerged.

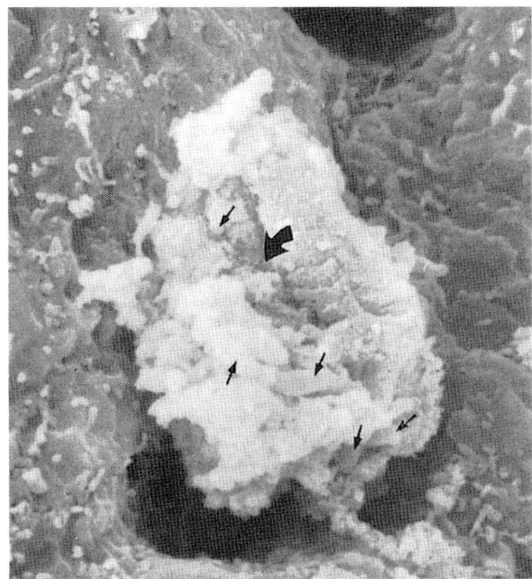

Fig. 14.4 Scanning electron microscope view at higher magnification than shown in Fig. 14.3. A leukocyte emerging from the pocket wall is covered with bacteria *(small arrows)*. The *large curved arrow* points to a phagosomal vacuole through which bacteria are being engulfed.

constitute a major protective mechanism against the extension of plaque into the gingival sulcus.

Live and dead leukocytes are found in saliva; this is discussed later in this chapter. The main port of entry of leukocytes into the oral cavity is the gingival sulcus.[105]

Saliva

In addition to GCF, saliva has protective functions and maintains the oral tissues in a physiologic state (Table 14.3). Saliva exerts a major influence on plaque by mechanically cleansing the exposed oral surfaces, buffering acids produced by bacteria, and modulating bacterial activity with immune mediators.[85] Saliva is now considered a main biologic fluid for the diagnosis of human health and diseases. Systemic and local disease markers are available through saliva. Available tests allow the individual to measure multi-omics outputs.[24] Functional and static assays are now available as biosensors of health and disease.

TABLE 14.3 Role of Saliva in Oral Health

Function	Salivary Components	Probable Mechanism
Lubrication	Glycoproteins, mucoids	Coating similar to gastric mucin
Physical protection	Glycoproteins, mucoids	Coating similar to gastric mucin
Cleansing	Physical flow	Clearance of debris and bacteria
Buffering	Bicarbonate and phosphate	Antacids
Tooth integrity maintenance	Minerals	Maturation, remineralization
	Glycoprotein pellicle	Mechanical protection
Antibacterial action	Immunoglobulin A	Control of bacterial colonization
	Lysozyme	Breaking of bacterial cell walls
	Lactoperoxidase	Oxidation of susceptible bacteria

Antibacterial Factors

Saliva carries inorganic and organic factors that influence bacteria and their products in the oral environment. Inorganic factors include ions and gases, bicarbonate, sodium, potassium, phosphates, calcium, fluorides, ammonium, and carbon dioxide. Organic factors include lysozyme, lactoferrin, myeloperoxidase, lactoperoxidase, defensins, peptides, and agglutinins such as glycoproteins, mucins, β2-macroglobulins, fibronectins,[50] and antibodies.

Lysozyme is a hydrolytic enzyme that cleaves the linkage between structural components of the glycopeptide muramic acid-containing region of the cell wall of certain bacteria in vitro. Lysozyme works on both gram-negative and gram-positive organisms[53]; its targets include *Veillonella* species and *Actinobacillus actinomycetemcomitans.* It works on the molecular level, protecting the oral cavity and repelling transient bacterial invaders.[55]

The *lactoperoxidase–thiocyanate system* in saliva has been shown to be bactericidal to some strains of *Lactobacillus* and *Streptococcus*[83,101] by preventing the accumulation of lysine and glutamic acid, both of which are essential for bacterial growth. Another antibacterial finding is lactoferrin, which is effective against *Actinobacillus* species.[57]

Myeloperoxidase, an enzyme that is similar to salivary peroxidase, is released by leukocytes; it is bactericidal for *Actinobacillus,*[82] but it has the added effect of inhibiting the attachment of *Actinomyces* strains to hydroxyapatite.[23]

Human alpha and beta-defensins (hBD)-1,-2,-3 are a family of low-molecular-weight antimicrobial peptides. Produced by a number of cells, including neutrophils, they amplify and combat bacterial[1] infections important to homeostasis.

Salivary Antibodies

As with GCF, saliva contains antibodies that are reactive with indigenous oral bacterial species. Although immunoglobulins G (IgG) and M (IgM) are present, the preponderant immunoglobulin found in saliva is *immunoglobulin A* (IgA), whereas IgG is more prevalent in GCF.[114] Major and minor salivary glands contribute all of the secretory IgA and lesser amounts of IgG and IgM. GCF contributes most of the IgG, complement, and PMNs that, in conjunction with IgG or IgM, inactivate or opsonize bacteria.

Salivary antibodies appear to be synthesized locally, because they react with bacteria that are indigenous to the mouth but not with organisms that are characteristic of the intestinal tract.[37,39] Bacteria found in saliva are frequently associated with IgA, and the bacterial deposits on teeth contain both IgA and IgG in quantities that are greater than 1% of their dry weight.[38] It has been shown that IgA antibodies present in parotid saliva can inhibit the attachment of oral *Streptococcus* species to epithelial cells.[33,125] Gibbons and colleagues[37–39] suggested that antibodies in secretions may impair the ability of bacteria to attach to mucosal or dental surfaces.

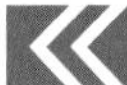

FLASH BACK

Saliva was known to have protective actions against infection through immunoglobulins only. Now it is clear that enzymes, cytokines, nucleotides, and live cells are part of the host armamentarium.

Enzymes

The *enzymes* that are normally found in saliva are derived from the salivary glands, bacteria, leukocytes, oral tissues, and ingested substances; the major enzyme is parotid amylase. Certain salivary enzymes have been reported in increased concentrations in periodontal disease: hyaluronidase and lipase,[18] β-glucuronidase and chondroitin sulfatase,[41] aspartate aminotransferase and alkaline phosphatase,[123] amino acid decarboxylases,[41] catalase, peroxidase, and collagenase.[62]

Proteolytic enzymes in the saliva are generated by both the host and oral bacteria. These enzymes have been recognized as contributors to the initiation and progression of periodontal disease.[49,77] To combat these enzymes, saliva contains antiproteases that inhibit cysteine proteases, such as cathepsins[54] and antileukoproteases that inhibit elastase.[89] Another antiprotease, which has been identified as a tissue inhibitor of matrix metalloproteinase, has been shown to inhibit the activity of collagen-degrading enzymes.[25]

High-molecular-weight mucinous glycoproteins in saliva bind specifically to many plaque-forming bacteria. The glycoprotein–bacteria interactions facilitate bacterial accumulation on the exposed tooth surface.[33,37–39,127] The specificity of these interactions has been demonstrated. The interbacterial matrix of human plaque appears to contain polymers that are similar to salivary glycoproteins and may aid in maintaining the integrity of plaque. In addition, these glycoproteins selectively adsorb to the hydroxyapatite to make up part of the acquired pellicle. Other salivary glycoproteins inhibit the adsorption of some bacteria to the tooth surface and to epithelial cells of the oral mucosa. This activity appears to be associated with the glycoproteins that possess blood group reactivity.[2,33,37,39,125] Another effect of mucin is the deletion of bacterial cells from the oral cavity via aggregation with mucin-rich films.

Glycoproteins and a glycolipid that is present on mammalian cell surfaces appear to serve as receptors for the attachment of some viruses and bacteria. Thus, the close similarity between the glycoproteins of salivary secretions and the components of the epithelial cell surface suggests that the secretions can competitively inhibit antigen sorption and that they therefore may limit pathologic alterations.

Salivary Buffers and Coagulation Factors

The maintenance of physiologic hydrogen ion concentration (pH) at the mucosal epithelial cell surface and the tooth surface is an important function of salivary buffers. The primary effect action of buffers has been investigated in relationship to dental caries. In saliva, the most important buffer is the bicarbonate–carbonic acid system.[76]

Saliva also contains coagulation factors (i.e., factors VIII, IX, and X; plasma thromboplastin antecedent; and Hageman factor) that hasten blood coagulation and protect wounds from bacterial invasion.[67] An active fibrinolytic enzyme may also be present.

Leukocytes

In addition to desquamated epithelial cells, saliva contains all forms of leukocytes, of which the principal cells are PMNs. Whole-blood PMNs are naïve and not activated, whereas the cells found in saliva have interacted with multiple antigens from the microbiome. The number of PMNs varies from person to person at different times of the day, and it is increased in the presence of gingivitis. PMNs reach the oral cavity by migrating through the lining of the gingival sulcus. Living PMNs in saliva are sometimes referred to as *orogranulocytes,* and their rate of migration into the oral cavity is termed the *orogranulocytic migratory rate.* A novel investigation presents a positive correlation between the rate of PMN migration and the severity of gingival inflammation, and it is therefore, a reliable index for the assessment of gingivitis.[110] In a high-throughput method, distinct subsets of neutrophils were found in oral mucosa, including naïve, parainflammatory, and proinflammatory cells.[34]

CLINICAL CORRELATION

What Is the Clinical Importance of Saliva?

Saliva has several important properties, including mechanical, chemical, biologic, and immunologic.[24] It is a viscous, clear, watery fluid secreted from salivary glands. It is a major biologic fluid for diagnosis and "omics" research. Diagnosing local and systemic conditions is possible through salivary markers. Low saliva is a risk factor for caries and periodontal disease. Xerostomia is defined as dry mouth resulting from reduced or absent saliva flow. Xerostomia is a symptom of various medical conditions, and it is a side effect of radiation to the head and neck and a wide variety of medications.

Role in Periodontal Pathology

Saliva modulates plaque initiation, maturation, and metabolism. Salivary flow and composition also influence calculus formation, periodontal disease, and caries. The removal of the salivary glands in experimental animals significantly increases the incidence of dental caries[40] and periodontal disease[46] in addition to delaying wound healing.[107]

In humans, increases in inflammatory gingival conditions, dental caries, rapid tooth destruction, and cervical or cemental caries are associated, at least partially, with decreased salivary gland secretion (xerostomia; Box 14.1). Xerostomia may result from sialolithiasis,

BOX 14.1 Hallmarks of Xerostomia

Features	Healthy	Xerostomia
Flow rate	1–2 mL	<0.1 mg/mL
Sensation	Normal	Dry mouth
Consistency and texture	Resilient and lubricated	Erythematous, sticky

sarcoidosis, Sjögren's syndrome, Mikulicz disease, irradiation, surgical removal of the salivary glands, and other factors.

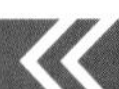

FLASH BACK

- Gingival tissue is constantly challenged by external factors.
- Epithelial surface, crevicular fluid, saliva, epithelial surfaces, immune cells, and mediators provide oral immunity.
- Oral diseases, including caries and periodontal diseases, benefit from oral immune components.

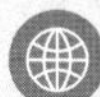

A Case Scenario is found on the companion website eBooks.Health.Elsevier.com.

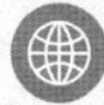

References for this chapter are found on the companion website eBooks.Health.Elsevier.com.

CHAPTER 15

Dental Biofilm-Induced Gingivitis and Its Management

Joseph P. Fiorellini | Dennis Sourvanos | David M. Kim | Yu-Cheng Chang | Marcelo Freire | Kevin W. Luan | Hector L. Sarmiento

CHAPTER OUTLINE

An increasing number of studies reveal that interactions between the host and microbes are coordinated, impacting human health and disease.[42] Local innate and specific immunity will maintain gingival health. Components of the innate immune response include epithelial cells and nonspecific cells within the epithelium, mucins, lysozyme, lactoferrin, lactoperoxidase, and various antimicrobial peptides, such as histatins, beta-defensins, and protease inhibitors. Epithelial cells (keratinocytes) themselves are reactive and express a variety of receptors, including toll-like receptors, and produce a variety of cytokines on activation.

The pathologic changes of gingivitis are initiated by a host response to oral microorganisms attached to the tooth and perhaps in or near the gingival sulcus. These organisms are capable of synthesizing products (e.g., collagenase, hyaluronidase, protease, chondroitin sulfatase, endotoxin) that cause damage to epithelial and connective tissue cells as well as to intercellular constituents, such as collagen, ground substance, and glycocalyx (cell coat). The resultant widening of the spaces between junctional epithelial cells during early gingivitis may permit injurious agents derived from bacteria or bacteria themselves to gain access to the connective tissue.[26,128,132] Microbial products activate cells, including monocytes and macrophages, to produce vasoactive substances, such as prostaglandin E2, interferon, tumor necrosis factor, and interleukin-1.[74,116] In addition, interleukin-1β alters the properties of gingival fibroblasts by delaying their death via a mechanism-blocking apoptosis. This stabilizes the gingival fibroblast population during inflammation.[158]

Morphologic and functional changes in the gingiva during plaque accumulation have been thoroughly investigated, especially in beagle dogs and humans.[114] A useful framework for the organization and consideration of these data has been devised on the basis of histopathologic, radiographic, and ultrastructural features and biochemical measurements.[115,117] The sequence of events that culminates in clinically apparent gingivitis is categorized as the *initial, early,* and *established* stages of the disease, with periodontitis designated as the *advanced stage* (Table 15.1).[116] One stage evolves into the next, with no clear-cut dividing lines.

Despite extensive research, we still cannot definitively distinguish between normal gingival tissue and the initial stage of gingivitis.[114] Most biopsies of clinically normal human gingiva contain inflammatory cells; these consist predominantly of T cells, with very few B cells or plasma cells.[114,133,134] These cells do not create tissue damage, but they appear to be important in the day-to-day host response to bacteria and other substances to which the gingiva is exposed.[114] Therefore, under normal conditions, a constant stream of neutrophils is migrating from the vessels of the gingival plexus through the junctional epithelium, to the gingival margin, and into the gingival sulcus and the oral cavity.[127]

Stage I Gingival Inflammation: The Initial Lesion

The first manifestations of gingival inflammation are vascular changes that consist of dilated capillaries and increased blood flow. These initial inflammatory changes occur in response to the microbial activation of resident leukocytes and the subsequent stimulation of endothelial cells. Clinically, this initial response of the gingiva to bacterial biofilm (i.e., subclinical gingivitis[75]) is not apparent.

TABLE 15.1 Stages of Gingivitis

Stage	Time (Days)	Blood Vessels	Junctional and Sulcular Epithelia	Predominant Immune Cells	Collagen	Clinical Findings
I. Initial lesion	2–4	Vascular dilation Vasculitis	Infiltration by PMNs	PMNs	Perivascular loss	Gingival fluid flow
II. Early lesion	4–7	Vascular proliferation	Same as stage I Rete pegs Atrophic areas	Lymphocytes	Increased loss around infiltrate	Erythema Bleeding on probing
III. Established lesion	14–21	Same as stage II, plus blood stasis	Same as stage II but more advanced	Plasma cells	Continued loss	Changes in color, size, texture, and so on

PMNs, Polymorphonuclear leukocytes (neutrophils).

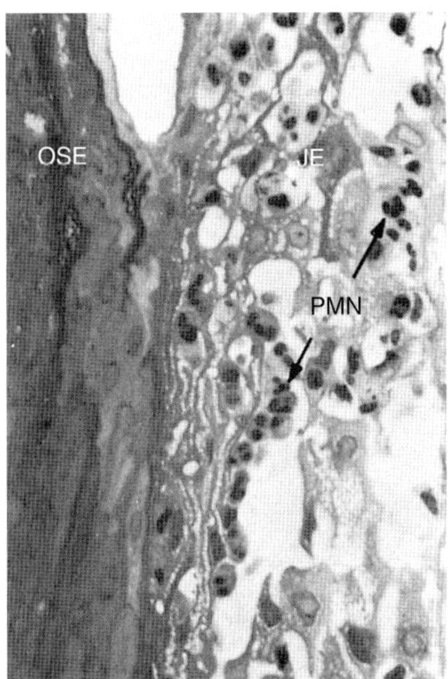

Fig. 15.1 Human biopsy sample, experimental gingivitis. After 4 days of plaque accumulation, the blood vessels immediately adjacent to the junctional epithelium are distended and contain polymorphonuclear leukocytes (neutrophils) *(PMNs).* Neutrophils have also migrated between the cells of the junctional epithelium *(JE). OSE,* Oral sulcular epithelium. (Magnification, ×500.) (From Payne WA, Page RC, Ogilvie AL, et al. Histopathologic features of the initial and early stages of experimental gingivitis in man. *J Periodontal Res.* 1975;10:51.)

Microscopically, some classic features of acute inflammation can be seen in the connective tissue beneath the junctional epithelium. Changes in blood vessel morphologic features (e.g., the widening of small capillaries or venules) and the adherence of neutrophils to vessel walls (margination) occur within 1 week and sometimes as early as 2 days after plaque has been allowed to accumulate (Fig. 15.1).[56,119] The etiopathogenesis of gingival diseases is linked to the local or systemic immune response, to innate or adaptive immunity, and to cellular or secretory factors. Leukocytes—mainly polymorphonuclear neutrophils (PMNs)—leave the capillaries by migrating through the walls via diapedesis and emigration (Fig. 15.2).[74,134,139] They are identified in increased quantities within the connective tissue, the junctional epithelium, and the gingival sulcus (Figs. 15.3 and 15.4).[12,14,73,110,119,129,130] Exudation of fluid from the gingival sulcus[56] and extravascular proteins is present.[65,66]

However, these findings are not accompanied by manifestations of tissue damage that are perceptible at the light microscopic or ultrastructural level; they do not form an infiltrate, and their presence is not considered to indicate pathologic change.[114]

Subtle changes can also be detected in the junctional epithelium and perivascular connective tissue at this early stage. For example, the perivascular connective tissue matrix becomes altered, and there is exudation and deposition of fibrin in the affected area.[114] In addition, lymphocytes soon begin to accumulate (see Fig. 15.2D). The increased migration of leukocytes and their accumulation within the gingival sulcus may be correlated with an increased flow of gingival fluid into the sulcus.[15]

The character and intensity of the host response determine whether this *initial lesion* resolves rapidly, with restoration of the tissue to a normal state; alternatively, it may evolve into a chronic inflammatory lesion. If the latter occurs, an infiltrate of macrophages and lymphoid cells appears within a few days.

Stage II Gingival Inflammation: The Early Lesion

The *early lesion* evolves from the *initial lesion* within about 1 week after the beginning of plaque accumulation.[113,119] Clinically, the early lesion may appear as early gingivitis, and it overlaps with and evolves from the initial lesion with no clear-cut dividing line. As time goes on, clinical signs of erythema may appear, mainly because of the proliferation of capillaries and the increased formation of capillary loops between rete pegs or ridges (Fig. 15.5). Bleeding on probing (BOP) may also be evident.[10] Gingival fluid flow and the numbers of transmigrating leukocytes reach their maximum between 6 and 12 days after the onset of clinical gingivitis.[75]

Microscopic examination of the gingiva reveals leukocyte infiltration in the connective tissue beneath the junctional epithelium, which consists mainly of lymphocytes (75%, with the majority being T cells)[119,131] but also includes some migrating neutrophils as well as macrophages, plasma cells, and mast cells. All of the changes seen in the initial lesion continue to intensify with the early lesion.[46,77,79,113,131] The junctional epithelium becomes densely infiltrated with neutrophils, as does the gingival sulcus, and may begin to show the development of rete pegs or ridges.

The amount of collagen destruction also increases[31,40,77]; 70% of the collagen is destroyed around the cellular infiltrate. The main fiber groups that are affected appear to be the circular and dentogingival fiber assemblies. Alterations in blood vessel morphologic features and vascular bed patterns have also been described.[56,61]

PMNs that have left the blood vessels in response to chemotactic stimuli from plaque components travel to the epithelium and cross

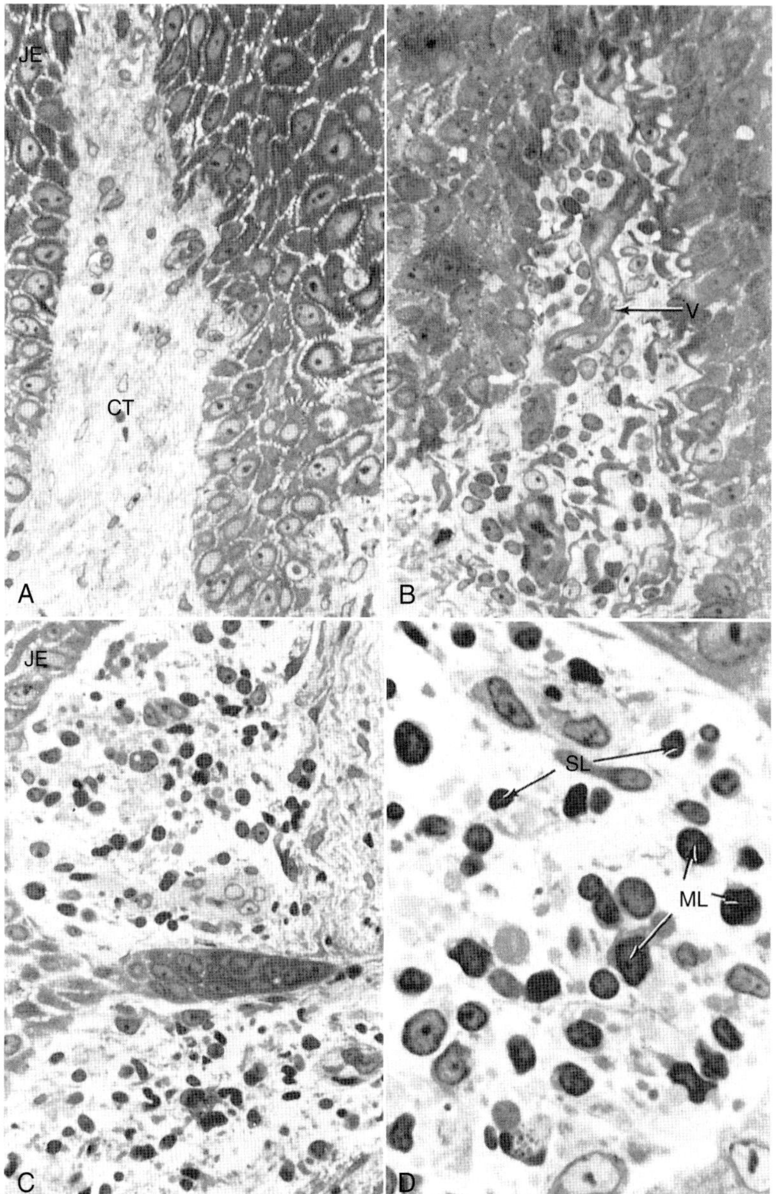

Fig. 15.2 Human biopsy, experimental gingivitis. (A) Control biopsy specimen from a patient with good oral hygiene and no detectable plaque accumulation. The junctional epithelium is on the *left*. The connective tissue *(CT)* shows few cells other than fibroblasts, blood vessels, and a dense background of collagen fibers (magnification, ×500.) (B) Biopsy specimen taken after 8 days of plaque accumulation. The connective tissue is infiltrated with inflammatory cells, which displace the collagen fibers. A distended blood vessel *(V)* is seen in the center (magnification, ×500). (C) After 8 days of plaque accumulation, the connective tissue next to the junctional epithelium *(JE)* at the base of the sulcus shows a mononuclear cell infiltrate and evidence of collagen degeneration (i.e., clear spaces around the cellular infiltrate (magnification, ×500). (D) The inflammatory cell infiltrate at higher magnification (×1250). After 8 days of plaque accumulation, numerous small *(SL)* and medium-sized *(ML)* lymphocytes are seen within the connective tissue. Most of the collagen fibers around these cells have disappeared, presumably as a result of enzymatic digestion. (From Payne WA, Page RC, Ogilvie AL, et al. Histopathologic features of the initial and early stages of experimental gingivitis in man. *J Periodontal Res.* 1975;10:51.)

the basement lamina; they are found in the epithelium, emerging in the pocket area (see Fig. 15.3). PMNs are attracted to bacteria and engulf them during the process of phagocytosis (Fig. 15.6). PMNs release their lysosomes in association with the ingestion of bacteria.[70] Fibroblasts show cytotoxic alterations,[118] with a decreased capacity for collagen production.

Meanwhile, collagen degradation is related to matrix metalloproteinases (MMPs). Different MMPs are responsible for extracellular matrix remodeling within 7 days of inflammation, which is directly related to MMP-2 and MMP-9 production and activation.[158]

Stage III Gingival Inflammation: The Established Lesion

Over time, the *established lesion* evolves. It is characterized by a predominance of plasma cells and B lymphocytes, and the creation

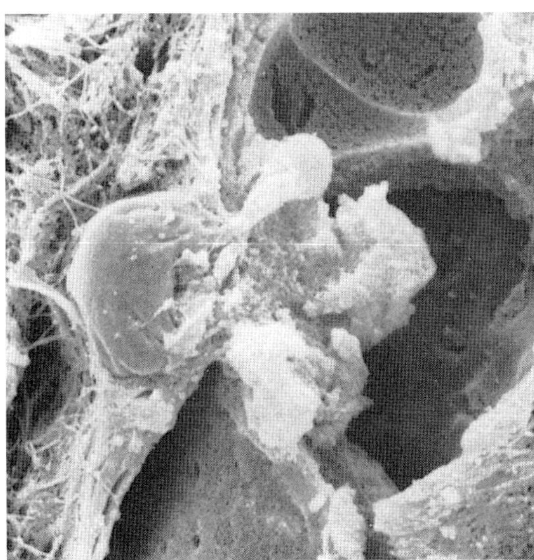

Fig. 15.3 Scanning electron micrograph showing a leukocyte traversing the vessel wall to enter into the gingival connective tissue.

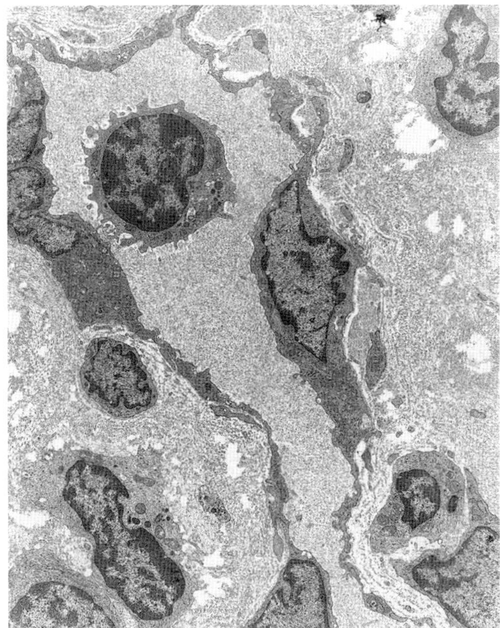

Fig. 15.4 Early human gingivitis lesion. There is an area of lamina propria subjacent to the crevicular epithelium that shows a capillary with several extravascular lymphocytes and one lymphocyte within the lumen. The specimen also exhibits a considerable loss of perivascular collagen density (magnification, ×2500). (Courtesy Dr. Charles Cobb, Kansas City, MO.)

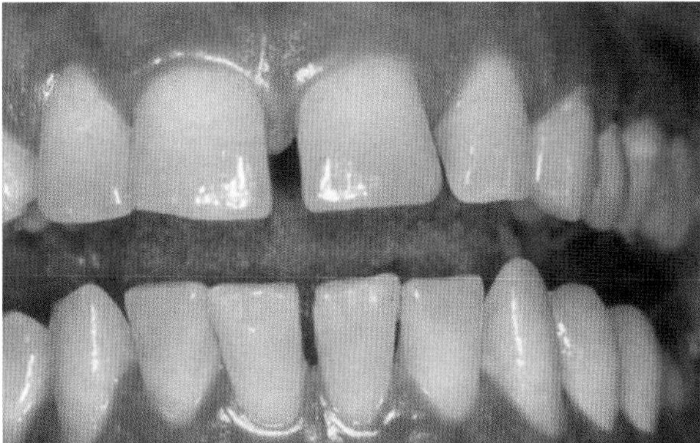

Fig. 15.5 Marginal gingivitis and irregular gingival contour.

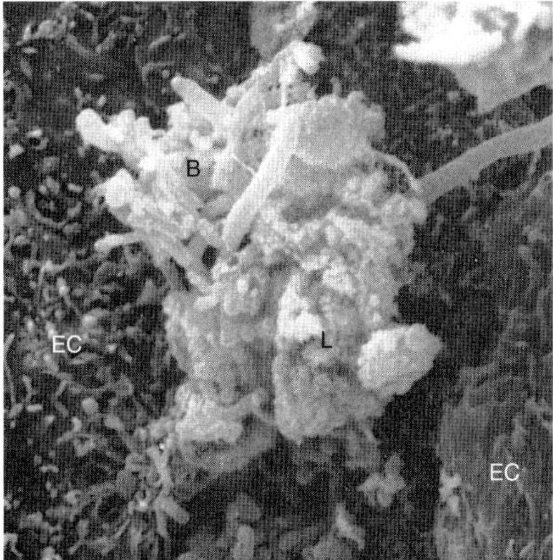

Fig. 15.6 Scanning electron micrograph of a leukocyte emerging to the pocket wall and covered with bacteria and extracellular lysosomes. *B,* Bacteria; *EC,* epithelial cells; *L,* lysosomes.

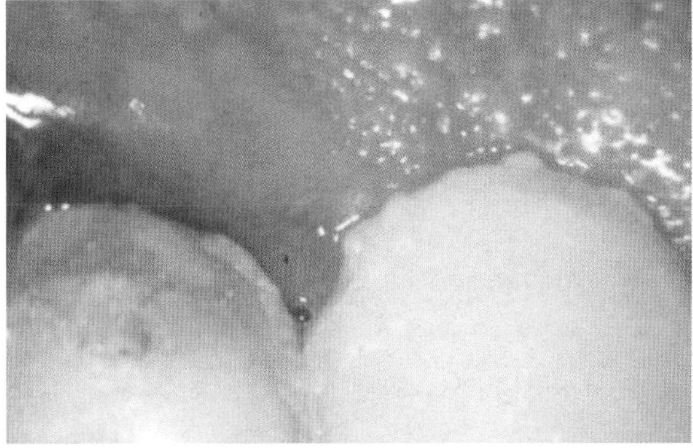

Fig. 15.7 Marginal supragingival plaque and gingivitis.

of a small gingival pocket lined with pocket epithelium.[130] The B cells that are found in the established lesion are predominantly of the immunoglobulin G1 and G3 subclasses.[114] This process is impacted by aging and other host factors.[39]

With chronic gingivitis, which occurs 2 to 3 weeks after the beginning of plaque accumulation, the blood vessels become engorged and congested, venous return is impaired, and the blood flow becomes sluggish (Fig. 15.7). The result is localized gingival *anoxemia,* which superimposes a somewhat bluish hue on the reddened gingiva.[53] The extravasation of erythrocytes into the connective tissue and the breakdown of hemoglobin into its component pigments can also deepen the color of the chronically inflamed gingiva. The established lesion can be described as moderately to severely inflamed gingiva.

In histologic sections, an intense and chronic inflammatory reaction is observed. Several detailed cytologic studies have been performed on chronically inflamed gingiva.[41,44,46,118,130,133,149] A key feature that differentiates established lesions is the increased number of plasma cells, which become the preponderant inflammatory cell type. Plasma cells invade the connective

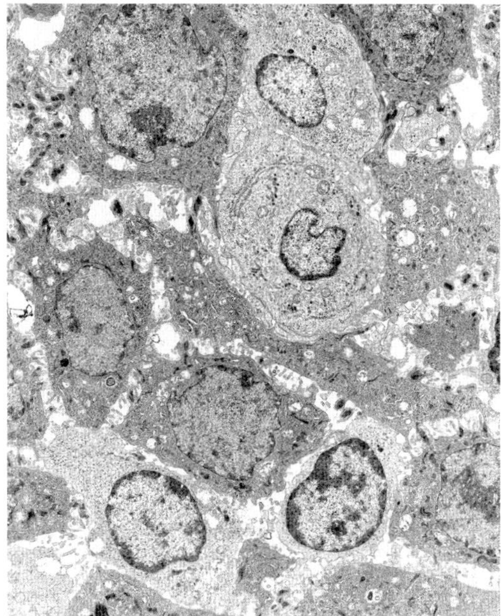

Fig. 15.8 Established gingivitis in a human subject. An area of crevicular epithelium exhibits enlarged intercellular spaces with numerous microvilli and desmosomal junctions. Several lymphocytes, both small and large, are seen migrating through the epithelial layer (magnification, ×3000).

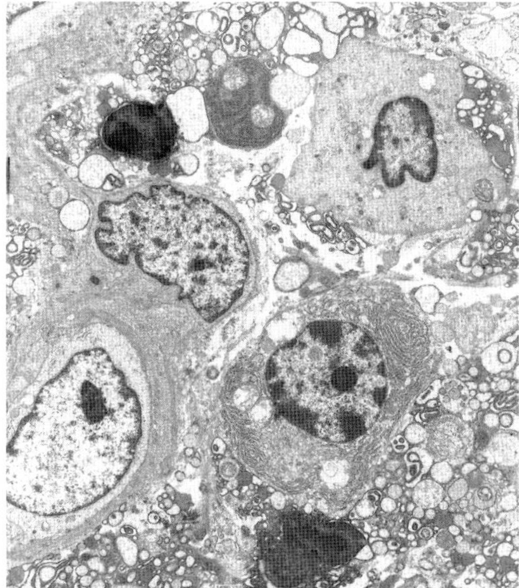

Fig. 15.9 Advanced gingivitis in a human subject. This specimen from the lamina propria exhibits plasma cell degeneration, with abundant cellular debris visible (magnification, ×3000). (Courtesy Dr. Charles Cobb, Kansas City, MO.)

tissue not only immediately below the junctional epithelium but also deep into the connective tissue, around the blood vessels, and between the bundles of collagen fibers.[21] The junctional epithelium reveals widened intercellular spaces that are filled with granular cellular debris, including lysosomes derived from disrupted neutrophils, lymphocytes, and monocytes (Fig. 15.8). The lysosomes contain acid hydrolases that can destroy tissue components. The junctional epithelium develops rete pegs or ridges that protrude into the connective tissue, and the basal lamina is destroyed in some areas. In the connective tissue, collagen fibers are destroyed around the infiltrate of intact and disrupted plasma cells, neutrophils, lymphocytes, monocytes, and mast cells (Fig. 15.9).

The predominance of plasma cells is thought to be a primary characteristic of established lesions. However, several studies of human experimental gingivitis have failed to demonstrate plasma cell predominance in the affected connective tissues,[22,23,133] including one study of 6 months' duration.[10] An increase in the proportion of plasma cells was evident with longstanding gingivitis, but the time for the development of classic "established lesions" may exceed 6 months.

An inverse relationship appears to exist between the number of intact collagen bundles and the number of inflammatory cells.[139] Collagenolytic activity is increased in inflamed gingival tissue[52] by the enzyme collagenase. While collagenase is normally present in gingival tissues,[18] in disease it is produced in high amounts by oral bacteria and innate immune cells, including PMNs.

Enzyme histochemistry studies have shown that chronically inflamed gingivae have elevated levels of acid and alkaline phosphatase,[160] β-glucuronidase, β-glucosidase, β-galactosidase, esterases,[78] aminopeptidase,[95,122] and cytochrome oxidase.[24] Neutral mucopolysaccharide levels are decreased,[149] presumably as a result of degradation of the ground substance.

Established lesions of two types appear to exist; some remain stable and do not progress for months or years,[86,95,145] and others seem to become more active and convert to progressively destructive lesions. In addition, established lesions appear to be reversible, in that the sequence of events that occurs in the tissues as a result of successful periodontal therapy seems to be essentially the reverse of the sequence of events observed as gingivitis develops. This reciprocal and reversible relationship is also true for the biofilm and microbiome. As oral hygiene habits change or metabolic stressors reduce, the microbiota reverts from that characteristically associated with destructive lesions, to that associated with periodontal health. This is accompanied by great decreases in the percentage of plasma cells and the lymphocyte population increases proportionately.[76,80]

Stage IV Gingival Inflammation: The Advanced Lesion

The extension of the lesion into the alveolar bone characterizes the fourth stage, which is known as the *advanced lesion*[118] or *phase of periodontal breakdown.*[75] This is described in detail in Chapter 21.

Microscopically, fibrosis of the gingiva is present and there is a widespread manifestation of inflammatory and immunopathologic tissue damage.[114] At the advanced stage, the presence of plasma cells dominates the connective tissue, and neutrophils continue dominating the junctional epithelium.

Patients with experimental gingivitis had significantly more plaque accumulation, higher interleukin-1β levels, and lower interleukin-8 concentrations at 28 days.[38]

Gingivitis will progress to periodontitis only in individuals who are susceptible. Patients who had sites with consistent bleeding (gingival index = 2) had 70% more attachment loss as compared with sites that were not consistently inflamed (gingival index = 0). Teeth with noninflamed sites consistently had a 50-year survival rate of 99.5%, whereas teeth with consistently inflamed gingiva had a 63.4% survival rate over 50 years. On the basis of this longitudinal study of the natural history of periodontitis in a well-maintained male population, persistent gingivitis represents a risk factor for periodontal attachment loss and tooth loss.[67] However, whether periodontitis can occur without a precursor of gingivitis is not known at this time.

Various systemic alterations are impacted by microbial metabolic changes and the host interactions described. Periodontal disease-related chronic inflammation impacts the vasculature, and the biofilm impacts the host directly via microbial invasion into tissues and/or through indirect mechanisms via the release of secreted mediators. For many conditions, the challenge is to establish a causal relationship and future investigations aim to identify "why" and "how" the microbiome transitions from a healthy to a pathogenic state. This will further lead to a dysbiosis, which triggers the host to shift from a reversible to an irreversible lesion in the context of inflammatory networks.[63]

Gingivitis

Experimental gingivitis studies provided the first empiric evidence that the accumulation of microbial biofilm on clean tooth surfaces results in the development of an inflammatory process in gingival tissues.[84,137] Research also shows that local inflammation persists as long as the microbial biofilm is present adjacent to the gingival tissues and that the inflammation resolves after meticulous removal of the biofilm.[137] Noting a reversibility of this gingivitis stage, it is considered a defensive process led by a series of host protective mechanisms that prevent inflammatory bone resorption.[16]

With the prevalence of gingivitis evident as worldwide, epidemiologic studies indicate that more than 82% of adolescents in the United States have overt gingivitis and signs of gingival bleeding. A similar or higher prevalence of gingivitis is reported for children and adolescents in other parts of the world.[4] A significant percentage of adults also show signs of gingivitis; more than half of the US adult population is estimated to exhibit gingival bleeding, and other populations have even higher levels of gingival inflammation.[3,5,6,8,125] Plaque remains the primary etiologic factor that causes gingivitis, but other factors can affect the development of periodontal disease. Experimental gingivitis studies suggest an important role of the host response in the development and degree of gingival inflammation.[154] Clinical features of gingivitis can be characterized by any of the following clinical signs: redness and sponginess of the gingival tissue, bleeding on provocation, changes in contour, and the presence of calculus or plaque with no radiographic evidence of crestal bone loss.[11] Histologic examination of inflamed gingival tissue reveals ulcerated epithelium. Inflammatory mediators negatively affect epithelial function as a protective barrier. Repair of this ulcerated epithelium depends on the proliferative or regenerative activity of the epithelial cells, and removal of the etiologic agents that triggered gingival breakdown is essential.

Oral Microbiome

Approximately, 800 bacterial species have been identified and the Human ORAL Microbiome Database (eHOMD: homd.org) is one of the most comprehensive repository databases for the oral and nasal cavities. To unravel the complex microbiome, new approaches have been employed. Novel technology 16S rRNAgene (16S) sequence has allowed elucidation of commensals and pathobionts. *Pophyromonas gingivalis*[104] was the first oral microbe to have its complete genome sequenced by Sanger sequencing. Subsequently, Bik and colleagues employed sequencing to determine the oral microbiome of 10 healthy individuals and discovered species-level data.[19] This was followed by 454 and shotgun sequencing, in which oral metagenomic studies[9] became more common and these sequences now reveal the landscape of the human oral microbiome. Sequencing is key to the field of oral microbiology because it allows the discovery of organisms that are not cultivable, and it enables the dissection of the polymicrobial community.

The scale and magnitude of the oral interface suggest that the host-microbe interactions impact disease susceptibility, microbial metabolism, and host immune responses. Tooth eruption and interactions with the oral microbiome impact periodontal niches (sulcular, gingival fluid, and periodontal pocket). There are differences in the biofilm attached to the tooth and root surfaces even millimeters apart. The human microbiome harbors thousands of pathways that[106] control metabolites and secrete molecules responsible for producing the signature that the host response interacts with. Metatranscriptomic studies of the healthy to gingivitis transition revealed a network of regulatory genes in proteolytic and nucleolytic processes that are key for microbial virulence.[106] The diversity of the 16S rRNA revealed that samples cluster according to disease severity and oral hygiene status. With the advent of metabolomics and proteomics, a new level of resolution is now possible; providing details on the function of microbes versus only their compositions. The transition from a commensal (habitant and healthy) microbiome to pathobionts (opportunistic and pathogenic) relates to nutritional backgrounds, genetic variations, niche anatomy, immune exposures, and other environmental factors. The biofilm members (composition) and the microbiome-derived metabolism (function) impact the salivary planktonic ecology, which in turn, impacts the host immune cell migration and sulcus permeability initiating a host response.

Course and Duration

Gingivitis can develop with sudden onset and have a short duration, and it can be painful. A less severe phase of this condition can also occur. Chronic gingivitis develops slowly and has a long duration. It is painless unless it is complicated by acute or subacute exacerbations, and it is the type that is most often encountered (Fig. 15.10). Chronic gingivitis is a fluctuating disease in which inflammation

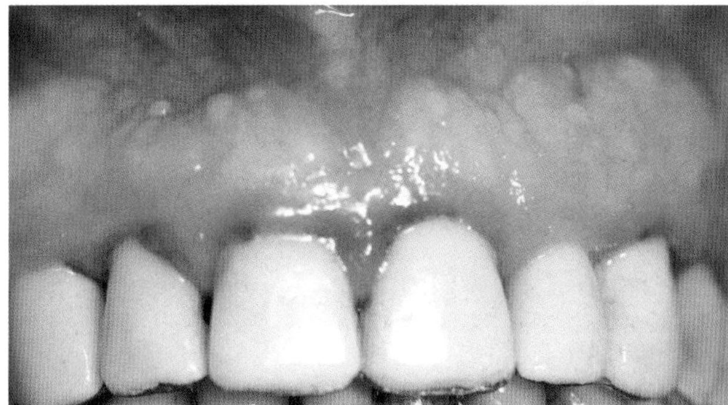

Fig. 15.10 Chronic gingivitis. The marginal and interdental gingivae are smooth, edematous, and discolored. Isolated areas of acute response are seen.

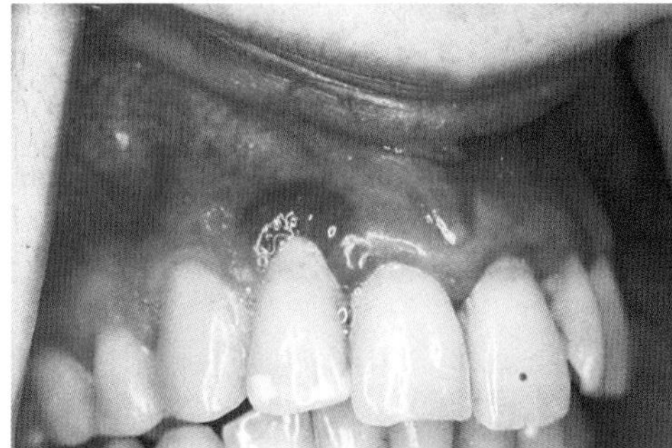

Fig. 15.11 Localized marginal gingivitis is confined to one or more areas of the marginal gingiva. Localized diffuse, intensely red area on the facial surface of tooth #7 and dark pink marginal changes in the remaining anterior teeth.

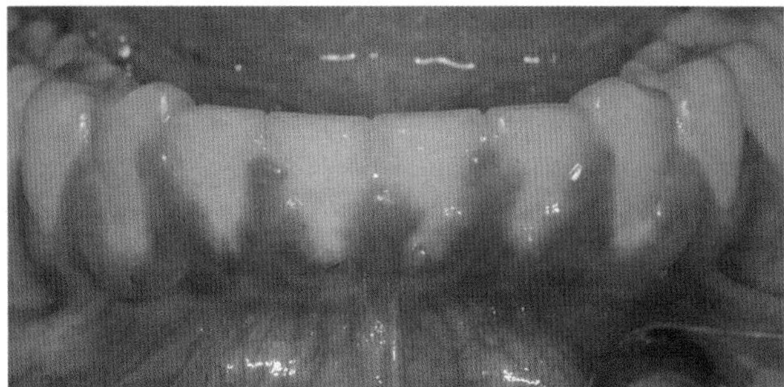

Fig. 15.12 Localized diffuse gingivitis extends from the margin to the mucobuccal fold in a limited area. Generalized marginal gingivitis in the lower jaw with areas of diffuse gingivitis.

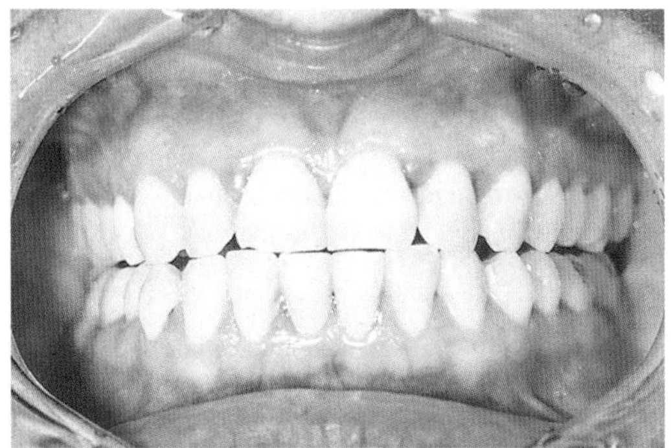

Fig. 15.13 Localized papillary gingivitis is confined to one or more interdental spaces in a limited area. Generalized papillary gingivitis.

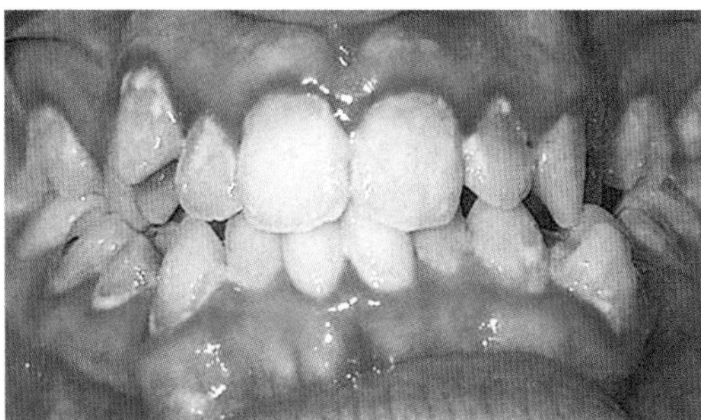

Fig. 15.14 Generalized marginal and papillary gingivitis. Generalized marginal gingivitis involves the gingival margins in relation to all the teeth. The interdental papillae are usually affected.

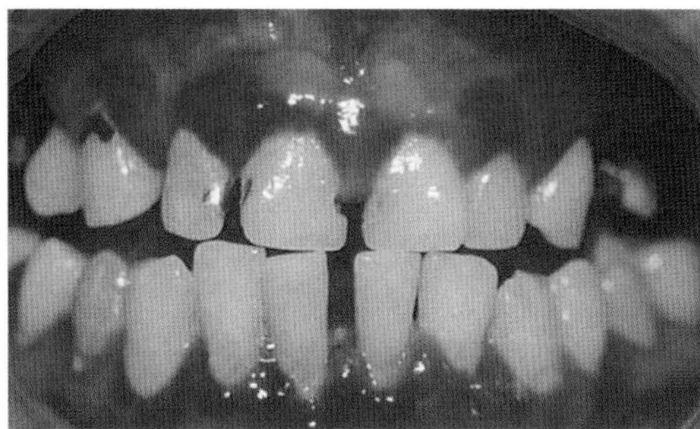

Fig. 15.15 Generalized diffuse gingivitis involves the entire gingiva. Because the alveolar mucosa and attached gingiva are affected, the mucogingival junction is sometimes obliterated. Generalized diffuse gingivitis involves the marginal, papillary, and attached gingivae.

TABLE 15.2 Hallmarks of Gingivitis

Feature	Healthy Gingiva	Gingivitis
Color	Coral pink	Red
Contour	Knife-edged and scalloped	Rolled with bulbous papillae
Consistency and texture	Firm and resilient with stippling of the attached gingiva	Edematous and with loss of stippling

persists or resolves and normal areas become inflamed.[57,69] Recurrent gingivitis reappears after having been eliminated by treatment or after disappearing spontaneously.

Description

Localized gingivitis is confined to the gingiva of a single tooth or group of teeth. Generalized gingivitis involves the entire mouth. Marginal gingivitis involves the gingival margin, and it can include a portion of the contiguous attached gingiva (Figs. 15.11 and 15.12). Papillary gingivitis involves the interdental papillae, and it often extends into the adjacent portion of the gingival margin. Papillae are involved more frequently than the gingival margin, and the earliest signs of gingivitis often occur in the papillae (Figs. 15.13 and 15.14). Diffuse gingivitis affects the gingival margin, the attached gingiva, and the interdental papillae (Fig. 15.15). Gingival disease in individual cases is described by combining the preceding terms as shown in Table 15.2.

2017 World Workshop Definition and Grading

A dental plaque biofilm-induced gingivitis site (GS) is defined as an inflammatory lesion resulting from interactions between the dental plaque biofilm and the host's immune-inflammatory response.[28] The 2017 World Workshop has recognized plaque biofilm-induced gingivitis as either a GS or a gingivitis case (GC).[28] The definitions are based on a comprehensive analysis of the clinical parameters (gingival crevicular fluid, gingival index, and gingival bleeding indices) and specific biomarkers in oral fluids (gingival crevicular fluid proteomics, salivary proteomics, microbiological markers, systemic inflammation markers, and genetic markers).[155] Differentiating between GS and GC allows the clinician-provider to incorporate a patient-centered approach towards precision dental medicine, to develop the appropriate assessment tools, and to reinforce oral home care instruction geared towards attaining clinical health.

Gingivitis Case

Intact Periodontium

The grading system for GC can be objectively identified by using the BOP score (BOP %) and further classified into categories of an intact periodontium, reduced periodontium, and having localized severity, or generalized severity.[155] The intact periodontium will present without clinical attachment loss or radiographic bone loss. Localized gingivitis in the intact periodontium can have a BOP % score ≥10% and ≤30% noting that patients may or may not potentially report symptoms of bleeding gums during routine oral home care. Although generalized gingivitis in the intact periodontium can also present without clinical attachment loss and radiographic bone loss, the typical BOP % grading score is greater than 30%. These patients typically self-report bleeding gums during routine care. After clinical examination, a periodontal assessment of an intact

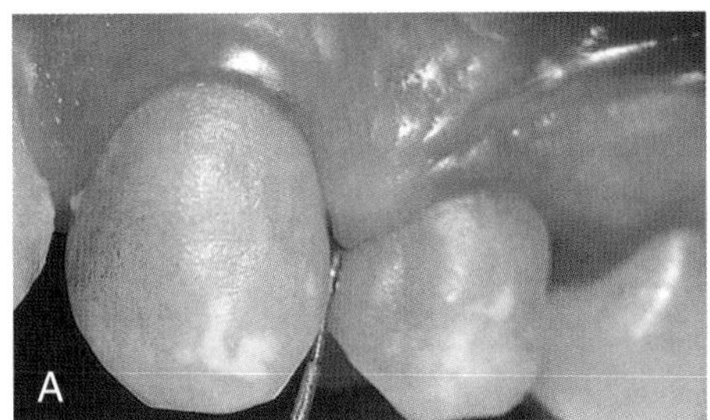

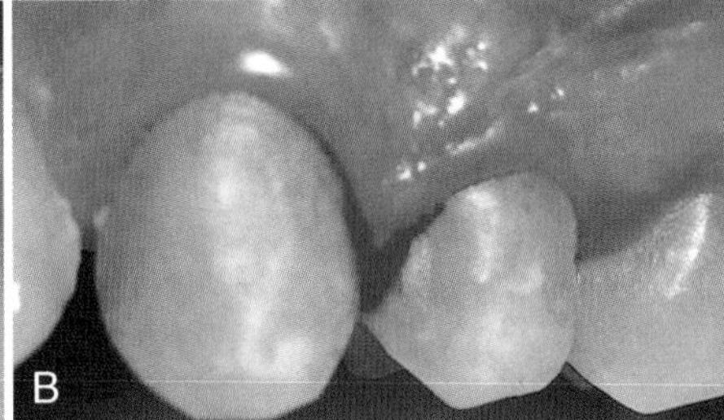

Fig. 15.16 Bleeding on probing. (A) To explore mild edematous gingivitis, a probe is introduced to the bottom of the gingival sulcus. (B) Bleeding appears after a few seconds.

periodontium with less than 10% BOP measurements (minimal inflammation) and without radiographic bone loss, can be appropriately assigned a status of clinical health.

Reduced Periodontium

The reduced periodontium patient can be broadly categorized as either not having a history of periodontitis or having successfully completed periodontal therapy while maintaining a state of periodontal stability. As reported by Trombelli and colleagues (2017), the GC on a reduced periodontium can typically present as gingival recession, or crown lengthening with BOP % ≥ 10%. Localized severity is defined as BOP ≥ 10% and ≤30%. Generalized severity shows as BOP greater than 30%. This grading system also considers the reduced periodontium patient who has been successfully treated for periodontitis presenting with probing attachment loss, possible radiographic bone loss, and BOP % ≥ 10%. The most significant consideration presenting without BOP in any site probing is ≥ 4 mm. Furthermore, while clinical periodontal health is defined as a state free from inflammatory periodontal disease, clinical gingival health on a reduced periodontium incorporates multiple factors under the new grading system. This is specifically characterized by an absence of BOP, erythema, edema in the presence of reduced clinical attachment, and possible reduced bone levels.[8]

Clinical Findings

A systematic approach is required for the evaluation of the clinical features of gingivitis. The clinician should focus on subtle tissue alterations because they may have diagnostic significance. A systematic clinical approach requires an orderly examination of the gingiva for color, contour, consistency, position, and ease and severity of bleeding and pain. This section discusses these clinical characteristics and the microscopic changes that are responsible for each.

Gingival Bleeding on Probing

The two earliest signs of gingival inflammation that precede established gingivitis are increased gingival crevicular fluid production and bleeding from the gingival sulcus on gentle probing (Fig. 15.16). Chapter 14 discusses gingival crevicular fluid in detail. Gingival bleeding varies in severity, duration, and ease of provocation. BOP is easily detected clinically and therefore is of value for early diagnosis and for the prevention of more advanced gingivitis. BOP appears earlier than a change in color or other visual signs of inflammation.[69,71,90] The use of bleeding rather than color changes to diagnose early gingival inflammation is advantageous, in that bleeding is a more objective sign that requires less subjective estimation by the examiner. An estimated 53.2 million (50.3%) US adults who are 30 years of age or older exhibit gingival bleeding.[5] Probing pocket depth measurements by themselves are of limited value in assessing the extent and severity of gingivitis. For example, gingival recession may result in a reduction of probing depth and cause inaccurate assessment of the periodontal status.[7] BOP is widely used by clinicians and epidemiologists to measure disease prevalence and progression, measure outcomes of treatment, and motivate patients to perform necessary home care.[48] See Chapter 6 for several gingival indices that are based on bleeding[2,27,98] and for more information on probing.

Gingival BOP indicates an inflammatory lesion in the epithelium and the connective tissue that exhibits specific histologic differences compared with healthy gingiva.[49] Although gingival BOP may not be a good diagnostic indicator of clinical attachment loss, its absence is an excellent negative predictor of future attachment loss.[67] The absence of gingival BOP is desirable and implies a low risk of future clinical attachment loss. Longitudinal findings revealed that sites with consistent bleeding (gingival index = 2) had 70% more attachment loss than sites that were noninflamed over a 26-year period in 565 male patients. Persistent gingivitis can be considered a risk factor for periodontal attachment loss that may lead to tooth loss.[68]

Numerous studies have shown that current cigarette smoking suppresses the gingival inflammatory response, and smoking was found to exert a strong, chronic, dose-dependent suppressive effect on gingival BOP in the Third National Health and Nutrition Examination Survey (NHANES III).[34] Research has revealed an increase in gingival BOP in patients who quit smoking,[100] and people who are committed to a smoking cessation program should be informed about the possibility of an increase in gingival bleeding associated with smoking cessation.

Gingival Bleeding Caused by Local Factors

Factors that contribute to plaque retention and may lead to gingivitis include anatomic and developmental tooth variations, caries, frenum pull, iatrogenic factors, malpositioned teeth, mouth breathing, overhangs, partial dentures, lack of attached gingiva, and recession. Orthodontic treatment and fixed retainers are associated with increased plaque retention and increased BOP.[72,148]

Chronic and Recurrent Bleeding

The most common cause of abnormal gingival BOP is chronic inflammation.[94] The bleeding is chronic or recurrent, and it is provoked by mechanical trauma (e.g., toothbrushing, toothpicks, food impaction) or by biting into solid foods (e.g., apples).

In gingival inflammation, histopathologic alterations that result in abnormal gingival bleeding include dilation and engorgement of the capillaries and thinning or ulceration of the sulcular epithelium (Fig. 15.17). Because the capillaries are engorged and closer to the surface and because the thinned, degenerated epithelium is less protective, stimuli that are normally innocuous cause rupture of the capillaries, and gingival bleeding occurs. Sites that bleed

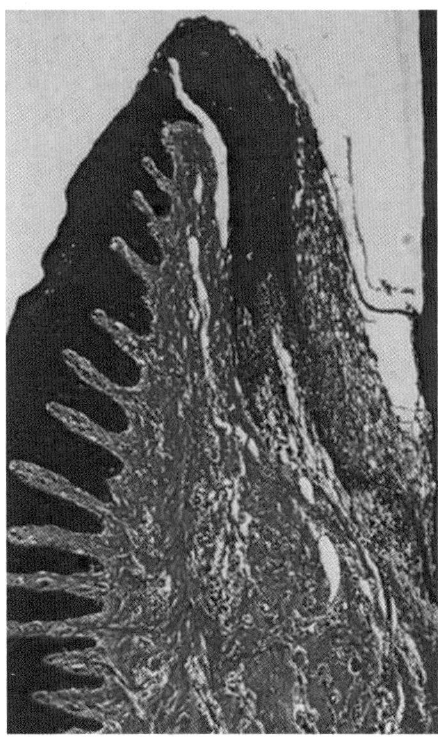

Fig. 15.17 Microscopic view of the interdental space in a human autopsy specimen. Note the inflammatory infiltrate and thinned epithelium in the area adjacent to the tooth and the collagenous tissue in the outer half of the section.

on probing have a greater area of inflamed connective tissue (i.e., cell-rich, collagen-poor tissue) than sites that do not bleed. In most cases, the cellular infiltrate of sites that bleed on probing is predominantly lymphocytic, which is a characteristic of stage II (early) gingivitis.[10,31,49]

Histologic evaluations of animal specimens have revealed that during the early stages of gingivitis, expression of the cytokines (i.e., matrix metalloproteinases [MMPs]) that are responsible for connective tissue breakdown is ubiquitous. Different MMPs play roles in this breakdown at different stages (e.g., a decrease of MMP-14 activity at day 7 of inflammation; immediate increase in MMP-2, especially with fibroblastic stimulation). MMP-9 expression peaked 5 days after gingivitis occurrence, which was also regulated by macrophages and neutrophils. Extracellular matrix remodeling was regulated with MMP-2 and MMP-9 production and activation by the host inflammatory response.[85] With the advancement of single-cell technologies, novel cell populations and cell heterogeneity are being discovered. Oral cell populations have been found in saliva, salivary glands, gingival tissues,[59] and in periodontal diseases.[159] These emerging concepts from single-cell transcriptomics and proteomics now open the opportunity to find pathogenic cellular populations within the tissues, improving understanding of the origin of diseases and dissecting dysbiotic molecular targets.

CLINICAL CORRELATION

Medications and Gingival Bleeding

- Drugs such as antiplatelet medications (e.g., aspirin) or anticoagulants (e.g., warfarin) that are prescribed for specific medical indications also increase the bleeding tendencies of gingival tissues.
- Women taking oral contraceptives are significantly more prone to gingivitis and therefore to gingival bleeding.

The severity of bleeding and the ease of its provocation depend on the intensity of inflammation. After the vessels are damaged and ruptured, interrelated mechanisms induce hemostasis.[142] The vessel walls contract, blood flow diminishes, blood platelets adhere to the edges of the tissue, and a fibrous clot is formed that contracts and results in approximation of the edges of the injured area. Bleeding recurs when the area is irritated.

In cases of moderate or advanced periodontitis, BOP is considered a sign of active tissue destruction. Acute episodes of gingival bleeding are caused by injury, and they can occur spontaneously in patients with gingival disease. Laceration of the gingiva by toothbrush bristles during aggressive toothbrushing or by sharp pieces of hard food can cause gingival bleeding, even in the absence of gingival disease. Gingival burns from hot foods or chemicals increase the ease of gingival bleeding.

Spontaneous bleeding or bleeding on slight provocation can occur with acute necrotizing ulcerative gingivitis. With this condition, engorged blood vessels in the inflamed connective tissue are exposed by ulceration of the necrotic surface epithelium.

Gingival Bleeding Associated With Systemic Changes

With some systemic disorders, gingival hemorrhage occurs spontaneously or after irritation (usually generalized), and it is excessive and difficult to control. These hemorrhagic diseases represent a wide variety of conditions that vary with regard to etiologic factors and clinical manifestations. Such conditions have the common feature of a hemostatic mechanism failure that results in abnormal bleeding in the skin, internal organs, and other tissues, including the oral mucosa.[140]

Hemorrhagic disorders in which abnormal gingival bleeding is encountered include vascular abnormalities (e.g., vitamin C deficiency, allergy such as Henoch–Schönlein purpura), platelet disorders[51] (e.g., thrombocytopenic purpura), hypoprothrombinemia (e.g., vitamin K deficiency), other coagulation defects (e.g., hemophilia, leukemia, Christmas disease), deficient platelet thromboplastic factor as a result of uremia,[91] multiple myeloma,[17] and postrubella purpura.[57] The effects of hormonal replacement therapy, oral contraceptives, pregnancy, and the menstrual cycle are also reported to affect gingival bleeding.[87,124,150,151] In women, long-term depression-related stress exposure may increase concentrations of interleukin-6 in gingival crevicular fluid and worsen periodontal conditions, producing elevated levels of gingival inflammation and increased pocket depths.[60]

CLINICAL CORRELATION

Pregnancy-Associated Gingivitis

Pregnancy-associated gingivitis affects many pregnant women and is primarily caused by the hormonal imbalances associated with pregnancy. It is characterized by mild to severe gingival inflammation along with pain and, in some cases, significant hyperplasia and bleeding. In most patients, the condition normally resolves by itself after delivery, when the hormonal levels return to normal.

Changes in sex hormones have long been established as significant modifying factors in gingivitis, especially among adolescents. Several reports have shown notable effects of fluctuating estrogen and progesterone levels on the periodontium, starting as early as puberty.[1,101] Diabetes is an endocrine condition with a well-characterized effect on gingivitis.[148] In diabetes, marked inflammation affects both epithelial and connective tissues, leading to a degeneration of the dermal papilla, an increase in the number of inflammatory cells, the destruction of reticulin fibers, and an accumulation of dense collagen fibers that causes fibrosis.[138]

Several medications have also been found to have adverse effects on the gingiva. For example, anticonvulsants, antihypertensive calcium channel blockers, and immunosuppressive drugs cause gingival enlargement (see Chapter 19), which can cause gingival inflammation and bleeding. The American Heart Association has recommended over-the-counter aspirin as a prophylactic and therapeutic agent for cardiovascular disease, and aspirin is often prescribed for other conditions such as rheumatoid arthritis, osteoarthritis, rheumatic fever, and other inflammatory joint diseases.[54] It is important to consider aspirin's effect on bleeding during a routine dental examination to avoid false-positive readings that could result in an inaccurate diagnosis.[126] Chapter 19 discusses periodontal involvement in hematologic disorders.

Color Changes in the Gingiva

The color of the gingiva is determined by several factors, including the number and size of blood vessels, the epithelial thickness, the quantity of keratinization, and the pigments in the epithelium.

Color Changes With Gingivitis

Change in color is an important clinical sign of gingival disease. The normal gingival color is coral pink, and it is produced by the tissue's vascularity and modified by the overlying epithelial layers. The gingiva becomes red when vascularization increases or the degree of epithelial keratinization is reduced or disappears. The color becomes pale when vascularization is reduced (in association with fibrosis of the corium) or epithelial keratinization increases. Chronic inflammation intensifies the red or bluish red color as a result of vascular proliferation and a reduction of keratinization. Venous stasis contributes a bluish hue. The gingival color changes with increasing chronicity of the inflammatory process. The changes start in the interdental papillae and gingival margin and then spread to the attached gingiva.

Proper diagnosis and treatment depend on understanding the tissue changes that alter the color of the gingiva at the clinical level. Color changes in acute gingival inflammation differ in both nature and distribution from those in patients with chronic gingivitis. The color changes can be marginal, diffuse, or patch-like, depending on the underlying acute condition. With acute necrotizing ulcerative gingivitis, the involvement is marginal; with herpetic gingivostomatitis, it is diffuse; and with acute reactions to chemical irritation, it is patch-like or diffuse.

CLINICAL CORRELATION

Mouth Breathing and Gingival Inflammation

Gingivitis in the maxillary buccal area of the oral cavity is a common finding in patients who are mouth breathers. The affected gingiva typically appears red, shiny, and edematous, which is thought to be related to the surface dehydration caused by mouth breathing.

Color changes vary with the intensity of inflammation. Initially, there is an increase in erythema. If the condition does not worsen, this is the only color change until the gingiva reverts to normal. With severe acute inflammation, the red color gradually becomes a dull, whitish gray. The gray discoloration produced by tissue necrosis is demarcated from the adjacent gingiva by a thin, sharply defined erythematous zone. Chapters 14 and 17 provides detailed descriptions of the clinical and pathologic features of the various forms of acute gingivitis.

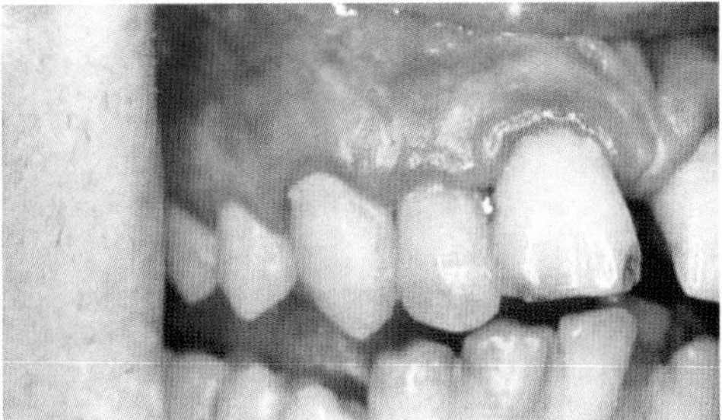

Fig. 15.18 Bismuth gingivitis. Note the linear black discoloration of the gingiva in a patient who is receiving bismuth therapy.

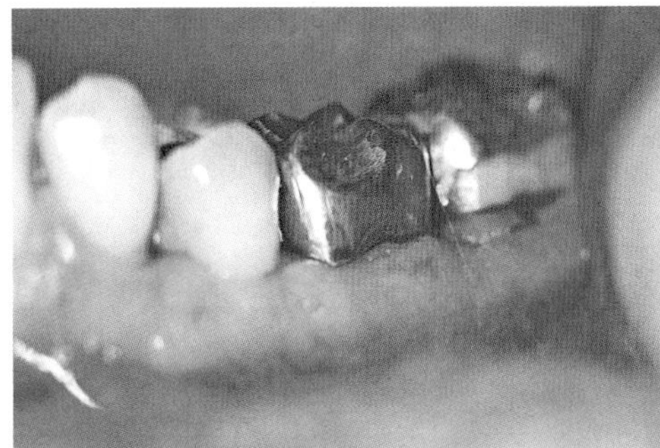

Fig. 15.19 Discoloration of the gingiva is caused by embedded metal particles (i.e., amalgam).

Various systemic alterations are impacted by microbial metabolic changes and host interactions described. Periodontal disease with chronic inflammation impacts the vasculature, and the biofilm impacts the host directly via microbial invasion and tissue establishment and/or through indirect mechanisms via the release of secreted mediators. For many conditions, the challenge is to establish a causal relationship and future investigations aim to identify "why" and "how" the microbiome transitions from healthy to pathogenic. This will further elucidate dysbiosis and the functions altered by the host to produce a reversible to an irreversible lesion in the context of inflammatory networks.[63]

Metallic Pigmentation

Heavy metals (i.e., bismuth, arsenic, mercury, lead, and silver) that are absorbed systemically as a result of therapeutic use or occupational or household exposures can discolor the gingiva and other areas of the oral mucosa.[39] These changes are rare, but they should be ruled out in suspected cases.

Metals typically produce a black or bluish line in the gingiva that follows the contour of the margin (Fig. 15.18). The pigmentation may also appear as isolated black blotches involving the interdental marginal and attached gingiva. This is different from the tattooing produced by the accidental embedding of amalgam or other metal fragments (Fig. 15.19).[25] Gingival pigmentation from systemically absorbed metals results from the perivascular precipitation of metallic sulfides in the subepithelial connective tissue.

Gingival pigmentation is not a result of systemic toxicity. It occurs only in areas of inflammation in which the increased permeability of irritated blood vessels permits the seepage of metal into the surrounding tissue. In addition to inflamed gingiva, mucosal areas that are irritated by biting or abnormal chewing habits (e.g., inner surface of lips, cheek at the level of the occlusal line, lateral border of the tongue) are common sites of pigmentation. Pigmentation can be eliminated by treating the inflammatory changes without necessarily discontinuing the metal-containing medication.

Color Changes Associated With Systemic Factors

Many systemic diseases can cause color changes in the oral mucosa, including the gingiva.[37] In general, these abnormal pigmentations are nonspecific, and they should stimulate further diagnostic efforts or referral to the appropriate specialist.[136]

Endogenous oral pigmentation can be caused by melanin, bilirubin, or iron.[89] Melanin oral pigmentation can be normal and is often found in highly pigmented ethnic groups (see Chapters 16 and 18). Diseases that increase melanin pigmentation include the following:

- Addison's disease is caused by adrenal dysfunction, and it produces isolated patches of discoloration that vary from bluish-black to brown.
- Peutz–Jeghers syndrome produces intestinal polyposis and melanin pigmentation in the oral mucosa and lips.
- Albright syndrome (i.e., polyostotic fibrous dysplasia) and von Recklinghausen disease (i.e., neurofibromatosis) produce areas of oral melanin pigmentation.

The skin and mucous membranes can also be stained by bile pigments. Jaundice is best detected by examination of the sclera, but the oral mucosa may also acquire a yellowish color. The deposition of iron in hemochromatosis may produce blue-gray pigmentation of the oral mucosa. Several endocrine and metabolic disturbances, including diabetes and pregnancy, can result in color changes. Blood dyscrasias, such as anemia, polycythemia, and leukemia also can induce color changes.

Exogenous factors that are capable of producing color changes in the gingiva include atmospheric irritants, such as coal and metal dust, and coloring agents in food and lozenges. Tobacco causes hyperkeratosis of the gingiva, and it can induce a significant increase in melanin pigmentation of the oral mucosa.[105] Localized bluish-black areas of pigment are often caused by amalgam implanted in the mucosa (see Fig. 15.19).

The need for esthetics in dentistry has increased, with a growing demand for a pleasing smile. This has made many individuals more aware of their gingival pigmentation, which may be apparent when smiling and speaking.[35,36] Traditionally, gingival depigmentation has been carried out with the use of nonsurgical and surgical procedures, including chemical, cryosurgical, and electrosurgical techniques. However, those techniques were met with skepticism because of their various degrees of success.

Lasers have been used to ablate cells that produce the melanin pigment; a nonspecific laser beam destroys the epithelial cells, including those at the basal layer. Selective ablation using a laser beam with a wavelength that is specifically absorbed by melanin effectively destroys the pigmented cells without damaging the nonpigmented cells. In both cases, radiation energy is transformed into ablation energy, resulting in cellular rupture and vaporization with minimal heating of the surrounding tissue.[146]

Changes in Gingival Consistency

Chronic and acute inflammation produce changes in the normal firm and resilient consistency of the gingiva. In patients with chronic gingivitis, destructive (i.e., edematous) and reparative (i.e., fibrotic) changes coexist, and the consistency of the gingiva is determined by their relative predominance (Figs. 15.20 and 15.21). Table 15.3

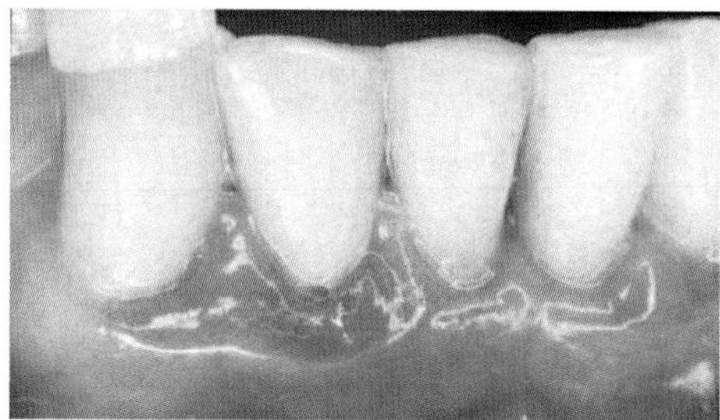

Fig. 15.20 Chronic gingivitis. Swelling, loss of stippling, and discoloration occur when inflammatory exudate and edema are the predominant microscopic changes. The gingiva is soft and friable and bleeds easily.

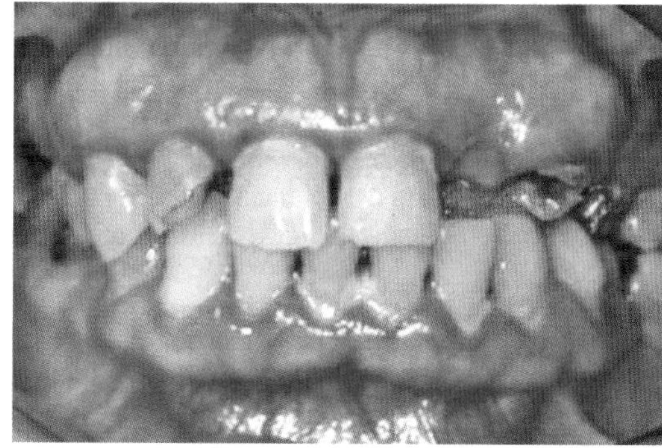

Fig. 15.21 Chronic gingivitis. Firm gingiva is produced when fibrosis predominates in the inflammatory process.

TABLE 15.3 Clinical and Histopathologic Changes in Gingival Consistency

Clinical Changes	Underlying Microscopic Features
Chronic Gingivitis	
1. Soggy puffiness that pits on pressure	1. Infiltration by fluid and cells of inflammatory exudate
2. Marked softness and friability, with ready fragmentation on exploration with probe and pinpoint surface areas of redness and desquamation	2. Degeneration of connective tissue and epithelium associated with injurious substances that provoke inflammation and inflammatory exudate; change in the connective tissue—epithelium relationship, with inflamed, engorged connective tissue expanding to within a few epithelial cells of the surface; thinning of epithelium and degeneration associated with edema and leukocyte invasion, separated by areas in which rete pegs are elongated to connective tissue
3. Firm, leathery consistency	3. Fibrosis and epithelial proliferation associated with long-standing chronic inflammation
Acute Gingivitis	
1. Diffuse puffiness and softening	1. Diffuse edema of acute inflammatory origin; fatty infiltration in xanthomatosis
2. Sloughing with grayish, flakelike particles of debris adhering to eroded surface	2. Necrosis with formation of pseudomembrane composed of bacteria, polymorphonuclear leukocytes, and degenerated epithelial cells in fibrinous meshwork
3. Vesicle formation	3. Intercellular and intracellular edema with degeneration of nucleus and cytoplasm and rupture of cell wall

summarizes the clinical alterations in the consistency of the gingiva and the microscopic changes that produce them.

Calcified Masses in the Gingiva

Calcified microscopic masses may be found in the gingiva.[20,97] They can occur alone or in groups, and they vary with regard to size, location, shape, and structure. Such masses may be calcified material that was removed from the tooth and traumatically displaced into the gingiva during scaling,[97] root remnants, cementum fragments, or cementicles. Chronic inflammation and fibrosis, an occasional foreign body, and giant-cell activity occur in reaction to the masses, which are sometimes enclosed in an osteoid-like matrix. Crystalline foreign bodies have also been described in the gingiva, but their origin has not been determined.[111]

Toothbrushing

Toothbrushing has various effects on the consistency of the gingiva, such as promoting keratinization of the oral epithelium, enhancing capillary gingival circulation, and thickening alveolar bone.[88,93,147] In animal studies, mechanical stimulation by toothbrushing was found to increase the proliferative activity of the junctional basal cells in dog gingiva by 2.5 times compared with the use of a scaler.[58] These findings may indicate that toothbrushing causes an increased turnover rate and desquamation of the junctional epithelial surfaces. This process may repair small breaks in the junctional epithelium and prevent direct access to the underlying tissue by periodontal pathogens.[153]

Changes in Gingival Surface Texture

The surface of normal gingiva usually exhibits numerous small depressions and elevations that give the tissue an orange-peel appearance referred to as stippling.[13] Stippling is restricted to the attached gingiva and is predominantly localized to the subpapillary area, but it extends to various degrees into the interdental papilla.[61] Although the biologic significance of gingival stippling is not known, some investigators conclude that the loss of stippling is an early sign of gingivitis.[62,112] However, clinicians must take into consideration that its pattern and extent vary in different mouth areas, among patients, and with age.

In patients with chronic inflammation, the gingival surface is smooth and shiny or firm and nodular, depending on whether the dominant changes are exudative or fibrotic. A smooth surface texture is also produced by epithelial atrophy in atrophic gingivitis, and peeling of the surface occurs with chronic desquamative gingivitis. Hyperkeratosis results in a leathery texture, and drug-induced gingival overgrowth produces a nodular surface.

CLINICAL CORRELATION

Stippling and Its Clinical Importance

Healthy, attached gingiva has a pitted orange-peel appearance on its surface. This surface feature, called stippling, is an external reflection of the underlying connective tissue projections into the overlying epithelium. The presence of stippling in the attached gingiva is indicative of gingival health, and this surface feature is usually lost when the tissue is edematous.

Changes in Gingival Position

Traumatic Lesions

A feature of gingival disease classification is the recognition of non–plaque-induced traumatic gingival lesions as distinct gingival conditions.[12] Traumatic lesions—whether chemical, physical, or thermal—are among the most common lesions in the mouth. Sources of chemical injuries include aspirin, hydrogen peroxide, silver nitrate, phenol, and endodontic materials. Physical injuries can include lip, oral, and tongue piercings, which can result in gingival recession. Thermal injuries can result from hot drinks and foods. In acute cases, the appearance of slough (i.e., necrotizing epithelium), erosion, or ulceration and accompanying erythema are common features. In chronic cases, permanent gingival defects usually take the form of gingival recession. Typically, the localized nature of the lesions and lack of symptoms readily eliminate them from the differential diagnosis of systemic conditions that may exist with erosive or ulcerative oral lesions.[123]

Gingival Recession

Gingival recession is a common finding. The prevalence, extent, and severity of gingival recession increase with age, and this condition is more prevalent among males.[5]

Positions of the Gingiva

By clinical definition, recession is an exposure of the root surface by an apical shift in the position of the gingiva. To understand recession, it helps to distinguish between the actual and apparent positions of the gingiva. The actual position is the level of the coronal end of the epithelial attachment on the tooth, whereas the apparent position is the level of the crest of the gingival margin (Fig. 15.22). The severity of recession is usually determined by the apparent position of the gingiva. However, the actual gingival position is used to determine the clinical attachment loss. For example, in periodontal disease, the inflamed pocket wall covers part of the denuded root; some of the recession is hidden, and some may be visible. The total amount of clinical attachment loss is the sum of the two. Recession refers to the location of the gingiva rather than to its condition. Receded gingiva can be inflamed, but it may be normal except for its position (Fig. 15.23). Recession can be localized to one tooth or a group of teeth, or it may be generalized throughout the mouth. Gingival recession increases with age; the incidence varies from 8% among children to 100% after 50 years of age.[161] This has led some investigators

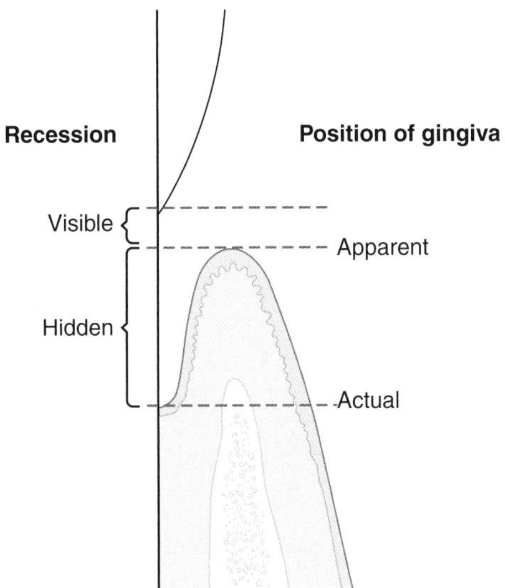

Fig. 15.22 Diagram of apparent and actual positions of the gingiva and visible and hidden recession.

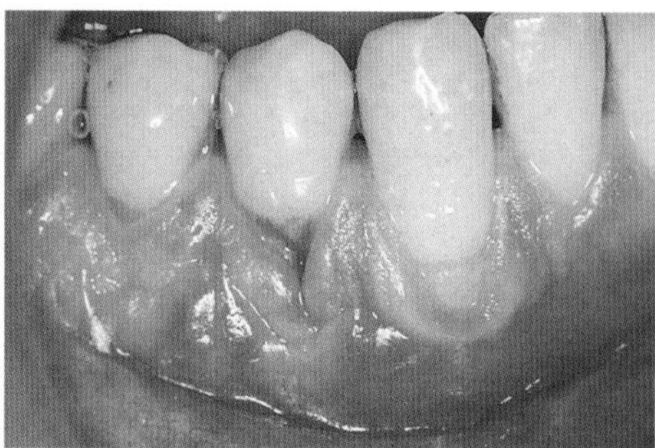

Fig. 15.23 Degrees of recession. Recession is slight in teeth #26 and #29 and marked in teeth #27 and #28. The change in gingival contour and the recession, as seen in tooth #28, are referred to as Stillman clefts.

to assume that recession might be a physiologic process related to aging. However, no convincing evidence has been presented for a physiologic shift of the gingival attachment.[82]

The gradual apical shift most likely results from the cumulative effect of minor pathologic involvement and repeated minor direct trauma to the gingiva. In some populations without access to dental care, however, recession can result from increasing periodontal disease.[55,83]

The following etiologic factors have been implicated in gingival recession: faulty toothbrushing technique (i.e., gingival abrasion), tooth malposition, friction from the soft tissues (i.e., gingival ablation),[141] gingival inflammation, abnormal frenum attachment, and iatrogenic dentistry. Trauma from occlusion has been suggested in the past, but its mechanism of action has never been demonstrated. For example, a deep overbite has been associated with gingival inflammation and recession. Excessive incisal overlap may result in a traumatic injury to the gingiva.

Orthodontic movement in a labial direction in monkeys has been shown to result in the loss of marginal bone and connective tissue attachment and in gingival recession.[143]

Standard oral hygiene procedures, including toothbrushing and flossing, frequently lead to transient and minimal gingival injury.[33,120] Although toothbrushing is important for gingival health, faulty technique or brushing with hard bristles can cause significant injury. This type of injury can manifest as lacerations, abrasions, keratosis, or recession, with the facial marginal gingiva being affected most often.[107] In these cases, recession tends to be more frequent and more severe in patients with clinically healthy gingiva, little bacterial plaque, and good oral hygiene.[47,108,109]

CLINICAL CORRELATION

Supracrestal Fibers (*Formerly Biologic Width*) and Gingival Inflammation

Supracrestal fibers are the circumferential rim of space around teeth where the junctional epithelium and the underlying connective tissue of the gingiva attach to the teeth. When restoring teeth, if the margins of the restorations violate the dimensions of supracrestal fibers, gingival inflammation ensues. If left untreated, it can lead to bone loss. Crown lengthening is a surgical procedure that is performed clinically (i.e., before restoration delivery) to intentionally create space for the supracrestal fibers to reestablish.

Susceptibility to recession is influenced by the position of teeth in the arch,[156] the root–bone angle, and the mesiodistal curvature of the tooth surface.[96] On rotated, tilted, or facially displaced teeth, the bony plate is thinned or reduced in height. Pressure from mastication or moderate toothbrushing damages the unsupported gingiva and produces recession. The effect of the angle of the root in the bone with recession is often observed in the maxillary molar area. If the lingual inclination of the palatal root is prominent or the buccal roots flare outward, the bone in the cervical area is thinned or shortened, and recession results from repeated trauma of the thin marginal gingiva.

The health of the gingival tissue also depends on properly designed and placed restorative materials. Pressure from a poorly designed partial denture, such as an ill-fitting denture clasp, can cause gingival trauma and recession.[162] Overhanging dental restorations have long been viewed as a contributing factor to gingivitis because of plaque retention. In addition, there is general agreement that placing restorative margins within the supracrestal fibers frequently leads to gingival inflammation, clinical attachment loss, and eventually bone loss. Clinically, the violation of supracrestal fibers typically manifests as gingival inflammation, deepened periodontal pockets, and gingival recession.

A relationship may exist between smoking and gingival recession (see Chapters 12 and 23). The multifactorial mechanisms probably include reduced gingival blood flow and an altered immune response, but current evidence is not conclusive.[50,121]

Clinical Significance

Several aspects of gingival recession make it clinically significant. Exposed root surfaces are susceptible to caries. Abrasion or erosion of the cementum exposed by recession leaves an underlying dentinal surface that can be sensitive. Hyperemia of the pulp and associated symptoms can result from excessive exposure of the root surface.[92] Interproximal recession creates oral hygiene problems resulting in plaque accumulation.

Changes in Gingival Contour

Changes in gingival contour are primarily associated with gingival enlargement (see Chapter 19), but changes may also occur with other conditions. Of historical interest are descriptions of indentations of the gingival margin referred to as Stillman clefts (see Fig. 15.23)[144] and McCall festoons. The term Stillman cleft has been used to describe a specific type of gingival recession that consists of a narrow, triangular-shaped gingival recession. As the recession progresses apically, the cleft becomes broader, thereby exposing the cementum of the root surface. When the lesion reaches the mucogingival junction, the apical border of oral mucosa is usually inflamed because of the difficulty in maintaining adequate plaque control at this site.

The term McCall festoon has been used to describe a rolled, thickened band of gingiva that is usually seen adjacent to the cuspids when recession approaches the mucogingival junction. Initially, Stillman clefts and McCall festoons were attributed to traumatic occlusion, and the recommended treatment was an occlusal adjustment. However, this association was never proved, and the indentations merely represent peculiar inflammatory changes of the marginal gingiva.[20]

Biofilm Management

The management of dental plaque biofilm-induced gingivitis is centered around the induced inflammatory response resulting from bacterial plaque accumulation at or below the gingival margin.[99] Routine mechanical debridement of this biofilm can be bolstered by a methodical strategy supportive for patient motivation and reinforcement through proper oral hygiene instruction. In addition, routine professional mechanical plaque removal is supportive to clinical gingival health as it can reestablish after the treatment of dental biofilm-induced gingivitis.[28] The significance of reinforced oral home care can be appreciated as the transition from periodontal health to gingivitis is reversible following treatment that resolves gingival inflammation.[28] Despite this relationship, it is relevant to note that the conversion from gingivitis to a state of periodontal disease is non-reversible. Empowering your patient population with oral health education that supports this transitionary phase and conversion state is vital to promoting appropriate home care management towards clinical health.

There are multiple factors that could put a patient at an increased susceptibility for biofilm plaque-induced gingivitis. The integration of an effective clinical assessment, adjunctive antimicrobial oral care products, nutritional dietary counseling, and effective tobacco cessation may be indicated as adjunctive therapeutics. Determining the state of clinical health begins with the information gathering stage and dental review for past history of gingivitis symptoms. This will allow for a thorough clinical evaluation, and to determine if there are any related medical conditions or contributing medications.[32] The reinforcement of nutritional counseling and tobacco cessation programs, specifically towards cigarettes, tobacco products, vape cartridges, and smokeless tobacco, all will contribute positively to attaining gingival health.[103,152]

The evolution of dental plaque biofilm management has been influenced by dental brushing devices and brushing modalities.[30,81] As a primary intervention, the dental toothbrush can be classified into categories of a manual non-motorized device, and a powered motorized device. Both are available in varying brush compositions and densities, noting that these characteristics are typically non-transferrable between makers.[102] Each manufacturer may have independent criteria for how they categorize their products as soft, medium, and hard, separate of whether the brush is a non-powered or powered device. Evidence-driven care will support that patients should brush their teeth at least twice a day for 2 minutes each session, with an appropriate dentifrice selection amongst other oral home care objectives.[29] Proper device adaptation and technique should be assessed during routine clinical care.[157] Reinforcing mechanical plaque removal in oral hygiene instruction is critical to ensuring optimal patient gingival health.

In addition to local aspects, various systemic alterations are impacted by microbial metabolic changes and host interactions described. Periodontal disease with chronic inflammation impacts the vasculature, and the biofilm impacts the host directly via microbial invasion and tissue establishment and/or through indirect mechanisms via the release of secreted mediators. For many conditions, the challenge is to establish a causal relationship and future investigations aim to identify "why" and "how" the microbiome transitions from healthy to pathogenic. This will further elucidate dysbiosis and the functions altered by the host to produce a reversible to an irreversible lesion in the context of inflammatory networks.[63]

The intervention of dental floss as a therapeutic modality is an equally important focus for the disruption of the plaque biofilm deposit. Interproximal mechanical debridement with dental floss will support the disruption of colonizing pathogenic microflora and is a large focus in gingivitis therapy.[29] Daily flossing is considered a necessary adjunct to brushing as this combination is highly effective in plaque biofilm disruption to areas that brushing cannot treat alone.[64] As an oral health provider, assess and guide patient instruction with consideration for dexterity. Alternative use of interdental and interproximal cleaning aids may be indicated as patients may become deterred and/or hesitant to utilize traditional floss modalities.

The adjunctive use of a well-formulated dentifrice and oral rinse for a routine oral home care routine can provide several benefits to a patient group. These chemotherapeutics for gingivitis prevention and therapy are integral to maintaining a homeostatic state of health as patients may have various levels of susceptibility to plaque biofilm deposits.[43] Consider recommendations that may include but are not limited to ingredients of fluoride, 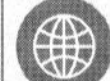 chlorhexidine gluconate, cetylpyridinium chloride, and saline. By endorsing a regular exposure to a properly indicated chemotherapeutic, the effects of plaque biofilm deposition can be significantly dampened, thus minimizing the inflammatory cascade that typically ensues course. Indications of these chemotherapeutics may be bacteriostatic, bactericidal, and pH-neutralizing. It is important to understand the indications for each product, how to appropriately prescribe dosing, and that they should not be considered interchangeable as adjunctive therapies for oral health.[45,135]

Case Scenarios are found on the companion website eBooks.Health.Elsevier.com

Suggested Readings

Alcaraz LD, et al. Identifying a healthy oral microbiome through metagenomics. *Clin Microbiol Infect*. 2012;18(suppl 4):54–57.

Bamashmous S, et al. Human variation in gingival inflammation. *Proc Natl Acad Sci U S A*. 2021;118(27).

Bik EM, et al. Bacterial diversity in the oral cavity of 10 healthy individuals. *Isme j*. 2010;4(8):962–974.

Chapple IL, et al. Primary prevention of periodontitis: managing gingivitis. *J Clin Periodontol*. 2015;42(suppl 16):S71–S76.

Chapple ILC, et al. Periodontal health and gingival diseases and conditions on an intact and a reduced periodontium: Consensus report of workgroup 1 of the 2017 World Workshop on the Classification of Periodontal and Peri-Implant Diseases and Conditions. *J Periodontol*. 2018;89(Suppl 1):S74–s84.

Daniel R, et al. Diabetes and periodontal disease. *J Pharm Bioallied Sci*. 2012;4(suppl 2):S280–S282.

Ebersole JL, et al. Transcriptome analysis of b cell immune functions in periodontitis: mucosal tissue responses to the oral microbiome in aging. *Front Immunol*. 2016;7:272.

Freire M, Nelson KE, Edlund A. The Oral Host-Microbial Interactome: An Ecological Chronometer of Health? *Trends Microbiol*. 2021;29(6): 551–561.

Friesen LR, et al. Comparative antiplaque effect of two antimicrobial dentifrices: laboratory and clinical evaluations. *J Clin Dent*. 2017;28:B6–11. 4 Spec No B.

Huang N, et al. SARS-CoV-2 infection of the oral cavity and saliva. *Nat Med*. 2021;27(5):892–903.

Kleinstein SE, Nelson KE, Freire M. Inflammatory networks linking oral microbiome with systemic health and disease. *J Dent Res*. 2020;99(10):1131–1139.

Kressin NR, et al. Increased preventive practices lead to greater tooth retention. *J Dent Res*. 2003;82(3):223–227.

Murakami S, et al. Dental plaque-induced gingival conditions. *J Periodontol*. 2018;89(suppl 1):S17–S27.

Neiva RF, et al. Effects of specific nutrients on periodontal disease onset, progression and treatment. *J Clin Periodontol*. 2003;30(7):579–589.

Nelson KE, et al. Complete genome sequence of the oral pathogenic Bacterium porphyromonas gingivalis strain W83. *J Bacteriol*. 2003;185(18): 5591–5601.

Nowicki EM, et al. Microbiota and metatranscriptome changes accompanying the onset of gingivitis. *mBio*. 2018;9(2).

Sharma N, et al. Adjunctive benefit of an essential oil-containing mouthrinse in reducing plaque and gingivitis in patients who brush and floss regularly: a six-month study. *J Am Dent Assoc*. 2004;135(4):496–504.

Tomar SL, Asma S. Smoking-attributable periodontitis in the United States: findings from NHANES III. National Health and Nutrition Examination Survey. *J Periodontol*. 2000;71(5):743–751.

Trombelli L, et al. Plaque-induced gingivitis: case definition and diagnostic considerations. *J Periodontol*. 2018;89(suppl 1):S46–s73.

Williams DW, et al. Human oral mucosa cell atlas reveals a stromal-neutrophil axis regulating tissue immunity. *Cell*. 2021;184(15):4090–4104. e15.

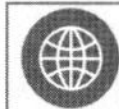
References for this chapter are found on the companion website eBooks.Health.Elsevier.com

CHAPTER 16

Select Systemic and Local Diseases That Affect the Gingiva

Alfredo Aguirre | Jill Marie Kramer | Rana Alshagroud

CHAPTER OUTLINE

A number of systemic and local conditions can manifest in the oral cavity. A subset of these have a particular affinity for the gingival tissues. The spectrum of systemic conditions affecting the gingiva range from autoimmune disorders to abnormalities of the fibrinolysis system, adrenal insufficiency, idiopathic conditions, and genetic diseases. Locally, the gingiva can give rise to reactive and neoplastic conditions, pharmacologically induced hyperpigmentation, autoimmune disorders, and metastatic tumors. The spectrum of autoimmune-mediated blistering and chronic ulcerative conditions that affect the gingiva are covered in a separate chapter (Chapter 18, Desquamative Gingivitis). This chapter will discuss select systemic and local conditions that are known to affect the gingiva. Gingival lesions may represent the first manifestation of serious systemic conditions or syndromes. Although lesions may be localized in nature, some may have aggressive growth potential, thereby requiring prompt attention. Thus, it is incumbent upon the clinician to recognize these conditions and establish a rigorous management strategy that includes appropriate testing and referral.

SYSTEMIC

Gingival Manifestations of Systemic Disease

Granulomatosis With Polyangiitis

Granulomatosis with polyangiitis (GPA, formerly known as Wegener granulomatosis) is a rare immune-mediated systemic disease characterized by necrotizing vasculitis of the upper and lower respiratory tract, kidneys, and small to medium arteries and veins.[95] Although the etiology of this condition is not known, epidemiological data suggest that GPA results from the interaction of genetic and environmental risk factors in susceptible populations.[88]

Clinical Features

At the time of diagnosis, most patients are over 20 years of age. There is no gender predilection and the overwhelming majority of patients are white. Two types of GPA are recognized, limited and generalized. In the limited presentation, the respiratory tract is affected with no renal involvement. If untreated, it may progress to the generalized form in which renal involvement is observed. Superficial GPA is a term used to characterize a subset of patients with this condition in which the disease is initially limited to the skin and mucosa. Patients with superficial GPA may exhibit a gradual progression to disseminated disease. At the onset of the disease most patients experience nonspecific symptoms of the upper respiratory tract, and oral lesions occur in approximately 10% of patients. The classic presentation of oral GPA is gingival hyperplasia with a granular surface exhibiting a red discoloration resulting in a "strawberry-like" appearance ("strawberry gingivitis"; Fig. 16.1).[220] "Strawberry gingivitis" typically precedes renal involvement in GPA cases.[210] The presence of palatal ulcers indicates a late stage of GPA, and is a harbinger of renal involvement.[220]

Histopathologic Features

Biopsy of the affected gingiva reveals the presence of an intense diffuse acute and chronic inflammatory cell infiltrate with a rich

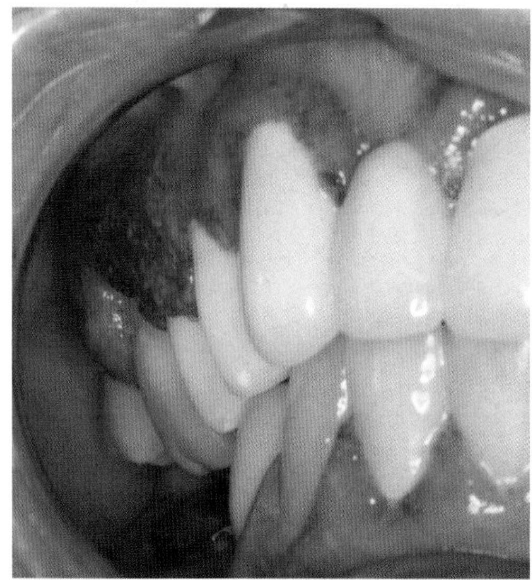

Fig. 16.1 Granulomatosis with polyangiitis. Erythematous festooning in the attached gingiva of lateral incisor and canine progresses to the classic "strawberry gingivitis" seen at the bicuspid-molar area.

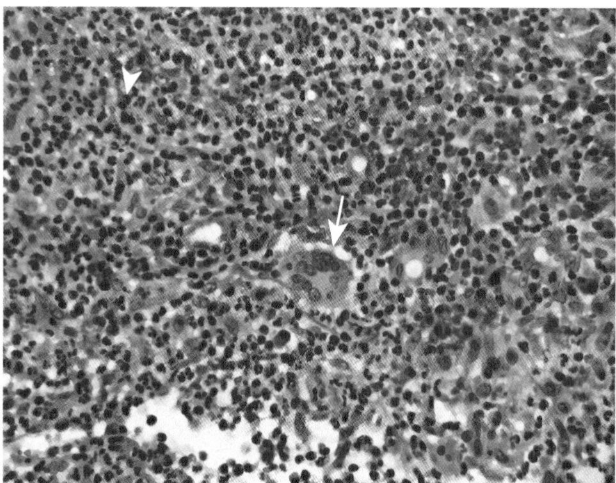

Fig. 16.2 Granulomatosis with polyangiitis. Medium power view showing multinucleated giant cells *(arrow)* amidst neutrophils, scattered eosinophils *(arrowhead)*, and lymphocytes (H&E, 5 μm; original magnification ×200).

vasculature, robust population of eosinophils, and interspersed multinucleated giant cells (Fig. 16.2). The classic leukocytoclastic vasculitis of GPA is difficult to identify in oral biopsies.[79]

Diagnosis

The 1990 American College of Rheumatology criteria for the classification of GPA includes nasal or oral inflammation, abnormal chest radiograph, urinary sediment, and granulomatous inflammation on biopsy.[139] The presence of two out of four of these criteria are sufficient for a diagnosis of GPA. Elevated levels of proteinase 3-antineutrophil cytoplasmic antibodies (PR3-ANCA; formerly known as c-ANCA) can be used to substantiate a diagnosis of GPA.[122]

Treatment and Prognosis

Early identification of the classic gingival involvement in GPA is essential to prevent severe renal damage that may lead to death. The therapeutic gold standard for GPA is aimed at achieving remission and consists of a combined regimen of corticosteroids and cyclophosphamide. Therapeutic plasma exchange reduces the risk of end–stage kidney disease in patients presenting with acute kidney failure. Other drugs, such as azathioprine (Azasan, Imuran), mycophenolate (CellCept), and methotrexate (Trexall) can be used.[244] Unfortunately, patients commonly experience significant side effects with these medications. These can be reduced with the use of pulse cyclophosphamide to induce remission, although this is associated with a higher risk of relapse. Rituximab is a good therapeutic alternative to induce and maintain remission.[244] A 10-year survival rate of 75% is achieved with conventional cyclophosphamide/corticosteroid therapy.[132]

KEY FACT

Granulomatosis with polyangiitis, although rare, has a significant impact on the well-being of affected patients. In the initial stages of the disease, the gingiva exhibits a characteristic erythematous hyperplasia named "strawberry gingivitis." This gingival finding precedes renal damage and thus, early recognition and diagnosis of this disease greatly reduce morbidity and mortality.

Plasminogen Deficiency

Plasminogen is a multifunctional protein with a molecular weight of 92 kDa that plays a central role in the fibrinolytic system.[83] Plasminogen is converted to plasmin, and the main substrate of plasmin is fibrin.[200] Plasminogen deficiency is a systemic autosomal recessive condition with a prevalence of 0.4% that mainly affects the eyes (ligneous conjunctivitis) and the gingiva (ligneous gingivitis).[65] However, the nervous system, skin, respiratory tract, female genital tract, gastrointestinal system, and genitourinary system can also be affected.[47] Plasminogen deficiency can be classified into two types: type 1 and type 2. In type 1 deficiency, patients have mutations in the gene that encodes plasminogen, termed *PLG*. This may lead to deficits in plasminogen levels and/or function. In type 2 deficiency, plasminogen levels are normal or slightly decreased but a marked reduction in activity is present.[47] Studies have shown that type 2 deficiency does not result in any clinical manifestations.[200] In patients with type 1 plasminogen deficiency, mucous membranes become thick and "woody" due to the persistence and buildup of fibrin. This "woody" appearance gave rise to the term "ligneous" (from the Latin *ligneous* which means related to wood).

Clinical Features

Plasminogen deficiency mainly affects the upper tarsal conjunctiva where creamy yellow to erythematous or white plaques and nodules form. The disease may be precipitated by infection, trauma, or surgery. Similar lesions present in the gingiva with intervening areas of ulceration and swelling (Fig. 16.3A and B).[203] These lesions tend to wax and wane and can be focal or diffuse in which they involve all quadrants. Rarely, plasminogen deficiency causes destructive periodontitis that may lead to rapid tooth loss.[18]

Histopathologic Features

Microscopic examination reveals an accumulation of eosinophilic acellular material resembling amyloid in the superficial lamina propria with adjacent granulation tissue and a variable density of inflammatory cells (Fig. 16.4). A negative Congo red stain rules out amyloidosis, a condition that is usually included in the microscopic differential diagnosis. Movat pentachrome or Fraser-Lendrum histochemical stains are confirmatory for fibrin.[56,81] Direct immunofluorescence reveals positive fibrin staining of the amorphous deposits.[223]

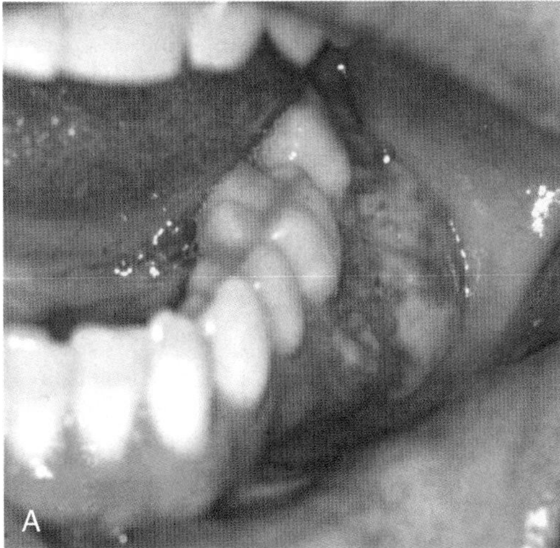

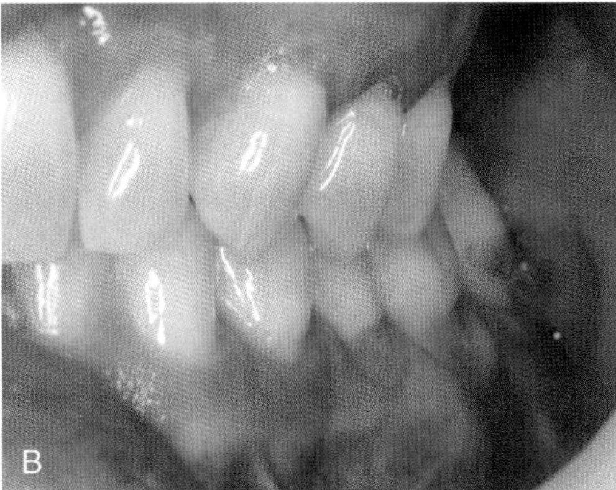

Fig. 16.3 (A) **Plasminogen deficiency.** Nodular mass with superficial yellowish plaques distal to # 20. (B) **Plasminogen deficiency.** Successful resolution of oral lesions after conservative treatment with warfarin-doxycycline-chlorhexidine. (*Courtesy of Dr. Sook Bin-Woo, Harvard School of Dental Medicine. USA.*)

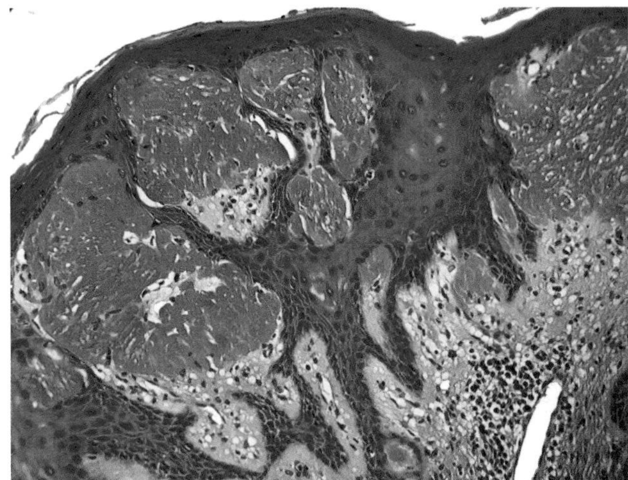

Fig. 16.4 Plasminogen deficiency. Amorphous eosinophilic material concentrating in the papillary and reticular lamina propria (H&E, 5 μm; original magnification ×200).

Diagnosis

Plasminogen deficiency can be diagnosed through either immunoassays to quantify plasminogen levels and/or functional assays to assess plasminogen activity. A common approach is to employ a functional assay first and in the event of an abnormal result, to perform an immunoassay.[223] Type 1 plasminogen deficiency is confirmed with genetic tests to identify mutations in *PLG,* and genetic testing is of value in distinguishing type 1 from type 2 deficiency.[155]

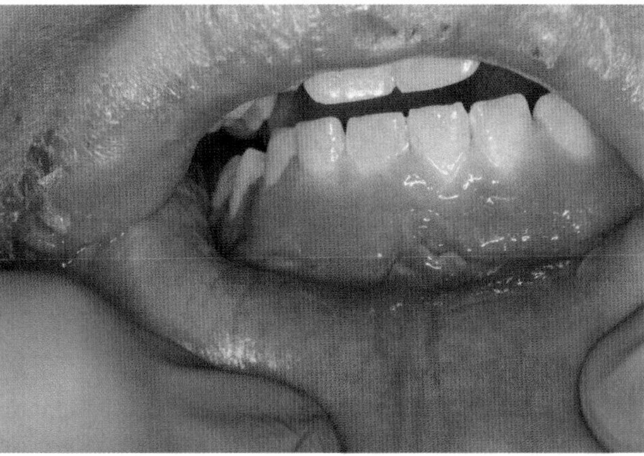

Fig. 16.5 Crohn's disease. A typical "epulis-fissuratum-like" lesion is seen in the mandibular mucobuccal fold along with erythema, mucogingivitis, and tags.

Treatment and Prognosis

As of today, there are no standardized treatment protocols or guidelines for affected individuals. Replacement therapy with human Glu-plasminogen has shown a significant clinical effect on conjunctival and gingival lesions.[205] A combination of warfarin, low-dose doxycycline, and chlorhexidine has also been used successfully.[77] Conservative treatment for mild to moderate gingival lesions is aimed at reducing local inflammation with meticulous oral hygiene. However, severe lesions should be excised followed by strict plaque control.[223]

Crohn's Disease

Inflammatory bowel disease (IBD) encompasses primarily two major categories of chronic inflammatory intestinal disorders: Crohn's disease (CD) and ulcerative colitis (UC). It is estimated that 1.5 million Americans suffer from IBD. Since UC is not commonly associated with gingival changes in the oral cavity, this section will focus primarily on CD. The annual incidence of CD ranges from 3.1 to 20.2 per 100,000 and has a prevalence of 201 per 100,000 population.[82] CD is considered a heterogeneous disorder with a multifactorial etiology where genetics and environmental factors interact to trigger the disease.[8]

Clinical Features

CD is characterized by transmural inflammation of any part of the intestine, extending from the anus to the oral cavity. This condition has a bimodal age distribution (20 and 50 years).[180] About 25% of patients with CD present with at least one extraintestinal manifestation (i.e., primary sclerosing cholangitis, ankylosing spondylitis, iritis/uveitis, pyoderma gangrenosum, erythema nodosum). In addition, asthma, bronchitis, pericarditis, psoriasis, rheumatoid arthritis, and multiple sclerosis can be seen associated with CD.[71,177] The oral lesions associated with CD are significant because as many as 35% harbinger asymptomatic intestinal involvement.[202,227] Oral findings include mucogingivitis, mucosal tags, linear ulcers in the mucobuccal fold with an "epulis fissuratum-like" appearance, cobblestone appearance, and labial swelling with vertical fissures (Fig. 16.5).[106,162] The gingiva of affected individuals exhibits segmental or diffuse erythema along with edematous hyperplastic

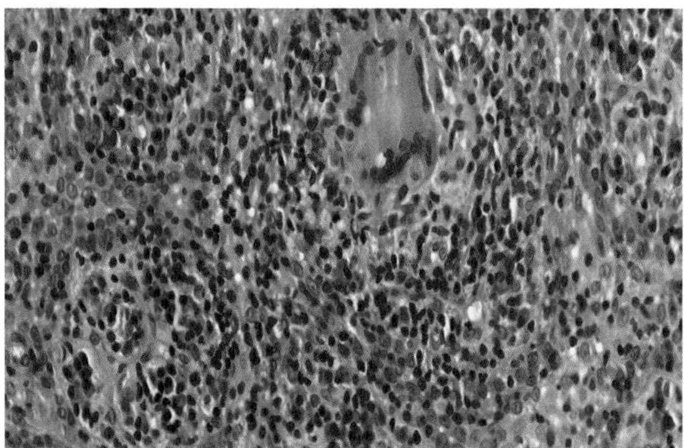

Fig. 16.6 Crohn's disease. Lymphohistiocytic granulomas with multinucleated giant cells (H&E, 5 μm; original magnification ×200).

fibrous lesions that occur in approximately 65% of patients. The mucogingival lesions show characteristic microscopic features suggesting that these are *bona fide* disease-specific manifestations of CD (see below, Microscopic Features section).[106] Classic involvement of the floor of the mouth consists of fleshy elevated bands with a "staghorn" appearance around Wharton's ducts.[42] Some studies have suggested that the prevalence of periodontitis is higher among patients with CD compared to controls.[32,101,219] In addition, periodontitis in the primary dentition may be suggestive of CD and could precede intestinal symptoms.[211]

Microscopic Features

The microscopic hallmark of CD is the presence of either discrete non-caseating granulomas or confluent granulomatous sheets of macrophages with multinucleated giant cells (Fig. 16.6). Sometimes fibrosis can be present.[254]

Diagnosis

The diagnosis of CD derives from the integration of clinical findings coupled with endoscopic, histologic, imaging, and/or biochemical testing. Identifying the complete extent of disease is important to developing a treatment plan.[240]

Treatment and Prognosis

The first-line therapy generally consists of corticosteroids for rapid palliation of symptoms along with initiation of anti-tumor necrosis factor α (TNFα) therapy such as infliximab, adalimumab, or certolizumab pegol. Other treatments may include immunosuppressants such as azathioprine, mercaptopurine, and methotrexate, or surgery.[62,233] Periods of clinical remission alternating with disease flares are characteristic. Within 10 years of diagnosis, 50% of patients will require surgery. Those with severe disease and concurrent rectal involvement will require a permanent stoma, as surgery is not curative in this patient group.[233] Healing of oral lesions can occur with the successful use of immunosuppressants.[250] Remission of symptomatic oral ulcers associated with CD can be accomplished with adalimumab or ustekinumab, drugs that target TNFα and IL-12 and IL-23, respectively.[24,126]

KEY FACT

The diagnosis of Crohn's disease may take a collaborative effort from a number of professionals. However, the mucogingivitis and "epulis fissuratum-like" lesions on the mucobuccal fold are characteristic and herald asymptomatic intestinal involvement in slightly more than a third of patients with this condition. Thus, dentists have an important role in the early diagnosis of this disease.

Sarcoidosis

Sarcoidosis is a multisystemic disease of unknown etiology that mainly affects the lungs (90% of cases) and other organs such as the eyes, skin, liver, spleen, and lymph nodes. In the United States, African Americans are three times more susceptible to sarcoidosis than whites (35.5/100,000 vs. 10.9/100,000). Sarcoidosis develops in genetically predisposed individuals after exposure to an environmental trigger. As of today, no specific gene has been linked to this disease.[120,146]

Clinical Features

Sarcoidosis is often diagnosed during a routine chest radiograph (up to 50% of patients). Sarcoidosis can be acute, subacute, or chronic. The acute phase is characterized by Lofgren syndrome (erythema nodosum and bilateral hilar adenopathy). Subacute sarcoidosis presents with weakness, fever, weight loss, arthralgia, and peripheral lymphadenopathy. Chronic sarcoidosis shows a slow onset with persistent lung involvement.[120] Oral lesions may be indicative of systemic involvement and can occur in any region of the mouth. They appear as asymptomatic, well-circumscribed, brown-red or violaceous papules, nodules, plaques, and erosions/ulcers. Gingivitis, gingival hyperplasia, or gingival recession are not unusual. Involvement of the jaw bones may lead to mobility and loss of teeth. Dental extractions may be associated with non-healing sockets. In addition, sarcoid involvement of parotid glands leads to salivary hypofunction.[4]

Microscopic Features

Multiple noncaseating "naked" granulomas (granulomas lacking significant lymphocyte aggregates) are seen in sarcoidosis. Schaumann bodies, asteroid bodies, Hamazaki–Wesenberg bodies, and calcium oxalate crystals may also be present. Because of the similarity in microscopic features, deep fungal and mycobacterial infections, as well as foreign body granulomas and CD, should be excluded with histochemical stains, polarized light examination, and microbial cultures.[4,164,236]

Diagnosis

The diagnosis of sarcoidosis relies on all of the following: (1) the presence of noncaseating granulomas on histopathologic examination, (2) compatible clinical presentation, and (3) exclusion of other causes of granulomatous inflammation.[60] Serum angiotensin-converting enzyme level was thought to be specific for sarcoidosis. However, a 40% sensitivity and a 15% false positivity rate render this test unreliable. The Kveim test (an intradermal injection of heat-sterilized splenic cells from patients with sarcoidosis) is also fraught with variable sensitivity and specificity as well as the potential to transmit a contagious disease.[236] Therefore, these tests are no longer indicated for the diagnosis of sarcoidosis.

Treatment and Prognosis

Corticosteroids (such as prednisone) are the first-line therapy for any type of sarcoidosis. The second line of therapy relies on steroid-sparing medications (mainly methotrexate). For refractory cases, the third line of therapy uses TNFα inhibitors, primarily infliximab.[87] Oral lesions may resolve after pharmacological therapy is initiated.[100] If systemic treatment fails to clear oral lesions, then surgical excision is warranted and loose teeth should be splinted.[224] Patients with salivary hypofunction should undergo preventive interventions to mitigate caries and fungal infection.[26] In half of affected patients, the

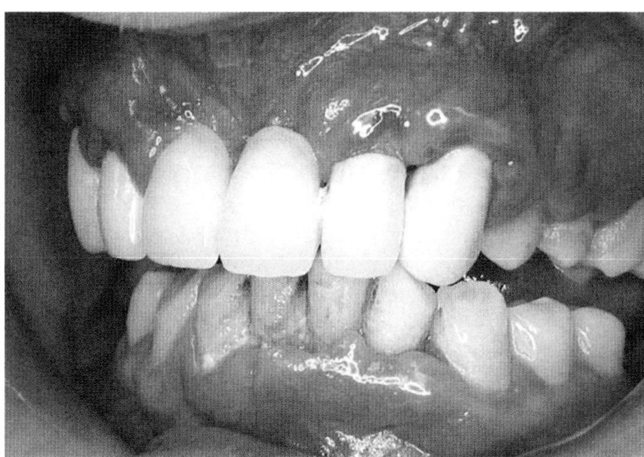

Fig. 16.7 Leukemia. Gingival enlargement and necrosis along with mucosal pallor. *(Courtesy of Dr. John Fantasia, Long Island Jewish Medical Center. USA.)*

disease resolves within 2 years, while for others it may take up to 5 years. Remission, however, is unlikely to occur after 5 years.[98] The mortality rate for Black patients with sarcoidosis is much higher than for White individuals (16 vs. 1.3 per million, respectively).[111]

Leukemia

Leukemias are a group of hematologic malignancies characterized by an abnormal proliferation of leukocytes. Leukemias can be classified according to their clinical behavior and histogenesis as either acute or chronic and as myelocytic or lymphocytic, respectively. Four major subtypes of leukemia are identified: acute lymphoblastic leukemia (ALL), acute myelogenous leukemia (AML), chronic lymphocytic leukemia (CLL), and chronic myelogenous leukemia (CML).[148] It is beyond the scope of this section to discuss in detail the characteristics of each type of leukemia. Thus, this section will focus mainly on AML, since 90% of this subtype presents with oral manifestations.[41] For a more detailed discussion on leukemia, the reader should consult specialized hematological literature.

Clinical Features

AML is the most common acute leukemia in adults, and it accounts for a substantial percentage of leukemias diagnosed in children and teenagers as well.[148] The systemic signs and symptoms associated with leukemia include fatigue, bruising, hemorrhage, fever, infections, and sometimes septicemia. Oral manifestations of AML are seen in slightly more than half of the patients and include petechiae, spontaneous bleeding, and ulcers. Gingival enlargement occurs in one-third of patients (Fig. 16.7). Mucosal pallor, high caries prevalence, and opportunistic herpetic and fungal infections are also observed.[41,54,75,191] Gingival infiltration represents the initial manifestation of AML in 5% of cases.[41] This collection of leukemic cells in tissue is known as myeloid sarcoma (formerly known as granulocytic sarcoma or chloroma). While not always associated with AML, myeloid sarcoma may precede or coincide with a diagnosis of AML or may be seen as the initial manifestation of an AML relapse.[125]

Microscopic Features

The connective tissue is completely infiltrated by sheets of myelomonocytic neoplastic cells showing myeloperoxidase expression with immunohistochemical stains. Myeloperoxidase is expressed by immature cells of the myeloid lineage.[119]

Diagnosis

Some cases of AML are diagnosed serendipitously on routine blood work. Others may become apparent because of infection, bleeding, or disseminated intravascular coagulation. Diagnosis relies on bone marrow examination. Cytomorphology, cytochemistry, immunophenotyping, cytogenetics, and molecular genetics are warranted to classify the subtype of AML precisely.[102] For those cases in which gingival enlargement is the first manifestation of AML, subsequent bone marrow evaluation is required for definitive diagnosis and to classify the AML subtype.[75]

Treatment and Prognosis

The mainstay of treatment for AML is chemotherapy, with or without concurrent targeted therapy (inhibitors and monoclonal antibodies).[72] Three prognostic risk groups (favorable, intermediate, and adverse) are recognized based on both cytogenetics and molecular findings. Treatment approaches depend on risk stratification, and hematopoietic cell transplant may be indicated in select cases.[182]

Rare Syndromes

Tuberous Sclerosis Complex

Tuberous sclerosis complex (TSC) is a multisystem, autosomal dominant genetic condition that affects 1 in 10,000 newborns.[181] TSC results from mutations in either the *TSC1* or *TSC2* genes leading to hyperactivation of the mTOR pathway. Dysregulated mTOR signaling results in increased cellular overgrowth that is characteristic of the syndrome.[186,197]

Clinical Features

The most common findings in TSC are benign tumors in the skin, brain, kidneys, lungs, and heart that lead to organ dysfunction. Seizures, cognitive disabilities, behavior problems, and autism are common. In addition, hypomelanotic macules ("ash leaf spots"), facial angiofibromas, forehead plaques, and ungual/subungual fibromas are present. Shagreen patches are also observed. These are irregularly shaped and thickened, slightly elevated, skin-colored, and occasionally slightly pigmented areas. Shagreen patches are usually on the lower back, and are comprised of excess fibrous tissue.[256] Oral lesions of TSC include fibromas presenting as confluent papules and nodules ranging in size from a few millimeters to 1 cm in diameter. The anterior gingiva is the most frequent site followed by the labial mucosa, maxillary labial frenum, palate, and tongue. Enamel pitting is also associated with TSC.[170,179]

Microscopic Features

Oral polypoid lesions associated with TSC show typical features of fibromas. These lesions are comprised of proliferating collagen fibers interspersed with fibroblasts and blood vessels.[217]

Diagnosis

The diagnosis of TSC is based on both genetic and clinical criteria. Genetic analyses are performed on suspected patients to identify pathogenic mutations that result in the inactivation of the tumor suppressor genes *TSC1* or *TSC2*. For the clinical criteria, 11 distinct major and 6 minor features are evaluated. The occurrence of two major features or one major feature with ≥2 minor features provides substantial evidence for a clinical diagnosis of TSC.[135,170,181]

Treatment and Prognosis

A multidisciplinary symptomatic treatment approach is recommended for TSC patients. The prognosis may be uncertain and

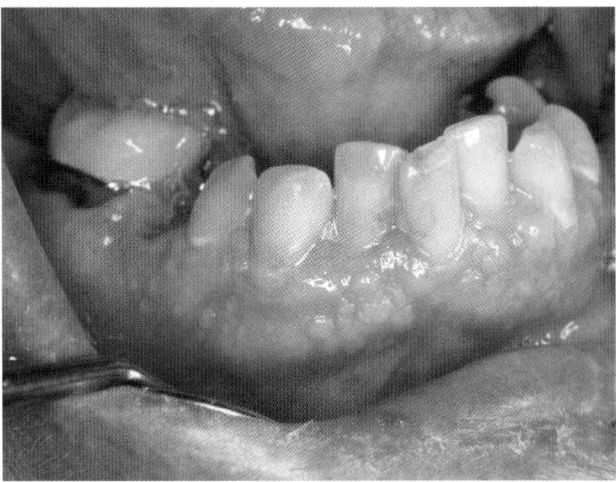

Fig. 16.8 Cowden syndrome. Multiple papules and nodules are present on the attached gingiva creating a cobblestone pattern.

requires a comprehensive evaluation and close follow-up in specialized institutions.[181]

Multiple Hamartoma Syndrome (Cowden Syndrome)

Cowden syndrome (CS) is an autosomal dominant genodermatosis. CS is considered a member of the spectrum of heritable disorders associated with the phosphatase and tensin homolog (PTEN) hamartoma tumor syndrome (PHTS) that are characterized by mutations in the *PTEN* tumor suppressor gene. Bannayan–Riley–Ruvalcaba syndrome, and Proteus and Proteus-like syndrome are also members of this family of disorders.[85,168]

Clinical Features

The prevalence of CS is estimated at 1:200,000 births.[179] *PTEN* mutations are reported in 25% to 80% of cases. The etiology of the remaining cases is still unknown.[213] CS is characterized by multiple hamartomas and an increased risk of malignancies. These include breast, thyroid, endometrial, colorectal, and renal cancers as well as melanoma.[178,213] Eighty percent of patients present with oral findings, and these may facilitate early clinical identification of CS patients. Oral lesions consist of multiple 1- to 3-mm whitish-pink papules or nodules, mainly affecting the gingiva, dorsal tongue, and buccal mucosa. Individual lesions may coalesce to create a cobblestone appearance (Fig. 16.8). In addition, a deep palatal vault, periodontitis, caries, and salivary hypofunction may be present.[179]

Microscopic Features

Papular and nodular lesions are surfaced by stratified squamous epithelium with or without hyperparakeratosis, papillomatosis, and acanthosis. Elongated, broad, and slender rete pegs may also be observed. The stroma shows a proliferation of collagen fibers with interspersed fibroblasts.[70]

Diagnosis

Twelve major and 10 minor criteria have been proposed for the diagnosis of CS.[178] The diagnosis requires either (1) three or more major criteria and should include either macrocephaly, Lhermitte–Duclos disease, or gastrointestinal hamartomas. Cancers of the breast, endometrium, and thyroid are also included or, (2) two major and three minor criteria. Minor criteria include autism spectrum disorder, colon cancer, and lipomas. Molecular testing for *PTEN* mutations is highly recommended.[178] Gingival nodulo-papular lesions may represent one of the earliest clinical signs of CS.[46]

Treatment and Prognosis

The mucocutaneous manifestations of CS are rarely life-threatening although follow-up is prudent. Oral lesions are typically asymptomatic and do not carry malignant potential, so treatment is not indicated.[179] The most important phase in the management of CS patients is to maintain a rigorous cancer surveillance program to detect neoplasms at their earliest stages to mitigate morbidity and mortality.[167]

Discoloration of the Gingiva Resulting From Systemic Disease

Numerous systemic diseases of diverse and distinct etiologies can result in discoloration of the gingiva. It is important for the clinician to expeditiously recognize these conditions in order to manage the patient appropriately and to facilitate referral to a specialist for further evaluation and care. This section will provide an overview of systemic conditions associated with gingival pigmentation.

Addison Disease

Addison disease (AD) is a primary adrenal insufficiency that is most commonly caused by autoimmunity.[21] Less commonly, AD is associated with an infectious etiology or is induced by drugs or neoplasia.[21] Vascular pathoses can also give rise to AD and several rare mutations are reported in the context of this condition.[21] AD results in the destruction of the adrenal gland, culminating in deficient production of adrenal cortex hormones.[21,27] Patients are staged based on the level of adrenal cortical insufficiency.[21] Symptoms of AD may be relatively nonspecific and thus the disease may be difficult to diagnose. While the cause of autoimmune AD is unclear at present, multiple factors likely contribute to disease onset and progression, such as environmental insults and genetics.[27] Specific polymorphisms are identified in the *HLA B8*, *DR3*, and *DR4* alleles that are thought to confer susceptibility to disease.[27] AD may be seen in association with other autoimmune conditions, including Type I diabetes and celiac disease.[21] Individuals with AD may experience adrenal or Addisonian crisis, an acute life-threatening emergency that occurs in patients with adrenal insufficiency which is often the first sign of disease.[66] This is typically precipitated by infection, although psychological and physical stress or cessation of glucocorticoid therapy can cause this condition.[66] Patients in adrenal crisis should receive parenteral hydrocortisone without delay.[66]

Clinical Features

Clinical features of AD are secondary to the attenuated production of glucocorticoids, mineralocorticoids, and androgens and subsequent increased adrenocorticotropic hormone (ACTH) levels.[21] Classical AD manifestations include weakness, fatigue, weight loss with decreased appetite, orthostatic hypotension and tachycardia, nausea, vomiting, and diarrhea.[21] Elevated ACTH stimulates melanocytes, resulting in hyperpigmentation or "bronzing" of the skin and mucosa in 80% to 94% of patients.[21] A diffuse brown pigmentation of the gingiva, tongue, buccal mucosa, hard palate, and lips is observed.[91,127] These alterations commonly progress during adult life.[91]

Diagnosis

AD is diagnosed based on several laboratory parameters. Measurements of ACTH, cortisol, plasma renin, and aldosterone concentrations in blood samples collected in the morning (at 8:00 a.m.) are required to confirm the diagnosis.[21] An increase in ACTH

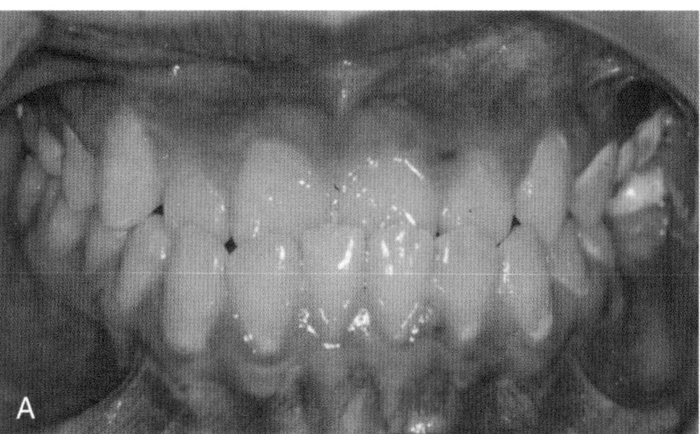

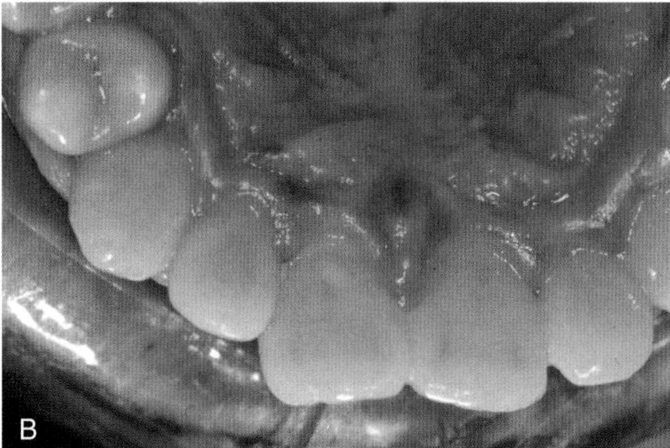

Fig. 16.9 Peutz–Jegher syndrome. (A) 11-year-old child with multiple melanotic macules on the vestibular attached gingiva. (B) Palatal gingiva and palatal mucosa also exhibit multiple melanotic macules. Extensive polyposis required partial colon removal. (*Courtesy of Dr. Mario E. Ramos, private practice. USA.*)

levels with concomitant low levels of cortisol are diagnostic for AD.[21] The conventional ACTH test, an intravenous injection of synthetic corticotropin, is the gold standard for assessing adrenal function.[21] Adrenal cortex and 21-OH autoantibodies are also quantified as part of the diagnostic workup.[21,27] An oral biopsy is not indicated for the diagnosis of this condition.

Treatment and Prognosis

Initial therapy for AD consists of corticosteroid replacement therapy.[21] Glucocorticoid and mineralocorticoid replacement therapy may also be indicated.[21] The hyperpigmentation of the skin and oral mucosa is reversible as a result of the replacement therapy.[140,161] The prognosis for patients with AD is excellent, as patients with AD who receive appropriate treatment have a normal life span.[21]

KEY FACT

The oral melanosis associated with Addison's disease is not specific and it is shared by a number of other conditions with diverse origins (i.e., smoking-associated melanosis, pharmacologically-induced melanosis, Peutz–Jegher syndrome, and Laugier–Hunziker syndrome). Laboratory evaluations of serum ACTH, cortisol, plasma renin, and aldosterone are valuable in reaching a precise diagnosis.

Peutz–Jegher Syndrome

Peutz–Jegher syndrome (PJS) is classified as a hamartomatous polyposis syndrome.[225] Most cases of PJS are caused by a germline mutation in the serine/threonine kinase gene *STK11/LBK*. This gene may function as a haploinsufficient tumor suppressor gene, although

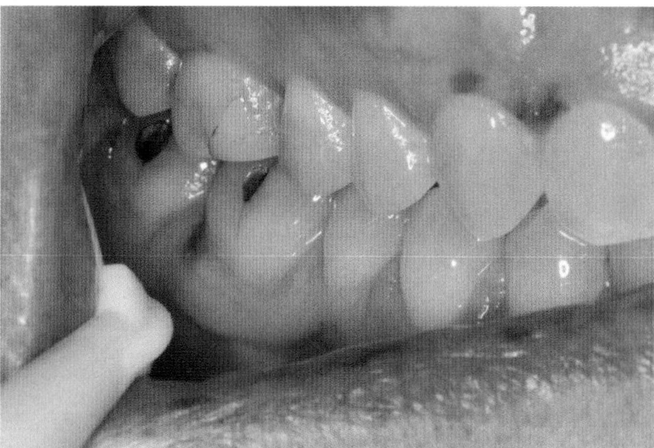

Fig. 16.10 Laugier-Hunziker syndrome. Fifty-four-year-old woman with multiple melanotic macules on the marginal and attached gingiva. Additional pigmented macules are also seen in the mandibular labial mucosa adjacent to the vermilion border.

the way in which mutations in *STK11/LBK* induce neoplasia remain incompletely understood.[159] PJS is a rare sporadic or autosomal dominant condition that typically manifests in childhood or early adulthood and occurs in approximately 1:200,000 individuals.[112,159] PJS affects all sexes and races equally.[112]

Clinical Features

PJS is characterized by mucocutaneous pigmentation and hamartomatous polyps.[242] Children typically present with polyps in the small intestine that may result in intussusceptions and bowel obstruction.[156] Adult patients with PJS have an increased risk of the development of malignancies involving the colon, stomach, small bowel, pancreas, breast, ovary, uterus, cervix, and testes.[19,159,225,242] Oral manifestations of PJS may be present at birth and typically become more prominent in childhood. The oral lesions are often the first to appear and may be the first sign of disease. These consist of peri- and intra-oral macules that are blue to dark brown in color. They are almost always observed on the lower lip and buccal mucosa, although they may extend to the upper lip, palate, and gingiva (Fig. 16.9A and B).[112,249] The macules typically range in size from 1 to 10 mm in diameter.[179] This pigmentation is reported in greater than 90% of patients with PJS and spots may fade during puberty.[19,112] Neither the oral nor cutaneous macules carry malignant potential; thus, a biopsy is not indicated.

Diagnosis

The clinical diagnosis of PJS is made when any one of the following is present: (1) two or more histologically confirmed PJS polyps, (2) PJS polyps in a person with a family history of PJS in close relative(s), (3) characteristic mucocutaneous pigmentation in a person with a family history of PJS in close relative(s), or (4) presence of PJS polyps in a person with characteristic mucocutaneous pigmentation.[19] While most patients diagnosed with PJS have the *STK11/LBK* mutation, genetic studies are not required for diagnosis.[11]

Treatment and Prognosis

Since PJS is associated with a heightened systemic risk of malignancy, extensive surveillance of these patients is recommended, although there are no established guidelines given the rarity of the disease.[19] Comprehensive management of PJS patients involves many different clinical specialties.[159,225] Currently, the underlying mechanisms that contribute to malignancy in PJS are poorly understood and there are no therapeutics available that address disease etiology.[19] Locally, laser ablation may be considered for esthetic reasons.[179]

KEY FACT

Distinct periorificial and intraoral macular pigmentation are characteristic of Peutz–Jegher syndrome and may represent the first manifestation of this disease. Due to the high likelihood of intestinal complications and malignant transformation in various organs, close follow-up of these patients and a multidisciplinary management approach is indicated.

Laugier-Hunziker Syndrome

Laugier-Hunziker syndrome (LHS) is characterized by macular hyperpigmentation of the skin and mucosa. LHS is a rare condition of unknown etiology that is not associated with any underlying systemic conditions. While some studies report a female disease predilection, a conflicting study found no gender differences.[160] LHS manifests most commonly in adults, with a few cases seen in children.[160,218] Cases arising within the same family are reported,[153] although genetic causes of LHS remain to be identified.

Clinical Features

Patients with LHS may exhibit widespread hyperpigmented areas on the skin of the face, conjunctiva, oral cavity, and oropharynx. About 50% of patients also display pigmentation of the fingernails and toenails that appear as longitudinal bands (melanonychia).[246,252] Lesions may be solitary or multifocal and are brown, gray, or black in appearance. Pigmentation is frequently observed on the lips, buccal mucosa, and hard palate, with the gingiva affected less commonly (Fig. 16.10).[246,252] One patient with LHS exhibited metachronous melanoacanthomas.[252] It is important to note that pigmentation associated with LHS can vary over time, as some lesions in one well-documented case become more prominent and others regressed during a 3-year period.[252]

Microscopic Features

Histologically, the lesions appear similar to an oral melanotic macule. Melanin incontinence may be observed. The architecture of rete ridges is identical to that of normal oral mucosa.[160,212,251,252] A biopsy is indicated to rule out other pathologies associated with oral pigmentation.

Diagnosis

There are no diagnostic tests to confirm the presence of LHS. Since LHS is a diagnosis of exclusion, patients should undergo an evaluation to rule out other disorders that mimic this condition, including AD and PJS.[152]

Treatment and Prognosis

Treatment for LHS is not required. If cosmetically objectionable, laser therapy successfully treats the pigmentation associated with this condition.[53,166]

HIV/AIDS-Associated Melanosis

HIV/AIDS-associated melanosis is a poorly understood condition that is seen in HIV seropositive individuals. Several studies report hyperpigmentation of the oral mucosa in the context of HIV/AIDS in both children and adults, although this is not considered to be an AIDS-defining feature of the disease.[50,52,222] While it is known that medication use can induce hyperpigmentation in HIV-positive individuals,[50,74] HIV-induced cytokine dysregulation and HIV-associated adrenocortical dysfunction may also be causative factors that mediate mucosal pigmentation.[50,74] Inflammatory cytokines, such as IL-1, IL-6, and TNFα are increased in HIV-positive patients and this may lead to heightened melanin production.[10,74] Levels of these cytokines increase with decreasing $CD4^+$ T cell counts, and patients with $CD4^+$ T cell counts of less than 200 cells/mm^3 are more likely to display oral hyperpigmentation.[74] HIV-associated oral melanin hyperpigmentation (HIV-OMP) typically appears 2 years after the diagnosis of HIV.[23,76] The prevalence of HIV-OMP varies by geographic region, as it is relatively low in Italy, Tanzania, and Kenya (approximately 5% of patients),[38,76,104] but is higher in Venezuela (38%) and India (26% to 30%).[30,187,215] One study showed an increase in oral pigmentation in patients receiving highly active antiretroviral therapy (HAART), as 15% of treatment-naïve HIV patients displayed oral pigmentation in contrast to 44% of HIV-positive individuals receiving HAART.[235] A study in children also provided evidence for a role of anti-retroviral therapy in mucosal hyperpigmentation. In HIV-positive children who were untreated, oral mucosal pigmentation was observed in 6% of cases.[222] These results are in contrast to those in children receiving this therapy for not more than 3 years. In this group, mucosal pigmentation was observed in 22% of study participants.[222]

Clinical Features

HIV-OMP is observed throughout the oral cavity, although the gingiva and buccal mucosa are the most commonly affected sites.[50,74] In most patients, the pigmentation is multifocal and no sex predilection is reported.[50,187] The pigmentation varies in intensity from light to dark.[50]

Microscopic Features

Microscopic features of HIV-OMP are not distinct and mimic those of melanotic macules and physiologic pigmentation.[74] HIV-OMP that occurs in the absence of HAART is characterized by increased production of melanin without an increase in the number of melanocytes.[74] In contrast, hyperpigmentation associated with the anti-retroviral drug zidovudine results from an increase in the number of melanocytes in the basal and suprabasal cell layers of the epidermis.[94] Studies in mice revealed increased production of melanin by melanocytes following zidovudine therapy that was reversible upon discontinuation of the drug.[171] Biopsy should be performed to rule out pigmented conditions that require treatment, such as oral mucosal melanoma.[74,149]

Diagnosis

Diagnosis of HIV relies on laboratory tests to detect antibodies specific for HIV-1 or HIV-2 or the HIV-1 p24 antigen.[49] An HIV-1 nucleic acid test is also conducted if very recent HIV exposure is suspected or reported.[49]

Treatment and Prognosis

HIV-OMP does not require treatment. HIV infection is managed with anti-retroviral therapy.[69] With the success of these therapies, the life span of HIV-positive patients has increased dramatically since 2000.[14] In the United States, the largest percentage increase in the rate of persons living with diagnosed HIV infection was among individuals aged 65 years and older.[39] Thus, patients undergoing retroviral therapy have a good prognosis and are living increasingly longer life spans.

Iatrogenic Discoloration of the Gingiva

Heavy Metal-Induced Pigmentation

Gingival pigmentation associated with heavy metal exposure is rare, but since this may cause considerable toxicity it is important for the clinician to be aware of this manifestation.[107] Ingestion or absorption of several different heavy metals can result in pigmentation of the oral mucosa, including bismuth, lead, mercury, silver, and gold.[158,192] Systemic absorption of these metals typically occurs through occupational exposure, inhalation, or accidental ingestion.[121,128,158] For example, exposure to lead may occur through ingestion of lead paint or by drinking water contaminated by lead pipes.[131] Occupational exposure is also reported.[192] Systemic exposure to silver (argyria) may result from ingestion or topical application of silver found in wound dressings.[243] Argyria may result from skin or mucosal exposure to a silver substrate or silver salt.[58] The systemic administration of gold to treat autoimmune conditions may cause chrysiasis.[58] Finally, acrodynia results from chronic mercury poisoning and is typically seen in young children who ingest mercury-containing products accidentally.[207] Food, particularly high fish consumption, is also a common source of mercury toxicity.[128] It is critical to identify patients with heavy metal toxicity in a timely manner, as heavy metal poisoning may lead to severe systemic injury, including damage to the nervous, respiratory, reproductive, and digestive tracts.[121]

Clinical Features

Clinical features of heavy metal absorption vary depending on the specific type of metal exposure. Bismuth-induced pigmentation is exceedingly rare and is reported as diffuse oral pigmentation along with a blue-back linear pigmentation at the marginal gingiva.[158] Systemic absorption of lead may result in the appearance of a linear gray pigmented band below the gingiva margin, referred to as Burton's line.[131,158,192] Argyria induces blue-black, blue-gray, or blue-green discoloration of the skin and oral mucosa.[58,129,141,238] Chrysiasis may lead to blue-gray or blue discoloration of the skin and rarely, gingival pigmentation.[58,123,158] Mercury deposition is described in periodontal tissues, leading to hyperpigmentation.[154]

Microscopic Features

Biopsies of oral tissues in patients with heavy metal-induced pigmentation reveal metal deposition in the lamina propria and increased melanin production.[93,154] Due to the distinctive clinical manifestations associated with heavy metal pigmentation, a biopsy is usually not indicated.

Diagnosis

Diagnosis of heavy metal toxicity is made based upon testing of blood, urine, skin, hair, or nails.[183] Additional tests to detect clinical sequelae of heavy metal poisoning may be helpful, such as studies to detect anemia and to assess liver and kidney function.[183]

Treatment and Prognosis

Treatment of heavy metal poisoning may be complex and often requires an interdisciplinary team of medical professionals.[183] Patients with heavy metal toxicity are typically treated with chelating agents. Specific chelation agents are indicated for each metal because each has a different reactivity from the chelators.[128] For example, dimercaptosuccinic acid (DMSA) and 2,3-dimercapto-propanesulphonate (DMPS) facilitate the removal of lead by the kidney.[128] Toxic levels of lead can be reduced by DMSA and sodium calcium EDTA.[128] Antioxidants may also be delivered concomitantly to mitigate toxicity.[121] Prompt treatment is critical for attaining good clinical outcomes and minimizing the risk of organ damage. While reports of pigment reduction following therapy are limited, one study described successful treatment of argyria following laser therapy.[105]

Drug-Induced Melanosis

Drug-induced melanosis is a relatively rare clinical finding that may be seen in association with a wide range of therapeutics, most commonly non-steroidal anti-inflammatory drugs, antiarrhythmic agents, tranquilizers, antibiotics, antimalarials, and chemotherapeutics.[5,165,201]

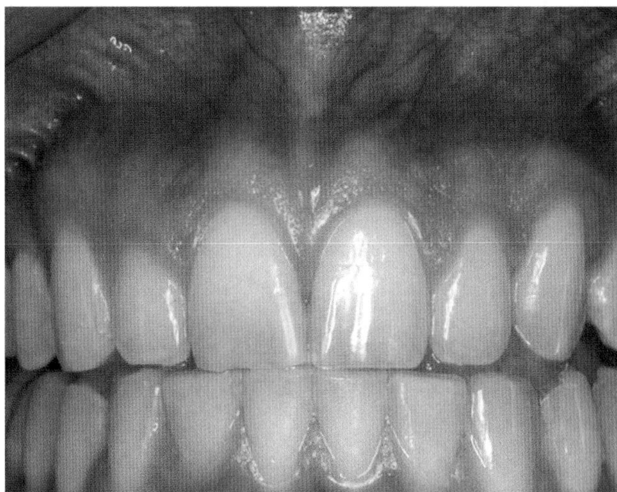

Fig. 16.11 Minocycline pigmentation. Green-gray discoloration of the alveolar mucosa developed in an individual who suffered from recalcitrant acne and was treated with minocycline. (*Courtesy of Dr. Kristin McNamara, College of Dentistry, The Ohio State University. USA.*)

More recently, reports implicate tyrosine kinase inhibitors as causative agents of drug-induced melanosis.[144,234] There are three primary mechanisms whereby drugs cause hyperpigmentation in the oral cavity: (1) increased numbers of melanocytes or melanin content, (2) deposition of the drug or substance in oral tissues as a foreign body that cannot be removed by macrophages—the drug may appear as free granules or it may chelate with melanin or iron, and (3) the drug may induce vascular damage. Red blood cells may accumulate in the lamina propria and subsequent lysis of these cells may result in iron accumulation leading to pigmentation.[165,234]

Clinical Features

Drug-induced pigmentation of oral tissues is either diffuse or multifocal.[234] Hyperpigmentation is documented on the gingiva, hard palate, lips, and buccal mucosa. Concomitant nail and skin pigmentation is also described.[234] Hyperpigmented areas may be homogenous or may appear as discrete macules.[234] The pigmentation may be uniform in color or may show variable intensity.[234] Pigmentation can result from both soft tissue alterations and deposition of the drug in the underlying alveolar bone.[248]

Microscopic Features

Histologic findings associated with drug-induced pigmentation may be relatively nonspecific and are often identical to those seen in oral melanotic macules. Histologic evaluation reveals normal-appearing oral epithelium, with no alteration in the number of melanocytes.[234] In addition to the evaluation of H&E-stained tissue, histochemical stains may aid in the diagnosis. Grocott (Gomori) methenamine-silver stain will stain melanin black and Perl's iron stain turns ferric iron blue. For certain drugs, namely minocycline, increased melanin deposition is observed, but the number of melanocytes remains unchanged (Fig. 16.11).[234] Additionally, pigmented granules are observed in the lamina propria.[234] In contrast, pigmentation induced by different classes of drugs (antimalarial drugs and tyrosine kinase inhibitors) does not alter melanin deposition or the number of melanocytes in the oral epithelium, although brown-yellow appearing granules are observed in the lamina propria.[234] Further evaluation revealed that these granules are consistent with drug products that are chelated to iron or that contain chemical groups of melanin or ferric iron.[234] Clinical correlation is often helpful to identify patients with drug-induced melanosis, although in some cases it is difficult to achieve this diagnosis with certainty.

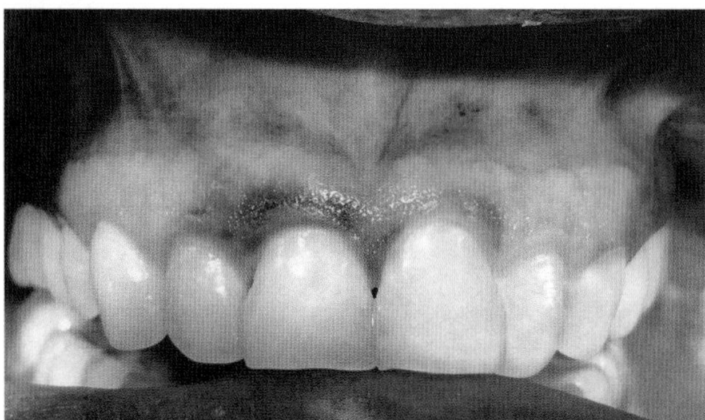

Fig. 16.12 Intentional tattooing. Bluish-purple pigmentation on the alveolar mucosa and attached gingiva extending from maxillary left to right bicuspids. Physiological pigmentation is observed on the attached gingiva of maxillary central incisors. (*Courtesy of Dr. Molly Rosebush, Louisiana State University. USA.*)

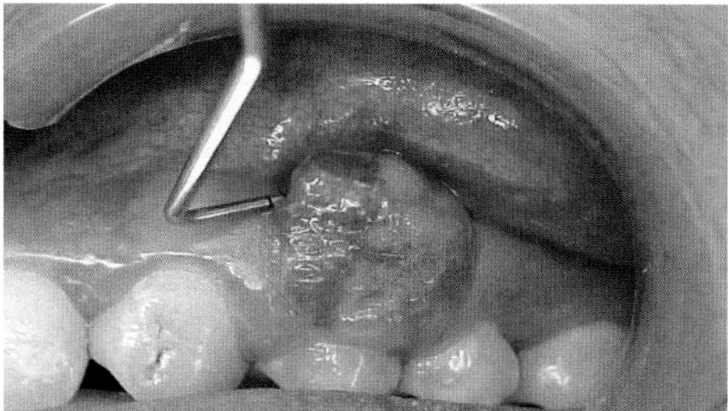

Fig. 16.13 Pyogenic granuloma. Ulcerated and hemorrhagic nodule on the attached and marginal gingiva. A biopsy is necessary to differentiate this lesion from other reactive and neoplastic conditions that share identical clinical presentations. (*Courtesy of Dr. Beatriz Aldape, National Autonomous University of Mexico. Mexico.*)

Treatment and Prognosis

Drug-induced pigmentation typically occurs slowly and becomes progressively more prominent over time.[165] The pigmentation usually fades if the drug is discontinued, although this does not always result in complete resolution of the hyperpigmentation.[165,234]

Intentional Gingival Tattoos

Intentional gingival tattoos are an integral part of many religious and cultural traditions, particularly in African countries.[189] Tattooing is done primarily for cosmetic reasons in order to make the teeth appear whiter. Some groups believe it can control gingival bleeding in periodontal disease, and it is also performed for repigmentation purposes in individuals with gingival vitiligo.[3,48,189]

Clinical Features

Clinically, gingival tattoos appear as diffuse bluish-gray or bluish-black gingival discolorations. They are seen almost exclusively in Black females who resided in African countries. Gingival tattoos are frequently located on the anterior maxillary facial gingiva and are typically limited to the vestibular aspect of the attached gingiva, extending symmetrically from the second premolar to the second premolar (Fig. 16.12). Rarely, they extend from the first molar to the first molar. Intraoral radiographs usually reveal a radiopaque material at the site of mucosal discoloration, although radiographic results may vary depending on the type of material used for tattooing. Radiographic findings are typically absent when a carbon-based material is used. Radiopacities are present when a heavy metal is incorporated in the tattooing material.[3,189] The characteristic color and distribution pattern of gingival pigmentation, along with compatible history, often allows for diagnosis based on the clinical appearance alone.

Microscopic Features

Histologic examination of gingival tattoo reveals randomly dispersed pigments throughout the connective tissue with characteristic perivascular deposits. Inflammation is typically absent in most cases.[86,189]

Treatment and Prognosis

No treatment is necessary.

LOCAL

Reactive Lesions of the Gingiva

Fibrous Hyperplasia

Focal fibrous hyperplasia (or irritation fibroma) is the most common benign reactive oral condition.[37,67] While gingival hyperplasia is rarely reported in association with certain drugs or syndromes,[25,103] this section will focus on focal fibrous hyperplasia that results primarily from local tissue irritation. The oral mucosa is subjected to many factors that induce hyperplastic changes, including plaque accumulation, trauma, improperly contoured dental restorations, and poorly fitting prostheses.[37,130,150]

Clinical Features

Focal fibrous hyperplasia is most commonly observed on the gingiva, although it may occur at any oral site.[67] The lesions range in size, from a few millimeters to a centimeter or greater.[67] Lesions may be sessile or pedunculated, fibrous or flaccid in consistency, and may vary in color from pink to red, depending on the degree of vascularization.[67] Fibrous hyperplasia of the gingiva is typically painless and appears as a firm nodular mass with a smooth, intact epithelial surface.[37] Denture-induced fibrous hyperplasia (also called denture fibroma or epulis fissuratum) is seen in association with ill-fitting dentures.[67]

Microscopic Features

A biopsy is indicated to establish the diagnosis since benign and malignant processes can mimic the clinical appearance of fibrous hyperplasia. Microscopically, fibrous hyperplasia is characterized by normal appearing epithelium that overlies a relatively hypovascular dense fibrous connective tissue.[37] In some cases, inflammatory cell infiltration and more prominent vasculature may be observed.[37] Increased mast cells and myofibroblasts are reported in the context of denture-induced fibrous hyperplasia.[130]

Treatment and Prognosis

Surgical excision is the recommended treatment and lesions typically do not recur.[226] If the source of irritation is identified this should be removed to facilitate healing. Dentures should be recontoured to mitigate chronic tissue irritation.[226]

Pyogenic Granuloma

Pyogenic granuloma (lobular capillary hemangioma or epulis gravidarum) is a common, benign vascular lesion.[199] The lesion was initially named because it was thought to represent an exuberant granulomatous reaction to an infectious or pyogenic agent.[199] While it is now understood that this is not the case, the original name is still retained. The etiology of pyogenic granuloma is incompletely understood, although several studies identify a role for hormones, localized trauma, and poor oral hygiene.[206,230] Pyogenic granulomas are observed in every age group, although

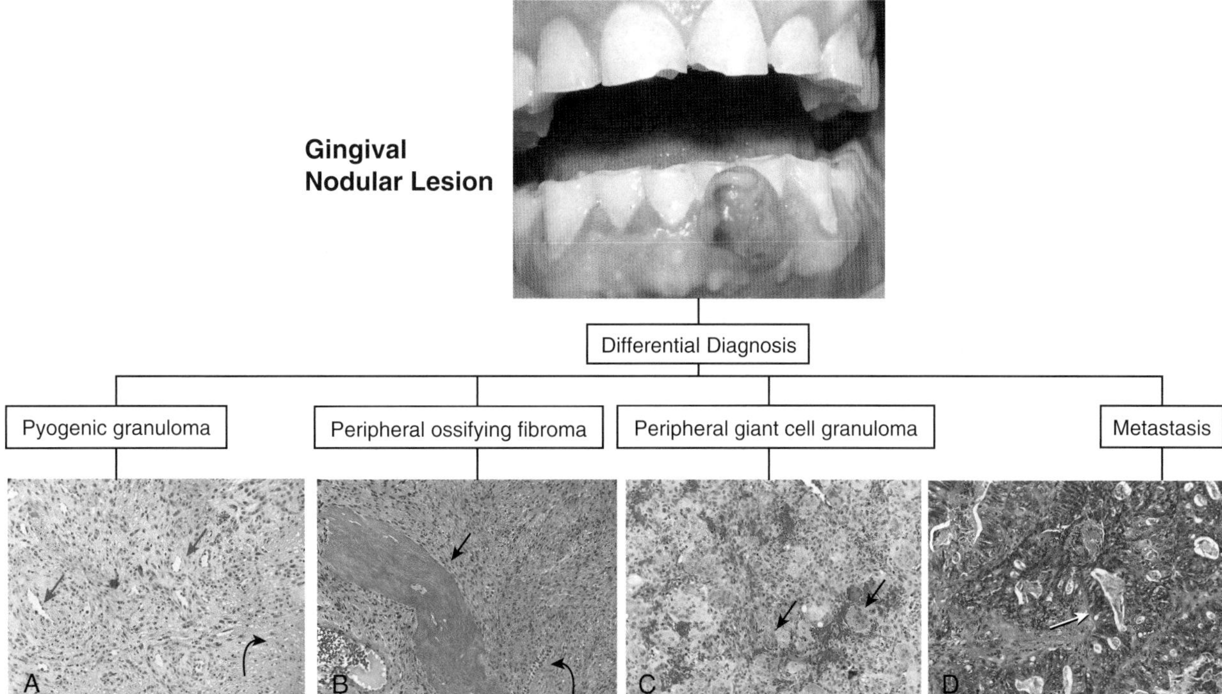

Fig. 16.14 Gingival nodular lesion. The clinical presentation of this gingival nodule can be shared by pyogenic granuloma, peripheral giant cell granuloma, peripheral ossifying fibroma, and metastasis. A biopsy is necessary to reach a diagnosis. The distinctive microscopic features of each one of these lesions are illustrated. (A) Pyogenic granuloma. Florid granulation tissue characterizes this lesion (*red arrow*, blood vessels, *curved black arrow*, fibrin mesh with neutrophils covering an area of ulceration). (B) Peripheral giant cell granuloma. Abundant multinucleated giant cells amidst a spindle to ovoid mesenchymal cell proliferation (*black arrows*, multinucleated giant cells). (C) Peripheral ossifying fibroma. Bone metaplasia (*black arrow*), occasional ribbons, and islands of odontogenic epithelium (*Curved black arrow*) amidst a hypercellular stroma. (D) Metastasis. Malignant glandular epithelium (*white arrow*) originating from an occult primary colon adenocarcinoma. (*Clinical picture courtesy of Dr. Beatriz Aldape, National Autonomous University of Mexico.*)

they tend to be most common in the second and third decades of life.[115,157,230] Pyogenic granulomas are observed in approximately 3% of pregnant women.[20] Studies suggest this may be due to hormonal changes, as progesterone, estrogen, and chorionic gonadotropin all induce increased vascular permeability and proliferation.[20] In the adult population, a 2:1 female to male predilection is reported.[37,230]

Clinical Features

Pyogenic granulomas arise most commonly on the anterior mandibular gingiva, although they can occur at any gingival location.[230] In pregnancy, the lips, buccal mucosa, and tongue are frequent sites of involvement.[230] Clinically, the lesions appear as an exophytic nodule that may be smooth or lobulated.[157] Ulceration is frequently observed.[230] Given the prominent vascular component, pyogenic granulomas often appear pinkish-red to purple in color.[157] Lesions may range in size from a few millimeters to several centimeters, and rapid growth is not uncommon (Fig. 16.13).[157]

Microscopic Features

A biopsy of suspected pyogenic granulomas is warranted to establish the diagnosis. Microscopically, the lesion exhibits a dense cellularity with a prominent vascular component.[157] Lobular collections of blood vessels are observed, consistent with an alternate name used for the lesion, lobular capillary hemangioma.[157] Pyogenic granulomas are often ulcerated, which appears histologically as an area of inflamed connective tissue devoid of surface epithelium.[157,230] Many different types of inflammatory cells may be present, including neutrophils, plasma cells, and lymphocytes (Fig. 16.14A).[157] In long-standing lesions, sclerotic changes may be observed, such as increased collagen deposition within the tissue.[157,230]

Treatment and Prognosis

The recommended treatment for pyogenic granuloma is surgical excision extending to the periosteum.[230] Lesions may recur, but this is relatively uncommon particularly if the initiating factor is removed.[226,230]

KEY FACT

Clinically, pyogenic granuloma, peripheral ossifying fibroma, and peripheral giant cell granuloma may appear similarly as nodular lesions on the gingiva. Excisional biopsy is the treatment of choice and is often curative if the underlying source of irritation is removed. Follow-up is warranted for peripheral ossifying fibroma and peripheral giant cell granuloma, as recurrence is reported.

Peripheral Ossifying Fibroma

Peripheral ossifying fibroma is less common than focal fibrous hyperplasia and pyogenic granuloma.[37,67] The etiology of the lesion is not well understood, although it is classified as a reactive process driven by cellular proliferation arising from the interdental papilla in response to a variety of factors including bacterial plaque, orthodontic appliances, and improperly contoured dental restorations.[138] Studies suggest that the lesion may arise from the proliferation of periodontal ligament cells, although this has not yet been established definitely.[172] This lesion occurs most frequently during the

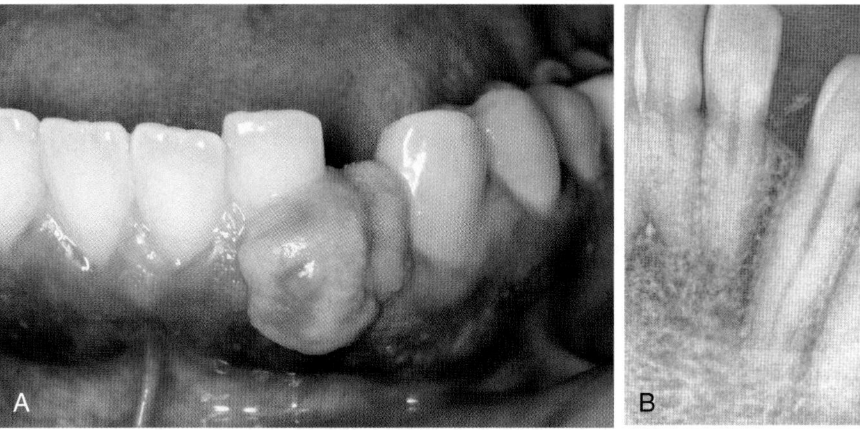

Fig. 16.15 Peripheral ossifying fibroma. (A) Pale nodular lesion on the gingiva. (B) The radiographic film identified calcifications in the soft tissue. Given the clinical presentation, the radiographic film is highly suggestive of peripheral ossifying fibroma. (*Courtesy of Dr. Kitrina Cordell and Dr. Ioannis Tsourounakis, School of Dentistry, Louisiana State University. USA.*)

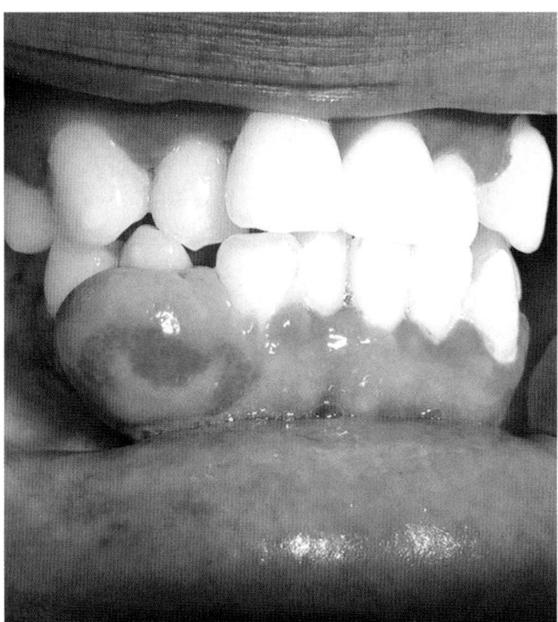

Fig. 16.16 Peripheral giant cell granuloma. Focal ulceration of an otherwise smooth nodule on attached and marginal gingiva has separated the mandibular right canine from the lateral incisor. (*Courtesy of Dr. Beatriz Aldape, National Autonomous University of Mexico. Mexico.*)

second, third, and fourth decades of life and is more prevalent in women.[37,138]

Clinical Features

Peripheral ossifying fibroma typically arises on the anterior gingiva and alveolar ridge,[67] although other intraoral sites are documented.[2] The lesion almost always presents as a painless, slow-growing solitary nodule.[138] Most lesions range from a few millimeters to 2 cm in size.[138] Lesions may be sessile or pedunculated, and in rare cases, erosion of the underlying bone is reported.[184] Peripheral ossifying fibroma is typically pale pink in appearance and is firm to hard in consistency (Fig. 16.15).[190]

Microscopic Features

A biopsy is indicated to confirm the diagnosis of peripheral ossifying fibroma. On histologic examination, lesions are poorly circumscribed and show proliferation of spindle cells within a fibrocellular stroma.[138,184] The presence of mineralized material is the distinctive feature of this lesion, and this may appear as mature or immature bone, or as cementum-like calcifications (see Fig. 16.14B).[138]

Treatment and Prognosis

Conservative surgical excision is the recommended management for peripheral ossifying fibroma. This lesion has a relatively high rate of recurrence, so it is imperative to perform a complete removal with periosteum.[117] Since these lesions tend to occur in the anterior gingiva, care must be taken to avoid mucogingival defects.[117]

Peripheral Giant Cell Granuloma

Peripheral giant cell granuloma (PGCG) also shows a predilection for the gingiva and alveolar mucosa and is seen less commonly than focal fibrous hyperplasia and pyogenic granulomas.[37,142] This lesion is reported over a wide age range but is most commonly seen in the fourth to sixth decades of life and no clear sex predilection is documented.[142] PGCG is classified as a reactive process. It is thought to originate from the periodontal ligament or periosteum in response to tissue irritation or trauma, such as extraction, implant placement, periodontal surgery, defective restorations, and orthodontic appliances.[13,142] It is important to establish the diagnosis of PGCG because the lesion may be indicative of hyperparathyroidism and thus the patient should be referred for further laboratory testing if clinically indicated.[137]

Clinical Features

PGCG typically presents as an asymptomatic, solitary, exophytic sessile or pedunculated lesion on the gingiva or alveolar ridge.[137,142,195] Erosion of bone is reported in one-third of cases.[55] The lesion is most often associated with teeth, although it is well-documented in edentulous areas in a minority of cases.[142] PGCG displays different colors on clinical exams and is usually described as red, purple, blue, or pink in appearance (Fig. 16.16).[142] Lesions typically have a smooth surface, although ulceration is reported in approximately one-third of cases.[142] Lesions may be soft or hard in consistency and are typically about one centimeter in size.[142,195]

Microscopic Features

A biopsy is required to establish the diagnosis of PGCG. Histologic evaluation reveals a non-encapsulated lesion with numerous multinucleated giant cells in a background of bland fibrocellular stroma (see Fig. 16.14C).[142,195] Abundant capillaries with extravasated red

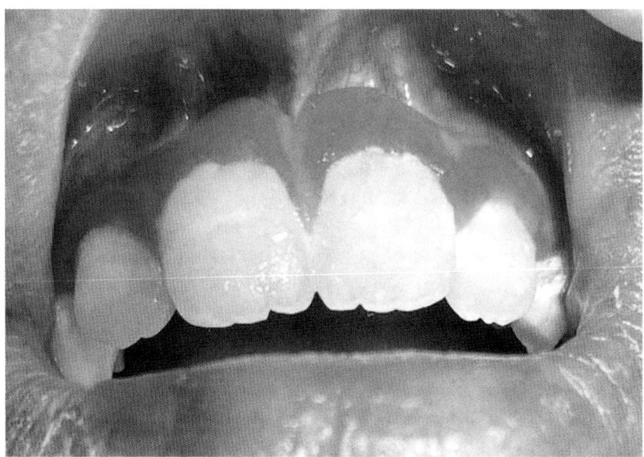

Fig. 16.17 Localized juvenile spongiotic gingival hyperplasia. Velvety red plaques on the marginal and attached gingiva. This is an unusually large segmental presentation. (*Courtesy of Dr. Yaser Alhazmi, College of Dentistry, Jazan University. Saudi Arabia.*)

blood cells are characteristically seen.[142] Inflammatory cells are also observed and are more numerous if ulceration is present.[142] PGCG can also exhibit mature bone or osteoid, and this is thought to be more common in recurrent lesions.[142]

Treatment and Prognosis

The recommended treatment for PGCG is wide surgical excision.[195] This lesion recurs in approximately 10% to 20% of cases,[55,142] and a recent study of several thousand cases found that the risk of recurrence can be mitigated if curettage is carried out at the time of excision.[55] Gingival defects may result and reconstructive surgery may be indicated to achieve an esthetic outcome following excision.[195]

Localized Juvenile Spongiotic Gingival Hyperplasia

Localized juvenile spongiotic gingival hyperplasia (LJSGH) was initially termed juvenile spongiotic gingivitis and was described as a reactive gingival lesion occurring in a pediatric population.[63] In 2008, Chang and colleagues described an additional 52 cases and proposed the name LJSGH.[51] This name has become somewhat controversial, as other groups have also identified cases in adults, and multifocal presentation is described in all ages.[63,209,229,239,245] Thus, the names spongiotic odontogenic gingivitis, spongiotic gingivitis with odontogenic metaplasia, and spongiotic gingival hyperplasia have been suggested as more appropriate designations for this condition.[209,229] Since the revised nomenclature has not been recognized formally in any classification criteria to date, we will use the original term (LJSGH) in this section while acknowledging that it does not encompass the clinical presentation of all cases.

Several small case series demonstrate LJSGH is observed primarily in young adults during the second decade of life with roughly equal sex predilection, although the original report noted a female disease predominance.[51,229,239,245] This lesion is not caused by human papilloma virus (HPV) infection and is not associated with sex hormones.[12,63] As the name implies, the lesion is almost always present on the gingiva and does not appear to be related to plaque accumulation.[51] While the etiology of LJSGH is poorly understood, immunohistochemical studies suggest it is derived from the junctional epithelium.[7] It is hypothesized that junctional epithelium exteriorized from the gingival sulcus may be exposed to irritants that would generate inflammation and subsequent hyperplasia of the tissue,[7] although further studies are needed to establish this conclusively.

Clinical Features

While our understanding of this condition continues to evolve, current studies demonstrate that LJSGH occurs most commonly on the anterior maxillary gingiva.[12,51,229,239,245] The lesion affects the attached and marginal gingiva and is typically localized, although multifocal cases are reported rarely.[51,63,209,229,245] The lesion is typically painless and manifests as a velvety red plaque or patch that is papillary in appearance and bleeds easily (Fig. 16.17).[51,63] LJSGH is usually less than one centimeter in size and may show an intermittent clinical course.[245]

Microscopic Features

Cases of suspected LJSGH should be biopsied to confirm the diagnosis. Histologic evaluation reveals an exophytic, papillary growth pattern.[51,229] Broad interconnecting bands of epithelial hyperplasia are described.[51] The epithelium is non-keratinized and may show atrophy, acanthosis, and elongated rete ridges.[63,229,245] Intracellular edema is observed.[51,245] Highly vascular connective tissue cores are a consistent feature, along with acute and chronic inflammatory cells.[51,209,229,245] An abrupt transition between lesion and normal tissue is a characteristic finding for LJSGH.[245]

Treatment and Prognosis

The recommended treatment for LJSGH varies depending on the clinical presentation. The lesion does not respond to conventional hygiene measures, such as brushing and flossing.[245] For asymptomatic lesions, observation alone may be appropriate.[245] Lesions that cause pain or discomfort or result in esthetic deficits should be removed.[245] Local ablative procedures, such as cryotherapy, are recommended since a recurrence rate of 25% is rep orted.[63,169,229]

Benign Tumors

Peripheral Odontogenic Tumors

Odontogenic cysts and tumors are relatively rare lesions that occur exclusively in the jawbone (intraosseous) and occasionally in the gingiva (peripheral or extraosseous). Odontogenic fibroma is considered the most common odontogenic lesion as it accounts for 50% of peripheral odontogenic lesions.[35] The second most common peripheral odontogenic tumor is ameloblastoma.[35] Other peripheral odontogenic lesions that may present on the gingiva include peripheral calcifying odontogenic cyst (COC), peripheral calcifying epithelial odontogenic tumor (CEOT), and odontoma. Since these are considerably rare, this section will be limited to a discussion of peripheral odontogenic fibroma and ameloblastoma.

Clinical Features

Peripheral odontogenic fibroma occurs most frequently in the second to the fourth decades of life. This lesion displays a predilection for the incisor-cuspid region.[193] The mandible is affected more frequently than the maxilla.[35] Clinically, the lesion appears as a sessile nodular mass covered by normal-colored mucosa. Rarely, peripheral odontogenic fibroma presents as diffuse or multifocal lesions. In addition, a very rare variant is identified that is associated with enamel hypoplasia/odontogenic fibroma-like hamartoma syndrome.[73] Peripheral odontogenic fibroma may show fine calcification on radiographic imaging. Typically, peripheral odontogenic

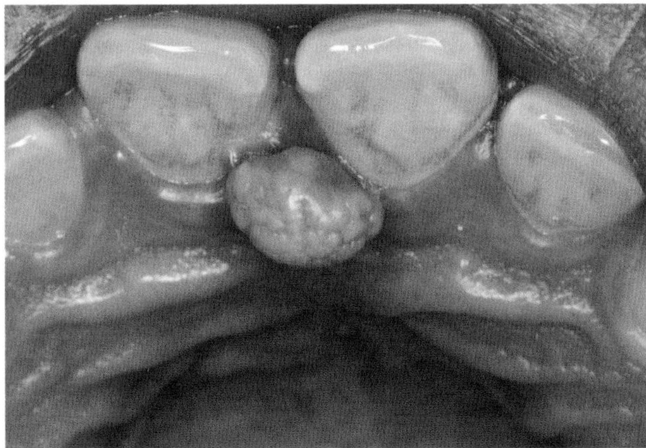

Fig. 16.18 Giant cell fibroma. Pink nodule with a papillary architecture that frequently evokes a clinical diagnosis of squamous papilloma. (*Courtesy of Dr. Kristin McNamara, College of Dentistry, The Ohio State University. USA.*)

fibroma does not involve the underlying bone. However, evidence of "saucerization" of the underlying alveolar bone may be seen.

Peripheral ameloblastomas have been reported in patients across a wide age range, although this neoplasm tends to arise in middle age. The posterior mandibular gingiva is the most common site for peripheral ameloblastoma. Peripheral ameloblastoma presents as a painless, sessile, or pedunculated gingival mass that is indistinguishable from other gingival lesions like fibrous hyperplasia or peripheral odontogenic fibroma. Radiographic studies demonstrate a soft tissue mass, which in some cases may show superficial erosion of the underlying alveolar bone.[84,193]

Microscopic Features

The microscopic features of these lesions are identical to their intraosseous counterparts.

Treatment and Prognosis

Most of these lesions behave in an indolent fashion, are treated with complete conservative surgical excision, and exhibit a low recurrence rate.[35] Peripheral odontogenic fibroma has a tendency to recur. Therefore follow-up of the patient is indicated.[193]

Giant Cell Fibroma

Giant cell fibroma is a benign fibrous proliferation of unknown etiology representing 2% to 4.7% of all oral fibrous lesions. This lesion is more common in young adults and shows a slight female predilection. The vast majority of cases occur in the gingiva.

Clinical Features

Giant cell fibroma occurs more frequently on the mandibular gingiva than on the maxillary. Other common sites include the tongue and the palate. Clinically, the lesion is asymptomatic and appears as a small pink nodule, usually less than 1 cm in diameter. The surface of the lesion often has a papillary architecture similar to a squamous papilloma (Fig. 16.18).[116,151] Retrocuspid papilla is a distinct developmental lesion that shares virtually identical histopathological features with the giant cell fibroma. Retrocuspid papillae are usually bilateral and occur on the lingual attached gingiva of mandibular cuspids. They are typically small, measuring less than 5 mm in diameter, and are the same color as the surrounding gingiva. They arise in children and young adults and tend to disappear with age, suggesting that retrocuspid papilla is a normal anatomical variation.[29]

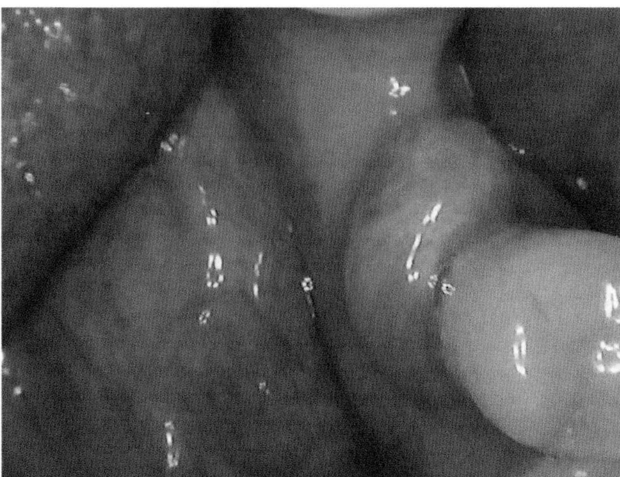

Fig. 16.19 Oral focal mucinosis. Occlusal view of a gingival smooth, light-pink nodule of the gingiva associated with the lingual and distal areas of tooth # 20. (*Courtesy of Dr. Lester Domingo, private practice, Miami, Florida. USA.*)

Microscopic Features

Microscopically, giant cell fibroma consists of a vascular fibrous connective tissue proliferation. Embedded within the connective tissue are multiple large stellate-shaped and multinucleated large fibroblasts. The rete ridges of the surface epithelium are usually delicate, tapered, and elongated.[110]

Treatment and Prognosis

The treatment of giant cell fibroma consists of conservative surgical excision and this is curative in most cases. Lesions located on the gingiva may show a tendency to recur.[116] Because of its typical clinical presentation, retrocuspid papilla requires no treatment.[29]

Gingival Fibrous Nodule

Gingival fibrous nodule is a relatively common but rarely reported oral mucosal condition. It represents a variation of normal rather than a disease. The typical location is the mandibular mucogingival line of the anterior labial gingiva.

Clinical Features

Gingival fibrous nodule presents as single or multiple asymptomatic small, exophytic, tumor-like nodule or nodules in the mandibular mucogingival line of the anterior labial gingiva. The mucosa covering the lesion is usually normal in color or slightly whitish. The lesion should be distinguished from retrocuspid papilla and mandibular gingival ridges. The clinical differential diagnosis includes fibroma, papilloma, focal epithelial hyperplasia, bony exostosis, gingival cyst, oral hamartomas associated with Cowden's syndrome, oral lesions of tuberous sclerosis, and oral nodules secondary to epidermolysis bullosa. However, the typical location and clinical presentation should easily segregate this lesion from other mimickers.[28,89]

Microscopic Features

A biopsy is rarely indicated but histologic examination reveals a nodular proliferation of hypovascular and hypocellular collagenized stroma.[28,89]

Treatment and Prognosis

The prognosis is excellent. However, some of these lesions may recur after removal so follow-up is warranted.[28,89]

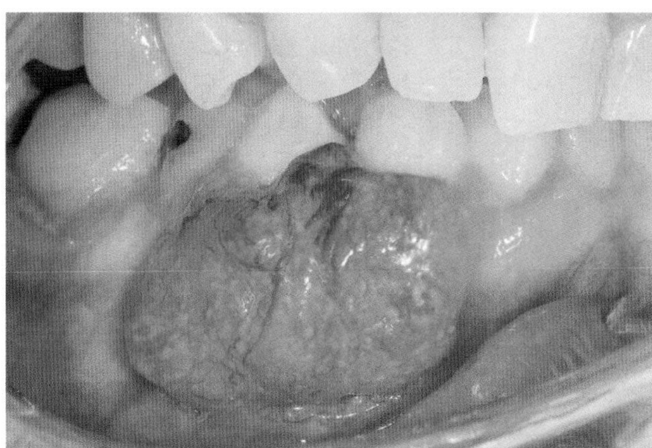

Fig. 16.20 Squamous cell carcinoma. Exophytic mass with focally hemorrhagic areas and subtle white granular surface. A presentation like this is reminiscent of a reactive gingival lesion such as pyogenic granuloma and peripheral giant cell granuloma. *(Courtesy of Dr. Howard Gross, private practice, Pennsylvania. USA and Dr. Scott Steward-Tharp, Emory University. USA)*

Oral Focal Mucinosis

Oral focal mucinosis is a rare tumor-like growth of unknown etiology. It is considered the oral counterpart of cutaneous focal mucinosis or cutaneous myxoid cyst.[232] The hallmark of the lesion is the overproduction of hyaluronic acid by fibroblasts. Oral focal mucinosis occurs in patients over a wide age range with a mean age of 45 years. It has a 2:1 female-to-male ratio. Almost 80% of the cases are found on the gingiva.

Clinical Features

Oral focal mucinosis presents as an asymptomatic smooth-surfaced, pink nodular mass ranging from a few millimeters to up to 2 cm in size (Fig. 16.19).

Microscopic Features

Microscopically, this lesion consists of a localized, nonencapsulated area of mucinous, myxomatous loose connective tissue containing spindle, ovoid, and stellate-shaped fibroblasts. Short bands of collagen fibers are embedded within the myxoid matrix. The surface epithelium is usually atrophic with inconspicuous rete ridges.

Treatment and Prognosis

The mainstay of treatment for oral focal mucinosis is surgical excision. The prognosis is excellent and recurrence is rare.[6,36,92]

Squamous Papilloma

Squamous papilloma is a common benign epithelial lesion caused by low-risk HPV types 6 and 11.[247,255] HPV induces squamous epithelial proliferation in a verrucopapillary pattern resulting in a clinical mass resembling a cauliflower. It can occur at any age and displays no sex predilection.

Clinical Features

Squamous papilloma can occur on any mucosal surface. However, the palate, tongue, and lips are most commonly involved, with gingiva lesions occurring less frequently. Typically, squamous papilloma appears as a painless exophytic mass with a rough pebbly surface. The color can vary from white, slightly red, to normal. Most squamous papillomas start as a small nodule that can rapidly increase in size to reach a dimension of about 0.5 cm. Eventually, the growth is arrested and the majority are 1 cm or less in diameter.[1]

Microscopic Features

The typical microscopic phenotype of squamous papilloma is that of a benign keratinized stratified squamous epithelial proliferation arranged in an exophytic papillary projection with fibrovascular cores. The epithelium can exhibit basal cell hyperplasia and mild epithelial atypia, especially in the context of inflammation. Koilocytes (virus-altered epithelial cells) are rarely seen.[1,221]

Treatment and Prognosis

Spontaneous regression is possible after several months or years. Surgical excision is the treatment of choice for oral squamous papilloma. Additional treatment modalities include cryosurgery, electrocautery, and laser ablation which is typically curative. However, frequent recurrences have been reported in HIV-positive patients. Interestingly, the prevalence of oral squamous cell papilloma is significantly increased in HIV patients undergoing HAART as compared to those who are not receiving this therapy.[9,175]

Malignant Tumors

Squamous Cell Carcinoma

Squamous cell carcinoma (SCC) is the most common malignant tumor of the oral cavity representing 90% of all malignancies that arise at this location.[44] Gingival SCC is infrequent and accounts for less than 10% of intraoral SCC.[78,143] Conventional SCC, which occurs mainly on the lateral surface of the tongue, has a strong association with tobacco and alcohol consumption. In contrast, these risk factors are weakly linked to gingival SCC.[99] Gingival SCC is diagnosed most frequently in the mandible of females[17,78] and can occur either *de novo* or from a preexisting leukoplakia, such as proliferative verrucous leukoplakia (PVL). PVL is a distinctive variant of leukoplakia that shows a striking predilection for females. It appears as multifocal and multicentric white lesions that often display a verruciform surface. PVL commonly involves the gingiva adjacent and sometimes circumferential to the teeth. PVL shows a spectrum of histopathology depending on the stage of disease. Early lesions show hyperkeratosis that progresses into verrucous hyperplasia, verrucous carcinoma, and finally to invasive SCC.[78,231,237]

Clinical Features

Typically, gingival SCC presents as an asymptomatic exophytic mass (Fig. 16.20). Less frequently, they may appear as an ulcerated lesion. The surface of the mass can be rough, irregular, granular, verrucous, and papillary with interspersed erythematous and leukoplakic areas. Gingival SCC can destroy the underlying bone, resulting in tooth mobility.[17,143,216] In its early stages, it may display a deceptively innocuous appearance that resembles gingivitis, periodontitis, and peri-implantitis. It may also mimic other reactive and benign conditions such as pyogenic granuloma and verruciform xanthoma.[78,99]

Histopathologic Features

Gingival SCC consists of islands and cords of invasive malignant keratinocytes arising from a dysplastic surface epithelium. The malignant keratinocytes exhibit cellular pleomorphism, nuclear hyperchromatism, increased nuclear-cytoplasmic ratio, prominent nucleoli, atypical mitoses, cellular desmosomes, intracellular keratinization, and keratin pearls. These features are used to assess the degree of differentiation and allow for the classification of SCC as either well-differentiated, moderately differentiated, or poorly differentiated. Most gingival SCC are moderately differentiated.[78] The degree of differentiation determines the

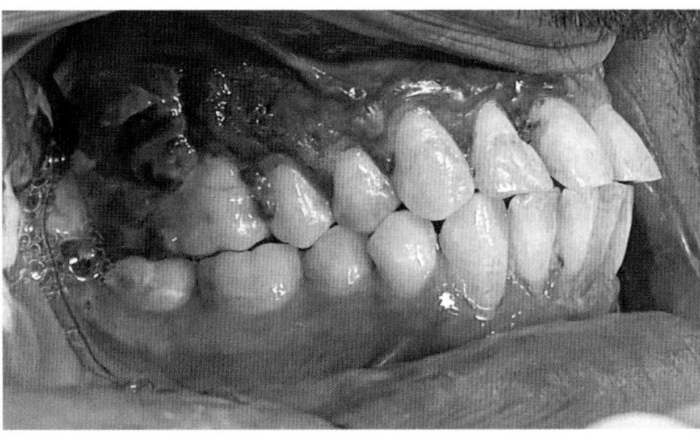

Fig. 16.21 Melanoma. Multiple pigmented exophytic tumor masses characteristic of an advanced nodular melanoma. Both the marginal and attached gingiva are involved. The anterior vestibular alveolar mucosa also shows peripheral pigmented patches representing radial growth.

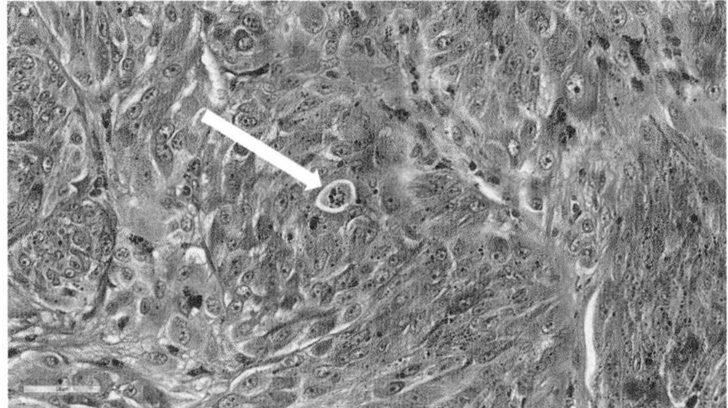

Fig. 16.22 Melanoma. High magnification showing nests of epithelioid to spindle tumor cells with prominent nucleoli, variation of nuclear and cellular size and intracellular melanin pigmentation. A mitotic figure is observed (*arrow*) (H&E, original magnification ×400).

grade of the tumor; well-differentiated SCC represents grade I (low-grade); moderately differentiated SCC characterizes grade II; poorly differentiated SCC represents grade III (high-grade). There are many factors that can affect the biological behavior of the tumor including the histopathological grading, extension of the lesion to the margin of the surgical resection, depth of invasion, bony invasion, perineural invasion, vascular invasion, and cervical metastasis.[40,173] Patients with SCC undergo comprehensive testing to establish the disease stage whereby the size of the tumor, lymph node involvement, and metastasis are evaluated. Patients are staged using a numeric system from 1 to 4, where 1 denotes the best prognosis and 4 the worst.

Treatment and Prognosis

The treatment of SCC depends on the clinical staging of the tumor. Generally, early diagnosis of localized SCC is associated with stage 1 and involves surgical resection. Optimally, wide negative surgical margins are achieved to prevent a recurrence. In contrast, a delayed diagnosis of SCC results in the diagnosis of the patient at a more advanced disease stage. That may require a more aggressive treatment approach that requires a combination of surgery (including cervical lymph node dissection), radiation therapy, and/or chemotherapy. The overall 5-year survival rate for oral SCC is around 50% and the disease stage is the best prognostic factor for intraoral SCC.[90]

KEY FACT

Squamous cell carcinomas of the gingiva are relatively uncommon, but these may cause significant morbidity or mortality if the diagnosis is delayed. Dysplastic lesions may progress to squamous cell carcinoma, so careful monitoring of dysplasia is recommended to detect malignant transformation. A biopsy is required to confirm the diagnosis and suspicious lesions should be biopsied promptly to facilitate appropriate patient management..

Mucosal Melanoma

Melanoma is a malignant neoplasm that arises from neoplastic melanocytes. While melanoma is the third most common malignant tumor of the skin, mucosal melanoma is much less common, accounting for 1% of malignant melanomas overall and approximately 10% of head and neck cases. Oral mucosal melanoma makes up less than 0.5% of all oral malignancies.[80,214] Mucosal melanoma is believed to arise from the melanocytes located in the basal cell layer of the mucosal epithelial lining. In contrast to cutaneous melanoma, mucosal melanoma has no association with ultraviolet light exposure and its exact etiology is unknown.[43] Various oncogenes and tumor suppressor genes are involved in oral mucosal melanoma notably, *c-KIT* mutations.[61] Approximately 50% of cutaneous melanoma have *BRAF* mutations.[68] In contrast, *BRAF* mutation is rarely observed in oral mucosal melanoma.[59] This discrepancy suggests that mucosal melanoma may represent a distinct entity with different etiopathogenesis.

Clinical Features

Mucosal melanoma occurs most commonly in adults in the fifth through seventh decades of life, with a slight male predilection.[147,188,214] Within the oral cavity, the hard palate and gingiva are the most frequent sites of involvement accounting for 70% to 80% of cases.[188,208] Mucosal melanomas are usually asymptomatic unless ulcerated. The majority of lesions begin as brown-black macules with heterogeneous pigmentation and irregular borders. Swelling, ulceration, and paresthesia are associated with advanced cases (Fig. 16.21). About 10% of cases are amelanotic or contain little pigmentation.[228] Due to their variable clinical appearance, the differential diagnosis of mucosal melanoma can include an array of pigmented lesions such as AD, blue nevus, Kaposi sarcoma, amalgam tattoo, melanotic macule, Peutz-Jegher syndrome, smoker's melanosis, and physiologic pigmentation.

Microscopic Features

Mucosal lentiginous melanoma is the most common histopathological expression of oral mucosal melanoma. In the early stages, atypical melanocytes proliferate radially at the epithelial-connective tissue interface. Subsequently, vertical growth of tumor cells ensues. The neoplastic melanocytes exhibit variable morphology including epithelioid, clear, pleomorphic, undifferentiated, plasmacytoid, and spindled phenotypes (Fig. 16.22). Immunohistochemical stains such as S-100, SOX10, HMB-45, and Melan-A, are sensitive melanocytic markers that are valuable in confirming the diagnosis of melanoma.[214]

Treatment and Prognosis

Mucosal melanoma is an aggressive malignancy associated with rapid local invasion and early metastatic spread. Therefore, wide surgical excision is the mainstay of treatment. Adjuvant radiotherapy has been useful in efforts to maximize locoregional control. The 5-year survival of mucosal melanoma range from 13% to 38%, with

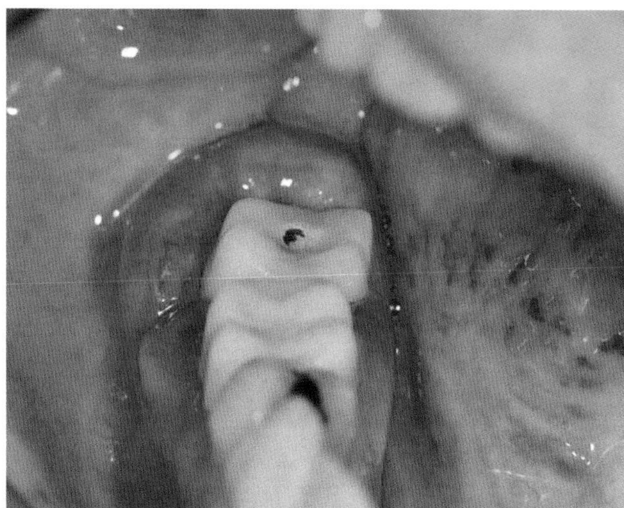

Fig. 16.23 Lymphoma. This presentation of lymphoma is suggestive of a reactive lesion (i.e., pyogenic granuloma, peripheral giant cell granuloma). However, the relatively uniform enlargement of the vestibular and lingual gingiva contrasts with the more localized and nodular presentation of a reactive lesion. (*Courtesy of Dr. Anupama Grandhi, School of Dentistry and School of Medicine, Loma Linda University. USA.*)

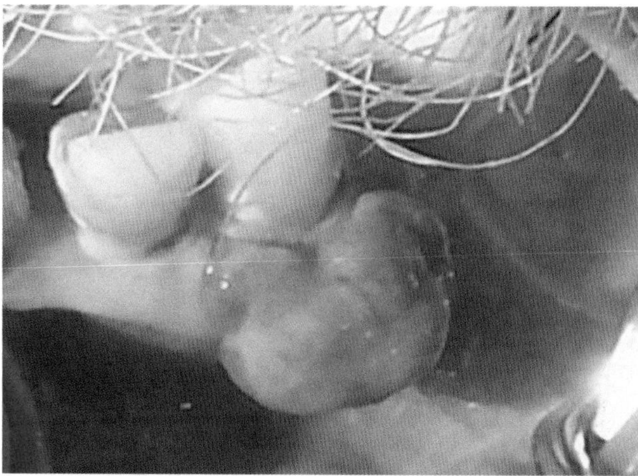

Fig. 16.24 Metastasis. A rather innocuous presentation of a multilobular, slow growing lesion that proved to be a metastatic hepatocarcinoma upon microscopic examination. (*Courtesy of Dr. Richard J. Vargo, A.T. Still University-Missouri School of Dentistry & Oral Health and Saint Louis University School of Medicine. USA.*)

even lower rates in amelanotic cases.[204] The overall prognosis of oral mucosal melanoma is poor, with most patients dying within a year. Some studies suggest that gingival lesions are associated with longer median survival rates than non-gingival lesions, however, there is limited evidence to support this notion. Distant metastases develop in 70% of patients, with the lung being the most common target, followed by the liver, bone, and brain.[31,80] Recently, immunotherapy with checkpoint inhibitors such as ipilimumab (anti-CTLA-4), nivolumab, and pembrolizumab (both target PD-1), have shown promising results for the treatment of cutaneous melanoma.[133] Although the effectiveness of these biologicals in the treatment of primary mucosal melanoma is modest, they have shown to delay disease progression and improve overall survival rates in patients with metastatic melanoma.[194]

KEY FACT

While the diagnosis of melanoma in the oral cavity is rare, it is critical to distinguish this malignancy from other pigmented lesions of the oral mucosa. Melanoma often appears as a diffuse, asymmetric pigmented lesion that may exhibit rapid growth. Mucosal melanoma is not associated with sun exposure. The recommended treatment for oral melanoma is radical surgical excision and the prognosis is poor.

Lymphoma

Lymphomas constitute a complex and heterogeneous group of lymphoreticular neoplasms with a spectrum of behavior ranging from relatively indolent to highly aggressive and potentially fatal.[196] In the most recent WHO classification, lymphomas were classified based on the stage of cell differentiation, cell lineage, cell origin, and underlying molecular mechanisms. Generally, they are classified as Hodgkin lymphoma and B-cell and T-cell non-Hodgkin lymphoma (NHL).[97] Extranodal Hodgkin lymphomas are rare. In contrast, about 20% to 30% of NHLs are found primarily in extranodal sites.[134] Only 2% of all extranodal lymphomas occur primarily in the oral cavity.[176] However, NHL is the second most common oral malignancy after SCC.[45]

Clinical Features

In the oral cavity, lymphoma can occur either in the soft tissues or in the jawbones. The most commonly affected sites in the oral cavity are the palate, gingiva, tongue, buccal mucosa, floor of mouth, and maxilla.[176,198] Most NHLs present in old adults, although younger patients may be affected, particularly if immunosuppressed. Soft tissue lesions present as discrete red to purplish swellings, sometimes ulcerated, with a boggy consistency. Gingival NHL most frequently causes destruction of the underlying bone and loosening of teeth. Bony lesions may result in delayed healing of extraction sites, vague pain or discomfort, dysesthesia, paresthesia, or trigeminal neuropathy.[253] NHL confined to gingival tissues should be differentiated from other gingival enlargements, as it may mimic benign reactive gingival growths such as pyogenic granuloma and PGCG (Fig. 16.23).[16,45] In the early stage, the radiographic changes may be subtle or nonexistent. As the disease progresses, it will show an ill-defined or ragged radiolucency, bony expansion, and eventually may perforate the cortex of the jaw.[241]

Microscopic Features

NHLs show diffuse effacement of the tissue by lymphocytes at different degrees of differentiation (depending on the lymphoma subtype). The histopathological findings of NHL on routine H&E analysis may be relatively nonspecific and often includes a broad differential diagnosis. Therefore, extensive immunohistochemical and molecular studies are needed to arrive at an accurate diagnosis. Diffuse large B-cell lymphoma is the most common type of lymphoma in the oral cavity.[22] Plasmablastic lymphoma is a distinctive type of lymphoma that occurs in immunosuppressed patients, especially those with HIV. Of note, plasmablastic lymphoma was initially described in the oral cavity.[64]

Treatment and Prognosis

The treatment and prognosis of lymphomas vary according to the subtype. However, most types of NHLs are treated with multiagent chemotherapy. The prognosis of a patient with NHL is based on multiple parameters such as the stage and grade of the disease, age of the patient, and the patient's overall health status.[118]

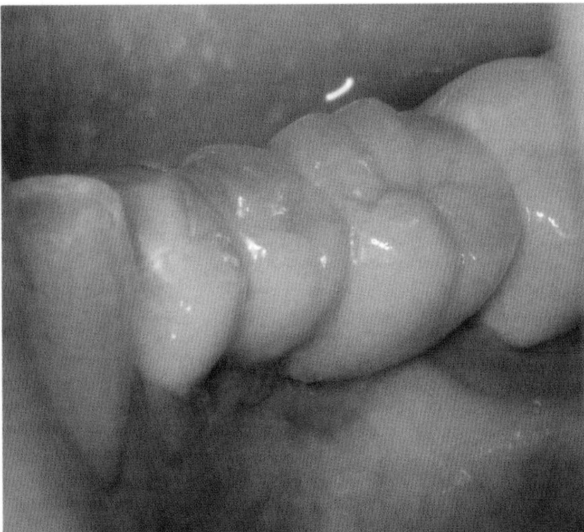

Fig. 16.25 Amalgam tattoo. Characteristic bluish-gray macule with diffuse borders on the lingual attached gingiva adjacent to complete crowns. Because of an abundance of caution, a biopsy of a lesion like this to rule out melanoma would be justified in the absence of radiographic films that document the presence of metallic particles in the soft tissue.

Metastatic Tumors

Metastatic tumors to the jaws and oral soft tissues are rare, accounting for approximately 1% of all oral malignancies.[113] Any carcinoma or sarcoma, regardless of the site of origin, can metastasize to the oral cavity, although carcinomas are the most common metastatic tumors observed in the orofacial region.[114,174] On histopathologic examination, most cases are adenocarcinomas.[124] In men, lung cancer is the most common primary tumor that metastasizes to the oral cavity, whereas for women, breast cancer is the most common primary.[114,174] The pathogenic mechanisms that govern the metastasis of primary tumor cells to the oral cavity are still poorly understood.[136] Metastasis to the oral cavity heralds the presence of a late-stage disseminated disease. Thus, the identification of oral metastases is crucial because disseminated metastatic lesions are associated with poor prognosis and about 25% of oral metastatic lesions represent the first sign of the disease.[145]

Clinical Features

The most common intraoral location for a metastasis is the gingiva, accounting for 54% of all cases.[136] The presence of inflammation (i.e., gingivitis, periodontitis, and peri-implantitis) may play a major role in creating a suitable environment for the establishment of metastatic malignant cells. Thus, the presence of chronic inflammation may explain, at least in part, the predilection of metastasis for the attached gingiva. Clinically, oral metastases may have an innocuous presentation that can result in diagnostic delay. Early gingival lesions may mimic hyperplastic or reactive processes, such as pyogenic granuloma, PGCG, peripheral ossifying fibroma, or fibrous epulis (Fig. 16.24). In some cases, the discovery of a metastatic lesion follows a dental extraction where the socket fails to heal.[114] Oral metastases can be seen in any age group, but middle-aged and older adults are affected most frequently, with a 2:1 male to female disease predilection.[136]

Microscopic Features

The microscopic features reflect the phenotype of the primary tumor (see Fig. 16.14D).

Treatment and Prognosis

The prognosis for patients with oral metastatic lesions is extremely poor and about 70% of the patients die within 1 year after the diagnosis.[57] Thus, the main goal of the treatment is to improve the patient's quality of life. However, the specific treatment approach depends on several factors such as the type of malignancy, biological behavior of the primary tumor, disease stage, and the age of the patient. Generally, a palliative approach is warranted.

Discoloration of the Gingiva

Amalgam Tattoo

Amalgam tattoo is considered to be the most common localized pigmented lesion of the oral mucosa. It occurs in approximately 0.4% to 0.9% of the adult population and results from the iatrogenic implantation of dental amalgam into mucosal tissues.[33] Amalgam can become impregnated in mildly injured or periodontally inflamed mucosa during the course of dental restorative procedures, tooth extractions, or endodontic surgery. Silver is the main element responsible for the tissue discoloration.

Clinical Features

While amalgam tattoos typically present on the gingiva and the alveolar mucosa, any oral tissue can be affected. It appears as a painless, blue-gray-black macule with a smooth surface. The borders may be well-defined, irregular, or diffuse (Fig. 16.25). The size of the lesion rarely exceeds 0.5 cm, although some as large as 3 cm in diameter have been reported.[34] Small particles are invisible in routine radiographs but large particles can be visualized as dense metallic radiopaque fragments.[33] The differential diagnosis for amalgam tattoo includes medication-induced pigmentation, blue nevus, and melanoma. Most amalgam tattoos are easily recognizable on clinical examination and thus, a biopsy is not indicated. However, those that display an unusual clinical presentation may necessitate a biopsy to confirm the diagnosis and rule out melanoma.

Microscopic Features

Microscopic examination of amalgam tattoo reveals black-brown spherical particles within the connective tissue. Silver contained within dental amalgam binds to argyrophilic reticulin fibers, particularly around nerve fibers and blood vessels. Generally, amalgam is composed of elements that are biocompatible and seldom evoke inflammation. In some cases, however, it can produce tissue fibrosis, chronic inflammation, and a granulomatous response.[34]

Treatment and Prognosis

Patients with amalgam tattoos have an excellent prognosis and no treatment is required.[34]

KEY FACT

The gingiva is the most common site for metastatic tumors in the oral cavity. In some cases, the patient is not aware of the underlying disease and the oral lesion is the first manifestation. In other cases, the patient may have a history of cancer, and this information should be included in the biopsy report to aid in the confirmation of the origin of the malignancy. Patients with widespread metastatic disease have a poor prognosis.

Smoker's Melanosis

Smoker's melanosis is a common oral condition. In some countries, smoking is considered to be the most common cause of oral pigmentation in light-skinned individuals. Many studies have shown a strong association between oral pigmentation and heavy smoking.[15,109] Melanin is produced by melanocytes in the oral mucosa as a protective response to harmful substances present in tobacco.[108] Although any oral mucosal site can be affected, cigarette smokers tend to develop pigmented areas on the anterior facial gingiva. In contrast, pigmentation in the commissure and buccal mucosa is seen more frequently in pipe smokers, while the hard palate of reverse smokers is most commonly affected. Smoker's melanosis is more frequent in females possibly due to the synergistic effect of sex hormones and tobacco smoke. Oral pigmentation is most pronounced during the first year of smoking and the degree of hyperpigmentation seems to correlate with the number of cigarettes smoked per day.

Clinical Features

Typically, smoker's melanosis presents either as a diffuse black-brown pigmentation or as discrete macules or plaques.[15] The clinical differential diagnosis includes physiologic pigmentation, medication-induced hyperpigmentation, chronic inflammation associated pigmentation, AD, Peutz–Jegher syndrome, and Laugier–Hunziker syndrome. In addition, endocrine disturbances, hemochromatosis, chronic pulmonary disease, melanotic macule, melanotic nevus, melanoacanthoma, and melanoma should be considered.[163]

Microscopic Features

Smoker's melanosis is not a premalignant lesion and biopsy is needed only for lesions with suspicious clinical characteristics. For example, lesions located on the hard palate and those with significant color changes or surface elevation should be biopsied. Microscopically, increased melanin pigmentation within the basal cells of the epithelium (termed basal cell melanosis) is the hallmark of smoker's melanosis. In addition, melanin incontinence and melanophages are present in the superficial lamina propria. Chronic inflammation is typically sparse and may be present in the subepithelial connective tissue.[185] These histopathological findings are not specific and are shared by many pigmented lesions. Therefore, clinical correlation and laboratory tests may be of value to exclude other pigmented lesions and establish the diagnosis.

Treatment and Prognosis

Smoking cessation often leads to gradual regression of mucosal pigmentation over a 3-year period.[15] Oral melanosis associated with smoking does not require treatment.

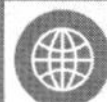
A Case Scenario is found on the companion website eBooks.Health.Elsevier.com.

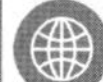
References for this chapter are found on the companion website eBooks.Health.Elsevier.com.

CHAPTER 17

Acute Gingival Infections and Management

Perry R. Klokkevold | Fermin A. Carranza

 For expanded discussions on gingival changes with healing and additional treatment considerations, please visit the companion website at eBooks.Health.Elsevier.com.

CHAPTER OUTLINE

Necrotizing Ulcerative Gingivitis

Necrotizing ulcerative gingivitis (NUG) is a severe inflammatory disease of the gingiva caused by bacteria that most often occurs in an impaired host with risk factors (e.g., poor oral hygiene, smoking, poor nutrition, compromised immune system).[38] NUG may occur in a mouth that is free of other gingival involvement or may be superimposed on underlying gingival or periodontal disease. Involvement can be limited to a single tooth, to several teeth, or it can be widespread throughout the mouth (Fig. 17.1). It manifests with characteristic clinical signs of necrosis and sloughing of the gingival tissues and may be accompanied by systemic symptoms as well.

Although the acronym *ANUG* (acute necrotizing ulcerative gingivitis) is frequently used, it is a misnomer.[75] Historically, NUG has been identified as an acute disease. However, the term *acute* is used as a clinical descriptor rather than a diagnostic term because chronic forms of the disease do not exist. The term *acute* has not been used in diagnosis since 1999.[38] Furthermore, a summary of acute periodontal lesions advocated the more simplified term *necrotizing gingivitis* rather than *necrotizing ulcerative gingivitis*, but the latter term continues to be used in this chapter.[37]

More advanced forms of necrotizing ulcerative disease can include destruction of the periodontal attachment apparatus, including bone,[54] especially in patients with long-standing disease or severe immunosuppression. When periodontal attachment and bone loss occurs, the condition is called *necrotizing ulcerative periodontitis* (NUP) (see Chapter 30).

Oral Signs and Symptoms

NUG is characterized by a sudden onset of symptoms, sometimes occurring after an episode of debilitating disease or acute respiratory tract infection. A change in living habits, protracted work without adequate rest, poor nutrition, tobacco use, and psychological stress are common features of patients' history.

Characteristic lesions are punched-out, craterlike depressions at the crest of the interdental papillae that subsequently extend to the marginal gingiva and rarely to the attached gingiva and oral mucosa. The surface of the gingival crater is covered by a gray pseudomembranous slough that is demarcated from the surrounding gingival mucosa by a pronounced linear erythema (see Fig. 17.1A). In some cases, the lesions are denuded of the surface pseudomembrane, exposing the gingival margin, which is red, shiny, and hemorrhagic. The characteristic lesions can progressively destroy the gingiva and underlying periodontal tissues (see Fig. 17.1B). Spontaneous gingival hemorrhage and pronounced bleeding after the slightest stimulation are characteristic clinical signs (see Fig. 17.1B and C). Fetid odor and increased salivation are also common characteristics of NUG.

NUG can be superimposed on gingivitis or periodontitis with periodontal pockets, but it does not lead to periodontal pocket formation because the necrotic changes involve the gingival and junctional epithelium; healthy epithelium is needed for periodontal pocket deepening (see Chapter 22).

 **KEY FACT**

Necrotizing ulcerative gingivitis can be superimposed on periodontitis with pockets, but NUG does not usually lead to pocket formation because the necrotic changes involve the gingival and junctional epithelium.

The lesions are extremely sensitive to touch, and the patient often complains of a constant radiating, gnawing pain that is intensified

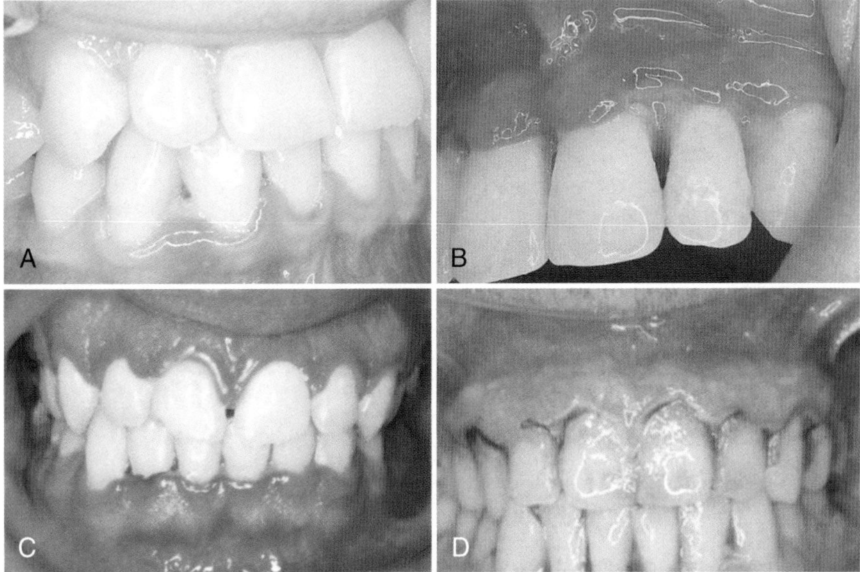

Fig. 17.1 Necrotizing ulcerative gingivitis. (A) Typical punched-out papilla between the mandibular canine and lateral incisor is covered by a grayish-white pseudomembrane. (B) More advanced case shows the destruction of the papillae, which results in an irregular marginal contour. (C) Typical lesions with spontaneous hemorrhage. (D) Generalized involvement of the papillae and the marginal gingiva with whitish necrotic lesions.

by spicy or hot foods and chewing. There is a foul metallic taste, and the patient is conscious of an excessive amount of pasty saliva.

Extraoral and Systemic Signs and Symptoms

Patients are usually ambulatory and have minimal systemic symptoms. Local lymphadenopathy and a slight elevation in temperature are common features of the mild and moderate stages of the disease. In severe cases, patients may present with high fever, increased pulse rate, leukocytosis, loss of appetite, and general lassitude. Systemic reactions are more severe in children. Insomnia, constipation, gastrointestinal disorders, headache, and mental depression sometimes accompany the condition.

In rare cases, severe sequelae, such as gangrenous stomatitis and noma, have been described.[5,6,23,42] These patients are almost exclusively encountered in populations in developing countries, especially children with systemic disease or malnutrition.[23,37,75]

Clinical Course

The clinical course varies among individuals. The severity of NUG often diminishes without treatment, leading to a subacute stage with milder clinical symptoms. Some patients experience repeated remissions and exacerbations, and the condition can recur in previously treated patients. If untreated, especially in an immunocompromised host, NUG can lead to progressive destruction of the periodontium and gingival recession accompanied by an increase in the severity of systemic complications.[40,67]

Histopathology

At the microscopic level, NUG is a nonspecific, acute necrotizing inflammation of the gingival margin that involves the stratified squamous epithelium and the underlying connective tissue. Comparable microscopic changes result from trauma, chemical irritation, or the application of caustic medications. The surface epithelium is destroyed, and replaced by a meshwork of fibrin, necrotic epithelial cells, polymorphonuclear leukocytes (PMNs, predominantly neutrophils), and various types of microorganisms (Fig. 17.2). This is the zone that appears clinically as the surface pseudomembrane. At the immediate border of the necrotic pseudomembrane, the epithelium is edematous, and the individual cells exhibit various degrees of hydropic degeneration. PMNs infiltrate the intercellular spaces.

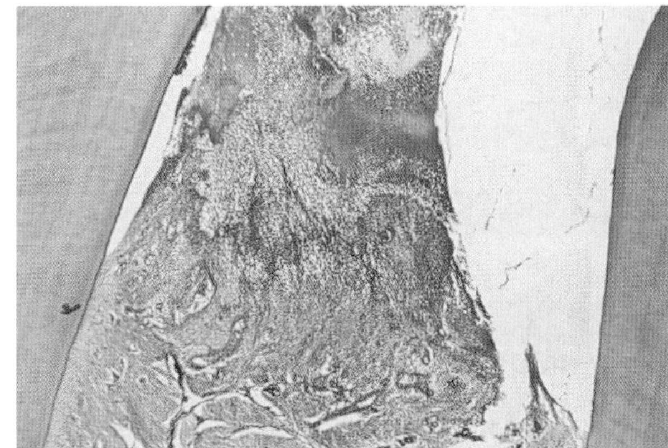

Fig. 17.2 In a survey section of interdental papilla in a patient with necrotizing ulcerative gingivitis, the necrotic tissue forms the gray marginal pseudomembrane *(top).* Ulceration and the accumulation of leukocytes and fibrin replace normal epithelium *(bottom).*

The underlying connective tissue is markedly hyperemic, with numerous engorged capillaries and a dense infiltration of PMNs. This acutely inflamed zone appears clinically as the linear erythema beneath the surface pseudomembrane. Numerous plasma cells can appear in the periphery of the infiltrate; this is interpreted as an area of established gingivitis on which the acute lesion became superimposed.[39] The epithelium and connective tissue alterations diminish with distance from the necrotic gingival margin, blending gradually with the uninvolved gingiva.

Relationship of Bacteria and the Necrotizing Ulcerative Gingivitis Lesion

Light and electron microscopy have been used to study the relationship of bacteria and the characteristic lesions of NUG. Light microscopy shows that the exudate on the surface of the necrotic lesions contains microorganisms that morphologically resemble cocci, fusiform bacilli, and spirochetes.[92] The layer between the necrotic and living tissue contains enormous numbers of fusiform bacilli and spirochetes in addition to leukocytes and fibrin. Spirochetes and other bacteria invade the underlying living tissue.[9,17,22,51]

Spirochetes have been found as deep as 300 μm from the surface. Most spirochetes in the deeper zones are morphologically different from cultivated strains of *Treponema microdentium.* They occur in nonnecrotic tissue before other types of bacteria, and they can achieve high-intercellular concentrations in the epithelium and connective tissue adjacent to the ulcerated lesion.[48]

Smears from the lesions (Fig. 17.3) show scattered bacteria (predominantly spirochetes and fusiform bacilli), desquamated epithelial cells, and occasional PMNs. Spirochetes and fusiform bacteria are usually seen with other oral spirochetes, vibrios, and filaments.

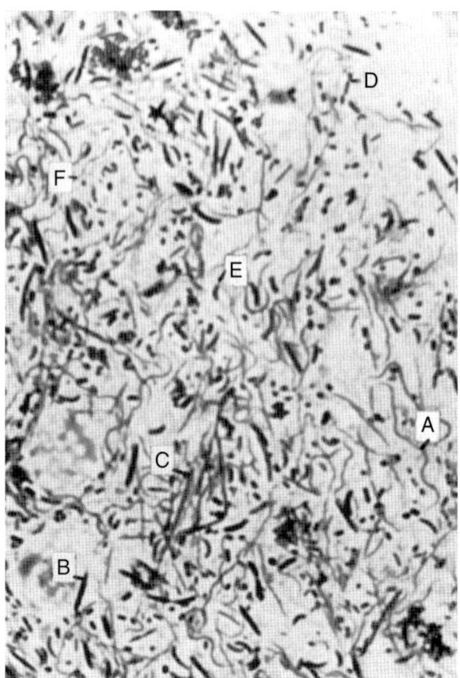

Fig. 17.3 A bacterial smear was obtained from a lesion in a patient with necrotizing ulcerative gingivitis. (A) *Spirochete.* (B) *Bacillus fusiformis.* (C) *Filamentous organism (i.e., actinomyces or leptotrichia)* (D) *Streptococcus.* (E) *Vibrio.* (F) *Treponema microdentium.*

Diagnosis

Diagnosis is based on clinical findings of gingival pain, ulceration, and bleeding. A bacterial smear is not necessary or definitive because the bacterial picture is not appreciably different from that of patients with marginal gingivitis, periodontal pockets, pericoronitis, or primary herpetic gingivostomatitis.[73] However, bacterial studies are useful for the differential diagnosis of NUG and other specific infections of the oral cavity, such as diphtheria, thrush, actinomycosis, and streptococcal stomatitis.

The microscopic examination of a biopsy specimen is not sufficiently specific to be diagnostic. It can be used to differentiate NUG from specific infections (e.g., tuberculosis) or neoplastic disease, but it does not differentiate NUG from other necrotizing conditions of nonspecific origin, such as those produced by trauma or caustic medications.

KEY FACT

A bacterial smear or culture is not necessary or definitive in the diagnosis of NUG because the bacterial flora is not appreciably different from that of patients with other common inflammatory conditions (e.g., gingivitis, periodontitis). However, bacterial studies are useful for the differential diagnosis of NUG when other specific infections of the oral cavity, such as diphtheria, thrush, actinomycosis, or streptococcal stomatitis, are suspected.

Differential Diagnosis

NUG should be differentiated from other conditions that resemble it in some respects, such as herpetic gingivostomatitis (Table 17.1), periodontitis, desquamative gingivitis (Table 17.2), streptococcal gingivostomatitis, aphthous stomatitis, gonococcal gingivostomatitis, diphtheritic and syphilitic lesions (Table 17.3), tuberculous gingival lesions, candidiasis, agranulocytosis, dermatoses (e.g., pemphigus, erythema multiforme, lichen planus), and stomatitis venenata (see Chapter 18).

Treatment options for these diseases vary dramatically, and misdiagnosis and improper treatment can exacerbate the condition. In the case of primary herpetic gingivostomatitis, early diagnosis can result in treatment with antiviral drugs that would be ineffective for NUG, whereas the treatment of a case of herpes with the debridement required for NUG could exacerbate the herpes.

Streptococcal gingivostomatitis is a rare condition that is characterized by a diffuse erythema of the gingiva and other areas of the oral mucosa.[57] In some cases, the extent is limited to marginal erythema with marginal hemorrhage. However, necrosis of the gingival margin is not a feature of this disease, and there is no fetid odor. Bacterial smears show a preponderance of streptococcal forms,

TABLE 17.1 Differentiation of Necrotizing Ulcerative Gingivitis and Primary Herpetic Gingivostomatitis

Necrotizing Ulcerative Gingivitis	Primary Herpetic Gingivostomatitis
Caused by interaction between host and bacteria, most often fusospirochetes	Caused by specific viral infection
Necrotizing condition	Diffuse erythema and vesicular eruption
Punched-out gingival margin; pseudomembrane that peels off and leaves raw areas	Vesicles that rupture and leave slightly depressed oval or spherical ulcer
Marginal gingiva affected; other oral tissues rarely affected	Diffuse involvement of gingiva; may include buccal mucosa and lips
Uncommon in children	Occurs more frequently in children
No definite duration	Duration of 7–10 days
No demonstrated immunity	Acute episode results in some degree of immunity
Contagion not demonstrated	Contagion

which were identified as *Streptococcus viridans,* but other studies report findings of group A β-hemolytic streptococci.[52]

Agranulocytosis is characterized by a marked decrease in the number of circulating PMNs, lesions of the throat and other mucous membranes, and may include ulceration and necrosis of the gingiva that can resemble that of NUG. This condition occurs most commonly after chemotherapy in cancer patients or in patients with leukemia. The oral condition of patients with agranulocytosis is primarily necrotizing, but it lacks the severe inflammatory reaction seen with NUG. Blood studies can differentiate between NUG and the gingival necrosis associated with agranulocytosis.

Vincent angina is a fusospirochetal infection of the oropharynx and throat that is distinguished from NUG, which affects the marginal gingiva. Patients with Vincent angina have a painful membranous ulceration of the throat, with edema and hyperemic patches breaking down to form ulcers that are covered with pseudomembranous material. The process can extend to the larynx and the middle ear.

TABLE 17.2 Differentiation of Necrotizing Ulcerative Gingivitis, Chronic Desquamative Gingivitis, and Chronic Periodontal Disease

Necrotizing Ulcerative Gingivitis	Desquamative Gingivitis	Chronic Destructive Periodontal Disease
Bacterial smears show fusospirochetal complex	Bacterial smears reveal numerous epithelial cells and few bacterial forms	Bacterial smears vary
Marginal gingiva affected	Diffuse involvement of marginal and attached gingivae and other areas of oral mucosa	Marginal gingiva affected
Acute history	Chronic history	Chronic history
Painful	May or may not be painful	Painless if uncomplicated
Pseudomembrane	Patchy desquamation of gingival epithelium	Usually no desquamation, but purulent material may appear from pockets
Papillary and marginal necrotic lesions	Papillae do not undergo necrosis	Papillae do not undergo noticeable necrosis
Affects adults of both genders and occasionally affects children	Affects adults, most often women	Usually found in adults, occasionally found in children
Characteristic fetid odor	No odor	Some odor, but not strikingly fetid

NUG in leukemia patients results from the reduced host defense mechanisms that occur with the disease. NUG can be superimposed on the gingival tissue alterations caused by leukemia. The differential diagnosis does not require distinguishing between NUG and leukemic gingival changes; instead, it is determined whether leukemia is a predisposing factor in the mouth of a patient with NUG. For example, if a patient with necrotizing involvement of the gingival margin also has diffuse discoloration and generalized edema of the attached gingiva, the possibility of an underlying systemically induced gingival change should be considered. Leukemia is one of the conditions that would need to be ruled out (see Chapter 25).

NUG in the patient with human immunodeficiency virus (HIV) infection has the same clinical features, although it often follows an extremely destructive course that leads to NUP, with a loss of soft tissue attachment and bone and the formation of bony sequestra (see Chapter 30).[34]

CLINICAL CORRELATION

A serious systemic disease or condition, such as leukemia or acquired immunodeficiency syndrome (AIDS), that renders the host immunocompromised can be the predisposing causative factor leading to acute gingival disease.

Etiology

Role of Bacteria

Plaut[69] in 1894 and Vincent[94] in 1896 postulated that NUG was caused by specific bacteria: fusiform bacilli and spirochetal organisms. Opinions still differ about whether bacteria are the primary causative factors of NUG. Several observations support this concept, including that spirochetal organisms and fusiform bacilli are always found in patients with the disease along with other organisms. Rosebury and colleagues[73] described a fusospirochetal complex that consists of *T. microdentium,* intermediate spirochetes, vibrios, fusiform bacilli, and filamentous organisms in addition to several *Borrelia* species.

Loesche and colleagues[53] described a predominant constant flora and a variable flora associated with NUG. The constant flora is composed of *Prevotella intermedia* in addition to the *Fusobacterium, Treponema,* and *Selenomonas* species. The variable flora consists of a heterogeneous array of bacterial types.

TABLE 17.3 Differentiation of Necrotizing Ulcerative Gingivitis, Diphtheria, and Secondary Stage of Syphilis

Necrotizing Ulcerative Gingivitis	Diphtheria	Secondary Stage of Syphilis (Mucous Patch)
Caused by interaction between host and bacteria, typically fusospirochetes	Caused by *Corynebacterium diphtheriae*	Caused by *Treponema pallidum*
Affects marginal gingiva	Rarely affects marginal gingiva	Rarely affects marginal gingiva
Membrane removal easy	Membrane removal difficult	Membrane not detachable
Painful condition	Less painful	Minimal pain
Marginal gingivae affected	Throat, fauces, and tonsils affected	Any part of mouth affected
Serologic findings normal	Serologic findings normal	Serologic findings abnormal[a]
Immunity not conferred	Immunity conferred by an attack	Immunity not conferred
Doubtful contagiousness	Contagious	Only direct contact can communicate disease
Antibiotic therapy relieves symptoms	Antibiotic treatment is effective	Antibiotic therapy has excellent results

[a]Wassermann test, Kahn test, and Venereal Disease Research Laboratories (VDRL) test.

Treatment with metronidazole results in a significant reduction of *Treponema* species, *P. intermedia,* and *Fusobacterium,* with resolution of the clinical symptoms.[20,53] The antibacterial spectrum of this drug provides evidence for the anaerobic members of the flora as etiologic agents. These bacteriologic findings have been supported by immunologic data[13] that demonstrated increased immunoglobulin G and M antibody titers for medium-sized spirochetes and *P. intermedia* in patients with NUG compared with titers in patients with gingivitis and healthy controls.

Role of the Host Response

The role of an impaired host response in NUG has long been recognized. Even in the early descriptions of the disease, NUG was associated with physical and emotional stress[15,75] and decreased resistance to infection. Regardless of whether specific bacteria are implicated in the cause of NUG, the presence of these organisms without other predisposing factors appears to be insufficient to cause the disease. The fusospirochetal flora is frequently found in patients who do not have NUG. And, although the numbers are much less, spirochetes and fusiform bacilli are found on normal edentulous mucosa as well.[74] Furthermore, exudates from NUG lesions inoculated subcutaneously into experimental animals produce fusospirochetal abscesses rather than typical NUG lesions.[72]

NUG has not been produced experimentally in humans or animals by inoculation of bacterial exudates from the lesions alone. In the animal model, local or systemic immunosuppression with glucocorticoids (e.g., ketoconazole) results in more characteristic lesions of NUG in infected animals. Swenson and Muhler used scillaren B, an amorphous glucoside, which reduced tissue resistance to create oral fusospirochetal infections in dogs.[88,89]

NUG is not found in well-nourished individuals with a fully functional immune system. All of the predisposing factors for NUG are associated with immunosuppression. Cogen and colleagues[14] described depression of host defense mechanisms, particularly in PMN chemotaxis and phagocytosis, in patients with NUG. Host-bacteria interactions are described in Chapter 11.

It is essential for the clinician to determine the predisposing factors that lead to immunodeficiency in patients with NUG to address the continued susceptibility of the patient and to determine whether an underlying systemic disease exists. Immunodeficiency may be related to various levels of nutritional deficiency, fatigue caused by chronic sleep deprivation, other health impairing habits (e.g., alcohol, drug abuse), psychosocial factors, or systemic disease. NUG can be the presenting symptom for patients with immunosuppression related to HIV infection.

Local Predisposing Factors

Preexisting gingivitis, injury to the gingiva, and smoking are important predisposing factors. Although NUG can appear in an otherwise disease-free mouth, it most often occurs superimposed on preexisting gingival disease and periodontal pockets. Deep periodontal pockets and pericoronal flaps are particularly vulnerable areas because they offer a favorable environment for the proliferation of anaerobic fusiform bacilli and spirochetes. Areas of the gingiva that are traumatized by opposing teeth in malocclusion (e.g., palatal surface behind the maxillary incisors, labial gingival surface of the mandibular incisors) can predispose the area to development of NUG in a susceptible individual.

The relationship between NUG and smoking has often been mentioned in the literature. Pindborg[67] reported that 98% of his patients with NUG were smokers and that the increasing frequency of this disease correlates with increasing exposure to tobacco smoke. The effect of smoking on periodontal disease in general has been the subject of numerous studies,[4,27,29,43,46,64] and smoking has been established as a high-risk factor for disease (see Chapter 23).

Systemic Predisposing Factors

NUG is not found in well-nourished individuals with a fully functional immune system. It is therefore important for the clinician to determine the predisposing factors for immunodeficiency. Immunodeficiency can be related to nutritional deficiency, psychosocial stress, fatigue caused by chronic sleep deficiency, other health impairing habits (e.g., alcoholism, drug abuse), and systemic disease (e.g., diabetes, debilitating infection).

Nutritional Deficiency

Necrotizing gingivitis has been produced in animals by giving them nutritionally deficient diets.[11,44,60,90,93] Several researchers found an increase in the fusospirochetal flora in the mouths of the experimental animals, but the bacteria were regarded as opportunists that proliferated only when the tissues were altered by the deficiency.

A poor diet has been cited as a predisposing factor for NUG and its sequelae in developing African countries, although the effects appear to primarily diminish the effectiveness of the immune response.[24,25,45] Nutritional deficiencies (e.g., vitamin C, vitamin B_2) accentuate the severity of the pathologic changes induced when the fusospirochetal bacterial complex is injected into animals.[87]

Debilitating Disease

Debilitating systemic disease can predispose patients to NUG. Systemic disturbances include chronic diseases (e.g., syphilis, cancer), severe gastrointestinal disorders (e.g., ulcerative colitis), blood dyscrasias (e.g., leukemia, anemia), and AIDS. Nutritional deficiency that results from debilitating disease can be an additional predisposing factor. Experimentally induced leukopenia in animals can produce ulcerative gangrenous stomatitis.[60,91,92] Ulceronecrotic lesions appear in the gingival margins of hamsters that are exposed to total body irradiation[56]; these lesions can be prevented with systemic antibiotics.[55]

Psychosomatic Factors

Psychological factors appear to be important in the cause of NUG. The disease often occurs in association with stressful situations (e.g., induction into the armed forces, academic examinations).[31] Psychological disturbances[33] and increased adrenocortical secretion[80] are common in patients with the disease.

A significant correlation between disease incidence and two personality traits—dominance and abasement—suggests there is an NUG-prone personality.[28] Data from a study evaluating the relationship between personality traits and stress with gingival inflammation and soft tissue pathology in military recruits found that gingival inflammation correlated significantly with personality traits (e.g., tolerance to change, anxiety).[61]

The mechanisms by which psychologic factors create or predispose an individual to gingival damage have not been established. However, alterations in digital and gingival capillary responses that suggest increased autonomic nervous activity have been demonstrated in patients with NUG.[30]

It can be concluded that opportunistic bacteria are the primary etiologic agents of NUG in patients who demonstrate immunosuppression. Stress, smoking, and preexisting gingivitis are common predisposing factors.

Epidemiology and Prevalence

The prevalence of NUG appears to have been rather low in the United States and Europe before 1914. During World Wars I and

II, numerous epidemics broke out among the Allied troops, but German soldiers did not seem to have been similarly affected. Epidemic-like outbreaks have also occurred among civilian populations. A study at a dental clinic in Prague, Czech Republic, reported the incidence of NUG as 0.08% among patients 15 to 19 years old, 0.05% among those 20 to 24 years old, and 0.02% among those 25 to 29 years old.[84] A recent case-controlled study of the British armed forces reported 0.11% prevalence of NUG among all military personnel, with smoking and poor periodontal health being strong risk indicators.[21]

NUG occurs in individuals of all ages, with the highest incidence reported for patients between the ages of 15 and 30 years.[19,47,84,87] It is not common among children in the United States, Canada, and Europe, but it has been reported in children from low-socioeconomic groups in underdeveloped countries.[42] In India, 54%[59] and 58%[68] of patients in two studies were younger than 10 years of age.

In a random school population in Nigeria, NUG occurred in 11.3% of children between the ages of 2 and 6 years.[81] In a Nigerian hospital population, it affected 23% of children who were younger than 10 years of age.[24] Studies of African populations typically report a higher prevalence of necrotizing periodontal disease among young children than in those older than 10 years.[1] NUG has been reported in several members of the same family in low socioeconomic groups. Twenty percent of households with children 2 to 6 years of age in a rural Nigerian city had one or more children with NUG.[81] It is more common among children with Down syndrome than among other children with mental deficiencies.[7]

Opinions differ with regard to whether NUG is more common during the winter,[47,65] summer, or fall[81] and whether there is a peak seasonal incidence.[18]

Communicability

NUG often occurs in groups in an epidemic pattern. At one time, it was considered **contagious**, and required reporting to the community health department, but it was later concluded not to be communicable.[71,77]

A distinction must be made between communicability and transmissibility when referring to the characteristics of disease. The term *transmissible* denotes a capacity for the maintenance of an infectious agent in successive passages through a susceptible animal host.[71] The term *communicable* signifies a capacity for the maintenance of infection by natural modes of spread, such as direct contact through drinking water, food, and eating utensils; by the airborne route; or by arthropod vectors. A disease that is communicable is described as *contagious*. It has been demonstrated that disease associated with the fusospirochetal bacterial complex is transmissible; however, *it is not communicable or contagious*.

Attempts to spread NUG from human to human have been unsuccessful.[78] King[45] traumatized an area in his own gingiva and introduced debris from a patient with a severe case of NUG. There was no response until he happened to fall ill shortly thereafter. After his illness, he observed the characteristic lesion in the experimental area. It can be inferred with reservation from this experiment that systemic debility is a prerequisite for the contagion of NUG.

Because NUG often occurs among groups that use the same kitchen facilities, it is a common impression that the disease is spread by bacteria on eating utensils. However, the growth of fusospirochetal organisms requires carefully controlled conditions and an anaerobic environment; they do not ordinarily survive on eating utensils.[16,36]

The occurrence of NUG in epidemic-like outbreaks does not necessarily mean that it is contagious. The affected groups may be afflicted by the disease as a result of common predisposing factors rather than because of its spread from person to person. In all likelihood, a predisposed immunocompromised host and the presence of appropriate bacteria are necessary for the production of this disease.

KEY FACT

Although certain bacteria (e.g., fusospirochetal complex) are likely responsible for the lesions observed in necrotizing ulcerative gingivitis, immunocompromise appears to be a necessary predisposing condition for the disease.

Management of Necrotizing Ulcerative Gingivitis

Treatment of NUG should include alleviation of the acute symptoms and correction of the underlying gingival or periodontal disease. The former is the simpler part of the treatment; the latter often requires more comprehensive procedures, follow-up, and patient education.

The treatment of NUG consists of (1) alleviation of the acute inflammation by reduction of the microbial load, and removal of necrotic tissue, (2) treatment of chronic disease either underlying the acute involvement or elsewhere in the oral cavity, (3) alleviation of generalized symptoms, such as fever and **malaise**, and (4) correction of systemic conditions or factors that contribute to the initiation or progression of gingival changes. Chapter 30 provides further information on the management and treatment of NUP in patients with AIDS.

Treatment of NUG should follow an orderly sequence, according to specific steps, at three clinical visits.

First Visit

On the first visit, the clinician should conduct a comprehensive evaluation of the patient, including a thorough medical history, with special attention to recent illness, living conditions, dietary background, cigarette smoking, type of employment, hours of rest, risk factors for HIV infection, and psychosocial parameters (e.g., stress, depression). The patient is questioned regarding the history of the acute disease, including its onset and duration, as follows:

- Is the disease recurrent?
- Are the recurrences associated with specific factors, such as menstruation, particular foods, exhaustion, or mental stress?
- Has there been any previous treatment? When and for how long?

The clinician should also inquire as to the type of treatment received and the patient's impression regarding the effectiveness of previous treatment.

The initial physical examination should include an assessment of general appearance, presence of halitosis, presence of skin lesions, vital signs including temperature, and palpation for the presence of enlarged lymph nodes, especially submaxillary and submental nodes.

The oral cavity is examined for the characteristic NUG lesions, distribution, and the possible involvement of the oropharyngeal region. Oral hygiene is evaluated, with special attention to the presence of pericoronal flaps, periodontal pockets, and local risk factors (e.g., poorly contoured and ill-fitting restorations, presence and distribution of **calculus**). Periodontal probing of NUG lesions is likely to be very painful, will not aid in the primary diagnosis, and may need to be deferred until after the acute lesions are resolved.

KEY FACT

The goals of initial therapy for necrotizing ulcerative gingivitis are reduction of the microbial load and removal of necrotic tissue to facilitate the healing process of repair and regeneration so that normal tissue barriers can be reestablished.

The goals of initial therapy are reduction of the microbial load and removal of necrotic tissue to the degree that repair and regeneration of normal tissue barriers can be reestablished. Treatment during the initial visit is confined to the acutely involved areas, which are isolated with cotton rolls and dried. A topical anesthetic is applied, and after 2 or 3 minutes, the areas are gently swabbed with a moistened cotton pellet to remove the pseudomembrane and nonattached surface debris. Bleeding may be profuse. Each cotton pellet is used in a small area, then discarded; sweeping motions over large areas with a single pellet are not recommended. After the area is cleansed with warm water, the superficial calculus is removed. Ultrasonic scalers are very useful for this purpose because they do not elicit pain, and the water jet and cavitation aid in lavage of the area.

Subgingival scaling and curettage are contraindicated at this time because these procedures may extend the infection into the deeper tissues and may also cause bacteremia. *Unless an emergency exists, procedures such as extraction or periodontal surgery are postponed until the patient has been symptom-free for 4 weeks to minimize the likelihood of exacerbating the acute symptoms.*

Antibiotics are effective in the treatment of patients with NUG.[44] Patients with moderate or severe NUG and local lymphadenopathy or other systemic signs or symptoms are placed on an antibiotic regimen of amoxicillin 500 mg orally every 6 hours for 10 days. For amoxicillin-sensitive patients, other antibiotics are prescribed, such as erythromycin (500 mg every 6 hours) or metronidazole (500 mg twice daily for 7 days). Systemic complications should subside in 1 to 3 days. *Antibiotics are not recommended in NUG patients who do not have systemic complications.*

Instructions to the Patient

The patient is discharged with the following instructions:

1. Avoid tobacco, alcohol, and condiments.
2. Rinse with a glassful of an equal mixture of 3% hydrogen peroxide and warm water every 2 hours and/or 0.12% chlorhexidine solution twice daily.
3. Get adequate rest. Pursue usual activities, but avoid excessive physical exertion or prolonged exposure to the sun, as in golfing, playing tennis, swimming, or sunbathing.
4. Confine toothbrushing to removal of surface debris with either a bland dentifrice or just water and an ultrasoft brush; overzealous brushing and the use of dental floss or interdental cleaners will be painful. Chlorhexidine mouthrinses are also helpful in controlling biofilm throughout the mouth.
5. An analgesic, such as a nonsteroidal antiinflammatory drug (NSAID; e.g., ibuprofen), is appropriate for pain relief.
6. Patients who have systemic complications, such as high fever, malaise, anorexia, or general debility, are given antibiotics and instructed to get plenty of bed rest, and drink lots of fluids.

Patients are asked to report back to the clinician in 1 to 2 days. They should be advised about the extent of total treatment required to resolve the condition and warned that treatment is not complete when pain stops. They should be informed of the presence of gingival or periodontal disease, which must be eliminated to reduce the likelihood of recurrence of the acute symptoms.

A large variety of drugs have been used in the treatment of NUG.[8] Topical drug therapy, however, is only an adjunctive measure; no drug when used alone can be considered complete therapy. Systemic antibiotics, when used, also reduce the oral bacterial flora and alleviate the oral symptoms,[95,96] but they are only an adjunct to the complete local treatment that the disease requires. If patients are treated by drugs or systemic antibiotics alone, the acute painful symptoms often reoccur after treatment is discontinued.

Second Visit

At the second visit, 1 or 2 days after the first visit, the patient is evaluated for amelioration of signs and symptoms. The patient's condition is usually improved; the pain is diminished or is no longer present. The gingival margins of the involved areas are erythematous but without a superficial pseudomembrane.

Scaling is performed if it is necessary and if sensitivity permits. Shrinkage of the gingiva may expose previously covered calculus, which is gently removed. Instructions to the patient are the same as those given previously.

Third Visit

At the next visit, approximately 5 days after the second visit, the patient is evaluated for resolution of symptoms, and a comprehensive plan for management of the patient's periodontal condition is formulated. The patient should be essentially symptom-free at this time. Some erythema may still be present in the involved areas, and the gingiva may be slightly painful on tactile stimulation (Fig. 17.4A and B). The patient is instructed in biofilm control procedures (see Chapter 50), which are essential for the success of the treatment and the maintenance of periodontal health. The patient is further counseled on nutrition, smoking cessation, and other conditions or habits associated with potential recurrence. The hydrogen peroxide rinses are discontinued, but chlorhexidine rinses may be maintained for an additional 2 or 3 weeks. Scaling and root planing is repeated if necessary. Unfortunately, patients often discontinue treatment because the acute condition has subsided; however, this is when comprehensive treatment of the chronic periodontal problem should begin. Patients need to be educated about the importance of comprehensive periodontal treatment and encouraged to complete it.

Appointments should be scheduled for treatment of gingivitis, periodontal pockets, and pericoronal flaps, as well as for elimination of all forms of local risk factors (see Chapter 24). The patient should be reevaluated approximately 4 to 6 weeks after treatment to determine compliance with oral hygiene, health habits, psychosocial factors, the potential need for reconstructive or esthetic surgery, and the interval of subsequent recall visits.

Role of Drugs

A large variety of drugs have been used for topical treatment of NUG. Topical drug therapy is only an adjunctive measure. *No drug when used alone can be considered complete treatment.*

Escharotic drugs, such as phenol, silver nitrate, chromic acid, or potassium bichromate, should not be used. They are necrotizing agents that alleviate pain by destroying the nerve endings of the ulcerated gingiva but also destroy young cells that are needed for repair whose loss would delay healing. Repeated use of these agents results in loss of gingival tissue that is not restored when the disease subsides.[32]

KEY FACT

No drug when used alone can be considered complete treatment for the resolution of acute gingival disease, such as NUG. Local therapy and elimination of risk factors are essential for complete resolution.

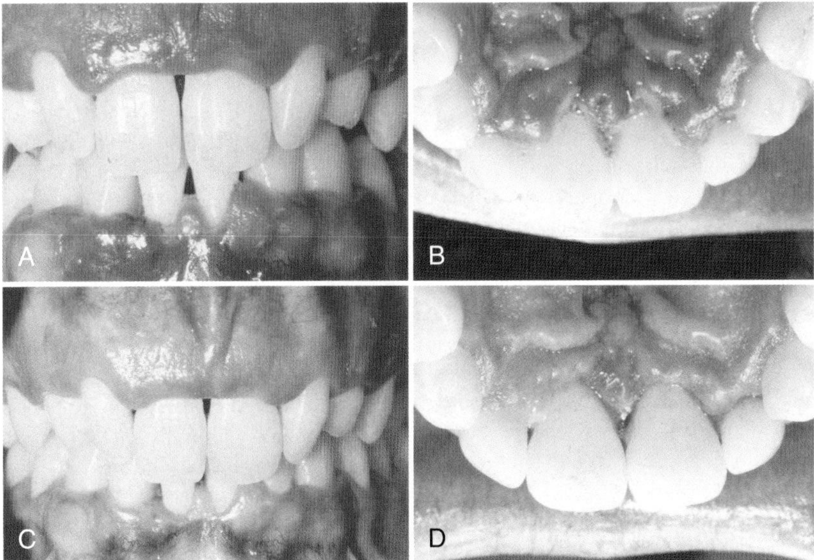

Fig. 17.4 (A) Initial view of the anterior gingival tissues in a 22-year-old white female smoker with acute necrotizing ulcerative gingivitis. (B) Palatal view of the same patient. (C) Facial view of the same patient, two days after initial scaling and cessation of smoking. (D) Palatal view of the same patient, two days after initial scaling and cessation of smoking. (*From Rose LF, Mealey BL, Genco RJ, Cohen DW.* Periodontics: Medicine, Surgery, and Implants. *Mosby: St. Louis; 2005.*)

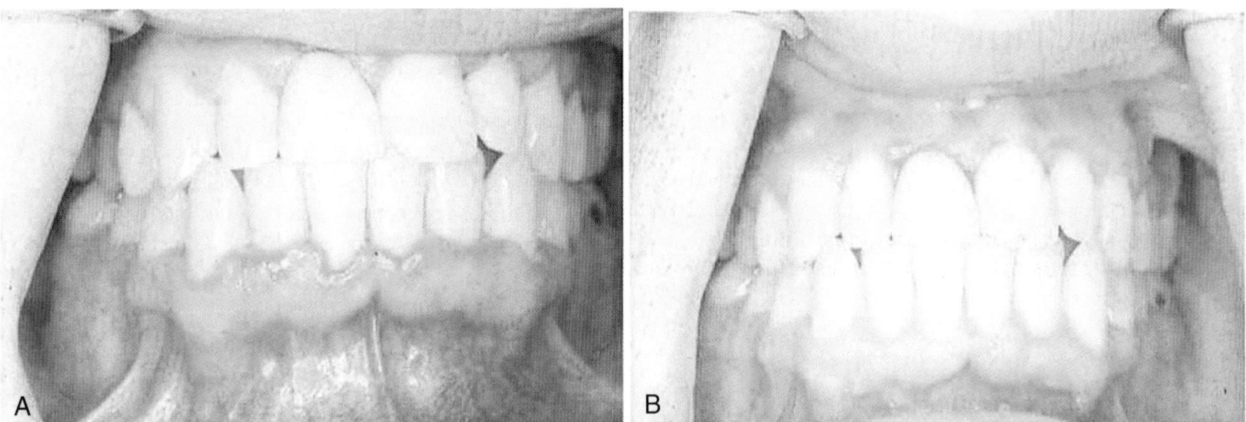

Fig. 17.5 Treatment of acute necrotizing ulcerative gingivitis. (A) Before treatment; notice the characteristic interdental lesions. (B) After treatment, showing restoration of healthy gingival contour.

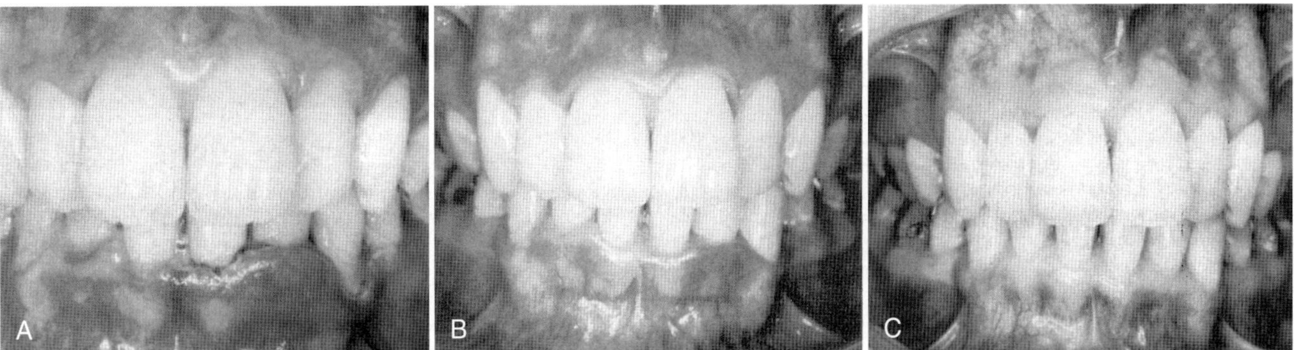

Fig. 17.6 Reshaping the gingiva in the treatment of acute necrotizing ulcerative gingivitis. (A) Before treatment. Bulbous gingiva and interdental necrosis are present in the mandibular anterior area. (B) After treatment. Gingival contours are still undesirable. (C) Final result. Physiological contours are obtained by reshaping the gingiva.

Persistent or Recurrent Cases

Adequate local therapy with optimal home care will resolve most cases of NUG. If a case of NUG persists despite therapy or if it recurs, the patient should be reevaluated with a focus on the following factors:

1. *Reassessment of differential diagnosis to rule out diseases that resemble NUG:* Several diseases and conditions (e.g., desquamative gingivitis) may initially manifest with an appearance similar to that of NUG. A renewed search for skin lesions and other signs or symptoms should be undertaken, with a biopsy if warranted (see Chapter 18.).
2. *Underlying systemic disease causing immunosuppression:* In particular, HIV infection may frequently manifest with symptoms of NUG or NUP. The patient should be reassessed for risk factors and may need counseling about testing for HIV or other suspected underlying systemic diseases (e.g., lymphoproliferative disease). The patient will likely need referral to their physician for further evaluation.
3. *Inadequate local therapy:* Too often, treatment is discontinued when the symptoms have subsided without elimination of the gingival disease and periodontal pockets that remain after the superficial acute condition is relieved. Remaining calculus and other local factors that predispose to gingival inflammation may contribute to recurrence. Recurrent acute involvement in the mandibular anterior area can be associated with persistent pericoronal inflammation arising from partial eruption and pericoronal inflammation of third molars.[62] Anterior involvement is less likely to recur after the third molar situation is corrected.
4. *Inadequate compliance:* Poor biofilm control, heavy use of tobacco, ineffective stress management, and continued malnutrition can also contribute to persistence or recurrence of NUG. The clinician should evaluate the quality and consistency of biofilm control. Further assessment and counseling on tobacco use will also determine the role of tobacco. If the clinician perceives that unresolved psychosocial factors are complicating health, the patient should be referred to an appropriate professional. A reassessment of the patient's nutritional state, with dietary analysis or nutritional testing, may be required.[45,50]

CLINICAL CORRELATION

Acute gingival disease may be a sign of a more serious systemic condition, such as acquired immunodeficiency disease or another condition that renders the host immunocompromised.

Primary Herpetic Gingivostomatitis

Primary herpetic gingivostomatitis is an infection of the oral cavity caused by herpes simplex virus (HSV) type 1.[19,57,58,76] It occurs most often among infants and children who are younger than 6 years of age,[10,76,79] but it is also seen in adolescents and adults. It occurs with equal frequency in male and female patients. In most individuals, however, the primary infection is asymptomatic.

As part of the primary infection, the virus ascends through the sensory and autonomic nerves, where it persists as latent HSV in neuronal ganglia that innervate the site. In approximately one-third of the world's population, secondary manifestations or recurrent herpetic episodes will occur. These recurrent outbreaks may be precipitated by dental treatment,[97] respiratory infection, sunlight exposure, fever, trauma, exposure to chemicals, or emotional stress in individuals with a history of herpes virus infection. Secondary manifestations include herpes labialis (Fig. 17.7), herpetic stomatitis, herpes genitalis, ocular herpes, and herpetic encephalitis. Secondary herpetic stomatitis can occur on the palate, on the gingiva (Fig. 17.8), or on the mucosa as a result of dental treatment that traumatizes or stimulates the latent virus in the ganglia that innervates the area. It may manifest as pain away from the site of treatment 2 to 4 days later. Careful inspection for characteristic vesicles can be diagnostic (see Fig. 17.7).

Clinical Features

Oral Signs and Symptoms

Primary herpetic gingivostomatitis appears as a diffuse, erythematous, shiny involvement of the gingiva and the adjacent oral mucosa, with various degrees of edema and gingival bleeding. During its initial stage, it is characterized by discrete, spherical, gray vesicles, which can occur on the gingiva, labial and buccal mucosae, soft palate, pharynx, sublingual mucosa, and tongue (Fig. 17.9). After approximately 24 hours, the vesicles rupture and form painful small ulcers with red elevated halo-like margins and depressed yellowish or grayish-white central portions. They occur in widely separated areas or in clusters where confluence occurs (Fig. 17.10).

Occasionally, primary herpetic gingivitis occurs without overt vesiculation. The clinical picture consists of diffuse, erythematous, shiny discoloration and edematous enlargement of the gingivae with a tendency to bleed.

The course of the disease is limited to 7 to 10 days. The diffuse gingival erythema and edema that appear early during the course of the disease persist for several days after the ulcerative lesions have healed. Scarring does not occur in the areas of healed ulcerations.

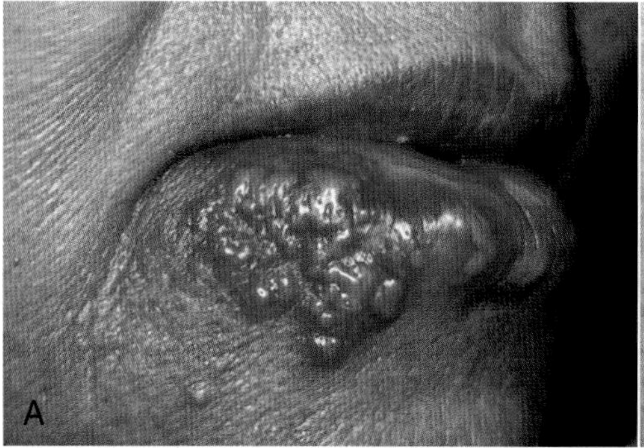

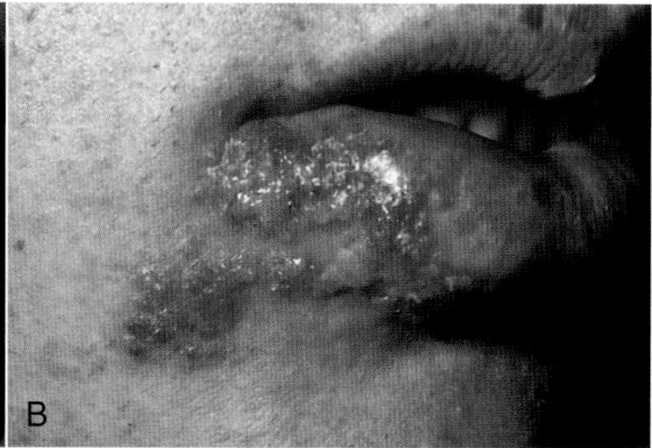

Fig. 17.7 Herpetic vesicles recurred in the lip. (A) Early stage. (B) Late stage, showing brownish crusted lesions. (*From Sapp JP, Eversole LR, Wysocki GP.* Contemporary Oral and Maxillofacial Pathology. *2nd ed. St Louis: Mosby; 2002.*)

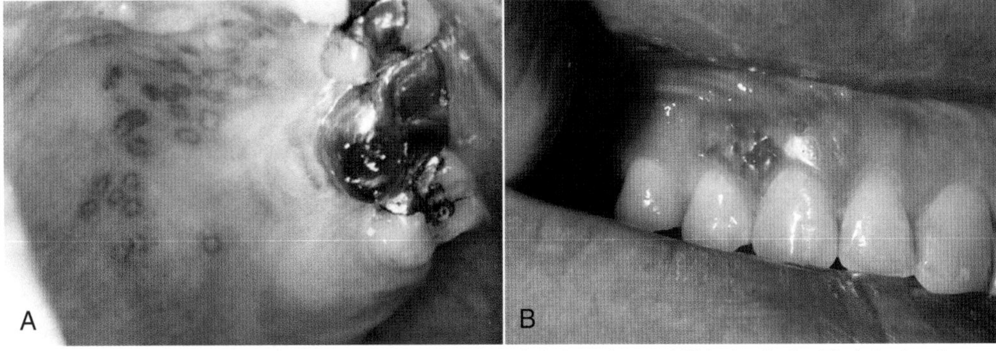

Fig. 17.8 Recurrent intraoral herpetic vesicles are seen (A) in the palate and (B) in the gingiva. The latter location is rare. (*From Sapp JP, Eversole LR, Wysocki GP.* Contemporary Oral and Maxillofacial Pathology. *2nd ed. St Louis: Mosby; 2002.*)

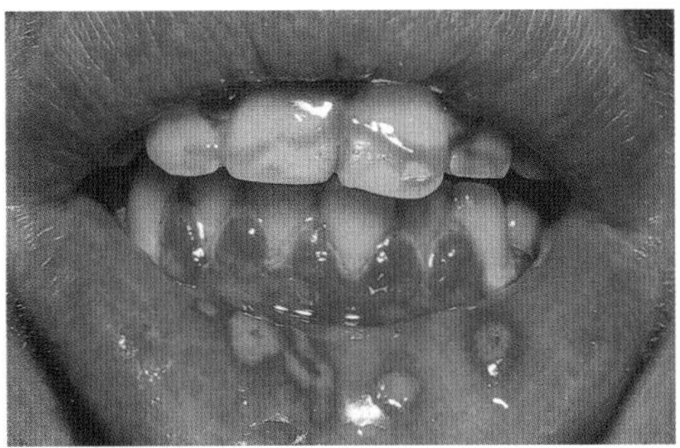

Fig. 17.9 Primary herpetic gingivostomatitis in a 12-year-old boy who has diffuse erythematous involvement of the gingiva and a spherical gray vesicle in the lip. (*Courtesy Dr. Heddie Sedano, University of California, Los Angeles, and University of Minnesota.*)

The disease is accompanied by generalized soreness of the oral cavity, which interferes with eating, drinking, and oral hygiene. The ruptured vesicles are the focal sites of pain; they are particularly sensitive to touch, thermal changes, foods such as condiments and fruit juices, and the action of coarse foods. In infants, the disease is marked by irritability and refusal to take food.

Extraoral and Systemic Signs and Symptoms

Cervical lymphadenitis, fever as high as 101°F to 105° F (38°C to 40.6° C) and generalized malaise are common.

History

Primary herpetic gingivostomatitis is the result of an acute infection by HSV. There is an acute onset of symptoms.

Histopathology

The virus targets the epithelial cells called *Tzanck cells*, which show ballooning degeneration that consists of acantholysis, nuclear clearing, and nuclear enlargement. Infected cells fuse to form multinucleated cells, and intercellular edema leads to the formation of intraepithelial vesicles that rupture and develop a secondary inflammatory response with a fibropurulent exudate (Fig. 17.11).[63] Discrete ulcerations that result from the rupture of the vesicles have a central portion of acute inflammation, with various degrees of purulent exudate surrounded by engorged blood vessels.

Diagnosis

It is critical to arrive at a diagnosis as early as possible for a patient with a primary herpetic infection. Treatment with antiviral medications can dramatically alter the course of the disease by reducing symptoms and potentially reducing recurrences. The diagnosis is usually established from the patient's history and the clinical findings. Material can be obtained from the lesions and submitted to the laboratory for confirmatory tests, including virus culture and immunological tests that involve the use of monoclonal antibodies or deoxyribonucleic acid hybridization techniques.[10,70] This should not delay treatment if strong clinical evidence exists for primary gingivostomatitis.

Differential Diagnosis

Primary herpetic gingivostomatitis should be differentiated from several conditions. Lesions of recurrent aphthous stomatitis (RAS)[26] range from occasional small (0.5 to 1 cm in diameter) well-defined, round or ovoid, shallow ulcers with a yellowish-gray central area surrounded by an erythematous halo, which heal in 7 to 10 days without scarring, to larger (1 to 3 cm in diameter), oval or irregular ulcers, which persist for weeks and heal with scarring (Fig. 17.12). The cause is unknown, although immunopathologic mechanisms appear to play a role.

RAS is a different clinical entity from primary herpetic gingivostomatitis. The ulcerations may look the same for the two conditions, but diffuse erythematous involvement of the gingiva and acute toxic systemic symptoms do not occur with RAS. A history of previous episodes of painful mucosal ulcerations suggests RAS rather than primary HSV.

Information about erythema multiforme, bullous lichen planus, and desquamative gingivitis can be found in Chapter 18.

Communicability

Primary herpetic gingivostomatitis is contagious.[12,52] Most adults have developed immunity to HSV as a result of infection during childhood, which in most cases is subclinical. For this reason, acute herpetic gingivostomatitis usually occurs in infants and children. Recurrent herpetic gingivostomatitis has been reported,[35] although it is not often clinically significant unless immunity is destroyed by debilitating systemic disease. Studies that have demonstrated HSV in periodontal pockets suggest more recurrence of viral replication than has previously been recognized.[85] Secondary herpetic infection of the skin, such as herpes labialis, does recur.[82]

CLINICAL CORRELATION

Acute herpetic gingivostomatitis usually occurs in infants and children because most adults have developed immunity to herpes simplex virus from childhood exposure, often with mild or no symptoms.

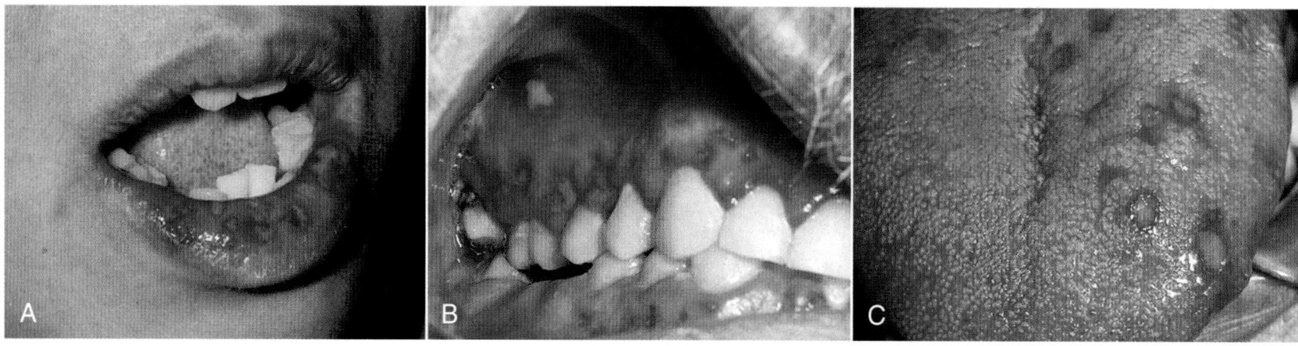

Fig. 17.10 Involvement of the lip (A), gingiva (B), and tongue (C) in primary herpetic gingivostomatitis. (*From Sapp JP, Eversole LR, Wysocki GP.* Contemporary Oral and Maxillofacial Pathology. *2nd ed. St Louis: Mosby; 2002.*)

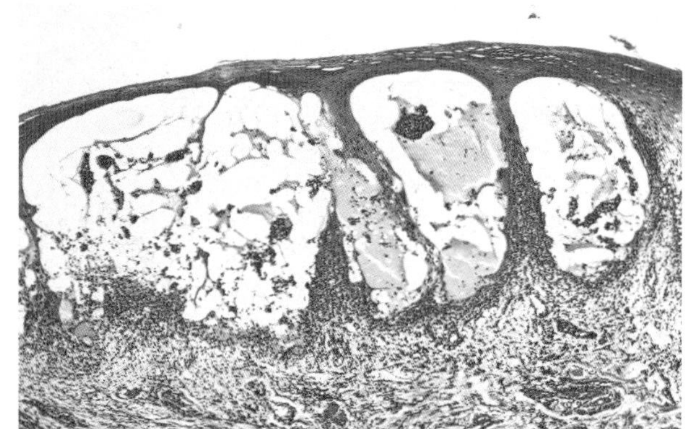

Fig. 17.11 Biopsy showing intraepithelial viral vesicles that contain fluid and debris, with a large number of viruses and virally altered epithelial cells (i.e., Tzanck cells). (*Courtesy Dr. Heddie Sedano, University of California, Los Angeles, and University of Minnesota.*)

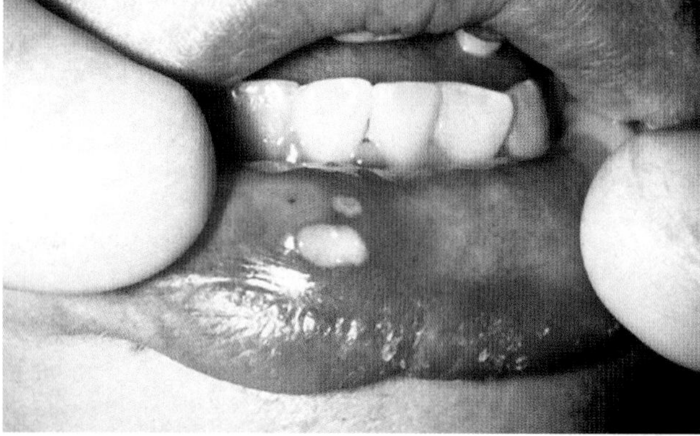

Fig. 17.12 Aphthous lesion in the lip. The depressed gray center is surrounded by an elevated red border. (*From Sapp JP, Eversole LR, Wysocki GP.* Contemporary Oral and Maxillofacial Pathology. *2nd ed. St Louis: Mosby; 2002.*)

Management of Primary Herpetic Gingivostomatitis

Treatment of primary herpetic gingivostomatitis consists of early diagnosis and immediate initiation of antiviral therapy. Historically, therapy for primary herpetic gingivostomatitis consisted of palliative care alone. However, since the development of antiviral therapy, the standard of care now includes the use of antiviral medications. In a randomized, double-blind, placebo-controlled study, Amir and colleagues[2] demonstrated that antiviral therapy with 15 mg/kg of an acyclovir suspension given five times daily for 7 days substantially changed the course of the disease without significant side effects. Acyclovir reduced the duration of symptoms, including fever, from 3 days to 1 day, decreased new extraoral lesions from 5.5 to 0 days, and reduced difficulty with eating from 7 to 4 days. Furthermore, viral shedding stopped at one day for the acyclovir group but persisted up to 5 days for the control group. Overall, oral lesions were present for only 4 days in the acyclovir group but persisted for 10 days in the control group. Although no clear clinical evidence indicates that this regimen will reduce recurrences, research data suggest that a greater number of latent virus copies incorporated into ganglia will increase the severity of recurrences.[2]

FLASH BACK

As part of the primary infection, the herpes simplex virus ascends through the sensory and autonomic nerves, where it persists as latent HSV in neuronal ganglia that innervate the site.

In summary, if primary herpetic gingivostomatitis is diagnosed within 3 days of onset, acyclovir suspension should be prescribed: 15 mg/kg five times daily for 7 days. If diagnosis occurs more than 3 days after onset in an immunocompetent patient, acyclovir therapy may have limited value. All patients, including those who present more than 3 days after disease onset, may receive palliative care, including removal of biofilm and food debris. An NSAID (e.g., ibuprofen) can be given systemically to reduce fever and pain. Patients may either take nutritional supplements, or use topical anesthetics (e.g., viscous lidocaine) before eating to aid in proper nutrition during the early phases of acute herpetic gingivostomatitis. Periodontal therapy should be postponed until the acute symptoms subside to avoid the possibility of exacerbation.

Local or systemic application of antibiotics is sometimes advised to prevent opportunistic bacterial or fungal infection of ulcerations, especially in the immunocompromised patient. If the condition does not resolve within 2 weeks, the patient should be referred to a physician for medical consultation.[49] The patient should be informed that herpetic gingivostomatitis is contagious at certain stages, such as when vesicles are present (highest viral titer). All individuals exposed to an infected patient should take precautions. Herpetic infection of a clinician's finger, referred to as *herpetic whitlow,* can occur if a seronegative clinician is exposed and becomes infected with herpes virus from a patient's herpetic lesions.[70,86]

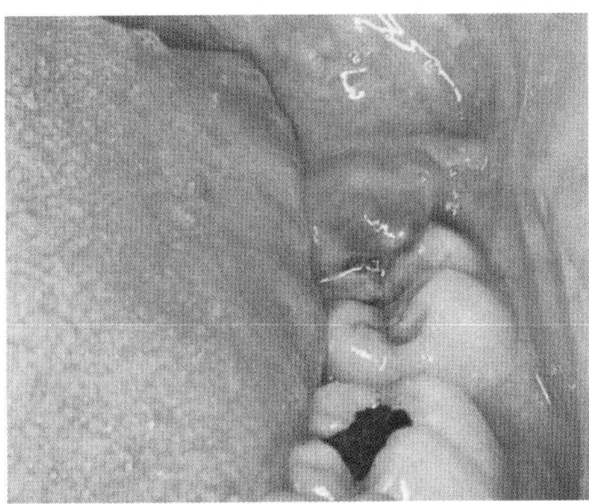

Fig. 17.13 Pericoronitis. An inflamed coronal flap covers the disto-occlusal surface of the impacted mandibular third molar. Note the swelling and redness. (*From Glickman I, Smulow J.* Periodontal Disease: Clinical, Radiographic and Histopathologic Features. *Philadelphia: Saunders; 1974.*)

Pericoronitis

The term *pericoronitis* refers to inflammation of the excess gingiva or flap of soft tissue that overlies the crown of an incompletely erupted tooth (Fig. 17.13). It occurs most often in the mandibular third molar area.[83] Pericoronitis can be acute, subacute, or chronic.

Clinical Features

The partially erupted or impacted mandibular third molar is the most common site of pericoronitis. The space between the crown of the tooth and the overlying gingival flap (i.e., operculum) is an ideal area for the accumulation of food debris and bacterial growth. Even in patients with no clinical signs or symptoms, the gingival flap is often chronically inflamed and infected, and it has various degrees of ulceration along its inner surface. Acute inflammatory involvement is a constant possibility; it may be exacerbated by trauma, occlusion, or a foreign body trapped underneath the tissue flap (e.g., popcorn husk, nut fragment).

Acute pericoronitis is identified by various degrees of inflammatory involvement of the pericoronal flap and adjacent structures and by systemic complications. The inflammatory fluid and cellular exudate increase the bulk of the flap, which can interfere with complete closure of the jaws. It can be traumatized by contact with the opposing dentition, thereby aggravating the inflammatory involvement.

The resultant clinical picture is a red, swollen, suppurating lesion that is exquisitely tender, with radiating pains to the ear, throat, and floor of the mouth. The patient is extremely uncomfortable as a result of pain, a foul taste, and an inability to close the jaws. Swelling of the cheek in the region of the angle of the jaw and lymphadenitis are common findings. Trismus may be a presenting complaint. The patient can have systemic complications such as fever, leukocytosis, and malaise.

Complications

Involvement can be localized in the form of a pericoronal abscess. It may spread posteriorly into the oropharyngeal area and medially to the base of the tongue, making it difficult for the patient to swallow. Depending on the severity and extent of the infection, there may be involvement of the submaxillary, posterior cervical, deep cervical, and retropharyngeal lymph nodes.[41,66] Peritonsillar abscess formation, cellulitis, and Ludwig angina are infrequent but potential sequelae of acute pericoronitis.

Management of Pericoronitis

The treatment of pericoronitis depends on several factors, including position and quality of the surrounding tissues, severity of the inflammation, presence and/or risk of systemic complications, and advisability of retaining the involved tooth. All pericoronal flaps, even in the absence of symptoms, should be viewed with suspicion. Strong consideration should be given to removal of any pericoronal flaps that persist as a preventive measure against subsequent acute involvement.

The initial treatment of acute pericoronitis consists of (1) gently flushing the area with warm water to remove debris and exudate and (2) swabbing with antiseptic after the pericoronal flap has been gently lifted away from the tooth with an instrument. The underlying debris is removed, and the area is flushed with warm water. The occlusion is evaluated to determine whether an opposing tooth is contacting the pericoronal flap. It may be necessary to reduce soft tissue surgically and/or adjust the opposing tooth as a palliative measure to alleviate pain. Antibiotics can be prescribed in severe cases and for patients who have clinical evidence of diffuse microbial infiltration of the tissue. If the pericoronal flap is swollen and fluctuant, an incision and drainage procedure may be indicated to establish drainage and relieve pressure.

Once the acute symptoms have subsided, the prognosis of the tooth can be evaluated. The decision is governed by the likelihood that the tooth will continue erupting into a functional position or that impaction and the factors predisposing to pericoronitis will persist. Bone loss on the distal surface of the second molar is a concern when third molars are impacted along the distal surface (see Chapter 56).[3] The problem is significantly greater if the third molars are extracted after the roots are formed or when the patient is older (i.e., mid-20s or later). To reduce the risk of bone loss around second molars, partially or completely impacted third molars should be extracted early in their development.

The quality of the soft tissues and the amount of space and vestibular depth are important factors to assess when deciding whether to retain or extract the tooth. If the decision is made to retain the tooth, the pericoronal flap is surgically reduced. It is necessary to reduce and reposition the tissue distal to the coronal aspect of the tooth, as well as remove the pericoronal flap on the occlusal surface. See Chapter 56 for a detailed description of distal surgical procedures and the proper management of tissues posterior to mandibular molars. Simply excising the occlusal portion of the pericoronal flap without managing the distal tissue leaves a deep periodontal pocket on the distal surface, which invites recurrence of acute pericoronal involvement. It is critical to leave the patient with a site that is cleansable and maintainable. As always, patient education and appropriate instruction in long-term maintenance of periodontal health is an essential part of successful therapy.

Conclusions

Acute gingival diseases are similar in that they typically manifest with painful intraoral or perioral lesions, and there is a need for urgent treatment to relieve symptoms. However, each case requires careful assessment and an accurate diagnosis, including identification of risk factors. The management of acute gingival disease entails alleviation of the acute symptoms and elimination of all etiologic factors, including periodontal disease. Treatment is not complete if periodontal pathologic changes or predisposing factors capable of causing them persist. In many cases, there are systemic risk factors that increase susceptibility to acute gingival disease that need to be identified and eliminated or reduced.

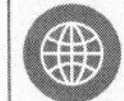

A Case Scenario is found on the companion website eBooks.Health.Elsevier.com.

Suggested Reading

Albandar JM, Tinoco EM. Global epidemiology of periodontal diseases in children and young persons. *Periodontol 2000*. 2002;29:153–176.

Dufty J, Gkranias N, Petrie A, McCormick R, Elmer T, Donos N. Prevalence and treatment of necrotizing ulcerative gingivitis (NUG) in the British Armed Forces: a case-control study. *Clin Oral Investig*. 2017;21(6):1935–1944. https://doi.org/10.1007/s00784-016-1979-9. PMID: 27830369. Epub 2016 Nov 9 .

Genco RJ, Borgnakke WS. Risk factors for periodontal disease. *Periodontol 2000*. 2013;62:59–94.

Herrera D, Alonso B, de Arriba L, et al. Acute periodontal lesions. *Periodontol 2000*. 2014;65:149–177.

Horning GM, Cohen ME. Necrotizing ulcerative gingivitis, periodontitis, and stomatitis: clinical staging and predisposing factors. *J Periodontol*. 1995;66:990–998.

Listgarten MA. Electron microscopic observations on the bacterial flora of acute necrotizing ulcerative gingivitis. *J Periodontol*. 1965;36:328–339.

Singh R, Devanna R, Tenglikar P, Gautam A, Anubhuti Kumari P. Evaluation of mandibular third molar position as a risk factor for pericoronitis: A CBCT study. *J Family Med Prim Care*. 2020;9(3):1599–1602. https://doi.org/10.4103/jfmpc.jfmpc_1101_19. PMID: 32509657. PMCID: PMC7266262 .

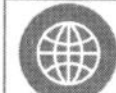
References for this chapter are found on the companion website eBooks.Health.Elsevier.com.

CHAPTER 18

Desquamative Gingivitis

Alfredo Aguirre | Jose Luis Tapia Vazquez | Yasmin Mair

CHAPTER OUTLINE

Chronic Desquamative Gingivitis

Although the condition was first recognized and reported in 1894,[185] the term *chronic desquamative gingivitis* was not coined by Prinz[141] until 1932. It describes a reaction characterized by intense erythema, desquamation, and ulceration of the free and attached gingiva (Fig. 18.1).[101]

Patients can be asymptomatic, but when symptomatic, their complaints range from a mild burning sensation to intense pain. Approximately 50% of desquamative gingivitis cases are localized to the gingiva, although patients can have involvement of the gingiva plus other intraoral and extraoral sites.[101,130]

The cause was initially unclear, with a variety of possibilities suggested. Because most cases were diagnosed in women during the fourth and fifth decades of life (although desquamative gingivitis can occur as early as puberty or as late as in the seventh or eighth decade), hormonal derangement was suspected. In 1960, McCarthy and colleagues[112] suggested that desquamative gingivitis was not a specific disease entity but was instead a *gingival response associated with a variety of conditions*. This concept has been supported by numerous immunopathologic studies.[93,101,132,153,174,187]

The use of clinical and laboratory parameters has revealed that approximately 75% of desquamative gingivitis cases have a dermatologic genesis.[131] Lichen planus and cicatricial pemphigoid account for 84% of the desquamative gingivitis cases.[94] However, many other mucocutaneous autoimmune conditions (e.g., bullous pemphigoid, pemphigus vulgaris, linear immunoglobulin A [IgA] disease, lichen planus pemphigoides, dermatitis herpetiformis [DH], lupus erythematosus, chronic ulcerative stomatitis, epidermolysis bullosa acquisita, dermatomyositis, mixed connective tissue disease, graft versus host disease, paraneoplastic forms) can manifest as desquamative gingivitis.[12–14]

Other conditions that must be considered in the differential diagnosis of desquamative gingivitis include chronic bacterial, fungal, and viral infections, reactions to medications, mouthwashes, chewing gum, and foreign body gingivitis. Although less common, Crohn disease, sarcoidosis, some leukemias, and factitious lesions have also been reported to manifest clinically as desquamative gingivitis.[101,164,193]

It is important to ascertain the disease responsible for desquamative gingivitis to establish the appropriate therapeutic approach. To achieve this goal, a clinical examination is coupled with a thorough history and routine histologic and immunofluorescence studies.[26,101,179,193] Despite a systematic diagnostic approach, the cause of desquamative gingivitis cannot be elucidated in up to one-third of cases.[146]

Diagnosis of Desquamative Gingivitis: A Systematic Approach

Desquamative gingivitis is a clinical term and not a diagnosis. After the condition is identified, a series of laboratory procedures should be used to arrive at a final diagnosis. The success of any therapeutic approach depends on the establishment of an accurate final diagnosis. The following sections describe a systematic approach to determining the disease that triggers desquamative gingivitis (Fig. 18.2).

Clinical History

A thorough clinical history is mandatory to begin the assessment of desquamative gingivitis.[101,131] Data regarding the symptoms associated with this condition and its historical aspects (e.g., lesion onset, whether it has worsened, habits that exacerbate it) provide the foundation for a thorough examination. Information about previous therapy to alleviate the condition should be documented.

Clinical Examination

The distribution pattern of the lesions (e.g., focal or multifocal, with or without confinement to gingival tissues) provides information that can begin to narrow the differential diagnosis.[26,101] A simple clinical maneuver such as the Nikolsky sign offers insight into the plausibility of a vesiculobullous disorder.[116]

CLINICAL CORRELATION

Nikolsky's sign is characterized by blister formation or peeling of the skin or mucosa when horizontal tangential pressure is applied to clinically normal tissues. This sign is typically seen in vesiculobullous diseases such as pemphigus vulgaris and mucous membrane pemphigoid.

Biopsy

Given the extent and number of lesions that may be present in an individual, an incisional biopsy is the best strategy for beginning the microscopic and immunologic evaluation.[26] An important consideration is the selection of the biopsy site. A perilesional incisional biopsy should avoid areas of ulceration because necrosis and epithelial denudation severely hamper the diagnostic process.[182]

After the tissue is excised from the oral cavity, the specimen can be bisected and then submitted for microscopic examination. Buffered formalin (10%) should be used to fix the tissue for conventional hematoxylin and eosin (H&E) evaluation. Michel's buffer (i.e., ammonium sulfate buffer, pH 7.0) is used as the transport solution for immunofluorescence assessment. An incisional biopsy of uninvolved (normal) mucosa typically shows the same immunofluorescent findings as the biopsy of the perilesional tissue. However, there are notable exceptions, such as lichen planus and chronic cutaneous lupus erythematosus, in which only the lesional tissue exhibits the corresponding immunologic markers (Table 18.1).[182]

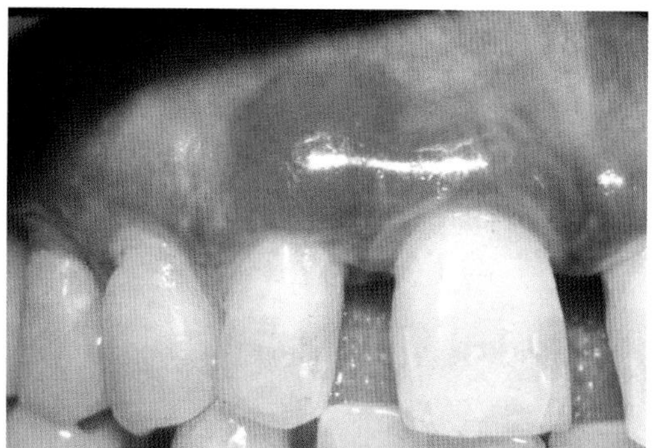

Fig. 18.1 In chronic desquamative gingivitis, irregular, conspicuous erythema involves the free and attached gingival tissues.

Microscopic Examination

Sections of approximately 5 μm of formalin-fixed, paraffin-embedded tissue stained with conventional H&E are obtained for light microscopy examination.[182]

Immunofluorescence

For *direct* immunofluorescence, unfixed frozen sections are incubated with a variety of fluorescein-labeled, antihuman serum (i.e., anti-IgG, anti-IgA, anti-IgM, antifibrin, and anti-C3). For *indirect* immunofluorescence, unfixed frozen sections of oral or esophageal mucosa from an animal, such as a monkey, are first incubated with the patient's serum to enable attachment of serum antibodies to the mucosal tissue. The tissue is then incubated with fluorescein-labeled antihuman serum. Immunofluorescence tests are positive if a fluorescent signal is observed in the epithelium, its associated basement membrane, or the underlying connective tissue (see Table 18.1).[182]

Management

After the diagnosis is established, the dentist must choose the optimal management strategy. The choice depends on the practitioner's experience, the systemic impact of the disease, and the systemic complications of the medications. A detailed consideration of these factors dictates three scenarios.

In the first scenario, the dental practitioner takes direct and exclusive responsibility for the treatment of the patient. This occurs with conditions such as erosive lichen planus, which is responsive to topical steroids (Fig. 18.3).

In the second scenario, the dentist collaborates with another health care provider to evaluate and treat a patient concurrently. The classic example is seen with cicatricial pemphigoid, in which dentists and ophthalmologists work together to provide treatment (Fig. 18.4). Although the dentist addresses the oral lesions, the ophthalmologist monitors the integrity of the ocular conjunctiva.

In the third scenario, the patient is immediately referred to a dermatologist for further evaluation and treatment. This occurs with conditions for which the systemic impact of the disease transcends the boundaries of the oral cavity and results in significant morbidity or mortality. Pemphigus vulgaris is an example of a condition that, after diagnosis by the dentist, requires immediate referral to a dermatologist (Fig. 18.5). The complications (e.g., diabetes mellitus, osteoporosis, methemoglobinemia) of chronically administered systemic medications that are indicated for the management of diseases, such as pemphigus vulgaris or nonresponsive mucous membrane pemphigoid (MMP), warrant referral to a dermatologist or a specialist in internal medicine.

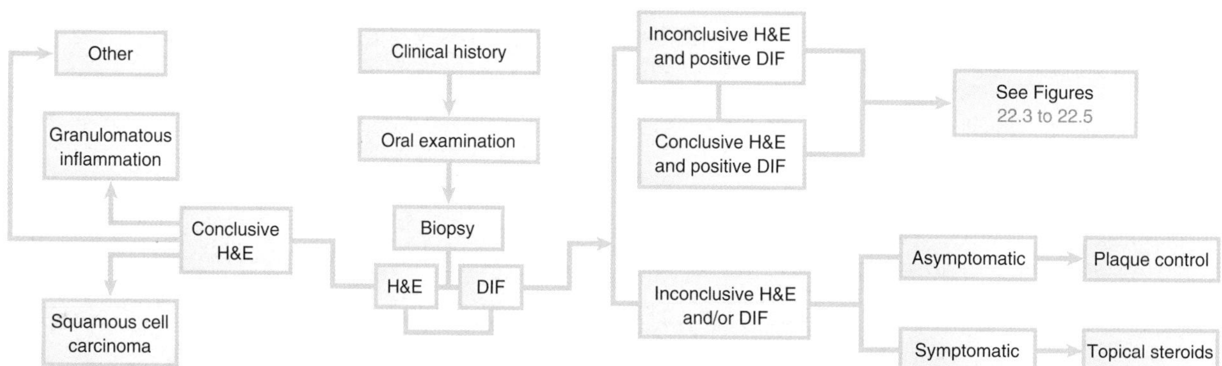

Fig. 18.2 The diagnostic approach for desquamative gingivitis includes hematoxylin and eosin *(H&E)* and direct immunofluorescence *(DIF)* evaluation of biopsy specimens.

TABLE 18.1 Diagnostic Findings for Conditions That Can Manifest as Desquamative Gingivitis

		DIRECT IMMUNOFLUORESCENCE		INDIRECT IMMUNOFLUORESCENCE
Disease	**Histopathology**	**Biopsy of Perilesional Mucosa**	**Biopsy of Uninvolved Mucosa**	**Serum**
Pemphigus	Intraepithelial clefting above the basal cell layer; basal cells have a characteristic tombstone appearance; acantholysis	Intercellular deposits in epithelium IgG in all cases and C3 in most cases	Same as for perilesional mucosa	Intercellular antibodies (IgG) in ≥90% of cases
Cicatricial pemphigoid	Subepithelial clefting with epithelial separation from the underlying lamina propria, leaving an intact basal layer	Linear deposits of C3 with or without IgG at the basement membrane zone in most cases	Same as for perilesional mucosa	Basement membrane zone antibodies (IgG) in 10% of cases
Bullous pemphigoid	Subepithelial clefting with epithelial separation from the underlying lamina propria, leaving an intact basal layer	Linear deposits of C3 with or without IgG at the basement membrane zone in most cases	Same as for perilesional mucosa	Basement membrane zone in 40%–70% of cases
Epidermolysis bullosa acquisita	Similar to bullous and cicatricial pemphigoid	Linear deposits of IgG and C3 at the basement membrane zone in most cases	Same as for perilesional mucosa	Basement membrane zone antibodies (IgG) in 25% of cases
Lichen planus	Hyperkeratosis, hydropic degeneration of the basal layer, and sawtooth rete pegs; lamina propria exhibits dense, bandlike infiltrate, primarily of T lymphocytes; colloid bodies	Fibrillar deposits of fibrin at the dermal–epidermal junction	Negative	Negative
Chronic ulcerative stomatitis	Similar to erosive lichen planus; hyperkeratosis, acanthosis, basal cell layer liquefaction, subepithelial clefting, and lymphohistiocytic chronic infiltrate in a bandlike configuration	IgG deposits in the nuclei of the basal layer of epithelial cells	Same as for perilesional mucosa	ANA specific for basal cells of stratified squamous epithelium
Linear IgA disease	Similar to erosive lichen planus	Linear deposits of IgA at the basement membrane zone	Same as for perilesional mucosa	IgA basement membrane zone antibodies (IgA) in 30% of cases
Dermatitis herpetiformis	Collection of neutrophils, eosinophils, and fibrin in the connective tissue papillae	IgA deposits in the dermal papillae in 85% of cases	IgA deposits in dermal papillae in 100% of cases	IgA endomysial antibodies in 70% of cases; gliadin antibodies in 30% of cases
Systemic lupus erythematosus	Hyperkeratosis, basal cell degeneration, epithelial atrophy, and perivascular inflammation	IgG or IgM with or without C3 deposits at the dermal–epidermal junction	Same as for perilesional mucosa	ANA in >95% of cases; DNA and ENA antibodies in >50% of cases
Chronic cutaneous erythematosus	Hyperkeratosis, basal cell degeneration, epithelial atrophy, and perivascular inflammation	IgG or IgM with or without C3 deposits at the dermal–epidermal junction	Negative	Usually negative
Subacute lupus erythematosus	Less inflammatory cell infiltrate than systemic and chronic cutaneous forms but with similar microscopic features	IgG or IgM with or without C3 deposits at the dermal-epidermal junction in 60% of cases; granular IgG deposits in basal cell cytoplasm in 30% of cases	Same as for perilesional mucosa	ANA in 60%–90% of cases; Ro (SSA) in 80% of cases; RF in 30% of cases; anti-RNP in 10% of cases

ANA, Antinuclear antibodies; *C3*, complement 3; *DNA*, deoxyribonucleic acid; *ENA*, extractable nuclear antigens; *IgA*, immunoglobulin A; *IgG*, immunoglobulin G; *IgM*, immunoglobulin M; *RF*, rheumatoid factor; *RNP*, ribonucleoprotein.

Adapted from Rinaggio J, Neiders ME, Aguirre A, Kumar V. Using immunofluorescence in the diagnosis of chronic ulcerative lesions of the oral mucosa. *Compend Contin Educ Dent.* 1999;20:943–944, 947–948, 950 passim quiz 962. PubMed PMID: 10650375.

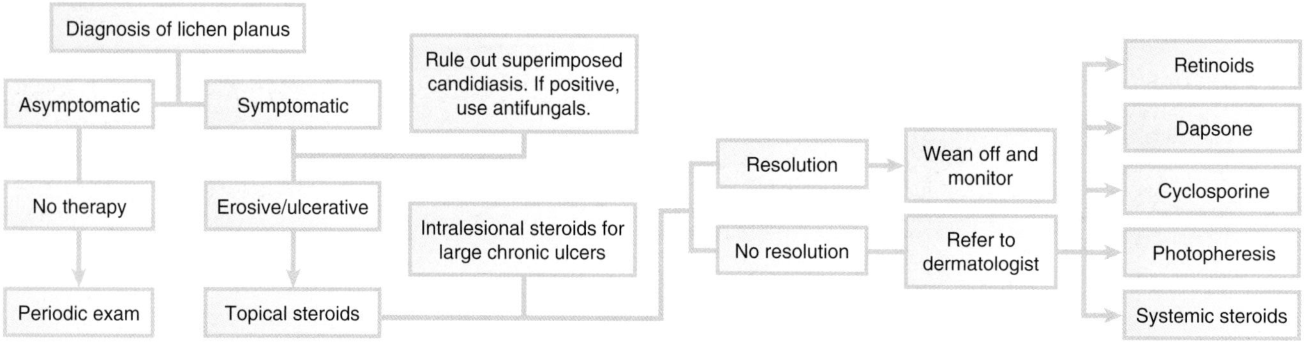

Fig. 18.3 Algorithm for the treatment of lichen planus.

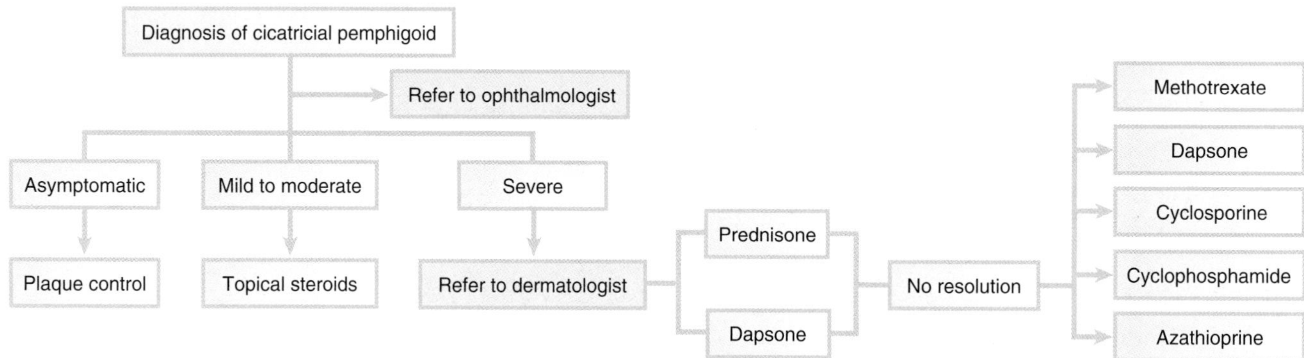

Fig. 18.4 Algorithm for the treatment of cicatricial pemphigoid.

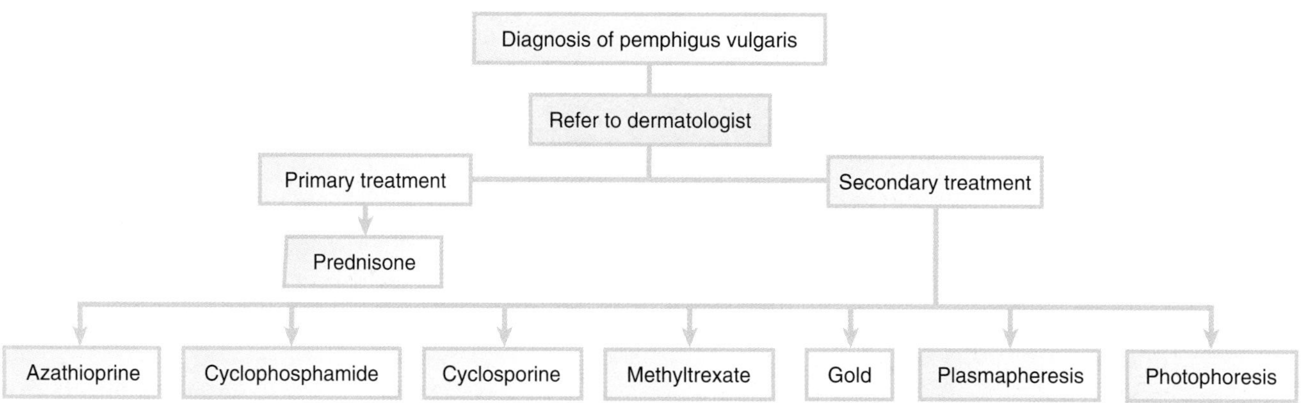

Fig. 18.5 Algorithm for the treatment of pemphigus vulgaris.

When oral treatment is provided, periodic evaluation is needed to monitor the patient's response to therapy. Initially, the patient should be evaluated at 2 to 4 weeks after beginning treatment to ensure that the condition is under control. Observation should continue until the patient is free of discomfort. Appointments every 3 to 6 months are then appropriate. Medication dosages are usually adjusted during this interval.

Table 18.2 summarizes suggested contemporary therapeutic approaches that can be used to treat selected conditions that can manifest as desquamative gingivitis. Dentists play an important role in the diagnosis and management of desquamative gingivitis. The importance of recognizing and properly diagnosing this condition is accentuated by the fact that a serious and life-threatening disease (i.e., squamous cell carcinoma) can mimic desquamative gingivitis.[149]

Diseases That Can Manifest as Desquamative Gingivitis

Lichen Planus

Lichen planus is an inflammatory mucocutaneous disorder that can involve the mucosal surfaces (e.g., oral cavity, genital tract, or other mucosae) and the skin, including the scalp and the nails.[152] Evidence suggests that lichen planus is an immunologically mediated mucocutaneous disorder in which host T lymphocytes play a central role.[13,76,87,110] Although the oral cavity can have lichen planus lesions with a distinct clinical configuration and distribution, the clinical presentation can simulate other mucocutaneous disorders. Oral lichen planus has a broad differential diagnosis.

TABLE 18.2 Therapeutic Approaches for Treating Selected Conditions That Manifest as Desquamative Gingivitis

	THERAPY		
Disease	**Mild Cases**	**Recalcitrant Cases**	**Severe or Refractory Cases**
Erosive lichen planus	Delivery of therapeutic agent is enhanced with use of vacuum-formed custom trays **Rx:** Lidex (0.05% fluocinonide) gel **Disp:** One tube (15 g) **Sig:** Apply to affected area pc and hs Monitoring of patient's oral cavity warranted because candidiasis may develop after a few weeks of topical steroid use; concomitant use of antifungal may be necessary **Rx:** Clotrimazole 10-mg troches **Disp:** 90 **Sig:** Dissolve in mouth tid, then expectorate for 30 consecutive days	**Rx:** Protopic (0.1% tacrolimus) ointment **Disp:** One tube (30 g) **Sig:** Apply to affected area bid **Rx:** Tacrolimus (0.1 mg per 100 mL of distilled water) **Disp:** Dilute one 0.5-mg capsule of tacrolimus in 500 mL of distilled water **Sig:** Rinse mouth with 15 mL for 2 min qid	Refer to dermatologist for management with systemic corticosteroids
Cicatricial pemphigoid	**Rx:** Lidex (0.05% fluocinonide) gel **Disp:** One tube (15 g) **Sig:** Apply to affected area pc and hs **Rx:** Temovate (0.05% clobetasol propionate) **Disp:** One tube (15 g) **Sig:** Apply to affected area qid		Refer to dermatologist for management with prednisone (20–30 mg/day); concomitant use of azathioprine may be needed; dapsone, sulfonamide, and tetracycline are other alternatives
Pemphigus	Refer to dermatologist for management with prednisone (20–30 mg/day); concomitant use of azathioprine may be needed		
Chronic ulcerative stomatitis	**Rx:** Lidex (0.05% fluocinonide) gel **Disp:** One tube (15 g) **Sig:** Apply to affected area qid **Rx:** Temovate (0.05% clobetasol propionate) **Disp:** One tube (15 g) **Sig:** Apply to affected area qid	Refer to dermatologist for management with hydroxychloroquine **Disp:** 200 mg tablets **Sig:** Take 200–400 mg a day	

bid, Twice daily; *g,* grams; *hs,* at bedtime; *IU,* international units; *mg,* milligrams; *pc,* after meals; *qid,* four times daily.

Numerous epidemiologic studies have found that oral lichen planus occurs in 0.1% to 4% of the population.[28,69,158] Most patients with oral lichen planus are middle-aged or older women; the disorder occurs with a 2:1 ratio of women to men. Children are rarely affected.[158] In a dental setting, cutaneous lichen planus is observed in about 15% to 30% of patients diagnosed with oral lichen planus.[28,107] Two-thirds of patients seen in dermatologic clinics exhibit oral lichen planus.[161]

KEY FACT

Lichen planus is a mucocutaneous disorder that classically manifests with bilateral, white striae on the buccal mucosae. The classic reticular subtype is asymptomatic, and no treatment is needed. Atrophic and erosive forms of oral lichen planus are associated with pain and a burning sensation, and topical corticosteroids are the mainstay of treatment. One percent of oral lichen planus cases may develop squamous cell carcinoma.

KEY FACT

Civatte bodies are eosinophilic globules typically seen at the junction of epithelium and connective tissue in lichen planus. They are derived from keratinocytes that are undergoing apoptosis.

KEY FACT

Direct immunofluorescence is a valuable tool for the diagnosis of lichen planus. Fibrinogen with a shaggy configuration along the basement membrane zone is typically seen in lichen planus. However, caution should be used when interpreting direct immunofluorescence findings because some premalignant and malignant oral lesions may yield fibrinogen positivity. Concurrent evaluation of H&E sections and clinical examination minimize the risk of misdiagnosis.

Oral Lesions

Although there are several clinical forms of oral lichen planus (i.e., reticular, papular, patch, atrophic, erosive, and bullous), the most common are the reticular and erosive subtypes. The typical reticular lesions are asymptomatic and bilateral, and they consist of interlacing white lines on the posterior region of the buccal mucosa. The lateral border and dorsum of the tongue, the hard palate, the alveolar ridge, and the gingiva may also be affected.[28] The reticular lesions can have an erythematous background, which is a feature associated with coexisting candidiasis. Oral lichen planus lesions follow a chronic course and have alternating, unpredictable periods of quiescence and flare-ups.

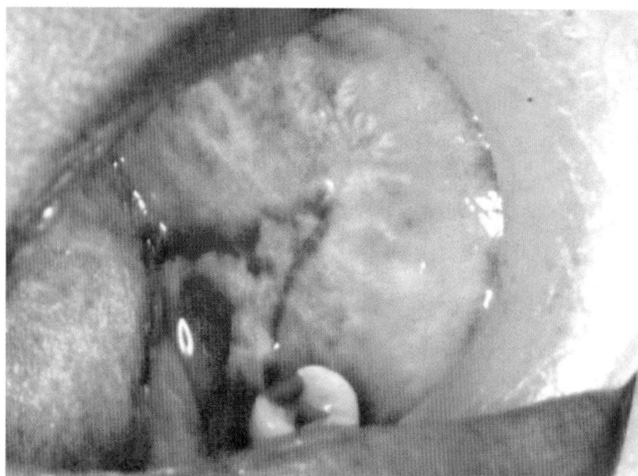

Fig. 18.6 In a case of erosive lichen planus, the large ulcerative lesion on the left buccal mucosa exhibits bordering erythema. The typical white striations of lichen planus are evident in the periphery of the ulcer.

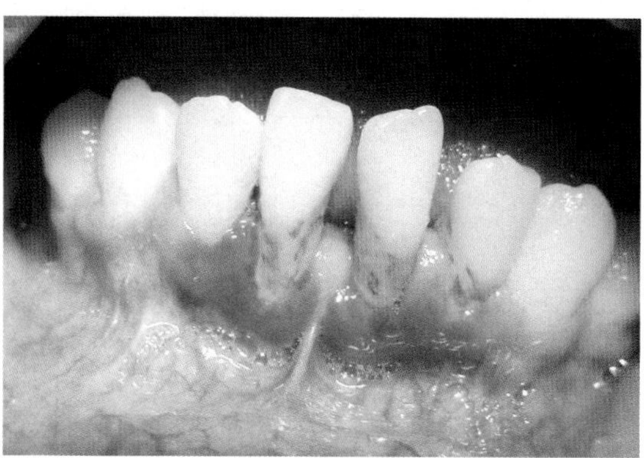

Fig. 18.7 Erosive lichen planus can manifest as desquamative gingivitis. The gingival tissues are erythematous, ulcerated, and painful. (*Courtesy Dr. Luis Gaitan, Oral Pathology Laboratory, Faculty of Odontology, National Autonomous University of Mexico, Mexico City, Mexico.*)

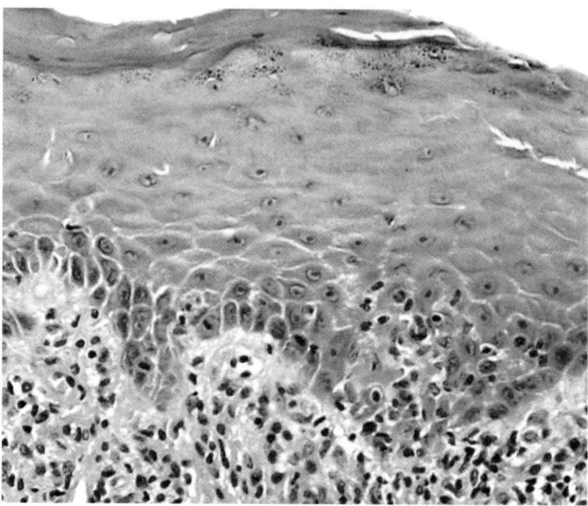

Fig. 18.8 Microscopic appearance of lichen planus. The biopsy specimen from a gingival lesion shows hyperkeratosis and mild hypergranulosis, along with focal basal cell degeneration, lymphocytic exocytosis, and thickening of the basement membrane. The rete pegs exhibit a slight serrated configuration. The papillary lamina propria shows a bandlike infiltrate of lymphohistiocytic chronic inflammatory cells. Hematoxylin and eosin stain; original magnification ×100.

The erosive subtype of lichen planus is often associated with pain. It manifests as atrophic, erythematous, and often ulcerated areas. Fine, white radiating striations are observed bordering the atrophic and ulcerated zones. These areas may be sensitive to heat, acid, and spicy foods (Fig. 18.6).

Gingival Lesions

Approximately 7% to 10% of patients with oral lichen planus have lesions restricted to the gingival tissue.[118,161] They may occur as one or more types of the following four distinctive patterns:

1. *Keratotic lesions.* The raised, white lesions can manifest as groups of individual papules, linear or reticular lesions, or plaque-like configurations.
2. *Erosive or ulcerative lesions.* The extensive erythematous areas with a patchy distribution can manifest as focal or diffuse hemorrhagic areas. The lesions are exacerbated by slight trauma (e.g., toothbrushing) (Fig. 18.7).
3. *Vesicular or bullous lesions.* The raised, fluid-filled lesions are uncommon and short lived on the gingiva, quickly rupturing and leaving ulcerations.
4. *Atrophic lesions.* Atrophy of the gingival tissues with ensuing epithelial thinning results in erythema that is confined to the gingiva.

Histopathology

Microscopically, three main features characterize oral lichen planus: (1) hyperkeratosis or parakeratosis; (2) hydropic degeneration of the basal layer; and (3) a dense, bandlike infiltrate, consisting primarily of T lymphocytes, in the lamina propria (Fig. 18.8). Classically, the epithelial rete ridges have a sawtooth configuration. Hydropic degeneration of the basal layer of the epithelium can be sufficiently extensive that the epithelium becomes thin and atrophic or detaches from the underlying connective tissue and produces a subepithelial vesicle or an ulcer. Colloid bodies (i.e., Civatte bodies) are often seen at the epithelium—connective tissue interface.[28]

The microscopic diagnosis of oral lichen planus is straightforward for the keratotic lesions, and biopsy specimens should be obtained from these areas if possible. However, classic histologic features may be obscured in areas of ulceration, making a conclusive diagnosis of oral lichen planus difficult if it is based solely on conventional microscopy. Electron microscopy studies indicate that separation of the basal lamina from the basal cell layer is an early manifestation of lichen planus.[74]

The pattern of oral lesions of lichen planus can change, and in unusual cases a second or third biopsy may be necessary to arrive at a definitive diagnosis. Controversy exists regarding the malignant potential of oral lichen planus. A meta-analysis and systematic review cited an average rate of 1.09% of oral cancer emerging in oral lichen planus.[61] Other researchers reject or question the connection between oral lichen planus and oral cancer.[53,78,105,143] Despite this controversy, biopsy and close follow-up are warranted for these patients.

Immunopathology

Direct immunofluorescence of lesional and perilesional oral lichen planus biopsy specimens reveals linear fibrillar (i.e., shaggy) deposits of fibrin in the basement membrane zone (Fig. 18.9), along with scattered immunoglobulin-staining cytoid bodies in the upper areas of the lamina propria (Fig. 18.10). Results of serum tests involving the use of indirect immunofluorescence are negative for patients with lichen planus (see Table 18.1).

Differential Diagnosis

The classic clinical presentation of oral lichen planus can be simulated by other conditions, mainly by lichenoid mucositis. If oral lichen planus is confined to the gingival tissues (i.e., erosive oral

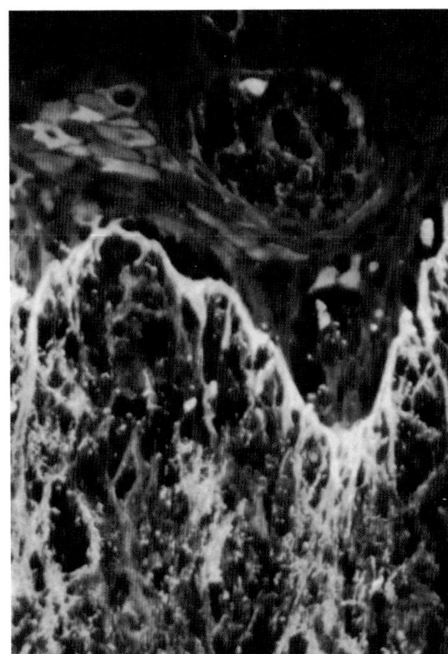

Fig. 18.9 Direct immunofluorescence staining of lichen planus. Fibrin deposits along the basement membrane of the epithelium exhibit a shaggy configuration.

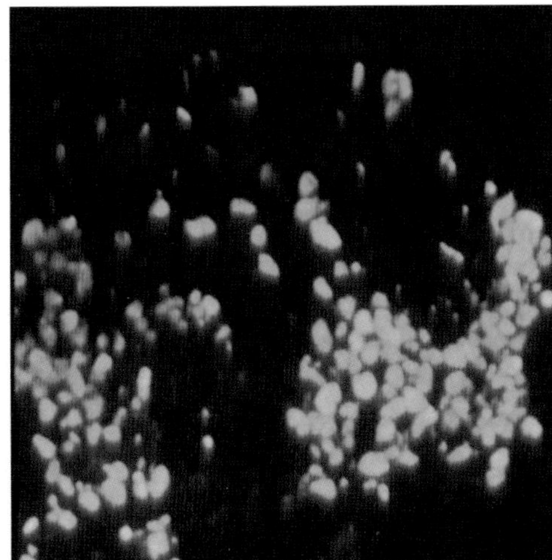

Fig. 18.10 Direct immunofluorescence staining of lichen planus. Clusters of cytoid bodies exhibit immunoglobulin M deposits in the lamina propria.

lichen planus), the identification of fine, white radiating striations bordering the erosive areas support a diagnosis of oral lichen planus. If the white striations are absent, the differential diagnosis should primarily include MMP and pemphigus vulgaris. Less common possibilities include linear immunoglobulin A disease (LAD), lichen planus pemphigoides, and chronic ulcerative stomatitis.

Treatment

The keratotic lesions of oral lichen planus are asymptomatic and do not require treatment after the microscopic diagnosis has been established. However, evaluation of the patient every 6 to 12 months is warranted to monitor suspicious clinical changes and to look for the emergence of an erosive component.

The erosive, bullous, or ulcerative lesions of oral lichen planus are treated with high-potency topical steroids, such as 0.05% fluocinonide gel (Lidex, three times daily). Lidex can also be mixed 1:1 with carboxymethylcellulose (Orabase) paste or another adhesive ointment. A gingival tray can be used to deliver 0.05% fluocinonide ointment or gel or 0.05% clobetasol propionate with 100,000 IU/mL of nystatin in Orabase (Fig. 18.11).

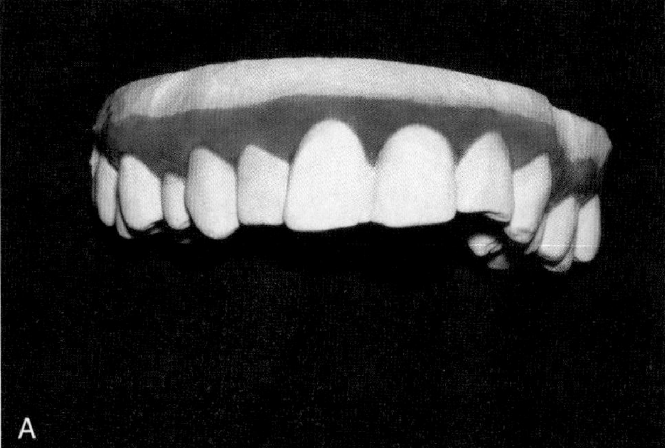

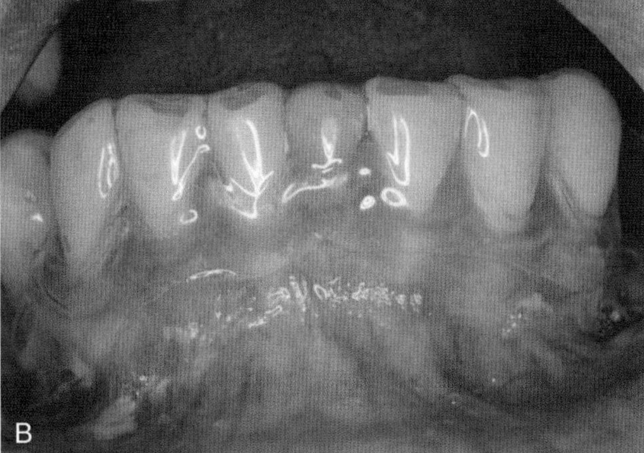

Fig. 18.11 (A) An alginate impression is obtained to create a stone model. A thin layer of block-out resin is applied on the gingival and alveolar mucosal areas with desquamative gingivitis to create a space to carry the medication. A trimmed maxillary stone model shows the block-out resin in place *(blue area)*. (B) A mandibular gingival tray is in place. Soft sheet material for vacuum-forming trays is prepared and trimmed to conform to the local anatomy.

Three daily 5-minute applications of the mixture appear to be effective for controlling erosive lichen planus.[68] Intralesional injections of triamcinolone acetonide (10 to 20 mg) or short-term regimens of 40 mg of prednisone daily for 5 days, followed by 10 to 20 mg daily for an additional two weeks, have also been used in more severe cases.[130] Because of the potential side effects, systemic steroids should be administered and monitored by a dermatologist.

Other treatment modalities (e.g., retinoids, hydroxychloroquine, cyclosporine, azathioprine, cyclophosphamide, free gingival grafts) have been used.[130,138] In recalcitrant cases, tacrolimus (0.1% Protopic ointment, twice daily) can be effective for controlling the lesions of erosive lichen planus.[88,109,122,167,178] Topical tacrolimus may also be indicated in patients with diabetes mellitus where the continuous use of corticosteroids may result in hyperglycemia.[75]

Because candidiasis is often associated with symptomatic oral lichen planus, and because topical steroid therapy promotes fungal growth, treatment should also include a topical antifungal agent.[18,64,79]

Pemphigoid

The term *pemphigoid* applies to several cutaneous, immune-mediated, subepithelial bullous diseases that are characterized by a

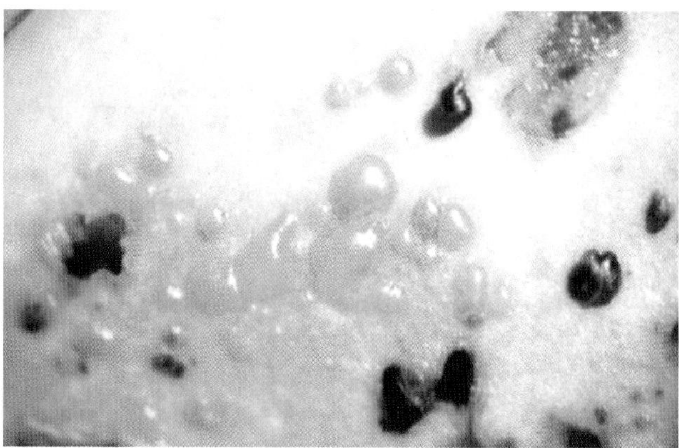

Fig. 18.12 Coalescing cutaneous bullae are seen in a case of bullous pemphigoid, and some of them are hemorrhagic. Rupture of the bullae leads to the formation of serpiginous ulcers.

separation of the basement membrane zone, including bullous pemphigoid, MMP, and pemphigoid (herpes) gestationis.[136,159] Among these conditions, bullous pemphigoid and MMP (i.e., benign MMP or cicatricial pemphigoid) have received considerable attention. Molecular findings for these two diseases indicate that they are separate entities.[159] However, considerable histologic and immunopathologic overlap exists between them, and differentiation may be impossible on the basis of the two criteria.[136]

In many cases, the clinical findings are probably the best way to discriminate between them. Accordingly, the term *bullous pemphigoid* is preferred when the disease is nonscarring and mainly affects the skin. The term *cicatricial pemphigoid* is favored when scarring occurs, and the disease is mainly confined to mucous membranes, although scarring may be absent with some subtypes of MMP.[189] Until more research allows a better understanding of this family of diseases, bullous pemphigoid and MMP are discussed separately.

Bullous Pemphigoid

Bullous pemphigoid (BP) is a chronic, autoimmune, subepidermal bullous disease with tense cutaneous bullae that rupture and become flaccid (Fig. 18.12). Recently, it has been suggested that some cases of BP can be drug-induced (i.e., checkpoint inhibitors and antihyperglycemic agents such as DPP4-inhibitors).[86] Although the skin lesions of bullous pemphigoid clinically resemble those of pemphigus, the microscopic picture is quite distinct.

Histopathology

There is no evidence of acantholysis in bullous pemphigoid, and the developing vesicles are subepithelial rather than intraepithelial. The epithelium separates from the underlying connective tissue at the basement membrane zone. Electron microscopic studies show horizontal splitting or replication of the basal lamina. The separating epithelium remains relatively intact, and the basal layer appears to be regular. The two major antigenic determinants of bullous pemphigoid are the 230-kDa protein plaque known as *bullous pemphigoid 1 (BP1)* and the 180-kDa collagen-like transmembrane protein known as *bullous pemphigoid 2 (BP2)*.[123,151]

Immunofluorescence

Immunologically, bullous pemphigoid is characterized by immunoglobulin G (IgG) and complement 3 (C3) immune deposits along the epithelial basement membranes and circulating IgG antibodies to the epithelial basement membrane.[85,127] Direct immunofluorescence studies are positive for 90% to 100% of these patients, whereas indirect immunofluorescence studies are positive for 60% to 90% of affected patients (see Table 18.1).[155]

Oral Lesions

Oral lesions of bullous pemphigoid have been reported to occur secondarily in about one-third of cases. The clinical presentation includes an erosive or desquamative gingivitis and occasional vesicular or bullous lesions.[171]

Treatment

Because the etiologic factors of bullous pemphigoid are unknown, treatment is designed to control its signs and symptoms.[85,127] The primary treatment is a moderate dose of systemic prednisone. Steroid-sparing strategies (i.e., prednisone plus other immunomodulatory drugs) are used when high doses of steroids are needed or when the steroid alone fails to control the disease.[44] The chimeric monoclonal antibody Rituximab has shown high rates of remission with an excellent safety profile.[137] For localized lesions of bullous pemphigoid, high-potency topical steroids or tetracycline with or without nicotinamide can be effective.[130]

Mucous Membrane Pemphigoid

MMP (i.e., cicatricial pemphigoid) is a chronic vesiculobullous autoimmune disorder of unknown cause that predominantly affects women during the fifth decade of life. It has rarely been reported in young children.[24,124,159] An undesirable side effect of anti-PD-1 checkpoint inhibitors is the development of MMP in some patients.[172]

Cicatricial pemphigoid involves the oral cavity, the conjunctiva, and the mucosa of the nose, vagina, rectum, esophagus, and urethra. In about 20% of patients the skin may also be involved.[120]

Investigations suggest that cicatricial pemphigoid encompasses a group of heterogeneous conditions with distinct clinical and molecular features.[42,119,156] An elaborate cascade of events is involved in the pathogenesis of cicatricial pemphigoid. Initially, antigen–antibody complexing occurs at the basement membrane zone, which is followed by complement activation and subsequent leukocyte recruitment. Proteolytic enzymes are then released and dissolve or cleave the basement membrane zone, usually at the level of the lamina lucida.[56]

The two major antigenic determinants for cicatricial pemphigoid are BP1 and BP2. Most cases of cicatricial pemphigoid are the result of an immune response directed against BP2; less often, this response is mounted against BP1, epiligrin (i.e., laminin 5, a lamina lucida protein in the basement membrane of stratified epithelium), and β_4 integrins.[10,23,42]

There is strong evidence of the existence of at least five subtypes of cicatricial pemphigoid: oral pemphigoid, anti-epiligrin pemphigoid, anti-BP antigen mucosal pemphigoid, ocular pemphigoid, and multiple-antigen pemphigoid.[159] The sera of ocular pemphigoid patients recognize the β_4 integrin subunit, whereas the sera of patients with oral pemphigoid recognize the α_6 unit.[144]

KEY FACT

Mucous membrane pemphigoid (MMP) is an autoimmune disorder characterized by ocular and oral lesions. Symblepharon (i.e., scarring resulting in adhesion of the eyelid to the eyeball) is a significant complication of MMP. The diagnosis is made by using hematoxylin and eosin (H&E) and direct immunofluorescence studies. The mainstay of treatment is corticosteroids.

Ocular Lesions

Among patients (mainly those with desquamative gingivitis) who first see a dentist, ocular involvement may later occur in approximately 25%.[128] In contrast, among patients who first see a

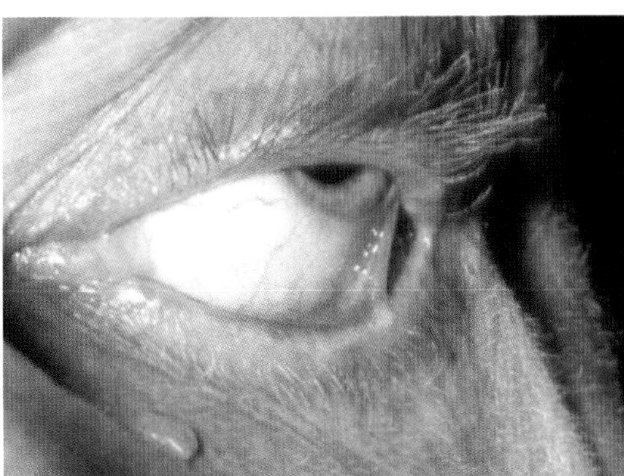

Fig. 18.13 In a patient with mucous membrane pemphigoid (i.e., cicatricial pemphigoid), the characteristic ocular lesion is a symblepharon, an adhesion of the eyelid to the eyeball. (*Courtesy Dr. Carl Allen, The Ohio State University, Columbus, OH.*)

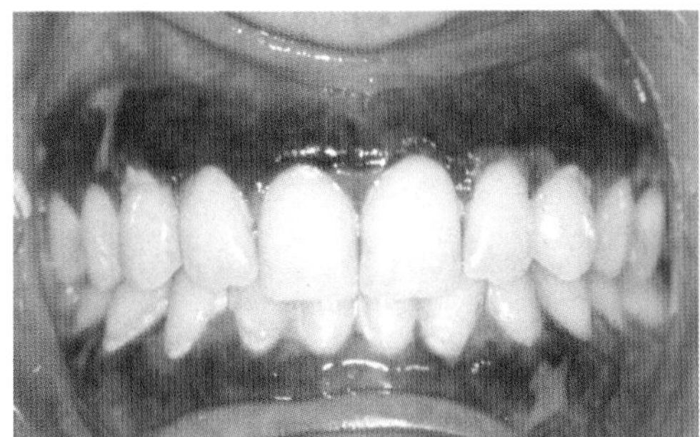

Fig. 18.14 When mucous membrane pemphigoid is confined to the gingival tissues, a typical desquamative gingivitis appearance is observed. (*Courtesy Dr. Stuart L. Fischman, State University of New York at Buffalo, Buffalo, NY.*)

dermatologist, 66% have conjunctival lesions; in ophthalmic studies, 100% of patients have ocular involvement.[62,98,120,121]

The initial lesion is characterized by unilateral conjunctivitis that becomes bilateral within two years. Subsequently, adhesions of the eyelid to the eyeball (i.e., symblepharon) may form (Fig. 18.13). Adhesions at the edges of the eyelids (i.e., ankyloblepharon) may lead to a narrowing of the palpebral fissure. Small vesicular lesions may develop on the conjunctiva, which can eventually produce scarring, corneal damage, and blindness.[67,121]

Oral Lesions

The most characteristic feature of oral involvement is desquamative gingivitis, typically with areas of erythema, desquamation, ulceration, and vesiculation of the attached gingiva (Fig. 18.14).[65,170] Vesiculobullous lesions can occur elsewhere in the mouth.[65] The bullae tend to have a relatively thick roof and rupture in 2 to 3 days after formation, leaving irregularly shaped areas of ulceration. Healing of these lesions can take up to 3 weeks or longer.

Histopathology

The microscopic appearance of the oral lesions, although not completely diagnostic of MMP, is sufficiently distinctive that a tentative diagnosis can be considered. A striking subepithelial vesiculation with the epithelium separated from the underlying lamina propria leaves an intact basal layer (Fig. 18.15). Separation of the epithelium and the connective tissue occurs at the basement membrane zone. Electron microscopic studies demonstrate a split in the basal lamina.[180] A mixed inflammatory infiltrate (i.e., lymphocytes, plasma cells, neutrophils, and scarce eosinophils) is observed in the underlying fibrous connective tissue.

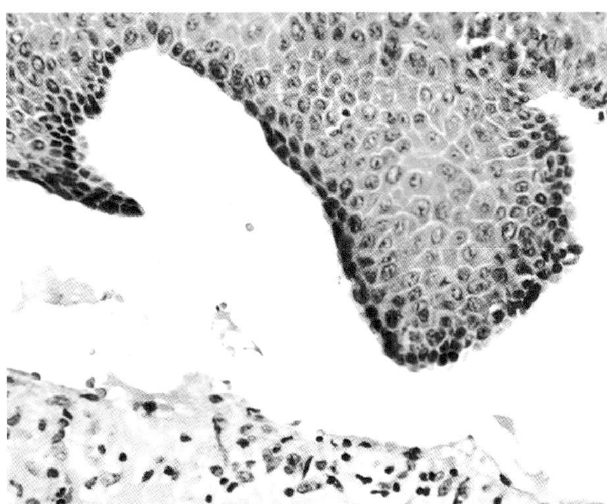

Fig. 18.15 Microscopic features of oral mucous membrane pemphigoid show a separation of the epithelium from the subjacent connective tissue (i.e., subepithelial clefting). An intact basal cell layer remains attached to the epithelium. Hematoxylin and eosin stain; original magnification ×100.

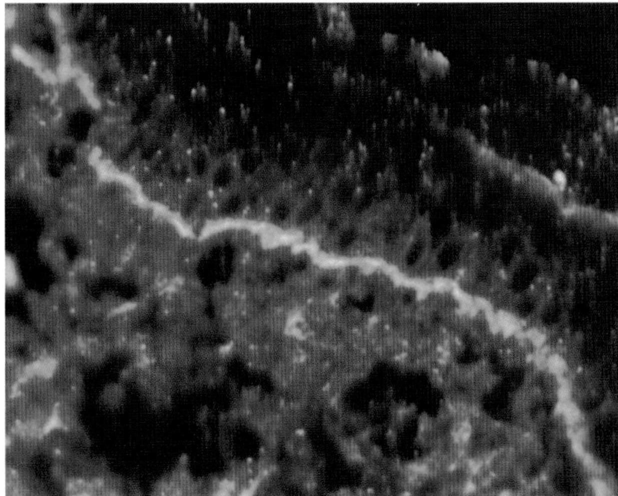

Fig. 18.16 Direct immunofluorescence staining of mucous membrane pemphigoid shows C3 deposits confined along the basement membrane.

Immunofluorescence

Positive findings along the basement membrane area have been reported with the use of direct and indirect immunofluorescence.[43,84,92] In biopsy tests using direct immunofluorescence, the main immunoreactants are IgG and C3, which are confined to the basement membrane (Fig. 18.16). Some studies indicate that a positive indirect immunofluorescence result is rare (<25%) for these patients.[114] The lack of indirect immunofluorescence findings may reflect an earlier diagnosis of MMP, thereby resulting in the identification of patients with less extensive disease.[2,96] In any event, circulating autoantibodies do not appear to play a role in the pathogenesis of the disease.

Differential Diagnosis

Several disease entities manifest with similar clinical and histologic (i.e., subepithelial bulla) features.[52] They include bullous pemphigoid, bullous lichen planus, DH, LAD, erythema multiforme (EM), herpes gestationis, and epidermolysis bullosa acquisita.

Pemphigus may be confined to the oral cavity during its early stage, and the vesicular and ulcerative lesions may resemble those of MMP. An erosive or desquamative gingivitis also can be seen in pemphigus as a rare manifestation. Biopsy studies can quickly rule out pemphigus by revealing the absence or presence of acantholytic changes.

In EM, there are obvious vesiculobullous lesions. However, the onset is usually acute rather than chronic, labial involvement is severe, and the gingivae are usually not affected. Desquamative gingivitis is an unusual finding in EM, although occasional vesicular lesions can develop. A biopsy study of an oral lesion reveals an unusual degeneration of the upper stratum spinosum that is characteristically seen in oral EM lesions.

Cicatricial pemphigoid must be differentiated from epidermolysis bullosa acquisita, which can manifest with similar histopathologic and immunopathologic features. When the biopsy is treated with salt to separate the dermis from the epidermis, basement membrane immunodeposits occur on the epidermal side with pemphigoid and on the dermal side with epidermolysis bullosa acquisita.[55]

Treatment

Topical steroids are the mainstay of treatment for MMP, particularly when lesions are localized. Fluocinonide (0.05%) and clobetasol propionate (0.05%) in an adhesive vehicle can be used three times daily for up to 6 months. When the oral lesions of MMP are confined to the gingival tissues, topical corticosteroids are effectively delivered with vacuum-formed custom trays or veneers.[159] Optimal oral hygiene is essential because local irritants on the tooth surface result in an exaggerated gingival inflammatory response. Gingival irritation from a dental prosthesis should be minimized.

If the disease is not severe and symptoms are mild, systemic corticosteroids may be omitted. If ocular involvement exists, systemic corticosteroids are indicated.

When lesions do not respond to steroids, systemic dapsone (4-4'-diaminodiphenylsulfone) has proved to be effective.[34,60,119,125] Because of the systemic side effects of dapsone, including hemolysis and methemoglobinemia (particularly in patients with glucose-6-phosphate dehydrogenase deficiency), referral to a dermatologist is often indicated.[133] Systemic steroids can be combined with azathioprine or cyclophosphamide.[9,162]

Biologic agents such as Rituximab (i.e., anti-CD20 monoclonal antibody) combined with an immunosuppressant (i.e., dapsone and/or sulfasalazine) have shown promising results in severe, refractory cases.[184] Some investigators advocate sulfonamides and tetracycline. Although surgery is not a treatment for MMP, it is used for some patients to prevent blindness and for esophageal and upper airways stenosis.[159] Connective tissue grafting to alleviate root surface sensitivity and to improve aesthetics has been used with success to manage gingival recession in a patient with cicatricial pemphigoid.[103]

Pemphigus Vulgaris

The pemphigus diseases are a group of autoimmune bullous disorders that produce cutaneous and mucous membrane blisters (Figs. 18.17 and 18.18). Pemphigus vulgaris is the most common of the pemphigus diseases, which also include pemphigus foliaceus, pemphigus vegetans, and pemphigus erythematosus.[150] Pemphigus vulgaris is a potentially lethal chronic condition with a 10% mortality rate and a worldwide annual incidence of 0.1 to 0.5 cases per 100,000 individuals.[14,150,160] A predilection for women, usually after the fourth decade of life, has been observed.[130] However, pemphigus vulgaris has also been reported in unusually young children and even in newborns.[32,63,150,166,191]

The epidermal and mucous membrane blisters occur when the cell-to-cell adhesion structures are damaged by the action of circulating autoantibodies and by the in vivo binding of the autoantibodies to the pemphigus vulgaris antigens, which are cell surface glycoproteins on keratinocytes. The pemphigus vulgaris glycoproteins

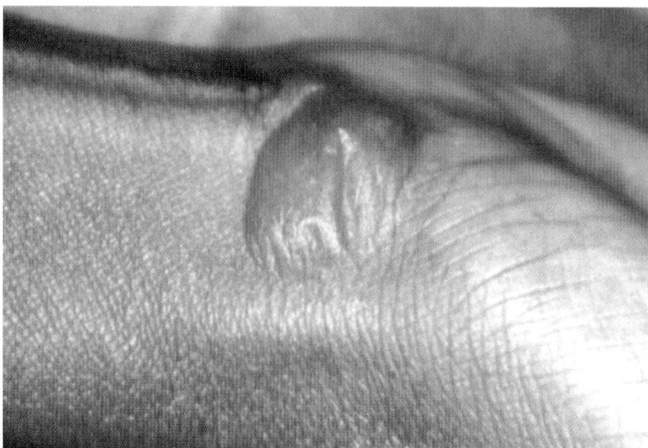

Fig. 18.17 Patient with pemphigus vulgaris exhibiting a large bulla on the flexor surface of the wrist.

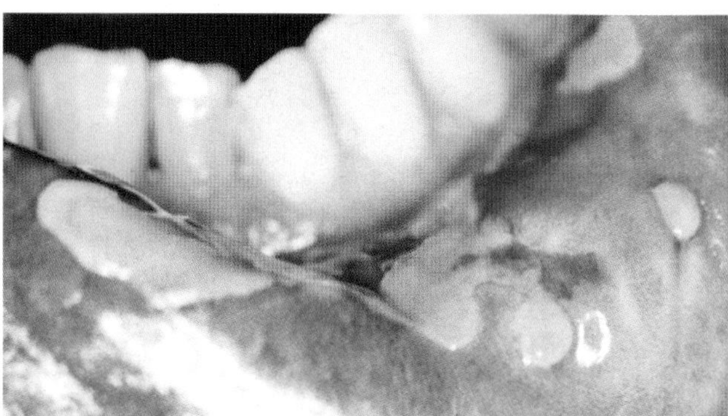

Fig. 18.18 Patient with pemphigus vulgaris of the oral cavity presenting multiple and coalescent areas of ulceration covered by pseudomembranes of necrotic epithelium. The patient had large ulcers on the labial mucosa, tongue, and soft palate.

are members of the desmoglein (DSG) subfamily of the cadherin superfamily of cell—cell adhesion molecules, which occur in desmosomes.[95] Whereas high levels of desmoglein 3 (DSG3) autoantibodies correlate with the severity of oral disease in patients with pemphigus vulgaris, elevated levels of desmoglein 1 (DSG1) autoantibodies are associated with severity of cutaneous disease.[73] Evidence suggests that DSG3, which is the gene that codes for pemphigus vulgaris, is located on chromosome 18.[190]

Most cases of pemphigus vulgaris are idiopathic. However, medications such as penicillamine and captopril can produce drug-induced pemphigus, which is usually reversible after withdrawal of the causative drug. Other triggering factors include UV radiation exposure, hepatitis B infection, dietary factors such as garlic, and vitamin D.[183] Paraneoplastic pemphigus is antigenically distinct from pemphigus vulgaris, and it is associated with underlying malignancies.[126]

In approximately 60% of patients with pemphigus vulgaris, the oral lesions are the first sign of the disease. The lesions may herald the dermatologic involvement by a year or more.[117,173]

KEY FACT

Pemphigus vulgaris (PV) is a severe autoimmune mucocutaneous disease that warrants immediate referral to a dermatologist or rheumatologist. This condition is potentially lethal if left untreated. Direct and indirect immunofluorescence studies along with H&E staining of biopsy specimens are used to diagnose PV. Systemic steroids are indicated to treat it.

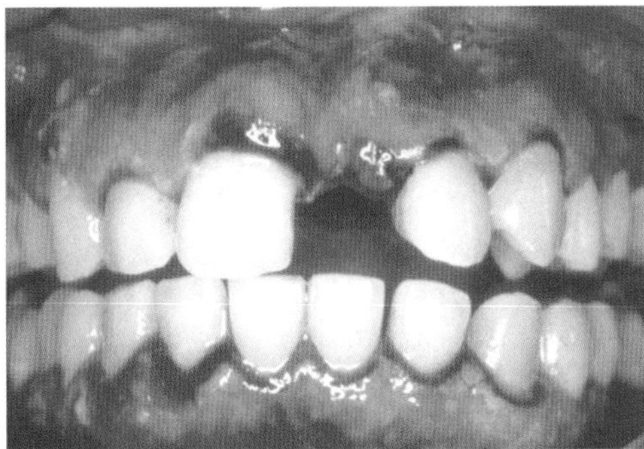

Fig. 18.19 Patient with pemphigus vulgaris confined to the gingivae. Clinically diagnosed as consistent with desquamative gingivitis. (*Courtesy Dr. Beatriz Aldape, Faculty of Odontology, National Autonomous University of Mexico, Mexico City, Mexico.*)

Oral Lesions

Oral lesions can range from small vesicles to large bullae. When the bullae rupture, they leave extensive areas of ulceration (Fig. 18.19). Virtually any region of the oral cavity can be involved, but multiple lesions often develop at sites of irritation or trauma. The soft palate is most often involved (80%), followed by the buccal mucosa (46%), the ventral aspect or dorsum of the tongue (20%), and the lower labial mucosa (10%). Oral lesions of pemphigus vulgaris are confined less often to the gingival tissues.[91] In these patients, erosive gingivitis or desquamative gingivitis is the sole manifestation of oral pemphigus.

Histopathology

The lesions of pemphigus demonstrate a characteristic intraepithelial separation that occurs above the basal cell layer. The intraepithelial vesiculation begins as a microscopic alteration (Fig. 18.20) and gradually results in a grossly visible, fluid-filled bulla. Occasionally, the entire superficial layers of epithelium are lost, leaving behind only the basal cells attached to the underlying lamina propria and conferring a characteristic tombstone appearance to the epithelial cells.

Acantholysis, which involves the separation of the epithelial cells of the lower stratum spinosum, takes place. It is characterized by round rather than polyhedral epithelial cells. The intercellular bridges are lost, and the nuclei are large and hyperchromatic.[40,97,194] The underlying connective tissue usually has a mild to moderate, chronic inflammatory cell infiltrate. As the vesicle or bulla ruptures, the ulcerated lesion becomes infiltrated with polymorphonuclear leukocytes, and the surface may show suppuration.

Immunofluorescence

Autoantibodies can be demonstrated in the oral mucosa of patients with oral pemphigus with the use of immunofluorescence techniques. For direct immunofluorescence, perilesional unfixed frozen sections are incubated with fluorescein-labeled human anti-IgG. For indirect immunofluorescence, unfixed frozen sections of oral or esophageal mucosa from an animal such as a monkey are first incubated with the patient's serum to allow attachment of serum antibodies to the mucosal tissue. The tissue is then incubated with fluorescein-labeled antihuman IgG serum. The test result is positive if immunofluorescence is observed in the intercellular spaces of the stratified squamous epithelium of the mucosa (Fig. 18.21).

The indirect technique is less sensitive than the direct technique, and it may be negative during the early stages of the disease, particularly in its localized forms (see Table 18.1). In most cases, however, the indirect immunofluorescence titers are helpful for monitoring of disease activity, and they have prognostic value.

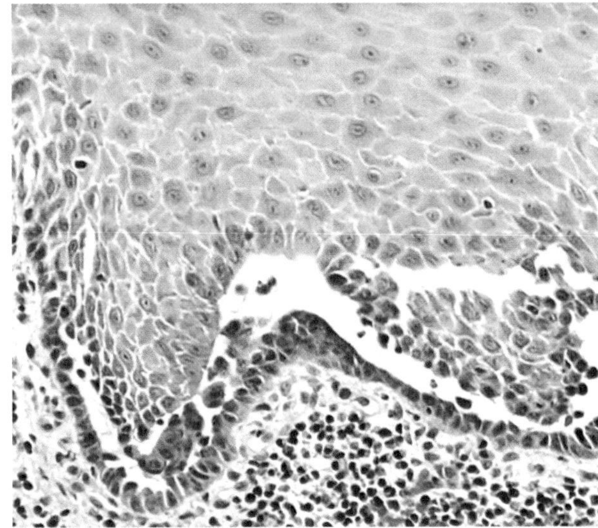

Fig. 18.20 Microscopic features of pemphigus vulgaris include typical intraepithelial clefting with a tombstone appearance of the basal cells, which remain attached to the subjacent basement membrane and fibrous connective tissue. Acantholysis of epithelial cells with the formation of Tzanck cells is seen in the intraepithelial cleft. (Hematoxylin and eosin stain; original magnification ×100.)

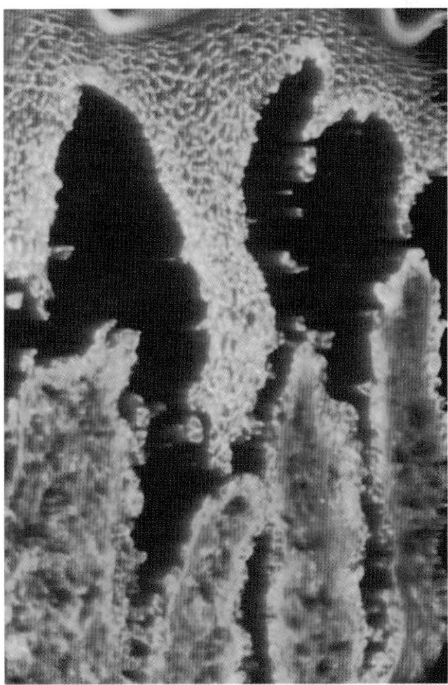

Fig. 18.21 Direct immunofluorescence staining of an oral pemphigus specimen shows the positive intercellular signal for immunoglobulin G deposits in keratinocytes of the stratified squamous epithelium.

Differential Diagnosis

The oral lesions of pemphigus vulgaris may be similar to those seen in EM. In patients with EM, however, recurrent active episodes of comparatively short duration are followed by long intervals that are free of skin and oral lesions. EM affects the lips with considerable severity. Microscopic examination with conventional H&E and direct immunofluorescence can discriminate between the oral lesions of pemphigus and those of EM. Pemphigus vulgaris shows characteristic intraepithelial clefting at the basal–spinous cell layers and interface with acantholysis, whereas EM shows microvesiculation of the superficial epithelial layers and numerous necrotic keratinocytes. Pemphigus vulgaris shows an intercellular and intraepithelial signal with direct immunofluorescence; EM exhibits negative immunofluorescence.

Pemphigoid may clinically resemble pemphigus. Microscopic examination and direct immunofluorescence studies are needed to establish a correct diagnosis. Bullous pemphigoid and MMP exhibit detachment of the epithelium from the underlying connective tissue (i.e., lifting off) rather than the acantholytic lesion characteristic of pemphigus.

Bullous lichen planus must also be considered during the differential diagnosis. The primary lesion of pemphigus may have a bullous character, and this may be followed by erosion, with its associated pain and discomfort. In patients with lichen planus, the characteristic reticular lesions are invariably associated with the bullae. Microscopic examination and direct immunofluorescence studies are necessary to differentiate this condition from pemphigus. Bullous lichen planus shows separation of the epithelium from the underlying fibrous connective tissue, sawtooth rete pegs, and a bandlike chronic inflammatory infiltrate in the lamina propria. Direct immunofluorescence reveals linear fibrillar deposits of fibrin in the basement membrane of bullous lichen planus, whereas pemphigus vulgaris has intercellular immunoglobulin deposition in the epithelium.

If the oral lesions of pemphigus vulgaris are restricted to the gingival tissues, erosive lichen planus, pemphigoid, LAD, and chronic ulcerative stomatitis should be ruled out.

Treatment

Guidelines for the treatment of pemphigus vulgaris are available.[81,115] The main therapy for pemphigus vulgaris is systemic corticosteroids with or without the addition of other immunosuppressive agents.[173] If the patient responds well to corticosteroids, the dosage can be gradually reduced, but a low maintenance dosage is usually necessary to prevent or minimize the recurrence of lesions. Many dermatologists monitor the dose of steroids by periodic evaluation of the titers of DSG3 and DSG1 antibodies. Increasing titers are often associated with an impending exacerbation and warrant an increase of the steroid dose. A decrease in titer justifies a reduction of the steroid dose.[27]

In patients who are not responsive to corticosteroids or who gradually adapt to them, steroid-sparing therapies are used. They are combinations of steroids plus other medications (e.g., azathioprine, cyclophosphamide, cyclosporine, dapsone, gold, methotrexate), as well as photoplasmapheresis and plasmapheresis.[130] The biologic Rituximab is used as an adjunct to treat pemphigus vulgaris.[29,54,163] However, when used in early stages of the disease, it may induce complete remission.[48,72]

The maintenance phase aims to control the disease with the lowest dose of medication. To minimize the risk of morbidity associated with the long-term use of steroids, alternate-day steroid therapy, steroid-sparing drugs, and topical steroids can be combined. Because topical steroids may promote the development of candidiasis, topical antifungal medication may also be needed.[108]

Minimization of oral irritation is important for patients with oral pemphigus vulgaris. Optimal oral hygiene is essential because there is usually widespread involvement of the marginal and attached gingivae and of other areas of the mouth, which can be exacerbated by plaque-associated gingivitis and periodontitis. Periodontal care is an important issue in the overall management of patients with pemphigus vulgaris. To prevent flare-ups, patients in the maintenance phase should receive prednisone before professional oral prophylaxis and periodontal surgery.[150] The fit and design of removable prosthetic appliances should receive special attention because even slight irritation from these prostheses can cause severe inflammation with vesiculation and ulceration.

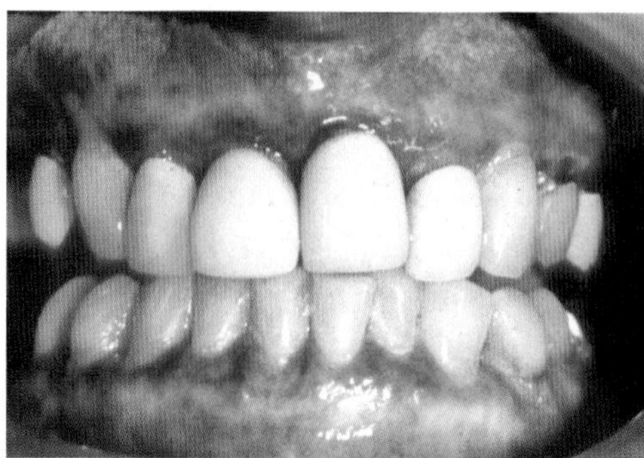

Fig. 18.22 Erythema and ulceration of the gingiva are consistent with a clinical diagnosis of chronic desquamative gingivitis. Direct and indirect immunofluorescence studies demonstrate stratified epithelium–specific antinuclear antibodies. (*Courtesy Dr. Douglas Damm, University of Kentucky, Lexington, KY.*)

Chronic Ulcerative Stomatitis

Chronic ulcerative stomatitis, which was first reported in 1990,[80] manifests with chronic oral ulcerations and has a predilection for women in the fourth decade of life. The erosions and ulcerations occur predominantly in the oral cavity, with only a few cases exhibiting cutaneous lesions.[31,99,192] Circulating specific IgG autoantibodies to ΔNp63α, an epithelial nuclear transcription factor that modulates epithelial cell growth, have been demonstrated.[22]

Oral Lesions

Painful, solitary, small blisters and erosions with surrounding erythema occur mainly on the buccal mucosae followed by the gingiva, tongue, labial mucosa, and the hard palate.[145] Because of the magnitude and clinical features of the gingival lesions, a diagnosis of desquamative gingivitis is considered (Fig. 18.22).

Histopathology

The microscopic features of chronic ulcerative stomatitis are similar to those observed in erosive lichen planus. Hyperkeratosis, acanthosis, and liquefaction of the basal cell layer with areas of subepithelial clefting are prominent features of the epithelium. The underlying lamina propria exhibits an admixture of T lymphocytes and plasma cells in a band-like configuration.[8,145]

Immunofluorescence

Direct immunofluorescence of normal and perilesional tissues reveals typical stratified epithelium–specific antinuclear antibodies (SES-ANA). They are nuclear deposits of IgG with a speckled pattern, and they are found mainly in the basal and parabasal cell layers of the normal epithelium (Fig. 18.23).[145] Deposition of complement 3 has been reported in some cases.[8,145] Fibrin deposits are visualized at the epithelial tissue–connective tissue interface. Indirect immunofluorescence studies involving the use of an esophageal substrate also reveal stratified epithelium–specific antinuclear antibodies.[175]

Diagnosis

Chronic ulcerative stomatitis is clinically similar to erosive lichen planus. Pemphigus vulgaris, MMP, LAD, bullous pemphigoid, and lupus erythematosus also have to be included in the differential diagnosis. Microscopic examination usually reduces the number of possibilities to chronic ulcerative stomatitis, LAD, and erosive lichen planus. Direct and indirect immunofluorescence studies are needed to arrive at the correct diagnosis.[142] An enzyme-linked immunosorbent assay (ELISA) has been developed, which may allow correlation of antibody titers with treatment response.[177]

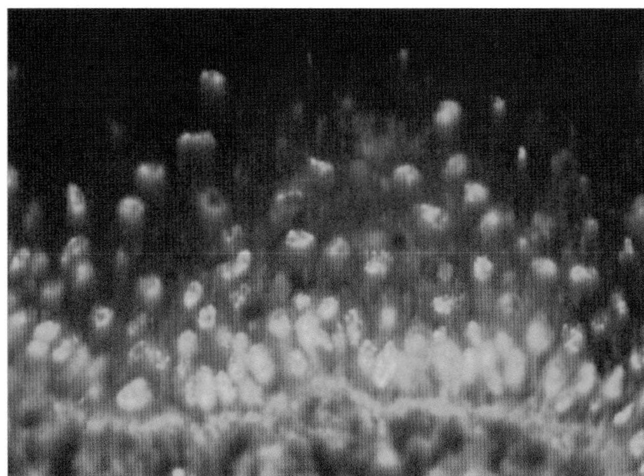

Fig. 18.23 Direct immunofluorescence study of chronic ulcerative stomatitis shows nuclear deposits of immunoglobulin G that are prominent in the basal cell layer and fade toward the superficial layers. (*Courtesy Dr. Douglas Damm, University of Kentucky, Lexington, KY.*)

KEY FACT

Chronic ulcerative stomatitis is an autoimmune condition that mainly affects oral mucosa. Its clinical and histologic features are similar to those of oral lichen planus. Despite the similarities, severe cases of chronic ulcerative stomatitis do not respond to corticosteroid treatment, but they are responsive to hydroxychloroquine.

Treatment

For mild cases, topical steroids (e.g., fluocinonide, clobetasol propionate) and topical tetracycline can produce clinical improvement, but recurrences are common.[102] For severe cases, a high dose of a systemic corticosteroid is needed to achieve remission. Unfortunately, reduction of the corticosteroid dose results in relapse of the lesions. Hydroxychloroquine sulfate at a dosage of 200 to 400 mg/day seems to be the treatment of choice to produce complete, long-lasting remission.[15,33,77,80] However, a long-term follow-up study demonstrated that combined therapy (i.e., small doses of corticosteroids and chloroquine) might be required because the initial good response to chloroquine ceases after several months or years of treatment.[31]

Linear Immunoglobulin A Disease

LAD (i.e., linear IgA dermatosis) is an uncommon mucocutaneous disorder with a predilection for women. The etiopathogenic aspects of LAD are not fully understood, although drug-induced LAD triggered by angiotensin-converting enzyme inhibitors and angioimmunoblastic T-cell lymphoma associated with LAD have been reported.[39,59]

LAD manifests as a pruritic vesiculobullous rash, usually during middle age or later, although younger individuals may also be affected. Characteristic plaques or crops with an annular manifestation surrounded by a peripheral rim of blisters affect the skin of the upper and lower trunk, the shoulders, the groin, and the lower limbs. The face and perineum may also be affected. Mucosal involvement, including that of the oral mucosa, ranges from 50% to 100% of the cases published.[25,35,82]

LAD can mimic lichen planus clinically and histologically. Immunofluorescence studies are needed to establish the correct diagnosis.[165]

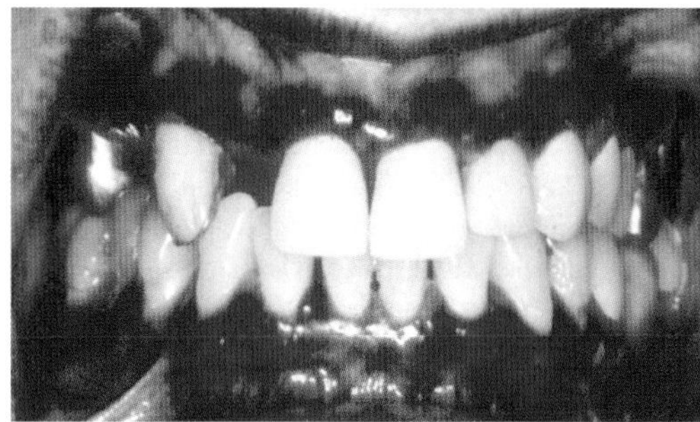

Fig. 18.24 In a patient with linear immunoglobulin A disease, intense erythema and ulceration of the gingiva are consistent with a diagnosis of desquamative gingivitis.

Oral Lesions

Oral manifestations of LAD consist of vesicles, painful ulcerations or erosions, and erosive gingivitis or cheilitis. The hard and soft palates are affected more often; the tonsillar pillars, buccal mucosa, tongue, and gingiva follow in frequency. Rarely, oral lesions may be the only manifestation of LAD for several years before cutaneous lesions occur.[21] The oral lesions of LAD have been clinically reported as desquamative gingivitis (Fig. 18.24).[45,134,139,140]

Histopathology

The microscopic features of LAD are similar to those observed with erosive lichen planus.

Immunofluorescence

Linear deposits of IgA are observed at the epithelial tissue–connective tissue interface.[188] They are different from the granular pattern that is observed with DH.

Differential Diagnosis

The differential diagnosis of LAD includes erosive lichen planus, chronic ulcerative stomatitis, pemphigus vulgaris, bullous pemphigoid, and lupus erythematosus. Microscopic examination and immunofluorescence studies are necessary to establish the correct diagnosis.

Treatment

The primary treatment of LAD involves a combination of sulfones and dapsone. Small amounts of prednisone (10 to 30 mg/day) can be added if the initial response is inadequate.[30] Alternatively, tetracycline (2 g/day) in combination with nicotinamide (1.5 g/day) has shown promising results.[135] Mycophenolate (500 mg twice daily) in combination with prednisolone (30 mg/day) resulted in the resolution of the refractory ulcerations associated with LAD.[100]

Dermatitis Herpetiformis

DH is a chronic condition characterized by severe pruritus in the skin resulting from an inflammatory response to gluten ingestion. DH usually develops in young adults between the ages of 20 and 30 years, and it has a slight predilection for men.[51] Evidence indicates that DH is a cutaneous manifestation of celiac disease, a gluten sensitivity enteropathy. Approximately 25% of patients with celiac disease have DH. The cause of celiac disease is obscure, but tissue transglutaminase seems to be the predominant autoantigen in the intestine, the skin, and sometimes the mucosae.[37] Tissue transglutaminase (TG3) immunoglobulin A targets tissue transglutaminases TG3 (papillary dermis of DH patients) and TG-2 (celiac disease patients) to form deposits in the skin and small bowel.[38,83] Circulating antibodies are also present in these patients.[83,147] Gluten enteropathy can be severe in about two-thirds of patients, and it is mild or subclinical in the remaining one-third. In severe cases, patients may complain of dysphagia, weakness, diarrhea, and weight loss.[83,111] Autoimmune thyroiditis, Sjogren's syndrome, and bullous pemphigoid have also been associated with DH.[5]

Clinically, DH manifests with bilateral and symmetric pruritic papules or vesicles that are primarily restricted to the extensor surfaces of the extremities. The sacrum, the buttocks, and occasionally the face and oral cavity can be affected.[17,51]

The term herpetic is derived from the initial manifestation of the disease, in which clusters of vesicles or papules arise on the skin. These vesicles or papules eventually resolve and are followed by hyperpigmentation of the skin, which ultimately wanes. The oral lesions of DH range from painful ulcerations preceded by the collapse of ephemeral vesicles or bullae to erythematous lesions.[129]

Histopathology

Microscopic examination of the initial lesions of DH reveals focal aggregates of neutrophils and eosinophils among deposits of fibrin at the apices of the dermal pegs.[195]

Immunofluorescence

Direct immunofluorescence demonstrates IgA and C3 at the dermal papillary apices in both perilesional tissue and normal, uninvolved tissue. In contrast, biopsies taken from lesional sites may fail to exhibit IgA or C3, producing false-negative results.[195] Although no circulating autoantibodies to epithelial basement membrane occur in DH, almost 80% of patients have anti-endomysial and gliadin antibodies.[16]

Treatment

A gluten-free diet is essential for the treatment of celiac disease and DH. Oral dapsone is usually needed for patients with newly detected DH to alleviate symptoms promptly.[21,37]

Lupus Erythematosus

Lupus erythematosus is an autoimmune disease with three clinical presentations: systemic, chronic cutaneous, and subacute cutaneous.

Systemic Lupus Erythematosus

Systemic lupus erythematosus (SLE) is a severe disease with a 10:1 predilection for women compared to men. SLE can affect the kidneys, heart, skin, and mucosa. The classic cutaneous lesions characterized by a rash on the malar area with a butterfly distribution are uncommon (Fig. 18.25).[41] The oral lesions of SLE are usually ulcerative or similar to those of lichen planus. Oral ulcerations occur in 36% of patients with SLE. In about 4% of patients, hyperkeratotic plaques reminiscent of lichen planus appear on the buccal mucosa and palate.[19]

Direct immunofluorescence of the perilesional and normal tissue reveals immunoglobulins and C3 deposits at the dermal-epidermal interface. Antinuclear antibodies are detected in more than 95% of cases, whereas deoxyribonucleic acid and extractable nuclear antigen antibodies are found in more than 50% of patients (see Table 18.1).

Chronic Cutaneous Lupus Erythematosus

Chronic cutaneous lupus erythematosus usually has no systemic signs or symptoms; lesions are limited to the skin or the mucosal surfaces. The skin lesions are referred to as discoid lupus erythematosus (DLE). DLE describes the chronic scarring, atrophy-producing lesion that may develop into hyperpigmentation or hypopigmentation of the healing area (Fig. 18.26). In the oral cavity, about 9% of patients with chronic cutaneous lupus erythematosus have lichen-planus–like plaques on the palate and the buccal mucosa.[6,19] The gingiva may be affected, and the condition can manifest as desquamative gingivitis (Fig. 18.27).

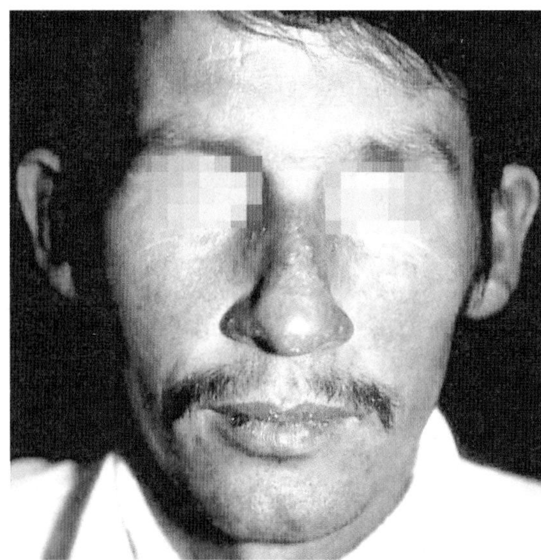

Fig. 18.25 Systemic lupus erythematosus produces erythema on the bridge of the nose with a butterfly pattern. (*Courtesy Department of Dermatology, Hospital General Manuel Gea González, Mexico City, Mexico.*)

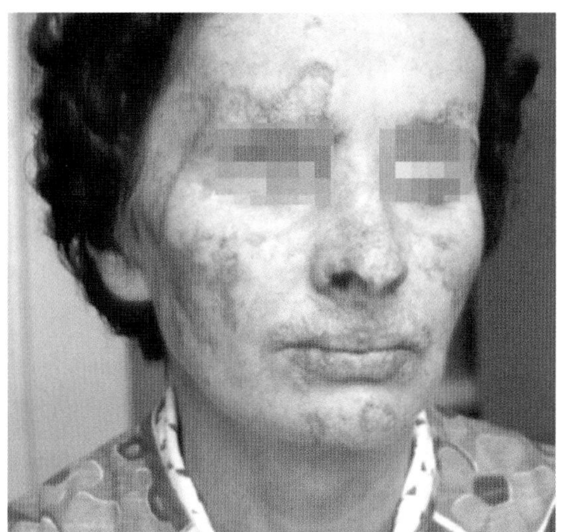

Fig. 18.26 In a patient with chronic cutaneous lupus erythematosus, there are multiple facial lesions with irregular hyperpigmented borders, some of which exhibit central scarring with cutaneous atrophy. Other lesions consist of hyperpigmented cutaneous patches.

Histopathology

The histopathology of the oral lesions of chronic cutaneous lupus erythematosus consists of hyperkeratosis, alternating acanthosis and atrophy, and hydropic degeneration of the basal layer of the epithelium. The lamina propria exhibits a chronic inflammatory cell infiltrate similar to that observed with lichen planus. However, a more diffuse and deeper inflammatory infiltrate with a perivascular pattern is typically observed.[169]

Immunofluorescence

Direct immunofluorescence study of lesional tissue reveals immunoglobulins and C3 deposits at the dermal-epidermal junction of the lesional or perilesional tissue but not in normal tissue. This seems to differentiate SLE from DLE. The indirect immunofluorescence

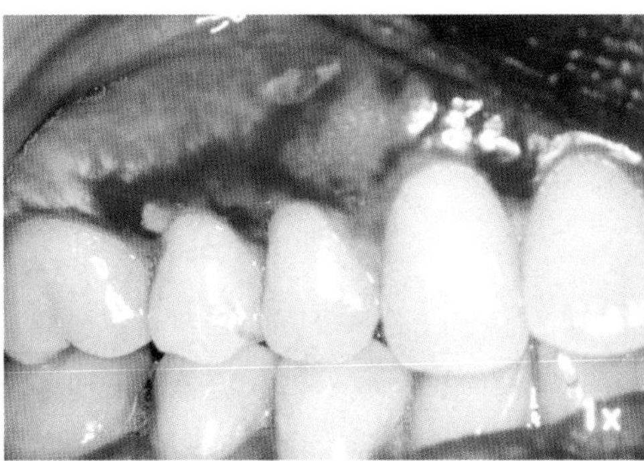

Fig. 18.27 Lupus erythematosus of the oral cavity can manifest as desquamative gingivitis. Intense erythema with ulceration is bordered by white radial lines. (*Courtesy Dr. Stuart L. Fischman, State University of New York at Buffalo, NY.*)

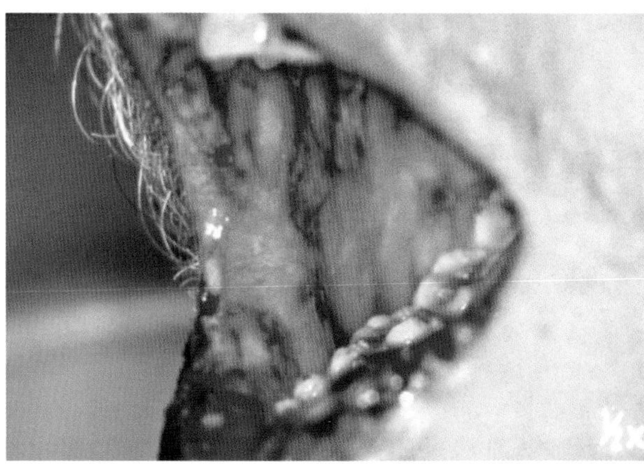

Fig. 18.28 In a patient with erythema multiforme, large, shallow, and painful ulcers involve the labial and buccal mucosae. Hemorrhagic crusting of the mandibular vermilion border of the lips is observed. (*Courtesy Dr. Stuart L. Fischman, State University of New York at Buffalo, NY.*)

method reveals antinuclear antibodies in more than 95% of patients, whereas deoxyribonucleic acid and extractable nuclear antigen circulating antibodies are found in more than 50% of patients.

Subacute Cutaneous Lupus Erythematosus

Patients with subacute cutaneous lupus erythematosus have cutaneous lesions that are similar to those of DLE but that lack the development of scarring and atrophy.[20] Arthritis and arthralgia, low-grade fever, malaise, and myalgia can occur in up to 50% of patients with subacute cutaneous lupus erythematosus.[20,181]

Direct immunofluorescence reveals immunoglobulins and C3 deposits at the dermal-epidermal junction in 60% of cases and granular IgG deposits in the cytoplasm of basal cells in 30% of cases. About 80% of patients with subacute cutaneous lupus erythematosus have Ro (SSA) antibodies to nuclear antigens, whereas 25% to 30% have La (SSB) antibodies to nuclear antigens. The test result for rheumatoid factor is positive in about 30% of these patients, positive for antinuclear antibodies in 60% to 90%, and positive for anti-ribonucleoprotein antibodies to nuclear antigens in 10% (see Table 18.1).

Differential Diagnosis

Erosive lichen planus, EM, and pemphigus vulgaris can simulate the lesions observed in patients with lupus erythematosus. The diagnosis of DLE confined to the oral cavity is difficult to make, but microscopic studies may suggest the characteristic histopathology.[4] Biopsy studies (i.e., H&E and direct immunofluorescence) help to differentiate lupus erythematosus from other erosive diseases.

Treatment

Therapy for SLE depends on the severity and extent of the disease. It can range from topical steroids to nonsteroidal anti-inflammatory drugs to moderate to high doses of prednisone for severe systemic organ involvement. Immunosuppressive drugs (e.g., cytotoxic agents such as cyclophosphamide and azathioprine) and plasmapheresis alone or with steroids can be useful.[130] Rituximab has produced dramatic, long-term remissions.[41] For chronic cutaneous lupus erythematosus, topical steroids are effective to manage the cutaneous and oral lesions. For patients whose disease is resistant to topical therapy, systemic antimalarial drugs can be used with good results.[128] For a comprehensive review of current management strategies and future directions for SLE, the reader is encouraged to consult Durcan's 2019 paper.[50]

Erythema Multiforme

EM is an acute bullous and macular inflammatory mucocutaneous disease that affects mainly young adults between the ages of 20 and 40 years; it is rarely seen in children (≤20%).[157] The genesis of the mucocutaneous lesions is thought to reside in the development of immune complex vasculitis. This is followed by complement fixation that leads to the leukocytoclastic destruction of vascular walls and small vessel occlusion. The culmination of these events produces ischemic necrosis of the epithelium and underlying connective tissue.[56]

Target (i.e., iris) lesions with central clearing are the hallmark of EM. It can be a mild (i.e., EM minor) or a severe and possibly life-threatening condition (i.e., EM major or Stevens–Johnson syndrome). An underdiagnosed type of EM is recurrent oral erythema multiforme (ROEM), with which most patients have chronic or recurrent oral lesions only.[7,49]

EM minor lasts approximately 4 weeks and exhibits moderate cutaneous and mucosal involvement. Stevens–Johnson syndrome can last a month or longer. It involves the skin, conjunctiva, oral mucosa, and genitalia, and it requires more aggressive therapy than EM minor. Some researchers consider toxic epidermal necrolysis to be the most severe form of EM, but other investigators think they are unrelated entities.[12]

The two most common etiologic factors for the development of EM are herpes simplex infection and drug reactions. Recent reports documented EM major and EM-like lesions in adult and pediatric individuals infected with COVID-19.[47,186] The most common causative drugs of EM are sulfonamides, penicillins, quinolones, chlormezanone, barbiturates, oxicam nonsteroidal anti-inflammatory drugs, anticonvulsant drugs, protease inhibitors, and allopurinol.[57]

Oral lesions in patients with EM are common, and they occur in more than 70% of patients with skin involvement.[58,106,113] In rare instances, EM is confined to the mouth.[7,104,164] The oral lesions consist of multiple, large, shallow, painful ulcers with an erythematous border. They affect the entire oral mucosa in approximately 20% of patients with EM. The lesions are so painful that chewing and swallowing are impaired (Fig. 18.28). The buccal mucosa and the tongue are the most frequently affected sites, followed by the labial mucosa. Areas that are less often affected include the floor of the mouth, the hard and soft palates, and the gingiva.[58] EM is rarely confined exclusively to the gingival tissues, prompting a clinical diagnosis of desquamative gingivitis.[11] Hemorrhagic crusting of the vermilion border of the lips may occur, which is helpful for arriving at a clinical diagnosis of EM.

Histopathology

Common microscopic findings of EM include the liquefaction degeneration of the upper epithelium and development of intraepithelial microvesicles without the acantholysis that occurs with pemphigus.[168] Acanthosis, pseudoepitheliomatous hyperplasia, and necrotic keratinocytes are observed in the epithelium. Degenerative changes also occur in the basement membrane. In some cases, the junction between the epithelium and the lamina propria is indistinct because of a dense inflammatory cell infiltrate. Edema of the lamina propria, vascular dilation, and congestion also occur. Deeper layers of the connective tissue stroma exhibit a perivascular chronic inflammatory cell infiltrate. However, neutrophils and eosinophils may also be seen.

Immunofluorescence

The immunofluorescence examination result is negative for patients with EM. Its value resides in ruling out other vesiculobullous and ulcerative disorders.

Treatment

There is no specific treatment for EM. For mild symptoms, systemic and local antihistamines, topical anesthetics, and debridement of lesions with an oxygenating agent are adequate. In patients with bullous or ulcerative lesions and severe symptoms, corticosteroids are considered the drug of choice, although their use is controversial and not completely accepted.[57]

Drug-Related Eruptions

An increase in the incidence of skin and oral manifestations of hypersensitivity to drugs occurred with the advent of sulfonamides, barbiturates, and various antibiotics. The cutaneous and oral lesions are attributed to the drug acting as an allergen that sensitizes the tissues.

Eruptions in the oral cavity that result from sensitivity to drugs that have been taken orally or parenterally are called stomatitis medicamentosa. The local reaction from the use of a medicament in the oral cavity (e.g., stomatitis resulting from topical penicillin use) is referred to as stomatitis venenata or contact stomatitis. In many cases, skin eruptions accompany the oral lesions.

Most drug eruptions in the oral cavity are multiform. Vesicular and bullous lesions occur most often, but pigmented or nonpigmented macular lesions are also frequently observed. Erosions, which are often followed by deep ulceration with purpuric lesions, can occur. The lesions are seen in different areas of the oral cavity, with the gingiva often being affected.[1,66]

The development of gingival lesions caused by contact allergy to the mercurial compounds in dental amalgam has been documented.[89] Because of financial considerations, biopsy and patch testing may be indicated before the indiscriminate replacement of dental amalgam restorations. Similarly, desquamative gingivitis has been reported with the use of tartar control toothpaste. Pyrophosphates and flavoring agents have been identified as the main causative agents of this unusual condition.[46] Oral reactions to cinnamon compounds (i.e., cinnamon oil, cinnamic acid, or cinnamic aldehyde) that are used to mask the taste of pyrophosphates in tartar control toothpaste include an intense erythema of the attached gingival tissues that is characteristic of plasma cell gingivitis (Fig. 18.29).[3,90]

A thorough clinical history usually discloses the source of gingival disturbance. Elimination of the offending agent (i.e., tartar control toothpaste) leads to resolution of the gingival lesions within a week, and challenge with the offending agent leads to recurrence of the oral lesions. If removal of the offending medication is not possible, topical corticosteroids and topical tacrolimus can be used to treat the lesions.[78]

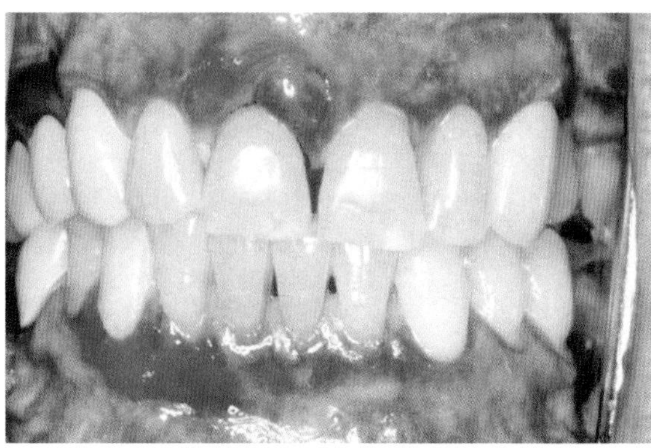

Fig. 18.29 Plasma cell gingivitis. The gingiva presents a band of moderate to severe inflammation that is reminiscent of desquamative gingivitis.

CLINICAL CORRELATION

Diseases That Mimic Desquamative Gingivitis

- Squamous cell carcinoma
- Wegener granulomatosis (strawberry gingivitis)
- Candidiasis
- Graft-versus-host disease
- Crohn's disease
- Foreign body gingivitis

Miscellaneous Conditions That Mimic Desquamative Gingivitis

Another group of heterogeneous conditions may masquerade as desquamative gingivitis. Factitious lesions, candidiasis, graft-versus-host disease, Wegener granulomatosis, foreign body gingivitis, Kindler syndrome, and squamous cell carcinoma can divert the attention of the clinician and provide a diagnostic challenge.

Factitious lesions are injuries that are consciously and intentionally produced without a clear motive, although guilt, seeking sympathy, or monetary compensation can be the driving forces for this abnormal behavior. Factitious desquamative gingivitis has been reported in the literature; it may be difficult to diagnose, and it may become apparent only after extensive and costly laboratory tests fail to reveal the genesis of the lesions.[114]

Candidiasis is rarely limited to the gingival tissues and can simulate desquamative gingivitis. Linear gingival erythema is a Candida-associated lesion in individuals who are infected with human immunodeficiency virus. It manifests as a ribbon-like red band of the gingival margins and is reminiscent of desquamative gingivitis.[154]

Graft-versus-host disease can occur in recipients of allogenic bone marrow transplants. The associated oral lesions occasionally resemble desquamative gingivitis (eFig. 18.1).

Wegener granulomatosis is a systemic disease that can manifest with striking alterations that are confined to the gingival tissues. Classically, the gingival tissues exhibit erythema and enlargement, and they are typically described as strawberry gums (eFig. 18.2).[36]

Foreign body gingivitis is clinically characterized by red or red and white chronic lesions that can be painful and that are reminiscent of desquamative gingivitis. This condition is more common among women approaching the fifth decade of life. Microscopic analysis reveals small (<5 μm in diameter) foreign bodies associated with a chronic inflammatory cell response that can exhibit granulomatous and lichenoid characteristics. Energy-dispersive radiographic microanalysis revealed that most of these foreign bodies originate from dental materials (i.e., abrasives, and restorative materials).[70,71]

Kindler syndrome, which involves cutaneous neonatal bullae, poikiloderma, photosensitivity, and acral atrophy, can manifest with oral lesions that are clinically consistent with desquamative gingivitis.[148]

A clinical diagnosis of desquamative gingivitis requires a series of diagnostic steps before a precise diagnosis can be obtained. The steps include a comprehensive clinical history, clinical-pathologic correlation, microscopic examination (e.g., H&E), and direct immunofluorescence studies.[180] The failure to systematically evaluate a patient with a clinical condition that is consistent with desquamative gingivitis can produce poor outcomes. This is particularly true when therapy for a putative desquamative gingivitis is established before a biopsy of the lesional tissue is obtained. Every year, in our laboratory, we see at least two examples of clinically diagnosed desquamative gingivitis for which microscopic and immunofluorescence studies were not performed to rule out the cause of the gingival lesions. The patients were monitored or prescribed topical steroids for several months before the lack of response of the gingival lesions impelled the clinician to obtain a biopsy, which revealed squamous cell carcinoma.[182] Clinicians should be alert to the possibility of squamous cell carcinoma of the gingival tissues with lesions that initially manifest as desquamative gingivitis.

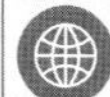
A Case Scenario is found on the companion website eBooks.Health.Elsevier.com.

References for this chapter are found on the companion website eBooks.Health.Elsevier.com.

CHAPTER 19

Gingival Enlargement and Management

Alpdogan Kantarci | Julie Teresa Marchesan | Kimon Divaris

CHAPTER OUTLINE

Inflammation of the periodontal tissues results in three outcomes: complete resolution of inflammation and restoration of tissue integrity (i.e., homeostasis), destruction of periodontal tissues, and loss of attachment (i.e., periodontitis) or fibrosis. A change in the dimensions of gingival tissue is *always* a pathologic event. Gingival enlargement can be transient and reversible or can be chronic and irreversible. Enlargement of the keratinized gingiva, a distinct group of pathologies leading to the overgrowth of the gingival structures and collectively known as "gingival enlargement," can manifest with various clinical characteristics. Fibrosis is mechanistically analogous to defense mechanisms at play against the progression of periodontal inflammation. During this process, fibroblasts stimulated by the presence of fibrin, growth factors, and cytokines may generate excessive amounts of collagen and noncollagenous proteins of the extracellular matrix. If this excessive matrix deposition is not sufficiently balanced by the enzymatic degradation of the matrix composition (e.g., collagen type I) by the matrix metalloproteinases (MMPs) and their tissue inhibitors (TIMPs), it can result in fibrotic changes of the soft tissues. In contrast to other tissues in which fibrosis is observed, gingival lesions present with clinical inflammation due to biofilm accumulation. In addition, maintenance of optimal oral hygiene is impaired due to disrupted tissue architecture. Thus, the gingival overgrowth lesions involve complex infecto-inflammatory pathogenetic mechanisms and are unique in their clinical manifestations.

Pathologic enlargements of gingival tissues were identified and linked to systemic conditions as early as the 18th century. Most common forms of gingival enlargement result from systemic use of medications. The first scientific report on drug-induced gingival overgrowth (DIGO) was published in 1939 when the anticonvulsant diphenylhydantoin was associated with gingival enlargement.[60] Later studies provided significant insights into the complex molecular and cellular mechanisms underlying gingival enlargement. Because many forms of gingival enlargement are related to systemic factors and conditions, understanding the pathogenesis of these clinical conditions is essential for designing better approaches to management, treatment, and optimizing care. This chapter discusses the clinical, etiologic, and pathologic aspects of gingival enlargement that are used to develop novel and targeted approaches to therapy. Neoplastic enlargements of gingival tissues associated with benign or malignant oral cancers are not covered in depth because this emerging field of oral pathology has evolved beyond the scope of this chapter and can be found in oral pathology textbooks that provide extensive coverage of oral tumors.

Terminology and Classification

Gingival enlargement and *gingival overgrowth* are terms frequently and interchangeably used with *hyperplasia*, *hypertrophy*, and *fibrosis*. **Hyperplasia** is an increase in the number of cells in tissues that results in increased tissue volume. **Hypertrophy** refers to increased tissue size and volume resulting from increased cell size. Although their pathogenetic mechanisms are different, hyperplasia and hypertrophy occur simultaneously when cellular involvement in hyperplasia triggers overgrowth. Therefore, all these processes are closely linked. **Fibrosis** is a pathologic process in which aberrant wound healing is associated with defective cell proliferation, cell-to-cell interactions, cell-to-matrix interactions, matrix deposition, and impaired immune system response. Thus, fibrosis can be defined as a pathologic lesion, whereas hyperplasia and hypertrophy can be viewed as pathologic processes. In gingival tissues, these processes are associated with various phases of inflammation. Hyperplastic, hypertrophic, and fibrotic changes are observed during gingival enlargement and cannot be accurately differentiated. Therefore, this chapter uses *gingival overgrowth* (GO) or *gingival enlargement* to refer to all pathologic forms in periodontal tissues.

Classification of GO is based on its etiologic factors. In its most common form, GO can result from inflammatory changes due to gingivitis, such as those seen in young patients undergoing orthodontic treatment. Gingivitis-related GO is reversible by restoring proper oral hygiene. More complex and fibrotic forms of GO result from the systemic use of medications and are collectively referred to as *drug-induced gingival overgrowth (DIGO)*. To date, three families of drugs were identified as etiological factors that can lead to DIGO: anticonvulsants, calcium channel blockers, and immunosuppressants. GO can also be associated with genetic syndromes, severe systemic diseases such as leukemia, and genetic mutations. Any form that cannot be classified among these GO forms is known as idiopathic GO. Enlargement of the gingiva can also be indirectly associated with changes in the dimensions of underlying osseous structures. Although not covered in depth in this chapter, neoplastic lesions in the oral cavity can manifest with fibrotic lesions and appear clinically similar to other GO forms. Regardless of the cause, all forms of gingival enlargement have distinct pathologic characteristics that should be carefully considered during their diagnosis, management, treatment, and maintenance. Since the underlying cause could be associated with non-dental conditions, GO lesions have a high recurrence potential. Therefore, it is important to identify the cause and contributing etiologic factors leading to different GO forms.

Diagnosis

Because GO is frequently associated with systemic conditions, the patient's general health and relevant drug use should be carefully managed. From the medical perspective, GO is one of the most serious pathologies in periodontal medicine. Therefore, it requires an accurate differential diagnosis to select a therapeutic approach tailored to the patient's systemic health status. Treatment options should be discussed with the patient's medical providers. In cases where the etiologic factor is a drug used for serious systemic reasons (e.g., solid-organ transplantation, epilepsy, cardiovascular diseases), cessation of the drug may not be possible. Therefore, an accurate diagnosis requires a thorough review of the patient's medical history.

Locally, the management of the GO cases is challenging. The excess gingival tissue can cover part or the entire crown of the tooth and can result in diastemas, tooth displacement, or tooth retention. Gingival enlargement can be localized or generalized. Generalized GO can affect marginal gingiva; localized forms can be confined to papillae. Classifications also distinguished between diffuse and discrete enlargements, which are sometimes difficult to differentiate. However, these categorizations can be critical for determining the correct cause of the pathology; therefore, they should be carefully recorded.

Several clinical indices exist for the quantification of the extent and severity of GO. For example, the degree of gingival enlargement can be scored as follows:

- Grade 0: no signs of gingival enlargement
- Grade I: enlargement confined to the interdental papilla
- Grade II: enlargement involves the papilla and marginal gingiva
- Grade III: enlargement covers three-fourths or more of the crown

This classification only focuses on the clinical volume changes with a limited identification of topography. However, it can be a practical method to distinguish the extent of clinical pathology. In addition to the clinical determination of the degree of severity, a more accurate assessment of GO can be made by models cast on the impressions. For example, a technique developed by Seymour and colleagues can be a valuable tool for precise determination of the severity and extent of GO, especially for research purposes and long-term follow-up.[23,35,57,93,101] Other indices used to assess the severity of GO included those developed by Angelopoulos and Goaz[3] and Pernu and coworkers.[81] More recently, three-dimensional scanning has been used to measure GO and compare the treatment outcomes with baseline.[110] There is no perfect and universal index to include all pathological elements of GO applicable to all forms of the pathologies. Therefore, regardless of the method used for measuring the extent and severity of GO lesions, an accurate assessment needs to be made for identifying the inflammatory and fibrotic components. Indices should be chosen based on the practicality of acquiring the necessary data and their utility in aiding clinicians to select the method of therapy (e.g., gingivectomy and gingivoplasty vs. nonsurgical treatment measures) and plan the maintenance phase.

Types of Gingival Enlargement

Inflammatory Enlargement of Gingiva Due to Gingivitis

Clinical Manifestations

All changes in gingival tissues manifest with some degree of inflammation. Gingival enlargement may be a direct outcome of gingivitis without any complicating factors or involvement of systemic conditions. When a patient with gingival enlargement is seen, the initial assessment should be made by careful visual examination of abnormalities of gingival contours, texture, and color, which are compared with normal standards. A detailed medical history should accompany visual inspection to exclude potential systemic factors and conditions. Dental irregularities, dysfunctional habits, and oral hygiene effectiveness should be considered in the evaluation, and clinical measurements should be recorded.

Clinical presentation of the gingivitis-associated inflammatory gingival enlargement can be observed as a slight ballooning of the interdental papilla and marginal gingiva at its initial stages. As it progresses, it involves swelling around the teeth, increasing in size until it covers part of the crowns. Its growth is slow and painless unless it is complicated by infection or trauma (Figs. 19.1 and 19.2). In severe cases, chronic inflammatory GO may present as a discrete sessile or pedunculated mass that resembles a tumor. It can be localized interproximal, on the marginal or attached gingiva, or may be generalized, sometimes presented with painful ulceration.

Etiology

Acute forms of inflammatory enlargement of the gingiva are usually caused by mechanical trauma, chemical or physical irritation, and can be resolved by removing the irritant. Therefore, a local factor should be sought. Mouth breathing, impacted food items, improperly placed or dislodged dental prostheses or appliances, and poor oral hygiene are usually responsible for acute inflammatory reactions in gingival tissues. Acute lesions are typically localized to marginal or papillary gingiva.

KEY FACT

The main etiological factor for acute inflammatory gingival enlargement is trauma. Traumatic lesions occur when a foreign substance (e.g., toothbrush bristle, popcorn kernel) is forcefully embedded into the gingiva, and the resident microbiota complicates the situation. Trauma-induced injuries result in a chronic process characterized by granulation tissue formation and fibrosis.

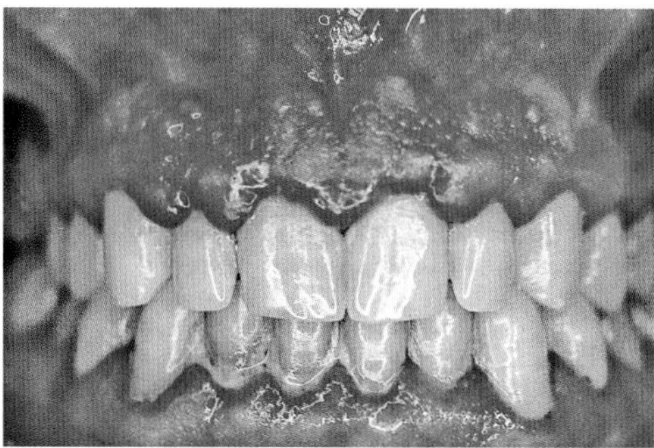

Fig. 19.1 Chronic inflammatory gingival enlargement localized to the anterior region.

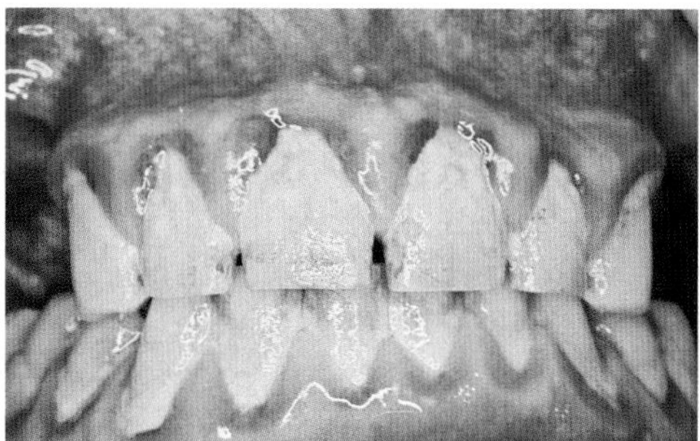

Fig. 19.2 Chronic inflammatory gingival enlargement.

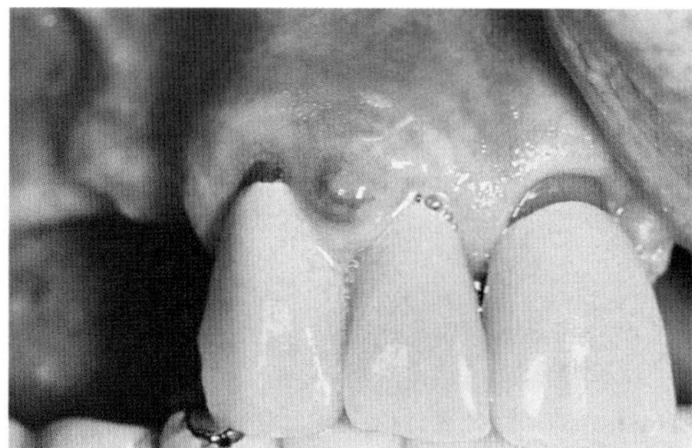

Fig. 19.3 Gingival abscess on the facial gingival surface in the space between the cuspid and the lateral incisor, unrelated to the gingival sulcus.

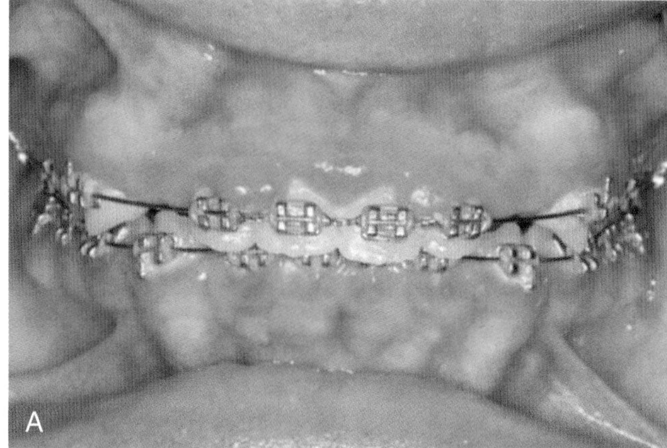

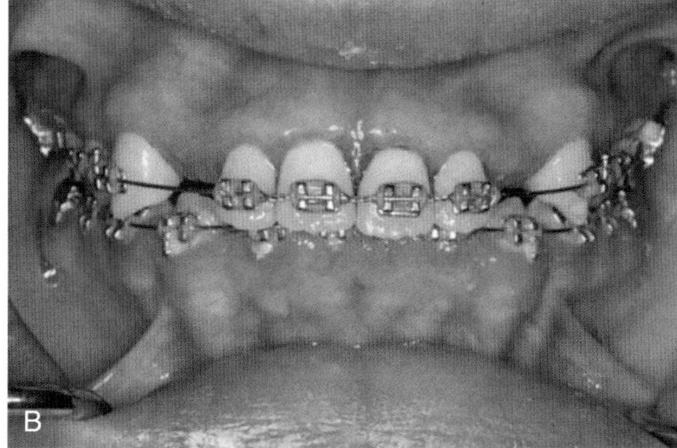

Fig. 19.4 Chronic inflammatory gingival overgrowth in a patient undergoing orthodontic treatment. (A) Baseline at the time when the appliances were placed. (B) After the orthodontic treatment is completed.

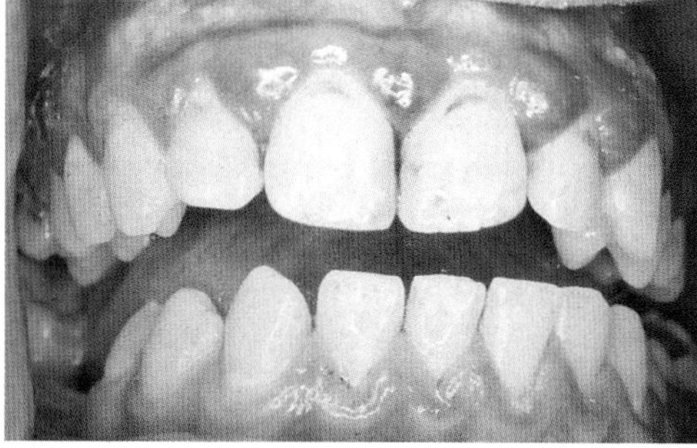

Fig. 19.5 Gingival enlargement in a mouth breather. The lesion is sharply circumscribed in the anterior marginal and papillary areas.

Acute inflammatory enlargement can lead to the formation of a gingival abscess. A gingival abscess is a localized, painful, rapidly expanding lesion (Fig. 19.3). It is typically limited to the marginal gingiva or the interdental papilla. In its early stages, it appears as a red swelling with a smooth, shiny surface. The lesion usually becomes fluctuant and pointed, with a surface orifice and a purulent exudate in 24 to 48 hours. Adjacent teeth may become sensitive to percussion. The lesion usually ruptures spontaneously. Histologically, because it involves an acute inflammatory process, the gingival abscess consists of a purulent exudate of diffuse infiltration of polymorphonuclear leukocytes, edema, and increased vascularization. The surface epithelium has various degrees of intracellular and extracellular edema, invasion by leukocytes, and sometimes ulceration. The lesion is confined to the gingiva to be distinguished from the periodontal abscess.

Chronic inflammatory GO is associated with microbial biofilm. The biofilm can be linked to a lack of proper oral hygiene, orthodontic appliances, faulty restoration margins, misaligned teeth, oral habits, an open bite, or other factors. Factors that favor plaque accumulation and retention include poor oral hygiene, irritation by anatomic abnormalities, and improper restorative and orthodontic appliances (Fig. 19.4).

Chronic gingivitis-associated GO is often seen in patients who are mouth-breathers. The gingiva appears red and edematous, with a diffuse surface shininess of the exposed area. The maxillary anterior region is commonly involved. The altered gingiva is demarcated from the adjacent, unexposed normal gingiva (Fig. 19.5). Irritation from surface dehydration was attributed to mouth breathing. However, comparable changes could not be reproduced by air-drying the gingiva of experimental animals, suggesting that the pathogenesis of mouth breathing–associated gingival changes is far more complex. Nevertheless, the use of animal models in understanding the pathogenesis of this particular pathology should be viewed with caution.

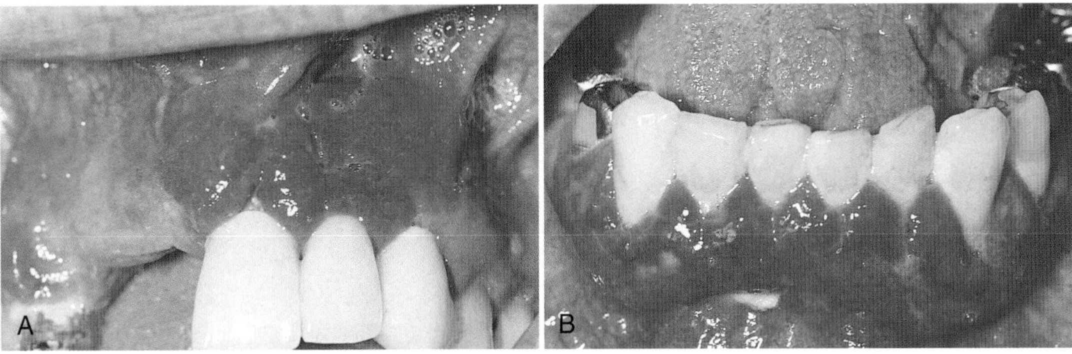

Fig. 19.6 Plasma cell gingivitis. (A) Diffuse lesions on the facial surface of the anterior maxilla. (B) Mandibular lesions. (*Courtesy Dr. Kim D. Zussman, Thousand Oaks, CA.*)

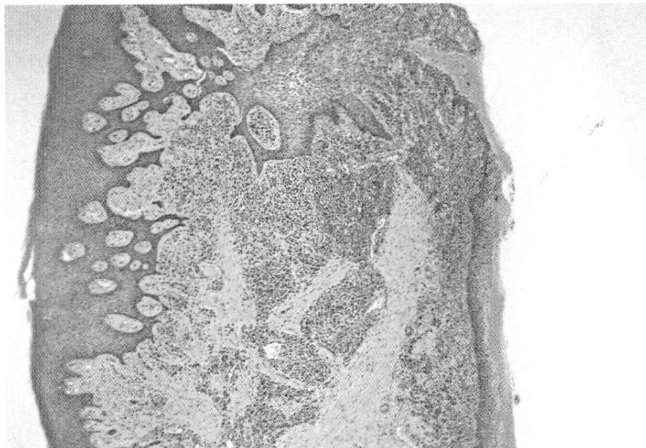

Fig. 19.7 Histological section of chronic inflammatory gingival enlargement shows the inflamed connective tissue core and strands of proliferating epithelium.

Histologically, plasma cells were detected in chronic gingivitis-associated GO cases leading to a definition of "plasma-cell gingivitis." However, it is unclear whether this form of GO is a distinct disease. It manifests as a mild marginal gingival enlargement that extends to the attached gingiva; the gingiva appears red, friable, and sometimes granular. It bleeds easily, and pseudopockets may be present, clinically indistinguishable from common forms of chronic gingivitis-associated GO except for its localization (Fig. 19.6). Plasma cell gingivitis was thought to be allergic in origin and possibly a reaction to chewing gum components, dentifrices, or various dietary items. Cessation of exposure to the allergen brings resolution of the lesion. However, no distinct etiology has been identified, leading to plasma-cell gingivitis.

While acute and chronic gingival enlargements can be associated with gingivitis, inflammatory lesions are observed in other GO forms. Therefore, the distinction should be made very early in treatment planning, the involvement of drugs, systemic conditions, and neoplastic lesions.

Histopathology

Inflammatory enlargement of the gingiva follows the inflammatory process sequence. As discussed, acute forms of the inflammatory GO are commonly due to traumatic factors where a full resolution is accomplished by removing the irritant and restoring oral hygiene. Histologically, inflammatory cell infiltration is observed. Chronic inflammatory GO lesions show the exudative and proliferative features of chronic inflammation (Fig. 19.7). Deep red or bluish-red lesions are soft and friable with a smooth, shiny surface that bleeds easily. They also have a preponderance of inflammatory cells and fluid, along with vascular engorgement, new capillary formation, and associated degenerative changes. Lesions that are relatively firm, resilient, and pink have a greater fibrotic component, with an abundance of fibroblasts and collagen fibers. The oral epithelium shows spongiosis and infiltration with inflammatory cells. Ultrastructurally, there are signs of damage in the lower spinous layers and the basal layers. The underlying connective tissue contains a dense infiltrate of plasma cells that extends to the oral epithelium, producing a dissecting type of injury. In rare instances, marked inflammatory gingival enlargements with a predominance of plasma cells can appear.

Treatment

Chronic enlargement of the gingiva due to gingivitis is reversible and can be resolved by removing the etiologic factors, including controlling the biofilm and any contributing environmental factors. In severe forms of inflammatory enlargement, surgical approaches may be required.

Drug-Induced Overgrowth of Gingiva

The most common forms of DIGO are caused by anticonvulsants, calcium channel blockers, and immunosuppressants prescribed to manage serious conditions. The prevalence of DIGO substantially varies for different medications and among studies. Three drugs associated with DIGO are phenytoin, nifedipine, and cyclosporine. An estimated 30% to 80% of the patients using various medications are at risk for overgrowth lesions. Genetic factors, drug dosage, and local factors can affect the development and severity of DIGO.[92,104]

DIGO is a serious and clinically challenging pathology. It frequently results in impaired oral hygiene, biofilm accumulation, and gingival inflammation. Increased prevalence of gingival infection and inflammation among patients with DIGO poses a risk for the general health of the patients.[20,24,71] Phenytoin, cyclosporine, and nifedipine are being replaced with alternatives. Still, they remain the drugs of choice in many countries to treat epilepsy-associated seizures, prevent organ transplant rejections, and control hypertension. More importantly, alternatives have also been linked to DIGO. To date, about 20 medications have been linked to DIGO. Thus, DIGO associated with medication use continues to be a clinical problem in dentistry and medicine.

DIGO lesions usually develop fast and become chronic over time (Fig. 19.8). The first signs of overgrowth can be observed as early as 3 months of drug use as a localized nodular enlargement of the interdental papilla. Because most of the medications associated with DIGO are prescribed for an extended time, the lesions expand and, in some cases, cover the crowns of the teeth. Severe forms of DIGO may

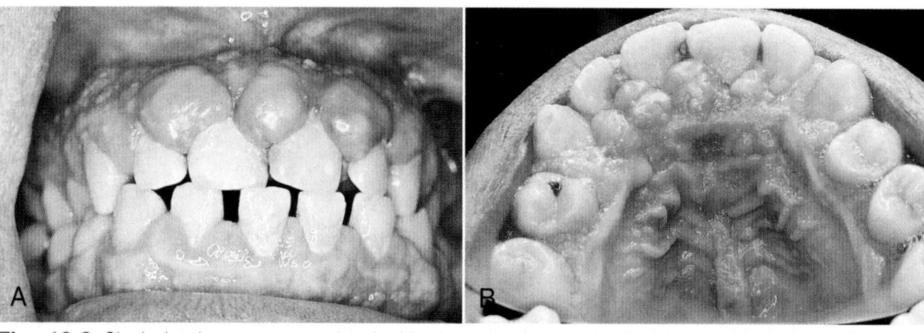

Fig. 19.8 Gingival enlargement associated with phenytoin therapy. (A) Facial view. (B) Occlusal view of the maxillary arch.

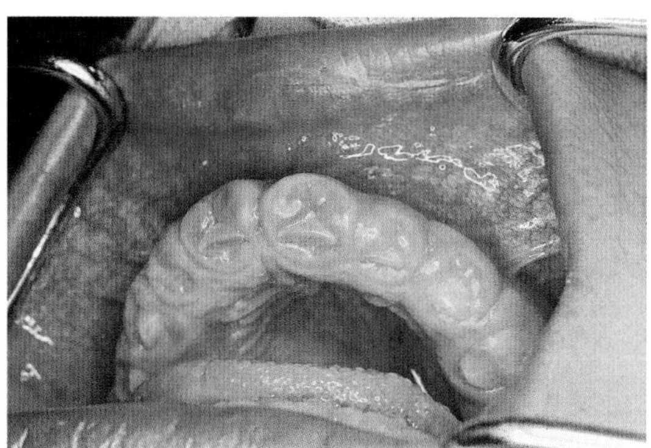

Fig. 19.9 Phenytoin-induced gingival enlargement.

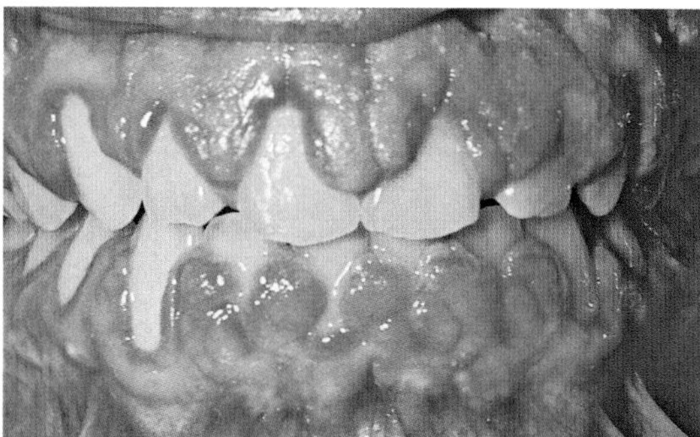

Fig. 19.10 Combined gingival enlargement resulted from the inflammatory involvement of a phenytoin-induced overgrowth.

result in complete coverage of dental surfaces (Fig. 19.9). Clinically, there are subtle differences in how lesions manifest depending on the type of medication used. Dental biofilm and bacterial infection frequently lead to inflamed tissues characterized by edema and bleeding (Fig. 19.10). The degree of fibrosis and inflammation depends on the dose, duration, and type of drug; oral hygiene; individual susceptibility, including genetic factors; and environmental influences.[103,105]

CLINICAL CORRELATION

Anticonvulsants, calcium channel blockers, and immunosuppressants are prescribed to patients with serious conditions, including but not limited to epilepsy, hypertension, and solid organ transplantation. Drug-induced GO is a major dental and medical problem due to impaired oral hygiene, biofilm accumulation, and gingival inflammation, posing a risk for the general health of these patients.

Anticonvulsants

Phenytoin (diphenylhydantoin) is the drug of choice for treating grand mal, temporal lobe, and psychomotor seizures, and it has been linked to GO for more than 70 years.[69]. Other anticonvulsant agents such as phenobarbital and valproic acid have been associated with gingival overgrowth less frequently than phenytoin.[63,87] The prevalence of phenytoin-induced GO is estimated to be around 50%[22] with a clinical onset as early as 1 month and increasing severity in 12 to 18 months.[1,14,30] Clinical localization of phenytoin-induced GO lesions is frequently the anterior buccal maxilla and mandible while the entire dentition may be affected and covered in extremely severe cases.[19,64] Phenytoin-induced GO is characterized by an enlargement of interdental papillae and increased thickening of the marginal tissues[3] causing esthetic and functional problems such as malposition of teeth, difficulty in speech, and impaired oral hygiene.[82]

Calcium Channel Blockers

Calcium channel blockers are a group of drugs commonly used to treat hypertension, angina pectoris, coronary artery spasm, and cardiac arrhythmia.[69] Benzothiazepine derivatives (diltiazem), phenylalkylamine derivatives (verapamil), and dihydropyridines (amlodipine, felodipine, isradipine, nicardipine, nifedipine, nitrendipine, oxodipine, nimodipine, and nisoldipine) are different types of calcium channel blockers. They have all been associated with some degree of DIGO.[13,15,17,28,65,72,91]

The first case of gingival overgrowth associated with the calcium channel blocker nifedipine was reported in 1984.[85] Prevalence of nifedipine-induced GO is highly variable, ranging from 6% to 83% of patients taking the medication.[7,36,37,97] Clinically, interdental papillae are affected, and overgrowth is limited to attached and marginal gingiva, usually observed on the anterior segments.[94] Nifedipine-induced GO may be accompanied by periodontitis and attachment loss differing from other forms of DIGO.

Immunosuppressants

Cyclosporine A has been used as the immunosuppressant of choice to prevent rejection of solid organ transplants, bone marrow transplantation, and treatment of autoimmune conditions.[46] The prevalence of cyclosporine A-induced GO has been around 30%, while this number can reach much higher, especially in pediatric populations.[59]

The first case of cyclosporine A-induced GO was reported in 1983.[86] Clinically, the lesions are more inflamed and bleed more than other DIGO forms and are frequently limited to buccal surfaces. The severity of the lesions can be similar to phenytoin and nifedipine, affecting the entire dentition and interfering with occlusion, mastication, and speech.[38]

Histopathology

Histologically, the lesions from different types of DIGO demonstrate significant variations.[105] Tissues from GO biopsies from

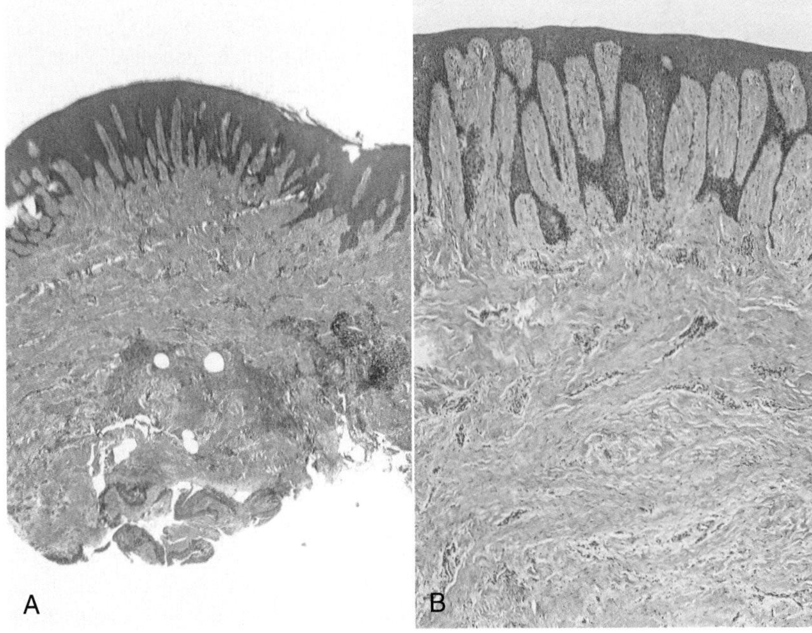

Fig. 19.11 Microscopic view of gingival enlargement associated with phenytoin therapy. (A) Hyperplasia and acanthosis of the epithelium and densely collagenous connective tissue are seen with evidence of inflammation in the area adjacent to the gingival sulcus. (B) The high-power view shows the extension of deep rete pegs into the connective tissue.

patients undergoing treatment with phenytoin present a thick stratified squamous epithelium with long thin rete pegs extending deep into the connective tissue.[4,19,33] Fibrosis is a common finding in these patients with minimal inflammatory cell infiltration.[104] The histologic characteristics of GO induced by calcium channel blockers are similar to phenytoin-induced lesions, including epithelial thickness, rete peg formation, and excessive matrix accumulation, but differs in histological attachment loss due to the accompanying periodontitis (Fig. 19.11). Cyclosporin A-induced GO also manifests with a thickened epithelium, rete peg formation, and irregular collagen fibers. These lesions, however, are characterized by more inflammatory infiltration and vascularization compared with DIGO associated with phenytoin and calcium channel blockers (Figs. 19.11 and 19.12).[86]

KEY FACT

DIGO lesions demonstrate a thick, stratified squamous epithelium with long, thin rete pegs extending deep into the connective tissue. Fibrosis is a common finding in patients with phenytoin-induced GO. Histologic characteristics of GO induced by calcium channel blockers are similar to those of phenytoin-induced lesions, including epithelial thickness, rete peg formation, and excessive matrix accumulation. Cyclosporin A-induced GO lesions have more inflammatory infiltration and increased vascularization than GO caused by phenytoin or calcium channel blockers.

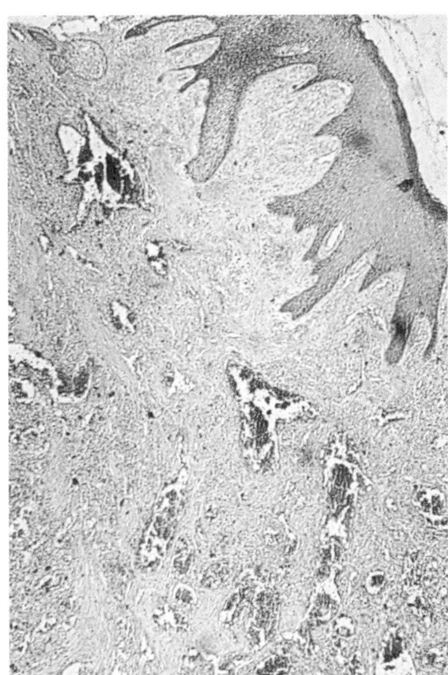

Fig. 19.12 Microscopic view of cyclosporine-associated gingival enlargement.

Pathogenesis of Drug-Induced Gingival Overgrowth

The pathogenesis of DIGO is complex. The main mechanism is mediated by the impaired function of gingival fibroblasts. Because gingival fibroblasts are responsible for matrix deposition in gingival tissues, extensive research has focused on these key cells and their function. Study findings vary, some pathways have not been validated in humans, and data are limited to in vitro and animal studies; however, the results suggest that DIGO-associated medications affect the extracellular matrix metabolism by decreasing collagenase activity and increasing the production of matrix proteins through a TGF-β1 and CCN2 (also known as connective tissue growth factor-CTGF)-mediated mechanism. Elevated levels of collagen synthesis characterize gingival fibroblasts from phenytoin-induced GO.[47] Fibroblasts may be susceptible to the development of DIGO.[47] Gingival fibroblasts from nifedipine-induced GO lesions have defective collagen production due to decreased levels of collagenase activity, which can result in excessive collagen deposition.[102]

Through interference with calcium metabolism, calcium channel blockers decrease calcium levels in gingival fibroblasts and T cells, affecting T-cell proliferation or activation and collagen biosynthesis.[7,102] Cyclosporine A directly impairs the collagen synthesis by gingival fibroblasts[68] with a specific rise in the levels of type I collagen.[90] Concomitantly, cyclosporine A leads to a decrease in the expression of matrix metalloproteinase-1 (MMP-1) and MMP-3.[12] In addition to collagen, the major extracellular matrix component of gingival tissues, the noncollagenous matrix is affected by the medications that result in DIGO. Glycosaminoglycan metabolism is impaired in patients with phenytoin-induced GO[32] and cyclosporin A-treated gingival fibroblasts.[77]

In addition to fibroblast metabolism and function, inflammatory regulation of tissue turnover is a major factor in DIGO pathogenesis. Fibroblast functions such as proliferation, differentiation, and extracellular matrix production are affected by cytokine levels and growth factors. GO lesions are characterized by increased levels of interleukin-6 (IL-6), IL-1β, platelet-derived growth factor subunit B (PDGFB), fibroblast growth factor 2 (FGF2), transforming growth factor-β (TGF-β), and connective tissue growth factor (CTG F).[6,16,31,49,51,74,76,83,88,89,105,107] Macrophages are the main source of these cytokines.[18,23,29,34,80]

TGF-β1-CTGF axis has been characterized in detail and presents as one of the critical and plausible mechanistic pathways leading to DIGO. TGF-β1 regulates cell proliferation and differentiation and can activate gene expression to synthesize extracellular matrix components, including collagen in CsA-induced GO.[54,88] TGF-β1 induces CTGF mRNA and protein expression in human gingival fibroblasts; the TGF-β1-CTGF pathway directly regulates fibrosis, gingival fibroblast lysyl oxidase, and collagen generation.[49] CTGF expression is increased in all forms of DIGO with the highest levels in phenytoin-induced GO, which are also characterized with the highest levels of fibrosis.[105]

CTGF expression is not limited to the connective tissue but is also demonstrated in the gingival epithelium, predominantly in the basal epithelial cells close to the connective tissue border.[56] In vitro studies demonstrated that CTGF can be directly produced by the gingival epithelial cells[56] illustrating a possible mechanism of fibrosis in the gingiva, which may be related to a cross-talk between epithelial and connective tissue cells. Studies have revealed a unique mechanism for TGF-β1—induced CTGF expression in gingival fibroblasts regulated by prostaglandin E_2, cAMP, mitogen-activated protein kinases (MAPK), and activation of JNK.[11] One of the key events demonstrated as a pathogenetic mechanism of DIGO is epithelial-mesenchymal transition induced by the medications at varying degrees. Highly fibrotic tissues are characterized by increased epithelial-mesenchymal transition through which epithelial cells in the gingiva acquire fibroblast function, and this process is regulated by the CTGF.[99] Molecular pathways of DIGO have been recently reviewed elsewhere.[104]

Treatment

Conventional approaches cannot prevent DIGO, but they can ease the clinical presentation by eliminating local factors, plaque control, and regular periodontal maintenance. The most effective treatment of DIGO is withdrawal or substitution of medications leading to the resolution of gingival lesions in 1 to 8 weeks after discontinuing the medication.[58] Changing nifedipine to another antihypertensive drug, isradipine, caused regression of gingival enlargement.[106] Tacrolimus, used as an alternative for cyclosporin A, resulted in the reversal of gingival enlargement.[53] However, most alternatives have also been linked to DIGO in recent years. In addition to withdrawal or substitution of medication, scaling and root planing reduces the severity of the clinical presentation of GO.[98] Nonsurgical treatment can eliminate the inflammatory component of DIGO, which can account for 40% of tissue enlargement, reducing the extent and need for surgical intervention.[57]

Because the anterior labial gingiva is frequently affected, surgery is commonly performed to solve esthetic and functional problems. Surgical elimination of DIGO lesions involves gingivectomy and gingivoplasty[52] and eliminates secondary complications due to inaccessibility of the tissues for proper oral hygiene. Surgical intervention enables the reduction of biofilm accumulation and gingivitis; therefore, it is the treatment of choice in DIGO after the phase I periodontal treatment. However, the recurrence rate is high and can be up to 40% 18 months after the surgery.[52] To prevent or reduce the recurrence, an optimal oral hygiene regimen is required. Patients should be given oral hygiene instructions, and periodontal prophylaxis and calculus removal should be done as needed during recall visits. On the other hand, DIGO due to phenytoin use may also be complicated by neurological impairment of manual dexterity of the patients in maintaining proper oral hygiene. This is especially a concern in pediatric patients undergoing anticonvulsant treatment and results in exacerbation of clinical complications. Pharmacologic strategies to replace these medications, especially using animal models, are being explored; however, clinical management of the DIGO will continue to present a challenge.[5]

CLINICAL CORRELATION

DIGO cannot be prevented, but it can be alleviated by eliminating local factors, plaque control, and regular periodontal maintenance. The most effective treatment for drug-induced gingival overgrowth is withdrawal or substitution of the medication. Nonsurgical treatment results in the elimination of the inflammatory component of DIGO. Surgical elimination of DIGO lesions involves gingivectomy and gingivoplasty. Unfortunately, the recurrence rate is high. Maintenance should include oral hygiene instructions, periodontal prophylaxis, and removal of calculus as needed.

Gingival Overgrowth Associated With Systemic Conditions

Changes in systemic health can lead to gingival enlargement. The causes and clinical features of GO associated with systemic conditions are diverse and usually manifest with amplification of existing biofilm-induced inflammation. These gingival pathologies are *conditioned enlargements* and include lesions related to hormonal and nutritional etiologic factors. Biofilm-induced gingival inflammation is a prerequisite that hormonal and nutritional changes modify. For example, pregnancy and puberty have been established as causes for hormonal changes. Nutritional factors are rare but have historically included deficits such as vitamin C [illegible]y. There is no conse[illegible]sus on how and whether these horm[illegible]ietary fluctuations an[illegible] conditions lead to GO; however, the role of biofilm and gingivitis is clear. It should be noted that the role of hormonal factors on gingival health is an ongoing research field.

Pregnancy-Associated Gingival Overgrowth

Clinical Manifestations

GO is a common feature in pregnancy. Clinically, it manifests as a single mass or multiple tumor-like masses at the gingival margin. Marginal gingival enlargement during pregnancy results from the aggravation of existing inflammation and its incidence has been

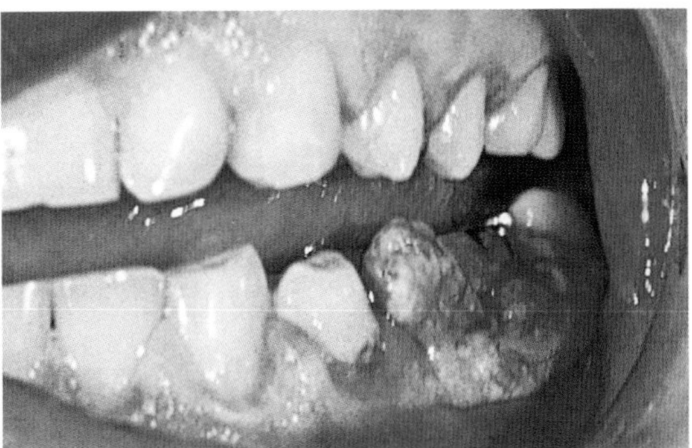

Fig. 19.13 Localized gingival enlargement in a 27-year-old pregnant patient.

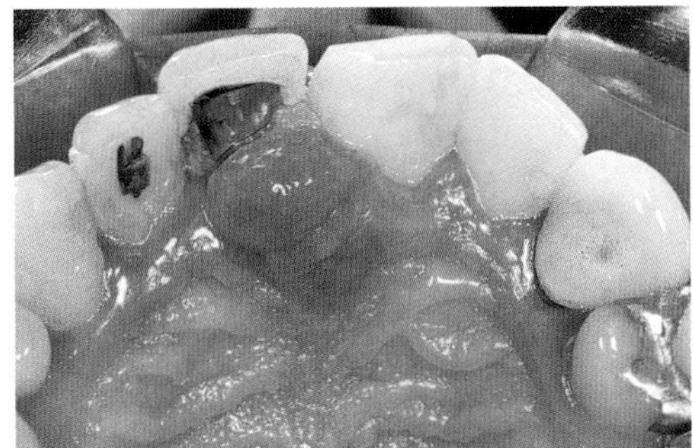

Fig. 19.14 Pyogenic granuloma. (*Courtesy Dr. Silvia Oreamuno, San Jose, Costa Rica.*)

reported as 10% to 70%. These lesions can be observed as single enlargements, which are referred to as *pregnancy tumors*. Pregnancy tumors are not neoplasms; they represent an inflammatory response to microbial plaque modified by the patient's altered host response. It usually appears after the third month of pregnancy, but it may occur earlier. The reported incidence is 1.8% to 5%.[66]

Overall, pregnancy-associated GO manifests with a highly varied clinical picture. Enlargement is usually generalized, but it tends to be more prominent interproximally than facial and lingual surfaces. The enlarged gingiva is bright red or magenta, soft, and friable, with a smooth and shiny surface. Bleeding occurs spontaneously or on slight provocation. The lesion appears as a discrete, mushroom-like, flattened spherical mass that protrudes from the gingival margin or, more often, from the interproximal space. It is attached by a sessile or pedunculated base (Fig. 19.13). It tends to expand laterally, and pressure from the tongue and the cheek perpetuates its flattened appearance. It is dusky red or magenta; it has a smooth, glistening surface that often exhibits numerous deep red pinpoint markings.

The superficial lesion of pregnancy-associated GO usually does not invade the underlying bone. The mass is generally firm, but it may have various degrees of softness and friability. It is typically painless unless its size and shape foster the accumulation of debris under its margin or interfere with occlusion, in which case painful ulceration may occur. Although the microscopic findings are characteristic of gingival enlargement during pregnancy, they are not pathognomonic.

Pyogenic granuloma is similar in clinical and microscopic appearance to the gingival enlargement seen during pregnancy. This lesion manifests as a tumor-like gingival enlargement and is considered an exaggerated response to minor trauma (Fig. 19.14). The exact nature of the systemic etiological factor has not been identified. The differential diagnosis is based on the patient's history.[10]

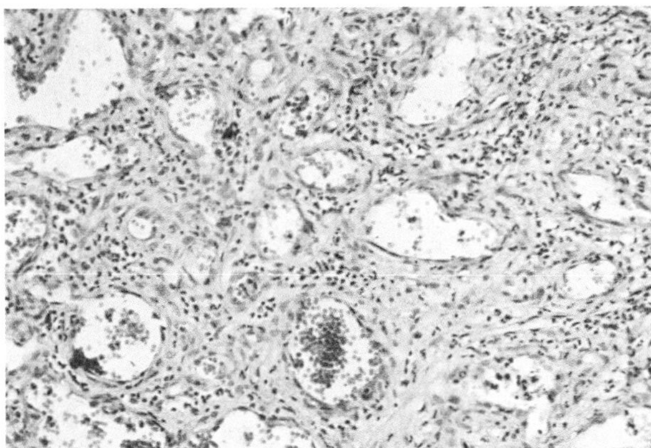

Fig. 19.15 Microscopic view of gingival enlargement in a pregnant patient.

Etiology

Hormonal changes have always been linked to periodontal tissue changes and pathology. For example, progesterone and estrogen levels increase 10 to 30 times by the end of the third trimester compared with the menstrual cycle.[2] Although mechanistic evidence is lacking, it is thought that these hormonal changes induce an increased vascular permeability, which leads to gingival edema and an increased inflammatory response to dental plaque. During this process, the impaired vascular response and inflammatory milieu can modify the subgingival microbiota. Although not specific, the increased abundance of periodontal pathogens, including *Prevotella intermedia, Prevotella melaninogenica,* and *Porphyromonas gingivalis,* has been linked to pregnancy-associated GO in vivo and in vitro,[61,62,84] demonstrating that the lesions are biofilm-associated.

Histopathology

Gingival enlargement in pregnancy is called angiogranuloma, referring to its strong clinical presentation with vascular changes and fibrotic process. Marginal and tumor-like enlargements consist of a central mass of connective tissue, with numerous diffused, newly formed, and engorged capillaries lined by cuboid endothelial cells (Fig. 19.15) and a moderately fibrous stroma with various degrees of edema and chronic inflammatory infiltrate. In addition, the stratified squamous epithelium is thickened, with prominent rete pegs and some degree of intracellular and extracellular edema, prominent intercellular bridges, and leukocytic infiltration.

Treatment

Like other forms of gingival changes associated with hormonal variations during pregnancy, GO lesions can be prevented by good oral hygiene in most cases. Therefore, oral care in pregnant women should be meticulous, and patients should be treated by removing calculus and biofilm. Severe cases may require surgical excision during the second trimester; however, removing the GO lesions without establishing an optimal oral hygiene regimen will likely lead to the recurrence of gingival enlargement. Although the spontaneous reduction in the size of gingival enlargement typically follows the termination of pregnancy, complete elimination of the residual inflammatory lesion and GO requires removal of all plaque deposits, elimination of factors that favor its accumulation, and in some fibrotic cases, surgical intervention after the pregnancy. Treatment of pyogenic granuloma consists of the surgical removal of the lesions and eliminating irritating local factors. In contrast with pregnancy-associated GO, the recurrence rate of pyogenic granuloma is about 15%.

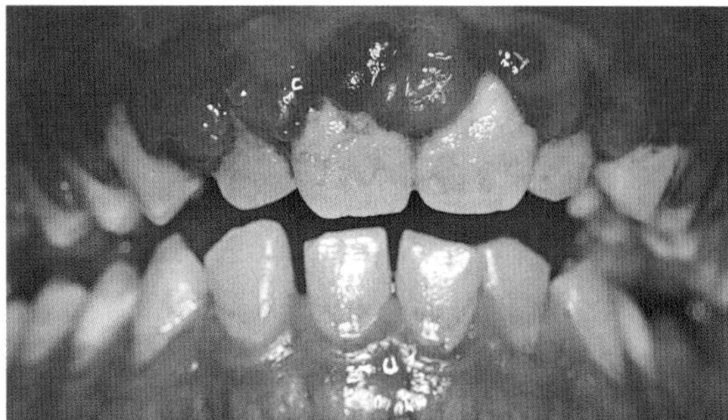

Fig. 19.16 Conditioned gingival enlargement during puberty.

Puberty-Associated Gingival Overgrowth

Clinical Manifestations

Enlargement of the gingiva can be seen during puberty. The lesions are not specific to any gender; both male and female adolescents may develop puberty-associated GO. Clinically, there is a strong association with biofilm accumulation. The lesions are usually marginal and interdental, and they are characterized by prominent bulbous interproximal papillae (Fig. 19.16). Often, only the facial gingivae are enlarged, and the lingual surfaces are relatively unaltered. The mechanical action of the tongue and the excursion of food prevent a heavy accumulation of local irritants on the lingual surfaces.

Etiology

Gingival enlargement during puberty has all the clinical features that are associated with the chronic inflammatory gingival disease. The degree of growth and its tendency to recur in the relatively scant plaque deposits distinguish puberty-associated GO from purely gingivitis-associated lesions, suggesting a profound impact on hormonal changes. In addition, the incidence of puberty-associated GO lesions declines with age,[100] further supporting the role of hormonal changes during puberty.

Studies of the subgingival microbiota of children between the ages of 11 and 14 and their association with clinical parameters implicated *Capnocytophaga* species in the initiation of pubertal gingivitis[41,73] Other studies have reported that hormonal changes coincide with an increase in *P. intermedia* and *Prevotella nigrescens.*[75,109] The etiologic role of the changes in microbiota, however, is not clear. In addition, it is not known whether changes in inflammatory conditions predispose to a shift in microbial species. The inflammatory lesions due to orthodontic appliances are also dominant during this age range. Therefore, it is unclear whether the age-alone hormonal changes during puberty or mechanical irritations due to external stimuli (e.g., orthodontic appliances) are the dominant driving factors in puberty-associated GO lesions.

Histopathology

The microscopic appearance of gingival enlargement during puberty is one of chronic inflammation with prominent edema. It cannot be distinguished from other forms of gingivitis-associated GO lesions.

Treatment

After puberty, enlargement undergoes spontaneous reduction, but it may not disappear completely until the plaque and calculus are removed.

Nutrition-Associated Gingival Overgrowth

Malnutrition has been historically associated with several oral lesions. GO has been observed in cases of chronic vitamin C deficiency in patients with scurvy. These lesions are no longer common, but GO is still considered a part of the classic description of scurvy.

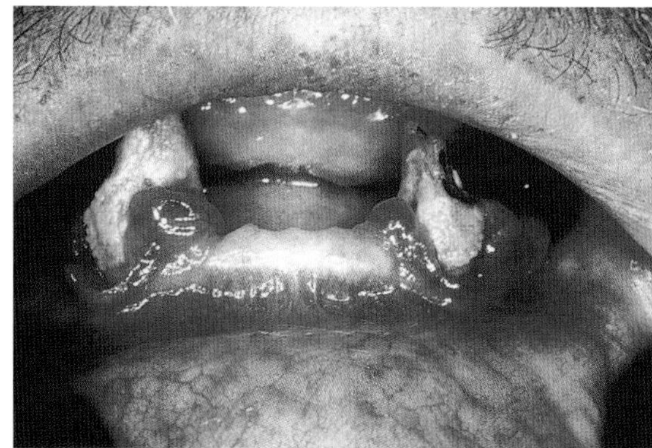

Fig. 19.17 Gingival enlargement in a patient with vitamin C deficiency. (*Courtesy Dr. Gerald Shklar, Boston, MA.*)

Clinical Manifestations

Gingival enlargement with vitamin C deficiency is marginal. The gingiva is bluish red, soft, and friable, and it has a smooth, shiny surface. Bleeding that occurs spontaneously or on slight provocation, and surface necrosis with pseudomembrane formations are common features.

Etiology

Acute vitamin C deficiency alone does not cause gingival inflammation, but it does cause hemorrhage, collagen degeneration, and edema of the gingival connective tissue. These changes modify the response of the gingiva to biofilm to the extent that the normal defensive delimiting reaction is inhibited, and the extent of the inflammation is exaggerated, thereby resulting in the massive gingival enlargement seen in patients with scurvy (Fig. 19.17).

Histopathology

The gingiva presents with a chronic inflammatory cell infiltration with an acute and superficial response in patients with vitamin C deficiency. There are scattered areas of hemorrhage with engorged capillaries. Marked diffuse edema, collagen degeneration, and a scarcity of collagen fibrils and fibroblasts are striking findings.

Treatment

Nutrition-associated GO lesions are rare. Changes in nutrition accompanied by nonsurgical treatment and good oral hygiene usually result in complete resolution of the pathology. However, in rare cases, surgical removal may be indicated.

Gingival Fibromatosis

Clinical Manifestations

Gingival fibromatosis (GF) can be hereditary or idiopathic. These lesions are rare and occur in highly fibrotic forms of GO.[40,108] Hereditary gingival fibromatosis (HGF) is the most common form, and it has been linked to several genetic loci, including mutations of the Son-of-Sevenless 1 *(SOS1)* and REI-silencing transcription factor *(REST)* genes[8,26,43,44,95,111,112] (Fig. 19.18). Idiopathic gingival fibromatosis (IGF) is a rare condition of undetermined cause, likely driven by yet to be discovered genetic defects or physiologic changes (Fig. 19.19).

In all forms of GF, the enlargement is highly fibrotic with minimal clinical inflammation. GF affects the attached gingiva, the

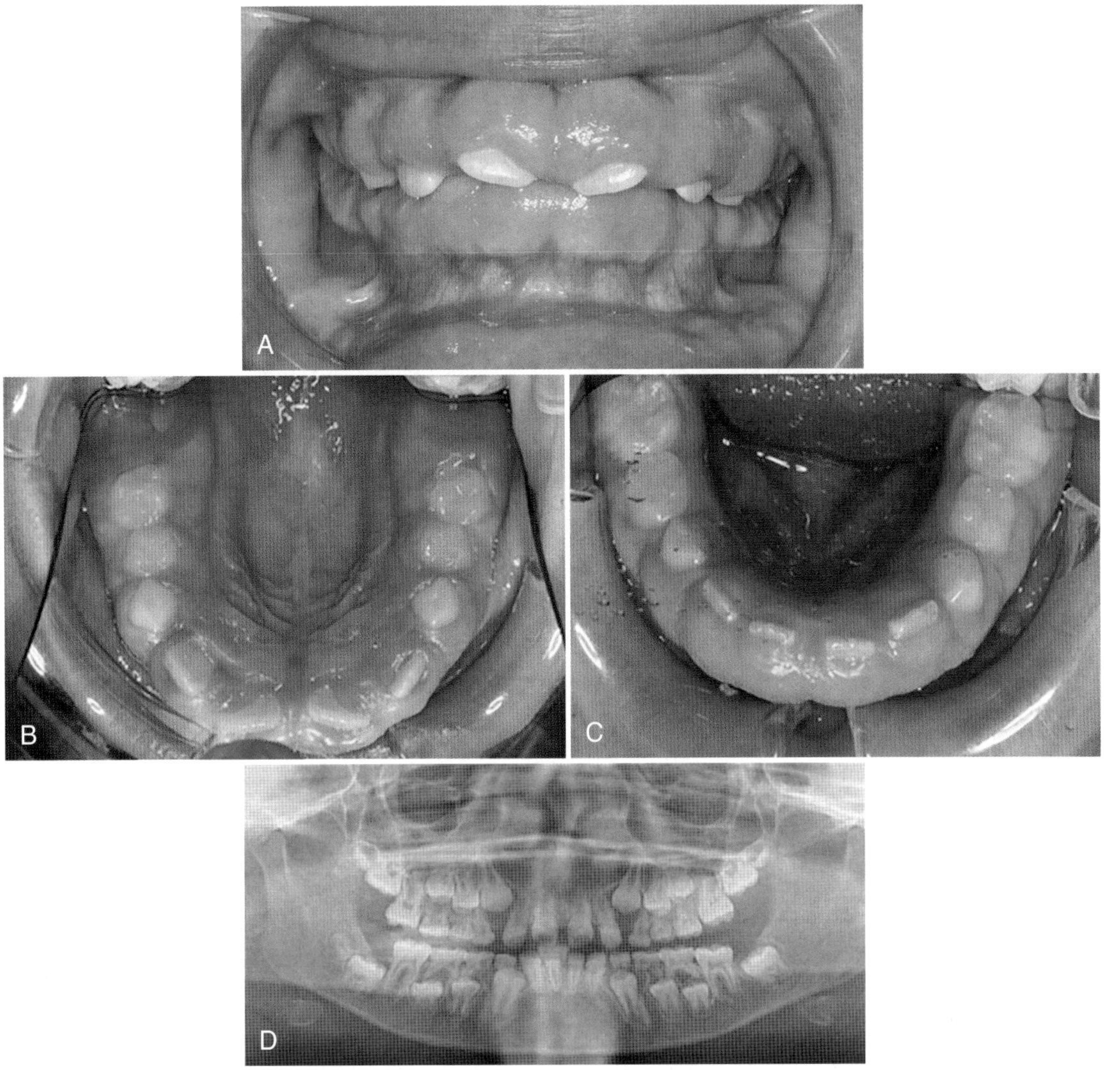

Fig. 19.18 Hereditary gingival fibromatosis. (A) Fibrotic gingival enlargement is generalized and covers the entire dentition. (B) Palatal view. (C) Lingual view. (D) Panoramic radiographic view showing the mixed dentition.

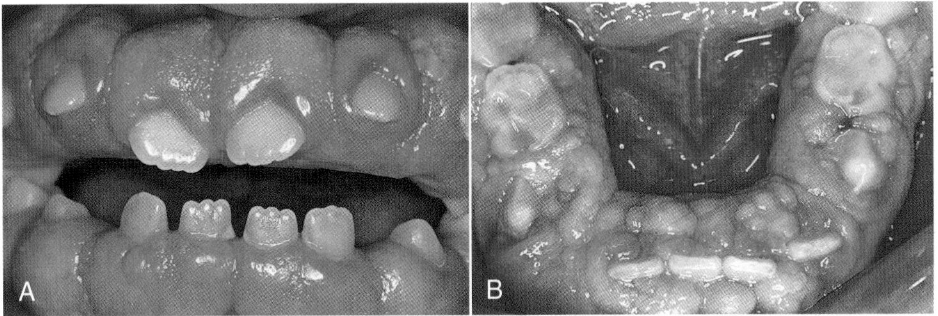

Fig. 19.19 Idiopathic gingival enlargement. (A) Facial view. (B) Occlusal view of the mandibular arch.

gingival margin, and the interdental papillae. As shown in Fig. 19.18, the facial and lingual surfaces of the mandible and maxilla usually are affected, but the involvement may be limited to either jaw. The fibrotic gingiva is pink, firm, and almost leathery, and it has a characteristic minutely pebbled surface. The teeth are almost completely covered in severe cases and the enlargement projects into the oral vestibule. The jaws appear distorted because of the bulbous enlargement of the gingiva. Secondary inflammatory changes are common at the gingival margin.

Etiology

The genetic basis of HGF is well established, with different populations having different contributing genetic loci and lead genes.[9,27,42,45,50,70,78,79,96,113,114] In some families, gingival enlargement is associated with the impairment of physical development. In addition, other syndromes are sometimes colocalized with GF including, generalized hypertrichosis terminalis (OMIM: 135400), Zimmermann-Laband syndrome (OMIM: 135500), amelogenesis imperfecta type IG (OMIM: 204690), hyaline fibromatosis syndrome (OMIM:

228600), among other syndromes.[39,48,67] Forms of GF that have not been linked to specific genetic causes are designated as idiopathic.

KEY FACT

The genetic basis of hereditary gingival fibromatosis is well established. In some families, gingival enlargement is associated with the impairment of physical development. Other syndromes can coexist with gingival fibromatosis. Idiopathic forms of gingival fibromatosis are those that have not been linked to specific genetic defects.

Although the genes associated with lesions of hereditary forms have been identified, the pathogenetic mechanisms linked to these genetic factors are not fully understood. The enlargement usually begins with the eruption of the primary or permanent dentition. It may regress after extraction, suggesting that the teeth or the biofilm may be initiating factors. The presence of bacterial plaque is a complicating factor. Gingival enlargement has been described in tuberous sclerosis, which is an inherited condition characterized by the triad of epilepsy, mental deficiency, and cutaneous angiofibromas.

Histopathology

GF presents with highly fibrotic lesions, with a bulbous increase in connective tissue that is relatively avascular and consists of densely arranged collagen bundles and numerous fibroblasts. The surface epithelium is thickened and acanthotic, with elongated rete pegs.[21,55,56] Histopathology is similar to phenytoin-induced GO with low levels of inflammatory infiltration. However, collagen bundle formation, dominance, and orientation are distinctive in areas where cellular structures are reduced.[21]

Treatment

Treatment of GO lesions manifesting as gingival fibromatosis requires gingivectomy and gingivoplasty. The high level of fibrosis may even require multiple surgical blades to be used during the gingivectomy procedures. In many cases, an underlying osseous growth accompanies the GF, which requires osteoplasty in addition to the gingivectomy and gingivoplasty. Postsurgical clinical management is challenging because of the high recurrence rate. The severity of lesions usually results in extreme crowding and misalignment of teeth. After removal of the fibromatosis lesions, patients may require orthodontic treatment and a meticulous oral hygiene program.[25]

Other Forms of Gingival Enlargement

Other forms of gingival enlargement can be due to a wide range of contributing factors and causes. In addition, as covered elsewhere in this book, GO may be linked to various systemic diseases. Although uncommon and occurring with different etiopathogenetic mechanisms, the GO associated with systemic diseases can be related to serious issues that must be considered in its clinical management. Therefore, these lesions should be carefully diagnosed.

In addition to the types of GO discussed in this chapter, the gingiva can be enlarged due to increases in the size of the underlying osseous and dental tissues. These *false enlargements* usually have no abnormal clinical features except for the massive increase in the size of the area. For example, enlargement of the bone subjacent to the gingival area occurs most often with tori and exostoses. Still, it can also occur with Paget disease, fibrous dysplasia, cherubism, central giant cell granuloma, ameloblastoma, osteoma, and osteosarcoma.

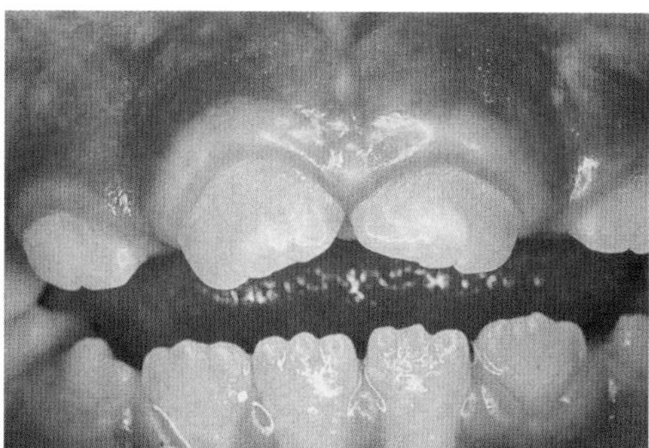

Fig. 19.20 Developmental gingival enlargement.

The gingival tissue can appear normal, or it can have unrelated inflammatory changes. Likewise, during the various stages of the eruption, particularly of the primary dentition, the labial gingiva can have a bulbous marginal distortion caused by the superimposition of the bulk of the gingiva on the normal prominence of the enamel in the gingival half of the crown. This enlargement is called *developmental enlargement,* and it often persists until the junctional epithelium has migrated from the enamel to the cementoenamel junction. In a strict sense, developmental gingival enlargements are physiologic, and they usually present no problems for patients. However, when the enlargement is complicated by marginal inflammation, the composite picture gives the impression of extensive gingival enlargement (Fig. 19.20).

On the other hand, neoplastic formations in gingival tissues can be clinically confused with fibrotic enlargements of the gingiva. Oral cancer accounts for less than 3% of all malignant tumors in the body, but it is the 6th most common cancer in males and the 12th most common in females. The gingiva is not a common site of oral malignancy, accounting for only 6% of oral cancers; however, neoplastic growth of the underlying alveolar bone should be carefully assessed.

Epulis is a generic term used to clinically designate all discrete tumors and tumor-like masses of the gingiva. It serves to locate the tumor but does not describe it. Most lesions referred to by this term are inflammatory rather than neoplastic. For example, fibromas arise from the gingival connective tissue or the periodontal ligament. They are slow-growing, spherical tumors that tend to be firm and nodular but may also be soft and vascular. Fibromas are usually pedunculated. Hard fibromas of the gingiva are rare; most lesions clinically diagnosed as fibromas are inflammatory enlargements. Histopathological analyses of fibromas demonstrate bundles of well-formed collagen fibers with scattered fibrocytes and various degrees of vascularity. The so-called giant cell fibroma contains multinucleated fibroblasts. In another variant, mineralized tissue (i.e., bone, cementum-like material, and dystrophic calcifications) can be found; this type of fibroma is called *peripheral ossifying fibroma.*

Similar to fibromas, papillomas are benign proliferations of surface epithelium that are in many cases associated with human papillomavirus (HPV) infection. Gingival papillomas appear as solitary wartlike or cauliflower-like protuberances (Fig. 19.21). They can be small and discrete or broad, hard elevations with minutely irregular surfaces. The lesions consist of finger-like projections of stratified squamous epithelium that are often hyperkeratotic, with central cores of fibrovascular connective tissue.

Peripheral giant cell granulomas of the gingiva arise interdentally or from the gingival margin. They occur most frequently on the labial surface, and they can be sessile or pedunculated. They vary in appearance from smooth, regularly outlined masses to irregularly shaped, multilobulated protuberances with surface indentations (Fig. 19.22). Ulceration of the margin is occasionally seen. The lesions are painless, vary in size, and can cover several teeth. They can be firm or spongy, and their color varies from pink to deep red or purplish-blue. Clinically, peripheral giant cell granulomas cannot be easily differentiated from other forms of gingival enlargement. Microscopic examination is required for definitive diagnosis. The word *peripheral* is needed to distinguish them from similar lesions within the jawbone (i.e., central giant cell granulomas).

In some cases, the giant cell granuloma of the gingiva is locally invasive and destroys the underlying bone (Fig. 19.23). Complete removal leads to an uneventful recovery. The lesion has multiple foci of multinuclear giant cells and hemosiderin particles in a connective tissue stroma. Areas of chronic inflammation are scattered throughout the lesion, with acute involvement occurring at the surface. The overlying epithelium is usually hyperplastic, with ulceration at the base. Bone destruction occasionally occurs within the lesion (Fig. 19.24).

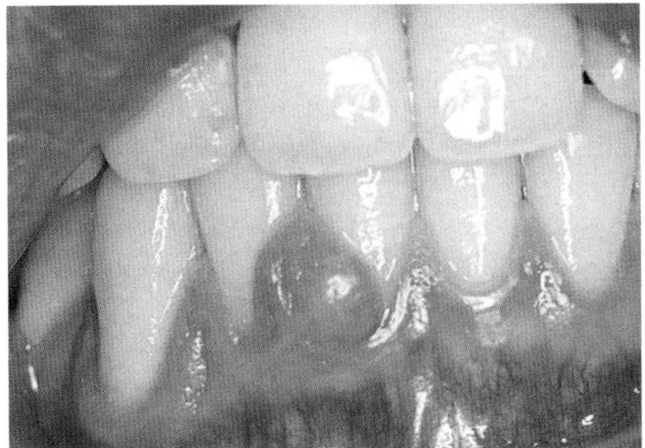

Fig. 19.21 Papilloma of the gingiva.

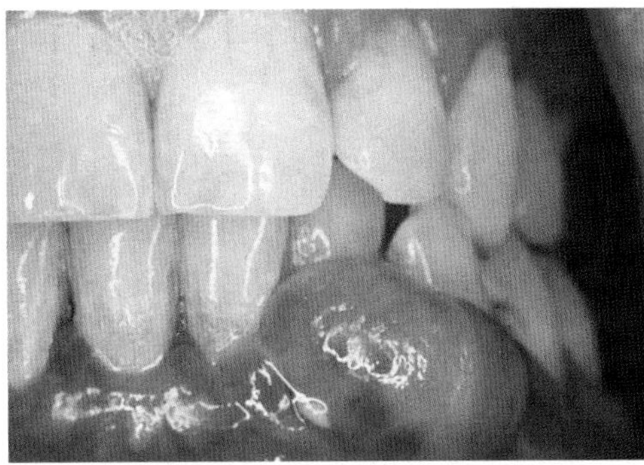

Fig. 19.22 Gingival giant cell granuloma.

Gingival cysts of microscopic proportions are common, but they seldom reach a clinically significant size. When they do, they appear as localized enlargements that may involve the marginal and attached gingiva. The cysts occur in the mandibular canine and premolar areas, most often on the lingual surface. They are painless, but with expansion, they can cause erosion of the surface of the alveolar bone. The gingival cyst should be differentiated from the lateral periodontal cyst, which arises within the alveolar bone adjacent to the root and is developmental in origin. Gingival cysts develop from odontogenic epithelium or surface or sulcular epithelium traumatically implanted in the area. An uneventful recovery follows removal. A gingival cyst cavity is lined by a thin, flattened epithelium with or without localized areas of thickening. Nonkeratinized stratified squamous epithelium, keratinized stratified squamous epithelium, or parakeratinized epithelium with palisading basal cells can be seen less frequently.

Squamous cell carcinoma is the most common malignant tumor of the gingiva. It may be *exophytic*, manifesting as an irregular outgrowth, or *ulcerative,* appearing as a flat, erosive lesion. It is often symptom-free, going unnoticed until complicated by inflammatory changes that can mask the neoplasm but cause pain; it sometimes becomes evident after tooth extraction. These masses are locally invasive, and they involve the underlying bone and periodontal ligament of adjoining teeth and the adjacent mucosa (Fig. 19.25). Metastasis is usually confined to the region above the clavicle; however, a more extensive involvement can include the lung, liver, or bone.

Malignant melanoma is a rare oral tumor that tends to occur in the hard palate and maxillary gingiva of the elderly. It is usually darkly pigmented, and it is often preceded by localized pigmentation. It can be flat or nodular, and it is characterized by rapid growth and early metastasis. It arises from melanoblasts in the gingiva, cheek, or palate. Infiltration into the underlying bone and metastasis to cervical and axillary lymph nodes is common.

Fibrosarcoma, lymphosarcoma, and reticulum cell sarcoma of the gingiva are rare; only isolated cases have been described in the literature. Kaposi's sarcoma often occurs in the oral cavity, particularly in the palate and the gingiva, of patients with acquired immunodeficiency syndrome. Tumor metastasis to the gingiva occurs infrequently.

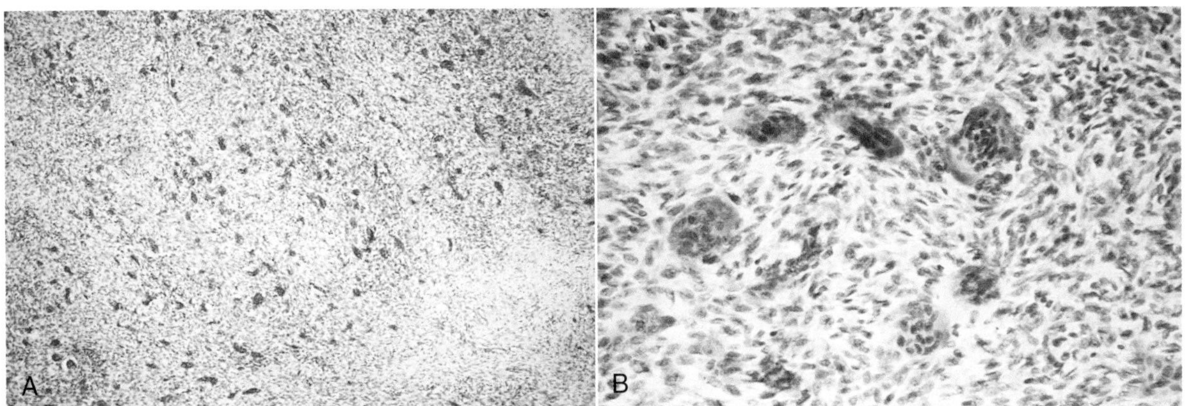

Fig. 19.23 (A) Microscopic survey of a peripheral giant cell granuloma. (B) A high-power microscopic study of the lesion demonstrates the giant cells and the intervening stroma.

KEY FACT

The low incidence of oral malignancy should not mislead the clinician. Ulcerations that do not respond to therapy in the usual manner and all gingival tumors and tumor-like lesions must be biopsied and submitted for microscopic diagnosis.

In most clinical cases of GO, the clinical appearance is complicated by inflammation, bleeding, and swelling, which further creates difficulty in identifying the cause and pathologic process. Thorough knowledge of GO and the patient's systemic and oral medical histories is critical for designing the treatment and maintaining outcomes. Because some GO forms are linked to systemic and severe diseases, this approach is essential for securing patient safety before treatment is initiated.

A Case Scenario is found on the companion website eBooks.Health.Elsevier.com.

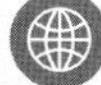
References for this chapter are found on the companion website eBooks.Health.Elsevier.com.

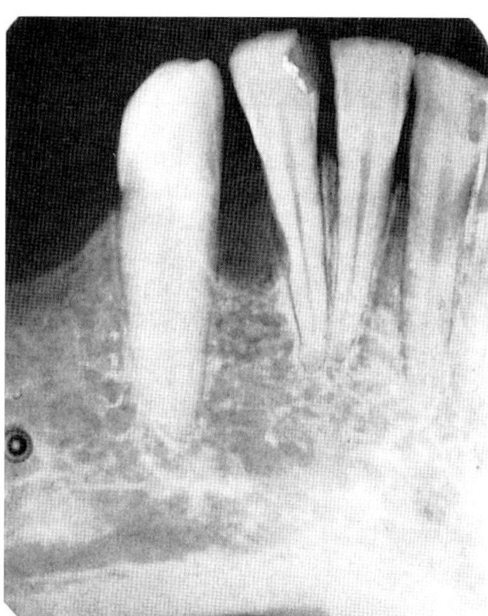

Fig. 19.24 Bone destruction in the interproximal space between the canine and the lateral incisor is caused by the extension of a peripheral giant cell reparative granuloma of the gingiva. (*Courtesy Dr. Sam Toll.*)

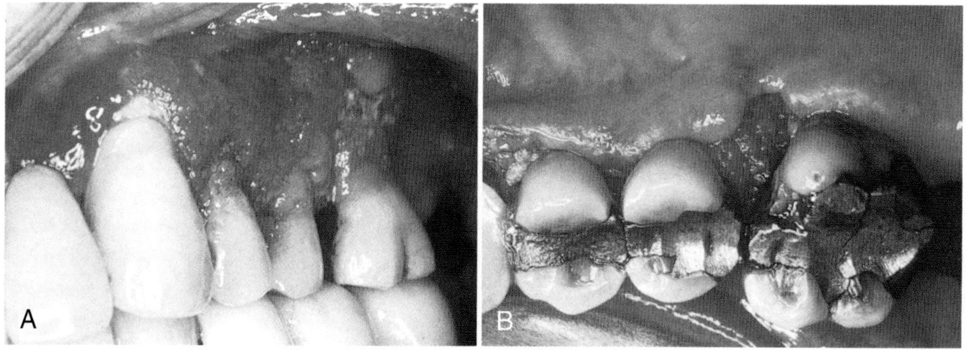

Fig. 19.25 Squamous cell carcinoma of the gingiva. (A) The facial view shows extensive verrucous involvement. (B) The palatal view shows mulberry-like tissue emerging between the second premolar and the first molar.

CHAPTER 20

Periodontal Health and Disease in Children and Adolescents

Daniela Rodrigues P. Silva

CHAPTER OUTLINE

Periodontal disease in adults is partly precipitated by gingival inflammation during the formative years of childhood and early adolescence. Gingivitis in children has received much less attention in terms of understanding the long-term impact that chronic inflammation of the periodontal tissues may have throughout life compared to caries disease. Without appropriate diagnosis and management, the nondestructive gingival inflammation of childhood may progress to more significant periodontal diseases seen in the adult population.

After first reviewing anatomic and physiologic changes in the periodontium and dentition, this chapter presents the gingival changes associated with childhood and adolescence. Periodontal diseases during these early periods of life are also discussed when associated with or without systemic diseases (see Chapters 16, 25, and 26).

Periodontium of the Primary Dentition

Periodontal Health

Periodontal health is defined as the absence of clinical inflammation that is typically associated with gingivitis, periodontitis, or any other periodontal conditions. Clinical gingival health is characterized by the absence of bleeding on probing, erythema and edema, patient symptoms, and attachment and bone loss.[24]

In the edentulous infant, the gingival tissues present with thick gingival mucosa and segmentations that correspond with the primary buds. A high labial frenum attachment is a normal finding in almost 85% of infants, which may diminish in size with normal development (Fig. 20.1).[81] During the primary dentition stage, the normal gingiva continues to be somewhat different from that found in adults. The tissues are pale pink, but they are pink to a lesser degree than the attached gingiva of adults because the thinness of the keratinized layer causes the underlying vessels in children to be more visible. Stippling appears at about 3 years of age and has been reported in 56% of children between ages 3 and 10 years, with little differences between maxillary and mandibular arches or between boys and girls throughout childhood (Fig. 20.2).[14]

The *interdental gingiva* is broad buccolingually and narrows mesiodistally, which is consistent with the morphology of the primary dentition. Its structure and composition are similar to those of the adult gingiva.

Gingival sulcular depth is shallower in the primary dentition than in the permanent dentition. Probing depths range from 1 to 2 mm, with an increase in depth from anterior to posterior.[12,34,85]

The *attached gingiva* varies in width anteroposteriorly, with a range of 3 to 6 mm. On the buccal surfaces, the width decreases from anterior to posterior, with some data indicating a narrowing over the canines (Fig. 20.3). The lingual attached gingiva shows an inverse relationship, with an increase in width from anterior to posterior.[34] The gingival width normally increases with age as children transition from the primary to the permanent dentition.[12,19,85] Interestingly, the junctional epithelium (JE) is thicker in the primary dentition than in the permanent dentition, which is thought to reduce the permeability of the tissues to bacterial toxins.[13]

Radiographically, the lamina dura is prominent in the primary dentition, with a wider periodontal space than in the permanent dentition. The marrow spaces of the bone are larger, and the crests of the interdental bony septa are flat, with bony crests within 1 to 2 mm of the cementoenamel junction (Fig. 20.4).[37]

Periodontal Changes Associated With Normal Development

Significant changes occur in the periodontium as the dentition changes from the primary to the permanent teeth. Most of the changes are associated with eruption and are physiologic in nature.

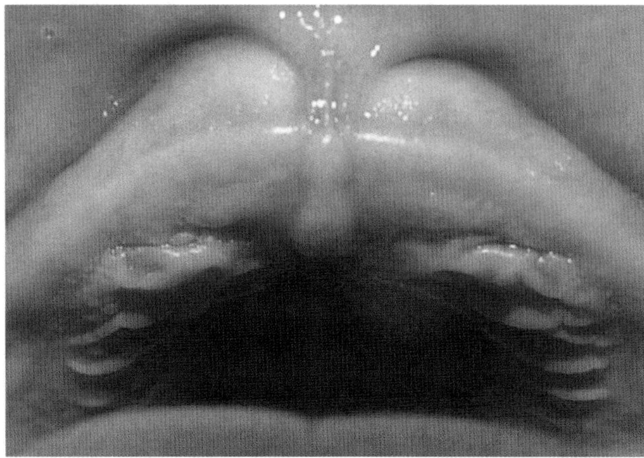

Fig. 20.1 Normal gingiva of an edentulous 1-month-old child showing high labial frenulum and pink and healthy tissues. (Copyright Dr. Daniela Silva. All rights reserved.)

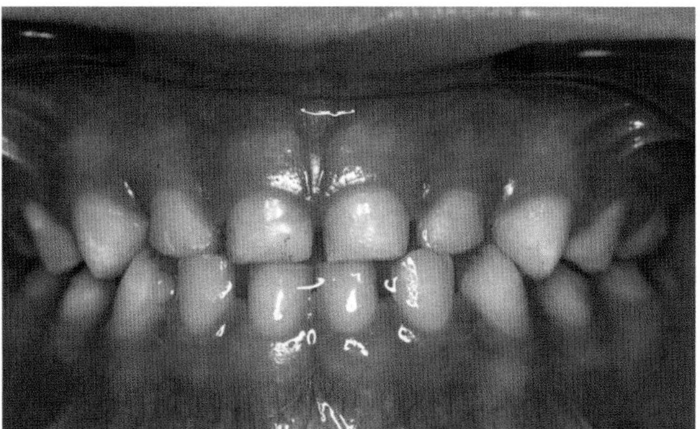

Fig. 20.2 Normal gingiva of a 4-year-old child showing light stippling and flattened interproximal gingiva in areas of physiologic spacing. (Copyright Dr. Daniela Silva. All rights reserved.)

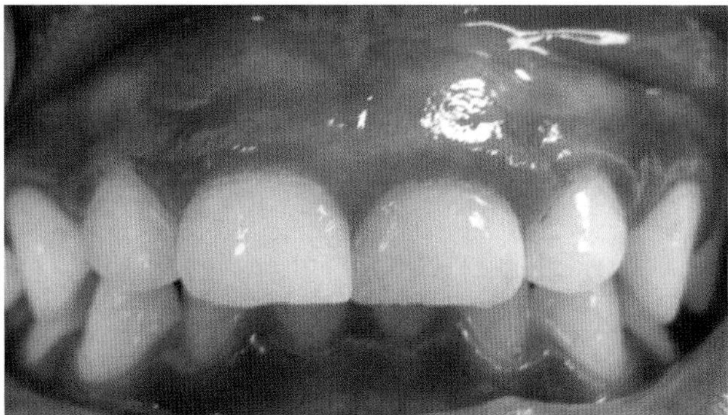

Fig. 20.3 Normal gingiva of a 4-year-old African-American child demonstrating the width of the attached gingiva, as illustrated by the pigmentation that occurs only in the attached area. (Copyright Dr. Daniela Silva. All rights reserved.)

These changes should be distinguished from gingival disease, which may occur simultaneously.

Tooth Eruption

Tooth eruption is a natural continuous physiological process under strong genetic control with minor influence from environmental factors. When teeth erupt, the continuity of the oral epithelium is disrupted. To compensate for this breach, a specialized structure around erupting teeth provides oral epithelium integrity and protects

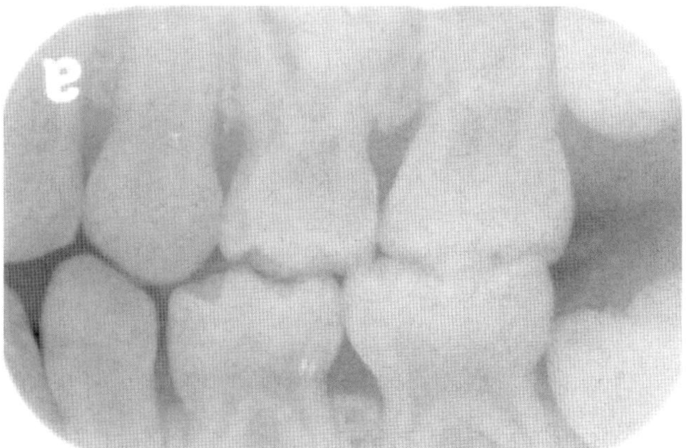

Fig. 20.4 Bitewing radiograph of a 6-year-old child illustrating the flattened interseptal bone, and bony crests within 1 to 2 mm of the cementoenamel junction. (Copyright Dr. Daniela Silva. All rights reserved.)

underlying tissues from bacterial invasion. This specialized structure is known as the JE. Epithelia exist in other parts of the body and are designed to protect underlying tissues from physical and chemical trauma; one mechanism by which this is accomplished is via a high rate of cell proliferation.[104]

According to a recent systematic review,[64] tooth eruption is closely intertwined with root formation and is executed through three defined stages. The first stage (pre-eruptive tooth movement) begins at the end of the early bell stage and lasts until the beginning of tooth root formation. In this stage, dental epithelial cells located at the apical region of the enamel organ in the developing tooth proliferate and invade further apically, sending signals to recruit dental follicle mesenchyme inside the tooth bud to become odontoblasts that produce the dentin. Growth of the tooth bud owing to the formation of the enamel and dentin at this stage continues until the tooth crown is complete, preparing the tooth to emerge into the oral cavity. The second stage (eruptive tooth movement) begins with the onset of tooth root formation and lasts until the crown appears in the oral cavity and reaches the occlusal plane. Eruptive tooth movement is subdivided into two phases: intraosseous and supraosseous. In this stage, the epithelial structure termed Hertwig's epithelial root sheath and the dental mesenchyme signal each other to achieve a rapid elongation of the tooth root. Subsequent bone resorption of the cortical shell on the coronal portion of the tooth bud by osteoclasts facilitates the tooth to emerge into the oral cavity. The third stage (posteruptive tooth movement) starts when the tooth reaches its occlusion and maintains its position within the alveolar bone to achieve proper occlusion. This stage requires continuous maturation of the periodontal attachment apparatus and maintenance of its related structures.[64]

As a tooth erupts, the gingival margin and the sulcus develop. At this point, the margin is rounded, edematous, and reddened (Fig. 20.5). During the period of active tooth eruption, it is normal for the marginal gingiva that surrounds partially erupted teeth to appear prominent; this is most evident in the maxillary anterior region. The prominence is caused by the height of the contour of the erupting tooth and mild inflammation from mastication. Poor oral hygiene can contribute to the development of significant gingivitis in unprotected gingival areas.

Before the eruption of a primary or permanent tooth, the gingiva reveals a bulge that is firm and pink or blanched as a result of the underlying tooth crown. An *eruption cyst* may occasionally be evident, and most of them occur in the maxilla and the first decade of life. This fluctuant mass may be filled with blood, and it generally

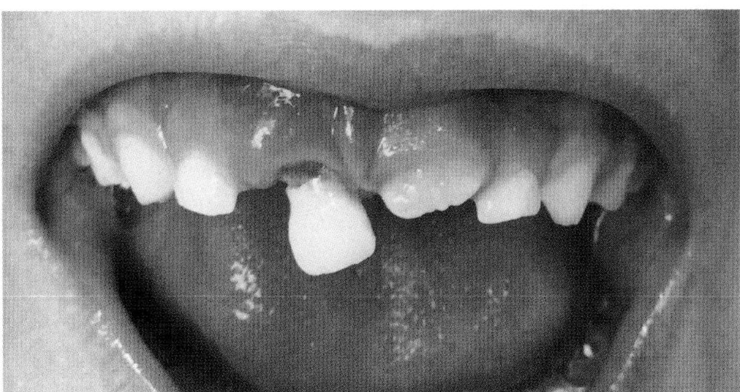

Fig. 20.5 Exfoliating upper primary right central incisor and erupting upper left permanent central incisor showing inflamed gingiva in both areas. (Copyright Dr. Daniela Silva. All rights reserved.)

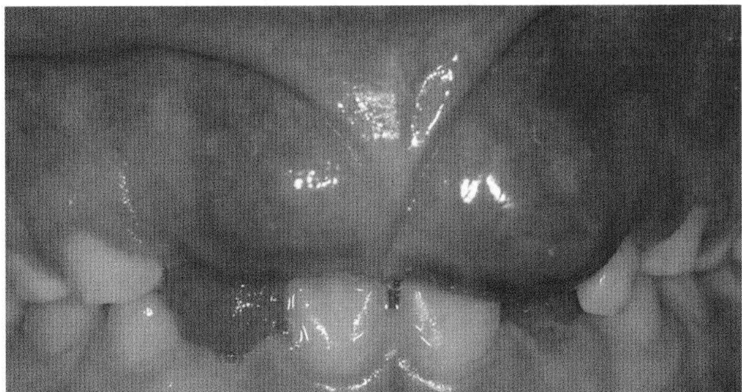

Fig. 20.6 Eruption cyst at upper central incisors area of an 8-year-old child. Transparent, bluish, blue, or blue-black swelling of alveolar mucosa over a tooth in eruption. (Copyright Dr. Daniela Silva. All rights reserved.)

presents as a bluish or deep red enlargement of the gingiva over the erupting tooth (Fig. 20.6). The most common sites of these cysts are the primary first molars and the permanent central incisors. Many resolve without treatment, but a simple excision or marsupialization could assist with the draining of fluids if the cyst is painful or interfere with mouth closure.[18]

Teething

The effect of primary tooth eruption on infant health has been debated for centuries, but there is little scientific evidence regarding the diagnosis and management of the teething child. The period associated with the eruption of the primary teeth in infants can be difficult and stressful for both the child and the parents. The timing of primary incisor eruption (i.e., 5 to 12 months old) coincides with the diminution of the passive humoral immunity conferred by the transfer of maternal antibodies via the placenta and the establishment of the child's own immunity.[45,82] Pain is a common feature of teething, as reported by parents and some health care providers. However, it is not the tooth that causes the pain but rather the follicle, which is a rich source of eicosanoids, cytokines, and growth factors and which results in a localized inflammatory response.[79,82]

Most medical and dental professionals agree that teething does not cause life-threatening illness, but they disagree about which symptoms may be associated with tooth eruption. A summary of the studies and systematic reviews of symptoms related to teething most commonly include decreased appetite, biting, drooling, gum rubbing, irritability, sucking, and abnormal temperature.[32,45,55,56,66,67,74,79,82,95,96] One of those studies found an association between fever and primary tooth eruption only when rectal temperature was evaluated.[66] However, there is no scientific evidence that any of the aforementioned symptoms can

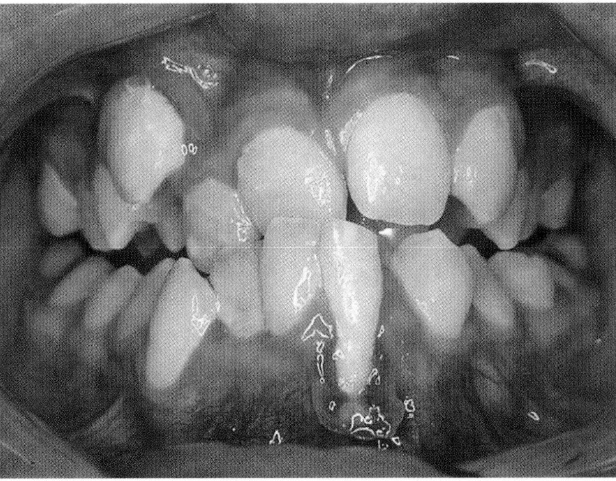

Fig. 20.7 Eleven-year-old with history of "idiopathic osteoporosis" with severe crowding, poor oral hygiene, and gingival recession on lower left incisor. (Courtesy of Dr. Yvonne Kapila. All rights reserved.)

be diagnostic of teething in a child without excluding the possibility of other systemic diseases.

A novel study looking for information on selected popular parenting websties worldwide found that the teething information followed those described in the literature, and they emphasized that symptoms such as fever, ear pulling, and loss of appetite could indicate unrecognized illness. A majority of the sites proposed the use of gum massage and chewing on an object as recommended by the American Academy of Pediatrics and the American Academy of Pediatric Dentistry (AAPD), and they also recommended OTC medications despite the lack of evidence regarding the effectiveness of these medications for a teething infant.[47,98]

Primary Tooth Exfoliation

As with tooth eruption, the process of tooth exfoliation involves changes in the periodontium. The depth of the gingival sulcus increases as the JE migrates down the resorbing root of an exfoliating tooth.[13] Microscopically, minor traumatic changes may demonstrate compression, ischemia, and the hyalinization of the periodontal ligament.[70] There may be changes in the permeability and integrity of the JE, thereby making the exfoliating tooth more susceptible to inflammation (see Fig. 20.5).[13]

During the process of exfoliation, teeth may change position, which may lead to changes in occlusion. Malalignment caused by spacing and changes in skeletal relationships related to erupting teeth may also contribute to significant trauma of the periodontal structures. With a more severe injury, crushing and necrosis of the periodontal ligament may occur. In most patients, these injuries are spontaneously resolved as the teeth exfoliate, erupt, and align through the normal growth and development processes.

Other Developmental Issues

Relation of Periodontal Status to Malocclusion

Data indicate an association between abnormal tooth position and gingivitis.[25,94] Crowding in the dentition (Fig. 20.7) can often make plaque and food removal more difficult, thereby leading to an increased incidence of gingivitis. Severe changes may include gingival enlargement (GE), discoloration, occasional ulceration, and the formation of deep pockets or pseudo pockets. Generally, gingival health can be restored with orthodontic correction, but a failure to align the teeth does not necessarily affect periodontal disease later in life.[25]

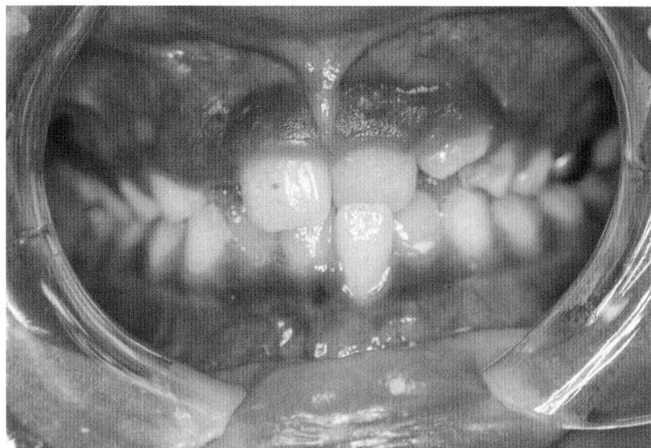

Fig. 20.8 Erupting lower permanent incisor in crossbite showing minimal attached gingiva and gingival recession. (Copyright Dr. Daniela Silva. All rights reserved.)

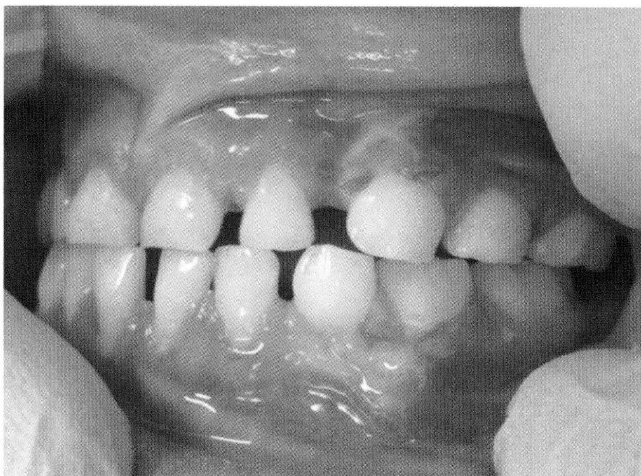

Fig. 20.9 Gingival recession on maxillary and mandibular left primary canine areas caused by self-inflicted trauma from the patient's fingernail. (Copyright Dr. Daniela Silva. All rights reserved.)

Mucogingival Deformities and Conditions

The prevalence of mucogingival problems and recession in children ranges from 1% to 19%, depending on the criteria used to assess the condition.[59] Evidence suggests that some mucogingival problems may start during the primary dentition as a consequence of developmental aberrations in eruption and deficiencies in the thickness of the periodontium.[59] A high frenum attachment may also be a factor in the development of mucogingival problems if there is excess tension at the marginal tissues.[73,86] Although erupting permanent lower incisors often show minimal attached gingiva, gingival width often increases as the teeth erupt and stimulate bone development.[19,84] During the mixed dentition stage, a recession is most often found on the facial aspect of mandibular permanent incisors secondary to rotations or labial positioning related to space problems, when the mandibular incisors present with minimal attached gingiva with frequent trauma (Fig. 20.8). While lack of keratinized tissue is a predisposing factor for gingival recession and inflammation, periodontal health can be maintained with optimal home care and professional maintenance despite this issue. The periodontal phenotype (gingival thickness, keratinized tissue width) can be assessed by measuring the gingival thickness through the use of a periodontal probe. The phenotype is classified as thin when the periodontal probe inserted into the sulcus is visible through the tissue and thick when the periodontal probe is not visible through the tissue.[91]

The maxillary canine region is also prone to localized gingival recession. Late-erupting canines in a crowded dentition may be displaced buccally, erupting into or near unattached gingiva or mucosa and increasing the risk of insufficient gingival tissue width and recession. Recession may also be associated with an anterior open bite as a result of the labial inclination of the teeth.[54] Orthodontic treatment and realignment may be necessary to protect the integrity of the attached gingiva. An interdisciplinary approach between the pediatric dentist/general dentist, the orthodontists, and the periodontist is a crucial step in the prognosis of the teeth that present with recession.

Mucogingival problems can also result from factitious habits, like self-inflicted trauma from a fingernail (Fig. 20.9) or excessive toothbrushing by either the parent or the child. Because the width of the attached gingiva increases with age, any of these problems may resolve spontaneously, thereby suggesting a cautious approach to treatment with judicious monitoring instead of immediate surgical intervention.[19,84]

Gingival Diseases

Dental Plaque Biofilm-Induced Gingivitis

Gingivitis is a reversible disease characterized by an inflammation of the gingiva that does not result in clinical attachment loss (CAL). Dental plaque biofilm-induced gingivitis usually is regarded as localized inflammation initiated by microbial biofilm accumulation on teeth and is considered one of the most common human inflammatory diseases, affecting almost 95% of the population.[24] Although gingivitis is considered to be "nearly universal" among children, current and early studies show that 50% of children by age 4 to 5 years have gingivitis, and it peaks at nearly 100% at puberty.[8,68] The initiation of gingivitis occurs if dental plaque accumulates over days or weeks without disruption or removal due to a loss of symbiosis between the biofilm and the host's immune-inflammatory response and the development of an incipient dysbiosis. Plaque-induced gingivitis begins at the gingival margin and may spread throughout the remaining gingival unit.[63] Its severity can be influenced by tooth anatomy, tooth position, alignment in the arch, existing restorations, and other tooth-related factors. Although studies have suggested that bacterial phylotypes associated with gingivitis are distinct from those associated with health or periodontitis, further studies are needed to clearly define the microbial community of gingivitis.[63]

Gingivitis is a clinical diagnosis with signs of inflammation, like erythema, edema, pain (soreness), heat, and loss of function. It can be simply, objectively, and accurately defined and graded based on a bleeding on probing score (BoP%). Ideally, it can be assessed as the proportion of bleeding sites stimulated by a standardized periodontal probe with controlled force at six sites (mesiobuccal, buccal, distobuccal, mesiolingual, lingual, distolingual).[91] Limitations on probing score might be very common in young pediatric patients due to uncooperative behavior; nevertheless, probing prior to the eruption of the first permanent molars is encouraged. When probing positioning and pressure into the sulcus are performed correctly, the patient should not feel discomfort. For healthy patients or those with special health care needs receiving dental treatment under sedation and/or general anesthesia, clinicians should take the opportunity afforded by sedation and perform periodontal probing. While probing, clinicians should rule out the presence of pseudo pockets associated with tooth exfoliation or partially erupted teeth.

Dental Plaque Biofilm-Induced Gingivitis is extremely common among children and adolescents, and it affects up to 70% of children who are more than 7 years old.[8,68] Inflammation is generally limited to the marginal gingiva, with undetectable connective tissue attachment or bone loss in most cases. Although gingivitis does not always progress to periodontitis, the diagnosis and management of gingival disease in children and adolescents is important, because periodontitis is always preceded by gingivitis.[8,68]

In children, as in adults, the primary cause of gingivitis is dental plaque, which is related to poor oral hygiene. The relationship between plaque and the gingival index, however, is weak and remains unclear. Although gingivitis is highly prevalent in children, its severity is generally less intense than what is found in adults.[13] Similar oral hygiene conditions produce less severe forms of disease among children as compared with adults.[68]

As children age, their tendency to develop gingivitis increases. The prevalence of the disease is lowest during the preschool years and increases throughout childhood, peaking during puberty. However, increases in the degree of gingival inflammation do not fully correlate with the amount of plaque, thereby suggesting the influence of other factors.

Clinical Features

The most prevalent type of gingival disease in childhood is *marginal gingivitis*. The gingival tissues exhibit changes in color, size, consistency, and surface texture that are similar to those of chronic inflammation in adults. Red, linear inflammation is accompanied by underlying chronic changes, including swelling, increased vascularization, and hyperplasia. Bleeding and increased pocket depth are not found as often in children as in adults, but they may be observed if severe gingival hypertrophy or hyperplasia occurs.[68]

Marginal gingivitis in children is characterized by a loss of collagen in the area around the JE and an infiltrate that consists mostly of lymphocytes, with small numbers of polymorphonuclear leukocytes, plasma cells, monocytes, and mast cells. Lesions generally have relatively few plasma cells, and they resemble the early nondestructive, nonprogressive lesions that are seen in adults. Furthermore, gingivitis in children differs from adult gingivitis in that the response is dominated by T lymphocytes, with few B lymphocytes and plasma cells in the infiltrate. This difference could explain why gingivitis in children rarely progresses to periodontitis.[53,77] Gingival histology of specimens from children also demonstrate other unique features that may contribute to a decreased tendency to progress to severe gingivitis. The JE of the primary dentition tends to be thicker than in the permanent dentition, which is thought to reduce the permeability of the gingival structures to bacterial toxins that initiate the inflammatory response.[13]

Microbiology of Disease

Because the intensity of gingival disease increases as a child develops into adulthood, it is important to understand the microbiology of the disease, which is discussed fully in Chapters 10 and 11. Interestingly, the composition of the oral microflora changes as the child matures.[2,13] Yang and colleagues analyzed samples of dental plaque in children and reported that 71% of 18- to 48-month-old children were infected with at least one periodontal pathogen. Sixty-eight percent were infected with *Porphyromonas gingivalis*, and 20% exhibited *Bacteroides forsythus (Tannerella forsythia)*.[102] A moderate correlation also has been found between *B. forsythus* in children and periodontal disease in their mothers. *B. forsythus* also has been associated with gingival bleeding in children.

In a similar study, 60% of children between the ages of 2 and 18 years had detectable levels of *P. gingivalis* in their plaque, and 75% showed similar levels of *Actinobacillus actinomycetemcomitans*.[93]

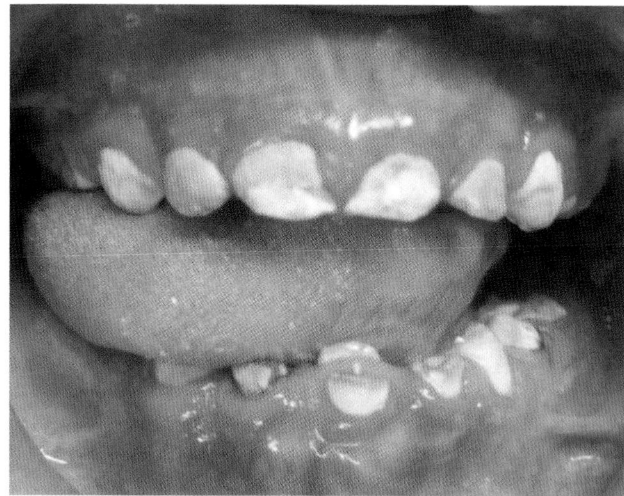

Fig. 20.10 Five-year-old male with history of liver transplant and gastric tube feeding showing generalized calculus deposit. (Copyright Dr. Daniela Silva. All rights reserved.)

The presence of *P. gingivalis* was most strongly associated with the progression of gingivitis and the onset of periodontitis in healthy children.[62,69]

Calculus

Calculus deposits are uncommon in infants and toddlers, but they may increase with age. Lingual surfaces of the mandibular incisors are the most common location of dental calculus, followed by buccal surfaces of maxillary molars. Several authors have reported that changes in the levels of sodium, ammonium, and bicarbonate were associated with an increase in salivary flow, and high salivary flow in these areas is responsible for calcium phosphate deposition. A clinical study looking at the prevalence of calculus formation between primary and mixed dentitions, its relation to the anatomy of the teeth, and biological indices, found that calculus is less frequently seen on flat surfaces compared to concave areas; probably because of a higher accumulation of dental plaque/biofilm, which may turn into calculus with time, is seen less often on flat surfaces.[2]

About 9% of 4- to 6-year-old children exhibit calculus deposits. By the age of 7 to 9 years, 18% of children present with calculus deposits, and by the age of 10 to 15 years, 33% to 43% have some calculus formation.[2] Within the category of special needs patients, children with cystic fibrosis[26] or chronic kidney disease[58] have a higher incidence of calculus deposits, which may be caused by increased calcium and phosphate concentrations in their saliva. Children who are fed exclusively with gastric or nasogastric tubes show significant signs of gingival diseases and calculus buildup as a result of a lack of function and increased oral pH (Fig. 20.10).[10,31]

Considering the multifactorial nature of calculus formation, changes in one or another causative factor may not be regarded as the only reason for the presence or absence of calculus. Histatin, cystatin, and particularly proline-rich proteins and statherin play important roles in the regulation of calculus formation via inhibition of hydroxyapatite crystal growth.[2] It is well known that dental plaque deposition precedes dental calculus accumulation; therefore, we should instruct our patients and caregivers on proper toothbrushing techniques and motivate them to take good oral care.

Eruption Gingivitis

Gingivitis associated with tooth eruption is so common that the term *eruption gingivitis* has come into common use. Tooth eruption per se does not cause gingivitis, however, inflammation associated with plaque accumulation around erupting teeth, perhaps secondary to discomfort caused by brushing these friable areas, may contribute to gingivitis.[8,13] The gingiva around erupting teeth may appear reddened because gingival margins have not yet keratinized fully, and sulcus development is incomplete. It is believed that microbes start colonizing the tooth surface and the newly formed JE immediately after the eruption. Events occurring during tooth formation and eruption could predispose to such colonization with specific bacteria and potentially contribute to the onset of gingivitis and/or periodontal diseases.

Exfoliating and severely carious primary teeth often contribute to gingivitis caused by plaque accumulation as a result of pain during brushing or food impaction in areas of cavitation. As a normal part of exfoliation, the JE migrates under the resorbing tooth, thereby increasing pocket depth and potentially creating a niche for pathogenic bacteria.[13] The discomfort of chewing on severely infected teeth often leads to unilateral chewing on the unaffected side.

Puberty Gingivitis

As mentioned previously, the incidence of marginal gingivitis increases as a child matures, peaking when they are 10 to 14 years old and then decreasing slightly after puberty.[13] Gingival disease that behaves in such a manner is often referred to as *pubertal (or puberty) gingivitis.*

The altered gingival response during this developmental stage is thought to be the result of hormonal changes that magnify the vascular and inflammatory response to dental plaque[13,63,68] and that modify the reactions of dental plaque microbes.[28] Estrogens reduce keratinization and effectiveness of epithelial barrier, stimulating proliferation of gingival fibroblasts and synthesis of periodontal connective tissue. Progesterone enhances blood circulation in capillary vessels, increases vascular permeability, and stimulates the production of prostaglandins. An increase in hormone production during puberty results in steroid hormone-related gingivitis, characterized by gingival bleeding, inflammation in interproximal areas, and microbial changes.[33,61]

The incidence and severity of gingivitis in adolescents are influenced by a variety of factors, including dental plaque biofilm levels, dental caries, mouth breathing, crowding of teeth, and tooth eruption. However, the dramatic increase in steroid hormone levels during puberty has a transient effect on the inflammatory status of the gingiva.[63] Many adolescents will show signs of puberty-associated gingivitis in the presence of relatively small amounts of plaque, which is key to identifying this condition.

Gingival Changes Related to Orthodontic Appliances

GE can be related to the presence of fixed orthodontic appliances, which complicate plaque removal (Fig. 20.11). While some studies clearly indicate poor oral hygiene as responsible for gingival growth, others demonstrate that gingival changes during orthodontic treatment are transient and do not imply any permanent alteration of the periodontal tissue.[25,38,95] These responses may depend on the quality and/or quantity of biofilm, the host's immune response to the aggression, metal corrosion, hormonal levels, the microbial baseline, and tooth movement.[38] The fact that most orthodontic treatment is provided to individuals during puberty when they are subject to the inflammatory changes associated with puberty gingivitis, may exacerbate the observed effect.

Mouth Breathing

The effect of mouth breathing on the oral cavity in children remains controversial, and research on this topic is scarce. An observational cross-sectional randomized study with 785 children and adolescents

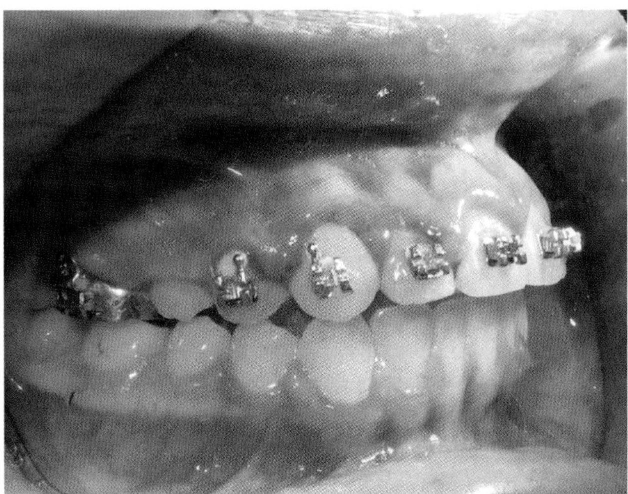

Fig. 20.11 Chronic marginal gingivitis secondary to orthodontic therapy and inadequate oral hygiene.

found that 17.7% were mouth breathers, and this breathing pattern did not influence gingival health status, but there was a significant increase in halitosis levels compared to nose breathers.[5] One review reported that mouth breathing and lip incompetence, which are together referred to as an *open mouth posture,* are often associated with increased plaque and gingival inflammation. The area of inflammation is often limited to the gingiva of the maxillary incisors. There is usually a clear line of demarcation where the gingiva is uncovered by the lip.[25]

Non-Dental Plaque Biofilm-Induced Gingival Diseases

Human gingiva, as well as other oral tissues, may exhibit several non-plaque-induced pathologic lesions, which may or may not be associated with a systemic condition or a medical disorder. Dentists are the key healthcare providers in establishing diagnoses and formulating treatment plans for patients affected by such lesions.[41] Intraoral soft-tissue lesions may be encountered in the pediatric population as they are in the adult population. The six most common pediatric intraoral lesions are primary herpetic gingivostomatitis (PHG), recurrent herpes simplex, recurrent aphthous stomatitis, candidiasis, angular cheilitis, and geographic tongue.[68]

Primary Herpetic Gingivostomatitis

PHG is the most common clinical manifestation of primary herpes simplex infection. It is an acute-onset viral infection that occurs early during childhood, with a heightened incidence between the ages of 6 months and 5 years. In children with primary herpetic infections, 99% are symptom-free or have symptoms that are attributed to *teething*. The remaining 1% can develop significant gingival inflammation and ulceration of the attached gingiva, tongue, palate, lips, and extraoral lesions[68] associated with other symptoms like cervical lymphadenopathy, malaise, low-grade fever, irritability, pain, and drooling (Fig. 20.12). The oral lesions may start as vesicles in the tongue and buccal and gingival mucosa, which rapidly rupture to become ulcers. The ulcers are usually 1 to 3 mm in size and may subsequently form a large, ulcerated area covered by a yellowish-gray membrane. The general course of the PHG is 10 to 14 days, which is usually preceded by an incubation period of 1 to 26 days, and healing generally occurs without scarring.[65] Complications are rare but do occur due to viral shedding. During this phase, eye infections (ocular herpes) and infections of the digits (herpetic whitlow) are not infrequent complications.

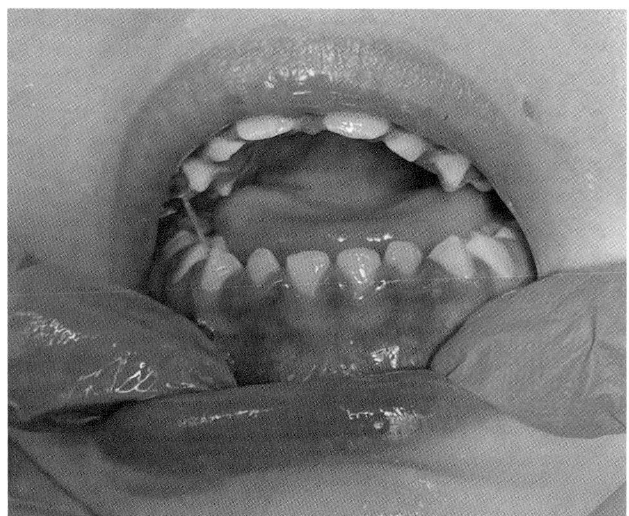

Fig. 20.12 Primary herpetic gingivostomatitis in a 23-month-old male with swollen gingiva and mild fever. The infection is mostly limited to the attached gingiva, tongue, palate, and lips. (Copyright Dr. Daniela Silva. All rights reserved.)

A systematic review on acyclovir as the treatment for PHG was not able to provide evidence that acyclovir is an effective treatment in reducing the number of oral lesions, preventing the development of new extraoral lesions, decreasing the number of individuals with difficulties experienced in eating and drinking and those who are admitted to the hospital under the age of 6 with PHG.[65] The most important measure is to control the child's fever, pain, and hydration with bland, nonacidic fluids. Hospitalization might be necessary in some severe cases.

Candidiasis

Candida albicans is by far the most commonly detected fungal organism on human mucosal surfaces. It is considered an opportunistic pathogen that lives as a benign commensal organism in the mouth of healthy individuals, adults, or children. Candidiasis results from an overgrowth of *C. albicans*, usually after a course of antibiotics, inhaler use, or as a result of congenital or acquired immunodeficiency. It is far less common in children than adults, and it is rarely associated with a healthy child. Oral candidiasis is the most frequently found HIV-related oral manifestation in children, and the second most common is gingivitis, which is not considered an HIV-related lesion but appears to have a significant incidence in HIV-positive patients.[52] There are controversies among studies indicating a positive correlation between *C. albicans* prevalence and early childhood caries (ECC) severity. A recent systematic review and meta-analysis noted a statistically significant difference between *C. albicans* prevalence in the oral cavity of children with ECC compared to those without ECC. Moreover, they found that individuals with oral *C. albicans* present were associated with a greater than five times odds of experiencing ECC.[17,99]

Hereditary Gingival Fibromatosis

Hereditary gingival fibromatosis (HGF), sometimes referred to as idiopathic gingival hyperplasia, is a rare, hereditary, benign disease characterized by slow and progressive fibrous hyperplasia of the gingiva, and it affects both mandibular and maxillary gingiva. It is mostly seen in children and adolescents and has a prevalence of 1:175,000 according to phenotype and 1:350,000 according to genotype.[20,21,48] HGF is commonly described as a non-syndromic disorder, but it can occasionally be part of a syndrome.

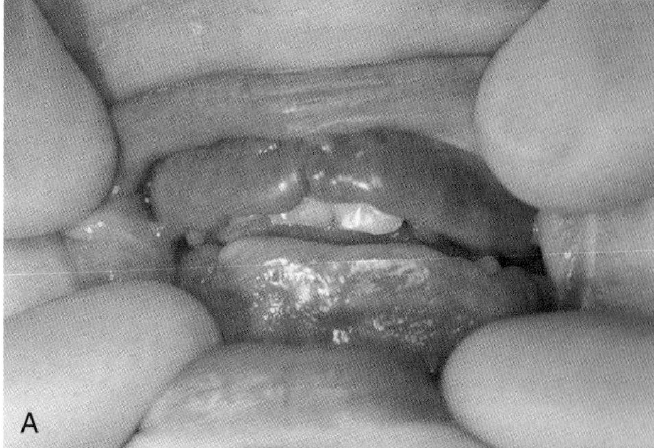

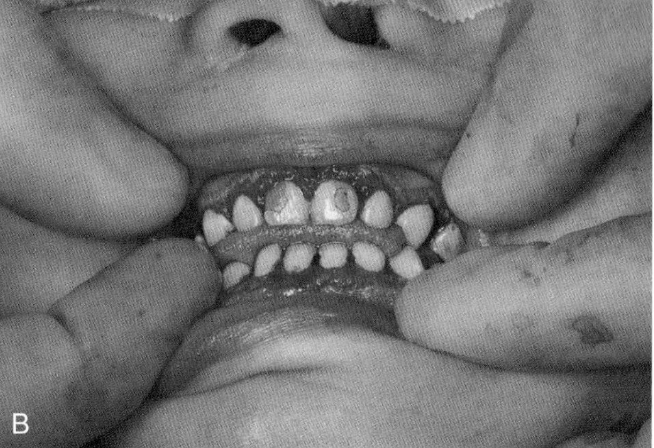

Fig. 20.13 (A) Three-year-old male with hereditary gingival fibromatosis. Asymptomatic enlargement of gingival tissue, normal pink color, firm, and fibrous consistency. (B) Three-year-old male with hereditary gingival fibromatosis, immediately after gingivectomy was performed with laser in the operatory room. (Courtesy of Dr. Flavio M. Soares. All rights reserved.)

The onset of the gingival overgrowth usually coincides with the eruption of the permanent incisors, while under rare circumstances, HGF can be present at birth. Breen et al. reported a 28-month-old child presenting with severe HGF, where only the incisal third of the lower primary incisors were visible, and all other primary teeth were easily palpable.[21] This patient had a family history of HF in an older brother, who had multiple surgical procedures for gingival reductions, and three unaffected sisters. Clinically, HGF causes a non-hemorrhagic, asymptomatic enlargement of the gingival tissues in various degrees; and it has a normal pink color, a firm, dense, and fibrous consistency, with significant stippling (Fig. 20.13A and B). Radiographic findings include retained, impacted/submerged teeth, or even delayed root resorption of the primary teeth. Bone involvement or bone loss is also frequently seen in children with HGF.[20,48]

HGF cannot be cured, but it can be controlled with varying degrees of success. Early diagnosis is very important in order to prevent gingival inflammation and potential attachment loss due to difficulty in oral hygiene. When the GE is minimal, professional cleaning and good home care may be sufficient. As the gingival tissue grows and starts affecting mastication, speech, or esthetics, surgical intervention—gingivectomy followed by gingivoplasty—might be required, and frequent follow-up is highly recommended. In a recent systematic review recurrence rate of GE after surgical treatment reached 34.92%.[20]

Localized Juvenile Spongiotic Gingival Hyperplasia

An additional condition that also appears to be unrelated to plaque accumulation is localized juvenile spongiotic gingival hyperplasia

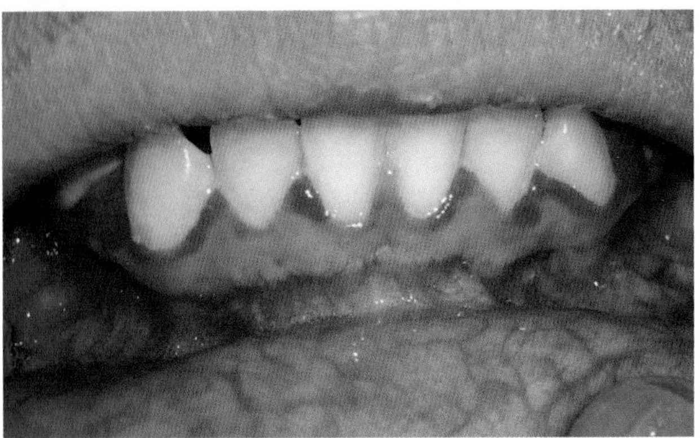

Fig. 20.14 Localized juvenile spongiotic gingival hyperplasia located on anterior labial mandibular area, covering the free gingival margins in a 13-year-old male. Papillary gingiva red, with gingival overgrowth prone to easy bleeding. (Copyright Dr. Daniela Silva. All rights reserved.)

(LJSGH). This condition was only identified in recent years by Darling et al. in 2007.[29] Its pathogenesis is not yet well defined, and most of the patients with this condition are between 8 and 14 years old. The lesions are most commonly located on the anterior labial maxillary area of the gingiva, covering the free gingival margin and attached gingiva, and present clinically as papillary, bright-red raised overgrowths; they are usually painless and associated with easy bleeding. LJSGH could also be associated with some environmental conditions such as tooth eruption, lip incompetence, and minor local trauma, e.g., the placement of orthodontic appliances.

Unlike puberty- and biofilm-related gingivitis, LJSGH is reported to not respond to conventional oral hygiene measures, such as brushing and flossing.[4,18,22,29,83,90,97] For cases of asymptomatic lesions, observation would be viable with spontaneous resolution after 3 to 6 months, and others recommend conservative surgical excision with recurrence having been reported to occur in 6% to 16.7% of the cases.[18,29,83,90,97]

A report of 52 microscopically identified cases found that the size of these lesions ranged from 2 to 10 mm in diameter, and most were localized single lesions. The epithelium was nonkeratinized and displayed prominent intercellular edema containing mostly acute, but some chronic inflammatory cells; highly vascular connective tissue cores were identified in connective tissue papilla (Fig. 20.14).[22]

An immunohistochemical study comparing the cytokeratin expression of the JE with that of the gingival epithelium (GE) proposed that, in the process of this "exteriorization," the epithelial cells of LJSGH retain their JE phenotype while beginning to show GE-related features, enabling them to adjust to their new location in the gingiva. The molecular changes precede the morphological ones, and, as the JE is typically thinner and less keratinized than the GE, it is more likely to be influenced by local irritants and become spongiotic.[4]

Periodontal Diseases in Children and Adolescents

Periodontitis is a multifactorial, microbially associated, host-mediated inflammatory disease characterized by progressive destruction of the periodontal attachment apparatus. It is a chronic inflammatory disease that can be successfully controlled, and teeth can be retained for life. Periodontitis can remain stable or enter periods of exacerbation. Therefore, precision dental medicine requires ongoing, individual risk assessment as part of optimal patient management.[24]

The AAPD recognizes that although the prevalence of destructive forms of periodontal disease is low amongst children and adolescents, this population can develop several forms of periodontal diseases and conditions associated with an underlying systemic or immunologic disorder.[8] Epidemiological studies of the formerly called aggressive periodontitis have used different study designs and a range of examination methods and case definitions, and this greatly complicates the study of disease prevalence in populations.[88] It is also known that the prevalence of periodontitis varies significantly between different geographic locations and between different races/ethnicities. Studies consistently show that (aggressive) periodontitis is most prevalent in African populations and their descendants. The disease prevalence in African populations is between 1% and 5%, and in Caucasians residing in North America, the disease affects 0.1% to 0.2% of Caucasians. The disease prevalence in South America is between 0.3% and 2.0%, and the disease prevalence in Asian populations is between 0.2% and 1.0%.[88]

As discussed previously, clinicians are encouraged to start probing regularly when the first permanent molars have fully erupted and the child is able to cooperate for this procedure in order to establish a baseline and detect early signs of periodontal disease. Ideally, it can be assessed as the proportion of bleeding sites stimulated by a standardized periodontal probe with controlled force at six sites (mesiobuccal, buccal, distobuccal, mesiolingual, lingual, distolingual). When probing into the sulcus, positioning the probe, and applying probe pressure correctly, the patient should not feel discomfort. While probing, clinicians should rule out the presence of pseudo pockets associated with tooth exfoliation or partially erupted teeth. For patients with special health care needs that are receiving dental treatment under oral sedation and/or general anesthesia, this gives clinicians an opportunity to perform periodontal probing more easily, in case it cannot be performed during regular appointments.

Rather than recording full-mouth probing depths in pediatric patients, clinicians may elect to focus on select teeth. For example, a rudimentary assessment of teeth #3, 8, 14, 19, 24, and 30 has been suggested,[25] with notes made regarding gingival health, bleeding on probing, and the presence of any calculus. This quick screening is generally sufficient for children up to the age of 11. Between the ages of 12 to 19, when most individuals have full permanent dentition, clinicians should also note pocket depths of more than 4 mm. By this stage of dental development, full-mouth pocket-depth probing may be warranted on the basis of general indicators of each patient's gingival health or risk of disease.

In 2017, the American Academy of Periodontology and the European Federation of Periodontology co-sponsored the World Workshop on the Classification of Periodontal and Peri-implant Diseases and Conditions. Due to concerns from clinicians, researchers, educators, and epidemiologists regarding their ability to properly distinguish between chronic and aggressive periodontitis, the World Workshop members proposed grouping these two forms of periodontitis into a single category, simply referred to as periodontitis.[8,91] One of the major highlights of this workshop included the recategorization of three forms of periodontitis (necrotizing periodontal diseases, periodontitis, and periodontitis as a manifestation of systemic diseases), the development of a multidimensional staging and grading system for periodontitis, and the new classification for peri-implant diseases and conditions.[91]

This new classification is extensively discussed in Chapter 21.

Periodontal probing depth (PPD) or probing attachment levels alone should not be used as evidence of gingival health or disease; rather they should be considered in conjunction with other important clinical parameters, such as BoP, predisposing factors—any agent that contributes to the accumulation of dental plaque, and modifying factors—any agent or condition that alters the way in which an individual responds to subgingival plaque accumulation (see

Chapters 23, 24, and 25 for a further discussion on this topic).[8,24] The workshop also identified a specific threshold for the values in BoP to define periodontal health and gingivitis (10% BoP in the absence of attachment loss) and gingival inflammation in a periodontitis patient (BoP >10% in the presence of attachment loss). Secondly, the classification workshop highlighted the need to establish CAL as the primary definition of periodontitis.[91]

Clinically, a patient is characterized as a periodontitis case if: (1) interdental CAL is detectable at ≥2 non-adjacent teeth; or (2) buccal or lingual CAL ≥3 mm with pocketing detectable at ≥2 teeth. Radiographic assessment is a critical component of clinical assessment of the periodontal tissues. A normal, anatomically intact periodontium would present an intact lamina dura, no evidence of bone loss, and a 1 to 3 mm distance from the most coronal portion of the alveolar bone crest to the cementoenamel junction (CEJ).[91]

The clinical entity previously referred to as aggressive periodontitis due to its rapid rate of progression is now categorized as Grade C periodontitis and represents the extreme end of a continuum of disease rates. This form is defined as a "generalized interproximal attachment loss, including at least three teeth that are not first molars and incisors," and is rare among children (Fig. 20.15A and B). The onset of this form of periodontitis generally occurs after the initiation of adolescence. The general prevalence is 0.13% among 14- to 17-year-old children[16]; however, individuals with Down syndrome demonstrate a higher prevalence.[6,19,75] A purported genetic influence in the overall disease process suggests that any signs of disease in a child with a family history of periodontitis should be investigated further.

Once the diagnosis is made, periodontitis cases need to be characterized by the newly introduced process of staging and grading.[8,91] Periodontitis stages are a simple description of the severity and complexity of management of individual cases, while periodontitis grades capture the risk of progression and the risk factor profile. With respect to previously utilized descriptions of periodontitis severity, the newly introduced system aims to identify, on one side of the spectrum, cases as early as possible through the identification of initial signs of attachment loss (stage I), and on the other side the more advanced cases requiring more advanced periodontal therapy (stage III) or complex periodontal and oral rehabilitation (stage IV). The identification of a periodontitis grade must involve the accumulated knowledge of direct or indirect evidence of disease progression or the presence of risk factors with clear evidence of modifying the prognosis and case management.[8]

Although the microbiology of this disease is discussed in Chapters 10 and 11, it is important to note that recent studies suggest the familial transmission of certain bacteria associated with periodontitis. Species such as *Tannerella forsythia, P. intermedia*, and *Prevotella nigrescens* are found more often in the children of individuals who have been shown to harbor these types of bacteria.[87] Both *Fusobacterium nucleatum* and *P. gingivalis* have been noted at significant levels in children of similarly affected parents.[15,46] The levels of these bacteria have been observed to increase with age, which suggests that *P. gingivalis* and *B. forsythus* may serve as early markers during screening for periodontal disease.[15,51,87] Thus, although periodontitis may not be highly prevalent in children, early colonization may underscore the importance of early detection, particularly for those at elevated risk for adult forms of the disease.

Several studies have suggested the involvement of *A. actinomycetemcomitans*[3,51,78] and *P. gingivalis*[3] in the pathogenesis of periodontitis. Both of these pathogens are relatively rare in healthy children, with a prevalence of 4.8%, but they are elevated in children with periodontitis, with a reported prevalence of 20%.[69] A recent study found a very strong association between generalized periodontitis and the prevalence and abundance of *A. actinomycetemcomitans*. They also observed *A. actinomycetemcomitans* as being very site-specific: it was more prevalent and abundant in diseased sites as compared with healthy sites in individuals with periodontitis.[78]

Therapeutic Considerations in the Pediatric Patient

Oral hygiene habits should be imprinted early during life, with instructions regarding proper technique and directions regarding the frequency of plaque removal procedures. These will form a foundation for a lifetime of dedication to periodontal health. Clinicians should be aware of the specific periodontal needs of children with particular abnormalities, such as gingival hyperplasia associated with immune suppression protocols used with organ transplants, antiseizure medications, and increased severity of periodontal disease in children with diabetes. Physically and mentally challenged children deserve special care to ensure that appropriate preventive techniques are available; these may include the use of electric toothbrushes and antibacterial mouthrinses.

In-office professional plaque control procedures can vary in accordance with a patient's stage of development. As noted previously, calculus deposits are uncommon in infants and toddlers. Supragingival plaque removal with the use of simple rubber-cup coronal polishing or a toothbrush is usually sufficient during the primary dentition.[25] If calculus deposits are evident, selective supragingival scaling may be performed. As the permanent teeth erupt, the prevalence of calculus deposits increases, often necessitating targeted subgingival scaling in addition to supragingival plaque removal.[25]

Toothbrushing can be considered a complex skill. It consists of two main components: motor skill (toothbrush grip and dexterity) and the cognitive aspect (understanding the process and its objective). In children, however, the dynamic process of developing manual dexterity affects the ability of a child to perform expected procedures. It is well known that oral health education alone does not necessarily lead to behavior changes. For children to have a more joyful learning process, education and entertainment should be combined; this can be achieved by making use of cost-effective media and tools. Individual oral hygiene training given to children has been shown to increase toothbrushing efficiency, but not in the long term.[103] Each child requires an individualized home care program based on their ability to actually perform the requested activities. For young children, plaque control should be a shared responsibility between children and their parents or caregivers. Instruction in plaque control should be delivered to parents and children in language and terms that both understand. For children who are less than 7 years old, parents or caregivers should be asked to assist with toothbrushing. Children may be encouraged to take a turn brushing their teeth using a simple scrub technique. However, parents should also take a turn to ensure the proper removal of plaque. By 7 years old, children generally possess the manual dexterity to brush their teeth on their own and may only require limited adult supervision. More refined brushing techniques can be introduced during adolescence.

Parents' and caregivers' oral hygiene habits have a significant influence on children's oral health behavior. An extensive survey performed with parents in the UK found that both children and parents place a large emphasis on the cosmetic benefit of toothbrushing. Parents who placed more emphasis on the short-term benefits of toothbrushing were more likely to miss brushing their child's teeth

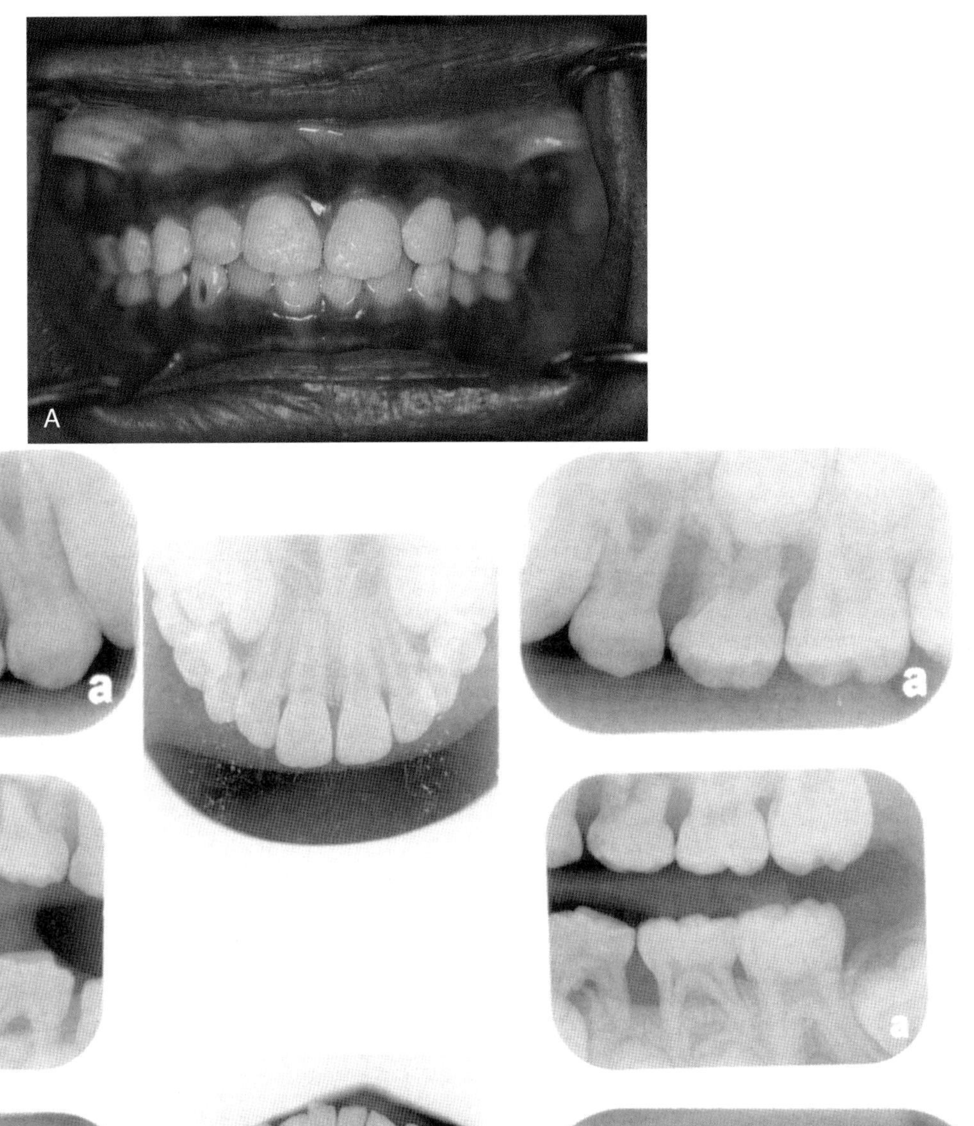

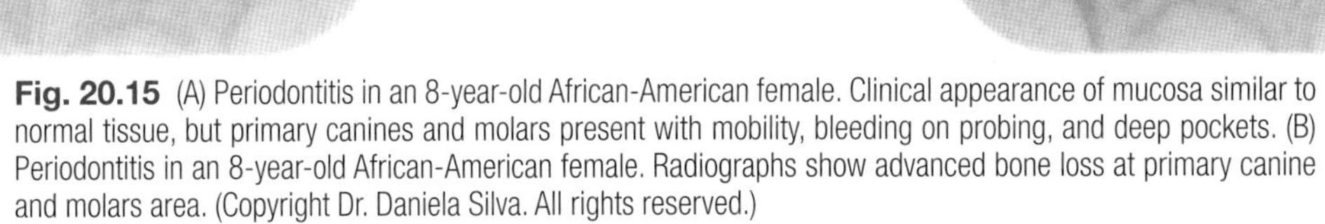

Fig. 20.15 (A) Periodontitis in an 8-year-old African-American female. Clinical appearance of mucosa similar to normal tissue, but primary canines and molars present with mobility, bleeding on probing, and deep pockets. (B) Periodontitis in an 8-year-old African-American female. Radiographs show advanced bone loss at primary canine and molars area. (Copyright Dr. Daniela Silva. All rights reserved.)

in the evening, but when brushing a child's teeth was "habitual" there was a significantly higher chance of brushing twice a day.[92]

Mechanical toothbrushes with rotary heads have been shown to be effective for plaque removal.[25] The use of these devices can be encouraged as soon as children are able to tolerate the vibrating sensation because many children initially dislike the feeling of the rotary movement. Mechanical toothbrushes are especially recommended for physically challenged children and individuals with fixed orthodontic appliances.[68,102] A Cochrane review on "powered versus manual toothbrushing for oral health" published in 2014 found that compared with manual toothbrushes, powered toothbrushes are more effective than manual brushes in reducing plaque and gingivitis in the long and short term.[101] An 11% reduction in plaque (Quigley Hein [Turesky] index) was shown at 1 to 3 months and a 21% reduction in plaque at longer than three months. With regard to gingivitis, a 6% reduction (Löe Silness index) was seen at one to three months and a greater reduction of 11% in the long term. The clinical importance of these findings remains unclear.

Nonetheless, only three trials were able to be used in the sensitivity analysis for trials at low risk of bias. And these trials were unable to demonstrate statistically significant differences between powered and manual toothbrushes, although the effect estimates for plaque and gingivitis at 1 to 3 months were higher than those for all trials.[100]

Flossing is usually not indicated for children during the primary dentition stage because most children have interdental spacing throughout most of their arches. However, as interdental contacts develop, flossing should be added to the home care routine. Studies have demonstrated both a decrease in gingival bleeding and the number of microbes associated with periodontal disease when tooth and tongue brushing is combined with flossing.[11,27] Again, limitations in manual dexterity may necessitate parental assistance with flossing during the mixed dentition stage. Adolescents with sufficient manual dexterity can be expected to floss on their own.[25] A recent Cochrane review on interproximal cleaning devices found that additional use of floss or interdental brushes compared to toothbrushing alone may reduce gingivitis or plaque, or both, and interdental brushes may be more effective than floss. The evidence is low to very low certainty, and the effect sizes observed may not be clinically important. The available evidence for cleaning sticks and oral irrigation aids is limited and inconsistent. Adverse events reported were minor; there were no serious adverse events and no evidence of a difference between study arms. The long-term significance of the findings is unclear as few of the studies evaluated pocket probing depth as a measure of periodontitis and none assessed interproximal caries.[99]

Antimicrobial mouthrinses for chemical plaque control are not indicated for very young children because of the risk of ingestion of chemical agents.[25] However, rinses may be indicated for older children who demonstrate the ability to expectorate after rinsing. In 2017, a Cochrane review on chlorhexidine mouthrinse found high-quality evidence of a large reduction in dental plaque with chlorhexidine used as an adjunct to mechanical oral hygiene procedures for 4 to 6 weeks and 6 months. There was no evidence that one concentration of chlorhexidine mouthrinse was more effective than another. Rinsing with chlorhexidine mouthrinse for 4 weeks or longer causes extrinsic tooth staining. In addition, other adverse effects such as calculus build-up, transient taste disturbance, and effects on the oral mucosa were reported in the included studies.[42]

Periodontitis as Manifestations of Systemic Conditions

Systemic diseases may share common risk factors that lead to an increased inflammatory response when there is an interruption in equilibrium. For example, the host response to oral bacteria may be altered by diabetes, rheumatoid arthritis, systemic lupus erythematous, and leukocyte adhesion deficiency (LAD) so that the degree of inflammation induced is greater than it would be in normal conditions.[36] Systemic diseases that result in periodontitis occur more frequently in children than adults.[3] Chapter 25 discusses some of the general systemic diseases and disorders that affect periodontal health in adults. The are many diseases and conditions that can affect the periodontal tissues, either by influencing the course of periodontitis (e.g., Papillon–Lefèvre syndrome, leukocyte adhesion deficiency, and hypophosphatasia [HPP]) or by affecting the periodontal supporting tissues independently of dental plaque biofilm-induced inflammation (e.g., diabetes mellitus). In this chapter, we will discuss only the most common diseases and conditions affecting the periodontal tissues in children and adolescents.

Endocrine Disorders

Diabetes Mellitus

Type 1 or insulin-dependent diabetes mellitus occurs more frequently in children and young adults than type 2 or non–insulin-dependent diabetes mellitus. As in adults with diabetes, gingival inflammation and periodontitis are more prevalent in affected children than in unaffected individuals, and the level of glycemic control may be more important in determining the severity of gingival inflammation than the quality of plaque control.[43,63,68] Clinical consequences include premature tooth loss and impaired immune response to the oral flora. There are no characteristic phenotypic features that are unique to periodontitis in patients with diabetes mellitus.

A recent systematic review and a meta-analysis on the periodontal risk markers in children and adolescents with type 1 diabetes (T1D) provided strong evidence that the severity of the plaque index, gingival index, bleeding on probing, PPD, and clinical attachment loss is increased in the population with T1D when compared to healthy children and adolescents.[1,43,49] A study comparing 350 children with T1D to 350 healthy controls found that the plaque index was significantly higher in permanent teeth than in primary teeth in both groups, but both dentitions presented higher gingival bleeding in the T1D group. The number of teeth with bleeding gingiva has an association with the mean HbA1c, body mass index (BMI), and duration of diabetes.[49]

Although destructive changes are rather rare in healthy children, periodontal destruction can be observed in children with diabetes, usually appearing around the time of puberty and becoming progressively worse as children mature into adulthood. Disease prevention and fastidious oral hygiene measures should be highly promoted.[43,49–51]

Hematologic Disorders and Immune Deficiencies

Leukemias

Leukemia is the most common pediatric malignancy accounting for about 30% of all pediatric cancers in children less than 15 years of age. Leukemia is a malignancy of the bone marrow characterized by a clonal expansion of hematopoietic cells with compromised differentiation, regulation, and apoptosis. Acute lymphocytic leukemia (ALL) accounts for the majority of cases among children who are less than 7 years old, with the highest incidence between 2 and 5 years of age.[94] Oral manifestations may occur in any of the leukemias, but they are more prevalent in acute (vs. chronic) and myeloid (vs. lymphoid) leukemias. Leukemia must be considered as part of the differential diagnosis for children who present with the hallmark features of lymphadenopathy, petechiae, mucosal ulcers, acute GE, gingival bleeding, and infection, or presenting with mucosa pallor due to anemia (Fig. 20.16).[72]

Gingival bleeding is a common sign in patients with leukemia and is the initial oral sign and/or symptom in 17.7% and 4.4% of patients with acute and chronic leukemias, respectively.[63] The bleeding is due to thrombocytopenia and clotting factor deficiencies and can present in preleukemic stages. Patients may also develop severe viral, fungal, and bacterial oral infections as a consequence of immunosuppression. Gingival hyperplasia results from leukemic infiltration of the gingiva, and it often improves markedly following appropriate chemotherapy.[76] Oral complications from chemotherapy include mucositis, gingival bleeding, xerostomia, candidiasis, and viral or bacterial infections.[94] Because the oral lesions are extremely painful, brushing has to be replaced by wiping with pads soaked in cold water, sodium bicarbonate, or non-alcohol chlorhexidine solutions. A lip moisturizer can be applied using a cotton tip applicator throughout the day. Regular oral examinations are recommended, and dental care should focus on maintaining dental health and treating the long-term effects of therapy.

Neutrophil-Associated Primary Immunodeficiency (PIDs)

As mentioned in greater detail in Chapter 11, neutrophil disorders impair defenses against infections, thereby making afflicted individuals susceptible to severe periodontal destruction. Neutrophils make up more than 95% of the total number of leukocytes in the gingival tissues and form the first line of defense against the subgingival biofilm.[40] Therefore, the diagnosis of the systemic disorder generally will have occurred before any signs of periodontal destruction appear. Many neutrophil disorders are genetic, including severe congenital neutropenia and cyclic neutropenia, glycogen storage disease, LAD, Papillon–Lefèvre syndrome, Chédiak-Higashi syndrome, and Cohen syndrome.[40,44] A recent systematic review on neutrophil disorders found that 71% to 97% of the patients present with severe levels of periodontitis, and mild periodontitis was described in 9% to 33% of the cases. The characteristics of periodontal disease in these patients were reported as alveolar bone loss in up to 90% of the cases, tooth mobility in up to 75% of cases, furcation involvement in up to 27% of cases, and gingival recession in up to 57% of cases. Affected patients often complain of pain, bleeding and swollen gums, loose teeth, bad breath, and difficulty eating (Fig. 20.17A and B).[39,40]

LAD represents a group of inherited disorders that affects 1 in 1 million individuals. The disease inhibits the normal extravasation of circulating neutrophils to sites of infection or inflammation. Few, if any, neutrophils can be found in extravascular sites in these patients, who display neutrophilia even in the absence of infection.[28,39] Clinical features usually present in infancy or early childhood and consist of recurrent bacterial infection of the skin, mouth, and respiratory tract together. LAD type I patients suffer from those recurrent infections and develop severe periodontitis early in life, affecting both primary and permanent dentitions.[28]

Even though periodontal changes are difficult to reverse in children with neutrophil disorders, disease management should include oral hygiene measures, mechanical debridement, antimicrobial therapy, teeth extraction, and supportive care for any resultant tissue destruction or tooth loss. The periodontal stability in such patients using these management approaches has been maintained for up to 9 years.[40] Treatment success is unpredictable as a result of the impact of systemic disease, and the early tooth loss could have devastating effects on mastication, esthetics, and quality of life.[8,44]

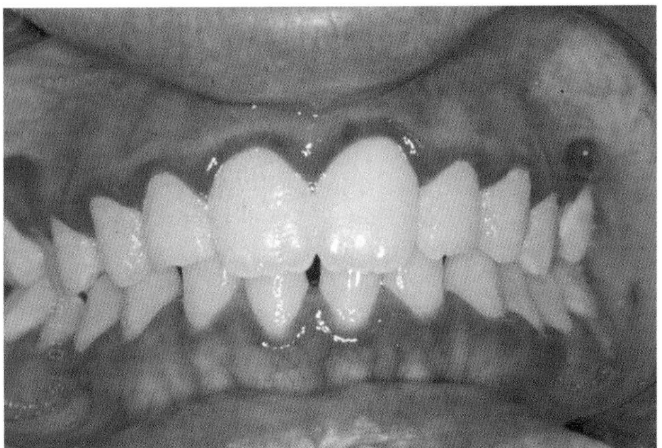

Fig. 20.16 Twelve-year-old male with acute lymphoblastic leukemia. Generalized redness of marginal gingiva, with spontaneous bleeding. (Copyright Dr. Daniela Silva. All rights reserved.)

Congenital Anomalies

Down Syndrome

Down syndrome is another congenital condition that would be diagnosed before the manifestation of periodontal disease. Afflicted individuals experience a high prevalence of periodontitis with different levels of severity during early adulthood. In children, the teeth most affected by the disease are the mandibular incisors and maxillary first molars; canines are the least affected teeth. The disease process is thought to be related to some kind of host susceptibility that results in an exaggerated immune-inflammatory response rather than a reaction to a specific causative microbe.[6,7,44] Studies performed on subjects with Down syndrome uncovered defective neutrophil chemotaxis, as well as increased production of inflammatory mediators and proteolytic enzymes, which can lead to significant tissue loss and the progression of periodontitis.[44,75]

The results of a recent meta-analysis revealed no statistically significant differences between patients with DS and control patients with regard to an oral hygiene index (OHI). To avoid clinical heterogeneity, the investigators compiled similar parameters in the meta-analysis. Although investigators in some studies used the OHI to diagnose periodontal disease, this index is an indicator of oral hygiene performance, which alone cannot be used to determine the presence of the disease.[75]

Hypophosphatasia

HPP is a rare, genetic, systemic, metabolic disease caused by the deficient activity of the tissue's nonspecific isoenzyme alkaline

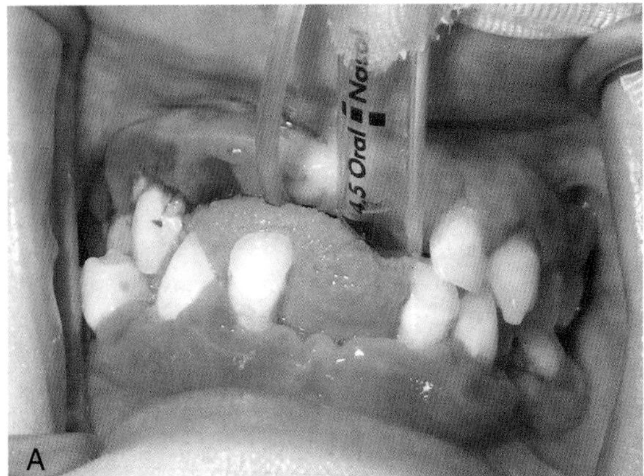

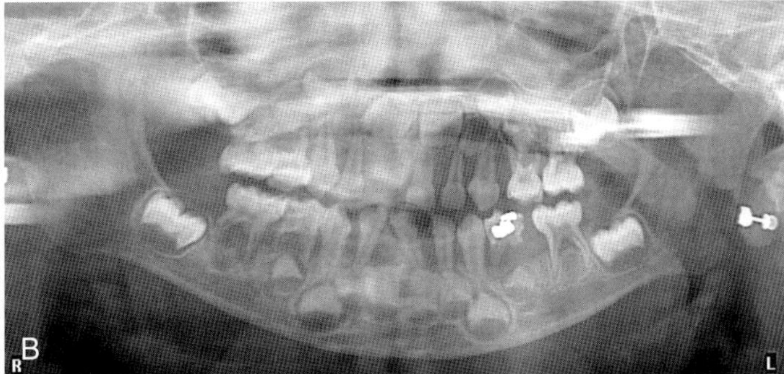

Fig. 20.17 (A) Four-year-old male with severe congenital neutropenia. Generalized periodontitis with painful, erythematous and edematous gingival tissue, and premature loss of primary teeth. (B) Panoramic image of 4-year-old male with severe congenital neutropenia. Generalized bone loss and premature loss of primary teeth. (Copyright Dr. Daniela Silva. All rights reserved.)

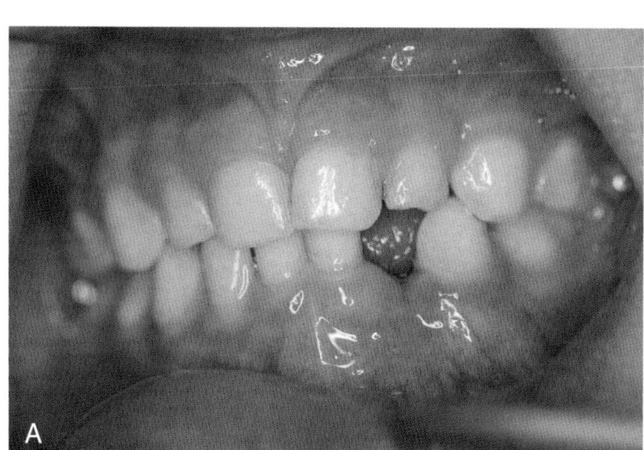

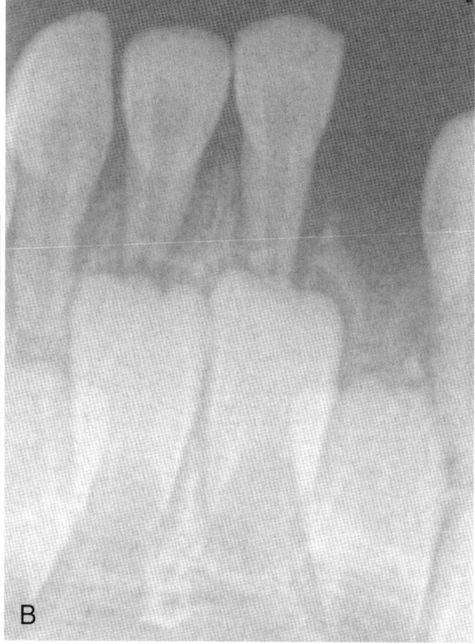

Fig. 20.18 (A) Three-year-old male with hypophosphatasia and premature loss of primary lower left incisor. Chlorhexidine stains around the gingival margins are present. (B) Lower occlusal radiograph of a 3-year-old male with hypophosphatasia and premature loss of primary lower left incisor. (Copyright Dr. Daniela Silva. All rights reserved.)

phosphatase, resulting in the extracellular accumulation of its substrate, which may be detected in blood and urine. The clinical manifestations of HPP have a wide spectrum of symptoms, including early loss of primary teeth (with intact roots) and alveolar bone mineralization defects, skeletal problems, muscle weakness, ambulatory difficulties, and pain (Fig. 20.18A and B).[16,89]

A recent systematic review included 511 individual cases of HPP, where 265 cases had a minimum follow-up of 1 year. The median age for this group was 4 years, and the median duration of follow-up was 7 years. Premature tooth loss, bone fracture, and pain were the most common manifestations, regardless of when the disease first manifests.[89]

Nutritional Influences—Malnutrition

The precise role of nutrition in the initiation or progression of periodontal disease remains to be elucidated. The one nutritional deficiency that has well-documented effects on periodontal tissue is the reduction of plasma ascorbic acid (vitamin C).[30,63] One of vitamin C's principal roles is stimulating collagen synthesis by increasing the transcription of procollagen genes. For this reason, vitamin C induces periodontal ligament differentiation and osteoblast differentiation. Severe vitamin C deficiency results in scurvy, and some of the clinical features of scurvy are hyperkeratosis, petechiae, ecchymosis, xerostomia, impaired wound healing, and inflamed and bleeding gums.[30,35] In the absence of frank scurvy, the effect of declining ascorbic acid levels on the gingiva can be difficult to detect clinically, and when it is detected, it usually has characteristics that are similar to plaque-induced gingivitis.[30]

Vitamins are defined as essential organic compounds that are catalysts for the body's metabolic reactions; they also function as electron donors, antioxidants, and transcription effectors. The bioavailability of those vitamins is regulated or influenced by other physiological factors, including the efficiency of gastrointestinal absorption and digestion. Clinical studies have demonstrated a significant association between vitamin D's endocrine effects and periodontal disease, where patients with generalized periodontitis have shown significantly elevated vitamin D-binding protein plasma levels.[23] Vitamin D may also have an impact on the periodontal immune response by decreasing interleukin (IL)-8 and IL-6 expression.[35]

Because vitamin deficiency may play a role in the development and progression of periodontitis and gingival bleeding, the 2017 EFP/ORCA Workshop concluded that dietary counseling on vitamin C and vitamin D intakes should be part of the information provided to our patients and caregivers.[23]

Obesity

Childhood obesity is a global epidemic; however, the understanding of this medical problem in children is far from being achieved due to the lack of comparable representative data from different countries. Obesity is a complex, multifactorial disease arising from excessive storage of fat, resulting from an interaction of social, behavioral, cultural, physiological, metabolic, and genetic factors.

Recent cross-sectional comparative studies[71,105] and meta-analyses consistently showed a statistically significant positive association between obesity and periodontitis in the pediatric population and adults.[57] Several hypotheses for biological interactions between obesity and periodontal diseases have been proposed. Theories suggest that obesity is known to induce a hyper-inflammatory state, with T-lymphocyte and monocyte/macrophage changes that could affect response to microbial challenges. It is also associated with cytokine production, adipokines, and other bioactive substances like reactive oxygen species that could contribute to increased gingival inflammation and/or periodontal breakdown associated with periodontal disease. Nevertheless, the specific molecular and cellular mechanisms are not yet clear.[57]

Drug-Induced Gingival Enlargement

GE, which is discussed in Chapter 19, may result from the use of certain drugs. Drugs primarily associated with gingival tissue enlargement include antiepileptic drugs (e.g., phenytoin and sodium valproate), immunosuppressive drugs (e.g., cyclosporine) for solid-organ transplanted patients, and the concomitant use of calcium

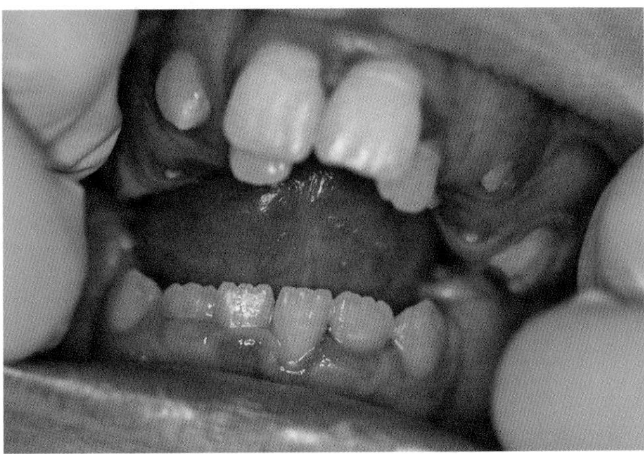

Fig. 20.19 Ten-year-old male with history of cerebral palsy, seizures, and phenytoin-induced gingival enlargement. (Copyright Dr. Daniela Silva. All rights reserved.)

channel blockers (e.g., verapamil, nifedipine, felodipine) used to offset the hypertensive side effect of cyclosporine (Fig. 20.19). A recent randomized clinical trial found an interesting and significant decrease in the incidence (21%) of phenytoin-induced gingival hyperplasia in children with epilepsy taking oral folic acid supplementation (0.5 mg/day) as compared with the control group (88%).[9] Although complicated by the plaque levels along the gingival margin, this form of gingival disease has features that are not typical of chronic marginal gingivitis.[68] The common clinical characteristics of drug-influenced GEs include variations in interpatient or intrapatient patterns or enlargement, a tendency to occur more often in the anterior areas, a higher prevalence in younger age groups, onset within 3 months of drug use (usually observed at the papilla), and it is not associated with attachment loss or tooth mobility.[60,63] In children, GE may be so severe that the overgrown gingival tissues interfere with normal oral functions and may cause delayed and/or ectopic tooth eruptions (resulting in poor plaque control and severe gingivitis), impaired speech, and esthetic problems, which may have serious consequences on their self-esteem.[80]

Regarding the management of drug-induced GE, a recent systematic review[60] on the different treatment modalities concluded that there is not enough evidence to recommend nonsurgical versus surgical interventions. The nonsurgical techniques include medication substitution, only if the new medication is anticipated to control the patient's underlying condition, as well as improving the drug-induced gingival hyperplasia, scaling and root planing, and/or antimicrobial and antibiotic therapies. Patients with more severe cases may cosmetically benefit from resection of the fibrotic gingival tissues using a scalpel or laser-assisted therapy. The risk of recurrence has been linked to different factors, such as age, gingival inflammation, and patient compliance with recall visits.

Conclusions

- The periodontium of the primary dentition differs from that of the permanent dentition.
- Normal development can result in changes to the periodontium.
- Plaque-induced gingivitis is very common in children, although it may be less intense than in adults.
- With the exception of localized aggressive periodontitis, children rarely show signs of periodontitis.
- It is evident that dental plaque causes gingival inflammation, and the extent and the severity of the inflammation are influenced by oral factors and systemic conditions.
- Plaque accumulates more rapidly at inflamed gingival sites than at non-inflamed sites
- Some systemic disorders that are commonly associated with periodontal disease present initially during childhood.
- Recommendations regarding home plaque control routines should be individualized according to each patient's periodontal disease status and developmental stage.
- Since early diagnosis ensures the greatest chance for successful treatment, it is paramount that children receive a periodontal examination as part of their routine dental visits.

Summary of Basic Periodontal Examination

1. Healthy: no attachment loss (identified as no CAL ≤ 3 mm) and no to minimal gingival inflammation (measured as <10% sites bleeding on probing).
2. Gingivitis: no attachment loss (identified as no CAL ≤ 3 mm) and presence of gingival inflammation (≥10% sites bleeding on probing).
   - Localized gingivitis: 10% to 30% bleeding sites
   - Generalized gingivitis: ≥30% bleeding sites
3. Periodontitis: CAL ≥ 3 mm in ≥2 non-adjacent teeth and radiographic bone loss ≥15% (for details on the staging and grading refer to Chapter 21).

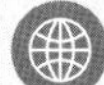 References for this chapter are found on the companion website eBooks.Health.Elsevier.com.

CHAPTER 21

Periodontitis

Henrik Dommisch | Moritz Kebschull

CHAPTER OUTLINE

Definition of Periodontitis

Periodontitis is defined as a complex inflammatory disease that affects the tooth-supporting structures, including the periodontal ligament and alveolar bone. In this context, the word "complex" describes not only the fact that there are multiple clinical symptoms that account for the disease, but also because of the multiple factors that lead to and influence periodontal inflammation. Periodontitis occurs most frequently in adults. Nonetheless, it may also be diagnosed in children and adolescents when associated with chronic plaque and calculus accumulation. Therefore, periodontitis should be understood as age-associated, but not age-dependent, complex chronic inflammation of the periodontal tissues. As described below, systemic and/or environmental factors (e.g., diabetes mellitus, smoking) modify the host immune response to the dental biofilm so that the periodontal destruction becomes more progressive.

Periodontitis is a highly prevalent progressing disease and is considered the sixth most common human disease which belongs to the group of chronic non-communicable diseases (CNCDs) (Figs. 21.1 and 21.2). It affects approximately 10%, 5% up to 12% of the world population.[61] In the past decade, it has been found that periodontitis exerts adverse effects on systemic health, and in this context, important pathological interdependencies with, for example, diabetes mellitus have been identified.[19,49,50,74,99] Also, it is known that systemic inflammatory markers, such as the C-reactive protein (CRP), are elevated in patients with periodontitis.[95,126] In general, periodontitis is considered a slowly progressing disease, but in the presence of severe systemic conditions and/or environmental factors, such as smoking, this inflammatory disease progresses more rapidly.

The former classification described two different major forms of periodontitis, aggressive and chronic periodontitis,[2] with aggressive periodontitis being defined as a rapidly progressing entity in systemically healthy subjects with a familiar aggregation (see "Historical Perspective" below).

The classical definition reflected periodontitis as "an infectious disease resulting in inflammation within the supporting tissues of the teeth, progressive attachment loss, and bone loss."[37] In the past decades, the etiopathologic factors that lead to periodontal inflammation, and subsequently, in the destruction of periodontal tissues, have been widely studied, and the interplay between the microbial environment and the individual host immune response gained attention in the scientific community (see below).

Periodontitis represents major clinical and etiologic characteristics of this complex disease: (1) microbial biofilm formation (dental plaque), (2) periodontal inflammation (gingival swelling, bleeding on probing), and (3) attachment as well as alveolar bone loss.

Besides the local immune response to the dental biofilm, periodontitis may also be associated with a number of systemic disorders and defined syndromes. In most cases, patients with systemic diseases, which lead to impaired host immunity, may also show periodontal destruction. On the other hand, periodontitis is a disease not only limited to the area of the oral cavity, but may be associated with severe systemic diseases such as cardiovascular disease, stroke, and diabetes mellitus.[35,49,71,96,99,107]

This chapter discusses clinical features that have been described for periodontitis in light of the current classification of periodontal and peri-implant diseases and conditions, and specifically, with respect to stages and grades of periodontitis.[18,94]

General Characteristics and Symptoms

Characteristic clinical findings in patients with untreated periodontitis may include the following symptoms:

- Supragingival and subgingival plaque (and calculus)
- Gingival swelling, redness, and loss of gingival stippling
- Altered gingival margins (rolled, flattened, cratered papillae, recessions)
- Pocket formation
- Bleeding on probing
- Attachment loss
- Bone loss (angular or horizontal)
- Root furcation involvement
- Increased tooth mobility
- Change in tooth position
- Tooth loss

The aforementioned signs and symptoms may all be simultaneously present or not. However, the main symptom of periodontitis is the loss of attachment.

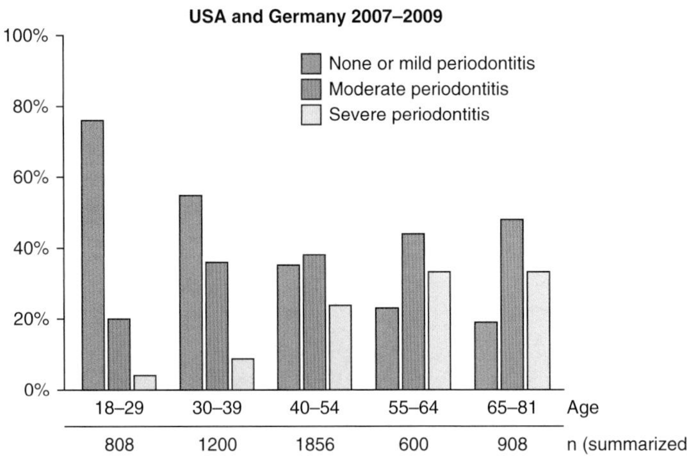

Fig. 21.1 Prevalence for periodontitis in the United States and Germany (2007–2009). (Combined data from Genco RJ, Falkner KL, Grossi S, et al. Validity of self-reported measures for surveillance of periodontal disease in two western New York population-based studies. *J Periodontol.* 2007;78:1439–1454; Holtfreter B, Schwahn C, Biffar R, Kocher T. Epidemiology of periodontal diseases in the Study of Health in Pomerania. *J Clin Periodontol.* 2009;36:114–123. Reviewed in Demmer RT, Papapanou PN. Epidemiologic patterns of chronic and aggressive periodontitis. *Periodontol 2000.* 2010;53:28–44.)

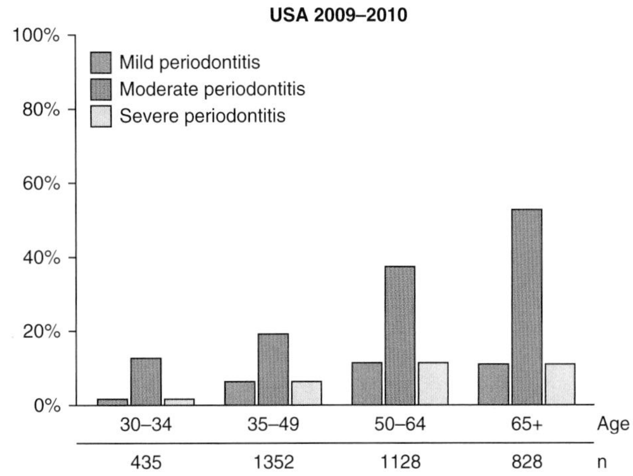

Fig. 21.2 Prevalence for periodontitis in the United States (2009–2010). (Combined data from Eke PI, Dye BA, Wei L, et al. CDC Periodontal Disease Surveillance Workgroup. James Beck GDRP. Prevalence of periodontitis in adults in the United States: 2009 and 2010. *J Dent Res.* 2012;91:914–920.)

Periodontitis can be clinically revealed by means of periodontal screening (e.g., periodontal screening index; PSI), diagnosed by an assessment of the clinical attachment level, and therewith, the detection of inflammatory changes in the marginal gingiva (Fig. 21.3). Measurements of periodontal probing pocket depth in combination with the location of the marginal gingiva allow conclusions regarding the loss of clinical attachment (Fig. 21.4). Dental radiographs reveal the extent of bone loss indicated by the distance between the cementoenamel junction and the alveolar bone crest (Fig. 21.5).

Periodontitis is commonly a slowly progressive complex disease without pain experience. Therefore, most patients are unaware that they have developed a chronic disease. For the majority of patients, gingival bleeding during oral hygiene procedures or eating may be the first sign of disease occurrence. Areas with advanced periodontal inflammation may show pus emersion from the periodontal pocket. As a result of gingival recession, patients may notice black triangles between teeth and/or tooth sensibility in response to temperature changes (cold and heat). In addition, food impaction may occur in the space of interdental triangles leading to increased patient discomfort and bad breath.

In cases with advanced attachment and bone loss, tooth mobility, tooth movement, fanned out or elongated front teeth, and, on rare occasions, tooth loss may be reported. In those cases with advanced disease progression, areas of localized dull pain or pain sensations radiating to other areas of the mouth and/or head may occur.

Systematic Diagnosis—Staging and Grading

The current classification scheme for periodontal and peri-implant diseases and conditions represents a systematic approach to defining both the disease phenotype (staging) and the disease progression (grading).[18] This scheme exhibits well-defined parameters that provide characteristics for staging and grading.

Staging

Staging corresponds to the description of the disease phenotype, and the classification scheme provides a table that displays three categories that define disease severity, complexity, and distribution. Differentiation between stages is based on parameters that define the severity and complexity of periodontitis. Severity and complexity need to be interpreted interdependently, and the combination of clinical features eventually results in a defined stage of disease. In this context, it is important to note that clinical findings and features that relate to disease severity and complexity need to be present at at least two independent periodontal sites. Periodontitis is, hence, not considered as a disease that affects one single site in the dentition. Here, other diagnostic considerations and examinations are mandatory to distinguish between periodontitis and other conditions related to the periodontium, such as vertical root fractures or endo-perio-lesions, that may occur at one single site only (also see Chapter 49). Periodontitis needs to be considered as a—in most cases—slowly progressive complex inflammatory disease that eventually affects the entire dentition, if not treated. Therefore, the diagnosis of a certain stage of periodontitis may only reflect a transient stage during disease progression at the examination time-point. If no treatment is provided to the patient, a higher stage of periodontitis will most likely be diagnosed at the time of re-examination several years later.

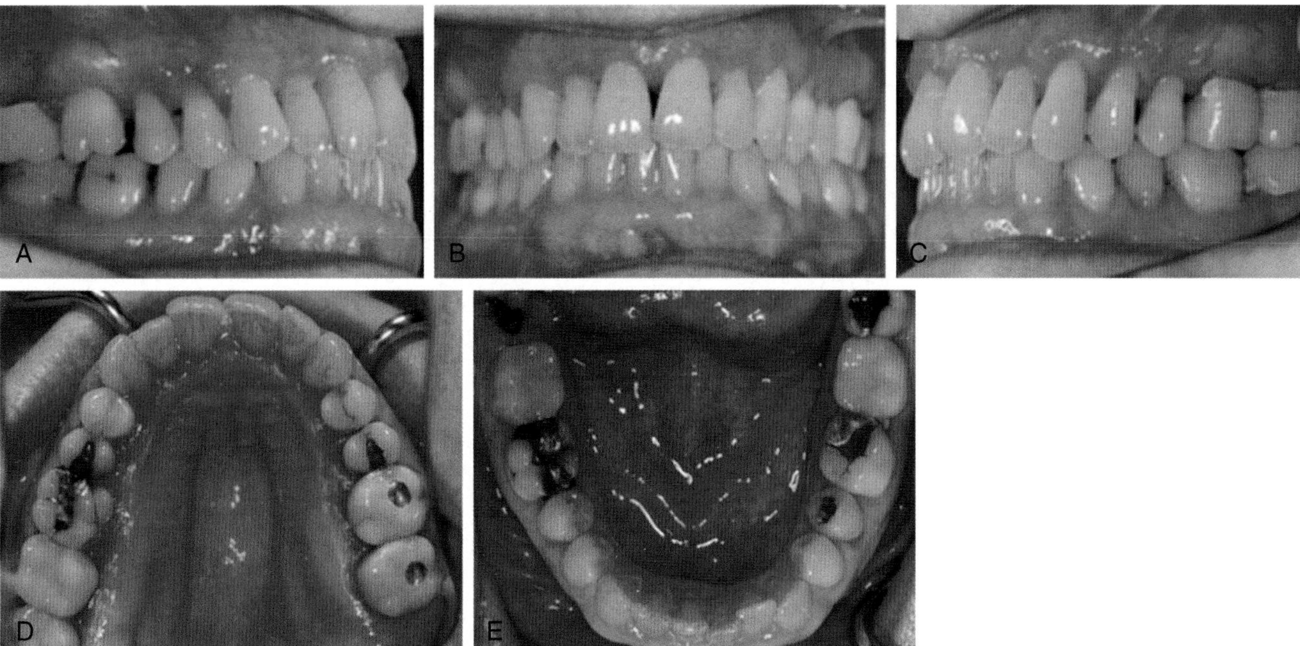

Fig. 21.3 Clinical features of generalized periodontitis (stage III, grade B) in a 49-year-old, medically healthy male patient. The patient reported smoking habits (15 cigarettes per day). At the first visit, the periodontal photo documentation displays untreated chronic periodontitis with abundant dental plaque and calculus deposits, gingival redness and swelling, and alteration of the gingival texture (loss of gingival stippling). The patient noticed multiple recessions. In this case, recessions were the result from loss of clinical attachment and alveolar bone. (A) Right lateral view; (B) frontal view; (C) left lateral view; (D) maxillary view; (E) mandibular view.

CLINICIAN'S CORNER

For defining the correct periodontal diagnosis, clinical findings and features that relate to disease severity and complexity need to be present at at least two independent periodontal sites. Periodontitis is considered as a disease that eventually affects the entire dentition, and the defined stages of disease are transient stages during the progression of periodontitis.

Severity of Periodontitis

In most cases, the severity and extent of periodontal destruction occur over time in combination with systemic disorders impairing and/or enhancing host immune responses. If untreated and/or oral hygiene behaviors remain unchanged, periodontitis eventually leads to tooth loss, and systemic conditions may be negatively influenced by the uncontrolled progression of periodontal inflammation. Relative to the degree of attachment and bone loss, disease severity is described by the definition of disease stages.

Periodontal disease severity is defined by three parameters: interproximal attachment loss (clinical attachment loss; CAL), alveolar bone loss, and tooth loss due to periodontitis (Table 21.1). These parameters initially determine the stage of the disease. Interpretation of the CAL, as well as the alveolar bone loss (BL), allow to distinguish between stage I, II, and III:

- **Stage I:** CAL = 1 to 2 mm and BL ≤ 15%;
- **Stage II:** CAL = 3 to 4 mm and BL = 15% to 33%
- **Stage III and IV:** CAL ≥ 5 mm and BL = 33% to 100%.

Determination of tooth loss due to periodontitis then allows further differentiation between stages. For stages I and II, no teeth should be missing or tooth loss occurred due to other reasons besides periodontitis such as caries, or traumatic or endodontic complications. If ≤4 or ≥5 teeth were lost due to periodontitis, a stage III or IV, respectively, needs to be considered:

- **Stage I and II:** no tooth loss due to periodontitis;
- **Stage III:** ≤4 teeth lost due to periodontitis;
- **Stage IV:** ≥5 teeth lost due to periodontitis.

Tooth loss is equal to 100% attachment loss, and therefore, teeth that were lost during the course of periodontitis are highly relevant to the interpretation of disease severity.

Complexity of Periodontitis

Complexity factors are defined to further differentiate between stages of periodontitis (see Table 21.1).

To describe disease complexity, the following local parameters need to be determined: probing pocket depth (PPD), furcation involvement (FI), horizontal and vertical BL, tooth mobility, mastication function, and ridge defects.

With respect to the complexity factors, stage I and stage II are differentiated by PPD, while a horizontally destroyed alveolar bone is characteristic for both stages:

- **Stage I:** PPD ≤4 mm, mostly horizontal BL;
- **Stage II:** PPD ≤5 mm, mostly horizontal BL.

The precise determination of complexity factors is important to distinguish stage III and stage IV. In certain cases, differentiation between stage III and IV is not possible solely based on severity factors. Thus, complexity factors eventually allow for clear differentiation.

In the case of stage III, deeper pocket probing depth and vertical bone loss with furcation involvement are clinical features in addition to stage II:

- **Stage III:**
  - PPD ≥6 mm;
  - Vertical bone loss ≥3 mm;

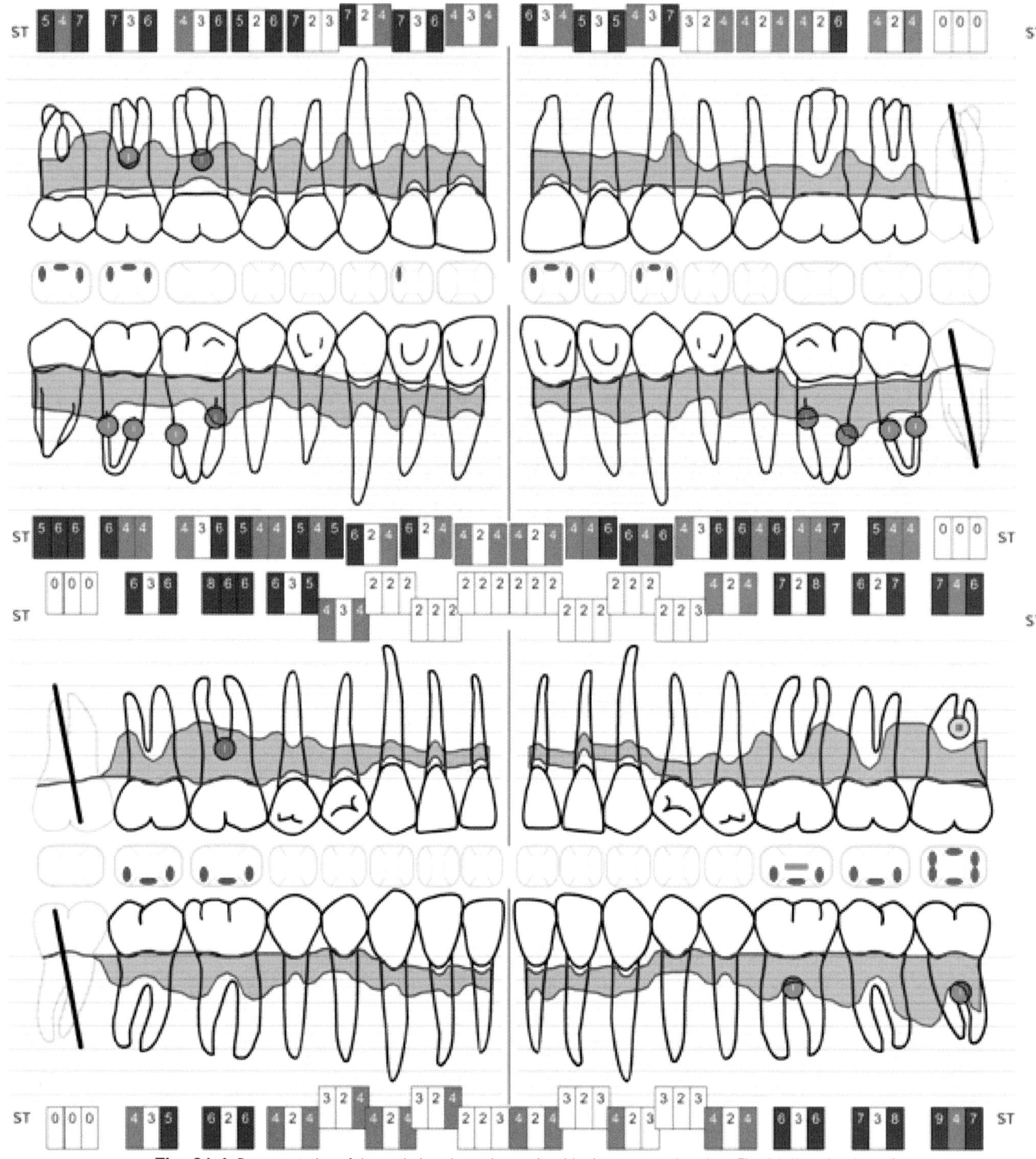

Fig. 21.4 Documentation of the periodontal attachment level in the same patient (see Fig. 21.1) at the time of the first visit. The red line displays the gingival margin reflecting recessions. Clinical attachment loss is illustrated by the filled *(blue)* area on the root surfaces. The deepest periodontal pocket was measured with 9 mm. Class I *(green)* and class II *(yellow)* furcation involvement were documented. Bleeding upon periodontal probing (gingival inflammation) is reflected by red dots. Due to the history of smoking, the bleeding on probing score was relatively low, although the patient presented advanced attachment loss. Tooth mobility is indicated by the green line (tooth #19).

- Furcation involvement: class II or III;
- Moderate ridge defects.

The diagnosis of stage IV periodontitis depends on all parameters defined for stage III as well as factors that predict the necessity for a complex rehabilitation.

In addition to stage III, those factors are:

- Masticatory dysfunction;
- Secondary occlusal trauma;
- Severe ridge defects;
- Bite collapse;
- Drifting;
- Flaring;
- Less than 20 remaining teeth (or 10 opposing pairs).

Disease Distribution

Periodontitis exhibits a site-specific clinical picture, where attachment and bone loss are not equally distributed throughout the entire dentition as well as around teeth. In most cases, interproximal bone

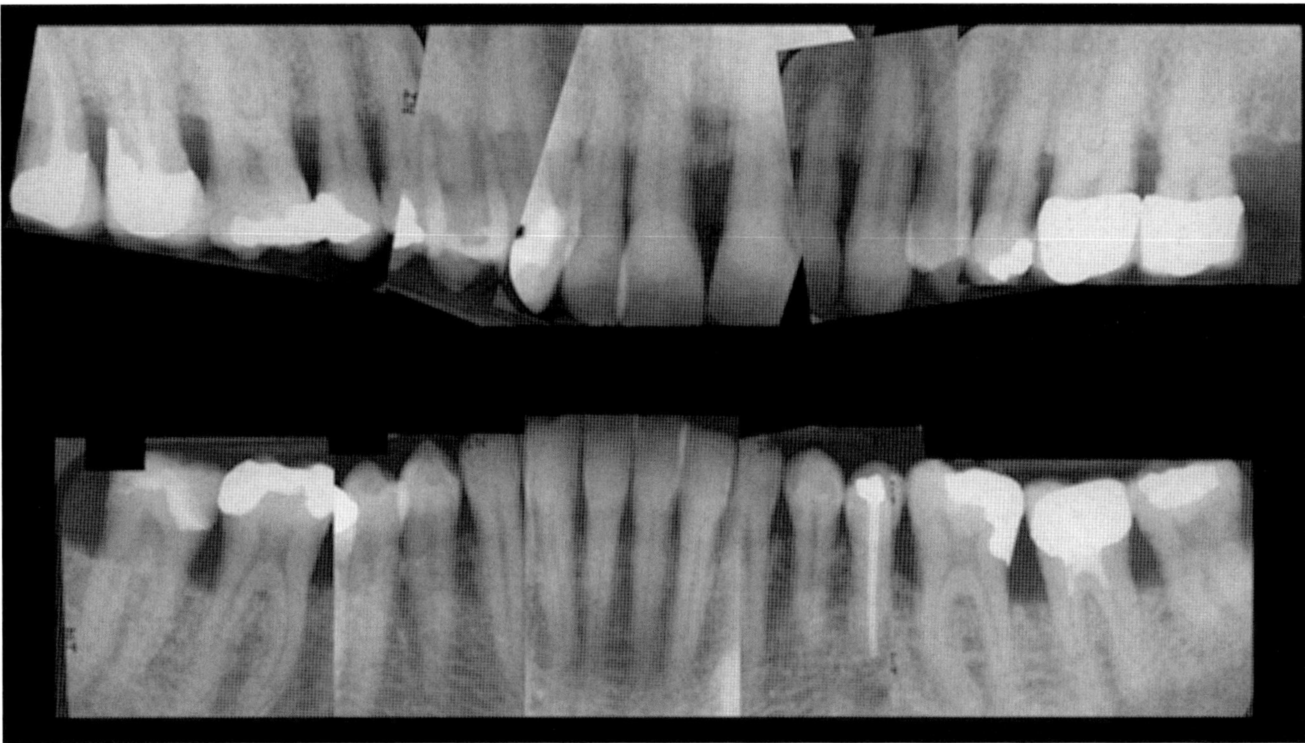

Fig. 21.5 Collage of the radiographic periodontal status (a total of 11 x-rays) at the time of diagnosis (compare Figs. 22.1 and 22.2). Generalized horizontal and localized angular, vertical bone loss on the mesial and distal sites of molars. Radiographs present deep subgingival restorations (teeth: #2 and #19), overhanging margins of restorations (teeth: #14 and #15), carious lesion (tooth #14), insufficient root canal treatment (tooth #18).

TABLE 21.1 Stages of Periodontitis

Periodontitis Stages		Stage I	Stage II	Stage III	Stage IV
Severity	**Interdental CAL** (site with greatest loss)	1–2 mm	3–4 mm	≥5 mm	≥5 mm
	Radiographic bone loss	Coronal third (<15%)	Coronal third (<15%–33%)	Middle third (33%–100%)	Up to apical third (33%–100%)
	Tooth loss	No tooth loss due to periodontitis		Tooth loss due to perio. ≤4 teeth	Tooth loss due to perio. ≥5 teeth
Complexity	Local	Maximum pocket depth ≤4 mm Mostly horizontal bone loss	Maximum pocket depth ≤5 mm Mostly horizontal bone loss	In addition to II: • PD ≥6 mm • vertical BL ≥3 mm • FI: II od. III • moderate ridge defects	In addition to III: Compl. rehabilitation • masticatory dysfunction • secondary occl. trauma • severe ridge defects • bite collapse, drifting, flaring • <20 teeth (10 opposing pairs)
Extent/ Distribution	Additional to stage as descriptor		for each stage: localized (<30% of teeth), generalized (>30% of teeth), or molar/incisor pattern		

loss occurs at few sites during disease development, and will eventually, be present at multiple periodontal sites. Local inflammation, pocket formation, attachment loss, and bone loss are the sequela of the direct exposure to the subgingival plaque (dental biofilm) and local inflammatory responses. Periodontal pocket formation, attachment, and bone loss may develop on one or more sites of a tooth, while other sites remain at a physiological attachment level.

Thus, periodontitis may show a localized or a generalized distribution pattern. If less than 30% of teeth are affected in the dentition, stages of periodontitis exhibit a localized distribution pattern, while a generalized pattern is present when more than 30% of teeth are affected (see Table 21.1):

- **Localized periodontitis:** <30% of teeth show attachment and bone loss;
- **Generalized periodontitis:** >30% of teeth show attachment and bone loss.

In young patients without restorations, periodontal bone loss most likely occurs interproximally at first incisors and/or first molars. This phenomenon of a molar/incisor-pattern indicates early disease onset, and it has been defined as localized juvenile periodontitis in former versions of the classification of periodontal diseases and conditions (Grade C/Rapid Progression—Historical Perspective).[2]

During periodontitis, the local inflammatory response may lead to different patterns of bone loss, including vertical (angular) and horizontal bone destruction. While vertical bone loss is associated with intrabony pocket formation, horizontal bone loss is usually associated with suprabony (supra-alveolar) pockets.

Disease Progression—Grading

Periodontitis may develop at any time in life. First clinical signs of inflammation may occur even during adolescence, not only if oral hygiene is neglected, and dental plaque and calculus were allowed to accumulate, but also due to hereditary genetic disorders or a specific genetic predisposition involving multiple forms of genetic alterations (e.g., variations of single nucleotide polymorphisms, epigenetic alterations). In most cases, the progression rate of periodontitis is slow so that symptoms of the disease appear around the age of forty or later in life. Onset and the rate of disease progression, however, may be influenced by a number of different modifiable (e.g., smoking) and non-modifiable (e.g., genetic disorders) factors. In this context, patients that develop a metabolic disorder, such as diabetes mellitus, may exhibit a much higher progression rate of periodontitis along with increased alveolar bone loss, periodontal bleeding, and pocketing.[99,125,131] Thus, diabetes mellitus and the degree of blood sugar control belong to the most important systemic factors that are directly correlated with periodontal disease.[110]

The progression pattern of periodontitis does not show equal degrees of attachment loss on each affected site over time. While some sites exhibit more rapid periodontal breakdown over time, the attachment level remains static at other sites in the dentition for longer time periods.[77] Interestingly, disease progression is more rapidly at interproximal sites compared to oral or buccal areas of neighboring teeth.[75,78] This phenomenon may be explained by the fact that these interproximal areas become wider along with disease progression, recession development, and the related increased probability of plaque accumulation and food impaction in those areas. Plaque control becomes more difficult, and interproximal furcation areas, interproximal caries, root caries, overhanging restoration margins, and tooth crowding may further promote interproximal attachment loss.

As periodontitis exhibits individual and heterogeneous progression patterns throughout the dentition, three different models have been proposed to describe the rate of disease progression and determine the degree of attachment loss over time,[122] as follows:

The continuous model:

- describes slow and continuous disease progression;
- sites exhibit a constant progression rate of attachment loss throughout the duration of the disease.

The random or episodic-burst model:

- describes the episodic occurrence of short progressive bursts of periodontal destruction followed by periods of stagnation;
- sites, teeth, and the chronology of bursts and stagnation are subject to random effects.

The asynchronous, multiple-burst model:

- describes the occurrence of periodontal destruction (bursts) during defined periods, which are asynchronously interrupted by periods of stagnation or remission for individual sites and teeth.

The grading procedure allows for the determination of periodontal disease progression. Upon defining the phenotype of the disease by identification of the disease stage, the probability of disease progression needs to be determined. For disease progression, direct and indirect evidence exist for each patient individually. It is important to understand that periodontitis is a progressive disease that leads to tooth loss if not treated. In the majority of cases, periodontal attachment loss will occur in a moderate manner.[86] Therefore, a moderate progression rate (grade B) is a priori considered for each patient with a stage of periodontitis.[94] During the grading procedure, evidence needs to be identified in order to determine the progression rate, which may be slow or rapid in individual cases (Table 21.2). Eventually, the grade of periodontitis determines the individual risk for future attachment loss, and in the same context, the grade is also an indicator of the individual supportive periodontal therapy (SPT) interval. The systematic grading procedure requires evaluation of the primary criteria for direct and indirect evidence of disease progression as well as identification of grade modifiers.[94]

TABLE 21.2 Grades of Periodontitis

Periodontitis Grades			Grade A Slow Progression	Grade B Moderate Progression	Grade C Rapid Progression
Primary criteria	Direct evidence for progression	Longitudinal data (x-rays of clinical attachment loss [CAL])	No evidence for bone loss over 5 years	<2 mm bone loss over 5 years	≥2 mm bone loss over 5 years
	Indirect evidence for progression	% bone loss / age	<0.25	0.25–1.0	>1.0
		Case phenotype	Massive biofilm deposits with low levels of destruction	Destruction commensurate with biofilm deposits	Destruction exceeds expectation given biofilm deposits; specific clinical pattern suggestive and/or early onset disease (e.g., molar/incisor pattern; lack of expected response to standard therapies)
Grade modifiers	Risk factors	Smoking	Nonsmoker	Smoker <10 cig/d	Smoker ≥10 cig/d
		Diabetes mellitus	Normoglycemic/ no diagnosis of DM	HbA1c <7%, patients with DM	HbA1c ≥7%, patients with DM

Direct Evidence for Disease Progression

The determination of direct evidence for disease progression involves either longitudinal data for radiographic bone loss or a continuously monitored CAL. The latter would only involve patients that were either referred with their entire clinical periodontal records or patients that have been already treated for periodontitis and subsequently, progressive periodontal breakdown occurred during SPT (non-stable periodontitis patient).[20] However, clinical recordings of CAL are not available for most of the referred or new patients. Conversely, it is likely that a new or referred patient has access to x-rays that monitor their current as well as former bony level around affected teeth. If those x-rays cover a time period of 5 years or more, it may be directly determined whether periodontitis has progressed. If no bone loss has occurred within the 5-year time period, it is most likely that the disease exhibits a slow progression pattern (grade A). In the case of interproximal bone loss of less than 2 mm within 5 years, a moderate progression pattern is most likely (grade B). In cases where ≥2 mm of interproximal bone loss is detected over the 5-year time period, a rapid rate of progression is evident (grade C, see Table 21.2). As a consequence of this highly reliable procedure to determine the disease progression rate, each patient should be asked for recent and past radiographic files.

Indirect Evidence for Disease Progression

In the clinical reality, patients may not possess or have access to their past radiographic files, and therefore, indirect evidence for disease progression must be determined during an examination of current radiographs. In order to find orientation, the percentage of the highest interproximal bone loss in relation to the root length is determined. The value in percent will then be further calculated in a quotient equation that includes that patient's age (% bone loss /age). In the consequence, the calculated value will provide the following thresholds and interpretations:

- a quotient <0.25 indicates a slot rate of progression (grade A);
- a quotient of 0.25 to 1.0 indicates a moderate rate of progression (grade B);
- a quotient of >1.0 indicates a rapid rate of progression (grade C).

Further, the case phenotype also adds to the interpretation of the progression type:

- Heavy biofilm deposits with low levels of destruction (grade A);
- Distribution and quantity of biofilm deposits commensurate with periodontal destruction (grade B9);
- Localized distribution and low quantity of biofilm deposits not commensurate with periodontal destruction, specific clinical patterns suggestive of periods of rapid progression, and/or early onset of the disease (e.g., molar/incisor pattern; lack of expected response to standard periodontal therapy) (grade C, see Table 21.2).[15]

LEARNING BOX 21.1

Grade C/Rapid Progression—Historical Perspective

In 1923, Gottlieb reported a patient with a fatal case of epidemic influenza and a disease that Gottlieb called "diffuse atrophy of the alveolar bone."[45] This disease was characterized by a loss of collagen fibers in the periodontal ligament and their replacement by loose connective tissue and extensive bone resorption, resulting in a widened periodontal space. The gingiva apparently was not involved. In 1928, Gottlieb attributed this condition to the inhibition of continuous cementum formation, which he considered essential for the maintenance of the periodontal fibers.[46] He then termed the disease "deep cementopathia" and hypothesized that this was a "disease of eruption" and that cementum initiated a foreign body response. As a result, it was postulated that the host attempted to exfoliate the tooth, resulting in the observed bone resorption and pocket formation.

In 1938, Wannenmacher described incisor–first molar involvement and called the disease "parodontitis marginalis progressiva"[134] Several explanations evolved for the etiology and pathogenesis of this type of disease. Many authors considered this to be a degenerative, noninflammatory disease process and therefore gave it the name "periodontosis."[44,92,127] Other investigators denied the existence of a degenerative type of periodontal disease and attributed the changes observed to trauma from occlusion.[16,84] Finally, in 1966, the World Workshop in Periodontics concluded that the concept of "periodontosis" as a degenerative entity was unsubstantiated and that the term should be eliminated from periodontal nomenclature.[104] The committee did recognize that a clinical entity different from "adult periodontitis" might occur among adolescents and young adults.

The term "juvenile periodontitis" was introduced by Chaput and colleagues in 1967 and by Butler in 1969.[13] In 1971, Baer defined it as "a disease of the periodontium occurring in an otherwise healthy adolescent which is characterized by a rapid loss of alveolar bone about more than one tooth of the permanent dentition.[4] The amount of destruction manifested is not commensurate with the amount of local irritants." In 1989 the World Workshop in Clinical Periodontics categorized this disease as localized juvenile periodontitis (LJP), a subset of the broad classification of early-onset periodontitis (EOP).[17] Under this classification system, age of onset and distribution of lesions were of primary importance when making a diagnosis of LJP.

In 1999, the World Workshop in Periodontics introduced a novel classification that was meant to eliminate the shortcomings of earlier endeavors in classifying periodontal disease. Most importantly, the new 1999 classification sought "to discard classification terminologies that were age-dependent or required knowledge of rates of progression."[2] In the 1999 classification scheme, several rapidly progressing periodontitis forms were united under the term "aggressive periodontitis."

A decade after the 1999 workshop, the evidence summarized in an entire *Periodontology 2000* volume pointed to the shortcoming that no distinctive differences between the two major entities of periodontitis, aggressive and chronic periodontitis, had been identified thus far on the pathophysiological level.[1,38,106,120,123]

Indeed, in a comprehensive assessment of the differences between chronic and aggressive periodontitis lesions on the transcriptomic level from 120 systemically healthy nonsmoking subjects with previously untreated moderate to severe aggressive or chronic periodontitis, diagnosed strictly according to the 1999 workshop criteria, only minor differences between both entities and substantial diagnostic imprecision were identified.[64] On the other hand, clustering of the same data identified two novel classes of periodontitis subjects with marked differences in disease severity and past progression.[62] Similar work based on microbiological data and radiological information confirmed that not all periodontitis is equal.[26]

These findings were among the reasons for the 2017 World Workshop that introduced a single periodontitis entity characterized by extent, severity, and progression.

Risk Factors—Modification of Grades

A number of different factors influence the etiopathogenesis of periodontitis. The composition of the oral microflora and the amount of dental biofilm (plaque) is a major etiologic factor. In this context, the extent of the periodontal destruction depends on the host's immune competence as well as genetic predispositions influencing the individual susceptibility to disease. In addition, both systemic diseases and environmental factors interfere with the development and progression of periodontitis. The below-described risk factors (microbial, local, systemic, immunologic, genetic, environmental, and behavioral) may either occur simultaneously or a selection of factors is present in patients with periodontitis. The degree of the individual risk factor contribution differs between patients so that is worthwhile to not only identify the risk factors but also to specify the degree of contribution of individual risk factors.

It may also be noted that the prior history of gingivitis and periodontitis should be considered as general predictors for the development and/or progression of periodontitis.[75] It is possible that the disease could not be successfully treated in the first place. The reason for an unsuccessful treatment outcome can be as simple as the patient's unwillingness (noncompliant patients) to understand the disease and/or perform proper oral hygiene. On the other hand, reasons for disease progression can also be more complex when non-modifiable factors, such as genetic predispositions/syndromes, severe immunologic disorders, other therapies (e.g., organ transplantations) that affect the patient's immune status, lack of dexterity, and/or other systemic diseases, are present. This highlights the complexity of not only the development but also the progression/re-occurrence of periodontitis. Several risk factors that contribute to the patient's susceptibility to periodontitis are discussed later in the chapter.

At this point, the grading algorithm allows to formally modify the grade of progression based on smoking and diabetes status only (see Table 21.2). It was envisioned by the working group of the 2017 World Workshop that these factors would eventually be complemented by additional factors, once more clearly established and/or measurable in clinical practice. Likely, precision dentistry tools such as diagnostic tests for microbiological and/or immunological markers of disease (see below) will be the next additions to the Grading table.

Smoking

Smoking is a major risk factor for the development and progression of periodontitis.[10,11,42] Periodontitis is influenced by smoking in a dose-dependent manner. The intake of more than 10 cigarettes per day tremendously increases the risk of disease progression when compared to nonsmokers and former smokers, respectively.[129] In addition, tobacco smoking not only increases the susceptibility to periodontitis but also contributes to a poorer response to periodontal therapy.[93]

Compared to nonsmokers, the following features are found in smokers[9,60,98,108]:

- increased periodontal pocket depth with more than 3 mm
- increased attachment loss
- more recessions
- increased loss of alveolar bone
- increased tooth loss
- fewer signs of gingivitis (less bleeding upon probing)
- greater incidence of furcation involvement.

Due to the consumption of tobacco, reactive oxygen (radicals) is released that chemically irritate periodontal tissues by DNA damage, lipid peroxidation of cell membranes, damage of endothelial cells, and induction of smooth muscle cell growth.[85]

Diabetes Mellitus

Periodontitis is known as the sixth complication of diabetes mellitus.[42,81] For diabetes mellitus and periodontitis, it is known that there is an interaction where both diseases mutually correlate to each other.[73] Patients with diabetes mellitus exhibit a higher risk to develop periodontitis, and the periodontal infection/inflammation may negatively interfere with the glycemic control of the diabetic patient.[99] A number of studies showed that prevalence, severity, and prognosis of periodontitis are associated with the incidence of diabetes mellitus. It was found that the average pocket depth as well as the clinical attachment loss was increased in patients with diabetes mellitus (independently from the type of diabetes mellitus).[27,66,99,109] Patients with poor glycemic control tend to experience more severe progression of periodontitis compared to patients with good glycemic control. Regarding the progression of severe periodontitis, no difference was found between patients with good glycemic control and nondiabetic patients.[131] With diabetes mellitus, advanced glycation end products (AGEs) may arise which lead to the release of free oxygen and pro-inflammatory mediators (cytokines). AGEs may also promote chemotaxis and adhesion of inflammatory cells to periodontal tissues, and increased apoptosis of fibroblasts and osteoblasts may occur.[48] Furthermore, patients with diabetes mellitus tend to show a higher body mass index, and therefore, increased concentrations of adipokines that directly influence inflammatory responses were found.[100] Hyperglycemia per se leads to the release of pro-inflammatory mediators in the bloodstream, which in turn promote increased glucose concentration.[99] Periodontal therapy may contribute to the glycemic control of the diabetic patient. It was shown that the systematic therapy of chronic periodontitis leads to a at least short-term reduction of glycated hemoglobin of approximately 0.3% up to 0.6% (HbA1c).[14,19,58,76,119] Each therapy regimen that contributes to achieving a reduction of glycated hemoglobin may decrease the risk of diabetes-related long-term consequences, such as myocardial infarction, microvascular complications, and many others.[99]

In the context of diabetes mellitus, a number of patients exhibit an increased body weight (obesity) which is also correlated with the prevalence and severity of periodontal attachment and bone loss.[87] The negative effect of a high body mass index with regards to the outcome of periodontal therapy was comparable to the negative effect that has been described for smokers.[124]

Microbiological Aspects

Plaque accumulation on the tooth and gingival surfaces (dental biofilm formation) at the dentogingival junction is considered the primary initiating agent in the etiology of gingivitis and periodontitis.[75] It is important to note that the scientific literature mainly used the former classification of periodontal diseases and conditions.[9] Thus, both termini aggressive and chronic periodontitis are mentioned when appropriate. As the dental biofilm develops, early signs of an inflammatory reaction occur in the gingival margin (gingivitis) without attachment loss. Generally, optimal plaque control leads to the complete resolution of this early gingival inflammation.[80] With neglected oral hygiene, on the other hand, inflammation will progress and eventually result in the loss of attachment around teeth.[75] Although not all patients with gingivitis develop periodontitis, it is known that all patients with periodontitis experienced prior gingivitis. The occurrence of periodontitis depends on the individual immune response that modifies the onset and progression of the disease.[75,91,96]

Attachment and bone loss are associated with an increase in the proportion of gram-negative organisms in the subgingival biofilm, with specific increases in organisms known to be pathogenic and virulent. *Porphyromonas gingivalis*, *Tannerella forsythia*, and *Treponema denticola*, otherwise known as the "red complex" bacteria, are frequently associated with ongoing attachment and bone loss in chronic periodontitis.[121] Development and progression of periodontitis may not depend on the presence of one specific bacterium or bacterial complex alone. It is assumed that chronic periodontitis is the sequelae of a multi-species infection with a number of different bacteria that influence the pro-inflammatory immune response of the host.[65,111] Furthermore, the concept of host-microbial interactions gained scientific attention in the past years. It has been found that increased numbers of periodontal pathogens contribute to the development of a dysbiotic microbial environment that is triggered by the inflammatory milieu in the periodontal pocket.[7,52] This concept describes a shift from a symbiotic microbial environment to the development of a dysbiosis within the biofilm involving so-called keystone pathogens, such as *P. gingivalis*, as a polymicrobial synergistic effect.[76–78] Periodontal pathogens like *P. gingivalis* may then invade the periodontal tissue, and therewith, induce further immune responses with increasing concentrations of pro-inflammatory mediators that may enhance periodontal breakdown. In addition, a number of periodontal pathogens are capable of producing proteases that directly affect the tissues and host immune responses.[96]

As the dental biofilm develops, early signs of an inflammatory reaction occur in the gingival margin (gingivitis) without attachment loss. Generally, optimal plaque control leads to the complete resolution of this early gingival inflammation. With neglected oral hygiene, on the other hand, inflammation will progress and eventually result in the loss of attachment around teeth.[75] Although not all patients with gingivitis develop periodontitis, it is known that all patients with periodontitis experienced prior gingivitis. The occurrence of periodontitis depends on the individual immune response that modifies the onset and progression of the disease.[75,91,96]

In addition to bacteria, it has recently been shown that a eukaryotic organism (*Entamoeba gingivalis*) also relates to periodontitis. *Entamoeba gingivalis* was found to be associated with periodontitis, and it could be demonstrated that may be one of the causal factors that lead to gingival inflammation and periodontal destruction.[5,6]

Local Factors

Plaque accumulation and biofilm development is the primary cause of periodontal inflammation and destruction. Therefore, factors that facilitate plaque accumulation or prevent plaque removal by oral hygiene procedures can be detrimental to the patient. Plaque-retentive factors are important in the development and progression of periodontitis because they retain microorganisms in proximity to the periodontal tissues, providing an ecologic niche for biofilm maturation. Calculus is considered the most important plaque-retentive factor because of its ability to retain and harbor plaque bacteria on its rough surface as well as inside.[59,118] As a consequence, calculus removal is essential for the maintenance of a healthy periodontium. In addition, tooth morphology may influence plaque retention. Roots may show grooves and/or concavities, and in some instances, enamel projections on the surface and/or furcation entrances. Those morphologic variations may facilitate plaque retention, subgingival calculus formation, and disease progression.[42,57,105] In addition, subgingival and overhanging margins of restorations, carious lesions that extend subgingivally, and furcations exposed by loss of bone promote plaque retention.[69,132]

Immunologic Factors

Periodontitis is a disease induced by bacteria organized in the dental biofilm. The onset, progression, and severity of the disease depend, however, on the individual host immune response.[41,91] Patients may show alterations of peripheral monocytes which relate to reduced reactivity of lymphocytes and/or enhanced B-cell response.[91,96,] Not only B-cells and macrophages, but also periodontal ligament cells, gingival fibroblasts, and epithelial cells synthesize pro-inflammatory mediators, such as interleukin-1 beta (IL-1 beta), IL-6, IL-8, prostaglandin-E2 (PGE2), tumor necrosis factor alpha (TNF-alpha), and many others, that modify innate and adaptive immune responses at periodontal sites.[89–96] Pro-inflammatory mediators regulate the synthesis and secretion of matrix metalloproteinases (MMPs) and receptor-activator-of-NF-kappaB-ligand (RANKL). In periodontal lesions, MMPs contribute to soft and hard tissue degradation during active inflammatory reactions.[88] RANKL binds to its receptor RANK on the cell surface of premature osteoclasts, and therewith, initiates osteoclast differentiation leading to degradation of alveolar bone.[88–90] Physiologically, osteoprotegerin (OPG) is the opponent of RANKL, and during periodontitis, an imbalance between OPG and RANKL promotes further bone degradation.[41]

In addition, reduced counts in neutrophils (PMNs) influence the degree of periodontal inflammation. Congenital neutropenia (Kostmann syndrome) leads not only to an increased susceptibility to infection in general but also to severe periodontitis. Patients with Kostmann syndrome show reduced levels of antimicrobial peptides, such as the cathelicidin LL-37 and neutrophil peptides (alpha-defensins), which impair their innate immune response.[15,102] LL-37 is an effective antimicrobial peptide that is synthesized from inactive precursors, and mutations in the Cathepsin C gene hinder cleavage, and therewith, activation of LL-37. Those genetic alterations contribute to the severity and progression of periodontitis (Papillon-Lefèvre syndrome; Haim-Munk syndrome).[25,56]

Systemic Associations

Periodontitis is a complex disease that may not only be limited to infection at local sites, but in several instances, periodontitis is also associated with other systemic disorders, such as Haim-Munk syndrome, Papillon-Lefèvre syndrome, Ehlers-Danlos syndrome, Kindlers syndrome, and the Cohen syndrome. Patients who suffer from diseases that impair host immune responses (e.g., HIV/AIDS) may also show periodontal destruction. Further, it is also known that osteoporosis, severe unbalanced diet, stress as well as dermatologic, hematologic, and neoplastic factors interfere with periodontal inflammatory responses.

In addition to defined syndromes, periodontitis is also associated with severe systemic diseases, such as diabetes mellitus, cardiovascular disorders, stroke, and lung disorders.[3,19,63,90,96,128,130,133]

Genetic Factors

Periodontitis is considered as a complex inflammatory disease influenced by local, systemic, and immunologic factors (see above). Each factor is in turn directly related to individual genetic conditions. It is important to note that the scientific literature mainly used the former classification of periodontal diseases and conditions.[2] Thus, both termini aggressive and chronic periodontitis are mentioned when appropriate.

Several genetic disorders are known to show periodontal destruction as one of their major symptoms. For example, the Papillon-Lefèvre syndrome is a well-known genetic disorder (defect on chromosome 11) that not only exhibits severe periodontitis but also palmoplantar hyperkeratosis.[36,55,70] Besides the Papillon-Lefèvre syndrome, the Haim-Munk syndrome, Ehlers-Danlos syndrome, Down syndrome, Kindlers syndrome, Cohen syndrome, and congenital neutropenia (Kostmann syndrome) are other genetic disorders that have been related to periodontal disease. These genetic conditions are extensively discussed in Chapter 9.

Periodontal disease has been found in different family members (twins, siblings) and generations of one family. Early twin studies suggested the involvement of genetic susceptibility factors in the etiopathogenesis of periodontitis.[82] In a number of studies, the prevalence of aggressive and chronic periodontitis has been investigated in families with a history of one or more family members with periodontitis. The data from those studies showed variable results with a likelihood for heritability of up to 50%. Variations are mainly due to different study designs as well as the number of evaluated individuals.[8,79,83,112]

In addition, other genetic variations (single nucleotide polymorphisms, SNPs; genetic copy number variations) that have so far not been identified as responsible for certain syndromes may also directly influence innate and adaptive immune responses as well as the structure of periodontal tissues. In recent years, the identification of genes that are relevant to the development of periodontitis led to new scientific concepts and findings. There are at least two different concepts (candidate genes and genome-wide associations) to identify genetic variances in relation to disease. In candidate gene studies, certain already known variances (SNPs) are correlated to a specific phenotype such as periodontitis. Therefore, a hypothesis is required in order to choose specific SNPs in relevant genes. The data from those studies showed variable results so that it is mostly not possible to draw clear conclusions. In this context, studies on SNPs in the IL-1 gene led to the early conclusion that alterations in sequences of immunologically relevant genes may explain the heritability of periodontitis.[68] Conflicting data in the literature, however, indicate inconclusive knowledge regarding SNPs in the IL-1 gene and their potential role during heritability and etiopathology of periodontitis.[72] Also, it seems not plausible that one single polymorphism in a specific gene sequence can cause a complex inflammatory disease, such as periodontitis, without causing any other symptoms relevant to the systemic health. Thus, genome-wide association studies (GWAS) became more relevant in the past years. Here, a high number of DNA-sequence variances are evaluated at the same time. In contrast to candidate gene studies, no hypotheses are required for GWAS so that there is no potential bias during analysis. In several GWAS, a number of new genes have been identified to be associated with periodontitis. One of the best-replicated genes is called ANRIL (antisense RNA in the Inc locus). ANRIL is not only associated with periodontitis but also with cardiovascular disease which underlies potential systemic interactions.[24,114–116] The role of ANRIL during the development of periodontitis is subject of ongoing investigations. It is known that it represents a non-coding regulatory RNA that is involved during the regulation of cell division and in affecting other genes that play a role in glucose and lipid metabolism (ADIPOR1, VAMP3, C11ORF10).[12,28,135] In addition to ANRIL, genetic variances (SNPs) in the sequences of the glucosyltransferase 6 domain containing 1 gene (GLT6D1), the plasminogen gene (PLA), the neuropeptide Y gene (NPY), BACH1 (linked with *ST8SIA1*), pseudogene *MTND1P5*, a nucleotide variant in *SIGLEC5*, and a nucleotide variant in *DEFB1A3* (potentially involved in innate immune processes) have been associated with periodontal disease.[22,39,88,89,113,117] Due to the technical and scientific progress it may be expected that more genes will be identified to be associated with periodontitis in the future. In addition, recent findings indicate natural genetic variations may affect the heritability of periodontitis among sexes.[40]

Other Factors

Psychological factors, such as stress and depression, also negatively influence the progression of periodontitis.[47] Patients with periodontitis often report the experience of family and/or work-related stress.[97] Positive correlations between cortisol levels and periodontal indices (plaque index, gingival index), bone loss, and missing teeth were recorded.[29,47,103] In addition, stress as an etiologic factor was even stronger associated with periodontitis when patients were smokers compared to nonsmokers.[21]

Science Transfer

In most cases, patients with periodontitis exhibit slow progressive attachment and bone loss that extends over decades. This attachment and bone loss is initiated by the interplay of inflammatory responses and the microbial infection with periodontal pathogenic gram-negative anaerobic bacteria organized in a well-structured dysbiotic biofilm, and therefore, control of the subgingival biofilm is an essential part of the therapy. Disease susceptibility and pronounced attachment and bone loss are reported for patients that suffer from systemic syndromes, diabetes mellitus, and/or other environmental factors (smoking, stress). In addition, genetic variances may influence the susceptibility to periodontitis.

Periodontitis can effectively be treated by a systematic periodontal therapy (therapy steps 1, 2, 3, and 4) that includes optimal long-term supragingival plaque and risk factor control (step 1), debridement of subgingival soft and hard deposits (step 2), and surgical pocket reduction (case-dependent either resective osseous surgery or regenerative surgery) (step 3; see Figs. 21.6 and 21.7). Depending on the individual periodontal risk, each patient should be re-motivated, re-instructed, and re-treated (if necessary) during a systematic supportive periodontal therapy regimen (step 4) (revisits every 3, 6, or 12 months; Fig. 21.8).

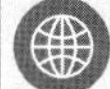
References for this chapter are found on the companion website eBooks.Health.Elsevier.com

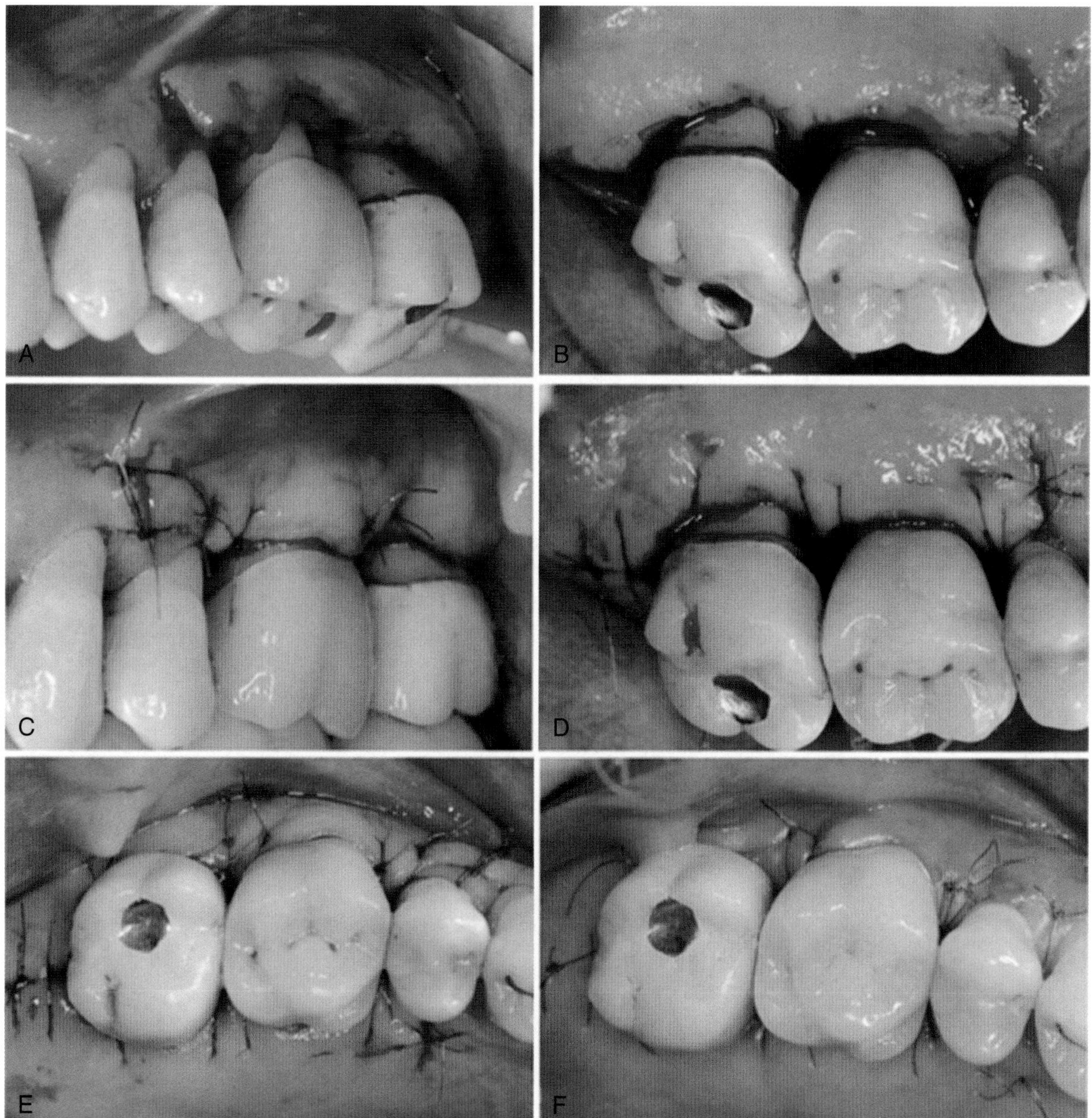

Fig. 21.6 Subsequent to the anti-infective therapy and periodontal reevaluation (therapy step 2), resective periodontal surgery (therapy step 3) was performed in the patient introduced in Figs. 21.3–21.5 Surgical method: apically repositioned flap. (A) Intrasucluar incision at buccal sites; notice: class I furcation involvement on tooth #14; (B) paramarginal incision at palatal sites, excision of a distal wedge; (C and D). suture using 5-0 Prolene, buccal and palatal view, respectively; (E) occlusal view after suturing; (F) occlusal view 1 week post surgery. Tooth #14 received endodontic therapy and crown restoration prior to periodontal surgery.

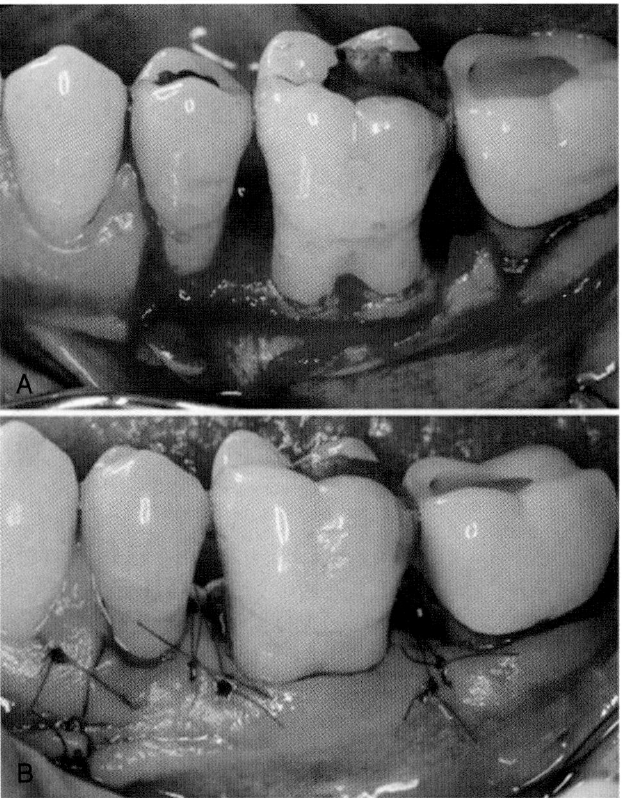

Fig. 21.7 Subsequent to the anti-infective therapy and periodontal reevaluation (therapy step 2), resective periodontal surgery (therapy step 3) was performed in the patient introduced in Figs. 21.3–21.6. Surgical method: apically repositioned flap. (A) Intrasulcular incision at buccal sites; notice: class I furcation involvement on tooth #19, and horizontal bone loss teeth #18 - #20; (B) suture using 5-0 Prolene, buccal view.

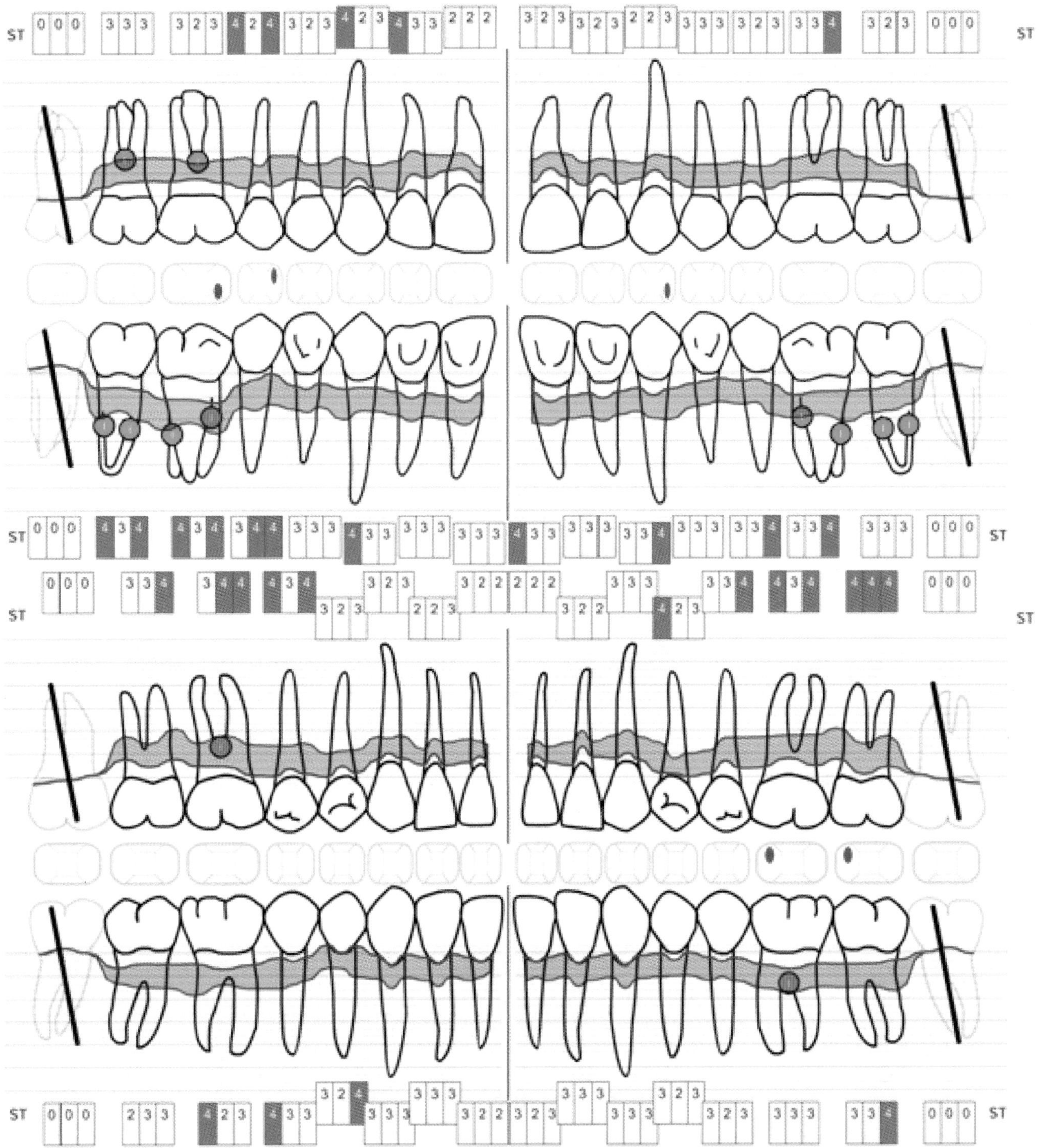

Fig. 21.8 Documentation of the periodontal attachment level in the same patient (see Figs. 21.1–21.5) after active periodontal therapy was completed and the supportive periodontal therapy (therapy step 4) was initiated. The red line displays the gingival margin reflecting recessions. Clinical attachment loss is illustrated by the filled *(blue)* area on the root surfaces. The deepest periodontal pocket was measured with 4 mm.

CHAPTER 22

The Periodontal Pocket Formation and Patterns of Bone Loss

Satheesh Elangovan | Fermin A. Carranza | Henry H. Takei | Paulo M. Camargo

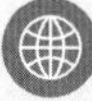

Editors' Note: An animation (slide show) has been added by the editors as a supplement to the chapter. It was produced by My Dental Hub as a patient education tool and covers the basic elements in a conceptual manner. It is not intended to be a procedural guide for dental professionals.

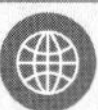

Videos for this chapter can be viewed on the companion website at eBooks.Health.Elsevier.com.

CHAPTER OUTLINE

The periodontal pocket, which is defined as a pathologically deepened gingival sulcus, is one of the most important clinical features of periodontal diseases. All types of periodontitis, as outlined in Chapter 5, share histopathologic features, such as tissue changes in the periodontal pocket, mechanisms of tissue destruction, and healing mechanisms. However, they differ with regard to their etiology, natural history, progression, and response to therapy.[47]

Classification

Deepening of the gingival sulcus may occur as a result of coronal movement of the gingival margin, apical displacement of the gingival attachment, or a combination of the two processes (Fig. 22.1). Therefore pockets can be classified as follows:

- *Gingival pocket* (also called "pseudo-pocket") is formed by gingival enlargement without destruction of the underlying periodontal tissues. The sulcus is deepened because of the increased bulk of the gingiva (Fig. 22.2A).
- *Periodontal pocket* is formed by loss of periodontal attachment, which can lead to loosening and exfoliation of the teeth. The remainder of this chapter refers to this type of pocket.

Based on the location of the base of the pocket in relation to the underlying bone, periodontal pockets can be classified into the following types:

- *Suprabony* (*supracrestal* or *supra-alveolar*) occurs when the bottom of the pocket is coronal to the underlying alveolar bone (see Fig. 22.2B).
- *Intrabony* (*infrabony, subcrestal,* or *intraalveolar*) occurs when the bottom of the pocket is apical to the level of the adjacent alveolar bone. With this second type, the lateral pocket wall lies between the tooth surface and the alveolar bone (see Fig. 22.2C).

Pockets can involve one, two, or more tooth surfaces, and they can be of different depths and types on different surfaces of the same tooth, and on proximal surfaces of the same interdental space.[40,61] Pockets can also be spiral (i.e., originating on one tooth surface and twisting around the tooth to involve one or more additional surfaces) (Fig. 22.3). These types of pockets are most common in furcation areas.

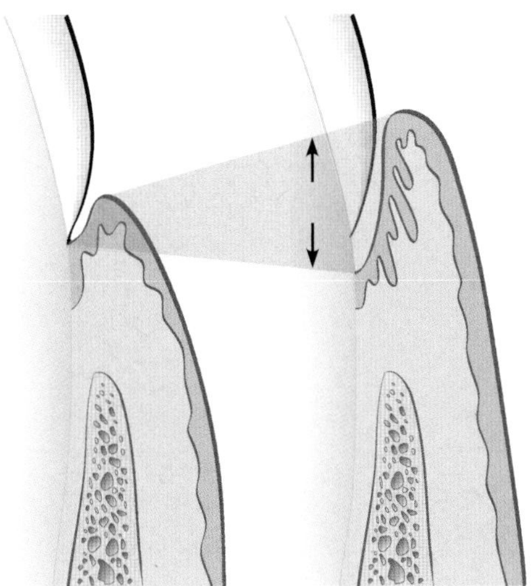

Fig. 22.1 Illustration of pocket formation that indicates expansion in two directions *(arrows)* from the normal gingival sulcus *(left)* to the periodontal pocket *(right)*.

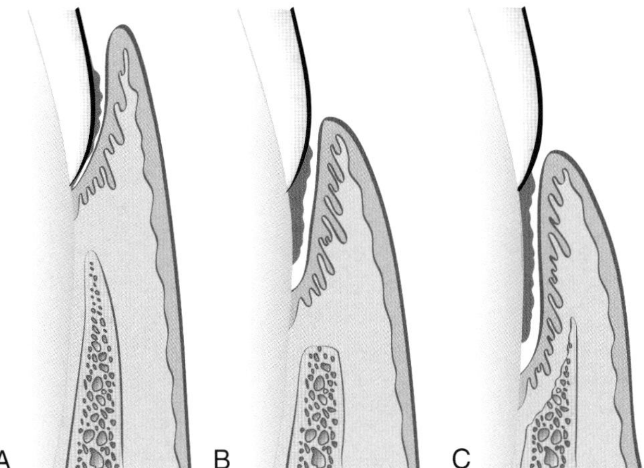

Fig. 22.2 Different types of periodontal pockets. (A) Gingival pocket. There is no destruction of the supporting periodontal tissues. (B) Suprabony pocket. The base of the pocket is coronal to the level of the underlying bone. Bone loss is horizontal. (C) Intrabony pocket. The base of the pocket is apical to the level of the adjacent bone. Bone loss is vertical.

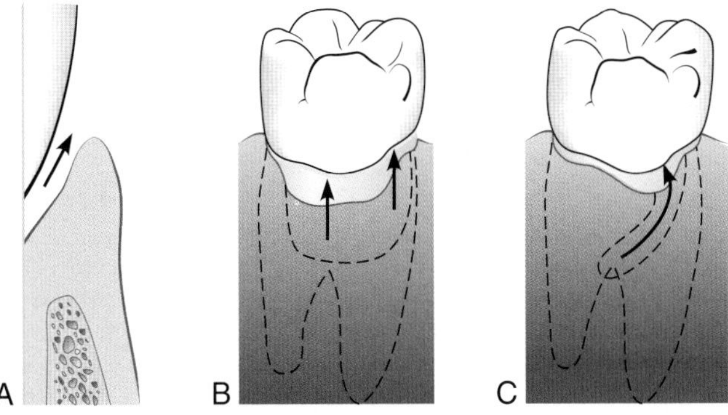

Fig. 22.3 Classification of pockets according to involved tooth surfaces. (A) Simple pocket. (B) Compound pocket. (C) Complex pocket.

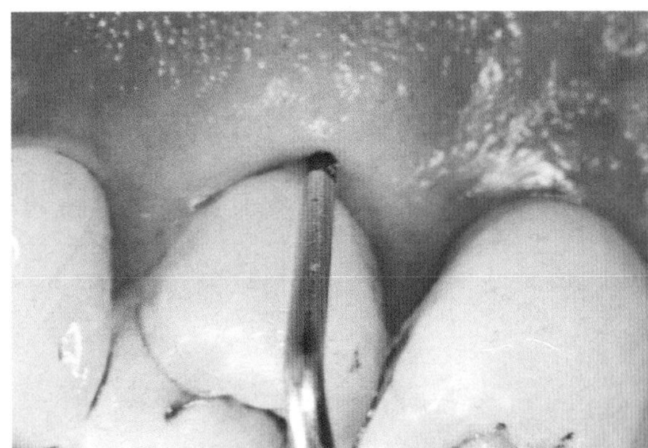

Fig. 22.4 Probing of a deep periodontal pocket. The entire length of the periodontal probe has been inserted to the base of the pocket in the palatal surface of the first premolar.

Clinical Features

Clinical signs that suggest the presence of periodontal pockets include a bluish-red thickened marginal gingiva, a bluish-red vertical zone from the gingival margin to the alveolar mucosa, gingival bleeding and suppuration, tooth mobility, diastema formation, and symptoms such as localized pain or pain "deep in the bone." The only reliable method of locating periodontal pockets and determining their extent is careful probing of the gingival margin along each tooth surface (Fig. 22.4 and Table 22.1). On the basis of depth alone, however, it is sometimes difficult to differentiate between a deep normal sulcus and a shallow periodontal pocket. In such borderline cases, pathologic changes in the gingiva distinguish the two conditions.

For a more detailed discussion of the clinical aspects of periodontal pockets, see Chapter 38.

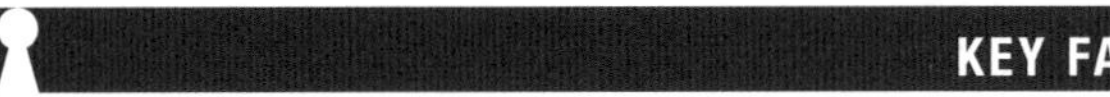

Sulcus Versus Periodontal Pocket

Gingival sulcus is the space between the neck of the tooth and the circumferential gingival tissue. Sulcus, when it deepens (as in periodontitis) due to the apical migration of **junctional epithelium**, accompanied by attachment loss, is referred to as a *periodontal pocket*.

Pathogenesis

The initial lesion in the development of periodontitis is the inflammation of the gingiva in response to a bacterial challenge. Changes involved in the transition from the normal gingival sulcus to the pathologic periodontal pocket are associated with different proportions of bacterial cells in dental plaque. Healthy gingiva is associated with few microorganisms, mostly coccoid cells and straight rods. Diseased gingiva is associated with increased numbers of spirochetes and motile rods.[69,71,73] However, the microbiota of diseased sites cannot be used as a predictor of future attachment or bone loss, because their presence alone is not sufficient for disease to start or progress.[54]

Pocket formation starts as an inflammatory change in the connective tissue wall of the gingival sulcus. The cellular and fluid

TABLE 22.1 Correlation of Clinical and Histopathologic Features of the Periodontal Pocket

Clinical Features	Histopathologic Features
1. The gingival wall of the pocket presents various degrees of bluish-red discoloration; flaccidity; a smooth, shiny surface; and pitting on pressure.	1. The discoloration is caused by circulatory stagnation; the flaccidity by the destruction of gingival fibers and surrounding tissues; the smooth, shiny surface by atrophy of the epithelium and edema; and the pitting on pressure by edema and degeneration.
2. Less frequently, the gingival wall may be pink and firm.	2. In such cases, fibrotic changes predominate over exudation and degeneration, particularly in relation to the outer surface of the pocket wall. However, despite the external appearance of health, the inner wall of the pocket invariably presents some degeneration and is often ulcerated (see Fig. 22.15).
3. Bleeding is elicited by gently probing the soft-tissue wall of the pocket.	3. Ease of bleeding results from increased vascularity, the thinning and degeneration of the epithelium, and the proximity of engorged vessels to the inner surface.
4. When explored with a probe, the inner aspect of the pocket is generally painful.	4. Pain on tactile stimulation is caused by the ulceration of the inner aspect of the pocket wall.
5. In many cases, pus may be expressed with the application of digital pressure.	5. Pus occurs in pockets with suppurative inflammation of the inner wall.

inflammatory exudate causes degeneration of the surrounding connective tissue, including the gingival fibers. Just apical to the junctional epithelium, collagen fibers are destroyed,[25,38] and the area is occupied by inflammatory cells and edema (Fig. 22.5).

Early concepts assumed that after the initial bacterial attack, periodontal tissue destruction continued to be linked to the presence of bacteria. More recently it was established that the host's immune-inflammatory response to the initial and persistent bacterial attack unleashes mechanisms that lead to collagen and bone destruction. These mechanisms are related to various cytokines, some of which are produced normally by cells in non-inflamed tissue and others by cells that are involved in the inflammatory process, such as polymorphonuclear leukocytes (PMNs), monocytes, and other cells, thereby leading to collagen and bone destruction. This chapter describes the histologic aspects of gingival inflammation and tissue destruction. For further information about the molecular biology aspects of these mechanisms of tissue destruction, please see Chapters 8 through 12 and eBooks.Health.Elsevier.com.

KEY FACT

Cytokines are proteins secreted by cells that interact with other cells and eventually lead to a specific cellular response. Cytokines can be proinflammatory or anti-inflammatory in nature. Proinflammatory cytokines such as interleukin-1 (IL-1) and tumor necrosis factor-alpha (TNF-α) are implicated strongly in the pathogenesis of the progression of periodontal diseases. Anti-inflammatory cytokines such as IL-4 and IL-10 counteract the effects of proinflammatory cytokines.

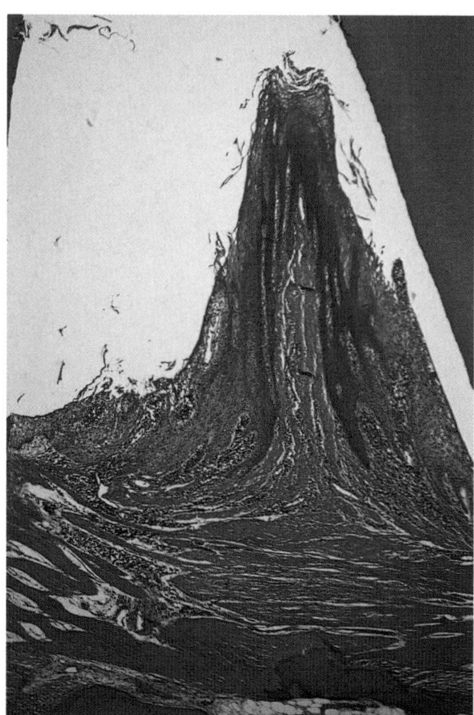

Fig. 22.5 Interdental papilla with suprabony pockets on proximal tooth surfaces. Note the densely inflamed connective tissue, with the infiltrate extending between the collagen fibers and the proliferating and ulcerated pocket epithelium.

The two mechanisms associated with collagen loss are as follows: (1) collagenases and other enzymes secreted by various cells in healthy and inflamed tissue, such as fibroblasts,[130] PMNs,[129] and macrophages,[98] destroy collagen (enzymes that degrade collagen and other matrix macromolecules into small peptides are called *matrix metalloproteinases*[132]); and (2) fibroblasts phagocytize collagen fibers by extending cytoplasmic processes to the ligament–cementum interface and degrade the inserted collagen fibrils and the fibrils of the cementum matrix.[25,26]

As a consequence of the loss of collagen, the apical cells of the junctional epithelium proliferate along the root surface and extend finger-like projections that are two or three cells in thickness (Fig. 22.6).

KEY FACT

Matrix Metalloproteinases and Tissue Inhibitors of Metalloproteinases

Matrix metalloproteinases (MMPs) are a group of proteases that play an important role in several biologic processes. Like any protease, they are involved in the degradation of proteins. Specifically, they are important players in extracellular matrix (ECM) degradation and are inhibited by tissue inhibitors of metalloproteinases (TIMPs). The balance between MMPs and TIMPs is critical for the maintenance of ECM remodeling in tissues, including the periodontium.

As a result of inflammation, PMNs invade the coronal end of the junctional epithelium in increasing numbers (Fig. 22.7). The PMNs are not joined to one another or to the epithelial cells by desmosomes. When the relative volume of PMNs reaches approximately 60% or more of the junctional epithelium, the tissue loses cohesiveness and detaches from the tooth surface. Thus the coronal portion of the junctional epithelium detaches from the root as the apical

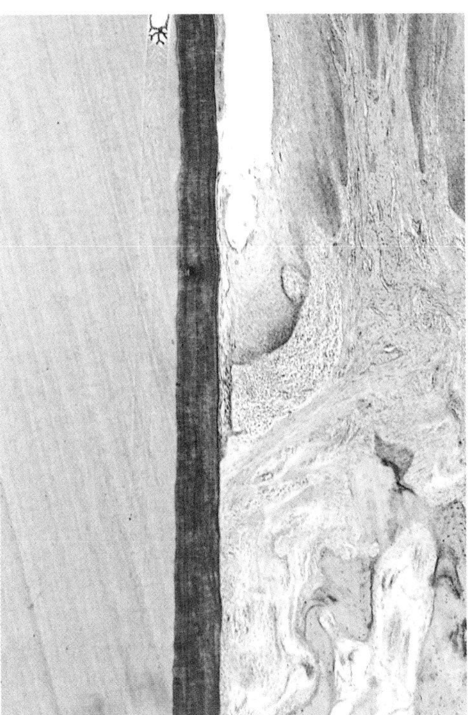

Fig. 22.6 Low-power view of the base of the periodontal pocket and apical area. Note the dense inflammatory infiltrate on the area of destroyed collagen fibers and the thin, finger-like extension of epithelium covering the cementum, which has been denuded of fibers.

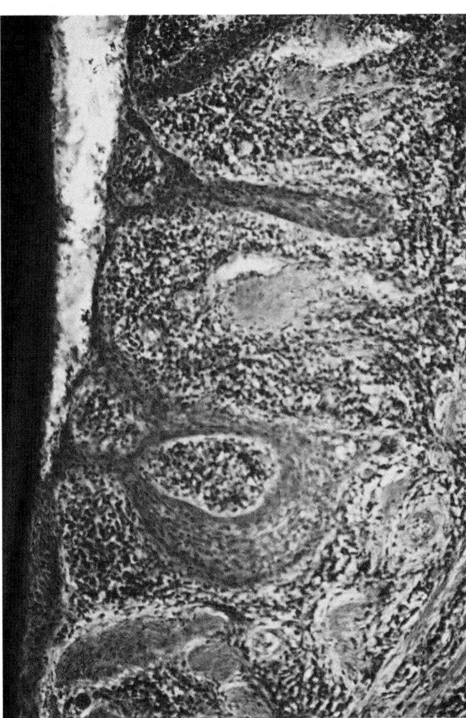

Fig. 22.7 Base of periodontal pocket showing extensive proliferation of lateral epithelium next to atrophic areas, dense inflammatory infiltrate, remnants of destroyed collagen fibers, and the junctional epithelium, which is apparently in a less altered state than the lateral pocket epithelium.

portion migrates, resulting in its apical shift; the oral sulcular epithelium gradually occupies an increasing portion of the sulcus (then a pocket) lining.[114]

Extension of the junctional epithelium along the root requires the presence of healthy epithelial cells. Marked degeneration or necrosis of the junctional epithelium impairs rather than accelerates pocket formation. (This occurs in necrotizing gingivitis, which results in an ulcer rather than pocket formation.)

Degenerative changes seen in the junctional epithelium at the base of periodontal pockets are usually less severe than those in the epithelium of the lateral pocket wall (see Fig. 22.7). Because the migration of the junctional epithelium requires healthy, viable cells, it is reasonable to assume that the degenerative changes seen in this area occur after the junctional epithelium reaches its position on the cementum.

The degree of leukocyte infiltration of the junctional epithelium is independent of the volume of inflamed connective tissue; thus this process may occur in gingiva with only slight signs of clinical inflammation.[112]

With continued inflammation, the gingiva increases in bulk, and the crest of the gingival margin extends coronally. The apical cells of the junctional epithelium continue to migrate along the root, and its coronal cells continue to separate from it. The epithelium of the lateral wall of the pocket proliferates to form bulbous, cord-like extensions into the inflamed connective tissue. Leukocytes and edema from the inflamed connective tissue infiltrate the epithelium that lines the pocket, resulting in various degrees of degeneration and necrosis.

The transformation of a gingival sulcus into a periodontal pocket creates an area in which plaque removal becomes impossible, and a feedback mechanism is established. The rationale for pocket reduction is based on the need to eliminate areas of plaque accumulation. For detailed information on pocket reduction surgeries, refer to Chapters 61 and 62.

Histopathology

Changes that occur during the initial stages of gingival inflammation are presented in Chapter 15. In this section, the microscopic features associated with an established pocket will be discussed.

Soft-Tissue Wall

The connective tissue will be edematous and densely infiltrated with plasma cells (approximately 80%), **lymphocytes**, and a scattering of PMNs.[144] The blood vessels will increase in number, will be dilated, and engorged, particularly in the subepithelial connective tissue layer.[11] The connective tissue exhibits varying degrees of degeneration. Single or multiple necrotic foci are occasionally present.[93] In addition to exudative and degenerative changes, the connective tissue shows proliferation of the endothelial cells, with newly formed capillaries, fibroblasts, and collagen fibers (see Fig. 22.5).

The junctional epithelium at the base of the pocket is usually much shorter than that of a normal sulcus. Although marked variations are found with regard to the length, width, and condition of the epithelial cells,[113] usually the coronoapical length of the junctional epithelium is reduced to only 50–100 μm.[7] The cells may be well formed and in good condition, or they may exhibit slight to marked degeneration (see Figs. 22.6 and 22.7).

The most severe degenerative changes in the periodontal pocket occur along the lateral wall (Fig. 22.8). The epithelium of the lateral wall of the pocket presents striking proliferative and degenerative changes. Epithelial buds or interlacing cords of epithelial cells project from the lateral wall into the adjacent inflamed connective tissue, and they may extend farther apically than the junctional epithelium (see Figs. 22.7 and 22.9A). These epithelial projections, as well as the remainder of the lateral epithelium, are densely infiltrated by leukocytes and edema from the inflamed connective tissue. The cells undergo vacuolar degeneration and rupture to form vesicles. Progressive degeneration and necrosis of the epithelium lead to ulceration of the lateral wall, exposure of the underlying inflamed connective tissue, and suppuration. In some cases, acute inflammation is superimposed on the underlying chronic changes.

A comparative study of gingival changes in rapidly progressing periodontitis with molar incisor involvement (previously termed as "aggressive periodontitis") and periodontitis revealed more pronounced degenerative changes in the epithelium of aggressive cases with more open intercellular spaces, including microclefts and necrotic areas.[54] The severity of the degenerative changes is not necessarily related to pocket depth. Ulceration of the lateral wall may occur in shallow pockets, and deep pockets are occasionally observed in which the lateral epithelium is relatively intact or shows only slight degeneration. The epithelium at the gingival crest of a periodontal pocket is generally intact and thickened, with prominent rete pegs.

For a detailed electron microscopic study of the pocket epithelium in experimentally induced pockets in dogs, see the article by Müller-Glauser and Schröder.[86]

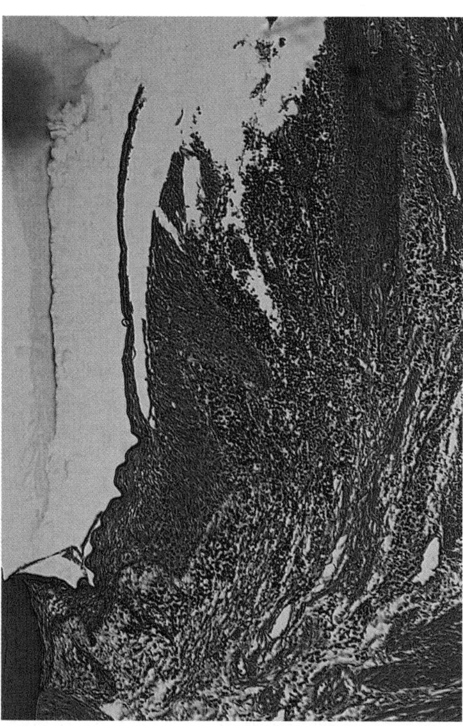

Fig. 22.8 View of the ulcerated lateral pocket wall of a periodontal pocket. Note the extension of epithelial cells and the dense accumulation of leukocytes within the epithelium and in the connective tissue.

KEY FACT

Features of Junctional Epithelium

- It acts as a physical barrier against plaque bacteria.
- It is stratified squamous nonkeratinized in nature, which develops by the union of oral epithelium and reduced enamel epithelium during tooth eruption.
- It is attached to the tooth by internal basal lamina and to the connective tissue by external basal lamina.
- It exhibits higher permeability to cells, gingival fluid, and host-defense molecules to flow through.
- It has higher rate of cellular proliferation and turnover.

Bacterial Invasion

Bacterial invasion of the apical and lateral areas of the pocket wall has been described in human periodontitis (previously named periodontitis). Filaments, rods, and coccoid organisms with predominant gram-negative cell walls have been found in intercellular spaces of the epithelium.[31,32] Hillmann and colleagues[54] have reported the presence of *Porphyromonas gingivalis* and *Prevotella intermedia* in the gingiva of aggressive periodontitis cases. *Aggregatibacter actinomycetemcomitans* has also been found in the tissues.[22,82,108]

Bacteria may invade the intercellular space under exfoliating epithelial cells, but they are also found between deeper epithelial cells as well as accumulating on the basement lamina. Some bacteria traverse the basement lamina and invade the subepithelial connective tissue (Figs. 22.10 and 22.11).[109]

The presence of bacteria in the gingival tissues has been interpreted by different investigators as bacterial invasion or as the "passive translocation" of plaque bacteria.[72] This important point has significant clinicopathologic implications and has not yet been clarified.[23,67,73]

Mechanisms of Tissue Destruction

The inflammatory response triggered by bacterial plaque unleashes a complex cascade of events aimed at destroying and removing bacteria, necrotic cells, and deleterious agents. However, this process is nonspecific; in an attempt to restore health, the host's cells (e.g., neutrophils, macrophages, fibroblasts, epithelial cells) produce proteinases, cytokines, and prostaglandins that can damage or destroy the host tissues.

Chapters 8 and 11 describe in detail these aspects of inflammation and the mechanisms of tissue destruction at the molecular level.

Microtopography of the Gingival Wall

Scanning electron microscopy has permitted the description of several areas in the soft-tissue (gingival) wall of the periodontal pocket in which different types of activity take place.[105] These areas are irregularly oval or elongated and adjacent to one another, and they measure about 50 to 200 μm. These findings suggest that the pocket wall is constantly changing as a result of the interaction between the host and the bacteria. The following areas have been noted:

1. *Areas of relative quiescence,* showing a relatively flat surface with minor depressions and mounds and occasional shedding of cells (Fig. 22.12A).
2. *Areas of bacterial accumulation,* which appear as depressions on the epithelial surface, with abundant debris and bacterial clumps penetrating into the enlarged intercellular spaces. These bacteria are mainly cocci, rods, and filaments, with a few spirochetes (see Fig. 22.12B).
3. *Areas of emergence of leukocytes,* in which leukocytes appear in the pocket wall through holes located in the intercellular spaces (Fig. 22.13).
4. *Areas of leukocyte–bacteria interaction,* in which numerous leukocytes are present and covered with bacteria in an apparent process of phagocytosis. Bacterial plaque associated with the epithelium is seen either as an organized matrix covered by a fibrin-like material in contact with the surface of cells or as bacteria penetrating into the intercellular spaces (see Fig. 22.12C).
5. *Areas of intense epithelial desquamation,* consisting of semiattached and folded epithelial squames, which are sometimes partially covered with bacteria (see Fig. 22.12D).
6. *Areas of ulceration,* with exposed connective tissue (Fig. 22.14).
7. *Areas of hemorrhage,* with numerous erythrocytes.

The transition from one area to another could result from bacteria accumulating in previously quiescent areas and triggering the

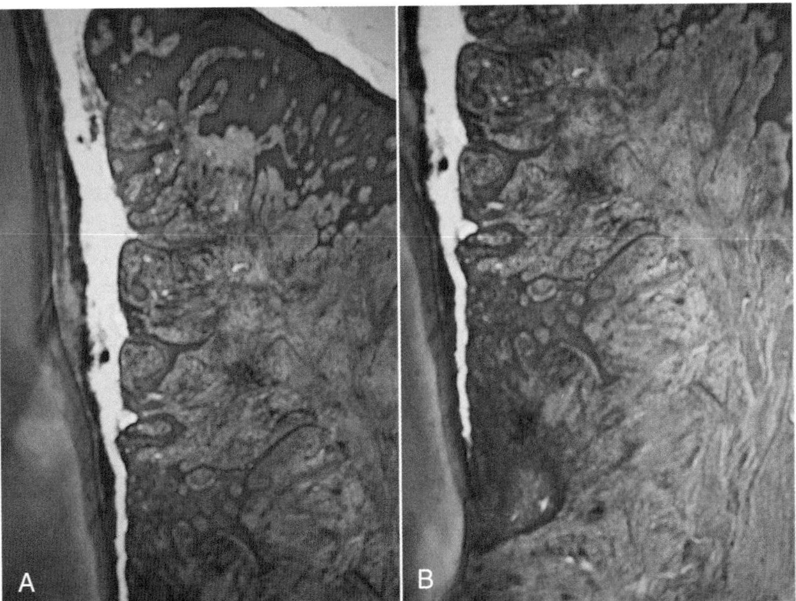

Fig. 22.9 (A) Lateral wall of a periodontal pocket showing epithelial proliferative and atrophic changes as well as marked inflammatory infiltrate and the destruction of collagen fibers. (B) Slightly apical view of the same patient showing the shortened junctional epithelium.

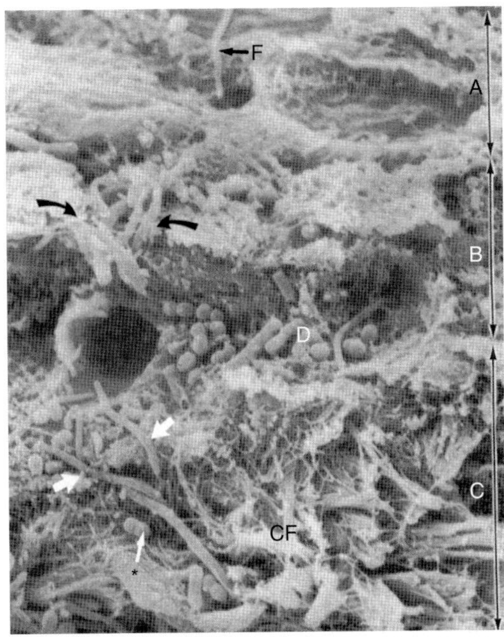

Fig. 22.10 Scanning electron micrograph of a section of pocket wall in advanced periodontitis in a human specimen showing bacterial penetration into the epithelium and connective tissue. Scanning electron microscope view of the surface of the pocket wall *(A)*, sectioned epithelium *(B)*, and sectioned connective tissue *(C)*. *Curved arrows* point to areas of bacterial penetration into the epithelium. *Thick white arrows* point to bacterial penetration into the connective tissue through a break in the continuity of the basal lamina. *CF,* Connective tissue fibers; *D,* accumulation of bacteria (rods, cocci, and filaments) on the basal lamina; *F,* filamentous organism on the surface of the epithelium. The *asterisk* points to coccobacillus in the connective tissue.

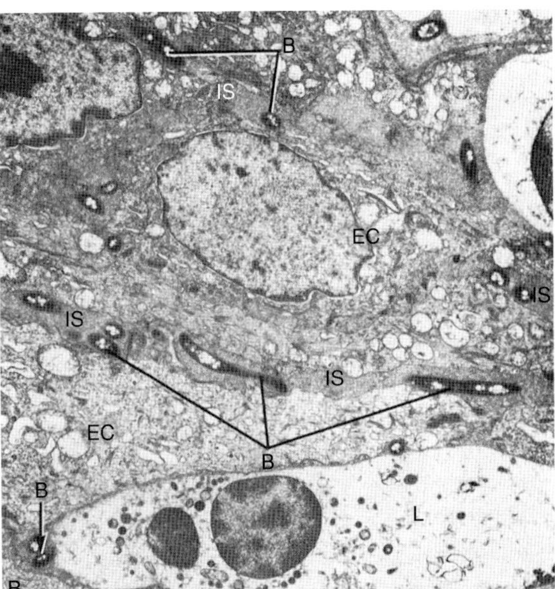

Fig. 22.11 Transmission electron micrograph of the epithelium in the periodontal pocket wall showing bacteria in the intercellular spaces. *B,* Bacteria; *EC,* epithelial cell; *IS,* intercellular space; *L,* leukocyte about to engulf bacteria. (Magnification ×8000.)

emergence of leukocytes and the leukocyte–bacteria interaction. This would lead to intense epithelial desquamation and finally to ulceration and hemorrhage.

Periodontal Pockets as Healing Lesions

Periodontal pockets are chronic inflammatory lesions and thus are constantly undergoing repair. Complete healing does not occur because of the persistence of the bacterial attack, which continues to stimulate an inflammatory response, thereby causing degeneration of the new tissue elements formed during the continuous effort at repair.

The condition of the soft-tissue wall of the periodontal pocket results from the interplay of the destructive and constructive tissue changes. Their balance determines clinical features such as color, consistency, and surface texture of the pocket wall. If the inflammatory fluid and cellular exudate predominate, the pocket wall is bluish-red, soft, spongy, and friable, with a smooth, shiny surface; at the clinical level, this is generally referred to as an *edematous pocket wall.* If there is a relative predominance of newly formed connective tissue cells and fibers, the pocket wall is more firm and pink and clinically referred to as a *fibrotic pocket wall* (see Table 22.1).

Edematous and fibrotic pockets represent opposite extremes of the same pathologic process rather than different disease entities. They are subject to constant modification, depending on the relative predominance of exudative and constructive changes.

Fibrotic pocket walls may be misleading, because they do not necessarily reflect what is taking place throughout the pocket wall. The most severe degenerative changes in periodontal tissues occur adjacent to the tooth surface and the subgingival plaque. In some cases, inflammation and ulceration on the inside of the pocket are walled off by fibrous tissue on the outer aspect (Fig. 22.15). Externally the pocket appears pink and fibrotic, despite the inflammatory changes occurring internally.

Pocket Contents

Periodontal pockets contain debris that consists principally of microorganisms and their products (enzymes, endotoxins, and other metabolic products), gingival fluid, food remnants, salivary mucin, desquamated epithelial cells, and leukocytes. Plaque-covered calculus usually projects from the tooth surface (Fig. 22.16). Purulent exudate, if present in the patient, consists of living, degenerated, and

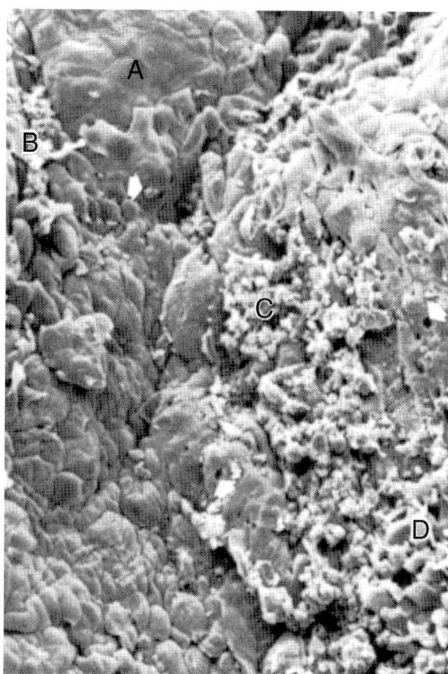

Fig. 22.12 Scanning electron frontal micrograph of the periodontal pocket wall. Different areas can be seen in the pocket wall surface. *A,* Area of quiescence. *B,* Bacterial accumulation. *C,* Bacterial–leukocyte interaction. *D,* Intense cellular desquamation. Arrows point to emerging leukocytes and holes left by leukocytes in the pocket wall. (Magnification ×800.)

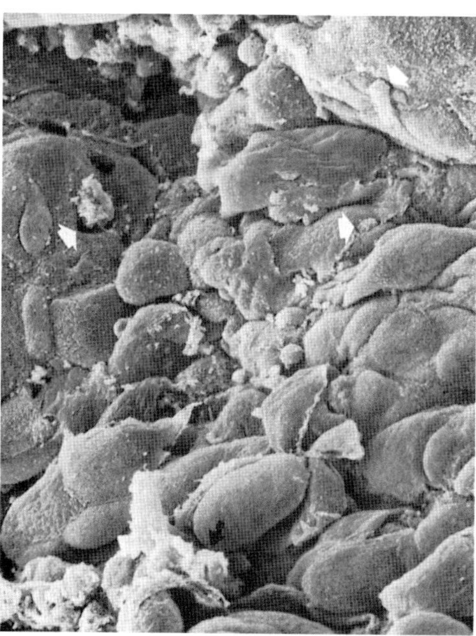

Fig. 22.13 Scanning electron micrograph of the periodontal pocket wall, frontal view, in a patient with advanced periodontitis. Note the desquamating epithelial cells and leukocytes *(white arrows)* emerging onto the pocket space. Scattered bacteria can also be seen *(black arrow).* (Magnification ×1500.)

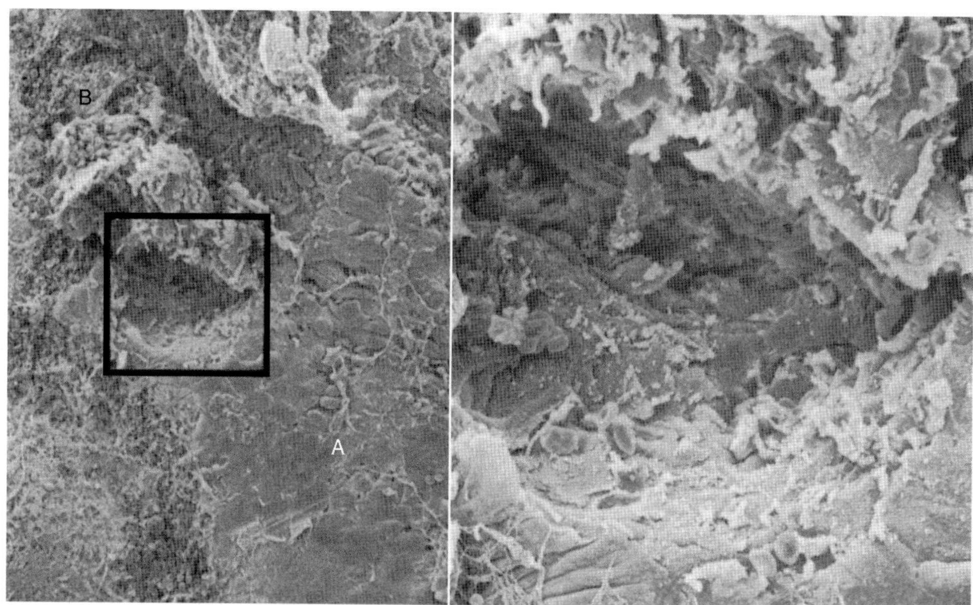

Fig. 22.14 Area of ulceration in the lateral wall of a deep periodontal pocket in a human specimen (magnification ×800) *(left). A,* Surface of pocket epithelium in a quiescent state. *B,* Area of hemorrhage. Scanning electron microscopy (magnification ×3000) of the square on the left *(right).* Connective tissue fibers and cells can be seen in the bottom of the ulcer.

necrotic leukocytes; living and dead bacteria; serum; and a scant amount of fibrin.[81] The contents of periodontal pockets, when filtered free of organisms and debris, have been demonstrated to be toxic when injected subcutaneously into experimental animals.[46]

Pus *is a common feature of periodontal diseases, but it is only a secondary sign.* The presence of pus or the ease with which it can be expressed from the pocket merely reflects the nature of the inflammatory changes in the pocket wall. It is not an indication of the depth of the pocket or the severity of the destruction of the supporting tissues. Extensive pus formation may occur in shallow pockets, whereas deep pockets may exhibit little or no pus. The localized accumulation of pus constitutes an abscess, which is discussed later in the online version of this chapter.

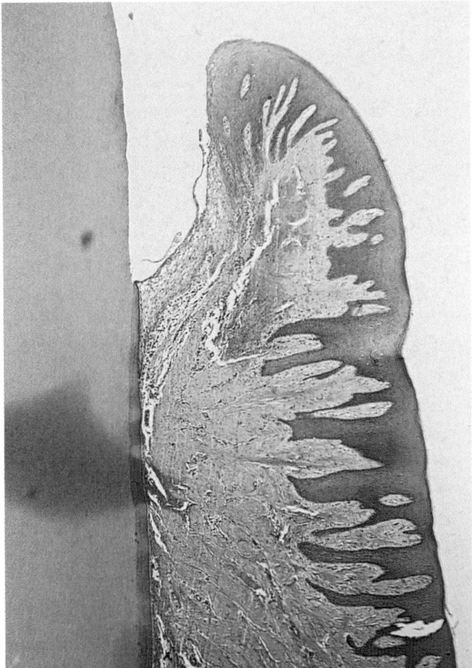

Fig. 22.15 Periodontal pocket wall. The inner half is inflamed and ulcerated; the outer half is densely collagenous.

KEY FACT

Gingival Crevicular Fluid

Gingival crevicular fluid (GCF) is an ultrafiltrate of blood, present in the gingival sulcus space, that contains several molecular components like bacterial degradation products, host tissue degradation products, and inflammatory mediators. Due to the location and ease of collection, several human clinical studies have been and are currently exploring and validating biomarkers of periodontal diseases in GCF. The implant equivalent of GCF is commonly referred to as periimplant sulcular fluid (PISF).

Root Surface Walls

The root surface wall of periodontal pockets often undergoes changes that are significant because they may perpetuate the periodontal infection, cause pain, and complicate periodontal treatment.[12]

As the pocket deepens, collagen fibers embedded in the cementum are destroyed, and cementum becomes exposed to the oral environment. Collagenous remnants of Sharpey fibers in the cementum undergo degeneration, creating an environment favorable to the penetration of bacteria. Viable bacteria have been found in the roots of 87% of periodontally diseased noncarious teeth.[2] Bacterial penetration into the cementum can be found as deep as the cementodentinal junction,[1,24] and it may also enter the dentinal tubules.[37,46] Penetration and the growth of bacteria lead to fragmentation and breakdown of the cementum surface and result in areas of necrotic cementum that are separated from the tooth by masses of bacteria.

Pathologic granules[10] have been observed with light and electron microscopy,[7,8] and they may represent areas of collagen

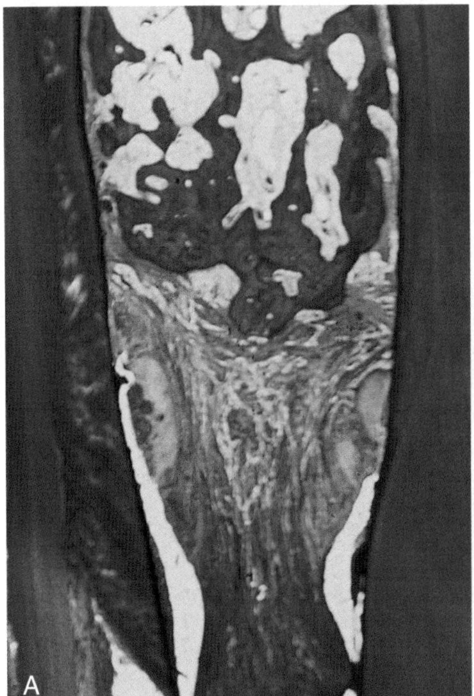

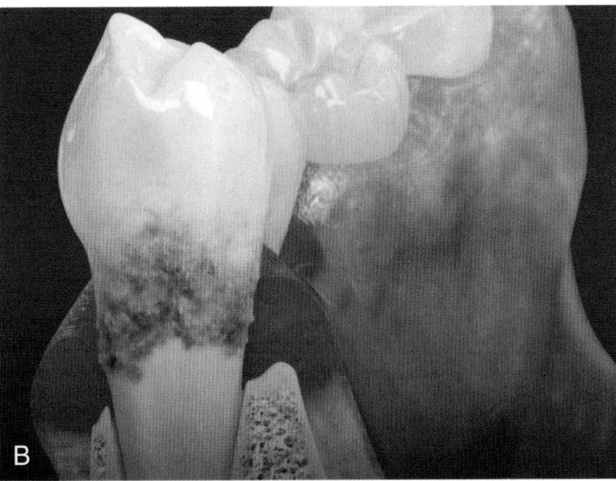

Fig. 22.16 (A) Interdental papilla with ulcerated suprabony periodontal pockets on its mesial and distal aspects. Calculus is present on the approximal tooth surfaces and within the gingiva. (B) A graphical illustration depicting gingival inflammation and bone loss adjacent to dental calculus formed on the root surface. ©Periopixel.

degeneration or areas in which collagen fibrils have not been fully mineralized initially.

In addition, bacterial products (e.g., endotoxins[5,6]) have also been detected in the cementum wall of periodontal pockets. When root fragments from teeth with periodontitis are placed in tissue culture, they induce irreversible morphologic changes in the cells of the culture. Such changes are not produced by normal roots.[50] Diseased root fragments also prevent the in vitro attachment of human gingival fibroblasts, whereas normal root surfaces allow the cells to attach freely.[4] When placed in the oral mucosa of the patient, diseased root fragments induce an inflammatory response, even if they have been autoclaved.[76]

KEY FACT

Bacterial Endotoxin

Endotoxins are lipopolysaccharide (LPS) in nature and are associated with the cell walls of gram-negative bacteria. LPS is highly immunogenic, which the innate immune system recognizes via Toll-like receptors (TLRs), leading to an immune response. LPS from *Porphyromonas gingivalis*, a key pathogen in periodontitis, plays an important role in both triggering and sustaining inflammation in the periodontium.

These changes manifest clinically as softening of the cementum surface; this is usually asymptomatic, but it can be painful when a probe or explorer penetrates the area. They also constitute a possible reservoir for reinfection of the area after treatment. During the course of treatment, these necrotic areas are removed by root planing until a hard, smooth surface is reached. Cementum is very thin in the cervical areas, and scaling and root planing often remove it entirely, exposing the underlying dentin. Sensitivity to cold may result until the pulp tissue forms secondary dentin. Recent studies indicate that endotoxins are not tightly bound to cementum and can be easily removed using ultrasonic instrumentation without having to completely remove the entire cementum layer.

Decalcification and Remineralization of Cementum

Areas of *increased mineralization*[118] are probably a result of an exchange of minerals and organic components at the cementum–saliva interface after exposure to the oral cavity. The mineral content of exposed cementum increases,[117] and the minerals that are increased in diseased root surfaces include calcium,[120] magnesium,[87,120] phosphorus,[87] and fluoride.[87] Microhardness, however, remains unchanged.[101,141] The development of a highly mineralized superficial layer may increase the tooth's resistance to decay.[4]

The hypermineralized zones are detectable by electron microscopy, and they are associated with increased perfection of the crystal structure and organic changes that are suggestive of a subsurface cuticle.[117,118] These zones have also been seen in microradiographic studies[119] as a layer that is generally 10- to 20-mm thick, with areas as thick as 50 mm. No decrease in mineralization was found in deeper areas, indicating that increased mineralization does not come from adjacent areas. A loss of or reduction in the crossbanding of collagen near the cementum surface[33,34] and a subsurface condensation of organic material of exogenous origin[117] have also been reported.

Areas of demineralization are often related to root caries. Exposure to oral fluid and bacterial plaque results in proteolysis of the embedded remnants of Sharpey fibers; the cementum may be softened, and it may undergo fragmentation and cavitation.[53] Unlike enamel caries, root surface caries tend to progress around rather than into the tooth.[85] Active root caries lesions appear as well-defined yellowish or light brown areas; they are frequently covered by plaque, and they have a softened or leathery consistency on probing. Inactive lesions are well-defined darker lesions with a smooth surface and a harder consistency on probing.[30]

The dominant microorganism in root surface caries is *Actinomyces viscosus,*[128] although its specific role in the development of the lesion has not been established.[30] Other bacteria, such as *Actinomyces naeslundii, Streptococcus mutans, Streptococcus salivarius, Streptococcus sanguinis,* and *Bacillus cereus,* have been found to induce root caries in animal models. Quirynen and colleagues[100] reported that when plaque levels and pocket depths decrease after periodontal therapy (both nonsurgical and surgical), a shift in oral bacteria occurs, leading to a reduction in periodontal pathogens, an increase in *S. mutans,* and the development of root caries.

A prevalence rate study of root caries among 20- to 64-year-old individuals revealed that 42% had one or more root caries lesions and that these lesions tended to increase with age.[59]

The tooth may not be painful, but exploration of the root surface reveals the presence of a defect, and penetration of the involved area with a probe may cause pain. Caries of the root may lead to pulpitis, sensitivity to sweets and thermal changes, or severe pain. Pathologic exposure of the pulp occurs in severe cases. Root caries may be the cause of toothache in patients with periodontitis and no evidence of coronal decay.

Caries of the cementum requires special attention when the pocket is treated. The necrotic cementum must be removed by scaling and root planing until firm tooth surface is reached, even if this entails extension into the dentin.

Areas of cellular resorption of cementum and dentin are common in roots that are unexposed by periodontitis.[123] These areas are of no particular significance because they are symptom free, and, as long as the root is covered by the periodontal ligament, they are likely to undergo repair. However, if the root is exposed by progressive pocket formation before repair occurs, these areas appear as isolated cavitations that penetrate into the dentin. These areas can be differentiated from caries of the cementum by their clear-cut outline and hard surface. They may be sources of considerable pain that require the placement of a restoration.

Surface Morphology of Tooth Wall[137]

The following zones can be found in the bottom of a periodontal pocket (Fig. 22.17):

1. *Cementum covered by calculus,* in which all of the changes described in the preceding paragraphs can be found.
2. *Attached plaque,* which covers calculus and extends apically from it to a variable degree (typically 100 to 500 μm).
3. The zone of *unattached plaque* that surrounds attached plaque and extends apically to it.
4. The zone of *attachment of the junctional epithelium to the tooth.* The extension of this zone, which in normal sulci is more than 500 μm, is usually reduced in periodontal pockets to less than 100 μm.
5. A zone of *semidestroyed connective tissue fibers* may be apical to the junctional epithelium[109] (see the Pathogenesis section earlier in this chapter).

Zones 3, 4, and 5 make up the "plaque-free zone" seen in extracted teeth.[9,15,55,107,137] The total width of the plaque-free zone varies according to the type of tooth (i.e., it is wider in the molars than in the incisors) and the depth of the pocket (i.e., it is narrower in deeper pockets).[106] It is important to remember that the term *plaque-free zone* refers only to attached plaque, because unattached plaque contains a variety of gram-positive and gram-negative morphotypes, including cocci, rods, filaments, fusiforms, and spirochetes. The most apical zone contains predominantly gram-negative rods and cocci.[134]

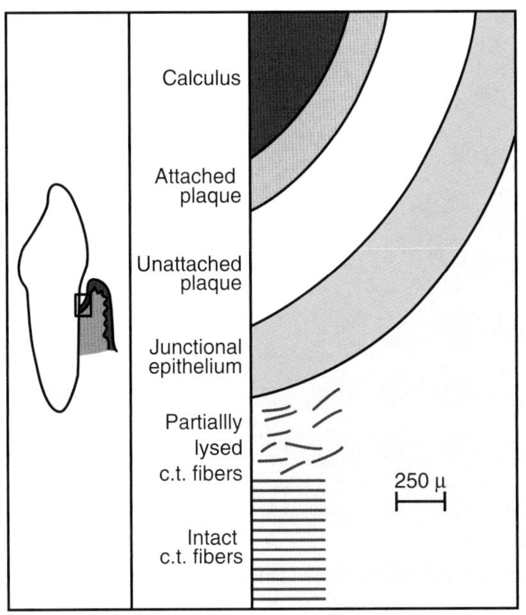

Fig. 22.17 Diagram of the area at the bottom of a pocket. *c.t.*, Connective tissue.

Periodontitis Activity

For many years the loss of attachment produced by periodontitis was thought to be a slow but continuously progressive phenomenon. More recently, as a result of studies of the specificity of plaque bacteria, the concept of periodontitis activity has evolved.

According to this concept, periodontal pockets go through periods of exacerbation and quiescence as a result of episodic bursts of activity followed by periods of remission. *Periods of quiescence* are characterized by a reduced inflammatory response and little or no loss of bone and connective tissue attachment. A buildup of unattached plaque, with its gram-negative, motile, and anaerobic bacteria (see Chapter 10), starts a *period of exacerbation* during which bone and connective tissue attachment are lost and the pocket deepens. This period may last for days, weeks, or months, and it is eventually followed by a period of remission or quiescence during which gram-positive bacteria proliferate and a more stable condition is established. On the basis of a study of radioiodine ^{125}I absorptiometry, McHenry and colleagues[80] confirmed that bone loss in patients with untreated periodontitis occurs in an episodic manner.

These periods of quiescence and exacerbation are also known as *periods of inactivity* and *periods of activity*. Clinically, active periods show bleeding, either spontaneously or with probing, and greater amounts of gingival exudate. Histologically, the pocket epithelium appears thin and ulcerated, and an infiltrate composed predominantly of plasma cells,[24] PMNs,[98] or both is seen. Bacterial samples from the pocket lumen that are analyzed with dark-field microscopy show high proportions of motile organisms and spirochetes.[73]

Methods to detect periods of activity or inactivity are currently being investigated (see ebooks.Health.Elsevier.com).

Site Specificity

Periodontal destruction does not occur in all parts of the mouth at the same time; rather it occurs on a few teeth at a time or even only on some aspects of some teeth at any given time. This is referred to as the *site specificity* of periodontitis. Sites of periodontal destruction are often found next to sites with little or no destruction. Therefore the severity of periodontitis increases with the development of new disease sites and with the increased breakdown of existing sites.

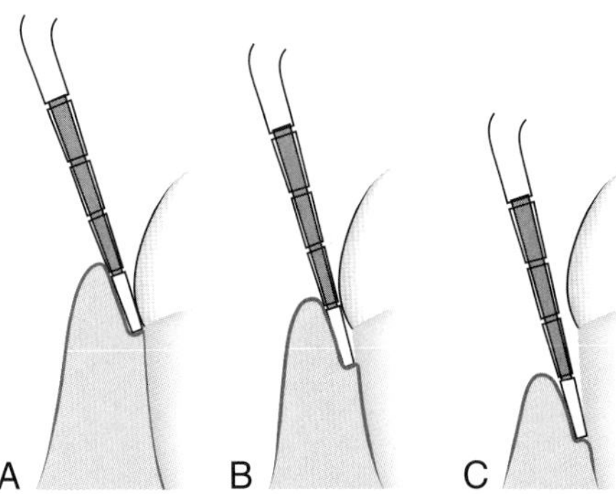

Fig. 22.18 Same pocket depth with different amounts of recession. (A) Gingival pocket with no recession. (B) Periodontal pocket of similar depth as shown in part A but with some degree of recession. (C) Pocket depth the same as shown in parts A and B but with still more recession.

Pulp Changes Associated With Periodontal Pockets

The spread of infection from periodontal pockets may cause pathologic changes in the pulp. Such changes may give rise to painful symptoms, or they may adversely affect the response of the pulp to restorative procedures. Involvement of the pulp in periodontitis occurs through either the apical foramen or the lateral pulp canals after pocket infection reaches them. Atrophic and inflammatory pulpal changes occur in such cases (see Chapter 49).

Relationship of Attachment Loss and Bone Loss to Pocket Depth

The severity of the attachment loss in pocket formation is generally but not always correlated with the depth of the pocket. This is because the degree of attachment loss depends on the location of the base of the pocket on the root surface, whereas pocket depth is the distance between the base of the pocket and the crest of the gingival margin. Pockets of the same depth may be associated with different degrees of attachment loss (Fig. 22.18), and pockets of different depths may be associated with the same amount of attachment loss (Fig. 22.19).

The severity of bone loss is generally but not always correlated with pocket depth. Extensive attachment and bone loss may be associated with shallow pockets if the attachment loss is accompanied by recession of the gingival margin, and slight bone loss can occur with deep pockets, if it is accompanied by gingival enlargement.

Area Between Base of Pocket and Alveolar Bone

Normally, the distance between the apical end of the junctional epithelium and the alveolar bone is relatively constant. The distance between the apical extent of calculus and the alveolar crest in human periodontal pockets is most constant, having a mean length of 1.97 mm (±33.16%).[126,136]

The distance from attached plaque to bone is never less than 0.5 mm and never more than 2.7 mm.[137–139] These findings suggest that the bone-resorbing activity induced by the bacteria is exerted within these distances. However, the presence of isolated bacteria or clumps of bacteria in the connective tissue[109] and on the bone surface[32] may modify these considerations.

Relationship of Pocket to Bone

In infrabony pockets, the base of the pocket is apical to the crest of the alveolar bone, and the pocket wall lies between the tooth and the

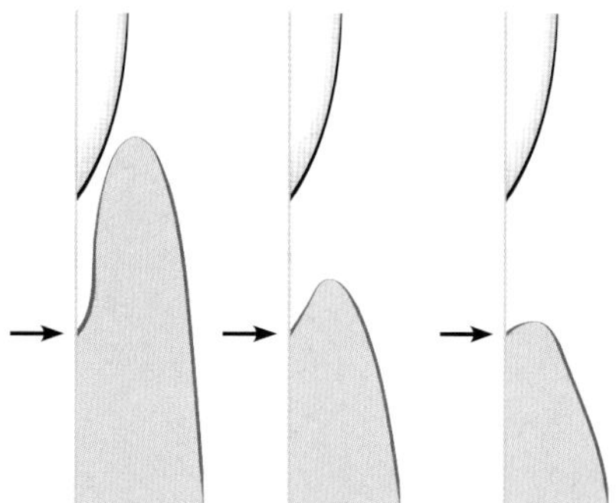

Fig. 22.19 Different pocket depths with the same amount of attachment loss. Arrows point to the bottom of the pocket. The distance between the arrow and the cementoenamel junction remains the same despite different pocket depths.

bone. The bone loss is therefore vertical. Alternatively, in suprabony pockets, the base is coronal to the crest of the alveolar bone, and the pocket wall lies coronal to the bone. The type of bone loss is always horizontal.

This creates some microscopic differences that have some therapeutic importance. They are the relationship of the soft-tissue wall of the pocket to the alveolar bone, the pattern of bone destruction, and the direction of the transseptal fibers of the periodontal ligament (Figs. 22.20–22.22).[19]

In suprabony pockets, the alveolar crest gradually attains a more apical position in relation to the tooth, but it retains its general morphology and architecture. The interdental fibers that run over the bone from one tooth to the other maintain their usual horizontal direction. In infrabony pockets, the morphology of the alveolar crest changes completely, with the formation of an angular bony defect. The interdental fibers in this case run over the bone in an oblique direction between the two teeth of the interdental space.[19,139] This may affect the function of the area and also necessitate a modification in treatment techniques (see Chapters 61–63).[16,19] Table 22.2 summarizes the distinguishing features of suprabony and infrabony pockets. The classification of infrabony pockets is discussed later in this chapter.

CLINICAL CORRELATION

Pocket Reduction Surgeries

Pocket reduction surgeries are aimed at reducing the probing pocket depths in patients with periodontitis. Depending on the disease presentation, one can take a resective or regenerative approach. Suprabony pockets are primarily treated by resective procedures such as gingivectomy or osseous surgery, whereas infrabony defects with multiple walls (that are contained) are amenable to regenerative approaches.

Bone Destruction Caused by the Extension of Gingival Inflammation

The cause of bone destruction in periodontitis is the extension of inflammation from the marginal gingiva into the supporting periodontal tissues. The inflammatory migration of the bone surface and the initial bone loss that follows mark the transition from gingivitis to periodontitis.

Periodontitis is always preceded by gingivitis, but not all gingivitis progresses to periodontitis. Some cases of gingivitis apparently never become periodontitis, and other cases go through a brief gingivitis phase and rapidly develop into periodontitis. The factors responsible for the extension of inflammation to the supporting structures, thereby initiating the conversion of gingivitis to periodontitis, are not clearly understood and are likely to be related to individual susceptibility to the insult presented by the bacterial biofilm or microbiologic changes that occur in the pocket environment and surrounding tissues.

As stated previously, the transition from gingivitis to periodontitis is associated with changes in the composition of the bacterial biofilm. In advanced stages of disease, the number of motile organisms and spirochetes increases, whereas the number of coccoid rods and straight rods decreases.[69] The cellular composition of the infiltrated connective tissue also changes with increasing severity of the lesion (see Chapter 8). Fibroblasts and lymphocytes predominate in stage 1 gingivitis, whereas the number of plasma cells and blast cells increases gradually as the disease progresses. Seymour and colleagues[121,122] have postulated a stage of "contained" gingivitis, in which T lymphocytes are preponderant; they suggest that, as the lesion becomes a B-lymphocyte lesion, it becomes progressively destructive.

Heijl and coworkers[52] were able to convert, in experimental animals, a confined, naturally occurring state of chronic gingivitis into progressive periodontitis by placing a silk ligature into the sulcus and tying it around the neck of the teeth. Placement of the ligature induced ulceration of the sulcular epithelium, a shift in the inflammatory infiltrate from predominantly plasma cells to polymorphonuclear leukocytes, and osteoclastic resorption of the alveolar crest. The recurrence of episodes of acute destruction over time may be one mechanism that leads to progressive bone loss in individuals with periodontitis.

The extension of the inflammatory process into the supporting structures of a tooth may be modified by the pathogenic potential of biofilm and the susceptibility/resistance of the host. The latter includes immunologic activity and other tissue-related mechanisms, such as the degree of fibrosis of the gingiva, probably the width of the attached gingiva, and the reactive fibrogenesis and osteogenesis that occur peripheral to the inflammatory lesion.[103] Some studies suggest that the quality of the host response to a similar bacterial insult varies, resulting in some individuals being more susceptible to the destructive aspects of periodontitis than others.

Histopathology

Gingival inflammation extends along the collagen fiber bundles and follows the course of the blood vessels through the loosely arranged tissues around them into the alveolar bone (see Fig. 22.25).[142] Although the inflammatory infiltrate is concentrated in the marginal periodontium, the reaction is a much more diffuse one, often reaching the bone and eliciting a response before evidence of crestal resorption or loss of attachment exists.[84] In the upper molar region, inflammation can extend to the maxillary sinus, resulting in thickening of the sinus mucosa.[83]

Interproximally, inflammation spreads to the loose connective tissue around the blood vessels, through the fibers, and then into the bone through vessel channels that perforate the crest of the interdental septum at the center of the crest (Fig. 22.26), toward the side of the crest (Fig. 22.27), or at the angle of the septum. In addition, inflammation may enter the bone through more than one channel. Less frequently, the inflammation spreads from the gingiva directly into the periodontal ligament and from there into the interdental septum (Fig. 22.28).[3]

Facially and lingually, inflammation from the gingiva spreads along the outer periosteal surface of the bone (see Fig. 22.28) and penetrates into the marrow spaces through vessel channels in the outer cortex.

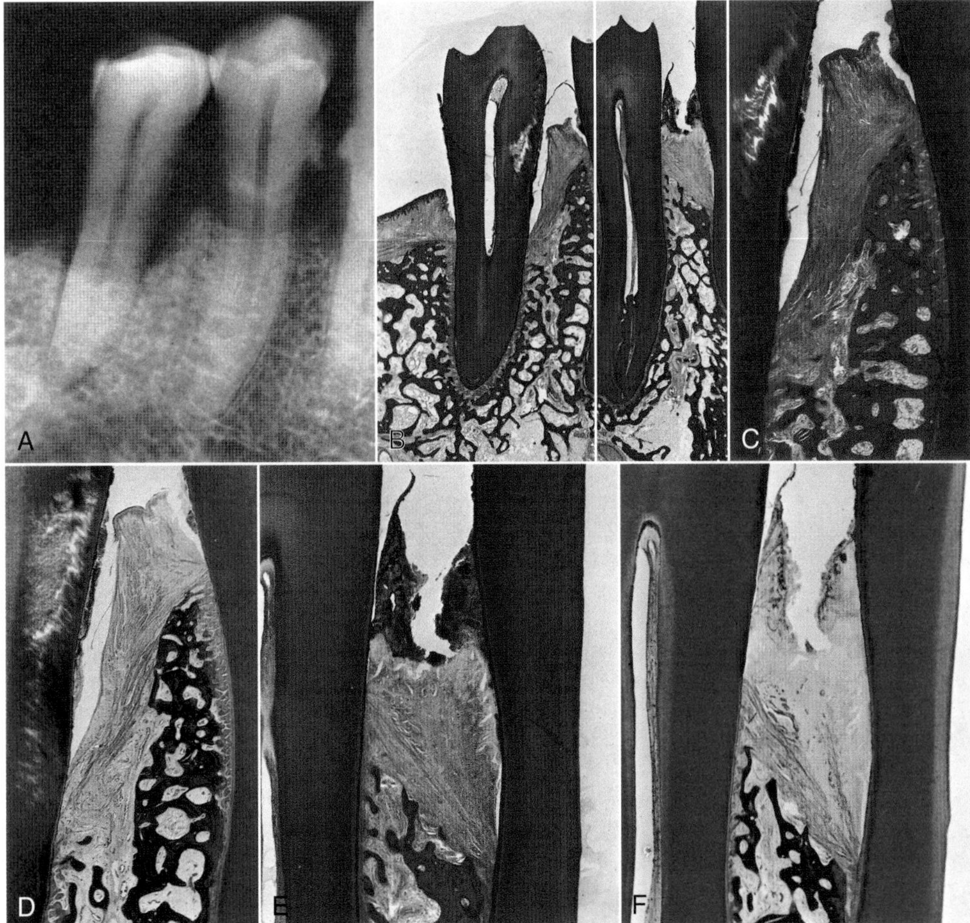

Fig. 22.20 Radiographic and microscopic features of intrabony pockets. (A) Radiograph of a mandibular canine and premolar area showing angular bone loss mesial to the second premolar. The type of bone loss between the first premolar and the canine is not radiographically apparent. (B) Mesiodistal histologic section of the teeth seen in part A showing an intrabony pocket mesial to the second premolar as well as suprabony pockets distal to the second premolar and mesial and distal to the first premolar. The mesial suprabony pocket of the first premolar appears to be coronal to a vertical bone loss. (C) Higher-power view of the area between the premolars. Note the angular bone loss and the transseptal fibers that cover the bone. (D) Higher-power view of the area between the premolars stained with Mallory connective tissue stain, clearly showing the direction of transseptal fibers. (E) Higher-power view of the area between the first premolar and the canine. Note the abundant calculus, the dense leukocytic infiltration of the gingiva, and the angulation of the transseptal fibers and bone. The pocket is still suprabony. (F) Mallory stain of a similar area to the one shown in part E. Note the destruction of the gingival fibers caused by inflammation and the angular fibers formed over angular bone loss and less affected by the inflammation. Transseptal fibers extend from the distal surface of the premolar over the crest of the alveolar bone into the intrabony pocket. Note the leukocytic infiltration of the transseptal fibers. (From Glickman I, Smulow J. *Periodontal Disease: Clinical, Radiographic and Histopathologic Features.* Philadelphia: Saunders; 1974.)

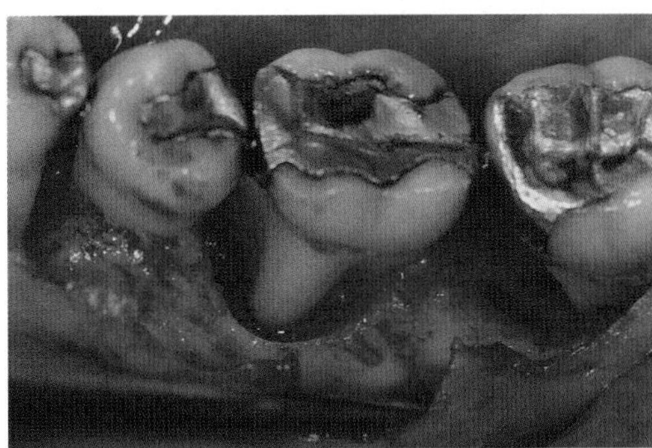

Fig. 22.21 After raising a flap for the treatment of the infrabony pockets, the vertical bone loss around the mesial roots of the mandibular first and second molars can be seen.

Along its course from the gingiva to the bone, the inflammation destroys the gingival and transeptal fibers, reducing them to disorganized granular fragments interspersed among the inflammatory cells and edema.[92] However, there is a continuous tendency to recreate transeptal fibers across the crest of the interdental septum farther along the root as the bone destruction progresses (Fig. 22.29). As a result, transeptal fibers are present, even in cases of extreme periodontal bone loss. The dense transeptal fibers form a firm covering over the bone that is encountered during periodontal flap surgery after the superficial granulation tissue is removed.[99]

After inflammation reaches the bone via extension from the gingiva (Fig. 22.30), it spreads into the marrow spaces and replaces the marrow with a leukocytic and fluid exudate, new blood vessels, and proliferating fibroblasts (Fig. 22.31). Multinuclear osteoclasts and

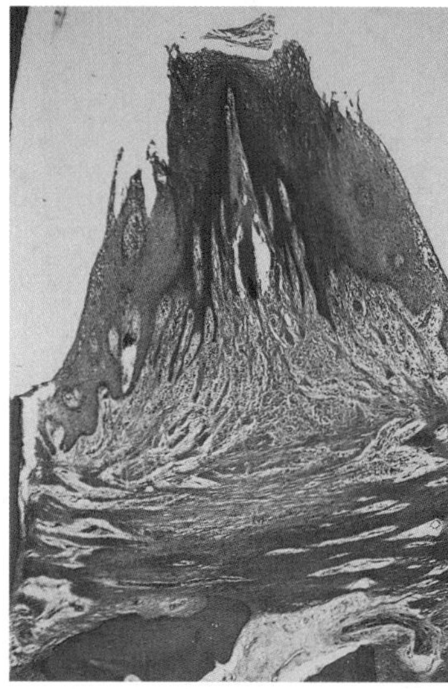

Fig. 22.22 Two suprabony pockets in an interdental space. Note the normal horizontal arrangement of the transseptal fibers.

TABLE 22.2 Distinguishing Features of Suprabony and Intrabony Periodontal Pockets

Suprabony Pocket	Intrabony Pocket
1. The base of the pocket is coronal to the level of the alveolar bone.	1. The base of the pocket is apical to the crest of the alveolar bone so that the bone is adjacent to the soft-tissue wall (see Fig. 22.2).
2. The pattern of destruction of the underlying bone is horizontal.	2. The pattern of bone destruction is vertical (angular) (see Figs. 22.20 and 22.21).
3. Interproximally, transseptal fibers that are restored during progressive periodontitis are arranged horizontally in the space between the base of the pocket and the alveolar bone (see Fig. 22.22).	3. Interproximally, transseptal fibers are oblique rather than horizontal. They extend from the cementum beneath the base of the pocket along the alveolar bone and over the crest to the cementum of the adjacent tooth (see Fig. 22.20).
4. On the facial and lingual surfaces, periodontal ligament fibers beneath the pocket follow their normal horizontal–oblique course between the tooth and the bone.	4. On the facial and lingual surfaces, periodontal ligament fibers follow the angular pattern of the adjacent bone. They extend from the cementum beneath the base of the pocket along the alveolar bone and over the crest to join with the outer periosteum.

mononuclear phagocytes increase in number, and the bone surfaces appear to be lined with Howship lacunae (Fig. 22.32).

In the marrow spaces, resorption proceeds from within and causes a thinning of the surrounding bony trabeculae and an enlargement of the marrow spaces; this is followed by the destruction of the bone and a reduction in bone height. Normally, fatty bone marrow is partially or totally replaced by a fibrous type of marrow in the vicinity of the resorption.

Bone destruction in periodontitis is not a process of bone necrosis.[62] It involves the activity of living cells along viable bone. With the exception of necrotic bone that is visible in distinct pathogenic processes such as necrotizing periodontitis and bisphosphonate-related osteonecrosis of the jaws, all bone present in areas with periodontitis is viable, live bone. In periodontitis, bone resorption may be related to the analogy of the bone attempting to run away from the infectious/inflammatory process; this may be seen as a host protection mechanism.

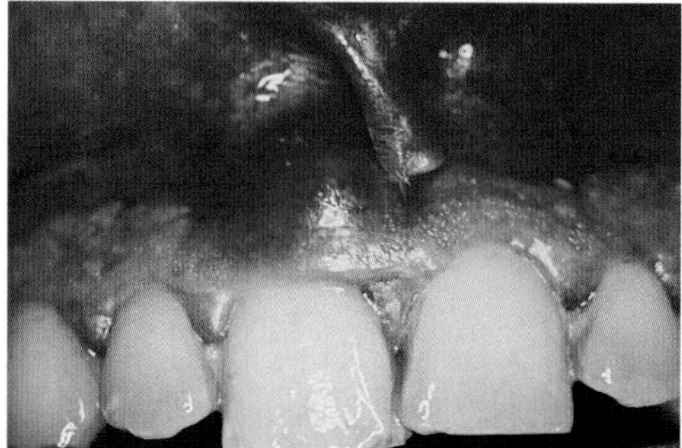

Fig. 22.23 Periodontal abscess on an upper right central incisor.

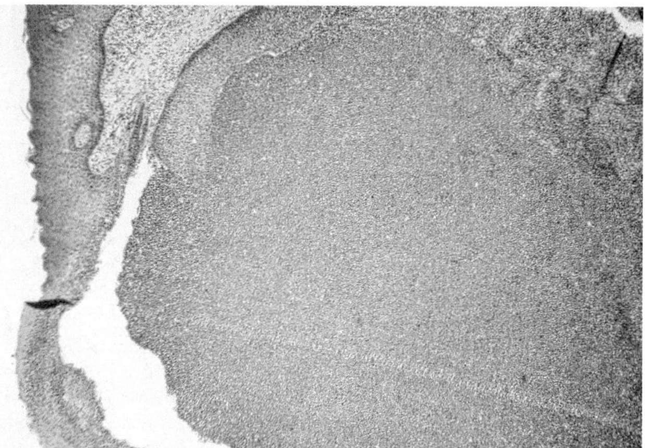

Fig. 22.24 Microscopic view of a periodontal abscess showing the dense accumulation of polymorphonuclear leukocytes covered by squamous epithelium.

The amount of inflammatory infiltrate correlates with the degree of bone loss but not with the number of osteoclasts. However, the distance from the apical border of the inflammatory infiltrate to the alveolar bone crest correlates with both the number of osteoclasts on the alveolar crest and the total number of osteoclasts.[102] Similar findings have been reported in experimentally induced periodontitis in animals.[68]

Radius of Action

Garant and Cho[35] suggested that locally produced bone resorption factors may need to be present in the proximity of the bone surface to exert their action. Page and Schroeder,[97] on the basis of Waerhaug's measurements made on human autopsy specimens,[138,139] postulated a range of effectiveness of about 1.5 to 2.5 mm in which bacterial biofilm can induce loss of bone. Beyond 2.5 mm, there is little or no effect; interproximal angular defects can appear only in spaces that are wider than 2.5 mm, because narrower spaces would end up with horizontal bone loss. Tal[131] corroborated this concept with measurements in human patients.

Large defects that greatly exceed a distance of 2.5 mm from the tooth surface (as described in periodontitis with molar-incisor pattern) may be caused by the presence of bacteria in the tissues.[20,35,110]

Rate of Bone Loss

In a study of Sri Lankan tea laborers with no oral hygiene and no dental care, Löe and colleagues[75] found the rate of bone loss

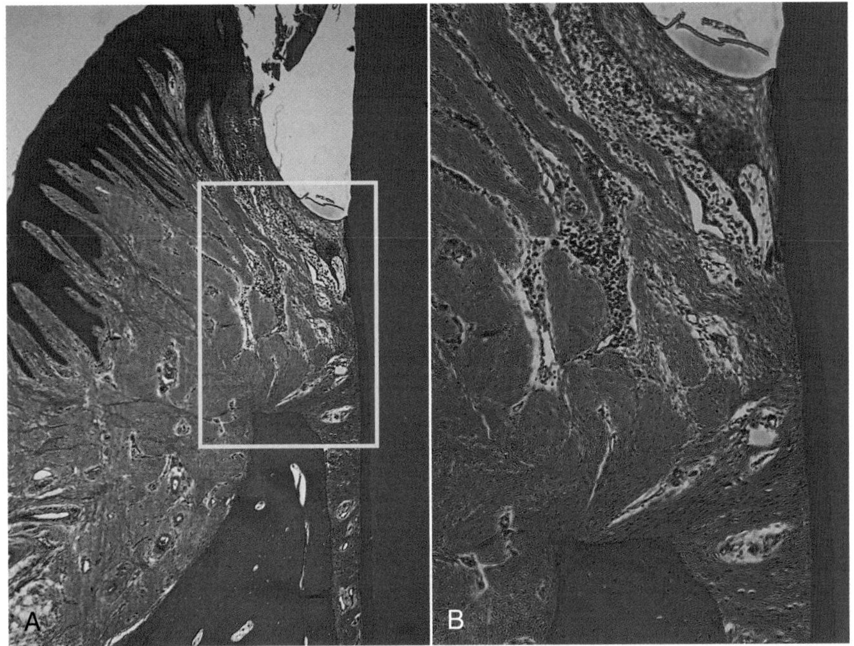

Fig. 22.25 (A) An area of inflammation extending from the gingiva into the suprabony area. (B) Extension of inflammation along the blood vessels and between collagen bundles.

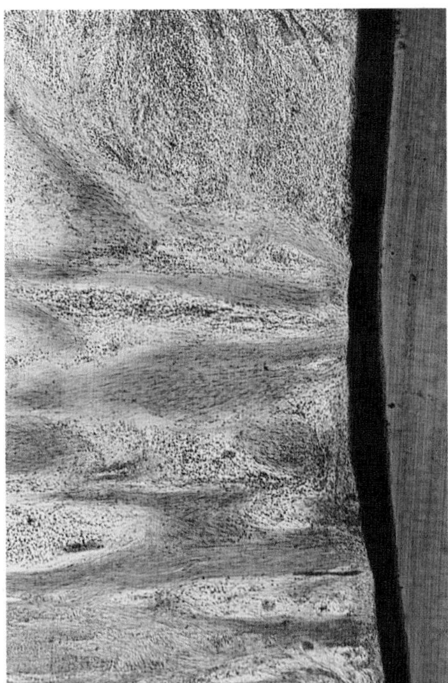

Fig. 22.26 Inflammation that extends from the pocket area *(top)* between the collagen fibers, which are partially destroyed.

averages about 0.2 mm per year for facial surfaces and about 0.3 mm per year for proximal surfaces when periodontitis was allowed to progress untreated.

However, the rate of bone loss may vary, depending on the type of disease present. Löe and colleagues[74] also identified the following three subgroups of patients with periodontitis on the basis of the interproximal loss of attachment and tooth mortality (loss of attachment can be equated with loss of bone, although attachment loss precedes bone loss by about 6 to 8 months[44]):

1. Approximately 8% of persons had a rapid progression of periodontitis that was characterized by a yearly loss of attachment of 0.1 mm to 1 mm.
2. Approximately 81% of individuals had moderately progressive periodontitis with a yearly loss of attachment of 0.05 mm to 0.5 mm.
3. The remaining 11% of persons had minimal or no progression of destructive disease with a yearly loss of attachment of 0.05 mm to 0.09 mm.

Periods of Destruction

Periodontal destruction occurs in an episodic, intermittent manner, with periods of inactivity or quiescence that alternate with destructive periods that result in the loss of collagen and alveolar bone and the deepening of the periodontal pocket.

Periods of destructive activity are associated with subgingival ulceration and an acute inflammatory reaction that results in the rapid loss of alveolar bone[97,115]; it has been hypothesized that this coincides with the conversion of a predominantly T-lymphocyte lesion to one with a predominantly B-lymphocyte–plasma cell infiltrate.[122] Microbiologically, these lesions are associated with an increase in the loose, unattached, motile, gram-negative, anaerobic pocket flora, whereas periods of remission coincide with the formation of a dense, unattached, nonmotile, gram-positive flora with a tendency to mineralize.[89]

It has also been suggested that the onset of periods of destruction coincide with tissue invasion by one or several bacterial species and that this is followed by an advanced local host defense that controls the attack.[110]

The dense network transseptal fiber that is attached interdentally from tooth to tooth is one of the barriers that protects the interdental bone from the inflammatory process. Even after these fibers are initially destroyed, they continually re-form and are the fibers found during periodontal flap surgery.

Mechanisms of Bone Destruction

The factors involved in bone destruction in periodontitis are bacterial and host mediated. The bacterial biofilm products induce the

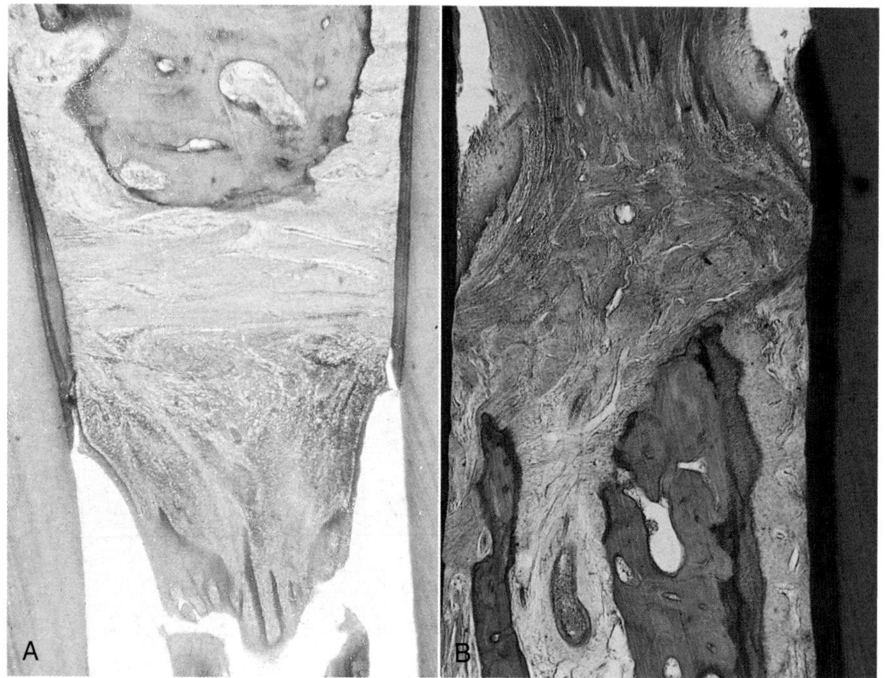

Fig. 22.27 (A) Extension of inflammation into the center of the interdental septum. Inflammation from the gingiva penetrates the transseptal fibers and enters the bone around the blood vessel in the center of the septum. (B) The cortical layer at the top of the septum has been destroyed, and the inflammation penetrates into the marrow spaces.

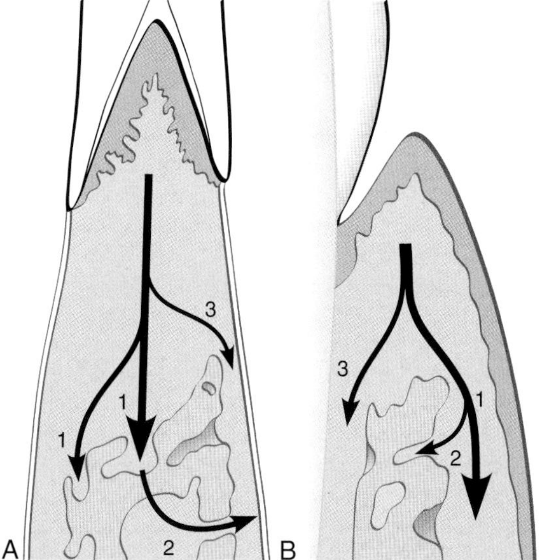

Fig. 22.28 Pathways of inflammation from the gingiva into the supporting periodontal tissues in a patient with periodontitis. (A) Interproximally, from the gingiva into the bone *(1)*, from the bone into the periodontal ligament *(2)*, and from the gingiva into the periodontal ligament *(3)*. (B) Facially and lingually, from the gingiva along the outer **periosteum** *(1)*, from the periosteum into the bone *(2)*, and from the gingiva into the periodontal ligament *(3)*.

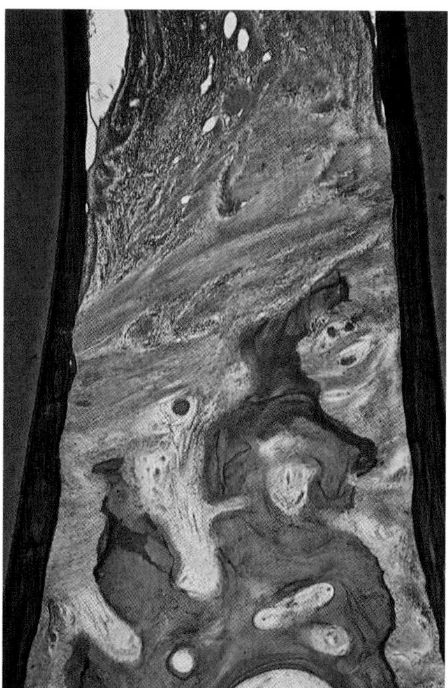

Fig. 22.29 Reformation of transseptal fibers. A mesiodistal section through the interdental septum shows gingival inflammation and bone loss. Recreated transseptal fibers can be seen above the bone margin, where they have been partially infiltrated by the inflammatory process.

differentiation of hematopoietic progenitor cells in bone marrow into osteoclasts and stimulate gingival cells to release mediators that have the same effect.[51,116] Bacterial biofilm products and inflammatory mediators can also act directly on osteoblasts or their progenitors, thereby inhibiting their action and reducing their numbers.

In addition, in patients with rapidly progressing diseases (e.g., periodontitis with molar incisor pattern), bacterial microcolonies or single bacterial cells have been found between collagen fibers and over the bone surface, suggesting a direct effect.[20,32,116]

Several host factors released by inflammatory cells are capable of inducing bone resorption in vitro, and they play a role in periodontitis. These include host-produced prostaglandins and their precursors, interleukin-1α, interleukin-β, and tumor necrosis factor alpha.

When injected intradermally, prostaglandin E_2 induces the vascular changes that are seen with inflammation; when injected

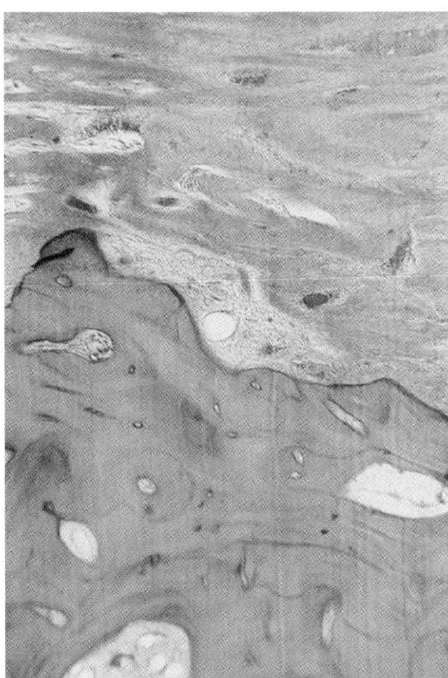

Fig. 22.30 Extension of inflammation has reached the crestal bone surface.

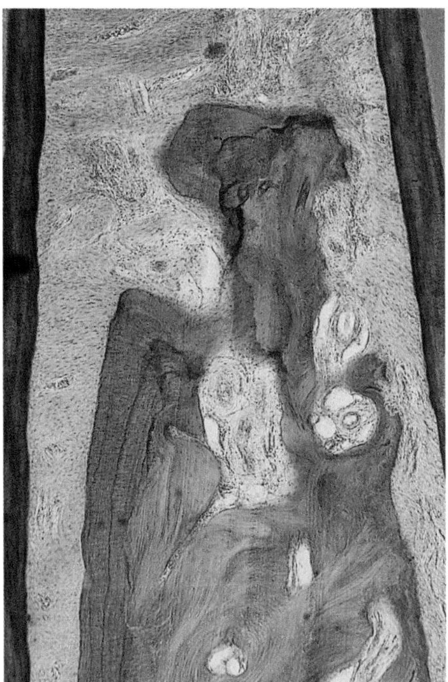

Fig. 22.31 Interdental septum in a human autopsy section. Extensive inflammatory infiltrate has invaded the marrow spaces, entering from both the mesial and distal aspects. Fatty bone marrow has been replaced by inflammatory cells and fibrous marrow.

over a bone surface, prostaglandin E_2 induces bone resorption in the absence of inflammatory cells, with few multinucleated osteoclasts.[45,60] In addition, nonsteroidal anti-inflammatory drugs (e.g., flurbiprofen, ibuprofen) inhibit prostaglandin E_2 production, thereby slowing bone loss in naturally occurring periodontitis in beagle dogs and humans. This effect disappears 6 months after the cessation of drug administration.[58,143] (For more information about the host-mediated mechanisms of bone destruction, see Chapter 11.)

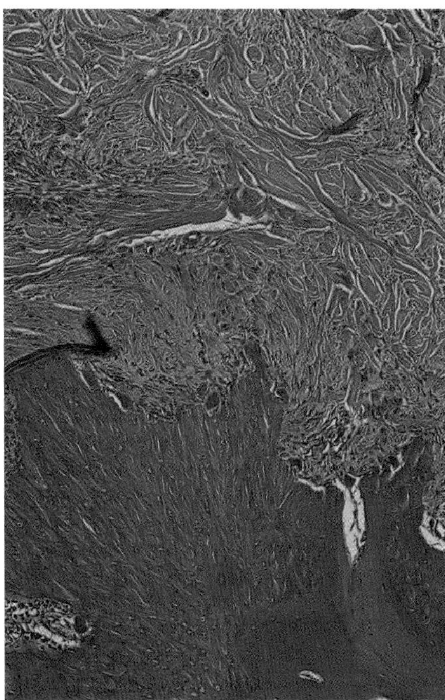

Fig. 22.32 Osteoclasts and Howship lacunae in the resorption of crestal bone.

Bone Formation in Periodontitis

Areas of bone formation are also found immediately adjacent to sites of active bone resorption and along trabecular surfaces at a distance from the inflammation in an apparent effort to reinforce the remaining bone (i.e., buttressing bone formation). This estrogenic response is clearly found in experimentally produced periodontal bone loss in animals.[21] In humans, it is less obvious, but it has been confirmed by histometric[17,18] and histologic studies.[39]

Autopsy specimens from individuals with untreated disease occasionally show areas in which bone resorption has ceased and new bone is being formed on previously eroded bone margins. This confirms the intermittent character of bone resorption in periodontitis, and it is consistent with the varied rates of progression observed clinically in individuals with untreated periodontitis.

The periods of remission and exacerbation (or inactivity and activity, respectively) appear to coincide with the quiescence or exacerbation of gingival inflammation as manifested by changes in the extent of bleeding, the amount of exudate, and the composition of bacterial biofilm (see Chapter 15).

The presence of bone formation in response to inflammation, even in those with active periodontitis, has an effect on the outcome of treatment. The basic aim of periodontal therapy is the elimination of inflammation to inhibit the stimulus for bone resorption and therefore to allow the inherent constructive tendencies to predominate.

Bone Destruction Caused by Trauma From Occlusion

Another cause of periodontal bone destruction is trauma from occlusion, which can occur in the absence or presence of inflammation (see Chapter 32).

In the absence of inflammation, the changes caused by trauma from occlusion vary from increased compression and tension of the periodontal ligament and increased osteoclasis of alveolar bone to necrosis of the periodontal ligament and bone and the resorption of bone and tooth structure. These changes are reversible in that they can be repaired if the offending forces are removed. However, persistent trauma from occlusion results in funnel-shaped widening of the crestal portion of the periodontal ligament with resorption of the adjacent bone.[70] These changes, which may cause the bony crest to have an angular shape, represent adaptation of the periodontal tissues aimed at "cushioning" increased occlusal forces; however, the modified bone shape may weaken tooth support and cause tooth mobility.

When it is combined with inflammation, trauma from occlusion may aggravate the bone destruction caused by the inflammation[70] and results in bizarre bone patterns.

Bone Destruction Caused by Systemic Disorders

Local and systemic factors regulate the physiologic equilibrium of bone. When a generalized tendency toward bone resorption exists, bone loss initiated by local inflammatory processes may be magnified.

This systemic influence on the response of alveolar bone, as envisioned by Glickman[38] during the early 1950s, considers a systemic regulatory influence in all cases of periodontitis. In addition to the virulence of biofilm bacteria, the nature of the systemic component rather than its presence or absence influences the severity of the periodontal destruction. This concept of a role played by systemic defense mechanisms has been validated by the studies of immune deficiencies and host modulation in severely destructive types of periodontitis.

Interest has increased concerning the possible relationship between periodontal bone loss and osteoporosis.[36] Osteoporosis is a physiologic condition of postmenopausal women that results in the loss of bone mineral content as well as structural bone changes. Periodontitis and osteoporosis share a number of risk factors (e.g., aging, smoking, certain diseases, medications that interfere with healing). Some studies show a relationship between skeletal density and oral bone density; between crestal height and residual ridge resorption; and among osteopenia and periodontitis, tooth mobility, and tooth loss.[48,56,57,111,135]

Periodontal bone loss may also occur with generalized skeletal disturbances (e.g., hyperparathyroidism, leukemia, histiocytosis X) via mechanisms that may be totally unrelated to the more common biofilm-induced, inflammatory periodontal lesion.

KEY FACT

In the absence of inflammation, the localized bone loss caused by trauma from occlusion is reversible (can be repaired), if the offending forces are removed.

Factors Determining Bone Morphology in Periodontitis

Normal Variation in Alveolar Bone

Considerable normal variation exists within the morphologic features of alveolar bone, and this affects the osseous contours resulting from periodontitis. The anatomic features that substantially affect the bone-destructive pattern of periodontitis include the following:

- Thickness, width, and crestal angulation of the interdental septa
- Thickness of the facial and lingual alveolar plates
- Presence of fenestrations and dehiscences
- Alignment of the teeth
- Root and root trunk anatomy
- Root position within the alveolar process
- Proximity with another tooth surface

For example, angular osseous defects cannot form in thin facial or lingual alveolar plates, which have little or no cancellous bone between the outer and inner cortical layers. In such cases, the entire crest of the plate is destroyed, and the height of the bone is reduced in a horizontal fashion (Fig. 22.33).

Exostoses

Exostoses are outgrowths of bone of varied size and shape. Palatal exostoses have been found in 40% of human skulls.[94] They can occur as small nodules, large nodules, sharp ridges, spike-like projections, or any combination of the above (Fig. 22.34).[88] Exostoses have been described in rare cases as developing after the placement of free gingival grafts.[94]

Trauma From Occlusion

Trauma from occlusion may be a factor in determining the dimension and shape of bone deformities. It may cause a thickening of the cervical margin of alveolar bone or a change in bone morphology (e.g., funnel-like crestal bone, buttressing bone) on which inflammatory changes may later be superimposed.

Buttressing Bone Formation

Bone formation sometimes occurs in an attempt to buttress bony trabeculae that are weakened by resorption. When this occurs within the jaw, it is termed *central buttressing bone formation.* When it occurs on the external surface, it is referred to as *peripheral buttressing bone formation.*[39] The latter may cause bulging of the bone contour, which sometimes accompanies the production of osseous craters and angular defects (Fig. 22.35).

Food Impaction

Interdental bone defects often occur where the proximal contact is light or absent. Physical pressure and the additional collection of bacteria from food impaction contribute to interproximal resorption and the development of reverse bone architecture. In some cases, the

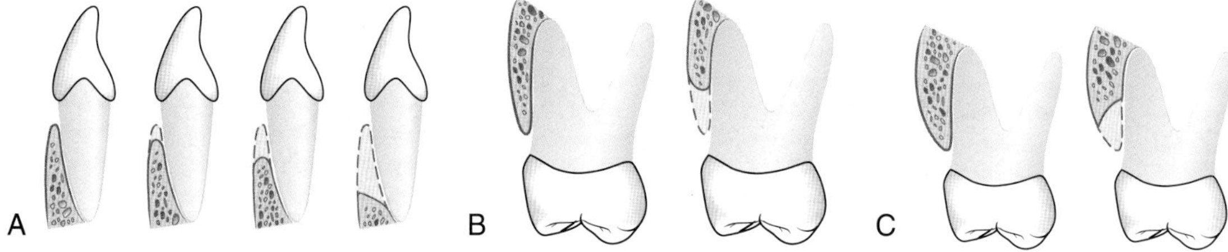

Fig. 22.33 (A) Lower incisor with thin labial bone. Bone loss can become vertical only when it reaches thicker bone in apical areas. (B) Upper molars with thin facial bone, where only horizontal bone loss can occur. (C) Upper molar with a thick facial bone that allows for vertical bone loss.

poor proximal relationship may result from a shift in tooth position as a result of extensive bone destruction that precedes food impaction. In patients with this condition, food impaction is a contributing factor rather than the cause of the bone defect.

Periodontitis With Molar Incisor Pattern of Involvement

Periodontitis with molar incisor pattern usually results in attachment and bone loss around incisors and first molars, particularly in cases where the disease is observed in teenagers (Fig. 22.36). Although such bone loss is usually horizontal in nature around incisors, a vertical or angular pattern of alveolar bone destruction is found around the first molars. The cause of the localized bone destruction associated with this type of periodontitis is unknown.

Bone Destruction Patterns in Periodontitis

Periodontitis alters the morphologic features of the bone in addition to reducing bone height. An understanding of the nature and pathogenesis of these alterations is essential for effective diagnosis and treatment.[96]

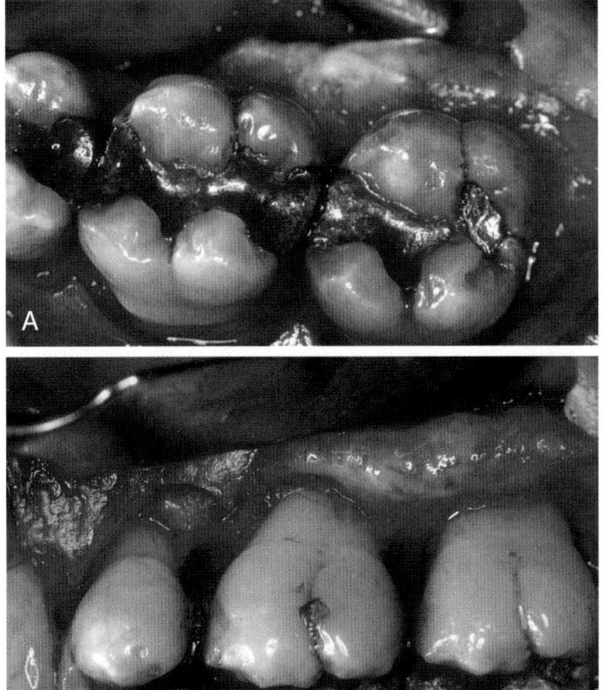

Fig. 22.34 Occlusal (A) and palatal (B) views of exostosis on the first and second molars.

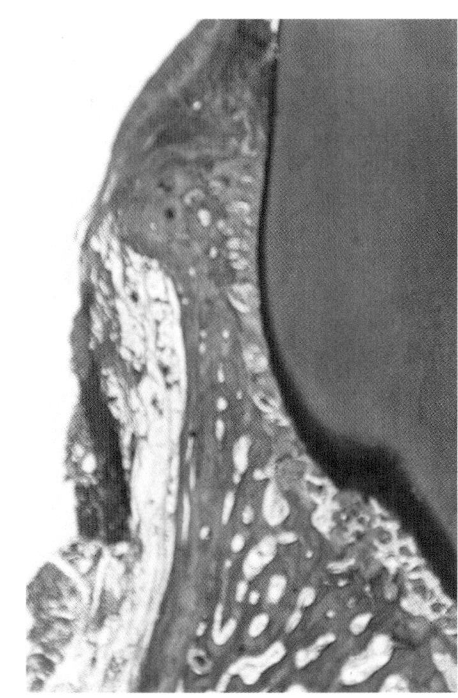

Fig. 22.35 Lipping of facial bone. There is a peripheral buttressing bone formation along the external surface of the facial bony plate and at the crest. Note the deformity in the bone produced by the buttressing bone formation and the bulging of the mucosa.

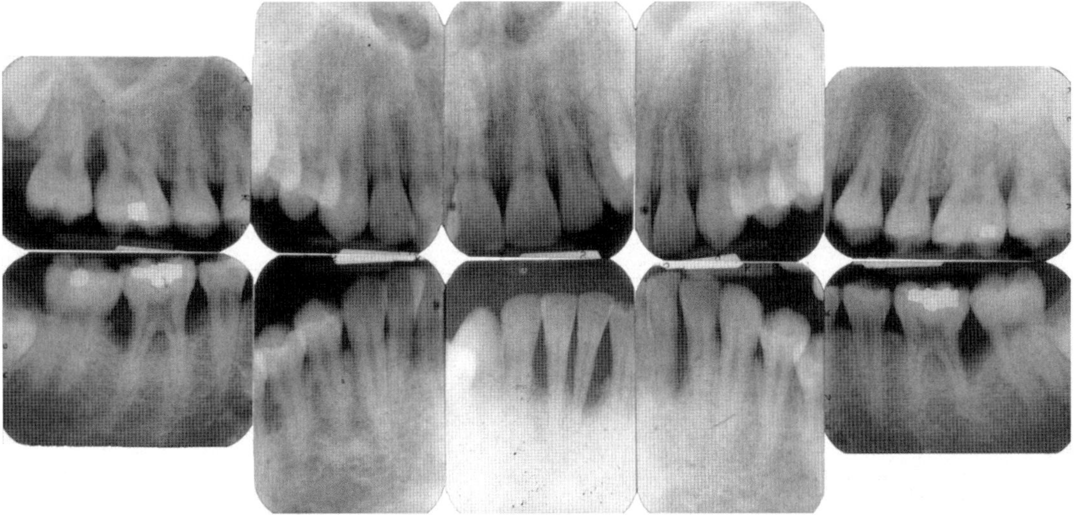

Fig. 22.36 Radiographs of a 15-year-old patient with molar-incisor pattern periodontitis (previously called "**localized aggressive periodontitis**") showing localized, vertical, angular bone loss associated with the maxillary and mandibular first molars and the mandibular central incisors.

Horizontal Bone Loss

Horizontal bone loss is the most common pattern of bone loss in periodontitis (Fig. 22.37A–B). The bone is reduced in height, but the bone margin remains approximately perpendicular to the tooth surface. The interdental septa and the facial and lingual plates are affected but not necessarily to an equal degree around the same tooth.

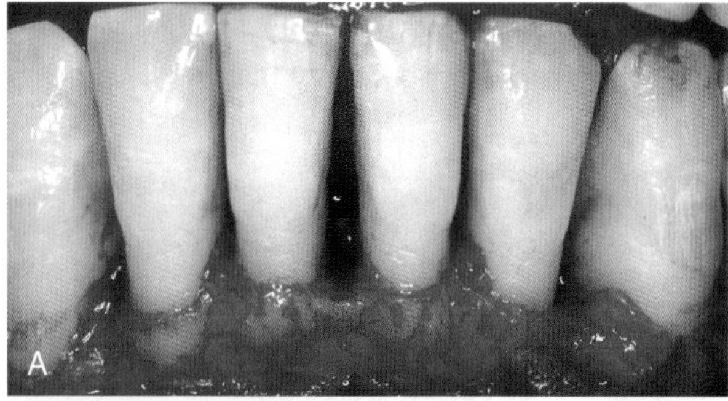

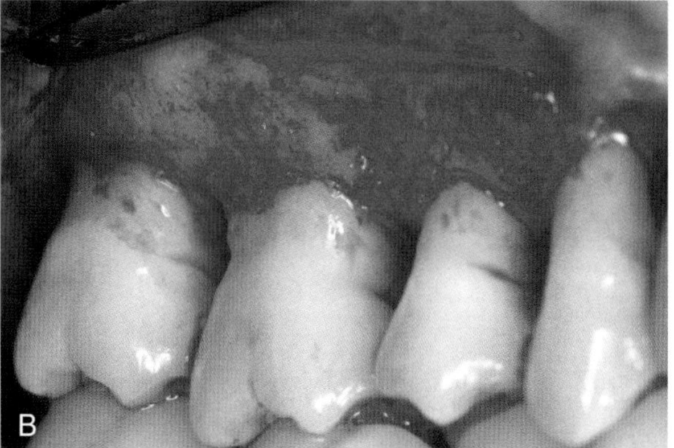

Fig. 22.37 Horizontal bone loss in the anterior (A) and posterior (B) areas. Notice the increased distance between the marginal bone and the cementoenamel junction; yet the overall bone contour is scalloped, indicating that bone resorption has affected the buccal and interproximal surfaces to a similar degree.

Vertical or Angular Defects

Different types of bone deformities can result from periodontitis. These usually occur in adults, but they have also been reported in human skulls with deciduous dentitions.[63] Their presence may be suggested on radiographs, but careful probing and surgical exposure of the areas are required to determine their exact conformation and dimensions.

Vertical or angular defects are those that occur in an oblique direction, leaving a hollowed-out trough in the bone alongside the root; the base of the defect is located apical to the surrounding bone (Figs. 22.38A–B and 22.39). In most instances, angular defects have accompanying infrabony periodontal pockets; infrabony pockets, on the other hand, must always have an underlying angular defect.

Goldman and Cohen classified angular defects on the basis of the number of osseous walls.[43] Angular defects may have one, two, or three walls (Figs. 22.40 and 22.41). Continuous defects that involved more than one surface of a tooth, in a shape that is similar to a trough, are called *circumferential defects* (Fig. 22.42). The number of walls in the apical portion of the defect is often greater than that in its occlusal portion, in which case the term *combined osseous defect* is used (Fig. 22.43).

Vertical defects that occur interdentally can generally be seen on the radiograph, although thick, bony plates may sometimes obscure them. Angular defects can also appear on facial and lingual or palatal surfaces, but these defects are more difficult to visualize on radiographs. Surgical exposure is the only sure way to determine the presence and configuration of vertical osseous defects.

Vertical defects increase with age.[91,95,145] Approximately 60% of people with interdental angular defects have only a single defect.[91] Vertical defects detected radiographically have been reported to

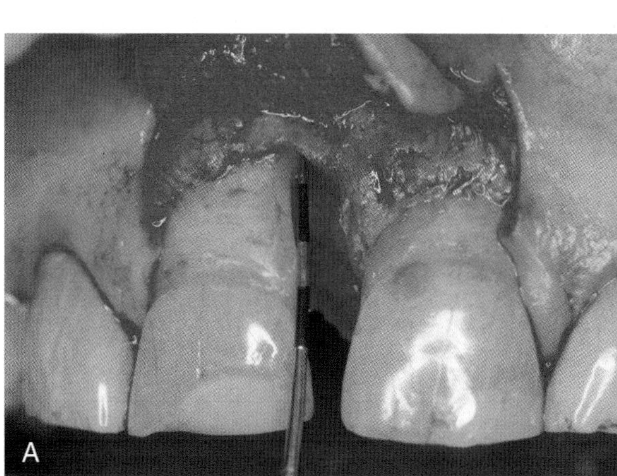

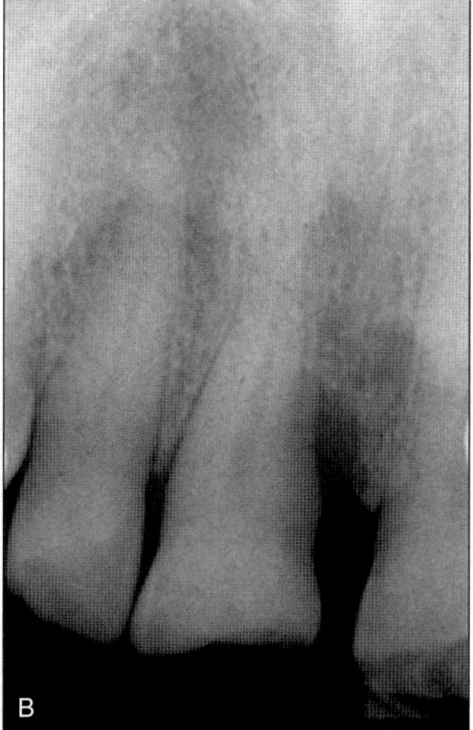

Fig. 22.38 Clinical (A) and radiographic (B) views of a vertical (angular) defect mesial of the upper right central incisor. Note the periodontal probe in a more apical position than the surrounding walls of the bony defect.

appear most often on the distal[91] and mesial surfaces.[95] However, three-wall defects are more frequently found on the mesial surfaces of the upper and lower molars.[64]

Osseous Craters

Osseous craters are a specific type of two-wall defect; they present as concavities in the crest of the interdental bone that is confined within the facial and lingual walls (Fig. 22.44). Craters have been found to make up about one-third (35.2%) of all defects and about two-thirds (62%) of all mandibular defects; they occur twice as often in posterior segments as in anterior segments.[77,78]

The heights of the facial and lingual crests of a crater have been found to be identical in 85% of cases, with the remaining 15% being almost equally divided between higher facial crests and higher lingual crests.[104]

The following reasons for the high frequency of interdental craters have been suggested[77,78,104]:

- The interdental area collects biofilm and is difficult to clean.
- The normal flat or even slightly concave buccolingual shape of the interdental septum in the lower molars may favor crater formation.
- Vascular patterns from the gingiva to the center of the crest may provide a pathway for inflammation.

Bulbous Bone Contours

Bulbous bone contours are bony enlargements that are caused by exostoses (see Fig.22.44), adaptation to function, or buttressing bone formation. They are found more frequently in the maxilla than in the mandible.

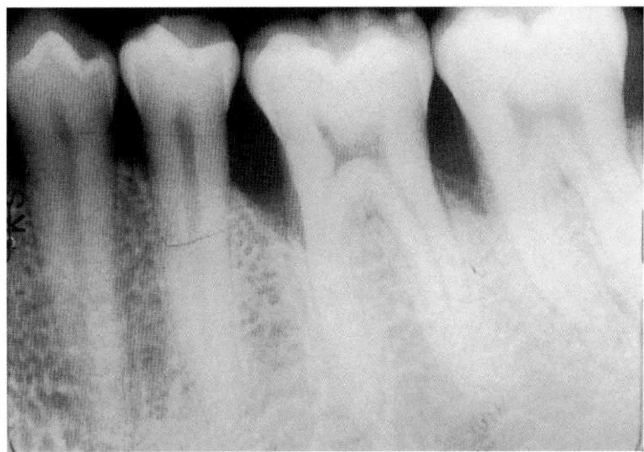

Fig. 22.39 Vertical (angular) defects mesial of the first and second molars.

Reversed Architecture

Reverse (or negative) alveolar bone architecture is the result of a loss of interdental bone, without a concomitant loss of radicular (buccal or lingual/palatal) bone, thereby reversing the normal (or positive) architecture (Fig. 22.45). Negative architecture is more common in the maxilla of patients with periodontitis.[91]

Ledges

Ledges are plateau-like bone margins that are caused by the resorption of thickened bony plates (Fig. 22.46).

Furcation Involvement

The term **furcation involvement** refers to the invasion of the bifurcation and trifurcation of multirooted teeth by periodontitis. The prevalence of furcation-involved molars is not clear.[28,95] Although some reports indicate that the mandibular first molars are the most common sites and that the maxillary premolars are the least common,[65] other studies have found a higher prevalence in the upper molars.[145] The number of furcation involvements increases with age.[65,66]

The denuded furcation may be visible clinically or covered by the wall of the pocket. The extent of the involvement is determined by exploration with a periodontal or Nabers probe (Fig. 22.47A–B).

Furcation involvements have been classified as **grades** I through IV according to the amount of tissue destruction. Grade I involves incipient bone loss; grade II involves partial bone loss (cul-de-sac); and grade III involves total bone loss with a through-and-through opening of the furcation, but the opening of the furcation is not visible due to the gingiva, which covers the orifice. Grade IV is similar to grade III but includes gingival recession that exposes the furcation to view. (See Chapter 61 for further discussion on furcation classification.)

Microscopically, furcation involvement presents no unique pathologic features. It is simply the apical extension of the periodontal pocket along a multirooted tooth. During its early stages, widening of the periodontal space occurs with cellular and fluid inflammatory exudation, and this is followed by epithelial proliferation into the furcation area from an adjoining periodontal pocket. Extension of the inflammation into the bone leads to resorption and a reduction in bone height. The bone-destructive pattern may produce horizontal loss, but angular osseous defects associated with

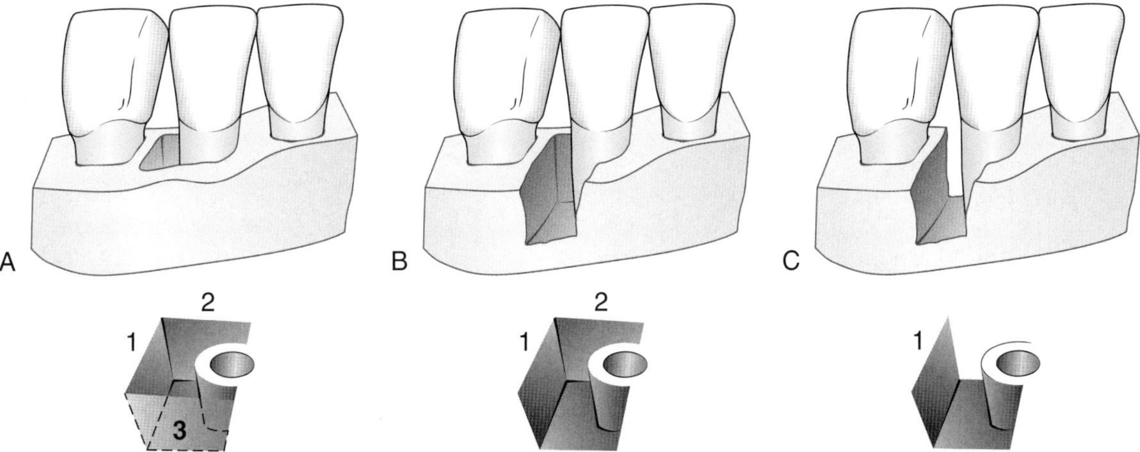

Fig. 22.40 Diagrammatic representation of one-, two-, and three-walled vertical defects on the right lateral incisor. (A) Three bony walls: distal *(1)*, lingual *(2)*, and facial *(3)*. (B) Two-wall defect: distal *(1)* and lingual *(2)*. (C) One-wall defect: distal wall only *(1)*.

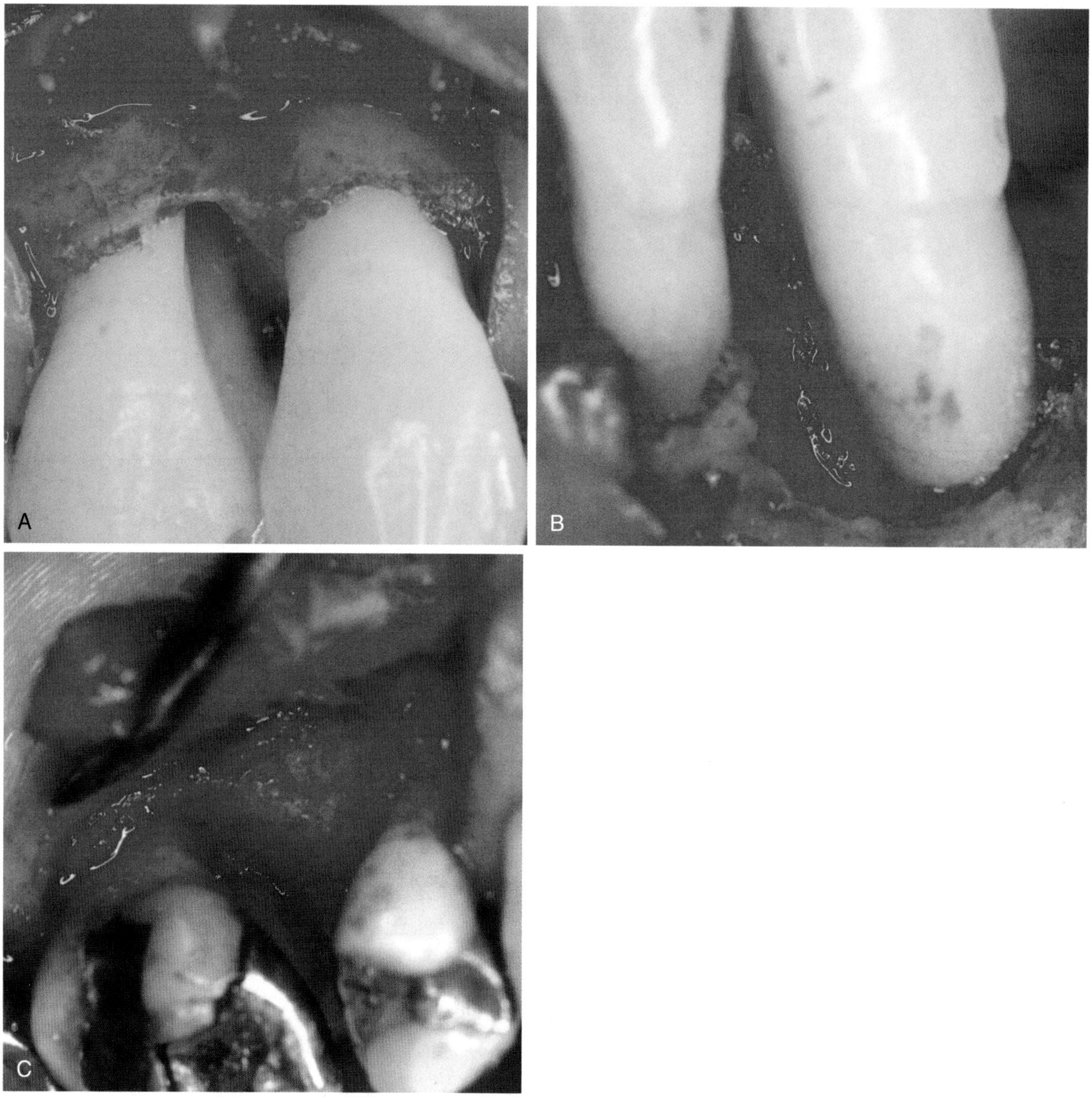

A

B

C

Fig. 22.41 Clinical examples of a three-wall defect mesial of the first bicuspid (A), two-wall defect mesial of the lower canine (buccal wall is missing) (B), and one-wall defect mesial of the first molar (buccal and lingual walls are missing) (C).

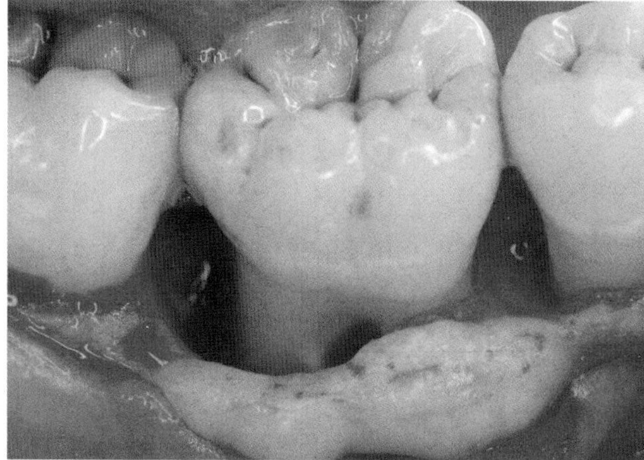

Fig. 22.42 Circumferential (troughlike) defect on the buccal and distal aspects of the first molar. Notice that the defect extends into the buccal furcation.

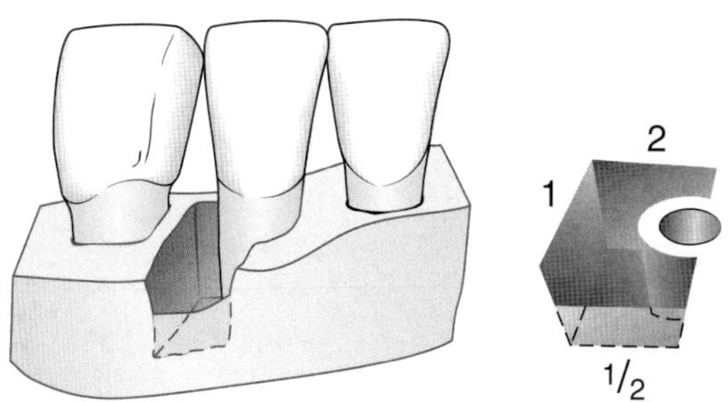

Fig. 22.43 Combined type of osseous defect. Because the facial wall is half the height of the distal *(1)* and lingual *(2)* walls, this is an osseous defect with three walls in its apical half and two walls in its occlusal half.

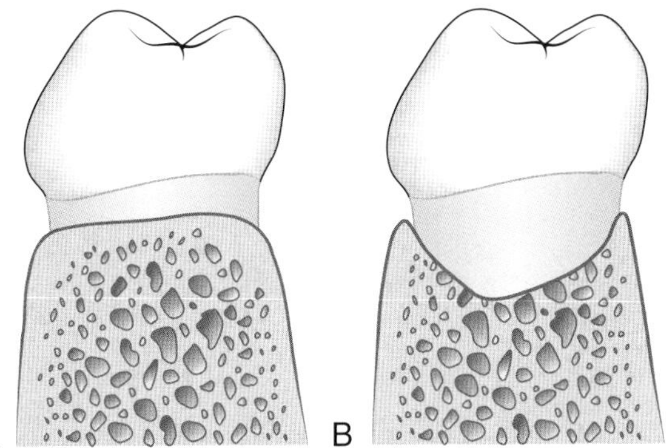

Fig. 22.44 (A) Diagrammatic representation of an osseous crater in a buccolingual section between two lower teeth. *Left,* Normal bone contour. *Right,* Osseous crater. (B) Clinical aspect of an osseous crater between the two bicuspids—notice the buccal and lingual bone walls.

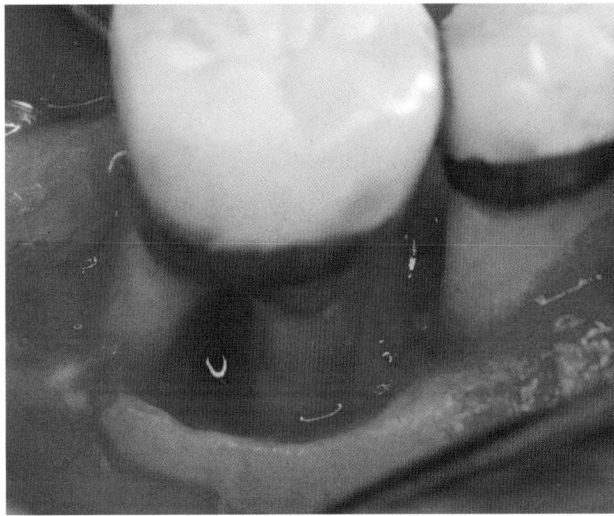

Fig. 22.46 Example of bone ledge on the lingual aspect of the bicuspid and molar.

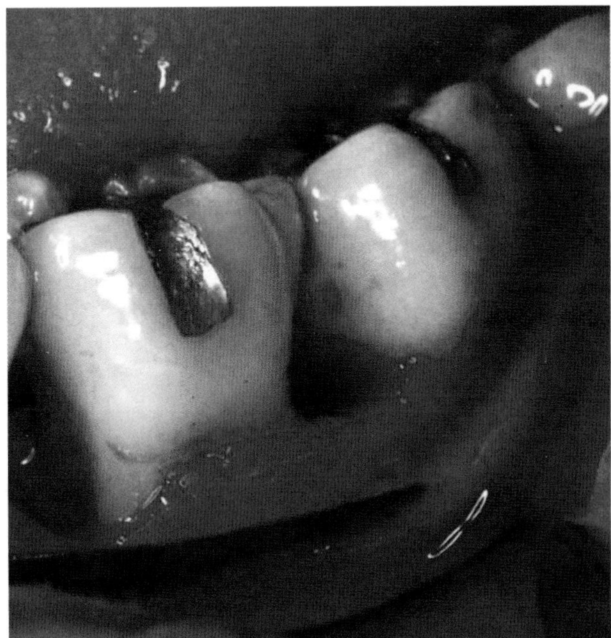

Fig. 22.45 Examples of positive (normal) and negative (reverse) osseous architecture on the lower left posterior segment. The interproximal bone level in the interdental space between the two bicuspids is more coronal than on the buccal aspect of both teeth, whereas the interproximal bone level in the interdental space between the second bicuspid and the first molar shows the bone level to be apical to the buccal bone.

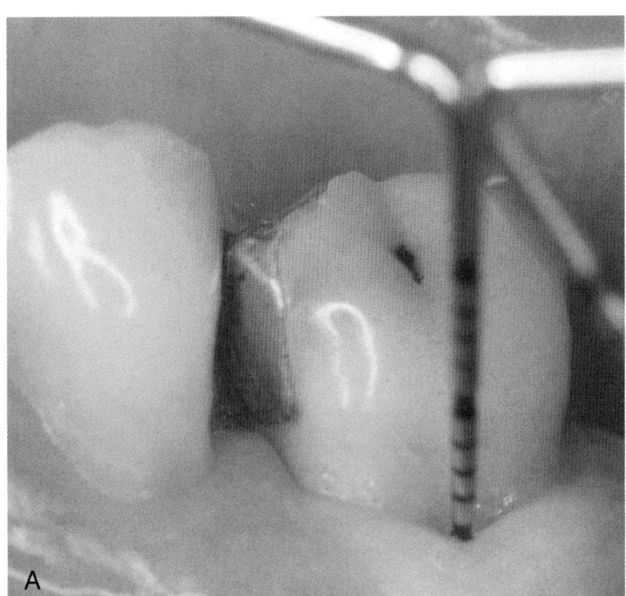

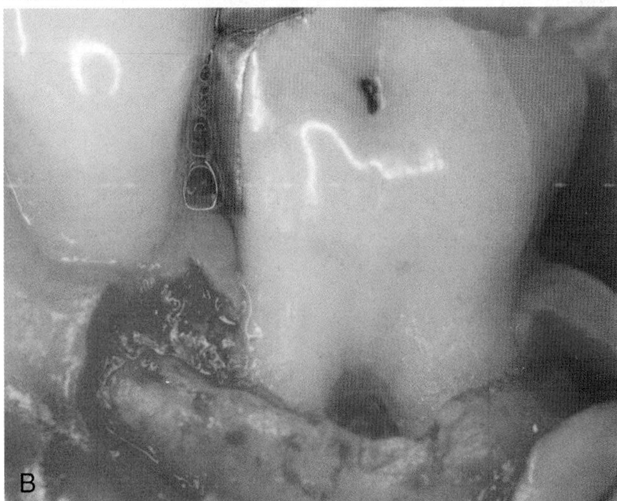

Fig. 22.47 Grade II furcation on the buccal aspect of the lower first molar. (A) Periodontal probe in place showing a 5-mm pocket. (B) After the flap was elevated, it revealed horizontal bone loss.

intrabony pockets may also exist (Fig. 22.48). Biofilm, calculus, and bacterial debris occupy the denuded furcation space.

The destructive pattern of a furcation involvement varies in different cases and with the degree of involvement. Bone loss around each individual root may be horizontal or angular, and frequently a crater develops in the interradicular area (Fig. 22.49A and B). Probing to determine the presence of these destructive patterns must be done horizontally and vertically around each involved root and in the crater area to establish the depth of the vertical component.

Furcation involvement is a stage of progressive periodontitis, and it has its same etiology. The difficulty and sometimes the impossibility[13,14] of controlling biofilm in furcations are responsible for the presence of extensive lesions in this area.[140]

The role of trauma from occlusion in the etiology of furcation lesions is controversial. Some assign a key role to trauma, thinking

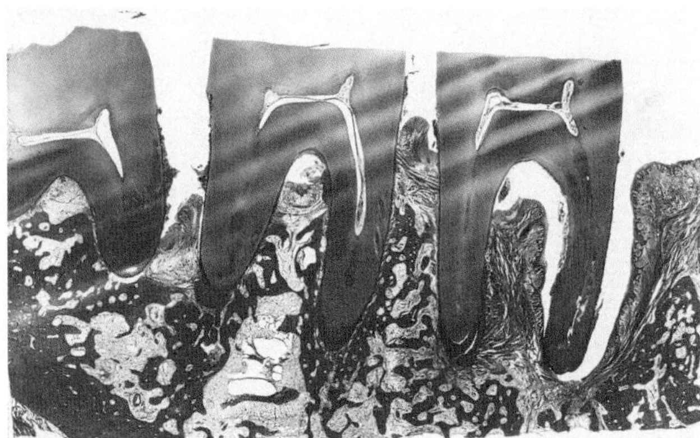

Fig. 22.48 Different degrees of furcation involvement in a human autopsy specimen. Furcation involvement is found in all three molars, with an advanced lesion in the second molar and an extremely severe lesion in the first molar that is combined with the exposure of the entire mesial root.

that furcation areas are most sensitive to injury from excessive occlusal forces.[41] Others deny the initiating effect of trauma and consider that inflammation and edema caused by biofilm in the furcation area tend to extrude the tooth, which then becomes traumatized and sensitive.[127,140]

Other factors that may play a role are the presence of enamel projections into the furcation,[79] which occurs in about 13% of multirooted teeth, and the proximity of the furcation to the cementoenamel junction, which occurs in about 75% of cases of furcation involvement.[66]

The presence of accessory pulpal canals in the furcation area may extend pulpal inflammation to the furcation.[49] This possibility should be carefully explored, particularly when mesial and distal bone retains its normal height. Accessory canals that connect the pulp chamber floor to the furcation have been found in 36% of maxillary first molars, 12% of maxillary second molars, 32% of mandibular first molars, and 24% of mandibular second molars.[133]

The diagnosis of furcation involvement is made by clinical examination and careful probing with a specially designed probe (see Chapters 38 and 61). Radiographic examination of the area is helpful, but lesions can be obscured by the angulation of the beam and the radiopacity of neighboring structures (see Chapter 39).

For more detailed clinical considerations involved with the diagnosis and treatment of furcation involvement, see Chapters 38, 39, and 61.

Conclusion

Periodontal pocketing is an important clinical manifestation of periodontal diseases. Understanding the pathogenesis and the histopathological features of pocket formation is central to the understanding of the pathogenesis of periodontal diseases. Equally important is the understanding of the anatomy, histology, and pattern of bone loss for the diagnosis of and prognosis for periodontitis in determining the therapy that must be rendered. In the final analysis, it is the loss of bone that will determine the retention, maintenance, or loss of the dentition in periodontitis.

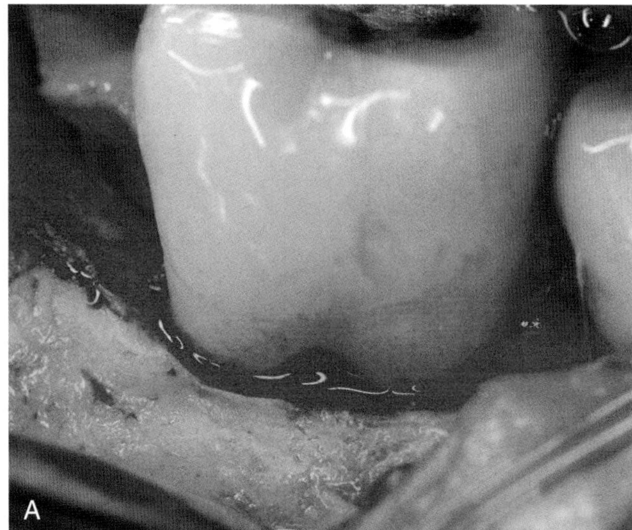

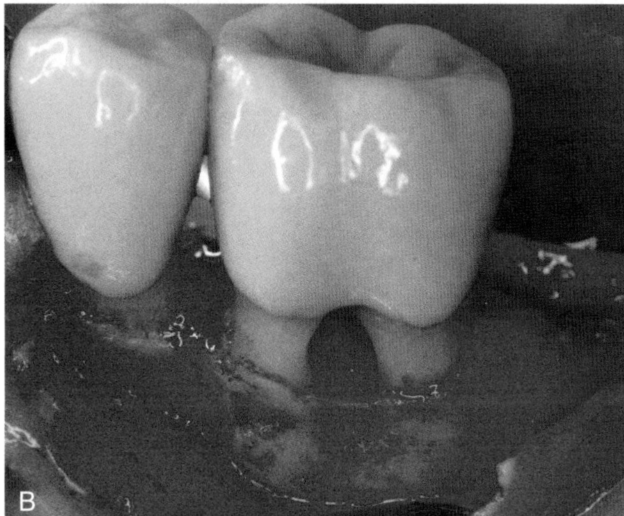

Fig. 22.49 Clinical examples of grade I furcation involvement (A) and grade II furcation involvement (B).

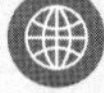
A Case Scenario is found on the companion website eBooks.Health.Elsevier.com.

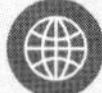
References for this chapter are found on the companion website eBooks.Health.Elsevier.com.

CHAPTER 23

Risk Factors of Periodontal Disease (Smoking)

Philip M. Preshaw | Leandro Chambrone | Richard Holliday

CHAPTER OUTLINE

The Smoking Epidemic

Many factors can increase the risk for periodontitis, including genetics, systemic diseases, such as diabetes, and local plaque biofilm-retentive factors. These are discussed elsewhere in this book. In the present chapter, we will focus on a single major risk factor for periodontitis, which is smoking. Smoking is highly prevalent and can be considered an epidemic in both upper- and lower-income countries. Smoking rates, however, have seen marked declines over the last few decades. Global estimated daily tobacco smoking prevalence rates (in individuals >15 years old) reduced from 43.0% in 2000 to 34.1% in 2015 for males and from 10.9% (2000) to 6.4% (2015) for females.[143] Despite this development, with population growth, the number of daily smokers worldwide has actually increased to 1.1 billion in 2015, upholding tobacco smoking's position as a major public health threat.[143] The highest prevalence rates (2015 estimates for those aged ≥15 years) are seen in high-income countries (24.6%) and upper-middle-income countries (23.4%) with lower rates estimated in lower-middle-income (17.4%) and low-income (11.6%) countries.[143]

The overall daily smoking prevalence rates for the United States were 20.9% in 2015 (23.8% for males, 18.1% for females) and for the United Kingdom were 20.8% (23.3% for males, 18.5% for females).[143] The World Health Organization (WHO) has set a target of a 30% relative reduction target between 2010 and 2025. The only WHO region expected to attain this is the Americas, with all regions showing a downward trend, except the Eastern Mediterranean region which is projected to see an increase in prevalence unless additional measures are implemented.[143]

A Global Perspective

- As many as 6.25 trillion cigarettes are smoked annually across the globe.[95]
- Tobacco kills 6 million people each year.[142]
- Only 30% of the world's population have access to smoking cessation services.[144]
- Only 22% of the world's population are protected by smoke-free laws.[144]

Smoking is harmful to almost every organ in the body and is associated with multiple diseases that reduce life expectancy and quality of life. Diseases associated with smoking include lung cancer, heart disease, stroke, emphysema, bronchitis, and cancers of the oral cavity, bladder, kidney, stomach, liver, and cervix. Approximately half of the long-term smokers will die early as a result of smoking, and those who die before the age of 70 years will lose an average of 20 years of life.[35] Most deaths from smoking are due to lung cancer, chronic obstructive pulmonary disease, and coronary heart disease.

Tobacco smoke contains thousands of noxious chemicals, and it comprises a gaseous phase and a solid (particulate) phase. The gas phase contains carbon monoxide, ammonia, formaldehyde, hydrogen cyanide, and many other toxic and irritant compounds, including more than 60 known carcinogens such as benzo(a)pyrene and dimethylnitrosamine. The particulate phase includes nicotine, "tar" (itself made up of many toxic chemicals), benzene, and benzo(a)pyrene. Tar is inhaled with the smoke. In its condensate form, it is the sticky brown substance that stains fingers and teeth yellow and brown. Nicotine, which is an alkaloid, is found within the tobacco leaf and evaporates when the cigarette is lighted. It is quickly absorbed in the lungs, and it reaches the brain within 10 to 19 seconds. Nicotine is highly addictive. It causes a rise in blood pressure, increased heart and respiratory rates, and peripheral vasoconstriction.

CLINICIAN'S CORNER

Smokeless Tobacco

Smokeless tobacco products are becoming increasingly popular and exist in many different forms. Tobacco can be ground/grated and presented with salt and water as "moist snuff," which is usually delivered as a small tea-bag-like sachet placed under the lip. Alternatively, tobacco can be ground to a powder ("dry snuff") that is inhaled into the nasal cavity. Finally, tobacco can be coarsely cut (chewing tobacco) and placed inside the cheek. Numerous smokeless tobacco varieties are popular in South Asian communities. The International Agency for Research on Cancer classifies smokeless tobacco as a cause of mouth, esophageal, and pancreatic cancer.[67]

Snus (or Swedish snuff) is a special type of smokeless tobacco that is popular in Sweden and increasingly the United States. It is banned across the rest of Europe. The manufacturers claim to use a special process to lower the levels of carcinogens in the product. Studies have shown a link to pancreatic cancer but not to mouth or lung cancer.[83]

All dental patients must be asked about their smoking status or tobacco usage. Current smoking status is the minimal information that must be recorded (e.g., "Patient is currently smoking *X* cigarettes per day"), but the importance of cumulative exposure to cigarette smoke means that it is more appropriate to record **pack-years** of smoking (Box 23.1). Biochemical tests can also be used to assess smoking status, including exhaled carbon monoxide and the measurement of cotinine (the major metabolite of nicotine) in serum, saliva, or urine. Cotinine is measured in preference to nicotine because the half-life of nicotine is short (≈1 to 2 hours),[103] whereas that of cotinine is approximately 20 hours.[69] Plasma and saliva cotinine concentrations in smokers are approximately 100 ng/mL[10,41] and the urine concentration is approximately 1200 ng/mL.[78] Nonsmokers usually have plasma and saliva cotinine concentrations of less than 2 ng/mL, unless they are passive smokers. Biochemical validation of nonsmoking uses cotinine levels of 1 to 6 ng/mL to confirm nonsmoking status depending on race/ethnicity.[10]

Smoking is a major risk factor for periodontitis, and it affects the prevalence, extent, and severity of the disease. In addition, smoking has an adverse impact on the clinical outcome of nonsurgical and surgical therapy as well as the long-term success of implant placement. With 41.9% of periodontitis cases in the United States reported as being *attributable* to smoking (discussed next),[134] it is essential to understand the impact of smoking on the initiation, progression, and management of the disease. This chapter discusses the effects of smoking on the prevalence, severity, etiology, and pathogenesis of periodontal disease as well as its impact on treatment. The reader is referred to several excellent reviews of the topic for detailed results of specific studies.[1,25,26,55,59,60,61,72,73,96,97,111,112,135,140]

BOX 23.1 Challenge of Assessing Smoking Status

Current Smokers

Ask about current smoking and past smoking. Many smokers are trying to quit, and therefore simply asking how many cigarettes they are smoking today may not give an accurate assessment of their lifetime exposure (e.g., a patient who is currently smoking 5 cigarettes per day may have been smoking 40 cigarettes per day until yesterday, when he or she decided to cut down). Try to get an indication of the patient's approximate level of smoking (e.g., the average number of cigarettes per day for a certain number of years). It can also be useful to calculate the number of pack-years:

$$\text{Pack} - \text{years} = \text{Number of packs smoked per day} \times \text{Number of years of smoking}$$

In other words, 1 pack-year is the cumulative exposure that corresponds with the smoking of 1 pack of 20 cigarettes per day for 1 year. For example, a smoker who has smoked 20 cigarettes per day for 15 years has 15 pack-years of smoking.

Former Smokers

Ask patients about their past smoking. Patients with periodontitis may have a significant smoking history that has had an impact on their periodontal status, even if they no longer smoke. Former smokers should always be congratulated for their achievement in quitting, but it is also very important to document the following:

- How much they used to smoke
- How many years they smoked
- When they quit

Is the Patient's Response Accurate?

The inaccurate or false reporting of smoking status is common; patients will tell you what they think you want to hear, or they may be embarrassed because they have not managed to cut down yet. Many patients report smoking 20 cigarettes per day because this is the number of cigarettes in a pack in most countries, so 20 may be a convenient response rather than an accurate response. Cultural factors may also influence responses.[124]

When Is a Smoker Not a Smoker?

- Smokers have smoked ≥100 cigarettes in their lifetime and currently smoke.
- Former smokers have smoked ≥100 cigarettes in their lifetime and do not currently smoke.
- Nonsmokers have not smoked ≥100 cigarettes in their lifetime and do not currently smoke.

It must be noted that many periodontal research studies have not used these definitions, and this can sometimes make it difficult to interpret the studies, particularly in the context of what constitutes a former smoker. For example, from an exposure point of view, there is a big difference between someone who smoked 5 cigarettes per day for 10 years and who quit 30 years ago as compared with someone who smoked 40 cigarettes per day for 20 years and quit 6 months ago. It is always best in clinical practice to gather full information about each patient's smoking history.

Effects of Smoking on the Prevalence and Severity of Periodontal Diseases

Gingivitis

Controlled clinical studies have demonstrated that, in human models of experimental gingivitis, the development of inflammation in response to plaque biofilm accumulation is reduced in smokers as compared with nonsmokers (Table 23.1).[18,34] In addition, cross-sectional studies have consistently demonstrated that smokers present with less gingival inflammation than nonsmokers.[11,12,16,104,105] These data suggest that smokers have a decreased expression of clinical inflammation in the presence of plaque biofilm accumulation as compared with nonsmokers. The microbiologic, immunologic, and

TABLE 23.1 Effects of Smoking on Gingivitis and Periodontitis

Periodontal Disease	Effects of Smoking
Gingivitis	↓ Gingival inflammation and bleeding on probing
Periodontitis	↑ Prevalence and severity of periodontal destruction ↑ Pocket depth, attachment loss, and bone loss ↑ Rate of periodontal destruction ↑ Prevalence of severe periodontitis ↑ Tooth loss ↑ Prevalence with increased number of cigarettes smoked per day ↓ Prevalence and severity with smoking cessation

↓, Decreased; ↑, increased.

physiologic factors that may account for this observation are discussed later.

Periodontitis

Although gingival inflammation in smokers appears to be reduced in response to plaque biofilm accumulation as compared with nonsmokers, an overwhelming body of evidence points to smoking as a major risk factor for increasing the prevalence and severity of periodontal destruction. Multiple cross-sectional and longitudinal studies have demonstrated that pocket depth, attachment loss, and alveolar bone loss are more prevalent and severe in patients who smoke as compared with nonsmokers.[72,73,111,135] An assessment of the relationship between cigarette smoking and periodontitis was performed on more than 12,000 dentate individuals who were more than 18 years old as part of the Third National Health and Nutrition Examination Survey.[134] Periodontitis was defined as one or more sites with clinical attachment loss of 4 mm or greater and pocket depth of 4 mm or greater. Smoking status was defined with the use of criteria established by the Centers for Disease Control and Prevention (see Box 23.1). Of the more than 12,000 individuals studied, 9.2% had periodontitis; this represented approximately 15 million cases of periodontitis in the United States. On average, smokers were four times as likely to have periodontitis as compared with **never smokers** after adjusting for age, gender, race/ethnicity, education, and income/poverty ratio. **Former smokers** were 1.7 times more likely to have periodontitis than persons who had never smoked. This study also demonstrated a dose-response relationship between cigarettes smoked per day and the odds of having periodontitis. In subjects smoking 9 or fewer cigarettes per day, the odds of having periodontitis were 2.8, whereas subjects who smoked 31 or more cigarettes per day were almost six times more likely to have periodontitis. In former smokers, the odds of having periodontitis declined with the number of years since quitting. These data indicated that approximately 42% of periodontitis cases (6.4 million cases) in the U.S. adult population were attributable to current smoking and that approximately 11% (1.7 million cases) were attributable to former smoking. These data highlight the serious threat to dental public health posed by cigarette smoking and raise questions about the best methods for managing periodontitis in patients who smoke (Box 23.2).

These data are consistent with the findings of other cross-sectional studies performed in the United States and Europe. The odds ratio for periodontitis in current smokers has been estimated to range from as low as 1.5 to as high as 7.3 compared to nonsmokers, depending on the observed severity of periodontitis.[97] A meta-analysis of data from six such studies involving 2361 subjects indicated that current smokers were almost three times more likely to have severe periodontitis than nonsmokers.[96] The detrimental impact of long-term smoking on the periodontal and dental status of older adults has been clearly demonstrated. Older adult smokers are approximately three times more likely to have severe periodontal disease,[9,82] and the number of years of tobacco use is a significant factor in tooth loss, coronal root caries, and periodontal disease.[70,71]

Smoking has also been shown to affect periodontal disease severity in younger individuals. Cigarette smoking is associated with increased severity of periodontitis in young adults,[123] and those who smoke are 3.8 times more likely to have periodontitis as compared with nonsmokers.[48] Longitudinal studies have demonstrated that young individuals who smoke more than 15 cigarettes per day showed the highest risk for tooth loss.[63] In addition, smokers are more than six times as likely as nonsmokers to demonstrate continued attachment loss.[62] Over a 10-year period, bone loss has been reported to be twice as rapid in smokers as in nonsmokers[19] and to proceed more rapidly even in the presence of excellent plaque control.[13] Less information is available about the effects of cigar and pipe smoking, but it appears that effects similar to those of cigarette smoking are observed with these forms of tobacco use.[5,42,43,80] The prevalence of moderate and severe periodontitis and the percentage of teeth with more than 5 mm of attachment loss were most severe in current cigarette smokers, but cigar and pipe smokers showed a severity of disease that was intermediate between that of current cigarette smokers and nonsmokers.[5] Tooth loss is also increased among cigar and pipe smokers as compared with nonsmokers.[80]

Former smokers have less risk for periodontitis than current smokers but more risk than nonsmokers, and the risk for

BOX 23.2 Should We Change How We Manage Periodontal Disease?

Fact 1: Smoking is a major risk factor for periodontal disease.
Fact 2: According to the literature, smoking may be responsible for more than half of periodontitis cases among adults in the United States.[134]
Fact 3: Depending on the study, approximately 10%–15% of adults in most populations examined have advanced periodontitis.

Questions

- Would there be a benefit at the population level for periodontal health if all smokers in the population quit smoking today?
- Would dental professionals be able to more successfully manage periodontitis in smokers if we focused more on smoking cessation as a primary treatment strategy for managing periodontitis?

These questions are intended to be controversial. It is clear that smoking has a huge deleterious impact on periodontal status, and smoking cessation *must* be a core part of periodontal treatment in patients with periodontitis who smoke. The answer to the first question is almost certainly a resounding yes, but this probably will never be able to be tested. The answer to the second question is more difficult. Certainly, smokers with periodontitis must be educated about the harm that they are causing to their periodontal tissues, and they must be encouraged and helped to quit smoking. Treatment outcomes are improved among smokers who quit as compared with those who continue to smoke.[108]

Two Final Points (These Are Contentious and Designed to Stimulate Discussion.)

- If more than half of the cases of periodontitis are attributable to smoking, then patients who smoke may be better served if dental professionals put more than half of their efforts into treating these patients via smoking cessation treatments (as opposed to other forms of periodontal therapy). Discuss!
- It is absurd for smokers in the Western world to worry about anything except stopping smoking.[102]

BOX 23.3 Helping Your Patients to Quit Smoking

Smoking cessation is a public health priority for governments around the world. Excellent online resources are available to provide information about the harmful effects of smoking and to help people to quit, including the following:

- http://www.cdc.gov/tobacco
- http://www.ash.org.uk
- http://smokefree.nhs.uk

Smoking cessation must be an integral part of the management of dental patients who smoke, and it is the responsibility of all dental health professionals to address this issue with their patients. The dental team is well placed to provide this treatment, because there are tangible smoking-related oral changes which can be used as prompts for a quit attempt and because they see patients on a regular basis as part of ongoing routine dental management.[62] Furthermore, interventions to help patients quit smoking in dental practices are effective, although the exact approach has yet to be strongly confirmed in the evidence base.[61] The whole dental team should therefore be involved in smoking cessation, but this is not always the case. Why? Some of the barriers to providing smoking cessation counseling in the dental practice are shown in Table 23.2.

Various methods for helping patients to quit smoking in the dental environment have been described, and these are typically referred to as *brief intervention programs.* One such program[11] is known as the 5 A's:

ASK Ask the patient about his or her smoking status (see Box 23.1).
This should be part of the medical history.

ADVISE Advise smokers of the associations between oral disease and smoking.
Be informative, honest, and helpful but not judgmental. The patient's response to this information will reveal his or her interest in quitting.

ASSESS Assess the patient's interest in and readiness to attempt smoking cessation.
Patients may not yet be in an action phase when it comes to quitting smoking, which is why it is always important to make these assessments every time you see the patient.

ASSIST Assist the patient with his or her quit attempt.
If you are trained, there are many techniques that can be used (see Box 23.4). Alternatively, assist the patient with seeking the help that he or she needs.

ARRANGE Arrange for a follow-up visit or a referral to professional smoking cessation services.
The most important aspect of this strategy is to keep in regular contact, particularly around the quit date and during the immediate period after the patient quits.

A simplified version of this is the 3 A's. This is a *very brief intervention* and can be particularly useful for the dental team.[94,110] The intervention is designed to be used at every clinical contact, and its very brief nature may help overcome some of the barriers presented by dental practices (the duration is <30 s). The focus is taken away from advising smokers to stop and shifts to offering support. The "advise" step deliberately leaves out the health benefits of stopping smoking or the harms of smoking. This minimizes the duration of the intervention and helps to avoid a defensive reaction or developing anxiety in the patient. The 3 A's technique is as follows:

ASK and record smoking status.
ADVISE how to stop.
ACT on the patient's response (prescribe, monitor, or refer).

Clearly, for the patient undergoing a comprehensive course of periodontal therapy over several visits, there may be more opportunity to focus on the harms of smoking and the personal benefits of quitting.

TABLE 23.2 Barriers Against and Stimuli for the Provision of Smoking Cessation Advice by the Dental Team in Dental Practice

	Barriers	Stimuli
Professional characteristics	Perceived lack of efficacy or lack of confidence in giving the advice	Self-efficacy
	Concerns about disturbing the patient-dentist relationship	Positive attitude toward giving advice as part of health care provider role
	Lack of knowledge about how to give the correct advice	Training
	Belief that counseling is unnecessary or perception that advising patients is frustrating and has a low success rate	Self-belief
	Dental team member may be a smoker himself or herself	Dental team member needs to quit!
Practice organization	Lack of time	Task delegation
	No organizational support in the practice to deliver advice	Focus on helping smokers quit
Health care system	No reimbursement	Health care system changes to encourage healthier lifestyles
	No referral options for further help	Local availability of smoking cessation services

Adapted from Rosseel JP, Jacobs JE, Hilberink SR, et al. What determines the provision of smoking cessation advice and counselling by dental care teams? *Br Dent J.* 2009;206:E13.[117]

periodontitis decreases with the increasing number of years since quitting smoking.[134] This suggests that the negative effects of smoking on the host are reversible with smoking cessation and therefore that smoking cessation programs must be an integral component of periodontal education and therapy (Box 23.3, Table 23.2). Several tobacco intervention approaches can be used when helping the patient deal with the physiologic factors (i.e., nicotine withdrawal symptoms) and the psychological factors associated with smoking cessation (Box 23.4).[98,114] Smoking cessation interventions can also be applied effectively in the dental setting with evidence revealing that these are well received by patients (Box 23.5).[62] Electronic cigarettes have also emerged and are being used by many smokers to help them quit (Box 23.6). However, the effects on oral health are yet to be fully established.

BOX 23.4 Overview of Smoking Cessation Approaches

Willpower Alone

This is the least effective method of smoking cessation, with only 3% of smokers managing to quit after 12 months.[2]

Self-Help Materials

The provision of self-help materials can increase quit rates compared to no intervention, although only by a small amount.[53] When included with any other intervention, there was no additional benefit.

Brief Intervention Program in Primary Care

A brief advice intervention delivered by a physician or dentist can increase the rate of quitting (12 months) by 40%–90%.[61,127] Assuming an unassisted quit rate of 3%, a brief intervention by a dentist could increase the quit rates to around 4.5%–6%. Although this cessation rate may seem low, if the dental team gave this brief advice to most of their smoking patients, a significant number of smokers in the whole population would be assisted to quit each year.

Nicotine Replacement Therapy

Nicotine replacement therapy (NRT) can increase the rate of quitting (12 months) by 50%–70%.[128] For example, in primary care settings in which brief advice is given, 12-month success rates can increase from around 5% to around 8% if NRT is also used. In an intensive setting such as a smoker's clinic, success rates increase from around 10% to up to 16%. NRT is not a magic cure, but it helps with cravings and withdrawal when a person quits smoking. Although NRT products do contain nicotine, they do not contain the toxic products such as tar and carbon monoxide that are found in cigarette smoke. NRT products include the following:

- Patches (available in different doses and worn for 16–24 h/day)
- Lozenges and gum (available in different flavors; should be chewed slowly to allow the nicotine to be absorbed through the mouth)
- Nasal spray (delivers nicotine solution via the nasal passages)
- Inhalator (a plastic mouthpiece with a supply of nicotine cartridges that fit on the end; nicotine is absorbed in the mouth by drawing on the inhalator like a cigarette).

Varenicline

A course of varenicline, at standard dose, can increase the rate of quitting (12 months) by 100%–150%.[21] Varenicline is a nicotine receptor partial agonist, and it aims to reduce both withdrawal symptoms and the pleasure people usually experience when they smoke.

Bupropion

Bupropion can increase the rate of quitting (12 months) by 50%–80%.[65] This medication is used as an antidepressant at higher doses, but it is effective for smoking cessation at lower doses. It is usually prescribed to be started 1–2 weeks before the quit date. There are serious potential drug interactions and unwanted effects.

Other Methods

Whatever works for the patient is good! In addition to combinations of the methods listed here, techniques for smoking cessation can include intensive counseling, motivational interviewing, cognitive behavioral therapy, hypnosis, and acupuncture. Many smokers are now also using e-cigarettes to help to quit smoking (see Box 23.6).

BOX 23.5 Do Smoking Cessation Interventions Work in Dental Settings?

Smoking cessation interventions have been shown to be effective in a wide range of settings from highly medicalized hospital-based programs to a wide range of community-based settings.

Within dental settings, there is evidence that behavioral interventions (such as the 5As or 3As approaches) can lead to just under a doubling in the quit rate at 6 months.[61] The certainty around this evidence is not strong with issues of potential biases in the studies and substantial heterogeneity.

Although rarely offered as part of usual care in dental settings, a small number of research studies have looked at the dental team providing some form of pharmacotherapy alongside the behavioral interventions.[61] These studies show promising results with a further increase in quit rates but further research is needed to determine the size of this additional benefit and the cost-effectiveness of the dental team delivering this "in-house".

What Do Patients Think About the Dental Team Giving Smoking Cessation Advice?

A recent interview-based study explored patients' perceptions of dentist-delivered smoking cessation advice.[62] Several themes emerged, including:

- Opportunistic nature—advice from the dental team was always viewed positively and described as an "olive branch" to building communication and shared understanding.
- Personal impact and tangible prompts—the aesthetic consequences of smoking (staining, drifting, tooth loss) were very impactful in helping patients to quit smoking.
- Positive context of cessation attempt—focusing on the improved outcomes of periodontal therapies was felt to be a better motivator for quitting, rather than focusing on the damage already done by smoking.

Beyond E-Cigarettes

The popularity of **e-cigarettes** took most people by surprise. But what's next?

Heated Tobacco Products (Heat-Not-Burn)

These products heat tobacco to ~500°C, producing an inhalable aerosol.[23] Although not a new idea, they have received recent attention. Prevalence rates however remain relatively low in most countries. For example, 0.2% of adults in England reported being a user in 2021.[141] Japan has notably higher rates with a prevalence of 2.7% reported, equivalent to nearly 4.4 million people (2018).[131]

Water Pipes (Hookah, Shisha)

Popular in some communities, these are likely to carry significant negative health risks. A good summary is produced by the National Center for Smoking Cessation and Training (NCSCT).[93]

Nicotine Gels

These gels allow nicotine to be absorbed through the skin. Currently, they are not very popular.

Oral Nicotine Pouches

A similar concept to snus, a range of products have been marketed since 2018. Typically, users hold the pouch between the upper lip and gum while the nicotine is released.

BOX 23.6 Electronic Cigarettes

Electronic cigarettes (e-cigarettes) are battery-powered devices that produce an aerosol that the user inhales. The e-cigarette usually contains a solution, called an "e-liquid," which is drawn through a heating element to produce the aerosol. The process of using an e-cigarette (often referred to as *vaping*) closely resembles tobacco smoking, making e-cigarettes a particularly attractive alternative to smokers. In contrast, this similarity to cigarette smoking has produced much of the controversy and concerns around e-cigarettes.

What Is in the E-liquid?

The e-liquid usually comprises three main components: diluents, nicotine, and flavorings. The diluents account for the majority of the solution and are usually propylene glycol or vegetable glycerin. Nicotine is included at a wide range of concentrations; two-thirds of users in Great Britain were using strengths between 1 and 12 mg/mL.[3] Flavorings are often added, as both nicotine and the diluents are largely tasteless. The large range of flavors can generally be divided into three main groups: tobacco, fruit, and menthol/mint.

Are E-cigarettes a Useful Smoking Cessation Aid?

E-cigarettes are a modern phenomenon introduced to the U.S. and European markets in 2006, with their popularity taking off around 2011. The evidence base is continually growing with several ongoing clinical trials. A Living Cochrane Collaboration systematic review currently (2021) concludes that nicotine e-cigarettes probably do help people to stop smoking for at least 6 months, and probably work better than using NRT or nicotine-free e-cigarettes.[54]

Are E-cigarettes Safe?

This has been the topic of many debates, and controversy still exists. Two substantial reports concluded that the hazard to health from long-term e-cigarette vapor inhalation was unlikely to exceed 5% of the harm from smoking tobacco.[88,118] Clinical trial data do not report any clear evidence of harm but these studies are short term with a maximum of 2 years' follow-up.[54]

What Are the Oral Health Effects?

There have been an increasing number of studies conducted over the last few years to explore potential oral health effects.[54] Laboratory in vitro studies report a range of cellular effects, but these are much less pronounced than those resulting from exposure to tobacco smoke. Some of the strongest evidence to date comes from microbiological studies which indicated that e-cigarette users have a distinct microbiome and that this might be more pathogenic (compared to nonusers). Evidence from clinical trials is limited and weak in design, usually being cross-sectional. Epidemiological studies have identified concerns over oral dryness, irritation, and gingival diseases. There are many challenges in interpreting research on this topic, for example, tobacco smoking is often a confounder and product development is rapid, meaning studies often become outdated. Future research is needed in this area, particularly in clinical trials and high-quality in vitro studies.

How Are E-cigarettes Regulated?

A range of regulatory approaches have been taken across the globe, from e-cigarettes being completely prohibited to being classified under general consumer product regulations.[23]

What Is the Bottom Line?

E-cigarettes are a consumer-led bottom-up public health initiative that has taken the realms of research, public health, regulation, and industry by surprise. They are popular with users (smokers/former smokers), with probably only a fraction of the health hazards of tobacco smoking. From a public health perspective, they have the potential to significantly reduce tobacco-related morbidity and mortality. There are limited data on the oral health risks but these are likely to be less than those associated with tobacco smoking.

Effects of Smoking on the Etiology and Pathogenesis of Periodontal Disease

The increased prevalence and severity of periodontal destruction associated with smoking suggests that the host–bacterial interactions normally seen with periodontitis are altered, resulting in more extensive periodontal breakdown (Table 23.3). This imbalance between bacterial challenge and host response may be caused by changes in the composition of the subgingival biofilm (e.g., increases in the numbers and virulence of pathogenic organisms), changes in the host response to the bacterial challenge, or a combination of both.

Microbiology

Several studies have explored the possible changes in the subgingival microbiome caused by smoking. Earlier studies tended to show little difference between smokers and nonsmokers. For example, Preber and colleagues (1992) took plaque samples from deep pockets (i.e., ≥6 mm) in 142 patients and found no differences in the counts of *Aggregatibacter actinomycetemcomitans*, *Porphyromonas gingivalis*, and *Prevotella intermedia*.[107] In a similar study of 615 patients involving the use of immunoassay, the prevalence of *A. actinomycetemcomitans*, *P. gingivalis*, *P. intermedia*, and *Eikenella corrodens* was not found to be significantly different between smokers and nonsmokers.[129]

By contrast, other studies have demonstrated differences in the microbial composition of subgingival biofilm of smokers and nonsmokers. A study of 798 subjects with different smoking histories found that smokers had significantly higher levels of *Tannerella forsythia* and that smokers were 2.3 times more likely to harbor *T. forsythia* as compared with nonsmokers and former smokers.[145] Of interest were observations that smokers did not respond to

TABLE 23.3 Effects of Smoking on the Etiology and Pathogenesis of Periodontal Disease

Etiologic Factor	Effects of Smoking
Microbiology	Increased complexity of the microbiome and colonization of periodontal pockets by periodontal pathogens
Immune–inflammatory response	Altered neutrophil chemotaxis, phagocytosis, and oxidative burst ↑ Tumor necrosis factor-α and prostaglandin E_2 in gingival crevicular fluid ↑ Neutrophil collagenase and elastase in gingival crevicular fluid ↑ Production of prostaglandin E_2 by monocytes in response to lipopolysaccharide
Physiology	↓ Gingival blood vessels with ↑ inflammation ↓ Gingival crevicular fluid flow and bleeding on probing with ↑ inflammation ↓ Subgingival temperature ↑ Time needed to recover from local anesthesia

↓, Decreased; ↑, increased.

mechanical therapy as well as nonsmokers did; this was associated with increased levels of *T. forsythia*, *A. actinomycetemcomitans*, and *P. gingivalis* remaining in the pockets after therapy in the smoking group as compared with nonsmokers.[45,46,49,113]

Many discrepancies between the findings of microbiologic studies are a function of the methodology involved, including bacterial counts versus proportions or prevalence of bacteria, the number of sites sampled and the pocket depths selected, the sampling technique, the disease status of the subject, and the methods of bacterial identification and data analysis. In an attempt to overcome some of these problems, one study sampled subgingival biofilm from all teeth with the exception of third molars in 272 adult subjects, including 50 current smokers, 98 former smokers, and 124 nonsmokers.[51] Using checkerboard DNA–DNA hybridization technology to screen for 29 different subgingival species, it was found that members of the orange and red complex species—including *Eikenella nodatum*, *Fusobacterium nucleatum* ss *vincentii*, *P. intermedia*, *Peptostreptococcus micros*, *Prevotella nigrescens*, *T. forsythia*, *P. gingivalis*, and *Treponema denticola*—were significantly more prevalent in current smokers than in nonsmokers and former smokers. The increased prevalence of these periodontal pathogens was caused by increased colonization of shallow sites (pocket depth ≤4 mm), with no differences among smokers, former smokers, and nonsmokers in pockets 4 mm or greater. In addition, these pathogenic bacteria were more prevalent in the maxilla than the mandible. These data suggest that smokers have a greater extent of colonization by periodontal pathogens than nonsmokers or former smokers, which may increase the risk of periodontal disease progression. Contemporary studies have drawn similar conclusions, with next-generation sequencing analysis of periodontally healthy smokers demonstrating a highly diverse, pathogen-rich, commensal-poor, anaerobic microbiome that is more similar to the microbiome observed in patients with advanced periodontitis than that observed in periodontally healthy nonsmokers, and which is primed for future development of periodontitis given appropriate ecologic and environmental changes.[87]

Immune–Inflammatory Responses

The immune response of the host to biofilm accumulation is essentially protective. In periodontal health, a balance exists between the bacterial challenge of the biofilm and the immune-inflammatory responses in the gingival tissues, with no resulting loss of periodontal support. By contrast, periodontitis is associated with an alteration in the host–bacterial balance that may be initiated by changes in the bacterial composition of the subgingival biofilm, changes in the host responses, other environmental changes, or a combination of these.

Smoking exerts a major effect on the immune-inflammatory response that results in an increase in the extent and severity of periodontal destruction. The deleterious effects of smoking appear to result from alterations in the immune-inflammatory response to bacterial challenge. The neutrophil is an important component of the host response to the bacterial challenge, and alterations in neutrophil number or function may result in localized and systemic infections. Critical functions of neutrophils include *chemotaxis* (directed locomotion from the bloodstream to the site of infection), *phagocytosis* (internalization of foreign particles such as bacteria), and *killing* via oxidative and nonoxidative mechanisms.

Neutrophils obtained from the peripheral blood, oral cavity, or saliva of smokers or exposed in vitro to whole tobacco smoke or nicotine have demonstrated functional alterations in chemotaxis, phagocytosis, and the oxidative burst.[40,76] In vitro studies of the effects of tobacco products on neutrophils have shown detrimental effects on cell movement as well as on the oxidative burst.[33,75,81,120,125] In addition, levels of antibody to the periodontal pathogens essential for phagocytosis and killing of bacteria, specifically immunoglobulin G_2, have been reported to be reduced in smokers as compared with nonsmokers with periodontitis,[22,47,49,132] thereby suggesting that smokers may have reduced protection against periodontal bacteria. By contrast, elevated levels of tumor necrosis factor–α have been demonstrated in the gingival crevicular fluid of smokers,[20] and elevated levels of prostaglandin E_2, neutrophil elastase, and matrix metalloproteinase-8 have also been found.[126] In vitro studies have also shown that exposure to nicotine increases the secretion of prostaglandin E_2 by monocytes in response to lipopolysaccharide.[100]

These data suggest that smoking alters the response of neutrophils to the bacterial challenge such that there are increases in the release of tissue-destructive enzymes, causing increased periodontal tissue destruction. Furthermore, immune-inflammatory responses in periodontitis are also likely modified as a result of epigenetic mechanisms (i.e., changes in expression of genes not arising from changes in the DNA sequence). For example, it has been shown that methylation of the *SOCS1* gene promoter (with possible alteration of gene expression) results from exposure to tobacco smoke but is not correlated with the severity of periodontitis in smokers.[35] It is clear that further research is needed to better understand the changes in immunologic, inflammatory, and (likely) epigenetic mechanisms that result in the more severe periodontal tissue destruction observed in smokers compared to nonsmokers.

Physiology

Previous studies have shown that certain clinical signs of inflammation (e.g., gingival redness, gingival bleeding) are less pronounced in smokers than in nonsmokers.[12,34] This may result from alterations in the vascular response of the gingival tissues. Although no significant differences in the vascular density of healthy gingiva have been observed between smokers and nonsmokers,[101] the response of the microcirculation to biofilm accumulation appears to be altered in smokers as compared with nonsmokers. With developing inflammation, increases in gingival crevicular fluid flow, bleeding on probing,[18] and gingival blood vessels[17] are lower in smokers than in nonsmokers. In addition, the oxygen concentration in healthy gingival tissues appears to be lower in smokers than in nonsmokers, although this condition is reversed in the presence of moderate inflammation.[52] Subgingival temperatures are lower in smokers than nonsmokers,[37] and recovery from the vasoconstriction caused by local anesthetic administration takes longer in smokers.[77,137] These data suggest that significant alterations are present in the gingival microvasculature of smokers as compared with nonsmokers and that these changes lead to decreased blood flow and decreased clinical signs of inflammation. This explains the long-observed phenomenon of a transient increase in gingival bleeding when a smoker quits; patients need to be warned about this phenomenon.

Is Nicotine the Bad Guy?

The role of nicotine in the detrimental health effects seen in smokers has never been more relevant with the increasing popularity of novel nicotine delivery devices (e.g., e-cigarettes). Nicotine is not carcinogenic,[56,66] and it is now largely accepted that nicotine has likely been unfairly blamed. A classic quote, with reference to lung cancer, is "smokers smoke for nicotine but are killed by tar."[119] The potential role of nicotine in periodontitis development is less clear. Nicotine has been the subject of many in vitro investigations with oral cells. A review of studies on this topic included 42 highly heterogeneous studies.[59] The review concluded that nicotine at the levels found in tobacco smokers, **nicotine replacement therapy** (NRT) users, and e-cigarette users, was unlikely to be directly cytotoxic. The higher levels seen in smokeless tobacco users may be high enough to achieve cytotoxicity. Data on other cellular processes such as attachment, proliferation and inflammatory mediator production was limited and contradictory.

Clinical studies are required to determine the clinical relevance of these in vitro results.

TABLE 23.4 Effects of Smoking on the Response to Periodontal Therapy

Therapy	Effects of Smoking
Nonsurgical	↓ Clinical response to root surface debridement ↓ Reduction in probing depth ↓ Gain in clinical attachment levels ↓ Negative impact of smoking with ↑ level of plaque control
Surgery and implants	↓ Probing depth reduction and ↓ gain in clinical attachment levels after access flap surgery ↑ Deterioration of furcations after surgery ↓ Gain in clinical attachment levels, ↓ bone fill, ↑ recession, and ↑ membrane exposure after guided tissue regeneration ↓ Root coverage after grafting procedures for localized gingival recession ↓ Probing depth reduction after bone graft procedures ↑ Risk for implant failure and periimplantitis
Maintenance care	↑ Probing depth and attachment loss during maintenance therapy ↑ Disease recurrence in smokers ↑ Need for retreatment in smokers ↑ Tooth loss in smokers after surgical therapy

↓, Decreased; ↑, increased.

Effects of Smoking on the Response to Periodontal Therapy

Nonsurgical Therapy

Numerous studies have indicated that current smokers do not respond as well to periodontal therapy as nonsmokers or former smokers do (Table 23.4). Most clinical research supports the observation that probing depth reductions are generally greater in nonsmokers than in smokers after nonsurgical periodontal therapy.[4,45,46,49,74,106,113] In addition, gains in clinical attachment as a result of nonsurgical treatment are less pronounced in smokers than in nonsmokers. In a study of patients with previously untreated advanced periodontitis, nonsurgical therapy resulted in significantly greater mean reductions in probing depth and bleeding on probing in nonsmokers than in smokers when evaluated 6 months after the completion of therapy.[113] Mean probing depth reductions of 2.5 mm for nonsmokers and 1.9 mm for smokers were observed in pockets that averaged 7 mm or more before treatment. In another study, the nonsurgical management of pockets of 5 mm or greater showed that smokers had less probing depth reduction than nonsmokers after 3 months (1.29 mm vs. 1.76 mm) as well as less gain in clinical attachment levels.[45] When a higher level of oral hygiene was achieved as part of nonsurgical care, the differences in the resolution of 4- to 6-mm pockets between nonsmokers and smokers became clinically less significant.[106]

Moreover, it has been demonstrated by a systematic review that the 6-month outcomes of nonsurgical periodontal therapy (i.e., probing depth reduction and clinical attachment level gain) of smoking patients may benefit from the adjunctive use of local antibiotics.[31] For deep pockets (probing depth >5 mm) these improvements were more manifest when treated with locally derived azithromycin, clarithromycin, or doxycycline gels (overall, pooled estimates suggested an additional probing depth reduction and attachment level gain of around 1 mm compared with sites submitted solely to nonsurgical therapy).[31] The same review also did not identify significant additional effects on probing depth reduction and attachment level gain when systemic antibiotics were combined with nonsurgical periodontal therapy.

It can be concluded that smokers respond less well to nonsurgical therapy than do nonsmokers. With excellent plaque biofilm control, these differences may be minimized, but the emphasis is on truly excellent plaque control. When comparing current smokers with former smokers and nonsmokers, the former and nonsmoking subjects appear to respond equally well to nonsurgical care,[45] thereby reinforcing the need for patients to be informed of the benefits of smoking cessation.

Surgical Therapy and Implants

The less favorable response of the periodontal tissues to nonsurgical therapy that is observed in current smokers is also observed after surgical therapy. In a longitudinal comparative study of the effects of four different treatment modalities (coronal scaling, root planing, modified Widman flap surgery, and osseous resection surgery), smokers (with "heavy" defined as ≥20 cigarettes per day and "light" defined as ≤19 cigarettes per day) consistently showed less pocket reduction and less gain in clinical attachment as compared with nonsmokers or former smokers.[74] These differences were evident immediately after the completion of therapy and continued throughout 7 years of supportive periodontal therapy. During the 7 years, deterioration at furcation areas was greater in heavy and light smokers than in former smokers and nonsmokers. Smoking has also been shown to have a negative impact on the outcomes of guided tissue regeneration[136,138] and the treatment of infrabony defects by bone grafts.[116] By 12 months after guided tissue regeneration therapy at deep infrabony defects, smokers demonstrated less than half the attachment gain that was observed in nonsmokers (2.1 mm vs. 5.2 mm).[136] In a second study, 73 smokers also showed less attachment gain than nonsmokers (1.2 mm vs. 3.2 mm), more gingival recession, and less bone infill of the defect. Similarly, after the use of bone grafts for the treatment of infrabony defects, smokers showed less reduction in probing depths as compared with nonsmokers.[116]

Open flap access surgery without regenerative or grafting procedures is a common surgical procedure used for accessing the root and bone surfaces. By 6 months after this procedure, smokers showed significantly less reduction of deep pockets (≥7 mm) than nonsmokers (3 mm for smokers vs. 4 mm for nonsmokers) and significantly less gain in clinical attachment (1.8 mm for smokers vs. 2.8 mm for nonsmokers), even though all of the patients received supportive periodontal therapy every month for 6 months.[122]

Tobacco smoking also affects the outcomes of periodontal plastic surgery.[26,29] For instance, a systematic review assessed the influence of smoking on the outcomes achieved by root coverage procedures.[26] This review identified that significantly greater root coverage and greater gains in clinical attachment levels were recorded for nonsmokers as compared with smokers after the treatment of gingival recession defects by subepithelial connective-tissue grafts. Furthermore, smokers showed significantly fewer sites with complete root coverage than were seen in nonsmokers.[29]

Recent evidence from human histologic clinical trials evaluating transitional implants showed that smoking had: (a) a detrimental impact on peri-implant bone healing (reduced bone-to-implant contact, bone density in the threaded area, and bone density outside the threaded area); and (b) reduced survival rates, especially for maxillary implants.[30]

Clinically, several meta-analyses have investigated the influence of smoking on the short- and long-term outcomes of implant therapy and have identified that smoking increases the risk of implant failure.[27,58,79,90,130] These studies used various definitions to define implant failure, including implant loss, implant bone loss, mobility, pain, and peri-implantitis. Overall, the risk for implant failure in smokers appears to be approximately double the risk for failure in nonsmokers, and the risks appear to be higher in maxillary implants and when implants are placed in poor-quality bone. Smoking has also been shown to be a risk factor for periimplantitis, with a majority of studies showing a significant increase in periimplant bone loss as compared with nonsmokers.[57] Collectively, these data indicate that implant failure is more common among smokers than nonsmokers. However, because numerous factors can influence implant success, further controlled clinical trials are needed to address the role of smoking as an independent variable in implant failure. Given the current evidence, all patients who are considering implant therapy should be informed about the benefits of smoking cessation and the risks of smoking for the development of periimplantitis and implant failure.

Maintenance Therapy

The detrimental effect of smoking on treatment outcomes appears to be long-lasting and independent of the frequency of maintenance therapy. After four modalities of therapy (scaling, scaling and root planing, modified Widman flap surgery, and osseous surgery), maintenance therapy was performed by a hygienist every 3 months for 7 years.[74] Smokers consistently had deeper pockets than nonsmokers and less gain in attachment when evaluated each year for the 7-year period. Even with more intensive maintenance therapy given every month for 6 months after flap surgery,[122] smokers had deeper and more residual pockets than nonsmokers, although no significant differences in plaque or bleeding on probing scores were found. These data suggest that the effects of smoking on the host response and the healing characteristics of the periodontal tissues may have a long-term effect on pocket resolution in smokers, possibly requiring more intensive management during the maintenance phase. Smokers also tend to experience more periodontal breakdown than nonsmokers after therapy.[80,86] In studies of patients who failed to respond to periodontal therapy, approximately 90% of these poorly responding patients were smokers.[84,85]

A systematic review that assessed the potential predictors of tooth loss during long-term periodontal maintenance care demonstrated that, although oral health and the prevention of tooth loss were achieved in the majority of patients, the long-term outcomes were also influenced by smoking.[24] Tobacco smoking was positively associated with tooth loss even when regular recall maintenance care was performed (overall, smokers had a risk of losing their teeth that was up to 380% higher than that of nonsmokers).[24] The authors of this review also highlighted the importance of quitting smoking in improving tooth survival over time, although it may not modify immediately the negative consequences of smoking.[24] Similarly, smoking has a detrimental effect on periimplant tissue status, even when patients are under strict periimplant preventive maintenance care.[36] It has been also demonstrated in a practice-based study that the smoking status may be highly associated with periimplant tissue loss around 10-mm implants restored with single crowns.[36] For instance, when comparing nonsmokers and light smokers (i.e., subjects who smoked <10 cigarettes per day), it was found that the majority of patients who experienced bone loss were smokers (88.9%), with an odds ratio of 39.64 (95% confidence interval, 8.62 to 182.27) for increased risk of bone loss.[36]

It is clear from these studies that (1) smokers may present with periodontal disease at an early age; (2) they may be difficult to treat effectively with conventional therapeutic strategies; (3) they may continue to have progressive or recurrent periodontitis; and (4) they may be at an increased risk of tooth loss or periimplant bone loss, even when adequate maintenance control is established. For these reasons, smoking cessation counseling must be a cornerstone of periodontal therapy in smokers.

Effects of Smoking Cessation on Periodontal Treatment Outcomes

The effect of smoking cessation on periodontal status has been studied in a large number of cross-sectional and cohort observational studies, in which the periodontal status of smokers, former smokers, and nonsmokers is compared.[7,8,13–15,19,38,48,50,71,99,133,134] Similarly, periodontal treatment outcomes have been assessed in smokers, former smokers, and nonsmokers.[46,64,74,89,109,121] Collectively, these studies have demonstrated that smokers have significantly worse periodontal status (i.e., deeper probing depths, more attachment loss and bone loss) than either former smokers or nonsmokers and usually have poorer treatment outcomes. The periodontal status of former smokers is intermediate to that of current smokers and nonsmokers, and it appears to usually be closer to that of nonsmokers.

There are very few intervention studies of the effect of smoking cessation on periodontal treatment outcomes (i.e., studies in which smokers were helped to quit and in which the effect on periodontal status was then assessed). Two short-term studies have indicated that smoking has a negative impact on the gingival vasculature and that these changes are reversible with smoking cessation.[91,92] Two interventional studies have assessed the impact of smoking cessation on outcomes after nonsurgical periodontal treatment.[108,115] The first study employed dental hygienists who were trained as smoking cessation advisers and who achieved a 20% quit rate at 12 months in a population of smokers who also had periodontitis. The hygienists used a variety of strategies to assist these smokers, including counseling, nicotine replacement therapy, and bupropion. All of the patients received nonsurgical therapy as treatment for their periodontitis in addition to smoking cessation counseling. Those individuals who successfully quit smoking for the entire 12 months of the study had the best response to the periodontal treatment. The treatment responses in the nonquitters and the failed quitters (i.e., the "oscillators" who initially quit but who then resumed smoking) were significantly poorer than those seen in the quitters, and they did not differ significantly from each other. The second study was a 12-month prospective single-blinded study in which smoking cessation advice, nicotine replacement therapy, and medication were provided at four consecutive appointments, once a week, by a multidisciplinary team that included doctors, psychologists, and a dentist, in addition to nonsurgical treatment of periodontitis.[115] The confirmed continuous quit rate at 12 months was 18.3%. At the end of the 12-month follow-up period, it was identified that the quitters had improved clinical attachment gain as compared with the nonquitters. In addition, a supplementary study that described a set of meta-analyses performed with individual patient data from these two trials reported a highly significant beneficial impact of quitting smoking, with quitters demonstrating 30% more sites with probing depth reductions of 2 mm or more as compared with nonquitters.[28] Equally, quitters had 22% fewer sites with residual probing depths of 4 mm or greater as compared with nonquitters at the end of the 12-month follow-up period.[28]

The benefit of smoking cessation on the periodontium is likely to be mediated through various pathways, such as a shift toward a less pathogenic microbiome, the recovery of the gingival microcirculation, and improvements in certain aspects of the immune-inflammatory responses. In support of this observation, in the interventional study described previously,[108] plaque samples were collected as the study progressed. It became clear that subgingival microbial profiles differed significantly between smokers and quitters at 6 and 12 months after smoking cessation.[44] At 6 and 12 months after treatment, the microbial community in smokers was similar to that observed at baseline (i.e., before periodontal treatment/smoking cessation counseling), whereas the quitters demonstrated significantly divergent profiles; changes in bacterial levels contributed to this shift. These data suggest a critical role of smoking cessation in the alteration of the subgingival biofilm. Further research is necessary to investigate the impact of quitting smoking on the immune-inflammatory mechanisms that drive tissue destruction in the periodontium.

In conclusion, smoking is a major risk factor for periodontitis, and smoking cessation should be an integral part of periodontal therapy among patients who smoke. Smoking cessation should be considered a priority for the management of periodontitis in smokers.

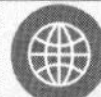
A Case Scenario is found on the companion website eBooks.Health.Elsevier.com.

Suggested Reading

Chaffee BW, Couch ET, Ryder M. The tobacco-using periodontal patient: role of the dental practitioner in tobacco cessation and periodontal disease management. *Periodontol*. 2016;2000 71:52-64.

Chambrone L, Preshaw PM, Rosa EF, et al. Effects of smoking cessation on the outcomes of non-surgical periodontal therapy: a systematic review and individual patient data meta-analysis. *J Clin Periodontol*. 2013;40:607–615.

Heasman L, Stacey F, Preshaw PM, et al. The effect of smoking on periodontal treatment response: a review of clinical evidence. *J Clin Periodontol*. 2006;33:241–253.

Holliday R, Hong B, McColl E, et al. Interventions for tobacco cessation delivered by dental professionals. *Cochrane Database of Syst Rev*. 2021:CD005084.

Holliday R, Chaffee BW, Jakubovics NS, et al. Electronic cigarettes and oral health. *J Dent Res*. epub ahead of print, 2021. https://doi.org/10.1177/00220345211002116. (Accessed 28 May 2021).

Holliday R, Campbell J, Preshaw PM. Effect of nicotine on human gingival, periodontal ligament and oral epithelial cells. A systematic review of the literature. *J Dent*. 2019;86:81–88.

Holliday R, McColl E, Bauld L, et al. Perceived influences on smoking behaviour and perceptions of dentist-delivered smoking cessation advice: a qualitative interview study. *Community Dent Oral Epidemiol*. 2020;48:433–439.

Ramseier CA, Woelber JP, Kitzmann, et al. Impact of risk factor control interventions for smoking cessation and promotion of healthy lifestyles in patients with periodontitis: a systematic review. *J Clin Periodontol*. 2020;47:90–106.

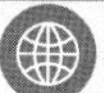
References for this chapter are found on the companion website at eBooks.Health.Elsevier.com.

CHAPTER 24

The Role of Dental Calculus and Other Local Predisposing Factors

Vivek Thumbigere-Math | James E. Hinrichs

CHAPTER OUTLINE

The primary cause of **gingival inflammation** is bacterial plaque. Other predisposing factors include calculus, faulty restorations, complications associated with orthodontic therapy, self-inflicted injuries, and the use of tobacco. These will be discussed in turn.

Calculus

Calculus consists of mineralized bacterial plaque that forms on the surfaces of natural teeth and dental prostheses.

Supragingival and Subgingival Calculus

Supragingival calculus is located coronal to the gingival margin and therefore is visible in the oral cavity. It is usually white or whitish-yellow in color; hard, with a claylike consistency; and easily detached from the tooth surface. After removal, it may rapidly recur, especially in the lingual area of the mandibular incisors. The color is influenced by contact with substances such as tobacco and food pigments. It may be localized on a single tooth or group of teeth, or it may be generalized throughout the mouth.

KEY FACT

Mechanical removal of subgingival plaque and calculus is considered the fundamental cornerstone of the treatment of chronic periodontitis.

The two most common locations for the development of supragingival calculus are the buccal surfaces of the maxillary molars (Fig. 24.1) and the lingual surfaces of the mandibular anterior teeth (Fig. 24.2).[40]

Saliva from the parotid gland flows over the facial surfaces of the upper molars via the parotid duct, whereas the submandibular duct and the lingual duct empty onto the lingual surfaces of the lower incisors from the submaxillary and sublingual glands, respectively. In extreme cases, calculus may form a bridge-like structure over the interdental papilla of adjacent teeth or cover the occlusal surface of teeth that are lacking functional antagonists.

Subgingival calculus is located below the crest of the marginal gingiva and therefore is not visible on routine clinical examination. The location and the extent of subgingival calculus may be evaluated by careful tactile perception with a delicate dental instrument such as an explorer. Clerehugh and colleagues[37] assessed the validity of the World Health Organization (WHO) no. 621 probe to detect and score subgingival calculus. Following clinical detection of subgingival calculus, teeth were extracted and microscopically scored for subgingival calculus. An agreement of 80% was found between the two scoring methods. Subgingival calculus is typically hard and dense; it frequently appears to be dark brown or greenish-black in color (Fig. 24.3), and it is firmly attached to the tooth surface. Supragingival calculus and subgingival calculus generally occur together, but one may be present without the other. Microscopic studies demonstrate that deposits of subgingival calculus usually extend nearly to the base of periodontal pockets in individuals with chronic periodontitis but do not reach the junctional epithelium.

When the gingival tissues recede, subgingival calculus becomes exposed and is therefore reclassified as supragingival (Fig. 24.4A). Thus, supragingival calculus can be composed of both the initial supragingival calculus and previous subgingival calculus. A reduction in gingival inflammation and probing depths with a gain in clinical attachment can be observed after the removal of subgingival plaque and calculus (see Fig. 24.4B; see Chapter 43).

CLINICAL CORRELATION

A reduction in gingival inflammation and probing depths accompanied by a gain in clinical attachment can be expected following thorough removal of subgingival plaque and calculus.

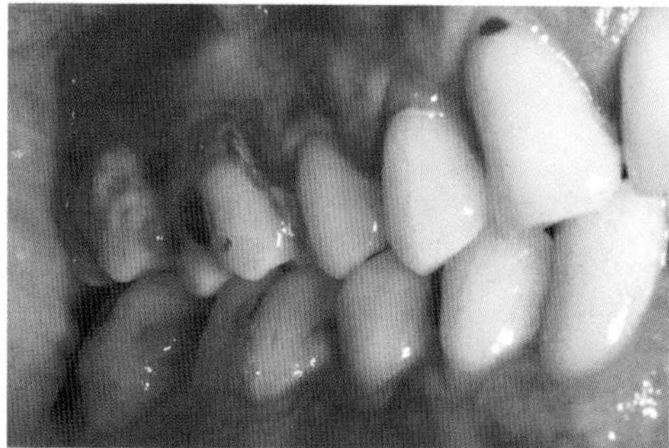

Fig. 24.1 Supragingival calculus is depicted on the buccal surfaces of maxillary molars adjacent to the orifice for the parotid duct.

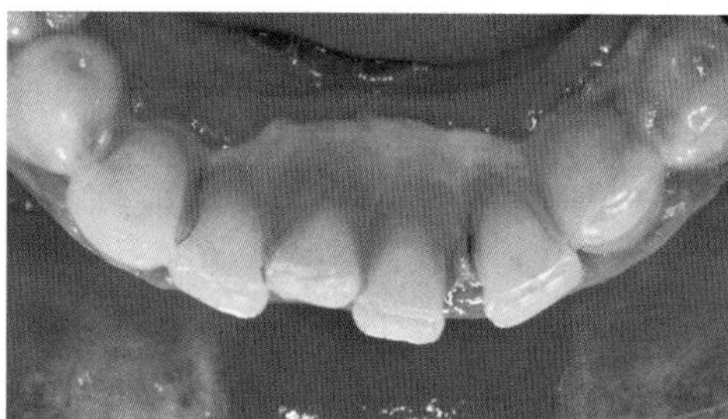

Fig. 24.2 Extensive supragingival calculus is present on the lingual surfaces of the lower anterior teeth.

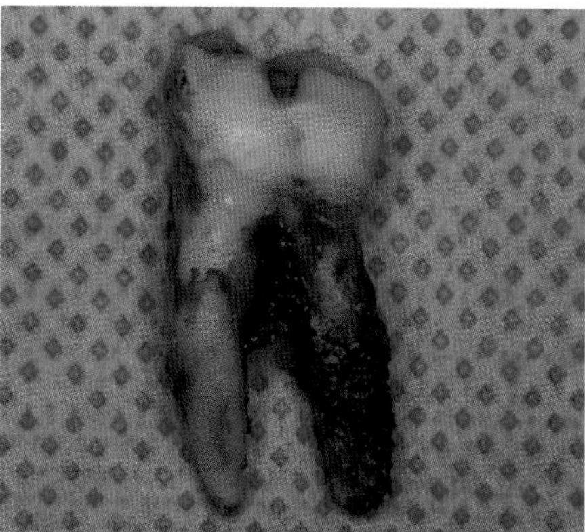

Fig. 24.3 Dark pigmented deposits of subgingival calculus are shown on the distal root of an extracted lower molar.

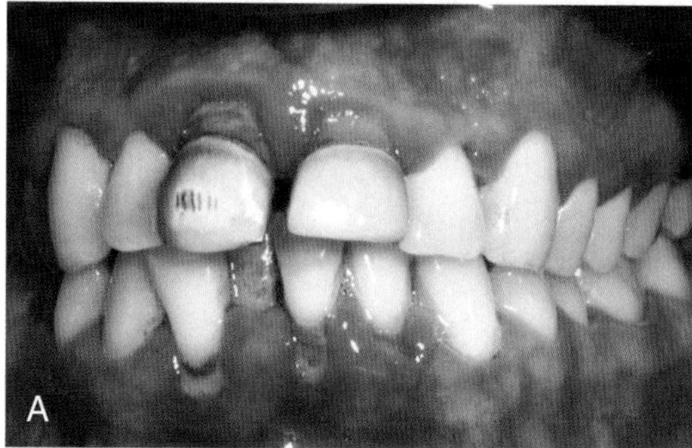

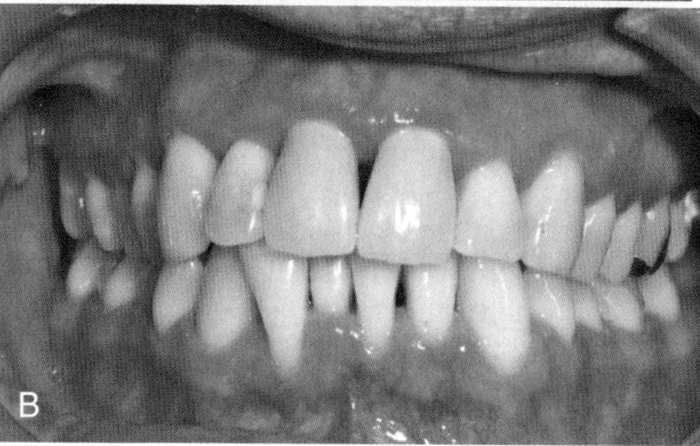

Fig. 24.4 (A) A 31-year-old white man with extensive supragingival and subgingival calculus deposits throughout his dentition is shown. (B) One year after receiving thorough scaling and root planing to remove supragingival and subgingival calculus deposits, followed by restorative care. Note the substantial reduction in gingival inflammation.

Prevalence

Anerud and colleagues[6] observed the periodontal status of a group of Sri Lankan tea laborers and a group of Norwegian academicians for a 15-year period. The Norwegian population had ready access to preventive dental care throughout their lives, whereas the Sri Lankan tea laborers did not. The formation of supragingival calculus was observed early in life in the Sri Lankan individuals, probably shortly after the teeth erupted. The first areas to exhibit calculus deposits were the facial aspects of maxillary molars and the lingual surfaces of mandibular incisors. The deposition of supragingival calculus continued as individuals aged, and it reached a maximal calculus score when the affected individuals were 25 to 30 years old.

At this time, most of the teeth were covered by calculus, although the facial surfaces had less calculus than the lingual or palatal surfaces. Calculus accumulation appeared to be symmetric, and by the age of 45 years, these individuals had only a few teeth (typically the premolars) without calculus deposits. Subgingival calculus appeared first either independently or on the interproximal aspects of areas where supragingival calculus already existed.[6] By the age of 30 years, all surfaces of all teeth had subgingival calculus without any pattern of predilection.

In contrast to the Sri Lankan group, the Norwegian academicians who received oral hygiene instructions and frequent preventive dental care throughout their lives exhibited a marked reduction in the accumulation of calculus. Approximately 80% of teenagers formed limited supragingival calculus on the facial surfaces of the upper first molars and the lingual surfaces of lower incisors. However, no additional calculus formation occurred on other teeth, and its presence did not increase with the individual's age.[6]

Both supragingival calculus and subgingival calculus may be seen on radiographs (see Chapter 39). Highly calcified interproximal calculus deposits are readily detectable as radiopaque projections that protrude into the interdental spaces (Fig. 24.5).

However, the sensitivity level of detecting calculus by radiographs is inconsistent.[30] The location of calculus does not indicate the bottom of the periodontal pocket, because the most apical plaque is not sufficiently calcified to be visible on radiographs.

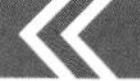

FLASH BACK

Whereas the presence of subgingival calculus can be observed on dental radiographs, the sensitivity of such detection is inconsistent.

Composition

Inorganic Content

Dental calculus is primarily composed of inorganic components (70% to 90%)[62] and the organic components constitute the rest. The major inorganic proportions of calculus are approximately 76% calcium phosphate ($Ca_3[PO_4]_2$), 3% calcium carbonate ($CaCO_3$), 4% magnesium phosphate ($Mg_3[PO_4]_2$), 2% carbon dioxide, and traces

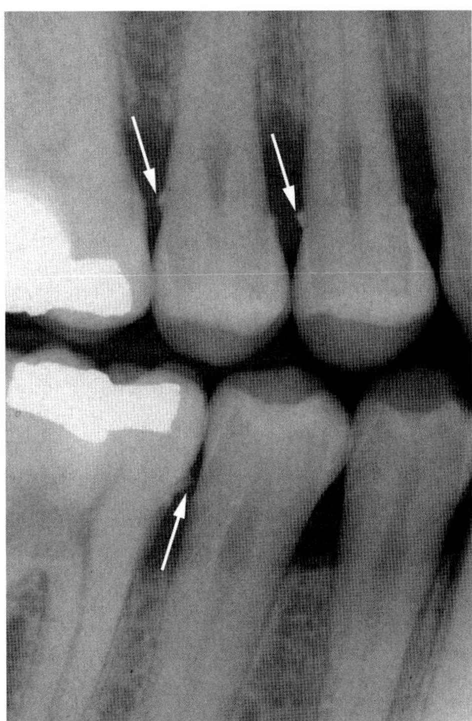

Fig. 24.5 A bitewing radiograph illustrating subgingival calculus deposits that are depicted as interproximal spurs *(arrows).*

of other elements such as sodium, zinc, strontium, bromine, copper, manganese, tungsten, gold, aluminum, silicon, iron, and fluorine.[135,209] The percentage of inorganic constituents in calculus is similar to that of other calcified tissues of the body (Table 24.1).

At least two-thirds of the inorganic component is crystalline in structure.[106] The four main crystal forms and their approximate percentages are as follows: hydroxyapatite, 58%; magnesium whitlockite, 21%; octacalcium phosphate, 12%; and brushite, 9%.

Two or more crystal forms are typically found in a sample of calculus. Hydroxyapatite and octacalcium phosphate are detected most frequently (i.e., in 97% to 100% of all supragingival calculus) and constitute the bulk of the specimen. Brushite is more common in the mandibular anterior region, and magnesium whitlockite is found in the posterior areas. The incidence of the four crystal forms varies with the age of the deposit.[20]

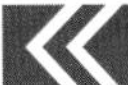 **FLASH BACK**

The four main crystalline inorganic forms of calculus are hydroxyapatite, magnesium whitlockite, octacalcium phosphate, and brushite.

Organic Content

The organic component of calculus consists of a mixture of protein–polysaccharide complexes, desquamated epithelial cells, leukocytes, and various types of microorganisms.[120]

Between 1.9% and 9.1% of the organic component is carbohydrate, which consists of galactose, glucose, rhamnose, mannose, glucuronic acid, galactosamine, and sometimes arabinose, galacturonic acid, and glucosamine.[112,118,189] All of these organic components are present in salivary glycoprotein, with the exception of arabinose and rhamnose. Salivary proteins account for 5.9% to 8.2% of the organic component of calculus and include most amino acids. Lipids account for 0.2% of the organic content in the form of neutral fats, free fatty acids, cholesterol, cholesterol esters, and phospholipids.[113]

TABLE 24.1 Calculus Versus Other Oral Hard Tissues

Structure	Inorganic Content (%)[a]
Dental calculus	70–90
Enamel	96
Dentin	45
Bone	60–70

[a]Organic components and water constitute the rest.

The composition of subgingival calculus is similar to that of supragingival calculus, with some differences. It has the same hydroxyapatite content but more magnesium whitlockite and less brushite and octacalcium phosphate.[170,194] The ratio of calcium to phosphate is higher in subgingival calculus, and the sodium content increases with the depth of periodontal pockets.[114] These altered compositions may be attributed to the fact that the origin of subgingival calculus is plasma, whereas supragingival calculus is partially composed of salivary constituents. Salivary proteins present in supragingival calculus are not found in subgingival calculus.[14] Dental calculus, salivary duct calculus, and calcified dental tissues are similar in inorganic composition.

Attachment to the Tooth Surface

Differences in the manner in which calculus is attached to the tooth surface affect the relative ease or difficulty encountered during its removal. Four modes of attachment have been described.[97,178,183,216] (1) Attachment by means of an organic pellicle on cementum is depicted in Fig. 24.6, and attachment on enamel is shown in Fig. 24.7. (2) Mechanical locking into surface irregularities, such as caries lesions or resorption lacunae, is illustrated in Fig. 24.8. (3) Close adaptation of the undersurface of calculus to depressions or gently sloping mounds of the unaltered cementum surface[189] is shown in Fig. 24.9. (4) Penetration of bacterial calculus into cementum is shown in Figs. 24.10 and 24.11.

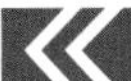 **FLASH BACK**

Four modes by which calculus may attach to cementum are (1) organic pellicle, (2) mechanical locking into surface irregularities, (3) close adaption to gentle depression or sloping mounts of unaltered cementum, and (4) bacterial penetration into cementum surface.

Formation

Calculus is *mineralized dental plaque.* The soft plaque is hardened by the precipitation of mineral salts, which usually starts between the 1st and 14th day of plaque formation. Calcification has been reported to occur within as little as 4 to 8 hours.[195] Calcifying plaques may become 50% mineralized in 2 days and 60% to 90% mineralized in 12 days.[134,174,182] All plaque does not necessarily undergo calcification. Early plaque contains a small amount of inorganic material, which increases as the plaque develops into calculus. Plaque that does not develop into calculus reaches a plateau of maximal mineral content within 2 days.[173] Microorganisms are not always essential in calculus formation because calculus readily occurs in germ-free rodents.[69]

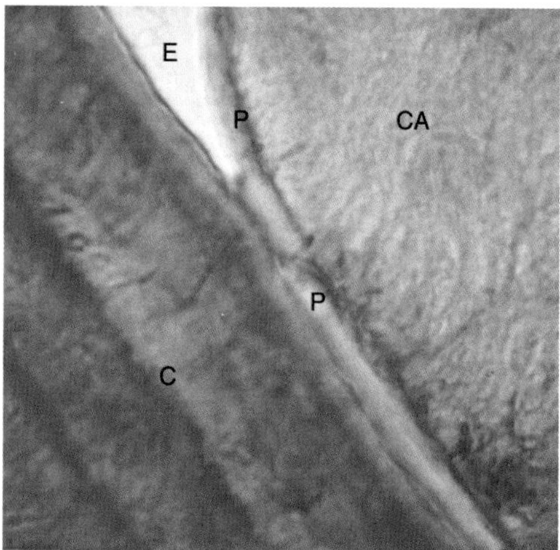

Fig. 24.6 Calculus attached to the pellicle on the enamel surface and the cementum. An enamel void *(E)* has been created during the preparation of the specimen. *C,* Cementum; *CA,* calculus; *P,* pellicle. (*Courtesy Dr. Erwin Schaffer, Minneapolis, MN.*)

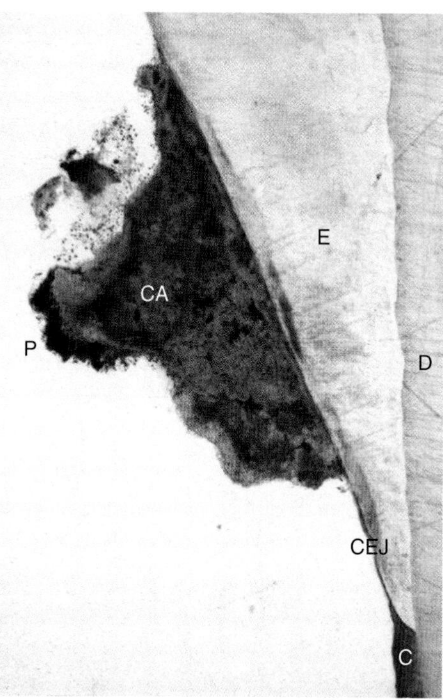

Fig. 24.7 Non-decalcified specimen with calculus *(CA)* attached to enamel *(E)* surface just coronal to the cementoenamel junction *(CEJ).* Note plaque *(P)* on the surface of the calculus; dentin *(D)* and cementum *(C)* are also identified. (*Courtesy Dr. Michael Rohrer, Minneapolis, MN.*)

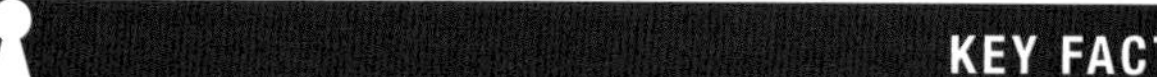

KEY FACT

Calculus by itself does not contribute directly to gingival inflammation. Like other retentive factors, such as open crown margin or an overhanging restoration, calculus retains dental plaque, which contributes to gingival inflammation.

Saliva is the primary source of mineralization for supragingival calculus, whereas the serum transudate called *gingival crevicular fluid* furnishes the minerals for subgingival calculus.[83,191] The calcium concentration or content in plaque is 2 to 20 times higher than in saliva.[20] Early plaque of heavy calculus formers contains more

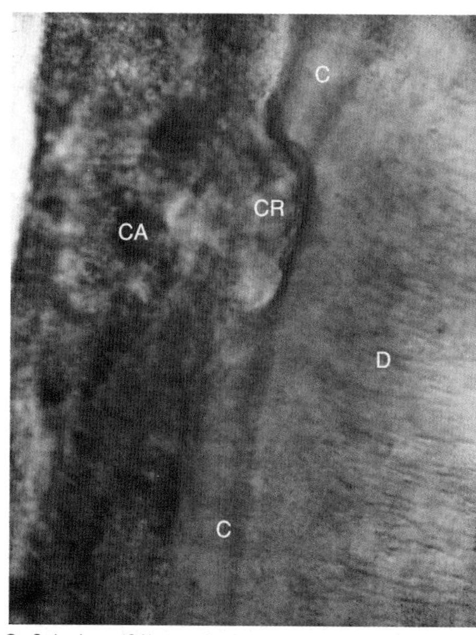

Fig. 24.8 Calculus *(CA)* attached to a cemental resorption area *(CR)* with cementum *(C)* adjacent to dentin *(D).* (*Courtesy Dr. Erwin Schaffer, Minneapolis, MN.*)

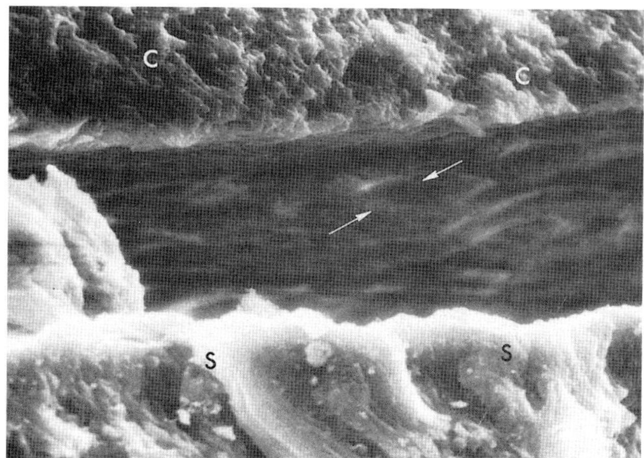

Fig. 24.9 Undersurface of subgingival calculus *(C)* previously attached to the cementum surface *(S).* Note the impression of cementum mounds in the calculus *(arrows).* (*Courtesy Dr. John Sottosanti, La Jolla, CA.*)

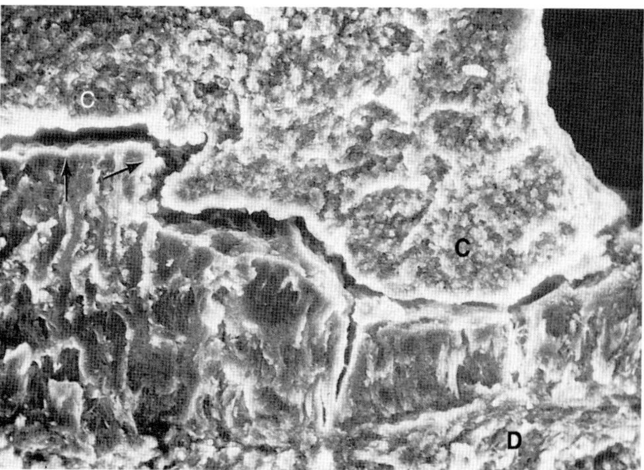

Fig. 24.10 Subgingival calculus *(C)* embedded beneath the cementum surface *(arrows)* and penetrating to the dentin *(D),* thereby making removal difficult. (*Courtesy Dr. John Sottosanti, La Jolla, CA.*)

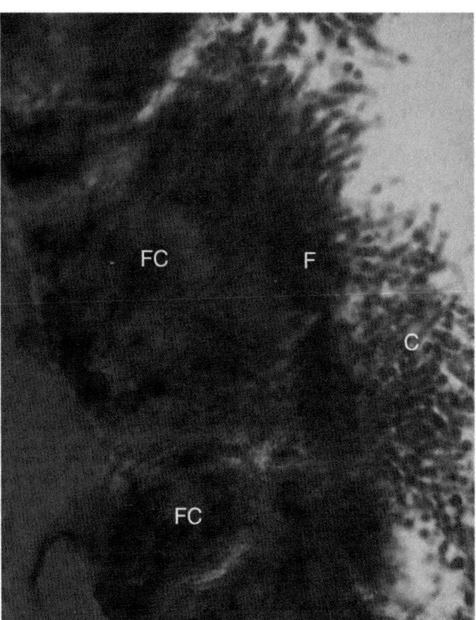

Fig. 24.11 Plaque and calculus on the tooth surface. Note the spherical areas of focal calcification[82] and the perpendicular alignment of the filamentous *(F)* organisms along the inner surface of plaque and cocci *(C)* on the outer surface. (*Courtesy Dr. Erwin Schaffer, Minneapolis, MN.*)

calcium, three times more phosphorus, and less potassium than that of noncalculus formers, suggesting that phosphorus may be more critical than calcium for plaque mineralization.[120] Calcification entails the binding of calcium ions to the carbohydrate–protein complexes of the organic matrix and the precipitation of crystalline calcium phosphate salts.[117] Crystals form initially in the intercellular matrix and on the bacterial surfaces and finally within the bacteria.[63,219]

The calcification of supragingival plaque and the attached component of subgingival plaque begins along the inner surface adjacent to the tooth structure. Separate foci of calcification increase in size and coalesce to form solid masses of calculus (see Fig. 24.11). For the initial mineralization process to occur, calcium phosphate supersaturation, certain membrane-associated components, and regulation of nuclear inhibitors are required.[85] Calcification may be accompanied by alterations in the bacterial content and staining qualities of the plaque. As calcification progresses, the number of filamentous bacteria increases, and the foci of calcification change from basophilic to eosinophilic. There is a reduction in the staining intensity of groups that exhibit a positive periodic acid–Schiff reaction.

Sulfhydryl and amino groups are also reduced and instead stain with toluidine blue, which is initially orthochromatic but becomes metachromatic and disappears.[206] Calculus is formed in layers, which are often separated by a thin cuticle that becomes embedded in the calculus as calcification progresses.[121]

The initiation of calcification and the rate of calculus accumulation vary among individuals, among tooth variety in the same dentition, and at different times in the same person.[135,198] On the basis of these differences, persons may be classified as *heavy, moderate,* or *slight* calculus formers or as noncalculus formers. The average daily increment in calculus formers is from 0.10% to 0.15% of dry weight calculus.[182,198] Calculus formation continues until it reaches a maximum, after which it may be reduced in amount. The time required to reach the maximal level has been reported to be between 10 weeks[38] and 6 months.[203]

The decline from maximal calculus accumulation, which is referred to as the *reversal phenomenon,* may be explained by the vulnerability of bulky calculus to mechanical wear from food and from the cheeks, lips, and tongue movement.

Theories Regarding the Mineralization of Calculus

The theoretical mechanisms by which plaque becomes mineralized can be stratified into two categories.[136]

1. Mineral precipitation results from a local rise in the degree of saturation of calcium and phosphate ions, which may be brought about in several ways:
   - *A rise in the pH of the saliva causes the precipitation of calcium phosphate salts by lowering the precipitation constant.* The pH may be elevated by the loss of carbon dioxide and the formation of ammonia by dental plaque bacteria or by protein degradation during stagnation.[19,77]
   - *Colloidal proteins in saliva bind calcium and phosphate ions and maintain a supersaturated solution with respect to calcium phosphate salts.* With the stagnation of saliva, colloids settle out, and the supersaturated state is no longer maintained, thereby leading to the precipitation of calcium phosphate salts.[155,172]
   - *Phosphatase liberated from dental plaque, desquamated epithelial cells, or bacteria precipitates calcium phosphate by hydrolyzing organic phosphates in saliva, thereby increasing the concentration of free phosphate ions.*[208] *Esterase* is another enzyme that is present in the cocci and filamentous organisms, leukocytes, macrophages, and desquamated epithelial cells of dental plaque.[12] Esterase may initiate calcification by hydrolyzing fatty esters into free fatty acids. The fatty acids form soaps with calcium and magnesium that are later converted into the less-soluble calcium phosphate salts.
2. Seeding agents induce small foci of calcification that enlarge and coalesce to form a calcified mass.[138] This concept has been referred to as the *epitactic concept* or, more appropriately, as *heterogeneous nucleation*. The seeding agents in calculus formation are not known, but it is suspected that the intercellular matrix of plaque plays an active role.[119,134,219] The carbohydrate–protein complexes may initiate calcification by removing calcium from the saliva (chelation) and binding with it to form nuclei that induce the subsequent deposition of minerals.[117,204]

Role of Microorganisms in the Mineralization of Calculus

Mineralization of plaque generally starts extracellularly around both gram-positive and gram-negative organisms, but it may also start intracellularly.[102] Filamentous organisms, diphtheroids, and *Bacterionema* and *Veillonella* species have the ability to form intracellular apatite crystals (see Fig. 24.11). Mineralization spreads until the matrix and the bacteria are calcified.[63,218]

Bacterial plaque may actively participate in the mineralization of calculus by forming phosphatases, which change the pH of the plaque and induce mineralization,[46,117] but the prevalent opinion is that these bacteria are only passively involved[63,165,208] and are simply calcified with other plaque components. The occurrence of calculus-like deposits in germ-free animals supports this opinion.[69] However, other experiments suggest that transmissible factors are involved in calculus formation and that penicillin in the diets of some of these animals reduces calculus formation.[13]

Etiologic Significance

Distinguishing between the effects of calculus and plaque on the gingiva is difficult, because calculus is always covered with a nonmineralized layer of plaque.[173] A positive correlation between the presence of calculus and the prevalence of gingivitis exists,[159] but

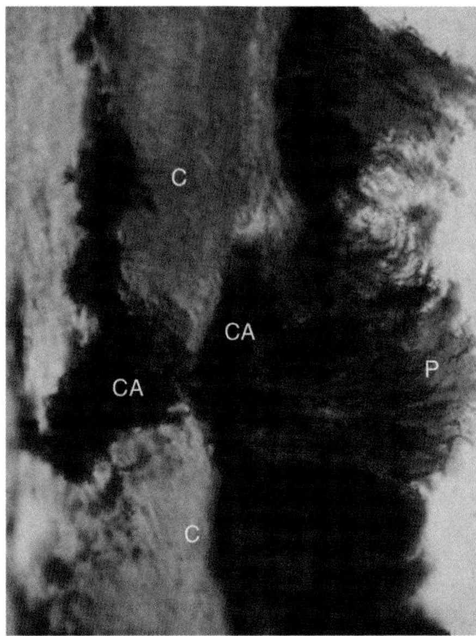

Fig. 24.12 Calculus *(CA)* penetrates the tooth surface and is embedded within the cementum *(C)*. Note the plaque *(P)* attached to the calculus. (*Courtesy Dr. Erwin Schaffer, Minneapolis, MN.*)

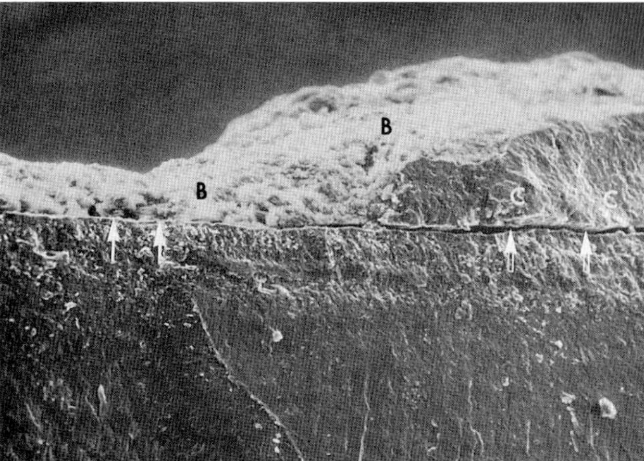

Fig. 24.13 Scanning electron microscope view of an extracted human tooth showing a cross-section of subgingival calculus *(C)* separated *(arrows)* from the cemental surface during processing of the specimen. Note the bacteria *(B)* attached to the calculus and the cemental surfaces. (*Courtesy Dr. John Sottosanti, La Jolla, CA.*)

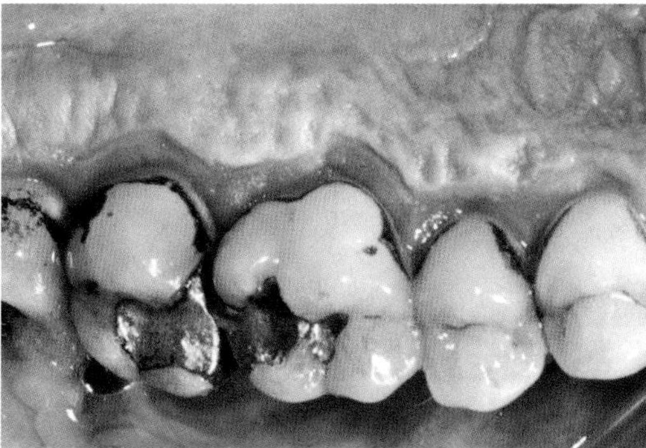

Fig. 24.14 Tobacco stains on the apical third of the clinical crown caused by cigarette smoking.

this correlation is not as great as that between plaque and gingivitis.[65] The initiation of periodontal disease in young people is closely related to plaque accumulation, whereas calculus accumulation is more prevalent in chronic periodontitis found in older adults.[65,109]

The incidence of calculus, gingivitis, and periodontal disease increases with age. It is extremely rare to find periodontal pockets in adults without at least some subgingival calculus being present, although the subgingival calculus may be of microscopic proportions.

Calculus does not contribute directly to gingival inflammation, but it provides a fixed nidus for the continued accumulation of bacterial plaque and its retention in close proximity to the gingiva (Fig. 24.12). Periodontal pathogens such as *Aggregatibacter actinomycetemcomitans, Porphyromonas gingivalis*, and *Treponema denticola* have been found within the structural channels and lacunae of supragingival and subgingival calculus.[139,140]

Subgingival calculus is likely to be the product rather than the cause of periodontal pockets. Plaque initiates gingival inflammation, which leads to pocket formation, and the pocket in turn provides a sheltered area for plaque and bacterial accumulation. The increased flow of gingival crevicular fluid associated with gingival inflammation provides the minerals that mineralize the continually accumulating plaque, resulting in the formation of subgingival calculus (Fig. 24.13). Over a 6-year period, Albandar and colleagues observed 156 teenagers with aggressive periodontitis.[4] They noted that areas with detectable subgingival calculus at the initiation of the study were much more likely to experience a loss of periodontal attachment than sites that did not initially exhibit subgingival calculus.

Although the bacterial plaque that coats the teeth is the main etiologic factor in the development of periodontal disease, the removal of subgingival plaque and calculus constitutes the cornerstone of periodontal therapy. Calculus plays an important role in maintaining and accentuating periodontal disease by keeping plaque in close contact with the gingival tissue and by creating areas where plaque removal is impossible. Therefore, the clinician must not only possess the clinical skill to remove the plaque and calculus, but he or she must also be very conscientious about performing this task.

Materia Alba, Food Debris, and Dental Stains

Materia alba is an accumulation of microorganisms, desquamated epithelial cells, leukocytes, and a mixture of salivary proteins and lipids, with few or no food particles; it lacks the regular internal pattern observed in plaque.[175] It is a yellow or grayish-white, soft, sticky deposit, and it is somewhat less adherent than dental plaque. The irritating effect of materia alba on the gingiva is caused by bacteria and their products.

Most food debris is rapidly liquefied by bacterial enzymes and cleared from the oral cavity by salivary flow and the mechanical action of the tongue, cheeks, and lips. The rate of clearance from the oral cavity varies with the type of food and the individual. Aqueous solutions are typically cleared within 15 minutes, whereas sticky foods may adhere for more than 1 hour.[104,202] Dental plaque is not a derivative of food debris, and food debris is not an important cause of gingivitis.[45,89]

Pigmented deposits on the tooth surface are called *dental stains.* Stains are primarily an aesthetic problem and do not cause inflammation of the gingiva. The use of tobacco products (Fig. 24.14), coffee, tea, certain mouthrinses, and pigments in foods can contribute to stain formation.[115,190]

Other Predisposing Factors

Iatrogenic Factors

Deficiencies in the quality of dental restorations or prostheses are contributing factors to gingival inflammation and periodontal destruction.

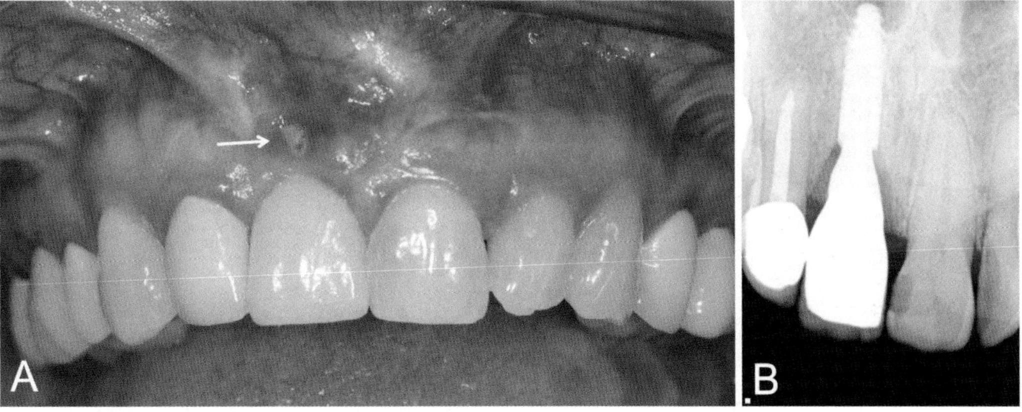

Fig. 24.15 (A) A fenestration defect *(arrow)* is noted after placement of a dental implant too far labial and apical, yielding inadequate bone and blood supply to support the surrounding gingiva. (B) Radiograph of the malpositioned dental implant.

Inadequate dental procedures that contribute to the deterioration of the periodontal tissues are referred to as *iatrogenic factors*. Iatrogenic endodontic complications that can adversely affect the periodontium include root perforations, vertical root fractures, and endodontic failures that may necessitate tooth extraction.[214,216] Immediate implant placement in conjunction with extraction can contribute to an excessive labial and apical position of the implant, whereby the blood supply of surrounding osseous and gingival tissues is compromised, yielding to gingival fenestration or dehiscence (Fig. 24.15).[196] In order to mitigate the risk of dental implant complications, evidence-based clinical guidelines encourage practitioners to consider cone-beam computed tomography (CBCT) for dental implant treatment planning while taking into account the cost, acceptable radiation dose, and risks versus benefits.[199]

Characteristics of dental restorations and removable partial dentures that are important to the maintenance of periodontal health include the location of the gingival margin for the restoration, the space between the margin of the restoration and the unprepared tooth, the contour of the restorations, the occlusion, the materials used in the restoration, the restorative procedure itself, and the design of the removable partial denture. These characteristics are described in this chapter as they relate to the etiology of periodontal disease. A more comprehensive review with special emphasis on the interrelationship between restorative procedures and the periodontal status is presented in Chapter 45.

Margins of Restorations

Overhanging margins of dental restorations contribute to the development of periodontal disease by (1) changing the ecologic balance of the gingival sulcus to an area that favors the growth of disease-associated organisms (predominantly gram-negative anaerobic species) at the expense of the health-associated organisms (predominantly gram-positive facultative species)[104] and (2) inhibiting the patient's access to remove accumulated plaque.

The frequency of overhanging margins on proximal restorations has varied in different studies from 16.5% to 75%.[22,61,82,145] A highly significant statistical relationship has been reported between marginal defects and reduced bone height.[22,70,82] Gilmore and Sheiham noted that persons with overhanging posterior restorations had an average of 0.22 mm reduced alveolar bone support adjacent to the surfaces with overhangs.[61] The removal of overhangs allows for the more effective control of plaque, thereby resulting in a reduction of gingival inflammation and a small increase in radiographic alveolar bone support (Fig. 24.16).[64,74,186]

The location of the gingival margin of a restoration is directly related to the health status of the adjacent periodontal tissues.[184] Numerous studies have shown a positive correlation between

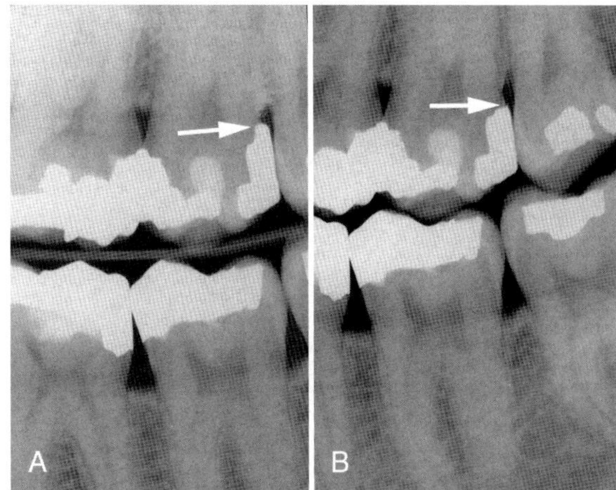

Fig. 24.16 (A) Radiograph of an amalgam overhang on the distal surface of the maxillary second molar that is a source of plaque retention and gingival irritation. (B) Radiograph depicts the removal of excessive amalgam.

restoration margins located apical to the marginal gingiva and the presence of gingival inflammation.[61,79,88,162,186] Subgingival margins are associated with large amounts of plaque, more severe gingivitis, deeper pockets, and a change in the composition of the subgingival microflora that closely resembles the microflora noted in chronic periodontitis.[101] Even high-quality restorations with clinically perfect margins, if placed subgingivally, will increase plaque accumulation, gingival inflammation,[101,104,132,137,163,185] and the rate of gingival crevicular fluid flow.[16,66] Margins placed at the level of the gingival crest induce less severe inflammation, whereas supragingival margins are associated with a degree of periodontal health similar to that seen with nonrestored interproximal surfaces.[55,184]

Roughness in the subgingival area is considered to be a major contributing factor to plaque buildup and subsequent gingival inflammation.[184] The subgingival zone is composed of the margin of the restoration, the luting material, and the prepared and unprepared tooth surfaces. Sources of marginal roughness include grooves and scratches in the surface of acrylic resin, porcelain, or gold restorations (Fig. 24.17); separation of the restoration margin and the luting material from the cervical finish line, thereby exposing the rough surface of the prepared tooth (Fig. 24.18); dissolution and disintegration of the luting material between the preparation and the restoration, thereby leaving a space; and inadequate marginal fit of the restoration.[184]

Subgingival margins typically have a gap of 20 to 40 μm between the margin of the restoration and the unprepared tooth.[181] Colonization of this gap by bacterial plaque undoubtedly contributes

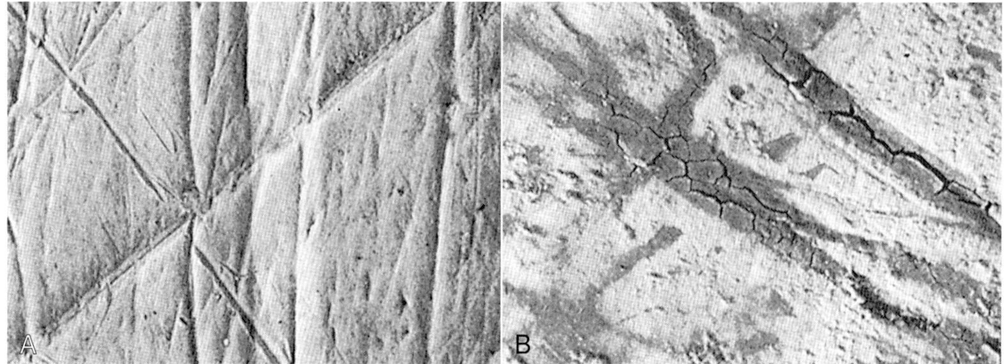

Fig. 24.17 (A) Polished gold alloy crown demonstrating surface scratches. (B) Gold alloy crown that had been in the patient's mouth for several years has scratches filled with deposits. (*From Silness J. Fixed prosthodontics and periodontal health.* Dent Clin North Am. *1980;24[2]:317–329.*)

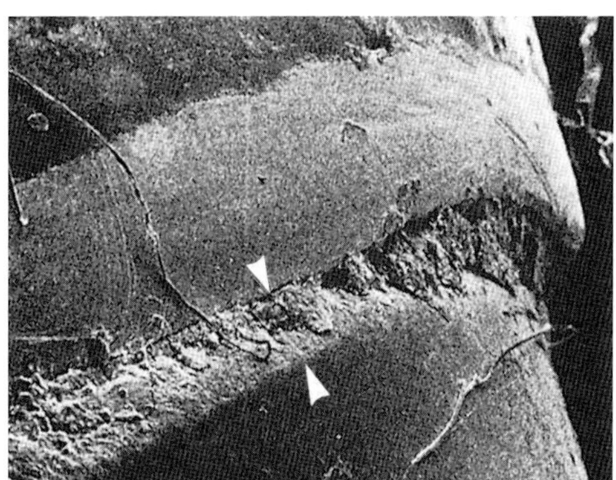

Fig. 24.18 After cementation, luting material prevents the approximation of the crown margin and the finishing line, thereby leaving part of the prepared tooth uncovered *(area between arrowheads).* (*From Silness J. Fixed prosthodontics and periodontal health.* Dent Clin North Am. *1980;24[2]:317–329.*)

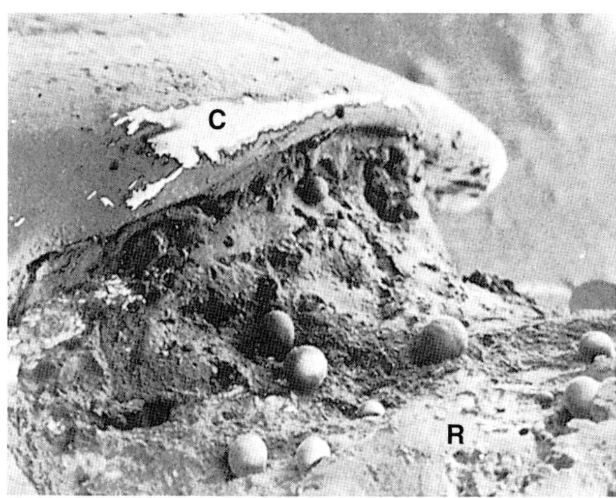

Fig. 24.19 A void has developed after dissolution and disintegration of the luting material. Spherical bodies are not identified. *C,* Crown; *R,* root. (*From Silness J. Fixed prosthodontics and periodontal health.* Dent Clin North Am. *1980;24[2]:317–329.*)

to the detrimental effect of margins placed in a subgingival environment (Fig. 24.19).

Retained Cement and Peri-Implantitis

Peri-implantitis is an inflammatory disease of the tissues around dental implants resulting in progressive bone loss (Fig. 24.20A and B), whereas peri-implant mucositis is a reversible inflammatory change of the soft tissues around implants without bone loss.[110] The prevalence of peri-implantitis among implant-supported prostheses/restorations ranges from 28% to 56%.[221]

The early diagnosis of this condition and its proper management are critical to the longevity of the implant and the supported prosthesis.

Complex microbiota colonize pristine peri-implant crevices within a week after implant placement, and the microbiota associated with failing implants is significantly different from that of healthy implants.[25,78,105,157,171] Classic studies that explored the composition of the peri-implant biofilm in disease have shown that peri-implantitis is an infection that is dominated by gram-negative bacteria with many similarities to the microbiota that is responsible for the development of periodontal diseases, including *Aggregatibacter actinomycetemcomitans, Porphyromonas gingivalis, Tannerella forsythia,* and *Fusobacterium* species.[157,164,171] The application of new microbiologic approaches has allowed for a broader characterization of the peri-implant microbiome, which has led to the identification of peri-implant-specific microbial lineages such as *Streptococcus mutans* and *Butyrivibrio fibrisolvens.*[100,130,171]

FLASH BACK

Peri-implantitis is frequently associated with crowns exhibiting retained excessive luting cement.

A larger proportion of black-pigmented bacteria are found at peri-implantitis sites in dentate patients as compared with edentulous patients. Presumably these peri-implantitis infectious organisms arise from the sulcular microbiota of the natural dentition.[9] Consequently, it is critical that practitioners evaluate the patient's periodontal status and provide appropriate periodontal therapy in conjunction with implant rehabilitation.

Local factors such as retained residual cement or inadequate seating of the implant abutment or prosthesis can lead to bone loss around an implant (see Fig. 24.20C–E). In a retrospective study, Wilson found that 81% of the implants diagnosed with peri-implantitis had residual cement associated with their cement-retained restorations.[211] The surgical removal of the residual cement resolved the infection and halted the peri-implantitis in 74% of the implants. A deeper crown margin makes it more difficult to remove excess cement. The greatest amount of residual cement was noted when the crown margin was 2 or 3 mm below the gingival margin.[111]

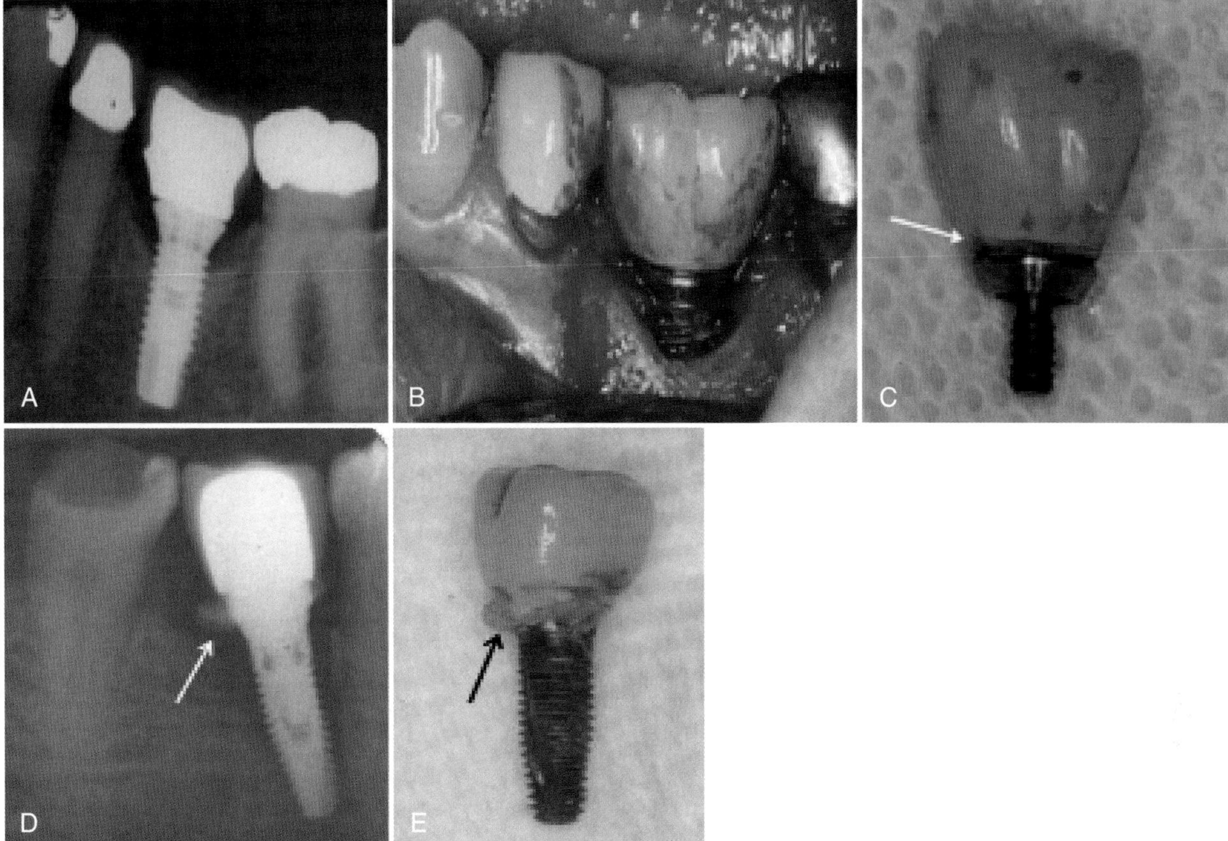

Fig. 24.20 (A) Radiograph of a moat-like bony defect at a peri-implantitis site associated with retained cement and a crown that is not fully seated. (B) Moat-like bony defect and retained excessive cement. (C) The *arrow* points to visibly retained excessive cement between the crown margin and the abutment that prevents the full seating of the crown and leads to hyperocclusion. (D) Radiograph of a peri-implantitis site shows bone loss associated with retained excessive cement *(arrow)*. (E) Retrieved implant restoration shows excessive cement remnants *(arrow)* on implant surface. (*Courtesy Dr. Emilie Vachon, Minneapolis, MN.*)

CLINICAL CORRELATION

The deeper a subgingival crown margin is placed, the higher the likelihood of poorer marginal integrity with accompanying gingival inflammation.

CLINICAL CORRELATION

Overcontoured crowns are more detrimental to periodontal health than undercontoured crowns.

The possible adverse effect of traumatic occlusion on implants has been correlated with early implant failures.[128] However, the relationship between traumatic occlusion and peri-implantitis is, to date, a controversial issue. In vivo experiments have shown that, in the absence of peri-implant inflammation, the application of excessive occlusal stress leads to only minor alterations in the marginal bone level.[95] Alternatively, the application of excessive occlusal forces in the presence of plaque-induced inflammation can significantly increase the rate of bone loss around implant-supported restorations.[35]

Contours and Open Contacts

Overcontoured crowns and restorations tend to accumulate plaque and handicap oral hygiene measures in addition to possibly preventing the self-cleaning mechanisms of the adjacent cheek, lips, and tongue (Fig. 24.21).[8,98,133,212] Restorations that fail to reestablish adequate interproximal embrasure spaces are associated with papillary inflammation. Undercontoured crowns that lack a protective height of contour do not retain as much plaque as overcontoured crowns and therefore may not be as detrimental during mastication as once thought.[212]

The contour of the occlusal surface as established by the marginal ridges and related developmental grooves normally serves to deflect food away from the interproximal spaces. The optimal cervico-occlusal location for a posterior contact is at the longest mesiodistal diameter of the tooth, which is generally just apical to the crest of the marginal ridge. The integrity and location of the proximal contacts along with the contour of the marginal ridges and developmental grooves typically prevent interproximal food impaction. *Food impaction* is the forceful wedging of food into the periodontium by occlusal forces. As the teeth wear down, their originally convex proximal surfaces become flattened, and the wedging effect of the opposing cusp is exaggerated. Cusps that tend to forcibly wedge food into interproximal embrasures are known as *plunger cusps*. The interproximal plunger cusp effect may also be observed when missing teeth are not replaced and the relationship between the proximal contacts of adjacent teeth is altered. An intact proximal contact precludes the forceful wedging of food into the interproximal embrasure space, whereas a light or open contact is conducive to impaction.

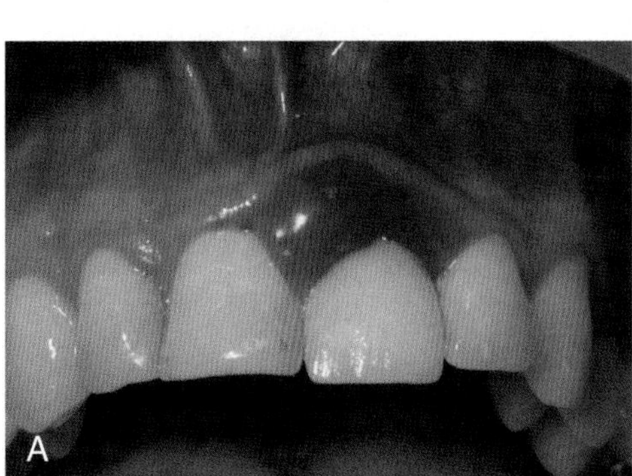
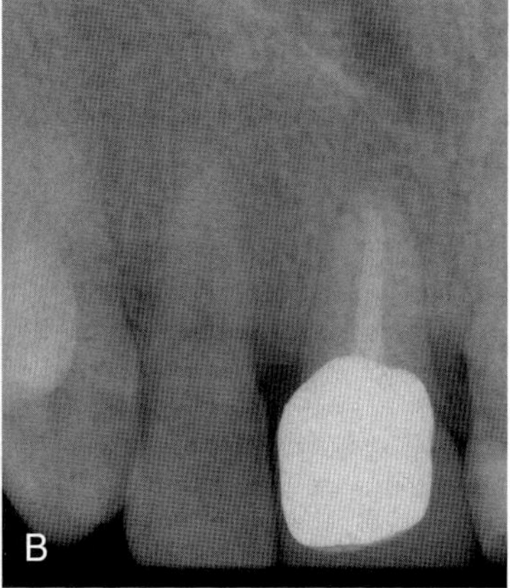

Fig. 24.21 (A) Inflamed marginal and papillary gingiva adjacent to an overcontoured porcelain-fused-to-metal crown on the maxillary left central incisor. (B) Radiograph of an ill-fitting porcelain-fused-to-metal crown.

FLASH BACK

Posterior teeth with open contact and food impaction exhibit greater probing depth and clinical attachment loss than contralateral control sites without food impaction.

The classic analysis of the factors that lead to food impaction was made by Hirschfeld,[76] who recognized the following factors: uneven occlusal wear, opening of the contact point as a result of loss of proximal support or from extrusion, congenital morphologic abnormalities, and improperly constructed restorations.

The presence of the previously mentioned abnormalities does not necessarily lead to food impaction and periodontal disease. A study of interproximal contacts and marginal ridge relationships[104] in three groups of periodontally healthy males revealed that 4.9% to 62.5% of the proximal contacts were defective and that 33.5% of adjacent marginal ridges were uneven.[144] However, greater probing depth and a loss of clinical attachment have been reported for sites that exhibited both an open contact and food impaction as compared with contralateral control sites without open contacts or food impaction.[84] Excessive anterior overbite is a common cause of food impaction on the lingual surfaces of the maxillary anterior teeth and the facial surfaces of the opposing mandibular teeth. These areas may be exemplified by attachment loss with gingival recession.

Materials

In general, restorative materials are not in themselves injurious to the periodontal tissues.[8,91] One exception to this may be self-curing acrylics (Fig. 24.22).[205]

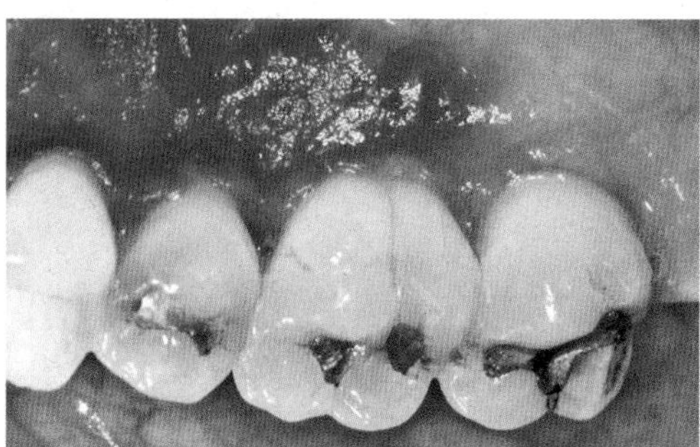

Fig. 24.22 Inflamed palatal gingiva associated with a maxillary provisional acrylic partial denture. Note the substantial difference in color of the inflamed gingiva adjacent to the premolars and the first molar as compared with the gingiva adjacent to the second molar.

Plaque that forms at the margins of restorations is similar to that found on adjacent nonrestored tooth surfaces. The composition of plaque formed on all types of restorative materials is similar, with the exception of that formed on silicate.[138] Although surface textures of restorative materials differ with regard to their capacity to retain plaque,[209] all can be adequately cleaned if they are polished and accessible to methods of oral hygiene.[141,187] The undersurface of pontics in fixed bridges should barely touch the mucosa. Access for oral hygiene is inhibited with excessive pontic-to-tissue contact, thereby contributing to plaque accumulation that will cause gingival inflammation and possibly the formation of pseudopockets.[53,184]

Design of Removable Partial Dentures

Several investigations have shown that, after the insertion of partial dentures, mobility of the abutment teeth, gingival inflammation, and periodontal pocket formation all increase.[21,32,177] This is because partial dentures favor the accumulation of plaque, particularly if they cover the gingival tissue. Partial dentures that are worn during both night and day induce more plaque formation than those worn only during the daytime.[21] These observations emphasize the need for careful and personalized oral hygiene instruction to avoid the harmful effects of partial dentures on the remaining teeth and the periodontium.[16] The presence of removable partial dentures induces not only quantitative changes in dental plaque[60] but also qualitative changes, thereby promoting the emergence of spirochetal microorganisms.[59]

Restorative Dentistry Procedures

The use of rubber dam clamps, matrix bands, and burs in such a manner as to lacerate the gingiva results in varying degrees of mechanical trauma and inflammation. Although such transient injuries generally undergo repair, they are needless sources of discomfort to the patient. The forceful packing of a gingival retraction cord into the sulcus to prepare the subgingival margins of a tooth or for the purpose of obtaining an impression may mechanically injure the periodontium and leave behind impacted debris that is capable of causing a foreign body reaction.

Malocclusion

The irregular alignment of teeth as found in cases of malocclusion may facilitate plaque accumulation and make plaque control more difficult. Several authors have found a positive correlation between crowding and periodontal disease,[31,148,193] whereas other investigators did not find such a correlation.[58] Uneven marginal ridges of

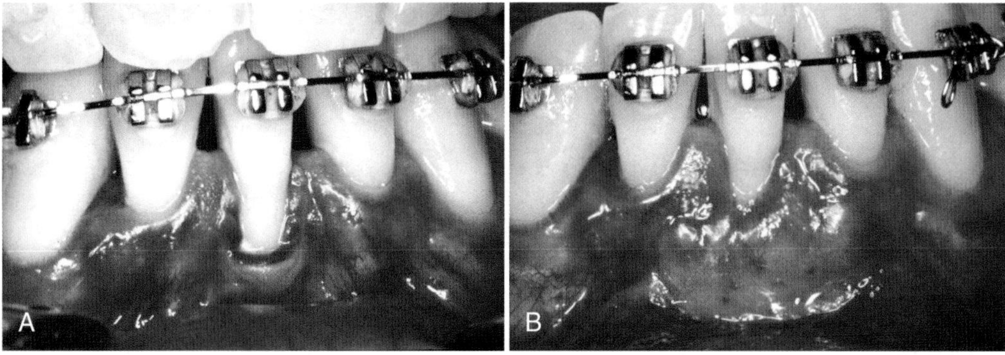

Fig. 24.23 (A) Lower incisor showing a prominent root with gingival recession and a lack of attached gingiva. (B) Appearance 3 months after the placement of a free gingival graft, which resulted in a gain in attached gingiva and a reduction in gingival recession.

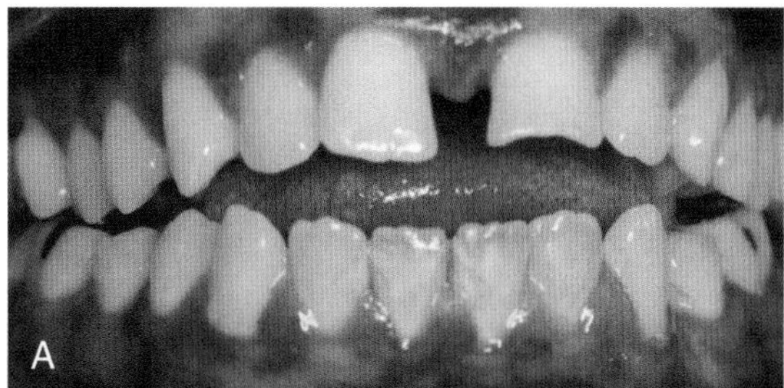

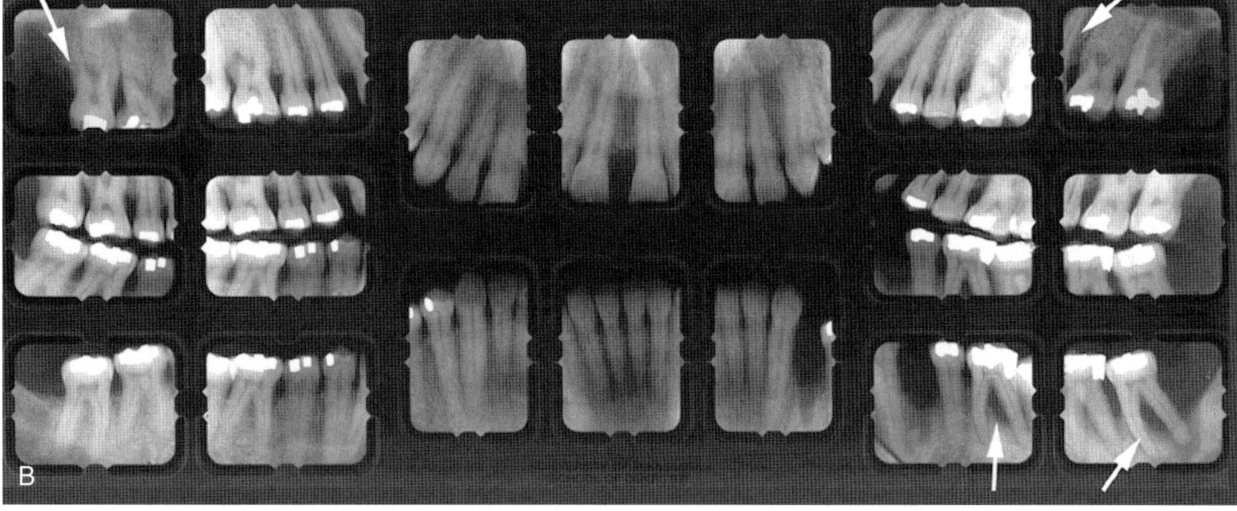

Fig. 24.24 (A) Anterior open bite with flared incisors as observed in association with a habit of tongue thrusting. (B) Radiographs show severe periodontal destruction *(arrows)* in the molar regions.

contiguous posterior teeth have been found to have a low correlation with pocket depth, loss of attachment, plaque, calculus, and gingival inflammation.[93] Roots of teeth that are prominent in the arch (Fig. 24.23)—such as in a buccal or lingual version or that are associated with a high frenal attachment and small quantities of attached gingiva—frequently exhibit recession.[1,127]

The failure to replace missing posterior teeth may have adverse consequences on the periodontal support for the remaining teeth.[34]

The following hypothetical scenario illustrates the possible ramifications of not replacing a missing posterior tooth. When the mandibular first molar is extracted, the initial change is a mesial drifting and tilting of the mandibular second and third molars with extrusion of the maxillary first molar. As the mandibular second molar tips mesially, its distal cusps extrude and act as plungers. The distal cusps of the mandibular second molar wedge between the maxillary first and second molars and open the contact by deflecting the maxillary second molar distally. Subsequently, food impaction may occur and may be accompanied by gingival inflammation with the eventual loss of the interproximal bone between the maxillary first and second molars. This example does not occur in all cases in which mandibular first molars are not replaced. However, the drifting and tilting of the remaining teeth with an accompanying alteration of the proximal contacts is generally a consequence of not replacing posterior teeth that have been extracted.

Tongue thrusting exerts excessive lateral pressure on the anterior teeth, which may result in the spreading and tilting of the anterior teeth (Fig. 24.24). Tongue thrusting is an important contributing factor to tooth migration and the development of an anterior open bite.[33] Mouth breathing may be observed in association with a habit of tongue thrusting and an anterior open bite. Marginal and papillary gingivitis is frequently encountered in the maxillary anterior sextant in cases that involve an anterior open bite with mouth breathing.

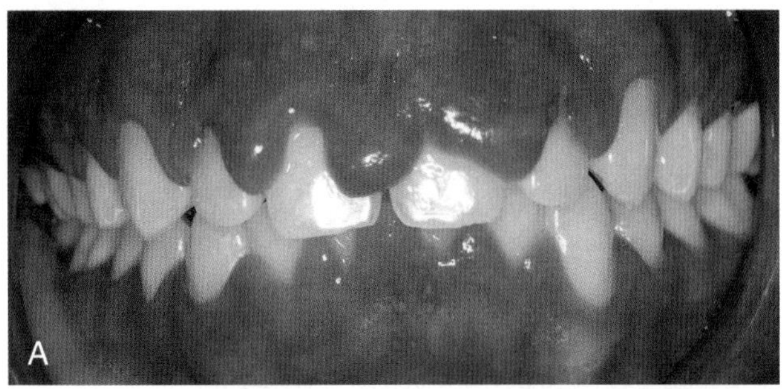

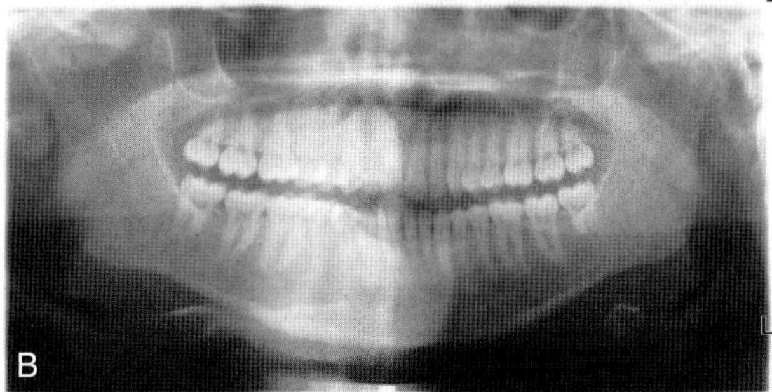

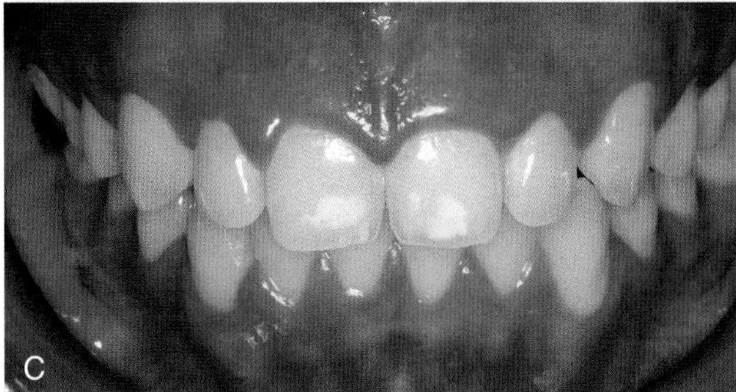

Fig. 24.25 (A) Gingival enlargement noted in a 17-year-old Somalian American who habitually utilizes mouth breathing habit and has a noncontributory medical history including no intake of any medications. (B) Radiographs show no evidence of alveolar bone destruction. (C) Significant reduction in gingival hyperplasia following oral prophylaxis and 6-week usage of 0.12% chlorhexidine mouthrinse and Vaseline application. Note: Surgical procedure was not performed due to insurance denial. (*Courtesy Dr. John Pizarek, Minneapolis, MN.*)

However, the role of mouth breathing as a local causative factor is unclear, because conflicting evidence has been reported.[5,80,81,193] Several case reports of gingival hyperplasia have been associated with mouth breathing (Fig. 24.25).[2,3,15] Although considered as inflammatory, the exact mechanism of gingival overgrowth in mouth breathers is unclear. It is thought to be due to alternate wetting and drying of the gingival surface. A diagnostic feature of this type of enlargement is the presence of significant overgrowth in the maxillary and mandibular anterior regions without any involvement of posterior regions.

Restorations that do not conform to the occlusal pattern of the mouth result in occlusal disharmonies that may cause injury to the supporting periodontal tissues. More issues involving deeper initial probing depths, worse prognoses, and greater mobility have been observed for teeth with occlusal discrepancies as compared with teeth without initial occlusal discrepancies.[72,142] Histologic features of the periodontium for a tooth that has been subjected to traumatic occlusion include a widened subcrestal periodontal ligament space, a reduction in the collagen content of the oblique and horizontal fibers, an increase in vascularity and leukocyte infiltration, and an increase in the number of osteoclasts on bordering alveolar bone.[18] However, these observations are generally apical and separate from

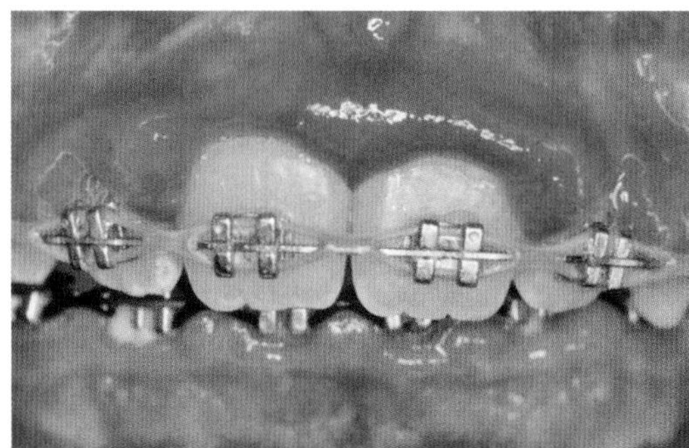

Fig. 24.26 Gingival inflammation and enlargement associated with an orthodontic appliance and poor oral hygiene.

the bacteria-induced inflammation that occurs at the base of the sulcus. On the basis of current human trials, it is still impossible to definitively answer the question, "Does occlusal trauma modify the progression of periodontal attachment loss that is associated with periodontal inflammation?"[179]

(See Chapters 32 and 35 for a more detailed explanation of periodontal trauma from occlusion and the periodontal response to external forces.)

Periodontal Complications Associated With Orthodontic Therapy

Orthodontic therapy may affect the periodontium by favoring plaque retention, by directly injuring the gingiva as a result of overextended bands, and by creating excessive forces, unfavorable forces, or both on the tooth and its supporting structures.

Plaque Retention and Composition

Orthodontic appliances tend to retain bacterial plaque and food debris, thereby resulting in gingivitis (Fig. 24.26), and they are also capable of modifying the gingival ecosystem. Scanning electron microscopic examination of the orthodontic bracket–tooth junction shows that excess bonding composite around the bracket base creates a critical site for plaque accumulation due to its rough surface texture and the presence of a distinct gap at the composite—enamel interface. A complex community of bacterial plaque may be noted on the excess composite material within 2 to 3 weeks after bonding.[192] An increase in *Prevotella melaninogenica, Prevotella intermedia,* and *Actinomyces odontolyticus* and a decrease in the proportion of facultative microorganisms was detected in the gingival sulcus after the placement of orthodontic bands.[43] More recently, *A. actinomycetemcomitans* was found in at least one site in 85% of children who were wearing orthodontic appliances.[146]

By contrast, only 15% of unbanded control subjects were positive for *A. actinomycetemcomitans*.

KEY FACT

Orthodontic treatment should not be commenced in the presence of uncontrolled periodontal disease because it will worsen the periodontal condition.

Gingival Trauma and Alveolar Bone Height

Orthodontic treatment is often started soon after the eruption of the permanent teeth, when the junctional epithelium is still adherent to the enamel surface. Orthodontic bands should not be forcefully placed beyond the level of attachment, because this will detach the gingiva from the tooth and result in the apical proliferation of the junctional epithelium with an increased incidence of gingival recession.[149]

KEY FACT

Adult patients planning to undergo orthodontic care should undergo pretreatment assessment for their periodontal status and potential risk for root resorption.

The mean alveolar bone loss per patient for adolescents who underwent 2 years of orthodontic care during a 5-year observation period ranged between 0.1 and 0.5 mm.[24] This small magnitude of alveolar bone loss was also noted in the control group and therefore is considered to be of little clinical significance. However, the degree of bone loss during adult orthodontic care may be higher than that observed in adolescents,[116] especially if the periodontal condition is not treated before the initiation of orthodontic therapy. Orthodontic treatment in adults with active periodontitis (evidenced by deep pockets and bleeding on probing) has been shown to accelerate the periodontal disease process.[10,48,215] *Therefore, orthodontic treatment should not be commenced in the presence of uncontrolled periodontal disease.*

Tissue Response to Orthodontic Forces

Orthodontic tooth movement is possible because the periodontal tissues are responsive to externally applied forces.[161,176] Alveolar bone is remodeled by osteoclasts that induce bone resorption in areas of pressure and by osteoblasts that form bone in areas of tension. Although moderate orthodontic forces ordinarily result in bone remodeling and repair, excessive force may produce necrosis of the periodontal ligament and the adjacent alveolar bone.[152–154] Excessive orthodontic forces also increase the risk of apical root resorption.[28,29] The prevalence of severe root resorption (i.e., resorption of more than one-third of the root length) during orthodontic therapy in adolescents has been reported to be 3%.[86] The incidence of moderate to severe root resorption for incisors among adults aged 20 to 45 years has been reported to be 2% before treatment and 24.5% after treatment.[116] Risk factors associated with root resorption during orthodontic treatment include the duration of treatment, the magnitude of the force applied, the direction of the tooth movement, and the continuous versus intermittent application of forces[151] (Fig. 24.27).

KEY FACT

It is important to avoid excessive force and too-rapid tooth movement during orthodontic treatment to prevent injury to the periodontium.

The use of elastics to close a diastema may result in severe attachment loss with possible tooth loss as the elastics migrate apically along the root surface (Fig. 24.28). The surgical exposure of impacted teeth and orthodontic-assisted eruption has the potential to compromise periodontal attachment on adjacent teeth (Fig. 24.29). However, the majority of impacted teeth that are surgically exposed and aided in their eruption by orthodontic treatment subsequently exhibited more than 90% of their attachment as being intact.[75]

It has been reported that the dentoalveolar gingival fibers that are located within the marginal and attached gingiva are stretched when teeth are rotated during orthodontic therapy.[44] The surgical severing or removal of these gingival fibers in combination with a brief period of retention may reduce the incidence of relapse after orthodontic treatment that is intended to realign rotated teeth.[27,129]

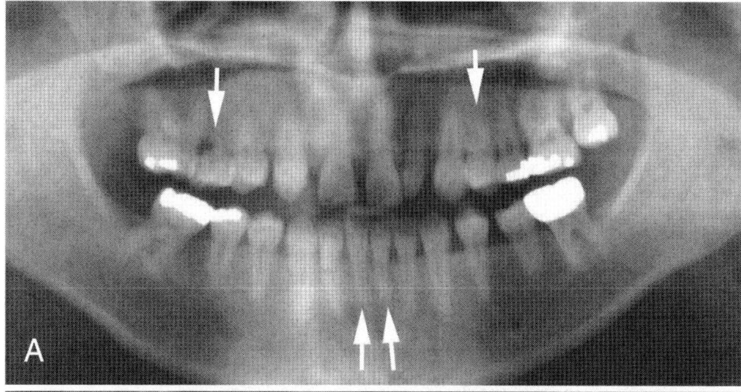

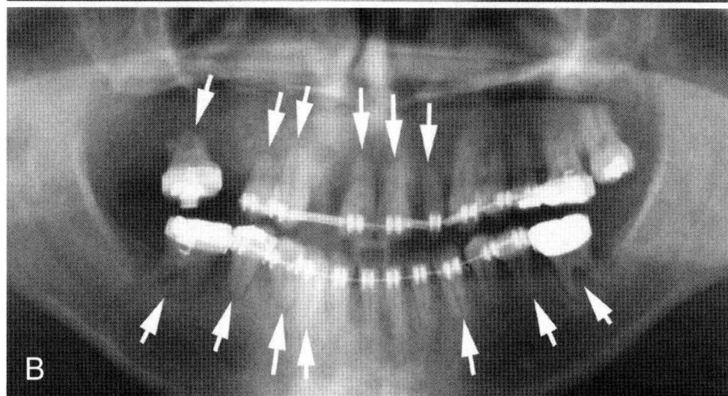

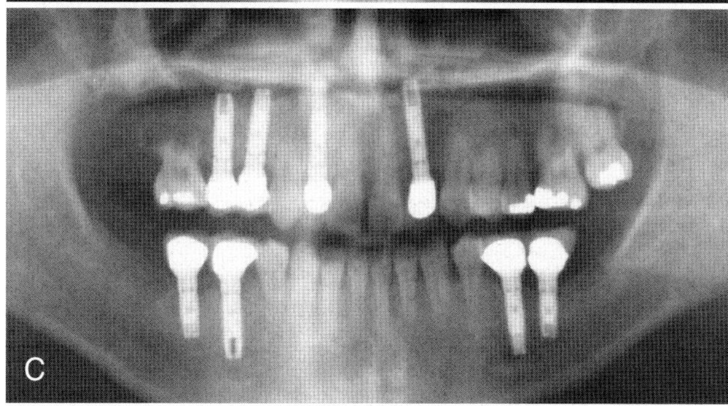

Fig. 24.27 (A) Panoramic radiograph illustrating that a limited degree of pretreatment root resorption *(arrows)* existed before orthodontic care. (B) Note that several roots have undergone severe resorption *(arrows)* during 4 years of intermittent orthodontic treatment. (C) The teeth that developed extensive root resorption with accompanying hypermobility have been extracted and replaced with implant-supported crowns.

Extraction of Impacted Third Molars

Numerous clinical studies have reported that the extraction of impacted third molars often results in the creation of vertical defects distal to the second molars.[11,99,124] This iatrogenic effect is unrelated to flap design,[156] and it appears to occur more often when third molars are extracted from individuals who are more than 25 years old.[11,99,124] Other factors that appear to play a role in the development of lesions on the distal surface of second molars—particularly in those who are more than 25 years old—include the presence of visible plaque, bleeding on probing, root resorption in the contact area between the second and third molars, the presence of a pathologically widened follicle, the inclination of the third molar, and the close proximity of the third molar to the second molar (Fig. 24.30).[99] Other potential iatrogenic adverse consequences of the removal of third molars include permanent paresthesia (i.e., numbness of the lip, tongue, and cheek), damage to adjacent teeth, mandibular fracture, maxillary tuberosity fracture, displacement of third molars and root tips, oro-antral communications or fistula, and temporomandibular joint complications.[26] Permanent paresthesia occurs at a frequency of approximately 1 of every 100,000 wisdom teeth removed in the United States.[56] The incidence of damage to second molar as a consequence of third molar extraction has been estimated to be 0.3% to 0.4%.[36] Although the incidence of mandibular fracture during or after third

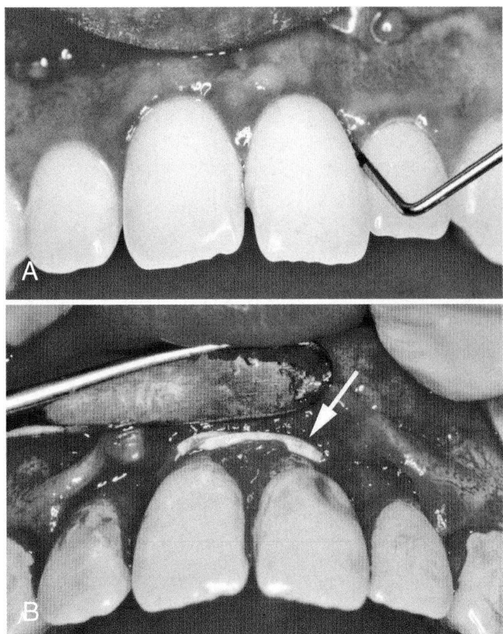

Fig. 24.28 (A) Maxillary central incisors for which an elastic ligature was used to close a midline diastema. Note the inflamed gingiva and the deep probing depths. (B) Reflection of a full-thickness mucoperiosteal flap reveals elastic ligature *(arrow)* and angular intrabony defects around the central incisors.

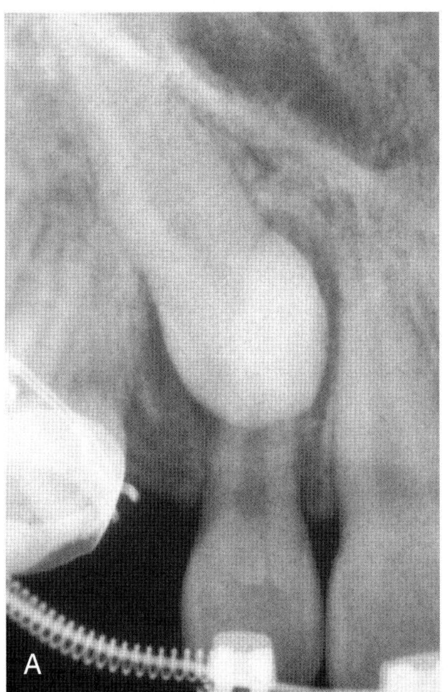

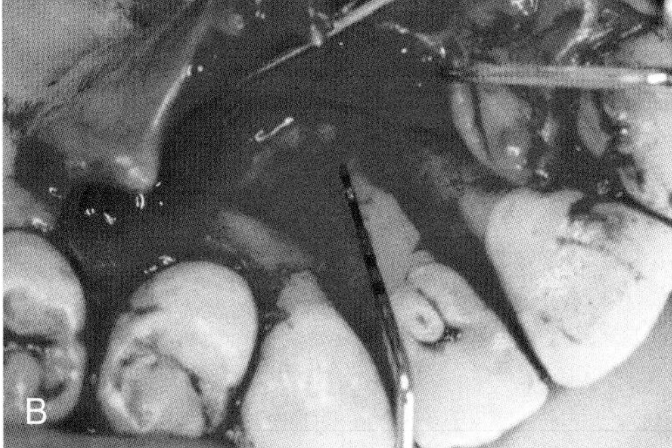

Fig. 24.29 (A) Radiograph of an impacted maxillary canine that required surgical exposure and orthodontic assistance to erupt. (B) A palatal flap is reflected to reveal bony dehiscence on the maxillary lateral incisor after orthodontic therapy.

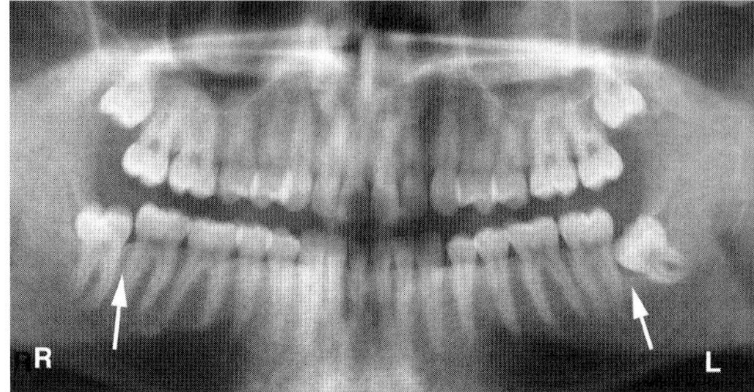

Fig. 24.30 Panoramic radiograph illustrating a mesially impacted lower left third molar with a widened follicle and no apparent bone on the distal interproximal surface of the second molar. Alternatively, the lower right third molar is vertically impacted and exhibits interproximal bone distal to the second molar and mesial to the third molar.

molar removal is low (0.003% to 0.005%)[108], it may pose important medicolegal and patient care implications. Iatrogenic displacement of a maxillary third molar into the maxillary sinus[147,213] and displacement of a mandibular third molar into the sublingual, submandibular, pterygomandibular, and lateral pharyngeal spaces[50,213] have been reported with unknown incidence rates.

FLASH BACK

Preoperative use of three-dimensional radiographs in conjunction with extraction of impacted third molars has the potential to minimize the risk of inferior alveolar nerve paresthesia or damage to the adjacent second molar.

For several decades, panoramic radiography has been the standard of choice to assess the state of third molar impaction, including angulation of the tooth, root morphology, root development, related pathology, and, most importantly, the relation between the tooth or roots and the mandibular canal. However, when an overprojection is observed between the impacted third molar and the mandibular canal, or when specific signs suggest a close contact between the third molar and the mandibular canal, CBCT is recommended to be more beneficial in proper treatment planning (Fig. 24.31).[126]

Habits and Self-Inflicted Injuries

Patients may not be aware of their self-inflicted injurious habits that may be important to the initiation and progression of their periodontal disease. Mechanical forms of trauma can stem from the improper use of a toothbrush, the wedging of toothpicks between the teeth, the application of fingernail pressure against the gingiva (Fig. 24.32), pizza burns, and other causes.[23] Sources of chemical irritation include the topical application of caustic medications such as aspirin or cocaine, allergic reactions to toothpaste or chewing gum, the use of chewing tobacco, and concentrated mouthrinses.[180] Accidental and iatrogenic gingival injuries may be caused by a variety of chemical, physical, and thermal sources, yet they are generally self-limited. Iatrogenic injuries are often acute, whereas factitious injuries tend to be more chronic in nature.[160]

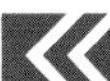

FLASH BACK

Sources of self-inflicted injuries include improper use of toothbrushes, wedging toothpicks between teeth, application of fingernail pressure against gingiva, and pizza burn. Chemical sources include topical application of caustic medications, such as aspirin or cocaine, allergic reaction to toothpaste or chewing gum, use of chewing tobacco, and concentrated mouthrinses.

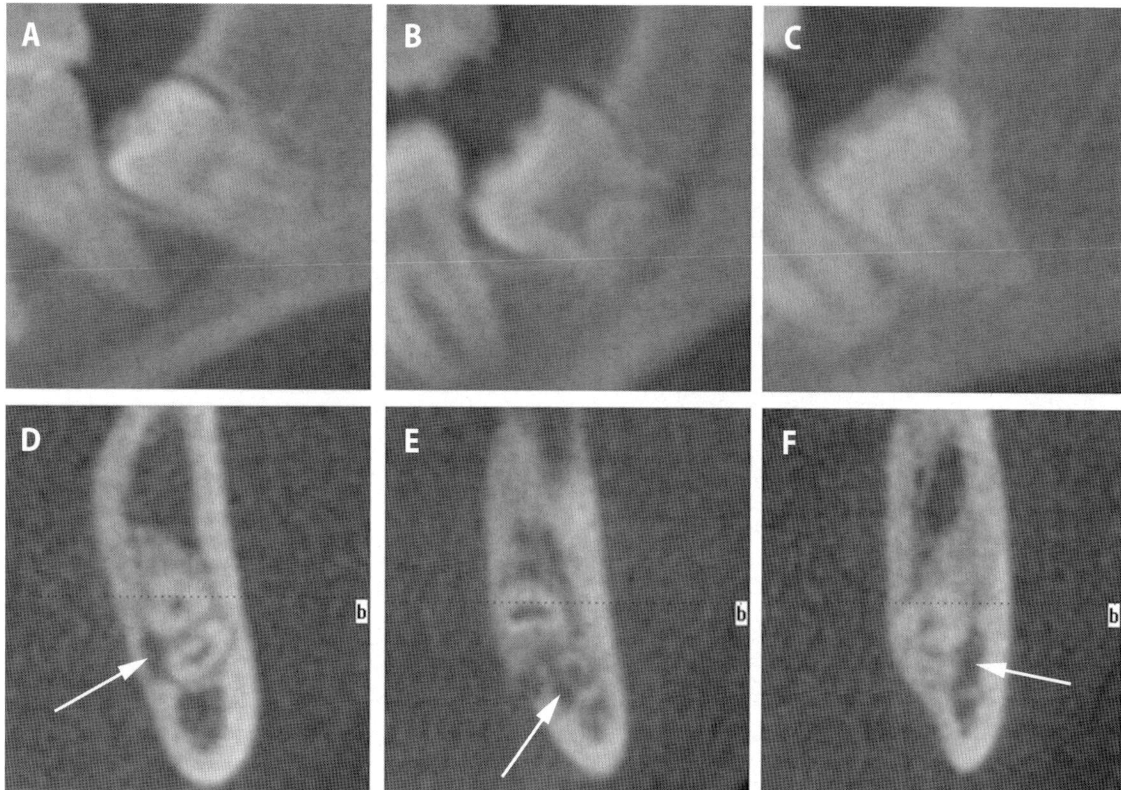

Fig. 24.31 Segmented panoramic images. (A and B) Overprojection between the impacted third molar and the mandibular canal. (C) Signs of close contact between the third molar and the mandibular canal. (D through F) Corresponding cone-beam computed tomographic images (*axial views*) of the impacted third molars reveal the path of the inferior alveolar nerve *(arrow)* (D) lingual to the root, (E) surrounded by three segments of the root, and (F) buccal to the root. (*Courtesy Dr. Mansur Ahmad, Minneapolis, MN.*)

Trauma Associated With Oral Jewelry

The use of piercing jewelry in the lip or tongue has become more common among teenagers and young adults (Fig. 24.33A). However, piercings are associated with potential complications including gingival injury or recession[73,103,107,217,220]; damage to teeth, restorations and fixed porcelain prostheses[51,57,73,107]; increased salivary flow[57,200]; interference with speech, mastication, or deglutition[87,201]; scar-tissue formation[200]; and development of metal hypersensitivities.[96]

Use of tongue- or lip-piercing jewelry is associated with localized gingival recession and periodontitis.

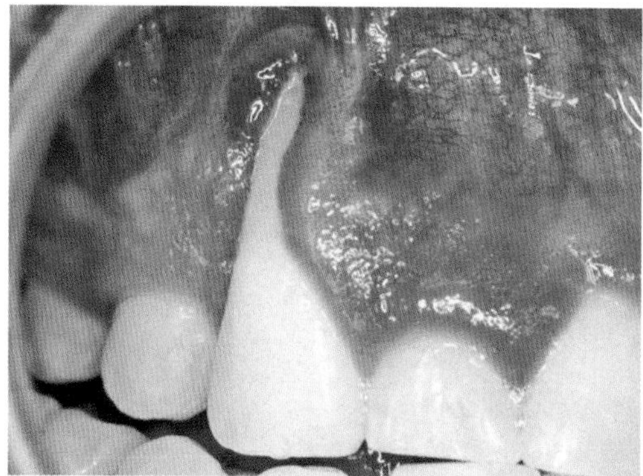

Fig. 24.32 Gingival recession on a maxillary canine caused by self-inflicted trauma from the patient's fingernail.

Whittle and Lamden[210] surveyed 62 dentists and found that 97% had seen patients with either lip- or tongue-piercing jewelry within the previous 12 months. The incidence of lingual recession with pocket formation (see Fig. 24.33B) and radiographic evidence of bone loss (see Fig. 24.33C) was 50% among subjects with a mean age of 22 years who wore lingual "barbells" for 2 years or longer.[41] Chipped lower anterior teeth were noted in 47% of the patients who wore tongue-piercing jewelry for 4 years or longer. Patients need to be informed of the risks of wearing oral jewelry and cautioned against such practices.

Toothbrush Trauma

Abrasions of the gingiva as well as alterations in tooth structure may result from aggressive toothbrushing in a horizontal or rotary fashion. The deleterious effect of excessively forceful brushing is accentuated when highly abrasive dentifrices are used. The gingival changes that are attributable to toothbrush trauma may be acute or chronic. The acute changes vary with regard to their appearance and duration, from scuffing of the epithelial surface to denudation of the underlying connective tissue with the formation of a painful gingival ulcer (Fig. 24.34). Diffuse erythema and denudation of the attached gingiva throughout the mouth may be a striking result of overzealous brushing. Signs of acute gingival abrasions are frequently noted when the patient first uses a new brush. Puncture lesions may be produced when heavy pressure is applied to firm bristles that are aligned perpendicular to the surface of the gingiva. A forcibly embedded toothbrush bristle can be retained in the gingiva and cause an acute gingival abscess.

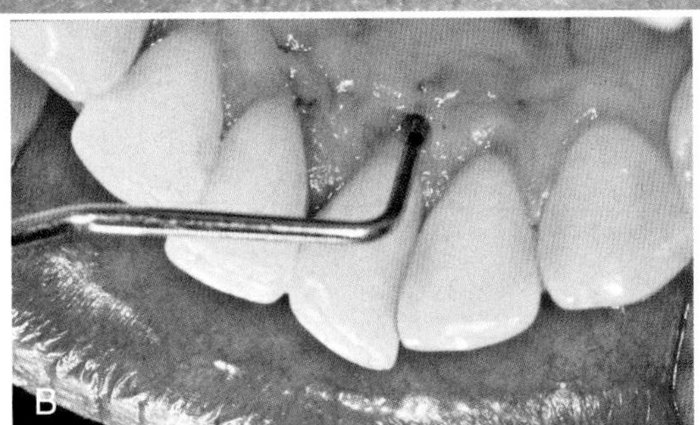

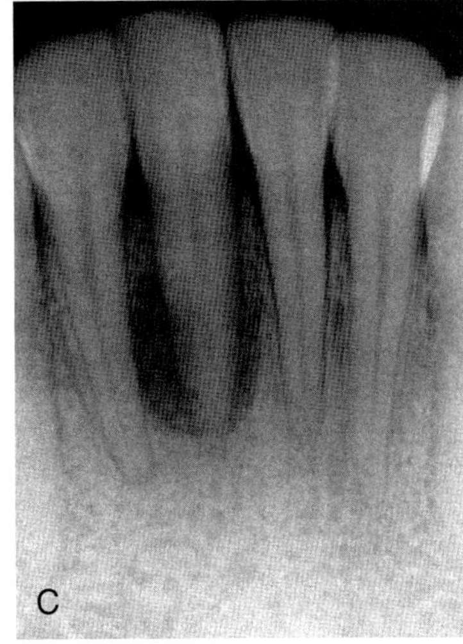

Fig. 24.33 (A) Tongue pierced with oral jewelry. (B) Probing depth of 8 mm with 10 mm of clinical attachment loss on the lingual surface of the lower central incisor adjacent to the oral jewelry in the pierced tongue. The central incisor was found to be vital. (C) Bone loss associated with a tongue pierced by oral jewelry. (*B, Courtesy Dr. Leonidas Batas, Thessaloniki, Greece.*)

Chronic toothbrush trauma results in gingival recession with denudation of the root surface. Interproximal attachment loss is generally a consequence of bacteria-induced periodontitis, whereas buccal and lingual attachment loss is frequently the result of toothbrush abrasion.[188] The improper use of dental floss may result in lacerations of the interdental papilla.

Chemical Irritation

Acute gingival inflammation may be caused by chemical irritation that results from either sensitivity or nonspecific tissue injury. In allergic inflammatory states, the gingival changes range from simple erythema to painful vesicle formation and ulceration. Severe reactions to ordinarily innocuous mouthwashes, dentifrices, and denture materials are often explainable on this basis.

Acute inflammation with ulceration may be produced by the nonspecific injurious effect of chemicals on the gingival tissues.

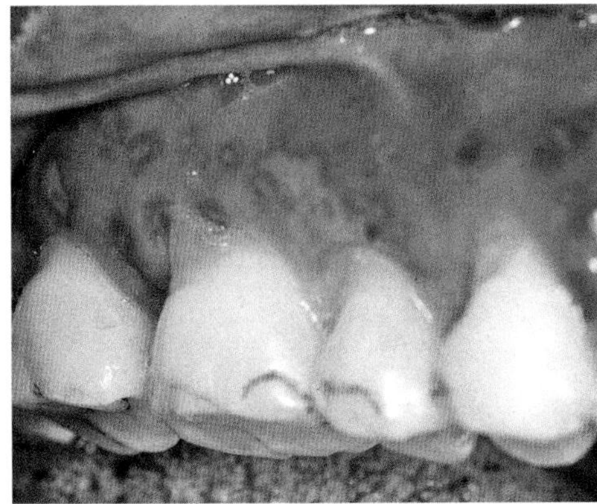

Fig. 24.34 The overzealous use of a toothbrush resulted in denudation of the gingival epithelial surface and exposure of the underlying connective tissue as a painful ulcer.

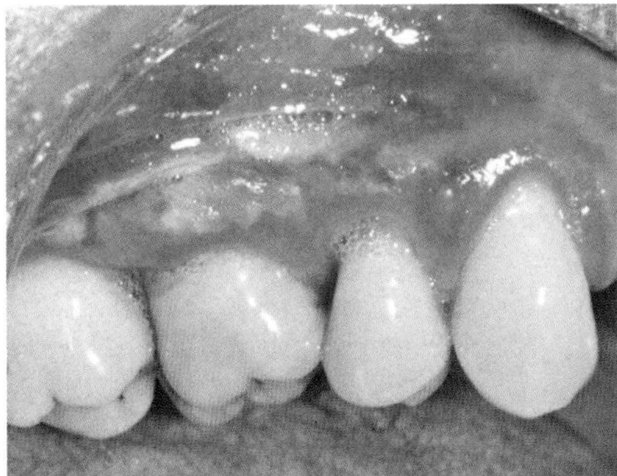

Fig. 24.35 Chemical burn caused by aspirin. Note the sloughing gingival tissue and the resultant recession.

The indiscriminate use of strong mouthwashes, the topical application of corrosive drugs such as aspirin (Fig. 24.35) or cocaine, and accidental contact with drugs such as phenol or silver nitrate are common examples of chemical exposures that cause irritation of the gingiva. A histologic view of an aspirin-induced chemical burn shows vacuoles with serous exudates and an inflammatory infiltrate in the connective tissue (Fig. 24.36).

Smokeless Tobacco

Snuff and chewing tobacco constitute the two main forms of smokeless tobacco. Snuff is a fine-cut form of tobacco that is available loosely packed or in small sachets. Chewing tobacco is a more coarse-cut tobacco that is available in the form of loose leaves, a solid block, a plug, or a twist of dried leaves. Chewing tobacco is typically placed in the mandibular buccal vestibule for several hours, during which time saliva and dilute tobacco are periodically expectorated.[207] The nicotine uptake of smokeless tobacco is similar to that of smoking cigarettes in that the consumption of a 34-g container of smokeless tobacco is approximately equal to 1.5 packs of cigarettes.[67] Many professional baseball players use chewing tobacco. The perceived benefits of chewing tobacco are those derived from nicotine, including improved mental alertness, diminished reaction time, muscle relaxation, and reduced anxiety and appetite.[68,166] A 1990 survey of 1109 professional baseball players in the United States reported that 39% of the players used smokeless tobacco, with 46% of the users exhibiting leukoplakia within the gingiva or the mucosa (Fig. 24.37).[49] Histologic features of oral leukoplakia associated with smokeless tobacco include (1) a chevron-like pattern of hyperkeratosis with focal areas of inflammation and (2) hyperplasia in the basal cell layer (Fig. 24.38). Increased incidences of gingival recession, cervical root abrasion, and root caries have been reported with the use of smokeless tobacco (Fig. 24.39).[143,167,168,197]

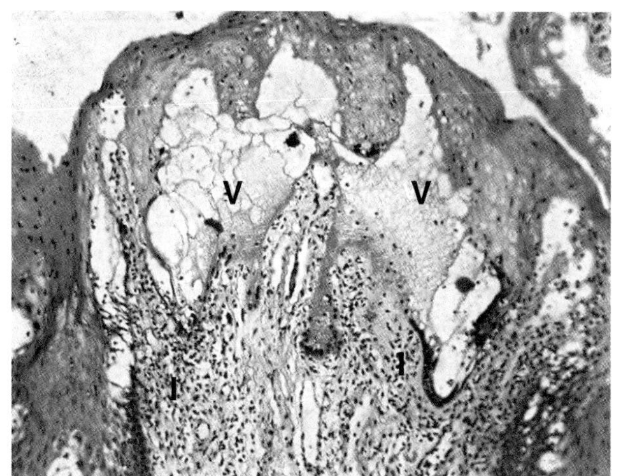

Fig. 24.36 Biopsy of an aspirin-induced chemical burn. Note the intraepithelial vesicles *(V)* and inflammatory infiltrate *(I)* within the underlying connective tissue.

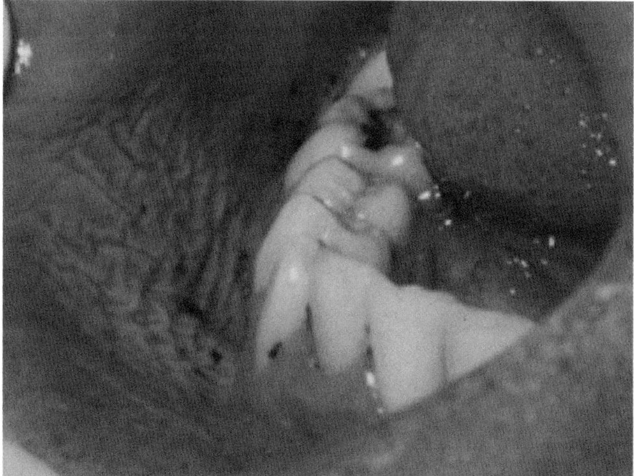

Fig. 24.37 Oral leukoplakia in the vestibule associated with the use of smokeless tobacco.

The incidence of gingival recession among adolescents who use smokeless tobacco has been reported to be 42%, compared with 17% among nonusers.[39,125,127,131] The Third National Health and Nutrition Examination Survey (NHANES III) investigated the adverse effect of smokeless tobacco on the periodontium and found double the incidence of severe periodontitis (odds ratio, 2.1; 95% confidence interval, 1.2 to 3.7) among 12,932 adults who used smokeless tobacco but who never smoked cigarettes.[52] However, Bergstrom and colleagues found similar incidences of severe periodontitis among both smokeless tobacco users and nonusers.[17] It can be concluded that the use of smokeless tobacco is associated with at least localized gingival recession, clinical attachment loss, leukoplakia, and possibly enhanced susceptibility to severe periodontitis.

Radiation Therapy

Radiation therapy has cytotoxic effects on both normal cells and malignant cells. A typical total dose of radiation for head and neck tumors is in the range of 5000 to 8000 centigray (cGy); 1 cGy is equal to 1 radiation absorbed dose (rad) and equivalent to 50 to 80 Sieverts (Sv).[150] The total dose of radiation is usually given in partial incremental doses, and this is referred to as *fractionation.* Fractionation helps to minimize the adverse effects of radiation while maximizing the death rate for the tumor cells.[54] Fractionated doses are typically administered in the range of 100 to 1000 cGy or 1 to 10 Sv per week.

Radiation treatment induces an obliterative endarteritis that results in soft tissue ischemia and fibrosis; irradiated bone becomes hypovascular and hypoxic.[122] Adverse effects of head and neck radiation therapy include dermatitis and mucositis of the irradiated area as well as muscle fibrosis and trismus, which may restrict access to the oral cavity.[169] The mucositis typically develops 5 to 7 days after radiation therapy is initiated. The severity of the mucositis can be reduced by asking the patient to avoid secondary sources of irritation (e.g., smoking, alcohol, spicy foods) to the mucous membrane. The use of a chlorhexidine digluconate mouthrinse may help to reduce the mucositis.[158] However, most chlorhexidine mouthrinses currently available in the United States have a high alcohol content that may act as an astringent, which dehydrates the mucosa and thus intensifies the pain. Saliva production is permanently impaired when salivary glands that are located within the portal of radiation receive 6000 cGy (60 Sv) or more.[123] Xerostomia results in greater plaque accumulation and a reduced buffering capacity of saliva. Effective oral hygiene, professional dental prophylactic cleanings, fluoride applications, and frequent dental examinations are essential to control caries and periodontal disease. The use of customized

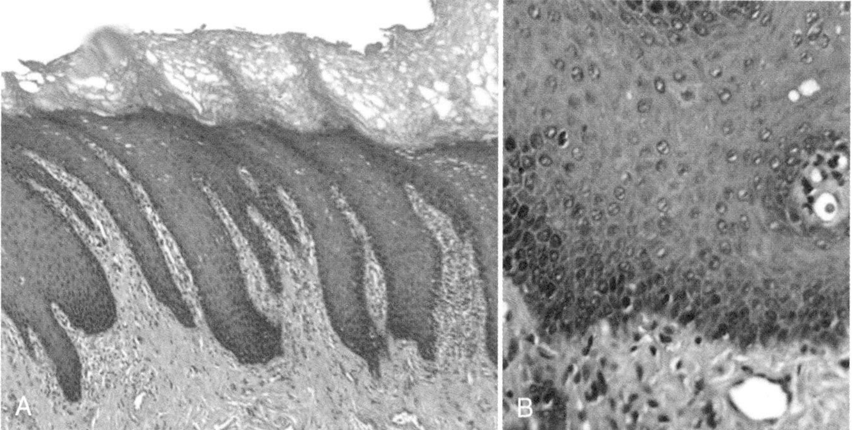

Fig. 24.38 (A) Histologic features of oral leukoplakia associated with smokeless tobacco. Note the chevron-like pattern of hyperkeratosis with focal areas of inflammation. (B) Hyperplasia in the basal cell layer.

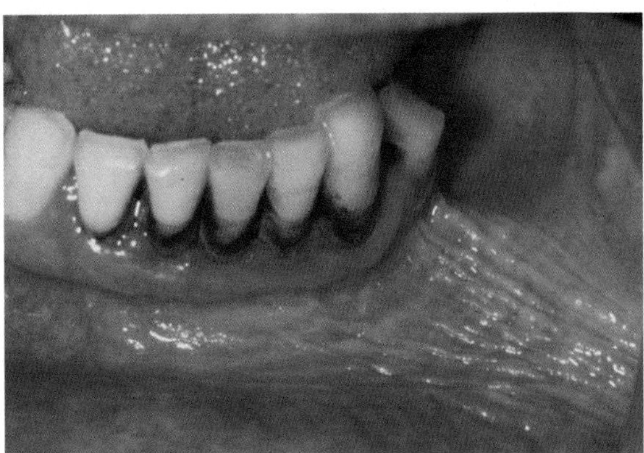

Fig. 24.39 Oral leukoplakia, recession, and clinical attachment loss associated with the use of smokeless tobacco.

trays appears to be a more effective method for fluoride application compared with the toothbrush.[92]

Among cancer patients who were treated with high-dose unilateral radiation, periodontal attachment loss and tooth loss were reported to be greater on the irradiated site compared with the nonradiated control side of the dentition.[47] Patients who are diagnosed with oral cancer and who require radiation therapy should ideally be assessed for dental needs (i.e., mucositis, xerostomia, faulty restorations, periapical lesion, coronal and cervical decay, and periodontal status) before the initiation of radiation treatment.[71] The treatment and prevention of trismus, oral fungal infections, odontogenic infections, osteoradionecrosis, decay, and periodontal disease are critical to minimize oral morbidity for these patients. Dental and periodontal infections have the potential to be severe risks for patients who have been treated with head and neck radiation. The risk of osteoradionecrosis for oncology patients can be minimized by evaluating their oral status, providing dental care, and allowing time for tissue repair before the commencement of radiotherapy.[94]

CLINICAL CORRELATION

Use of smokeless tobacco has been associated with localized gingival leukoplakia, recession, clinical attachment loss, and increased susceptibility to severe periodontitis.

Oral conditions that increase the risk of osteoradionecrosis for patients about to undergo radiation therapy for oral malignancies include periodontal probing depths of more than 5 mm, dental plaque score of more than 40%, and alveolar bone loss of more than 60%.[90] Nonrestorable teeth and teeth with significant periodontal problems should be extracted before radiation therapy to reduce the risk of postradiotherapy osteoradionecrosis (see Chapter 25 for more detail regarding the periodontal management of medically compromised patients).[94]

The risk of osteoradionecrosis must be evaluated before the performance of atraumatic extractions or limited periodontal surgical procedures in previously irradiated sites. Therefore, the dentist may choose to consult with the patient's oncologist before the initiation of dental therapy. A randomized multicenter clinical trial questioned the merit of using hyperbaric oxygen therapy to treat osteoradionecrosis because, at 1 year after treatment, only 19% of test subjects had responded to hyperbaric oxygen therapy, compared with 32% of placebo subjects.[7] The administration of the combination of pentoxifylline with vitamin E as antioxidant therapy currently shows the greatest promise for revascularization and treatment of osteoradionecrosis sites.[42]

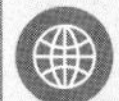

Case Scenarios are found on the companion website eBooks.Health.Elsevier.com.

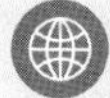

References for this chapter are found on the companion website eBooks.Health.Elsevier.com.

SECTION V: CONDITIONS AFFECTING THE PERIODONTAL PATIENT

CHAPTER 25

Influence of Systemic Conditions on the Periodontium

Perry R. Klokkevold | Brian L. Mealey | Yvonne L. Hernandez-Kapila

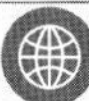

For expanded discussions on female sex hormones, genetic disorders, and nutritional influences on periodontal disease as well as online-only content on hyperparathyroidism, anemia, thrombocytopenia, antibody deficiency disorders, and other systemic conditions, please visit the companion website at eBooks.Health.Elsevier.com.

CHAPTER OUTLINE

Many systemic diseases, disorders, and conditions have been implicated as risk indicators or risk factors in periodontal disease. Clinical and basic science research over the past several decades has led to an improved understanding of and appreciation for the complexity and pathogenesis of periodontal diseases.[200] Although there is clear evidence for a bacterial etiology and there are specific bacteria (periodontal pathogens) associated with destructive periodontal disease, the presence of these pathogens does not invariably cause disease. Their absence, on the other hand, appears to be consistent with periodontal health. The role of bacteria in disease etiology and pathogenesis is discussed in Chapters 8, 10, 11, and 15.[237]

Perhaps the most significant advance in our understanding of the pathogenesis of periodontitis is that the host response varies among individuals and that an altered, deficient, or exaggerated host immune response to bacterial pathogens may lead to more severe forms of the disease.[13] In other words, the individual host immune response to periodontal pathogens is very important and likely explains many of the differences in disease severity observed from one individual to the next. Furthermore, systemic diseases, disorders, and conditions alter host tissues and physiology, which may impair the host's barrier function and immune defense against periodontal pathogens, thereby creating the opportunity for destructive periodontal disease to progress.

Evidence also suggests that periodontal infections can adversely affect systemic health with manifestations such as coronary heart disease, stroke, diabetes, preterm labor, low-birth-weight delivery, and respiratory disease.[65,133,148,178,209,211,283] The role of periodontal infections on these systemic health conditions is discussed in Chapter 26.

The relationships between periodontal infections and host defense are complex. A number of environmental, physical, and psychosocial factors have the potential to alter periodontal tissues and the host immune response, thereby resulting in more severe periodontal disease expression. It is important to recognize that the systemic diseases, disorders, or conditions themselves do not cause periodontitis; rather, they may predispose, accelerate, or otherwise increase the disease's progression. This chapter discusses important systemic diseases, disorders, and conditions that have the potential to influence periodontal health.

Endocrine Disorders and Hormonal Changes

Endocrine diseases such as diabetes and hormonal fluctuations that are associated with puberty and pregnancy are well-known examples of systemic conditions that adversely affect the condition of the periodontium. Endocrine disturbances and hormone fluctuations affect the periodontal tissues directly, modify the tissue response to local factors, and produce anatomic changes in the gingiva that may favor plaque accumulation and disease progression. This section describes the evidence that supports the relationships among endocrine disorders, hormonal changes, and periodontal disease.

Diabetes Mellitus

Diabetes mellitus is an extremely important disease from a periodontal standpoint. It is a complex metabolic disorder characterized by chronic hyperglycemia. Diminished insulin production, impaired insulin action, or a combination of both result in the inability of glucose to be transported from the bloodstream into the tissues, which in turn results in high blood glucose levels and the excretion of sugar in the urine. Lipid and protein metabolism are altered in diabetes as well. Uncontrolled diabetes (chronic hyperglycemia) is associated with several long-term complications, including microvascular diseases (retinopathy, nephropathy, or neuropathy), macrovascular diseases (cardiovascular and cerebrovascular conditions), increased susceptibility to infections, and poor wound healing. An estimated 34.2 million people of all ages, or 10.5% of the US population, have diabetes.[45] The prevalence for those 18 years old or older is 34.1 million or 13%. About 7.3 million (21.4%) of these individuals are undiagnosed. For those individuals 65 years old and older, the prevalence of diabetes is 26.8% with 5.4% of them being unaware they have the disease (undiagnosed). Approximately 88 million American adults have prediabetes.

There are two major types of diabetes, type 1 and type 2, with several less common secondary types. *Type 1 diabetes mellitus,* which was formerly known as *insulin-dependent diabetes mellitus,* is caused by a cell-mediated autoimmune destruction of the insulin-producing beta cells of the islets of Langerhans in the pancreas, which results in insulin deficiency. Type 1 diabetes accounts for 5% to 10% of all cases of diabetes and most often occurs in children and young adults. This type of diabetes results from a lack of insulin production, and it is very unstable and difficult to control. It has a marked tendency toward ketosis and coma, it is not preceded by obesity, and it requires the injection of insulin to be controlled. Patients with type 1 diabetes mellitus present with the symptoms that are traditionally associated with diabetes, including polyphagia, polydipsia, polyuria, and predisposition to infections.

Type 2 diabetes mellitus, which was formerly known as *non–insulin-dependent diabetes mellitus,* is caused by peripheral resistance to insulin action, impaired insulin secretion, and increased glucose production in the liver. The insulin-producing beta cells in the pancreas are not destroyed by cell-mediated autoimmune reaction. It typically begins as insulin resistance, which leads to the reduced production of insulin in the pancreas as the demand increases. Type 2 diabetes is the most common form of diabetes, and it accounts for 90% to 95% of all diagnosed cases in adults. Individuals are often not aware they have the disease until severe symptoms or complications occur. Type 2 diabetes generally occurs in obese individuals, and it can often be controlled by diet and oral hypoglycemic agents. Ketosis and coma are uncommon. Type 2 diabetes can manifest with the same symptoms as type 1 diabetes but typically in a less severe form.

An additional category of diabetes is *hyperglycemia* secondary to other diseases or conditions. A prime example of this type of hyperglycemia is gestational diabetes associated with pregnancy. *Gestational diabetes* develops in 2% to 10% of all pregnancies but disappears after delivery. Women who have had gestational diabetes are at increased risk of developing type 2 diabetes. Other secondary types of diabetes are those associated with diseases that involve the pancreas and the destruction of the insulin-producing cells. Endocrine diseases (e.g., acromegaly, Cushing syndrome), tumors, pancreatectomy, and drugs or chemicals that cause altered insulin levels are included in this group. Experimentally induced types of diabetes generally belong in this category rather than in the categories of type 1 or 2 diabetes mellitus.

KEY FACT

Diabetes mellitus is an extremely important disease that impacts multiple systems including periodontal health. It is a complex metabolic disorder characterized by chronic hyperglycemia. Uncontrolled diabetes is associated with long-term complications, including microvascular diseases (retinopathy, nephropathy, or neuropathy), macrovascular diseases (cardiovascular and cerebrovascular conditions), increased susceptibility to infections, and poor wound healing. An estimated 25.8 million individuals (both children and adults)—8.3% of the US population—have diabetes.[44] Approximately 7 million of these individuals are unaware that they have the disease.

Oral Manifestations

Numerous oral changes have been described in patients with diabetes, including cheilosis, mucosal drying and cracking, burning mouth and tongue, diminished salivary flow, and alterations in the flora of the oral cavity, with greater predominance of *Candida albicans,* hemolytic streptococci, and staphylococci.[1,23,105,173] An increased rate of dental caries has also been observed in patients with poorly controlled diabetes.[80,90] It is important to note that these changes are not always present, that they are not specific, and that they are not pathognomonic for diabetes.[176] Furthermore, these changes are less likely to be observed in patients with well-controlled diabetes. Individuals with controlled diabetes have a normal tissue response, a normally developed dentition, a normal defense against infections, and no increase in the incidence of caries.[256]

The influence of diabetes on the periodontium has been thoroughly investigated. Although it is difficult to make definitive conclusions about the specific effects of diabetes on the periodontium, a variety of changes have been described, including a tendency toward an enlarged gingiva, sessile or pedunculated gingival polyps, polypoid gingival proliferations, abscess formation, periodontitis, and loosened teeth (Fig. 25.1).[120] Perhaps the most striking changes in patients with uncontrolled diabetes are the reductions in the defense mechanisms and the increased susceptibility to infections, which lead to destructive periodontal disease. In fact, periodontal disease is considered to be the sixth complication of diabetes.[163] Periodontitis in patients with type 1 diabetes appears to start after the age of 12 years, and it has a fivefold increased prevalence in teenagers.[53] The prevalence of periodontitis has been reported as 9.8% in 13- to 18-year-old patients, and it increases to 39% in those who are 19 years old and older.

The extensive literature on this subject and the overall impression of clinicians indicate that *periodontal disease in patients with diabetes follows no consistent or distinct pattern.* Severe gingival inflammation, deep periodontal pockets, rapid bone loss, and frequent periodontal abscesses often occur in patients with poorly controlled diabetes and poor oral hygiene (Figs. 25.2 and 25.3).[3] Children with type 1 diabetes tend to have more destruction around

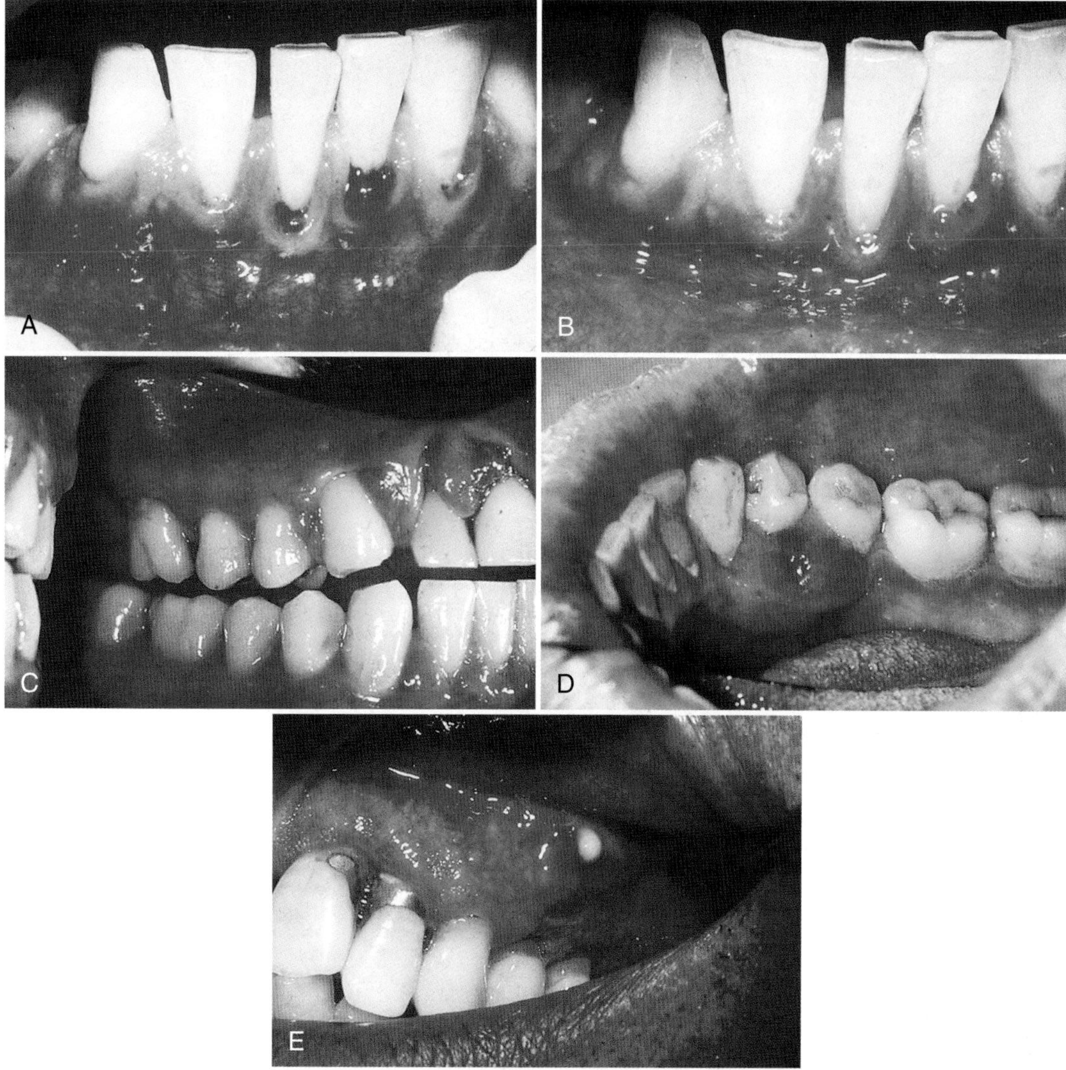

Fig. 25.1 Periodontal condition in patients with diabetes. (A) Adult with diabetes (blood glucose level >400 mg/dL). Note the gingival inflammation, spontaneous bleeding, and edema. (B) The same patient as shown in A. Improved control of diabetes was noted after 4 days of insulin therapy (blood glucose level <100 mg/dL). The clinical periodontal condition has improved without local therapy. (C) Adult patient with uncontrolled diabetes. Note the enlarged, smooth, erythematous gingival margins and papilla in the anterior area. (D) The same patient as shown in C. This is a lingual view of the right mandibular area. Note the inflamed and swollen tissues in the anterior and premolar areas. (E) Adult patient with uncontrolled diabetes. There is a suppurating abscess on the buccal surface of the maxillary premolars.

the first molars and incisors, but this destruction becomes more generalized at older ages.[51] In patients with juvenile diabetes, extensive periodontal destruction often occurs as a consequence of having more severe disease at a younger age.

Other investigators have reported that the rate of periodontal destruction appears to be similar for those with diabetes and those without diabetes up to the age of 30 years.[96,250] Older patients with diabetes have a greater degree of periodontal destruction, possibly related to more disease destruction over time. Patients who have had overt diabetes for more than 10 years have a greater loss of periodontal support than those with a diabetic history of less than 10 years.[96] This destruction may also be related to the diminished tissue integrity, which continues to deteriorate over time (see Altered Collagen Metabolism).

Although some studies have not found a correlation between the diabetic state and the periodontal condition, the majority of well-controlled studies show a higher prevalence and severity of periodontal disease in individuals with diabetes compared with nondiabetic persons with similar local factors.[15,23,42,54,116,190,192,194,253] Findings include a greater loss of attachment, increased bleeding on probing, and increased tooth mobility. A study of risk indicators for a group of 1426 patients between the ages of 25 and 74 years revealed that individuals with diabetes were twice as likely to exhibit attachment loss as nondiabetic individuals.[113] The lack of consistency across studies is most likely related to the different degrees of diabetic involvement, variations in the level of disease control and the diversity of indices, and patient sampling from one study to another.

Studies have suggested that uncontrolled or poorly controlled diabetes is associated with an increased susceptibility to and severity of infections, including periodontitis.[17,226] Adults who are 45 years of age or older with poorly controlled diabetes (i.e., with a glycated hemoglobin level >9%) were 2.9 times more likely to have severe periodontitis than those without diabetes. The likelihood was even greater (4.6 times) among smokers with poorly controlled diabetes.[45] As with other systemic conditions associated

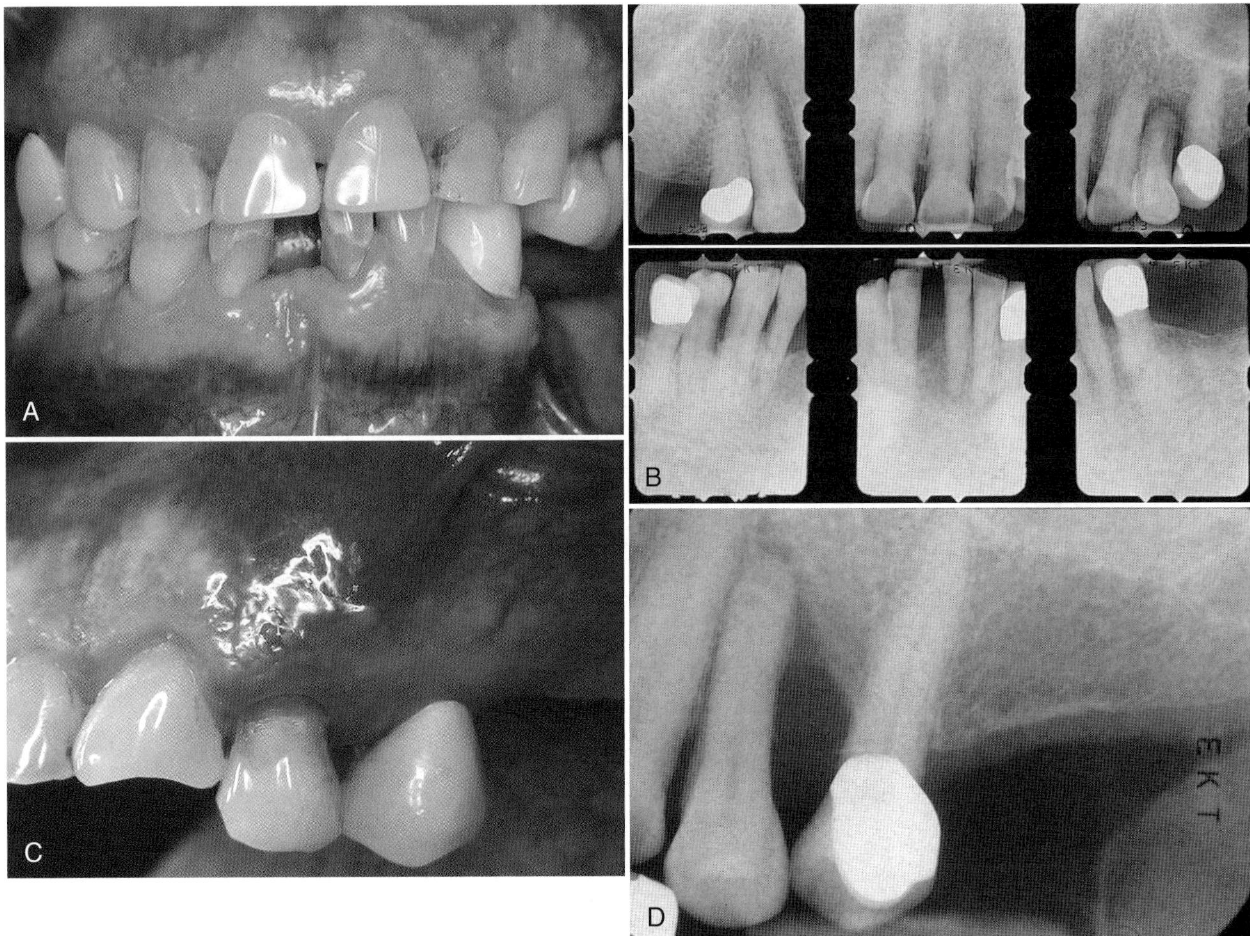

Fig. 25.2 A 60-year-old patient with a long-term history of type 2 diabetes. (A) Anterior retracted view of the patient's dental and periodontal condition. Note the missing posterior teeth, the supereruption of the premolars, and the mild generalized gingival inflammation. (B) Periapical radiographs of the remaining teeth. Note the mild generalized bone loss with localized areas of severe bone loss. The failure to replace the posterior teeth adds to the occlusal burden of the remaining dentition. (C) Clinical photograph of the maxillary premolar area presenting with abscess. Notice the diffuse erythema and inflammation surrounding the abscess area. (D) Periapical radiograph of the maxillary premolar showing extensive bone loss associated with abscess.

with periodontitis, diabetes mellitus does not cause gingivitis or periodontitis, but evidence indicates that it alters the response of the periodontal tissues to local factors, thereby hastening bone loss and delaying postsurgical healing. Frequent periodontal abscesses appear to be an important feature of periodontal disease in patients with diabetes.

Approximately 40% of adult Pima Indians in Arizona have type 2 diabetes. A comparison of individuals with and without diabetes in this Native American tribe showed a clear increase in the prevalence of destructive periodontitis as well as a 15% increase in edentulousness among patients with diabetes.[239] The risk of developing destructive periodontitis was increased threefold in these individuals.[77]

Bacterial Pathogens

The glucose content of gingival fluid and blood is higher in individuals with diabetes than in those without diabetes with similar plaque and gingival index scores.[83] The increased glucose in the gingival fluid and blood of patients with diabetes could change the environment of the microflora, thereby inducing qualitative changes in bacteria that may contribute to the severity of periodontal disease observed in those with poorly controlled diabetes.

Patients with type 1 diabetes mellitus and periodontitis have been reported to have a subgingival flora that is composed mainly of *Capnocytophaga*, anaerobic vibrios, and *Actinomyces* species. *Porphyromonas gingivalis, Prevotella intermedia,* and *Aggregatibacter actinomycetemcomitans*, which are common in periodontal lesions of individuals without diabetes, are present in low numbers in those with the disease.[115,174] However, other studies have found scarce *Capnocytophaga* and abundant *A. actinomycetemcomitans* and black-pigmented *Bacteroides* as well as *P. intermedia, Prevotella melaninogenica,* and *Campylobacter rectus*.[173,229] Black-pigmented species—especially *P. gingivalis, P. intermedia,* and *C. rectus*—are prominent in severe periodontal lesions of Pima Indians with type 2 diabetes.[93,286] Although these results may suggest an altered flora in the periodontal pockets of patients with diabetes, the exact role of these microorganisms has not been determined. To date, there is insufficient evidence to support the role of a specific altered microflora that is responsible for periodontal disease destruction in patients with diabetes.

Polymorphonuclear Leukocyte Function

The increased susceptibility of patients with diabetes to infection has been hypothesized as being caused by polymorphonuclear leukocyte (PMN) deficiencies that result in impaired chemotaxis, defective phagocytosis, or impaired adherence.[177,253] In patients with poorly controlled diabetes, the functions of PMNs, monocytes,

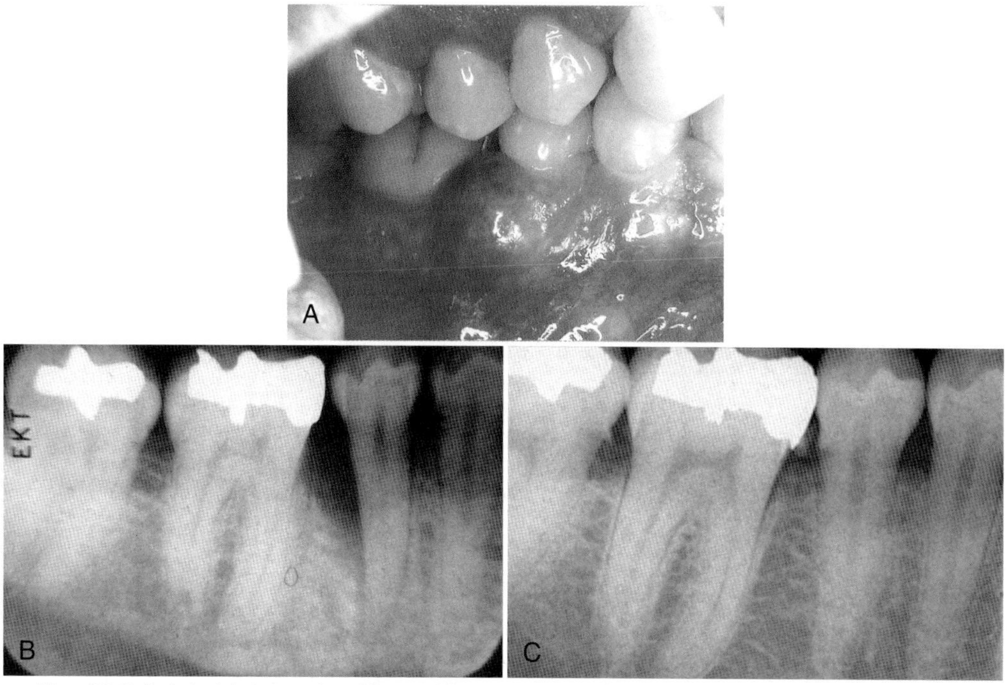

Fig. 25.3 Periodontal abscess in a 28-year-old patient with poorly controlled type 1 diabetes. (A) The patient presented with pain and abscess a few weeks after scaling and root planing of the area. (B) Radiograph of the mandibular right premolar area demonstrating severe localized destruction of bone in the area of periodontal abscess. (C) Radiograph of the mandibular right premolar area taken 2 months before the presentation of the abscess. Note the presence of calculus and the level of interproximal bone before the abscess occurred.

and macrophages are impaired.[124] As a result, the primary defense mounted by PMNs against periodontal pathogens is diminished, and bacterial proliferation is more likely. No alteration of immunoglobulin A (IgA), G (IgG), or M (IgM) has been found in patients with diabetes.[219]

Altered Collagen Metabolism

Chronic hyperglycemia impairs collagen structure and function, which may directly impact the integrity of the periodontium. Decreased collagen synthesis, osteoporosis, and a reduction in alveolar bone height have been demonstrated in diabetic animals.[97,233] Chronic hyperglycemia adversely affects the synthesis, maturation, and maintenance of collagen and extracellular matrix. In the hyperglycemic state, numerous proteins and matrix molecules undergo a nonenzymatic glycosylation, thereby resulting in *advanced glycation end-products (AGEs)*. The formation of AGEs occurs at normal glucose levels as well; however, in hyperglycemic environments, AGE formation is excessive. Many types of molecules are affected, including proteins, lipids, and carbohydrates. Collagen is cross-linked by AGE formation, which makes the collagen less soluble and less likely to be normally repaired or replaced. Cellular migration through cross-linked collagen is impeded, and, perhaps more importantly, tissue integrity is impaired as a result of damaged collagen that remains in the tissues for longer periods (i.e., collagen is not renewed at a normal rate).[113] As a result, collagen in the tissues of patients with poorly controlled diabetes is older and more susceptible to pathogenic breakdown (i.e., less resistant to destruction by periodontal infections).

AGEs and receptors for AGEs (RAGEs) play a central role in the classic complications of diabetes,[36] and they may play a significant role in the progression of periodontal disease as well. Poor glycemic control, with the associated increase in AGEs, renders the periodontal tissues more susceptible to destruction.[232] The cumulative effects of altered cellular response to local factors, impaired tissue integrity, and altered collagen metabolism undoubtedly play a significant role in the susceptibility of patients with diabetes to infections and destructive periodontal disease.

CLINICAL CORRELATION

Chronic hyperglycemia impairs collagen structure and function. Chronic hyperglycemia causes proteins and matrix molecules to undergo a nonenzymatic glycosylation, thereby resulting in advanced glycation end-products (AGEs). AGEs and receptors for AGEs (RAGEs) play a central role in the classic complications of diabetes, and they most likely play a significant role in the progression of periodontal disease as well.

Metabolic Syndrome

Obesity is a global concern with serious health consequences including diabetes mellitus and cardiovascular disease. It is believed that the condition of excess adipose tissue contributes to an increased systemic proinflammatory response in these individuals. Metabolic syndrome is a term used to describe a condition of abdominal obesity combined with two or more of the following metabolic disturbances: hypertension, dyslipidemia, and hyperglycemia. Individuals diagnosed with metabolic syndrome are at increased risk for developing type 2 diabetes[230] and cardiovascular disease.

Recent evidence suggests that obesity, obesity-related characteristics, and metabolic syndrome in particular may be risk indicators for the severity and progression of periodontitis.[10,158,189,209,273] Previous studies have documented the relationship between obesity and periodontitis as well as obesity-related characteristics such as body mass index and future progression of periodontal disease.[104] A systematic review that included the results from five prospective studies evaluating the association between weight gain and the incidence of periodontitis in adults found a clear positive relationship:

subjects who became overweight and obese had a higher risk of developing periodontitis when compared with those who did not gain weight.[188] The authors cautioned that the evidence was limited and that more prospective, longitudinal research is needed to establish obesity as a risk factor for periodontitis.

The association between periodontitis and metabolic syndrome is thought to be the result of systemic oxidative stress and an increased inflammatory response.[149] It may be explained by common risk factors such as obesity and obesity-related habits including diet, exercise, and poor oral hygiene.[142] Obesity is associated with increased cytokine production as well as T-cell and monocyte/macrophage dysfunction, factors known to contribute to periodontitis. The proinflammatory cytokines interleukin-6 (IL-6) and tumor necrosis factor alpha (TNF-α), which are elevated in obese individuals, are thought to be produced by activated macrophages that have infiltrated adipose tissue.[142] Although these associations are highly suggestive, the specific mechanisms and relationship between metabolic syndrome and periodontitis remain unknown. More well-designed studies are needed to better understand this relationship.

Female Sex Hormones

Gingival alterations during puberty, pregnancy, and menopause are associated with physiologic hormonal changes in the female patient. During puberty and pregnancy, these changes are characterized by nonspecific inflammatory reactions with a predominant vascular component, which leads clinically to a marked hemorrhagic tendency. Oral changes during menopause may include thinning of the oral mucosa, gingival recession, xerostomia, altered taste, and burning mouth.

The changes associated with each phase of the female life cycle from puberty to menopause are briefly addressed in the online materials associated with this book. See Chapter 28 for a detailed description of these changes, including management considerations for the periodontal manifestations of hormonal changes in the female patient.

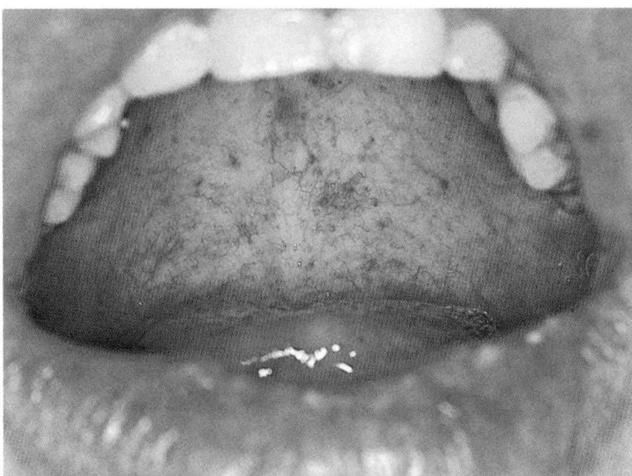

Fig. 25.4 Petechiae evident on the soft palate of a patient with an underlying bleeding disorder (thrombocytopenia).

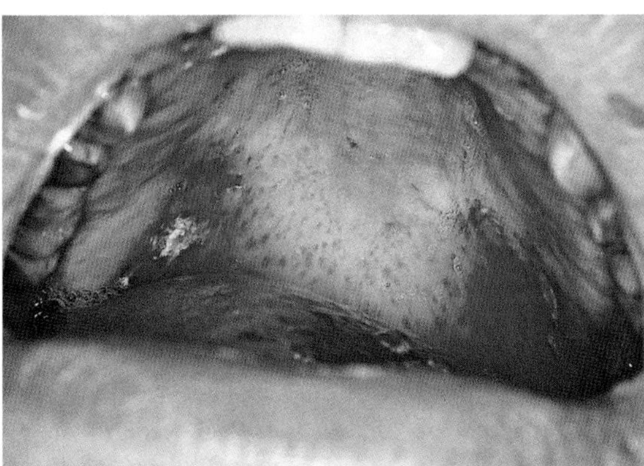

Fig. 25.5 Ecchymosis that is evident on the lateral aspects of the soft palate and tonsillar pillars of a patient with chemotherapy-induced thrombocytopenia.

Hematologic Disorders and Immune Deficiencies

All blood cells play an essential role in the maintenance of a healthy periodontium. White blood cells (WBCs) are involved in inflammatory reactions, and they are responsible for cellular defense against microorganisms as well as for proinflammatory cytokine release. Red blood cells (RBCs) are responsible for gas exchange and nutrient supply to the periodontal tissues and platelets, and they are necessary for normal hemostasis as well as for the recruitment of cells during inflammation and wound healing. Consequently, disorders of any blood cells or blood-forming organs can have a profound effect on the periodontium.

Certain oral changes (e.g., hemorrhage) may suggest the existence of a blood dyscrasia. However, a specific diagnosis requires a complete physical examination and a thorough hematologic study. Comparable oral changes occur in more than one form of blood dyscrasia, and secondary inflammatory changes produce a wide range of variation in the oral signs.

Gingival and periodontal disturbances associated with blood dyscrasias must be viewed in terms of fundamental interrelationships among the oral tissues, the blood cells, and the blood-forming organs rather than in terms of a simple association of dramatic oral changes with hematologic disease. Hemorrhagic tendencies occur when the normal hemostatic mechanisms are disturbed. Abnormal bleeding from the gingiva or other areas of the oral mucosa that is difficult to control is an important clinical sign that suggests a hematologic disorder. Petechiae (Fig. 25.4) and ecchymosis (Fig. 25.5), observed most often in the soft palate area, are signs of an underlying bleeding disorder. It is essential to diagnose the specific etiology to appropriately address any bleeding or immunologic disorder.

Deficiencies in the host immune response may lead to severely destructive periodontal lesions. These deficiencies may be primary (inherited) or secondary (acquired) and may be caused by either immunosuppressive drug therapy or the pathologic destruction of the lymphoid system. Leukemia, Hodgkin disease, lymphomas, and multiple myeloma may result in secondary immunodeficiency disorders. This section discusses common hematologic and certain immunodeficiency disorders that are not related to the human immunodeficiency virus or acquired immunodeficiency syndrome. See Chapter 27 for a detailed discussion of patients with human immunodeficiency virus infection.

KEY FACT

Clinicians must be aware that certain oral manifestations (e.g., hemorrhage, ecchymosis) can suggest the existence of a systemic disorder. Atypical gingival and periodontal findings should be assessed in terms of the interrelationships among oral tissues, blood cells, and blood-forming organs rather than in terms of a simple association of dramatic oral changes with hematologic disease. Determining a specific systemic diagnosis requires a complete physical examination and a thorough hematologic study. Patients should be referred to a medical doctor for comprehensive workup.

Leukocyte (Neutrophil) Disorders

Disorders that affect the production or function of leukocytes may result in severe periodontal destruction. PMNs (i.e., neutrophils) in particular play a critical role in bacterial infections, because PMNs are the first line of defense (see Chapters 8, 11, and 12). A quantitative deficiency of leukocytes (e.g., neutropenia, agranulocytosis) is typically associated with a more generalized periodontal destruction that affects all teeth.

Neutropenia

Neutropenia is a blood disorder that results in low levels of circulating neutrophils. It is a serious condition that may be caused by diseases, medications, chemicals, infections, idiopathic conditions, or hereditary disorders. It may be chronic or cyclic and severe or benign. It affects as many as one in three patients who are receiving chemotherapy for cancer. An absolute neutrophil count (ANC) of 1000 to 1500 cells/μL is diagnostic for mild neutropenia. An ANC of 500 to 1000 cells/μL is considered moderate neutropenia, and an ANC of less than 500 cells/μL indicates severe neutropenia. Infections are sometimes difficult to manage and may be life threatening, particularly with severe neutropenia.

Agranulocytosis

Agranulocytosis is a more severe neutropenia that involves not only neutrophils but also basophils and eosinophils. It is defined as an ANC of less than 100 cells/μL. It is characterized by a reduction in the number of circulating granulocytes, and it results in severe infections, including ulcerative necrotizing lesions of the oral mucosa, the skin, and the gastrointestinal and genitourinary tracts. Less severe forms of the disease are called *neutropenia* or *granulocytopenia.*

Drug idiosyncrasy is the most common cause of agranulocytosis, but, in some cases, its cause cannot be explained. Agranulocytosis has been reported after the administration of drugs such as aminopyrine, barbiturates and their derivatives, benzene ring derivatives, sulfonamides, gold salts, and arsenical agents.[146,161,181,212] It generally occurs as an acute disease. It may be chronic or periodic, with recurring neutropenic cycles (e.g., cyclic neutropenia).[251]

The onset of disease is accompanied by fever, malaise, general weakness, and sore throat. Ulceration in the oral cavity, the oropharynx, and the throat is characteristic. The mucosa exhibits isolated necrotic patches that are black and gray and that are sharply demarcated from the adjacent uninvolved areas.[135,168] The absence of a notable inflammatory reaction caused by a lack of granulocytes is a striking feature. The gingival margin may or may not be involved. Gingival hemorrhage, necrosis, increased salivation, and fetid odor are accompanying clinical features. With cyclic neutropenia, the gingival changes recur with recurrent exacerbation of the disease.[55] The occurrence of generalized periodontitis stage 4, grade C (generalized aggressive periodontitis) has been described in patients with cyclic neutropenia (Fig. 25.6).[236]

Because infection is a common feature of agranulocytosis, the differential diagnosis involves consideration of such conditions as necrotizing ulcerative gingivitis, noma, acute necrotizing inflammation of the tonsils, and diphtheria. Definitive diagnosis depends on the hematologic findings of pronounced leukopenia and the almost complete absence of neutrophils.

Leukemia

Leukemia is an important disease to understand and appreciate because of its seriousness and its periodontal manifestations. The leukemias are malignant neoplasias of WBC precursors that are characterized by the following: (1) diffuse replacement of the bone marrow with proliferating leukemic cells; (2) abnormal numbers and forms of immature WBCs in the circulating blood; and (3) widespread infiltrates in the liver, spleen, lymph nodes, and other body sites.[215]

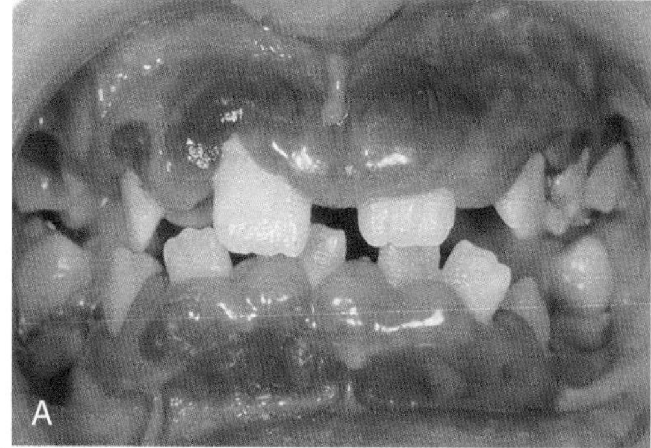

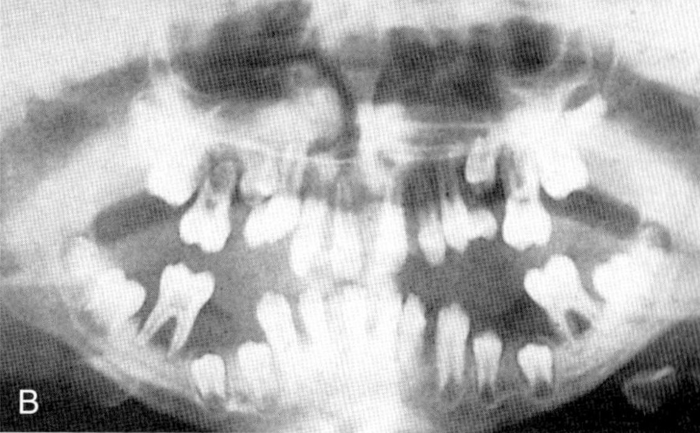

Fig. 25.6 Generalized periodontitis stage 4, grade C (aggressive periodontitis) in 10-year-old boy with cyclic neutropenia and agammaglobulinemia. (A) Clinical presentation of the periodontal condition. Note the severe swelling and inflammation of the marginal and papillary gingiva. There is gross migration of teeth caused by a loss of bone support. (B) Panoramic radiograph demonstrating severe bone loss around all permanent teeth that have erupted into the oral cavity.

According to the cell type involved, leukemias are classified as *lymphocytic* or *myelogenous.* A subgroup of the myelogenous leukemias are the *monocytic* leukemias. The term *lymphocytic* indicates that the malignant change occurs in cells that normally form lymphocytes. The term *myelogenous* indicates that the malignant change occurs in cells that normally form RBCs, some types of WBCs, and platelets. According to their evolution, leukemias can be *acute* (which is rapidly fatal), *subacute,* or *chronic.* In acute leukemia, the primitive blast cells released into the peripheral circulation are immature and nonfunctional; in chronic leukemia, the abnormal cells tend to be more mature and to have normal morphologic characteristics and functions when released into the circulation.

All leukemias tend to displace normal components of the bone marrow elements with leukemic cells, thereby resulting in the reduced production of normal RBCs, WBCs, and platelets, which leads to anemia, *leukopenia* (a reduction in the number of *nonmalignant* WBCs), and thrombocytopenia. Anemia results in poor tissue oxygenation, which makes tissues more friable and susceptible to breakdown. A reduction of normal WBCs in the circulation leads to a poor cellular defense and an increased susceptibility to infections. *Thrombocytopenia* leads to bleeding tendency, which can occur in any tissue but which in particular affects the oral cavity, especially the gingival sulcus (Fig. 25.7). Some patients may have normal blood counts while leukemic cells reside primarily in the bone marrow. This type of disease is called *aleukemic leukemia.*[102]

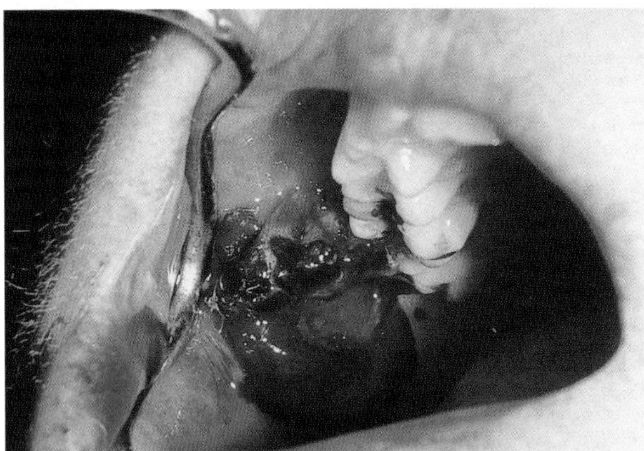

Fig. 25.7 Spontaneous bleeding from the gingival sulcus in a patient with thrombocytopenia. Normal coagulation is evident by the appearance of the large clot that forms in the mouth. However, platelets are inadequate to establish hemostasis at the site of hemorrhage.

The Periodontium in Leukemic Patients

Oral and periodontal manifestations of leukemia may include leukemic infiltration, bleeding, oral ulcerations, and infections. The expression of these signs is more common with acute and subacute forms of leukemia than with chronic forms.

Leukemic Infiltration

Leukemic cells can infiltrate the gingiva and, less frequently, the alveolar bone. Gingival infiltration often results in *leukemic gingival enlargement* (see Chapter 19).

A study of 1076 adult patients with leukemia showed that 3.6% of the patients with teeth had leukemic gingival proliferative lesions, with the highest incidence seen in patients with acute monocytic leukemia (66.7%), followed by those with acute myelocytic–monocytic leukemia (18.7%) and acute myelocytic leukemia (3.7%).[68] It should be noted, however, that monocytic leukemia is an extremely rare form of the disease. Leukemic gingival enlargement is not found in edentulous patients or in patients with chronic leukemia, suggesting that it represents the accumulation of immature leukemic blast cells in the gingiva adjacent to tooth surfaces with bacterial plaque. Leukemic gingival enlargement consists of a basic infiltration of the gingival corium by leukemic cells that increases the gingival thickness and creates gingival pockets in which bacterial plaque accumulates, thereby initiating a secondary inflammatory lesion that contributes to the enlargement of the gingiva. It may be localized to the interdental papilla area (Fig. 25.8), or it may expand to include the marginal gingiva and partially cover the crowns of the teeth (Fig. 25.9C and D). Clinically, the gingiva appears bluish-red and cyanotic, with a rounding and tenseness of the gingival margin. The abnormal accumulation of leukemic cells in the dermal and subcutaneous connective tissue is called *leukemia cutis,* and it forms elevated and flat macules and papules (see Fig. 25.9A and B).[69,215]

Microscopically, the gingiva exhibits a dense, diffuse infiltration of predominantly immature leukocytes in the attached and marginal gingiva. Occasionally, mitotic figures indicative of ectopic hematopoiesis may be seen. The normal connective tissue components of the gingiva are displaced by the leukemic cells (Fig. 25.10). The nature of the cells depends on the type of leukemia. The cellular accumulation is denser in the entire reticular connective tissue layer. In almost all cases, the papillary layer contains comparatively few leukocytes. The blood vessels are distended and contain predominantly leukemic cells, and the RBCs are reduced in number. The epithelium shows a variety of changes, and it may be thinned or hyperplastic. Common findings include degeneration associated with intercellular and intracellular edema and leukocytic infiltration with diminished surface keratinization.

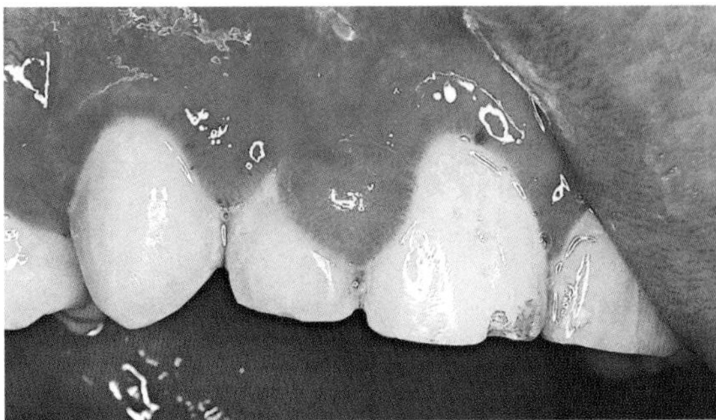

Fig. 25.8 Leukemic infiltration that causes localized gingival swelling of the interdental papillae between the maxillary lateral and central incisors. Note the tense induration of the area.

The microscopic picture of the marginal gingiva differs from that of other gingival locations in that it usually exhibits a notable inflammatory component in addition to the leukemic cells. Scattered foci of plasma cells and lymphocytes with edema and degeneration are common findings. The inner aspect of the marginal gingiva is usually ulcerated, and marginal necrosis with pseudomembrane formation may also be seen.

The periodontal ligament and alveolar bone may also be involved in acute and subacute leukemia. The periodontal ligament may be infiltrated with mature and immature leukocytes. The marrow of the alveolar bone exhibits a variety of changes, such as localized areas of necrosis, thrombosis of the blood vessels, infiltration with mature and immature leukocytes, occasional RBCs, and the replacement of the fatty marrow with fibrous tissue.

In leukemic mice, the presence of infiltrate in marrow spaces and the periodontal ligament results in osteoporosis of the alveolar bone with destruction of the supporting bone and disappearance of the periodontal fibers (Fig. 25.11).[34,43]

Bleeding

Gingival hemorrhage is a common finding in leukemic patients (see Fig. 25.7), even in the absence of clinically detectable gingivitis. Bleeding gingiva can be an early sign of leukemia. It is caused by the thrombocytopenia that results from the replacement of bone marrow cells with leukemic cells and from the inhibition of normal stem cell function by leukemic cells or their products.[215] This bleeding tendency can also manifest in the skin and throughout the oral mucosa, where petechiae are often found, with or without leukemic infiltrates. A more diffuse submucosal bleeding manifests as ecchymosis (see Fig. 25.5). Oral bleeding has been reported as a presenting sign in 17.7% of patients with acute leukemia and in 4.4% of patients with chronic leukemia.[163] Bleeding may also be a side effect of the chemotherapeutic agents used to treat leukemia.

Oral Ulceration and Infection

In patients with leukemia, the response to bacterial plaque or other local irritation is altered. The cellular component of the inflammatory exudate differs both quantitatively and qualitatively from that found in nonleukemic individuals in that there is a pronounced infiltration of immature leukemic cells in addition to the usual inflammatory cells. As a result, the normal inflammatory response may be diminished.

Granulocytopenia (diminished WBC count) results from the displacement of normal bone marrow cells by leukemic cells, which increases the host susceptibility to opportunistic microorganisms and leads to ulcerations and infections. Discrete, punched-out ulcers

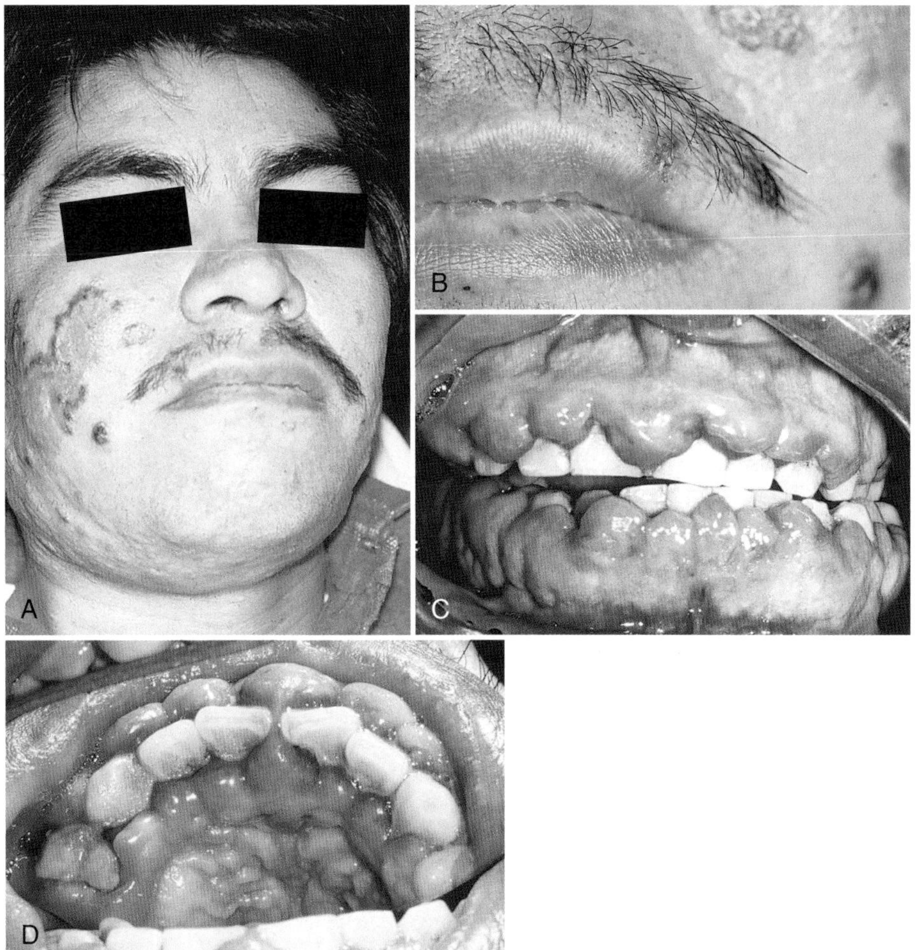

Fig. 25.9 Adult male with acute myelocytic leukemia. (A) A view of the patient's face. Note the elevated, flat macules and papules (leukemia cutis) on the right cheek. (B) Close-up view of skin lesions. (C) An intraoral view showing pronounced gingival enlargements of the entire gingival margin and interdental papilla areas of both arches. (D) Occlusal view of the maxillary anterior teeth. Note the marked enlargement in both the facial and the palatal aspects. (*Courtesy Dr. Spencer Woolfe, Dublin, Ireland.*)

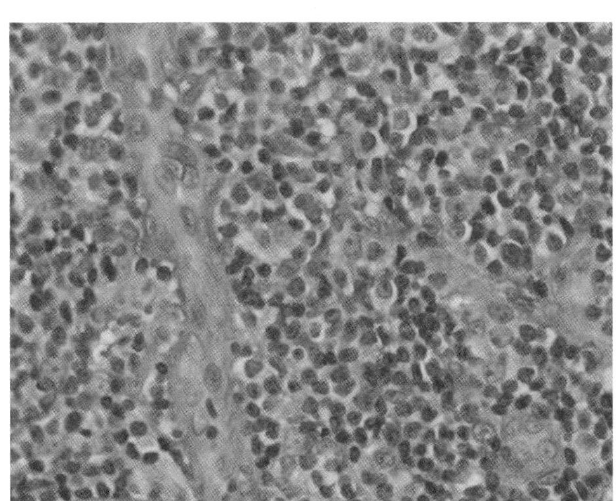

Fig. 25.10 Human histologic appearance of leukemic infiltrate with dense diffuse infiltration of predominantly immature leukocytes. The normal connective tissue components of the gingiva are displaced by the leukemic cells. The cellular accumulation is denser in the entire reticular connective tissue layer. (*Courtesy Dr. Russell Christensen, University of California, Los Angeles, CA.*)

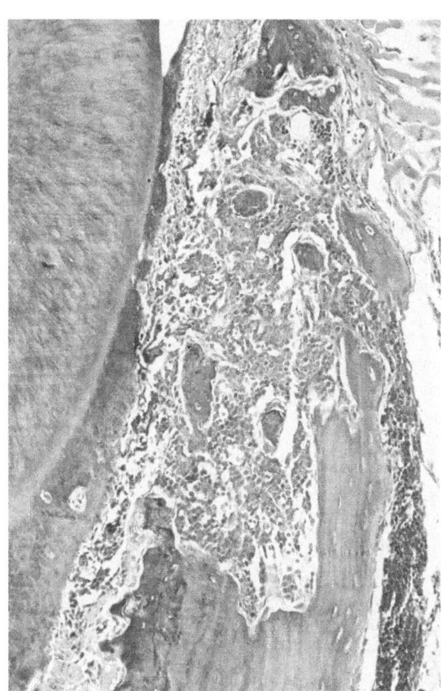

Fig. 25.11 Leukemic infiltrate in alveolar bone in a leukemic mouse. Note the leukemic infiltrate causing destruction of the bone and a loss of the periodontal ligament.

that penetrate deeply into the submucosa and are covered by a firmly attached white slough can be found on the oral mucosa.[17] These lesions occur in sites of trauma (e.g., the buccal mucosa) in relation to the line of occlusion or on the palate. Patients with a history of herpesvirus infection may develop recurrent herpetic oral ulcers (often in multiple sites) and large, atypical forms, especially after chemotherapy is instituted (Fig. 25.12).[109]

A gingival (bacterial) infection in leukemic patients can be the result of an exogenous bacterial infection or an existing bacterial infection (e.g., gingival or periodontal disease). Acute gingivitis and lesions that resemble necrotizing ulcerative gingivitis are more frequent and more severe in patients with terminal cases of acute leukemia (Figs. 25.13 and 25.14).[23] The inflamed gingiva in patients with leukemia differs clinically from that found in nonleukemic individuals. The gingiva is a peculiar bluish-red, it is spongelike and friable, and it bleeds persistently on the slightest provocation or even spontaneously in leukemic patients. This greatly altered and degenerated tissue is extremely susceptible to bacterial infection, which can be so severe as to cause acute gingival necrosis with pseudomembrane formation (Fig. 25.15) or bone exposure (Fig. 25.16). These are secondary oral changes that are superimposed on the oral tissues that have been altered by the blood dyscrasia. They produce associated disturbances that may be a source of considerable difficulty to the patient, such as systemic toxic effects, loss of appetite, nausea, blood loss from persistent gingival bleeding, and constant gnawing pain. Eliminating or reducing local factors (e.g., bacterial plaque) can minimize the severe oral changes associated with leukemia. In some patients with severe acute leukemia, symptoms may be relieved only by treatment that leads to the remission of the disease.

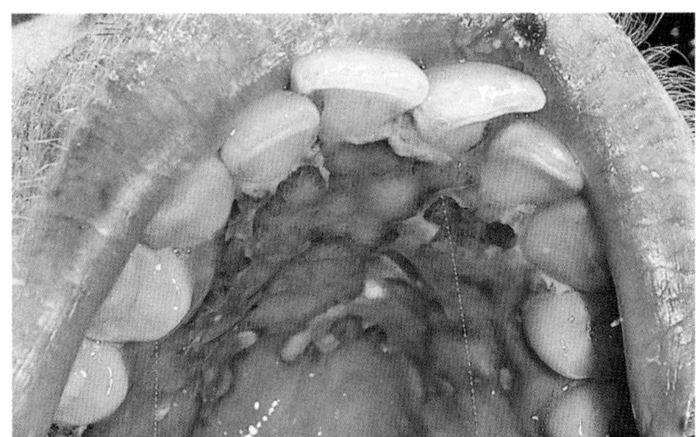

Fig. 25.12 Large ulcerations on the palate of a patient with granulocytopenia secondary to leukemia. These atypical ulcerations are caused by a herpesvirus opportunistic infection. Notice the smaller, discrete, round ulcerations that have coalesced into the larger lesion.

In those with chronic leukemia, oral changes that suggest a hematologic disturbance are rare. The microscopic changes of chronic leukemia may consist of replacing the normal fatty marrow of the jaws with islands of mature lymphocytes or lymphocytic infiltration of the marginal gingiva without dramatic clinical manifestations.

The existence of leukemia is sometimes revealed by a gingival biopsy performed to clarify the nature of a troublesome gingival condition. In such cases, the gingival findings must be corroborated by medical examination and hematologic study. In patients with diagnosed leukemia, gingival biopsy may indicate the extent to which leukemic infiltration is responsible for the altered clinical

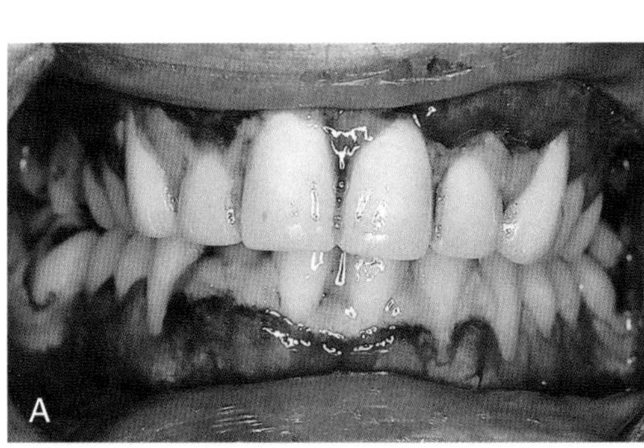

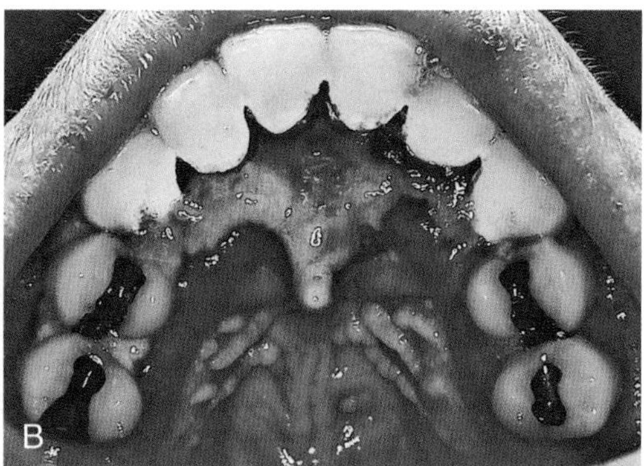

Fig. 25.13 Adult female with acute myelocytic leukemia. (A) Anterior view of a patient with acute myelocytic leukemia. The interdental papillae are necrotic, with highly inflamed and swollen gingival tissue at the base of the lesions. (B) Palatal view demonstrating extensive necrosis of the interdental and palatal tissues behind the maxillary incisors.

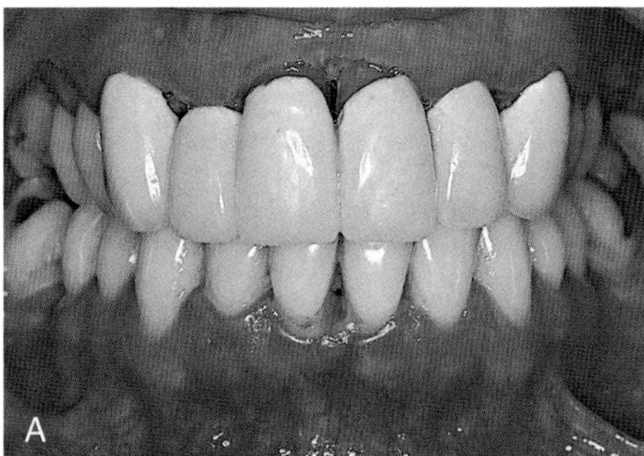

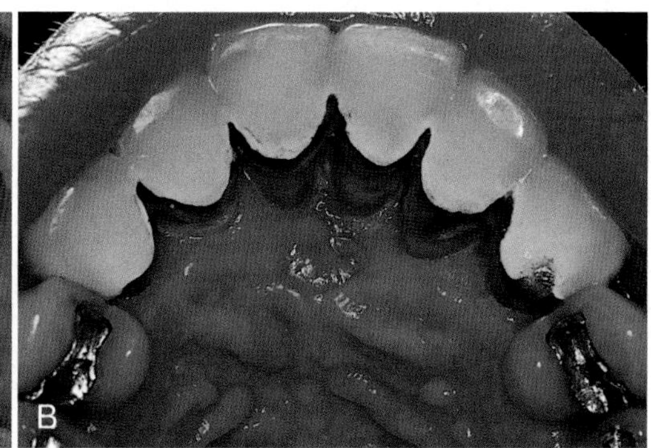

Fig. 25.14 The same patient as shown in Fig. 25.13 after chemotherapy that resulted in the remission of her leukemia. (A) An anterior view reveals dramatic improvement in gingival health after the remission of leukemia. Note the loss of interdental papillae as well as gingival recession in the anterior areas. (B) A palatal view shows the extensive loss of gingival tissue around the maxillary incisors.

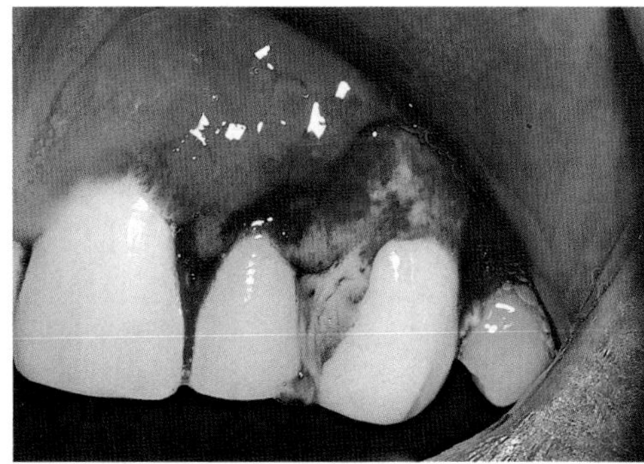

Fig. 25.15 An opportunistic bacterial infection of the gingiva in a patient who has been hospitalized with leukemia. The gingival tissue is highly inflamed, bleeding, and necrotic, with pseudomembrane formation.

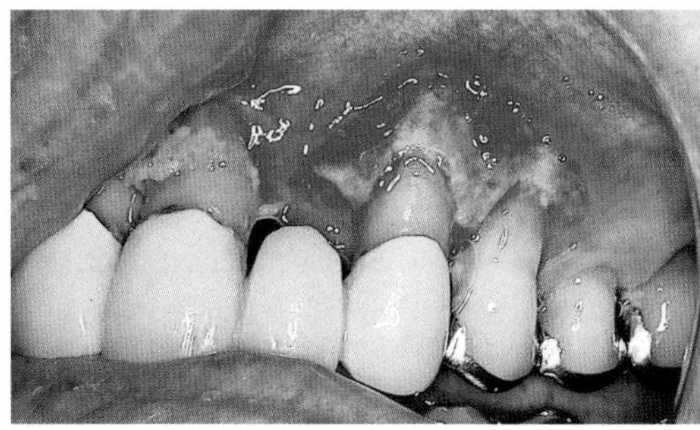

Fig. 25.16 An opportunistic bacterial infection in an immunosuppressed patient caused the complete destruction of the gingiva, thus exposing the underlying alveolar bone.

appearance of the gingiva. *Although such findings are of interest, their benefit to the patient is insufficient to warrant routine gingival biopsy studies in patients with leukemia.* Furthermore, it is important to note that the absence of leukemic involvement in a gingival biopsy specimen does not rule out the possibility of leukemia. A gingival biopsy in a patient with chronic leukemia may reveal typical gingival inflammation without any suggestion of a hematologic disturbance.

See the online material for discussion of additional blood dyscrasias and their influence on periodontal health.

Anemia

Anemia is a deficiency in the quantity or quality of the blood as manifested by a reduction in the number of erythrocytes and in the amount of hemoglobin. Anemia may be the result of blood loss, defective blood formation, or increased RBC destruction. Anemias are classified according to cellular morphology and hemoglobin content as follows: (1) macrocytic hyperchromic anemia (pernicious anemia); (2) microcytic hypochromic anemia (iron deficiency anemia); (3) sickle cell anemia; and (4) normocytic–normochromic anemia (hemolytic or aplastic anemia).

Pernicious anemia results in tongue changes in 75% of patients. The tongue appears red, smooth, and shiny as a result of atrophy of the papillae (eFig. 25.5). There is also marked pallor of the gingiva (eFig. 25.6). *Iron deficiency anemia* induces similar tongue and gingival changes. A syndrome that consists of glossitis and ulceration of the oral mucosa and oropharynx and that induces dysphagia (Plummer–Vinson syndrome) has been described in patients with iron deficiency anemia. *Sickle cell anemia* is a hereditary form of chronic hemolytic anemia that occurs almost exclusively in blacks. It is characterized by pallor, jaundice, weakness, rheumatoid manifestations, and leg ulcers. Oral changes include generalized osteoporosis of the jaws, with a peculiar stepladder alignment of the trabeculae of the interdental septa, along with pallor and yellowish discoloration of the oral mucosa. Periodontal infections may precipitate sickle cell crisis.[206] *Aplastic anemia* results from a failure of the bone marrow to produce erythrocytes. The etiology is usually the effect of toxic drugs on the marrow or the displacement of RBCs by leukemic cells. Oral changes include pale discoloration of the oral mucosa and increased susceptibility to infection because of the concomitant neutropenia.

Thrombocytopenia

Thrombocytopenia is a term that is used to describe the condition of a reduced platelet count that results from either a lack of platelet production or an increased loss of platelets. *Purpura* refers to the purplish appearance of the skin or mucous membranes where bleeding has occurred as a result of decreased platelets. *Thrombocytopenic purpura* may be idiopathic (i.e., of unknown etiology, as with Werlhof disease), or it may occur secondary to some known etiologic factor that is responsible for a reduced amount of functioning marrow and a resultant reduction in the number of circulating platelets. Such etiologic factors include aplasia of the marrow, displacement of the megakaryocytes in the marrow (as with leukemia), replacement of the marrow by tumor, and destruction of the marrow by irradiation or radium or by drugs such as benzene, aminopyrine, or arsenical agents.

Thrombocytopenic purpura is characterized by a low platelet count, a prolonged clot retraction and bleeding time, and a normal or slightly prolonged clotting time. There is spontaneous bleeding into the skin or from the mucous membranes. Petechiae and hemorrhagic vesicles occur in the oral cavity, particularly in the palate, the tonsillar pillars, and the buccal mucosa. The gingivae are swollen, soft, and friable. Bleeding occurs spontaneously or with the slightest provocation, and it is difficult to control. *Gingival changes represent an abnormal response to local irritation.* The severity of the gingival condition is dramatically alleviated by removal of the local factors (eFig. 25.7).

Antibody Deficiency Disorders

Agammaglobulinemia, or *hypogammaglobulinemia*, is an immune deficiency that results from inadequate antibody production caused by a deficiency in B cells. It can be congenital (X-linked or Bruton agammaglobulinemia) or acquired (common variable immunodeficiency).

Congenital agammaglobulinemia is caused by an X-linked, recessive gene (Bruton tyrosine kinase). It affects approximately 1 of every 100,000 individuals. Because the defect is recessive and linked to the X chromosome, only males have the disease. The gene is responsible for B-cell development. In the absence of mature B cells, patients lack lymphoid tissue and fail to develop plasma cells. Thus, the production of antibodies is deficient. Germinal centers where B cells proliferate and differentiate are poorly developed in all lymphoid tissues. The tonsils, adenoids, and peripheral lymph nodes are small or absent.

Acquired or *late-onset* agammaglobulinemia is most often known as *common variable immunodeficiency disease* (CVID). The disorder is characterized by the onset of recurrent bacterial infections during the second and third decades of life as a result of drastic decreases in immunoglobulin and antibody levels. The basic immunologic defect of CVID is the failure of B-lymphocyte differentiation into plasma cells. In contrast to patients with the X-linked form of the disease, patients with CVID typically have an enlarged spleen and swollen glands or lymph nodes. Along with other autoimmune problems, some patients develop autoantibodies against their blood cells. Causes of the disease are unknown. Unlike the X-linked early-onset form of the disease, CVID is not genetically determined, and both males and females are susceptible.

T-cell function remains normal in individuals with agammaglobulinemia. The disease, whether congenital or acquired, is characterized by recurrent bacterial infections, especially ear, sinus, and lung infections. Patients are also susceptible to periodontal infections. Periodontitis, stage 3 or 4, grade C (aggressive periodontitis) is a common finding in children who are diagnosed with agammaglobulinemia (see Fig. 25.6).

Genetic Disorders

Systemic conditions that are associated with or that predispose an individual to periodontal destruction include genetic disorders that result in an inadequate number or reduced function of circulating neutrophils. This underscores the importance of the neutrophil in the protection of the periodontium against infection. Severe periodontitis has been observed in individuals with primary neutrophil disorders such as neutropenia, agranulocytosis, Chédiak–Higashi syndrome, and lazy leukocyte syndrome. In addition, severe periodontitis has been observed in individuals who exhibit secondary neutrophil impairment, such as those with Down syndrome, Papillon–Lefèvre syndrome, and inflammatory bowel disease.

See the online material for this chapter as well as for Chapter 9 for detailed descriptions of the periodontal manifestations of these genetic disorders and syndromes.

Chédiak–Higashi Syndrome

Chédiak–Higashi syndrome is a rare disease that affects the production of organelles found in almost every cell. It affects mostly the melanocytes, platelets, and phagocytes. It causes partial albinism, mild bleeding disorders, and recurrent bacterial infections. Neutrophils contain abnormal, giant lysosomes that can fuse with the phagosome, but their ability to release their contents is impaired. As a result, the killing of ingested microorganisms is delayed. Patients with Chédiak–Higashi syndrome are susceptible to repeated infections that can be serious and life threatening. Periodontitis stage 3 or 4, grade C (aggressive periodontitis) has been described in these patients. Chédiak–Higashi syndrome has been described as a genetically transmitted disease in ranch-raised mink (see Chapter 9).[12,202]

Lazy Leukocyte Syndrome

Lazy leukocyte syndrome is characterized by susceptibility to severe microbial infections, neutropenia, defective chemotactic response by neutrophils, and an abnormal inflammatory response.[202] Those who are diagnosed with lazy leukocyte syndrome are susceptible to periodontitis grade C (aggressive periodontitis) with destruction of bone and early tooth loss.

Leukocyte Adhesion Deficiency

Leukocyte adhesion deficiency (LAD) is a very rare genetic disorder; only a few hundred cases have been diagnosed. Because LAD is an inherited disease, it is categorized as a primary immunodeficiency that is most often diagnosed at birth. Many children with LAD do not survive.

LAD results from an inability to produce or a failure to normally express an important cell surface integrin (CD18), which is necessary for leukocytes to adhere to the vessel wall at the site of infection. When leukocytes cannot effectively adhere to the vessel wall near the site of infection, they cannot migrate to the infection. As a result, bacterial infections are able to continue to destroy host tissues unimpeded by the normal host immune response. Infections act similarly to those observed in neutropenic patients, because phagocytes are unable to reach the site of infection.

Cases of periodontal disease that are attributed to LAD are rare. They begin during or immediately after the eruption of the primary teeth. Extremely acute inflammation and proliferation of the gingival tissues with rapid destruction of the bone are found. Profound defects in peripheral blood neutrophils and monocytes and an absence of neutrophils in the gingival tissues have been noted in patients with LAD.[201,202] These patients also have frequent respiratory tract infections and sometimes otitis media. Both the primary and the permanent teeth are affected, often resulting in early tooth loss.[270]

Papillon–Lefèvre Syndrome

Papillon–Lefèvre syndrome, which was first described by French physicians Papillon and Lefèvre in 1924,[200] is a very rare inherited condition that appears to follow an autosomal-recessive pattern. Parents are not affected, and both must carry the autosomal genes for the syndrome to appear in their offspring. It may occur in siblings, and it has no gender predilection. The estimated frequency is 1 to 4 cases per 1 million individuals. Rare cases of adult onset of this syndrome, with only mild periodontal lesions, have also been described.[38]

The syndrome is characterized by hyperkeratotic skin lesions, severe destruction of the periodontium, and, in some cases, calcification of the dura.[43,80] The cutaneous and periodontal changes usually appear together when the patient is between the ages of 2 and 4 years. The skin lesions consist of hyperkeratosis and ichthyosis of localized areas on the palms, soles, knees, and elbows (eFig. 25.8).

Periodontal involvement consists of early inflammatory changes that lead to bone loss and exfoliation of teeth. The primary teeth are lost by 5 or 6 years of age. The permanent dentition then erupts normally, but within a few years the permanent teeth are also lost as a result of destructive periodontal disease (eFig. 25.9). At a very early age (usually 15 to 20 years), patients are often edentulous except for the third molars. These may be lost as well a few years after eruption. Tooth extraction sites heal uneventfully.[81]

There are few case reports of successful tooth retention in patients with Papillon–Lefèvre syndrome.[258,272] The successful retention of permanent teeth may be associated with timing of treatment (i.e., antibiotics and the extraction of erupted teeth) in relation to the severity of syndrome symptoms.[272] The extraction of all primary teeth followed by a period of edentulousness may partially explain the lack of recurrent infection. In their review of the literature, Wiebe and colleagues reported that the symptoms of Papillon–Lefèvre syndrome diminish with age and that teeth that erupt later may not be lost.[272]

The microscopic changes reported include marked chronic inflammation of the lateral wall of the pocket with a predominantly plasma cell infiltrate, considerable osteoclastic activity with an apparent lack of osteoblastic activity, and an extremely thin cementum.[169] Bacterial flora studies of biofilm (plaque) in a patient with Papillon–Lefèvre syndrome revealed a similarity to bacterial flora in patients with (chronic) periodontitis.[161] Spirochete-rich zones in the apical portion of the pockets as well as spirochete adherence to the cementum and microcolony formation of *Mycoplasma* species have been reported with Papillon–Lefèvre syndrome.[130] Gram-negative cocci and rods appear at the apical border of the plaque.[266] Although Schroeder and colleagues[235] failed to show defects in peripheral blood neutrophils in a 10-year-old boy with Papillon–Lefèvre syndrome, others have implicated neutrophil defects as a contributing factor. Firatli and colleagues[84] reported depressed chemotaxis of peripheral neutrophils and suggested that this explained the pathogenesis of the Papillon–Lefèvre syndrome. Ghaffer and colleagues found significantly depressed neutrophil function in probands with

Papillon–Lefèvre syndrome with respect to phagocytic and lytic activity.[95]

Down Syndrome

Down syndrome (mongolism, trisomy 21) is a congenital disease caused by a chromosomal abnormality and is characterized by mental deficiency and growth retardation. The prevalence of periodontal disease in patients with Down syndrome is high, occurring in almost 100% of patients who are younger than 30 years of age.[57,64] Although plaque, calculus, and local irritants (e.g., diastemata, crowding of teeth, high frenum attachments, malocclusion) are present and oral hygiene is poor, the severity of periodontal destruction exceeds that explainable by local factors alone.[53–55,216,235]

Periodontal disease in those with Down syndrome is characterized by the formation of deep periodontal pockets associated with substantial plaque accumulation and moderate gingivitis (eFig. 25.10). These findings are usually generalized, although they tend to be more severe in the lower anterior region. Moderate recession is sometimes seen in this region as well. The disease progresses rapidly. The high prevalence and increased severity of periodontal destruction associated with Down syndrome is most likely explained by poor PMN chemotaxis, phagocytosis, and intracellular killing.[13,14,57,61,108,125,134]

Stress and Psychosomatic Disorders

Psychologic conditions, particularly psychosocial stress, have been implicated as risk indicators for periodontal disease.[10,65,91] The most notable example is the documented relationship between stress (e.g., experienced by soldiers at war or by students during examinations) and acute necrotizing ulcerative gingivitis (see Chapters 17). The presence of necrotizing ulcerative gingivitis among soldiers stressed by wartime conditions in the trenches led to one of the early diagnostic terms used to describe this condition: "trench mouth." Despite this well-known association between stress and necrotizing ulcerative gingivitis, confirming the connection between psychologic conditions and other forms of periodontal disease (e.g., periodontitis) has been elusive. These relationships are difficult to elucidate, because, as with many common diseases, the etiology and pathogenesis of periodontal disease is multifactorial, and the role of individual risk factors is difficult to define.

Some studies have failed to recognize a relationship between psychologic conditions and periodontal disease despite specific efforts to identify them. In a study of 80 patients (40 with aggressive periodontitis and 40 with chronic periodontitis), Monteiro da Silva and colleagues failed to find a relationship between psychologic factors and periodontal disease.[187] The researchers were able to identify depression and smoking as marginally significant in the aggressive periodontitis grade C group. Their inability to find a relationship may be attributed to a lack of significant differences in psychologic characteristics between the two groups in the study. In an earlier study, the same researchers identified depression and loneliness as significant factors associated with aggressive periodontal disease in 50 patients as compared with 50 periodontally healthy individuals and 50 individuals with periodontitis.[186] Another challenge when defining the relationship between psychosocial status and periodontitis is the myriad confounding factors and the difficulty of controlling for them.[71]

Psychosocial Stress, Depression, and Coping

Several clinical studies and a systematic review of the subject have documented a positive relationship between psychosocial stress and chronic periodontal disease.[204] In case–control studies, individuals with stable lifestyles (based on family structure and employment status) and minimal negative life events had less periodontal disease destruction than individuals with less stable lifestyles (e.g., unmarried, unemployed) and more negative life events.[61] It is now becoming apparent that the effect is not simply a matter of the presence or absence of stress; rather, the type of stress and the ability of the individual to cope with stress correlate with destructive periodontal disease.

All individuals experience stress, but these events do not invariably result in destructive periodontitis. The types of stress that lead to periodontal destruction appear to be more chronic or long term and less likely to be controlled by the individual. Life events such as the loss of a loved one (e.g., spouse, family member), a failed relationship, loss of employment, and financial difficulties are examples of stressful life events that are typically not controllable by the individual or not perceived by the individual as being under his or her control, thereby resulting in a feeling of helplessness. The duration of the stressful life event also has an influence on the total impact of the stress-induced disease destruction.

Financial stress is an example of a long-term, constant pressure that may exacerbate periodontal destruction in susceptible individuals. Genco and colleagues[92] found that individuals with high levels of financial stress and poor coping skills had twice as much periodontal disease as those with minimal stress and good coping skills. Psychologic tests were used to identify and weigh the causes of stress (e.g., children, spouse, finances, single life, work) and to measure individual coping skills. Individuals with problem-focused (practical) coping skills fared better than individuals with emotion-focused (avoidance) coping skills with respect to periodontal disease. As part of their analysis, the researchers also found that chronic stress and inadequate coping could lead to changes in daily habits, such as poor oral hygiene, clenching, and grinding, as well as physiologic changes such as decreased saliva flow and suppressed immunity.

When comparing 89 patients with periodontal disease to 63 periodontally healthy individuals, Wimmer and colleagues[277] found that patients with defensive (emotional) coping skills were more likely to refuse responsibility and to downplay their condition. All patients completed a comprehensive stress assessment questionnaire (given in German) to evaluate their coping behavior. Patients with periodontal disease were less likely to use active coping skills (i.e., situation control) and more likely to cope with stress by averting blame (emotional) than were periodontally healthy individuals.

These studies support the concept that one of the most important aspects related to the influence of stress on periodontal disease destruction is the manner in which the individual copes with the stress. Emotional coping methods appear to render the host more susceptible to the destructive effects of periodontal disease than do practical coping methods. Furthermore, emotional coping is more common in situations that must be accepted and among individuals who feel helpless in the situation.

KEY FACT

The effect of psychosocial stress on the manifestation of disease (i.e., periodontitis) is not simply a matter of the presence or absence of stress; rather, the type of stress and the ability of the individual to cope with stress correlate with destructive periodontal disease.

Stress-Induced Immunosuppression

Stress and psychosomatic disorders most likely impact periodontal health via changes in the individual's behavior and through complex interactions among the nervous, endocrine, and immune systems. Individuals under stress may have poorer oral hygiene; they may start or increase the clenching and grinding of their teeth; and they may smoke more frequently. All of these behavioral changes increase their susceptibility to periodontal disease destruction. Likewise, individuals who are under stress may be less likely to seek professional care.

In addition to the many behavioral changes that may influence periodontal disease destruction, psychosocial stress may also impact the disease through alterations in the immune system. The influence of stress on the immune system and systemic health conditions (e.g., cardiovascular disease) is well known. Stress-related immune system changes clearly have the potential to affect the pathogenesis of periodontal disease as well. One possible mechanism involves the production of cortisol. Stress increases cortisol production from the adrenal cortex by stimulating an increase in the release of adrenocorticotropic hormone from the pituitary gland. Increased cortisol suppresses the immune response directly through the suppression of neutrophil activity, immunoglobulin G production, and salivary IgA secretion. All of these immune responses are critical for the normal immunoinflammatory response to periodontal pathogens (see Chapters 8, 11, and 12). The resulting stress-induced immunosuppression increases the potential for destruction by periodontal pathogens. Stress may also affect the cellular immune response directly through an increased release of neurotransmitters, including epinephrine, norepinephrine, neurokinin, and substance P, which interact directly with lymphocytes, neutrophils, monocytes, and macrophages via receptors that cause an increase in their tissue-destructive function. Thus, in a manner similar to cortisol production, the stress-induced release of these neurotransmitters results in an upregulated immune response that increases the potential for destruction by the cellular response to periodontal pathogens.

It is important to remember that, although stress may predispose an individual to more destruction from periodontitis, the presence of periodontal pathogens remains as the essential etiologic factor. In other words, stress alone does not cause or lead to periodontitis in the absence of periodontal pathogens.

Influence of Stress on Periodontal Therapy Outcomes

Psychologic conditions such as stress and depression may also influence the outcome of periodontal therapy. In a large-scale retrospective study of 1299 dental records from a health maintenance organization database, 85 individuals with depression had post-therapy outcomes that were less favorable (below median) than the outcomes of individuals without depression.[76] More than half of these records (697) were complete enough for a comprehensive evaluation that included both periodontal diagnosis and psychologic profiles. The authors concluded that depression might have a negative effect on periodontal treatment outcomes.

A study investigating the relationship between psychologic stress and wound repair in patients after routine surgery (in this case, inguinal hernia open incision repair) revealed that stress impairs the inflammatory response and matrix degradation.[33] Forty-seven adults were given a standardized questionnaire to assess their psychologic stress before surgery. Wound fluids were collected during the first 20 hours after surgery to measure inflammatory markers: IL-1, IL-6, and matrix metalloproteinase-9 (MMP-9). Greater psychologic stress was significantly associated with lower levels of IL-1 and MMP-9 as well as with a significantly more painful, poorer, and slower recovery.

Another study compared the psychiatric characteristics of individuals with different outcomes to periodontal therapy.[11] Two groups were compared to evaluate the psychologic characteristics of 11 individuals who were responsive to periodontal treatment compared with 11 individuals who were not responsive to periodontal treatment. The members of the responsive group had more rigid personalities, whereas those in the nonresponsive group had more passive, dependent personalities. Furthermore, the nonresponsive group reported more stressful life events having occurred in their past.

These studies suggest that both stressful life events and the individual's personality and coping skills are factors to consider when assessing the risk of periodontal disease destruction and the potential for successful periodontal therapy. If patients with emotional or defensive coping skills are identified, care should be taken to ensure that they receive information in a manner that does not elicit a defensive reaction.

Psychiatric Influence of Self-Inflicted Injury

Psychosomatic disorders may result in harmful effects to the health of tissues in the oral cavity through the development of habits that are injurious to the periodontium. Neurotic habits such as grinding or clenching the teeth, nibbling on foreign objects (e.g., pencils, pipes), nail biting, and excessive use of tobacco are all potentially injurious to the teeth and the periodontium. Self-inflicted gingival injuries, such as gingival recession, have been described in both children and adults (Fig. 25.17). However, these types of self-inflicted, factitious injuries do not appear to be common among psychiatric patients.[228]

Nutritional Influences

Some clinicians enthusiastically adhere to the theory in periodontal disease that assigns a key role to nutritional deficiencies and imbalances. Previous research did not support this view, but numerous problems in experimental design and data interpretation could be responsible for making these research findings inadequate.[5,227] The majority of opinions and research findings regarding the effects of nutrition on oral and periodontal tissues point to the following:

1. *There are no nutritional deficiencies that by themselves can cause gingivitis or periodontitis.* However, nutritional deficiencies can affect the condition of the periodontium and thereby may accentuate the deleterious effects of plaque-induced inflammation in susceptible individuals. Theoretically, one may presume that an individual with a nutritional deficiency is less able

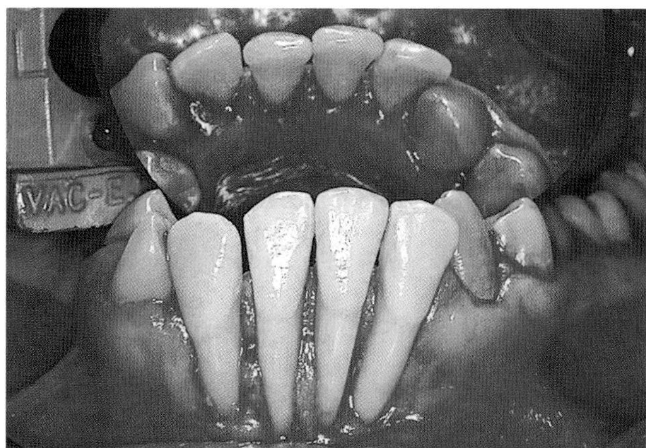

Fig. 25.17 Severe gingival recession localized to the labial surface of all mandibular incisors. This finding was discovered in an uncooperative, institutionalized adult with mental disorders who had been placed under general anesthesia. The patient was known to pace around the home with all four fingers inside his lower lip.

to defend against a bacterial challenge as compared with a nutritionally competent individual.

2. *There are nutritional deficiencies that produce changes in the oral cavity.* These changes include alterations of the tissues of the lips, oral mucosa, gingiva, and bone. These alterations are considered to be the periodontal and oral manifestations of nutritional disease.

The role of nutrition in periodontal disease may be related to the effect of nutrition on inflammation. A 2009 review of the literature evaluating the effect of nutritional factors on inflammation demonstrated that subtle shifts in nutritional status are associated with the prevalence of periodontitis.[48] More specifically, the authors reported that the results of contemporary animal and human studies have demonstrated the role of specific micronutrients in the modulation of the host's inflammatory response by reducing inflammatory biomarkers, which may in turn be responsible for periodontal destruction. The evidence for the effect of nutrition on inflammation is significant. Data suggest that diets that contain foods rich in antioxidants are beneficial, whereas foods that contain high levels of refined carbohydrates are detrimental to the inflammatory process.[48]

See the online material for a review of the existing knowledge of the effects of vitamin and protein deficiencies on changes in the periodontium.

Medications

Some medications that are prescribed to cure, manage, or prevent diseases have adverse effects on periodontal tissues, wound healing, or the host immune response. Bisphosphonates are a class of medications widely prescribed for the treatment of osteoporosis and various types of cancer. Corticosteroids have long been prescribed to suppress the immune system for the control and management of autoimmune disease, during cancer treatment, and as an antirejection medication after organ transplantation. This section discusses the effect of bisphosphonates and corticosteroids on the periodontium. Readers are referred to Chapter 67 for additional information about these and other important medications.

Bisphosphonates

Bisphosphonate medications are primarily used to treat cancer (via intravenous [IV] administration) and osteoporosis (via oral administration). They act by inhibiting osteoclastic activity, which leads to less bone resorption, less bone remodeling, and less bone turnover.[225] The use of bisphosphonates in cancer treatment is aimed at preventing the often-lethal imbalance of osteoclastic activity. For the treatment of osteoporosis, the goal is simply to harness osteoclastic activity to minimize or prevent bone loss and, in many cases, to increase bone mass by creating an advantage for osteoblastic activity. The major differences in the use of bisphosphonates for cancer versus osteoporosis are the potency and route of administration of the specific bisphosphonate medication used. Potency is influenced by the chemical properties as well as by the binding and release pharmacokinetic properties of these agents as they apply to bone. Specifically, the strength of binding and the ease of release of bisphosphonates with hydroxyapatite make these drugs more or less potent.

Bisphosphonates were first synthesized during the 1950s as a substitute for pyrophosphate, a compound used in detergent. The ability of bisphosphonates to increase bone mass was discovered after animal studies that took place in 1966, but the potential advantage of using bisphosphonates in humans with low bone mass was not appreciated until 1984.[267] The US Food and Drug Administration approved the use of alendronate for osteoporosis in 1995.

Pyrophosphate

OH OH
P=P—O—P=O
OH OH

Generic bisphosphonate

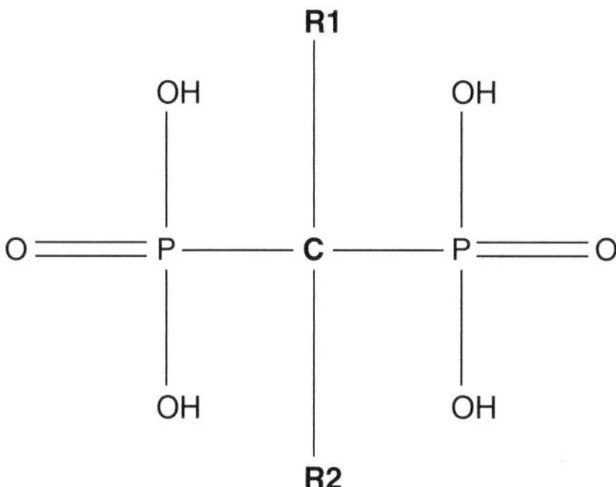

R1 Enhances binding to hydroxyapatite
-C- Enhances chemical stability
R2 Determines antiresorptive potency

Fig. 25.18 Chemical structure of a bisphosphonate molecule. Two phosphate groups are covalently bonded with a central carbon. The carbon also has two side chains, R1 and R2.

The chemical structure of bisphosphonate consists of two phosphate groups covalently bonded to a central carbon (Fig. 25.18). In addition to the two phosphate groups, the central carbon also has two side chains, R1 and R2. Both the short R1 side chain and the long R2 side chain influence the chemical properties and pharmacokinetics. The long R2 side chain also influences the mode of action and determines the strength or potency of the medication. Bisphosphonates inhibit osteoclasts by two mechanisms that depend on whether the R2 side chain contains nitrogen. Nonaminobisphosphonates are metabolized by osteoclasts to form an adenosine triphosphate analog that interferes with energy production and causes osteoclast apoptosis. Aminobisphosphonates (i.e., risedronate, zoledronate, ibandronate, and alendronate) are more potent and have multiple effects on osteoclasts, including: (1) inactivation of adenosine triphosphate; (2) osteoclast cytoskeletal disruption; (3) impairment of osteoclast recruitment; and (4) induction of osteoblasts to produce osteoclast-inhibiting factor.[197] Bisphosphonates also inhibit bone metabolism via antiangiogenic activity.[37]

Table 25.1 lists some of the common bisphosphonate medications used for osteoporosis and cancer treatment that are currently available in the United States.

Bisphosphonates and other antiresorptive medications including denosumab have been implicated in osteonecrosis of the jaw (ONJ), a serious condition that is characterized by non-healing and often painful exposure of nonvital and often sequestrating bone in the jaws.[136]

There is growing evidence that bisphosphonates also affect soft tissues and that they may contribute to ONJ via inhibition of soft tissue healing.[150] An in vitro study by Kim and colleagues suggested that bisphosphonates may act on oral keratinocytes to impair wound healing by inhibiting epithelial migration and wound closure.[139]

TABLE 25.1 Current Nonaminobisphosphonate and Aminobisphosphonate Medications and Common Therapeutic Uses

Generic Name	Commercial Name	Route of Administration	Therapeutic Use	Nitrogen-Containing R2 Side Chain	Relative Antiresorptive Potency
Etidronate	Didronel	PO	Paget disease	No	1
Tiludronate	Skelid	PO	Paget disease	No	10
Risedronate	Actonel	PO	Osteoporosis, Paget disease	Yes	5000
Ibandronate	Boniva	PO	Osteoporosis	Yes	10,000
Alendronate	Fosamax	PO	Osteoporosis, Paget disease	Yes	1000
Pamidronate	Aredia	IV	Paget disease, cancer	Yes	100
Zoledronate	Zometa	IV	Cancer	Yes	10,000+
Zoledronate	Reclast	IV	Osteoporosis	Yes	Same as Zometa but given as a single treatment, annually or biennially

IV, Intravenous; *PO*, by mouth.

Interestingly, the effects of bisphosphonates on oral mucosal cells and bone cells share the common mechanism of interference with products of the mevalonate pathway, which may be more significant to the overall problem than the reported apoptosis effects on osteoclasts. The inhibition of farnesyl pyrophosphate synthase leads to inhibition of the mevalonate pathway end product, geranylgeranyl pyrophosphate (Fig. 25.19). This bisphosphonate-inhibited pathway is required for many essential cellular functions in a variety of tissues. In the case of soft tissues, the bisphosphonate-induced senescence of human oral keratinocytes was found to be mediated, at least in part, by inhibition of the mevalonate pathway. Similarly, Fisher and colleagues reported that bisphosphonates inhibit bone resorption via prevention of protein prenylation in osteoclasts that is caused by the inhibition of farnesyl pyrophosphate synthase, resulting in interference with the production of geranylgeranyl pyrophosphate.

Bisphosphonates have a high affinity for hydroxyapatite. They are rapidly absorbed in bone, especially in areas of high activity, which may help to explain why bisphosphonate-induced osteonecrosis is found only in the jaws.[267] The bisphosphonate molecule gets incorporated into bone without being metabolized or modified. During the osteoclastic resorption of bone, the trapped bisphosphonate is released and able to affect osteoclasts again. As a result, the half-life of bisphosphonates in the bone is estimated to be 10 years or longer.

ONJ associated with bisphosphonates was first described in 2003 by Marx in a report of 36 patients with avascular necrosis of the jaw who had been treated with IV bisphosphonate for malignant tumors.[170] Several case series reporting an association between bisphosphonates and ONJ were published subsequently.[172,223] Various terms have been used to describe this type of ONJ, including *avascular necrosis, bisphosphonate-associated ONJ, bisphosphonate-induced ONJ,* and *bisphosphonate-related ONJ (BRONJ).*[267] Today, with the widespread recognition of BRONJ, it is important to remember that necrotic bone exposure of the jaw (ONJ) is a condition with multiple possible etiopathogenic factors, including systemic medications, radiation, infection, trauma, direct chemical toxicity, and other idiopathic mechanisms; clinicians should carefully consider all factors before making a diagnosis of BRONJ.[8] Denosumab (Prolia, Xgeva), an antiresorptive medication used to treat osteoporosis and bone metastasis by inhibiting osteoclast activity, has also been implicated in ONJ.[30] Other antiresorptive agents have been associated with ONJ, hence the current term, antiresorptive agent-induced osteonecrosis of the jaw (ARONJ).[117]

Clinically, ARONJ manifests as exposed alveolar bone that occurs spontaneously or after a traumatic event such as a dental procedure (Figs. 25.20 and 25.21). The sites may be painful, with surrounding soft tissue induration and inflammation. Infection with drainage may be present. Radiographically, lesions appear radiolucent, with sclerosis of the lamina dura, a loss of the lamina dura, or a widening of the periodontal ligament in areas where teeth are present. Histologically, bone appears necrotic, with empty lacunae demonstrating a lack of living osteocytes. In advanced cases, pathologic fracture may be present through the area of exposed or necrotic bone.

The high potency of nitrogen-containing bisphosphonates—especially those administered intravenously for cancer treatment (e.g., zoledronate)—may explain the high incidence of ARONJ in these patients compared with osteoporotic patients taking oral bisphosphonates. The incidence among patients who are being treated for cancer has been reported to range from 2.5% to 5.4%[271] or from 1% to 10%[37] and as much as 1% to 15%.[136] Estimating the incidence among patients who are taking oral bisphosphonates for osteoporosis is more difficult due to the large number of patients taking this prescription medication and a lack of good reporting or documentation for these patients. Some reports estimate the incidence of ARONJ from oral bisphosphonates to range from 0.007% to 0.04%,[267] whereas other reports suggest a slightly higher incidence that ranges from 0.004% to 0.11%.[243] Clearly, the incidence among patients taking oral bisphosphonates appears to be low.

It has been observed that ARONJ lesions occur most often in areas with dense bone and thin overlying mucosa, such as tori, bony exostoses, and the mylohyoid ridge.[172,222,223] Lesions are found more commonly in the mandible than in the maxilla at a 2:1 ratio.[221] Work by Schaudinn and colleagues suggests that there may be a toxic threshold of accumulated bisphosphonate in the bone that leads to the induction of ARONJ lesions and that measuring or calculating the concentration in bone may be a means of assessing an individual's risk for the development of ARONJ.[228]

In addition to bisphosphonate therapy, other factors are thought to increase individual susceptibility to ARONJ. Potential risk factors that may contribute to ARONJ include systemic corticosteroid therapy, smoking, alcohol, poor oral hygiene, chemotherapy, radiotherapy, diabetes, and hematologic disease.[31]

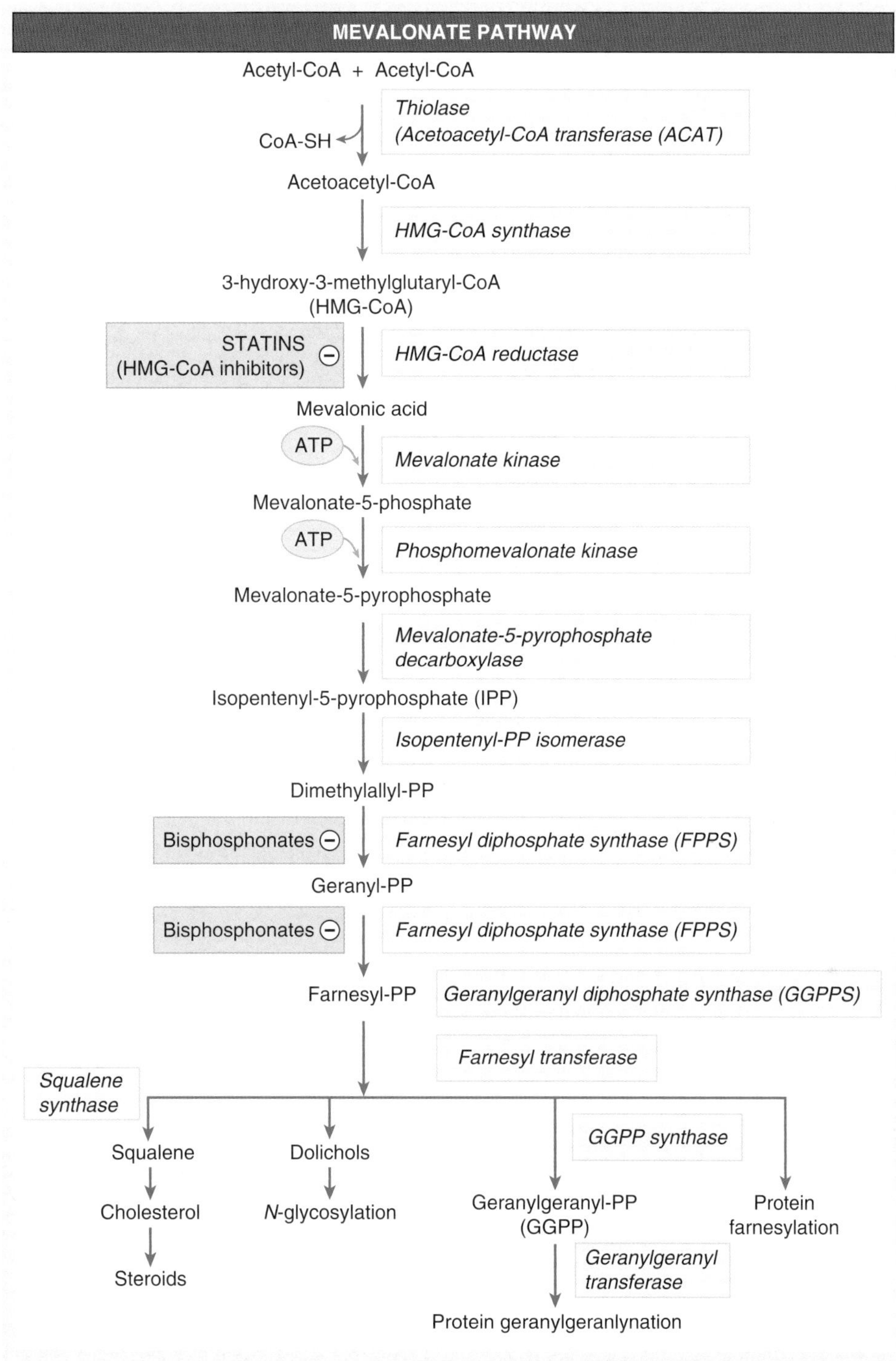

Fig. 25.19 Mevalonate pathway. Bisphosphonates interfere with the farnesyl pyrophosphate synthase enzyme, which leads to the inhibition of geranylgeranyl pyrophosphate, an important end product for cellular functions.

The precipitating factors or trauma-inducing events that lead to ARONJ are reported to include extractions, root canal treatment, periodontal infections, periodontal surgery, and dental implant surgery; however, some cases appear to be idiopathic, with spontaneous exposures.[172] In a retrospective evaluation of patients treated with IV bisphosphonates for metastatic bone cancer from 1996 to 2006, Estilo and colleagues[79] found that the type of cancer, the duration of bisphosphonate therapy, sequential IV bisphosphonate treatment with pamidronate followed by zoledronate, comorbid osteoarthritis, rheumatoid arthritis, and benign hematologic conditions were significantly associated with an increased likelihood of ONJ. In their study, the systemic administration of corticosteroids was not found to be associated with an increased risk of ARONJ.[79]

As stated previously, patients who are being treated for cancer with IV bisphosphonates are at greater risk than patients being treated for osteoporosis with oral bisphosphonates. Dental health care providers should evaluate patients carefully, consider the risks, communicate with medical health care providers, inform patients, and consider treatment options and risks carefully.

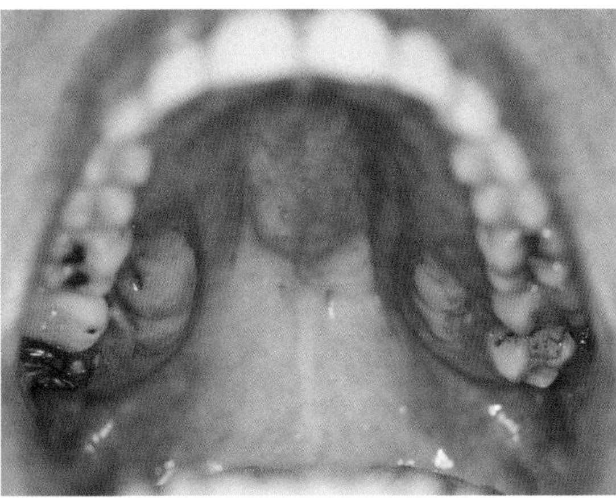

Fig. 25.20 Clinical photograph of exposed bone on the palatal surface of the maxilla adjacent to the molar root in a 60-year-old female with bisphosphonate-induced osteonecrosis of the bone (maxilla). The bone exposures were noted after about 1 year of treatment with bisphosphonate (Aredia and Zometa). (*Courtesy Drs. Eric S. Sung and Evelyn M. Chung, University of California, Los Angeles, CA.*)

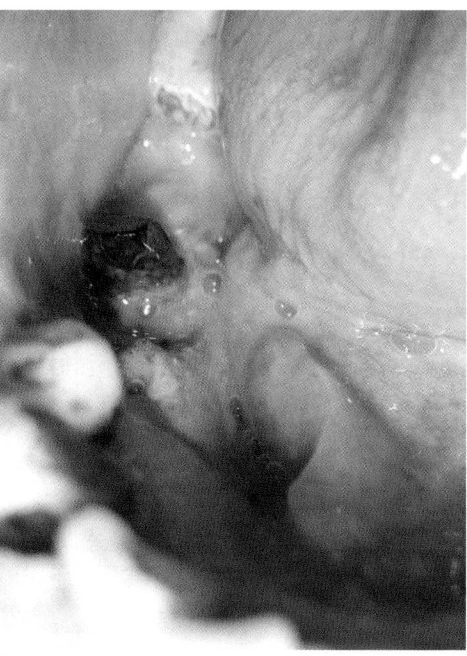

Fig. 25.21 Clinical photograph of exposed bone on the lingual surface of the posterior mandible of a 70-year-old male with bisphosphonate-induced osteonecrosis of the bone (mandible). The bone exposure was noted after 3 years of bisphosphonate treatment (Aredia and Zometa) for multiple myeloma. (*Courtesy Drs. Eric S. Sung and Evelyn M. Chung, University of California, Los Angeles, CA.*)

KEY FACT

The effects of bisphosphonates on oral hard and soft tissue cells share the common mechanism of interference with products of the mevalonate pathway, which may be more significant to the overall problem than the reported apoptosis effects on osteoclasts. The inhibition of farnesyl pyrophosphate synthase leads to the inhibition of the mevalonate pathway end product, geranylgeranyl pyrophosphate (see Fig. 25.19). This bisphosphonate-inhibited pathway is required for many essential cellular functions in a variety of tissues.

Bisphosphonates and Periodontal Bone Loss

Not surprisingly, the bone-preserving action of bisphosphonates has been studied and advocated for use in the prevention of bone loss from periodontal disease.[255] Several animal studies have shown that bisphosphonates, either applied topically or administered systemically, have the potential to prevent the alveolar bone loss caused by periodontitis.[46,108,180,182,198,241,274] The use of bisphosphonates for bone regeneration has been proposed as well.[255] Although some studies have demonstrated bone preservation with low doses of bisphosphonate, higher doses and longer administration may have a neutral or detrimental effect on bone loss caused by periodontitis.[38,46] In a 2- to 3-year follow-up report of four female patients with periodontitis treated with etidronate (200 mg daily for periods of 2 weeks with 10-week off-drug periods), the potential of this agent to prevent periodontal bone loss was reported.[252] In a 2-year, randomized, placebo-controlled clinical trial of 335 patients treated with alendronate (70 mg once weekly), no significant difference in alveolar bone loss or alveolar bone density was found.[128] Interestingly, alendronate was found to significantly reduce bone loss relative to controls in a subset of this group (i.e., patients with low mandibular bone mineral density [BMD] at baseline), suggesting that the effect may be more perceptible in cases with less bone mass or less bone density. In another clinical trial of 24 patients (12 experimental and 12 control), alendronate was shown to have a significant positive (bone-preserving) effect on bone density in jaws.[74] The BMD of the maxilla and mandible was measured for all patients with the use of dual-energy x-ray absorptiometry (DEXA) at baseline and after 6 months of treatment (10 mg daily for 6 months).

Corticosteroids

In humans, the systemic administration of cortisone and adrenocorticotropic hormone appears to have no effect on the incidence or severity of gingival and periodontal disease. However, renal transplantation patients receiving immunosuppressive therapy (either prednisone or methylprednisolone combined with either azathioprine or cyclophosphamide) have significantly less gingival inflammation than control subjects with similar amounts of plaque.[22,134,147,196,259]

Exogenous cortisone may have an adverse effect on bone quality and physiology. The systemic administration of cortisone in experimental animals resulted in the osteoporosis of alveolar bone.[99] There was capillary dilation and engorgement with hemorrhage into the periodontal ligament and gingival connective tissue, degeneration and a reduction in the number of collagen fibers in the periodontal ligament, and increased destruction of the periodontal tissues associated with inflammation.[101]

Stress increases circulating cortisol levels through stimulation of the adrenal glands (i.e., the hypothalamic–pituitary–adrenal axis). This increased exposure to endogenous cortisol may have adverse effects on the periodontium by diminishing the immune response to periodontal bacteria (see the section about Psychosocial Stress, Depression, and Coping).

See the online material for discussion of additional systemic conditions and their influence on periodontal health.

Other Systemic Conditions

Osteoporosis

Osteoporosis is a disease that is characterized by low bone mass and structural deterioration leading to an increased risk of bone fracture. It affects approximately 10 million people in the United States. The condition has a higher predilection for females (80%) compared with males (20%). An additional 34 million individuals in the

United States are estimated to have osteopenia or low bone density. The loss of bone mass and the incidence of osteoporosis increases with age for both men and women, with women being affected earlier than men. The rate of bone loss is greatest for women during the perimenopausal years, when estrogen levels decrease.

A BMD test is used to measure an individual's bone mass. BMD is measured with the use of a DEXA scan. The DEXA value or T-score is a comparison of the patient's BMD with that of a healthy 30-year-old adult with peak bone mass. The World Health Organization defines osteoporosis and osteopenia by measures of standard deviation rather than comparison with a normal, healthy, young adult. Thus, a T-score between +1 and −1 is considered normal, whereas a T-score between −1 and −2.5 indicates low bone density or osteopenia and a T-score of less than −2.5 (i.e., more than 2.5 standard deviations below normal) is diagnostic for osteoporosis (eTable 25.1).

One of the most significant consequences of osteoporosis is the increased risk of bone fracture. All bones affected by osteoporosis are susceptible to fracture, but fractures of the pelvis and vertebrae carry the most serious risk of morbidity and mortality. Studies have reported that approximately 20% of patients with hip fractures die within a year and that 50% experience significant disability (e.g., an inability to walk unassisted).[152]

Although it is logical to surmise a relationship between osteoporosis and periodontitis, it has been a challenging hypothesis to prove. One of the difficulties is the fact that both osteoporosis and periodontitis are chronic, multifactorial diseases that result in bone loss, and bone loss in each condition is exacerbated by local and systemic factors.[193] Gender, genetic predisposition, inactivity, deficient diets (e.g., deficient in calcium or vitamin D), alcohol, smoking, hormones, and medications put individuals at risk for osteoporosis, with some of these factors putting them at risk for the progression of periodontitis as well. Variations in populations studied, measurements used to assess disease, and study design have also hindered the ability to clearly define a relationship between osteoporosis and periodontitis.

Attempts to use tooth loss as an indirect measure of periodontitis in individuals with osteoporosis have offered mixed conclusions. Several studies have reported greater tooth loss, more alveolar bone loss, and edentulism in individuals with osteoporosis.[63,70,114,285] However, some other studies have suggested that tooth loss is not correlated with osteoporosis or BMD.[29,2,183] One large study of 1365 Caucasian postmenopausal females that investigated systemic BMD (lumbar spine and proximal femur) and tooth loss found no significant correlation.[72] Part of the challenge and the reason for conflicting results in these studies may be differences in measurement methods. Another problem with translating any tooth loss study conclusions to address the question of whether osteoporosis contributes to periodontitis is that the cause of tooth loss in these studies is often unknown (i.e., tooth loss may or may not be related to periodontal disease).

Studies that attempt to correlate osteoporosis with periodontitis are fraught with similar if not greater challenges. Again, some studies have concluded or suggested that osteoporosis does contribute to the progression of periodontitis,[125,141,184,257] whereas others refute this conclusion.[75,162] One study by Elders and colleagues failed to show a correlation between lumbar BMD and clinical parameters of periodontitis in a dentate group of 286 females between the ages of 46 and 55 years.[75] The researchers used intraoral periodontal examinations (i.e., probing depth, bleeding on probing, and missing teeth) and bitewing radiographs to assess clinical parameters of periodontitis and interproximal alveolar bone loss. This study included edentulous subjects as well, but no significant difference in BMD was found between edentulous (60) and dentate (226) subjects, suggesting that neither periodontitis nor tooth loss was related to osteoporosis. The mean age of the subjects in this study was relatively young, which may have contributed to the lack of correlation.[94]

Most studies citing a positive correlation between osteoporosis or BMD and periodontitis are cross-sectional studies of postmenopausal females. Klemetti and colleagues evaluated 227 healthy postmenopausal women between the ages of 48 and 56 years and found that women with higher skeletal BMD were more likely to retain their teeth in the presence of periodontitis (i.e., deep periodontal pockets) compared with women with osteoporosis.[141] Tezal and colleagues concluded that skeletal BMD (measured by DEXA at multiple sites) is related to alveolar bone loss and, to a lesser extent, to clinical attachment loss, thereby implicating postmenopausal osteopenia as a risk indicator for periodontal disease in 70 postmenopausal white women between the ages of 51 and 78 years.[257] Periodontal parameters included probing depth, supragingival plaque, calculus, bleeding on probing, clinical attachment loss, and interproximal alveolar bone loss. Analysis was adjusted for age, age at menopause, estrogen supplementation, cigarette smoking, body mass, and supragingival plaque. Inagaki and colleagues evaluated the association between periodontal conditions, tooth loss, and metacarpal BMD in a cross-sectional study of 356 Japanese women: 171 premenopausal women (mean age, 37.9 years) and 185 postmenopausal women (mean age, 63.3 years). The authors concluded that periodontal status and tooth loss after menopause could be a useful indicator of metacarpal BMD loss in Japanese women.[125] These cross-sectional studies are suggestive but do not consider the periodontal condition or existence of periodontitis before the onset of osteoporosis or the loss of systemic BMD.

The effect of estrogen deficiency and osteopenia or osteoporosis on periodontitis is not known, but it may be an important factor to consider. Reinhardt and colleagues[214] conducted a 2-year, prospective, longitudinal study of postmenopausal women (59 with moderate or advanced periodontitis and 16 with no periodontitis) to evaluate the effect of estrogen (serum estradiol) levels on periodontitis in these patients. Clinical measurements—including supragingival plaque, bleeding on probing, and relative clinical attachment—were taken at baseline and every 6 months for 2 years. The authors concluded that estrogen deficiency and osteopenia or osteoporosis together are risk factors for alveolar bone loss in postmenopausal women with a history of periodontitis.[214] Lerner[153] also proposed that estrogen deficiency may play a significant role in the progression of periodontitis in osteopenic or osteoporotic women, citing the fact that the cytokines thought to be involved in inflammation-induced remodeling are very similar to those suggested to play crucial roles in postmenopausal osteoporosis. In patients with periodontal disease and concomitant postmenopausal osteoporosis, the possibility exists that the lack of estrogen influences the activities of bone cells and immune cells in such a way that the progression of alveolar bone loss is enhanced.[153] In fact, there are numerous studies that report less risk for tooth loss and improved oral health among postmenopausal women receiving hormone replacement therapy.[7,19,26,111,112,251] More prospective, longitudinal studies evaluating the effect of estrogen and osteopenia or osteoporosis on periodontitis are needed to improve the current understanding.

Congenital Heart Disease

Congenital heart disease occurs in about 1% of live births. Approximately 40% of individuals born with heart defects would die without treatment. However, the prognosis has been dramatically improved with advances in cardiac surgery. Cardiac defects can involve the heart, the adjacent vessels, or a combination of both.

The most striking feature of congenital heart disease is cyanosis caused by the shunting of deoxygenated blood from the right to the left, which results in the return of poorly oxygenated blood to the systemic circulation. In severe cases, cyanosis is obvious at birth, particularly in the presence of tetralogy of Fallot. Chronic hypoxia causes impaired development, compensatory polycythemia (i.e., an increase in RBCs and hemoglobin), and clubbing edema of toes and fingers (eFig. 25.11). Polycythemia is significant because it can result in hemorrhagic or thrombotic tendencies. Patients with congenital heart defects are often at risk for infective endocarditis as a result of turbulent blood flow in the heart and the associated cardiovascular defects. The need for prophylactic antibiotics should be evaluated before dental therapy.

In addition to the obvious cyanosis of the lips and the oral mucosa, oral abnormalities associated with cyanotic congenital heart disease include delayed eruption of both primary and permanent dentitions, increased positional abnormalities, and enamel hypoplasia. The teeth often have a bluish-white appearance with an increased pulp vascular volume. Gingival disease and other oral symptoms have been reported in children with congenital heart disease.[28,132] Reports seem to indicate more severe caries and periodontal disease in patients with cyanotic congenital heart defects. However, the apparent increase in dental disease may be attributed to poor oral hygiene and a general lack of dental care rather than a disease-related etiology.

Tetralogy of Fallot

As its name implies, tetralogy of Fallot is characterized by four cardiac defects: (1) ventricular septal defect, (2) pulmonary stenosis, (3) malposition of the aorta to the right, and (4) compensatory right ventricular enlargement. Clinical features include severe cyanosis, audible heart murmurs, and breathlessness. Cyanosis and breathlessness cause cerebral anoxia and syncope. Oral changes include a purplish-red discoloration of the lips and the gingiva. Severe marginal gingivitis and periodontal destruction have been reported (eFig. 25.12). The discoloration of the lips and the gingiva corresponds to the general degree of cyanosis and returns to normal after corrective heart surgery. The tongue appears coated, fissured, and edematous, and there is extreme reddening of the fungiform and filiform papillae. The number of subepithelial capillaries is increased, but this also returns to normal after heart surgery.[85]

Eisenmenger Syndrome

Among patients with ventricular septal defects, about half of those with large defects (i.e., > 1.5 cm in diameter) develop Eisenmenger syndrome. This syndrome is distinguished by a greater blood flow from the stronger left ventricle to the right ventricle (backward flow) through the septal defect. This causes increased pulmonary blood flow, which in turn leads to progressive pulmonary fibrosis, small vessel occlusion, and high pulmonary vascular resistance. With increasing pulmonary resistance, the right ventricle hypertrophies, the shunt becomes bidirectional, and ultimately blood flow is reversed (i.e., it flows from right to left). The increased vascular resistance builds pressure in the right ventricle, thereby causing right ventricular hypertrophy and a reversal in the direction of the blood flow, which results in a right-to-left shunt.

The natural history of a patient with untreated Eisenmenger syndrome is a gradual increase in cyanosis over many years that eventually leads to cardiac failure. Cyanosis of the lips, cheeks, and buccal mucous membranes is observed in these patients, but it is much less severe than in those with tetralogy of Fallot. Severe, generalized periodontitis has been reported in patients with Eisenmenger syndrome.[51] However, as in patients with other types of congenital heart disease, the incidence of periodontal disease reported in those with Eisenmenger syndrome may be related more to poor oral hygiene and a general lack of dental care than to any specific, syndrome-related etiology.

Hypophosphatasia

Hypophosphatasia is a rare familial skeletal disease that is characterized by rickets, poor cranial bone formation, craniostenosis, and the premature loss of the primary teeth, particularly the incisors. Patients have a low level of serum alkaline phosphatase, and phosphoethanolamine is present in serum and urine.

Teeth are lost with no clinical evidence of gingival inflammation, and they show reduced cementum formation.[24] In patients with minimal bone abnormalities, the premature loss of the deciduous teeth may be the only symptom of hypophosphatasia. In adolescents, this disease resembles localized (juvenile/aggressive) periodontitis, grade C.[284]

Metal Intoxication

The ingestion of metals such as mercury, lead, and bismuth in medicinal compounds and through industrial contact may result in oral manifestations caused by either intoxication or absorption without evidence of toxicity.

Bismuth Intoxication

Chronic bismuth intoxication is characterized by gastrointestinal disturbances, nausea, vomiting, and jaundice as well as by an ulcerative gingivostomatitis, generally with pigmentation and accompanied by a metallic taste and burning sensation of the oral mucosa. The tongue may be sore and inflamed. Urticaria, different types of exanthematous eruptions, bullous and purpuric lesions, herpes zoster–like eruptions, and pigmentation of the skin and mucous membranes are among the dermatologic lesions attributed to bismuth intoxication. Acute bismuth intoxication, which is seen less frequently, is accompanied by methemoglobin formation, cyanosis, and dyspnea.[119]

Bismuth pigmentation in the oral cavity usually appears as a narrow, bluish-black discoloration of the gingival margin in areas of preexisting gingival inflammation (eFig. 25.13). Such pigmentation results from the precipitation of particles of bismuth sulfide associated with vascular changes in inflammation; it is not evidence of intoxication but simply indicates the presence of bismuth in the bloodstream. Bismuth pigmentation in the oral cavity also occurs in cases of intoxication; it assumes a linear form if the marginal gingiva is inflamed.

Lead Intoxication

Lead is slowly absorbed, and toxic symptoms are not particularly definitive when they do occur.[129] There is a pallor of the face and lips and gastrointestinal symptoms that consist of nausea, vomiting, loss of appetite, and abdominal colic. Peripheral neuritis, psychologic disorders, and encephalitis have been reported. Oral signs include salivation, coated tongue, a peculiar sweetish taste, gingival pigmentation, and ulceration. Gingival pigmentation is linear (Burtonian line), steel gray, and associated with local inflammation. Oral signs may occur without toxic symptoms.

Mercury Intoxication

Mercury intoxication is characterized by headache, insomnia, cardiovascular symptoms, pronounced salivation (ptyalism), and a metallic taste.[4] Gingival pigmentation in linear form results from the deposition of mercuric sulfide. The chemical also acts as an irritant, which accentuates the preexisting inflammation and often leads to notable ulceration of the gingiva and the adjacent mucosa as well as the destruction of the underlying bone. Mercurial pigmentation of the gingiva also occurs in areas of local irritation in patients without symptoms of intoxication.

Other Chemicals

Other chemicals (e.g., phosphorus, arsenic, chromium) may cause necrosis of the alveolar bone, with loosening and exfoliation of the teeth.[154,234] Inflammation and ulceration of the gingiva are usually associated with the destruction of the underlying tissues. Benzene intoxication is accompanied by gingival bleeding and ulceration with the destruction of the underlying bone.[234]

Conclusions

Today, we have a better appreciation for the complexity and significance of interrelationships between periodontal infections and host defense. Genetic, environmental, physical, and psychosocial factors have the potential to alter periodontal tissues and the host immune response, thereby resulting in more severe periodontal disease. It is important to recognize that the systemic diseases, disorders, or conditions themselves do not cause periodontitis; rather, they may predispose, accelerate, or otherwise increase disease progression. This chapter reviewed important systemic diseases, disorders, and conditions that influence periodontal health.

A Case Scenario is found on the companion website eBooks.Health.Elsevier.com.

Suggested Reading

Atabay VE, Lutfioğlu M, Avci B, et al. Obesity and oxidative stress in patients with different periodontal status: a case-control study. *J Periodontal Res*. 2017;52:51–60.

Borgioli A, Viviani C, Duvina M, et al. Biphosphonates-related osteonecrosis of the jaw: clinical and physiopathological considerations. *Ther Clin Risk Manag*. 2009;5:217–227.

Brozoski MA, Traina AA, Deboni MC, et al. Bisphosphonate-related osteonecrosis of the jaw. *Rev Bras Reumatol*. 2012;52(2):265–270.

Deas DE, Mackey SA, McDonnell HT. Systemic disease and periodontitis: manifestations of neutrophil dysfunction. *Periodontol 2000*. 2003;32:82–104.

Genco RJ. Current view of risk factors for periodontal diseases. *J Periodontol*. 1996;67:1041–1049.

Genco RJ, Ho AW, Grossi SG, et al. Relationship of stress, distress and inadequate coping behaviors to periodontal disease. *J Periodontol*. 1999;70:711–723.

Gorman A, Kaye EK, Apovian C, et al. Overweight and obesity predict time to periodontal disease progression in men. *J Clin Periodontol*. 2012;39:107–114.

Iacopino AM. Periodontitis and diabetes interrelationships: role of inflammation. *Ann Periodontol*. 2001;6:125–137.

Lamster IB, Pagan M. Periodontal disease and the metabolic syndrome. *Int Dent J*. 2017;67:67–77.

Loe H. Periodontal disease. The sixth complication of diabetes mellitus. *Diabetes Care*. 1993;16:329–334.

Mealey BL. Influence of periodontal infections on systemic health. *Periodontol 2000*. 1999;21:197–209.

Nascimento GG, Leite FR, Do LG, et al. Is weight gain associated with the incidence of periodontitis? A systematic review and meta-analysis. *J Clin Periodontol*. 2015;42:495–505.

Nascimento GG, Peres KG, Mittinty MN, et al. Obesity and periodontal outcomes: a population-based cohort study in Brazil. *J Periodontol*. 2017;88:50–58.

Peruzzo DC, Benatti BB, Ambrosano GM, et al. A systematic review of stress and psychological factors as possible risk factors for periodontal disease. *J Periodontol*. 2007;78:1491–1504.

Ruggiero SL, Dodson TB, Assael LA, et al. American Association of Oral and Maxillofacial Surgeons position paper on bisphosphonate-related osteonecrosis of the jaws—2009 update. *J Oral Maxillofac Surg*. 2009;67(suppl 5):2–12.

Wilkins LM, Kaye EK, Wang HY, et al. Influence of obesity on periodontitis progression is conditional on interleukin-1 inflammatory genetic variation. *J Periodontol*. 2017;88:59–68.

Wimmer G, Janda M, Wieselmann-Penkner K, et al. Coping with stress: its influence on periodontal disease. *J Periodontol*. 2002;73:1343–1351.

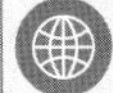
References for this chapter are found on the companion website eBooks.Health.Elsevier.com.

CHAPTER 26

Impact of Periodontal Infection on Systemic Health

Brian L. Mealey | *Perry R. Klokkevold* | *Yvonne L. Hernandez-Kapila*

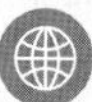

For online-only content on periodontal disease and pregnancy outcome, periodontal disease and chronic obstructive pulmonary disease, and periodontal disease and acute respiratory infections, please visit the companion website at eBooks.Health.Elsevier.com.

CHAPTER OUTLINE

Knowledge of the pathogenesis of periodontal diseases has evolved markedly over the last 50 years.[148] Periodontal disease is an inflammatory disease initiated by bacterial pathogens. Environmental, physical, social, and host stresses may affect and modify disease expression through a multitude of pathways. Certain systemic conditions can affect the initiation and progression of gingivitis and periodontitis. Systemic disorders that affect neutrophil, monocyte, macrophage, and lymphocyte function result in the altered production or activity of host inflammatory mediators.[148,218] These alterations may manifest clinically as the early onset of periodontal destruction or as a more rapid rate of destruction than would occur in the absence of such disorders.

Evidence has also shed light on the converse side of the relationship between systemic health and oral health: the potential effects of inflammatory periodontal diseases on a wide range of organ systems.[137a] This field of periodontal medicine addresses the following important questions:

- How does the inflammatory response to bacterial infection of the periodontium affect tissues and organ systems distant from the oral cavity?
- Is periodontal infection a risk factor for systemic diseases or conditions that affect human health?

Pathobiology of Periodontitis

Our understanding of the pathogenesis of periodontitis has changed remarkably over the last 40 years.[148,218,225] The nonspecific accumulation of bacterial plaque was once thought to be the cause of periodontal destruction, but it is now recognized that periodontitis is an infectious disease associated with a relatively small number of predominantly gram-negative microorganisms that exist in a subgingival biofilm.[99] Furthermore, the importance of the host in disease initiation and progression is clearly recognized. Although pathogenic bacteria are necessary for periodontal disease, they are not sufficient alone to cause the disease. A susceptible host is also imperative. In a host who has relatively low susceptibility to disease, bacterial pathogens may have minimal clinical effect. This may be due to a particularly effective host immunoinflammatory response that eliminates pathogenic organisms while minimizing destruction of native tissues. Conversely, in a host with relatively high disease susceptibility, marked destruction of periodontal tissues may result.

KEY FACT

Whereas pathogenic bacteria are necessary for periodontal disease, bacteria alone are not sufficient to cause disease. A susceptible host is imperative. In a host with relatively low susceptibility, bacterial pathogens may have little or no clinical effect.

Recognizing the importance of host susceptibility opens a door to understanding the differences in the onset, natural history, and progression of periodontitis found throughout the scientific literature. Because of differences in host susceptibility, not all individuals are equally vulnerable to the destructive effects of periodontal pathogens and the immunoinflammatory response to those organisms. Thus, patients may not necessarily have similar disease expression despite the presence of similar bacteria. Likewise, the response to periodontal treatment may vary depending on the wound-healing capacity and susceptibility of the host to further disease progression. The importance of host susceptibility is clearly evident in the medical literature. For example, respiratory tract pathogens may have a minimal effect on many individuals, but in a susceptible host such as an elderly patient, these same pathogens may cause life-threatening respiratory tract illnesses.

There are many systemic conditions that can modify the host's susceptibility to periodontitis. For example, patients with immune suppression may not be able to mount an effective host response to subgingival microorganisms, thereby resulting in more rapid and severe periodontal destruction. Conversely, individuals with a significant increase in the production of proinflammatory mediators may respond to periodontal pathogens with an exuberant inflammatory response that results in the destruction of periodontal tissues. Although the potential impact of many systemic disorders on the periodontium is well documented, evidence suggests that periodontal infection may significantly enhance the risk for certain systemic diseases or alter the natural course of systemic conditions.[160,189,208,227,260,308] Although more than 50 different systemic conditions have been associated with periodontal diseases, the evidence base is quite large for many of these conditions and smaller for others. For example, conditions in which the influences of periodontal infection are well documented include coronary heart disease (CHD) and CHD-related events such as angina, infarction, atherosclerosis, and other vascular conditions; stroke; diabetes mellitus; preterm labor, low-birth-weight delivery, and preeclampsia; and respiratory conditions, such as chronic obstructive pulmonary disease (COPD; Box 26.1).[160,189,226] A smaller but growing evidence base supports an association between poor oral health, tooth loss, or periodontitis and conditions such as chronic kidney disease and renal insufficiency[47,83,84,153,154,266]; certain forms of cancer[7,85,200,201,287] affecting the liver, pancreas, and colorectal region; rheumatoid arthritis[23,59,60]; and altered cognitive function, dementia, and Alzheimer disease.[137,140,160,278,281,324] This chapter focuses on those conditions with the strongest evidence base, recognizing that ongoing research will further elucidate relationships between inflammatory periodontal diseases and systemic health.

BOX 26.1 Organ Systems and Conditions Possibly Influenced by Periodontal Infection

Cardiovascular and Cerebrovascular Systems
Atherosclerosis
Coronary heart disease
Angina
Myocardial infarction
Cerebrovascular accident (stroke)
Erectile dysfunction
Anemia

Endocrine System
Metabolic syndrome
Diabetes mellitus

Reproductive System
Preterm and low-birth-weight infants
Preeclampsia

Respiratory System
Chronic obstructive pulmonary disease
Acute bacterial pneumonia

Kidney Diseases
Renal insufficiency
Chronic kidney disease
End-stage kidney disease

Autoimmune Diseases
Rheumatoid arthritis
Ankylosing spondylitis

Cognitive Function
Dementia
Alzheimer disease

Cancers
Colorectal
Pancreatic
Hepatocellular
Others

Focal Infection Theory Revisited

Research in the area of periodontal medicine marks a resurgence in the concept of focal infection. In 1900, British physician William Hunter first developed the idea that oral microorganisms were responsible for a wide range of systemic conditions that were not easily recognized as being infectious in nature.[214,309] He claimed that restoration of carious teeth, instead of extraction, resulted in the trapping of infectious agents under restorations. In addition to caries, pulpal necrosis, and periapical abscesses, Hunter identified gingivitis and periodontitis as foci of infection. He advocated the extraction of teeth with these conditions to eliminate the source of sepsis. Hunter thought that teeth were prone to septic infection primarily because of their structure and their relationship to alveolar bone. He stated that the degree of systemic effect produced by oral sepsis depended on the virulence of the oral infection and the individual's degree of resistance. He also thought that oral organisms had specific actions on different tissues and that these organisms acted by producing toxins, thereby resulting in low-grade "subinfections" that produced systemic effects over prolonged periods. Finally, Hunter thought that the connection between oral sepsis and resulting systemic conditions could be shown via removal of the causative sepsis through tooth extraction and observation of the improvement in systemic health. Because it explained a wide range of disorders for which there was no known explanation at the time, Hunter's theory became widely accepted in Britain and eventually in the United States, leading to the wholesale extraction of teeth.

The focal infection theory fell into disrepute during the 1940s and 1950s, when widespread extraction—often of the entire dentition—failed to reduce or eliminate the systemic conditions to which the supposedly infected dentition had been linked.[308] The theory, while offering a possible explanation for perplexing systemic disorders, had been based on very little (if any) scientific evidence. Hunter and other advocates of the theory were unable to explain how focal oral sepsis produced these systemic maladies. They were also unable to elucidate possible interactive mechanisms between oral and systemic health. Furthermore, the suggested intervention of tooth extraction often had no effect on the systemic conditions for which patients sought relief. However, Hunter's ideas did encourage extensive research in the areas of microbiology and immunology.

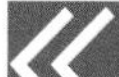

FLASH BACK

The focal infection theory fell into disrepute during the 1940s and 1950s, when widespread extraction—often of the entire dentition—failed to reduce or eliminate the systemic conditions. The theory, while offering a possible explanation for perplexing systemic disorders, had been based on very little (if any) scientific evidence.

Evidence-Based Clinical Practice

Many of the precepts of the focal infection theory are being revived today in light of recent research demonstrating links between oral and systemic health. However, as expressed by Newman, for the "hypothesis not to fall into disrepute for a second time, there must be no unsubstantiated attributions, no theories without evidence."[214] Today's era of evidence-based medicine and dentistry provides an excellent environment in which to examine the possible relationships between oral infection and systemic disorders. To establish a relationship between conditions A and B, different levels of evidence must be examined. All scientific evidence is not given the same weight.[116,195,215] The stronger the evidence, the more likely it is that a true relationship exists between the conditions. Table 26.1 describes these various levels of evidence.

For example, when examining the relationship between elevated cholesterol levels and CHD-related events, the literature might initially consist entirely of *case reports* or similar anecdotal information in which individual patients with recent myocardial infarction (MI) are found to have elevated cholesterol levels. These anecdotal reports suggest a possible relationship between elevated cholesterol and MI, but the evidence is weak. The case reports may lead to *cross-sectional studies,* in which a large patient population is examined to determine whether those individuals who had an MI have higher cholesterol levels than other individuals (control patients) who did not have an MI. Ideally, these cross-sectional studies are controlled for other potential causes or factors associated with MI, such as age, gender, and smoking history. In other words, the patients with a previous MI would be retrospectively matched with patients of similar age, gender, and smoking history, and their cholesterol levels would then be examined for similarities or differences. Significantly higher cholesterol levels in patients with a previous MI compared with those without MI offer stronger evidence than case reports; such evidence further substantiates a possible link between elevated cholesterol and MI.

Even stronger evidence is provided by *longitudinal studies,* in which patient populations are examined over time. For example, a group of patients might periodically have their cholesterol levels evaluated over several years. If individuals with elevated cholesterol levels have a significantly higher rate of MI over time compared with patients with normal cholesterol levels, then even stronger evidence is available to substantiate the link between cholesterol and MI. Finally, *intervention trials* may be designed to alter the potentially causative condition and to determine the effect of this change on the resultant condition. For example, patients with elevated cholesterol levels may be divided into two groups: a group that uses a cholesterol-lowering drug or diet and a control group that uses no intervention. These two groups might also be compared with a third group of patients with normal cholesterol

TABLE 26.1 Evaluation of Evidence

Type of Evidence	Strength of Evidence	Description
Case report	+/–	• Provides relatively weak retrospective anecdotal evidence • May suggest that further study is needed
Cross-sectional study	+	• Compares groups of subjects at a single point in time • Stronger than a case report • Fairly easy to conduct • Relatively inexpensive to conduct
Longitudinal study	++	• Follows groups of subjects over time • Stronger than a cross-sectional study • Studies with a control group much stronger than studies without controls • More difficult and expensive to conduct
Intervention trial	+++	• Examines the effects of some intervention • Studies with a control group (i.e., placebo) much stronger than studies without controls • Strongest form of evidence is the randomized controlled intervention trial • Difficult and expensive to conduct
Systematic review	++++	• Systematically evaluates evidence from multiple studies, especially randomized controlled trials • Uses clearly defined guidelines for the selection of evidence to be included or excluded from the review • Examines for heterogeneity in the overall data to indicate variations in study design, sample populations, and assessment methodologies

levels. Over time, the rate of MI in each group would be determined. If the group receiving the cholesterol-lowering regimen has a significantly lower rate of MI than the group with continued elevations in cholesterol level, strong evidence of a link between cholesterol and MI is established.

Finally, the highest level of evidence is the *systematic review*. A systematic review is not a standard literature review in which the articles selected for review are based on the desires and search methods chosen by the author, often for convenience. In a systematic review, the topic in question is selected before the review begins. For example, the authors may state the question as follows: "As compared with subjects not taking cholesterol-lowering medications, do subjects taking such medications demonstrate a difference in the rate of myocardial infarction?" A specific search strategy is then determined to reveal as much potential data as possible to answer the stated question. The authors state specifically why research papers were included or excluded from the review. If possible, the data are subjected to meta-analysis, a statistical method that combines the results of multiple studies that address a similar research hypothesis. This provides a more robust evaluation of the overall data than one can glean from individual research articles.

At each level of evidence, it is important to determine whether a biologically plausible link exists between conditions A and B. For example, if case reports, cross-sectional studies, longitudinal studies, and intervention trials all support a link between cholesterol levels and MI, the following questions remain:

- How is cholesterol related to MI?
- What are the mechanisms by which cholesterol affects the cardiovascular system and thus increases the risk for MI?

These studies evaluate the mechanisms by which conditions A and B might be linked and provide explanatory data that further substantiate the association between the two conditions.

The focal infection theory, as proposed and defended during the early part of the 20th century, was based on almost no evidence. Only the occasional case report and other anecdotes were available to substantiate the theory. Although explanatory mechanisms were proposed, none were validated with scientific research. This theory predated current concepts of evidence-based clinical practice and led to the unnecessary extraction of millions of teeth. Currently, when reexamining the potential associations between oral infections and systemic conditions, it is important (1) to determine what evidence is available; (2) to determine what evidence is still needed to substantiate the associations; and (3) to validate the possible mechanisms of association. This chapter reviews current knowledge that relates periodontal infection to overall systemic health.

Subgingival Environment as a Reservoir for Bacteria

The subgingival microbial biofilm in patients with periodontitis provides a significant and persistent gram-negative bacterial challenge to the host that is met with a potent immunoinflammatory response.[219] These organisms and their products, such as lipopolysaccharides (LPSs), have ready access to the periodontal tissues and to the circulation via the sulcular epithelium, which is frequently ulcerated and discontinuous. Even with treatment, complete eradication of these organisms is difficult, and their reemergence is often rapid. The total surface area of pocket epithelium in contact with subgingival bacteria and their products in a patient with generalized moderate periodontitis has been estimated to be approximately the size of the palm of an adult hand, with even larger areas of exposure in cases of more advanced periodontal destruction.[225] Bacteremias are common after mechanical periodontal therapy, and they also occur frequently during normal daily function and oral hygiene procedures.[72,163,188] Just as the periodontal tissues mount an immunoinflammatory response to bacteria and their products, systemic challenge with these agents also induces a major vascular response.[66,108,242] There is emerging evidence that the host response is similarly shaped by microbially and environmentally mediated epigenetic programs that exert a signature on the periodontium and thereby impact periodontal disease pathogenesis.[10] This host response may offer explanatory mechanisms for the interactions between periodontal infection and a variety of systemic disorders.

KEY FACT

The subgingival microbiota in patients with periodontitis provides a significant and persistent gram-negative bacterial challenge to the host. These organisms and their products, such as LPSs, have access to the periodontal tissues and to the circulation via ulcerations in the sulcular epithelium.

Periodontal Disease and Mortality

The ultimate medical outcome measure is mortality. A number of studies suggest that an increased mortality rate from various causes is associated with inflammatory periodontal diseases.[7,47,70,87,129,159,248] The Normative Aging Study examined 2280 healthy men every 3 years for longer than 30 years after baseline clinical, radiographic, laboratory, and electrocardiographic examinations. A subset of this population was examined in the Veterans Affairs Dental Longitudinal Study to determine age-related changes in the oral cavity and identify risk factors for oral disease. Clinical examinations were performed, and alveolar bone level measurements were determined from full-mouth radiographs. The mean percentage of alveolar bone loss and mean probing depth were determined for each patient. From the original sample of 804 dentate, medically healthy patients, a total of 166 died during the study.[87] Periodontal status at the baseline examination was a significant predictor of mortality independent of other factors such as smoking, alcohol use, cholesterol levels, blood pressure, family history of heart disease, education level, and body mass. For those patients with the most alveolar bone loss (>21% alveolar bone loss at baseline), the risk of dying during the follow-up period was 70% higher than for all other patients. Interestingly, alveolar bone loss increased the risk of mortality more than smoking (52% increased risk), which is a well-known risk factor for mortality. A later evaluation of these same patients confirmed a higher incidence of CHD-related events such as MI and unstable angina among men younger than 60 years of age with alveolar bone loss compared with those without bone loss.[70]

In a prospective cohort study of 1400 dentate men from Northern Ireland, patients were divided into thirds (tertiles) based on average periodontal attachment loss.[159] Those with the highest levels of periodontal attachment loss had a significantly higher risk of death compared with those with the least attachment loss. The mortality rate over a 9-year period was 15.7% in those with the greatest attachment loss and 7.9% in those with the lowest level of periodontal attachment loss. In these studies, periodontitis preceded and increased the risk of mortality. However, this finding only establishes an association; it does not confirm causation. It is possible that periodontal disease reflects other health behaviors not evaluated in this study rather than acting as a specific cause of mortality. In other words, patients with poor periodontal health may also have other risk factors that increase mortality rate (e.g., smoking).

When examining research that suggests oral health status is a possible risk factor for systemic conditions, it is important to recognize when other known risk factors for those systemic conditions have been accounted for in the analysis. Host susceptibility factors that place individuals at risk for periodontitis may also place them at risk for systemic diseases, such as cardiovascular disease. In these patients, the association may actually be among the risk factors rather than among the diseases. For example, periodontitis and cardiovascular disease share such risk factors as smoking, age, race, male gender, and stress. Genetic risk factors may also be shared.[149] In the Veterans Affairs Dental Longitudinal Study, smoking was an independent risk factor for mortality. When the data were examined to determine whether periodontal status was a risk factor, smoking status and other known risk factors for mortality were removed from the equation to allow for the independent evaluation of periodontal status. Other studies support an association between poor oral health and an increased risk of mortality.[248] In a prospective longitudinal study of patients with type 2 diabetes, those with severe periodontitis had 3.2 times the risk of death from ischemic heart disease or kidney disease as patients without periodontitis or with only slight periodontitis, after adjusting for other risk factors, including age, sex, duration of diabetes, glycemic control, macroalbuminuria, body mass index, serum cholesterol concentration, hypertension, and current smoking.[248]

Periodontal Disease and Oncogenesis

Microbiota and Cancer

Links between the microbiome and specific microbiota and carcinogenesis have been postulated for years. Recent emerging data derived from novel omic and imaging approaches and epidemiologic studies in several cancers, including oral and head and neck cancer, are shedding new light on this link.[204,256,259,265,275]

The human microbiome maintains a dynamic relationship with the human host.[51] If the microbiome experiences an ecological imbalance, also known as dysbiosis, disease processes can emerge.[32,42] Alternatively, changes in the human host, such as changes in the host adaptive immunity, can alter the associated microbiome.[330] Numerous studies have reported that microbial dysbiosis is linked to cancer.[204,256,275,315] For example, imbalances in the gut microbiota promote altered host-microbial interactions that mediate colorectal cancer tumorigenesis.[151,186,217] In addition, genomic analysis of the microbiome of colorectal cancer patients have revealed a significant enrichment in *Fusobacterium* species with depletion in species from the phyla Bacteroidetes and Firmicutes relative to normal healthy controls.[148,283] Others reported that alterations in the oral microbiota are strongly associated with oral cancer and head and neck cancer.[255,265]

The role of specific bacteria in carcinogenesis is being elucidated through the extensive work undertaken to understand the relationship between *Helicobacter/H. pylori* and gastric cancer, now classified as a causal agent by the International Agency of Cancer Res earch.[1,144,178] The case with *H. pylori* and gastric cancer effectively led to a paradigm shift regarding the relationship between bacterial microbes and cancer. Several lines of evidence have emerged implicating specific bacteria in the etiology of different cancers, such as *H. pylori* in gastric cancer,[1,144,173,178] *Chlamydia trachomatis* in cervical cancer,[177] *Salmonella typhi* in gallbladder cancer,[212] *Bacteroides fragilis, Eubacteria, Bifidobacterium,* and *Fusobacterium nucleatum (F. nucleatum)* in colon cancer,[150,151,299] and *F. nucleatum, Porphyromonas gingivalis,* and *Aggregatibacter actinomycetemcomitans* in pancreatic cancer.[78,207]

Periodontal Disease and Cancer

Periodontal disease is associated with an increased risk for oral cancer.[196] Bacterial pathogens in the oral cavity responsible for chronic inflammation, and chronic immune cell infiltration are an accompanying feature of oral and head and neck cancer.[4,114,115,138,229,284,306] The leading bacteria at sites with periodontal destruction include members of the red complex, namely *Porphyromonas/P. gingivalis, Tannerella/T. forsythia,* and *Treponema/T. denticola.*[276] Also, *F. nucleatum* is one of the most abundant oral bacteria present in periodontal disease biofilms. *F. nucleatum* has strong intermicrobial binding properties with most oral biofilm colonizers, and it can help other bacteria cross host-epithelial and -endothelial barriers.[80,103,147,269] *P. gingivalis* and *F. nucleatum* have been implicated in the pathogenesis of several chronic diseases and cancer. Indeed, although the relationship between these bacteria and cancer have been reported in colon and pancreatic cancer,[150,151,202,204,245] involvement of these oral pathogens in the etiology and progression of oral cancer, and in potential mechanistic contributions to oral cancer is emerging.[7,20,306]

Epidemiological data suggest that there is an association between tooth loss, periodontal disease, or periodontal microbial pathogens and cancer.[7,15,119,196,200,202,205,304,306,322] For example, risk of pancreatic cancer is increased in people with tooth loss or periodontal disease.[3] In addition, in a large European cohort study, participants with elevated antibody titers to the periodontal pathogen, *P. gingivalis*, had a 2.14 times greater risk for pancreatic cancer compared to those with undetectable or low antibody levels.[203,269] Tooth loss and periodontal disease have also been associated with oral or head and neck cancer.[5,7,15,255] However, knowledge about the direct link between periodontal pathogens and oral cancer and the mechanisms involved are limited.

Several mechanisms and processes have been postulated for the causal role of pathogenic bacteria and microbial dysbiosis in cancer and the host, including modulation of the host-immune response, heightened inflammation, altered metabolism, and altered host-cell signaling.[9,18,31,48,89,124,134,151,152,217,245,246] A direct relationship between *F. nucleatum* and colorectal cancer was demonstrated whereby the fusobacterial adhesin FadA binds to E-cadherin on colon cancer cells and activates beta-catenin signaling.[245] Other studies found that *P. gingivalis* and *F. nucleatum* seem to promote migration and invasion of oral cancer cells by triggering an epithelial to mesenchymal transition, acquisition of stemness properties, and cytokine signaling.[101,102,123,124,301] *P. gingivalis* can also promote invasion in oral squamous cell carcinoma[102] and esophageal cancer.[86] The specific carcinogenic mechanisms induced or potentiated by pathogenic oral bacteria on the host or cancer are also emerging.[136,204,235a,235b,304,306]

Commensal bacteria are critically important to maintaining a healthy microbiome and a dynamic relationship with the human host.[30] However, in cancer, the role that commensal bacteria play is even much less explored, yet studies suggest that their involvement may be important. In a recent study, comparisons of the microbial content of saliva from pancreatic cancer cases versus healthy controls resulted in the identification of two commensal bacteria (*Neisseria elongata* and *Streptococcus mitis*) that, combined, could distinguish cancer cases and controls with 96.4% sensitivity and 82.1% specificity.[81] In another study, levels of antibodies to commensal oral bacteria were generally lower in cancer cases than controls, and individuals with overall higher antibody levels had a significantly lower risk of subsequent pancreatic cancer.[38] In oral cancer, specific commensal bacteria are also more abundant in healthy control versus tumor tissues.[7,265] Thus, commensal bacteria seem to be important in distinguishing cancer from a healthy phenotype, but the exact mechanisms involved are not known.

As new evidence emerges, the links between the microbiome, specific microbes, and carcinogenesis will continue to unfold. This new knowledge may help seed the development of novel treatment approaches for cancer that lead to a paradigm shift focused on antimicrobial-based therapies for cancer.

The role of the microbiota in specific cancers, including head and neck, oral, gastric, pancreatic, intestinal, and lung cancer are discussed in the e-only online version.

Periodontal disease has been associated with prostate, breast, and uterine cancer as well. However, further studies are needed to determine the strength of this association and potential underlying mechanisms.

Prostate Cancer

Periodontal disease has been associated with prostate cancer.[62,113,119,201] For instance, Hujoel et al. reported a 1.81-fold increased risk for prostate cancer in patients with periodontal disease compared to patients without it.[119] This was the highest-fold risk from all the cancers studied. Recently, the presence of oral bacterial DNA (i.e., *Prevotella intermedia, P. gingivalis*, and *T. denticola*) was found in expressed-prostatic secretion of patients with periodontitis.[76] Interestingly, patients with periodontitis and prostate inflammation had greater levels of prostate-specific antigen compared with either disease alone, and periodontal treatment decreased prostate-specific antigen levels in those patients, improving prostate inflammation symptoms.[11,135] These data support the concept of a bacteremia mechanism, whereby oral pathogens would reach the prostate via the circulation then colonize and infect this tissue. This infection would, then, lead to a chronic inflammatory response in the prostate, which, in turn, would induce neoplastic transformation; growing evidence implicates chronic prostate inflammation as one of the main contributors for prostate cancer.[62,67,271,280] Specifically, Simons et al. provide direct evidence that bacterial-induced prostate inflammation accelerates prostate cancer progression and sheds light on how changes in the prostate microenvironment caused by prostate inflammation may accelerate tumor progression.[271]

Breast Cancer

Literature is still inconsistent with regard to associations between periodontitis and breast cancer. For instance, in 2011, a longitudinal prospective study in Sweden with more than 3000 subjects between 30 and 40 years of age reported that chronic periodontitis patients were 2.3 times more likely to be diagnosed with general breast cancer compared to those with a healthy periodontium.[277] However, the conclusions were limited by the fact that the authors did not clinically examine the patients for periodontitis, but instead used missing molars as a proxy to distinguish patients with or without periodontitis. Since caries can also lead to tooth loss, periodontitis may have been overestimated in these patients. Similarly, Sfreddo et al. reported that women diagnosed with periodontitis had two- to three-fold more chances of having invasive ductal breast carcinoma than healthy patients, even after adjusting for confounding variables.[261] In this study, patients were subjected to full-mouth periodontal examinations to diagnose periodontitis. Recently, a meta-analysis study with more than 1.5 million participants investigated the association between periodontitis and general breast cancer and found a 1.2-fold increased risk for general breast cancer in periodontitis cases compared to controls.[263] Interestingly, no significant association was found among patients with periodontitis and history of periodontal therapy and general breast cancer. If this association is accurate, this report suggests that periodontitis therapy can decrease the higher risk of having general breast cancer. In contrast, Mai et al. evaluated 1337 postmenopausal women and found no significant association between the incidence of invasive general breast cancer and either alveolar bone loss or presence of periodontal pathogens.[174,175] Hujoel et al. also reported no significant association between periodontitis and higher risk of general breast cancer (hazard ratio = 1.32; 95% confidence interval: 0.74 to 2.28).[119] Thus, more studies are needed to determine the potential association between periodontitis and breast cancer and the possible underlying mechanism.

Although the association between periodontitis and breast cancer is unclear, Parhi et al. recently tested whether an *F. nucleatum* bacteremia could lead to tumorigenesis and increase the aggressiveness of triple-negative breast cancer in mice.[228] The authors observed a 100-fold increase in abundance in bacteria 24 hours after the intravenous injection of the bacterium within breast cancer tissues (triple-negative breast cancer cell line; autochthonous tumor 3 [AT3]) compared to normal tissues. They reported that *F. nucleatum* colonizes the triple-negative breast tumor tissue, accelerates tumor growth and progression, and inhibits tumor immune-modulator cells, such as T, B, and natural killer cells, thus indicating that *F. nucleatum* via a bacteremia can reach breast tumor tissue and induce tumor growth and progression. However, it is not known whether this bacterial accumulation is driven by the bacterium itself or by an enhanced permeability and retention effect.

Uterine Cancers

Few studies have examined the correlation between periodontitis and uterine cancer. In a study by Arora et al. that examined twins (to control for confounding factors), periodontitis was positively associated with increased risk of uterine corpus cancer (hazard ratio = 2.20).[17] Interestingly, Han et al. demonstrated that intravenous tail vein injection with *F. nucleatum* led to uterine bacterial colonization, proliferation, and intrauterine infection.[104] Nevertheless, this result may be due to the tail vain draining more to the uterus than other tissues, thus resulting in higher uterine colonization of the bacterium compared to other tissues. In this context, gingival inoculation may be more suitable to replicate periodontal bacteremia and evaluate whether uterine colonization by periodontal pathogens is, indeed, possible. Interestingly, recent reports have detected periodontal pathogens in placental/uterine tissue and/or associated with multiple adverse pregnancy outcomes, indicating that uterine colonization by periodontal pathogens is, indeed, possible and potentially related to birth outcomes. However, further studies are needed to better understand how periodontitis may be associated with uterine cancer and whether *F. nucleatum* intrauterine infection can lead to uterine cancer.[2,49,82,104,300,319]

Head and Neck and Oral Cancer

Head and neck cancer is a devastating disease, often disfiguring and debilitating affected patients. It is the sixth most common cancer worldwide and comprises cancers of the oral cavity, larynx, hypopharynx, oropharynx, paranasal sinuses and nasal cavity, and salivary glands.[37,132] In 2018, head and neck cancer accounted for approximately 706,000 new cases and 358,000 deaths worldwide.[37] In the United States, head and neck cancer accounts for 3% of all cancers and approximately 65,000 Americans are diagnosed with head and neck cancer annually.[37,91,166]

Oral squamous cell carcinoma (OSCC) is the most common type of cancer in the head and neck region and accounts for greater than 370,000 new cases worldwide annually, thereby levying a major public health burden.[283] Additionally, OSCC is the sixth most common cancer in the world. Oral cancers affect 54,010 people annually within the United States, resulting in over 10,000 deaths each year.[268] OSCC affects tissues of the oral cavity, which include the lips, tongue, floor of the mouth, gingiva, buccal mucosa, and hard palate. OSCC frequently arises from a precancerous lesion called oral leukoplakia, which exhibits varying degrees of oral epithelial dysplasia (OED).[303] Clinically, OED may take the form of leukoplakia (a white patch), erythroplakia (a red patch), or some combination of the two. Transformation rates from OED to OSCC range from ~10% to 32% for low- and high-grade lesions, respectively, and may be as high as 90% in a subtype called proliferative leukoplakia.[38,46,192,254,270]

The 5-year survival rates for oral and oropharyngeal cancer have remained largely unchanged for decades with oral cancer rates increasing approximately 15% from the mid 1970s until the latest National Cancer Institute Survey in 2004.[36] Recent data from the Surveillance, Epidemiology, and End Results (SEER) Program show that oral cavity and pharyngeal cancer patients diagnosed with localized, pre-metastatic disease have 5-year survival rates of up to 85%. However, once these cancers metastasize either locally (e.g., to the cervical lymph nodes in the neck) or distantly (e.g., outside of the head and neck region), the 5-year survival rates fall precipitously to about 67% and 40%, respectively. These trends were nearly identical in patients with cancers arising on the tongue, the most common intraoral site for oral cancer (82%, 68%, and 40%, respectively). When stratified by race, Black people are disproportionately affected and have even worse survival outcomes in all three categories. Additionally, higher increases in oral cancer rates are seen in Hispanic and Black men.[238] Although these oral and pharyngeal sites are accessible for self-inspection or during medical and dental exams, these cancers can sometimes be confused with more common intraoral benign lesions. As a result, 60% of oral and oropharyngeal cancers are diagnosed at advanced stages (i.e., following locoregional metastasis), which significantly decreases the prognosis for both survival and quality of life.[237]

Treatment for oral cancer typically involves surgery, radiation, and/or chemotherapy. Given the anatomic complexity of the head and neck and oral cavity, complete surgical excision of OSCC tumors is not always possible, increasing the likelihood of persistent disease, local recurrences, and/or metastases. OSCC and its treatments are also associated with high morbidity due to loss of function affecting speech, ability to eat, taste, salivary flow, and facial deficiencies.

The known primary risk factors for OSCC include tobacco and alcohol use. Unlike the oropharynx in which ~70% of cases are associated with infection by high-risk human papilloma virus (HPV) subtypes, only a small percentage of OSCC (less than 5%) are associated with high-risk HPV infection.[69] However, these risk factors alone are not sufficient to explain the incidence and the mechanisms of OSCC tumorigenesis, and it is likely that other factors play important roles in OSCC tumor development, progression, and metastasis. Recent evidence indicates that specific oral microbial pathogens and shifts in the oral microbiome are important for cancer pathogenesis, including OSCC carcinogenesis.[125,136,204,256,259,265,275,292]

It is well established that disease processes can emerge as a result of an imbalance in the microbiome, also known as dysbiosis.[32,42,51] Numerous studies have reported that microbial dysbiosis is linked to cancer,[204,256,259,275] including colorectal cancer and OSCC[51,65,66] Genomic analysis of the microbiomes in colorectal cancer patients revealed a significant enrichment in *Fusobacterium* species with depletion in species from the phyla Bacteroidetes and Firmicutes,[150,285] including *Streptococci* species. Similarly, reports show that there are distinct microbial communities associated with primary and metastatic OSCC, and these exhibit a high Fusobacterial and low Streptococcal signature, whereas controls exhibit opposite profiles.[265] Bacterial pathogens in the oral cavity responsible for chronic inflammation are also an accompanying feature of OSCC.[115,229,306] Epidemiological data suggest an association between cancer and tooth loss, periodontal disease, and periodontopathic bacteria, such as *P. gingivalis, T. forsythia, T. denticola*, and *F. nucleatum* and cancer.[7,15,119,120,200,304]

Mechanisms utilized by pathogenic oral bacteria to promote OED development and/or drive transformation to OSCC are not well understood. Several processes have been postulated, including modulation of host-immune responses, heightened inflammation, epithelial barrier dysfunction, altered metabolism, altered host-cell signaling, altered cell-extracellular matrix interactions, disruption of deoxyribonucleic acid (DNA)-repair mechanisms, and epigenetic modulation (Fig. 26.1).[9,18,136,151,217,245,259] With the development of high-throughput omic approaches to interrogate the genetic, proteomic, microbiome, and metabolomic changes that characterize oral carcinogenesis, there may be advances in better understanding the pathogenesis of the disease and identifying critical control points for development of novel treatment approaches for improving patient outcomes.

Gastrointestinal Cancers (Gastric, Pancreatic, Colon)

Gastrointestinal cancer is one of the most common causes of cancer worldwide. Gastrointestinal cancer is often subdivided by anatomical location—esophagus, stomach, liver, gallbladder, pancreas, colon, rectum, and anus. Combined, gastrointestinal cancers accounted for almost 5 million new cases and more than 3.5 million deaths worldwide in 2018.[119] In 2020, more than 330,000 Americans are expected to be diagnosed with gastrointestinal cancer and more than 155,000 deaths of gastrointestinal cancer are expected in the United States.[118,136]

In terms of gastrointestinal cancer, Zhang et al. meta-analyzed 10 cohort studies and demonstrated a 23% increased risk for overall gastrointestinal cancer in periodontitis patients, compared to normal patients (hazard ratio = 1.23, 95% confidence interval: 1.10 to 1.37).[331] The study also found 59% increased mortality from gastrointestinal cancer in patients with periodontitis compared to healthy patients (hazard ratio = 1.59, 95% confidence interval: 1.16 to 2.16). In the meta-analysis of gastric cancer, Zhang et al. found a 12% increased risk of gastric cancer (hazard ratio = 1.12, 95% confidence interval: 0.88 to 1.42) and a 28% increased mortality rate for gastric cancer in patients with periodontitis compared to healthy patients (hazard ratio = 1.28, 95% confidence interval: 0.71 to 3.37).[331] Another meta-analysis study showed that patients with tooth loss, a marker for severe periodontitis, have increased risk for gastric cancer. Since tooth loss is not a unique marker for periodontitis, these data should be interpreted with caution.[320]

The oral microbiome has been examined in the context of gastric cancer. Interestingly, Salazar et al. demonstrated that plaque colonization by periodontal pathogens (*P. gingivalis, T. forsythia, T. denticola*, and *A. actinomycetemcomitans*) was associated with an increased risk of precancerous lesions in gastric tissues, suggesting that periodontal pathogens may play a role in gastric cancer pathogenesis.[42] However, most patients included in this study were Hispanic (45.4%) females (63.0%) with a mean age of 57 years and a high prevalence of smoking. Thus these results may be more relevant to this demographic.

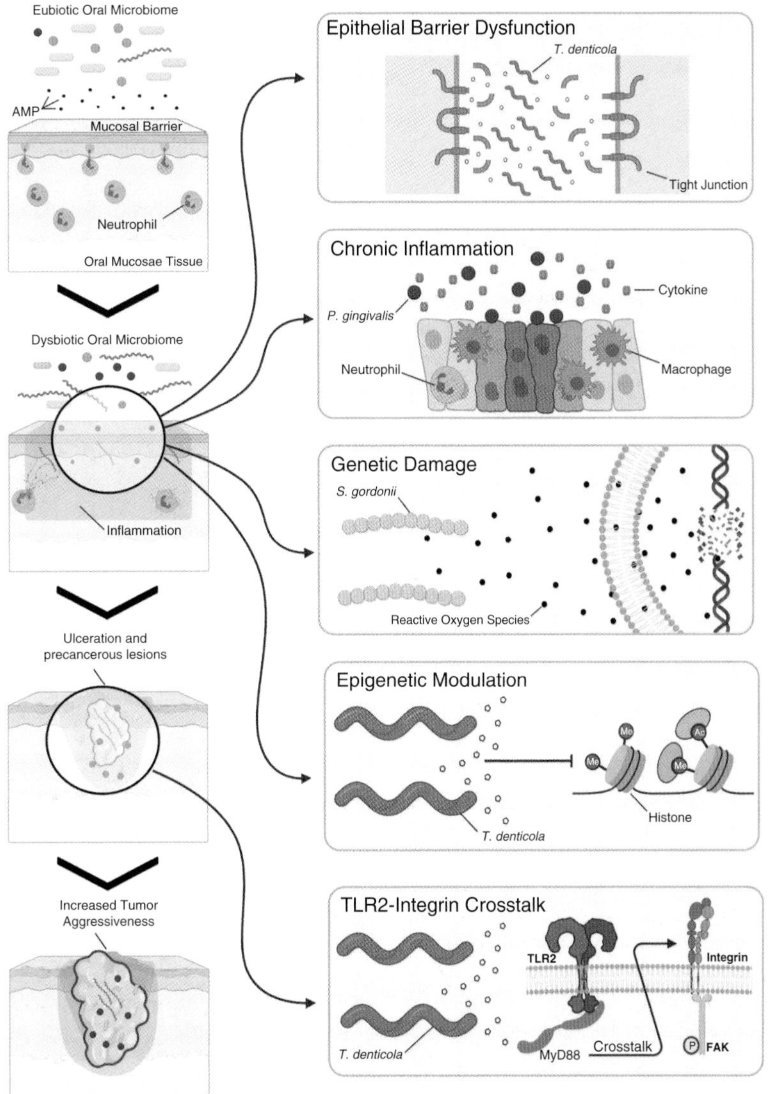

Fig. 26.1 Mechanisms of oral microbiome dysbiosis that promote carcinogenesis. Epithelial barrier disruption, bacterial invasion, chronic inflammation, genetic and epigenetic modulation, and altered tumor cell migration and signaling are mechanisms by which an oral microbiome dysbiosis can promote carcinogenesis.

Regarding pancreatic cancer, a prospective study with more than 700 patients reported that the presence of *P. gingivalis* and *A. actinomycetemcomitans* in the oral cavity was associated with a 60% increased risk of pancreatic cancer (hazard ratio = 1.60% to 95% confidence interval: 1.15 to 2.22).[78] The study reported that patients positive for the presence of *P. gingivalis* in the oral cavity had a 59% greater risk of developing pancreatic cancer than those who were negative for the pathogen. Even after excluding pancreatic cancer cases that occurred less than 2 years after oral samples were obtained, no significant changes were found in the risk factor, demonstrating that it is unlikely that the oral dysbiosis occurred after or concurrently with pancreatic cancer.[78,126] Similarly, a prospective cohort study found that patients with higher levels of *P. gingivalis* antibodies in the blood (>200 ng/mL) had a twofold greater risk of developing pancreatic cancer than those with lower levels of the same antibody.[203] Zhang et al. found a 25% increased risk of having pancreatic cancer (hazard ratio = 1.25, 95% confidence interval: 0.84 to 1.85) and a remarkable 120% increased mortality rate for pancreatic cancer in patients with periodontitis compared to those without periodontitis (hazard ratio = 2.20, 95% confidence interval: 1.44 to 3.37).[331]

In terms of colon cancer, a prospective study of 17,904 women and 24,582 men found increased risks for colon precursor lesions (i.e., serrated polyps and conventional adenomas) with a hazard ratio = 1.17 (95% confidence interval: 1.06 to 1.29) and 1.11 (95% confidence interval: 1.02 to 1.19), respectively, in patients with chronic periodontitis compared to healthy patients. Losing teeth (≥4 teeth) increased the risk for colon cancer by 20% for those with serrated polyps (odds ratio, 1.20, 95% confidence interval: 1.03 to 1.39).[161] In contrast, in a meta-analysis, Zhang et al. found no significant difference for risk of colon cancer, but found a 66% increased mortality rate for colon cancer in patients with periodontitis compared to those without periodontitis (hazard ratio = 1.66, 95% confidence interval: 0.44 to 6.27).[331]

Accumulating evidence demonstrates that periodontal disease is associated with gastrointestinal carcinogenesis. Further, various pathogenic members of the oral microbiota (*P. gingivalis, T. forsythia, T. denticola*, and *A. actinomycetemcomitans*) have been linked to cancers of the gastrointestinal tract.

Periodontal Disease, Coronary Heart Disease, and Atherosclerosis

To further explore the association between periodontal disease and CHD or atherosclerosis, investigators have studied specific systemic disorders and medical outcomes to determine their relationship to periodontal status. The proceedings of the first international Workshop on Periodontitis and Systemic Disease held by the American Academy of Periodontology (AAP) and the European Federation of Periodontology (EFP) were published in 2013, a major focus of which was the relationship between periodontitis and atherosclerotic cardiovascular disease.[63,71,239,253] CHD-related events are a major cause of death. MI has been associated with acute systemic bacterial and viral infections and is sometimes preceded by influenza-like symptoms.[180,279,] Is it possible that oral infection is similarly related to MI? Traditional risk factors such as smoking, dyslipidemia, hypertension, and diabetes mellitus do not explain the presence of coronary atherosclerosis in a large number of patients. Localized infection that results in a chronic inflammatory reaction has been suggested as a mechanism underlying CHD in these individuals.[193]

In cross-sectional studies of patients with acute MI or confirmed CHD who were compared with age- and gender-matched control patients, patients with MI had significantly worse dental health (e.g., periodontitis, periapical lesions, caries, pericoronitis) than controls.[128,181,182] This association between poor dental health and MI was independent of known risk factors for heart disease, such as age, cholesterol levels, hypertension, diabetes, and smoking. Because atherosclerosis is a major determinant of CHD-related events, dental health has also been related to coronary atheromatosis. Mattila and colleagues[183] performed oral radiographic examinations and diagnostic coronary angiography on men with known CHD and found a significant correlation between the severity of dental disease and the degree of coronary atheromatosis. This relationship remained significant after accounting for other known risk factors for coronary artery disease. Similarly, Malthaner and colleagues[176] found an increased risk of angiographically defined coronary artery disease in patients with greater bone loss and attachment loss; however, after adjusting for other known cardiovascular risk factors, the relationship between periodontal status and coronary artery disease was no longer statistically significant. There is evidence that the extent of periodontal disease may be associated with CHD. For example, there may be a greater risk for CHD-related events, such as MI, in patients who have periodontitis affecting a greater number of teeth in the mouth compared with those who have periodontitis involving fewer teeth.[16]

Cross-sectional studies thus suggest a possible link between oral health and CHD; however, such studies cannot determine causality in this relationship. Rather, dental diseases may be indicators of general health practices. For example, periodontal disease and CHD are both related to lifestyle and share numerous risk factors, including smoking, diabetes, and low socioeconomic status. Bacterial infections have significant effects on endothelial cells, blood coagulation, lipid metabolism, and monocytes and macrophages.

Longitudinal studies provide compelling data regarding this relationship. In a 7-year follow-up study of the patients from the study by Mattila and colleagues, dental disease was significantly related to the incidence of new fatal and nonfatal coronary events as well as overall mortality.[184] In a prospective study of a national sample of adults, patients with periodontitis had a 25% increased risk for CHD compared with those with no or minimal periodontal disease, after adjusting for other known risk factors.[68] Among males between the ages of 25 and 49 years, periodontitis increased the risk of CHD by 70%. The level of oral hygiene was also associated with heart disease. Patients with poor oral hygiene, as indicated by higher debris and calculus scores, had a twofold increased risk for CHD.

In another large prospective study, 1147 men were followed for 18 years.[27] During that time, 207 men (18%) developed CHD. When periodontal status at baseline was related to the presence or absence of CHD-related events during the follow-up period, a significant relationship was found. Patients with more than 20% mean bone loss had a 50% increased risk of CHD compared with those with less than 20% bone loss. The extent of sites with probing depths greater than 3 mm was strongly related to the incidence of CHD. Patients with probing depths greater than 3 mm on at least half of their teeth had a twofold increased risk, whereas those with probing depths of greater than 3 mm on all of their teeth had more than a threefold increased risk of CHD. This study and others in which the periodontal condition was known to have preceded the CHD-related events have supported the concept that periodontal disease is a risk factor for CHD, independent of other classic risk factors. Not all studies, however, support this concept; some show little independent effect of periodontal status on the risk for CHD after adjusting for commonly accepted cardiovascular risk factors.[117,118] It is particularly difficult to control for smoking as a confounding variable in these studies, because it is such an important risk factor for both periodontal disease and cardiovascular disease. This confounding influence of smoking makes it difficult to clarify the significance of the relationship between the diseases.

Perhaps the best evidence available comes from systematic reviews of studies examining the relationship between periodontal infection and cardiovascular disease. A systematic review and meta-analysis of data from 15 studies showed a significant 14% to 222% increase in the risk of CHD-related events in patients with periodontal disease as compared with those without periodontal disease.[22] A similar systematic review of longitudinal cohort and case–control studies showed a significant increase in the risk of incident MI, angina, or CHD-related death in patients with periodontitis in five of the six studies reported.[71] This increased risk was noted mainly in younger patients (i.e., <65 years old). Janket and colleagues[127] performed a meta-analysis of periodontal disease as a risk factor for future cardiovascular events and found an overall 19% increased risk of such events among individuals with periodontitis. The increase in risk was greater (44%) among people younger than 65 years of age. Although this increased risk is fairly modest, the extensive prevalence of periodontal disease in the population may increase the significance of the risk from a public health perspective. Extensive systematic reviews by Scannapieco and colleagues[249] and by an American Heart Association working group[162] concluded that a moderate degree of evidence exists to support an association between periodontal disease and atherosclerosis, MI, and cardiovascular disease independent of known confounders; however, causality is unclear. The results of the 2103 AAP/EFP Workshop on Periodontitis and Systemic Diseases concluded that "there is consistent and strong epidemiologic evidence that periodontitis imparts increased risk for future cardiovascular disease," but whereas many studies support multiple biologic mechanisms to explain this relationship, "intervention trials to date are not adequate to draw further conclusions."[298] That is, insufficient evidence exists to show that the treatment of periodontal disease has any impact on the risk of heart disease.

KEY FACT

There is consistent and strong epidemiologic evidence that periodontitis imparts increased risk for future cardiovascular disease.

Effects of Periodontal Infection

There are numerous mechanisms—both direct and indirect—through which periodontal infection may affect the onset or progression of atherosclerosis and CHD.[141,239,253] Periodontitis and

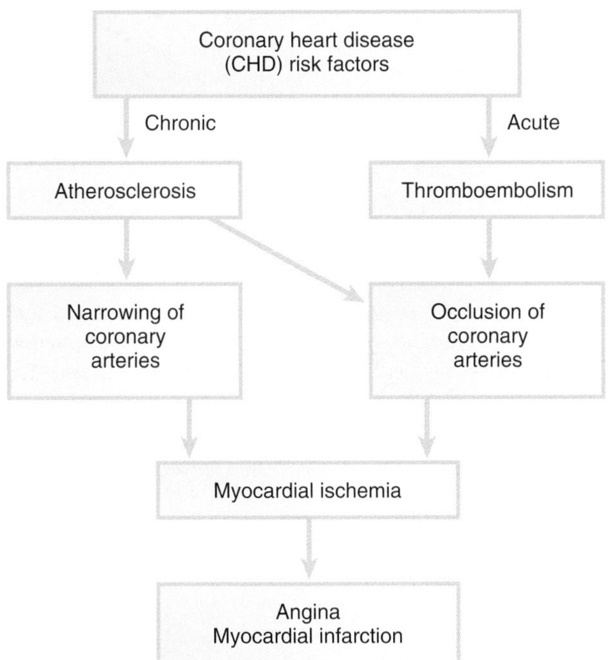

Fig. 26.2 Acute and chronic pathways to ischemic heart disease. Coronary heart disease–related events, such as angina and myocardial infarction, may be precipitated by either pathway or both pathways.

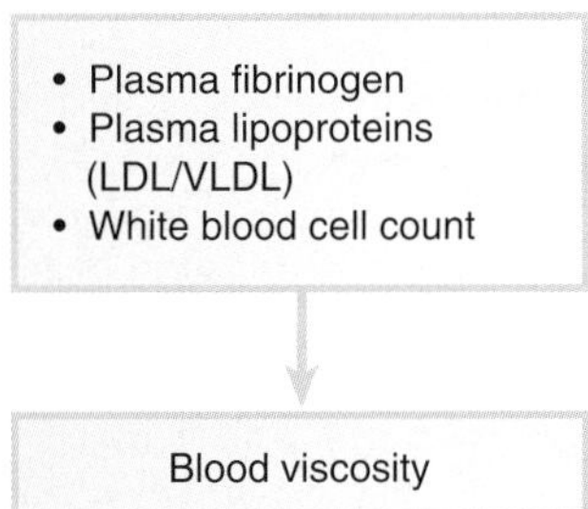

Fig. 26.3 Factors that affect blood viscosity in health. *LDL,* Low-density lipoprotein; *VLDL,* very-low-density lipoprotein.

atherosclerosis both have complex etiologic factors that combine genetic and environmental influences. In addition to smoking, the diseases share many risk factors and have distinct similarities with regard to their basic pathogenic mechanisms.

Ischemic Heart Disease

Ischemic heart disease is associated with the processes of atherogenesis and thrombogenesis (Fig. 26.2). Damage to the vascular endothelium, with a subsequent inflammatory reaction, plays a major role in atherosclerosis and ischemic organ damage.[298] Increased viscosity of blood may promote ischemic heart disease and cerebrovascular accident (stroke) by increasing the risk of thrombus formation.[170] Fibrinogen is a major factor in the promotion of this hypercoagulable state. *Fibrinogen* is the precursor to fibrin, and increased fibrinogen levels increase blood viscosity. Increased plasma fibrinogen is a recognized risk factor for cardiovascular events and peripheral vascular disease (Fig. 26.3).[169] An elevated white blood cell count is also a predictor of heart disease and stroke, and circulating leukocytes may promote the occlusion of blood vessels. Coagulation factor VIII (von Willebrand factor) has likewise been associated with a risk of ischemic heart disease.[240]

Systemic Infections

Systemic infections are known to induce a hypercoagulable state and increase blood viscosity (Fig. 26.4). Fibrinogen levels and white blood cell counts are often increased in patients with periodontal disease.[52,157]

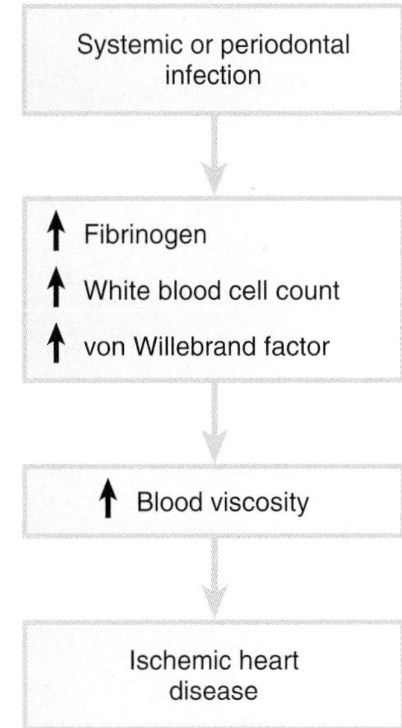

Fig. 26.4 The effect of infection on blood viscosity. Increased plasma fibrinogen and von Willebrand factor cause hypercoagulability. When they are combined with an increased white blood cell count, the blood viscosity increases, thereby increasing the risk of coronary ischemia.

Individuals with poor oral health may also have significant elevations in coagulation factor VIII/von Willebrand factor antigen, thereby increasing the risk of thrombus formation. Thus, periodontal infection may also promote increased blood viscosity and thrombogenesis, which leads to an increased risk for central and peripheral vascular disease.

Daily Activity

Routine daily activities, such as mastication and oral hygiene procedures result in frequent bacteremia with oral organisms.[163] Periodontal disease may predispose the patient to an increased incidence of bacteremia, including the presence of virulent gram-negative organisms associated with periodontitis. There is a greater risk of bacteremia after toothbrushing in patients with higher levels of plaque, calculus, and gingivitis as compared with those with minimal plaque and gingival inflammation.[164] In fact, patients with generalized gingival bleeding after brushing showed an almost eightfold increase in their incidence of bacteremia as compared with those having minimal gingival bleeding. An estimated 8% of all cases of infective endocarditis are associated with periodontal or dental disease without a preceding dental procedure.[72] The periodontium, when affected by periodontitis, also acts as a reservoir of endotoxins (LPSs) from gram-negative organisms. Endotoxins in the subgingival biofilm can pass readily into the systemic circulation during normal daily function, thereby inducing damage to the vascular endothelium and precipitating negative cardiovascular effects. In a study of the incidence of endotoxemia after simple chewing, patients with periodontitis were four times more likely to have endotoxin present in the bloodstream than patients without periodontitis. Furthermore, the concentration of endotoxin in the bloodstream was more than fourfold greater in those with periodontitis as compared with healthy patients.[88]

Thrombogenesis

Platelet aggregation plays a major role in thrombogenesis, and most cases of acute MI are precipitated by thromboembolism. Oral organisms may be involved in coronary thrombogenesis. Platelets selectively bind some strains of *Streptococcus sanguinis,* which is a common component of supragingival plaque, and *P. gingivalis,* which is a pathogen closely associated with periodontitis.[109,110] The aggregation of platelets is induced by the *platelet aggregation–associated protein* (PAAP) expressed on some strains of these bacteria.[244] In animal models, intravenous infusion of PAAP-positive bacterial strains resulted in alterations of heart rate, blood pressure, cardiac contractility, and electrocardiogram readings consistent with MI. Platelet accumulation also occurred in the lungs and led to tachypnea. No such changes were seen with the infusion of PAAP-negative strains. PAAP-positive bacteria caused aggregation of circulating platelets, which resulted in the formation of thromboemboli and resultant cardiac and pulmonary changes. Thus, periodontitis-associated bacteremia with certain strains of *S. sanguinis* and *P. gingivalis* may promote acute thromboembolic events via interaction with circulating platelets.

Atherosclerosis

Atherosclerosis is a focal thickening of the arterial *intima,* the innermost layer lining the vessel lumen, and the *media,* the thick layer under the intima that consists of smooth muscle, collagen, and elastic fibers (Fig. 26.5).[244] The formation of atherosclerotic plaques is precipitated by damage to vascular endothelium that results in an inflammatory response in which circulating monocytes adhere to the vascular endothelium. Damage to vascular endothelium can occur because of the presence of intravascular microorganisms and their products; chemical damage, often resulting from elements of tobacco and other exogenous toxins; and increased shear force along the vascular lining, such as that occurring in hypertension. The adherence of monocytes to the damaged vascular endothelium is mediated by several adhesion molecules on the endothelial cell surface, including intercellular adhesion molecule-1 (ICAM-1), endothelial leukocyte adhesion molecule-1 (ELAM-1), and vascular cell adhesion molecule-1 (VCAM-1).[28,145] These adhesion molecules are upregulated by a number of factors, including bacterial LPSs, prostaglandins, and proinflammatory cytokines. After binding to the endothelial cell lining, monocytes penetrate the endothelium and migrate under the arterial intima. The monocytes ingest circulating low-density lipoprotein in its oxidized state and become engorged, thereby forming the foam cells that are characteristic of atheromatous plaque. After entering the arterial media, monocytes may also transform to macrophages.

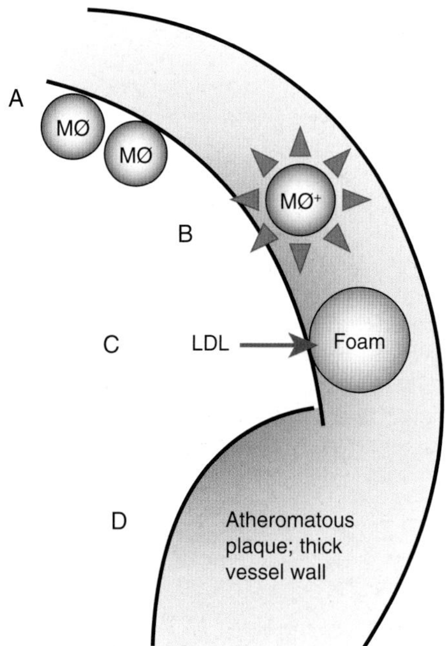

Fig. 26.5 Pathogenesis of atherosclerosis. (A) Monocytes and macrophages *(MØ)* adhere to the vascular endothelium. (B) Monocytes and macrophages penetrate into the arterial media and produce proinflammatory cytokines and **growth factors**. (C) The ingestion of oxidized low-density lipoprotein *(LDL)* enlarges monocytes to form foam cells. (D) Smooth muscle proliferation and plaque formation thicken vessel walls and narrow the lumen. *MØ⁺*, Hyperinflammatory monocyte/macrophage phenotype.

A host of proinflammatory cytokines such as interleukin-1 (IL-1), tumor necrosis factor alpha (TNF-α), and prostaglandin E_2 (PGE_2) are then produced, and they propagate the atheromatous lesion. Mitogenic factors, such as fibroblast growth factor and platelet-derived growth factor stimulate smooth muscle and collagen proliferation within the media, thereby thickening the arterial wall.[169] Atheromatous plaque formation and thickening of the vessel wall narrow the lumen and dramatically decrease blood flow through the vessel.[244] Arterial thrombosis often occurs after an atheromatous plaque ruptures. Plaque rupture exposes circulating blood to arterial collagen and tissue factor from monocytes and macrophages that activate platelets and the coagulation pathway. Platelet and fibrin accumulation forms a thrombus that may occlude the vessel and result in an ischemic event, such as angina or MI. The thrombus may separate from the vessel wall and form an embolus, which may also occlude vessels, again leading to an acute event such as MI or cerebral infarction (stroke).

Role of Periodontal Disease in Atherosclerotic Myocardial or Cerebral Ischemia

In animal models, gram-negative bacteria and associated LPSs cause infiltration of inflammatory cells into the arterial wall, proliferation of arterial smooth muscle, and intravascular coagulation. These changes are identical to those seen with naturally occurring atheromatosis. There is strong evidence that periodontal bacteria disseminate from the oral cavity to the systemic vasculature, can be found within distant tissues, and can live within those affected tissues.[239] Furthermore, in animal models, dissemination of periodontal bacteria can induce atherosclerosis in distant vessels. Patients with periodontitis are at increased risk for thickening of the walls of the major coronary arteries.[27] In several studies of atheromas obtained from humans during endarterectomy, more than half of the lesions contained periodontal pathogens, and many atheromas contained multiple different periodontal species.[50,106,327] Periodontal diseases result in chronic systemic exposure to products of these organisms. Low-level bacteremia may initiate host responses that alter coagulability, endothelial and vessel wall integrity, and platelet function, thereby resulting in atherogenic changes and possible thromboembolic events (Fig. 26.6).

CLINICAL CORRELATION

There is strong evidence that periodontal bacteria disseminate from the oral cavity to the systemic vasculature, can be found within distant tissues, and can live within those affected tissues.

Research has clearly shown a wide variation in host response to bacterial challenge. Some individuals with heavy plaque accumulation and high proportions of pathogenic organisms appear relatively resistant to bone and attachment loss. Others develop extensive periodontal destruction in the presence of small amounts of plaque and low proportions of putative pathogens. Patients with an abnormally exuberant inflammatory response often have a hyperinflammatory monocyte and macrophage phenotype (MØ⁺). Monocytes and macrophages from these individuals secrete significantly increased levels of proinflammatory mediators (e.g., IL-1, TNF-α, PGE_2) in response to bacterial LPSs compared with patients with a normal monocyte and macrophage phenotype. Patients with aggressive periodontitis, refractory periodontitis, and type 1 diabetes mellitus often possess the MØ⁺ phenotype,[29] which appears to be under both genetic and environmental control.

The monocyte and macrophage cell line is intimately involved in the pathogenesis of both periodontal disease and atherosclerosis. Diet-induced elevations in serum low-density lipoprotein levels upregulate monocyte and macrophage responsiveness to bacterial LPSs. Thus, elevated low-density lipoprotein, which is a known risk factor for atherosclerosis and CHD, may increase the secretion of destructive and

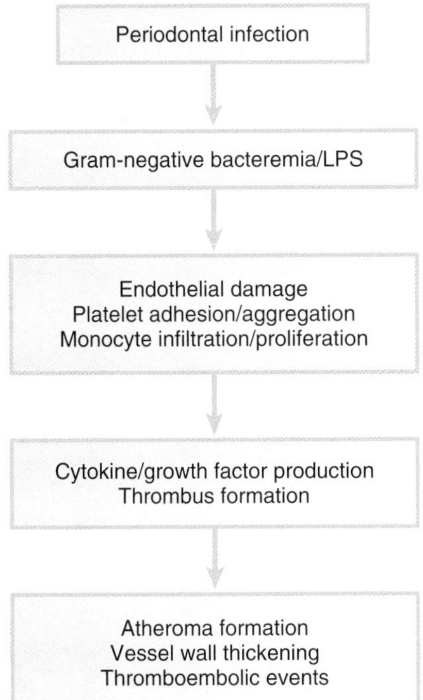

Fig. 26.6 The influence of periodontal infection on atherosclerosis. Periodontal pathogens and their products result in damage to the vascular endothelium. Monocytes and macrophages enter the vessel wall and produce cytokines that further increase the inflammatory response and propagate the atheromatous lesion. Growth factor production leads to smooth muscle proliferation in the vessel wall. Damaged endothelium also activates platelets, thereby resulting in platelet aggregation and potentiating thromboembolic events. *LPS,* Lipopolysaccharide.

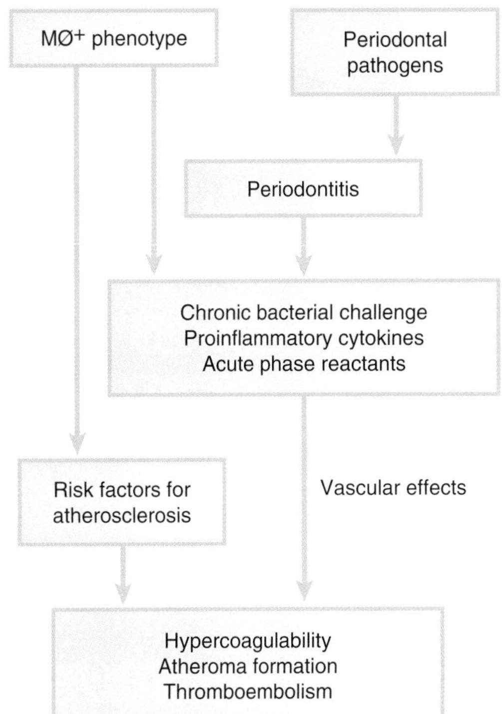

Fig. 26.7 The cardiovascular and periodontal consequences of the hyperresponsive monocyte/macrophage phenotype *(MØ+).* In combination with other risk factors, the MØ+ phenotype predisposes individuals to both atherosclerosis and periodontitis. Bacterial products and inflammatory mediators associated with periodontitis affect vascular endothelium, monocytes and macrophages, platelets, and smooth muscle and may increase blood coagulability. This may further increase atherosclerosis and may result in thromboembolism and ischemic events.

inflammatory cytokines by monocytes and macrophages. This may result not only in the propagation of atheromatous lesions, but also in enhanced periodontal destruction in the presence of pathogenic organisms. This is one example of a potential shared mechanism in the pathogenesis of cardiovascular and periodontal diseases. The presence of an MØ+ phenotype may place patients at risk for both CHD and periodontitis (Fig. 26.7). Periodontal infections may contribute to atherosclerosis and thromboembolic events by repeatedly challenging the vascular endothelium and arterial wall with bacterial LPSs and proinflammatory cytokines. Vascular monocytes and macrophages in patients with an MØ+ phenotype meet this challenge with an abnormally elevated inflammatory response that may directly contribute to atherosclerosis and may precipitate thromboembolic events.[189]

Cardiovascular diseases have a major systemic inflammatory component, further emphasizing possible similarities with inflammatory periodontal diseases.[244] As such, the detection of systemic inflammatory markers plays an increasingly important role in risk assessment for vascular events, such as MI and cerebral infarction. Acute-phase proteins, such as *C-reactive protein* (CRP) and fibrinogen, are produced in the liver in response to inflammatory or infectious stimuli and act as inflammatory markers.[242] CRP induces monocytes and macrophages to produce tissue factor, which stimulates the coagulation pathway and increases blood coagulability. Increased fibrinogen levels may contribute to this process. CRP also stimulates the complement cascade, further exacerbating inflammation.

Elevations in serum CRP and fibrinogen levels are well-accepted risk factors for cardiovascular disease.[241,242] Research has focused on periodontitis as a potential trigger for systemic inflammation. Serum CRP and fibrinogen levels are often elevated in patients with periodontitis as compared with patients without periodontitis.[57,165,311] These acute-phase proteins may act as intermediary steps in the pathway from periodontal infection to cardiovascular disease (see Figs. 26.6 and 26.7). Thus, periodontal diseases may have both direct effects on the major blood vessels (e.g., atheroma formation) and indirect effects that stimulate changes in the cardiovascular system (e.g., elevation of systemic inflammatory responses).

Interesting supportive evidence for these mechanisms can be derived from intervention trials in which serum levels of inflammatory mediators and markers are assessed before and after treatment that is aimed at decreasing periodontal inflammation. For example, in patients with chronic periodontitis, serum levels of IL-6 and CRP are reduced after scaling and root planing.[64] A systematic review and meta-analysis of 25 intervention studies examining periodontitis patients with and without periodontal treatment demonstrated that periodontal treatment was associated with a significant reduction in serum levels of CRP, IL-6, fibrinogen, and TNF-α.[291] Inflammatory periodontal disease (compared with periodontal health) is also associated with altered vascular endothelial function.[65] Altered vascular endothelial function is a major risk factor for acute thrombotic events. After scaling and root planing with a resultant decrease in periodontal inflammation, markers of vascular health improve significantly over time.[65,297] The functional assessment of vascular endothelial function also returns to normal after scaling and root planing.[257,297] These results suggest that periodontal inflammation adversely affects the health of the vascular endothelium, whereas a reduction in inflammation improves endothelial health. Whether these changes directly impact the risk of acute cardiovascular events remains to be determined in prospective controlled clinical intervention trials over long periods; such studies do not currently exist.

Role of Periodontal Disease in Erectile Dysfunction

Erectile dysfunction (ED) is associated with endothelial dysfunction, and elevated levels of oxidative stress and systemic inflammation are common to both periodontal disease and ED. Studies have shown a relationship between ED and periodontitis. In a large case–control study of almost 200,000 male patients in Taiwan, those with ED were significantly more likely to have chronic periodontitis than those without ED, with an overall significant odds ratio of 3.35 after adjusting for confounding variables.[142] Other studies have supported these findings in smaller populations in other countries,[223,264,326] and a systematic review of four studies found a significant association between periodontitis and ED, with an odds ratio of 3.07.[305] An intervention trial was conducted in 120 patients with ED and chronic periodontitis; 60 patients received scaling and root planing, and 60 control patients received no periodontal treatment.[6] Three months later, the treatment group had significant improvement in ED, whereas the control group had no change. These preliminary studies suggest a relationship between periodontitis and ED, but more research is needed to understand the mechanisms of interaction.

Periodontal Disease and Stroke

Ischemic cerebral infarction, or stroke, is often preceded by systemic bacterial or viral infection. In one study, patients with cerebral ischemia were five times more likely to have had a systemic infection within 1 week before the ischemic event than nonischemic control patients.[96] Recent infection was a significant risk factor for cerebral ischemia; it was independent of other known risk factors, such as hypertension, history of a previous stroke, diabetes, smoking, and CHD. Interestingly, the presence of systemic infection before the stroke resulted in significantly greater ischemia and a more severe postischemic neurologic defect than stroke not preceded by infection.[97] Stroke patients with a preceding infection had slightly higher levels of plasma fibrinogen and significantly higher levels of CRP compared with those without infection.

Periodontal Infection Associated With Stroke

Stroke is classified as either hemorrhagic or nonhemorrhagic. Nonhemorrhagic stroke, or ischemic stroke, is usually caused by thromboembolic events and cerebrovascular atherosclerosis, whereas hemorrhagic stroke often results from a vascular bleed, such as an aneurysm. Periodontal disease has been associated primarily with an increased risk of nonhemorrhagic stroke. Numerous studies have shown that periodontal disease is associated with an increased risk of stroke. In a case–control study, patients with severe periodontitis had a 4.3-times higher risk of stroke than patients with mild or no periodontitis.[95] Severe periodontitis was a risk factor in men but not women, and in those younger but not older than 65 years of age. In a longitudinal study of 1137 dentate men who were followed for a mean of 24 years, patients with greater than 20% mean radiographic bone loss at baseline were more than three times as likely to have a stroke than patients with less than 20% bone loss.[133] There was a stronger effect of periodontitis on the risk for stroke among men younger than 65 years of age compared with older patients. Both large epidemiologic studies and systematic reviews of the evidence have suggested an approximate threefold increased risk of stroke in patients with periodontitis.[127,312]

As previously discussed, periodontal infection may contribute directly to the pathogenesis of atherosclerosis by providing a persistent bacterial challenge to the arterial endothelium, thereby contributing to the monocyte- and macrophage-driven inflammatory process that results in atheromatosis and narrowing of the vessel lumen. Furthermore, periodontal infection may stimulate a series of indirect systemic effects, such as elevated production of fibrinogen and CRP, which increases the risk of stroke (see Figs. 26.5 and 26.6). Finally, bacteremia with PAAP-positive bacterial strains from supragingival and subgingival plaque can increase platelet aggregation, thereby contributing to thrombus formation and subsequent thromboembolism, which is the leading cause of stroke.[189]

CLINICAL CORRELATION

Periodontal infection may contribute directly to the pathogenesis of atherosclerosis by providing a persistent bacterial challenge to the arterial endothelium, thereby contributing to the monocyte- and macrophage-driven inflammatory process that results in atheromatosis and narrowing of the vessel lumen.

Periodontal Disease and Diabetes Mellitus

The relationship between diabetes mellitus and periodontal disease has been extensively examined. It is clear from epidemiologic research that diabetes increases the risk for and severity of periodontal diseases.[191] The biologic mechanisms through which diabetes influences the periodontium are discussed in this chapter. The increased prevalence and severity of periodontitis typically seen in patients with diabetes—especially those with poor metabolic control—has led to the designation of periodontal disease as the "sixth complication" of diabetes.[171] In addition to the five "classic" complications of diabetes (Box 26.2), the American Diabetes Association has officially recognized that periodontal disease is common among patients with diabetes, and its Standards of Care include taking a history of current or past dental infections as part of the physician's examination.[12] Since 2009, the American Diabetes Association's Standards of Medical Care in Diabetes have specifically recommended that physicians refer patients with diabetes to a dentist for a comprehensive dental and periodontal examination.[13]

Many studies have examined the effects of diabetes on the periodontium, whereas others have examined the effect of periodontal infection on the control of diabetes.[191] Such studies are difficult to perform because of the influence of ongoing medical management of diabetes during the study. The following questions remain:

- Does the presence or severity of periodontal disease affect the metabolic state of diabetic patients?
- Does periodontal treatment aimed at reducing the bacterial challenge and minimizing inflammation have a measurable effect on glycemic (blood glucose) control?

A review of four studies including more than 22,000 patients found that the incidence of type 2 diabetes (i.e., new diagnoses) was significantly greater in individuals with periodontal disease than in those without periodontal disease.[35] In a longitudinal study of patients with type 2 diabetes, severe periodontitis was associated with the significant worsening of glycemic control over time.[288] Individuals with severe periodontitis at the baseline examination had a greater incidence of worsening glycemic control over a 2- to 4-year period as compared with those without periodontitis at

BOX 26.2 Complications of Diabetes Mellitus

1. Retinopathy
2. Nephropathy
3. Neuropathy
4. Macrovascular disease
5. Altered wound healing
6. Periodontal disease

From Löe H. Periodontal disease: the sixth complication of diabetes mellitus. *Diabetes Care.* 1993;16(Suppl 1):329.

baseline. In this study, periodontitis was known to have preceded the worsening of glycemic control. Periodontitis has also been associated with the classic complications of diabetes. Diabetic adults with severe periodontitis at baseline had a significantly greater incidence of kidney and macrovascular complications over the subsequent 1 to 11 years than did diabetic adults with only gingivitis or mild periodontitis.[296] This was true despite both groups' having similar glycemic control. One or more cardiovascular complications occurred in 82% of patients with severe periodontitis versus 21% of patients without severe periodontitis. Again, severe periodontitis preceded the onset of clinical diabetic complications in these patients.

Among diabetic patients with periodontitis, periodontal therapy may have beneficial effects on glycemic control.[74,191,262,272,290] A large number of studies, starting as far back as 1960,[309] have examined the impact of periodontal therapy on glycemic control in patients with diabetes. Most of these studies compared scaling and root planing (with or without adjunctive systemic antibiotics) with no periodontal therapy and followed patients for several months to assess changes in glycemic control measured by glycated hemoglobin (HbA1c) values. Others included in the treatment regimen not only scaling and root planing but also extraction of periodontally hopeless teeth and even periodontal surgery. Many of these studies showed a significant improvement in glycemic control, as determined by reductions in HbA1c values, in the periodontal treatment group compared with the nontreatment group.[99,146,206] Other studies showed minimal change in glycemic control in periodontally treated patients.[8,53,75,274] Greater improvement in glycemic control after periodontal therapy may be seen in patients with poorer glycemic control at the time of therapy. For example, after scaling and root planing in type 2 diabetes patients, the average improvement in HbA1c was almost three times greater in patients whose pretreatment HbA1c was less than 9% compared to those with baseline HbA1c of greater than 9%.[235]

When studies of similar treatment regimens demonstrate conflicting results, systematic reviews with meta-analyses of the data are essential to aid the clinician in evaluating the evidence. Numerous systematic reviews and meta-analyses have consistently shown that periodontal therapy is associated with a statistically significant and clinically relevant improvement in glycemic control in patients with diabetes and periodontitis.[74,262,290] However, clinicians must understand that individual patients may or may not have outcomes similar to the average outcome in any given study or systematic review. That is, treatment results vary from patient to patient, and clinicians should not expect the same result in all patients. These studies suggest that periodontal therapy is most likely to result in short-term improvement in glycemia in those diabetic patients with severe periodontitis and poor metabolic control who demonstrate marked reduction in periodontal inflammation after treatment. Conversely, individuals with moderately well-controlled or well-controlled diabetes and periodontitis who have less reduction in inflammation may demonstrate no or only minimal changes in glycemic control.

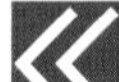

FLASH BACK

Periodontal disease was designated as the "sixth complication" of diabetes because of the increased prevalence and severity of periodontitis typically seen in patients with diabetes, especially those with poor metabolic control.

Most of the studies evaluating the treatment of periodontal disease and its impact on glycemic control have been performed in patients with type 2 diabetes. However, research suggests that periodontal therapy may have a smaller impact on glycemic control in patients with type 1 diabetes than in those with type 2 disease.[40] In a study of periodontitis patients with type 1 or type 2 diabetes, periodontal therapy was associated with a significant improvement in glycemic control overall in those with type 2 diabetes but not in those with type 1 disease, despite improvement in the periodontal condition of both groups.[40]

It is common to observe wide interindividual variability in response to various medical management approaches in patients with type 1 diabetes. Similarly, wide variability in the impact of periodontal therapy on glycemic control can be expected in the type 1 diabetic population. For example, a study of periodontal therapy in 65 people with type 1 diabetes and chronic periodontitis showed highly variable responses.[294] Although there was an overall improvement in periodontal health after therapy, approximately 35% of patients had an improvement in glycemic control after treatment, 37% had no significant change, and 28% showed a worsening of glycemic control. In this study, patients were divided into those with better baseline glycemic control (i.e., glycated hemoglobin values <8.5%) and those with poorer glycemic control (i.e., glycated hemoglobin values ≥8.5%). Interestingly, twice as many patients showed improved glycemic control among those whose glycemic control before periodontal treatment was poor compared with those among whom baseline glycemic control was good. Therefore, the clinician may anticipate a greater glycemic response to periodontal therapy among those patients with type 1 diabetes whose glycemic control is relatively poor than among those whose glycemic control is already good before periodontal treatment.

Periodontal Infection Associated With Glycemic Control in Diabetes

An understanding of the effects of other infections is useful to delineate the mechanisms by which periodontal infection influences glycemia. It is well known that systemic inflammation plays a major role in insulin sensitivity and glucose dynamics. As discussed previously, periodontal diseases can induce or perpetuate an elevated systemic chronic inflammatory state, which is reflected in increased serum CRP, IL-6, and fibrinogen levels seen in many people with periodontitis.[64,165,289] Inflammation induces insulin resistance, and such resistance often accompanies systemic infections. For example, acute nonperiodontal bacterial and viral infections have been shown to increase insulin resistance and aggravate glycemic control.[247,321] This occurs in individuals either with or without diabetes. Systemic infections increase tissue resistance to insulin through a variety of mechanisms, thereby preventing glucose from entering target cells, causing elevated blood glucose levels, and requiring increased pancreatic insulin production to maintain normoglycemia. Insulin resistance may persist for weeks or even months after the patient has recovered clinically from the illness. In an individual with type 2 diabetes who already has significant insulin resistance, further tissue resistance to insulin as a result of infection may considerably exacerbate poor glycemic control.

It is possible that chronic gram-negative periodontal infections may also result in increased insulin resistance and poor glycemic control.[98,289] In patients with periodontitis, persistent systemic challenge with periodontopathic bacteria and their products results in an upregulation of the immunoinflammatory response, with elevation in serum levels of proinflammatory mediators, such as IL-1β, TNF-α, and IL-6, similar to well-recognized systemic infections but on a more persistent, chronic basis (Fig. 26.8). Increased serum levels of several cytokines, including TNF-α and IL-6, are associated with increased insulin resistance. This mechanism would explain the worsening of glycemic control associated with severe periodontitis. Periodontal treatment designed to decrease the bacterial insult and reduce inflammation may result in decreased systemic inflammation, restoring insulin sensitivity over time and thereby resulting in improved metabolic control. The improved glycemic control seen in

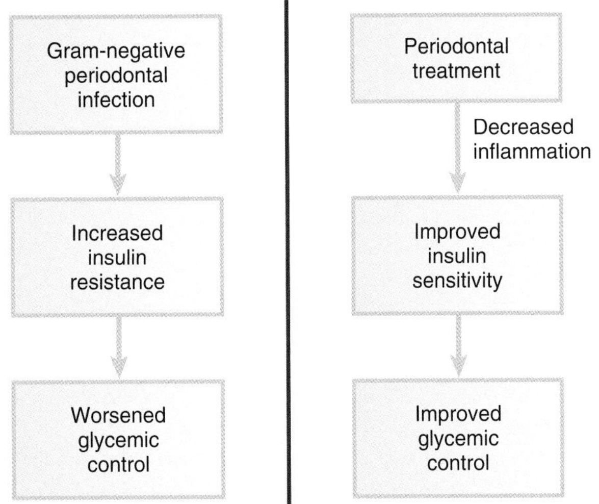

Fig. 26.8 Potential effects of periodontal infection and periodontal therapy on glycemia in patients with diabetes.

many studies of periodontal therapy would support such a hypothesis. This mechanism may also explain differences in the glycemic response to periodontal therapy between individuals with type 1 and type 2 diabetes.[40] Because type 2 diabetes is strongly associated with insulin resistance, periodontal therapy that reduces systemic inflammation may improve insulin sensitivity and result in improved glycemic control. Conversely, type 1 diabetes is not strongly associated with insulin resistance, so reduced inflammation after periodontal therapy may not have a major effect on insulin sensitivity in patients with type 1 disease, which would minimize the impact of periodontal treatment in these patients.

Periodontal Disease and Asthma

Evidence evaluating the relationship between periodontal disease and asthma is now emerging. In a large case–control study of 220 adults, half with severe asthma and half without asthma, after adjusting for age, smoking habit, education level, and body mass index, people with periodontitis were 4.8 times more likely to have severe asthma than those without periodontitis.[94] Although this study does not demonstrate causation, it suggests a possible link between inflammatory periodontal disease and asthma in adults.

A large study of over 450 patients examining the relationship between periodontitis and asthma found that patients with severe asthma were four times more likely to have periodontitis than those without asthma.[166] A systematic review of 21 studies evaluating the association between asthma and periodontal diseases found significantly less gingival inflammation in patients without asthma compared to those with asthma. However, the relationship between asthma and parameters of periodontitis, such as probing depth and clinical attachment levels, was unclear, with conflicting results between studies.[210] More research is needed to clarify the relationship between asthma and periodontal diseases.

Periodontal Disease and Rheumatoid Arthritis

An association between periodontitis and rheumatoid arthritis (RA) has been a topic of research for decades.[23,194] Both are chronic destructive conditions in which inflammation plays the primary role. Both show distinct heterogeneity in expression and progression. Some patients with RA have mild symptoms that can be easily controlled with nonsteroidal anti-inflammatory agents; similarly, some periodontitis patients respond well to relatively simple periodontal procedures and good oral hygiene. Conversely, some patients with RA or periodontitis are less responsive to such therapies and demonstrate progressive destruction of the associated tissues. Studies consistently show a strong and statistically significant association between the prevalence of RA and periodontitis.[23] Proinflammatory cytokine profiles are similar in RA and periodontitis, and matrix metalloproteinase enzymes play a major role in tissue destruction found in both conditions. RA and periodontitis have similar mechanistic activation of osteoclasts through the nF-kappa B ligand (RANKL)/osteoprotegerin (OPG) axis.

In RA, an inflammatory infiltration of the joint synovial membranes leads to synovitis and eventual damage to the joint structures that compromise joint function. The cause of that inflammation has been the subject of much research, and bacterial infection of the joint has long been postulated. DNA from numerous periodontal bacteria has been detected in joint spaces.[139] Among these, *P. gingivalis* has unique properties that may directly link it to RA.

Proteins can be modified by a process called citrullination in which the peptidyl arginine residue of the protein is converted to citrulline by the peptidylarginine deiminase (PADI) class of enzymes. These altered proteins are called "citrullinated proteins." They are commonly found in inflamed tissues, and they can elicit a profound autoimmune response resulting in production of anti-citrullinated protein antibodies. Anti-citrullinated protein antibodies play a predominant role in RA. Elevated levels of anti-citrullinated protein antibodies occur years before clinical onset of RA, and higher antibody levels are associated with more severe RA over time.[236] In fact, the prevalence of anti-citrullinated protein antibodies in RA patients is much higher than the prevalence of rheumatoid factor (RF), the autoantibody most closely associated with RA.

P. gingivalis in strongly implicated in periodontal inflammation. *P. gingivalis* is also unique in its ability to produce PADI, resulting in citrullination of proteins. This may then prime the immune response to respond rapidly and robustly to the presence of citrullinated proteins present in other tissues, such as the synovium, by producing high levels of anti-citrullinated protein antibodies. Translocation of *P. gingivalis* from the oral cavity to the joint space via the bloodstream may result in production of PADI by the bacteria, which can then directly citrullinate proteins, such as fibrinogen and fibrin, in the joint synovium. This then stimulates rapid local production of anti-citrullinated protein antibodies in the synovium, leading to complement activation, stimulation of proinflammatory cytokine production, and activation of osteoclasts.[243] While these mechanisms may provide a possible link between periodontal diseases and RA, a causal relationship cannot be established without extensive confirmatory research.

Periodontal Medicine in Clinical Practice

The concept of periodontal diseases as localized entities that affect only the teeth and the supporting apparatus is oversimplified. Rather than being confined to the periodontium, inflammatory periodontal diseases may have wide-ranging systemic effects. In most people, these effects are relatively inconsequential, or at least not clinically evident. In susceptible individuals, however, periodontal infection may act as an independent risk factor for systemic disease, and it may be involved in the basic pathogenic mechanisms of these conditions. Furthermore, periodontal infection may exacerbate existing systemic disorders.

Periodontal Disease and Systemic Health

Proper use of the knowledge of potential relationships between periodontal disease and systemic health requires the dental professional to recognize the oral cavity as one of many interrelated organ systems. A palm-sized infection on the leg of a pregnant woman would be of major concern to the patient and her health care provider, given the potential negative consequences of this localized infection on fetal and maternal health. Similarly, a suppurating infection on the foot of a person with diabetes would be cause for immediate evaluation and aggressive treatment, considering the effects of such infections on the metabolic control of diabetes.

Periodontal infection must be viewed in a similar manner. Periodontitis is a gram-negative infection that often results in severe inflammation, and it potentially involves the intravascular dissemination of microorganisms and their products throughout the body. However, periodontitis tends to be a "silent" disease until destruction results in acute oral symptoms. Most patients—and many medical professionals—do not recognize the potential infection that may exist within the oral cavity.

Patient Education

Patient education is a priority. Just a few decades ago, the factors involved in CHD were unclear. At present, however, it would be difficult to find an individual who was unfamiliar with the link between cholesterol and heart disease. This change was precipitated by research that clearly demonstrated the increased risk for heart disease among individuals with high cholesterol levels, followed by intensive education efforts to spread the message from the scientific community to the public at large. It is important to recognize that high cholesterol levels have not been shown to *cause* heart disease in all individuals; rather, they significantly *increase the risk* of disease. Cholesterol has also been demonstrated to have a biologically plausible role in the pathogenesis of CHD.

Similarly, patient education efforts in the realm of periodontal medicine must emphasize the inflammatory nature of periodontal infections, the increased risk for systemic disease associated with the infection, and the biologically plausible role that periodontal infection may play in systemic disease. Few individuals had their cholesterol levels evaluated until knowledge of the link between cholesterol and heart disease became widespread. Likewise, an increased appreciation of the potential effects of periodontal infection on systemic health may result in increased patient demand for periodontal evaluation.

Enhanced community awareness may be derived from newspapers, magazines, and other lay sources. However, the most reliable origin of information should be dental and medical professionals, through daily contact with patients. A pregnant woman usually knows that infections may adversely affect her pregnancy. Individuals with diabetes generally know that infections impair glycemic control. However, many of these patients do not know that occult periodontal infections can have the same effect as more clinically evident infections. The dentist is responsible for diagnosing periodontal infections, providing appropriate treatment, and preventing disease recurrence or progression. Because many medical professionals are unfamiliar with the oral cavity and oral health research, dentists must reach out to the medical community to improve patient care through education and communication.[190] Likewise, patients must be educated about disease prevention. Just as patients know that lowering their cholesterol levels may decrease their risk for heart disease, similar knowledge regarding the prevention of periodontal infection should be emphasized. A physician would be remiss if he or she did not provide education about decreasing cholesterol level, losing weight, and ceasing a smoking habit to a patient at risk for CHD. Likewise, controlling the risk factor of periodontal infection requires the dentist to emphasize personal and professional preventive measures that are focused on oral hygiene and regular recall.

Conclusions

Does periodontal disease *cause* CHD, COPD, or adverse pregnancy outcomes? This question may be answered only by use of the evidence that is currently available, with the full knowledge that conclusions may change as future evidence dictates. Periodontal disease may increase the risk for many systemic disorders. Biologically plausible mechanisms support the role of periodontal infection in these conditions, but it should not be presented as the cause of such systemic diseases, any more than cholesterol should be said to cause heart disease. Periodontal infection is one of many potential risk factors for a number of systemic conditions. Fortunately, it is a readily modifiable risk factor, unlike age, gender, and genetic influences.

The focal infection theory of the early 20th century was widely and appropriately discredited when treatment based on the theory, which consisted almost solely of tooth extraction, had no effect on the underlying diseases that oral sepsis supposedly caused. Similarly, the clinical utility of our current knowledge base is only now evolving. Future research will further delineate the role of periodontal infection in systemic health. The associations between periodontal infection and conditions such as LBW delivery, diabetes, cardiovascular and cerebrovascular diseases, and respiratory diseases may be further substantiated. Longitudinal studies and intervention trials are needed before any causative role can be assigned.

The field of periodontal medicine offers new insights into the concept of the oral cavity as one system that is interconnected with the whole human body. For many years, the dental profession has recognized the effects of systemic conditions on the oral cavity. Only now, however, are dental professionals beginning to understand more fully the impact of the periodontium on systemic health.

Finally, it is important to appreciate the differences between the science and the art of dental practice as they relate to periodontal medicine. Science is based, in general, on means and standard deviations or standard errors. Thus, science may determine that, on average, diabetic patients with periodontal disease have poorer glycemic control than diabetic patients who are periodontally healthy. However, the patient who is sitting in the dental chair at any given time may or may not be a "mean" patient; in other words, she may or may not demonstrate the same relationship that science has determined to exist as an average within the population. She may lie somewhere within or outside the standard deviation. She may have extremely poor glycemic control that is directly related to her extensive periodontal inflammation; she may have average glycemic control; or she may have good glycemic control. The clinical practice of periodontal medicine recognizes that, while using an evidence-based approach is absolutely key to modern dentistry, each patient is an individual, and he or she may not always fit the average determined by science.

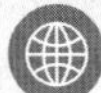 A Case Scenario is found on the companion website eBooks.Health.Elsevier.com.

Suggested Reading

Almiñana-Pastor PJ, Boronat-Catalá M, Micó-Martinez P, Bellot-Arcís C, Lopez-Roldan A, Alpiste-Illueca FM. Epigenetics and periodontics: A systematic review. *Med Oral Patol Oral Cir Bucal*. 2019;24(5):e659–e672. https://doi.org/10.4317/medoral.23008. PubMed PMID: 31433392. PMID: PMCID: PMC6764711.

Bartold PM, Lopez-Olivia I. Periodontitis and rheumatoid arthritis: An update 2012-2017. *Periodontology 2000*. 2020;83:189–212.

Hooper SJ, Wilson MJ, Crean SJ. Exploring the link between microorganisms and oral cancer: a systematic review of the literature. *Head Neck*. 2009;31(9):1228–1239. https://doi.org/10.1002/hed.21140.

Hujoel PP, Drangsholt M, Spiekerman C, Weiss NS. An exploration of the periodontitis-cancer association. *Ann Epidemiol*. 2003;13(5):312–316. https://doi.org/10.1016/s1047-2797(02)00425-8.

Irfan M, Delgado RZR, Frias-Lopez J. The Oral Microbiome and Cancer. *Front Immunol*. 2020;11:591088. https://doi.org/10.3389/fimmu.2020.591088.

Jacob JA. Study Links Periodontal Disease Bacteria to Pancreatic Cancer Risk. *JAMA*. 2016;315(24):2653–2654. https://doi.org/10.1001/jama.2016.6295.

Kaur S, White S, Bartold PM. Periodontal disease and rheumatoid arthritis: a systematic review. *J Dent Res*. 2013;92:399–408.

Kebschull M, Demmer RT, Papapanou PN. "Gum bug, leave my heart alone"—epidemiologic and mechanistic evidence linking periodontal infections and atherosclerosis. *J Dent Res*. 2010;89:879–902.

Lee W-C, Fu E, Li C-H, et al. Association between periodontitis and pulmonary function based on the Third National Health and Nutrition Examination Survey (NHANES III). *J Clin Periodontol* 47: 788-795.

Linden GJ, Lyons A, Scannapieco FA. Periodontal systemic associations: review of the evidence. *J Periodontol*. 2013;84(suppl 4):S8–S19.

Lopes MP, Cruz AA, Xavier MT, et al. *Prevotella intermedia* and periodontitis are associated with severe asthma. *J Periodontol*. 2020;91:46–54.

Mealey BL. The interactions between physicians and dentists in managing the care of patients with diabetes mellitus. *J Am Dent Assoc*. 2008;139(suppl):4s–7s.

Mercado FB, Marshall RI, Bartold PM. Inter-relationships between rheumatoid arthritis and periodontal disease. A review. *J Clin Periodontol*. 2003;30:761–772.

Michaud DS, Fu Z, Shi J, Chung M. Periodontal Disease, Tooth Loss, and Cancer Risk. *Epidemiol Rev*. 2017;39(1):49–58. https://doi.org/10.1093/epirev/mxx006.

Moraschini V, Calasans-Maia JA, Calasans-Maia MD. Association between asthma and periodontal disease: a systematic review and meta-analysis. *J Periodontol*. 2018;89:440–455.

Offenbacher S, Barros SP, Beck JD. Rethinking periodontal inflammation. *J Periodontol*. 2008;79:1577–1584.

Rantapaa-Dahlqvist S, de Jong BAW, Berglin E, et al. Autoantibodies against cyclic citrullinated peptide and IgA rheumatoid factor predict development of rheumatoid arthritis. *Arthritis Rheum*. 2003;48:2741–2749.

Scannapieco FA, Bush RB, Paju S. Associations between periodontal disease and risk for nosocomial bacterial pneumonia and chronic obstructive pulmonary disease: a systematic review. *Ann Periodontol*. 2003;8:54–69.

Takeuchi K, Matsumoto K, Furuta M, et al. Periodontitis is associated with chronic obstructive pulmonary disease. *J Dent Res*. 2019;98:534–540.

Tonetti MS, VanDyke TE. Periodontitis and atherosclerotic cardiovascular disease: consensus report of the Joint EFP/AAP Workshop on Periodontitis and Systemic Diseases. *J Periodontol*. 2013;84(suppl 4):S24–S29.

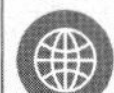 References for this chapter are found on the companion website eBooks.Health.Elsevier.com.

CHAPTER 27

Pathology and Management of Periodontal Problems Associated With Viral Infection, Including HIV, COVID, and Others

April Guadalupe Martinez | Purnima S. Kumar | Yvonne L. Hernandez-Kapila

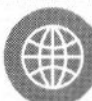

For expanded discussion on virus isolation and identification, modifications for virus propagation, antiviral development, and pathogenesis studies, viroinformatics, testing for HIV, sequencing, HIV and salivary gland disorders, preventative measures for COVID-19, HAART therapy, oral and periodontal manifestations of HIV, and necrotizing ulcerative gingivitis, please visit the companion website at eBooks.Health.Elsevier.com.

CHAPTER OUTLINE

Introduction

The human oral microbiome consists of a complex community that spans all three domains of life (*Archaea*, *Bacteria*, *Eukarya*), including eukaryotic RNA and deoxyribonucleic acid (DNA) viruses and prokaryotic viruses. These acellular molecular complexes are found in almost every ecosystem and are believed to be the most abundant entities on Earth. Although the size of the human oral virome is not known, quantitative biological studies estimate that the more well-described bacterial microorganisms are similar in number to human cells while the ratio of viral-like particles to human cells approximates 100:1.[1] Despite the oral cavity being one of the most diverse and dynamic environments of the human body, a deficit in our understanding of viruses that inhabit it is evident.

Viruses can cause acute, persistent, or latent infections as they have the capacity to integrate into the human genome as seen with endogenous retroviruses. Conversely, viruses also play a role in the formation of our commensal microbiome which begins shortly after birth and continuously develops throughout our lifetime.[2] Due to early life variables, antibiotic use, host genetics, and the distinct selective pressures present between body sites there are compositional variations of the human microbiome within this holobiont complex.[3,4] For example, the genomic composition on a coronal surface of a tooth between two individuals would be more similar than between either individual's tongue surface. As more distinct oral niches harboring viruses are identified through the progression in sequencing technology, future research can begin to evaluate how the human oral virome affects the acquisition of host-associated microbiomes.

Coexistence with our diverse microbiome equips us with crucial biological functions and traits to protect us from invasion by transient or pathogenic microorganisms. Dysbiosis in the bacterial community has been markedly documented to be associated with numerous diseases including inflammatory bowel disease, rheumatoid arthritis, diabetes mellitus, asthma, and cancer.[5–7] Oral diseases such as dental caries, periodontitis, and oral mucosal diseases also arise from microbial dysbiosis.[8] Viruses have been described as drivers of oral blisters, ulcers, and tumors and will be briefly described in this chapter. The pathophysiology of these oral conditions have remained focused on a bacterial or fungal origin but with the emergence of metagenomics, the roles of viruses are now being reevaluated.

Various models centering around the disruption of the host-microbe homeostasis currently exist to illustrate the etiology of periodontitis. Even as these models have developed throughout the decades it has been a challenge to fully describe all the epidemiological and clinical presentations of periodontitis. Certain characteristics of the episodic-burst model of periodontitis first proposed by Socransky in 1984 can be supported when proposing viral reactivation and synergy as potential drivers of periodontal disease.[9] It has been postulated that enhanced bacterial pathogenicity may result from the reactivation of common herpes viruses and their intimate topographic relationship with putative periodontopathogens within diseased periodontal pockets.[40] Viruses may compound the destructive inflammatory process by modulation of the host immune response which affects a similar cytokine and chemokine profile found in patients with periodontitis. Studies with murine models and human subgingival plaque demonstrate that a dysbiosis within the oral virome is aggravated with disease progression.[88,338] Including viruses in these models can elucidate novel mechanisms that underlie the breakdown of the periodontal host-microbe homeostasis.

Eukaryotic viruses are not the only members of the virome that can influence human health as prokaryotic viruses (bacteriophages) can indirectly affect human hosts by modulating bacterial composition and fitness.[337] Bacteriophages are the natural predators of bacteria and have a defined role in the management of biofilms. Isolation of bacteriophages in various oral niches has been achieved and these metagenomic analyses demonstrate bacteriophages as the more abundant and diverse branch of the human virome.[295,335] After the human gut, the oral cavity harbors the second-largest microbial community. Studies of bacteriophages within the human gut demonstrated that their relative abundance and diversity correlate with intestinal inflammation and enteric bacterial dysbiosis associated with conditions such as inflammatory bowel disease.[95,213] The prophage form of bacteriophages has also been implicated in dampening the antibacterial host immune response while enhancing bacterial virulence, thus prolonging and aggravating certain bacterial infections. Currently, only a few bacteriophages have been characterized and known to infect putative periodontopathogens, but a shift in the composition of this community in diseased states has already been documented.[338]

Shortly after the discovery of the destructive effects of bacteriophages, they were proposed as therapeutic agents against bacterial infections prior to the discovery of antibiotics. The success of phage therapy was overshadowed by antibiotics as phages have a narrow host range and were difficult to isolate, but now are currently appealing as antibiotic resistance continues to rise. Successful bacteriophage-based antibiofilm strategies in animal models have been employed in biofilm-mediated conditions as the rise of antibiotic resistance limits the efficacy of standard-of-care treatment.[341] Development of phage therapy shows an effective reduction in planktonic bacteria and biofilm communities as bacteriophages influence the dynamics of biofilm formation and dispersal. Thus, bacteriophages may be a promising approach for the management of the primary etiology of periodontal inflammation, that is, dental plaque.

Viral Complex

Bacterial cells are visible under optical microscopes as they are unicellular organisms that typically measure 0.5 to 3 μm in diameter. However, in order to view viruses, electron microscopy (EM) or x-ray crystallography must be employed as their typical size ranges from 10 to 200 nm. These techniques allow researchers to delineate viral morphology and the protein subunit arrangement. Characteristic morphological features are distinguishable through EM as accelerated, monochromic electrons are used to irradiate viruses that are stained with heavy metals or dried in a vacuum (Fig. 27.1A). Details of the interior architecture of viruses in more physiological states are achievable through cryogenic EM.[16] Diagnosis of viral diseases utilizing EM is advantageous as it is independent of pathogen-specific reagents, however, due to its narrow field of view, high viral particle concentrations are required for detection. More recent advancements in atomic force microscopy techniques have allowed researchers to visualize viruses *in situ* emerging from infected, living cells while maintaining a high resolution of the fine structural components of the viral particle.[189]

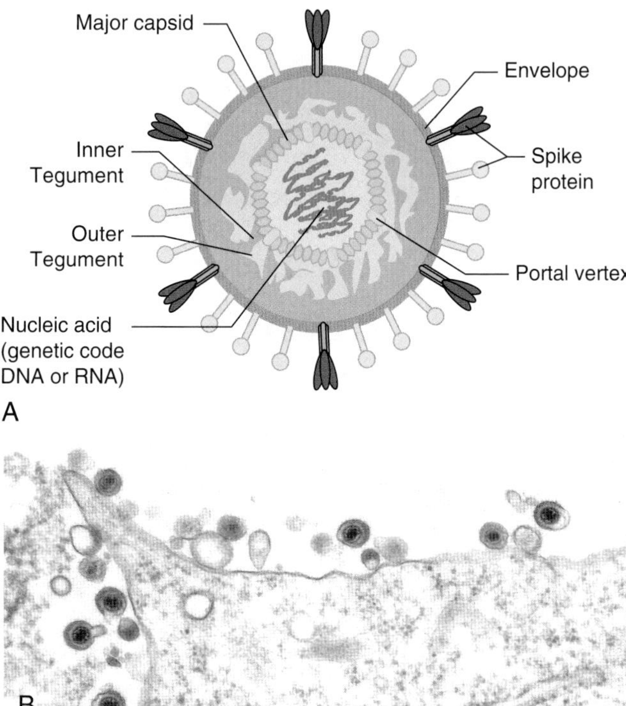

Fig. 27.1 (A) Depiction of an icosahedral virion with common structural elements which can aid in replication, transmission, and evasion mechanisms. (B) This electron microscopic image depicted numbers of human herpesvirus-8 (HHV-8) particles, the causative agent of Kaposi sarcoma, which had been grown in cell culture. These extracellular particles are composed of an inner nucleocapsid, surrounded by an envelope with a layer of tegument opposed to the envelope. (A, Copyright © 2022. Ryutaro Kuraji. B, From Centers for Disease Control and Prevention/Cynthia Goldsmith and Jodi Black, Public Health Image Library (PHIL), https://phil.cdc.gov/Details.aspx?pid=22885.)

Similar to bacterial cells, viruses contain genetic material. First introduced in 1971, the Baltimore classification system organizes viruses on genomic trends. This animal virus-centric classification system sorts a virus into seven categories based on the distinct mechanism a virus produces mRNA.[180] Through these seven categories one is able to determine if the nucleic acid a virus possesses is a single- or double-strand of RNA or DNA which is encased by an outer shell of proteins collectively known as a capsid. The genome size varies between viruses and is independent of their size.[27] The simplest virus carries enough RNA or DNA to encode four proteins while the most complex can encode up to 200 proteins. These small genomes are capable of encoding the identical protein subunits that self-assemble through electrostatic and hydrophobic forces to form their capsid. The main purpose of this capsid is to protect the fragile nucleic acid from the harsh external environment that the viral particle encounters and successfully transport the genetic material into the host cell. Ultimately, the formation of the capsid determines the virus' morphology, reproduction, and infectivity.

Viruses are classified into four main morphological types: helical, icosahedral, enveloped, and complex. Animal viruses with icosahedral morphologies predominate and include human papillomavirus, hepatitis B virus, and herpesvirus. Additional structures may be acquired from the host plasma membrane to form a viral envelope that is studded with virus-coded, glycosylated membrane proteins. For example, herpesviruses display a multilayered icosahedral architecture, which includes an envelope spiked with glycoproteins, a layer of proteins embedded in the viral matrix, a capsid shell, and a large DNA genome (see Fig. 27.1B). Attachment to the host cell is mediated by viral proteins, glycans, or lipids that bind to specific host surface molecules. These same viral components of the capsid or envelope determine the host range and antigenic composition of the viral particle.

TABLE 27.1 Cytopathic Effects of Viruses That Colonize Oral Cavity

Virus	Oral Manifestation	CPE in Cell Cultures	Tissue Tropism	Identification
Cytomegalovirus	Oral ulcers	Rounding and enlargement	Epithelium, Fibroblasts, Endothelium, Monocytes	CPE
Herpes simplex virus	Oral ulcers	Intranuclear inclusion bodies	Epithelium, Fibroblasts, Neurons	IF & Neutralization
Epstein-Barr virus	Hairy leukoplakia, oral ulcers	Intranuclear inclusion bodies	Epithelium, Fibroblasts, $CD21^+$ B lymphocytes	IF
HIV-1	Hairy leukoplakia, necrotizing ulcerative periodontitis, aphthous ulcer	Multinucleated giant cells	Epithelium, Fibroblasts, $CD4^+$ T cells	IF & Neutralization

CPE, Cytopathic effect; *HIV*, human immunodeficiency virus.

Cell Cultures

Despite molecular advancements, cell culturing remains a useful approach as it has the capacity to isolate a wide variety of viruses and provide viable isolates for further characterization. In addition to viral screening, culturing cells derived from multicellular animal, plant, fungi or bacterial cells allow clinicians and researchers the ability to characterize viral infectivity and virulence. Standard cell lines found in virology laboratories include primary rhesus monkey kidney (RhMK) cells, human lung fibroblasts (MRC-5), and human epithelial (Hep-2) cells which are used to isolate enteroviruses, herpesviruses, and adenoviruses, respectively.[136] The study of viruses using cell lines can only occur if these cell lines are susceptible to viral infection and permissible for viral replication. Since no one cell line can support the growth of all relevant viruses several cell lines must be applied or genetically modified.[112,293]

The replication of many human pathogenic viruses is associated with cellular transformation and eventually cellular destruction. Evidence of viral presence can be demonstrated microscopically through degenerative morphological changes in cell lines collectively known as cytopathic effects (CPE). Typical CPEs usually are visible between 1 and 3 weeks post-incubation and include swelling or shrinking of cells, cytoplasmic granulation, syncytium formation, and cellular lysis (Table 27.1). The type or severity of the CPE is dependent on the cell line involved, the length of incubation, and type of virus studied. Some CPEs are distinct enough to allow viruses to be identified at the genus level, such as herpes simplex virus (HSV) and CMV infections (Fig. 27.2), whereas enteroviruses demonstrate nonspecific CPEs.[7,345]

Molecular Techniques

Molecular approaches are utilized in order to bypass the inherent limitation of cell cultures, such as long incubation times, delayed or indistinguishable CPE appearance and inability to support viral reproduction. Viral presence can be recognized by detecting viral antigens or antiviral antibodies through immunofluorescence, enzyme-linked immunosorbent (ELISA), agglutination, hemagglutination, or lateral flow assays. These methods may not differentiate between infectious and noninfectious viral particles nor quantify viral particles with great precision but can serotype viral species effectively based on antigen structure. Suspected human immunodeficiency virus (HIV) infections are commonly verified in a clinical setting using ELISA reactions, Western blot (WB) analysis, and lateral flow assays to confirm both presence of viral antigens and the determination of antiviral antibodies.

Viral analysis can also be conducted by monitoring viral nucleic acids through qualitative and quantitative PCR techniques that are characterized as practical, rapid and highly specific, and sensitive. Employing quantitative PCR assays at different time points can reveal the dynamics of viral proliferation, viral response to treatment, and the distinction between latent and active infections.[343] Commercial PCR assays are available for quantitative analysis; however, these assays are usually limited to clinically important viruses, such as enteroviruses, hepatitis B and C viruses, HSV, and HIV-1.[78,79] Protocols exist for oral samples from pooled saliva and oral mucosal swabs for these commercial assays as viral infections can be diagnosed and monitored with results comparable to serum analysis.[41,181,361] Studies using PCR methods to analyze whole saliva, oral mucosa, gingival crevicular fluid, and dental plaque samples for specific viral species in patients with periodontitis sustain the proposed association of these acellular entities and periodontal destruction.

Limitations of PCR assays for viral detection are largely due to the high mutation rate of viral genomes, particularly that of RNA viruses, which encode RNA-dependent RNA polymerases that replicate their genomes.[70,120] The lack of a proofreading mechanism produces progeny that possess on average 1 to 2 mutations from parental viruses, which may confer an increase in viral fitness.[333] The continuous need to update primer sequences to stay on pace with new viral strains can be inconvenient; however, unadjusted primers can lead to false positives as they might anneal incorrectly. Likewise, the design process of primers for new viral strains becomes a complex task as reliable detection is only possible when sequences do not overlap with any host or other viral off-target sequences (eBox 27.1). Conversely, additional mutations can often be deleterious and lower the fitness of RNA progeny. Researchers and clinicians illustrate this drawback by enhancing viral mutation rates in RNA viruses through an exogenous mutagen which resulted in lethal mutagenesis.[55,99]

Next-Generation Sequencing

The classical and molecular techniques described remain the gold standard for viral research and clinical diagnostics. However, in recent decades, next-generation sequencing (NGS) has expanded the survey of known bacteria, fungi, and viruses in a variety of ecosystems.[224,330] In the same manner, applications of metagenomics with NGS techniques have increased the breadth of the human virome at an accelerated rate to move beyond pathogenic viruses and include previously unrecognized resident viruses that inhabit our bodies without causing clinical symptoms. Furthermore, NGS technologies prove to be a powerful application for phylogenomic and metagenomic studies as complete or partial genomic sequences extracted from oral biofilms are frequently reported of novel oral bacteriophages shedding light on their potential role in bacterial and biofilm regulation.[56,73,290,355]

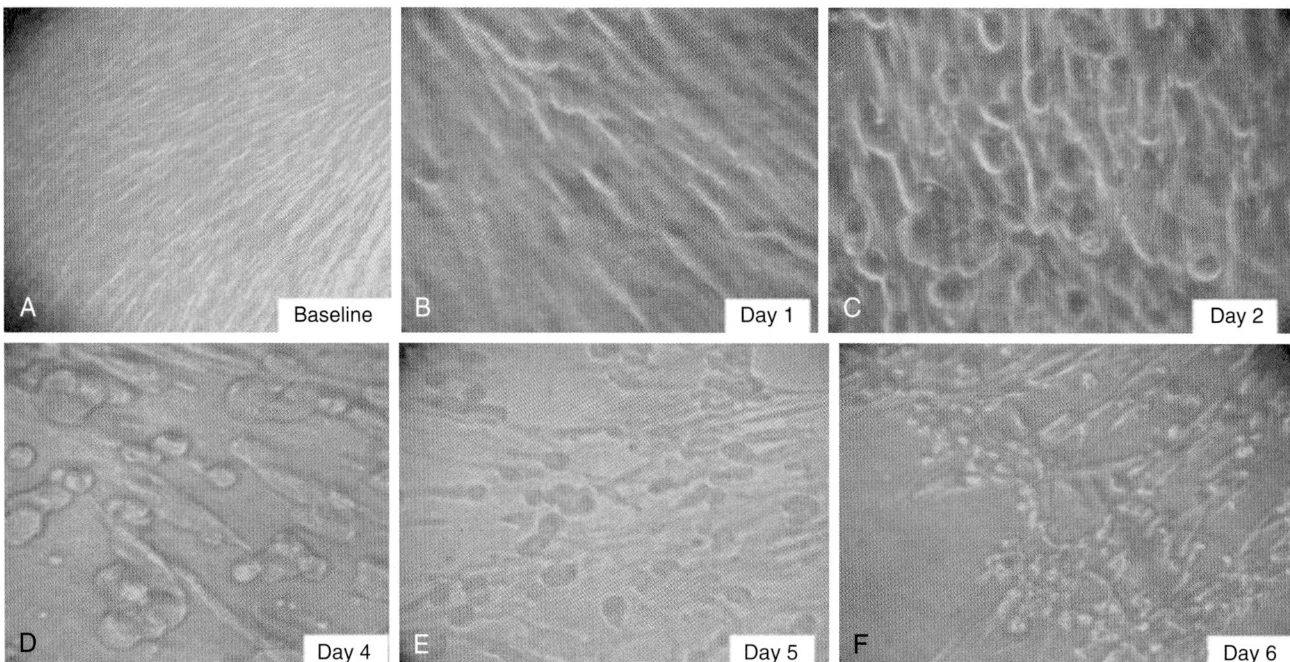

Fig. 27.2 Progression of cytopathic effects of cytomegalovirus infected gingival fibroblasts. Panels A through F depict the temporal progression of virus effects on the cellular morphology from baseline through day 6. (Adapted from Contreras A, Mardirossian A, Slots J. Herpesviruses in HIV-periodontitis. *J Clin Periodontol.* 2001;28:96–102.)

Viral Transmission

Due to their dependency on host cellular machinery, all successful viruses are able to establish themselves in a host population so that virus propagation is ensured. Despite its importance, no single mode of transmission is used by all viruses nor are all viruses bound to only one exclusive mode of transmission (Fig. 27.3). Viruses can alternate between lytic and latent life cycles dependent on intrinsic and environmental factors to enhance survival and transmission. Eventually, progeny virus particles must egress from infected cells as free particles into the external environment or spread from cell to cell without exposure to the extracellular milieu. The oral cavity's close relationship with the external environment, the array of cell types, and access to various organ systems are characteristics that make it a major portal of entry for infectious and transient microbial species. Intraoral tissues can be directly exposed to viruses through eating, drinking, kissing, and sexual contact. Indirect exposure mainly occurs in the form of saliva-contaminated droplets or aerosols expelled by an infected individual.

The presence of viral particles within the oral cavity does not necessarily indicate an active infection or predict the route of transmission used. Virus, host, and environmental factors influence transmission success by determining the infectivity of viruses, the contagiousness of the carrier, susceptibility of the recipient, and environmental stress on the virus. These determinants have different relative effects on each mode of transmission used by viruses and may instead result in intraoral tissues acting as reservoirs for the large breadth of oral viruses detected.[308] Although not all viruses are able to infect intraoral tissues, the physiological conditions of these tissues influence the viral load, translocation, and transmissibility of these viruses. In addition to viruses that are capable of infecting intraoral tissues, it is important to remain mindful of invading bacterial species that harbor their own constellation of viruses.

Oral Viral Ecology

Oral tissues are sensitive indicators of nutritional deficiencies, endocrine imbalances, anemias, gastrointestinal disturbances, and communicable diseases. Early life stresses in the form of malnutrition or hazardous environmental exposures are recorded in enamel and dentin defects. Indication of the current health status of individuals can be determined by examining the alveolar bone, gingiva, and tongue. Similarly, the highly individualistic indigenous microbial flora that lines hard and soft tissues of the oral cavity can imply past and present host and exogenous challenges within its genomic and transcriptomic profile.[18] Exogenous viral challenges on microbial and host defenses result in a constant flux in the oral microbial signature as microbial succession and acquisition occur through horizontal transmission.

Some viruses that reproduce in the lungs, nasal mucosa, or salivary glands are shed into the oral cavity. Transmission may occur through aerosols, contaminated hands, kissing, or spitting. Saliva that forms aerosol also contains both pathogenic bacteria (*Staphylococcus* species, *Porphymonas gingivalis*) and viruses (HIV, HSV, Epstein-Barr virus [EBV], hepatitis B virus) which are involved in the development of caries and periodontitis. Both the direct exchange and aerosolized particles can carry 108 virus-like particles (VLPs) per milliliter of saliva, which is mainly composed of bacteriophages of the taxon *Caudovirales* with limited homologs of herpesviruses and circoviruses.[247] Perhaps the best-known eukaryotic virus that is transmitted via saliva is Epstein Barr virus which results in mononucleosis, or "kissing disease."

Whole or aerosolized saliva exposure most frequently occurs within households and in dental settings. Tremendous effort has been implemented to limit the transmission of infectious diseases within dental clinics. These safeguards allow dental practitioners to conduct procedures with minimized risk of transmission of infectious pathogens from the patient to themselves, their dental team, or future patients. It would be impractical to enforce all infection control safeguards outside of dental offices. For this reason, cariogenic or periodontal pathogens are more likely to spread within the community and between individuals that share a household.

Currently, there is a limited understanding of which viruses humans are exposed to mainly due to the lack of available homologs to aid in the identification of virome constituents. However, studies of identifiable

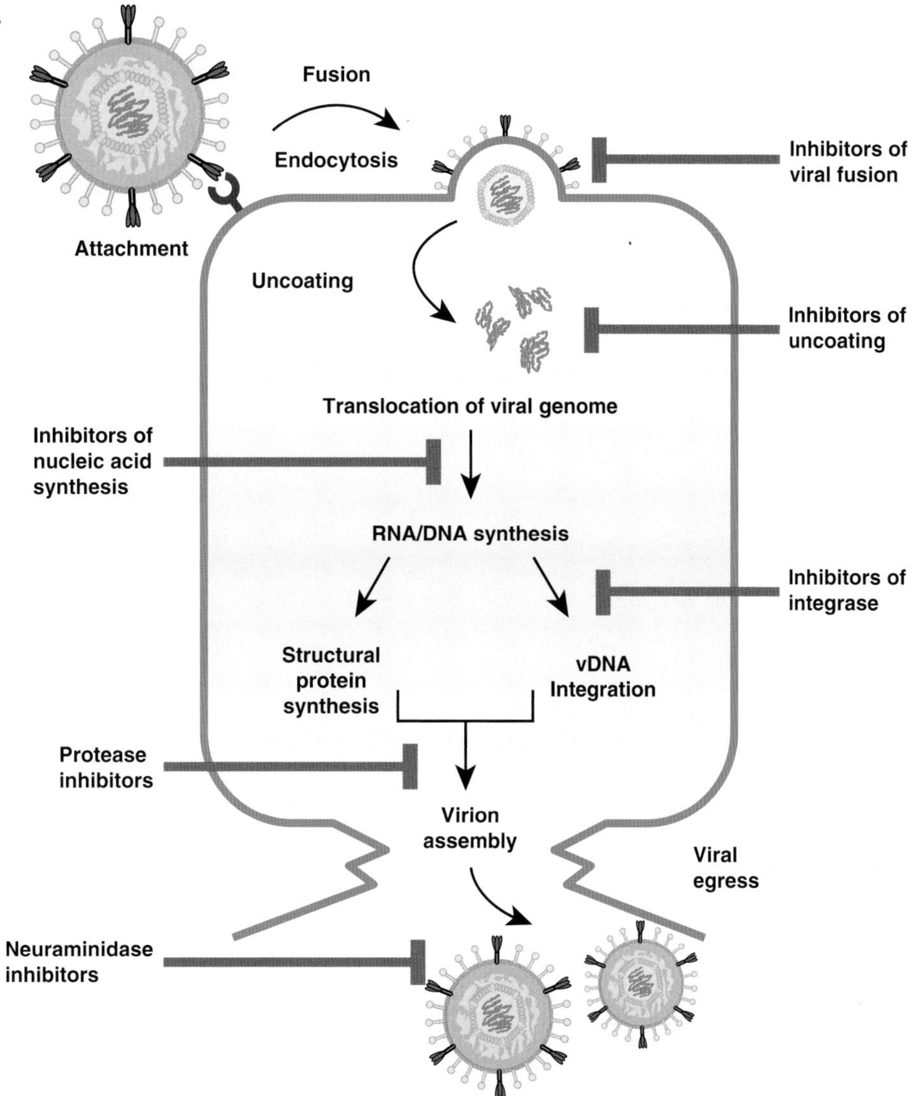

Fig. 27.3 Mechanism of virus infection to host cells. (Copyright © 2022. Ryutaro Kuraji.)

viruses from salivary samples suggest that shared environments are a significant determinant of the oral virome in humans.[247] In addition, the oral virome appears to maintain a personal signature and is persistent as nearly 20% of viruses could be identified throughout a 60-day period while less than 12% of viruses could be identified for less than 4 days in that same study period.[1] The vast majority of homologs identified in salivary samples between cohabitants and unrelated individuals were bacteriophages with host assignments to the phyla Proteobacteria or Firmicutes (Fig. 27.4). Another research group based in Spain obtained a similar viral composition from young Spanish adults (18 to 25 years of age) and proposed that there may be a small universal core of oral viruses within healthy individuals which include bacteriophages from the *Siphoviridae* and *Myoviridae* family, *Streptococcus* phages and *Herpesviridae*.[235] This proposed universal core of viruses certainly follows similar trends of oral bacterial composition as *Firmicutes* dominate subgingival and salivary microbiota in healthy individuals.[153] These preliminary findings in healthy individuals suggest a beneficial or mutualistic role in oral health for a large portion of bacteriophages identified.

Shifts in viral ecology are influenced by both intimate and non-intimate close contacts, which can occur in a matter of days or weeks.

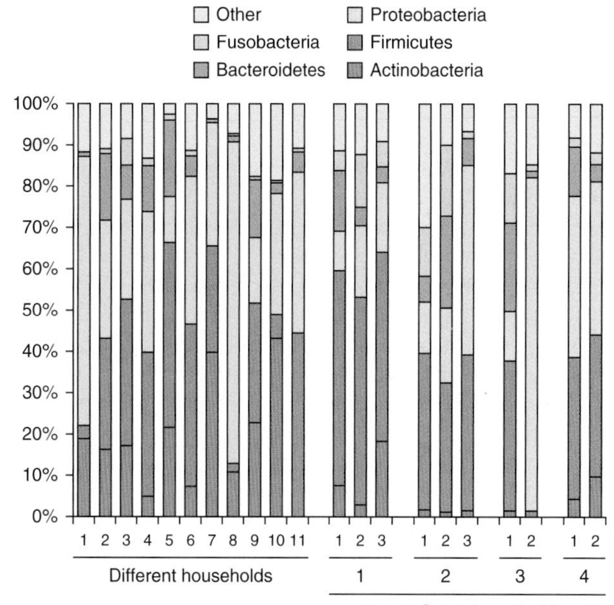

Fig. 27.4 Homologs identified in salivary samples between cohabitants and unrelated individuals.

Saliva

Of the diverse oral niches present, saliva is an important component of the oral mucosal immune system which limits entry to microbial species. Human whole saliva consists of salivary gland secretions, gingival crevicular fluids, secretory mucosa from the pharynx, desquamated epithelial cells, and microbial metabolites. The antimicrobial defense system found within saliva is largely composed of salivary proteins that vary between individuals.[273] Specific antiviral salivary proteins have been identified and can influence the viral load detected.[182] Although these salivary proteins are present in low concentrations, they can be involved in both innate and acquired immune functions resulting in a synergistic molecular defense network. Local concentrations of salivary proteins may be elevated near the periodontal sulcus or oral wounds suggesting their primary role is in inflammatory reactions.

Alternatively, saliva possesses both chemical and physical components that aid the development of pathogenic processes, such as periodontitis and viral reactivation. The formation of plaque is aided by salivary proteins, carbohydrates, and lipids by supplementing binding sites for biofilm-promoting bacteria and viruses on hard and soft tissue surfaces. Remodeling of microbial diversity and metabolic functions within the maturing biofilm creates ideal conditions and provides metabolites required for viral reactivation and replication.[128] These altered conditions along with a dampened immune state may lead to an elevated viral load in saliva which can then function as a vehicle for infectious viral transmission.

Salivary Proteins

Secretory IgA found at mucosal surfaces can neutralize viruses by inhibition of fusion, internalization, and attachment as the ratio of IgA to virus increases. Outside its extracellular functions, mucosal IgA can inhibit in vitro viral replication of respiratory viruses within epithelial cells.[190] Although HIV is detected in whole saliva samples at various levels, the possibility of HIV transmission via saliva are isolated events as salivary antibodies to HIV are detected and secretory IgA can neutralize certain strains of HIV.[274,296] Mucins secreted by salivary glands, MUC5B and MUC7, display inhibitory effects against bacterial and fungal species while playing a key role in the reduction of HIV transmission via saliva.[22,106] In opposition to viral inhibition, an active glycoprotein factor of unknown origin in saliva from healthy donors acts on oral fibroblasts in vitro triggering an increase in HSV-1 susceptibility.[366] These findings reflect the complex physiology of salivary secretions that is influenced by their genetic, immunological, and microbial components.

Salivary secretion, flow rate, and composition can further be dependent on gland conditions, nutritional status, gender, age, or emotional state. Whole salivary samples between healthy individuals document baseline variability of nonspecific and specific immune response proteins such as secretory IgA.[28,208,251] Patients with damage to major salivary glands, such as in primary Sjögren syndrome have compromised salivary flow leading to significantly more frequent dental visits for oral conditions, such as dental caries, oral ulceration, and periodontitis.[44] Increased presentations of oral ulcerations and periodontitis have previously been associated with the reactivation of EBV, which can be promoted by whole saliva and TGF-β1 extracted from patients with primary Sjögren's syndrome.[202] Reduced salivary secretions of the parotid gland are observed during a deficiency in vitamin D (<12 ng/mL) as the vitamin is necessary for the production of proteins that modulate extracellular calcium in the secretion process.[91] Studies have supported a strong association of lowered circulating levels of vitamin D with chronic periodontitis (CP), which highlights its roles in bone maintenance and the immune response.[178] Maintaining adequate levels of vitamin D is relevant to the oral virome as it upregulates the production of cathelicidin LL-35 (an antimicrobial peptide) in neutrophils, monocytes, salivary glands, and gingival tissue during viral infections, such as herpes simplex-1, HIV-1, and influenza.[151]

Nonoral and environmental conditions can also result in changes in salivary composition and flow rate. A generalized phenomenon of diabetic patients is elevated levels of salivary and serum immunoglobulins in which salivary IgA levels are influenced by glycemic control.[8] These elevated levels of IgA are maintained in diabetic patients with moderate periodontitis but begin to display a decrease in IgA secretions similar to nondiabetic patients when diagnosed with more aggressive forms of periodontitis.[96] In a longitudinal cohort study of seropositive-HIV women there was a significantly increased risk of HIV-1 shedding in saliva with decreased CD4 cell count, generalized gingival bleeding sites, and incidence of diabetes.[205] A history of smoking in patients with periodontitis also affects salivary composition as total protein and mineral concentrations are consistently reduced.[367] Although the salivary changes that smoking or diabetes mellitus imposes may not directly reactivate viral strains, studies have demonstrated that patients with diabetes mellitus type 2 have a higher prevalence of herpesvirus infections compared to a healthy cohort in Poland.[71] Smoking appears to have limited effects on viruses as it has been weakly associated with reactivating EBV in a cohort study in China that surveyed nasopharyngeal cancer risk.[123]

Deciphering the compositional complexity of saliva remains a worthwhile endeavor with studies indicating that salivary constituents may be effective indicators of both local and systemic disorders.[32] In the context of periodontitis, reliable salivary biomarkers to determine the severity of disease and proper treatment are still being investigated but remain focused on antibacterial effects.[90] The role of saliva in viral transmission and infectivity can only be fully described when all salivary components are characterized with susceptibility-enhancing or antiviral properties.

CLINICAL CORRELATION

It is prudent to note any changes in salivary flow rate or consistency and screen patients for any undiagnosed medical conditions. Patients can also be routinely screened for these medical conditions as more accurate salivary diagnostic biomarkers are identified. Periodontal patients with unmanaged immunocompromising conditions present an altered oral environment with factors that promote reactivation or induce lytic replication of viruses within the oral cavity. Thus, successful management of systemic conditions affecting baseline salivary measurements can regulate viral load and transmission of viruses that cause oral conditions or are associated with the progression of periodontitis.

Viruses

Eukaryotic Viruses

In the absence of viruses, all life would have a restricted evolutionary potential and weakened biological fitness. Since the beginning of human evolution, viruses have developed a complex relationship with the human holobiont. Evidence of extinct retroviruses survives within 8% of the human genome due to ancient germline infections that provide RNAs and proteins potentially able to trans-regulate human genes and influence the host immunity.[100] Human viruses are able to maintain a long-standing relationship with humans as many enter a latent phase, such as HIV, which has an average asymptomatic period

TABLE 27.2 Papillomavirus

Virus	Characteristics	Disease Association	Oral Pathos
Papillomavirus (types 6, 11, 16, 18, 31, 36, and 42)	Epithelial cell proliferation with specificity principally in the anogenital area, the urethra, the skin, the larynx, tracheobronchial region, and the oral mucosa	Genital and cutaneous warts, cervical and anogenital cancers, condylomata acuminate (sexually transmitted disease), and recurrent respiratory papillomatosis	Unspecified oral ulcers Recurrent oral aphthous stomatitis Focal epithelial hyperplasia Oral squamous cell carcinoma/verrucous carcinoma Oral leukoplakia Oral lichen planus

of 8 to 10 years in which time its carrier may transmit the virus to any number of contacts. Despite enhancing our immunity and being silent passengers, the mention of viruses connotes morbidity and mortality as eukaryotic viruses have the potential to promote cellular degradation, dysregulation, and carcinogenesis.

Characterization of the oral virome becomes essential as the oral cavity is the direct gateway to not only the gastrointestinal or respiratory tract but it also provides access to the circulatory system. Arguably, the oral cavity and gut contain the most functionally active microbiomes that affect human health. Although linked anatomically, the oral cavity and gut possess distinct microbial signatures that perform divergent functions.[277] However, alterations in the oral microbiome by periodontal treatment or oral administration of periodontopathogens have been linked to downstream gut microbiome changes.[14] The connection between the oral virome and systemic diseases still needs further exploration but viruses within the herpesvirus, human papillomavirus, and retrovirus family are ulcerogenic and tumorigenic agents in the human mouth. The presence and influence of these viruses within periodontal lesions suggest that viruses play a role in the development and progression of periodontitis.

Papillomaviruses

Human papillomaviruses (HPVs) are a family of small, non-enveloped, double-stranded DNA viruses with cutaneous and mucosal tropism, causing the most common sexually transmitted disease (Table 27.2). At present, over 150 HPV types have been identified and only a small number of high-risk HPV types are commonly associated with the development of cancer. Types 16 and HPV 18 together account for 70% of invasive cervical cancers while HPV 16 is strongly associated with oropharyngeal squamous cell carcinoma (OPSCC).[109,139] However, most HPV infections are transient with no clinical symptoms although a minority of infections result in clinical disease, such as warts or malignancies. Initial studies recognized sexual behavior, HIV-related immunosuppression, age, and smoking as predominant risk factors for oral HPV infection.[157] Regardless of behavior, detection rates of any type of HPV within normal oral mucosa average to 4.5%.[158] Oral HPV infection can result in different clinical presentations, including benign, papillomatous, hyperplastic, verrucous, and carcinomatous lesions.

Management of HPV-induced oral lesions typically involves surgical removal of the lesion by scalpel, laser ablations, electrocautery, or cryotherapy. HPV-driven oral lesions such as squamous papilloma, verruca vulgaris, and focal epithelial hyperplasia have low recurrence rates. Other lesions particularly HPV-associated oral epithelial dysplasia and oral warts associated with HIV are refractory with multiple therapy attempts. Immunosuppressed status increases vulnerability to HPV-related disease and within these lesions, multiple HPV types are detected compared to a single infection type pattern seen in healthy patients.[336] For recurrent lesions, surgical excision followed by interferon and antiviral cidofovir therapy are indicated.[12]

HPV has been isolated from inflamed periodontal tissues as HPV persists within the basal layer of stratified epithelium, which is found in ulcerated gingival sulcular epithelium. Indicators of micro-abrasions associated with oral inflammation, such as high interproximal plaque index and gingival bleeding index are significantly correlated with the detection of oral HPV of any type.[58] An association between HPV and periodontitis is biologically plausible due to the synergistic effects of extensive exposure of damaged crevicular epithelium and the ecological proximity to periodontopathogens.[292] A positive relationship between oral HPV infection and periodontitis with a low degree of evidence was calculated as studies have conflicting results.[5] Analysis from oral rinse samples collected from Hispanic adults (n = 740) demonstrated that PD greater than 6 are higher predictors of oral HPV infection along with the diagnosis of severe periodontitis.[219] Meanwhile a larger study of US adults (n = 6004) with similar detection methodology was unable to determine any association between oral HPV infection and periodontitis.[348] Based on these findings, the oral mucosa may represent an infection reservoir for HPV; however, the primary involvement of HPV in the progression of periodontitis should be excluded at this time.

Herpesviruses

Over 150 herpesviruses have been identified, all consisting of large, double-stranded linear DNA viruses surrounded by an icosahedral capsid, tegument, and lipid envelope studded with viral glycoproteins. Only eight human herpesviruses with distinct biologic and clinical characteristics have been described: HSV-1, HSV-2, varicella-zoster virus, EBV, hCMV, human herpesvirus-6, human herpesvirus-7, and human herpesvirus-8 (Table 27.3). Without exception, herpesviruses establish a lifelong infection and are divided into three subfamilies (α, β, and γ) according to biological properties and particularly the cell types in which they establish latency.

Herpesviruses are typically spread by close contact between infectious and susceptible hosts as they are fragile viruses that cannot survive independently for much time in the external environment. Human herpesviruses can spread in a variety of ways: transmitted directly from mother to child in breast milk (CMV) and spread among family members and close contact via saliva (HSV-1, CMV, EBV, HHV-6, -7, and -8). Of these viruses, HHV-6 and -7 are the most successful, infecting almost everyone worldwide. The prevalence of asymptomatic infections of EBV, CMV, and HSV-1 lies between 50% and 90% of the population, whereas the prevalence of herpesvirus-associated malignancies continues to rise.[148]

Latency and active replication have been demonstrated to occur within various microenvironments of the oral cavity and the different cell types that comprise the periodontium. This state of dormancy can be disturbed by a number of environmental stresses that lead to the reactivation of viral replication, cellular lysis, viral transmission, and eventually clinical symptoms. In the oral cavity, an infection with herpesviruses can present itself as a primary herpetic stomatitis, herpes labialis (cold sores), chickenpox (varicella), or shingles (zoster). Herpesvirus active infections can remain asymptomatic but still give rise to viral shedding, or they can cause illness

TABLE 27.3 Herpesvirus

Virus	Characteristics	Disease Association	Oral Pathos
Herpes simplex virus-1	Latency in sensory ganglia Causes orolabial disease	Herpetic gingivostomatitis Recurrent orolabial lesions Herpetic whitlow Keratoconjunctivitis Eczema herpeticum Pharyngitis Mononucleosis-like syndrome Encephalitis Neonatal infection	Adult herpetic gingivostomatitis HIV-/AIDS-related oral ulcers Recurrent oral aphthous stomatitis Behçet syndrome Oral pemphigus vulgaris Erythema multiforme Dry socket after tooth extraction
Herpes simplex virus-2	Latency in sensory ganglia Causes genital and newborn infections	Genital infection Aseptic meningitis Sacral autonomic nervous system dysfunction	—
Varicella-Zoster virus	Latency in sensory ganglia Only three major genotypes of the wild-type virus are known More than 90% are infected before adolescence in an unvaccinated population	Varicella (chickenpox) Herpes zoster (shingles) Central nervous system involvement pneumonia Secondary bacterial infections Death Available varicella vaccines include a single-antigen vaccine and a combination vaccine against measles-mumps-rubella-varicella	Recurrent oral aphthous stomatitis Osteomyelitis herpes zoster (Ramsay Hunt Syndrome)
Epstein-Barr virus	Identified initially in 1964 from African Burkitt lymphoma Infects epithelial cells with a cytolytic infection and B lymphocytes with a latent infection	Infectious mononucleosis Hairy leukoplakia of the tongue Burkitt lymphoma B lymphoproliferative disease Hodgkin lymphoma X-linked lymphoproliferative disease Nasal T-cell lymphoma Nasopharyngeal carcinoma Gastric carcinoma Parotid carcinoma Leiomyosarcoma	Recurrent oral aphthous stomatitis Erythema multiforme Various epithelial type tumors, such as lymphoepithelioma-like carcinoma, salivary gland lymphoepithelial carcinoma, Warthin tumor (cystadenolymphoma) of the parotid gland, oral squamous cell carcinoma, tonsillar carcinoma, oral undifferentiated carcinomas, and oral hairy leukoplakia Various lymphoid type tumors, such as Hodgkin lymphoma, T-cell/natural killer cell lymphoma, Burkitt lymphoma, cyclosporine-related posttransplant lymphoproliferative disorder, oral post-transplant lymphoproliferative disorder/B-cell lymphoma, follicular lymphoid hyperplasia, and plasmablastic lymphoma Infectious mononucleosis
Human cytomegalovirus	Infects mainly T lymphocytes and macrophages The gB protein in the virion envelope participates in the virus-cell interaction and is a major target of the immune response	Preterm birth Preeclampsia Transplant rejection Immunosenescence Hemorrhagic retinal necrosis (patients with HIV) Encephalitis Infectious mononucleosis Atherosclerosis Gastrointestinal disease Pneumonia	HIV-/AIDS-related oral ulcers Recurrent oral aphthous stomatitis Behçet syndrome Oral pemphigus vulgaris Erythema multiforme Cyclosporine-steroid associated lymphoproliferative disorder Benign infantile hemangioendothelioma Kaposi sarcoma Occasionally infectious mononucleosis Sialadenitis Osteomyelitis
Human herpesvirus-6	Cell tropism for T lymphocytes and the neural cells Frequently shed in the saliva of healthy donors	Roseola infantum (sixth disease) Meningitis Encephalitis Possibly multiple sclerosis	Uvulopalatoglossal junctional ulcers Oral squamous cell carcinoma Oral leukoplakia Oral lichen planus
Human herpesvirus-7	Latency in macrophages and T lymphocytes Frequently shed in the saliva of healthy donors	Exanthema subitem Macular–papular rashes Transplant–recipient pathogens	—
Human herpesvirus-8	Six genetic subtypes with marked clustering to geographic area B lymphocytes and monocytes serve as reservoirs	Kaposi sarcoma Multicentric Castleman disease Primary effusion lymphoma Mononucleosis-like illness Aplastic anemia (Unlike Epstein-Barr virus, herpesvirus-8 is not involved in epithelial tumors)	Recurrent oral aphthous stomatitis Kaposi sarcoma

AIDS, Acquired immunodeficiency syndrome; *HIV*, human immunodeficiency virus.

that ranges from classic infectious diseases to benign and malignant tumors, especially in immunocompromised hosts (e.g., patients with acquired immunodeficiency syndrome [AIDS], organ transplant recipients).

During lytic and latent viral life cycles, herpesviruses express proteins that modulate innate and adaptive immune systems and alter the cellular environment. Direct CPEs on fibroblasts, keratinocytes, endothelial cells, inflammatory cells, and osteocytes occur during active herpesvirus infections. Lytic proteins have been shown to increase proinflammatory cytokine expression to promote osteoclastogenesis which is seen in periapical bone lesions.[261] Overlap of cytokines and chemokines that are actively involved in periodontal lesions are associated with herpesvirus infections. Co-infection with bacterial periodontopathogens within periodontal lesions may facilitate the initiation or progression of periodontitis. In addition, the resolution of periodontitis may be hampered by herpesviruses as they infect fibroblasts that affect tissue turnover and repair.[177]

Epstein-Barr Virus

EBV is classified into the γ-herpesviruses subfamily due to its very restrictive host range. Along with HHV-8, γ-herpesviruses are oncogenic viruses associated with Burkitt and Hodgkin lymphoma. Persistent infection and latency of EBV occur in epithelial cells of the oropharynx and in B-cells. It is estimated that more than 90% of adult humans present with a latent infection of EBV and are subject to EBV reactivation causing classic mononucleosis and several life-threatening diseases.[138,217] The mechanisms which promote and regulate the reactivation of EBV are still being uncovered and are critical for potential prophylactic treatment.

Close contact behaviors like kissing or sharing personal objects such as eating utensils, toothbrushes, food and drinks with an infected individual can lead to the spread of EBV. Transmission of the virus through saliva indicates a productive infection within the oropharynx directly from desquamated epithelial cells or B-cells. The rate of shedding of EBV is influenced by the propensity of a single B-cell to infect epithelial cells, which have been estimated to be 1 to 5 cells.[107] Additionally, the levels of EBV detected within salivary samples are variable within individuals with no distinction between low, intermediate, and high shedding rates between individuals. A complex of three glycoproteins (gpH/gpL/gp42) mediates the transition between cell tropism and lymphatic circulation or epithelial latency in asymptomatic carriers.[23] Lymphoproliferative disorders or immunosuppressive conditions can reactivate the virus and result in salivary samples that contain elevated levels of viral load in symptomatic individuals that are infectious.[263]

EBV generally infects silently during childhood but may manifest as infectious mononucleosis in adolescents or young adults.[267] Infection and latency of EBV in B-cells results in an exaggerated $CD8^+$ T-cell response leading to the acute syndrome characterized by a tetrad of symptoms: fever, fatigue, sore throat, and lymphadenopathy. Although periodontal cells are susceptible to EBV, it is mature B cells that are required for primary infection as seen in agammaglobulinemia patients.[80] In 1985, EBV replication was observed in oral hairy leukoplakia, which first suggested viral replication within oral epithelial cells. Unlike receptor-mediated infection of B cells, cell-to-cell infection from EBV-coated B-cells is the main pathway for epithelial cell infection.[283] Circulating B cells can shuttle EBV to the epithelial lining of the periodontium and approximate the virus to putative periodontopathogens.

Manifestations of epithelial malignancies indicate that epithelial cells play a role in the persistence and infection of EBV, albeit to a lesser degree than B cells. Upon epithelial cell infection, EBV is amplified for cell-to-cell spread with viral replication occurring in the upper differentiated layers. EBV is frequently isolated in a latent episomal state from nasopharyngeal epithelial cells, and in a lytic state within oral hairy leukoplakia plaques.[101] Oral hairy leukoplakia is caused by the Epstein–Barr virus, and it is the only Epstein–Barr virus lesion with which viral shedding in saliva is common.[212] Oral hairy leukoplakia primarily occurs in persons with HIV infection.[101] It is found on the lateral borders of the tongue, it frequently has a bilateral distribution, and it may extend to the ventrum. The lesion is characterized by an asymptomatic, poorly demarcated, keratotic area that ranges in size from a few millimeters to several centimeters (Fig. 27.5). Often, characteristic vertical striations are present, and these impart a corrugated appearance; the surface may also be shaggy and appear hairy when dried. The lesion does not rub off, and it may resemble other keratotic oral lesions.

Detection of Epstein–Barr virus within epithelial cells that are in healthy conditions is rare. However, epithelial cells within the periodontium are challenging the tenet that latency of EBV occurs mainly in lymphoid tissue, such as Waldeyer ring. Periodontal epithelium, specifically the junctional epithelium, is commonly infected with EBV where one in vivo study found 13.2% of healthy and 30% of inflamed epithelium expressing elevated latent transcripts (i.e., EBNA1, EBNA2, LMP2, and LMP1) and low levels of lytic transactivator BZFL-1.[334] The close proximity and a shared integrin profile to B-cells within adjacent connective tissue may enhance the permissibility of junctional epithelium to EBV infection. Thus, an oral reservoir of latent EBV can exist in the periodontal epithelium with the potential to shed infectious viral particles as the lytic transactivator is expressed but at low levels.

Along with the presence in the periodontal epithelium, oral fluid samples further implicate EBV in the development or progression of periodontitis. Viral load within salivary samples may reflect the status of periodontal inflammation as there is a significant elevated difference of EBV in patients with periodontitis compared

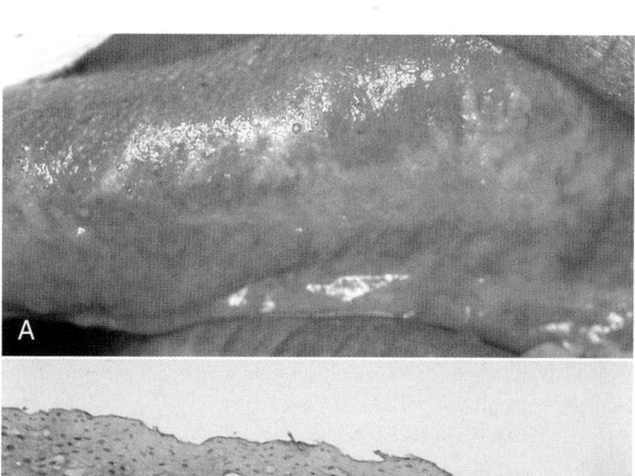

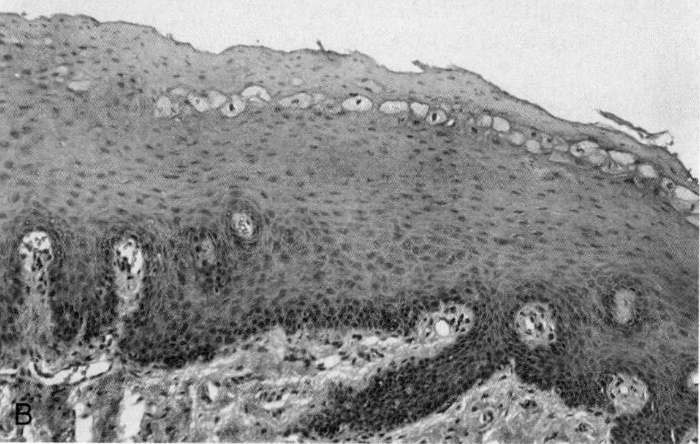

Fig. 27.5 Oral hairy leukoplakia on the left lateral border of the tongue. (A) Clinical view. (B) Biopsy confirmation of oral hairy leukoplakia. Note the ballooned epithelial cells near the surface of the epithelium.

to healthy patients.[129,150,271] A similar association of EBV levels in gingival crevicular fluid to the severity of periodontitis has been documented.[154,282] However, an established association using these samples has not been achieved as several studies report a lack of association between EBV and periodontitis.[221,225,313]

During sampling of ulcerated gingival tissue and subgingival plaque, EBV in both latent and lytic forms is present. Subgingival plaque from deepened pockets (≥5 mm) in Japanese patients with CP had higher detection rates of EBV (66%) than shallow pockets (48%) and healthy pockets (45%).[145] Within the same cohort, 44% of measured deep pockets were coinfected with EBV and *P. gingivalis*, while shallow and healthy pockets had a significantly lowered coinfection rate of 14% and 13%, respectively. The increase in periodontal pocket depths reflects the degradation of the periodontal connective tissue from dysregulated release of collagenases and host immune response. In these advanced stages of periodontitis, dual infection of EBV and CMV is found more frequently within deep periodontal pockets and associated with bacterial periodontopathogens.[272] HIV-infected patients that present with advanced periodontitis and necrotic gingiva are coinfected with EBV in 57% of periodontitis lesions.[50]

The high prevalence of EBV seen in ulcerated periodontal pockets demonstrates the potential contributions that the virus has on the multifactorial pathogenesis of periodontitis. Disruption of the innate immune response to bacterial challenges occurs during coinfection with herpesviruses. Architectural and functional changes occur within key periodontal inflammatory cells as herpesvirus-like viral bodies are identified within these cells in juvenile periodontitis lesions.[33] The immune landscape a herpesvirus produces favors the survival of pathogenic bacteria as TNF-α receptor synthesis and phagocytic activity is downregulated even in the presence of lipopolysaccharides.[97,268] A failure to recruit natural killer cells and CD4$^+$ T-cells results from an EBV encoded viral microRNA that targets fibroblast production of the chemokine CXCL-11.[353] Regulation of these antiviral cytokines and innate inflammatory cells aids in achieving latency and is dependent on virus-encoded latency proteins and promoters.

Viruses can further destabilize the immune response by secreting cytokine homologs, or "virokines," to mimic the immunosuppressive action of host proteins. During its lytic phase, Epstein Barr-virus codes for an IL-10 homolog that can downregulate MHC class II surface proteins by inhibiting IFN-γ expression, which is required to induce CD4$^+$ T-cell activation.[61]

Neutrophils, the predominant inflammatory cell in periodontitis, are also affected by virus-encoded IL-10 as it inhibits TLR-induced ROS production. A combination of virus-encoded IL-10 and viral DNase activity degrade neutrophil extracellular traps allowing the escape of periodontopathogens to stimulate a hyper-response in the trapped neutrophils within local tissues.[62]

Interactions between EBV and *P. gingivalis* can accelerate the destructive nature of periodontitis as synergistic modulation of the local immune response within periodontal pockets occurs.[147,269,302] Gram-negative LPS and lytic transactivator Zta are potent inducers of IL-8 that promote local neutrophil infiltration and proinflammatory cytokine production.[126,145] Periodontal epithelial cells that line deep periodontal pockets express elevated levels of chemokine CCL20 in monoinfections of EBV or *P. gingivalis*.[334] However, in dual infected pockets the monocyte chemoattractant levels were consistently higher than epithelial cells infected with just one pathogen. *P. gingivalis* can stimulate the production of visfatin in periodontal ligament cells and fibroblasts to promote B-cell maturation, IL-1β, TNF-α, and IL-6 secretion.[59] A significant increase in visfatin within GCF is associated with *P. gingivalis* in CP patients and elevated EBV levels regardless of periodontal status.[222]

In addition to the synergistic effects seen in co-infected periodontal pocket sites, periodontopathogens may interact with EBV to cause the reactivation of these viruses within the periodontium. Determination of which life cycle stage EBV undergoes during detection is made by measuring the expression of latency transcripts (EBNA1, BNA 2, LMP1, and LMP2), transactivator BZLF-1 and lytic transcripts. A potent lytic inducer of EBV via the activation of BZLF-1 is the short-chain fatty acid, butyric acid which is seen in high concentrations within the gingival crevicular fluid of periodontally inflamed pockets.[211] The high concentration of butyric acid may be attributed to its fermentation from periodontopathogens, such as *P. gingivalis* and *F. nucleatum*.[175] The close association between EBV and these butyric acid-producing periodontopathogens, suggests that tissues of the periodontium and the microbiome associated with it provide EBV with an environment that facilitates its replication and latency (Fig. 27.6). Regulation of EBV's life cycle within the periodontium, thus becomes critical not only for the progression of periodontitis but for other EBV-related malignancies (eBox 27.2).

Cytomegalovirus

Cytomegalovirus is classified into the β-herpesviruses subfamily due to its long replicative cycle and restricted host range. Cytomegalovirus is transmitted via close interpersonal contact with body fluids, including blood, semen, breast milk, urine, and saliva. The ubiquity of cytomegalovirus infection is reflected in an 80% worldwide seroprevalence in immunocompetent adults that increases with age.[311,368] Primary infection, re-infection, or reactivation of cytomegalovirus typically manifests as asymptomatic in immunocompetent hosts. However, with an immature or compromised immune system, such as in neonates, transplant recipients, or HIV-infected individuals the true pathogenic potential of cytomegalovirus may be realized.

Transmission of cytomegalovirus from mother to fetus can occur anytime during gestation. Primary maternal cytomegalovirus infections account for 35% of congenital cytomegalovirus infections and are the most likely to cause significant harm to a fetus.[45] Cytomegalovirus disrupts organ and tissue development, most frequently that of the central nervous system. Only a small cohort of neonates have apparent clinical manifestations of congenital cytomegalovirus. Depending on the trimester cytomegalovirus is contracted, congenital cytomegalovirus can cause permanent physical sequelae, such as hearing loss, visual impairment, mental retardation, and increased infant mortality.[204]

Outside the central nervous system, branchial arch derivatives are vulnerable to cytomegalovirus infection during critical stages of their organogenesis. Dental anomalies resembling an amelogenesis phenotype in primary dentition were documented to manifest in 40% of children who suffered from a more severe form of congenital cytomegalovirus infection.[312] The presentation of cytomegalovirus-mediated effect on the development and maturation of enamel can extend to anomalies of permanent incisors or first molars in infants that remain ill in the first six months of life. Diligent preventative dental care should be recommended for patients with congenital cytomegalovirus infections due to the increased risk of caries and the need for orthodontic treatment due to potential developmental delays. The ability to infect tissues surrounding a tooth germ and alter tooth morphology has led to a theory that cytomegalovirus holds the potential to increase the susceptibility to the development of periodontitis.[132,303]

Considerable morbidity and mortality are associated with the reactivation of cytomegalovirus in older adults and in HIV-infected individuals. Nearly all HIV-infected individuals present with cytomegalovirus antibodies and the proportion of

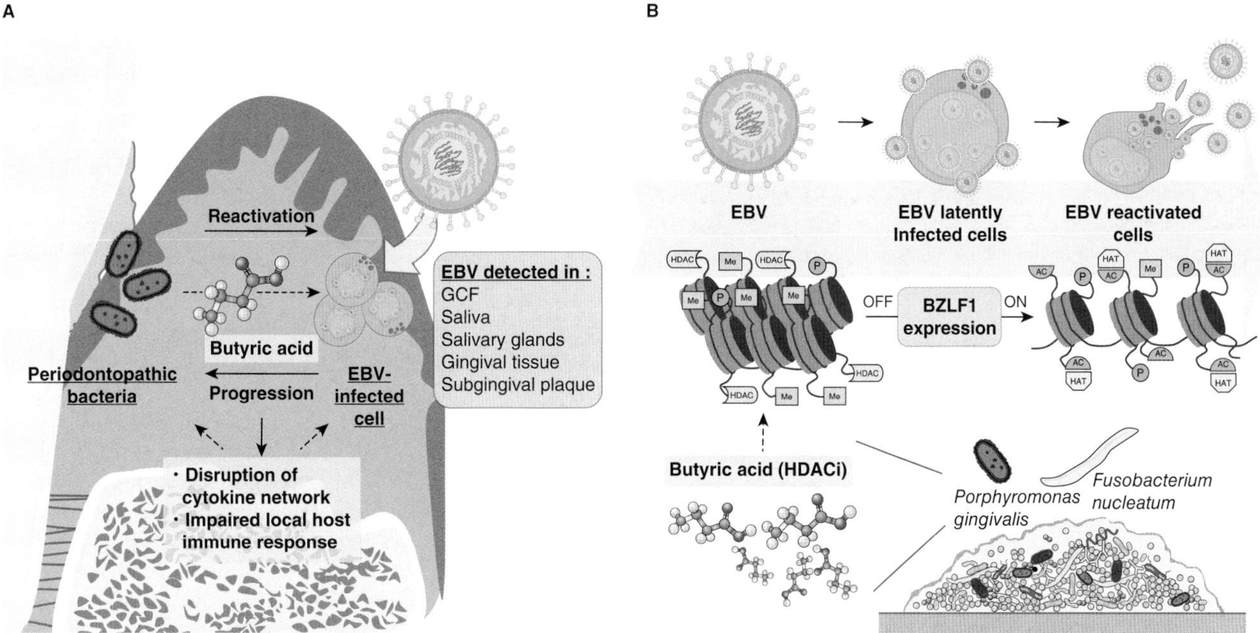

Fig. 27.6 Role of Epstein-Barr virus *(EBV)* in the progression of periodontal disease. (A) Environmental proximity of periodontal pathogens and EBV within the periodontium. (B) Epigenetic modulation of EBV via butyric acid leading to lytic EBV. (Copyright © 2022. Ryutaro Kuraji.)

cytomegalovirus-specific CD8 T-cells exceeds that of HIV-specific T-cells.[163] Cardiovascular pathologies in HIV-infected individuals are associated with cytomegalovirus infections and include CMV-retinitis and carotid artery stiffness.[127] These manifestations are correlated with the $CD4^+$ T-cell levels that fall below 50 to 100/μL and decrease in frequency with antiviral and protease inhibitor therapies of HIV.

Persistent cytomegalovirus replication occurs in oral structures, such as the salivary glands and oral manifestations may present. Approximately 30% of HIV-infected individuals with an asymptomatic infection shed cytomegalovirus through salivary secretions compared to only 1% to 2% of immunocompetent individuals.[176] Oral manifestations of cytomegalovirus infections are a rare occurrence but are characterized as painful necrotic oral mucosal ulcerations with a punched-out appearance, and nonindurated borders that affect the lips, gingiva, tongue, or buccal mucosa.[141] Herpesviruses are often found in various oral and labial ulcers in HIV-infected individuals as up to 53% of the ulcerogenic viral agents identified were of cytomegalovirus alone compared to 19% of the herpes-simplex virus.[86] Evaluation for CMV-retinitis or disseminated cytomegalovirus in HIV-infected individuals is recommended when such oral lesions develop as they may be the initial manifestation of AIDS.

Like other herpesviruses, cytomegalovirus can establish itself as a life-long infection in an exposed host. The tissue tropism of cytomegalovirus within humans is extensive as it can reside within epithelial cells, fibroblasts, endothelial cells, smooth muscle cells, and monocytes.[301] Systemic clinical manifestations of cytomegalovirus can be corroborated with salivary viral load levels.[344] Additionally, detection in saliva, gingival crevicular fluid, and subgingival plaque demonstrate an association of cytomegalovirus with periodontal inflammation status.[21,51,160] In a meta-analysis of 26 studies of periodontal patients, a statistically significant increased odds for periodontitis (OR 5.31; 95% CI 3.15 to 8.97) with the detection of subgingival cytomegalovirus was reported.[25] Given its ubiquitous nature, there have been reports that fail to measure a significant association between oral cytomegalovirus levels and systemic or periodontal disease. There are instances where elevated levels of cytomegalovirus are seen in periodontally healthy sites compared to periodontally diseased sites.[209]

Isolation of cytomegalovirus within advanced or necrotic periodontal lesions is often accompanied by gram-negative periodontopathogens.[67,270,286] In the subgingival plaque of Sudanese adolescents detection of putative periodontopathogens (*Aggregatibacter actinomycetemcomitans, P. gingivalis, T. forsythia,* and *T. denticola*) and two herpesviruses (EBV and cytomegalovirus) were documented in all healthy and diseased states at various levels.[75] A significant association was noted for *A. actinomycetemcomitans, P. gingivalis* and cytomegalovirus, and aggressive periodontitis; however, the strongest dual infection association belonged to *A. actinomycetemcomitans* and cytomegalovirus (OR 39.1; 95% CI 2.0, 754.6). Subgingival plaque from Jamaican adolescents presented with similar strong associations for aggressive periodontitis (OR 51.4; 95% CI 5.4,486.5) and attachment loss (OR 3.9; 95% CI 1.3, 12.0) in a dual infection with *P. gingivalis* and cytomegalovirus.[187] Thus, dual infection with cytomegalovirus may allude to additive or synergistic effects of herpesviruses in aggressive periodontitis-diseased sites.

Gingival and periodontal diseases associated with HIV-infected individuals can present with elevated levels of cytomegalovirus. Individuals who present with acute necrotizing ulcerative gingivitis (ANUG) possess a combination of predisposing factors that include HIV infection, malnutrition, smoking, or psychophysical stress. The role of herpesviruses in ANUG has been analyzed in Nigerian children 3 to 14 years of age who present with malnutrition and past history of viral infection. In these children, cytomegalovirus appeared in 59% of lesions followed by EBV in 27% of lesions.[52] ANUG in the developed world is more commonly seen in young adults and HIV-infected individuals suggesting that cytomegalovirus and possibly other herpesviruses contribute to the development of ANUG in malnourished individuals. Likewise, herpesviruses are more commonly detected in HIV-periodontitis lesions than in periodontitis lesions of non-HIV individuals. Again, cytomegalovirus was the most common herpesvirus detected in HIV-associated periodontitis lesions (81%) and non-HIV periodontitis lesions (50%).[53] Other HIV-infection-related conditions that present with cytomegalovirus co-infection are acute periodontitis and osteomyelitis.[19,67] Treatment of these lesions requires debridement, local antimicrobial therapy, immediate follow-up care, and long-term maintenance.

CLINICAL CORRELATION

Proper management of oral manifestations and periodontal lesions associated with cytomegalovirus is crucial for the immunocompromised patient, especially those that are HIV-infected. Reactivated cytomegalovirus infections may be the first clinical manifestation of a progressing immunocompromised state and perhaps the first evidence of AIDS.

Ganciclovir administered intravenously is the treatment of choice for oral ulcerations associated with cytomegalovirus which typically resolve in 14 days.[163] Cytomegalovirus reactivation associated with HIV-infected individuals may require a longer duration and increased dosage of intravenous ganciclovir. Ganciclovir-resistant cytomegalovirus strains may develop and foscarnet can be an alternative treatment provided for patients.[114]

Of the established risk factors of periodontitis, interactions between bacterial periodontopathogens are plausible for cytomegalovirus to influence this inflammatory state; however, a molecular mechanism has not been described. Aiding in bacterial colonization has been noted in other viral co-infections by altering host cell-surface receptors and promoting bacterial internalization with viral agglutination.[11,218] Specific to cytomegalovirus, enterococcal adherence to renal epithelial cells in renal transplant patients increased as the viral infection promoted expression of a plasmid-encoded surface protein that enhanced the enterococcal binding substance.[133]

Modulation of the immune host response by cytomegalovirus may influence *A. actinomycetemcomitans* and *P. gingivalis* in ulcerated periodontal pockets. All of these pathogens invade and disrupt epithelial cells and potentially benefit from chemotaxis upregulation and inhibition of apoptosis in neutrophils modulated by cytomegalovirus.[102,245] Upregulation of interleukin-1β and tumor necrosis factor-α by cytomegalovirus-infected macrophages may lead to increased metalloproteinases within the periodontal pocket.[24] Immune evasion mechanisms employed by cytomegalovirus may favor local immunosuppression that can help bacterial growth in periodontal lesions.

Severe Acute Respiratory Syndrome Coronavirus

An outbreak of a viral respiratory illness originating from Wuhan, China, in late 2019 had its causative agent identified as a novel species from the genus betacoronavirus. Novel Severe Acute Respiratory Syndrome Coronavirus-2 (SARS-CoV-2) is the third documented case of zoonotic coronavirus in the early twenty-first century along with SARS-CoV-1 and Middle Eastern Respiratory Syndrome Coronavirus (MERS-CoV). In March 2020, the crisis was declared a pandemic as the RNA virus is responsible for more than 250 million cases worldwide that can result in diffuse alveolar damage, thromboembolism, and nonspecific shock injury in multiple organs.[35]

The primary receptor for SARS-CoV-2 cell entry are angiotensin-converting enzyme 2 (ACE2) receptors that are highly expressed in respiratory tract cells and various oral epithelial tissues such as the tongue, minor salivary ducts, and gingiva (Fig. 27.7).[125,167,264] Numerous studies have reported oral manifestations in patients with coronavirus disease 2019 (COVID-19) which include taste disorders, mucosal lesions, xerostomia, or sialadenitis that may result directly from SARS-CoV-2 infection or represent secondary signs of infection (Table 27.4).[36,46,47,309] Discrepancies of clinical manifestations of COVID-19 patients seem to be mediated by differential immune response rather than viral load.[89] This realization led to proposals that inflammatory conditions, such as the periodontal status of COVID-19 patients, are risk factors for the progression of SARS-CoV-2 infection severity.[118,265]

SARS CoV-2 Transmission

Attempts to decelerate the momentum of the COVID-19 pandemic focused on limiting transmission that occurs mainly by exposure to infected aerosolized particles, droplet inhalation, and contact with infected individuals.[246] Transmission by close contact is defined as being within 1 m of a known SARS-CoV-2 infected individual for over 15 minutes over a 24-hour period. The incubation period

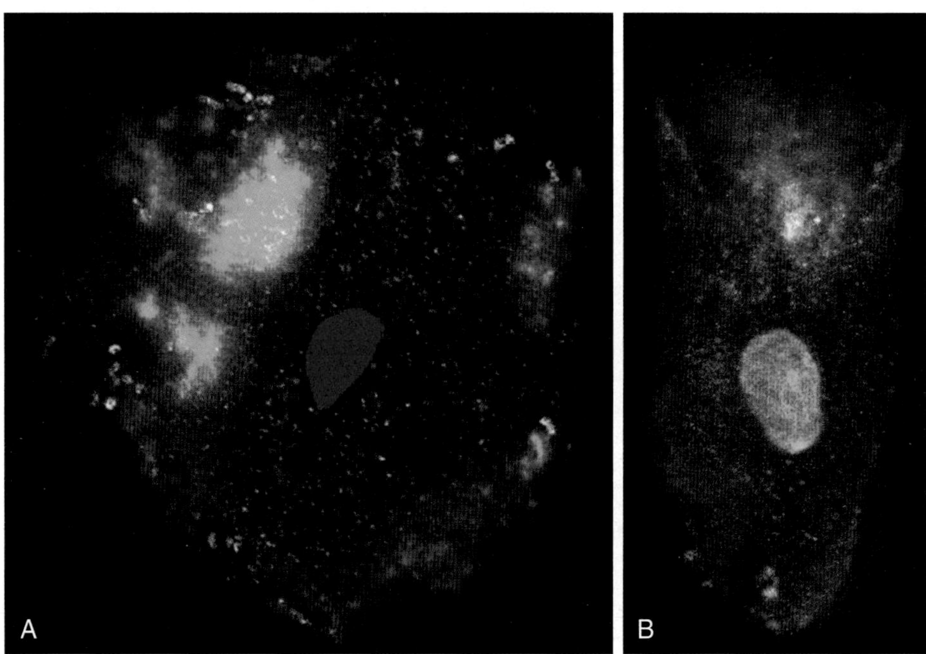

Fig. 27.7 3D confocal microscopic images of ACE-2 *(gray)* expressing salivary cells infected by SARS-CoV-2 that demonstrate detectable SARs-CoV-2 spike *(red)* expression in pan-cytokeratin positive (pCK; *green*) cells. *SARS-CoV-2,* Severe acute respiratory syndrome coronavirus-2. A and B depict two salivary cells collected from mildly symptomatic individuals who were positive for SARS-CoV-2 and were analyzed for entry factor expression. (Courtesy Kevin Byrd, Yu Mikami, and Ricard Boucher.)

TABLE 27.4 SARS CoV-2

Virus	Characteristics	Disease Association	Oral Pathos
SARS CoV-2	Cell entry utilizing broadly expressed ACE2 receptors Rapid replication in alveolar epithelial cells of respiratory tract More transmissible than SARS-CoV and MERS-CoV	Pneumonia Myocarditis Thromboembolism Disseminated intravascular coagulation Hemorrhagic colitis Hepatomegaly Acute kidney damage Encephalopathy Erythematous rashes Conjunctivitis	Dysgeusia Irregular ulcers Petechiae Candidiasis Erythema multiforme Dry mouth Sialadenitis Desquamative gingivitis

ACE2, Angiotensin-converting enzyme 2; *MERS-CoV,* Middle Eastern respiratory syndrome coronavirus; *SARS-CoV-2,* severe acute respiratory syndrome coronavirus-2.

for SARS-CoV-2 ranges from 2 to 14 days and transmission of the virus may occur during or after this period. A large proportion of transmission of SARS-CoV-2 appears to be through exposure to infected aerosols produced by presymptomatic and asymptomatic individuals during breathing or speaking.[31] Infected tissues of the oral cavity may play a role in presymptomatic and asymptomatic spread as sources of cellular and acellular SARS-CoV-2 are commonly isolated in saliva.[125]

The high percentage of asymptomatic carriers and unequivocal presence of SARS-CoV-2 in saliva evokes the risk of SARS-CoV-2 infection during dental clinical treatments that generate aerosols. Limitations on various dental instruments such as high- or low-speed handpieces, ultrasonic scalers, and air-water sprays had been recommended at the early-stages of the COVID-19 pandemic to diminish possible airborne transmission. Persistence of SARS-CoV-2 within the oral cavity has been identified as oral tissues are enriched with ACE2 receptors and pose a risk for prolonged virus shedding even after respiratory symptoms.[13,364] Despite the high viral loads in saliva, these viral particles may not be infectious as intraoral innate immune mechanisms such as oral epithelial cells produced β-defensins provide antiviral protection against other pathogenic coronaviruses like SARS-CoV-1 and MERS-CoV.[363]

KEY FACT

The World Health Organization (WHO) developed a set of recommendations for aerosol-generating procedures (AGPs) within dental settings. A fit-tested N95 or FFP2 respirator is recommended when AGPs are performed along with fluid-resistant gowns, gloves, and eye protection (goggles or face shield) as personal protective equipment for dental surgery. All other universal infection control guidelines should be maintained such as performing proper hand hygiene. Although reports have suggested the possibility of transmission of SARS-CoV-2 through AGPs during dental procedures, an accurate **risk assessment** is limited and transmissions from AGPs have not been frequently reported.[134]

Mouth-SARS-CoV-2 Connection

A high density of ACE2 receptors and a high frequency of oral symptoms associated with COVID-19 suggest a greater role of the oral cavity in the pathogenesis of SARS-CoV-2 infection. The palate, tongue, gingiva, and lips represent the most frequent locations for oral COVID-19 symptoms that were present in 25% of mild to moderate cases in a cohort of over 600 patients.[214] These oral lesions healed within 3 to 21 days, either spontaneously or through topical treatment and oral hygiene.[81] Studies that have documented the onset of these oral mucosal lesions associate mild COVID-19 cases to oral symptoms that develop before or at the same time as initial respiratory symptoms, whereas lesions developed 7 to 24 days after respiratory symptoms were associated with COVID-19 hospitalizations.[6] One hallmark prodromal symptom that is present in over half (54%) of patients presenting with mild to moderate SARS-CoV-2 infections as the sudden loss of taste (dysgeusia/ageusia) occurs prior to the onset of general COVID-19 symptoms.[266] Characterizing oral prodromal symptoms of COVID-19 can alert individuals and dental practitioners of a progressing infection for which treatment in a timely manner is crucial.

Biomarkers commonly associated with periodontitis are postulated to facilitate the entry of SARS-CoV-2 into the cells of the oral mucosa. ACE2 receptors are expressed by epithelial cells, fibroblasts, T-cells, and B-cells on the surface of the tongue, buccal mucosa, palate, and gingiva.[13,125] Elevated furin and cathepsin L proteases in the gingival crevicular fluid of periodontally inflamed tissues may amplify cleavage of spike glycoprotein of SARS-CoV-2 which mediates ACE2 receptor binding and endosomal fusion.[15] Overexpression of galectin-3, a carbohydrate-binding protein, by pulmonary and oral epithelial cells during periodontitis and COVID-19 leads to hyperinflammation and increased viral attachment to epithelial tissues.[146] Ultimately, these biomarkers signal gingival epithelium ulceration that occurs in periodontitis which further exposes the periodontium as a site of active SARS-CoV-2 infection and potentially a reservoir.[83]

Etiological agents and risk factors associated with COVID-19 indicate a potential relationship to periodontitis. The exact shared mechanisms between these two conditions are still sought after as COVID-19 patients with periodontitis are at a higher risk for complications (OR = 3.67; 95% CI 1.46 to 9.27) and ICU admission (OR = 3.54; 95% CI 1.39 to 9.05).[184] Respiratory symptoms are exacerbated as SARS-CoV-2 interacts with both the lung and oral microbiome that modulates cytokine and immune cell regulation. Aspiration of *P. gingivalis* and *F. nucleatum* have previously been implicated in the pathogenesis of respiratory illness and may stimulate ACE2 expression in the lungs during a SARS-CoV-2 infection due to cellular recognition of bacterial **adhesion** molecules and **endotoxins** (LPS).[161,318] Protein-protein interaction analysis revealed overexpression of 18 *Prevotella* species proteins that directly interact with host proteins that directly upregulate NF-κB which is correlated with the progression and viral survival of SARS-CoV-2 infection.[63,149]

Identifying and providing treatment for aspirated periodontopathogens may directly attenuate the severity of a SARS-CoV-2 infection. Likewise, inflamed periodontal states in COVID-19 patients would subside as symptoms of COVID-19 resolved.[81] However, a direct mechanism of action for periodontal manifestations (gingival pain, spontaneous bleeding, desquamative gingivitis, and necrotizing periodontal disease) that have been described since the advent of the COVID-19 pandemic is still left to be characterized. Potential mechanisms are plausible as many structures of the oral cavity (tongue, salivary glands, and gingival epithelium) are thought to be reservoirs of SARS-CoV-2.[13,125] Additionally, dysregulation in the functions of periodontal structures occurs during infection of SARS-CoV-2 which may further aggravate the bacterial dysbiosis that is essential in the development of periodontitis.[279]

The most apparent connection between COVID-19 and periodontitis is the hyperinflammatory response that may result in adverse outcomes. Chronic inflammatory conditions commonly associated with periodontitis such as diabetes, obesity, and cardiovascular disease also constitute high-risk factors for severe forms of COVID-19.[104] In these conditions, the low- to moderate-grade inflammation and bacterial dysbiosis can create an environment for heightened SARS-CoV-2 virulence. More specifically, the keystone cytokines (IL-6, IL-1β, IL-8, TNF-α, INF-γ) released by immune cells in periodontitis stimulated by periodontopathogens overlap with the cytokines involved in the cytokine storm described in severe forms of COVID-19 manifestations.[262] Although there is no established mechanism on how periodontitis directly affects systemic inflammation, these cytokines can enter the systemic circulation when transferred from the gingival crevicular fluid to saliva.

CLINICAL CORRELATION

An increased risk for secondary **pneumonia** can result from aspiration of oral bacterial pathogens that accumulate due to poor oral hygiene in hospital settings.[278] Frequent and thorough oral health care measures should be recommended by health care providers during the early period of hospitalization to protect COVID-19 patients from secondary infections and alleviate any respiratory symptoms present. Dental plaque management can be enforced using either mechanical or chemical controls to reduce the respiratory **pathogen** loads. Oral hygiene provided should include:

- Brushing teeth, gums, and tongue two times per day
- Moistening oral mucosa and lips every 2–4 hours
- Rinsing mouth with 0.5%–1.5% hydrogen peroxide, 2% chlorhexidine twice per day, 0.5%–1.5% povidone-iodine, or chlorine dioxide oral rinses

Human Immunodeficiency Virus

AIDS is characterized by profound impairment of the immune system (Table 27.5). The condition was first reported in 1981, and a viral pathogen, the *HIV*, was identified in 1984.[256] The condition was originally thought to be restricted to male homosexuals. Subsequently, it was also identified in male and female heterosexuals and bisexuals who participated in unprotected sexual activities or who abused injected drugs.[223] Currently, sexual activity and drug abuse remain the primary means of transmission.

HIV has a strong affinity for cells of the immune system, most specifically those that carry the CD4 cell surface receptor molecule. Thus helper T-cells (T4 cells) are most profoundly affected, but monocytes, macrophages, Langerhans cells, and some neuronal and glial brain cells may also be involved. Viral replication occurs continuously in the lymphoreticular tissues of the lymph nodes, the spleen, the gut-associated lymphoid cells, and the macrophages.[346,347]

Combined therapeutic regimens that consist of antiretroviral agents and protease-inhibiting drugs have resulted in marked improvement in the health status of HIV-infected individuals and occasionally a reduction in viral plasma loads to below detectable levels (i.e., <50 copies/mL), although the infection may still be transmissible.[87,362] Evidence indicates that the virus is never completely eradicated; rather, it is sequestered at low levels in resting CD4 cells, even in individuals with no detectable plasma viral RNA.[84] These findings suggest that effective combination drug therapy may be necessary for the lifetime of infected individuals. Long-term control of the infection may be difficult because the antiviral agents that are currently used have many adverse side effects and drug-resistant variant viral strains readily develop.[346] In addition, growing evidence suggests that oral pathogenic microorganisms (including putative periodontal pathogens) may help to induce HIV recrudescence by reactivating latently infected dendritic cells, macrophages, or **T cells**.[122]

The number of individuals living with AIDS in the United States has greatly increased as a result of the development of multidrug HAART, which combines various types of antiretroviral drugs, protease inhibitors, and fusion inhibitors.[135] The median period between initial HIV infection and outright AIDS is approximately 15 years, and the life expectancy of persons living with AIDS has been significantly

TABLE 27.5 Human Immunodeficiency Virus

Virus	Characteristics	Disease Association	Oral Pathos
HIV-1	Global infection Infects cells that contain CD4 receptors, such as T-helper lymphocytes and cells of the macrophage lineage	Rank order of AIDS-defining pathoses is as follows: Pneumocystis pneumonia (43%) Esophageal candidiasis (15%) Wasting (11%) Kaposi sarcoma (11%) Disseminated mycobacterium avium infection (5%) Mycobacterium tuberculosis infection (5%) Cytomegalovirus disease (4%) HIV-associated dementia (4%) Recurrent bacterial pneumonia (3%) Toxoplasmosis (3%) Oral hairy leukoplakia	Plasmablastic lymphoma Kaposi sarcoma Xerostomia (Sjögren syndrome) Sialadenitis Osteomyelitis
HIV-2	Infection occurring mainly in West Central Africa (Guinea-Bissau)	HIV-2 is associated with similar types of diseases as HIV-1 but is generally less virulent	Oral hairy leukoplakia Plasmablastic lymphoma Kaposi sarcoma Xerostomia (Sjögren syndrome) Sialadenitis Osteomyelitis

AIDS, Acquired immunodeficiency syndrome; *HIV*, human immunodeficiency virus.

prolonged with current anti-HIV drug therapy.[34] Infected individuals treated with HAART may experience a marked rise in CD4 cell levels and a decreased plasma viral load. CD4 counts may reach normal levels, and viral load may decrease to a point below the level of detection.[239] Despite this improvement, these individuals are still considered to have AIDS, because the virus is apparently sequestered somewhere in the body. Patients remain potentially infectious to others, and viral activity may resume if medications are discontinued or if severe coinfections with sexually transmitted diseases or other diseases occur.[327] Some evidence suggests that severe oral infections, including periodontal diseases, may sometimes represent a significant coinfection.

HIV Pathogenesis

A few weeks to a few months after initial exposure, some HIV-infected individuals may experience acute symptoms, such as the sudden onset of an acute mononucleosis-like illness that is characterized by malaise, fatigue, fever, myalgia, erythematous cutaneous eruption, oral candidiasis, oral ulcerations, and thrombocytopenia.[328] This acute phase may last for up to 2 weeks, with seroconversion occurring 3 to 8 weeks later. However, antigenic viremia may sometimes be present for an extended time before seroconversion occurs.[170] Some individuals experience asymptomatic HIV infection, whereas others may become asymptomatic after the initial acute infection. In either case, infected individuals eventually become seropositive for HIV antibodies, but the mean time from infection until the development of AIDS is now estimated to be up to 15 years or more.[130]

In patients with untreated or inadequately treated HIV infection, the overall effect is the gradual impairment of the immune system via interference with T4 cells and other immune cell functions.[347] Evidence indicates that innate immune response may play a role in controlling HIV replication. Chemokine receptor type 5 (CCR5) is found on the surface of CD4 cells, and it often serves as a point of entry for HIV into the cell. A genetic variation associated with the expression of CCR5 and its ligand has been found to decrease an individual's susceptibility to HIV infection and delay clinical progression independent of their effects on viral replication. This may partially explain the lack of progression of HIV infection in some individuals, and it may ultimately lead to a cure.[316]

B lymphocytes are not infected, but the altered function of infected T4 lymphocytes secondarily results in B-cell dysregulation and altered neutrophil function.[173] This may place HIV-positive individuals at increased risk for malignancy and disseminated infections with microorganisms such as viruses, mycobacterioses, and mycoses.[240] HIV-positive individuals are also at increased risk for adverse drug reactions as a result of altered antigenic regulation.[231]

Epithelial cells of the mucosa may become infected, and they may allow the virus to access the bloodstream. Some evidence suggests that oral epithelial cells may harbor HIV virions and infect $CD4^+$ cells by direct cell-to-cell transfer or by transporting and releasing low levels of infectious virions.[325] Most evidence, however, indicates that oral transmucosal viral transmission occurs after mild or severe traumatic injury or puncture of the mucous membranes. This allows for the infection of circulating host defense cells, such as lymphocytes, macrophages, and dendritic cells.[298]

HIV has been detected in most body fluids, although it is found in high quantities only in blood, semen, and cerebrospinal fluid. Transmission occurs almost exclusively by sexual contact, illicit use of injection drugs, or exposure to blood or blood products. Transmission is more likely to occur through contact with HIV-infected individuals harboring a high plasma load of the virus.[232] HIV transmission has also been reported to occur through organ transplantation and artificial insemination.[48] Some short-term studies have suggested that HIV-positive individuals who have been successfully treated with antiretroviral therapy (i.e., who have no detectable viral load) cease to be infectious to others.[250] However, incomplete adherence to antiretroviral therapy could further increase the risk of transmission. Unprotected sex in this scenario creates a risk of HIV transmission that is four times greater than that associated with condom use.

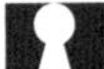

KEY FACT

Compliance, especially with universal precautions, will eliminate or minimize risks to both patients and the dental staff. Immunocompromised patients are potentially at risk for acquiring as well as transmitting infections in the dental office and other health care facilities.

Gingival and Periodontal Diseases

Considerable research has focused on the nature and incidence of periodontal diseases in HIV-infected individuals. Some studies suggest that CP is more common in this patient population, but others do not. However, some unusual types of periodontal diseases do seem to occur with greater frequency among HIV-positive individuals.[103,162,238,254]

Linear Gingival Erythema

A persistent, linear, easily bleeding, erythematous gingivitis has been described in some HIV-positive patients. The intensity of the erythema is disproportionate to the amount of plaque present. There is no ulceration, pocketing, or attachment loss, and the condition does not respond predictably to conventional periodontal therapy.[324] Lesions that are clinically identical to linear gingival erythema (LGE) were observed before the advent of HIV in association with severely immunocompromised individuals or in those with NUG.

LGE may or may not serve as a precursor to rapidly progressive NUP (Figs. 27.8 and 27.9).[92] The microflora of LGE may closely mimic that of periodontitis rather than gingivitis. However, *Candida* infection has been implicated as a major etiologic factor, and human herpesviruses have been proposed as possible triggers or cofactors.[258] Linear gingivitis lesions may be localized or generalized in nature. The erythematous gingivitis may be limited to marginal tissue, extend into attached gingiva in a punctate or diffuse erythema, or extend into the alveolar mucosa.

Others have reported that LGE is most often found in HIV-positive individuals whose $CD4^+$ counts are depressed (200 to 500 cells/mm^3 or <200 cells/mm^3) or whose viral loads are elevated, suggesting that it may represent an early marker of progressive immunodeficiency or even the transition to outright AIDS.[307]

LGE-like lesions can sometimes be adequately managed by following the therapeutic principles associated with marginal gingivitis. However, as mentioned previously, it has been suggested that gingivitis lesions that respond to conventional therapy do not represent LGE. The affected sites should be scaled and polished. Subgingival irrigation with chlorhexidine or 10% povidone-iodine may be beneficial. The patient should be carefully instructed regarding the performance of meticulous

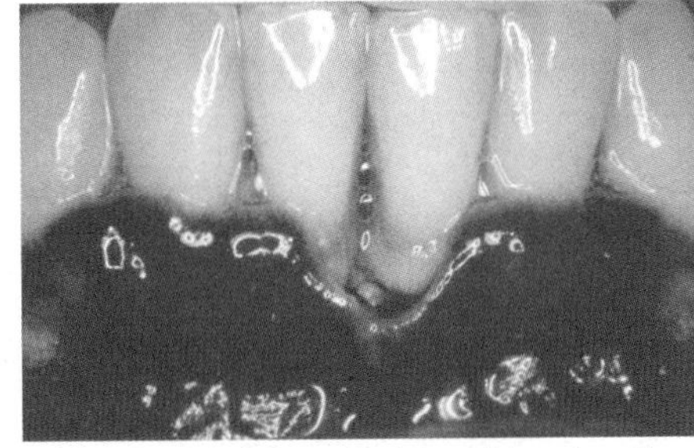

Fig. 27.8 Linear gingival erythema and necrotizing ulcerative gingivitis in a patient with acquired immunodeficiency syndrome.

oral hygiene procedures. The condition should be reevaluated 2 to 3 weeks after initial therapy. If the patient is compliant with home care procedures and the lesions persist, the possibility of a candidal infection should be considered. It is doubtful that topical antifungal rinses will reach the base of the gingival crevices. Consequently, the treatment of choice may be the empiric administration of a systemic antifungal agent, such as fluconazole, for 7 to 10 days.[119]

CLINICAL CORRELATION

It is important to remember that LGE is often refractory to treatment. If so, the patient should be carefully monitored for developing signs of more severe periodontal conditions (e.g., NUG, NUP, NUS). The patient should be placed on a 2–3-month recall maintenance interval and re-treated as necessary.

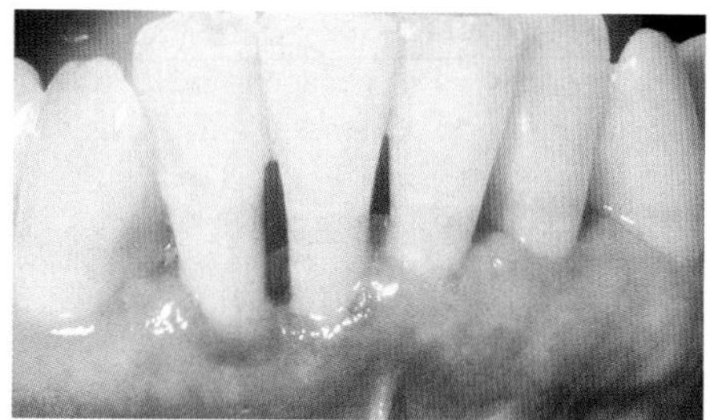

Fig. 27.9 Mild linear gingival erythema. The patient had a T4 count of 9 and a viral load that was too numerous to count.

Systemic antibiotics, such as metronidazole or amoxicillin may be prescribed for patients with moderate to severe tissue destruction, localized lymphadenopathy, or systemic symptoms. Metronidazole may be the antibiotic of choice because it has been demonstrated to be effective for the treatment of NUG, and its narrow bactericidal spectrum may minimize the risk of secondary opportunistic infections, such as candidiasis.[356] The use of prophylactic antifungal medication should be considered if antibiotics are prescribed.

Necrotizing Ulcerative Periodontitis

A necrotizing, ulcerative, rapidly progressive form of periodontitis occurs more frequently among HIV-positive individuals, although such lesions were described long before the onset of the AIDS epidemic. NUP appears to represent an extension of NUG in which bone loss and periodontal attachment loss occur.[216]

NUP is characterized by soft-tissue necrosis, rapid periodontal destruction, and interproximal bone loss (Figs. 27.10 and 27.11).[244] Lesions may occur anywhere in the dental arches; they are usually localized to a few teeth, although generalized NUP is sometimes present after marked $CD4^+$ cell depletion. Bone is often exposed, which results in necrosis and subsequent sequestration. NUP is severely painful at onset, and immediate treatment is necessary. Occasionally, however, patients undergo spontaneous resolution of the necrotizing lesions, which leave painless, deep, interproximal craters that are difficult to clean and that may lead to conventional periodontitis.[93]

Therapy for NUP includes local debridement; scaling and root planing; in-office irrigation with an effective antimicrobial agent, such as chlorhexidine gluconate or povidone-iodine (Betadine);

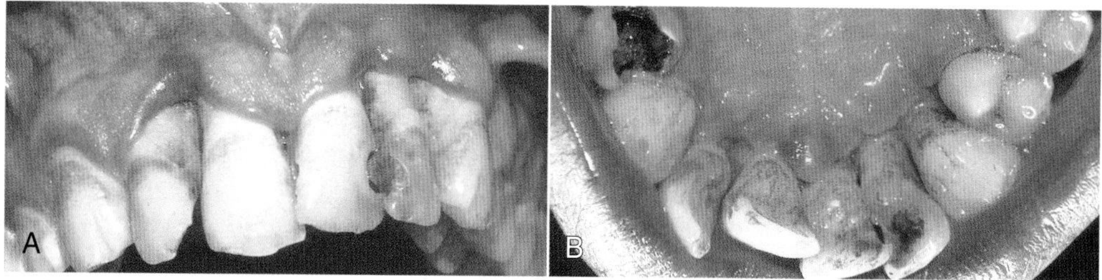

Fig. 27.10 Necrotizing ulcerative periodontitis in an otherwise healthy 19-year-old man without human immunodeficiency virus. (A) Anterior maxilla. (B) Palatal view.

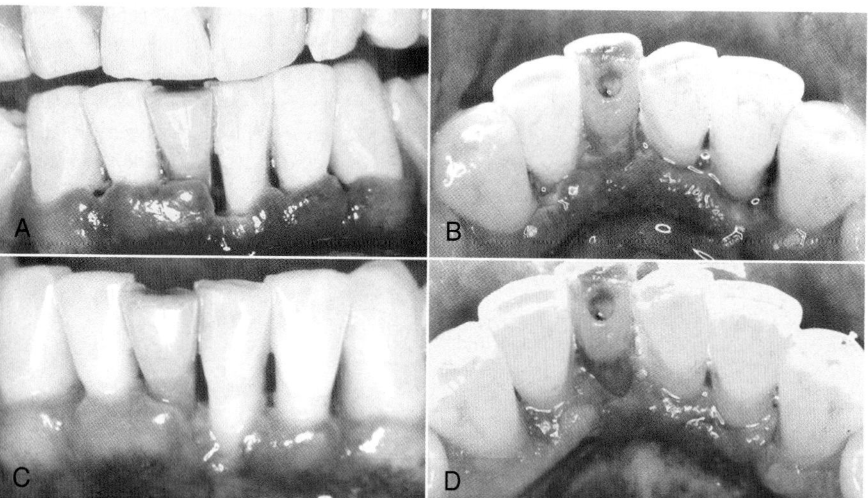

Fig. 27.11 Early necrotizing ulcerative periodontitis in a patient with acquired immunodeficiency syndrome. (A) Facial view. (B) Lingual view. (C) Facial view of the complete resolution of necrotizing ulcerative periodontitis after treatment. (D) Lingual view.

and the establishment of meticulous oral hygiene, including the home use of antimicrobial rinses or irrigation.[228,243] This therapeutic approach is based on reports that involved only a small number of patients.

In patients with severe NUP, antibiotic therapy may be necessary, but it should be used with caution in HIV-infected patients to avoid an opportunistic and potentially serious localized candidiasis or even candidal septicemia.[198] If an antibiotic is necessary, metronidazole (250 mg, with two tablets taken immediately and then two tablets taken four times daily for 5 to 7 days) is the drug of choice. The prophylactic prescription of a topical or systemic antifungal agent is prudent if an antibiotic is used.

Chronic Periodontitis

A number of longitudinal studies and prevalence studies have suggested that HIV-positive individuals are more likely to experience CP than the general population.[191,207,255] Most studies, however, do not take into account the level of oral hygiene, the presence of preexisting gingivitis, poor diet, the age of the patient, smoking, other periodontal disease risk factors, the degree of immunodeficiency in the population studied, or whether the individuals in the study are injection drug users (IDUs); these confounding factors cloud the issue.

Despite these limitations, most studies of CP in HIV-positive individuals report that the incidence is similar to that found in the general population. In addition, the periodontal pathogenic organisms that are routinely found in conventional CP are also found in HIV-associated CP. However, numerous studies have also reported a high prevalence of microorganisms in HIV-associated CP that are not found in the general population, including *Acinetobacter baumannii, Candida* spp., *Clostridium difficile, Clostridium clostridioforme, Entamoeba gingivalis, Enterobacter* spp., *Enterococcus faecalis, Enterococcus avium, Klebsiella pneumoniae, Mycoplasma salivarium,* and *Pseudomonas aeruginosa.*[64,324] Whether or not these rare organisms influence periodontal pathogenesis has not been determined. However, it is certainly possible that these microorganisms may alter the subgingival biofilm environment and cause an HIV-infected individual to experience more rapid CP progression. Many of these organisms are also associated with systemic diseases, thereby suggesting the possibility that CP in HIV-positive individuals may increase the risk for nosocomial infections as well as the development of antimicrobial resistance in affected individuals.

In previous studies, Shugars and colleagues reported that HIV RNA was detectable in the saliva of some seropositive individuals and that both salivary and plasma levels were higher in those with HIV-associated periodontal diseases, leading some to suggest that periodontal infections may contribute to HIV viremia.[228]

A well-controlled study indicated that gingival recession and early attachment loss are more common in HIV groups than in matched groups from the general population.[258] This appears to affirm that immunocompromised individuals are slightly more susceptible to CP than those with robust immune systems. In support of this theory, there was a 30% decrease reported in the prevalence of CP among patients with AIDS who were receiving HAART.[39] The majority of HIV-positive individuals experience gingivitis and CP in a manner similar to the general population. However, several studies have suggested that proinflammatory cytokines are increased in HIV-positive individuals, which suggests that CP may tend to be more severe in this population should it be present.[356]

With proper home care and appropriate periodontal treatment and maintenance, HIV-positive individuals can anticipate reasonably good periodontal health throughout the course of their disease.[142] This indicates that HIV-infected patients are potential candidates for conventional periodontal treatment procedures, including surgery and implant placement. Treatment decisions should be based on the overall health status of the patient, the degree of periodontal involvement, and the motivation and ability of the patient to perform effective oral hygiene.

It is imperative for the patient to maintain meticulous personal oral hygiene. In addition, periodontal maintenance recall visits should be conducted at short intervals (i.e., every 2 to 3 months), and any progressive periodontal disease should be treated vigorously.[356] Systemic antibiotic therapy should be administered with caution. Blood and other medical laboratory tests may be required to monitor the patient's overall health status, and close consultation and coordination with the patient's physician are necessary.

Health Status

The patient's health status should be determined from the health history, the physical evaluation, and consultation with the patient's physician. Treatment decisions will vary, depending on the patient's state of health. For example, delayed wound healing and an increased risk of postoperative infection are possible complicating factors in patients with AIDS, but neither concern should significantly alter treatment planning for an otherwise healthy, asymptomatic, HIV-infected patient with a normal or near-normal CD4 count and a low viral load.[110,248]

It is important to obtain information about the patient's immune status with questions, such as the following:

- What is the $CD4^+$ T4 lymphocyte level?
- What is the current viral load?
- How do current $CD4^+$ T4 cell and viral load counts differ from previous evaluations? How often are such tests performed?
- How long ago was the HIV infection identified? Is it possible to identify the approximate date of original exposure?
- Is there a history of drug abuse, sexually transmitted diseases, multiple infections, or other factors that may alter immune response? For example, does the patient have a history of chronic hepatitis B, hepatitis C, neutropenia, thrombocytopenia, nutritional deficiency, or adrenocortical insufficiency?
- What medications is the patient taking?
- Does the patient describe or present with possible adverse side effects from medications?

Infection Control Measures

The clinical management of HIV-infected periodontal patients requires strict adherence to established methods of infection control, which should be based on guidance from the American Dental Association and the CDC. Compliance, especially with universal precautions, will eliminate or minimize risks to both patients and the dental staff. Immunocompromised patients are potentially at risk for acquiring as well as transmitting infections in the dental office and other health care facilities.

Bacteriophages

Viral infection of bacteria and archaea is mediated by prokaryotic viruses known as bacteriophages. Considered the most abundant biological entity, bacteriophages are isolated in various environments in coexistence with their bacterial host as a free virion or dormant prophage. Bacteriophages play a crucial role in human health and disease as they are capable of modulating the ecology of the microbiota in which they reside.[74] As more bacteriophages are fully characterized they can be utilized to identify bacterial strains, detect bacterial pathogens and treat antibiotic-resistant bacterial strains.[351] Bacteriophages residing in the oral cavity infect commensal oral bacteria, primary colonizers of dental plaque, and periodontopathogens, and hold the potential to serve as a therapeutic for periodontitis.

At present, the taxonomic classification of the 19 families of bacteriophages is based on viral genome composition, morphology, host range, infectious cycle, and shared genomic sequencing.[299] Bacteriophage capsid morphology may be icosahedral, filamentous, or pleomorphic. Icosahedral capsids are further classified by tail morphology or the absence of a tail structure. The bacteriophage tail serves as an adhesive system that protects the viral genome from environmental insult during delivery to host cytoplasm. Bacteriophage-derived enzymes, called depolymerases, form part of the tail spike proteins of bacteriophages and are responsible for the depolymerization of bacterial capsules, facilitating bacteriophage adsorption.[155] *Caudovirales* is the most studied order of bacteriophages that consists of approximately 96% tailed bacteriophages (Fig. 27.12).[4]

Regulation of bacterial population and biodiversity results from the lytic or lysogenic life cycle that the bacteriophage undergoes. Adsorption involves the recognition and attachment to a highly unique region of the bacterial cell wall, capsule, surface receptor, or appendages and dictates the host range of bacteriophages, which typically involves only a single host species or strain.[185] Once engaged, lytic bacteriophages hijack bacterial cell machinery to replicate and eventually lyse the cell as they spread to other susceptible bacteria. Temperate bacteriophages integrate their genome into the bacterial chromosome as a prophage, replicate with the host bacteria and then repackage themselves to induce the release of new virions that propagate infection. Temperate bacteriophages play an important role in lateral gene transfer which may allow for the acquisition of antibiotic resistance in bacteria.

Oral Bacteriophage Ecology

Metagenomic surveys of bacteriophages indicate that our current genomic databases are insufficient to fully characterize the bacteriophage ecology within the oral cavity. Community composition of bacteriophages is influenced by bacterial abundance, density, and between different environments.[349] Similar to bacterial distribution, oral bacteriophage distribution is not random. Specific niche tropism for the buccal mucosa, dorsum of the tongue, and gingiva is demonstrated by the strong preference for the microbiota of the tongue of the *Haemophilus* bacteriophage, BcepMu. While other oral bacteriophages of *Haemophilus* species displayed a generalized tropism for all three sites.[317] It is hypothesized that bacteriophages with generalized distribution are capable of infecting more resistant strains of a bacterial species, whereas highly susceptible bacteria are infected by bacteriophages with more narrow host ranges.

A survey of the oral bacteriophage composition revealed a stable and highly personalized population with a significant portion belonging to the *Caudovirales* order.[2] Subgingival plaque taken from inflamed periodontal pockets have a reduction in bacteriophage richness and diversity within *Caudovirales* families isolated.[174,236,339] Dominance of *Siphoviridae* temperate bacteriophages in health is replaced by a surge in *Myoviridae* lytic bacteriophages in subgingival plaque during active periodontal disease.[174] This shift towards a high abundance of lytic bacteriophages within plaque during disease states may reflect the bacterial composition change that occurs[186] and imply that bacteriophages play a role in enhancing the collective virulence within the developing biofilm.

CRISPR/Cas Identification

An adaptive defense mechanism was developed in bacterial hosts to combat against previously encountered bacteriophages that regulate the bacterial population. Bacteria that carry the CRISPR-cas system can be screened for bacteriophage-like elements and CRISPR spacers which reflect bacteriophage DNA fragments that are now incorporated into CRISPR memory arrays. CRISPR loci are profiled using DNA and RNA sequencing and meta-omics techniques.[199]

Limitations in the current genomic data bank have led to modifications in the organization of the identification of novel bacteriophages. In order to place two bacteriophages in the same species they must share greater than 90% nucleotide identity through metagenomic readings, thus identifying novel oral bacteriophages has been a challenge due to the limited number of reads from the oral cavity. The use of various detection techniques allows for an increase in bacteriophage reads to characterize the oral bacteriophage community more clearly. Application of CRISPR loci profiling in dental plaque from periodontally healthy individuals was used to identify bacteriophages at the species level, which included a high abundance of Streptococcus prophages (UCN34, IS7493), Actinomyces bacteriophage AV-1, Streptococcus bacteriophage DP-1, Enterobacteria bacteriophage P7 and Enterobacteria

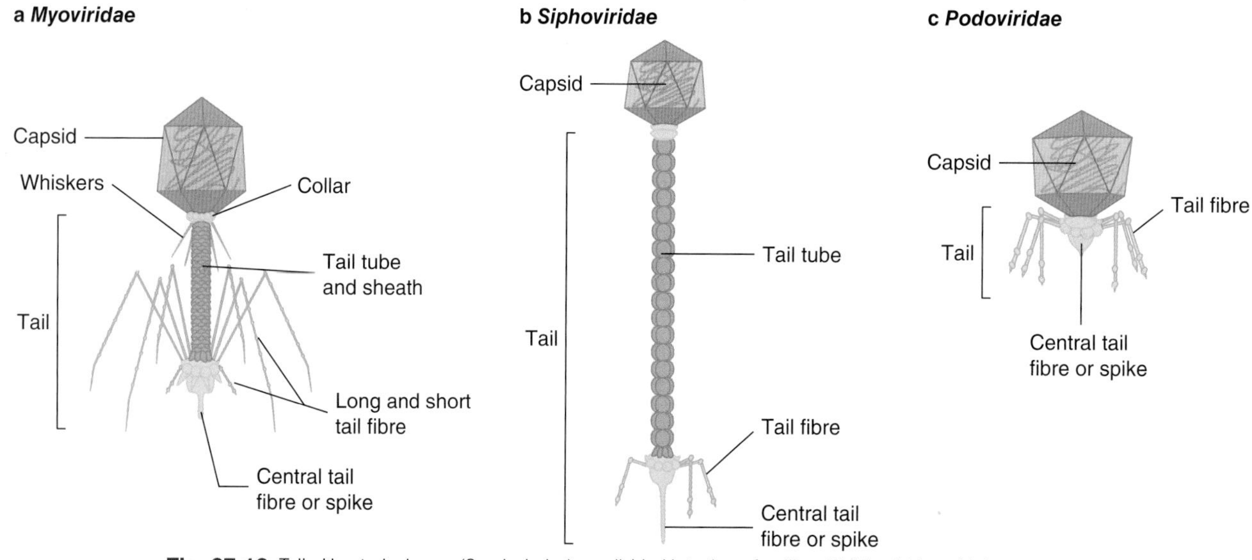

Fig. 27.12 Tailed bacteriophages (Caudovirales) are divided into three families. (A) Myoviridae with long contractile tails. (B) Siphoviridae with long noncontractile tails. (C) Podoviridae with short noncontractile tails. (Copyright © 2022. Ryutaro Kuraji.)

bacteriophage λ.[203] Identification of bacteriophages using CRISPR-cas systems demonstrated bacteriophage ecology is characteristic for each individual despite approximately 50% of contigs remaining without homologous sequences.

CRISPR-cas systems can act as a catalog of bacteriophage-host interactions and document bacterial host resistance to certain bacteriophages. A transposon encoding tetracycline resistance from the Enterobacteria bacteriophage P7 was isolated though CRISPR loci profiling in dental plaque in healthy individuals.[203] Ampicillin, colistin, and β-lactam resistance genes are frequently described in the Myoviridae family to which that bacteriophage P7 belongs.[331] A further understanding of the development and transfer of these resistance genes requires a deeper understanding of the CRISPR-cas system. In doing so, interventions can be developed to those important determinants that affect periodontal health.

Bacteriophages of Oral Pathogens

The oral cavity is host to bacteriophages that inhabit all its niches and infect both commensal and pathogenic bacterial community members. Known bacteriophages of the oral cavity commonly infect members of the bacterial phyla Actinobacteria, Bacteroidetes, Firmicutes, Fusobacteria, and Proteobacteria.

Oral streptococci are the most abundant member of the commensal oral flora but produce lactate that is associated with the development of dental caries. A few streptococcus species (*S. mitis, S. oralis, S. sanguinis*) are the primary colonizers that initiate the formation of dental plaque. Approximately 50 bacteriophages infect *S. mitis*, *S. mutans*, *S. oralis*, *S. salivarius,* and *S. sobrinus.*[9] Only a small portion of these streptococcus bacteriophages have been characterized. Notably, siphovirus SM1 that lyses its host *S. mitis* resulted in the release of a phage-encoded platelet binding factor that links bacterial cells to platelets in endocarditis isolates.[195] Fewer bacteriophages infecting caries-associated Lactobacillus species have been isolated.[194]

Bacteria implicated in dental plaque development and periodontitis are infected by several bacteriophages that demonstrate mutualistic relationships (Box 27.1). *Actinomyces* species and *Corynebacterium* species are involved in plaque formation and provide a scaffold in biofilms, respectively. A bacteriophage of *Actinomyces* allows for the extracellular release of bacterial DNA that contributes to plaque development.[287] Three lytic bacteriophages have been isolated from the bacterial "bridge" of oral biofilms each resulting in different infection outcomes. FnpΦ02 displayed slow lysis of *F. nucleatum*;[179] however, FNU1 is reported to significantly reduce *F. nucleatum* biofilm mass.[143] *Actinobacillus actinomycetemcomitans* isolated from active periodontal pockets in juvenile periodontitis consistently had bacteriophages adsorbed onto the bacterial cell surface, suggesting an association between periodontal breakdown and bacteriophage infection of *A. actinomycetemcomitans*.[249] The arsenal of virulence factors for *A. actinomycetemcomitans* may be attributed to temperate *Myoviridae* that, in vitro, transfers antibiotic resistance genes, induce serotype conversion, and stimulates the production of leukotoxins.[315] Another identified temperate *Myoviridae* bacteriophage infecting *Treponema denticola* designated as φtd1 was found as integrated prophage DNA and upregulated expression of prophage genes during biofilm growth.[196] Unlike the documented herpesvirus-*Porphymonas gingivalis* relationship,[304] forty bacteriophages are linked to commensal *Porphyromonas* species but no bacteriophages have been isolated to *P. gingivalis*.[342]

Bacteriophage-Mediated Biofilm Dynamics

Biofilms are ubiquitous complex microbial communities that shelter microbial cells from the relentless environmental and chemical stress found within the oral cavity. After adhering to hard tissue surfaces, microbial members are encased in a self-producing matrix of extracellular polymeric substances (EPS). Formation of oral biofilms is a concerted effort that involves more than the periodontopathogens isolated in periodontally inflamed tissues. Physiological changes in a multi-species biofilm allow microbial members to share metabolic resources and develop resistance to antimicrobial agents.[166] As the natural predators of bacteria, bacteriophages may attempt biofilm degradation but face resistance to entry or coexist with their host and aid in the formation and reorganization of oral biofilms, which initiate periodontal tissue destruction as depicted in Fig. 27.13.

Bacteriophages can enhance aggregation and interactions between microbial members which is typically possible through direct cellular contact or linkage within EPS. Production of a highly structured and significantly more antibiotic-resistant biofilm results from bacteriophage φ2 infections that induce a phenotype change in *Pseudomonas fluorescens* leading to an overproduction of alginate and loss of motility.[115] A high volume of oral bacteriophages infect the early colonizers of dental plaque that interact through cell surface structures to contribute to biofilm formation.[197] Exposure to *Actinomyces* bacteriophages may mediate physical contact with *Streptococcus* species acting as appendages since *Actinomyces* mutant strains resistant to its bacteriophage lost the ability to co-aggregate with *Streptococcus*.[323] In the absence of these *Actinomyces* bacteriophages, the development of oral biofilms may be delayed and more susceptible to the host immune response.

The mechanical and chemical strength of the biofilm matrix is attributed to the mixture of EPS, extracellular DNA (eDNA), proteins, and lipoteichoic acid that embed microbial members. Within *Pseudomonas* biofilms, filamentous bacteriophages are embedded in the biofilm matrix promoting a liquid crystal phenotype that is more viscous and stress-tolerant.[276] Release of eDNA by both lytic and temperate bacteriophages provides structural integrity and nutritional support for microbial members.[37] Temperate bacteriophage xhp1 infects *Actinomyces odontolyticus* in subgingival plaque and during its prophage form can

BOX 27.1 Bacteriophage-Host Interaction Network

Interaction networks allow for the delineation of the true impact bacteriophages have on the microbial shift seen in periodontal disease states. The first oral bacteriophage-host interaction network was computed through analysis of a CRISPR-cas system in 40 dental plaque and salivary samples of periodontally healthy and diseased individuals.[339] The majority of the bacteriophages isolated possess a narrow host range or a one-to-one infection model. Cross-infective bacteriophages represented a small portion of bacteriophages, mainly infecting the biofilm-promoting bacterial species of *Streptococcus* and *Actinomyces.* A regulatory role has been proposed for a smaller subset of the cross-infective bacteriophages of both periodontopathogens (*Campylobacter, Fusobacterium,* and *Prevotella*) and commensal bacteria. Those bacteriophages that have the ability to cross-infect between hosts of distinct species can potentially modulate the bacterial dysbiosis prevalent in the development of periodontitis. The study of bacteriophage-bacteria interactions has provided key insights into bacteriophage infection that could lead to the development of novel antibacterial therapies.

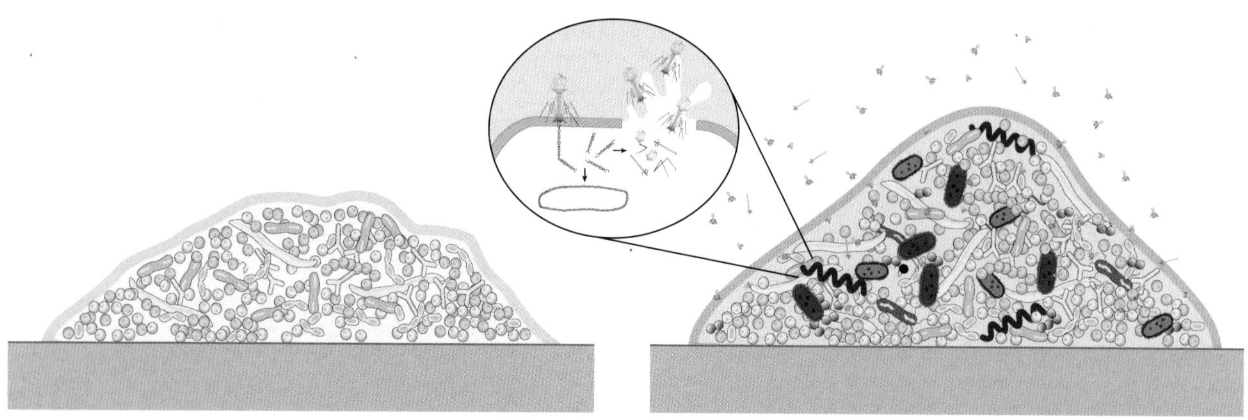

Fig. 27.13 Surface interactions or infiltration of lytic or lysogenic bacteriophages into biofilms can aid in its development and maturation through a variety of mechanisms. (Copyright © 2022. Ryutaro Kuraji.)

induce the spontaneous release of host eDNA compared to bacteriophage-cured stains.[288] Additionally, temporal regulation of bacteriophage-mediated lysis during the early stages of biofilm formation tends to promote larger biomass of biofilms with the release of eDNA.[94] The robust nature of oral biofilms becomes more difficult to depict as interactions between bacteriophages and hosts in multi-species biofilms result in higher diversity of EPS and heterogeneity of the biofilm.

Bacteriophages as Therapeutic Agents

Shortly after their discovery in 1915, a cocktail of bacteriophages relieved symptoms of severe dysentery in a 12-year-old boy within a few days. The application of bacteriophages to treat persistent bacterial and biofilm infections was termed phage therapy but soon fell out of favor with the advent of penicillin. However, attraction towards phage therapy is on the rise as it may help overcome the main drawbacks to current antibiotic therapy. In contrast to antibiotics, bacteriophages have a low impact on the commensal microbiome since they are strain specific and replicate only where host bacteria reside (Fig. 27.14).[3] Resistance to phage therapy is still a possibility but can be more easily resolved due to the extensive supply of novel bacteriophages in nature. Once bacteriophage databases are further developed, tailoring a bacteriophage cocktail to match a patient's specific bacterial infection will make personalized phage therapy a potential reality (Box 27.2).

CLINICAL CORRELATION

After the selection of a bacteriophage cocktail, the determination of proper dosage and timing is imperative to improve the antibiofilm efficacy of phage therapy. Similar to antibiotics, if proper dosage is not determined, repeated phage treatment can result in increased biofilm thickness and appearance of bacteriophage-resistant microcolonies.[116] However, these same microcolonies prove to be more susceptible to dual-antimicrobial treatment, which includes phage and antibiotic therapy. More pertinent to the treatment of oral biofilms is that after mechanical scraping, biofilms become significantly more susceptible to bacteriophage predation.[193] Both in vivo models and compassionate clinical phage therapy treatments resulted in satisfactory clearance of infection only with prior mechanical debridement of the predominately mono-species Staphylococcal biofilms followed by phage therapy.[230,280] These results suggest that a disturbed extracellular biofilm matrix allows for increased penetration of species-specific bacteriophages. Subsequently, treatment of periodontitis with phage therapy may first appear as adjunctive therapy to local or systemic antibiotics and non-surgical treatment procedures that include the debridement of dental plaque.

Acknowledgment

Terry D. Rees for his earlier contributions to this topic.

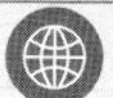
References for this chapter are found on the companion website eBooks.Health.Elsevier.com.

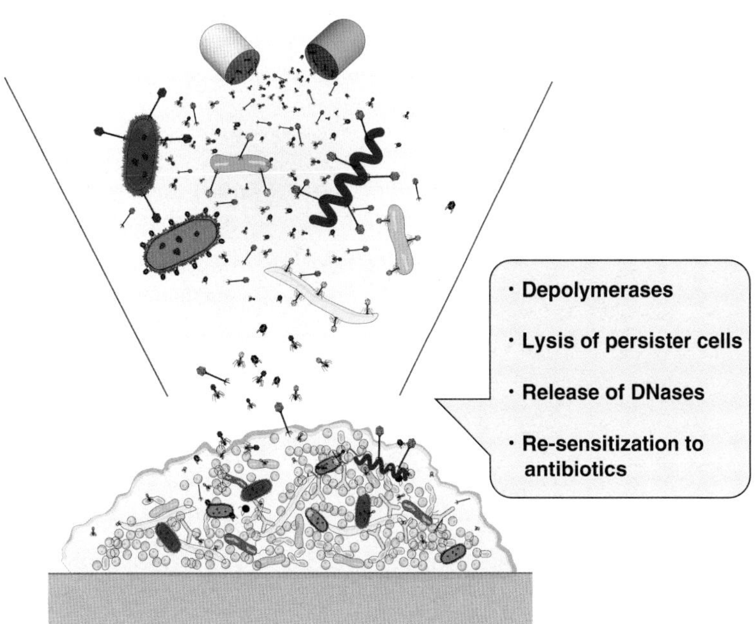

Fig. 27.14 Phage therapy selects for mechanisms employed by bacteriophages that result in the lysis of specific bacteria in mono-species biofilms or the disruption of multi-species biofilms. (Copyright © 2022. Ryutaro Kuraji.)

BOX 27.2 Phage Cocktail Formulation

Multi-species biofilms predominate the oral cavity and are present on teeth, prostheses, gingiva, and tongue. Polymicrobial infections complicate selecting the appropriate therapeutic strategy to undertake that addresses both host response and interbacterial interactions. Reports of resistance to the current management of periodontitis is on the rise and includes the use of local and systemic antibiotics.[252] Proposed strategies to reduce the risk of bacterial antimicrobial resistance include: prescribing dual-antimicrobial drugs with complementary effects, combination treatment with mechanical debridement and focus on therapeutic rather than prophylactic use.

Phage therapy has demonstrated its potential as a promising contender for oral polymicrobial infections in both in vitro and in vivo studies due to the relatively high abundance of phages and their specificity for bacterial pathogens.[229,241] Cocktail phage therapy is the formulation of multiple bacteriophages that target pathogenic bacteria in a synergistic manner while sparing commensals. In order to achieve the full potential of cocktail phage therapy further characterization of oral bacteriophages and multi-species biofilm dynamics is required. There are a limited number of bacteriophages currently identified at the species level that can be effective against subgingival plaque pathogens, such as for *A. actinomycetemcomitans*, *Enterococcus faecalis,* and *S. mutans*.[317] Due to the high number of identified *Streptococcal* bacteriophages, patents on phage therapy for oral infections are already established.[65,85]

Successful management of the bacterial species in a polymicrobial biofilm with cocktail phage therapy also reduces the emergence of bacteriophage-resistant bacteria and the reinstatement of biofilms that cause recurring infections.[359] Bacteriophages selected for cocktails that target different cell receptors aid in extending host range and reduce the incidence of **bacterial resistance**.[49,241] Another way to effectively disrupt biofilms and prevent bacteriophage resistance is by combining phage therapy with antibiotics simultaneously or sequentially.[332] Synthetic bacteriophages that are fabricated can be infused to cocktail phage therapy to resensitize bacteria to carbapenems by targeting β-lactamase genes in susceptible bacteria.[358] All the different modalities that bacteriophages can take on make phage therapy promising in the management of the primary etiology of periodontal inflammation—dental plaque.

Resilience to antimicrobial agents is a necessary characteristic for oral biofilms. Due to the viscidity of extracellular polymeric substance (EPS), oral plaque displays a reduced susceptibility to cationic antimicrobials, such as chlorhexidine.[289] Reinstatement of oral biofilms after antimicrobial treatment is realized by persister cells found in the deep layers of the biofilm which allow innate tolerance towards antimicrobial agents due to their dormant metabolic state.[144] Curiously, horizontal gene flux within biofilms is facilitated by bacteriophages and contributes to the expression of antibiotic-resistance genes. Even in the absence of prior exposure, tetracycline resistance genes are expressed by *Streptococci* species in subgingival plaque of both healthy and periodontitis patients.[10] The prevalence of these antibiotic resistance genes may derive from bacteriophages such as *Enterococci* P7 and *Actinomyces* Aaϕ23 that express a transposon encoding tetracycline resistance in the subgingival plaque of healthy individuals.[203,350] Thus, the effectiveness of phage therapy is dependent on the spatial structure, microbial species, and bacteriophage composition.

Penetration into the dense biofilm matrix is a major hurdle for which bacteriophages have developed mechanisms for its degradation. Release of extracellular DNA (eDNA) is an important factor through the various stages of biofilm development in various bacterial strains.[314,320] Bacteria often produce DNases to evade immobilization from neutrophil extracellular traps that contain neutrophil DNA filaments.[30] Similarly, bacteriophages encode DNases that degrade DNA filaments that reinforce the matrix scaffold and inadvertently halt the transfer of virulent bacterial genes occurring within biofilms.[29] Commonly found on the tail structures of bacteriophages are EPS depolymerases that aid in adsorption while soluble EPS depolymerases aid in bacteriophage movement through the biofilm matrix.[156] The susceptibility of biofilms to EPS depolymerases is dependent on the bacterial species that are embedded. Depolymerases (Dpo) of bacteriophage Petty demonstrated a 20% reduction of biofilm biomass of *Acinetobacter* species;[117] however, Dpo7 of *Staphylococcal* bacteriophages can reduce biomass of multiple bacterial strains by 53%–85%.[105]

Continued

BOX 27.2 Phage Cocktail Formulation—cont'd

Following the degradation of eDNA and EPS, bacteriophages are able to diffuse throughout the biofilm to continue their life cycle. In fact, confocal microscopy demonstrates that bacteriophage-infected hosts mainly appear in regions with lowered amounts of biofilm matrix present, emphasizing bacteriophage influence on the spatial organization of the biofilm.[193] Bacteriophages are also seen infecting those persister cells in the deep layers of the biofilms, albeit at lower concentrations.[322] Population dynamics within biofilms begin to achieve homeostasis once persister cells are bacteriophage-infected, which allows repopulation of susceptible cells as bacteriophages are clustered in the deep layers.[300] It is evident that in a multi-species biofilm, various bacteriophages are necessary for the growth and regulation of biofilm structure and physiology. Effective bacteriophage infection in biofilms also is time dependent as young developing biofilms are more likely saturated with susceptible bacteriophages than older mature biofilms with less susceptibility to bacteriophages.[242]

CHAPTER 28

Periodontal Therapy in the Female Patient

Joan Otomo-Corgel

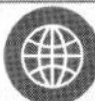 For online-only content on menopause, please visit the companion website at eBooks.Health.Elsevier.com.

CHAPTER OUTLINE

Throughout a woman's life, hormonal influences affect therapeutic decision-making in periodontics. Historically, therapies have been gender-biased. Research has provided a keener appreciation of the unique systemic influences on oral, periodontal, and implant tissues. Oral health care professionals have a greater awareness of and can better deal with hormonal influences associated with the reproductive process. Periodontal and oral tissue responses can be altered, creating diagnostic and therapeutic dilemmas. The clinician should recognize, customize, and appropriately alter periodontal therapy according to the individual woman's needs based on her stage of life.

Sex steroids exert profound biologic effects on immune function and bone metabolism.[144] Estrogen can significantly affect the periodontium, including maturation of gingival epithelium, osteoblastic differentiation of periodontal ligament cells, and bone formation.[143]

This chapter reviews the phases of the female reproductive cycle from puberty through menopause. Periodontal manifestations, systemic effects, and clinical management are addressed.

Puberty

Puberty occurs, on average, between the ages of 11 to 14 in most girls. The production of sex hormones (i.e., estrogen and progesterone) increases and then remains relatively constant during the remainder of the reproductive phase. The prevalence of gingivitis increases without an increase in the amount of plaque. Gram-negative anaerobes, especially *Prevotella intermedia*, have been associated with puberty gingivitis. Kornman and Loesche[74] postulated that this anaerobic organism may use ovarian hormones as a substitute for vitamin K as a growth factor. Levels of black-pigmented *Bacteroides*, especially *P. intermedia* (formerly known as *Bacteroides intermedius*), are thought to increase with increased levels of gonadotropic hormones in puberty. *Capnocytophaga* species also increase in incidence and proportion. These organisms have been implicated in the increased bleeding tendency observed during puberty.

Studies of pubertal gingivitis indicate proportionately elevated numbers of motile rods, spirochetes, and *P. intermedia.*[52,67,101] Statistically significant increases in gingival inflammation and the proportions of *P. intermedia* and *Prevotella nigrescens* have been seen in pubertal gingivitis.[105] A study of 11- to 17-year-old adolescents found higher levels of *Actinobacillus actinomycetemcomitans* and *Fusobacterium nucleatum*, which were associated with bleeding indices, probing depth, and attachment loss.[88]

During puberty, periodontal tissues can have an exaggerated response to local factors. A hyperplastic reaction of the gingiva can occur in areas where food debris, materia alba, plaque, and calculus are deposited. The inflamed tissues become erythematous, lobulated, and retractable. Bleeding may occur easily with mechanical debridement of the gingival tissues. Histologically, the appearance is consistent with inflammatory hyperplasia.

During the reproductive years, women tend to have a more vigorous immune response, including higher immunoglobulin concentrations, stronger primary and secondary responses, increased resistance to the induction of immunologic tolerance, and a greater ability to reject tumors and homografts.[141] Allergy, sensitivity, and asthma occur more often in young men, but after puberty, women become more susceptible than their male counterparts.

KEY FACT

Sex steroids exert profound biologic effects on immune function and bone metabolism. Estrogen can have a significant impact on the periodontium, including maturation of gingival epithelium, osteoblastic differentiation of periodontal ligament cells, and bone formation. During puberty, periodontal tissues can have an exaggerated response to local factors. A hyperplastic reaction of the gingiva can occur. Inflamed tissues become erythematous, lobulated, retractable, and bleed easily. Histologically, the appearance is consistent with inflammatory hyperplasia.

Management

During puberty, the education of the parent or caregiver is part of successful periodontal therapy. Preventive care, including a vigorous program of oral hygiene, is also vital.[6] Milder gingivitis cases respond well to scaling and root planing, with frequent oral hygiene reinforcement. Severe cases of gingivitis may require microbial culturing, antimicrobial mouthwashes and local site delivery, or antibiotic therapy. Periodontal maintenance appointments may need to be more frequent when periodontal instability is identified.

The clinician should recognize the periodontal manifestations and intraoral lesions associated with systemic diseases (e.g., diabetes).[27,111] Thorough review of the patient's medical history and medical referral should occur when deemed necessary. The clinician should be aware of the effects of chronic regurgitation of gastric contents on intraoral tissues; this age group is susceptible to eating disorders such as bulimia and anorexia nervosa.[18] *Perimolysis* (i.e., smooth erosion of enamel and dentin), typically on the lingual surfaces of maxillary anterior teeth, varies with the duration and frequency of the behavior.[20] Enlargement of the parotid glands (occasionally sublingual glands) has been estimated to occur in 10% to 50% of patients who binge and purge.[93] A diminished salivary flow rate may be identified, which can increase oral mucous membrane sensitivity, gingival erythema, and caries susceptibility.

Menses

Periodontal Manifestations

During the reproductive years, the ovarian cycle is controlled by the anterior pituitary gland. The gonadotropin follicle-stimulating hormone (FSH) and luteinizing hormone (LH) are produced by the anterior pituitary gland. The secretion of gonadotropins also depends on the hypothalamus. Ongoing changes in the concentration of the gonadotropins and ovarian hormones occur during the monthly menstrual cycle (Fig. 28.1). Under the influence of FSH and LH, estrogen and progesterone are steroid hormones produced by the ovaries during the menstrual cycle. During the reproductive cycle, the purpose of estrogen and progesterone is to prepare the uterus for the implantation of an egg.

The monthly reproductive cycle has two phases. The first phase is referred to as the *follicular phase.* Levels of FSH are elevated, and estradiol (E2), the major form of estrogen, is synthesized by the developing follicle and peaks approximately 2 days before ovulation. Estrogen stimulates the egg to move down the fallopian tubes (i.e., ovulation) and stimulates the proliferation of the stroma cells, blood vessels, and glands of the endometrium.

The second phase is called the *luteal phase*. The developing corpus luteum synthesizes estradiol and progesterone. Estrogen peaks at 0.2 ng/mL and progesterone at 10.0 ng/mL to complete the rebuilding of the endometrium for implantation of a fertilized egg. If the egg is not fertilized, the corpus luteum involutes, ovarian hormone levels drop, and menstruation ensues. It has been postulated that ovarian hormones increase inflammation in gingival tissues and exaggerate the response to local irritants. Gingival inflammation seems to be aggravated by an imbalance or increase in sex hormones.[60] Menstrual cycle irregularity is a risk indicator for periodontal disease before menopause.[53] Numerous in vitro and in vivo studies have demonstrated that sex hormones affect and modify the actions of cells of the immune system.

Evidence suggests that the interaction between estrogen and cells of the immune system can have nonimmune regulatory effects.[9,26] Possible mechanisms have been suggested for the increase in hormonal gingival interaction in the menstrual cycle. Tumor necrosis factor alpha (TNF-α), which fluctuates during the menstrual cycle;[16] elevated prostaglandin E_2 (PGE_2) synthesis;[98] and angiogenetic factors, endothelial growth factors, and receptors may be modulated by progesterone and estrogen, contributing to increases in gingival inflammation during certain stages of the menstrual cycle.[70]

Progesterone has been associated with increased permeability of the microvasculature, altering the rate and pattern of collagen production in the gingiva,[89] increasing folate metabolism,[116,158] and altering the immune response. During menses, progesterone increases from the second week, peaks at approximately 10 days, and dramatically drops before menstruation (based on a 28-day cycle; individual cycles vary). Progesterone plays a role in stimulating the production of prostaglandins that mediate the body's response to inflammation. PGE_2 is one of the major secretory products of monocytes, and the level is increased in inflamed gingiva. Miyagi and colleagues[97] found that the chemotaxis of polymorphonuclear leukocytes (PMNs) was enhanced by progesterone but reduced by estradiol. Testosterone did not have a measurable effect on PMN chemotaxis. The researchers suggested that the altered PMN chemotaxis associated with gingival inflammation might be caused by the effects of sex hormones. Physiologic, experimental, and clinical data confirm differences in immune responses between the two sexes.[170]

Gingival tissues have been reported to be more edematous during menses and erythematous before the onset of menses in some women. One study reported higher gingival indices during ovulation and before menstruation despite reported increases in oral symptoms during menses.[90] An increase of gingival exudate has been observed during the menstrual period and is sometimes associated with a minor increase in tooth mobility.[48] The incidence of postextraction osteitis is also higher during the initiation of menses. No significant hematologic laboratory findings accompany this, other than a slightly reduced platelet count and a slight increase in clotting time.

When the progesterone level is highest (during the luteal phase of the cycle), intraoral recurrent aphthous ulcers,[40] herpes labialis lesions, and candidal infections occur in some women in a cyclic pattern. Because the esophageal sphincter is relaxed by progesterone, women may be more susceptible to gastroesophageal reflux disease (GERD) during this time of the cycle. Symptoms of GERD include heartburn, regurgitation, and chest pain, and when reflux is severe, some patients develop unexplained coughing, hoarseness, sore throat, gingivitis, or asthma.[133]

Management

During the peak level of progesterone (about 7 to 10 days before menstruation), premenstrual syndrome (PMS) may also occur. There appears to be no significant difference in estrogen and progesterone levels between women with PMS and those without PMS. However, women with PMS seem to have lower levels of certain neurotransmitters such as enkephalins, endorphins, γ-aminobutyric acid (GABA), and serotonin. Depression, irritability, mood swings, and difficulty with

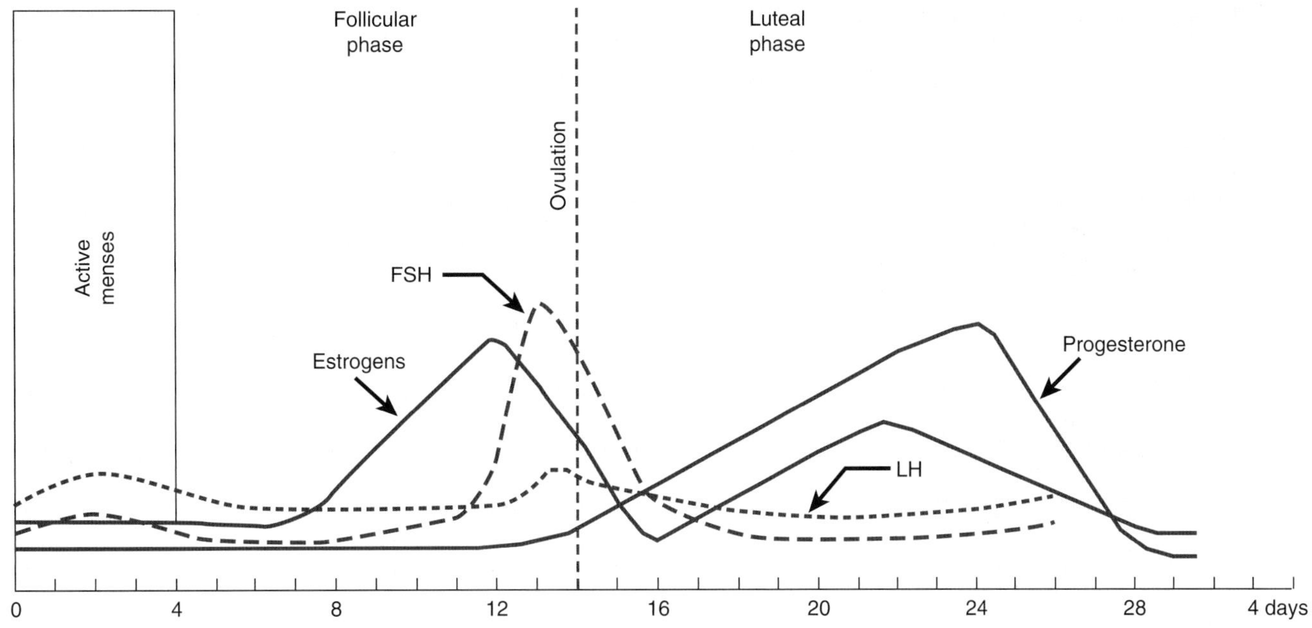

Fig. 28.1 Female menstrual cycle, showing the peak levels of progesterone and estrogen compared with follicle-stimulating hormone *(FSH)* and luteinizing hormone *(LH)*.

memory and concentration are symptoms of neurotransmitter reduction. Patients are more sensitive and less tolerant of procedures, have a heightened gag reflex, and can have an exaggerated response to pain.

Increased gingival bleeding and tenderness associated with the menstrual cycle require closer periodontal monitoring. Periodontal maintenance should be titrated to the individual patient's need, and if problematic, 3- to 4-month intervals should be recommended. An antimicrobial oral rinse before cyclic inflammation may be indicated. Emphasis should be placed on oral hygiene. For the patient with a history of excessive postoperative hemorrhage or menstrual flow, scheduling surgical visits after cyclic menstruation is prudent. Anemia is common, and appropriate consultation with a physician and laboratory tests, when indicated, should be maintained.

During PMS, many women exhibit physical symptoms that include fatigue, sweet and salty food cravings, abdominal bloating, swollen hands or feet, headaches, breast tenderness, nausea, and gastrointestinal upset. GERD may make it more uncomfortable for the patient to lie fully supine, especially after a meal, and she may have a more sensitive gag reflex. The clinician should be aware that nonsteroidal antiinflammatory drugs (NSAIDs), infection, and acidic foods exacerbate GERD. Patients with GERD may take over-the-counter antacids, H_2-receptor antagonists (e.g., cimetidine, famotidine, nizatidine, ranitidine), prokinetic agents (e.g., cisapride, metoclopramide), or proton pump inhibitors (e.g., lansoprazole, omeprazole, pantoprazole, rabeprazole).[134] These medications interact with some antibiotics and antifungals, and a review of their pharmacology is necessary. Fluoride rinses and trays, frequent periodontal debridement, and avoidance of mouthwashes with high alcohol content can reduce the associated gingival and caries sequelae.

PMS is often treated with antidepressants. Selective serotonin reuptake inhibitors (SSRIs) usually are the first-line choice because they have fewer side effects than other antidepressants, do not require blood monitoring, and are safe if overdosed. Women with PMS taking the SSRI fluoxetine had a 70% response rate. Fluoxetine was ranked the fifth most dispensed prescription (i.e., new and refills) in the United States in 1998, but when the patent was lifted, sales slowed. However, overall SSRIs ranked second in total dollar sales in the 2000s. Sertraline was ranked twelfth and is the drug of choice for the treatment of PMS.[179]

The clinician should be aware that patients taking fluoxetine have increased side effects with highly protein-bound drugs (e.g., aspirin), and the half-life of diazepam and other central nervous system (CNS) depressants is increased. Other common SSRIs are fluvoxamine, paroxetine, and citalopram. Other prescribed antidepressants include selective serotonin-norepinephrine reuptake inhibitors (SNRIs), tricyclics, trazodone, mirtazapine, nefazodone, and maprotiline.

KEY FACT

Increased gingival bleeding and tenderness associated with the menstrual cycle require close periodontal monitoring. Periodontal maintenance should be adjusted to the individual patient's needs. If problematic, 3- to 4-month recall intervals should be recommended.

The PMS patient may be difficult to treat because of emotional and physiologic sensitivity. The dentist should treat the gingival and oral mucosal tissues gently. Gauze pads or cotton rolls should be moistened with a lubricant, chlorhexidine rinse, or water before placing them in the aphtha-prone patient. Careful retraction of the oral mucosa, cheeks, and lips is necessary in patients prone to aphthous or herpetic lesions. Because the hypoglycemic threshold is elevated, the clinician should advise the patient to have a light snack before her appointment. Of menstruating women, 70% have PMS symptoms, but only 5% meet the strict diagnostic criteria.

Because women's oral health is more vulnerable during the menstrual cycle, dysbiotic changes in the microbial ecosystem could cause a transient deterioration of oral health if oral hygiene is not maintained.[14]

Pregnancy

Periodontal Manifestations

The link between pregnancy and periodontal inflammation has been known for many years. In 1778, Vermeeren discussed "tooth pains" in pregnancy. In 1818, Pitcarin[124] described gingival hyperplasia in pregnancy. Despite awareness regarding pregnancy and its

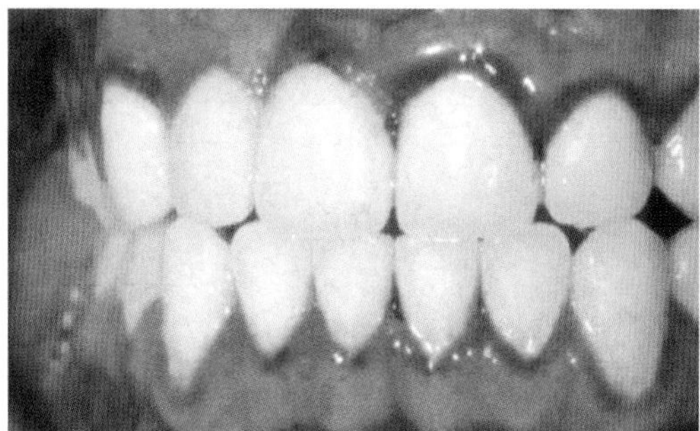

Fig. 28.2 Moderate form of pregnancy gingivitis.

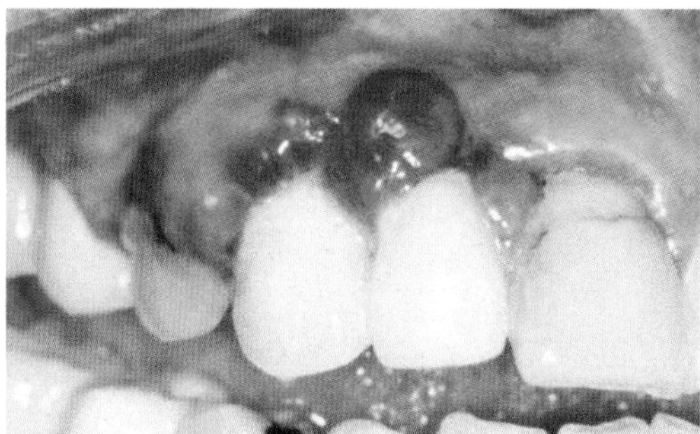

Fig. 28.3 Pyogenic granuloma of pregnancy (i.e., pregnancy tumor).

effect on periodontal disease, only recently has evidence indicated an inverse relationship with systemic health. Research confirms that periodontal disease alters the systemic health of the patient and may potentially adversely affect the well-being of the fetus by elevating the risk for preterm low-birth-weight (PLBW) infants.

In 1877, Pinard[123] recorded the first case of pregnancy gingivitis. Only recently has periodontal research begun to focus on causative mechanisms. Pregnancy gingivitis is extremely common, occurring in 30% to 100% of pregnant women.[55,79,80,87,138] It is characterized by erythema, edema, hyperplasia, and increased bleeding. Histologically, the description is the same as for gingivitis. However, the etiologic factors are different despite clinical and histologic similarities. Cases range from mild to severe inflammation (Fig. 28.2), which can progress to severe hyperplasia, pain, and bleeding (Figs. 28.3 and 28.4).

Other growths that resemble pregnancy granulomas must be ruled out, such as central giant cell granulomas or underlying systemic diseases. Periodontal status before pregnancy may influence the progression or severity as the circulating hormones fluctuate. The anterior region of the mouth is affected more often, and interproximal sites tend to be most involved.[31] Increased tissue edema can lead to increased pocket depths and may be associated with transient tooth mobility.[114] Anterior site inflammation can be exacerbated by increased mouth breathing, primarily in the third trimester, from pregnancy rhinitis. The gingiva is the most common site involved (approximately 70% of cases), followed by the tongue and lips, buccal mucosa, and palate.[138] An increase in attachment loss can represent active periodontal infection accelerated by pregnancy.[80]

Pyogenic granulomas (i.e., pregnancy tumors or pregnancy epulis) occur in 0.2% to 9.6% of pregnancies. They are clinically and histologically indistinguishable from pyogenic granulomas occurring in nonpregnant women or in men. Pyogenic granulomas appear most often during the second or third month of pregnancy. Clinically, they bleed easily and become hyperplastic and nodular. When excised, the lesions usually do not leave a large defect. They may be sessile or pedunculated and ulcerated, ranging in color from purplish red to deep blue, depending on the vascularity of the lesion and degree of venous stasis.[12] The lesion classically occurs in an area of gingivitis and is associated with poor oral hygiene and calculus. Alveolar bone loss is usually not associated with pyogenic granulomas of pregnancy.

Role of Pregnancy Hormones

Subgingival Plaque Composition

Epidemiologic studies indicate a relationship between the level of home care and the severity of gingival inflammation. It appears that the association between signs of gingival inflammation and the amount of plaque is greater after parturition than during pregnancy. An alteration in the compositions of subgingival plaque occurs during pregnancy. Kornman and Loesche[75] found that during the second trimester, gingivitis and gingival bleeding increased without an increase in plaque levels. Bacterial anaerobic/aerobic ratios increased in addition to proportions of *Bacteroides melaninogenicus* and *P. intermedia* (2.2% to 10.1%). The study authors suggested that estradiol or progesterone could substitute for menadione (vitamin K) as an essential growth factor for *P. intermedia* but not *Porphyromonas gingivalis* or *Eikenella corrodens.* There was also an increase in *P. gingivalis* during the 21st through 27th weeks of gestation, but this was not statistically significant. The relative increase in the numbers of *P. intermedia* may be a more sensitive indicator of an altered systemic hormonal situation than clinical parameters of gingivitis.[148]

One study concluded that subgingival levels of bacteria associated with periodontitis did not change. *P. gingivalis* and *Tannerella forsythia* counts were higher and associated with bleeding on probing at week 12.[2] Bacterial challenge to the gingival tissues, quantitatively (plaque scores) and qualitatively (*P. gingivalis*), appears to affect the level of gingival inflammation observed during pregnancy.[21]

Periodontal Disease and Preterm, Low-Birth-Weight Infants

Although several studies support a causal relationship regarding the hypothesis that periodontitis during pregnancy poses an increased risk of adverse pregnancy outcomes, there are conflicting results. Variations in study results may result from confounding factors, effect modifiers, populations studied, the timing of intervention or evaluation, and the severity of periodontal disease based on different definitions. The majority of high-quality randomized controlled trials reveal that nonsurgical periodontal therapy during the second trimester of gestation does not improve pregnancy outcomes. From a biologic standpoint, this can be partially explained by the fact that therapy rendered at the fourth to sixth month of pregnancy is too late to prevent placental colonization by periodontal pathogens and consequently incapable of affecting pathogen-induced injury at the feto-placental unit. Thus, interventions during the preconception period may be more meaningful.[175]

Several systematic reviews indicate that periodontal disease[14,140,160,165,173] adversely affects pregnancy outcomes. Intervention trials have shown a positive effect with periodontal therapy and reduction of adverse pregnancy outcomes,[14,56,64,85,86,110] but three large multicenter trials in the United States did not support these results.[95,107,149] Studies indicate that routine nonsurgical periodontal therapy after the first trimester is not associated with adverse pregnancy outcomes.[95]

Initially, Offenbacher and colleagues[109] provided evidence that untreated periodontal disease in pregnant women could be a significant risk factor for preterm (<37 weeks' gestation) and low birth-weight (<2500 g) infants. The relationship between genitourinary

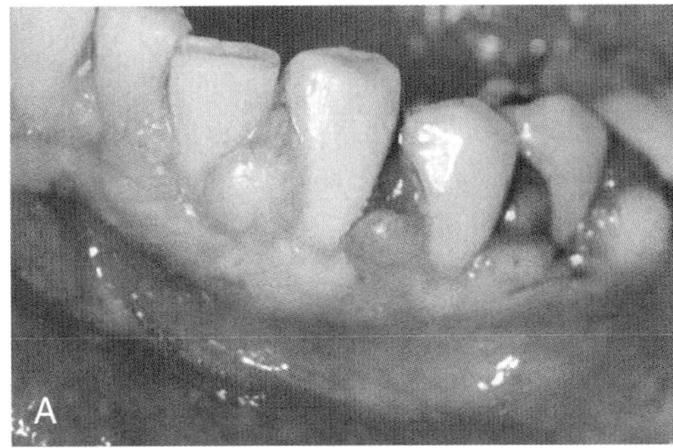

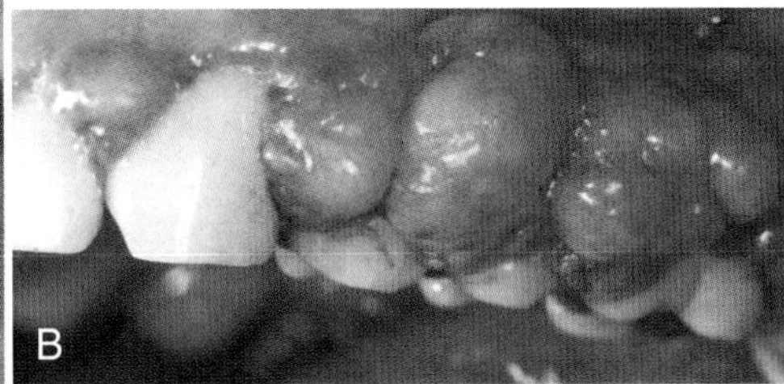

Fig. 28.4 Severe pregnancy gingivitis with hyperplasia can occur in patients with poorly controlled non–insulin-dependent diabetes mellitus. (A) Moderate gingival enlargement. (B) Severe gingival enlargement.

tract infection and PLBW infants is well documented in human and animal studies. Periodontal researchers, suspecting periodontal disease as another source of infection, found that otherwise low-risk mothers of PLBW infants had significantly more periodontal attachment loss than control mothers having normal-weight infants at birth.

Current opinion is that the correlation of periodontal disease with PLBW birth may result from infection and is mediated indirectly, principally by the translocation of bacterial products such as endotoxin (i.e., lipopolysaccharide [LPS]) and the action of maternally produced inflammatory mediators.[43] Jared and coworkers[62] found that fetal exposure to oral pathogens in utero increased the risk of neonatal intensive care unit admission and extended length of stay. Concentrations of biologically active molecules, such as PGE_2 and TNF-α, which usually are involved in normal parturition, are raised to artificially high levels by the infection process, which can foster premature labor.[4]

Gram-negative bacteria in periodontal diseases may permit their selective overgrowth or invasion within the genitourinary tract. Han and associates[54] documented hematogenous spread of oral bacteria to the amnion, and Madianos and colleagues[91] showed that oral bacteria crossed the placental barrier and triggered an immune response by the fetus.

Gingival crevicular fluid (GCF) levels of PGE_2 were positively associated with intraamniotic PGE_2 levels (P = .018), suggesting that gram-negative periodontal infection presents a systemic challenge sufficient to initiate the onset of premature labor as a source of LPS or through stimulation of secondary inflammatory mediators such as PGE_2 and interleukin-1 beta (IL-1β).[28] Offenbacher and coworkers[108] suggested a dose-response relationship for increasing GCF PGE_2 as a marker of current periodontal disease activity and decreasing birth weight.

Four organisms associated with mature plaque and progressing periodontitis—*T. forsythia, P. gingivalis, A. actinomycetemcomitans,* and *Treponema denticola*—were detected at higher levels in PLBW mothers compared with normal-birth-weight controls. Despite research supporting the association of periodontal disease and PLBW,[29,30] more studies with improved methodology are needed to assess the validity of the association.

KEY FACT

Current opinion suggests a possible association between periodontal disease and preterm, low-birth-weight (PLBW) infants, but further investigation is warranted. Adverse pregnancy events can result from an infection that is mediated by one of two major pathways: (1) directly by oral **microorganisms** or (2) indirectly, principally by the translocation of bacterial products such as endotoxin (i.e., lipopolysaccharide) and the action of maternally produced inflammatory mediators.

Preeclampsia

A systematic review of preeclampsia and periodontitis indicated an increased risk during pregnancy. Preeclampsia is a life-threatening condition in late pregnancy that is characterized by high blood pressure and excess protein in the urine. High C-reactive protein levels also are associated with preeclampsia in this population.[32,136,146,164]

Maternal Immunoresponse

The maternal immune system is thought to be suppressed during pregnancy. This response may allow the fetus to survive as an allograft. Documentation of immunosuppressive factors in the sera of pregnant women shows a marked increase of monocytes (which in large numbers inhibit in vitro proliferative responses to mitogens, allogenic cells, and soluble antigen),[162] and pregnancy-specific β_1-glycoproteins contribute to diminished lymphocyte responsiveness to mitogens and antigens.[13] The ratio of peripheral helper T cells to suppressor T cells (CD4/CD8) decreases throughout pregnancy.[8,128]

The changes in maternal immunoresponsiveness suggest an increased susceptibility to developing gingival inflammation. In one study, the gingival index was higher, but percentages of T3 (CD3), T4 (CD4), and B cells appeared to decrease in peripheral blood and gingival tissues during pregnancy compared with a control group.[1] Other studies report decreased PMN (i.e., neutrophil) chemotaxis, depression of cell-mediated immunity, phagocytosis, and decreased T-cell response with elevated ovarian hormone levels, especially progesterone.[126] Decreased in vitro responses of peripheral blood lymphocytes to several mitogens and to a preparation of *P. intermedia* have been reported.[15,84,114] Evidence suggests a decrease in the absolute numbers of $CD4^+$ cells in peripheral blood during pregnancy compared with postpartum.[99,107]

Lapp and colleagues[78] suggested that high levels of progesterone during pregnancy affect the development of localized inflammation by downregulation of IL-6 production, rendering the gingiva less efficient at resisting the inflammatory challenges produced by bacteria. Progesterone mediates a series of immune adaptations that preferentially promote continued pregnancy.[142] Another study indicated that live preterm birth was associated with decreased levels of immunoglobulin G (IgG) antibody to periodontal pathogens in women with periodontitis when assessed during the second trimester but was not associated with birth outcomes.[34]

Ovarian hormones stimulate the production of prostaglandins, particularly PGE_1 and PGE_2, which are potent mediators of the inflammatory response. With the prostaglandin acting as an immunosuppressant, gingival inflammation can increase when the mediator level is high.[37,112] Kinnby and coworkers[71] found that high progesterone levels during pregnancy influenced plasminogen activator inhibitor type 2 (PAI-2) and disturbed the balance of the fibrinolytic system. Because PAI-2 is an important inhibitor of tissue proteolysis, this research implies that components of the fibrinolytic system may be involved in the development of pregnancy gingivitis.

During pregnancy, sex hormone levels rise dramatically (Box 28.1). Progesterone reaches levels of 100 ng/mL, 10 times the peak luteal phase of menses. Estradiol in the plasma may reach levels 30 times higher than during the reproductive cycle. In early pregnancy and during the normal ovarian cycle, the corpus luteum is the major source of estrogen and progesterone. During pregnancy, the placenta begins to produce estrogens and progesterone.

Estrogen regulates cellular proliferation, differentiation, and keratinization, whereas progesterone influences the permeability of the microvasculature,[81,82] alters the rate and pattern of collagen production, and increases the metabolic breakdown of folate (necessary for tissue maintenance).[177] High concentrations of sex hormones in gingival tissues, saliva, serum, and GCF also can exaggerate the response.

Regulation of most cellular processes by hormones occurs through the interaction of these products with intracellular receptors. The resulting effects depend on the concentration of unbound hormone diffused through the cell membrane. Vittek and associates[167] demonstrated specific estrogen and progesterone receptors in gingival tissues, providing direct biochemical evidence that this tissue functions as a target organ for sex hormones. Muramatsu and Takaesu[103] found increasing concentrations of sex hormones in saliva from the first month and peaking in the ninth month of gestation, along with increasing percentages of *P. intermedia.* Probing depth, the number of gingival sites with bleeding, and redness increased until 1 month after delivery. Evidence indicates sex hormone concentration, which may substitute vitamin K as a growth factor for anaerobic bacteria in GCF, may provide a growth media for periodontal pathogens.[74]

BOX 28.1 Causes of Gingival Responses to Elevated Estrogen and Progesterone During Pregnancy

Subgingival Plaque Composition
- Increase in anaerobic/aerobic ratio
- Higher concentrations of *Prevotella intermedia* (i.e., substitutes sex hormone for vitamin K growth factor)
- Higher concentrations of *Bacteroides melaninogenicus*
- Higher concentrations of *Porphyromonas gingivalis*

Maternal Immunoresponse
- Depression of cell-mediated immunity
- Decrease in neutrophil chemotaxis
- Depression of antibody and T-cell responses
- Decrease in ratio of peripheral helper T cells to suppressor-cytotoxic T cells (i.e., CD4/CD8 ratio)
- Cytotoxicity directed against macrophages and B cells can diminish immunoresponsiveness
- Decrease in absolute numbers of $CD3^+$, $CD4^+$, and $CD19^+$ cells in peripheral blood during pregnancy versus postpartum

Stimulation of prostaglandin production

Sex Hormone Concentration

Estrogen
- Increases cellular proliferation in blood vessels (e.g., in the endometrium)
- Decreases keratinization while increasing epithelial glycogen
- Specific receptors are found in gingival tissues

Progesterone
- Increases vascular dilation and increases permeability, resulting in edema and accumulation of inflammatory cells
- Increases proliferation of newly formed capillaries in gingival tissues (i.e., increased bleeding tendency)
- Alters rate and pattern of collagen production
- Increases metabolic breakdown of folate (i.e., folate deficiency can inhibit tissue repair)
- Specific receptors are found in gingival tissues
- Decreases plasminogen activator inhibitor type 2, increasing tissue proteolysis

Estrogen and Progesterone
- Affect ground substance of connective tissue by increasing fluidity
- Concentrations increase in saliva and fluid, with increased concentrations in serum

Other Oral Manifestations of Pregnancy

Perimolysis (i.e., acid erosion of teeth) can occur if morning sickness or esophageal reflux is severe and involves repeated vomiting of the gastric contents. Severe reflux can cause scarring of the esophageal sphincter, and the patient may become more susceptible to GERD later in life.

Xerostomia is a frequent complaint among pregnant women. One study found this persistent dryness in 44% of pregnant participants.[35]

A rare finding in pregnancy is *ptyalism* (i.e., sialorrhea). Excessive secretion of saliva usually begins at 2 to 3 weeks gestation and may abate at the end of the first trimester. The cause of ptyalism has not been identified, but it may result from the inability of a nauseated gravid woman to swallow normal amounts of saliva, rather than from a true increase in saliva production.[25]

Because pregnancy places the woman in an immunocompromised state, the clinician must be aware of her total health. Gestational diabetes, leukemia, and other medical conditions may appear during pregnancy.

Clinical Management

A thorough medical history is an imperative component of the periodontal examination, especially for the pregnant patient. Because of immunologic alterations, increased blood volume (i.e., ruling out mitral valve prolapse and heart murmurs), and fetal interactions, the clinician must diligently and consistently monitor the patient's medical and periodontal stability. Medical history discussion should include pregnancy complications, previous miscarriages, and recent history of cramping, spotting, or pernicious vomiting. The patient's obstetrician should be contacted to discuss her medical status, periodontal or dental needs, and the proposed treatment plan.

Establishing a healthy oral environment and maintaining optimal oral hygiene are primary objectives for the pregnant patient. A preventive periodontal program consisting of nutritional counseling and rigorous plaque control measures in the dental office and at home should be reinforced. Women of childbearing age, especially those trying to conceive, should be informed of the possible impact of inflammation on the unborn.

Plaque Control

The increased tendency for gingival inflammation during pregnancy should be clearly explained to the patient so that acceptable oral hygiene techniques may be taught, reinforced, and monitored throughout pregnancy. Scaling, polishing, and root planing can be performed whenever necessary during pregnancy. Some practitioners avoid the use of high-alcohol-content antimicrobial rinses for pregnant women and prefer to use non–alcohol-based oral rinses.

Prenatal Fluoride

Prescribing prenatal fluoride supplements has been an area of controversy. Although two studies have claimed beneficial results,[44,45] others suggest that the clinical efficacy of prenatal fluoride supplements is uncertain and the mechanism by which they might impart cariostasis is unclear.[31] The American Dental Association (ADA) does not recommend the use of prenatal fluoride because its efficacy has not been demonstrated. The American Academy of Pediatric Dentistry also supports this position. The American Academy of Pediatrics has no stated position on prescribing prenatal fluorides.

Treatment

Elective Dental Treatment

Other than good plaque control, it is prudent to avoid elective dental care if possible during the first trimester and the last half of the third trimester. The first trimester is the period of organogenesis when the fetus is highly susceptible to environmental influences. In the last half of the third trimester, a hazard of premature delivery exists because the uterus is very sensitive to external stimuli. Prolonged chairtime may need to be avoided because the woman is most uncomfortable at this time.

Supine hypotensive syndrome may occur. In a semi-reclining or supine position, the great vessels, particularly the inferior vena cava, are compressed by the gravid uterus. By interfering with venous return, this compression causes maternal hypotension, decreased cardiac output, and eventual loss of consciousness. Supine hypotensive syndrome can usually be reversed by turning the patient on her left side, which removes pressure on the vena cava and allows blood to return from the lower extremities and pelvic area. A preventive 6-inch soft wedge (i.e., rolled towel) should be placed on the patient's right side when she is reclined for clinical treatment.

Early in the second trimester is the safest period for providing routine dental care. The emphasis at this time is on controlling active disease and eliminating potential problems that can arise in late pregnancy. Major elective oral or periodontal surgery may be postponed until after delivery. Pregnancy tumors that are painful, interfere with mastication, or continue to bleed or suppurate after mechanical debridement may require excision and biopsy before delivery.

COVID

Because there are no current guidelines regarding the management of oral lesions and dental emergencies during the COVID-19 pandemic, the clinician should follow the CDC's Interium Infection Prevention and Control Recommendations for HealthCare Personnel During the Coronavirus Disease 2019 (COVID-19) Pandemic.[24] The clinician must consider what is medically necessary and what is in the best interest of the patient as well as the outcome of the unborn.[151]

It is hypothesized that when the inflammatory cascade is activated during pregnancy, interventions targeting this pathway may be ineffective in reducing the rate of preterm birth. Treatment during pregnancy may be too late; it is possible that treatment before pregnancy (in nulliparous women) or in the period between pregnancies (for multiparous women, especially those with a history of preterm birth) may yield more promising results.[46]

The American Academy of Periodontology (www.perio.org) developed a position statement regarding the need to provide proper periodontal therapy for pregnant patients (Fig. 28.5). Because of research indicating a possible impact on the fetus, acute infection, abscesses, or other potential disseminating sources of sepsis may warrant prompt intervention irrespective of the stage of pregnancy.[3] A consensus report of a Joint European Workshop of Periodontology and an American Academy of Periodontology Workshop stated that "although periodontal therapy has been shown to be safe and leads to improved periodontal conditions in pregnant women, case-related periodontal therapy, without systemic antibiotics does not reduce overall rates of preterm birth and low birth weight."[139]

CLINICAL CORRELATION

It is prudent to avoid elective dental care during the first trimester and the last half of the third trimester. The first trimester is the period of organogenesis, and the fetus is highly susceptible to environmental influences. During the last half of the third trimester, the fetus is vulnerable to premature delivery. The uterus is very sensitive to external stimuli. The second trimester is the safest period for providing routine dental care.

Dental Radiographs

The safety of dental radiography during pregnancy has been well established, provided items such as high-speed film, filtration, collimation, and lead aprons are used. However, it is most desirable not to have any irradiation during pregnancy, especially during the first trimester, because the developing fetus is particularly susceptible to radiation damage.[83] When radiographs are needed for diagnosis, the most important aid for the patient is the protective lead apron. Studies have shown that when an apron is used during contemporary dental radiography, gonadal and fetal radiation is virtually unmeasurable.[11]

Even with the obvious safety of dental radiography, x-ray films should be taken selectively during pregnancy and only when necessary and appropriate to aid in diagnosis and treatment. In most cases, only bitewing, panoramic, or selected periapical films are indicated.

Medications

Drug therapy for the pregnant patient is controversial because drugs can affect the fetus by diffusion across the placenta. Prescriptions should be used only for the duration absolutely essential for the pregnant patient's well-being and only after careful consideration of potential side effects. The classification system established by the U.S. Food and Drug Administration (FDA) in 1979 to rate fetal risk levels associated with many prescription drugs provides safety guidelines (Box 28.2). The prudent practitioner should consult references,

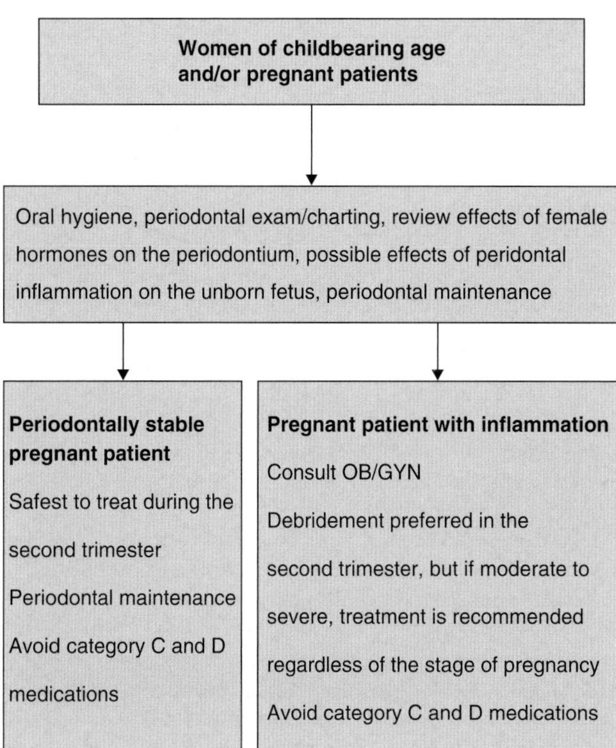

Fig. 28.5 Treatment algorithm for the pregnant patient.

BOX 28.2 FDA Drug Classification System Based on Potential to Cause Birth Defects

A: Controlled studies enrolling women fail to demonstrate a risk to the fetus in the first trimester (there is no evidence of risk in later trimesters), and the possibility of fetal harm appears remote.
B: Animal reproduction studies have not demonstrated a fetal risk, but there are no controlled studies in pregnant women; or animal reproduction studies have shown an adverse effect (other than decreased fertility) that was not confirmed in controlled studies in women in the first trimester (there is no evidence of risk in later trimesters).
C: Studies in animals have revealed adverse effects on the fetus (i.e., teratogenic, embryocidal, or other), and there are no controlled studies in women, or studies in women and animals are not available. Drugs should be given only if the potential benefit justifies the potential risk to the fetus.
D: There is positive evidence of human fetal risk, but the benefits of use in pregnant women may be acceptable despite the risk (e.g., the drug is needed in a life-threatening situation or for a serious disease for which safer drugs cannot be used or are ineffective).
X: Studies in animals or humans have demonstrated fetal abnormalities, or there is evidence of fetal risk based on human experience or both, and the risk of using the drug in pregnant women clearly outweighs any possible benefit. The drug is contraindicated in women who are or may become pregnant.

such as Briggs and colleagues' *Drugs in Pregnancy and Lactation*[19] and Olin's *Drug Facts and Comparisons,*[113] for information on the FDA pregnancy risk factors associated with prescription drugs.

Ideally, no drug should be administered during pregnancy, especially in the first trimester.[83] However, it is sometimes impossible to adhere to this rule. Fortunately, most common drugs in dental practice can be given during pregnancy with relative safety, although there are a few important exceptions. Tables 28.1–28.3 provide guidelines for anesthetic and analgesic, antibiotic, and sedative-hypnotic drugs, respectively.[129,159]

Antibiotics are often needed in periodontal therapy. The effect of a particular medication on the fetus depends on the type of antimicrobial, dosage, trimester, and duration of the course of therapy.[115] Research regarding subgingival irrigation and local site delivery in relation to the developing fetus is inadequate.

Breastfeeding

Usually, there is a risk that the drug can enter breast milk and be transferred to the nursing infant, on whom exposure could have adverse effects (Tables 28.4 and 28.5). Unfortunately, there is little conclusive information about drug dosage and effects through breast milk; however, retrospective clinical studies and empiric observations coupled with known pharmacologic pathways allow recommendations to be made.[83] The amount of drug excreted in breast milk is usually not more than 1% to 2% of the maternal dose; therefore it is highly unlikely that most drugs have any pharmacologic significance for the infant.[172]

The mother should take prescribed drugs just after breastfeeding and then avoid nursing for 4 hours or more if possible[83,150] to decrease the drug concentration in breast milk.

Oral Contraceptives

Women may have responses to oral contraceptives (OCs) similar to those seen in pregnant patients. Mullally and associates found that current users of OCs had poorer periodontal health.[102] An

TABLE 28.1 Local Anesthetic and Analgesic Administration During Pregnancy

Drug	FDA Category	During Pregnancy
Local Anesthetics[a]		
Lidocaine	B	Yes
Mepivacaine	C	Use with caution; consult physician
Prilocaine	B	Yes
Bupivacaine	C	Use with caution; consult physician
Etidocaine	B	Yes
Procaine	C	Use with caution; consult physician
Articaine	B	Yes; no blocks
Analgesics		
Aspirin	C/D, third trimester	Caution; avoid in third trimester
Acetaminophen	B	Yes
Ibuprofen	B/D, third trimester	Use with caution; avoid in third trimester
Codeine[b]	C	Use with caution; consult physician
Hydrocodone[b]	B	Use with caution; consult physician
Oxycodone[b]	B	Use with caution; consult physician
Propoxyphene	C	Use with caution; consult physician

[a]Can use vasoconstrictors if necessary.
[b]Avoid prolonged use.
FDA, U.S. Food and Drug Administration.

exaggerated response to local irritants occurs in gingival tissues, especially when used for longer durations.[125] Inflammation ranges from mild edema and erythema to severe inflammation with hemorrhagic or hyperplasic gingival tissues. It has been reported that more exudate is present in the inflamed gingival tissues of OC users than in those of pregnant women.[147,178]

Investigators have suggested several mechanisms for the heightened response in gingival tissues. Kalkwarf[68] reported that the response might be caused by an altered microvasculature, increased gingival permeability, and increased synthesis of prostaglandin. Levels of PGE, a potent mediator of inflammation,[38] appear to rise significantly with increasing levels of sex hormones. Jensen and colleagues[66] found dramatic microbial changes in pregnant and OC groups compared with a nonpregnant group. A 16-fold increase in *Bacteroides* species was seen in the OC group versus the nonpregnant group, despite no statistically significant clinical differences in the gingival index or GCF flow. The study authors found that the increased female sex hormones substituting for the naphthoquinone requirement of certain *Bacteroides* species was most likely responsible for this increase.

OC-associated gingival inflammation may become chronic (vs. the acute inflammation of pregnancy) because of the extended periods that women are exposed to elevated levels of estrogen

TABLE 28.2 Antibiotic Administration During Pregnancy

Drugs	FDA Category	During Pregnancy	Risks
Penicillin	B	Yes	Diarrhea
Erythromycin	B	Yes; avoid estolate form	Intrahepatic jaundice in mother
Clindamycin	B	Yes, with caution	Drug concentrated in fetal bone, spleen, lung, and liver
Cephalosporins	B	Yes	Limited information
Tetracycline	D	Avoid	Depression of bone growth, enamel hypoplasia, gray-brown tooth discoloration
Ciprofloxacin	C	Avoid	Possible developing cartilage erosion
Metronidazole	B	Avoid; controversial	Theoretic carcinogenic data in animals
Gentamicin	C	Caution; consult physician	Limited information
Ototoxicity			
Vancomycin	C	Caution; consult physician	Limited information
Clarithromycin	D	Avoid; use only if potential benefit justifies risk to fetus	Limited information Adverse effects on pregnancy, outcome, and embryo and fetal development in animals

FDA, U.S. Food and Drug Administration.

TABLE 28.3 Sedative-Hypnotic Drug Administration During Pregnancy

Drugs	FDA Category	During Pregnancy
Benzodiazepines	D	Avoid
Barbiturates	D	Avoid
Nitrous oxide	Not assigned	Avoid in first trimester; otherwise use with caution; consult physician

FDA, U.S. Food and Drug Administration.

TABLE 28.4 Local Anesthetic and Analgesic Administration During Breastfeeding

Drug	During Breastfeeding
Local Anesthetics	
Lidocaine	Yes
Mepivacaine	Yes
Prilocaine	Yes
Bupivacaine	Yes
Etidocaine	Yes
Procaine	Yes
Analgesics	
Aspirin	Avoid
Acetaminophen	Yes
Ibuprofen	Yes
Codeine	Yes
Hydrocodone	No data
Oxycodone	Yes
Propoxyphene	Yes

TABLE 28.5 Antibiotic and Sedative-Hypnotic Administration During Breastfeeding

Drugs	During Breastfeeding
Antibiotics[a]	
Penicillins	Yes
Erythromycin	Yes
Clindamycin	Yes, with caution
Cephalosporins	Yes
Tetracycline	Avoid
Ciprofloxacin	Avoid
Metronidazole	Avoid
Gentamicin	Avoid
Vancomycin	Avoid
Sedative-Hypnotics	
Benzodiazepines	Avoid
Barbiturates	Avoid
Nitrous oxide	Yes

[a]Antibiotics carry a risk of diarrhea and sensitization in the mother and infant.

and progesterone.[73,118] Some have reported that the inflammation increases with prolonged use of OCs. Kalkwarf[68] did not find that duration of use made a significant difference, but the brands used resulted in different responses. Further studies are needed to elucidate the effects of dosage, duration, and type of OC on the periodontium. The concentration of female sex hormones in current OCs is significantly less than that of the 1970s while providing the same level of contraceptive efficacy.

Salivary composition changed notably in patients taking OCs in studies from the 1970s. Decreased concentrations of protein, sialic acid, hexosamine fucose, hydrogen ions, and total electrolytes have been reported. Salivary flow rates were increased in one report[92] and decreased in 30% of subjects in another report.[27]

The dental literature reports that women taking OCs experience a twofold to threefold increase in the incidence of localized osteitis after extraction of mandibular third molars.[153] The higher incidence of osteitis among these patients may be attributed to the effects of OCs (i.e., estrogens) on clotting factors. However, several studies refute these findings.[17] Evidence is inconclusive on osteitis after third molar extraction and OC use. A spotty melanotic pigmentation of the skin may occur with OC use. This suggests a relationship between the use of OCs and the occurrence of gingival melanosis,[57] especially in fair-skinned individuals.

Management

The medical history should include OCs along with other medications, and a discussion should include questions regarding OCs with women of childbearing age. The patient should be informed of the oral and periodontal side effects of OCs and the need for meticulous home care and compliance with periodontal maintenance. Treatment of gingival inflammation exaggerated by OCs should include establishing an oral hygiene program and eliminating local predisposing factors. Periodontal surgery may be indicated if resolution after initial therapy (i.e., scaling and root planing) is inadequate. It may be advisable to perform extraction of teeth (especially third molars) on nonestrogenic days of the OC cycle (i.e., days 23 to 28) to reduce the risk of a postoperative localized osteitis;[41] however, evidence of this association is inconclusive and warrants further investigation.

Although results from animal studies have demonstrated that antibiotic interference adversely affects contraceptive sex hormone levels, several human studies have failed to support such an interaction.[10,42,104,106,145] This issue is controversial, and it is currently questionable if antibiotics could render OCs ineffective in preventing pregnancy. In 1991, an ADA report stated that all women of childbearing age should be informed of the possible reduced efficacy of steroid OCs during antibiotic therapy and advised women to use additional forms of contraception during short-term antibiotic therapy.[7] During long-term antibiotic therapy, women should consult their physician about using high-dose OC preparations. Although only research regarding oral manifestations attributed to OCs has been reported in the literature, the same effects presumably occur with the use of contraceptive implants. Similarly, the remote possibility of reduced efficacy of contraceptive implants with concurrent antibiotic use exists, and women can follow the same precautions as with OC use.

Menopause

Female life expectancy is 80+ years, and many women live 40% of their lives in menopause. This cohort represents a large number of the patients who are seen in clinical practices. Dental clinicians must be aware of the effects of reduced hormones on the periodontal tissues and the systemic changes that may manifest.

Clinical Management

It is the clinician's responsibility to review the patient's medical history and keep the information up to date. Because of possible alterations in oral soft and osseous tissues during perimenopause and after menopause, appropriate questioning regarding hormonal changes should take place and be documented.

The clinician, however, must understand the patient's medication history with regard to bisphosphonate, monoclonal antibodies, or other prescriptions used to treat osteoporosis as well as their impact on the outcomes of periodontal and implant therapy.

Conclusions

Clinical periodontal therapy includes an understanding of the clinician's role in the total health and well-being of female patients. Dentists do not treat localized infections without affecting other systems and the fetus or the breastfed infant. The periodontal and systemic difficulties of female patients can alter conventional therapy.

The cyclic nature of the female sex hormones often is reflected in the gingival tissues as initial signs and symptoms. Medical histories and discussions should include thoughtful investigation of the individual patient's problems and needs. Questioning should reflect hormonal stability and medications associated with regulation. Patients should be educated regarding the profound effects sex hormones have on periodontal and oral tissues and the consistent need for home and office removal of local irritants.

Research regarding female issues and medical/periodontal therapy is in process. In the near future, information about the specific management and causes of sex hormone-mediated infections will enhance dentists' ability to provide quality care to their patients.

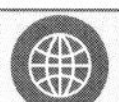
A Case Scenario is found on the companion website eBooks.Health.Elsevier.com.

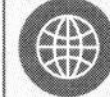
References for this chapter are found on the companion website eBooks.Health.Elsevier.com.

CHAPTER 29

Aging and Periodontal Health: A Long-Term Relationship

Evelyn Chung | Reeva Mincer | Ting-Ling Chang

CHAPTER OUTLINE

Introduction

Throughout the world, the proportion of the elderly population to the younger population is increasing. By 2050, over 21% of the world population will be over the age of 65 and will exceed the number of children for the first time in history.[67] The prevalence of aging-associated medical conditions has increased due to the longer life expectancy in more developed countries.[19,23] Similarly, older people are retaining more of their dentition into their eighth and ninth decades of life. The World Health Organization and other international dental associations stress the importance of oral health and have made it a priority for each person to retain more than 20 teeth by age 80.[64] This patient population presents with unique challenges not found in younger populations. Because of the entwining relationship between systemic and oral health, how oral health care providers approach the overall periodontal planning and treatment differ from that of the younger population groups. This chapter presents information about the relationship between aging, systemic conditions, and oral health.

Immunosenescence and the Periodontium

If people are retaining more of their teeth longer, then there may be more risk of periodontal disease. It has been reported that there may be an increase in loss of periodontal support with age, but only a small portion of patients actually experience severe periodontal destruction.[5,6,11] Older studies reported that the occurrence and severity of periodontitis were more associated with accumulated exposure rather than just the biologic effect of aging, but newer studies indicate that aging may increase the susceptibility to periodontal disease.[103] Aging alone may lead to physiological loss of periodontal attachment and even alveolar bone that is not necessarily pathological. But in the presence of periodontal inflammation, these parameters are exacerbated and can lead to functional loss.[48] It is possible to consider that aging results in changes in the immune response. This is commonly referred to as "immunosenescence." It is a progressive modification of the immune system that leads to greater susceptibility to infections, neoplasia, and autoimmune manifestations as a result of prolonged antigenic stimulation.[59]

This phenomenon is usually coupled with a progressive increase in inflammation, often referred to as "inflammaging."[29] The term, "inflammaging" has been gaining popularity to describe the development of chronic inflammatory states often seen in older patients, but not necessarily associated with infection.[31] There are elevated levels of pro-inflammatory cytokines, clotting factors, and acute-phase proteins in the steady state.[28] It has been hypothesized that the responses in the innate and adaptive immune systems are reduced in the aging population leading to an overall increase in the inflammatory environment. These responses are not indicative of immunodeficiency, but rather a dysregulation of the immune response.[37] Periodontitis has been considered as a possible contributor to chronic inflammatory conditions seen in the elderly population.[10]

Interestingly this condition is seen in both successful and unsuccessful aging populations, which leads to the hypothesis that there may be a threshold between immunosenescence, inflammaging, and successful aging.[30] Successful aging is defined as a low probability of disease and disease-related disability, high cognitive and physical functional capacity, and active engagement with life.[77] From a periodontal standpoint, this would include older people with intact dentition, limited attachment loss, and good function. The combined effect of aging and the presence of inflammation may lead to increases in periodontal destruction and disability (Fig. 29.1).[41] In other words, the age-altered changes in the immune system can make the aging periodontium more susceptible to periodontitis than in younger populations.[28,58,101] This does not only apply to periodontitis, but to a number of systemic diseases as well.[34,41,60]

Nonimmune Factors and Periodontitis

Nonimmune sources of periodontal deterioration associated with aging have also been proposed. It has been reported that there is a deterioration of type I collagen in periodontal tissues over time.[9] There is progressive atrophy seen in tooth-supporting structures over time. In a study done by Lim et al.,[53] the PDL space of mice was found to have decreased proliferation, loss in density, and disorientation of collagen fibers. There was also decreased bone formation that correlated with an overall decrease in osteoblastic

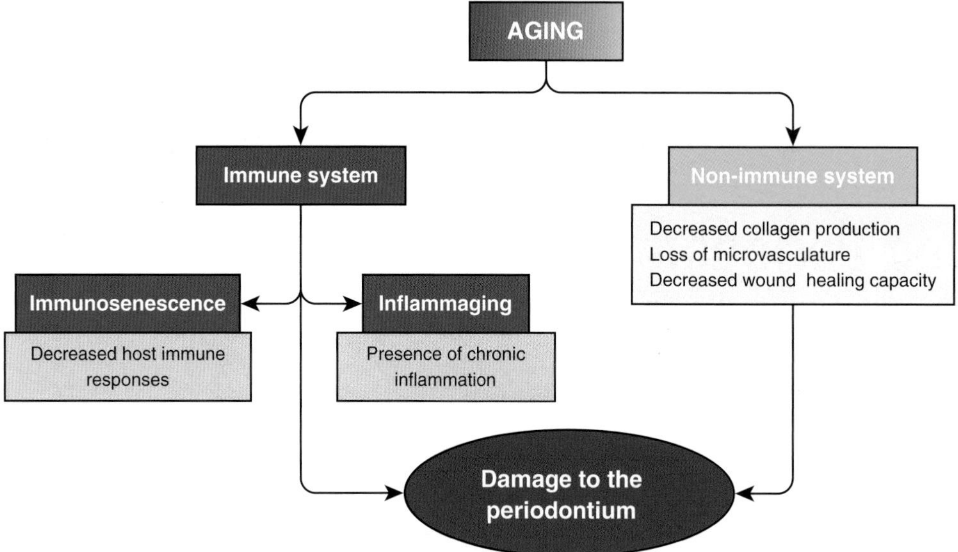

Fig. 29.1 Interaction of immunosenescence, inflammaging, and decreases in nonimmune response can result in loss of periodontal attachment and support.

precursor cells. The decrease in the number of collagen fibers leads to a reduction in elasticity and vascularity. There is also a reduction in metabolic rate. Overall, the regenerative potential of the PDL decreases with age.[105]

It has been commonly reported that people heal more slowly with increasing age. Controlling for confounding factors to actually determine the relationship between aging and delayed wound healing is a challenge. Older skin has been associated with reductions in vascularization, collagen density, and production. In the oral cavity, it presents as gingival recession, reductions in bone height, and thinning of the epithelium. A clinical study done by Engeland et al. in 2006 reported that older patients' palatal mucosal wounds took a statistically significantly longer time to heal than in younger patients and that older women took longer to heal than older men in the same age group. The study also found that patients taking common antihypertensive medications, such as alpha and beta blockers, diuretics, and other medications had smaller wounds in the first 2 days of healing than patients not on these medications.[26] This last finding correlates with the interaction between systemic disease and periodontal disease.

In a study looking at cultures of human gingival fibroblasts, aged fibroblasts showed significant decreases in collagen cell proliferation, migration, and remodeling than younger fibroblasts.[15] The mucosa is less resilient with aging due to a reduction in the microvasculature and decreased epithelial thickness.[16,50] It follows then that there would be deficiencies in wound healing in aged periodontal tissues. Delayed and reduced wound healing capacity means that damaged gingival tissues may not be able to compensate for continuous exposure to inflammatory insults, which then could ultimately result in damage to the periodontium in the aging population (see Fig. 29.1).

Systemic Diseases and Periodontal Considerations

Aging is associated with an increased prevalence of systemic diseases and a subsequent increase in medical therapies. The inevitable decline in physiologic functions, such as salivary flow, manual dexterity, and cognition can lead to detriments in maintaining periodontal health and eventual tooth loss. Studies have linked masticatory disability and the number of missing teeth as risk factors for mortality.[38] Periodontal disease is a chronic disease and its effects accumulate with time and aging. Poor oral health can contribute to increased morbidity and mortality in patients with systemic diseases, such as cardiovascular diseases, diabetes, osteoporosis, and dementia. Oral organisms from cavitated and periodontally infected teeth have been linked to serious systemic infections, such as endocarditis, brain abscesses, joint and bone infections, and sepsis. Bacteremia from an oral source may trigger inflammatory or immunological responses that can cause damage to tissues in distant sites. The chronic inflammatory component of periodontal disease is similar to systemic inflammation in the aging population, previously referred to as "inflammaging."[29] Uncontrolled periodontal disease may have a greater impact on the medical implications of the aging population. The strength of the causative relationship has not been successfully substantiated.

Systemic diseases can also have an impact on the periodontal health of the older patient population. Common disabilities associated with older adults, such as cardiovascular diseases, diabetes, osteoporosis, and cognitive impairments can negatively affect periodontal health due to deterioration of performance of effective oral hygiene as well as from the systemic effects of the disease, and side effects of medications used to treat these diseases. This section will discuss common systemic diseases associated with aging and their relationship with periodontal disease.

Cardiovascular Disease

Poor dental health has often been associated with an increased risk of myocardial infarction and exacerbation of coronary artery disease. Since atherosclerosis and cardiovascular diseases are one of the most common causes of death in the elderly population, there is a great interest in the roles of chronic inflammation and periodontal disease in the pathological process.[22] The proposed mechanisms are multifactorial and a discussion of the actual pathology is covered in Chapter 26. It is likely though that periodontal bacteria, as well as inflammation induced by these bacteria, may contribute to the pathogenesis of atherosclerosis by the increased presence of inflammatory cytokines and prostaglandins in the periodontal tissues and gingival crevicular fluid. These mediators enter the systemic circulation to directly stimulate inflammation.[40,82] This process can also include antibody production against the bacteria that cross-react with host antigens, promoting atherosclerosis.[97] *Porphyromonas gingivalis* has been associated with chronic periodontal disease and detected within atherosclerotic plaques. But other studies indicate that it may not be the invasive aggressor, but a persistent species inducing an inflammatory response and tissue destruction in patients with chronic periodontitis.[36]

Significant increases in levels of C reactive protein have been observed in patients with coronary artery disease and chronic periodontitis.[83] A longitudinal study that followed older men over a 3-year period reported that those with a diagnosis of periodontitis were at greater risk of recurrent acute coronary syndrome.[74] The positive correlation between elevated titers of different periodontal pathogens and patients with a history of acute myocardial infarction strengthens the association between chronic periodontal disease and coronary heart disease. However, controlling or preventing periodontitis in the aging population has not been strongly shown to prevent the recurrence of cardiovascular disease.[39,52] Since both conditions are common in the older patient populations, the coupling may be considered a possible complicating factor of aging.

In addition to atherosclerosis, aortic valve disease is a growing problem in the aging population. It is estimated that 25% of people over the age of 65 have some degree of atherosclerosis.[54] Standard treatment for aortic valve disease is surgical valve replacement (SAVR) but comes with its own morbidity and mortality in this age group. Transcatheter aortic valve replacement (TAVR) has emerged as a less invasive option for valve replacement in patients over the age of 65 (Figs. 29.2 and 29.3).[35,46] It allows a new bioprosthetic valve to be inserted within the native diseased aortic valve. The transfemoral approach is the most common. This is less invasive than SAVR which requires open heart surgery through a median sternotomy and the patient being placed on a heart-lung machine. The American Heart Association recommends that in patients over the age of 65 and in need of aortic valve replacement should consider TAVR over SAVR due to lower risk of major bleeding and pain, lower risk of transient or permanent atrial fibrillation, shorter hospital stay, and more rapid return to normal activity. TAVR is the recommendation of choice for patients over the age of 80 as well. Procedure rates have increased the most in patients over the age of 75.[7] Infective endocarditis (IE) after TAVR has been reported to be less than IE after SAVR, but the mortality with IE after TAVR seems to be higher.[43,99] One study by Regueiro et al. reported that IE after TAVR was associated with an in-hospital mortality of rate of 36%.[73] This is probably due to a higher incidence of other comorbidities associated with the patient population. Although the majority of IE after TAVR is associated with *Enterococci* and *Staphylococcus aureus,* orotracheal intubation can also be a risk factor for increased risk of IE after TAVR.[4,61] It has also been shown that oral bacteria, such as *Streptococcus mutans* and *Aggregatibacter actinmycetemcomitans* were found in infected heart valves.[65] These findings suggest that oral bacteria may play a role in valvular disease, and there may be a need for patients to have preventive periodontal therapy prior to valve replacement surgery.[63,88,93] Antibiotic prophylaxis should be considered in patients with any prosthetic valve, including TAVR due to the morbidity associated with this older, at-risk patient population.

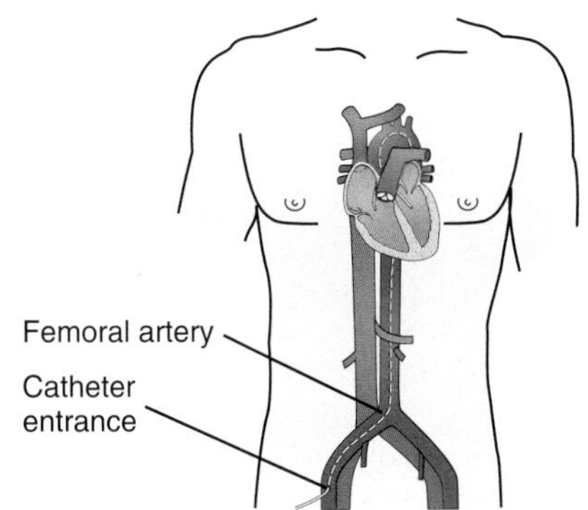

Fig. 29.2 Transfemoral approach for transcatheter aortic valve replacement. (From Elsevier. *Buck's Step-by-Step Medical Coding.* 2019 ed. St. Louis: Elsevier; 2019.)

In order to minimize the risk of stroke following a valve replacement, adjuvant anticoagulation originally consisted of dual antiplatelet therapy with aspirin and clopidogrel for 6 months after TAVR, but updated guidelines by the American College of Cardiology and American Heart Association recommend only 3 months of anticoagulation after both SAVR and TAVR patients at low risk of bleeding.[68] Long-term anticoagulation benefit still needs to be determined in terms of valve durability and valvular hemodynamics (Table 29.1).

Type 2 Non-Insulin-Dependent Diabetes Mellitus

More than 25% of the US population over the age of 65 has diabetes,[18] a higher prevalence than any other group. Unfortunately, the number of people over the age of 65 with diagnosed type 2 non-insulin-dependent diabetes mellitus (NIDDM) is expected to increase threefold by 2050.[66] Poorly controlled NIDDM increases the risk of cardiovascular complications due to microvascular damage. Literature consistently reports that NIDDM is a systemic risk factor for periodontal disease and periodontal disease is stated to be the sixth complication of diabetes.[17,55] There have been many studies

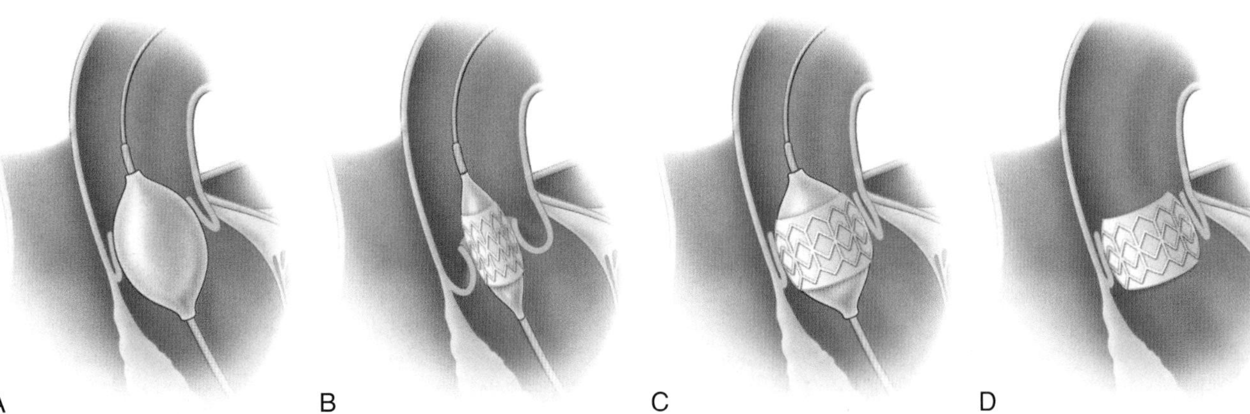

Fig. 29.3 Transcatheter aortic valve replacement in the heart. (From Chabner D. *The Language of Medicine.* 11th ed. St. Louis: Elsevier; 2017.)

TABLE 29.1 List of Common Anticoagulants That Elderly Patients May be Prescribed

Drug Name	Brand Name	Drug Class	Indications	Dental Implications
Warfarin	Coumadin	Vitamin K antagonist	Prevention of clot, DVT, pulmonary embolus, atrial fibrillation, heart valve replacement, recent myocardial infarction	Prolonged bleeding time; no indication to stop of INR <3 unless MD recommendation
Dabigatran	Pradaxa	Selective direct and reversible thrombin inhibitor	Stroke prevention in nonvalvular AF, VTE treatment and prevention	No need to discontinue and use local measures
Rivaroxaban	Xarelto	Direct Factor Xa inhibitor	Stroke prevention in nonvalvular AF, VTE treatment and prevention	No need to discontinue and use local measures
Apixaban	Eliquis	Direct Factor Xa inhibitor	Stroke prevention in nonvalvular AF, VTE treatment and prevention	No need to discontinue and use local measures
Edoxaban	Savaysa	Direct Factor Xa inhibitor	Stroke prevention due to AF, DVT, and PE treatment and prevention	No need to discontinue and use local measures
Betrixaban	Bevyxxa	Direct Factor Xa inhibitor	DVT prevention, PE prevention	No need to discontinue and use local measures
Clopidogrel	Plavix	Platelet aggregation inhibitor	Treatment of ACS, CVA, thromboembolism prevention	Prolonged bleeding time, may discontinue with MD recommendation
Aspirin	Ecotrin, Bayer	Platelet aggregation inhibitor, NSAID	Treatment of ACS, AMI, CVA, thromboembolism prevention	Prolonged bleeding time, not reversible, may discontinue with MD recommendation

ACS, Acute coronary syndrome; *AF*, atrial fibrillation; *AMI*, acute myocardial infarction; *CVA*, cerebrovascular accident; *DVT*, deep vein thrombus; *VTE*, venous thromboembolism.

linking poorly controlled periodontal disease to poor glycemic control in NIDDM. The study done in 1998 on elderly patients with NIDDM by Collin et al.[20] correlated poorly controlled periodontal disease with higher levels of glycosylated hemoglobin, further underscoring this relationship. NIDDM patients are more likely to have poorer periodontal health than patients without diabetes. Poor control of NIDDM has been associated with worse periodontal health.[25] Noninvasive periodontal therapy has been shown to significantly reduce the HbA1c levels in elderly patients with periodontal disease and NIDDM.[56] Patients with well-controlled NIDDM and receiving noninvasive periodontal therapy had a greater reduction in HbA1c than in the poorly controlled diabetic group. This shows that controlling periodontal disease may play a significant role in the control of NIDDM. Immunoaging reduces the ability to fight against infection, so the additive effect of controlling inflammation through nonsurgical periodontal therapy and diabetic control will have a beneficial effect on both conditions.

Osteoporosis

Osteoporosis is one of the most common chronic metabolic bone diseases, which is becoming more prevalent due to a longer life span. Osteoporosis and periodontal disease are frequent conditions that affect bone mass and may share risk factors. Systemic bony changes could negatively affect periodontal disease.[57] In periodontal disease, there is destruction and resorption of alveolar bone due to infection and inflammation. Bone remodeling capacity is reduced in patients with osteoporosis, resulting in potentially decreased recovery response in patients with periodontitis.[94]

Bisphosphonate (BP) therapy has been used to treat osteoporosis to decrease osteoclastic activity. A study by Jeffcoat in 2006 associated BP therapy with decreased alveolar bone loss in the periodontium of postmenopausal women, suggesting that oral BP therapy may be useful in periodontal disease.[42] In another study done in 2016 by Penoni et al., participants that were not treated for osteoporosis showed more clinical attachment loss and worse periodontal conditions compared to women with normal bone density and women being treated for osteoporosis.[70] This association seems to support the hypothesis that osteoporosis and periodontal disease are related.

Within the last 15 years, the use of intravenous BP (IVBP) therapy and other types of drugs have been used to successfully treat osteoporosis (Table 29.2).[12] IVBP is usually given as a once-yearly 30-minute infusion. It has been shown to increase bone density and reduce fracture risk. However, many papers have reported patients taking IVBP developing medication-related osteonecrosis of the jaw (MRONJ) after completing invasive dental procedures.[27,44,51] There should be careful consideration of surgical intervention in the management of periodontal disease or placement of dental implants in this patient population.

Another medication gaining popularity in treating osteoporosis is denosumab. It is a monoclonal antibody with a high affinity for the receptor activator of the nuclear factor-κB ligand (RANKL). Unlike BPs which affect osteoclastic function, denosumab inhibits the formation of osteoclasts, reduces bone resorption, and increases bone density.[21] More importantly, though, is that denosumab does not imbed in bone tissue and has a short half-life of only 12.5 days compared to IVBP which can have a half-life of 10 to 12 years.[76,95] However, there are studies that have reported incidences of MRONJ in patients taking denosumab.[1,49] Even though the risk of developing MRONJ is relatively low in patients on BP and/or denosumab, both are considered risk factors for developing MRONJ following invasive dental surgical procedures.[78]

Vitamin D assists in promoting the remodeling of bone and deficiencies can lead to decreased bone mineralization and loss of bone structure.[75] In the elderly population, this could lead to or exacerbate osteoporosis.[69,90] It also has an important role in stimulating the nonspecific immune response to fight against infectious diseases. Therefore, a deficiency in vitamin D can affect periodontal disease via deficient immunomodulation and decreased bone mineralization.[3] As oral health practitioners, awareness of the dental patient's

TABLE 29.2 List of Common Medications Used for Patients With Osteoporosis

Drug Name	Brand Name	Drug Class	Form	Dosage/Frequency
Alendronate	Fosamax	Bisphosphonate	Oral	Varies 70-mg tablet once a week, 5–10-mg tablet daily
Ibandronate	Boniva	Bisphosphonate	Oral	150-mg tablet once a month
Residronate	Actonel	Bisphosphonate	Oral	See form
Zoledronic acid	Reclast	Bisphosphonate	Intravenous injection	5-mg injection over 15 min every 2 years
Denosumab	Prolia	RANKL[a] inhibitor	Subcutaneous injection	60-mg once every 6 months
Raloxifene	Evista	SERM[b]	Oral	60-mg tablet once a day
Romosozumab	Evenity	Sclerostin inhibitor	Subcutaneous injection	210-mg once a month for 12 months
Teriparatide	Forteo	PTH[c] analogue	Subcutaneous injection	20-mcg once a day for up to 2 years

[a]Prevents the binding of receptor activator of nuclear factor-κB with its ligand to stimulate osteoclastic activity.
[b]Selective estrogen receptor modulators to mimic estrogen benefits on stimulating osteoblastic activity.
[c]Parathyroid hormone analogue that helps to promote growth of new bone.

systemic bone health status, including vitamin D levels, may be important to understand and manage their periodontal status.

Dementia

Dementia is a deterioration in cognitive function that affects memory, thinking, orientation, comprehension, learning capacity, language, and judgment. It is one of the major causes of disability among the older population worldwide. It is estimated that 5% to 8% of people over the age of 60 have dementia and this number will continue to grow as the total elderly population grows. A study conducted at the University of Michigan reported that as high as 1 out of 7 people over the age of 70 had some extent of dementia.[71] Alzheimer disease (AD) is the most well-known and common cause of dementia and is one of the leading causes of morbidity in the elderly population.[98] The exact cause or even the pathophysiology of AD has not been completely explained as it is multifactorial, which includes poor nutrition and inflammation.

Tooth loss in both older men and women has been related to an increased risk of developing dementia and cognitive decline.[8] Having fewer teeth impairs masticatory function, which could influence dietary choices and nutritional intake. Poor nutrition has been associated with increased progression of dementia.[79] Maintaining a healthy periodontium is critical in the retention of dentition so that elderly patients can retain their dentition longer for better mastication of nutritious foods.

It has also been well established that dementia is a predictor of poor oral health.[84] It has been challenging to determine whether the progression of cognitive decline is due to the progression of periodontal disease or whether it is due to dementia rendering patients incapable of maintaining their oral hygiene. In a 2006 Swedish twin study, authors reported that the twin that had worse periodontal disease and lost more teeth had a higher risk of developing AD.[33] These results were similarly repeated in studies done in Japan, Korea, and the United States.[45,47,89] Periodontal disease has been well established as a possible source of systemic chronic inflammation due to oral bacteria entering the circulatory system. Both animal and clinical evidence have shown that inflammation may be involved in the pathogenesis of AD.[2] Periodontal-derived pro-inflammatory molecules and bacteria can reach the brain through circulation. *Treponema* bacteria, a gram-negative pathogen associated with periodontal disease, has been more frequently found in deceased AD patient brains than in non-AD brains.[75] It has been hypothesized that the inflammatory changes that occur as a result of the presence of bacteria contribute to the production of amyloid. Peripheral inflammation and infections can increase the amyloid production in the brain faster than it can be cleared.[100] The beta-amyloid 42 protein is thought to be toxic to brain tissue by disrupting cell function. Regardless of the progression of dementia being a result of periodontal disease or a decrease in oral hygiene, control of periodontitis and retention of healthy dentition can play a significant role in the progression of dementia in the elderly population.

Advanced dementia patients and bedridden elderly patients with compromised ability to maintain their oral hygiene habits are at increased risk for aspiration pneumonia (AP). This is one of the leading causes of morbidity and mortality among elderly long-term care residents, which include dementia patients.[80] Mortality is highest in the most severely demented patients.[96] In a prospective study that looked at prognostic factors in elderly dementia patients and mortality rate from AP, 50% of the patients over the age of 75 died within 6 months of hospitalization.[13] As dementia progresses, the decrease in mastication and swallowing efficiency, as well as progressive loss of protective reflexes combined with the accumulation of oral bacteria, increases the risk of AP.[81] A prospective study that collected blood samples and bronchotracheal secretions from older patients admitted to hospitals due to AP found the presence of oral gram-negative bacillus isolates in the lungs.[24] Improvements in oral care have greatly reduced the incidence of pneumonia in elderly nursing home patients.[32] This scenario highlights the importance of good oral hygiene in the elderly dementia population as it may affect cognitive decline, and stop the loss of dentition due to lack of proper hygiene that can compromise the patient's ability to masticate nutritious foods. Lack of good nutrition may contribute to further cognitive decline.

Periodontal Treatment Planning Considerations

Periodontal treatment planning for older patients should focus on correct diagnosis, etiology, treatment options, and prognosis. Systemic diseases, multiple medications, and cognitive and functional decline, all play significant roles in the success of periodontal treatment and maintenance.[102] The ultimate goal should consist of the preservation of function and the elimination or prevention of disease. The frailer or more functionally compromised the elderly patient becomes, the more treatment goals should be geared toward control and care versus total cure.

A nonsurgical approach should be the first line of treatment, but surgical treatment can be considered depending on the extent and nature of the periodontal disease. Reducing the bacterial load through mechanical debridement and daily oral hygiene maintenance can slow the progression or development of periodontal disease. Medical therapy can also be incorporated into the regimen so long as there are minimal negative drug interactions with medications patients are taking for the treatment of systemic diseases. Patients who are unable to adequately remove plaque daily may benefit from antiplaque agents, such as chlorhexidine, topical antibiotics, and over-the-counter mouthrinses.[62,92,102] Chlorhexidine mouthrinse can be particularly useful in older patients that have difficulty removing plaque and take antihypertensive medications that cause gingival hyperplasia.[92] If a surgical approach is indicated, care should be taken to minimize additional root exposure if possible. If patients cannot maintain their hygiene due to noncompliance or impairment, then palliative treatment may be the optimal approach.[85]

Approximately 30% of the population over 65 years of age experience some notable degree of dry mouth, whether due to systemic conditions or medications.[86] Xerostomia can significantly affect a person's ability to talk, eat and swallow foods and overall quality of life. Saliva has antimicrobial properties that inhibit the adherence and growth of viruses and bacteria on oral mucosa. Dry mouth can lead to increased accumulation of plaque, food retention, atrophic mucosa, nonspecific gingival inflammation, and generalized oral erythema.[72] Not only are there soft tissue consequences to xerostomia, but patients will also be at increased risk of developing dental caries. For older patients, where gingival recession may be more common, they would be at increased risk of developing root caries. Mouthrinses, topical fluoride application, and more frequent periodontal recall intervals would be helpful in the early detection and intervention of periodontal decline and dental caries.[14,87,91,104]

The importance of controlling bacterial load through mechanical debridement has a significant impact not only on the periodontium but also on the control of systemic conditions. Therefore, periodontal treatment planning for this patient population should be focused not only on oral care and maintenance but also as a contributing role in the overall management of patients' systemic conditions.

Conclusions

The goal of clinically managing periodontal disease in older adults is based on specific, individualized care. With an emphasis on quality-of-life issues, the goal of periodontal treatment for older patients is to preserve function and eliminate or prevent the progression of inflammatory disease. Worsening periodontal disease can have a negative impact on various systemic conditions and cognitive decline, especially in the aging population. Periodontal treatment for older patients should also consider systemic diseases, medications, and cognitive and functional status, as these factors can affect the treatment choice and outcome.

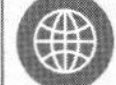
References for this chapter are found on the companion website eBooks.Health.Elsevier.com.

CHAPTER 30

Acute Periodontal Infections and Management

Perry R. Klokkevold | Fermin A. Carranza

CHAPTER OUTLINE

Necrotizing ulcerative periodontitis (NUP) may be an extension of *necrotizing ulcerative gingivitis (NUG)* into the periodontal structures that leads to periodontal attachment loss and bone loss. Alternatively, NUP and NUG may be different diseases. To date, there is little evidence to support the progression of NUG to NUP or to establish a relationship between the two conditions as a single disease entity. However, numerous clinical descriptions and case reports of NUP clearly demonstrate many clinical similarities between the two conditions. Until a distinction between NUG and NUP can be proved or disproved, it has been suggested that NUG and NUP be classified together under the broader category of *necrotizing periodontal diseases,* although with differing levels of severity.[1,16,17,24]

NUG has been recognized and described in the literature for more than a century.[27] The features of NUG are presented in Chapter 17. The lesions of NUG are confined to the gingiva without a loss of periodontal attachment or alveolar bone support; this is the feature that distinguishes NUG from NUP.

The term *necrotizing ulcerative periodontitis* was first adopted at the 1989 World Workshop in Clinical Periodontics.[3] It was changed from the 1986 term *necrotizing ulcerative gingivoperiodontitis,* which represented the condition of recurrent NUG that progresses to a chronic form of periodontitis that includes attachment and bone loss. The adoption of NUP as a disease entity occurred in 1989 when there was a heightened awareness and an increase in the number of necrotizing periodontitis cases being diagnosed and described in the literature. Specifically, more cases of NUP were being described among immunocompromised patients, especially those who tested positive for the human immunodeficiency virus (HIV) or who were diagnosed with acquired immunodeficiency syndrome (AIDS). In 1999, the subclassifications of NUG and NUP were included as separate diagnoses under the broader classification of "necrotizing ulcerative periodontal diseases."[1] These diagnoses and terms continue to be used in the new 2017 classification of periodontal and peri-implant diseases and conditions.[3,4,16,17]

Clinical Features

Clinical cases of NUP are defined by necrosis and ulceration of the coronal portion of the interdental papillae and gingival margin, with a painful, bright-red marginal gingiva that bleeds easily. This is similar to the clinical features of NUG. The distinguishing feature of NUP is the *destructive progression* of the disease, which includes periodontal attachment and bone loss. Deep interdental osseous craters typify periodontal lesions of NUP (Fig. 30.1). However, "conventional" periodontal pockets with deep probing depth are not found, because the ulcerative and necrotizing nature of the gingival lesion destroys the marginal epithelium and connective tissue, resulting in gingival recession. In periodontitis, periodontal pockets are formed because the junctional epithelial cells remain viable and can therefore migrate apically to cover areas of lost connective-tissue attachment (see Chapter 22). The necrosis of the junctional epithelium in patients with NUG and NUP creates an ulcer that prevents this epithelial migration. Consequently, a periodontal pocket cannot form. Advanced lesions of NUP lead to severe bone loss and tooth mobility, and may ultimately lead to tooth loss. In addition to these manifestations, as with cases of NUG, patients with NUP may present with oral malodor, fever, malaise, or lymphadenopathy.

KEY FACT

Necrotizing ulcerative gingivitis (NUG) and necrotizing ulcerative periodontitis (NUP) cases are defined by necrosis and ulceration of the coronal portion of the interdental papillae. Gingival margins are bright red and bleed easily. Lesions are painful. The feature that distinguishes NUP from NUG is the destructive progression of NUP, including periodontal attachment and bone loss.

Microscopic Findings

In a study involving the use of transmission electron microscopy and scanning electron microscopy of the microbial plaque overlying the

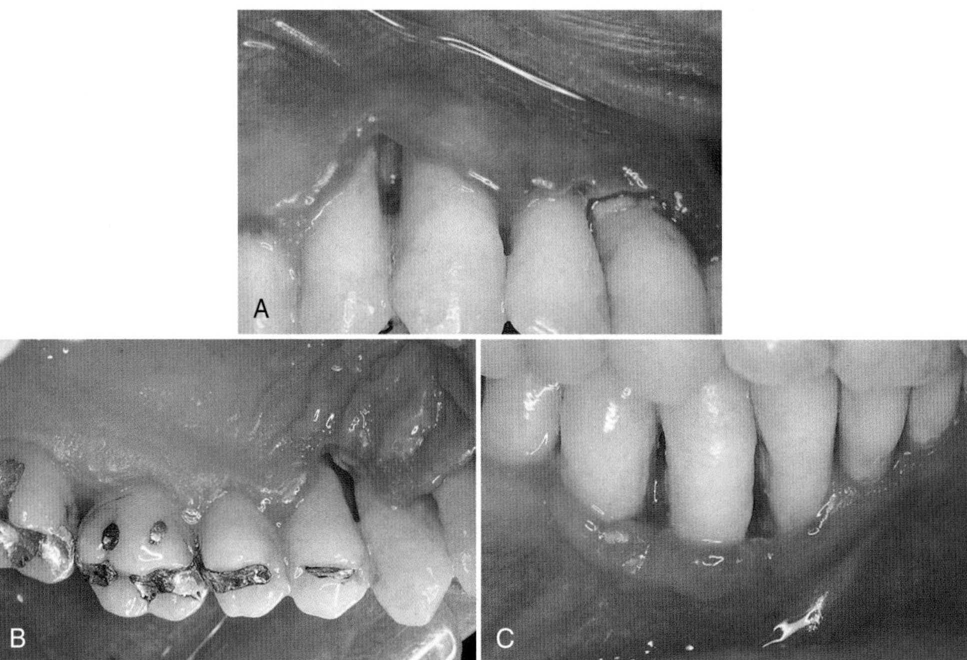

Fig. 30.1 Necrotizing ulcerative periodontitis in a 45-year-old, HIV-negative, white, male patient. (A) Buccal view of the maxillary cuspid–bicuspid area. (B) Palatal view of the same area shown in part A. (C) Buccal view of the mandibular anteriors. Note the deep craters associated with bone loss.

necrotic gingival papillae, Cobb and colleagues[5] demonstrated striking histologic similarities between NUP in HIV-positive patients and previous descriptions of NUG in HIV-negative patients.[21] Microscopic examination revealed a surface biofilm composed of a mixed microbial flora with different morphotypes and a subsurface flora with dense aggregations of spirochetes (i.e., the bacterial zone). Below the bacterial layers were dense aggregations of polymorphonuclear leukocytes (PMNs) (i.e., the neutrophil-rich zone) and necrotic cells (the necrotic zone). The biopsy technique used in this study did not allow for the observation of the deepest layer and thus was not able to identify the spirochetal infiltration zone, which is classically described in NUG lesions. In addition to the NUG-like microscopic features of NUP described in this study, high levels of yeasts and herpes-like viruses were observed. This latter finding is most likely indicative of the conditions afforded to opportunistic microbes in the immunocompromised host (i.e., HIV-positive patients).

Patients with HIV/AIDS

Gingival and periodontal lesions with distinctive features are frequently found in patients with HIV infection and AIDS. Many of these lesions are atypical manifestations of inflammatory periodontal diseases that arise during the course of HIV infection and as a result of the patient's concomitant immunocompromised state. Linear gingival erythema, NUG, and NUP are the most common HIV-associated periodontal conditions reported in the literature.[25] Chapter 27 provides detailed descriptions of the pathology and management of periodontal problems associated with viral infections, including HIV and others.

NUP lesions found in patients with HIV or AIDS can present with features similar to those seen in HIV-negative patients. Alternatively, NUP lesions in patients with HIV or AIDS can be much more destructive and frequently result in complications that are extremely rare among patients without HIV or AIDS. For example, periodontal attachment and bone loss associated with NUP in an HIV-positive patient may be extremely rapid. Winkler and colleagues[35] described cases of NUP in HIV-positive patients with teeth that lost more than 90% of periodontal attachment and 10 mm of bone over a 3- to 6-month period. Ultimately, many of these lesions resulted in tooth loss. Other complications reported in this population included the progression of the lesions to involve large areas of soft-tissue necrosis, with the exposure of bone and the sequestration of bone fragments. This type of severe, progressive lesion with extension into the vestibular area and the palate is referred to as *necrotizing ulcerative stomatitis*.[15a]

The reported prevalence of NUP among patients with HIV infection varies.[7,12,25,27] Riley and colleagues[20] described only two cases of NUP in 200 HIV-positive patients (1%), whereas Glick and colleagues[14] found a prevalence of 6.3% for NUP cases in a prospective study of 700 HIV-positive patients. Variations in reported findings may be related to differences in the populations studied (e.g., intravenous drug users versus homosexuals versus patients with hemophilia) and differences in the immune status of the study subjects.

Necrotizing forms of periodontitis appear to be more prevalent among patients with more severe immunosuppression.[25,26] Case reports have depicted NUP as a progressive extension of HIV periodontitis (i.e., periodontitis to necrotic progression).[21] Glick and colleagues[14,15] found a high correlation between the diagnosis of NUP and immunosuppression in HIV-positive patients. The patients who presented with NUP were 20.8 times more likely to have CD4+ counts of less than 200 cells/mm^3 as compared with HIV-positive patients without NUP. The authors consider a diagnosis of NUP to be a marker of immune deterioration and a predictor of the diagnosis of AIDS.[14] Others have suggested that NUP may be used as an indicator of HIV infection in undiagnosed patients. Shangase and colleagues[32] reported that a diagnosis of NUG or NUP in systemically healthy, asymptomatic South African patients was strongly correlated with HIV infection. Of patients presenting with NUG or NUP, 39 of 56 (69.6%) were subsequently found to be infected with HIV (see Chapter 27).

CLINICAL CORRELATION

Periodontal attachment and bone loss associated with NUP in an immunocompromised host (i.e., HIV-positive or AIDS) may be extremely rapid. NUP lesions in these patients are likely to be much more destructive and may also be associated with complications that are extremely rare among patients without HIV or AIDS.

Etiology of Necrotizing Ulcerative Periodontitis

The etiology of NUP has not been determined, although a mixed fusiform–spirochete bacterial flora appears to play a key role, since clinical improvement is often observed following debridement and antibiotics.[17] Because bacterial pathogens are not solely responsible for causing the disease, some predisposing "host" factors appear to be necessary. Numerous predisposing factors have been attributed to NUG, including poor oral hygiene, preexisting periodontal disease, smoking, viral infections, immunocompromised status, psychosocial stress, and malnutrition. One case report attributed heavy tobacco use as the most significant contributing factor associated with NUP in a 21-year-old who had been smoking >20 cigarettes/day and chewing tobacco since the age of 7 years.[36] The most relevant predisposing factors for NUP are those that alter the host's immune response, and usually more than one factor is necessary to cause the onset of disease.[17]

Microbial Flora

Assessment of the microbial flora of NUP lesions is almost exclusively limited to studies involving patients with HIV or AIDS, with some conflicting evidence. Murray and colleagues[24] reported that cases of NUP in HIV-positive patients demonstrated significantly greater numbers of the opportunistic fungus *Candida albicans* and a higher prevalence of *Aggregatibacter actinomycetemcomitans, Prevotella intermedia, Porphyromonas gingivalis, Fusobacterium nucleatum,* and *Campylobacter* species as compared with HIV-negative controls. In addition, they reported a low or variable level of spirochetes, which is inconsistent with the flora associated with NUG. Citing differences in microbial flora, they refuted the notion that the destructive lesions seen in HIV-positive patients were related to NUG lesions; they suggested that the flora of NUP lesions in HIV-positive patients is comparable to that of periodontitis lesions, thus supporting their concept that necrotizing periodontitis in the HIV-positive patient is an aggressive manifestation of periodontitis in the immunocompromised host.

In contrast with these findings, Cobb and colleagues[5] reported that the microbial composition of NUP lesions in HIV-positive patients was very similar to that of NUG lesions with distinct, identifiable zones, as discussed previously. Researchers used electron microscopy to describe a mixed microbial flora with various morphotypes in 81.3% of specimens. The subsurface microbial flora featured dense aggregations of spirochetes in 87.5% of specimens. The authors also reported opportunistic yeasts and herpes-like viruses in 65.6% and 56.5% of NUP lesions, respectively. The differences between these reports may be explained by the limitations of obtaining viable cultures of spirochetes,[24] as compared with the more complete sample assessment with electron microscopic observation of spirochetes.[5]

In a review article, Feller and Lemmer suggested that spirochetes, herpesviruses, candida, and HIV all have potentially pathogenic roles in NUP lesions in the HIV-seropositive individual.[13] Spirochetes have the ability to modulate the host's innate and adaptive immune responses and to stimulate inflammatory reactions,[9] which may reduce the local immune competence and facilitate the development of necrotizing disease.[13] Activated herpesviruses have the capacity to deregulate the host's immune system, which may lead to an increase in the colonization and activity of other pathogenic microorganisms. *C. albicans* has been reported to produce eicosanoids, leading to the release of proinflammatory mediators, which may facilitate spirochete colonization and invasion and promote the development of necrotizing periodontal diseases.[12,13]

KEY FACT

Patients with NUP are more likely to be immunocompromised. Although a mixed fusiform–spirochete bacterial infection appears to play a key role in the etiology of NUP, bacterial pathogens are not solely responsible. Predisposing "host" compromising factors appear to be necessary. Factors that have been attributed to NUG include poor oral hygiene, preexisting periodontal disease, smoking, viral infections, immunocompromised status, psychosocial stress, and malnutrition. These risk factors apply to NUP lesions as well, yet the most relevant predisposing factors for NUP appear to be those that alter the host's immune response, such as HIV infection and AIDS.

Immunocompromised Status

Evidently, both NUG and NUP lesions are more prevalent among patients with compromised or suppressed immune systems. Numerous studies—particularly those evaluating patients with HIV or AIDS—support the concept that a diminished host response is present in those individuals who have been diagnosed with necrotizing ulcerative periodontal diseases.[35] Whereas a compromised immune system (i.e., "immune compromise") in the HIV-infected patient is driven by impaired T-cell function and altered T-cell ratios, evidence indicates that other forms of compromised immunity predispose individuals to NUG and NUP as well.

Cutler and colleagues[7] described the impaired bactericidal activity of PMNs in two children with NUP. In a comparative assay of PMNs and periodontal pathogens, two brothers who were 9 and 14 years old showed significant depression of PMN phagocytosis and killing function as compared with gender- and age-matched controls. Furthermore, Batista and colleagues[2] reported periodontal findings and NUP in an adolescent patient with a rare genetic disease (multifactorial congenital immunodeficiency) that causes the impaired secretion of immunoglobulin; the oral lesions resolved with the administration of intravenous immunoglobulin.

Psychological Stress

Most studies evaluating the role of stress on necrotizing periodontal disease have involved subjects with NUG[8,18,33,34] and thus have not specifically addressed the role of stress on NUP. Patients with NUG have been found to have had significantly more anxiety, higher depression scores, a greater magnitude of recent stressful events, more overall distress and adjustments related to these events, and more negative life events.[6,15] Although the role of stress in the development of NUP has not been reported specifically, the many similarities between NUG and NUP would suggest that similar relationships to stress may exist.

The mechanisms that predispose an individual with stress to necrotizing ulcerative periodontal diseases have not been established. However, it is well known that stress increases the systemic cortisol levels, and sustained increases in cortisone have a suppressive effect on the immune response. In an investigation of 474 military personnel, Shannon and colleagues[33] found that urinary levels of 17-hydroxycorticosteroid were higher among subjects with NUG than in all other subjects who had been diagnosed with periodontal health, gingivitis, or periodontitis. This finding was subsequently confirmed in a different population.[21] Experimentally, noma-like lesions have been produced in rats by administering cortisone[31] and causing mechanical injury to the gingiva[30] and in hamsters via total body irradiation.[23] Thus, stress-induced immunosuppression may be one mechanism that impairs the host response and leads to necrotizing periodontal disease. The scientific evidence supporting an etiologic role of stress in periodontitis is not as clear (see Chapter 25).

Malnutrition

Direct evidence of the relationship between malnutrition and necrotizing periodontal disease is limited to descriptions of necrotizing infections in severely malnourished children. Lesions that resemble NUG but that progress to become *gangrenous stomatitis* or noma have been described in children with severe malnutrition in underdeveloped countries. Jimenez and Baer[20] reported cases of NUG among malnourished children and adolescents between the ages of 2 and 14 years in Colombia. In the advanced stages, NUG lesions extended from the gingiva to other areas of the oral cavity, becoming gangrenous stomatitis (noma) and causing exposure, necrosis, and sequestration of the alveolar bone. Later, Jimenez and colleagues reported that 44 of the 45 cases of necrotizing disease (NUG = 29, NUP = 7, and noma = 9) documented from 1965 to 2000 were from a low socioeconomic group and that malnutrition was associated with nearly all of the necrotizing conditions (29/29 NUG cases, 6/7 NUP cases, and 9/9 noma cases).[19] In a study of socioeconomically deprived Nigerian children with NUG (153 cases), Enwonwu and colleagues confirmed malnutrition by measuring circulating micronutrients.[11] As compared with neighborhood counterparts, the children with NUG and micronutrient deficiencies demonstrated dysregulated cytokine production with a complex interplay of elevated proinflammatory and anti-inflammatory mediators.

KEY FACT

A fusiform–spirochete infection, along with a host's weakened immune system, seem to play a major role in the pathogenesis of necrotizing ulcerative periodontitis.

A possible explanation is that malnutrition, particularly when extreme, contributes to a diminished host resistance to infection and necrotizing disease. It is well documented that many of the host defenses—including phagocytosis; cell-mediated immunity; and complement, antibody, and cytokine production and function—are impaired in malnourished individuals.[8] The depletion of nutrients to cells and tissues results in immunosuppression and increases disease susceptibility. Thus, it is reasonable to conclude that malnutrition can predispose an individual to opportunistic infections or intensify the severity of existing oral infections.

Management of Necrotizing Ulcerative Periodontitis

NUP is a rare disease, especially in developed countries. Most patients diagnosed with NUP have diseases or conditions that impair their host immune response, such as patients with HIV infection or AIDS. Regardless of the specific etiology, these patients often have an underlying predisposing systemic factor(s) that renders them susceptible to NUP. For this reason, patients presenting with NUP should be treated in consultation with their physician.

A comprehensive medical evaluation and diagnosis of any condition that may be contributing to an altered host immune response should be completed. Clinicians should check all patients who present with NUP to ascertain whether or not they are HIV positive. It is also important to rule out any hematologic disease (e.g., leukemia) before initiating treatment of any case that has a similar presentation to NUP (see Figs. 25.13 and 25.15 in Chapter 25).

Treatment of patients diagnosed with NUP pose a significant challenge for clinicians, not only because they are infrequently encountered, but also because they may not respond favorably to conventional periodontal therapy. Early diagnosis and treatment of NUP is crucial because the disease can progress rapidly and may lead to tooth exfoliation. The rapid and severe loss of periodontal support associated with these cases leaves the clinician faced with uncertainty about treatment outcomes and difficulty in making decisions about whether to save affected teeth or extract them. Additionally, the osseous defects that occur during the late stages of the disease are extremely difficult to resolve.

Treatment can be initiated only after a thorough medical history and examination has been undertaken to identify the existence of any systemic diseases. Modifiable factors, such as smoking, malnutrition, and heavy biofilm, that increase the risk of NUP must also be identified and addressed to improve chances of treatment success. Similar to the treatment of NUG, the treatment for NUP includes local debridement of lesions with scaling and root planing, lavage, and instructions for good oral hygiene. It may be necessary to use local anesthesia during the debridement because lesions are frequently painful. The use of ultrasonic instrumentation with profuse irrigation may enhance debridement and flushing of deep lesions. Achieving good oral hygiene may be challenging until the lesions and associated pain resolve.

Antimicrobial adjuncts, such as chlorhexidine, added to the oral hygiene regimen may aid in the daily reduction of bacterial loads. Locally applied topical antimicrobials and systemic antibiotics, as well as systemic analgesics, should be used as indicated by signs and symptoms.

Patients with NUP often harbor bacteria, fungi, viruses, and other nonoral microorganisms, complicating the selection of antimicrobial therapy. Superinfection or overgrowth of fungi and viruses may be propagated by antibiotic therapy. Antifungal and/or antiviral agents may be considered against these infections prophylactically or after they are diagnosed. Because oral hygiene for these patients is complicated by the painful lesions, alternative methods should be encouraged. Irrigation with diluted cleansing and antibacterial agents can beneficial.

Ultimately, the successful treatment of NUP may depend on the resolution or treatment of the underlying systemic condition (e.g., immune compromise) that predisposed the individual to the disease. Evaluation and treatment of patients with known systemic conditions, such as HIV infection, should be coordinated with the patient's physician.

Conclusion

NUP and NUG share many clinical and microbiologic features, but NUP is distinguished by a more severe condition with periodontal attachment and bone loss. Some individuals with NUP have severe and rapidly progressive disease. It appears that an impaired immune response and a lowered host resistance to infection are significant factors in the onset and progression of NUP. The best example of an immunocompromised host with a predisposition for NUP is the patient with HIV or AIDS. As with the other infection-related complications of HIV and AIDS, the immunocompromised status of the affected patient renders them vulnerable to opportunistic periodontal infections, including NUP. Several predisposing factors have been identified in cases of NUG that may also play a role in NUP, including smoking, viral infections, psychosocial stress, and malnutrition. Although none of these factors alone is sufficient to cause necrotizing disease, when they occur together with an immunocompromised status, there is a potential to adversely influence the host's response or resistance to infection.

A Case Scenario is found on the companion website eBooks.Health.Elsevier.com.

Suggested Reading

Batista Jr EL, Novaes Jr AB, Calvano LM, et al. Necrotizing ulcerative periodontitis associated with severe congenital immunodeficiency in a prepubescent subject: clinical findings and response to intravenous immunoglobulin treatment. *J Clin Periodontol*. 1999;26(8):499–504.

Cobb CM, Ferguson BL, Keselyak NT, et al. A TEM/SEM study of the microbial plaque overlying the necrotic gingival papillae of HIV-seropositive, necrotizing ulcerative periodontitis. *J Periodontal Res*. 2003;38(2):147–155.

Enwonwu CO, Phillips RS, Savage KO. Inflammatory cytokine profile and circulating cortisol levels in malnourished children with necrotizing ulcerative gingivitis. *Eur Cytokine Netw*. 2005;16(3):240–248.

Feller L, Lemmer J. Necrotizing periodontal diseases in HIV-seropositive subjects: pathogenic mechanisms. *J Int Acad Periodontol*. 2008;10(1):10–15.

Herrera D, Retamal-Valdes B, Alonso B, Feres M. Acute periodontal lesions (periodontal abscesses and necrotizing periodontal diseases) and endo-periodontal lesions. *J Periodontol*. 2018;89(Suppl 1):S85–S102. https://doi.org/10.1002/JPER.16-0642. PMID: 29926942.

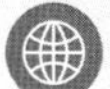
References for this chapter are found on the companion website eBooks.Health.Elsevier.com.

CHAPTER 31

Halitosis (Breath Malodor)

Wim Teughels | Jesica Dadamio | Jits Robben | Christel Dekeyser | Marc Quirynen

For online-only content on extraoral causes of breath malodor and the portable volatile sulfur monitor, as well as expanded discussions on the epidemiology and etiology of malodor, fundamentals of malodor detection, diagnosis of malodor, including organoleptic rating and gas chromatography, and chlorhexidine use in treating malodor, go to the companion website eBooks.Health.Elsevier.com.

CHAPTER OUTLINE

Semantics and Classification

Breath odor can be defined as the subjective perception after smelling someone's breath (organoleptic rating). It can be pleasant, unpleasant, or even disturbing, if not repulsive. If unpleasant, the terms *breath malodor, halitosis, bad breath,* or *fetor ex ore* can be applied. Breath malodor is a common complaint in the general population. One in four persons has bad breath at any given time in his or her life. It has a significant socioeconomic impact but, unfortunately, has been neglected until fairly recently by scientists and clinicians, and it is still rarely covered in the medical curricula. Halitosis can lead to personal discomfort and social embarrassment, and it remains one of the biggest taboos of society.

To minimize the confusing number of terms used in the literature, in 2014 a Consensus Workshop[167] proposed the use of the term *halitosis* together with a slight simplification of the previous International Classification of Halitosis proposed by Yaegaki and colleagues.[217] The three main categories of halitosis are genuine halitosis, pseudohalitosis, and halitophobia. *Genuine halitosis* is the term that is used when the breath malodor really exists and can be diagnosed organoleptically or by measurement of the responsible compounds. A distinction should be made between physiologic and pathologic halitosis (Fig. 31.1).

Transient disturbing odors caused by food intake (e.g., garlic, onions, certain spices) or smoking do not reveal a health problem and are common examples of physiologic halitosis. The same is true for "morning" bad breath, as habitually experienced on awakening. This malodor is caused by decreased salivary flow and increased putrefaction during the night, and it spontaneously disappears after breakfast or after oral hygiene measures. A persistent breath malodor, by definition, does reflect some pathology (pathologic halitosis). The causes of this condition are discussed later in the chapter. When the origin of pathologic halitosis can be found in the oral cavity, one speaks of intraoral halitosis or oral malodor. In case the origin of the halitosis lies outside of the oral cavity, the term *extraoral halitosis* applies. Extraoral halitosis can be further subdivided into *blood-borne* and *non–blood-borne* subtypes. When an obvious breath malodor cannot be perceived but the patient is convinced that he or she suffers from it, this is called *pseudohalitosis.* If the patient still believes that bad breath is present after treatment of genuine halitosis or a diagnosis of pseudohalitosis, one should consider halitophobia, which is a recognized psychiatric condition.[167,217]

Important Terms for the Diagnosis of Bad Breath

Term	Definition
Genuine halitosis	Malodor that can be verified objectively
Physiologic halitosis	Malodor that is transient and caused by physiologic factors, such as food intake or smoking
Intraoral halitosis or oral malodor	Obvious malodor originating from the oral cavity
Extraoral halitosis	Malodor originating from pathologic conditions outside the oral cavity
Pseudohalitosis	Malodor that cannot be perceived objectively, even though the patient complains of its existence. This condition can be improved by oral hygiene instruction and counseling.
Halitophobia	No malodor that can be perceived objectively after treatment of halitosis or pseudohalitosis, even though the patient persists in believing that halitosis exists

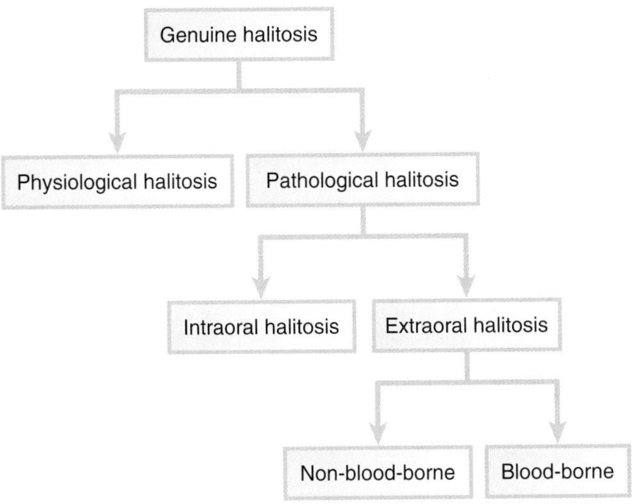

Fig. 31.1 Genuine halitosis: classification.

Etiology

In most patients, breath malodor originates from the oral cavity. Tongue coating is the predominant cause of oral malodor. Furthermore, periodontal diseases (gingivitis and periodontitis) are the second most important causative factors.[31,126,127,138,218,219]

A large-scale study including 2000 patients with halitosis complaints showed that for those patients whose bad breath could be objectively detected, the cause was mostly found within the oral cavity (90%). Tongue coating (51%), gingivitis or periodontitis (13%), or a combination (22%) accounted for the majority of the cases.[138] Because a large part of the population has tongue coating or gingivitis-periodontitis, the risk always exists that an intraoral condition is too easily considered as the cause, whereas more important pathologic conditions are overlooked. Indeed, for a minority of patients (4% in the same study), extraoral causes could be identified, including ear, nose, and throat (ENT) disorders, systemic diseases (e.g., diabetes), metabolic or hormonal changes, hepatic or renal insufficiency, bronchial and pulmonary diseases, or gastroenterologic disorders.[31,114,133,138,200]

Causes of Intraoral Halitosis

Tongue coating, poor oral hygiene, gingivitis, and periodontitis are the predominant causative factors.[138,166] In these cases, the term *intraoral halitosis* or *oral malodor* applies. It is the result of the degradation of organic substrates by anaerobic bacteria. During the process of bacterial putrefaction, peptides and proteins present in saliva, food debris, gingival crevicular fluid, interdental plaque, shed epithelial cells, postnasal drip, and blood are hydrolyzed to sulfide-containing and non–sulfide-containing amino acids, which can be further metabolized. The proteolytic degradation of sulfur-containing amino acids (cysteine, cystine, and methionine) by gram-negative bacteria produces sulfur-containing gases such as hydrogen sulfide (H_2S) and methylmercaptan (CH_3SH).[210]

The most commonly involved bacteria are *Porphyromonas gingivalis, Prevotella intermedia, Prevotella nigrescens, Aggregatibacter actinomycetemcomitans, Campylobacter rectus, Fusobacterium nucleatum, Peptostreptococcus micros, Tannerella forsythia, Eubacterium* spp., and spirochetes. A study by Niles and Gaffar[116] made clear that these gram-negative species in particular cause an unpleasant smell by the production of sulfur compounds. Recently, Foo and colleagues[44] presented an overview of the correlation of VSCs and oral bacteria. Based on previous selected studies the authors could establish significant correlations among *Porphyromonas, Prevotella, Campylobacter, Peptostreptococcus, T. forsythia, Eubacterium* and *Solobacterium*, and VSC compounds (Fig. 31.2). Because of the large microbial diversity found in the oral cavity, to which patients with halitosis are not the exception, it is suggested that breath malodor is the result of complex interactions among several bacterial species. One study indicated that some gram-positive microorganisms, such as *Streptococcus salivarius*, also contribute to oral malodor production by deglycosylating salivary glycoproteins, thus exposing their protein core to further degradation by gram-negative microorganisms.[181] The presence of *Solobacterium moorei,* a gram-positive bacterium, has also been linked to oral malodor.[58,59,71,198]

Thus, for oral malodor, the unpleasant smell of the breath mainly originates from VSCs, especially hydrogen sulfide, methylmercaptan, and (less significantly) dimethyl sulfide—$(CH_3)_2S$—as first discovered by Tonzetich.[194] Other compounds, such as the diamines indole and skatole, the polyamines putrescine and cadaverine, and the carboxylic acids acetic, butyric, and propionic acid, are also formed by proteolytic degradation of non–sulfur-containing amino acids by oral microorganisms.[51]

Tongue and Tongue Coating

The dorsal tongue mucosa, with an area of 25 cm^2, has a very irregular surface topography.[22,165] The innumerable depressions in the tongue surface are ideal niches for bacterial adhesion and growth, sheltered from cleaning actions.[28,218] Moreover, desquamated cells and food remnants also remain trapped in these retention sites and consequently can be putrefied by the bacteria.[11] A fissured tongue (deep fissures on the dorsum, also called *scrotal tongue* or *lingua plicata*) and a hairy tongue (*lingua villosa*) have an even rougher surface (Fig. 31.3).

Accumulated food remnants intermingled with exfoliated cells and bacteria form a coating on the tongue dorsum. The latter cannot be easily removed because of retention by the irregular surface of the tongue dorsum (see Fig. 31.3). As such, the two factors essential for putrefaction (bacteria and their nutrients) are united. Several investigators have identified the dorsal posterior surface of the tongue as the primary source of oral malodor.[11,21,28,152] Indeed, high correlations have been reported between tongue coating and odor formation.[11,24,100,218]

In both healthy individuals and patients with periodontitis, with or without complaints of intraoral halitosis, a significant positive correlation was found between the presence or amount of tongue coating and levels of VSCs[100,139] and/or organoleptic scores of the mouth odor.[28] In a group of 2000 patients visiting a multidisciplinary halitosis clinic,[138,207] significant correlations were found between organoleptic scores and tongue coating ($R = 0.52$; $P < .001$). In another study,[121] it was also observed that the amount of tongue coating was significantly greater in the halitosis-positive group compared with the halitosis-negative group. Morita and Wang[103] found that the volume of tongue coating and percentage of sites with bleeding on probing were significantly associated with oral malodor.[103] In 1992, Yaegaki and Sanada demonstrated that even in patients with periodontal disease, 60% of the VSCs were produced from the tongue surface.[218,219]

Research has shown that the strongest determinant of the presence of tongue coating is suboptimal oral hygiene. Other influencing factors were periodontal status, presence of a denture, smoking, and dietary habits.[206]

Periodontal Infections

A relationship between periodontitis and oral malodor has been shown. Though periodontally healthy patients can suffer from halitosis, not all patients with gingivitis and/or periodontitis complain about bad breath, and some disagreement exists in the literature as to what extent oral malodor and periodontal disease are related.[11,153,178] Bacteria associated with gingivitis and periodontitis are able to produce VSCs.[77,110,116,126,127,194]

	Total VSCs	Hydrogen sulfide	Methyl mercaptan	Dimethyl sulfide
Genera				
Peptostreptococcus	○	○	○	
Alloprevotella	○	○	○	
Eubacterium nodatum	○	○	○	○
Stomatobaculum	○	○		
Granulicatella	○			
Bergeyella	○	○	○	
Campylobacter	○			
Prevotella		○	○	○
Leptotrichia		○		○
Veillonella				○
Candidatus_Saccharimonas				○
Hemophilus		○		
Gemella		○		
Parvimonas			○	
Solobacterium			○	
Pseudomonas			○	
Species				
Prevotella tannerae		○		
Hemophilus_parainfluenzae		○		
Leptotrichia FP036		○		
Leptotrichia wadei		○		
Streptococcus unclassified		○		
Actinomyces odontolyticus_lingnae		○		
Hemophilus unclassified		○		
Porphyromonas gingivalis	○	○	○	
Tanerella forsythia	○	○		
Prevetella intermedia	○	○	○	
Prevotella nigrescens	○	○	○	
Treponema denticola	○	○		

Color scale: **1.0**, 0.8, 0.6, 0.4, 0.2, 0, −0.2, −0.4, −0.6, −0.8, −1.0

Fig. 31.2 Correlation of volatile sulfur compounds (VSCs) with oral bacteria. The figure depicts the genera and species of bacteria whose relative abundances significantly correlated with the concentration of VSCs value based on the Spearman correlation analysis from selected studies.[188,220,222] The color scale represents the Spearman correlation coefficient range from −1 to +1. (From Foo LH, Balan P, Pang LM, et al: Role of the oral microbiome, metabolic pathways, and novel diagnostic tools in intraoral halitosis: a comprehensive update. *Crit Rev Microbiol.* 2021;47(3):359-375.)

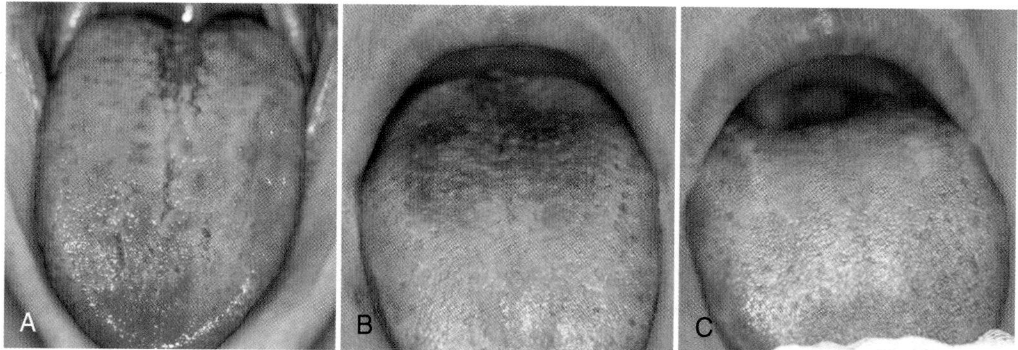

Fig. 31.3 (A–C) Clinical pictures of heavily coated tongues.

Several studies have shown that VSC levels in the mouth correlate positively with the depth of periodontal pockets—the deeper the pocket, the more bacteria, particularly anaerobic species—and that the amount of VSCs in the breath increases with the number, depth, and bleeding tendency of the periodontal pockets.[21,29,125,138,219] VSCs aggravate the periodontitis process by increasing the permeability of the pocket and mucosal epithelium, therefore exposing the underlying connective tissues of the periodontium to bacterial metabolites. Methylmercaptan enhances interstitial collagenase production, interleukin-1 production by mononuclear cells, and cathepsin B production, thus further mediating connective tissue breakdown.[88,144] It was shown that human gingival fibroblasts developed an affected cytoskeleton when exposed to methylmercaptan.[13,144] Furthermore, the reaction of hydrogen sulfide with collagen can alter the protein structure, thereby rendering the periodontal ligament and bone collagen more susceptible to destruction by proteases.[115] Investigators have shown, in cases of gingivitis and periodontitis, a decrease in the content of acid-soluble and total collagen in the affected tissues.[164] These findings suggest that increased production of VSCs may accelerate the progression of periodontal disease. Toxic VSCs are able to damage the periodontal tissues and create even more loss of attachment. A mutual reinforcement of the loss of periodontal attachment and production of VSCs occurs, resulting in a vicious cycle.[29]

Some studies, however, have shown that when the presence of tongue coating is taken into account, the correlation between periodontitis and oral malodor is much lower, thus indicating that tongue coating remains a key factor for halitosis. The prevalence of tongue coating is six times higher in patients with periodontitis, and the same bacterial species associated with periodontal disease can also be found in large numbers on the dorsum of the tongue, particularly when tongue coating is present.[218] The reported association between periodontitis and oral malodor may thus primarily be indirectly due to the effects of periodontal disease on tongue coating. It may also explain why other studies did not find a correlation.[11,178]

A systematic review with a meta-regression analysis demonstrated the association between periodontitis and halitosis based on the evidence derived from five cross-sectional studies, with a collective sample size of 7184 subjects. Subjects with periodontitis have 3.2 times higher odds of oral malodor. Interestingly, the authors concluded that the magnitude of the association was greater in studies that used the organoleptic test for halitosis detection, but the association vanished in those that used the VSC test.[172] The absence of increased levels of sulfuric compounds in breath does not rule out halitosis.[85] Prospective longitudinal studies are needed to assess the temporality of the events.

Other relevant malodorous pathologic manifestations of the periodontium are pericoronitis (the soft tissue "cap" being retentive for microorganisms and debris), major recurrent oral ulcerations, herpetic gingivitis, and necrotizing gingivitis-periodontitis. Microbiologic observations indicate that ulcers infected with gram-negative anaerobes (e.g., *Prevotella* and *Porphyromonas* spp.) are significantly more malodorous than noninfected ulcers.[12]

CLINICIAN'S CORNER

What is the influence of bad breath in patients with periodontitis?

The increased production of volatile sulfur compounds in people with bad breath may accelerate the progression of periodontal disease. For example, it is known that methylmercaptan and hydrogen sulfide can adversely affect collagen structure and gingival fibroblasts.

Dental Disorders

Possible causes within the dentition are deep carious lesions with food impaction and putrefaction, extraction wounds filled with blood clots, and purulent discharge leading to important putrefaction. Other causes include interdental food impaction in large interdental areas and crowding of teeth, favoring food entrapment and accumulation of debris. Acrylic dentures, especially when kept continuously in the mouth at night or not regularly cleaned, can lead to infections (e.g., candidiasis), which produce a typical smell. The denture surface facing the gingiva is porous and retentive for bacteria, yeasts, and debris, compounds needed for putrefaction.

Dry Mouth

Saliva has an important cleaning function in the oral cavity. Patients with xerostomia often present with large amounts of plaque on teeth and extensive tongue coating. The increased microbial load and the escape of VSCs when salivary flow is reduced explain the strong breath malodor.[76] Several studies link stress with VSC levels, but it is not clear whether this can simply be explained by a reduction of salivary flow.[82,135] Other causes of xerostomia are medications,[102] alcohol abuse,[43] Sjögren syndrome (a common autoimmune rheumatic disease),[95] and diabetes.[208]

Extraoral Causes

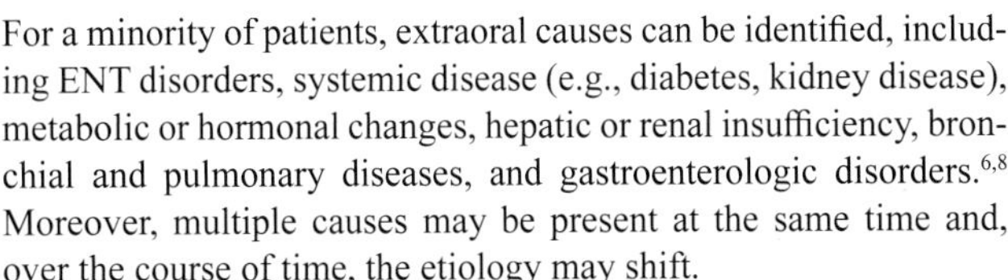

For a minority of patients, extraoral causes can be identified, including ENT disorders, systemic disease (e.g., diabetes, kidney disease), metabolic or hormonal changes, hepatic or renal insufficiency, bronchial and pulmonary diseases, and gastroenterologic disorders.[6,8] Moreover, multiple causes may be present at the same time and, over the course of time, the etiology may shift.

Extraoral halitosis can be subdivided into two types—non–blood-borne halitosis and blood-borne halitosis.[191] Non–blood-borne halitosis is less well researched, and most information about it comes from case reports. Non–blood-borne halitosis encompasses, for example, throat infections, nasal infections, infections of the respiratory system, lung diseases, and stomach disorders.

Blood-borne halitosis is the result of bad-smelling metabolites that can be formed or absorbed at any place in the body (e.g., liver, gut) and transported by the bloodstream to the lungs. Exhalation of these volatiles in the alveolar air then causes halitosis, at least when the concentrations of the bad-smelling metabolites are sufficiently high. The crevicular fluid reflects the circulating molecules in the blood and can thus also play a relevant role but, due to the small amount, probably not a very dominant one.

The extraoral causes are much more difficult to detect, although they can sometimes be recognized by a typical odor. Uncontrolled diabetes mellitus can be associated with a sweet odor of ketones, liver disease can be revealed by a sulfur odor, and kidney failure can be characterized by a fishy odor because of the presence of dimethylamine and trimethylamine.[133]

CLINICIAN'S CORNER

What is the most important cause of halitosis? Tongue coating is the most important cause of halitosis. The innumerable depressions in the tongue surface are ideal niches for bacterial adhesion and growth; additionally, desquamated cells and food remnants also remain trapped in these retention sites. The degradation of organic substrates by anaerobic bacteria results in the production of a range of unpleasant-smelling volatile compounds.

Mutations in *SELENBP1*

Mutations in *SELENBP1* have been attributed to be the underlying cause of a novel autosomal recessive malodor syndrome. Blood-borne extraoral halitosis was diagnosed in five patients with breath smelling like cabbage. Increased levels of methyl mercaptan and dimethyl sulfide were the main odorous compounds in their breath and were responsible for the malodor.[131]

Medications

At least nine medications have been identified as potential sources of bloodborne extraoral halitosis.[196] Dimethyl sulfoxide, cysteamine, and suplatast tosilate are known to be metabolized to dimethyl sulfide. Nitrates used to treat or prevent heart disease are metabolized to nitrite by the anaerobic bacteria. Some of this nitrite will reduce to nitric oxide, which can react with VSCs. Carbon disulfide can arise as a product of the metabolism of disulfiram (Antabuse). For drugs such as chloral hydrate, paraldehyde, and phenothiazide, the mode of action responsible of their association with halitosis is unclear. More recently, a systematic review extended the list to include other drug types such as anticholinergics, antidepressants, antifungals, chemotherapeutic agents, and dietary supplements (fish oil, selenium, and rose hip powder) as potential sources of extra-oral halitosis. Complaint rates varied enormously (0.5% for antidepressants to 100% for cysteamine and PX-12, a chemotherapeutic agent). Care must be taken with this information considering that most of the studies presented a high risk of bias—most of the reports did not include objective assessment of the halitosis complaints and did not consider the influence of intraoral halitosis.[105]

Pseudohalitosis or Halitophobia

If a patient presents with complaints but no objective halitosis can be detected, one speaks of pseudohalitosis or *imaginary breath odor,* which can lead to *halitophobia.*[123] The latter is the case when, even after repeated diagnosis of an absence of bad breath, the patient cannot accept the absence of halitosis. This condition has been associated with obsessive-compulsive disorder and hypochondria. Well-established personality disorder questionnaires (e.g., Symptom Checklist 90) allow the clinician to assess the patient's tendency for illusional breath malodor.[32,34,36] Having a psychologist or psychiatrist at the malodor consultation can be especially helpful for such patients. Because of the complexity of this disorder, a malodor consultation is thus preferably multidisciplinary, combining the knowledge of a periodontologist or dentist, ENT specialist, internist (if necessary), and psychologist or psychiatrist. In a study of 2000 patients, 16% were diagnosed with pseudohalitosis or halitophobia.[138]

KEY FACT

Only in a few cases is the cause of bad breath found outside the oral cavity. Thus, dentists play an important role in the diagnosis and treatment of halitosis.

Diagnosis of Malodor

Preconsultation Approach

A proper diagnostic approach starts with providing the correct information to the patient before the appointment. It is recommended that the patient not eat garlic, onions, or spices for 2 days before the consultation because they can cause bad breath and body odor that can last from several hours to 2 days.[57] To remove confounding odors, the patient is also instructed to refrain from alcohol, coffee, and smoking during the 12-hour period before the consultation. For the same reason, it is advisable for the patient not to use chewing gum, mints, drops, or mouthrinses during the 8 hours preceding the appointment. On the day of the consultation, the use of fragranced shampoo, body lotion, and perfume should also be avoided so as not to disturb the organoleptic ratings. All of the above apply both for the patient and for the diagnostician. Some of these guidelines are crucial not only for the organoleptic rating, but also for a correct interpretation of the results obtained with certain breath analyzers (see later).

In most halitosis consultations, the patient is asked not to eat or drink on the morning of the examination. However, if breakfast is consumed, morning bad breath can be excluded.

The patient should be encouraged to bring a companion to the consultations who can identify whether the perceived odor is the one previously noticed.

Course of a Halitosis Consultation

- Preconsultation patient information
- Anamnesis
- Organoleptic rating
- Examination of the breath with portable sulfur monitor
- Oropharyngeal examination
- Explanation of halitosis and instructions for oral hygiene
- If necessary, explanation of additional therapy

Anamnesis

Each consultation should start with thorough questioning about the breath malodor, eating habits, and medical and dental history. This can be done with a questionnaire that the patient fills out in the waiting room and/or replies verbally at the beginning of the consultation, depending on the preference of the examiner and the practical possibilities. To start with, the patient should be asked about the frequency of the halitosis (e.g., constantly, every day), the time of appearance during the day (e.g., after meals can indicate a stomach hernia), when the problem first appeared, and whether others have identified the problem (to exclude imaginary breath odor). In addition, the medical history has to be recorded, with an emphasis on medications and systemic diseases of the lungs, liver, kidneys, stomach, and pancreas.

Concerning the ENT history, attention should be paid to the presence of nasal obstruction, mouth breathing, postnasal drip, allergy, tonsillitis, dysphagia, and previous ENT encounters. The dental history includes questions assessing the frequency of dental visits, use of mouthrinses, presence and maintenance of a dental prosthesis, and frequency of and instruments used for toothbrushing, interdental cleaning, and tongue brushing and scraping. Finally, the patient is asked about smoking, drinking, and dietary habits.

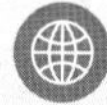

Examinations

After obtaining a thorough anamnesis, the clinician checks whether an unpleasant odor can be perceived and inspects the mouth to detect possible causes of bad breath. Different ways exist to examine the breath. The easiest and least expensive way is to smell the breath (organoleptic rating). However, several devices are on the market that mainly detect VSCs.

Organoleptic Rating

Despite the fact that devices able to analyze breath samples have existed for more than 40 years, organoleptic assessment by a judge is still the gold standard in the examination of breath malodor and therefore the most often used method. It reflects the everyday situation when halitosis is noticed and, initially, can be carried out by anyone. Moreover, the human nose can smell 10,000 different odors, many more than any device on the market.[57,61] In a specialized consultation, the organoleptic evaluation is performed by one (or more when possible) trained and preferably calibrated judges. The judge sniffs the expired air and assesses whether it is unpleasant by using an intensity rating.[158,167] Scoring is normally done according to the intensity scale of Rosenberg, where 0 represents the absence of odor, 1 is a barely noticeable odor, 2 is slight malodor, 3 is moderate malodor, 4 is strong malodor, and 5 is severe malodor.[158] In this six-point system, 0 indicates a concentration of odorant below a threshold, 1 to 4 indicate increasing occupancy of receptor binding sites, and 5 is assumed to be close to saturation.[52,53] To avoid bias, it is advisable that the organoleptic assessment precedes all other measurements.

In an organoleptic assessment, the judge smells a series of air samples (Fig. 31.4), as follows:

1. *Nasal breath odor:* The subject expires through the nose while keeping the mouth closed. When the nasal expiration is malodorous yet the air expired through the mouth is not, an ENT problem can be suspected. In that case, the procedure can be repeated one nostril at a time to obtain more details about the origin of the malodor.
2. *Oral cavity odor (passive):* The subject opens the mouth and refrains from breathing while the judge places his or her nose close to the mouth opening (approximately 10 cm from the patient's mouth).
3. *Oral cavity odor (active):* The patient counts from 1 to 10. This reveals the same as described earlier, but favors oral malodor because of drying of the palatal and tongue mucosa.
4. *Tongue coating:* The judge smells a tongue scraping from the posterior part of the tongue, obtained with an odorless plastic spoon or tongue scraper, at a distance of approximately 5 cm from his or her nose. This odor resembles that emanating from the tongue dorsum.

Although the organoleptic assessment is still the gold standard for diagnosis of halitosis, the method also has some important drawbacks. The assessment can, for example, be influenced by several aspects, such as the position of the head, hunger, and experience of the judge. Odor judges are also supposed to rest their nose for several minutes between tests to avoid habituation. The most important disadvantage of the method, however, is that it clearly has a degree of subjectivity. Researchers are trying to improve the reliability and reproducibility of the organoleptic method.[53] When using a panel of odor judges instead of only one judge, the reliability is already considered to increase.[217] Furthermore, the agreement among judges may be improved by standardization of the sense of smell using an odor solution kit for measuring the olfactory response.[228] Training is also considered to reduce odor judges' errors.[108]

Negative Pressure or Kim Method

The organoleptic method performed as described above can be a source of stress for the patients because of the proximity of the judge when sniffing the breath. In an attempt to improve this shortcoming, the use of a privacy screen or performing the test starting at a longer distance (1 m) have been used previously.[9,217] Kim and colleagues[73] have proposed a method for air sample collection that allows the organoleptic evaluation to be performed away from the patient. With this technique, a sample of mouth air is collected with a gas-tight syringe through negative pressure (hence, the given name of the procedure). The air sample is expelled into a plastic nonsmelling cup with the help of a needle. The judge holds the cup over the nose to rate the sample also according to the intensity scale of Rosenberg[158] (Fig. 31.5).

In a large study of 476 patients with halitosis complaints, breath samples collected with the negative-pressure method (NP) showed significant correlation with those evaluated with the classic method and with instrumental evaluations by means of the Halimeter and OralChroma (CHM-1 and -2). The method also showed high sensitivity (80.1%) and specificity (94.2%).[84] Even though the same considerations regarding minimizing odor interferences must be maintained, this method presents the advantage of being less affected by the presence of other odorants, as in case of body odor or the use of scented cosmetic products by the patient. Another relevant feature of the method is the possibility of assessing the exact same sample by more than one odor judge. A breath odor evaluation by an odor judge panel requires consecutive sampling and/or sequential measurements that might vary in concentration and even

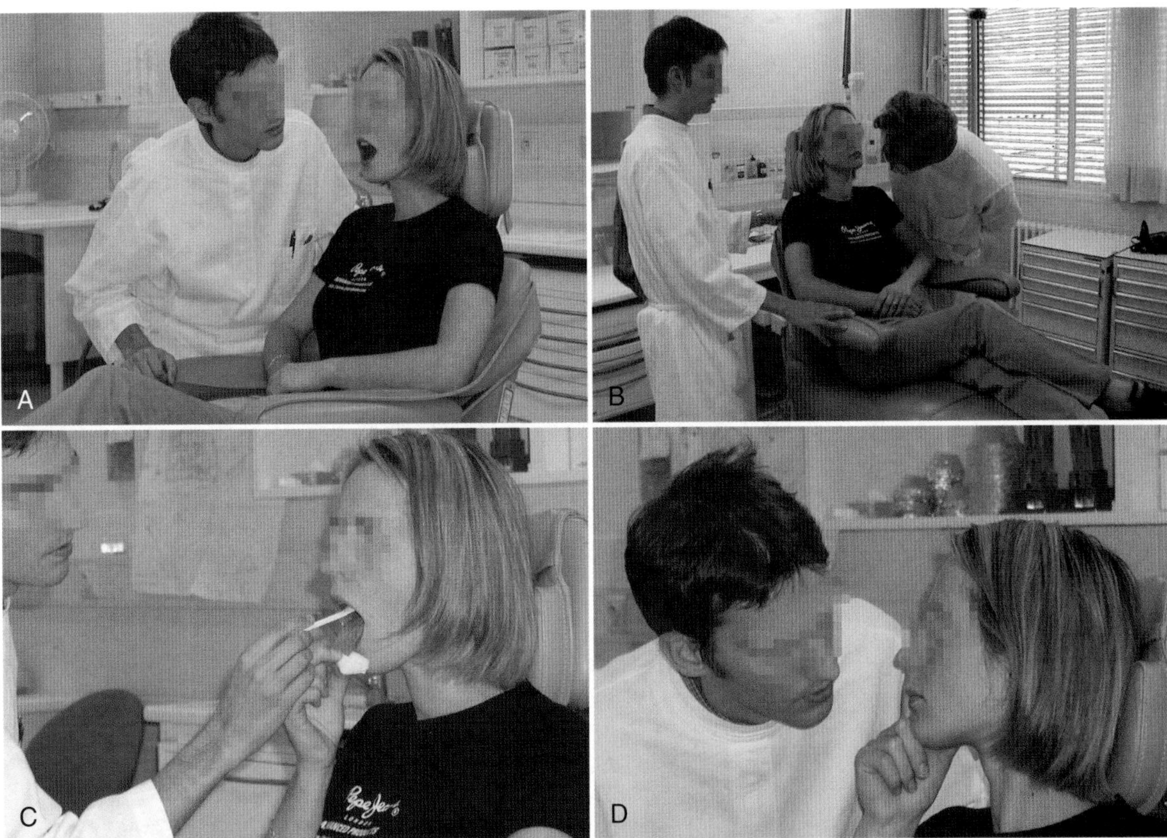

Fig. 31.4 (A) Organoleptic assessment of the oral cavity odor while the patient refrains from breathing. (B) Assessment of the oral cavity odor when the patient counts out loud from 1 to 10. (C) A sample of the tongue coating is taken to smell afterward. (D) The nasal odor is rated.

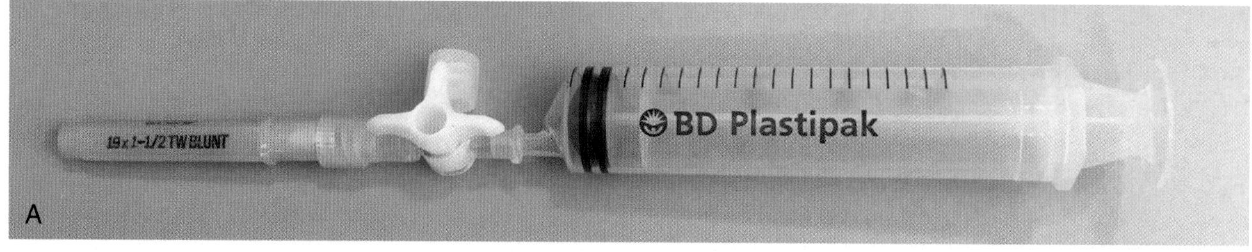

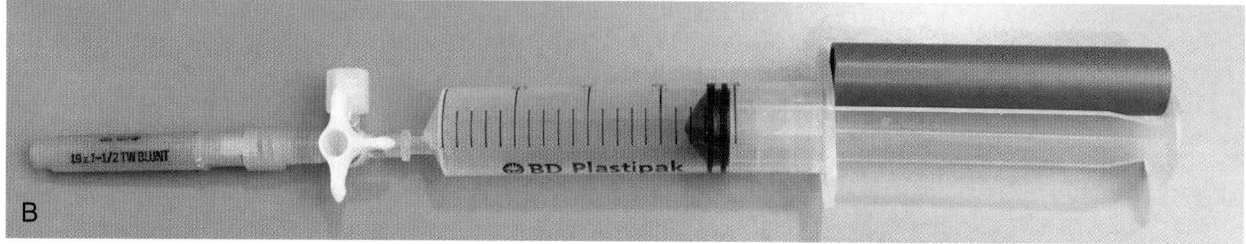

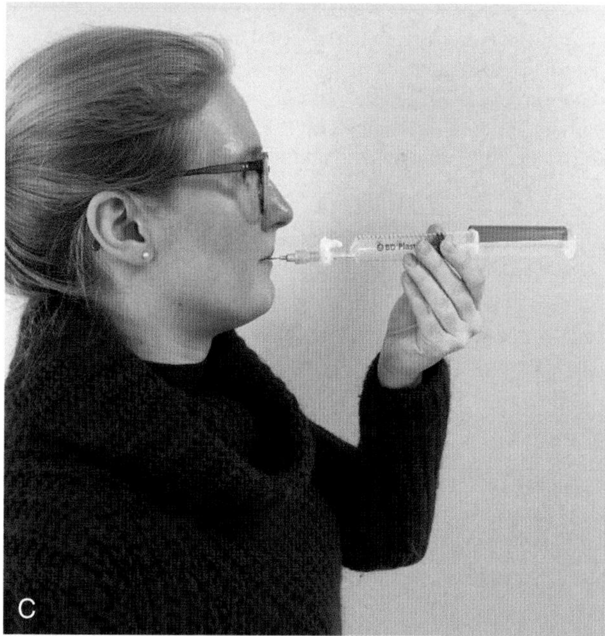

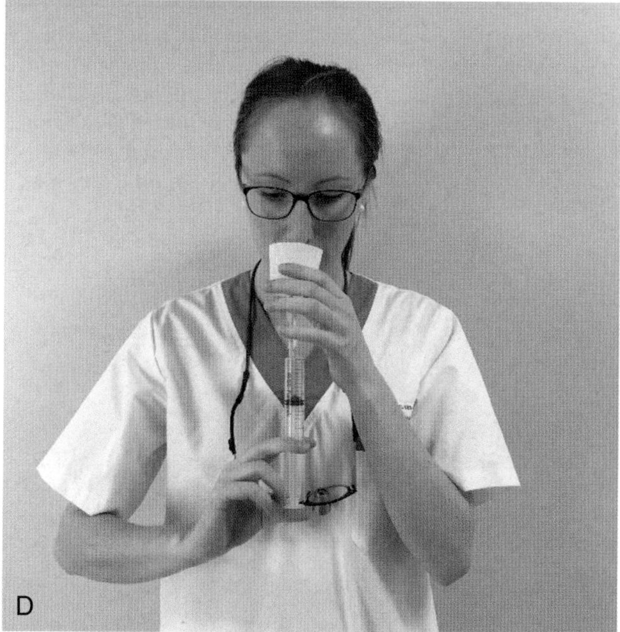

Fig. 31.5 (A) Syringe with valve and blunt needle attached. (B) The valve is closed and, by pulling the plunger and keeping this in place with a plastic tube, a vacuum is created. (C) Mouth air collection. (D) Smelling of the sample by the judge. (Note: These pictures were taken with permission of those depicted. Those shown are the first author (IL) and a colleague.) (From Laleman I, Dadamio J, De Geest S, et al: Instrumental assessment of halitosis for the general dental practitioner. *J Breath Res.* 2014;8(1):017103.)

composition.[158] The main disadvantage from this method is that it cannot be used for the evaluation of a sample of nasal air. Therefore, in the case of halitosis of extraoral origin, some relevant information could be overlooked.

Portable Volatile Sulfur Monitor

The Halimeter (Interscan, Chatsworth, CA) is an electronic device that detects the presence of VSCs such as hydrogen sulfide and methylmercaptan in the breath. The instrument cannot discriminate among the different sulfur compounds. The sensitivity for methylmercaptan is five times lower than for hydrogen sulfide, and the device is almost insensitive to dimethyl sulfide.[45] Moreover, ethanol and other compounds often used in a clinical practice can affect the measurements.

Following manufacturer's recommendations, the patient has to keep the mouth closed for 3 minutes before sampling. The mouth air is aspirated by inserting a drinking straw fixed on the flexible tube of the instrument (Fig. 31.6). The straw is kept inside the mouth, preferably above the posterior part of the tongue dorsum, not touching the oral mucosa or the tongue, while the subject keeps the mouth slightly open and breathes through the nose. The sulfur meter uses a voltametric sensor that generates a signal when exposed to

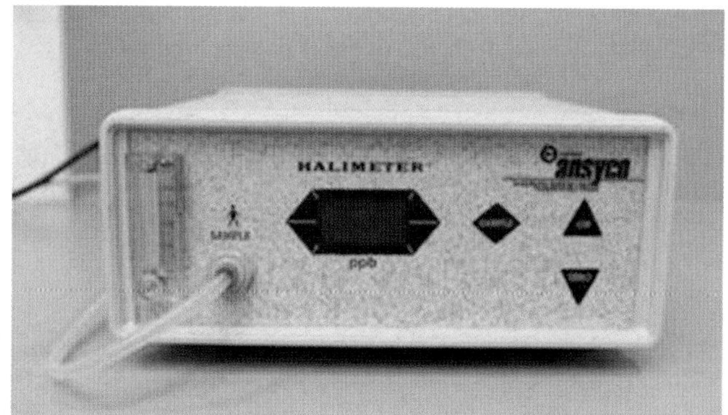

Fig. 31.6 Halimeter.

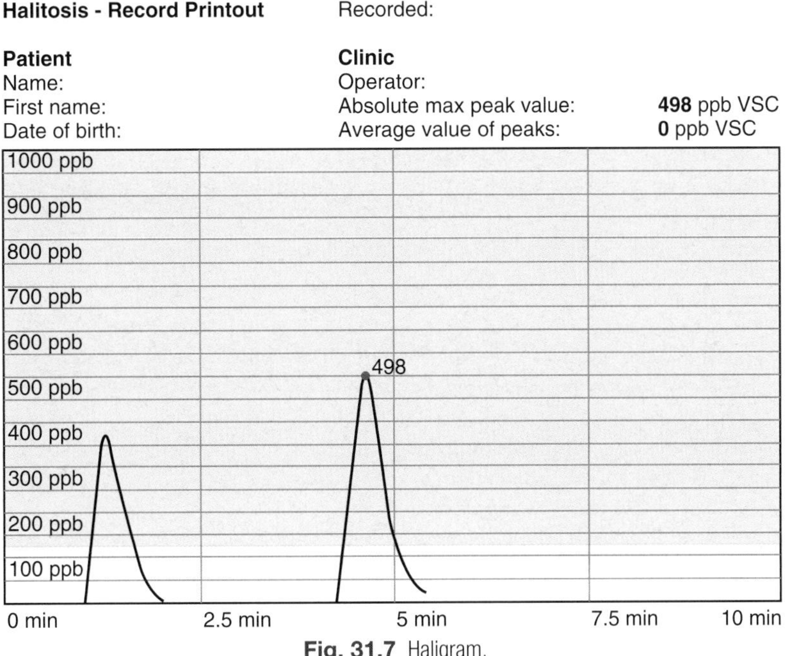

Fig. 31.7 Haligram.

sulfur-containing gases. For early models, using a recorder or specific software that gives the response as a function of time, a graphic presentation, called a *haligram*, could be obtained (Fig. 31.7). For the new model (Halimeter PLUS), this is no longer needed and the haligram is displayed directly in the front screen of the device. For the most optimal results, the manufacturer recommends performing three measurements and using the average value. For the older models, it is important to allow the meter to restabilize before repeating measurements. As for the more recent models, the device does it automatically. Independently of the model, the monitor needs regular calibration and replacement of the sensor biannually.

The Halimeter is easy to use as a chairside test and is less expensive than other portable devices. Patients are usually less embarrassed by this examination than by an organoleptic assessment. Moreover, the absence of odor in cases of halitophobia can be more convincingly proven than by an organoleptic assessment. Several studies have shown good correlations between the organoleptic measurement and the Halimeter.[156,159] An important drawback of the device is that it detects only sulfur compounds and thus is useful only for intraoral causes of halitosis. The absence of VSCs does not prove that no breath odor is present.

A wide range of threshold limits for halitosis has been proposed. Yaegaki and Sanade[218] recommended a value of 75 ppb as the limit for social acceptance, whereas the Halimeter's manufacturer proposes 150 ppb. Following this recommendation, the sensitivity and specificity of the device for the organoleptic score have been calculated to be 63% and 98%, respectively. Previous studies from our group showed that a reduction in this threshold to 120 ppb improves the sensitivity of the device without detriment to specificity.[207] In patients with oral malodor, VSC concentrations can easily reach 300 to 400 ppb.

Gas Chromatography

A gas chromatograph can analyze air, saliva, and/or crevicular fluid (Fig. 31.8). About 100 compounds have been isolated from the head space of saliva and tongue coating, including ketones, alkanes, sulfur-containing compounds, and phenyl compounds.[20] In the expired air of a person, at least 150 compounds can be found.[129,203,205] The most important advantage of the technique is that when coupled with mass spectrometry, it can detect virtually any compound when using adequate materials and conditions. Moreover, it has very high sensitivity and specificity.

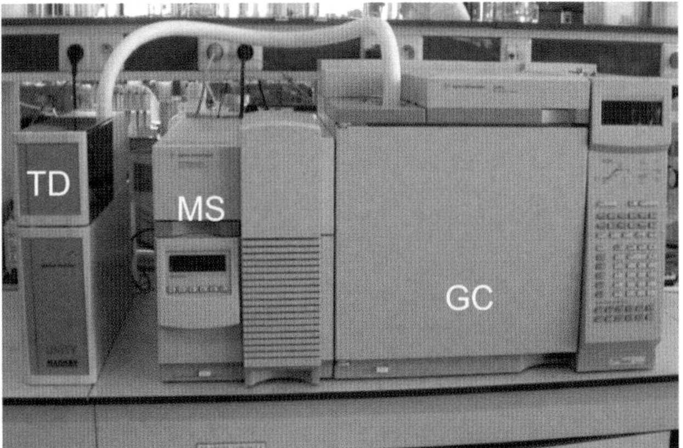

Fig. 31.8 Gas chromatography machinery, including thermal desorber *(TD)* to release molecules trapped in special collectors, gas chromatograph *(GC)* for separation of molecules, and mass spectrometer *(MS)* for identification of molecules.

Elaborate gas chromatography is available only in specialized centers but is especially useful for identifying nonoral causes.[64,128,184,202] However, it is expensive and requires trained personnel.

A small portable gas chromatograph (OralChroma, Nissha FIS, Japan) has been introduced, which makes this technique available for periodontal clinics (Fig. 31.9). More recently, the second generation of this portable gas chromatograph was introduced, the OralChroma CHM-2. The CHM-2 is a bit smaller than the first-generation OralChroma, the measurements only take half the time, and it comes with optimized software. The CHM-2 has shown similar clinical utility than its predecessor, with a reported sensitivity and specificity of 68.4% and 70.6%, respectively.[86]

Sample collection is done by use of a disposable syringe, which is inserted two thirds of the way into the oral cavity. The patient must close the mouth for 30 seconds before sample collection, and afterward the sample is injected into the gas chromatograph.

The analysis starts automatically. A software packet, OralChroma Data Manager, collects the data from the OralChroma and graphically displays the sensor responses on a computer screen. After 8 or 4 minutes for the OralChroma CHM-1 or CHM-2, respectively, the process is completed, and the concentrations of the three gases are displayed as either ng/10 mL or ppb (nmol/mol) (Fig. 31.10). The accompanying software packet gives a clear overview of the VSC measurement. However, with the OralChroma CHM-1, sometimes these graphics are not correct because the place of the VSCs is incorrectly assigned in the chromatogram. The latter can be corrected by analyzing the chromatograph.[190,192] For the CHM-2, the software uses four baseline points instead of two, which seems to have a positive impact on the peak resolution.[86]

The OralChroma has the capacity to measure the concentration of the three key sulfur compounds—hydrogen sulfide, methylmercaptan, and dimethyl sulfide—separately. This can be helpful for a differential diagnosis. A high concentration of methylmercaptan compared with hydrogen sulfide indicates, for example, periodontitis.[219] If only hydrogen sulfide is increased, a problem with oral hygiene may exist. Dimethyl sulfide can indicate an extraoral cause.[189] Just like the Halimeter, the OralChroma cannot detect compounds other than sulfur compounds, and some intraoral and extraoral causes can thus be overlooked. The apparatus needs calibration and the sensor and column need to be replaced every 2 years.[207]

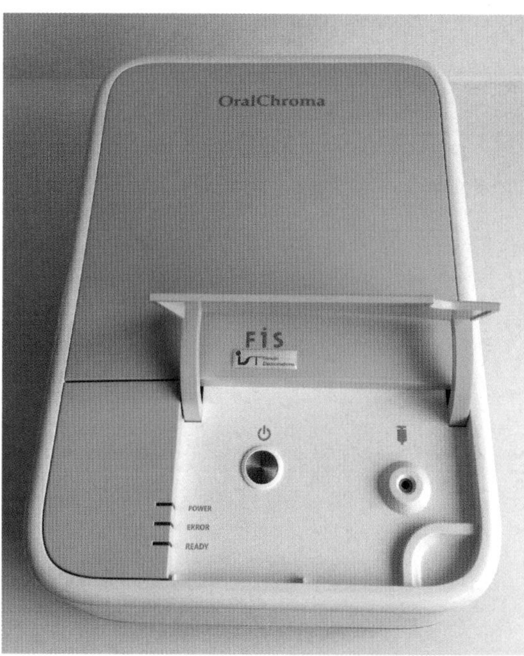

Fig. 31.9 OralChroma (CHM-2).

Halimeter Versus Oral Chroma

Halimeter	OralChroma
Easy to handle	Easy to handle, more expensive
Displays results immediately (Less than 1 min)	Takes 4 min (CHM-2[a]) or 8 min (CHM-1) before measurements are shown.
Cannot discriminate among different gases	Can discriminate among hydrogen sulfide, methylmercaptan, and dimethyl sulfide
Maintenance needed	Maintenance needed

[a]Software dependent.

Dark-Field or Phase-Contrast Microscopy

Oral malodor is typically associated with a higher incidence of motile organisms and spirochetes, so shifts in their proportions allow for the monitoring of the therapeutic progress. Another advantage of direct microscopy is that the patient becomes aware of bacteria present in plaque, tongue coating, and saliva. Too often, patients confuse plaque with food remnants.

Oropharyngeal Examination

The oropharyngeal examination includes inspection of deep carious lesions, interdental food impaction, wounds, bleeding of the gums, periodontal pockets, tongue coating, dry mouth, and the tonsils and pharynx (for tonsillitis and pharyngitis).

The tongue coating can be scored with regard to thickness and surface. Several methods have been proposed for thickness. Gross and coworkers in 1975[56] proposed an index ranging from 0 (no coating) to 3 (severe coating). Miyazaki and colleagues[100] (Fig. 31.11A) assessed tongue coating status according to area: 0 = none visible, 1 = less than one third of the tongue dorsum covered, 2 = less than two thirds, and 3 = more than two thirds.

Winkel and coworkers[213] considered both the extension and thickness of the tongue coating. The dorsum of the tongue is divided into six areas, three in the posterior and three in the anterior of the tongue (see Fig. 31.11B). The tongue coating in each sextant is scored as follows: 0 = no coating, 1 = light coating, and 2 = severe

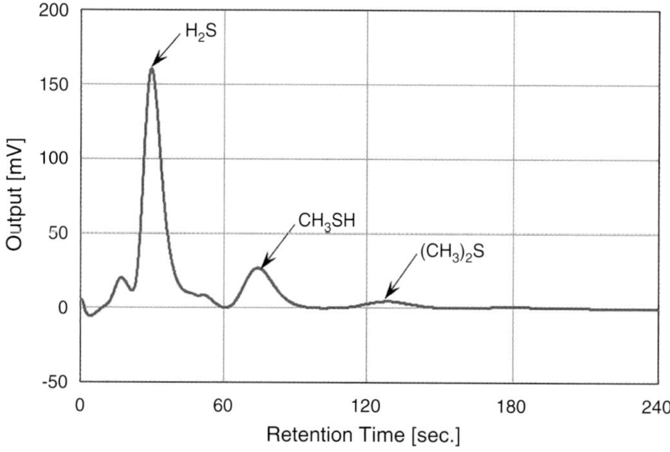

Fig. 31.10 Graphic from the OralChroma (CHM-2). The first peak indicates the level of hydrogen sulfide *(H_2S)*, the second the level of methylmercaptan *(CH_3SH)*, and the third the level of dimethyl sulfide *($[CH_3]_2S$)*.

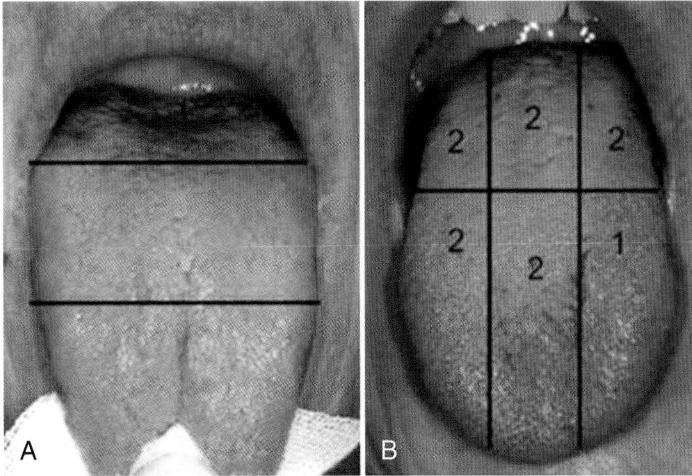

Fig. 31.11 (A) Miyazaki tongue coating index. Score 0 = none visible, score 1 = less than one third of the tongue dorsum covered, score 2 = less than two thirds, and score 3 = more than two thirds. Here score 2 applies because less than two thirds of the tongue dorsum is covered. (B) Winkel tongue coating index. Divide the dorsum of the tongue into six areas, three in the posterior and three in the anterior part of the tongue. The tongue coating in each sextant is scored as 0 = no coating, 1 = light coating, and 2 = severe coating.

coating. A score of 1 is given when the pink color underneath the coating is still visible; when this is not the case, 2 is given.

Attention should be paid to the morphology of the tongue. For example, the clinician should note whether the tongue looks normal or rough or has a deep sulcus or large papillae vallatae.[213]

Self-Examination

Smelling one's own breath by expiring into the hands in front of the mouth is not relevant because the nose becomes used to the odor,[183] and the smell of the skin and soap used for handwashing may interfere. Moreover, studies have shown that self-assessment of oral malodor is notoriously unreliable, and one should be careful with such information obtained from the patient.[9,35]

CLINICIAN'S CORNER

When one of your patients complains of bad breath and he or she is periodontally healthy but has a thick tongue coating, what can you do?

You give the patient oral hygiene instruction and stress the importance of using a tongue scraper. Optionally, a mouthrinse can be advised, with active ingredients of proven efficacy such as chlorhexidine, cetylpyridinium chloride, or a zinc formulation.

A high-performance chemiresistive electronic nose (CEN) showed enhanced sensitive detection of H_2S, NH_3, and NO in an 80% relative humidity (RH) atmosphere (similar to the composition of exhaled breath). It is a promising candidate as an inexpensive and noninvasive diagnostic tool for monitoring halitosis, kidney disorders, and asthma.[101]

Oral malodor has been evaluated with an array of six metal oxide semiconductor sensors sensitive to sulfur (hydrogen sulfide, methylmercaptan) and nonsulfur compounds (ammonia, trimethylamine, propionic acid, butylaldehyde, butylacetate, toluene, and heptane) and pattern recognition software by Nonaka and colleagues. The e-nose showed a higher accuracy than the VSC measured by gas chromatography when compared to the organoleptic assessment.[119]

Preclinical experimental assessments by Kim and colleagues have shown that it is possible to distinguish the breath of healthy subjects from simulated halitosis obtained by injecting hydrogen sulfide deliberately when using nanosensors.[74]

Nakhleh and colleagues[112] proposed the use of an array of sensors, using subsets with affinity for sulfuric and nonsulfuric volatiles that can react to the sample simultaneously. Once their responses are recorded and processed toward a pattern recognition application, they can be compared to a database of patterns obtained previously. Such a system would overcome the main limitation of the currently available devices that, as mentioned before, are limited to the detection of sulfuric compounds. The same authors have already developed a set of 20 sensors able to discriminate successfully among 17 systemic diseases by analysis of the exhaled breath.[111]

Treatment of Intraoral Halitosis or Oral Malodor

In general, the treatment of halitosis should preferably be cause-related. Because intraoral halitosis is caused by the metabolic degradation of available proteins to malodorous gases by certain oral microorganisms, the following general treatment strategies can be applied:

- Mechanical reduction of intraoral nutrients (substrates) and microorganisms
- Chemical reduction of oral microbial load
- Rendering malodorous gases nonvolatile
- Masking the malodor

Treatment should be centered on reducing the bacterial load and micronutrients by effective mechanical oral hygiene procedures, including tongue scraping. Periodontal disease should be treated and controlled and, as an auxiliary aid, oral rinses containing chlorhexidine and other ingredients may further reduce the oral malodor. If breath malodor persists after these approaches, other sources of the malodor, such as the tonsils, lung disease, gastrointestinal disease, or metabolic abnormalities (e.g., diabetes), should be investigated.

Mechanical Reduction of Intraoral Nutrients and Microorganisms

Because of the extensive accumulation of bacteria on the dorsum of the tongue, tongue cleaning should be emphasized.[18,160,218] Previous investigations demonstrated that tongue cleaning reduces both the amount of coating (and thus bacterial nutrients) and number of bacteria and thereby improves oral malodor effectively.[28,49,50,56,142] Other reports have indicated that the reduction of the microbial load on the tongue after cleaning is negligible and that the reduced malodor probably results from the reduction of bacterial nutrients.[4,38,97,137]

Cleaning of the tongue is best when performed before toothbrushing and can be done with a normal toothbrush, but preferably with a tongue scraper if a coating is established.[122,124] Even though there is no clear evidence of the superiority of one method over the other, in our experience the visualization of the deposit when removed by means of a scraper has a positive effect in patient motivation. Tongue cleaning using a tongue scraper reduces halitosis levels by 75% after 1 week.[124] This should be gentle cleaning to prevent soft tissue damage. It is best to clean as far backward as possible; the posterior portion of the tongue has the most coating.[157] Tongue cleaning should be repeated until almost no coating material can be removed.[19] The gagging reflex is often elicited, especially when using brushes[137]; practice helps prevent this.[17] It can also be helpful to pull the tongue out with a gauze pad. Tongue cleaning has the additional benefit of improving taste sensation.[137,214] In 2015, a novel tongue-cleaning device (TS1, TSpro GmbH, Karlsruhe, Germany) appeared on the market. This appliance can be used to perform professional tongue cleaning when connected to the suction device of a dental unit. The TS1 acceptance by children was high, and even better than a manual toothbrush.[149] Adult acceptance was optimal and did not differ from a manual tongue cleaner. The gag reflex was the major influence in acceptance of the treatment. The TS1 was able to remove the tongue coating as well as a manual tongue cleaner.[148]

Interdental cleaning and toothbrushing are essential mechanical means of dental plaque control. Both remove residual food particles and organisms that cause putrefaction. Clinical studies have shown that the mechanical action of toothbrushing alone has no appreciable influence on the concentration of VSCs.[185] In a short-term study, Tonzetich and Ng[195] showed a short-term effect on bad breath after brushing with a sodium monofluorophosphate toothpaste. However, the effect was half of that observed when combined with tongue brushing (73% and 30% reduction in VSCs, respectively).[195]

When chronic oral malodor arises as a consequence of periodontitis, professional periodontal therapy is needed.[11,21,125,219] A one-stage, full-mouth disinfection, combining scaling and root planing with the application of chlorhexidine, reduced organoleptic malodor levels up to 90% in one study.[139] In another study by the same investigators, initial periodontal therapy had only a weak impact on VSC levels, except when combined with a mouthrinse containing chlorhexidine.[140] In 2017, a randomized clinical trial assessed the effect of one-stage, full-mouth disinfection and conventional quadrant scaling in halitosis parameters in individuals with advanced chronic periodontitis. Both forms of nonsurgical periodontal therapy were effective in reducing organoleptic scores and CH_3SH levels. The greater reduction observed for the one-stage, full-mouth disinfection group could be attributed to the effect of the chlorhexidine included in the protocol that was not part of the conventional quadrant scaling.[174]

Chewing gum may control bad breath temporarily because it can stimulate salivary flow.[146] The salivary flow itself also has a mechanical cleaning capability. Not surprisingly, therefore, subjects with extremely low salivary flow rate have higher VSC ratings and tongue coating scores than those with normal saliva production.[79] Waler[209] showed that chewing gum without any active ingredient can reduce halitosis modestly. Muniz and colleagues[107] reviewed the effect of chewing gum in halitosis parameters and concluded that chewing gum containing active ingredients was better than placebo chewing gum. Even though no potential side effects were reported in any of the included studies, chewing for longer than 3 hours/day can contribute to muscle imbalance of the jaw and pain associated with temporomandibular malfunction.

Chemical Reduction of Oral Microbial Load

Together with toothbrushing, mouthrinsing has become a common oral hygiene practice.[47] Formulations have been modified to include antimicrobial and oxidizing agents, affecting the process of oral malodor formation. The active ingredients usually include antimicrobial agents such as chlorhexidine, cetylpyridinium chloride (CPC), essential oils, chlorine dioxide, triclosan, amine fluoride, stannous fluoride, hydrogen peroxide, and baking soda. Some of these agents have only a temporary effect on the total number of microorganisms in the oral cavity.

Chlorhexidine

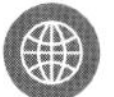

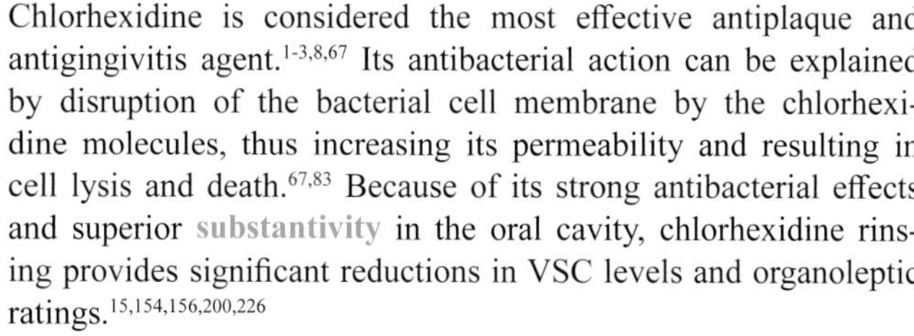

Chlorhexidine is considered the most effective antiplaque and antigingivitis agent.[1-3,8,67] Its antibacterial action can be explained by disruption of the bacterial cell membrane by the chlorhexidine molecules, thus increasing its permeability and resulting in cell lysis and death.[67,83] Because of its strong antibacterial effects and superior substantivity in the oral cavity, chlorhexidine rinsing provides significant reductions in VSC levels and organoleptic ratings.[15,154,156,200,226]

When chlorhexidine (CHX) concentrations were reduced to 0.025% and combined with 0.3% zinc acetate (CB12, MEDA OTC, Sweden), a significant reduction of malodor parameters was observed in a double-blind, controlled, cross-over study by Seemann and colleagues.[168] This long-term study confirmed the effectiveness previously reported in short-term studies[37,162] and added evidence to the synergic effect between the two main ingredients of the formulation. A 6-month follow-up study evaluating the same mouthrinse in 46 subjects with intraoral halitosis reported a 68% reduction in VSC levels and reductions in the organoleptic scores in one or two categories.[5] Unfortunately, as noted in some trials, chlorhexidine at a concentration of 0.2% or higher also has some disadvantages, such as increased tooth and tongue staining, unpleasant taste, and some temporary reductions in taste sensation.[39]

Essential Oils

Previous studies evaluated the short-term effect (3 hours) of a Listerine rinse (which contains essential oils) compared with a placebo rinse.[130] Listerine was found to be only moderately effective against oral malodor (±25% reduction vs. 10% for placebo of VSCs after 30 minutes) and caused a sustained reduction in the levels of odorigenic bacteria. Similar VSC reductions were found after rinsing for 4 days.[15] A recent review[33] concluded that despite some discrepancies, the results of in vitro studies support the effect of essential oils, but unfortunately with a lack of in vivo confirmation. It is interesting to note that the compounds with the highest antimicrobial activities are also less commonly used in formulations. Their strong smell translates to a lower acceptance by patients.[33]

Chlorine Dioxide

Chlorine dioxide (ClO_2) is a powerful oxidizing agent that can eliminate bad breath by oxidation of hydrogen sulfide, methylmercaptan, and the amino acids methionine and cysteine. Studies have demonstrated that a single use of a chlorine dioxide–containing oral rinse slightly reduced mouth odor.[41,42] After rinsing for 7 days with an experimental mouthwash containing ClO_2, Shinada and colleagues[171] reported reduced VSC levels in the experimental group compared with those in the control group. Reductions in plaque, tongue coating, and the counts of *F. nucleatum* in saliva were also observed. Long-term studies (3 weeks) by Lee and colleagues[90,91] reported clinically relevant improvements in oral malodor after twice-daily use of the same ClO_2- containing rinse for its unflavored and flavored formulations.

Two-Phase, Oil-Water Rinse

Rosenberg and colleagues[154] designed a two-phase, oil-water rinse containing CPC. The efficacy of oil-water-CPC formulations is thought to result from the adhesion of a high proportion of oral microorganisms to the oil droplets that is further enhanced by the CPC. A twice-daily rinse with this product (before bedtime and in the morning) showed reductions in both VSC levels and organoleptic ratings. These reductions were superior to those seen with Listerine and were significantly superior to placebo.[80,154] Currently, CPC is being used in the formulation of an alcohol-free mouthrinse and tongue spray (BreathRx). Saad and colleagues reported reductions in H_2S and malodor levels compared with water up to 180 minutes after use of the mouthrinse. A mouth spray has shown to reduce the organoleptic score and bacterial load significantly in comparison with a control. However, after 6 hours, the impact on the malodor indicators was small.[161]

Triclosan

Triclosan, a broad-spectrum antibacterial agent, has been found to be effective against most oral bacteria and has good compatibility with other compounds used for oral home care. A pilot study demonstrated that an experimental mouthrinse containing 0.15% triclosan and 0.84% zinc (Zn^{2+}) produced a stronger and more prolonged reduction in mouth odor than Listerine rinse.[145] The anti-VSC effect of triclosan, however, seems strongly dependent on the solubilizing agents.[225] Flavoring oils or anionic detergents and copolymers are added to increase the oral retention and decrease the rate of release in toothpaste formulations containing triclosan. The effects of these formulations in oral malodor have been illustrated in several studies.[63,117,118,169,170] Significant reductions of breath scores were observed after a single use as well as after a week of use (28% and >50%, respectively), with a similar effect on VSC levels (57% reduction after 1 week of using the paste). In vitro and ex vivo studies from Haraszthy and colleagues have demonstrated superior antimicrobial activity of triclosan-copolymer dentifrice when compared to other formulations. The triclosan-copolymer dentifrice significantly inhibited oral pathogens, such as *A. actinomycetemcomitans, Eikenella corrodens,* and *F. nucleatum.*[60]

A mouthrinse formulation combining triclosan and two other active ingredients with known effect on halitosis were shown to reduce VSC levels up to 5 hours after use in a morning bad breath model (27.5% peak reduction in the first hour).[98]

Amine Fluoride and Stannous Fluoride

The association of amine fluoride with stannous fluoride resulted in encouraging reductions of morning breath odor, even when oral hygiene was insufficient.[136] More recent evidence supporting the use of this rinse has been reported. The formulation showed not only short-term but also long-term effects on malodor indicators in patients with obvious malodor.[25]

Stannous fluoride has also been shown to be effective in the management of oral malodor as a component of a dentifrice, reducing both organoleptic scores and VSC levels.[48] A superior short-term and overnight benefit of a stannous-containing dentifrice versus a control dentifrice on morning bad breath was demonstrated in a meta-analysis.[40] In 2019, a systematic review of the evidence supporting the use of stannous fluoride toothpaste in oral health concluded that stannous fluoride reduces the level of halitosis to a larger extent than comparative toothpastes.[68]

Hydrogen Peroxide

Suarez and colleagues[185] reported that rinsing with 3% hydrogen peroxide (H_2O_2) produced impressive reductions (±90%) in sulfur gases that persisted for 8 hours. More recently, the bacterial count of the tongue showed a statistically significant decrease when brushing the tongue for 10 seconds using 3% H_2O_2.[46] Because this randomized controlled study involved only volunteers not reporting malodor complaints and assessed only the short-term effect after a single use, a future interventional study would be necessary to evaluate the efficacy of this disinfectant in tongue coating removal.

Oxidizing Lozenges

Greenstein and associates[55] reported that sucking a lozenge with oxidizing properties reduced tongue dorsum malodor for 3 hours. This antimalodor effect may be caused by the activity of dehydroascorbic acid, which is generated by peroxide-mediated oxidation of ascorbate in the lozenges.

Baking Soda

Baking soda dentifrices have been shown to confer a significant odor-reducing benefit for up to 3 hours.[14,116] The mechanism whereby baking soda produces its inhibition of oral malodor is related to its bactericidal effects.[134] Chewing gum containing baking soda was able to reduce organoleptic scores significantly in comparison to a control group.[199]

Conversion of Volatile Sulfur Compounds

Metal Salt Solutions

Metal ions with an affinity for sulfur are efficient in capturing the sulfur-containing gases. Zinc is an ion with two positive charges (Zn^{2+}), which will bind to the twice-negatively loaded sulfur radicals and thus reduce the expression of VSCs. The same applies for other metal ions such as stannous compounds, mercury, and copper. Clinically, the VSC inhibitory effect was copper chloride > stannous fluoride > zinc chloride ($CuCl_2 > SnF_2 > ZnCl_2$). In vitro, the inhibitory effect was mercury chloride = copper chloride = cadmium chloride > zinc chloride > stannous fluoride > tin chloride > lead chloride ($HgCl_2 = CuCl_2 = CdCl_2 > ZnCl_2 > SnF_2 > SnCl_2 > PbCl_2$).[227]

Compared with other metal ions, Zn^{2+} is relatively nontoxic and noncumulative and gives no visible discoloration. Thus, Zn^{2+} has been one of the most-studied ingredients for the control of oral malodor.[209,227] Schmidt and Tarbet[163] reported that a rinse containing zinc chloride was remarkably more effective than a saline rinse (or no treatment) in reducing the levels of both VSCs (±80% reduction) and organoleptic scores (±40% reduction) for 3 hours.

As mentioned, Halita, a rinse containing 0.05% chlorhexidine, 0.05% CPC, and 0.14% zinc lactate, has been found to be even more efficient than a 0.2% chlorhexidine formulation in reducing VSC levels and organoleptic ratings.[141,201] The special effects of Halita may result from the VSC conversion ability of Zn^{2+} in addition to its antimicrobial action. The combination of Zn^{2+} and chlorhexidine seems to act synergistically.[226]

Similar observations have been reported for a chlorhexidine-free mouthrinse. The addition of zinc ions to a basic formulation containing amino fluoride and stannous fluoride caused short- and long-term reduction of oral malodor indicators in volunteers with morning bad breath,[211,212] as well as in volunteers with obvious halitosis.[25]

In a study by Hoshi and van Steenberghe,[62] a zinc citrate–triclosan toothpaste applied to the tongue dorsum appeared to control morning breath malodor for 4 hours. If the flavor oil was removed, however, the antimalodor efficacy of the active ingredients decreased. Another clinical study reported up to a 41% reduction in

VSC levels after 7 days' use of a dentifrice containing triclosan and a copolymer, but the benefit compared with a placebo was relatively small (17% reduction).[118] Similar reductions were also found in two other more recent studies.[63,117]

Chewing gum can be formulated with antibacterial agents, such as fluoride or chlorhexidine, which helps reduce oral malodor through mechanical and chemical approaches. Waler[209] compared different concentrations of Zn^{2+} in a chewing gum and found that a 2-mg Zn^{2+} acetate–containing chewing gum that remained in the mouth for 5 minutes resulted in an immediate reduction in VSC levels of up to 45%, but the long-term effect was not mentioned.

A single brushing with the experimental zinc toothpaste (0.5–0.7% zinc as zinc citrate and polyvinyl methyl ether/maleic acid [PVM/MA] copolymer) was more effective than the existing marketed zinc toothpaste (0.1–0.3% zinc as zinc gluconate) in reducing VSC levels in volunteers with morning bad breath. The effect was attributed to the higher dose and higher availability of the zinc ions obtained with the copolymer.[224]

The most recent report on the effectiveness of zinc lactate–containing mouthwash showed reduced organoleptic scores and VSC over a period of 3 hours in subjects in periodontal maintenance. The amount and time of use of the rinse did not have an impact on the outcome. The effect was attributed to the neutralizing capacity of the zinc ions because the short-term evaluation did not allow for an antimicrobial effect.[66]

Potential New Strategies to Alleviate Intraoral Halitosis

The number of products claiming to be able control, combat, or solve the problem of halitosis has increased significantly in the past decade, but with only limited research supporting their rationale of use, as pointed out in previous systematic reviews.[7,39,175] Alternative therapies listed below, although promising, need to be evaluated in long-term follow-up studies before they can be taken into full consideration by professionals treating the condition.[215]

Probiotics

Probiotics are "living organisms which, when administered in adequate amounts, confer a health benefit for the host." Their use has been approved by the World Health Organization (WHO) and the Food and Agriculture Organization of the United Nations (FAO). The rationale for probiotic use is to restore the microbial balance by adding beneficial species. Probiotics can modulate the host inflammatory response or have direct and indirect effects against pathogenic bacteria.[87,193]

The probiotic effect of *Streptococcus salivarius* strain K12, *Weissella cibaria*, and *Streptococcus thermophilus* on halitosis parameters has been reported by in vitro studies. In regard to clinical studies, evidence supporting the use of probiotics to manage intraoral halitosis has been promising but not conclusive. A positive effect, evidenced by a reduction of organoleptic scores, has been reported in three different studies. However, with respect to the effect on VSC levels, the results were more heterogeneous.[215] A recent systematic review with meta-analysis concluded that this inconsistency could be due to heterogeneity of the probiotic strains used among the studies, test subjects, and overall absence of standardized probiotic strategies as a critical source of bias.[223]

Herbal Substances

Green tea polyphenolic catechins have an impact on oral health via antiseptic, antioxidative, and antiinflammatory activity. *Epigallocatechin gallate* is the main deodorizing agent among the tea catechins. The chemical reaction between epigallocatechin and methylmercaptan results in a nonvolatile product.[221] They are also able to suppress *mgl,* the gene encoding L-methionine-α-deamino-γ-mercaptomethane lyase, responsible for CH_3SH production by oral anaerobes.[216] Green tea can decrease the adhesion of *S. moorei* and *P. gingivalis* to oral epithelial cells and can as inhibit *Solobacterium moorei* by interrupting the bacterial cell membrane integrity.[71,104] Antibacterial activity of tannin and Zn^{2+} present in green tea are also thought to contribute to the antimalodor effect. Tsunoda and associates[197] investigated the beneficial effect of chewing gum containing tea extracts for its deodorizing mechanism. Short-term effects observed by Lodhia and colleagues[93] when they applied green tea powder on the back of the tongue were less conclusive than those reported by Porciani and Grandini,[132] which could demonstrate a significant immediate effect when using tablets containing green tea extract. Recently, a systematic review reported a study with a "high level of evidences" using mouth rinses containing green tea extract for a period of 4 weeks.[186] After 4 weeks, significant differences with baseline and with respect to the placebo group were reported. The insignificant effect during short-term evaluations was attributed to a possible washout effect, masking the ability of green tea catechins to render nonvolatile compounds.[143] A few other studies have reported the effects of other herbal compounds, with less remarkable results.[215]

Masking the Malodor

Treatment with mouth rinses and sprays or lozenges containing volatiles with a pleasant odor has only a short-term effect.[146,147] Typical examples are mint-containing lozenges and the aroma of rinses without antibacterial components.[25]

Another pathway is to increase the solubility of malodorous compounds in the saliva by increasing the secretion of saliva; a larger volume allows the retention of larger amounts of soluble VSCs.[77] The latter can also be achieved by ensuring proper liquid intake or using chewing gum; chewing triggers the periodontal-parotid reflex, at least when the lower (pre)molars are still present.

Conclusion

Breath malodor has important socioeconomic consequences and can reveal important diseases. A proper diagnosis and determination of the etiology allow initiation of the proper causative treatment. Although tongue coating and (less frequently) periodontitis and gingivitis are the most common causes of malodor, a clinician cannot take the risk of overlooking other, more challenging diseases. This can be done with a multidisciplinary consultation or, if this is not feasible, a trial therapy to deal quickly with intraoral causes (e.g., full-mouth, one-stage disinfection, including the use of proper mouthrinses, tongue scrapers, and toothpastes). For more detailed information, the reader is encouraged to consult review articles.[54,85,167]

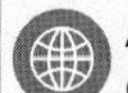
A Case Scenario is found on the companion website eBooks.Health.Elsevier.com.

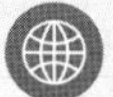
References for this chapter are found on the companion website eBooks.Health.Elsevier.com.

CHAPTER 32

Periodontal Response to External Forces

Flavia Q. Pirih | Paulo M. Camargo | Henry H. Takei | Fermin A. Carranza

CHAPTER OUTLINE

Adaptive Capacity of the Periodontium to Occlusal Forces

The periodontal ligament has a cushioning effect on forces applied to teeth as a means to accommodate forces exerted on the crown. Due to the elastic nature of the periodontal ligament, all teeth with normal bone support present with physiologic mobility in all directions. Physiologic tooth mobility varies among individuals and within the dentition of the same individual. In the absence of excessive occlusal forces or of reduced bone support induced by inflammatory periodontal disease, tooth mobility remains unchanged due to the fact that physiologic forces are not able to induce changes to the periodontal tissues.[3]

When there is an increase in occlusal forces, changes occur in the periodontium in order to accommodate such forces. Changes in the periodontium depend on the magnitude, direction, duration, and frequency of increased occlusal forces (Box 32.1).

When the *magnitude* of occlusal forces is increased, the periodontium responds with a widening of the periodontal ligament space, an increase in the number and width of periodontal ligament fibers, and an increase in the density of alveolar bone.

Changing the *direction* of occlusal forces causes a reorientation of the stresses and strains within the periodontium (Fig. 32.1).[23] The principal fibers of the periodontal ligament are arranged so that they best accommodate occlusal forces along the long axis of the tooth.

LEARNING BOX 32.1

When there is an increase in occlusal forces, changes occur in the periodontium in order to accommodate such forces. Changes in the periodontium depend on the magnitude, direction, duration, and frequency of increased occlusal forces.

Lateral (horizontal) and *torque* (rotational) forces are more likely to injure the periodontium.

The response of alveolar bone is also affected by the *duration* and *frequency* of occlusal forces. Constant pressure on the bone is more injurious than intermittent forces. The more frequent the application of an intermittent force, the more injurious the force is to the periodontium.

Trauma From Occlusion

Trauma from occlusion is defined as microscopic alterations of periodontal structures in the area of the periodontal ligament that manifest clinically in the elevation of tooth mobility. As mentioned earlier, an inherent "margin of safety" that is common to all tissues permits some variation in occlusion without adversely affecting the periodontium. However, when occlusal forces exceed the adaptive capacity of the tissues, tissue injury results.[43,44] The resultant injury is termed *trauma from occlusion,* which is also known as *occlusal trauma.*

Thus trauma from occlusion refers to the *tissue injury* rather than the *occlusal force.* An occlusion that produces such an injury is called a *traumatic occlusion.*[2] Excessive occlusal forces may also disrupt the function of the masticatory musculature and can cause painful spasms, injury to the temporomandibular joints, or produce excessive tooth wear. However, the term *trauma from occlusion* is generally used in connection with injury to the periodontium.

LEARNING BOX 32.2

Trauma from occlusion refers to the *tissue injury* rather than the *occlusal force.* An occlusion that produces such an injury is called a *traumatic occlusion.*

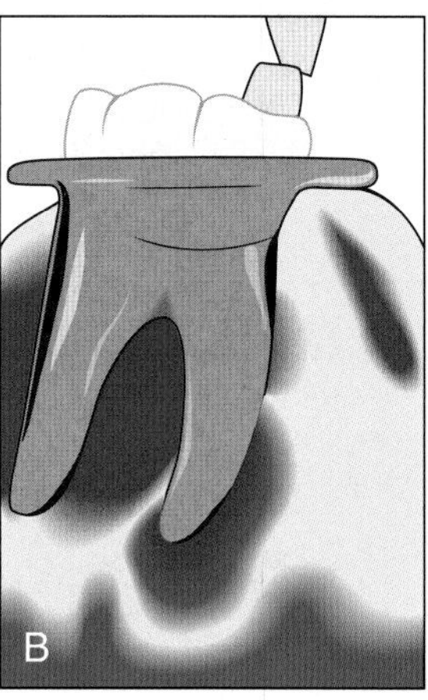

Fig. 32.1 Stress patterns around the roots changed by shifting the direction of occlusal forces (experimental model using photoelastic analysis). (A) Buccal view of an Ivorine molar subjected to an axial force. The *shaded fringes* indicate that the internal stresses are at the root apices. (B) Buccal view of an Ivorine molar subjected to a mesial tilting force. The *shaded fringes* indicate that the internal stresses are along the mesial surface and at the apex of the mesial root.

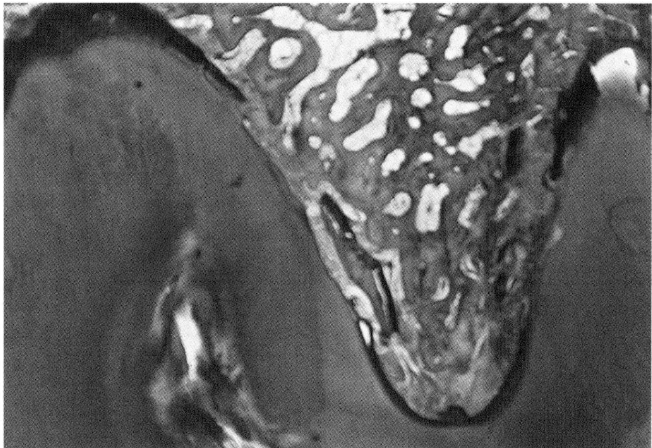

Fig. 32.2 Cemental tear, presumably caused by acute trauma from occlusion in a human autopsy specimen. Note the repair process depositing bone on the displaced, torn cementum and recreating a periodontal ligament.

Classification of Trauma From Occlusion

Trauma from occlusion can be classified according to the injurious occlusal force(s) mode of onset (acute and chronic) or according to the capacity of the periodontium to resist to occlusal forces (primary and secondary).

Acute and Chronic Trauma From Occlusion

Acute trauma from occlusion refers to periodontal changes associated with an abrupt occlusal impact such as that produced by biting on a hard object (e.g., an olive pit). In addition, restorations or prosthetic appliances that interfere with or alter the direction of occlusal forces on the teeth may also induce acute trauma. Acute trauma results in tooth pain, sensitivity to percussion, and increased tooth mobility. If the force is dissipated by a shift in the position of the tooth or by the wearing away or correction of the restoration, then the injury heals, and the symptoms subside. Otherwise, periodontal injury may worsen and develop into necrosis accompanied by periodontalabscess formation, or it may persist as a symptom-free chronic condition. Acute trauma can also produce cemental tears (Fig. 32.2).

LEARNING BOX 32.3

Acute trauma from occlusion refers to periodontal changes associated with an abrupt occlusal impact such as that produced by biting on a hard object (e.g., an olive pit). In addition, restorations or prosthetic appliances that interfere with or alter the direction of occlusal forces on the teeth may also induce acute trauma. Acute trauma results in tooth pain, sensitivity to percussion, and increased tooth mobility.

Chronic trauma from occlusion refers to periodontal changes associated with gradual changes in occlusion produced by tooth wear, drifting movement, and extrusion of the teeth in combination with parafunctional habits (e.g., bruxism, clenching) rather than as a sequela of acute periodontal trauma. Chronic trauma from occlusion is more common than the acute form and of greater clinical significance. The features of chronic trauma from occlusion and their significance are discussed in the following sections.

The criterion that determines if an occlusion is traumatic is whether it produces periodontal injury; the criterion is *not* based on how the teeth occlude. Any occlusion that produces periodontal injury is traumatic. Malocclusion is not necessary to produce trauma; periodontal injury may occur when the occlusion appears normal. The dentition may be anatomically and aesthetically acceptable but functionally injurious. Similarly, not all malocclusions are necessarily injurious to the periodontium. Traumatic occlusal relationships are referred to by such terms as *occlusal disharmony, functional imbalance,* and *occlusal dystrophy.* These terms refer to the effect of the occlusion on the periodontium rather than to the position of the teeth. Because trauma from occlusion refers to the tissue injury rather than the occlusion, an increased occlusal force is not traumatic if the periodontium can accommodate it.

LEARNING BOX 32.4

Chronic trauma from occlusion refers to periodontal changes associated with gradual changes in occlusion produced by tooth wear, drifting movement, and extrusion of the teeth in combination with parafunctional habits (e.g., bruxism, clenching) rather than as a sequela of acute periodontal trauma. Chronic trauma from occlusion is more common than the acute form and of greater clinical significance.

Primary and Secondary Trauma From Occlusion

As mentioned previously, trauma from occlusion can also be classified into primary and secondary trauma from occlusion according to the capacity of the periodontium to resist occlusal forces. In other words, trauma from occlusion may be caused by alterations in occlusal forces, a reduced capacity of the periodontium to withstand occlusal forces, or both. When trauma from occlusion is the result of alterations in occlusal forces, it is called *primary trauma from occlusion.* When it results from the reduced ability of the tissues to resist the occlusal forces, it is known as *secondary trauma from occlusion.*

Primary trauma from occlusion occurs if trauma from occlusion is considered the primary etiologic factor in periodontal destruction and if the only local alteration to which a tooth is subjected is a result of occlusion. Examples include periodontal injury produced around teeth with a previously healthy periodontium after the following: (1) the insertion of a "high filling"; (2) the insertion of a prosthetic replacement that creates excessive forces on abutment and antagonistic teeth; (3) the drifting movement or extrusion of the teeth into spaces created by unreplaced missing teeth; or (4) the orthodontic movement of teeth into functionally unacceptable positions. Most

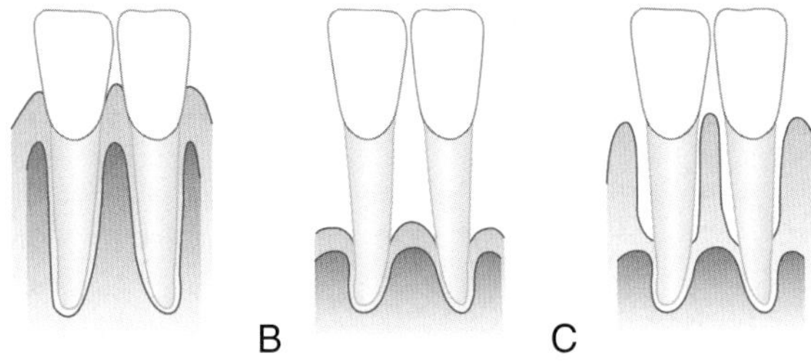

Fig. 32.3 Traumatic forces can occur on (A) normal periodontium with normal height of bone, (B) normal periodontium with reduced height of bone, or (C) marginal periodontitis with reduced height of bone.

studies of the effect of trauma from occlusion involving experimental animals have examined the primary type of trauma. Changes produced by primary trauma do not alter the level of connective tissue attachment and do not initiate pocket formation. This is probably because the supracrestal gingival fibers are not affected and therefore prevent the apical migration of the junctional epithelium.[48]

LEARNING BOX 32.5

Primary trauma from occlusion occurs if trauma from occlusion is considered the primary etiologic factor in periodontal destruction and if the only local alteration to which a tooth is subjected is a result of occlusion.

Secondary trauma from occlusion occurs when the adaptive capacity of the tissues to withstand occlusal forces is impaired by bone loss that results from marginal inflammation. This reduces the periodontal attachment area and alters the leverage on the remaining tissues. The periodontium becomes more vulnerable to injury, and previously well-tolerated occlusal forces become traumatic.

Fig. 32.3 depicts three situations on which excessive occlusal forces can be superimposed:

1. Normal periodontium with normal height of bone
2. Normal periodontium with reduced height of bone
3. Marginal periodontitis with reduced height of bone

The first case is an example of primary trauma from occlusion, whereas the last two represent secondary trauma from occlusion. The effects of trauma from occlusion in these different situations are analyzed in the following discussion.

It has been found in experimental animals that systemic disorders can reduce tissue resistance and that previously tolerable forces may become excessive.[21,51,61] This could theoretically represent another mechanism by which tissue resistance to increased forces is lowered, thereby resulting in secondary trauma from occlusion.

Stages of Tissue Response to Increased Occlusal Forces

Tissue response occurs in three stages[4,8]: injury, repair, and adaptive remodeling of the periodontium.

Stage I: Injury

Tissue injury is produced by excessive occlusal forces. The body then attempts to repair the injury and restore the periodontium. This can occur if the forces are diminished or if the tooth drifts away from them. If the offending force is chronic, however, the periodontium is remodeled to cushion its impact. The ligament is widened at the expense of the bone, which results in angular bone defects without periodontal pockets, and the tooth becomes loose.

Under the forces of occlusion, a tooth rotates around a fulcrum, or axis of rotation, which in single-rooted teeth is located in the junction between the middle third and the apical third of the clinical root and in multirooted teeth in the middle of the interradicular bone (Fig. 32.4). This creates areas of pressure and tension on opposite sides of the fulcrum. Different lesions are produced by different degrees of pressure and tension. If jiggling forces are exerted, these different lesions may coexist in the same area.

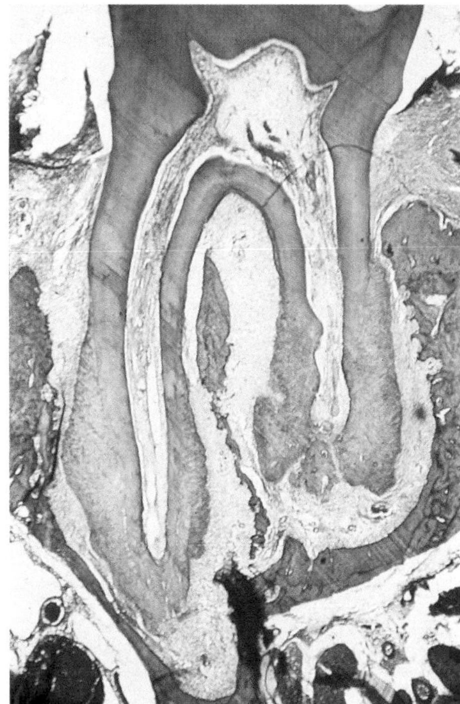

Fig. 32.4 Areas of tension and pressure in opposite sites of the periodontal ligament caused by experimentally induced orthodontic movement in a rat molar.

Slightly excessive pressure stimulates resorption of the alveolar bone, with a resultant widening of the periodontal ligament space. *Slightly excessive tension* causes elongation of the periodontal ligament fibers and the apposition of alveolar bone. In areas of increased pressure, the blood vessels are numerous and reduced in size; in areas of increased tension, they are enlarged.[67]

Greater pressure produces a gradation of changes in the periodontal ligament, starting with compression of the fibers, which produces areas of hyalinization.[54–56] Subsequent injury to the fibroblasts and other connective tissue cells leads to necrosis of areas of the ligament.[52,56] Vascular changes are also produced: within 30 minutes, impairment and stasis of blood flow occur; at 2 to 3 hours, blood vessels appear to be packed with erythrocytes, which start to fragment; and between 1 and 7 days, disintegration of the blood vessel walls and release of the contents into the surrounding tissue occur.[53,63] In addition, increased resorption of alveolar bone and resorption of the tooth surface occur.[29,34]

Severe tension causes widening of the periodontal ligament, thrombosis, hemorrhage, tearing of the periodontal ligament, and resorption of alveolar bone.

Pressure severe enough to force the root against bone causes necrosis of the periodontal ligament and bone. The bone is resorbed by a viable periodontal ligament adjacent to necrotic areas and from marrow spaces; this process is called *undermining resorption*.[25,43]

The areas of the periodontium that are most susceptible to injury from excessive occlusal forces are the furcations.[22]

Injury to the periodontium produces a temporary depression in mitotic activity, in the rate of proliferation and differentiation of fibroblasts,[62] in collagen formation, and in bone formation.[29,58,60,62] These return to normal levels after the dissipation of the forces.

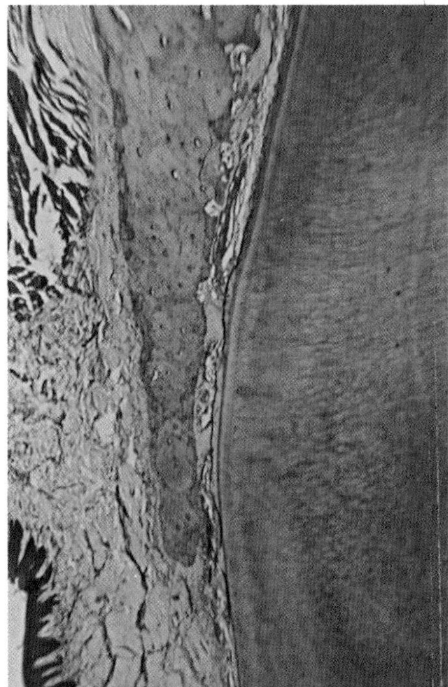

Fig. 32.5 Experimental occlusal trauma in rats. Note the area of necrosis of the marginal periodontal ligament and resorption and remodeling in the more apical periodontal sites.

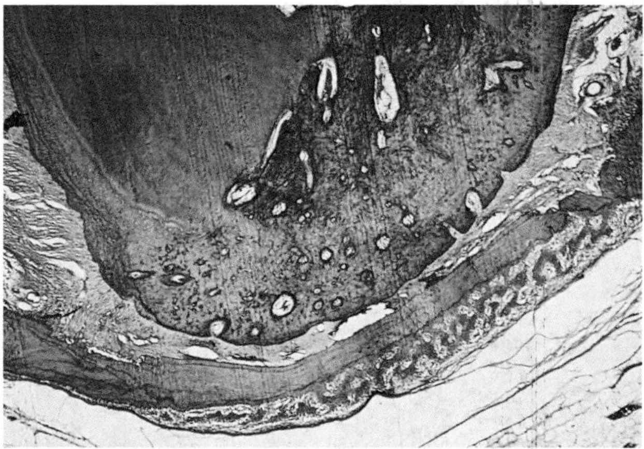

Fig. 32.6 Apical area of a premolar subjected to experimental occlusal trauma in a dog causing intrusion of the tooth and areas of necrosis in the periodontal ligament. Note the active bone formation on the outer aspect of the bone and the resorptive activity in the periphery of the necrotic site.

Stage II: Repair

Repair occurs constantly in the normal periodontium, and trauma from occlusion stimulates increased reparative activity. The damaged tissues are removed, and new connective tissue cells and fibers, bone, and cementum are formed in an attempt to restore the injured periodontium (Fig. 32.5). Forces remain traumatic only as long as the damage produced exceeds the reparative capacity of the tissues.

When bone is resorbed by excessive occlusal forces, the body attempts to reinforce the thinned bony trabeculae with new bone (Fig. 32.6). This attempt to compensate for lost bone is called *buttressing bone formation,* and it is an important feature of the reparative process associated with trauma from occlusion.[16] It also occurs when bone is destroyed by inflammation or osteolytic tumors.

Buttressing bone formation occurs within the jaw (central buttressing) and on the bone surface (peripheral buttressing). During *central buttressing,* the endosteal cells deposit new bone, which restores the bony trabeculae and reduces the size of the marrow spaces. *Peripheral buttressing* occurs on the facial and lingual surfaces of the alveolar plate. Depending on its severity, peripheral buttressing may produce a shelflike thickening of the alveolar margin, which is referred to as *lipping* (Fig. 32.7), or a pronounced bulge in the contour of the facial and lingual bone.[8,16]

Cartilage-like material sometimes develops in the periodontal ligament space as an aftermath of the trauma.[13] The formation of crystals from erythrocytes has also been demonstrated.[57]

Stage III: Adaptive Remodeling of the Periodontium

If the repair process cannot keep pace with the destruction caused by the occlusion, the periodontium is remodeled in an effort to create a structural relationship in which the forces are no longer injurious to the tissues.[18] *This results in a widened periodontal ligament, which is funnel shaped at the crest, and angular defects in the bone with no pocket formation. The involved teeth become loose.*[67] Increased vascularization has also been reported.[9]

The three stages in the evolution of traumatic lesions have been differentiated histometrically by the relative amounts of periodontal bone surface undergoing resorption or formation (Fig. 32.8).[5,8] The injury phase shows an increase in areas of resorption and a decrease in bone formation, whereas the repair phase demonstrates decreased resorption and increased bone formation. After adaptive remodeling of the periodontium, resorption and formation return to normal.

Effects of Insufficient Occlusal Force

Insufficient occlusal force may also be injurious to the supporting periodontal tissues.[6,36] Insufficient stimulation causes thinning of the periodontal ligament, atrophy of the fibers, osteoporosis of the alveolar bone, and a reduction in bone height. Hypofunction can result from an open-bite relationship, an absence of functional antagonists, or unilateral chewing habits that neglect one side of the mouth.

Reversibility of Traumatic Lesions

Trauma from occlusion is reversible. When trauma is artificially induced in experimental animals, the teeth move away or intrude into the jaw. When the impact of the artificially created force is relieved, the tissues undergo repair. Although trauma from occlusion is reversible under such conditions, it does not always correct itself, and therefore it is not always temporary or is of limited clinical significance. The injurious force must be relieved for repair to occur.[22,49] If conditions in humans do not permit the teeth to escape from or adapt to excessive occlusal force, periodontal damage persists and worsens.

The presence of inflammation in the periodontium as a result of plaque accumulation may impair the reversibility of traumatic lesions.[30,49]

Effects of Excessive Occlusal Forces on Dental Pulp

The effects of excessive occlusal forces on the dental pulp have not been established. Some clinicians report the disappearance of pulpal symptoms after the correction of excessive occlusal forces. Pulpal reactions have been noted in animals subjected to increased occlusal forces,[7,35] but these did not occur when the forces were minimal and occurred over short periods.[35]

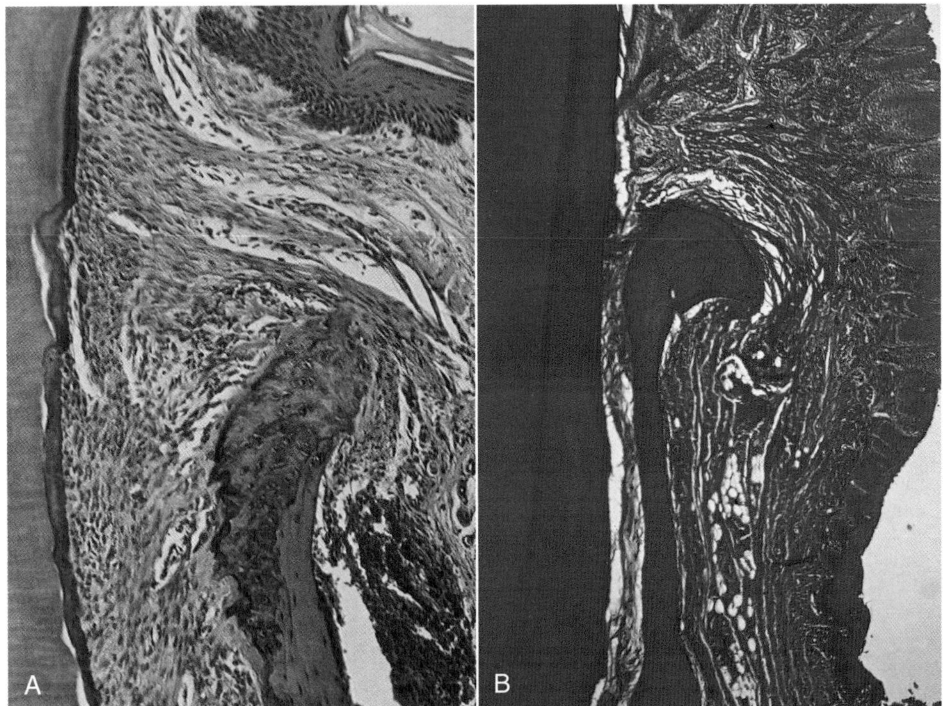

Fig. 32.7 (A) Widening of the periodontal ligament space in the cervical area and a change in the shape of the marginal alveolar bone as a result of chronic prolonged trauma from occlusion in rats. (B) Comparable changes in the shape of the marginal bone found in a human autopsy case.

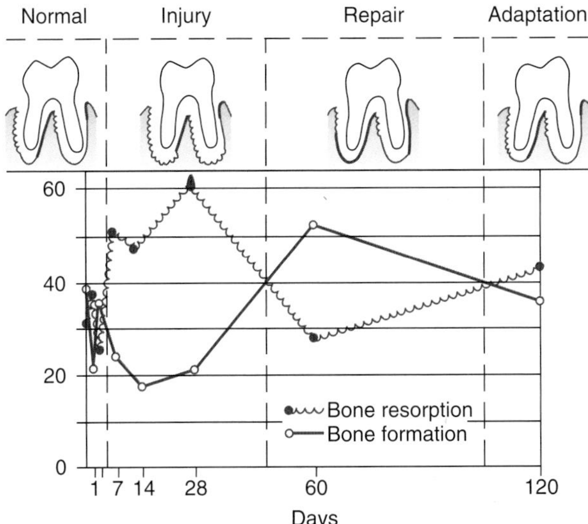

Fig. 32.8 Evolution of traumatic lesions as depicted experimentally in rats by variations in relative amounts of areas of bone formation and bone resorption in periodontal bone surfaces. The horizontal axis shows the number of days after the initiation of traumatic interference. The vertical axis shows the percentage of bone surface undergoing resorption or formation. The stages in the evolution of the lesions are represented in the top drawings, which show the average amount of bone activity for each group.[4]

LEARNING BOX 32.6

Secondary trauma from occlusion occurs when the adaptive capacity of the tissues to withstand occlusal forces is impaired by bone loss that results from marginal inflammation. This reduces the periodontal attachment area and alters the leverage on the remaining tissues. The periodontium becomes more vulnerable to injury, and previously well-tolerated occlusal forces become traumatic.

Relationship Between Plaque-Induced Periodontal Diseases and Trauma From Occlusion

The clinical impressions of early investigators and clinicians assigned an important role to trauma from occlusion in the etiology of periodontal lesions. Since then, numerous studies have been performed that have attempted to determine the mechanisms by which trauma from occlusion may affect periodontal disease.

Initial studies involved the placement of high crowns or restorations on the teeth of dogs or monkeys, thereby resulting in a continuous or intermittent force in one direction.[2,20] These investigations provided an orthodontic type of force and gave clear descriptions of changes that were occurring in pressure zones and tension zones. These procedures usually resulted in tooth displacement and consolidation in a new, nontraumatized position.

Trauma from occlusion in humans, however, is the result of forces that act alternatively in opposing directions. These were analyzed in experimental animals with "jiggling forces," which were usually produced by a high crown in combination with an orthodontic appliance that would bring the traumatized tooth back to its original position when the force was dissipated by separating the teeth. With another method, the teeth were separated by wooden or elastic material wedged interproximally to displace a tooth toward the opposite proximal side. After 48 hours, the wedge was removed, and the procedure was repeated on the opposite side.

These studies resulted in a combination of changes produced by pressure and tension on both sides of the tooth, with an increase in the width of the ligament and increased tooth mobility. None of these methods caused gingival inflammation or pocket formation, and the results essentially represented different degrees of functional adaptation to increased forces.[48,67] To mimic the problem in humans more closely, studies were then conducted on the effect produced by jiggling trauma and simultaneous plaque-induced gingival inflammation.

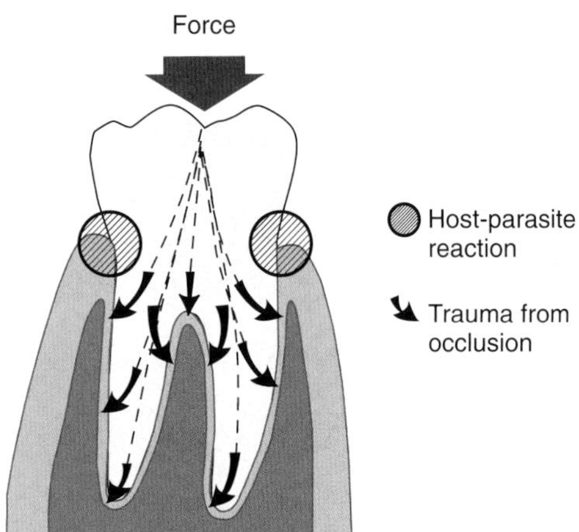

Fig. 32.9 The reaction between dental plaque and the host takes place in the gingival sulcus region. Trauma from occlusion appears in the tissues that are supporting the tooth.

The accumulation of bacterial plaque that initiates gingivitis and results in periodontal pocket formation affects the marginal gingiva, but trauma from occlusion occurs in the supporting tissues and does not affect the gingiva (Fig. 32.9). The marginal gingiva is unaffected by trauma from occlusion because its blood supply is not affected, even when the vessels of the periodontal ligament are obliterated by excessive occlusal forces.[24] It has been repeatedly proved that trauma from occlusion does not cause pockets or gingivitis[2,20,50,65,66,68,69] and that it also does not increase gingival fluid flow.[27,33,36,41,42,50] The 2017 World Workshop also concluded that occlusal trauma does not initiate periodontitis.[70]

Furthermore, experimental trauma in dogs does not influence the bacterial repopulation of pockets after scaling and root planing.[31] However, mobile teeth in humans harbor significantly higher proportions of *Campylobacter rectus* and *Peptostreptococcus micros* than do nonmobile teeth.[26]

As long as inflammation is confined to the gingiva, the inflammatory process is not affected by occlusal forces.[32] When inflammation extends from the gingiva into the supporting periodontal tissues (i.e., when gingivitis becomes periodontitis), plaque-induced inflammation enters the zone that is influenced by occlusion, which Glickman has called the *zone of co-destruction.*[14,15,17]

Two groups have studied this topic experimentally, with conflicting results, probably because of the different methods used. The Eastman Dental Center group in Rochester, New York, used squirrel monkeys, produced trauma by repetitive interdental wedging, and added mild to moderate gingival inflammation; experimental times were up to 10 weeks. They reported that the presence of trauma did not increase the loss of attachment induced by periodontitis.[42,45–47] The University of Gothenburg group in Sweden used beagle dogs, produced trauma by placing cap splints and orthodontic appliances, and induced severe gingival inflammation; experimental times were up to 1 year. This group found that occlusal stresses increase the periodontal destruction induced by periodontitis.[11,12,39]

When trauma from occlusion is eliminated, a substantial reversal of bone loss occurs, except in the presence of periodontitis. This indicates that inflammation inhibits the potential for bone regeneration.[30,38,48,49] Thus it is important to eliminate the marginal inflammatory component in cases of trauma from occlusion, because the presence of inflammation affects bone regeneration after the removal of the traumatizing contacts.[30] It has also been shown in experimental animals that trauma from occlusion does not induce progressive destruction of the periodontal tissues in regions that are kept healthy after the elimination of preexisting periodontitis.[11] In addition, a recent systematic review evaluated human studies and concluded that there is limited evidence that trauma from occlusion is associated with periodontitis and that there is also limited evidence to support occlusal adjustment improves the periodontal condition of patients with periodontitis.[69] Another systematic review also concluded that there is insufficient evidence to presume that occlusal adjustment is necessary to reduce the progression of periodontitis; however, adverse effects have also not been observed. Therefore the decision to perform an occlusal adjustment in conjunction with periodontal treatment should take into consideration patient comfort and tooth function.[71]

Trauma from occlusion also tends to change the shape of the alveolar crest. The change in shape consists of a widening of the marginal periodontal ligament space, a narrowing of the interproximal alveolar bone, and a shelflike thickening of the alveolar margin.[9,39,42] Therefore although trauma from occlusion does not alter the inflammatory process, it changes the architecture of the area around the inflamed site.[17,39] Thus in the absence of inflammation, the response to trauma from occlusion is limited to adaptation to the increased forces. In the presence of inflammation, however, the changes in the shape of the alveolar crest may be conducive to angular bone loss, and existing pockets may become intrabony.

Other theories that have been proposed to explain the interaction of trauma and inflammation include the following:

- Trauma from occlusion may alter the pathway of the extension of gingival inflammation to the underlying tissues. This may be favored by the reduced collagen density and the increased number of leukocytes, osteoclasts, and blood vessels in the coronal portion of increasingly mobile teeth.[3] Inflammation may then proceed to the periodontal ligament rather than to the bone. Resulting bone loss would be angular, and pockets could become intrabony.[1,17,19,40]
- Trauma-induced areas of root resorption uncovered by apical migration of the inflamed gingival attachment may offer a favorable environment for the formation and attachment of plaque and calculus and therefore may be responsible for the development of deeper lesions.[59]
- Supragingival plaque can become subgingival if the tooth is tilted orthodontically or if it migrates into an edentulous area, which results in the transformation of a suprabony pocket into an intrabony pocket.[10,12,17]
- Increased mobility of traumatically loosened teeth may have a pumping effect on plaque metabolites, thereby increasing their diffusion.[64]

LEARNING BOX 32.7

Despite conflicting scientific data and speculations generated based on such data on the role of trauma from occlusion in periodontitis, two points are not contested: (1) changes related to trauma from occlusion (bone loss and tooth mobility) are reversible if they occurred in the absence of periodontitis; (2) in situations where both plaque-induced periodontitis and trauma from occlusion are present, elimination of the former will prevent further apical migration of the attachment unit, despite the presence of trauma from occlusion. Therefore, in terms of patient care, all facts support the priority that should be given to eliminating the bacterial plaque portion of the disease process.

Clinical and Radiographic Signs of Trauma from Occlusion Alone

The most common clinical sign of trauma to the periodontium is *increased tooth mobility.* During the injury stage of trauma from

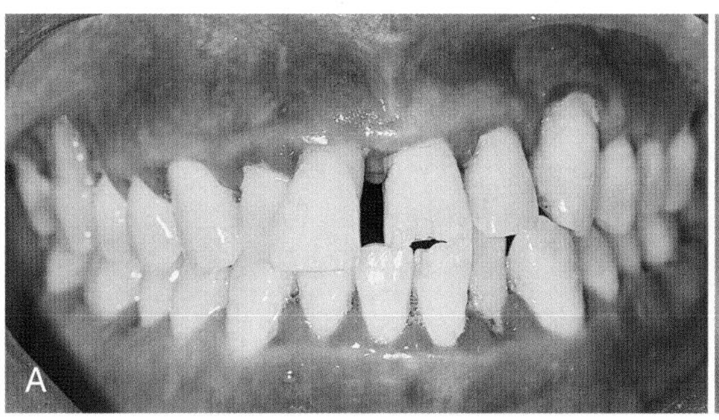

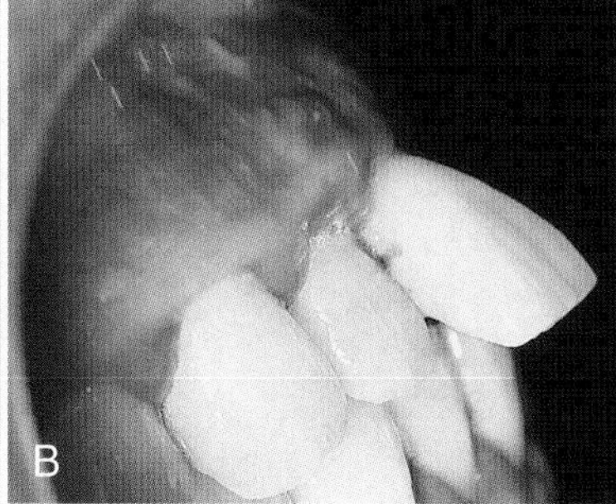

Fig. 32.10 Labial migration of the maxillary central incisors, especially the right incisor. (A) Frontal view. (B) Lateral view.

occlusion, the destruction of periodontal fibers occurs, which increases tooth mobility. During the final stage, the accommodation of the periodontium to increased forces entails a widening of the periodontal ligament, which also leads to increased tooth mobility. Although this tooth mobility is greater than the so-called normal mobility, it cannot be considered pathologic, because it is an adaptation and not a disease process. If it does become progressively worse, it can then be considered pathologic.

Other causes of increased tooth mobility include advanced bone loss, inflammation of the periodontal ligament of periodontal or periapical origin, and some systemic causes (e.g., pregnancy). The destruction of surrounding alveolar bone, such as occurs with osteomyelitis or jaw tumors, may also increase tooth mobility.

Radiographic signs of trauma from occlusion may include the following:

1. Increased width of the periodontal space, often with thickening of the lamina dura along the lateral aspect of the root, in the apical region, and in bifurcation areas. These changes do not *necessarily* indicate destructive changes, because they may result from thickening and strengthening of the periodontal ligament and alveolar bone, thereby constituting a favorable response to increased occlusal forces.
2. A vertical rather than horizontal destruction of the interdental septum.
3. Radiolucency and condensation of the alveolar bone.
4. Root resorption.

In summary, trauma from occlusion does not initiate gingivitis or periodontal pockets, but it may constitute an additional risk factor for the progression and severity of the disease. An understanding of the effect of trauma from occlusion on the periodontium is useful during the clinical management of periodontal problems.

Pathologic Tooth Migration

Pathologic migration refers to tooth displacement that results when the balance among the factors that maintain physiologic tooth position is disturbed by periodontal disease. Pathologic migration is relatively common. It may be an early sign of disease, or it may occur in association with gingival inflammation and pocket formation as the disease progresses.

Pathologic migration occurs most frequently in the anterior region, but posterior teeth may also be affected. The teeth may move in any direction, and the migration is usually accompanied by mobility and rotation. Pathologic migration in the occlusal or incisal direction is termed *extrusion.* All degrees of pathologic migration are encountered, and one or more teeth may be affected (Fig. 32.10). It is important to detect migration during its early stages and to prevent more serious involvement by eliminating the causative factors. Even during the early stage, some degree of bone loss occurs.

Pathogenesis

Two major factors play a role in maintaining the normal position of the teeth: the health and normal height of the periodontal attachment apparatus and the forces exerted on the teeth. The latter includes the forces of occlusion and pressure from the lips, cheeks, and tongue. Factors that are important in relation to the forces of occlusion include the following: (1) tooth morphologic features and cuspal inclination; (2) the presence of a full complement of teeth; (3) a physiologic tendency toward mesial migration; (4) the nature and location of contact point relationships; (5) proximal, incisal, and occlusal attrition; and (6) the axial inclination of the teeth. Alterations in any of these factors start an interrelated sequence of changes in the environment of a single tooth or group of teeth that may result in pathologic migration. Thus, pathologic migration occurs under conditions that weaken the periodontal support, that increase or modify the forces exerted on the teeth, or both.

Weakened Periodontal Support

The inflammatory destruction of the periodontium in patients with periodontitis creates an imbalance between the forces that maintain the tooth in position and the occlusal and muscular forces the tooth ordinarily needs to bear. The tooth with weakened support is unable to maintain its normal position in the arch and moves away from the opposing force unless it is restrained by proximal contact. The force that moves the weakly supported tooth may be created by factors such as occlusal contacts or pressure from the tongue.

It is important to understand that the abnormality of pathologic migration rests with the weakened periodontium; the force itself is not necessarily abnormal. Forces that are acceptable to an intact periodontium become injurious when periodontal support is reduced, as in the tooth with abnormal proximal contacts. Abnormally located proximal contacts convert the normal anterior component of force to a wedging force that causes occlusal or incisal movement of the tooth. The wedging force, which can be withstood by the intact periodontium, causes the tooth to extrude when the periodontal support is weakened by disease. *As its position changes, the tooth is subjected to abnormal occlusal forces, which aggravate the periodontal destruction and the tooth migration.*

Pathologic migration may continue after a tooth no longer contacts its antagonist. Pressures from the tongue, the food bolus during mastication, and the proliferating granulation tissue provide the force.

Pathologic migration is also an early sign of localized aggressive periodontitis. Weakened by the loss of periodontal support, the maxillary and mandibular anterior incisors drift labially and extrude, thereby creating diastemata between the teeth.

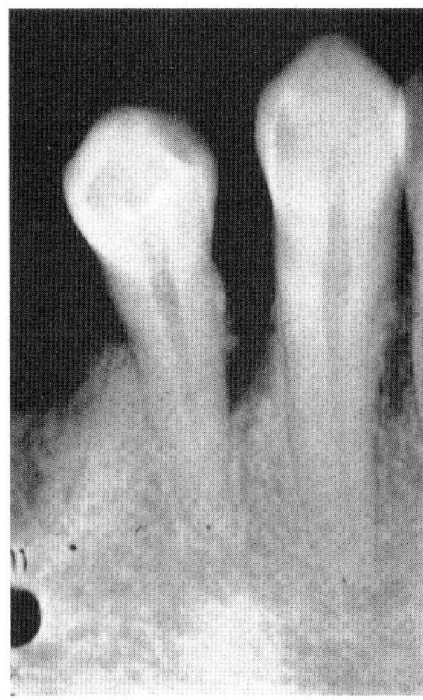

Fig. 32.11 Calculus and bone loss on the mesial surface of a canine that has drifted distally.

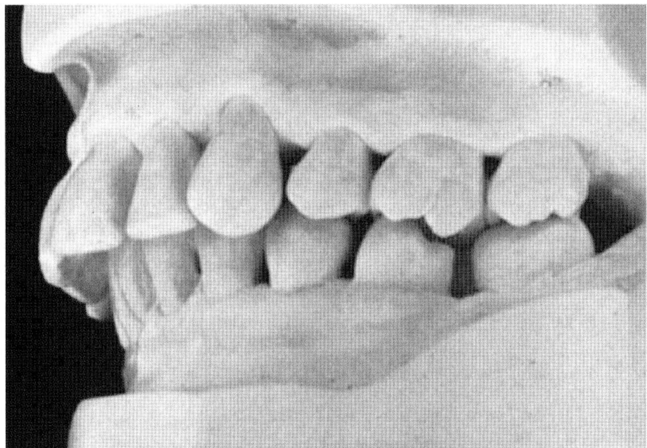

Fig. 32.12 Maxillary first molar that has tilted and extruded into the space created by a missing mandibular tooth.

Changes in the Forces Exerted on the Teeth

Changes in the magnitude, direction, or frequency of the forces exerted on the teeth can induce the pathologic migration of a tooth or group of teeth. These forces do not have to be abnormal to cause migration if the periodontium is sufficiently weakened. Changes in the forces may result from unreplaced missing teeth or other causes.

Unreplaced Missing Teeth

The drifting of teeth into the spaces created by unreplaced missing teeth often occurs. Drifting differs from pathologic migration in that it does not result from the destruction of the periodontal tissues. However, it usually creates conditions that lead to periodontal disease, and thus the initial tooth movement is aggravated by a loss of periodontal support (Fig. 32.11).

Drifting generally occurs in a mesial direction in combination with tilting or extrusion beyond the occlusal plane. The premolars frequently drift distally (Fig. 32.12). Although drifting is a common sequela when missing teeth are not replaced, it does not always occur (Fig. 32.13).

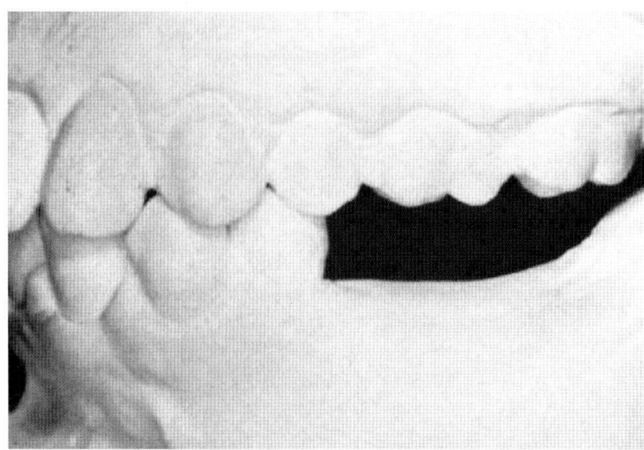

Fig. 32.13 No drifting or extrusion is present here, despite the 4-year absence of the mandibular teeth.

Failure to Replace First Molars

The pattern of changes that may follow the failure to replace missing first molars is characteristic. In extreme cases, it consists of the following:

1. The second and third molars tilt mesially, which results in a decrease in vertical dimension (Fig. 32.14).
2. The premolars move distally, and the mandibular incisors tilt or drift lingually. While drifting distally, the mandibular premolars lose their intercuspating relationship with the maxillary teeth, and they may tilt distally.
3. Anterior overbite is increased. The mandibular incisors strike the maxillary incisors near the gingiva or traumatize the gingiva.
4. The maxillary incisors are pushed labially and laterally (Fig. 32.15).
5. The anterior teeth extrude because the incisal apposition has largely disappeared.
6. Diastemata are created by the separation of the anterior teeth (see Fig. 32.14).

The disturbed proximal contact relationships lead to food impaction, plaque accumulation that results in gingival inflammation, and pocket formation, which are followed by bone loss and tooth mobility. Occlusal disharmonies created by the altered tooth positions traumatize the supporting tissues of the periodontium and aggravate the destruction caused by the inflammation. The reduction in periodontal support leads to the further migration of the teeth and the mutilation of the occlusion.

Other Causes

Trauma from occlusion may cause a shift in tooth position either by itself or in combination with inflammatory periodontal disease. The direction of movement depends on the occlusal force.

Pressure from the tongue may cause drifting of the teeth in the absence of periodontal disease, or it may contribute to the pathologic migration of teeth with reduced periodontal support (Fig. 32.16).

When tooth support has been weakened by periodontal destruction, *pressure from the granulation tissue of periodontal pockets* has been mentioned as contributing to pathologic migration.[28,37] The teeth may return to their original positions after the pockets are eliminated, but if more destruction has occurred on one side of a tooth than on the other, the healing tissues tend to pull in the direction of less destruction.

Summary

It is important to understand the etiology of the changes that occur in the periodontal tissues from both the clinical and histologic perspectives. Whatever the etiology, the periodontal

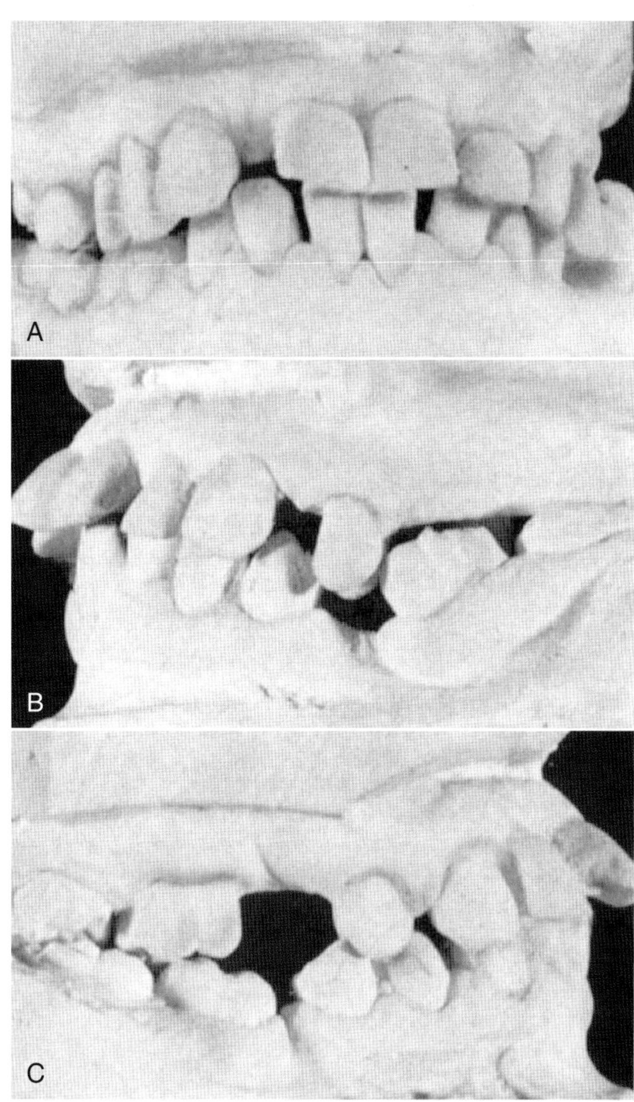

Fig. 32.14 Examples of the mutilation of occlusion associated with unreplaced missing teeth. Note pronounced pathologic migration, disturbed proximal contacts, and functional relationships with closing of the bite.

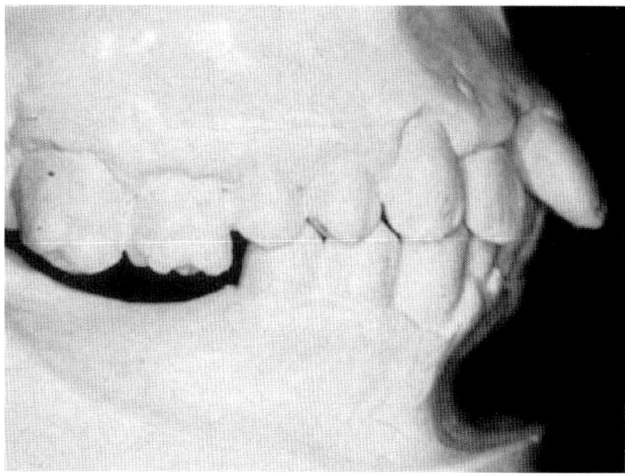

Fig. 32.15 Maxillary incisors pushed labially in a patient with bilateral unreplaced mandibular molars. Note the extrusion of the maxillary molars.

tissues have a tremendous adaptive ability to accommodate both the microbial and the traumatic occlusal factors within a certain limit. It is the combination of both and the patient's ability to resist these factors that may complicate the diagnosis and treatment plan of the clinical cases that are presented.

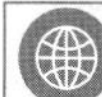
A Case Scenario is found on the companion website eBooks.Health.Elsevier.com.

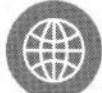
References for this chapter are found on the companion website eBooks.Health.Elsevier.com.

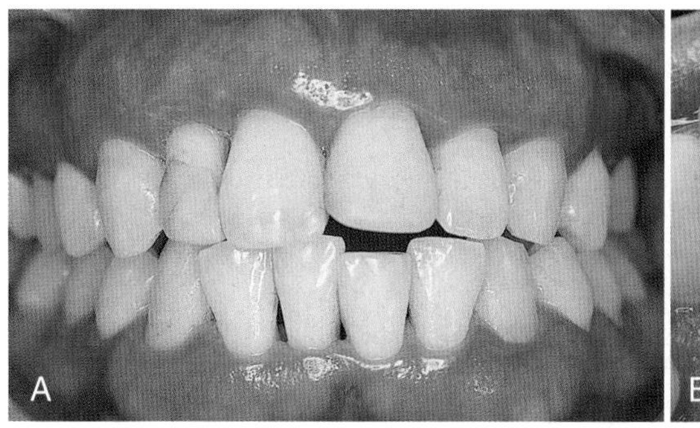

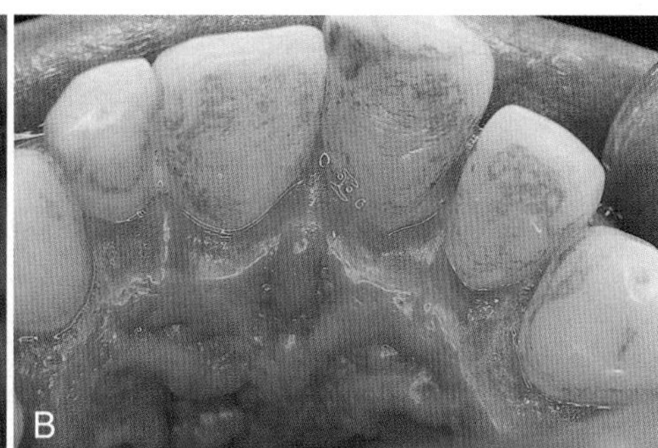

Fig. 32.16 Pathologic migration associated with tongue pressure. (A) Facial view. (B) Palatal view. (*From Fan J, Caton JG. Occlusal trauma and excessive occlusal forces: narrative review, case definitions, and diagnostic considerations.* J Periodontol. *2018;89[Suppl 1]:S214–S222.*)

CHAPTER 33

Sleep-Related Breathing Disorders

Adrian Karl Zacher 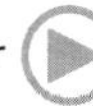 | *Michael J. McDevitt*

 For online-only content on the diagnosis of obstructive sleep apnea, device design, and compliance with therapy, please visit the companion website at eBooks.Health.Elsevier.com.

CHAPTER OUTLINE

New and Evolving Role of the Dentist

Everyone sleeps, and no one thinks much about sleep until something goes wrong. When sleep does go wrong—and it can in many ways—the effects can be more than just feeling a little tired in the morning. This chapter explores the exciting and evolving role of the dentist with an interest in sleep-related breathing disorders (SRBDs) who helps patients to breathe, sleep, and ultimately function better each day.

Snoring and sleep apnea (i.e., cessation of breathing) are points along a spectrum that extends from benign or simple snoring with no sleep disturbance to obstructive sleep apnea (OSA) with excessive daytime sleepiness and the physiologic consequences of recurrent asphyxia.[27] Over the years, there have been many dubious claims made regarding snoring cures. However, knowledge has greatly improved,[19] and much can be done to manage OSA and its associated consequences. It is in the provision of oral devices for OSA that a key role for suitably trained dentists is developing.

Sleep apnea can be caused by the lack of a central drive to breathe. The central, mixed, and complex types of apnea are reviewed later in this chapter.

Professor Colin Sullivan invented the mainstay therapy for sleep apnea: positive airway pressure (PAP) therapy. He was also an internationally renowned key opinion leader who advocated[8] for dentists as part of a multidisciplinary team, to play a critical role in four areas:

1. Treating adults with oral devices for snoring and mild to moderate OSA to slow the progression of the disease
2. Identifying at-risk children and adults by looking at their upper airway on a regular basis
3. Treating children with rapid maxillary expansion and avoiding deleterious orthodontic treatments
4. Recognizing the need for bimaxillary osteotomy in young adults requiring maxillofacial correction

Sleep-Related Breathing Disorders and the Periodontium

The prevalence of impaired breathing in patients may be as high as four times more likely among those who are experiencing periodontitis or have shown to be susceptible to periodontal disease, while periodontitis occurs twice as frequently among patients affected by SRBD.[1,58] Periodontitis is best understood as an inflammatory bone disease[66] most similar to rheumatoid arthritis.[4,54,11] Sleep disturbances, especially when occurring in stressed individuals, are associated with elevated systemic inflammation as does periodontitis.[17,41,50] The occurrence of periodontitis among individuals with an SRBD is significant, and the severity of both conditions run parallel.[5,57,63] As essential members of the health care team, dentists must determine if both conditions are being experienced by any patient presenting with either.

Whereas a qualified physician is responsible for diagnosing OSA, the dentist can identify and differentiate between clinical signs of possible airway issues, often before the patient becomes suspicious of the health risk. Information shared by the patient regarding his or her overall health status should be reviewed and correlated with clinical observations of oral indicators of attempted compensation by the patient for a significant degree of airway obstruction or resistance.

The value of early recognition and intervention cannot be overstated. The deleterious effects of SRBD and resultant periods of asphyxia on cardiovascular health, endocrine function, neurologic function, and masticatory system integrity add to the urgency for dentists to include recognition protocols during initial and recurring evaluations of their patients. A multidisciplinary team approach[33] that incorporates respect for each team member's professional role is essential to make an accurate diagnosis and facilitate provision of the most appropriate treatment.

The following sections discuss sleep, apnea, and the dentist's role in the provision of oral devices, which is one of the increasingly favored OSA treatment options.

Dental Identification of Signs and Symptoms

Review of Health Status and Systems

The frequency with which dentists see their patients places them in a unique position to recognize the symptoms of OSA. At the beginning of every dental appointment, the dentist or a member of the dental team should conduct an effective review and record the patient's health status. In addition to addressing specific items that might have been discussed previously, questions about breathing issues can alert the dentist to look for clinical indicators of SRBD. Identification of clinical signs can reframe future discussions of the patient's overall health to prevent overlooking possible correlations with observations. For example, snoring or gasping reported to the patient by his or her bed partner may correlate with unexpected mobility of occluding anterior teeth. Important conditions or factors that may be reported by a patient include the following:

- Hypertension
- Gastroesophageal reflux disease
- Excessive daytime sleepiness
- Cardiovascular disease, including arrhythmias
- Type 2 diabetes
- Hypothyroidism
- Obesity
- Sudden onset of snoring
- Awareness of snoring or SRBD
- Use of a snore appliance from a dentist or another source

Dental Signs and Symptoms of Obstructed Breathing

Neither the clinical indicators nor the health or breathing status reported by the patient can define the degree or implications of an SRBD for the dentist. Developing a list of observations to discuss with the patient allows him or her to confirm the possibility of a breathing disorder and communicate the signs to the physician for further assessment and diagnosis.

Sleep Bruxism

Patients commonly report SRBD and sleep bruxism. The evidence of what was only a suspected association because no evidence existed has now established a strong and compelling relationship.[14,31,47] The bruxing patient's repeated patterns of mandibular movement are primarily mediated by the central nervous system. It has been hypothesized that the advancement of the mandible during movement of the mandible opens the oropharynx, relieving some of the consequences of SRBD.[35,36] Most of the literature reporting sleep bruxism is focused on obstructive sleep apnea, another expression of an SRBD, upper airway resistance syndrome, has now been identified as encouraging bruxism in individual patients.[43] The evidence for the potential role of the excessive occlusal forces, especially from clenching the teeth, on the rate and location of inflammatory bone damage during periods of disease activity of periodontitis is presented in Chapter 32 of this textbook.

Clinical Signs and Symptoms

- Wear patterns on opposing incisors can suggest that the patient positions the mandible anteriorly to open the airway.[60,61]
- The mobility of the anterior teeth may be more than that estimated on the basis of the patient's health and the support available from periodontal structures.
- In the periodontitis-susceptible patient, progressive bone loss may be located or exaggerated in sites of unusual wear or mobility. The possible role of occlusal trauma in the amplification of the consequences of periodontitis is described in the online version of Chapters 32, 34 and 35 of this textbook (eBooks.Health.Elsevier.com).
- Tongue crenulations (i.e., scalloped borders) suggest that the patient is depressing the tongue forward against the mandibular teeth regularly to open the oral airway.
- Development of an anterior or lateral open-bite relationship of the opposing teeth may result from tongue posturing.
- Sleep bruxism may develop or increase.
- Dimpling of the cusps and lingual surfaces of the teeth can indicate related gastroesophageal reflux.
- The development of orofacial pain, temporomandibular joint (TMJ) dysfunction symptoms, masticatory muscle fatigue noticed on awakening, or morning headache can be related to the positioning of the mandible to open the patient's airway. This topic is addressed in the online version of Chapter 34 of this textbook (eBooks.Health.Elsevier.com), where comprehensive diagnostic references can also be found.
- During evaluation of the oropharynx, prominent tonsils, a large uvula, or a narrow or tongue-obstructed airway may be seen. The patient's age can contribute to the loss of pharyngeal muscle tone.
- Mouth breathing while sleeping can manifest as drying of the surface of the gingiva and greater adherence of dental biofilms. The increased difficulty of a patient with a drier mouth, xerostomia, has been shown to undermine effectiveness of both personal and professional periodontal therapies.[30] Xerostomia upon awakening has been reported to be experienced over twice as often in patients with SRBD as compared to controls (45% vs. 20.4%).[52] SRBD should be considered by dentists as a probable contributor to our patients' dry mouths along with the previously identified medicinal agents and aging.[51,68]

Sleep, Breathing, and Apnea

A basic understanding of sleep physiology, normal sleep cycles, and the variety of sleep disorders can provide the dentist with the means for effective communication with patients and their physicians.

Sleep is classically defined as a cyclic, temporary, and physiologic loss of consciousness that is readily, promptly, and completely reversed with appropriate stimuli. Not being able to breathe would seem to qualify as an appropriate stimulus, but affected individuals are rarely aware of any difficulty. Normal sleep progresses through different stages that are typically depicted on a hypnogram (Fig. 33.1).

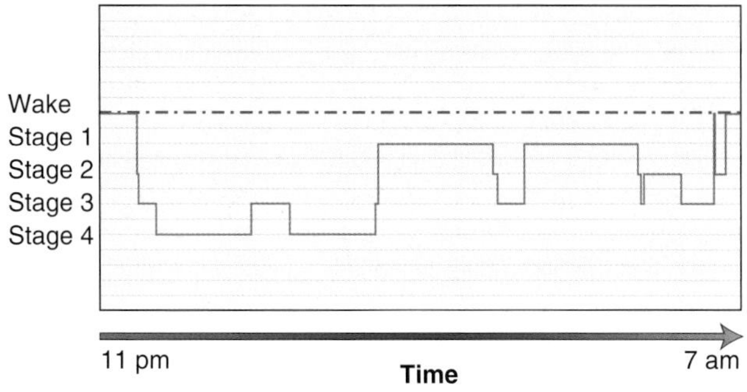

Fig. 33.1 Simplified hypnogram of a normal adult's sleep. (*Courtesy Adrian Zacher, 2013.* Snorer.com.)

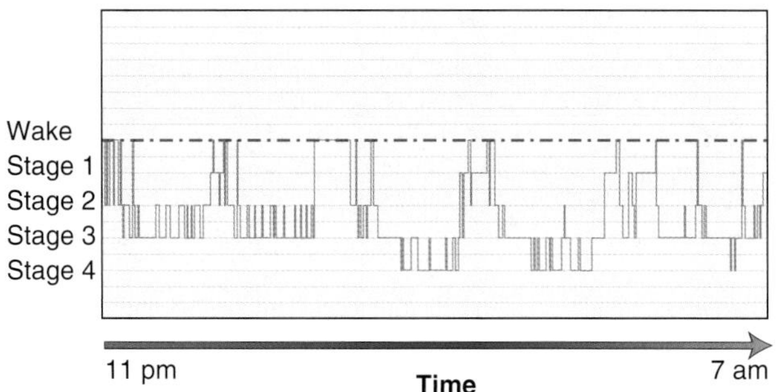

Fig. 33.2 Simplified hypnogram of an adult's fragmented sleep. (*Courtesy Adrian Zacher, 2013.* Snorer.com.)

Snoring is a vibratory noise that is generated by the back of the relaxed tongue, pharynx, and soft palate. Further loss of tone or narrowing produces louder snoring and labored inspiration. Still, further narrowing can cause complete collapse of the airway. This obstruction is known as an ***apneic episode***.

There comes a point at which the increased inspiratory effort or oxygen desaturation that may accompany the apneic episode is sensed by the sleeping brain and a transient arousal is provoked. This is a brief awakening to breathe before the individual returns to sleep. These arousals can be seen in Fig. 33.2 as decreased duration periods and increasingly frequent interruptions in the descent into deeper, more refreshing sleep. Disregarding complaints about the snoring noise, these repetitive arousals occur for the most part without the individual being aware, sometimes several hundred times a night.

Each apneic episode can last from a few seconds to approximately 2 minutes. The individual's descent into the deeper and more restorative slow-wave stages of sleep is interrupted because he or she has partially awakened to restore the airway. Sleep becomes highly fragmented, and the consequent daytime sleepiness known as ***hypersomnolence*** increases the individual's risk of accidents at home, at work, and on the road.[71]

OSA has a significant impact on an individual's quality of life.[15] If left untreated, it has neurologic and physiologic consequences,[49] including increased morbidity and mortality[46] and, particularly for men, impaired cardiovascular[72] and metabolic[24] function.

Prevalence of Obstructive Sleep Apnea

Sleep apnea affects many people, but it continues to be largely unrecognized. Estimates suggest that 24% of men and 9% of women who are 30 to 60 years old with an average body mass index of 25 to 28 kg/m^2 are affected.[70] When considered in the context of the concurrent metabolic dysfunction epidemic (which is manifested in obesity, cardiovascular disease,[34,40] and type 2 diabetes in men[18,55,56]),

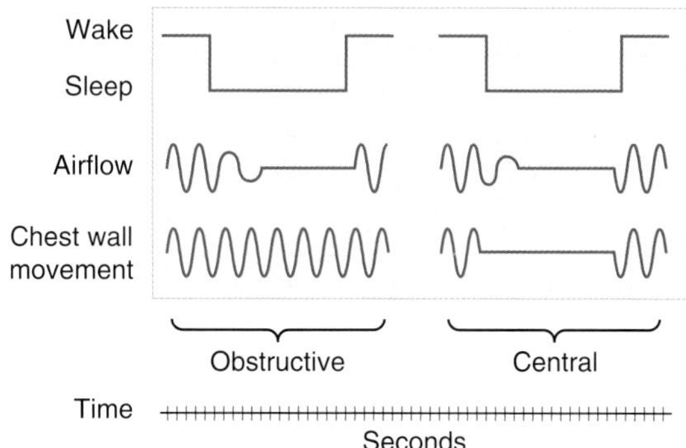

Fig. 33.3 Obstructive versus central apnea. (*Courtesy Learning Center, ResMed, San Diego, CA.*)

the prevalence of sleep apnea becomes alarming. The International Diabetes Federation urges health care professionals to ensure that a person diagnosed with OSA is evaluated for type 2 diabetes and vice versa.[59]

Central, Mixed, and Complex Apnea

In contrast to OSA, central sleep apnea (CSA) occurs without physical obstruction of the airway. CSA is caused by disorders that are characterized by the intermittent loss of the respiratory drive. Fig. 33.3 shows the lack of chest wall movement in a patient with CSA. Cheyne-Stokes respirations as a form of CSA are most often seen in patients with heart failure. Mixed apnea is a combination of OSA and CSA. Complex apnea occurs when CSA events emerge in response to PAP therapy for OSA.[23]

This chapter is confined to OSA because it is by far the most common form of apnea, and it is in the provision of oral devices, also known as *mandibular repositioning devices* (MRDs), for OSA that the suitably trained dentist can play a role.[28]

Chronic Disease

The maintenance of a separate silo approach and viewing one aspect of an individual's symptomatology in isolation can be considered flawed thinking. OSA in isolation and as a potential component of metabolic syndrome (i.e., syndrome Z[67]) requires a multidisciplinary approach to chronic disease management. The World Health Organization[69] states that chronic diseases are projected to be the leading cause of disability; if they are not successfully prevented and managed, they will become the most expensive problems for health care systems.

Diagnosis of Obstructive Sleep Apnea

Snoring is a symptom of a partially impeded airway, the walls of which are vibrating as the air passes. How frequently the walls of the airway vibrate (i.e., snoring noise) or collapse (i.e., apnea events of varying duration) indicates the severity of OSA.

A multidisciplinary team approach is necessary for the diagnosis and treatment of OSA. Dentists are experts when it comes to the mouth and should be recognized as such. For OSA treatment, dentists need to build relationships with physicians so they can provide an appropriate dental solution for a medical condition. However, it is important to recognize that the diagnosis of OSA is not within the purview of dentistry.[10]

The closest thing to internationally accepted practice parameters, which are those issued by the American Academy of Sleep Medicine,[20] state that the "presence or absence and severity of OSA must be determined before initiating treatment." In practice, this

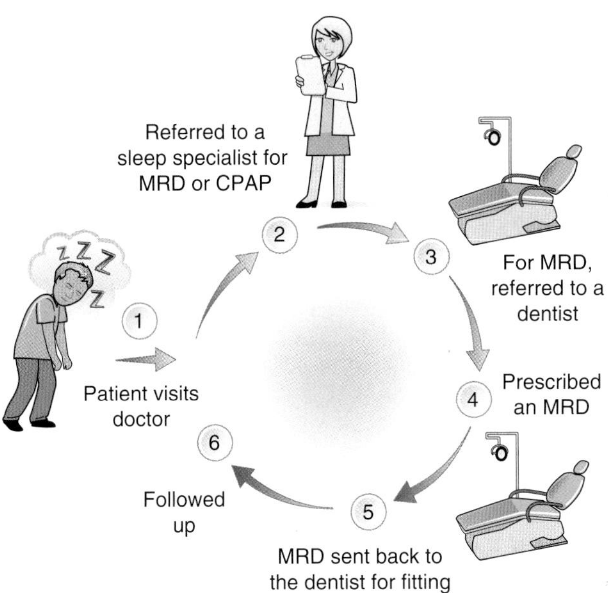

Fig. 33.4 Obstructive sleep apnea diagnosis and treatment route. *CPAP*, Continuous positive airway pressure; *MRD*, mandibular repositioning device. *(Courtesy ResMed, San Diego, CA, 2011.)*

means that a dentist must not initiate treatment with an oral device unless the patient has been assessed, medically diagnosed, and then referred to the dentist (Fig. 33.4).

If OSA is suspected, a referral is made for a sleep study. This can involve spending a night in a sleep laboratory or at home with an electronic monitoring device to wear while sleeping. A sleep laboratory is essentially a bedroom with monitoring equipment.

In a sleep laboratory, the patient undergoes *polysomnography* (PSG), during which multiple parameters are monitored while the patient is asleep. These parameters include, but are not limited to, sound, video, oxygen saturation, respiratory effort, electrocardiography, electroencephalography, and body position. Attended overnight PSG is an expensive assessment to perform, and availability and access vary based on geography.

Several screening protocols have been proposed over the years.[26,32] In January 2012, the California Dental Association[12] determined that it was appropriate for dentists to screen patients for the signs and symptoms of SRBD and to work with physicians to diagnose and treat it. The association also stated that SRBD is a medical condition and that its diagnosis is outside of the scope of dentistry.

Whether a PSG is essential to diagnose OSA is being questioned.[48] Since 2009 in the United Kingdom, a general dental practitioner working as part of a multidisciplinary team (including a sleep medicine specialist) can, in certain defined circumstances, screen, recognize the need for, and initiate treatment with an MRD without a prior medical diagnosis.[64] Currently in the United States, PSG and home study monitor results need to be interpreted by a physician.

The role of home sleep apnea testing and who should interpret the data that it produces are points of contention that fuel the debate surrounding PSG. The need for mandatory PSG may be questioned in response to the following:

- Increasingly valid and competitively priced home sleep apnea testing equipment
- Increase in the number of patients requiring assessment
- Perception that PSG is the point of contention in the treatment process
- Realization that oral devices are appropriate for milder forms of OSA and that dentists are uniquely positioned to provide them because they may see patients more frequently than sleep medicine specialists
- Realization that a trained dentist, as part of a multidisciplinary team, can filter referrals to the sleep medicine specialist

Apnea	Cessation of airflow > 10 seconds
Hypopnea	> 50% reduction in airflow for > 10 seconds
Apnea hypopnea index (AHI)	Number of apneas and hypopneas per hour of sleep
Severity	Normal: AHI < 5 Mild: AHI 5–15 Moderate: AHI 15–30 Severe: AHI > 30
Sleep apnea syndrome (SAS)	AHI > 5 with symptoms
Cheyne–Stokes respiration	> 3 consecutive cyclical crescendo-decrescendo changes in breathing amplitude during 10 consecutive minutes and/or an AHI > 5

Fig. 33.5 Sleep-related disorders in adults: definitions and diagnostic criteria.

A sleep laboratory's main function is to diagnose OSA and then offer treatment to those who are likely to benefit from it. If the symptoms are fairly disabling and the diagnosis is confirmed by a sleep study, PAP therapy is routinely offered. Increasingly, around the world, oral devices are becoming a first-line treatment for mild to moderate OSA when they can be prescribed and monitored by a multidisciplinary team. Fig. 33.5 provides definitions and diagnostic criteria for SRBD.[62]

Treatment Options for Obstructive Sleep Apnea

Otolaryngology or Oromaxillofacial Surgery

Surgical options for snoring and OSA are largely outside of the scope of this text. However, when physical obstructions to the airway (e.g., tonsils, deviated septum, nasal polyps) are present, surgical correction may improve breathing. For example, if adenotonsillar hypertrophy exists, childhood correction is considered advantageous.[39]

Limited evidence for adult palatal surgery, which is known as *uvulopalatopharyngoplasty,* exists; this surgery should be considered only after PAP therapy has failed.[9] Maxillary or bimaxillary orthognathic surgery is rarely considered, whereas tracheotomy is an effective option of last resort because it completely bypasses the affected area.

Positive Airway Pressure

PAP (Fig. 33.6) is considered the first-line treatment for OSA, and it is effective in helping the patient to overcome daytime sleepiness symptoms. Individuals with severe sleep apnea do well with this therapy, despite the forbidding appearance. Possibly considered an arduous therapy, it involves wearing a mask over the nose (and sometimes the mouth and nose) at night while being connected to a quiet blower. It works by slightly pressurizing the upper airway, thereby pneumatically splinting it open and preventing it from collapsing. PAP is particularly useful when there is a need for rapid control of OSA.

The sleep laboratory may also suggest that oral device therapy is appropriate. This depends on the severity of the OSA and the existence of other comorbidities. Oral devices can be used to provide therapy for sleep apnea of any severity; however, effective results are considered less certain with increasing severity.[25] PAP and MRD therapies are complementary; in patients with moderate OSA, the two modalities in some circumstances can be considered equally appropriate. Fig. 33.7 illustrates this point in broad terms. Treatment of severe sleep apnea with an oral device necessitates careful patient monitoring because things such as small weight changes can negate the effect.[45]

The technology of PAP and oral devices is fast developing, with particular focus on improving the patient's ability to tolerate their use and minimize their side effects. PAP development focuses on telemonitoring, better mask design, the inclusion of air humidifiers, and the sensitive electronically controlled variation of air pressure in response to inspiration and expiration. Oral devices have become increasingly adjustable and thinner, and they can be designed to minimize some common side effects, such as hypersalivation and incisor sensitivity. Future developments in oral devices may focus on objective compliance monitoring and treatment efficacy.

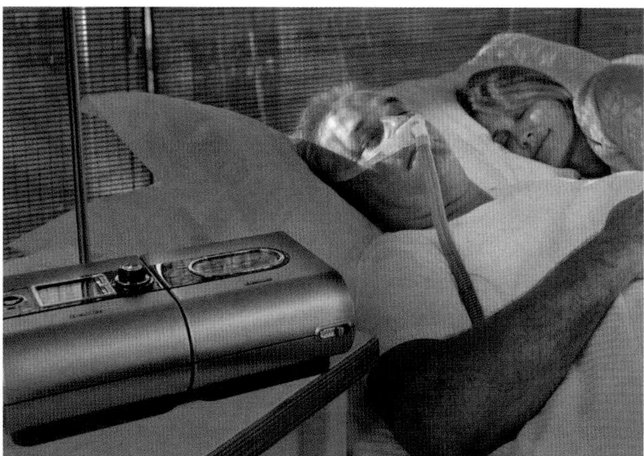

Fig. 33.6 Positive airway pressure therapy (*Courtesy ResMed, San Diego, CA, 2011.*)

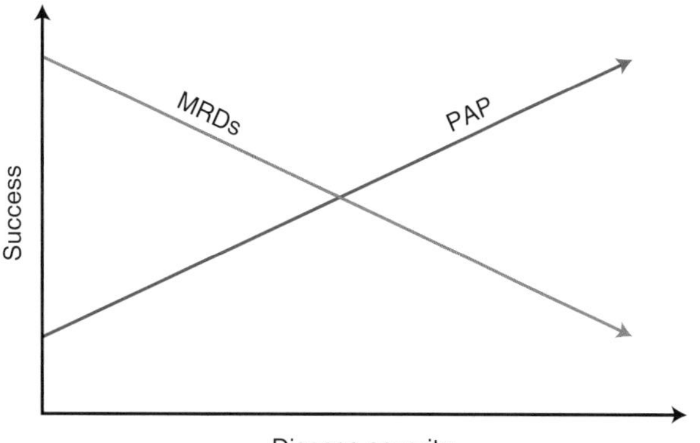

Fig. 33.7 Complementary therapies. *MRD,* Mandibular repositioning device; *PAP,* positive airway pressure. (*Courtesy Adrian Zacher, 2013,* Snorer.com.)

Oral Devices for Mandibular Repositioning

The developing role of dentistry in the provision of oral devices for snoring and OSA has given rise to concerns about training and professional indemnity. Dentists may be asked to place antisnoring devices; consequently, state boards of dentistry (and insurance providers) are issuing position statements regarding whether the provision of these devices falls within the practice of dentistry. These statements will determine whether the devices are within the scope of the assistance normally provided.

Dentists should check with their state boards of dentistry and professional indemnity insurers to clarify the situation. Most insurers suggest that dentists are well placed to construct oral devices if they have appropriate training to do so. However, the treatment of snoring and OSA does not routinely fall within the definition of the practice of dentistry and therefore would fall outside of the scope of assistance normally provided by the insurer.

Dentists should undergo a documented training course in the provision of antisnoring devices that includes training in appropriate screening for OSA. Candidates for oral devices should be properly assessed for the signs and symptoms of OSA in accordance with contemporary standards, and the assessment should be documented. If the patient exhibits signs or symptoms of OSA, there must be a referral for a medical assessment. Patients should be advised about the risks and benefits of antisnoring devices, including the potential impact on the occlusion, periodontium, and TMJs. Documentary evidence of the consent process must be retained. When OSA exists, an antisnoring device should be supplied only as part of an integrated treatment plan provided by a multidisciplinary team that includes the dentist.

Devices Pertinent to the Dentist

Oral devices for snoring and OSA aim to maintain the upper airway during sleep. Tongue-retaining devices and MRDs do this either directly, by acting on the tongue and holding it in a forward position, or indirectly, by forward repositioning of the mandible, which maintains upper airway patency (Fig. 33.8). MRDs are the most researched type of oral device for OSA, and they are the focus of this chapter.

Custom-made adjustable devices typically are associated with better treatment outcomes[65] compared with universal "boil and bite" MRDs. Adjustable MRDs are more likely to provide successful therapy in patients with moderate to severe OSA than nonadjustable MRDs.[38]

Predictor Devices

Sleep medicine specialists charged with caring for patients with OSA understandably desire certainty that the patient has been effectively treated. This has historically represented a legitimate concern

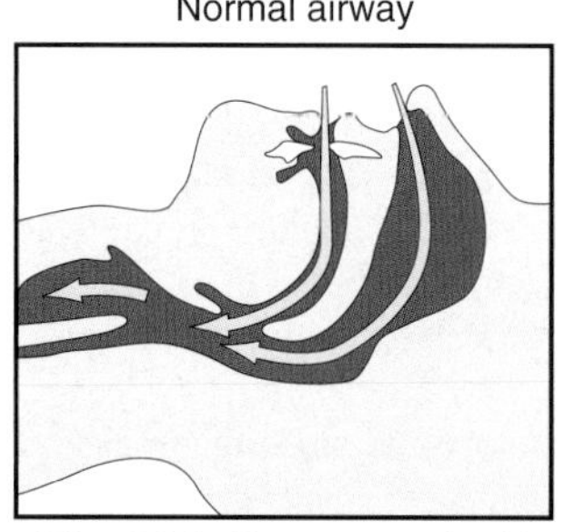

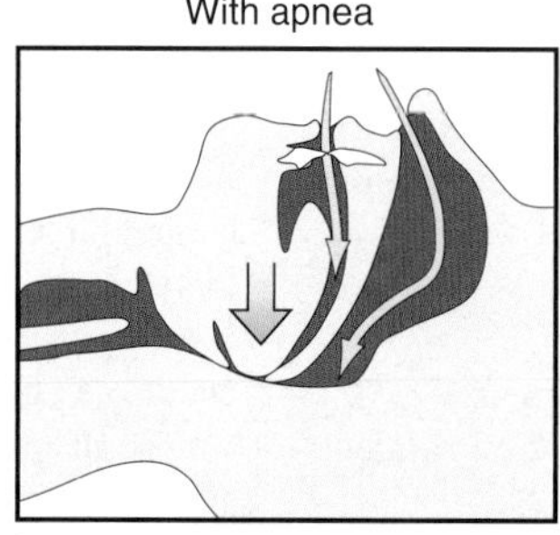

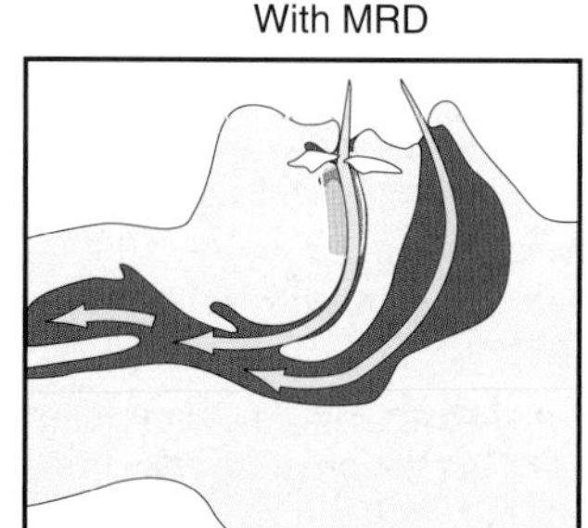

Fig. 33.8 Airway status: healthy and apneic, with a mandibular repositioning device *(MRD).* (*Courtesy ResMed, San Diego, CA, 2011.*)

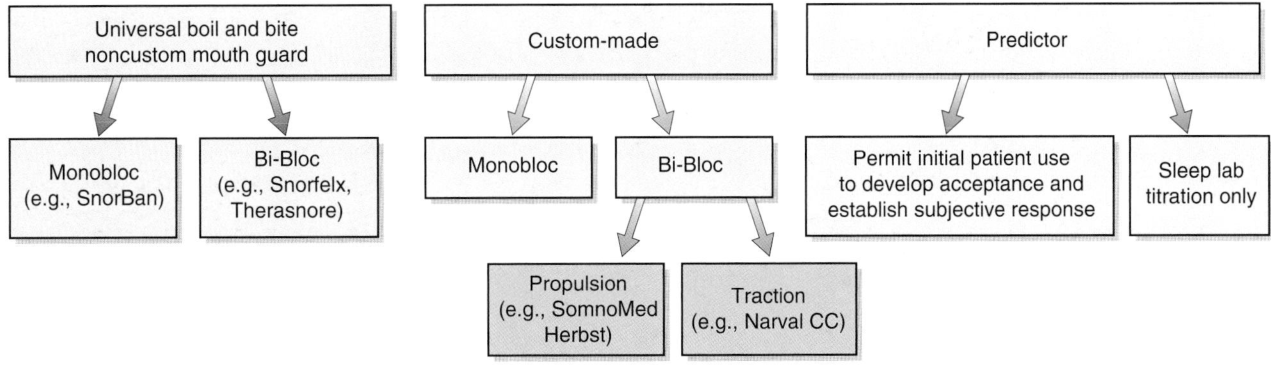

Fig. 33.9 Mandibular repositioning device taxonomy. *OSA*, Obstructive sleep apnea. (*Courtesy Adrian Zacher, 2013*, Snorer.com.)

when considering an MRD for a patient with OSA and has resulted in MRDs being confined to use for mild to moderate OSA. Predictor devices, which are sometimes known as titration *devices,*[16] are intended to do the following:

- Establish whether the patient can tolerate an intraoral device and whether it is subjectively effective
- Objectively determine whether mandibular repositioning delivers adequate therapy
- Provide a prescription jaw relationship for custom MRD manufacture if the outcome is positive

The use of predictor devices has been an area of MRD technologic innovation during recent years. In this role, it is important that predictor devices not be confused with thermoplastic universal treatment devices. Predictor devices are expressly designed for use for a limited number of nights; their use is self-limited, and they sacrifice patient convenience for functionality. Basic taxonomy for the oral devices of MRDs is shown in Fig. 33.9.

Characteristics of the Ideal Oral Device

From an individual wearer's perspective, any intraoral device feels foreign and invasive. The individual may seek treatment largely to please his or her partner and may perceive little or no personal benefit because hypersomnolence symptoms correlate poorly with OSA severity.[15] Affected individuals may have forgotten what it feels like to be fully awake.

Side effects of early devices included hypersalivation or dry mouth when worn, dental sensitivity, and perhaps a claustrophobic locking of the jaws in a protrusive position and a morning postwear TMJ ache. For these reasons, early oral devices required development. Some MRD manufacturers have reduced or eliminated these side effects, but there is no single perfect device.[3] Knowledge of a range of MRDs to suit different individuals is necessary. The characteristics of the ideal MRD vary for each patient, and some characteristics may preclude others. Table 33.1 presents several options.

Recognizing that a child may benefit from an SRBD investigation is important. MRDs are *not* recommended for children unless they are under the supervision of an orthodontist who is working as part of a multidisciplinary team.

Communication

Effective communication among the referring sleep laboratory, the patient, and the patient's general dental practitioner is essential and should begin before the patient is seen (Box 33.1).

Sleep Laboratory and Primary Care Physician Communication

The OSA diagnosis and the requirement for revaluation should be confirmed. Relevant medical history information should be exchanged. The existence of positional apnea (i.e., apnea that worsens when sleeping supine) should also be documented.

Patient Communication

Valid informed consent for treatment (including a risk-benefit analysis, information about side effects, and therapy limitations) and permission to get dental records from the general dental practitioner should be obtained.

General Dental Practitioner

With reference to the patient's existing dental records, a recent orthopantomogram may be valuable.

General Indications and Contraindications

When a patient who has been diagnosed with OSA is referred to a dentist, assessment to determine the suitability of MRD therapy is based on an individual analysis of indications and contraindications. It is essential to obtain valid informed consent and baseline records and to retain pre-MRD therapy casts. Uncontrolled epilepsy is an absolute contraindication.

All MRDs, which are also known as *mandibular advancement devices* (MADs) or *oral appliances,* protrude the mandible, but each MRD has a unique feature set. In 2010, Ahrens stated that "no [one] MAD design most effectively influences subjectively perceived treatment efficacy, but efficacy depends on many factors, including materials and method used for fabrication, type of MAD (monobloc or twin block [bi-bloc]), and the degree of protrusion."[2] Understanding the differences among these devices enables the dentist to prescribe appropriately, with knowledge of the indications, features, and design limitations, allowing him or her to maximize treatment efficacy and minimize unwanted side effects.

Temporomandibular Joint Dysfunction

Severe TMJ dysfunction, limited opening, and reports of jaw locking should be considered contraindications. A limited protrusive range (i.e., <5 mm) suggests a low likelihood of OSA treatment efficacy with an MRD.

Although basic assessment for TMJ dysfunction is essential, consideration of the validity of certain TMJ theories and diagnostic

TABLE 33.1 Characteristics of the Ideal Mandibular Repositioning Device

Acceptance, Adherence, and Efficacy	Mitigation of Side Effects	Practical Considerations
Constructed of two separate pieces; to give the patient time to accept wearing the device, one half is worn alone before the complete device is worn	Metal-free; no parts that can fatigue, fracture, and then be inhaled or ingested to create a galvanic reaction with other dental restorations	Low cost
Enables titration anteroposteriorly for tolerability and effect	Minimal bulk for less impact on phonetic function and reduced hypersalivation	Easy to fit for the patient and dental practitioner
Enables starting titration from zero protrusion to improve comfort throughout the titration process	Does not dictate a protrusive path or final protruded position for the temporomandibular joints	Can be titrated in the sleep laboratory without waking the patient
Encourages the mouth to close and prevents the mouth from falling open at sleep onset	No unwanted orthodontic effects (e.g., incisor tilting)	Instant device; no impressions or laboratory work required
Permits lip seal and encourages nasal breathing		Minimal follow-up appointments
Enables titration of the vertical opening (i.e., <5 mm measured at the incisors) considered optimal for acceptance and adherence[53]		Easy to modify
Easy to clean		Does not necessitate a remake if a dental restoration is necessary
Permits lateral movement where there is evidence of parafunction		
Does not encroach on tongue space or impede forward movement of the tongue		
Includes compliance and efficacy monitoring		
Is it worn and does it work?		

From Adrian Zacher, 2013. https://snorer.training

BOX 33.1 The Take-Home Message

1. Has the presence (and severity) or absence of obstructive sleep apnea been established?
2. Is the patient at least partially dentate? Does he or she have sufficient alveolar bone to withstand lateral loads?
3. Are you satisfied that there is no severe periodontal condition that the device would prejudice? Does the patient possess the competence to maintain his or her oral hygiene?
4. Are you satisfied there is no gross temporomandibular disorder?
5. Have you ensured that there is no pronounced gag reflex?
6. Does the patient have a competent nasal airway?
7. Does the patient comprehend the costs of therapy?
8. Have the patient's expectations of therapy been managed appropriately?

tools is necessary. Thorough record-keeping is advised. Referral to a dental practitioner who has advanced training in the diagnosis and management of TMJ dysfunction may be indicated if symptoms are identified at the initial evaluation or if they develop at any time during treatment. Reports of diffuse tenderness, ear canal stuffiness, clicks, significant deviation with opening or protruding, or pain associated with these movements necessitate referral to an expert. Refer to Chapter 34 in this text for further understanding of both functional and dysfunctional movement of each of a patient's TMJ. Masticatory muscle relationships and symptoms of and/or discomfort related to TMJ disharmonies are discussed in the context of differential diagnosis.

Dentate State

The individual must have sound teeth. Edentulous patients are unable to use MRDs because they function by retaining the teeth, and retention is used to reposition the mandible anteriorly. The minimum number and distribution of teeth varies by device. Placement of the adjustment mechanism routinely needs to be on the teeth and not in an edentulous area. To avoid excessive lateral load, the 8 to 10 teeth distributed around the arch serve as a general guide. The shape and inclination of the teeth can affect retention of the MRD and the dentist's ability to provide effective MRD therapy; the presence of no teeth or grossly undercut teeth can be problematic. Difficulty taking impressions in the setting of a pronounced gag reflex suggests that the patient will have difficulty adhering to MRD therapy.

Periodontal Condition and Tooth Mobility

A healthy periodontium with evidence of effective oral hygiene is essential before therapy with an MRD commences. Anything worn in the mouth can compromise oral hygiene if it is not kept clean.

Bruxism

Management of sleep bruxism is an important role for the dentist. Bruxism is not necessarily a contraindication to MRD therapy. An assessment for TMJ dysfunction is recommended. The bruxing individual should be advised that their parafunction will both limit their choice of MRD and negatively affect the life expectancy of the MRD.

Gastroesophageal Reflux Disease

Dentinal pooling that results from gastroesophageal reflux disease can be a symptom of OSA, and it is one that a dentist is ideally positioned to recognize.

Mandibular Repositioning Device Therapy

Long-term complications of MRD therapy are not well-documented. Given the intricacies of determining which device is most likely to be successful, the role of titration, and the management of complications, the dentist should seek advanced training before supplying MRDs.

Complete periodontal assessment should precede the decision to fit a patient with an MRD. Management of inflammation can be more difficult with an MRD, which the patient must use consistently when sleeping. Bacterial biofilm formation and retention are likely to be increased on the tissues and the device, and additional instruction and encouragement regarding effective bacterial biofilm removal are often necessary. Careful and frequent monitoring of the periodontal status with ongoing use of the MRD is essential to confirm sustained health and tooth stability, to recognize negative changes, especially signs of bone loss due to the host inflammatory response to chronic biofilm retention, particularly on proximal surfaces,[66] and to recommend intervention and consideration of an alternative treatment modality.

Device Design and Compliance

Application Considerations

eTable 33.1 proposes factors to consider when selecting an adjustable custom-made MRD for a patient, and eBox 33.1 provides definitions of terms.

Bulk, Xerostomia, and Hypersalivation

Logically, the least presence in the mouth the MRD represents, the easier the patient will tolerate it. Depending on the bulk of the device and the patient's ability to close the mouth while wearing it, dry mouth (i.e., xerostomia) and hypersalivation are common initial responses to MRD wear. These conditions normally resolve over the first few weeks as the patient adapts to the device. A non-bulky MRD that permits lip seal is therefore considered superior and may encourage nasal breathing.

Initial Protrusive Position

To overcome an inherent design limitation, some MRDs must start from approximately 50% to 70% of the patient's maximum protrusion. Ideally, the MRD should start from zero protrusion and be gradually protruded to maximize acceptance and minimize unnecessary protrusion to achieve effect.

Tongue Space Invasion

An MRD protrudes the jaw and effectively pulls the tongue away from the back of the throat. Placing a mechanism where the tongue is to be placed can be considered counterproductive.

Adjustable Protrusion: Placement of the Mechanism

MRDs can be broadly subdivided into those that place the mechanism in the buccal sulcus, incisally, or inside the tongue space. Proponents of each type vociferously defend its design logic. Recommending the suitability of one MRD over another requires a comprehensive assessment of the individual in context with proposed indications and contraindications.

Freedom of Lateral Movement

When evidence of bruxism is found during an examination, the use of an MRD that permits lateral movement and can withstand the forces imposed on it is advisable. Mechanisms that may fatigue and fracture should be considered carefully.

Durability and Ease of Cleaning

An inherently robust design and fabrication method is important because the device will be used to maintain an unconscious individual's airway. The consequences of metal fatigue should be considered. Complex mechanisms and materials that absorb saliva may present difficulty when it comes to cleaning and adversely affect the MRD's useful life.

Effect of Vertical Opening

Interincisal opening of more than 5 mm has been associated with lower patient adherence, perhaps because of discomfort.[53] However, a product trend based on empiric reporting suggests that an increased occlusal vertical dimension may be more comfortable in certain patients and permit the tongue to flow over the occlusal surfaces (i.e., allow the tongue to expand laterally). This may be relevant for patients with macroglossia or micrognathia.

Macroglossia and Micrognathia

Adding to an already crowded oral cavity makes wearing the MRD a challenge for the patient. Empiric evidence suggests that permitting the tongue to expand over the occlusal surface by increasing the vertical dimension (with protrusion of the mandible) in selected cases can be beneficial.

Side Effects

Maximizing the positive effects of MRD therapy while minimizing the side effects is the unstated aim of MRD design. The following sections highlight the primary side effects. Common side effects include incisor tilting, which should be discussed with the patient. Placing detected undesired tooth movement in context with OSA treatment benefits requires a risk-benefit analysis with consideration of treatment alternatives at review appointments. Valid informed consent is advisable.

Hypersalivation or Xerostomia

Immediate short-term side effects of wearing MRDs include hypersalivation or xerostomia (i.e., dry mouth) if lip seal is impossible due to vertical opening or bulk, or both.

Undesired Orthodontic Effects

Tooth movement may complicate MRD therapy and "may be predictable on the basis of initial characteristics in dental occlusion and the design."[44] Some degree of retroclination of the upper incisors and proclination of the lower incisors is thought to occur with most MRDs.[13] It may manifest during long-term use as a mild reduction in overjet or overbite,[6] and it may be undetectable by the patient. Occasionally, dental changes occur that require remedial dentistry to restore the occlusion. After wearing an MRD, some patients may experience a temporary sensation of bite change. Empiric reporting has led to the creation of morning-wear devices that can lessen this effect. The morning-wear device can be designed to reverse the lateral load applied to the teeth by the MRD and the potential overbite and overjet changes.

Change in Occlusal Relationship

Obtaining valid informed consent and retaining pre-MRD therapy study casts are highly recommended because a change in the occlusal relationship may be observed in rare instances. Careful and frequent dental follow-up appointments are suggested. Communication with the patient regarding detected changes that he or she may be unaware of is recommended, and these should be discussed in the context of a risk-benefit assessment and consideration of alternative treatment modalities.

A posterior open bite may develop in some MRD users for unknown reasons. Theories include:

- The device frees the bite. The MRD can eliminate interdigitation with opposing teeth and the influence of physiologic TMJ

function on tooth position, either or both of which can destabilize the occlusion.
- The condylar head is moved anteriorly and may move separate from the meniscus.
- Premature incisal contact results from inclination that appears as a posterior open bite.

Temporomandibular Joint Ache

An aggressive titration rate (i.e., increasing protrusion) or commencing MRD therapy in an excessively protruded or incorrect position (i.e., bite registration is not observed when the laboratory constructs the device) can cause TMJ ache. Frequent evaluation with gradual incremental titration from a minimal or zero protrusion starting point is advisable. TMJ ache can occur even with proper fitting and management, and the dentist should always ask the patient to communicate even seemingly minor and transient symptoms because they may indicate a developing complication.

Tooth Pain

Diffuse, low-level discomfort of the teeth may be reported.

Recording the Jaw Relationship

What

A protrusive bite registration can be considered a three-dimensional prescription to be given to the MRD manufacturer. It relates the position of the jaws, and this is the position to which the MRD is constructed. It can be merely a wax horseshoe shape into which the patient bites, or it can be a more sophisticated product with added functionality (e.g., George Gauge, IST [Intra-oral Snoring Therapy], Airway Metrics).

Why

Every patient is unique; consequently, an approach of "*x* millimeters of protrusion to be effective" will not work. When registering the protrusive bite, the intention is to record the relationship of the jaws in a position that is 50% to 70% of the maximum comfortable protrusion in anticipation that this will be close to the final effective position. The MRD will be constructed to this position, but therapy can ideally commence with less or no protrusion. The ideal bite registration position relates to and minimizes the vertical opening to permit lip seal and encourages nasal breathing. MRD designs vary, as does the impact of an incorrectly constructed or used protrusive bite registration.

How

Various products can assist the dentist with providing accurate bite registrations, including orthodontic bite forks, the George Gauge, and the IST bite fork. Alternatives include wax or putty. YouTube videos show how these products can best be used. Determining the optimal protrusion was discussed earlier in this chapter.

When or If

It is necessary to provide a protrusive bite registration for MRD construction to ensure that an even and balanced contact exists between the occlusal surfaces. Some MRDs have incisal contact only (e.g., Thornton Adjustable Positioner, MDSA), but a bite registration is still required. It is essential that deviation to the left or right on protrusion is reflected in the MRD.

Other Factors

Factors to communicate to the laboratory include the following:
- When the dental midlines do not coincide
- When the dental and facial midlines do not coincide
- When there is an acute condylar angle (commonly associated with skeletal class II)
- When there is a steep curve of Spee that leads to posterior interference on protrusion
- Overerupted or unopposed molars that may interfere with protrusion
- Marked facial or condylar asymmetry

Some MRD manufacturers may also ask for the following information:
- A record of the maximum comfortable protrusion
- A record of the maximum opening (measured interincisally)
- Whether the device should include all the molar teeth

It is important to ensure that the vertical space between the most posterior molar teeth is sufficient to include two devices (i.e., upper and lower) of adequate material thickness for robustness.

Fitting

The dentist must ensure that both parts of the device are appropriately retentive and that when the MRD design incorporates posterior support, it is even and balanced. The gingiva must not blanch where it is covered. It is essential to establish that the patient can insert and remove the individual parts and subsequently the complete device. He or she must understand how the pieces of the device interrelate to achieve effect. This discussion should include the requirement for titration and regular follow-up appointments.

Determining the Optimal Protrusion

Establishing optimal jaw advancement, which is also known as *protrusion,* to deliver OSA therapy is challenging. Each patient has a unique maximum response to protrusion, which must be balanced against increasing the load on the teeth and TMJs. This process, which is known as *titration*, must be performed while providing sufficient time for the wearer to adapt to the device, and it must be balanced against the individual's desire and his or her bed partner's desire for rapid resolution.

Increased protrusion yields improved resolution of OSA symptoms, but subjective and objective symptom improvements are poorly correlated.[22] A nonlinear dose-response relationship exists between protrusion and response (eFig. 33.1).[29] Increased protrusion improves response until a certain patient-specific optimum has been established. Protrusion beyond this position yields no further benefit and may even diminish response.

Titration is complicated by the interindividual heterogeneous response (i.e., difference between patient A and patient B regarding response and protrusion) and the detrimental effects of increasing the load directed toward the teeth and TMJs, which is concomitant with increased protrusion.

Several MRD titration protocols exist, and there is no consensus regarding what is optimal.[16] A multiparametric titration protocol as described by Dieltjens is suggested as ideal.[16] Subjective titration should be performed by the dental practitioner over time in response to patient and partner reporting, provided that the patient has had time to adapt to the device. The patient's maximum tolerable protrusion is established before further titration is performed in an objective assessment environment. Protrusion can be set up to the patient's physiologic or tolerable limit.

Dental Evaluation

The dentist should provide regular follow-up appointments to monitor patients for side effects and possible complications, particularly during the early weeks and months of therapy; to promote compliance;[21] and to titrate subjective or objective improvement in the patient's symptoms. An alternate type of MRD can also be considered.

Conclusions

Around the world, the future of sleep medicine is being debated. In the United States, the American Academy of Sleep Medicine published a white paper on its website.[7] The aim of this publication was to devise "frameworks for health care delivery such as the patient-centered medical home (PCMH), patient registries, and new outcomes measures and tools for the diagnosis and treatment of sleep disorders." With the rise in awareness of how obesity, cardiology, diabetes, and OSA are interrelated, sleep laboratories may in the future evolve into metabolism centers.

In 1997, Loube and Strauss[42] concluded that "future efforts at enhancing cooperation between dentists and sleep disorders physicians in the treatment of OSA with oral appliances should be promoted as a means of standardizing treatment." Empowering appropriately trained team members to perform functions that they are well-positioned to undertake seems logical and, in the face of an epidemic and a global financial crisis, necessary.

The role of dentistry in sleep medicine is developing to include increased emphasis on screening, and it may include patient evaluation (e.g., monitoring MRD compliance and objective efficacy). It may also include blood pressure and weight monitoring in an effort to recognize the best time to transition from an oral device to PAP.

The correlation of clinical indicators (e.g., incisal wear, tooth mobility) as signs of an SRBD with a patient's hypertension, for example, can help the physician develop a broad-based strategy of intervention.

Perspective is essential and can be gained through working as part of a multidisciplinary team. Tooth movement that in isolation may appear to be significant can be considered relatively unimportant when placed in the context of breathing and sleeping.

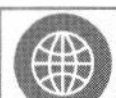
A Case Scenario is found on the companion website eBooks.Health.Elsevier.com.

References for this chapter are found on the companion website at eBooks.Health.Elsevier.com.

CHAPTER 34

Masticatory System Disorders That Influence the Periodontium

Michael J. McDevitt

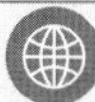
For online-only content about the biomechanics of the masticatory system as well as expanded discussions of the muscles and nerves of the masticatory system, dysfunction and deterioration, orofacial pain, and clinical examination, please visit the companion website at eBooks.Health.Elsevier.com.

CHAPTER OUTLINE

The masticatory system consists of the temporomandibular joints (TMJs), the masticatory muscles, the teeth in occlusion, and the neurologic and vascular supplies that support all of these structures. Research suggests that masticatory system disorders include many varied conditions with multiple possible contributing factors rather than different manifestations of a single disease or syndrome.[3,88,135] The ability to understand the anatomy and function of the masticatory system and to correctly interpret relevant diagnostic information is a prerequisite to fulfilling comprehensive standards of care. Our diagnostic process must have a broad enough base and be inclusive enough to determine the most appropriate cause of masticatory dysfunction.[145]

Temporomandibular Joint

Harmonious function of the TMJs is a product of the coordination of the muscles of mastication by intricate mechanisms of neurologic control. Understanding the dynamics and the relationship of the TMJ to the associated muscles and nerves provides the working knowledge required for effective assessment and diagnosis.

The TMJ is one of the most complex joints in the human body. It is capable of providing both hinging (rotation) and gliding (translation) movements, and it is able to resist incredible forces of mastication. The TMJ is formed by the head of the condyle of the mandible as it fits into the articular fossa of the temporal bone (Fig. 34.1). The body of the mandible effectively connects both condyles so that neither condyle functions independently of the other. Interposed between the head of the condyle and the articular surface of the temporal bone is the articular disc, which consists of dense connective tissue; this results in a compound joint with two joint cavities (Fig. 34.2). The articulating surfaces of the osseous structures are essentially convex in a healthy situation, so the biconcave configuration of the articular disc compensates for the opposing convexities. The articular surfaces of the condyles and the temporal bones consist of fibrous connective tissue, which renders them resistant to breakdown and capable of repair. Deep to the superficial connective tissue layer, articular cartilage provides the cellular and structural basis for the response to the functional loading and movement of the TMJs.[88,145,200] The discal ligaments and attachments to the capsule, along with the disc itself, become the means of separating the joint into superior and inferior joint spaces (see Figs. 34.1 and 34.2). Synovial lubrication of the articular surfaces is a function of the production of synovial fluid by endothelial cells along the borders of each joint cavity and at the anterior extent of the retrodiscal tissues.[46,47,88,145,195,197,200]

Muscles and Nerves of the Masticatory System

The muscles and nerves of the masticatory system are extensively reviewed elsewhere. They are only briefly discussed here for the purpose of understanding the mechanisms involved. Appropriate references are provided for further reading.

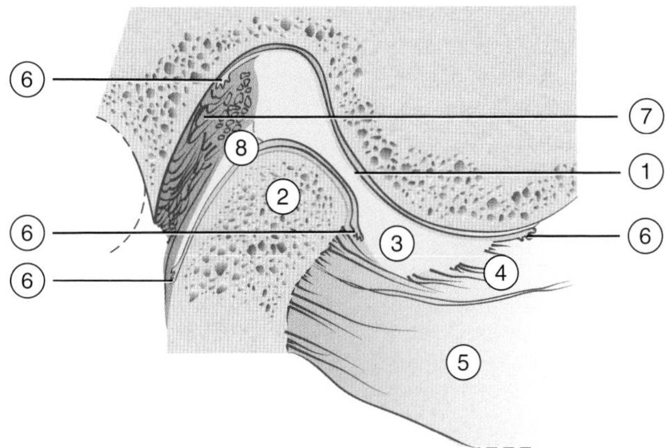

Fig. 34.1 Lateral view of a cross-section through the temporomandibular joint. *1*, Posterior slope of the articular eminence of the temporal bone; *2*, head of the condyle; *3*, articular disc (note the biconcave shape); *4*, superior lateral pterygoid muscle (note the attachment to both the head of the condyle and the articular disc); *5*, inferior lateral pterygoid muscle; *6*, synovial tissue; *7*, retrodiscal tissue; and *8*, discal ligament attachment to the posterior surface of the head of the condyle. (*Modified from Dawson PE.* Evaluation, Diagnosis, and Treatment of Occlusal Problems. *2nd ed. St. Louis: Mosby; 1989.*)

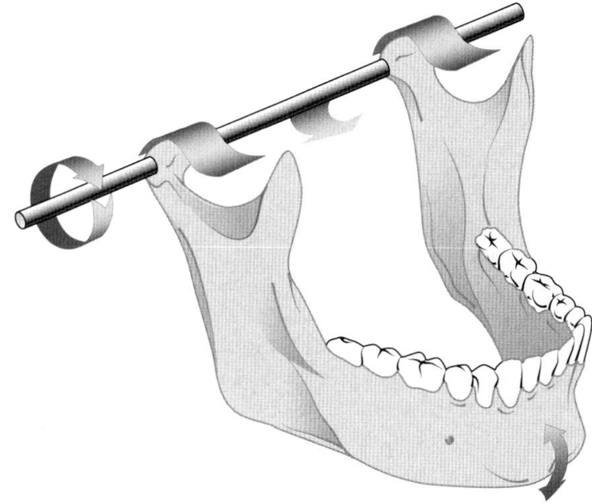

Fig. 34.3 When they are in centric relation, the condyles can rotate on a fixed axis. As long as the rotational axis stays fixed at the most superior position against the eminentiae, the mandible can open or close and still be in centric relation. If the condyle axis moves forward, it is no longer in centric relation. (*From Dawson PE.* Evaluation, Diagnosis, and Treatment of Occlusal Problems. *2nd ed. St. Louis: Mosby; 1989.*)

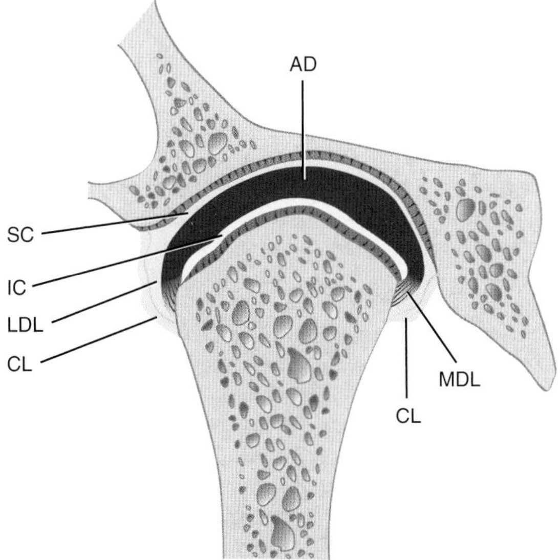

Fig. 34.2 Anterior view of the temporomandibular joint showing the collateral ligaments. *AD,* Articular disc; *CL,* capsular ligament; *IC,* inferior joint cavity; *LDL,* lateral discal ligament; *MDL,* medial discal ligament; *SC,* superior joint cavity. (*From Okeson JP.* Management of Temporomandibular Joint Disorders and Occlusion. *4th ed. St. Louis: Mosby; 1998.*)

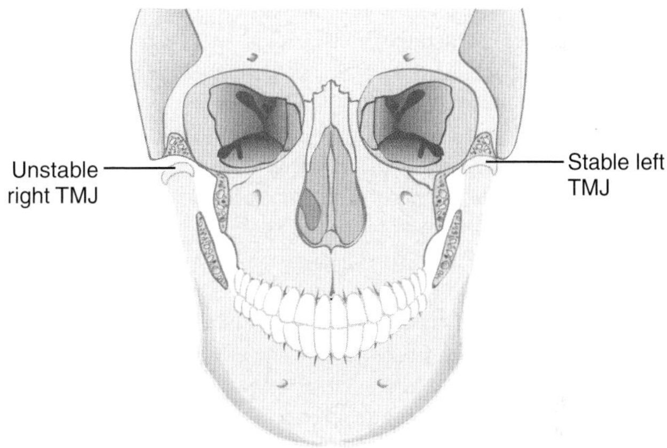

Fig. 34.4 Example of orthopedic instability. Note that, with the teeth in their stable position (i.e., maximum intercuspation), the left temporomandibular joint *(TMJ)* is in a stable relationship with the fossa. The right temporomandibular joint, however, is not in a stable position with the fossa. When the elevator muscles contract, the right condyle moves superiorly to seek a more stable relationship with the articular disc and fossa (i.e., the musculoskeletally stable position). This type of loading can lead to an intracapsular disorder. (*From Okeson JP.* Management of Temporomandibular Joint Disorders and Occlusion. *4th ed. St. Louis: Mosby; 1998.*)

Centric Relation

The mandible is suspended from the cranial base by ligaments and muscles. The understanding of mandibular movement begins with an initial reference point for each condyle, which is usually referred to as *centric relation*; this clinically determined relationship of the mandible to the maxilla occurs when both condyle–disc assemblies are in their most superior position in the maxillary (or glenoid) fossa and against the slope of the articular eminence of the temporal bone. Verification of centric relation is obtained by loading the TMJs bilaterally with the teeth apart via the bimanual mandibular manipulation technique advocated by Dawson and others.[46,45,47,186] When both condyles are in this relationship, rotation or hinging action occurs around an axis defined by the medial poles of each condyle (Fig. 34.3).

The term *centric relation* is limited to the rotation axis through both condyles while they are seated in their respective glenoid fossae. The only occlusal consideration relative to centric relation occurs when rotation of the mandible initiates the first contact of opposing occlusal surfaces. The term *initial contact* in centric relation can be used to define this relationship (see Chapter 35). If the contraction of elevator muscles occurs at the point of initial occlusal contact and results in the distraction of one or both condyle–disc assemblies from their seated relationship, then centric relation is no longer occurring.[46,47,48]

For TMJs to maintain orthopedic stability, the condyles must remain fully seated in their respective fossae when the teeth occlude in maximal intercuspation. Orthopedic instability occurs when the occlusal relationships are such that the contraction of elevator muscles is required to achieve stable occlusion in the maximal intercuspal position, which results in the unseating of one or both condyles from their respective fossae (Fig. 34.4).

The strain on the discal ligaments caused by a loaded joint being displaced from the fossa can lead to internal derangement of that joint, which will be described later in this chapter. Postural and parafunctional stress can also be sources of the orthopedic instability of a TMJ.

An individual's susceptibility to masticatory system disorders determines whether that person adapts with minimal consequence or develops dysfunction or degeneration.[29,46,47,145,186]

Dysfunction and Deterioration

Ideally, function never exceeds the integrity or adaptive limits of the structural elements of the masticatory system. Clinical experience shows that the tolerance of the components of the masticatory system can be exceeded by both acute trauma and chronic trauma. *Acute trauma* to the head and neck region can range from a distinct event, such as an accident or a blow to the face, to a sustained overuse experience, such as a long dental appointment. Acute trauma can serve as an initiating event that leads to a chronic condition, so accurate documentation and careful monitoring may prove extremely valuable should symptoms or dysfunction persist.[15,22,50]

Chronic trauma is defined as any experience that repeatedly exceeds the tolerances of the affected masticatory system structure. Postural stresses and parafunctional occlusal habits, with or without occlusal discrepancies, may produce musculoskeletal disharmony and orthopedic instability of the TMJ.

The general terms for occlusal parafunction used in this text include *bruxism,* which is the grinding of the teeth, and *clenching,* which is when a person holds the teeth firmly together with significant force. Bruxism is usually confirmed by the observation of excessive tooth wear. The clenching type of parafunction can be distinguished from the grinding of the teeth, and it seems to be more often associated with masticatory system disorders than does bruxism.[34,65,67,87,149,156] Sleep bruxism may include both tooth grinding and clenching, and it seems to occur primarily during stage 1 and stage 2 (i.e., non-rapid eye movement) sleep. These episodes often occur in association with short brain and cardiac reactivations called "microarousals." Rhythmic masticatory muscle activity is relatively common among nonbruxers, but the frequency and intensity of the muscle contraction is substantially greater for the sleep bruxer. The central pattern generator of the primate brain stem does not modulate or reduce muscle contraction during sleep as it does during waking hours. In addition, the amplification of oral parafunction has been reported in association with a patient's intake of selective serotonin reuptake inhibitors (e.g., Prozac).[13,46,47,145,157,188]

Sleep bruxism has gained increasing importance to dentists as the prevalence of sleep-related breathing disorders is diagnosed among our patients at a greater frequency than in the past by the patients' physicians, though it can often be suggested by symptoms a dentist has identified. The research into the association between sleep bruxism and masticatory system disharmonies and pain has resulted in mixed findings with both strong and weak correlations reported.[2,144] There is additional evidence that awake bruxism interacts with sleep bruxism and increases the presence of painful TMDs.[163]

The importance of the medical implications of sleep-related breathing disorders has apparently contributed to the development of a variety of interventions to reduce the potential of comorbidities of this condition among dental patients. When continuous positive airway pressure (CPAP) or other interventions are not successful, dentists are often asked to provide a mandibular advancement appliance to encourage opening of a patient's pharyngeal airway.[143] Though initial symptoms of discomfort and TMJ disharmonies may occur, some studies suggest minimal long-term negative consequence of the continued use of mandibular advancement appliances.[202] Conversely, other researchers found the inconsistent use of a mandibular advancement appliance due to TMD symptoms to the extent that appliance use was discontinued over time as similar symptoms developed.[141] Dental and skeletal changes have resulted from long-term use of these appliances, adding further evidence for continuous close supervision by the patients and by their sleep physician.[170,171] Chapters 32 and 35 in this textbook provide an in-depth discussion and presentation of the multifaceted role a dentist may assume in identifying and treating the consequences to oral structures and elements of the masticatory system.

Discrimination between occlusal function-related and parafunction-related masticatory system disorders and those with other etiologies requires exacting standards of occlusal evaluation. If sufficient evidence exists to suspect that the occlusal relationships in function or parafunction may have exceeded the tolerances of that individual's masticatory system, responsible intervention or monitoring can be initiated.[47,70,149,154]

Disruption of the relationship or alignment of the condyle, the disc, and the articular surface of the temporal bone is typically called an *intracapsular disorder* or an *internal derangement of the TMJ.* The articular disc can be displaced as a result of an acute blow to the jaw, chronic trauma, or the uncoordinated contraction of the lateral pterygoid muscle. When the disc cannot return to its normal relationship to the condyle with full closure of the mouth, it is considered to be displaced or dislocated.

Orofacial Pain

Discomfort associated with masticatory system disorders falls under the larger umbrella of orofacial pain. Pain associated with TMJ dysfunction is most frequently muscular in origin,[46] and it may be amplified by both occlusal parafunction and stress.[68] Although pain itself is a complex entity,[182] a working knowledge of even the uncommon sources of pain perceived in the region of the masticatory system is essential to providing comprehensive diagnosis and treatment.

Sources of dental or periodontal pain should be identified by clinical, radiographic, and historic information. Nondental sources of pain include TMJ structures, muscles, cervical structures, neuropathies, vascular inflammation, all types of headache, sleep disorders, systemic disorders, and psychoimmune neurologic sources.[146] A survey of 45,700 American households revealed that 22% of respondents had experienced some type of orofacial pain during the previous 6 months, thereby establishing a meaningful probability that the periodontal patient's list of symptoms includes pain.[12]

Box 34.1 provides the current list of possible sources of orofacial pain. This list was prepared by the American Academy of Orofacial Pain.[146]

Headache pain is perceived primarily within the trigeminal nerve pathways, although other cranial and cervical nerves may offer painful sensory input.[88,146,172] Pain that originates in masticatory system structures, which are also innervated by the trigeminal nerve, requires diagnostic differentiation from headache pain.[173] Headache can present in myriad forms, and it can influence the perception of pain and the diagnosis of the origin of pain.[88,146]

Pain of dental and periodontal origin must be clearly defined and differentiated from heart attack, sinus pain, and myofascial pain.[145,146] Pain that originates in pulpal or periodontal nociceptors can be differentiated with a comprehensive clinical and radiographic evaluation. Orofacial pain that originates in the TMJs or

BOX 34.1 Differential Diagnosis of Orofacial Pain

Intracranial Pain Disorders[74,80,88,126,146,151]
Neoplasm, aneurysm, abscess, hemorrhage, hematoma, edema

Primary Headache Disorders (Neurovascular Disorders)[96,129]
Migraine, migraine variants, cluster headache, paroxysmal hemicrania, cranial arteritis, carotidynia, tension-type headache[6,98,104,145]

Neurogenic Pain Disorders[126,129]
Paroxysmal neuralgias: Trigeminal, glossopharyngeal, nervus intermedius, and superior laryngeal neuralgias[176]
Continuous pain disorders: Deafferentation pain syndromes (peripheral neuritis, postherpetic neuritis, posttraumatic and postsurgical neuralgia, neuralgia-inducing cavitation osteonecrosis[19,20])
Sympathetically maintained pain[24]

Intraoral Pain Disorders
Dental pulp, periodontium, mucogingival tissues, tongue[16,114,126,199]

Temporomandibular Disorders
Masticatory muscle, temporomandibular joint, associated structures

Associated Structures[39,43,137,145,146]
Ears, eyes, nose, paranasal sinuses, throat, lymph nodes, salivary glands, neck

Axis II Mental Disorders
Somatoform disorders
Pain syndromes of psychogenic origin

Compiled by the American Academy of Orofacial Pain.

the muscles of mastication can result from a neoplasm, macrotrauma, repeated microtrauma, systemic disease, or anatomic predisposition.

Sleep-related breathing disorders may also play a role in a patient's orofacial pain through various potential mechanisms.[10] Sleep bruxism has been associated with hypoxia and arousals during sleep disruption.[28,59,191,192] Pain tolerance appears to be diminished with sleep deprivation.[4,179] Oral appliances that have been prescribed for sleep-disordered breathing have the potential to cause at least transient symptoms of TMDs as a result of the mandibular advancement that needs to be experienced for them to be effective.[49,54] Oral appliances prescribed for sleep bruxism may represent an additional airway obstruction for the patient with obstructive sleep apnea.[63] In light of the increasing emphasis on the effects of sleep-disordered breathing in both medicine and dentistry, Chapter 33 has been developed for this text to serve as a reference for the reader.

Comprehensive Evaluation

Patient History and Interview

The written history and personal interview should be designed to invite open-ended responses and reflection by the patient on past experiences and the current condition. Standard dental or medical history forms may require modification to include questions about any history of limited or painful jaw movement, noise in either joint, and masticatory muscle symptoms (Box 34.2). Asking the patient about quality of sleep, restfulness upon awakening and throughout the day, and their positions during sleep can be very helpful. An astute TMD specialist has found patients may sleep with pressure on their mandibles and chins with greater frequency than expected. The weight of the cranium and upper torso can readily overload the masticatory systems and contribute to TMD and pain.[130] These issues should be documented with regard to timing, duration, frequency, and relationship to any history of trauma.[146]

BOX 34.2 Examples of Questions About the Masticatory System to Include in the Patient History

Are you now experiencing or have you ever experienced:

1. Pain in either jaw joint or pain when opening or closing your mouth?[11]
2. Acute or direct trauma to the face, jaw, head, or neck, such as during an accident?
3. Any locking or restricted movement of either jaw joint?[53,180]
4. The inability to bite or close the teeth together completely without discomfort in one or both jaw joints?
5. Earache without infection, especially if it is recurring?
6. Ringing or rushing sounds in either ear?
7. Any type of neuralgia (nerve pain), especially with trigger points?[126,190]
8. Tooth pain without a diagnosed dental problem or after tooth removal?[127,128,183]
9. Fibromyalgia (muscle pain)?[44,153,159,178]
10. Sleep apnea or any sleep disturbance?
11. Any sounds, such as clicks or pops, in either jaw joint, especially when opening or while eating?
12. Chronic or frequently recurring headaches, especially migraines or cluster headaches?[6]
13. Shingles or any painful infection of the face or neck?
14. Having to "adjust" the jaw or manipulate the jaw joint with your hand to be able to open or close your mouth?
15. An occupation or activity that requires a regular stressful posture, such as cradling a telephone between the head and shoulder, working at a computer, playing a musical instrument, or scuba diving?[184,203]
16. An awareness of frequently keeping your teeth together, maintaining a clenched jaw, or holding your jaw in an assumed position, such as holding a pipe?
17. Lyme disease?[74]
18. Neck muscles that are often tired or sore?
19. A sleep position or posture that maintains pressure on your lower jaw?
20. Have you ever been diagnosed with or suspected of snoring or have other symptoms of compromised breathing when you sleep?"
21. Do you now wear or have you ever worn an appliance in your mouth while you sleep?"

Clinical Examination

The clinical examination continues the interview process through the co-discovery of the patient's masticatory system status. The dentist leads the patient to understand the meaning of signs and symptoms of dysfunction or deterioration and seeks opportunities to expand the patient's responses to questions.

The physical examination actually begins during the interview, when asymmetries in facial form, head posture, and mandibular movement patterns can be observed. The clinical evaluation of the various structures of the masticatory system, although individual to each practitioner, should afford the patient opportunities for understanding and include the following[13,46,145]:

1. The observation and measurement of the full range of motion of the mandible
2. The auscultation and light palpation of each TMJ in its full range of motion
3. The load testing of each TMJ
4. The palpation of each muscle of mastication and the related head and neck muscles

5. The evaluation of all of the soft tissues of the face, oral cavity, and oropharynx
6. Periodontal and dental examinations
7. Complete occlusal analysis, including accurately mounted diagnostic models

Imaging

When the clinical evaluation, panoramic radiographs, and patient history indicate the possibility of structural masticatory system disorders or the possible presence of pathology (especially neoplasm), appropriate imaging of the TMJ is warranted.[112] The state-of-the-art technique for the imaging of soft tissue, especially the articular disc, is magnetic resonance imaging. The current highest standard for the imaging of hard tissue, such as the condyle or the temporal bone, is computed tomography (CT). Cone-beam CT has become much more readily available to dentistry, with software systems able to display the data gathered as both anteroposterior and cross-sectional depictions of the condyle and cranial structures with image quality that is the same as or better than spiral CT. Less radiation exposure and lower cost to the patient are both reasons to favor cone-beam CT over conventional CT. The interpretation of magnetic resonance and CT images usually requires specialized training for the clinician or access to a radiologist. Arthrography is still being used for certain diagnostic situations, such as the suspected perforation of the articular disc, and nuclear medicine has developed protocols to image the TMJ to determine if active deterioration is occurring.[13,21,76,79,92,106,124,152]

Although plain-film tomography is occasionally a feature of some of the newer radiographic equipment, the technique that is most readily available to a majority of practitioners is panoramic radiography. The image produced depicts only general relationships and gross anatomy, so the information provided should be used only for screening purposes. When pathology or marked deformation is suggested by a panoramic radiograph, further diagnostic imaging and procedures may be warranted.[21,88]

Diagnostic Decision-Making

The complete evaluation of every patient's periodontal status must include the diagnostic components required to reveal any form of masticatory system disorder. The existence of factors that are responsible for the historical, current, or potential impairment of masticatory system function can be integrated into a comprehensive treatment plan. Patients who require substantial periodontal therapy or who have advanced periodontal disease may be at increased risk for masticatory system disorders, so diagnostic processes must remain consistently thorough and inclusive for all patients.[29,166] For the patient who presents with a symptomatic masticatory system disorder, the diagnostic strategy would logically begin with the inclusion of all potential sources of pain or dysfunction and be followed by the systematic exclusion of possible causative or contributing factors, beginning with the least likely. When no symptoms are reported, the history and clinical examination still need to be thorough, because some patients tend to tolerate modest dysfunction or mild transient discomfort. The diagnostic strategy for the patient who presents with minimal or no signs and symptoms of masticatory system disorders is to attempt to confirm a stable condition while identifying risk factors. The careful documentation of past or current trauma and disharmony provides the basis for the trend analysis and anticipation of possible future problems.[35,36,52,66,77,110,129,135,136,138,187]

Consistent professional maintenance care has been clearly demonstrated to be a key ingredient in the successful management of a patient's periodontal condition.[77,129] By complementing any treatment sequence, these appointments afford dentists the opportunity at every stage of comprehensive care to provide continuing evaluation of the status of the entire masticatory system and to provide timely and appropriate intervention when needed (see Chapter 70).

Acknowledgments

I would like to acknowledge the encouragement and the recommendation of references provided by Dr. Henry Gremillion during the revision of this chapter.

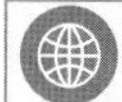
A Case Scenario is found on the companion website eBooks.Health.Elsevier.com.

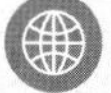
References for this chapter are found on the companion website eBooks.Health.Elsevier.com.

CHAPTER 35

Role of Occlusion and TMD in Periodontal Disease Management

Michael J. McDevitt

CHAPTER OUTLINE

Among the numerous local and systemic factors with the potential to influence the progression of periodontitis, the patient's occlusion remains a variable that requires an exact diagnosis. All of the disciplines of dentistry include the comprehensive analysis of occlusal relationships for determination of appropriate care.

The functional demands of the occlusion may fall within or substantially exceed the tolerances and the adaptability of the patient's periodontium and masticatory system. The full range of knowledge and skill needed to analyze all aspects of occlusal anatomy and function is beyond the scope of this chapter, which does present practical guidelines for the assessment and management of the occlusion specific to a patient's unique susceptibility to periodontitis. Harmony or disharmonies of the masticatory system must also be determined as accurate assessment of the occlusion is virtually impossible when the patient presents with or develops temporomandibular dysfunction and/or pain.

Pathogenesis

The host-driven inflammatory response of each patient to a pathogenic bacterial biofilm[58] is so specific that the patient is his or her only reference for the interpretation of possible contributing factors to the progressive loss of supporting bone. Destructive events can be episodic and are site specific.

A dentist's diagnostic responsibility includes careful measurement of periodontal structures in the entire circumference of each tooth, accurate documentation, and timely reassessment. Periodontal deterioration that occurs rapidly or that is excessive for a person's age should prompt the clinician to investigate all variables that can amplify the patient's periodontitis. If a local factor, such as an occlusal relationship, can influence the course of the disease, its analysis must be as precise as any other aspect of the periodontal examination.

Evidence-Based Decision Making

In a perfect world, all diagnostic and therapeutic decisions would reflect evidence from multiple prospective clinical trials that have been subject to systematic review. Prospective human investigations of occlusal trauma are considered unethical, and periodontics has conscientiously struggled to reach discipline-wide consensus regarding the interaction of a patient's occlusion with his or her periodontal status.[23] To be clinically applicable, the investigation's methodology must parallel the clinical diagnosis and treatment of an individual with periodontitis.[26]

Historically, data management and statistical credibility and methodology within retrospective studies limited the ability of dedicated researchers to interpret the role of occlusion in an individual's periodontitis experience.[28,57,64] The grouping of data points, especially for large study populations, departs from the site specificity that periodontal diagnosis requires. If occlusal trauma is affecting a tooth, the effect on the periodontium is site specific for only that tooth. Treatment for a patient with periodontitis would never be based on an average of diagnostic references, but rather on his or her unique susceptibility, anatomy, occlusion, and history.

KEY FACT

The role of occlusal trauma and its possible influence on the progression of periodontitis is tooth specific.

In 2001, Nunn and Harrell[52] reported the retrospective findings for a group of patients with periodontitis. The analysis was based on measurement of the loss of attachment of each tooth and the presence or absence of occlusal interferences. This study and a similar investigation confirmed that trauma from occlusion amplified the loss of attachment. Harrell and Nunn[27] also reported that eliminating

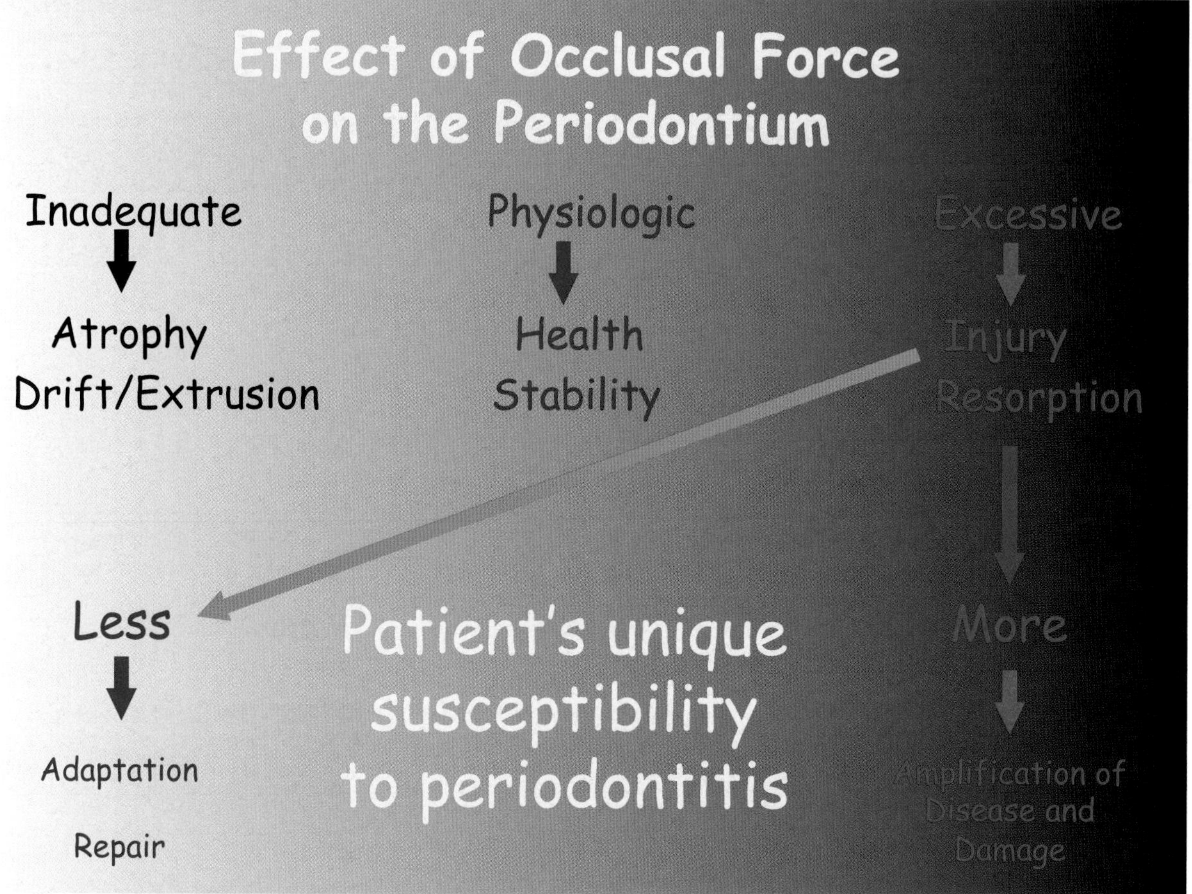

Fig. 35.1 The degree of occlusal force is depicted as a spectrum of white to black, representing none to excessive force.

occlusal interferences had a positive influence on the outcome of treatment when trauma from occlusion was found to be a contributing local factor. The positive influence of occlusal adjustment on the outcome of surgical and nonsurgical periodontal therapies was also reported by Burgett.[10] Evidence supports the possibility that trauma from occlusion can amplify damage to an inflamed periodontium.

KEY FACT

Occlusal trauma can amplify (not cause) localized loss of attachment from inflammatory bone damage.

Although animal studies do not carry the evidence-based hierarchic weight of ideally structured clinical trials, several newer studies seem to support the potential for excessive occlusal forces to amplify damage from inflammatory periodontitis. In two studies using a periodontitis-induced rat model, occlusal trauma resulted in readily identifiable changes in the periodontal ligament of the experimental group compared with the controls. Greater numbers of osteoclasts, perhaps related to increased receptor activator of nuclear factor-κB ligand (RANKL) expression, supported the observation of greater alveolar bone loss in the inflammation plus trauma group. That group also demonstrated increased numbers of immune complexes, which may be a product of the damaged periodontal ligament collagen fibers' greater permeability.[48,69] An in vitro study of human periodontal ligament fibroblasts from healthy individuals and chronic periodontitis patients also supported the observation of significant differences in healthy and diseased periodontal ligament fibroblasts when subjected to compression. Several matrix metalloproteins, interleukin-l6 (IL-16) and IL-21, and other inflammation-associated proteins were expressed by the diseased, compressed fibroblasts compared with healthy fibroblasts, suggesting the diseased fibroblasts could produce additional damage to the periodontium of patients with chronic periodontitis.[19]

Interest in occlusion in the discipline of periodontics appears to be increasing, especially with the rapid growth of the replacement of missing teeth with implants. Despite some conflicting reports in the literature, common ground for consensus exists, as shown in Fig. 35.1.

Occlusal force has an effect on the periodontium (see Chapters 32 and 34) and that susceptibility to periodontitis is unique to each patient. Occlusal forces occur across a broad spectrum. No or minimal occlusal contact on a tooth results in disuse atrophy of the periodontium, which can result in instability of that tooth. Harmonious occlusal force on a tooth stimulates the physiologic arrangement of the periodontal attachment fibers and osseous architecture and encourages stability. Forces that exceed the tolerance of the periodontium result in resorption of the bone and disruption of the attachment.[30,46,50] In the healthy person, the periodontium around teeth that are subject to excessive occlusal force experiences adaptation and repair or remodeling with no loss of attachment, which often occurs with orthodontics.

For the patient who is losing bone as a result of periodontitis, coupling the ongoing inflammatory disease with excessive occlusal force can amplify destruction and damage to the periodontium of affected teeth.[52] If this conclusion is valid, the clinician has the responsibility to correlate the periodontal status of each tooth with its occlusal responsibilities and possible occlusal excesses.

Terminology

The following is a list of key descriptive terms, as used in this chapter, and their common synonyms:

Centric relation: Position of the mandible when both condyle-disc assemblies are in their most superior positions in their respective glenoid fossae and against the slope of the articular eminences of each respective temporal bone.

Disclusion: Separation of certain teeth caused by the guidance provided by other teeth during an excursion. When anterior guidance provides separation of posterior teeth during an excursion, posterior disclusion is achieved.

Excursive movement: Any movement of the mandible away from maximum intercuspation.

Guidance: The pattern of opposing tooth contact during excursive movements of the mandible.

Initial contact in centric relation: The first occlusal contact in the centric relation closure arc.

Interference: Any occlusal contact in the centric relation closure arc or in any excursion that prevents the remaining occlusal surfaces from achieving stable contact or functioning harmoniously or that encourages masticatory system disharmony; also called an *occlusal discrepancy.*

Lateral excursion: Movement of the mandible laterally to the right or to left from maximal intercuspation.

Maximal intercuspation: Position of the mandible when there is maximal interdigitation and occlusal contact between the maxillary and mandibular teeth; also called *centric occlusion* and *intercuspal position.*

Nonworking side: The side of either arch that corresponds with the side of the mandible moving toward the midline during a lateral excursion; also called the *balancing side.*

Protrusion: Movement of the mandible anteriorly from maximal intercuspation.

Retrusion: Movement of the mandible posteriorly relative to a more anterior position.

Working side: The side of either dental arch that corresponds with the side of the mandible moving away from the midline during a lateral excursion.

Occlusal Function and Dysfunction

Excellent sources for a comprehensive understanding of dental anatomy and function include textbooks by Ash and Nelson,[7] McNeill,[43] and Dawson.[15,16] Trauma from occlusion is determined by whether the composite of all occlusal forces on a specific tooth exceeds the tolerance or adaptability of its periodontium. Identification of masticatory system disharmonies begins with an appreciation of physiologic norms; this allows the clinician to recognize dysfunctional relationships, which can influence the accuracy of the diagnosis.[16,50,54]

Centric relation is a term used to describe the position of both condyles when they are fully seated in the fossae of their respective temporomandibular joints (TMJs). Rotation of the mandible around an axis through both condyles is called the *centric relation closure arc* (see Chapter 34). This is strictly a skeletal relationship until tooth contact occurs. Maximal intercuspation occurs when opposing teeth make contact, with optimal interdigitation, at the most stable end point of mandibular closure. Stability is enhanced by the simultaneous bilateral contact of multiple posterior teeth with occlusal forces in the long axis of most posterior teeth. If the initial tooth contact in the centric relation arc of closure occurs simultaneously with maximal intercuspation, the teeth do not displace the condyles. Conversely, if the teeth are firm and any contact occurs before maximal intercuspation, incline relationships of opposing occlusal surfaces guide the mandible into intercuspal position, thereby requiring one or both condyles to become dislocated from their fossa.[16,52] If the teeth are mobile and contact first in the centric relation closure arc, then *they may move away from opposing teeth rather than cause condylar displacement.*

Cusp-fossa or cusp–marginal ridge relationships of the posterior teeth provide resistance to vertical loading and functional stability for the patient's dentition. When occlusal forces load teeth in their long axis, the periodontium is the most resistant and supportive.[15,16] The anterior teeth can be stable with little occlusal loading in centric occlusion if they are favorably influenced by the oral musculature. If the anterior teeth are in contact in maximal intercuspation, they are coupled.

Movement of the mandible from centric occlusion is called an *excursion.* Movement forward is called a *protrusive excursion,* and movement to either side is called a *lateral excursion.* If the mandible can move posteriorly, it is called *retrusion.* There is evidence that the contact of posterior teeth in excursions can overload those teeth, which results in negative dental, periodontal, muscular, and TMJ consequences.[1,11,16,54,72–74] The ideal relationship may be a light coupling of the anterior teeth in centric occlusion with immediate separation (i.e., disclusion) of all posterior teeth in all excursions.[73]

During a lateral excursion, posterior teeth that make contact on the same side as the direction of mandibular movement are described as having a working contact. Posterior teeth that make contact on the side opposite the direction of the lateral excursion are described as having a nonworking contact. Although nonworking contacts are classically associated with negative consequences,[74] the analysis of working contacts and the function of anterior teeth are critically important. Contacts that are disruptive to mandibular movement or stressful to individual teeth are called *occlusal interferences* or *discrepancies.* Dentists' ability to analyze the occlusion to identify contacts that can amplify a patient's periodontitis, thereby affecting certain teeth, is strategic to making the correct diagnosis.[71]

Inflammation disrupts the integrity of the attachment apparatus, which results in less resistance to force from opposing teeth. When bone loss has occurred, less root surface area is supported,[3,29] and there are fewer sensory fibers in the periodontal ligament, which limits the protective muscle modulation of the occlusal forces.[61] The clinician must differentiate among inflammation-caused intolerance to occlusal forces, normal forces on teeth with reduced periodontal support, excessive occlusal forces, and well-tolerated forces on teeth affected by periodontitis.

Parafunction

Bruxism can cause occlusal forces on teeth that are susceptible to periodontitis to be increased in intensity or frequency, thereby magnifying the potential amplification of damage.[12,34,35,67] Daytime or awake occlusal parafunction is commonly limited to clenching the teeth during incidents that require a person's focused effort or mental concentration. Patients can be engaged in identification of daytime teeth clenching, as was the case in a study of sleep bruxism and myofascial pain. Awake clenching was reported by 58 of the 60 participants.[62] Selection criteria for a study must be very exacting because self-reports of sleep bruxism by patients is usually unreliable.[59] Patients' identification of their parafunction can help them to understand its importance, and it supports the clinical experience that daytime clenching can be a frequent contributor to a patient's increased susceptibility to bone loss in sites of inflammatory periodontitis.

Nighttime or sleep bruxing of the teeth can take the form of grinding the teeth during various excursions or clenching the teeth. Sleep bruxism is probably an extension of the rhythmic masticatory muscle activity that is also observed in nonbruxers. Why nuclei in the brain stem allow bruxing to occur in some individuals while others are spared is unclear.[12,34,35]

Bruxing is associated with the greater frequency and persistence of TMJ dysfunction, orofacial pain, and possibly periodontal attachment loss.[67] The sensory input of teeth that are subject to bruxism is probably dampened, which may interfere with the diagnosis and treatment.[56] There seems to be limited influence on bruxing tendencies from occlusal interferences.[37] An exception was discovered in a clinical study of 30 bruxers and 30 nonbruxers; there was a significant difference in nonworking interferences in the bruxing population compared with their absence in the nonbruxing group.[63] When these findings are viewed along with those reported by Youdelis and Mann decades ago, the correlation of bruxing and site-specific inflammatory bone damage appears meaningful.[74]

Gerber and Lynd studied selective serotonin reuptake inhibitor–induced movement disorders.[22] They found that selective serotonin reuptake inhibitors such as Prozac encouraged bruxism.

Evidence is emerging that sleep-disordered breathing can influence or be associated with inflammatory diseases such as periodontitis.[9,18,25] A strong relationship between obstructive sleep apnea and sleep bruxism has now been firmly established; the reported data and observations support a definite association.[13,32,41,55,65,66] A patient with periodontitis with clinical evidence of occlusal trauma may be experiencing the consequences of sleep-disordered breathing. Chapter 33 provides an overview of sleep-disordered breathing, offering a reference for the dentist who is seeking to develop skill in the recognition of oral signs of sleep-disordered breathing to complement his or her diagnostic skills in evaluation of a patient's occlusion. If an occlusal appliance is being considered to address the periodontal implications of excessive occlusal force experienced by a periodontitis-susceptible patient, compliance may be problematic for a person with sleep-disordered breathing, because the appliance can contribute to airway obstruction.[20] Sleep and awake bruxism are also strongly related to increased incidence and symptoms of masticatory system disharmonies and stress.[2,53,60] Even mild to moderate sleep apnea encourages sleep bruxism as can upper airway syndrome.[47]

Clinical Examination

Before clinical evaluation, a conversation with the patient can help to provide a more complete diagnosis. With minimal symptoms, a patient may not associate loose teeth or significant dental wear with TMJ dysfunction or orofacial pain with occlusal function or parafunction. They are more likely to be aware of sleep-related breathing disorders with the frequently attendant bruxing, but if not previously diagnosed and otherwise aware of the clinical signs and symptoms detectable by their dentist, the oral examination may suggest reasons to pursue a medical evaluation. The list of questions in Chapter 34 and inquiries specific to the condition of the patient's teeth can help the clinician to open the lines of communication and set the tone for patient education during the clinical examination.

"Do you now wear or have you ever worn an appliance in your mouth while you sleep?" Comprehensive evaluation of occlusal anatomy and relationships is accomplished by the analysis of many factors in the clinical setting and by mounted diagnostic casts.

Clinical evaluation of the occlusion is sequenced to support the patient's learning. It should always include a clinical assessment of masticatory system function and identification of disharmonies.

BOX 35.1 Temporomandibular Disorder Screening Evaluation

1. Maximal interincisal opening (range, 40–50 mm)
2. Opening or closing pathway
3. Range of lateral and protrusive excursions (7–9 mm)
4. Auscultation for temporomandibular joint sounds
5. Palpation for temporomandibular joint tenderness or tissue displacement
6. Palpation for muscle tenderness
7. Load testing of the patient's temporomandibular joints

Temporomandibular Disorders Screening and Evaluation

Complete assessment of the masticatory system and identification of temporomandibular disorders are described in Chapter 34 and should be part of a patient's initial comprehensive examination. The temporomandibular disorder screening and clinical evaluation then become part of subsequent examinations.

The patient's range of motion is observed, maximal opening and the lateral and protrusive excursions are measured, and any deviation from the midline during opening and closing is defined. Light finger pressure applied over each TMJ can detect deflection of the tissue while the patient opens and closes the mouth; deflection suggests condyle-disc discoordination. Tenderness on palpation can indicate TMJ capsulitis. Listening to the joint with a stethoscope or a Doppler instrument during opening and closing can detect sounds that are consistent with uncoordinated condyle-disc relationships, arthritic changes, and other diagnostic sounds.[16]

Palpation of the muscles of mastication and the related head and neck musculature can reveal muscle tension or spasm related to compensation for occlusal or TMJ disharmonies.[16,54] Load testing of the TMJ is described in Chapter 34. Significant discoveries revealed during the screening examination summarized in Box 35.1 should lead the clinician to complete the comprehensive evaluation.

Testing for the Mobility of Teeth

Two basic methods are used to assess the firmness or looseness of a tooth. Classically, a dental instrument is used to exert pressure in the facial or lingual direction, and the dentist places his or her finger on the opposite side of the tooth to feel and see movement if it occurs (see Chapters 32 and 38). Recording a numeric value (range, 0 to 3) for the degree of mobility allows the clinician to track changes that may occur in response to therapy.

The other method is to test for the movement of teeth that are subject to pressure generated by the patient. Fremitus, vibration, or micromovement of a tooth can be felt when patients tap their teeth together. When the patient mimics clenching the teeth and then attempts to move the mandible in excursions, tooth movement can be observed. The patient placing a finger where the clinician felt tooth movement helps the patient to appreciate the looseness of his or her teeth (Fig. 35.2).

If the mobility of the teeth exceeds what is expected on the basis of the loss of support or the level of inflammation observed, trauma from occlusion is included in the diagnosis. The assimilation of all of the occlusal and periodontal diagnostic references can lead the clinician to conclude that even without mobility, there may be evidence of amplified periodontal damage as a result of unfavorable occlusal forces. Periodontitis susceptibility evidenced in previous or ongoing disease and damage and bruxism are both clearly identified as risk indicators for peri-implantitis. Partially dentate patients with dental implant tooth replacement restorations should have initial and ongoing tooth mobility carefully analyzed and documented

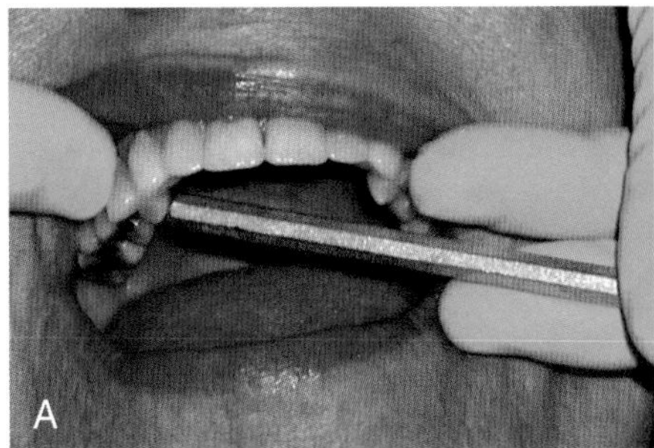

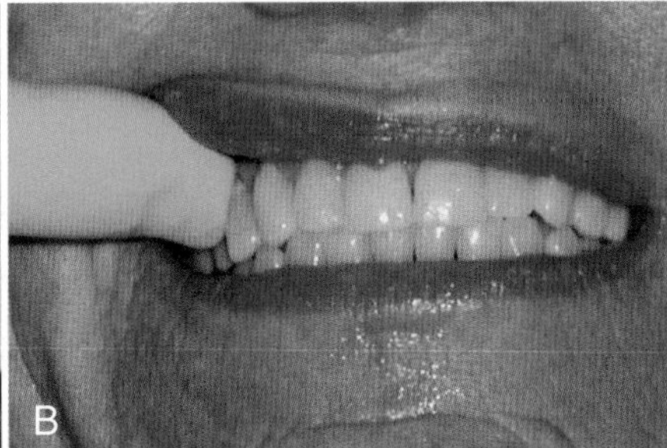

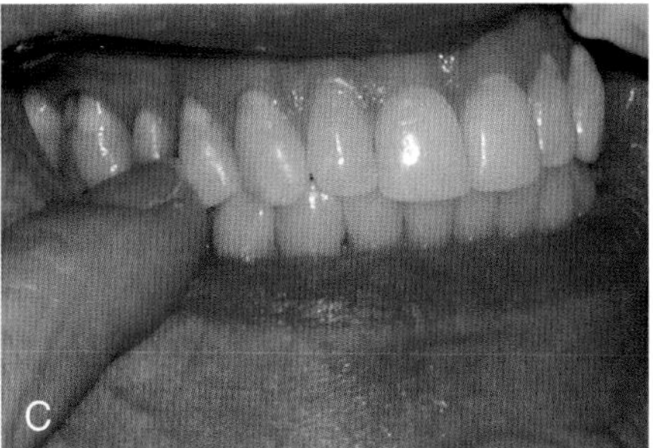

Fig. 35.2 (A) Tactile and visual testing for mobility is done with a dental instrument by the dentist. (B) Tactile and visual testing for mobility is done with the patient clenching and while beginning right lateral excursion by the dentist. (C) The patient feels movement of her tooth when lateral excursion is attempted while the teeth are clenched.

to determine if implant fixtures might be excessively loaded, especially in the presence of any peri-implant inflammation.[14]

KEY FACT

An inflamed periodontium often contributes to the mobility of a tooth.

Centric Relation Assessment

Bimanual manipulation of the mandible in the axis of rotation of the condyles in their respective glenoid fossae has become a standard method of assessing centric relation.[7,15,16,54] This method is illustrated in Fig. 35.3, and it involves gentle guidance rather than the forced positioning of the mandible. This technique is essential for load testing of the TMJs, and it is effective for generating centric relation records for mounting diagnostic casts. Telling the patient that he or she will feel modest lifting pressure on the inferior borders of the mandible and a light depressing force in the mental region often allows for relatively free and comfortable hinging of the mandible.[15,16] If hinging is uncomfortable or not repeatable, muscle deprogramming (see Chapter 34) may be beneficial. Other methods for guiding the condyles toward a seated position (e.g., leaf gauges, anterior bite stops) can be effective.[16]

Asking the patient to identify the first tooth to touch in the centric relation arc of closure may indicate that interferences to closure into maximal intercuspation exist. Asking the patient to close further may demonstrate a slide from centric relation to centric occlusion because teeth are firm enough to dislocate one or both condyles.[54] Drying the occlusal surfaces, positioning marking paper, and then guiding the patient to the initial contact in centric relation allows marking of occlusal contact points, thereby identifying any interference. Asking the patient to then close into maximal intercuspation marks the points or surfaces that contact during the slide. An early occlusal contact in centric relation before closure to centric occlusion is obtained that does not cause a slide may indicate the early contact that occurs on teeth that are mobile enough to move, allowing maximal intercuspation to be gained without condylar accommodation (Fig. 35.4). Confirmation of permissive intercuspation is a product of marking the teeth clinically and comparing the marks with the ones on mounted diagnostic casts, which demonstrates that mobile teeth can move out of the way to allow others to contact.

Evaluation of Excursions

Marking the teeth in all excursions reveals the pathways of contact of opposing occlusal or incisal surfaces during function, and it may identify interferences to harmonious function.[7,16,43] Movement of any teeth during marking may lessen the intensity of the marks and the assessed severity of the forces experienced by the affected teeth.

Vectors of force and steepness of the opposing inclines are studied to determine whether the force is excessive. Interpreting contacts on a tooth-by-tooth basis can suggest or deny occlusal trauma as a contributing factor to the loss of attachment of each affected tooth. When patients are engaged in the evaluation of their occlusion, they can be given suggestions to observe certain habits, such as clenching their teeth during the day or sleeping with pressure on their mandible. As they contribute to their own diagnosis, patients become better prepared to make informed choices about treatment options.

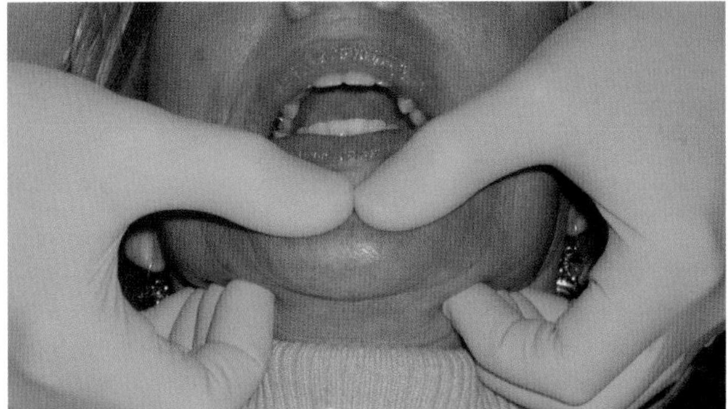

Fig. 35.3 Bimanual manipulation is used to hinge the mandible in centric relation and to load test the temporomandibular joints.

Articulated Diagnostic Casts

When the maxillary diagnostic cast is mounted on an articulator with a facebow transfer technique, the occlusal surfaces become oriented to the axis of rotation of the patient's condyles. The centric relation transfer record orients the mandibular teeth to the maxillary teeth in centric relation.[15,16] Study of the accurately mounted diagnostic casts can reveal occlusal discrepancies between initial contact in the centric relation closure arc and maximal intercuspation and occlusal disharmonies in excursions. Mobile teeth may produce a mark on a solid model but little or no mark in that patient's mouth during clinical assessment. Accuracy of the observations made on the models should be confirmed clinically to whatever degree possible.

Occlusal Therapy

Effective nonsurgical therapy usually reduces inflammation within the periodontium and results in some healing of attachment,[49] which often results in mobile teeth becoming more stable. If the clinician concludes that inflammation has been optimally controlled and that occlusal forces on individual teeth still exceed the tolerance of the periodontium, the basis for intervention is established.

The harmonious function of both TMJs and their associated muscles is required for occlusal stability. When there is sufficient evidence of excessive occlusal forces on the patient's teeth or when masticatory system disharmony exists and the patient desires a more stable occlusion, an occlusal appliance is prescribed.

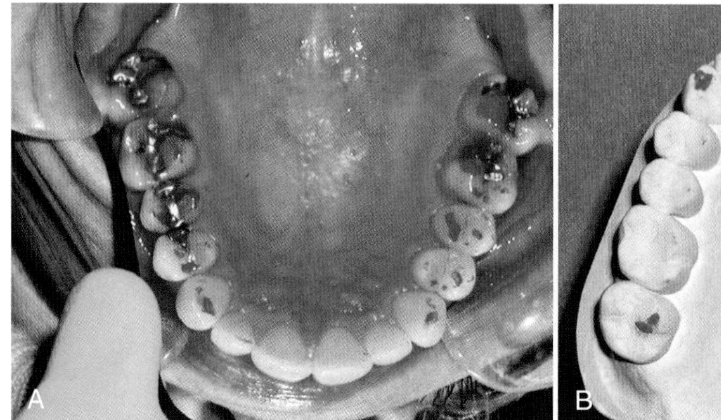
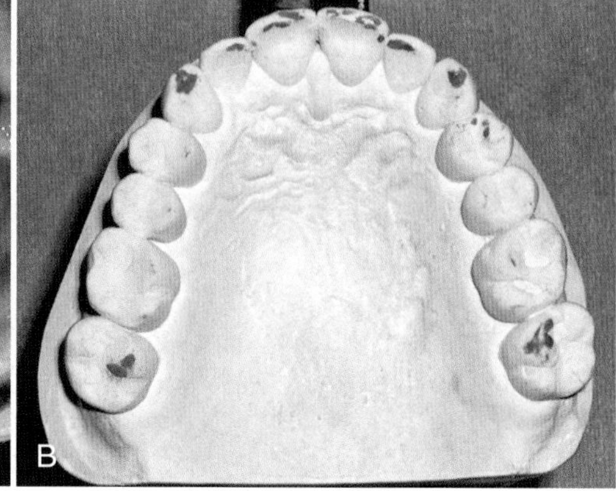

Fig. 35.4 (A) Teeth are marked clinically in maximal intercuspation and in excursions while clenching. (B) Teeth are marked in centric relation and maximal intercuspation on a diagnostic cast mounted in centric relation. Marks only on the second molars indicate that they were mobile and that they moved to permit the contact of other teeth.

Chapter 34 reviews TMJ anatomy; this can provide a better understanding of the goals of therapy.

KEY FACT

Optimal resolution of inflammation is necessary to accurately interpret tooth mobility.

Occlusal Appliance Therapy

A well-designed and accurately fitted appliance can benefit masticatory system function while encouraging loose teeth in both arches to tighten as the supporting periodontium heals. The bilateral simultaneous contact of all opposing posterior teeth in centric relation, shallow anterior guidance, and the immediate disclusion of all posterior teeth in every excursion are essential elements of maxillary and mandibular occlusal appliances (Figs. 35.5 and 35.6).

Teeth that are opposing an appliance should be loaded as close as possible to their long axis. Maxillary appliances engage a portion of the hard palate, which provides substantial bracing of teeth and resistance to vertical and lateral forces. A horseshoe-shaped maxillary appliance relies on other, possibly compromised teeth to attempt to protect the most mobile teeth. Soft or partial coverage appliances are contraindicated for long-term protection and stabilization.[49] The protective role of occlusal appliances was addressed in the 8-year study by McGuire.[42] Occlusal appliances are not expected to cure bruxism,[39] but they are often prescribed for patients with habitual parafunction as a compensating or protective intervention to limit masticatory system disharmony, damage to the teeth, and overstressing of implants.[33]

Temporomandibular Disorder Interventions

Because occlusal equilibration, orthodontics, and restoration of occluding surfaces are irreversible, their application to initially address TMD is contraindicated, especially when reversible intervention has not been used.[31,38] There is clear evidence that a multidisciplinary approach to TMD is very desirable with the dentist as a key member and often the initial diagnostician among the health professionals capable of an important role in addressing a patient's symptoms.[21,24,36] Oral appliances fabricated and accurately fitted to address TMJ disharmonies and dysfunction and craniofacial pain which may be associated with that diagnosis have a favorable record of being helpful with a patient's symptoms.[4,40,51] Physical therapy can usually be prescribed by a dentist addressing a painful TMD situation, and that mode of treatment has proven to be an effective adjunct or a helpful stand-alone intervention.[6,70] Comprehensive advanced training by dental or medical professionals may allow them to be able to aid the patient with masticatory myofascial pain with botulinum toxin injections.[45] A thorough explanation of risks and potential benefits must precede this intervention, which makes training essential, because unfavorable consequences may result from this treatment modality.[17] When persistence or magnitude of a patient's temporomandibular disorder, especially with pain, exceeds the knowledge and skill of a restorative dentist or a periodontist, referral to a TMD specialist or an oral surgeon may be indicated. Although surgical intervention is often considered to be undesirable, surgeons with TMD treatment training and experience can offer a patient a potential for a solution, which would otherwise be unavailable.[5]

Occlusal Adjustment

As teeth tighten from consistent use of the appliance, occlusal interferences may become more evident, and greater discrepancy between the initial dental contact and maximal intercuspation may be observed. Interferences with harmonious excursive movement of the mandible may also become more obvious. When the clinician confirms that the interferences correlate with a greater than expected loss of attachment, direct intervention in the patient's occlusion is considered. With the patient's full understanding and consent, occlusal adjustment or selective reshaping of the occluding surfaces of the teeth can reduce the magnitude of occlusal interferences or direct the forces to be more compatible with the long axes of the affected teeth.

Clinical analysis of the occlusion should be combined with a detailed analysis of diagnostic casts mounted in centric relation on an adjustable articulator. Accurately mounted duplicate models can be used to accomplish a trial occlusal adjustment to determine safety and efficacy for a patient.[16,43] Scheduling patients so that they leave their appliances on the teeth in each arch overnight and in place until they are seated in the dental chair allows assessment of their teeth at maximal firmness, when interferences are most readily identifiable. Teeth usually progressively tighten with continued compliance with the appliance and repeated careful occlusal adjustment.

Other methods that can be used to alter occlusal relationships include orthodontics and restorative dentistry. Provisional restoration of teeth is another method of improving occlusal contacts and stability, and it often simplifies the process of occlusal adjustment and final restoration.

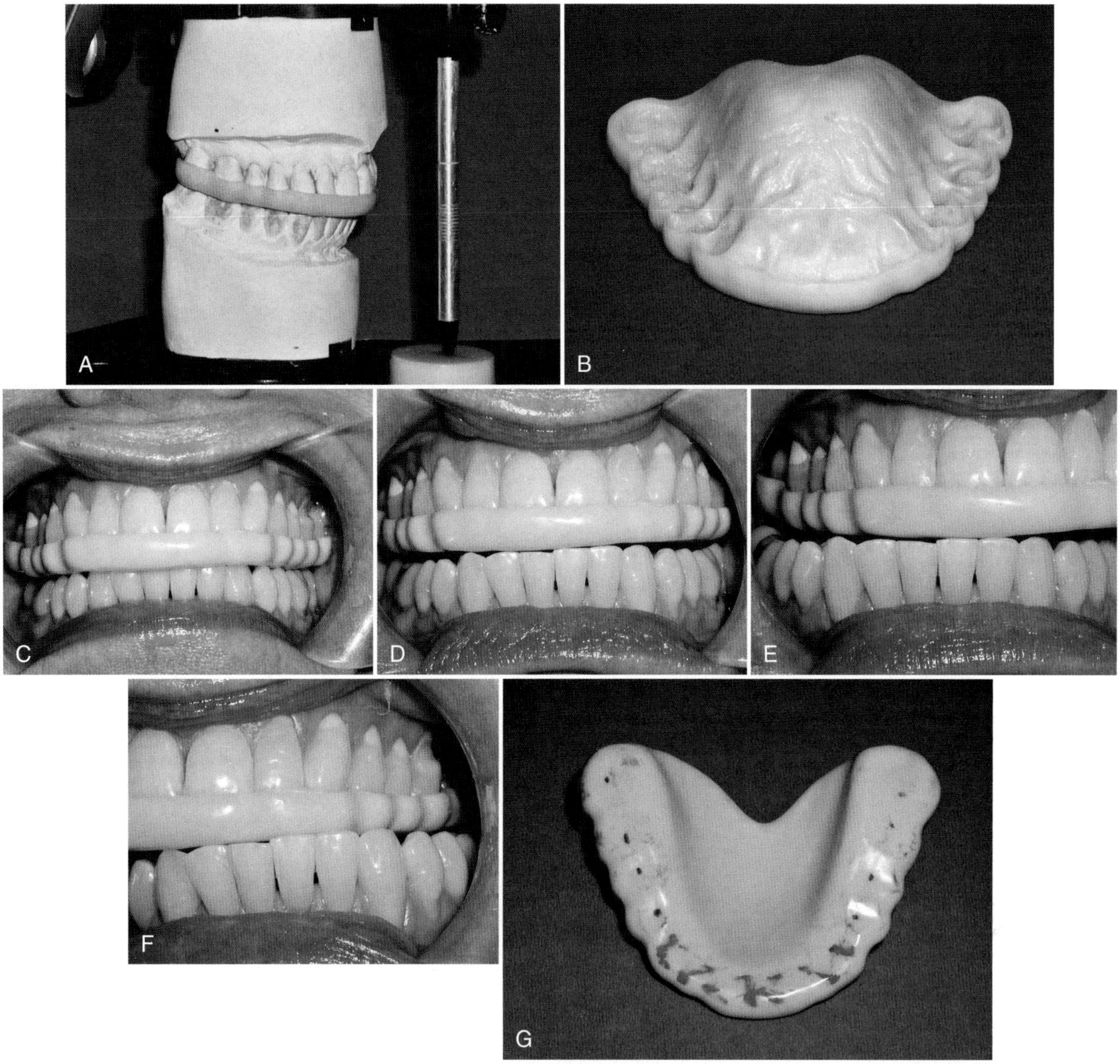

Fig. 35.5 (A) An occlusal appliance is fabricated on accurately mounted diagnostic casts. (B) The entire dental and palatal surface has been carefully relined to promote an optimal stabilizing influence on mobile teeth. (C) There is bilateral, simultaneous contact of the cuspids and all posterior teeth in centric relation, fabricated to enhance axial loading of opposing mandibular teeth. (D) There is smooth, relatively flat anterior guidance with immediate and sustained disclusion of all posterior teeth in protrusion. (E) There is smooth, relatively flat anterior guidance with immediate and sustained disclusion of all posterior teeth in right lateral excursions. (F) There is extreme left lateral excursion with smooth, harmonious transitions across the anterior teeth to maintain the disclusion of all posterior teeth. (G) Marks created by the opposing dentition demonstrate bilateral, simultaneous contact in centric relation and the immediate disclusion of the opposing posterior teeth in all excursions.

Occlusal Stability for Restorative Dentistry

A stable occlusion is considered a prerequisite for any restorative therapy (Box 35.2). Implants to replace the teeth of a partially dentate patient add to the occlusal considerations. Osseointegration of implants eliminates micromovement, which can allow teeth to accommodate occlusal forces. The extent and timing of occlusal loading and the guidance requirement for each tooth and for each implant must be carefully harmonized (see Chapter 85). This is especially critical if any of the teeth are mobile or the patient bruxes to a significant degree.[68] If bruxism is suspected or the functional forces are considered to be excessive, the occlusal appliance as described may be a valuable application.[33,44]

Conclusions

Confirmation of the appropriateness of occlusal therapy is the product of a thorough evaluation of the patient's occlusion and his or her masticatory system. The sequence of occlusal treatment begins with antiinflammatory therapy and progresses through reversible appliance therapy before any irreversible options are considered. This provides the clinician with the most careful approach to assessing and treating the occlusion of a patient with periodontitis.

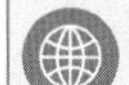
A Case Scenario is found on the companion website eBooks.Health.Elsevier.com.

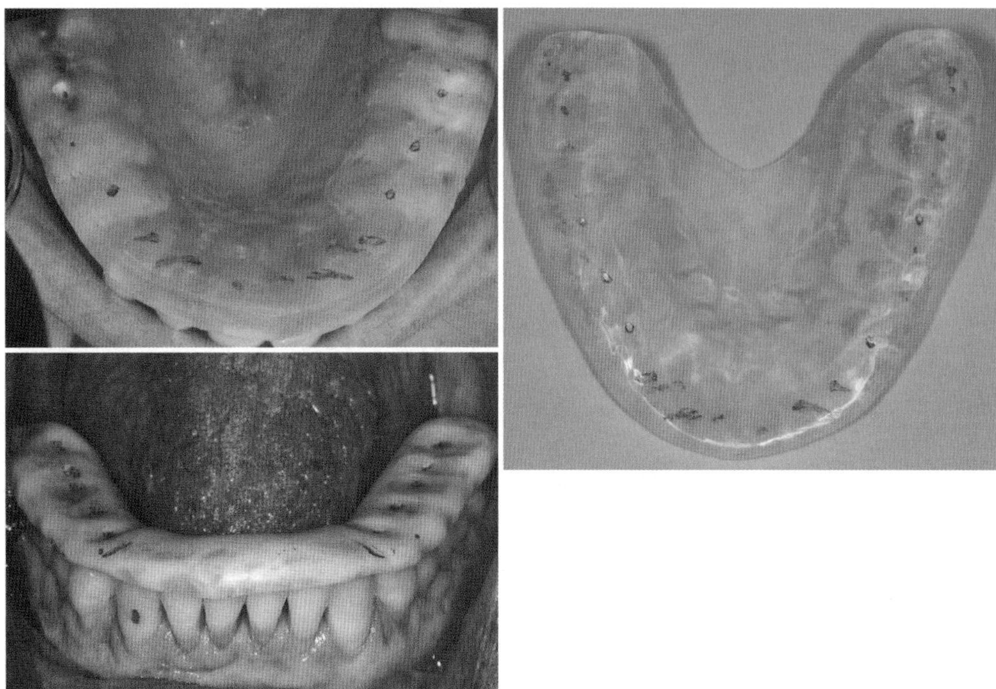

Fig. 35.6 A mandibular occlusal appliance is fabricated after surgery to provide a stabilizing influence for the incisors in particular and to demonstrate occlusal attributes similar to those of the maxillary appliance.

BOX 35.2 Requirements for Occlusal Stability

1. Forces on an individual tooth that do not exceed the support and resistance of the tooth's periodontium and that are vertically oriented to the long axis of each tooth as much as possible
2. Even and simultaneous contact of all posterior teeth in the centric relation closure or in maximal intercuspation, with minimal difference between the two
3. Little or no contact of the anterior teeth in centric occlusion, although such contact is readily available to provide guidance in excursion and to produce posterior disclusion
4. Harmonious excursive movement of the mandible within the patient's envelope of function and with complete absence of occlusal interference

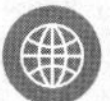

References for this chapter are found on the companion website eBooks.Health.Elsevier.com.

CHAPTER 36

Levels of Clinical Significance

Philippe P. Hujoel

CHAPTER OUTLINE

In one study of periodontal tissue regeneration, investigators reported that treatment that resulted in a gain of 1.2 mm in clinical attachment level and a reduction of 1 mm in probing pocket depth "may not have a great clinical impact."[5] In another study of a local antimicrobial, the investigators reported that a treatment that resulted in a gain of 0.0 mm in clinical attachment level and a reduction of 0.2 mm in probing depth had such clinical significance that it should "be used universally."[32] The American Dental Association defined a substantial effect as a mean change in attachment level greater than 0.6 mm.[28] These examples illustrate that different individuals will reach different decisions regarding what is meant by the term **clinical significance**. As a result, the term **clinically significant** has become more useful to marketers than to clinicians.

The term *clinically significant* could be made more relevant by recognizing (1) the nature of the benefits (tangible/intangible) and (2) the size of the treatment effect (large/small). The presence or absence of these two criteria can be used to classify clinical significance into four levels. Before doing so, each classification term is described.

Tangible Versus Intangible Benefits

Controversies remain as to whether outcomes tested in clinical trials designed for drug approval are tangible to the patient.[8,33] Some will argue that the clinical significance of a treatment should depend exclusively on whether the benefits identified are tangible or intangible to the patient who undergoes the procedure.

Tangible benefits are treatment outcomes that reflect how a patient feels, functions, or survives. The word *tangible* is defined as "capable of being precisely identified or realized by the mind." Examples of tangible benefits could include improved quality of life in relation to oral health,[15,16] a decrease in self-reported symptoms (e.g., bleeding) after brushing, prevention of tooth loss, or elimination of a painful periodontal abscess. These examples of treatment benefits can precisely be identified or realized by the *patient's mind*—that is, they are tangible. Tangible benefits can also be referred to as "clinically relevant" or "clinically meaningful" benefits. Patient Reported Outcome Measures (PROMs) adequately capture tangible benefits that patients perceive from an intervention and are becoming an important component of clinical studies. For more information on PROMs in periodontics, refer to Chapter 1.

KEY FACT

The issues with surrogate endpoints were recognized when the first randomized controlled trial in periodontics was published.[4] Almost half a century later, these issues remain largely unaddressed.

Intangible benefits cannot be realized or perceived by the patient's mind. Changes in probing attachment level because of scaling, changes in enamel mineralization level because of fluoride application, and changes in the size of a periapical radiolucency because of root canal treatment are examples of changes that the patient's mind cannot identify or realize; thus they are described as intangible treatment benefits. Intangible treatment benefits can often be measured objectively by the clinician or by laboratory methods.

The first and most important step in assessing the clinical significance of a treatment is to determine whether the documented treatment benefits are tangible or intangible. This distinction is important because intangible benefits often do not translate into tangible benefits. A medication that lowers elevated blood lipid levels (an intangible benefit) may shorten lifespan (a tangible patient harm). A treatment that increases bone density (an intangible benefit) can increase fracture risk (a tangible patient harm).[11] A treatment that provides extensive periodontal bone regeneration (an intangible benefit) may lead to tooth loss (a tangible harm).[14] A treatment that has been shown to provide tangible benefits has a higher level of clinical significance than a treatment for which only evidence of intangible benefits exists. The finding that implant-supported dentures improve quality of life[1] has a higher level of clinical significance than the finding that scaling increases probing attachment levels. The finding that an endodontic treatment reliably eliminates tooth pain has a higher level of clinical significance than the finding that chlorhexidine reduces *Streptococcus mutans* levels.

CLINICAL CORRELATION

We do not have high-level evidence on all periodontal treatments. Obtaining such information will be helpful in documenting their treatment efficacy as we move into the 21st century, as future economic policies may channel limited health care resources to treatments with a proven tangible benefit.

Size of the Treatment Effect

A second important criterion for assessing clinical significance is the size of the treatment effect. The size of the treatment effect is a comparison of the success rates of the experimental treatment and the control treatment. This comparison can be a subtraction of the success rates, a division of the success rates, or some other mathematical operation. The size of the treatment effect, regardless of how it is calculated, has long been recognized as an important part of assessing clinical significance. The larger the likelihood of obtaining an expected benefit of a treatment (relative to a control treatment), the more clinically significant the treatment is. We suggest that the number needed to treat (NNT) may be a good measure to separate large and small treatment effects.

The likelihood of obtaining a treatment benefit (relative to the control) largely determines the methodological and analytic rigor required to establish treatment effectiveness. At one extreme, in all-or-none situations, reliable evidence may result from observations of a small number of patients. For example, no concurrent controlled trials were conducted to assess the effectiveness of general anesthesia. Determining the effectiveness of treatments that achieve a dramatic and immediate effect is straightforward, and only essential scientific principles (e.g., consistency of observations across different operators) are considered sufficient evidence of treatment effectiveness. Reportedly, the words "Gentleman, this is no humbug" were sufficient to convince an audience that general anesthesia was effective.

KEY FACT

As in medicine, randomized controlled trials conducted in periodontics have primarily focused on surrogate endpoints. Having true endpoints in future randomized controlled trials will enhance the clinical applicability and relevance of their results. As mentioned earlier, including PROMs in clinical trials is gradually becoming a norm.

At another extreme, if the likelihood of obtaining an expected treatment benefit is small, substantial rigor in both design and analysis of controlled clinical trials is required. The benefits of mammography screening for early detection of breast cancer, of one "clot-buster" drug over another after a myocardial event, and of local antibiotics in the treatment of periodontitis are all so small that large randomized controlled trials (RCTs) are required to provide reliable evidence as to whether small benefits indeed are associated with treatment.

The likelihood of obtaining a treatment benefit is a determinant of clinical significance; the larger the likelihood, the more confident a patient can feel that a treatment will be successful. Although it is possible to have a clear, unequivocal definition of what constitutes a tangible benefit associated with treatment, it is not possible to have a similar rigorous definition of what can be considered a large likelihood. We define a "large treatment effect" as an NNT of five, which under fortuitous and very unusual circumstances can be reliably identified with nonexperimental study designs.[7,29]

CLINICAL CORRELATION

Many periodontal treatments result in small changes in clinical attachment levels or probing depths and consequently lead to questions regarding the clinical significance of periodontal therapy. For instance, one systematic review reported by the American Dental Association (ADA) indicated that the addition of metronidazole to scaling and root planing provided an additional gain of 0.18 mm in attachment level. The ADA refers to such an effect as a "zero effect."[28] Small to zero treatment effects are common in clinical trials in medicine.

Defining Four Levels of Clinical Significance

Based on the nature of the benefit (tangible/intangible) and the size of the treatment effect (large/small), four levels of clinical significance can be defined (Table 36.1). In order of decreasing levels of significance, these are numbered from 1 to 4.

Clinical Significance Level 1

Treatments of clinical significance level 1 are the "magic bullets" or "miracle cures," in which the treatment provides a tangible benefit and a large treatment effect. Examples include the use of vitamin C to treat scurvy, bone marrow transplantation to treat leukemia, and a very-low-carbohydrate diet to prevent all forms of dental decay. In all three examples, the benefits of the treatment are tangible and the size of the treatment effect is large.

Understanding the biologic mechanisms of a treatment is not required to establish that the treatment has clinical significance level 1. Lemon juice was identified as an effective method to prevent scurvy in 1601, but it was not until the beginning of the 20th century that vitamin C was isolated.[25] The dangers of carbohydrates in dental decay were recognized millennia before potential mechanisms of action were understood. Digitalis was discovered as a treatment for "dropsy" long before physicians became aware of the drug's cardiac effects.[31] Lithium is an effective drug for bipolar disorder, but its mechanism of action remains largely unknown.[27] In contrast, hormone replacement therapy (HRT), for which the biologic mechanisms explaining how the drug provided benefits were supposedly so well understood, resulted in more harm than good.[12]

TABLE 36.1 Definition of Levels of Significance Based on Size and Nature of the Benefit

		SIZE OF THE BENEFIT	
Clinical Significance		**Large[c]**	**Small[d]**
Nature of the benefit	Tangible[a]	Level 1	Level 2
	Intangible[b]	Level 3	Level 4

[a]Tangible benefits are outcomes that directly measure how a patient feels, functions, or survives.
[b]Intangible benefits are outcomes that are not perceivable by the patient's mind.
[c]A large benefit is defined as one that can reliably be identified using epidemiologic methodology.
[d]A small benefit is defined as one that requires randomized controlled trials for reliable identification.

KEY FACT

The size of the anticipated treatment effect has a profound impact on the planning of randomized clinical trials. The smaller the treatment effect, the larger the number of patients who will need to be recruited.

Treatments of clinical significance level 1 are not always immediately accepted or widely used. It took the British Navy 264 years from the time of the observations of Captain James until a universal preventive policy was established to prevent scurvy.[3] The lack of appreciation for this treatment of clinical significance level 1 was unfortunate.

It is estimated that 5000 lives a year were needlessly lost from scurvy during this period: that is a total of nearly 800,000. In the 200 years from 1600 to 1800 nearly 1,000,000 men died of an easily preventable disease. There are, in the whole of human history, few more notable examples of official indifference and stupidity producing such disastrous consequence to human life.[24]

Although it is easy to determine clinical significance level 1 in retrospect, it may be difficult to recognize at the time of discovery.

Clinical Significance Level 2

Treatments of clinical significance level 2 are those that have demonstrated a tangible benefit but for which the likelihood of obtaining the benefit from treatment is small. As the size of the benefit of one therapy over another decreases, RCTs, large in size and rigorous in execution and analysis, are required to provide unequivocal evidence that the treatment provides tangible patient benefits. Examples of such treatments include the advantage of tissue plasminogen activator (t-PA) over streptokinase[30] and the benefits of penciclovir in the treatment of herpetic lesions.[12]

Determining the clinical relevance of treatments of clinical significance level 2 is an individual choice in which issues such as cost and side effects often play a more important role. For example, administering antibiotics to 25 individuals could prevent 1 person from experiencing early implant loss.[6] Is a 4% increased survival probability of dental implants worth the potential side effects of antibiotics? Different individuals, different governments, and different health insurance companies may decide differently on this important question.

The use of penciclovir in the treatment of herpetic lesions provides another example of a drug of clinical significance level 2. When applying a 1% penciclovir cream, 70% of patients reported lesion healing by day 6. When applying placebo cream, 59% of patients reported lesion healing by day 6.[21] Is an 11% increased probability of lesion healing (NNT of 9) by day 6 of sufficient magnitude to refer to the treatment as "clinically relevant"? Once again, the answer to this question is highly subjective; the cream might be worth its weight in gold to a teenager when prom night is approaching, but it may be clinically irrelevant to an adult. By using the terminology "clinical significance level 2," the concept of small, tangible patient benefit can quickly be communicated without becoming trapped in meaningless discussions regarding the clinical relevance of small benefits.

KEY FACT

An all-or-none situation is defined as one of the following two scenarios in evidence-based medicine: either when all patients experienced an adverse tangible outcome before the treatment became available, but some do not experience this adverse outcome, or when some patients experienced the tangible adverse outcome before the treatment became available but none now experience it. All-or-none situations reflect the highest level of evidence.[19]

Clinical Significance Level 3

Treatments of clinical significance level 3 are the magic bullets or miracle cures in the surrogate world, in which the beneficial but intangible effects are so convincing that the need for RCTs may appear unethical. Examples of such treatments include highly active antiretroviral therapy (HAART) in patients with acquired immunodeficiency syndrome (AIDS),[18] imatinib (Gleevec) in the treatment of chronic myeloid leukemia,[31] and chlorhexidine varnish in the prevention of caries.[26] In periodontics, examples of treatments of clinical significance level 3 could be complete restoration of periodontal attachment and bone around teeth that had extensive destruction of the periodontal apparatus, and reconstruction of voluminous amounts of bone on an atrophic mandible for the purpose of placing dental implants.

With a treatment that has the label "clinical significance level 3," there is always uncertainty as to whether the intangible benefits translate into real, tangible patient benefits. For instance, bone marrow transplantation to the periodontal defect indeed resulted in regenerating prodigious amounts of bone, but about 50% of the teeth were lost due to root resorption.[14] Nonetheless, the larger the effect size observed on the surrogate, the more likely the surrogate benefit translates into a real, tangible patient benefit.[9]

CLINICAL CORRELATION

It is easy to overlook all-or-none situations in dentistry. For instance, root caries in periodontal patients can be prevented with a very-low-carbohydrate diet.[13] Such a conclusion can be made because carbohydrates and dental caries reflect an all-or-none situation.

For certain treatments, such as HAART for AIDS or Gleevec for chronic leukemia, the opportunity may exist to avoid RCTs, and treatments of clinical significance level 3 can become those of level 1 by means of epidemiologic studies in which large secular changes are observed in the incidence of true endpoints since the introduction of the novel treatment. For example, drastic changes in the viral load of human immunodeficiency virus (HIV) have been shown to lead to large reductions in the risk of AIDS and death. Using historical controls, it was shown that HAART treatment reduced AIDS risk by 38% and mortality risk by 34%.[17] A large surrogate benefit (clinical significance level 3) translated into a large survival benefit (clinical significance level 1).

However, assuming that large, intangible treatment benefits invariably translate into tangible benefits remains dangerous, no matter how large the effect on the surrogate endpoint. A 40% chlorhexidine varnish used for the prevention of caries was reported to result in a 99.9% reduction in mutans streptococci counts in all 20 subjects treated, and the counts remained below detectable levels for at least 4 weeks in nine subjects. In contrast, the placebo varnish sealant led to only a 32% mutans streptococci reduction, and none of the 20 subjects had mutans streptococci below detectable levels for 4 weeks.[19] Based on these data, it was reported that "Chlorzoin will wipe out dental decay much like smallpox." A subsequent RCT in 1240 children at high risk for caries did not translate into a reduction of large cavities in the teeth: the Chlorzoin group had 6.8 D3 lesions (standard deviation, 6.2), and the placebo group had 6.4 D3 lesions (standard deviation, 6.4)—in other words, fewer lesions.[29] It has become clear since then that most forms of chlorhexidine are contraindicated in the treatment of caries.[10] A large treatment effect on a surrogate in this instance did not translate into a tangible benefit.

Clinical Significance Level 4

Treatments of clinical significance level 4 are those that have reliable evidence on small, intangible treatment benefits. Because the treatment effects are small, epidemiologic studies are incapable of identifying treatments of clinical significance level 4. In other words, rigorously conducted RCTs are necessary to reliably identify a small surrogate benefit. Examples of treatments of clinical significance level 4 include those that cause a small decrease in lipid level, a small drop in blood pressure, or a small decrease in pocket depth. A large leap of faith is often required to jump from the observation that small changes in surrogate endpoints translate into real, tangible benefits.

Clofibrate, used to lower lipid levels, is an example of a drug of clinical significance level 4. Clofibrate reduced mean cholesterol levels from 324 to 224 mg and mean triglyceride levels from 271 to 125 (which can be argued are "not so small" mean changes).[2] Clofibrate was the most widely prescribed lipid-lowering agent in the United States, but uncertainty remained as to whether it actually provided a tangible patient benefit. Advertisements that were widely used in medical journals accurately reflected the clinical uncertainty surrounding the use of this drug. A textbox within the advertisements stated, "It has not been established whether the drug-induced lowering of serum cholesterol or lipid levels has a detrimental, beneficial, or no effect on mortality and morbidity due to atherosclerosis or coronary heart disease. Several years will be required before current investigations will yield an answer to this question." A subsequent World Health Organization (WHO) cooperative trial on clofibrate revealed the wisdom of this disclaimer. The trial outcome showed that clofibrate resulted in excess mortality of 47%, providing yet another example of a misleading surrogate.[22]

Treatment of clinical significance level 4 may cause more harm than good.[20] This observation has significant consequences in periodontics, because approved periodontal therapies are commonly of clinical significance level 4 and information on their long-term safety and lack of harm is minimal.

Summary

Two important determinants of clinical significance are the nature of benefit (tangible versus intangible) and the likelihood of obtaining the benefit (when compared to the control treatment). These two characteristics can be used to define four hierarchic levels of clinical significance. Treatments that provide a tangible patient benefit (levels 1 and 2) are of greater value and should correspond to a higher level of clinical significance than treatments with evidence of only intangible benefits (levels 3 and 4). Similarly, treatments with a large likelihood of clinical improvement (levels 1 and 3) are clinically more significant than treatments with a small likelihood of clinical improvement (levels 2 and 4). Providing four hierarchical levels of clinical significance may help clinicians and patients communicate more effectively regarding the clinical significance of a treatment. In particular, dental clinicians should inform their periodontal patients that no unequivocal evidence is available, showing that periodontal treatments provide tangible patient benefit. We hope that we provide tangible benefits to our patients, but the RCTs are lacking to ensure that we really do.

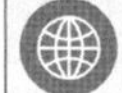

References for this chapter are found on the companion website eBooks.Health.Elsevier.com.

CHAPTER 37

Electronic Dental Records and the Role of Health Information Technology in Dentistry

Thankam P. Thyvalikakath | Radhakrishnan Nagarajan | Corey Stein | Joel M. White | Titus Schleyer | Grace Gomez Felix Gomez | Shuning Li | Anushri Singh Rajapuri | Lucy Bickett

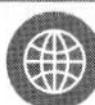
For online-only content on generation of big data and establishing data warehouses, assessing quality of electronic dental and health record data, and machine learning, artificial intelligence, and augmented intelligence, please visit the companion website at eBooks.Health.Elsevier.com.

CHAPTER OUTLINE

Electronic Dental Record Use in Dental Practices

Over the last 20 years, the use of **electronic dental records** (EDRs) in dental practices has risen significantly worldwide, and especially in the Unites States.[36,73] Early on in the 1980s, dental practices used computerized systems primarily for administrative functions such as patient accounting and billing (94%), insurance processing (90.9%), and patient scheduling (83%).[48] However, only 37% of dental practices reported using a computer to maintain patient records at that time. Studies on EDR use in the UK, Wales, and Sweden reported similar figures.[36,91,18]

More recent studies have pointed to a marked increase in EDR use for clinical documentation.[48,71,73] By 2010, US dental practices were using EDRs to acquire and store radiographs (68%), intraoral photos and videos (67%), examination forms (54%), progress notes (54%), and dental charting (50%).[48] Most practices maintained a hybrid system for patient records utilizing both paper records and EDR. As opposed to 2% in 2006, by 2012, about 15% of practices maintained completely paperless records.[70]

Figs. 37.1–37.3 illustrate how clinical information is stored in US solo and group practices and Scandinavian group dental practices.[70] These figures clearly show that more dental practices in Scandinavian countries stored clinical information on the computer than in the Unites States. Meanwhile, nearly all dental schools in the Unites States and Europe use primarily commercial EDR systems in some capacity.[33,92]

Commonly Used Electronic Dental Records

Four systems currently hold about 75% of the market for EDRs in the Unites States: Dentrix Dental Systems (Henry Schein) (37%), EagleSoft (Patterson Dental) (18%), and SoftDent and PracticeWorks (CareStream) (20%).[48,70,73] In addition, about 100 other companies, most of them relatively small, develop and market EDR systems in the Unites States. Notable among them are the Windows-based Mogo and web-based Curve Dental and Dental Symphony. While no public reports about EDRs commonly used in Europe exist, Al Dente (Nordenta, Horning, Denmark), Dental Suite (Plandent, Helsinki), and Opus (Planmeca, Helsinki) appear to dominate in Scandinavian countries.

On-premises Client Servers Versus Cloud-based Systems

EDR data are stored continuously and electronically over time in either on-premises client-servers or remote servers (cloud). On-premises client-server EDR systems are the more commonly used. The on-premises

US solo practices
Appointments
Treatment plan
Completed treatment
Intraoral images
Extraoral images
Radiographs
Dental status
Dental history
Perio charting
Diagnosis
Medical history
Progress notes
Chief Complaint
100 90 80 70 60 50 40 30 20 10 0 10 20 30 40 50 60 70 80 90 100
Percentage of offices using paper
Percentage of offices using paper and computer, or computer
Paper only
Computer only
Both
Not at all

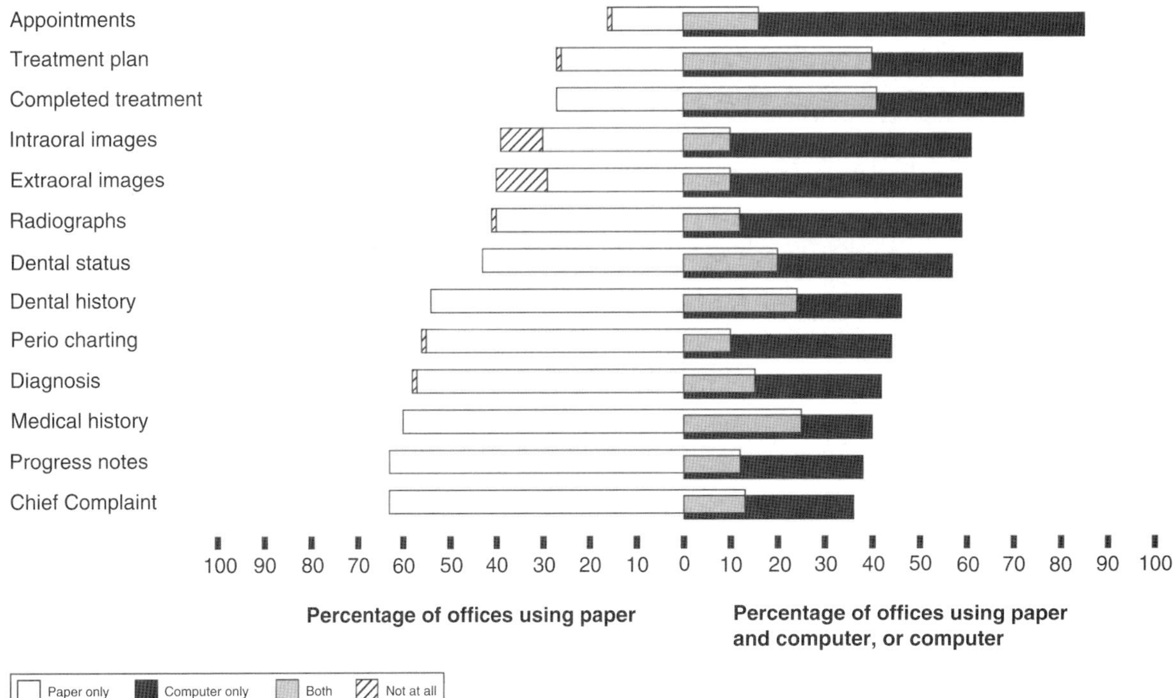

Fig. 37.1 Types of major clinical information stored on paper, a computer, or both by US solo practices. (*From Schleyer T, Song M, Gilbert GH, et al. Electronic dental record use and clinical information management patterns among practitioner-investigators in The Dental Practice-Based Research Network.* J Am Dent Assoc. *2013;144[1]:49–58. doi: 10.14219/jada.archive.2013.0013. PMID:* 23283926; *PMCID: PMC3539217*)

US group practices
Appointments
Treatment plan
Completed treatment
Intraoral images
Extraoral images
Radiographs
Dental status
Dental history
Perio charting
Diagnosis
Medical history
Progress notes
Chief Complaint
100 90 80 70 60 50 40 30 20 10 0 10 20 30 40 50 60 70 80 90 100
Percentage of offices using paper
Percentage of offices using paper and computer, or computer
Paper only
Computer only
Both
Not at all

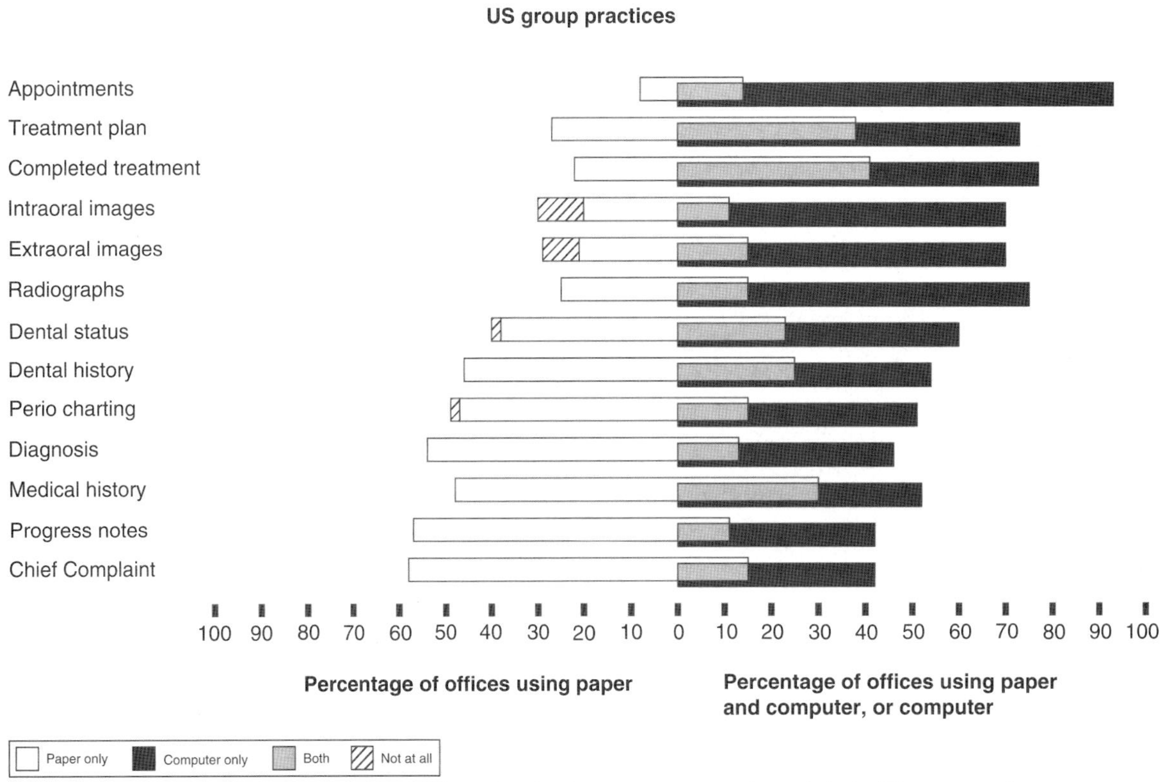

Fig. 37.2 Types of major clinical information stored on paper, a computer, or both by US group practices. (*From Schleyer T, Song M, Gilbert GH, et al. Electronic dental record use and clinical information management patterns among practitioner-investigators in The Dental Practice-Based Research Network.* J Am Dent Assoc. *2013;144[1]:49–58. doi: 10.14219/jada.archive.2013.0013. PMID:* 23283926; *PMCID: PMC3539217.*)

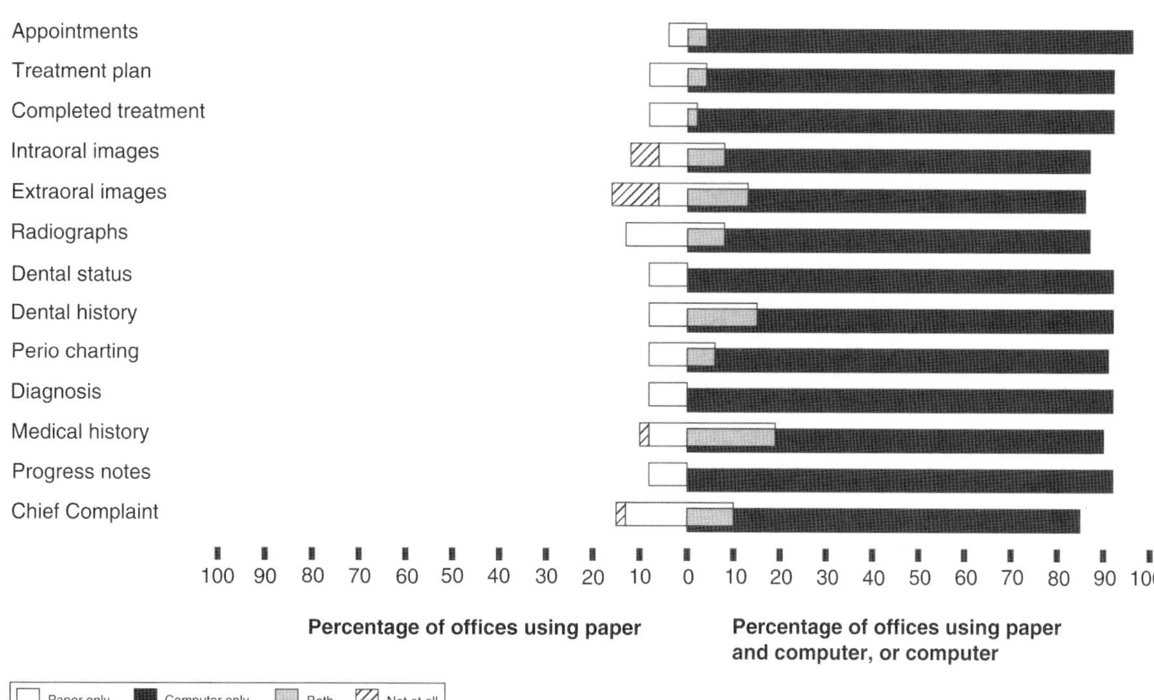

Fig. 37.3 Types of major clinical information stored on paper, a computer, or both by Scandinavian group. (*From Schleyer T, Song M, Gilbert GH, et al. Electronic dental record use and clinical information management patterns among practitioner-investigators in The Dental Practice-Based Research Network.* J Am Dent Assoc. *2013;144[1]:49–58. doi: 10.14219/jada.archive.2013.0013. PMID:* 23283926*; PMCID: PMC3539217.*)

client-servers have exceptionally high costs due to the amount of hardware needed for implementations. In addition, there is a high responsibility for data security measures due to the onsite location. Backup of data for on-premises client-servers is through hard drives, magnetic tapes, CDs, and other storage devices, which are highly vulnerable to theft and damage. Since the backups and the server are at the same location, they could be affected by an accident or disaster at the same time. Cloud-based EDR systems are getting more and more attention now due to some compelling advantages: cost reduction in hardware, software, and services components; elimination of installation and maintenance costs; higher data security mechanisms that utilize multiple encryption mechanisms, authentication, digital signature; and better interoperability for providers with multiple practices. Cloud-based Systems are located remotely from the dental facility, and the stored data can be accessed via the internet anytime. The cloud-based system can provide mobility and flexibility for patient treatment since dental practitioners can access patient data from different office locations or their mobile phones. The backups for cloud-based systems are kept off-site on multiple servers. Edits made to EDRs are saved instantaneously.

Functionalities and Components Available in Electronic Dental Records

An EDR typically includes patient registration, medical and medication history, extraoral and intraoral exam, hard and soft tissue charting, treatment planning, patient education, visit documentation, imaging, and scheduling. In this section, we review selected examples of these functions.

Patient Registration

Fig. 37.4 shows the data captured during patient registration: the patient's name, gender, birth date, identification numbers (social security number and driver's license), and address and contact information. Typically, offices with more than one clinician assign a provider (shown in the second panel of Fig. 37.4 on the right-hand side). This provider assignment facilitates the ability to list all patients for a particular provider.

Registration also includes an important data field on the right-hand side, the chart number. Dentrix assigns a patient chart number automatically as soon as this record is saved. This chart number is the identifier that links all parts of the electronic record for a particular patient together. It is a unique, internal identifier with which all information items of one patient are "stamped."

Another Dentrix feature is that most information on the registration screen is stored in separate fields, called "structured data." Structured data fields can be summarized and analyzed on their own or in combination, enabling some of the powerful reporting and analysis functions found in EDRs

Periodontal Chart

The sample periodontal chart shown in Fig. 37.5 shows not only the pocket depth and clinical attachment loss, but it also shows a graphical presentation of the periodontal changes over time. This presentation is difficult to achieve using paper-based periodontal charts. More detailed information on the components of a comprehensive periodontal examination is presented in Chapter 38.

Emerging Patient Care Data Acquisition Types

The emergence of digital technologies in the dental office[30] offers clinicians new diagnostic data capturing tools with superior capabilities for enhancing treatment planning and predictability.[30] Here, we discuss selected tools and their functionalities, such as cone-beam computed tomography, intra-oral scanners, and 3D printing.

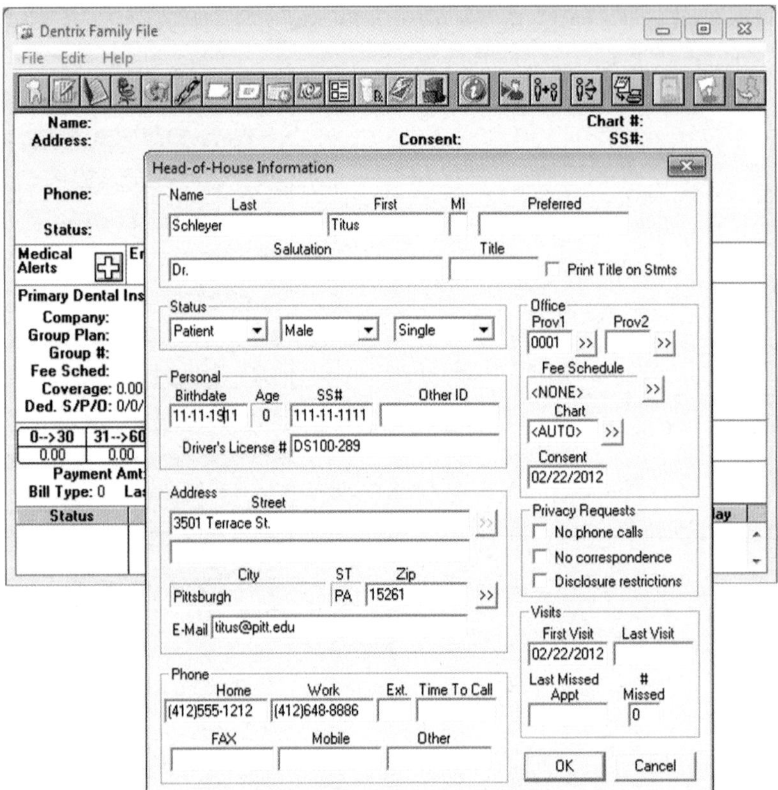

Fig. 37.4 Patient registration screenshot from Dentrix.

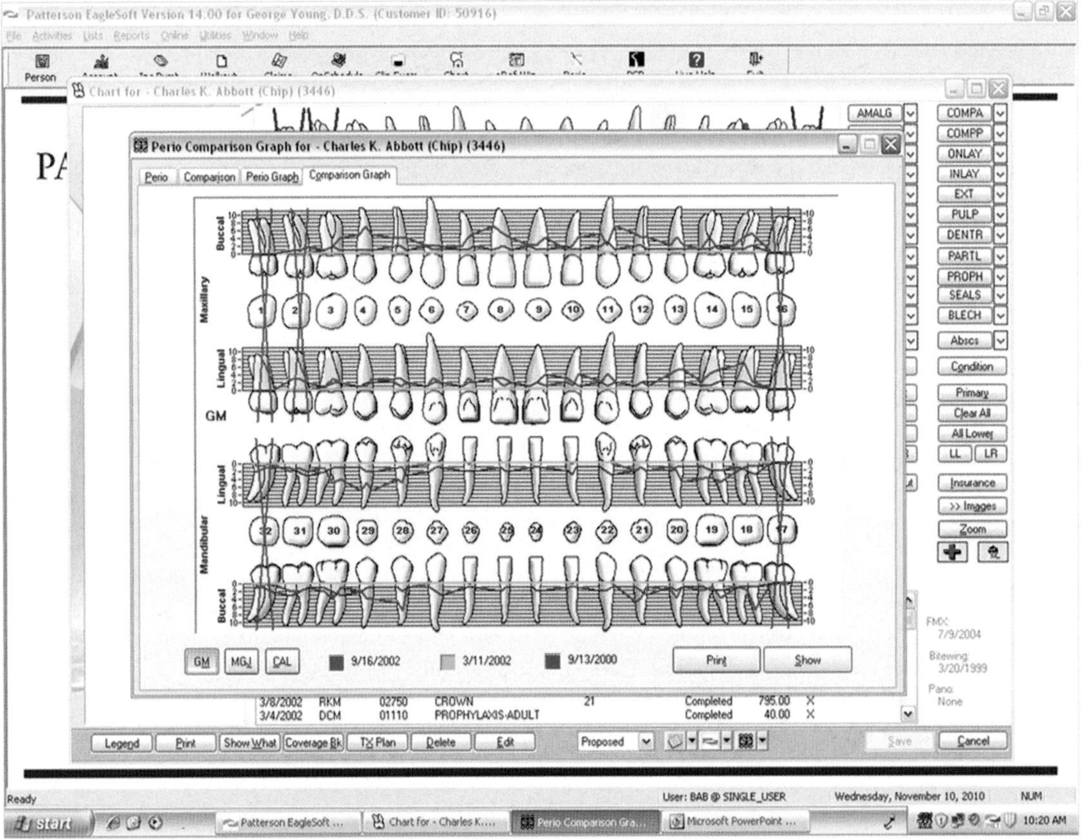

Fig. 37.5 Screenshot of the periodontal chart in EagleSoft.

Cone-beam computed tomography (CBCT) imaging: CBCT imaging is becoming more common in dental practices compared to the early part of this century.[30,89] In a single scan, a 3D rendering is produced of dentition, other hard and soft tissues, and nerve pathways. Individual slices of radiographic data can be visualized in all dimensions to provide more information for interpreting diagnoses and treatment planning. CBCTs allow more accurate representations of an individual's oral-facial structures including bone architecture and quality or any pathology that may be present. See Chapter 39 for detailed information on the use of CBCT in periodontics.

Intraoral scanners and cameras: Intraoral scanners and cameras have also become more common data-collecting tools in clinical practice.[30] Providers are capturing visual observations to monitor findings or to aid with patient education. In addition, intraoral scans provide a digital impression allowing greater accuracy and versatility of the information captured. These digital impressions are used to monitor changes in dentition and soft tissue, evaluate occlusions, and capture restorative and surgical information. The use of digital scanning to fabricate dental restorations has increased substantially since 2010.[87] Many clinicians often employ intraoral scans to aid in various laboratory design processes due to the heightened accuracy and ease of exchanging digital data. Currently, many dentists offer same-day restorations by utilizing intraoral scanners, design software, and other tools to mill restorative materials (composite, porcelain, zirconia). 3D facial scans and photogrammetry have also been employed to completely digitize laboratory workflows for even greater accuracy during the fabrication of prostheses and treatment appliances. These scanners can provide digital representations and produce detail up to 6 to 10 microns.[87]

The data captured from the intraoral scans also permits digital planning and manipulation of models. Restorative designs and surgical guides are being fabricated by software that can take only minutes to produce. Orthodontic software also uses this data to facilitate predictable aligner-therapies. Many software tools are now capable of merging the data captured from the CBCT images with intraoral scans. By "stitching" the image files together, the surgical and prosthetic components of a treatment are better integrated with added layers of precision. Implant therapies, orthognathic procedures, and other surgical reconstructions are more commonly planned by merging these files. Surgical guides are often fabricated to relay the digital plan from the computer to the treatment itself. They provide the clinician with surgical instructions and help execute more precise clinical outcomes. Enhancing the thoroughness of pre-operative and intra-operative surgical plans also allow for more minimally invasive treatments with greater prognoses.

3D printing: The emergence of "in-office" 3D printing (and software) has allowed these guides to be custom designed for the patient's treatment as well as the specifications of the clinicians' armamentarium.[89] For example, if an implant is planned to be placed at a more precise location, a patient's intraoral scan merged with a CBCT can be used to fabricate a surgical guide to align the surgery restoration most accurately. In addition, the guide would only be compatible with the implant drill armamentarium chosen by the surgeon. Other popular uses of the 3D images include printing occlusal appliances, aligners, restorative/surgical guides, and miscellaneous models.

Digital dentistry and its 3D components[89] continue to mature, albeit with some versatility limitations. Open file formats (.stl, DICOM) are universal and permit interoperability among different hardware components, while other closed-environment systems require hardware exclusive to a specific manufacturer. In addition, many of the closed-frame architectures offer users a very clean, easy-to-use digital workflow. However, too many disparate data sources and file types can hinder the ability to exchange, utilize, and store patient information among different technologies within the community of digital dentistry.

Utilizing Electronic Dental Record Data for Clinical Research and Patient Care

EDR data can be a strong alternative or can be synergistic to traditional research methods. They can be used for many studies, including epidemiology, patient care outcomes, and comparative effectiveness.[81,87] Using EDR data for research allows the study of actual patient populations instead of the research study populations, thus generating study results that apply to real-world clinical settings and patients. Limitations such as the poor quality of clinical data, lack of standards for clinical findings and diagnoses, and lack of interoperability of EDRs hamper the ability to synthesize patient data for research in dentistry. Nevertheless, recent studies have repurposed the available clinical data to study population health, assess risk determinants and progression of diseases, and monitor the quality of care provided.[27,42,70,76,87,88] Most of the valuable information in EDR are located within unstructured clinician notes. With the advancements in Natural Language Processing programs, now meaningful information that are buried within these treatment notes can be extracted and used for clinical and research purposes.[15,64,66,77]

In summary, the secondary use of clinical data for research (by aggregating) overrides the considerable cost of conducting a prospective clinical study to assess study treatment outcomes, interventions' effectiveness, and inform public health policies.[94]

Role of Electronic Dental Records in Precision Medicine and Dentistry

Electronic medical records and EDR came into existence independently and over time, they evolved as two separate entities and even now, they lack the connectivity between the two. Connecting the two records has several advantages for dentists, including, getting access to patient's complete medical history, prevention of potential drug interactions and performance of a thorough oral health risk assessment based on patients' systemic conditions.[69] Without having access to medical records, it is impossible for dentists to cross-check the completeness of patients' self-reported medical history. In a recent assessment, it was found that close to 15% and 30% of patients misreported their diabetes and hypertension conditions to dentists, respectively.[7] Similarly, high disagreement was observed regarding patients' reporting of cardiovascular conditions versus their conditions recorded in their medical records.[6] Significant efforts are underway to connect these two systems and a handful of studies that utilized such integrated databases point to its research utility in answering key clinical questions.[13,32] Big (biological) data from proteomic, metabolomic, or microbiome analyses when integrated with clinical data in EHR along with longitudinal patient data obtained from wearables and biosensors will provide the necessary data warehouse for delivering precision healthcare[24]. Therefore, in the near future, it is very clear that EHR will play an important role in precision dentistry (Fig. 37.6). For more information on this topic, refer to Chapter 1.

Benefits of Using Electronic Dental Records

Despite barriers and challenges to using EDR for patient care, tremendous opportunities exist for using EDRs to improve patient care. As mentioned in the introduction, EDRs can provide significant benefits to clinicians and researchers. Using EDRs, clinicians can track their patients' treatment progress and risks for various diseases. Other benefits include timely access to patient records, access to patient records regardless of geographic location, simultaneous access by multiple users, the ability to generate best evidence from patient data, and built-in decision support systems to reduce errors such as medication errors and drug-drug interactions. For researchers, digitization of patient data creates opportunities to dissect and analyze data in ways that were impossible before.[80] The reuse of electronic patient data for dental research is a significant opportunity to help build a "Learning Health Care System." Advantages of using EDR data for research include conducting studies of significant statistical power due to large sample sizes, obtaining well-matched controls, ascertaining important potential confounders, identifying patients with rare diseases, saving study time, collecting data in real time, and generating systematic data documentation.

Barriers to Using Electronic Dental Records

In spite of the rapid adoption of EDR, several barriers exist to using EDR effectively for patient care. They include limited functionality, suboptimal usability, steep learning curve, insufficient operational reliability, and cost and infection control issues.

Limited functionality for communication and collaboration: Dental personnel collaborates extensively during patient care.[35] However, existing EDRs provide limited support for collaboration and communication among dental team members. In addition, breakdowns related to technology interrupt the workflow, cause rework, and increase the number of steps in work processes.

Suboptimal usability and steep learning curve: Several studies have reported poor usability of existing EDRs.[7,32,33,69,73,91,92] Two examples of usability problems are the separation of patient information across multiple screens and the frequent mismatch between system design and task flow. As a result, users must shift their attention from patients to EDRs to navigate through the information and avoid making mistakes. Users believed they spent longer time interacting with EDRs than with paper records, resulting in less face time with their patients.[90]

Insufficient reliability of EDR and infection control issues: System crashes during patient care that lead to loss of patient data and time[33,73] are an example of insufficient operational reliability of EDRs. Infection control issues are primarily due to the fact that the keyboard and mouse are the primary mechanisms for interacting with a computer. Many practices use auxiliary personnel as remote controls for the EDR. While this workaround is effective, it reduces efficiency and increases the chance of errors.

Challenges to Realizing the Full Potential of Electronic Dental Records

Standards for the information content of EDRs: As expressed by the adage "dentists and patients forget but good records remember," complete and comprehensive patient records are essential to support effective decision-making and outcomes research.[59] Currently, no standards exist on what clinical information dental records should or must contain. As more and more dentists adopt EDR to deliver patient care,[70] it is essential that we address what patient information should be documented and how it should be structured.[4,5] During the last three decades, state, national, and international dental organizations have produced many guidelines and/or standards for essential components of the dental record. Common information categories recommended include personal/demographic information, the reason for visit, dental history, medical history, clinical examination information, diagnosis, treatment plan, and informed information. However, these recommendations are very general, and dental records vary significantly in how they meet them.[73] Currently, significant efforts are pursued toward developing a standard information model for EDRs.[4,5]

Data representation and interoperability: Dentistry lacks a standard terminology for documenting and describing dental findings and diagnoses. The World Health Organization's International Classification of Disease coding system or ICD is limited concerning oral and dental diagnoses. Several terminologies, such as SNODENT[28] and the EZcodes,[37] are being developed and evaluated as standard diagnostic codes for dentistry. However, standard terminologies alone will not solve the problem of data representation and interoperability. We need to consider how dental data in their totality can be represented on the computer to be easily stored, exchanged, and analyzed. Patient records typically consist of free text, numbers, standardized codes, radiographic, histological, and clinical images. While structured data can be represented and analyzed unambiguously, that is not true for free text data and images. Concepts in dental records must be represented to facilitate semantic interoperability and the exchange of information across different systems. Ontologies are a powerful way to create computer-based representations that fulfill that goal.[79]

Clinical Decision Support Systems

Clinical decision support systems (CDSS) are "information systems that improve clinical decision-making."[26] They are designed to provide relevant and current evidence to clinicians to improve patient care and reduce errors in practice. CDSSs analyze patient characteristics against a computerized knowledge base and generate patient-specific recommendations. Critical patient data are either entered by clinicians and/or patients or retrieved from the EHR. Patient-specific recommendations are delivered to clinicians through the EHR, email communications, text messages, or printouts placed in the patient charts. As Garg et al. have found, many decision-support systems demonstrably improve practitioner performance.[26]

Decision support system types: The theoretical foundations and the applications of decision-support have been extensively studied in medicine.[51] Research on medical decision-support has included studies on human diagnostic problem solving, the development of several types of algorithms to encode decision-support processes (e.g., rule-based systems, Bayesian Belief systems, and neural networks), and evaluating their performance in the clinics. These systems could be of two types: the open-loop system or the closed-loop system. Open-loop systems provide recommendations but do not act on their own. For example, alerts and reminders are part of open-loop systems. Closed-loop systems act on their own without the clinicians' intervention. During the last three decades, dentistry also saw many decision support systems,[95] but their use is not common. These systems addressed dental emergencies and trauma, radiographic interpretation of lesions, analysis of cephalograms in orthodontics, pulpal diagnosis, and design of partial denture in restorative dentistry.

Risk-based decision support systems for periodontal disease: In periodontology, risk-based decision support systems are the most common type of CDSSs. The PreViser Risk Calculator (PRC) (PreViser Corp., Mount Vernon, WA) developed by Page et al.,[61] UniFe developed by Trombelli et al., and DentoRisk

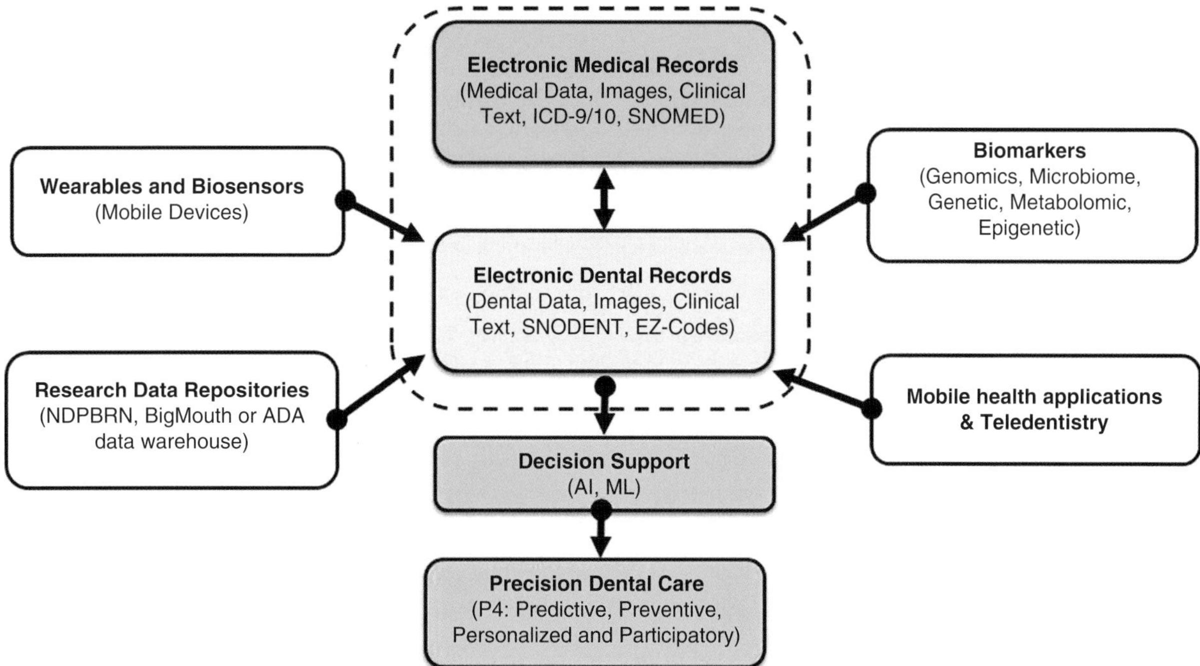

Fig. 37.6 Flowchart showing the role of Electronic Dental Records in conjunction with data from diverse sources and Decision Support systems for facilitating precision dental care. Artificial Intelligence *(AI)*, Machine Learning *(ML)*, American Dental Association *(ADA)* and NDPBRN denote, artificial intelligence, machine learning, American Dental Association and national dental practice-based research network, respectively. ICD9/10, SNOMED, SNODENT and EZ-Codes are structured medical and dental diagnostic terminologies. ICD stands for International Classification of Diseases. For more information on precision dental care, refer to Chapter 1.

(DentoSystem Scandinavia AB, Stockholm, Sweden) developed by Lindskog et al. are examples of risk assessment tools for periodontal disease. The PRC is a Web-based tool developed based on the scientific evidence of the importance of risk factors for periodontal disease. The tool calculates the patient's disease score and risk score based on a mathematical algorithm that assigns relative weights to nine factors: patient age; smoking history; diagnosis of diabetes; history of periodontal surgery; pocket depth; furcation involvement; restorations or calculus below the gingival margin; and radiographic bone lesions. The disease score ranges from 0 (no disease) to 100 (severe periodontitis), and the risk score from 1 (lowest) to 5 (highest). Further discussion of periodontal risk calculators is in Chapter 40.

Barriers to the adoption of clinical decision support systems: There are several reasons for the slow implementation of CDSSs: standalone systems that are not integrated with the clinicians' workflow, lack of formal evaluation, challenges in developing standards for representing data, lack of studies on the clinicians' decision-making process and the clinicians' skepticism on the value of CDSSs for patient care. Investigators emphasize the need for vigorous studies to integrate decision support systems into the clinicians' clinical workflow to improve patient care.[44,50,61,72,95]

Factors that improve the adoption of clinical decision support systems: Several important lessons on the implementation of CDSSs are available from the extensive literature in medical informatics. In syntheses of research on decision support, Bates et al.[9] and Kawamoto et al.[38] identified several factors that facilitate the adoption of decision support systems by practitioners. They include: delivering decision support to the individual making the decision at the time the decision is made; fitting the system into the user's workflow; focusing on usability for the clinician; and not requiring additional data entry unless absolutely necessary. It is also essential to evaluate the impact of these systems during the early phases of development and keep their knowledge bases up-to-date.

To summarize, CDSSs can improve clinical care and patient outcomes by delivering the best evidence to the clinician at the point of care. However, most systems are developed in isolation with limited impact on patient care. These systems must be implemented in electronic patient records to achieve improvements in patient care. Finally, more studies are needed to learn how to best influence clinician behavior through these systems.

Mobile (m)-Health Applications and Teledentistry

Mobile (m)-Health Applications to Triage Emergencies and/or to Screen for Oral Health

The advancements of smartphones and widespread internet connectivity have allowed mobile health (m-health) applications to intervene when routine, in-person care is less available. Patients and individuals with no dental knowledge can efficiently utilize web-based mobile technologies to communicate and relay oral health information over the internet. Using smartphones, tablets, and laptops, individuals can capture a digital report of symptoms, descriptors, as well as high-definition images for a dentist to evaluate and triage patient care remotely. Allied health and dental professionals also use mobile health applications to exchange patient information and treatment recommendations with off-site dentists when accessing a traditional examination may be unavailable. Employing these technologies in communities with geographical or socioeconomic barriers is helping bridge many of the disparities that prevent individuals from receiving optimal oral health care. These remote, virtual consultations extend the availability of dental care while expediting both routine and emergent treatment.

Teledentistry: Embedded in the Oral Health Care Standard

Teledentistry is rapidly becoming an integral part of managing patients' oral health needs for consultation and assessment of presented cases. In addition, by aligning with telehealth practices for general and specialty medicines, teledentistry is positioned to continue to expand its impact on oral health throughout the country and the world. In some scenarios, for example, in rural and remote areas, teledentistry may be the optimum or only means of evaluating dentistry patients for treatment referral.[23]

Technology advancements for oral health combined with state-of-the-art inter-organizational communications provide convenience to patients not available through traditional in-person visits.[23] The initiative for the merger of the EHR and the EDR further delineates technological advancements inherent in the success of teledentistry efforts.

If managed effectively, a teledentistry appointment can eliminate unnecessary travel costs and inconvenience.[23] In addition, teledentistry appointments allow providers the same flexibility patients receive, creating a mutually satisfying and fruitful experience. Furthermore, due to additional compliance guidelines implemented specifically for teledentistry, these appointments can be guaranteed to deliver the same treatment as a traditional in-person visit.[58] Further, studies reflect cost reduction for patients' oral healthcare evaluations without sacrificing quality care because of the teledentistry option.[23]

The Coronavirus Disease 2019 (COVID-19) pandemic created a critical need for teledentistry unlike any other event in recent history. Although several practices, agencies, and higher education institutions had begun some form of the practice, many institutions were forced to rapidly develop plans to implement teledentistry programs at the onset and throughout the pandemic. Otherwise, patients with a critical need for oral healthcare would have gone without evaluations and subsequent treatment due to quarantining and lockdown mandates.

Future of Electronic Dental Records and Health Information Technology in Dentistry

The adoption of EDRs has the potential not just to support clinical care, but also to advance research and improve patient outcomes. In addition, EDRs offer the opportunity to move from a reparative to a preventive approach to treating oral diseases. Many dental diseases, including periodontal disease, are currently being managed using a reparative model, under which dentists and hygienists concentrate on the clinically obvious that requires immediate intervention, focusing less attention on preventing future disease.[20,61] Using this model, the treatment is essentially the same for all patients with similar clinical presentations. EDR with integrated decision support systems can help with identifying patients at high risk, as well as with providing individualized recommendations. However, despite emerging evidence of these systems' validity and clinical utility on treatment in dentistry and, specifically, periodontology, little evidence suggests that these approaches are adopted broadly in general practice.[84] Leveraging the full functionalities of these systems will require significant work as well as trained informatics personnel. Dental informatics is an **interdisciplinary** field that applies computer and information science knowledge and methods to improve information management during clinical care, research, and dental education. Until now, the challenge for dentistry was to transition from paper to electronic dental records in an elementary fashion. Often, EDRs were designed as close or exact replicas of paper records.

However, going forward, this approach will be insufficient. Dentistry now faces the challenge of making sense of electronic data collected, facilitate clinical care and research, and improve outcomes. Trained dental informaticians, clinicians, educators, and researchers must collaborate to accomplish this goal. Dentistry, just as other healthcare disciplines, is an information-intensive domain. The future success of dentistry depends on how we best use information technology to make sense of data and improve patient care. Informatics holds the key to that success.

Suggested Readings

Bates D, Kuperman G, Wang S, et al. Ten commandments for effective clinical decision support: making the practice of evidence-based medicine a reality. *JAMA*. 2003;10(6):523–530.

Kalenderian E, Ramoni R, White J, et al. The development of a dental diagnostic terminology. *J Dent Edu*. 2010;75(1):68–76.

Page R, Krall E, Martin J, Mancl L, Garcia R. Validity and accuracy of a risk calculator in predicting periodontal disease. *J Am Dent Assoc*. 2002;133(5):569–576.

Schleyer T, Song M, Gilbert G, et al. Electronic dental record use and clinical information management patterns among practitioner-investigators in the dental practice-based research network. *JADA*. 2013;144(1):49–58.

Thyvalikakath TP, Duncan WD, Siddiqui Z, et al. Leveraging electronic dental record data for clinical research in the national dental PBRN practices. *Appl Clin Inform*. 2020;11(2):305–314.

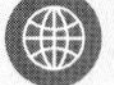
References for this chapter are found on the companion website eBooks.Health.Elsevier.com.

CHAPTER 38

Periodontal Examination

Satheesh Elangovan | Jonathan H. Do | Henry H. Takei | Fermin A. Carranza | Gustavo Avila-Ortiz

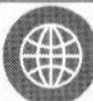
For online-only content on probing, use of clinical indices in dental practice, and mechanisms of tooth wear, please visit the companion website at eBooks.Health.Elsevier.com.

CHAPTER OUTLINE

Proper diagnosis is essential to effective treatment. Periodontal diagnosis is primarily aimed at determining whether the disease is present, as well as its severity and extent. An accurate diagnosis can also provide valuable information pertaining to the underlying pathologic processes and their causes, which is fundamental to formulating a personalized treatment plan. In other chapters of this book, detailed descriptions of the different diseases that can affect the periodontium and associated treatment modalities are provided.

The periodontal diagnosis is determined after careful analysis of the case history and evaluation of the clinical signs and symptoms, as well as the results of various diagnostic procedures (e.g., probing, mobility assessment, radiographs, blood tests, and biopsies).

The interest should be in the patient who has the disease and not simply the disease itself. Diagnosis must therefore include a general evaluation of the patient and an overall consideration of the oral cavity. For example, the 2018 periodontal disease classification system endorses this view and utilizes a holistic approach to arrive at the diagnosis of periodontitis, one of the most prevalent human diseases.

Diagnostic procedures must be systematic and organized for specific purposes. It is not enough to assemble facts. Findings must be pieced together so that they provide a meaningful explanation of the patient's periodontal status. The following is a recommended sequence of procedures for the diagnosis of periodontal diseases and conditions.

Overall Appraisal of the Patient

From the first interaction, the clinician should attempt to make an overall appraisal of the patient. This includes consideration of the patient's mental and emotional status, temperament, attitude, and physiologic age. An example is the observation of a patient's gait when walking in the clinic. This observation could provide valuable information on the patient's neurological status and the existence of physical inabilities that could potentially affect the patient's oral hygiene practices.

Health History

A thorough health/medical history should be obtained at the first visit. This information can be supplemented and updated by pertinent questioning on subsequent visits. The health history can be obtained verbally by questioning the patient and recording his or her responses in the patient's health record or by means of a questionnaire that the patient completes prior to the appointment. Fig. 38.1 shows the health history form recommended by the American Dental Association.

The importance of the health history should be clearly explained because patients often omit relevant information that they cannot relate to their dental problems or that they are not willing to share. In some situations, it is prudent to communicate with the patient's medical provider to obtain a complete history prior to treatment. The patient should be made aware of the following: (1) the possible impact of certain systemic diseases, conditions, behavioral factors, and medications on periodontal diseases and conditions, their treatment, and treatment outcomes; (2) certain conditions may require special precautions or modifications of the treatment procedure (see Chapter 25); and (3) the impact that oral infections may have on systemic health (see Chapter 26).

The health history should include the following information:

1. Vital signs and other morphometric assessments: Including blood pressure readings, heart rate, and temperature, as well as height and weight measures to determine the patient's body mass index (BMI).
2. The date of the last physical exam and the frequency of physical exams and physician visits. If the patient is under current medical care, the nature and duration of the problem(s) and associated therapy should be discussed. The name, address, and telephone number of the physician's practice should be recorded, because direct communication may be necessary.
3. Details regarding previous hospitalizations and surgical operations, including the diagnosis, the type of operation, and any untoward events (e.g., anesthetic, hemorrhagic, or infectious complications), should be obtained.
4. All medical problems, including cardiovascular, hematologic, and endocrine conditions, infectious diseases, high-risk behavior for human immunodeficiency virus infection, and possible occupational disease, should be identified and recorded.
5. Abnormal bleeding, such as nosebleeds, prolonged bleeding time after minor skin cuts, spontaneous ecchymosis, a tendency toward excessive bruising, and profuse menstrual bleeding, should be noted. These symptoms should be cross-checked with the medications that the patient takes on a regular basis.
6. Specifically for females, information regarding the onset of puberty, menopause, menstrual disorders, hysterectomy, pregnancies, and miscarriages should be recorded.
7. Need for antibiotic prophylaxis should be assessed.
8. A list of all medications being currently taken and whether they were prescribed or obtained over-the-counter should be included. All possible effects and drug interactions of these medications should be carefully analyzed to determine their effect, if any, on the oral tissues. It is of paramount importance to avoid administering other medications that would interact adversely with them. A special inquiry should be made regarding the dosage and duration of therapy with anticoagulants and corticosteroids. Patients who are taking any medications in the family of drugs called bisphosphonates (e.g., Alendronate, zolendronic acid), which are often prescribed for osteoporosis, should be cautioned about possible complications related to osteonecrosis of the jaw prior to undergoing any intervention involving trauma to bone tissue.
9. The patient's history of allergies should be recorded, including hay fever, asthma, sensitivity to foods, drugs (e.g., aspirin, codeine, barbiturates, sulfonamides, antibiotics, procaine, laxatives), and dental materials (e.g., latex, eugenol, acrylic resins).
10. Pertinent information regarding family history should be gathered, including bleeding disorders, cardiovascular disease, diabetes, and periodontal diseases.
11. Detailed information on current and history of alcohol, recreational drugs, and tobacco use and the desire to quit should be obtained.

For patients who are on medications (e.g., bisphosphonates and anticoagulants) or patients who do not know the current status of their systemic disease, such as diabetes, hypertension, or immunodeficiency, a medical consultation is often required before any periodontal treatment can be rendered.

Dental History

Chief Complaint and Current Illness

Some patients may be unaware of existing periodontal diseases and conditions. However, many patients presenting with severe diseases usually report profuse gingival bleeding, tooth mobility, spreading of the teeth with the appearance of spaces where none existed before, "longer" teeth, a foul taste in the mouth, or an itchy feeling in the gums that is relieved by digging with a toothpick. Some patients may also present with pain of varied types and duration, including constant, dull, gnawing pain; sensitivity when chewing; dull pain after eating; burning sensation in the gums; deep radiating pain in the jaws; spontaneous acute throbbing pain; sensitivity to hot and cold foods and beverages; or extreme sensitivity to inhaled air.

The dental history should include reference to the following:

1. The frequency of past visits to the dentist, the date of the most recent visit, and the nature of the treatment, including whether it was a dental prophylaxis, periodontal maintenance, or root debridement (scaling and root planing) by a dentist or hygienist.
2. The patient's oral hygiene habits, including toothbrushing frequency, time of day, method, type of toothbrush and dentifrice, and interval when brushes are replaced. Other methods for oral care, such as mouthwashes, interdental brushes, dental floss, water irrigation, and other devices.
3. Any previous or current orthodontic treatment, including its duration and the approximate date of completion.
4. If the patient is experiencing gingival or dental pain, information on the manner in which the pain is provoked, its nature, and duration.
5. Presence of any gingival bleeding, including when it first occurred; whether it occurs spontaneously, on brushing or eating, at night, or with regular periodicity; whether it is associated with the menstrual period or other specific factors; and its duration and the manner in which it is stopped.
6. Bad taste in the mouth, as well as halitosis and areas of food impaction.
7. Presence of tooth mobility, which is often described by patients as "loose" teeth. Tooth mobility may be associated with functional limitations (e.g., masticatory impairment).
8. Detect the existence of parafunctional habits, such as grinding or clenching of the teeth during the day or at night. Some leading questions to ascertain this information are: Do the teeth or jaw muscles feel "sore" in the morning? Do you have other habits, such as tobacco smoking or chewing, nail biting, or biting on objects?
9. Discuss the patient's history of previous periodontal problems, including the nature of the condition and, if it was previously treated, the type of treatment received (surgical and/or nonsurgical) and the approximate period of disease resolution. If, in the opinion of the patient, the present problem is a recurrence of a previous disease, what does he or she think caused it?
10. Note whether the patient wears any tooth-, mucosa- or implant-supported prostheses for tooth replacement. Does the removable prosthesis substantially enhance function and esthetics or

Health History Form

ADA. American Dental Association www.ada.org

E-mail: Today's Date:

As required by law, our office adheres to written policies and procedures to protect the privacy of information about you that we create, receive or maintain. Your answers are for our records only and will be kept confidential subject to applicable laws. Please note that you will be asked some questions about your responses to this questionnaire and there may be additional questions concerning your health. This information is vital to allow us to provide appropriate care for you. This office does not use this information to discriminate.

Name: (Last / First / Middle) — Home Phone: *Include area code* ( ) — Business/Cell Phone: *Include area code* ( )

Address: (Mailing address) — City: — State: — Zip:

Occupation: — Height: — Weight: — Date of birth: — Sex: M F

SS# or Patient ID: — Emergency Contact: — Relationship: — Home Phone: ( ) — Cell Phone: ( ) *Include area codes*

If you are completing this form for another person, what is your relationship to that person?

Your Name — Relationship

Do you have any of the following diseases or problems: ***(Check DK if you Don't Know the answer to the question)***

	Yes	No	DK
Active tuberculosis	☐	☐	☐
Persistent cough greater than a 3-week duration	☐	☐	☐
Cough that produces blood	☐	☐	☐
Been exposed to anyone with tuberculosis	☐	☐	☐

If you answer yes to any of the 4 items above, please stop and return this form to the receptionist.

Dental Information *For the following questions, please mark (X) your responses to the following questions.*

	Yes	No	DK
Do your gums bleed when you brush or floss?	☐	☐	☐
Are your teeth sensitive to cold, hot, sweets or pressure?	☐	☐	☐
Does food or floss catch between your teeth?	☐	☐	☐
Is your mouth dry?	☐	☐	☐
Have you had any periodontal (gum) treatments?	☐	☐	☐
Have you ever had orthodontic (braces) treatment?	☐	☐	☐
Have you had any problems associated with previous dental treatment?	☐	☐	☐
Is your home water supply fluoridated?	☐	☐	☐
Do you drink bottled or filtered water?	☐	☐	☐
If yes, how often? Circle one: DAILY / WEEKLY / OCCASIONALLY			
Are you currently experiencing dental pain or discomfort?	☐	☐	☐

	Yes	No	DK
Do you have earaches or neck pains?	☐	☐	☐
Do you have any clicking, popping or discomfort in the jaw?	☐	☐	☐
Do you brux or grind your teeth?	☐	☐	☐
Do you have sores or ulcers in your mouth?	☐	☐	☐
Do you wear dentures or partials?	☐	☐	☐
Do you participate in active recreational activities?	☐	☐	☐
Have you ever had a serious injury to your head or mouth?	☐	☐	☐

Date of your last dental exam:
What was done at that time?

Date of last dental x-rays:

What is the reason for your dental visit today?

How do you feel about your smile?

Medical Information *Please mark (X) your response to indicate if you have or have not had any of the following diseases or problems.*

	Yes	No	DK
Are you now under the care of a physician?	☐	☐	☐

Physician Name: — Phone: *Include area code* ( )

Address/City/State/Zip:

	Yes	No	DK
Are you in good health?	☐	☐	☐
Has there been any change in your general health within the past year?	☐	☐	☐

If yes, what condition is being treated?

Date of last physical exam:

	Yes	No	DK
Have you had a serious illness, operation or been hospitalized in the past 5 years?	☐	☐	☐

If yes, what was the illness or problem?

	Yes	No	DK
Are you taking or have you recently taken any prescription or over-the-counter medicine(s)?	☐	☐	☐

If so, please list all, including vitamins, natural or herbal preparations, and/or diet supplements:

Form S500

Fig. 38.1 Medical history form from the American Dental Association. (From ©American Dental Association. Reprinted with permission.)

(Continued)

Medical Information *Please mark (X) your response to indicate if you have or have not had any of the following diseases or problems.*

(Check DK if you Don't Know the answer to the question) Yes No DK

Do you wear contact lenses? ☐ ☐ ☐

Joint Replacement. Have you had an orthopedic total joint (hip, knee, elbow, finger) replacement? ☐ ☐ ☐
Date: ________ If yes, have you had any complications?________

Are you taking or scheduled to begin taking either of the medications, alendronate (Fosamax®) or risedronate (Actonel®) for osteoporosis or Paget's disease? ☐ ☐ ☐

Since 2001, were you treated or are you presently scheduled to begin treatment with the intravenous bisphosphonates (Aredia® or Zometa®) for bone pain, hypercalcemia or skeletal complications resulting from Paget's disease, multiple myeloma or metastatic cancer? ☐ ☐ ☐
Date Treatment began: ________

Yes No DK

Do you use controlled substances (drugs)? ☐ ☐ ☐

Do you use tobacco (smoking, snuff, chew, bidis)? ☐ ☐ ☐
If so, how interested are you in stopping?
(Circle one) VERY / SOMEWHAT / NOT INTERESTED

Do you drink alcoholic beverages? ☐ ☐ ☐
If yes, how much alcohol did you drink in the last 24 hours? ________
If yes, how much do you typically drink In a week? ________

WOMEN ONLY Are you:
Pregnant? ☐ ☐ ☐
Number of weeks: ________
Taking birth control pills or hormonal replacement? ☐ ☐ ☐
Nursing? ☐ ☐ ☐

Allergies - Are you allergic to or have you had a reaction to: Yes No DK
To all **yes** responses, specify type of reaction.

Allergy	Yes	No	DK	Allergy	Yes	No	DK
Local anesthetics ________	☐	☐	☐	Metals ________	☐	☐	☐
Aspirin ________	☐	☐	☐	Latex (rubber) ________	☐	☐	☐
Penicillin or other antibiotics ________	☐	☐	☐	Iodine ________	☐	☐	☐
Barbiturates, sedatives, or sleeping pills ________	☐	☐	☐	Hay fever/seasonal ________	☐	☐	☐
Sulfa drugs ________	☐	☐	☐	Animals ________	☐	☐	☐
Codeine or other narcotics ________	☐	☐	☐	Food ________	☐	☐	☐
				Other ________	☐	☐	☐

Please mark (X) your response to indicate if you have or have not had any of the following diseases or problems.

Condition	Yes	No	DK
Artificial (prosthetic) heart valve	☐	☐	☐
Previous infective endocarditis	☐	☐	☐
Damaged valves in transplanted heart	☐	☐	☐
Congenital heart disease (CHD)			
Unrepaired, cyanotic CHD	☐	☐	☐
Repaired (completely) in last 6 months	☐	☐	☐
Repaired CHD with residual defects	☐	☐	☐

Except for the conditions listed above, antibiotic prophylaxis is no longer recommended for any other form of CHD.

Condition	Yes	No	DK	Condition	Yes	No	DK
Cardiovascular disease.	☐	☐	☐	Mitral valve prolapse	☐	☐	☐
Angina	☐	☐	☐	Pacemaker	☐	☐	☐
Arteriosclerosis	☐	☐	☐	Rheumatic fever	☐	☐	☐
Congestive heart failure	☐	☐	☐	Rheumatic heart disease	☐	☐	☐
Damaged heart valves	☐	☐	☐	Abnormal bleeding	☐	☐	☐
Heart attack	☐	☐	☐	Anemia	☐	☐	☐
Heart murmur	☐	☐	☐	Blood transfusion	☐	☐	☐
Low blood pressure	☐	☐	☐	If yes, date: ________			
High blood pressure	☐	☐	☐	Hemophilia	☐	☐	☐
Other congenital heart defects	☐	☐	☐	AIDS or HIV infection	☐	☐	☐
				Arthritis	☐	☐	☐

Condition	Yes	No	DK	Condition	Yes	No	DK
Autoimmune disease	☐	☐	☐	Hepatitis, jaundice or liver disease	☐	☐	☐
Rheumatoid arthritis	☐	☐	☐	Epilepsy	☐	☐	☐
Systemic lupus erythematosus.	☐	☐	☐	Fainting spells or seizures	☐	☐	☐
Asthma	☐	☐	☐	Neurological disorders	☐	☐	☐
Bronchitis	☐	☐	☐	If yes, specify: ________			
Emphysema	☐	☐	☐	Sleep disorder	☐	☐	☐
Sinus trouble	☐	☐	☐	Mental health disorders	☐	☐	☐
Tuberculosis	☐	☐	☐	Specify: ________			
Cancer/Chemotherapy/ Radiation Treatment	☐	☐	☐	Recurrent infections	☐	☐	☐
Chest pain upon exertion	☐	☐	☐	Type of infection: ________			
Chronic pain	☐	☐	☐	Kidney problems	☐	☐	☐
Diabetes Type I or II	☐	☐	☐	Night sweats	☐	☐	☐
Eating disorder	☐	☐	☐	Osteoporosis	☐	☐	☐
Malnutrition	☐	☐	☐	Persistent swollen glands in neck	☐	☐	☐
Gastrointestinal disease	☐	☐	☐	Severe headaches/ migraines	☐	☐	☐
G.E. Reflux/persistent heartburn	☐	☐	☐	Severe or rapid weight loss	☐	☐	☐
Ulcers	☐	☐	☐	Sexually transmitted disease	☐	☐	☐
Thyroid problems	☐	☐	☐	Excessive urination	☐	☐	☐
Stroke	☐	☐	☐				
Glaucoma	☐	☐	☐				

Has a physician or previous dentist recommended that you take antibiotics prior to your dental treatment? ☐ ☐ ☐

Name of physician or dentist making recommendation: Phone:

Do you have any disease, condition, or problem not listed above that you think I should know about? ☐ ☐ ☐
Please explain:

NOTE: Both doctor and patient are encouraged to discuss any and all relevant patient health issues prior to treatment.
I certify that I have read and understand the above and that the information given on this form is accurate. I understand the importance of a truthful health history and that my dentist and his/her staff will rely on this information for treating me. I acknowledge that my questions, if any, about inquiries set forth above have been answered to my satisfaction. I will not hold my dentist, or any other member of his/her staff, responsible for any action they take or do not take because of errors or omissions that I may have made in the completion of this form.

Signature of Patient/Legal Guardian: Date:

FOR COMPLETION BY DENTIST

Comments: ________

Fig. 38.1 *Continued.*

is it detrimental to the existing dentition and/or the surrounding soft tissues?

11. Ascertain whether the patient faced any complications or unpleasant experiences with dental or periodontal treatment in the past. A previous bad clinical episode can impart anxiety and trigger dental fear in patients, which could have a direct negative impact on future treatment, particularly at the patient management level. Additionally, knowing if a patient has had an adverse reaction to local anesthesia, syncopal episodes, or other medical conditions in the dental chair can aid the clinician to better prepare and effectively manage the patient in future appointments while minimizing risks.

LEARNING BOX 38.1

A detailed periodontal examination must be preceded by obtaining a thorough medical and dental history.

Photographic Documentation and Study Models

An important element of the periodontal examination is the documentation of clinical findings. Digital photographic documentation is useful for record-keeping, education of both the clinician and the patient, communication with referrals and colleagues, and planning and treatment of patients with high esthetic demands. Photographs can provide details that a clinician may not otherwise remember, or even perceive while performing an intraoral exam, and allow the clinician to evaluate extra- and intraoral structures after the patient leaves and to monitor tissue changes over time. If possible, prior to initiating the clinical examination, a set of intraoral photos should be taken before the tissue is probed and manipulated to obtain an undisturbed baseline of the patient's mouth with intact gingiva and biofilm (Fig. 38.2). These initial photos, when presented to the patient on a large-screen monitor, can be extremely powerful in educating and helping the patient to understand the conditions of his or her mouth; the presence and location of biofilm, inflammation, and any tissue abnormality; and the need for improvement of oral hygiene habits (Fig. 38.3).

Similar to photographic documentation, a set of dental models can be a valuable diagnostic and patient-education tool. Models may be obtained with a conventional physical impression or through digital scanning and subsequent 3D printing. The three-dimensional nature of dental models may allow the clinician to not only study the case more precisely but also explain dynamic concepts, such as occlusion, to patients, as a complement to radiographs and photographs. Models may also be used to fabricate appliances like night guard, a protective palatal stent for autogenous soft tissue graft donor sites, or a surgical guide for implant placement.

LEARNING BOX 38.2

Intraoral photographs should be taken before the tissue is probed and manipulated to obtain an undisturbed baseline of the patient's periodontal status.

Clinical Examination

Examination of Extraoral Structures

A clinical examination should begin with an evaluation of the extraoral structures for abnormalities. The temporomandibular joints should be assessed for pain, crepitus, clicking, and range of motion.

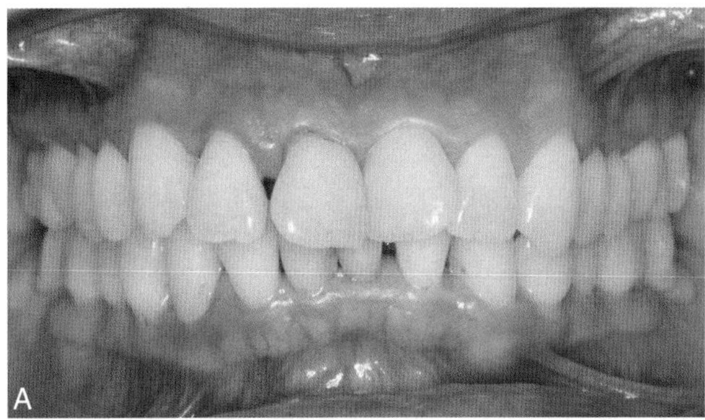

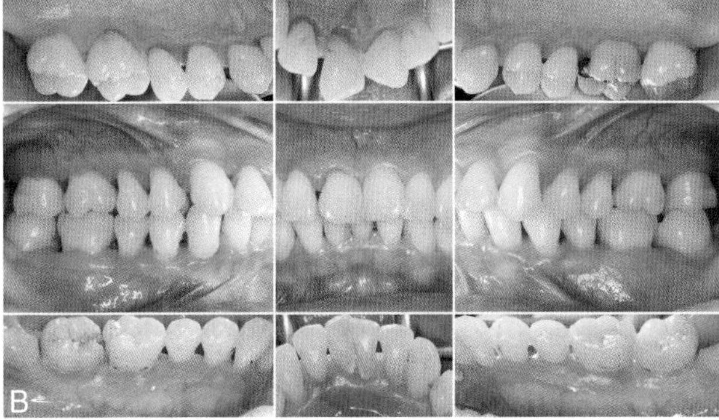

Fig. 38.2 At a minimum, an initial set of intraoral photographs contains nine images: (A) The retracted frontal image is a direct shot. (B) The two buccal shots are flipped horizontally and compiled with the remaining seven images to create a composite of the whole dentition. (Copyright Jonathan H. Do, DDS. All rights reserved.)

Masticatory muscles and salivary glands should be palpated for pain and tenderness.

Because periodontal and periapical pathosis and other oral diseases may result in lymph node changes, the clinician should routinely examine and evaluate the lymph nodes of the head and neck. Lymph nodes can become enlarged or indurated as a result of an acute infectious episode, malignant metastases, or residual fibrotic changes. Inflamed nodes typically become enlarged, palpable, tender, and fairly immobile. The overlying skin may be red and warm. Primary herpetic gingivostomatitis, necrotizing ulcerative gingivitis, and acute periodontal abscesses may produce lymph node enlargement. After successful therapy, lymph nodes typically return to normal in a matter of days to weeks.

Examination of the Oral Cavity

The entire oral cavity should be carefully examined, beginning with signs of oral hygiene efficiency. The cleanliness of the oral cavity may be visually appraised in terms of the extent of accumulated food debris, biofilm, calculus, and tooth surface stains, as well as biofilm coating of the dorsum of the tongue (Fig. 38.4). Oral malodor, which is also termed *fetor ex ore, fetor oris,* or *halitosis,* is a foul or offensive odor that emanates from the oral cavity. When present, mouth odors may be of diagnostic significance, and their origin may be either oral or extraoral (such as the gastrointestinal tract).[63] Problems related to oral malodor are discussed in detail in Chapter 31 of this book.

The lips, the vestibule, the buccal mucosa (i.e., cheeks), the floor of the mouth, the tongue, the palate, and the oropharyngeal region should be evaluated for abnormalities. The oral mucosa in the apical region of the alveolar ridge may be palpated for tenderness to detect periapical and periodontal abscesses. It is important to follow a consistent topographical sequence to ensure that all intraoral regions are thoroughly assessed during every exam.

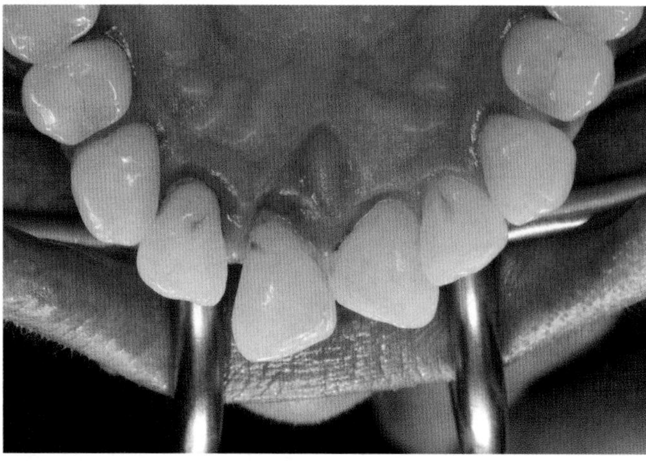

Fig. 38.3 An image capturing the palatal surfaces of the anterior maxilla is presented on a 27-inch computer screen to help a patient understand her periodontal status. (Copyright Jonathan H. Do, DDS. All rights reserved.)

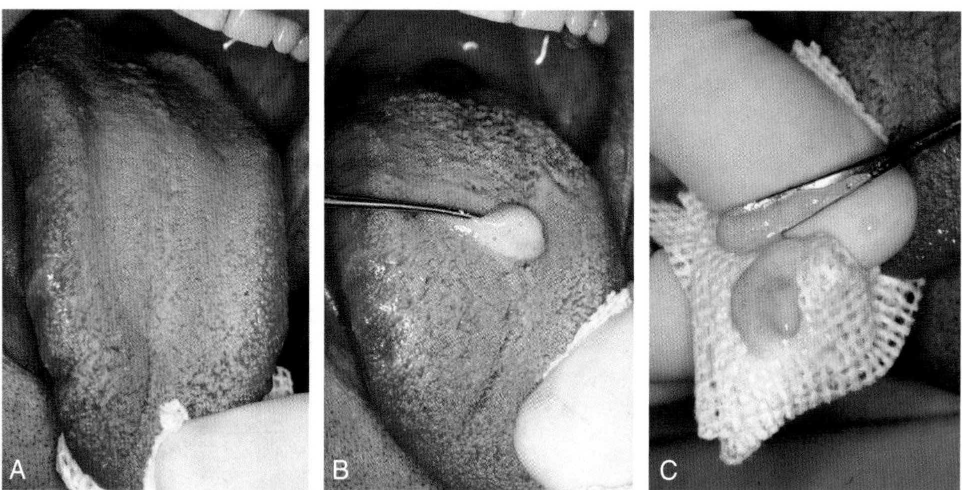

Fig. 38.4 Biofilm coating of the dorsum surface of the tongue (A) can be a source of oral malodor. When the tongue is heavily coated, the biofilm may need to be scraped off with a spatula or a tongue scraper (B and C).

KEY FACT

Although not all relevant findings may be related to periodontal problems, the examiner should be competent to detect all deviations from normality that are present in the oral cavity and, if necessary, make the appropriate dental or medical referral.

Assessment of Oral Hygiene Performance

Prior to initiating the periodontal examination *per se,* it is important to assess the patient's oral hygiene performance. This can be done in a simple and unbiased manner by giving the patient a toothbrush and a piece of floss and asking the patient to perform plaque removal as they would normally do on a day-to-day basis. This exercise can provide very valuable information regarding technical efficiency, dexterity and time spent, which can be further utilized for patient education purposes.

Examination of the Periodontium

The periodontal examination should be systematic and not immediately begin with the insertion of the periodontal probe into the gingival crevice, which can be uncomfortable and traumatic for a patient and may induce bleeding that could make visualization of inflammatory changes in the soft tissue challenging. Therefore the periodontal examination should begin with a thorough and careful visual evaluation of the gingival margin to assess biofilm and calculus accumulation, inflammatory changes in the soft tissue (Fig. 38.5), as well as alterations of the normal soft tissue contours and position, such as gingival recession defects and tooth mobility. Once a thorough visual periodontal assessment has been completed, the gingiva, the gingival crevice, and the subgingival tooth surface are carefully probed (tactile periodontal examination). Thorough probing of the gingival crevice and tactile assessment of the surrounding tissues provides a wealth of valuable information, such as probing depth measures, bleeding on probing, the position of the gingival margin respective to the CEJ and clinical attachment loss, which are essential parameters for the diagnosis and treatment of periodontal diseases and conditions (e.g., periodontitis).

LEARNING BOX 38.3

Examination of the periodontium consists of two parts: visual examination and tactile examination.

Visual Periodontal Examination

Visual examination begins with drying the tissue and taking a survey of biofilm and calculus accumulation to assess oral hygiene, as well as clinical signs of inflammation (e.g., erythema and edema) and apical migration of the gingival margin to assess the presence, extent, and severity of disease.

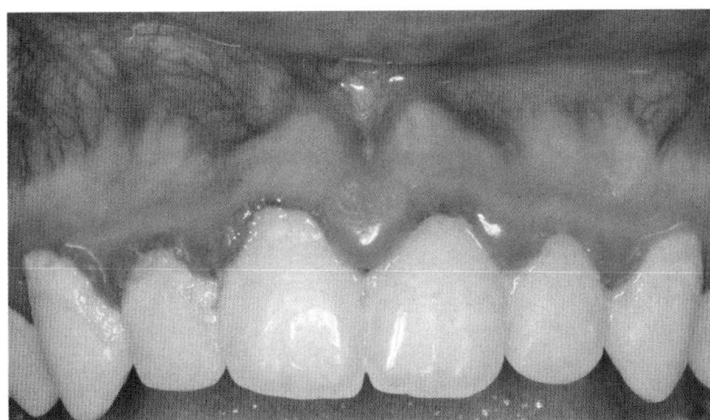

Fig. 38.5 The inflammatory response in the marginal gingiva is typically the result of biofilm accumulation on the tooth surface along the gingival margin. (Copyright Jonathan H. Do, DDS. All rights reserved.)

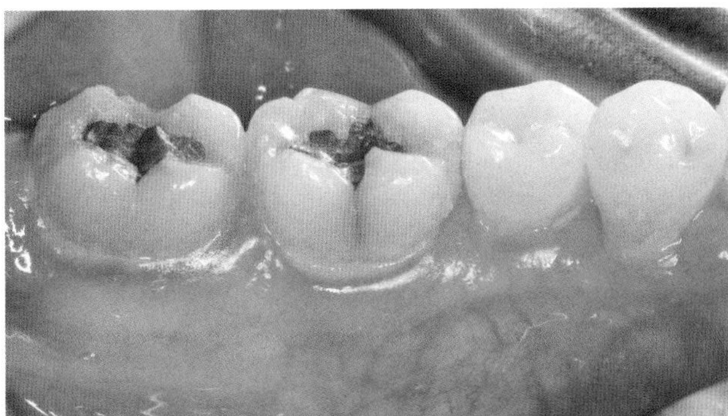

Fig. 38.6 Biofilm frequently accumulates on tooth surfaces in concavities along the gingival margin and interproximal spaces. (Copyright Jonathan H. Do, DDS. All rights reserved.)

Visual Examination of Biofilm and Calculus

There are many methods available for assessing biofilm and calculus accumulation.[18] The presence of biofilm and supragingival calculus can be observed directly. Biofilm frequently accumulates in concavities along the gingival margins and in embrasure spaces, especially in difficult-to-reach areas, such as the distal surface of the distal-most tooth in the quadrant and the lingual surfaces of mandibular posterior teeth (Fig. 38.6). Supragingival calculus tends to accumulate on the lingual surfaces of the mandibular anterior teeth and the buccal surfaces of the maxillary molars, mainly due to the presence of the Wharton and Stensen salivary ducts, respectively, and ineffective biofilm removal. The amount and location of biofilm and supragingival calculus may provide insights into the effectiveness of the patient's biofilm control as well as possible inflammatory changes in the tissue. Biofilm on the buccal and facial surfaces of teeth closest to the midline is most accessible for removal. The presence of biofilm in these areas is generally suggestive of inadequate oral hygiene (see Fig. 38.5). The absence of biofilm may not necessarily indicate that the patient practices good oral hygiene or that the disease is absent, as many patients thoroughly brush their teeth before seeing a dentist. The presence or absence of biofilm should be correlated with the presence and severity or absence of gingival inflammation, as well as the presence of subgingival deposits.

The presence of subgingival calculus may not be easily detected. Sometimes, subgingival calculus may be identified along the gingival margin with gentle separation of the mucosa or may even be visible through the soft tissue in sites exhibiting a thin gingival phenotype (Fig. 38.7). However, subgingival calculus is usually

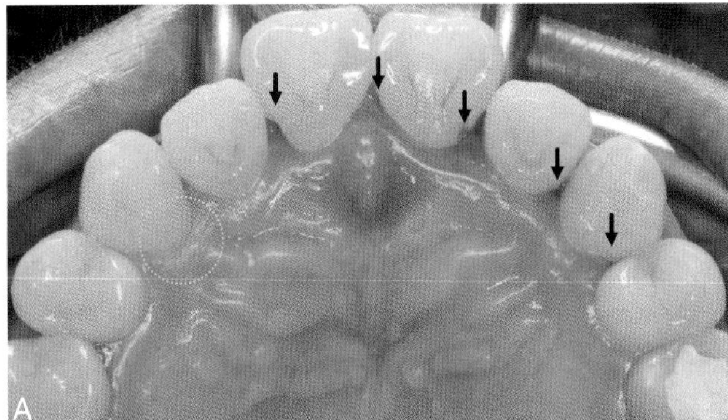

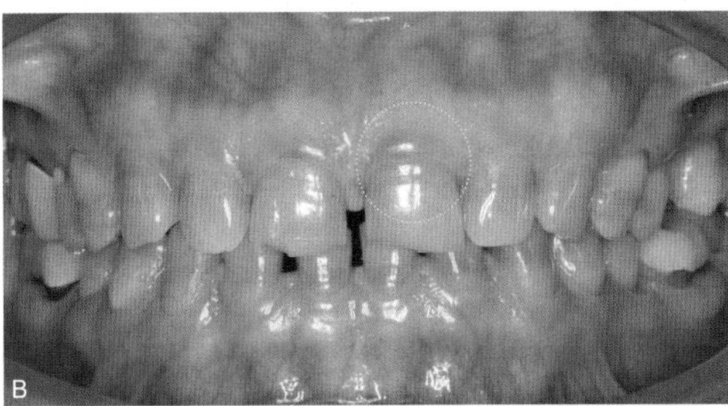

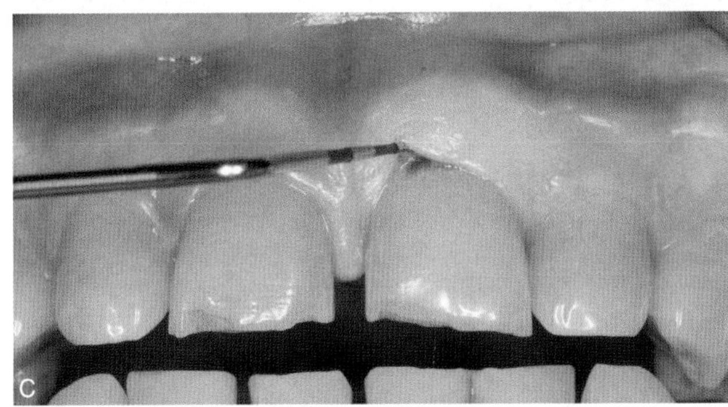

Fig. 38.7 (A) Subgingival calculus can be visible on the tooth surface *(arrows)* along the gingival margin. Its presence is associated with inflammatory changes in the tissue. In places where biofilm and calculus are absent, the gingiva is usually pink, firm, and stippled *(circle)*. (B) Subgingival calculus may be visible through the marginal gingiva. (C) Retraction of the gingiva confirms its presence. (Copyright Jonathan H. Do, DDS. All rights reserved.)

detected by careful tactile examination of the root surface using an instrument (e.g., periodontal probe or explorer). The presence of signs of gingival inflammation (e.g., discoloration and swelling) may provide clues to the location of subgingival calculus deposits.

Although radiographs may sometimes reveal heavy calculus deposits interproximally and even on the facial and lingual surfaces, they cannot be relied on for thorough calculus detection.

Visual Examination of the Gingiva

The gingiva is the collar of fibrous soft tissue that invests the cervical region of a tooth and is contiguous with its periodontal ligament and the alveolar mucosa. It extends from the gingival margin to the mucogingival junction. On the palate, where the mucogingival junction is absent, the gingiva extends apically and merges seamlessly with the masticatory mucosa that invests the hard palate.

Gingival width is the distance from the gingival margin to the mucogingival junction. The mucogingival junction can be determined by stretching the lip and cheek or by placing a probe

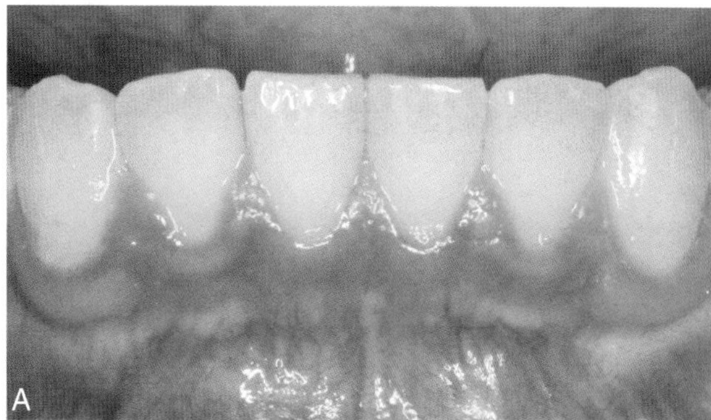

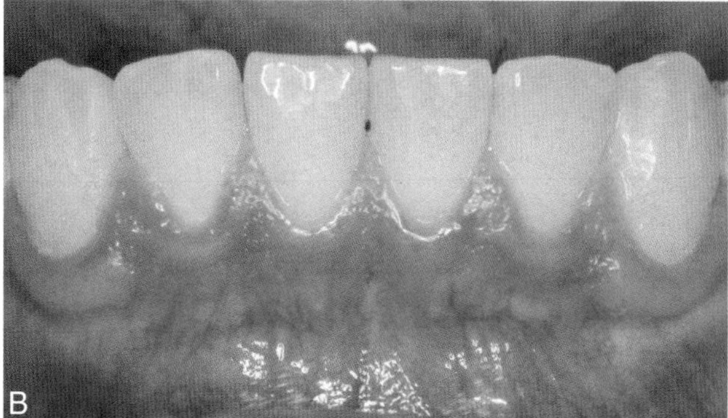

Fig. 38.8 Saliva obscures details. (A) The gingiva appears smooth when covered in saliva. (B) Once dried, stippling is visible, and erythema and edema become more obvious. (Copyright Jonathan H. Do, DDS. All rights reserved.)

horizontally in the vestibule and rolling toward the mucosa coronally. The mucogingival junction is where the mucosa stops rolling or moving. All teeth are surrounded by a variable amount of gingival width. However, there may be sites where keratinized tissue is minimal and cannot be clinically appreciated, giving the impression that the soft tissue margin is lined by non-keratinized mucosa.

As previously mentioned, visual evaluation of the gingiva requires the tissue to be dried before accurate observations can be made, as the presence of saliva can hide important details (Fig. 38.8). Once the gingiva is thoroughly dried, it can be evaluated for inflammatory changes. Although not always the case, when there is adequate gingival width, subtle inflammatory changes in the marginal gingiva may be best detected by comparing the marginal gingiva to the gingival tissue 2 or 3 mm apical to the gingival margin, where the tissue is likely to be healthier (Fig. 38.9). Local inflammatory changes tend to be correlated with the presence and severity of biofilm and calculus. If supragingival biofilm and calculus deposits are insignificant in sites exhibiting signs of inflammation, the presence of subgingival calculus or other contributing factors should be carefully investigated.

The appearance of the soft tissues investing a tooth and the underlying alveolar bone may vary from site to site and from individual to individual, depending on the location and the specific anatomical features of the area, as well as genetic and environmental determinants. Generally, healthy gingiva is coral pink or salmon pink in color. The gingival contour consists of sharp, thin, knife-edge margins with scalloped gingival architecture and sharp papillae. The surface texture of healthy gingiva is matte and may be stippled. The presence of stippling can vary across individuals and sites within the same individual. The absence of stippling does not necessarily imply inflammatory changes in the tissue.

In the presence of inflammatory disease, the color of the gingiva may be erythematous (reddish) or cyanotic (bluish). Instead of having knife-edge margins and sharp papillae gingival contours, inflamed gingival tissue typically has rolled margins and bulbous papillae. The surface of the gingiva in the presence of inflammation tends to be smooth and shiny, mainly due to tissue edema. Table 38.1 summarizes clinical findings of healthy and inflamed gingiva. Chapter 15 further discusses the clinical features of gingival inflammation.

In some individuals, the gingiva may be pigmented and exhibit a dark appearance (e.g., gingival melanosis). Even so, if healthy, it should exhibit the other features associated with gingival health. Likewise, in the presence of inflammation and disease, pigmented gingiva should exhibit many of the characteristics of gingival inflammation (Fig. 38.10).

Gingival Recession

The location of the gingival margin around teeth should be evaluated and recorded. In the absence of attachment loss, the gingival margin is normally located coronal to the cementoenamel junction. In these instances, measuring the exact distance between the gingival margin and the cementoenamel junction can be challenging as it is a purely tactile, blinded assessment. Gingival recession is defined as the apical migration of the gingival margin. The presence of recession indicates that attachment loss has occurred but not necessarily that inflammation is present. Depending on the extent of attachment loss and the anatomical features of the teeth and the periodontium at a specific site, the gingival margin may remain in a supragingival location, which is not common but certainly possible, or have shifted apically into a juxta- or subgingival location. When the cementoenamel junction is supragingival, recession depth can be measured using a standardized periodontal probe as the distance from the cementoenamel junction to the gingival margin. At sites exhibiting gingival recession defects, the amount of recession should be recorded. Additionally, the presence of biofilm and calculus, inflammatory changes in the gingiva, width of the keratinized tissue, and gingival thickness (phenotype) should be carefully evaluated and accounted for to establish a proper diagnosis and treatment plan (Fig. 38.11).[14]

LEARNING BOX 38.4

Periodontal examination begins with a visual evaluation of the gingival margin for the presence of biofilm and calculus accretion and signs of gingival inflammation.

Tactile Periodontal Examination

Tactile periodontal examination begins with the evaluation of the consistency of the gingiva and its adaptation to the tooth, as well as the presence of marginal bleeding and suppuration. The gingival crevice is probed to evaluate the subgingival environment. The tooth surface should be carefully probed for aberrations, concavities, furcation defects, and subgingival calculus. The response of the gingival tissue to probing is measured in terms of resistance to and depth of probe penetration, as well as bleeding, suppuration, and pain upon probing.

Tactile Examination of the Marginal Gingiva

The marginal gingiva is palpated with a periodontal probe to assess its consistency and adaptation to the tooth. Healthy gingiva is typically firm, resilient, and well-adapted to the tooth due to the presence of dense, well-organized collagen fiber bundles in the lamina propria of the gingiva. When inflamed, the gingiva normally appears edematous, spongy, and loosely adapted to the tooth surface due to the degradation of collagen and the influx of inflammatory cells and fluid into the lamina propria (Fig. 38.12). In cases of chronic inflammation and in smokers, the gingival tissue may clinically appear fibrotic yet inflamed at the microscopic level.

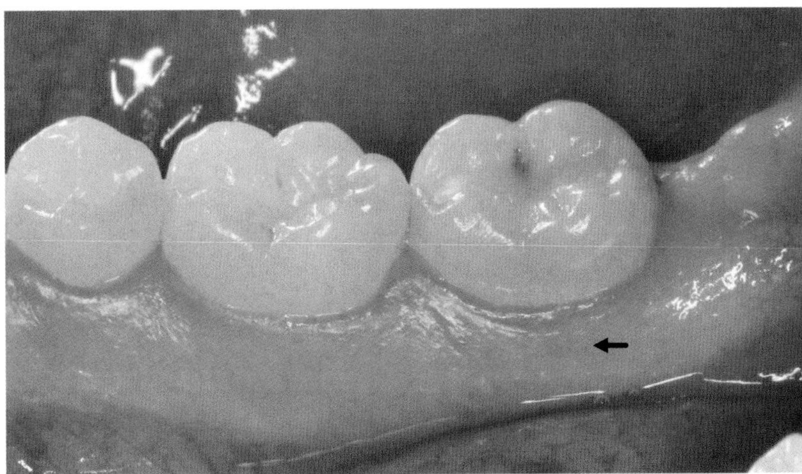

Fig. 38.9 When compared to the gingival tissue located at 2 to 3 mm apical to the gingival margin *(arrow)*, it is obvious that the marginal gingiva is erythematous and edematous. (Copyright Jonathan H. Do, DDS. All rights reserved.)

TABLE 38.1 Clinical Findings of Gingiva: Healthy Versus Inflamed

Gingiva: Healthy	Gingiva: Inflammation
• Color: coral pink or salmon pink	• Color: erythematous, cyanotic
• Consistency: firm, tight, well adapted	• Consistency: edematous, spongy, loosely adapted
• Contour: scalloped, sharp papillae, knife-edge margin	• Contour: bulbous, swollen papillae, rolled margin
• Surface texture: stippled, matte	• Surface texture: smooth, shiny
• Marginal bleeding: absent or slight	• Marginal bleeding: moderate or severe
• Probing depth: 1–3 mm	• Probing depth: >3 mm
• Noticeable tissue resistance to probe penetration	• Minimal tissue resistance to probe penetration
• Bleeding on probing: absent or slight	• Bleeding on probing: moderate to severe
• Discomfort on probing: absent or slight	• Could present with moderate to severe pain
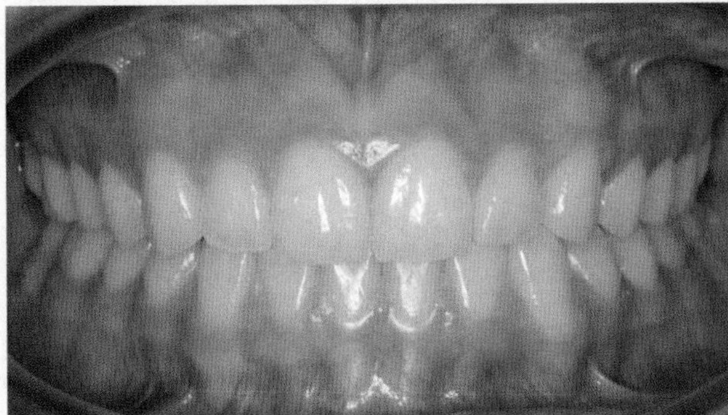	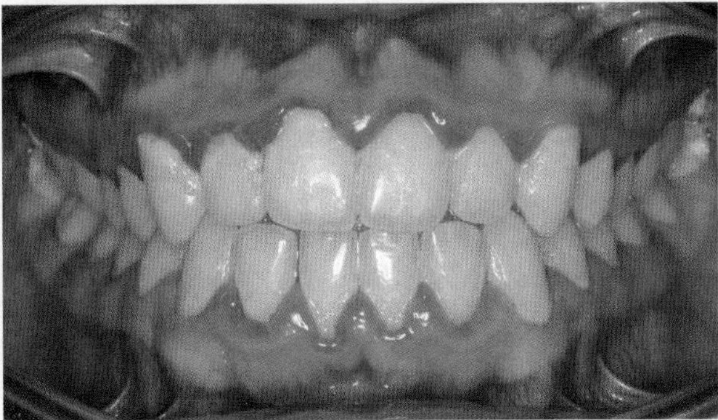

Marginal Bleeding

Marginal bleeding is normally associated with inflammatory changes in the coronal aspect of the gingiva. Marginal bleeding can be evaluated by running an instrument, such as a probe or rubber tip, along the gingival margin. Under pressure, healthy gingival tissue normally blanches and does not bleed, whereas in the presence of gingival inflammation, marginal bleeding is triggered. The ease and severity of marginal bleeding are usually correlated with the actual severity of gingival inflammation, although bleeding can be masked in some instances (e.g., smokers).

Suppuration

The palpation of the marginal gingiva with a probe or digitally, by placing the ball of the index finger on the gingiva apical to the margin and pushing coronally toward the gingival margin (Fig. 38.13), may trigger the release of a white-yellowish exudate from the gingival crevice. The presence of an abundance of neutrophils in the gingival fluid transforms it into a purulent exudate.[4] Suppuration does not occur in all periodontal pockets, but pressure may reveal it in pockets where its presence is not suspected. Several studies[8,11,13,30] have evaluated the association between suppuration and the progression of periodontitis and have reported that this sign is present in a very low percentage of diseased sites (i.e., 3% to 5%).[4] Therefore absence of suppuration does not indicate absence of disease.

Tactile Examination of the Gingival Crevice

The periodontal probe should be inserted into the gingival sulcus vertically with the tip of the probe touching and sliding down along the tooth surface to the bottom of the crevice. The probe should be "walked" circumferentially around each surface of each tooth to detect the areas of

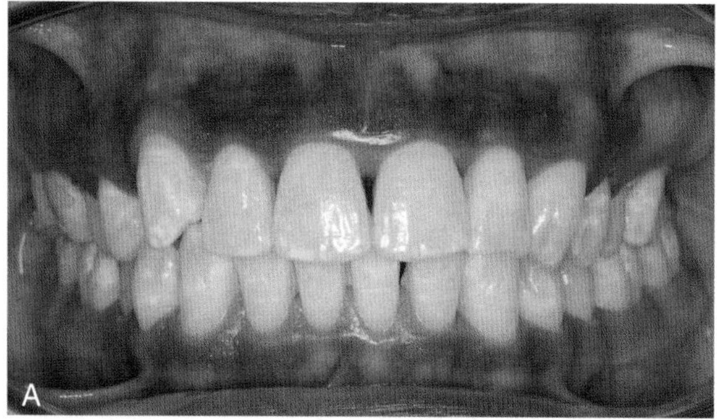

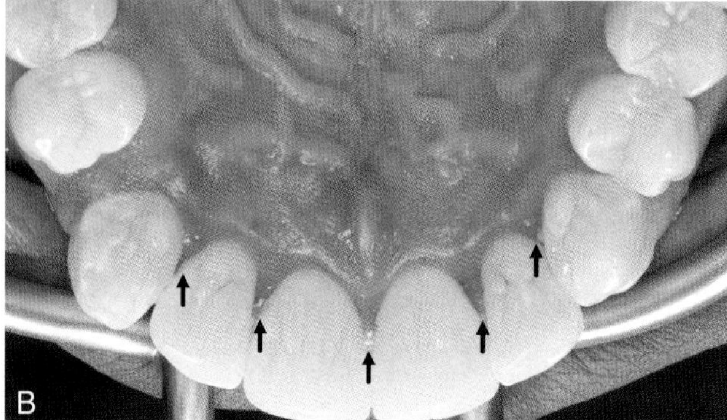

Fig. 38.10 Edema, papillary *(arrows)* and marginal erythema in a patient with physiologic pigmentation. Frontal view (A) and palatal view (B). (Copyright Jonathan H. Do, DDS. All rights reserved.)

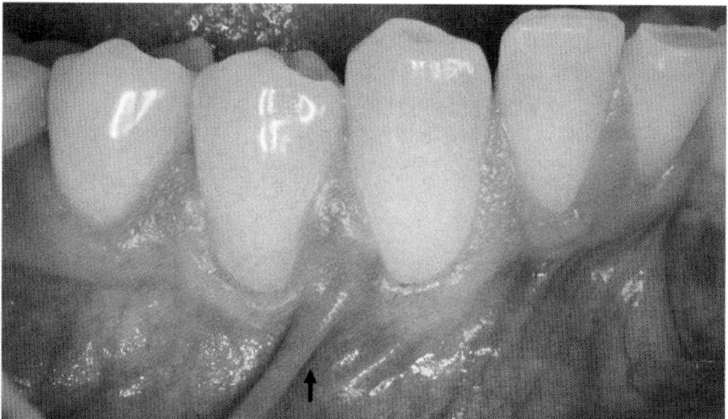

Fig. 38.11 The canine and first premolar exhibit gingival recession defects and minimal keratinized tissue. Both teeth are at risk of further recession depth increase due to the presence of gingival inflammation and a frenum pull *(arrow)*. (Copyright Jonathan H. Do, DDS. All rights reserved.)

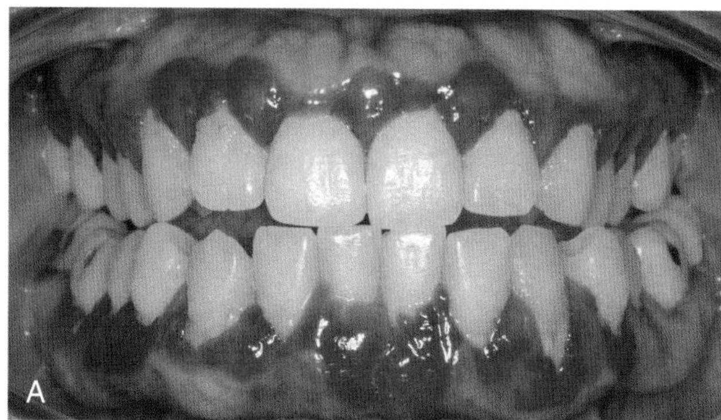

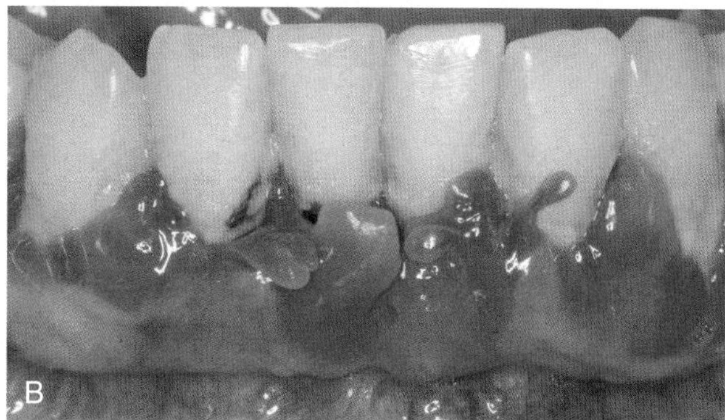

Fig. 38.12 The severely inflamed gingiva is loosely adapted to the tooth. The marginal gingiva is easily retracted to reveal heavy subgingival biofilm and calculus. Maxillary and mandibular frontal view (A) and mandibular frontal view (B). (Copyright Jonathan H. Do, DDS. All rights reserved.)

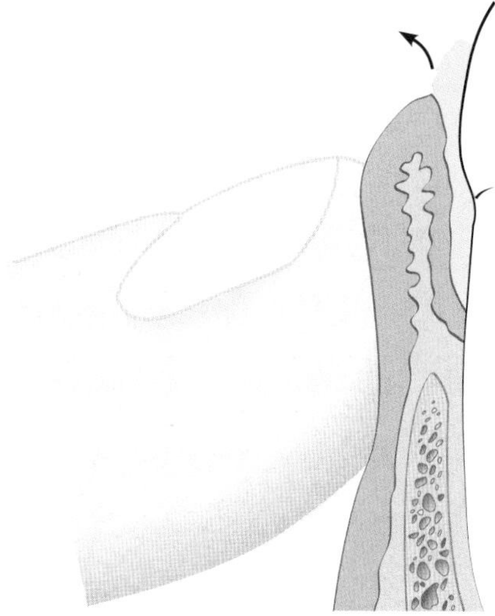

Fig. 38.13 Purulent exudate expressed from a periodontal pocket by digital pressure.

deepest penetration, instead of making "pinpoint assessments." As the probe tip slides down along the tooth surface, attention should be paid to the tactile feel of both the gingival tissue and the tooth surface. As aforementioned, healthy gingival tissue usually feels tight and resists probe penetration. The tightness of the tissue progressively increases as the instrument moves apically, and the probe will come to a stop. In healthy tissue, the tip of the probe typically stops within the junctional epithelium. If the gingival tissue is severely inflamed, the probe does not find as much resistance and it "falls" to the depth of the gingival crevice, penetrating into the connective tissue region.

As the probe tip slides along the tooth surface, if there is no anatomical irregularity or subgingival calculus, the tooth surface will feel smooth. On the contrary, if the tooth surface feels rough and/or if the advancement of the probe tip is impeded, the presence of subgingival calculus should be suspected. The probe may need to be moved axially away from the tooth to navigate around the calculus in order for it to penetrate to depth. As previously mentioned in this chapter, the presence of subgingival calculus is usually associated with inflammatory changes in the gingival tissue (see Fig. 38.7), the absence of gingival tightness, and the presence of bleeding on probing. For a thorough assessment of the extent and location of subgingival calculus around the dentition, tactile examination using specific instruments (e.g., Old Dominion 11/12 explorer) is recommended.

LEARNING BOX 38.5

When probing, the probe tip should be in contact with the tooth surface as it slides down along the tooth surface to reach the apical end of the gingival crevice. This allows for detection of tooth surface irregularities, furcation invasion, and subgingival calculus.

Additionally, attention should be directed to the detection of periodontal bone defects (e.g., interdental craters and furcation defects) and root surface abnormalities (e.g., cemental tears and enamel pearls). Periodontal defects tend to be associated with deep probing depths and gingival inflammation. To detect an *interdental crater*, the probe should be placed obliquely from both the facial and lingual surfaces to explore the deepest point of the pocket located beneath the contact point. Regarding furcation defects, the use of specially designed probes (e.g., Nabers probe) allows for an easier and more accurate exploration of the horizontal component of lesions affecting the furcation of multi-rooted teeth.

LEARNING BOX 38.6

Thorough probing of the gingival crevice and the surrounding tissues provides a wealth of valuable information beyond probing depth and bleeding on probing that is essential to the diagnosis and treatment of periodontal diseases and conditions.

Probing Depth

There are two different pocket depths: (1) the biologic or histologic depth and (2) the clinical or probing depth (Fig. 38.14).[27]

Biologic depth is the distance between the gingival margin and the base of the gingival sulcular epithelium (i.e., the coronal boundary of the junctional epithelium). This can be measured only in carefully prepared and adequately oriented histologic sections.

Probing depth is the distance from the gingival margin to the bottom of the probeable crevice (i.e., where the probe tip stops). For details on periodontal probes commonly used in contemporary clinical practice, see Chapter 51.

Probe penetration can vary depending on the force applied, the shape and size of the probe tip, the direction of penetration, the tooth contours, and the resistance of the tissues, which is typically related to the degree of tissue inflammation.[4] Probing depth is generally ≤3 mm in gingival health and greater than 3 mm in the presence of gingival inflammation. Several studies have been conducted to determine the depth of penetration of a probe in a sulcus or pocket. Armitage and colleagues[6] used beagle dogs to evaluate the penetration of a probe with the use of a standardized force of 25 g. They reported that in healthy gingiva, the probe penetrated the junctional epithelium to about two-thirds of its length; in gingivitis cases, it stopped 0.1 mm short of its apical end; and in cases of periodontitis, the probe tip consistently went past the most apical cells of the junctional epithelium and into the connective tissue compartment (Fig. 38.15). In human periodontal pockets, it has been demonstrated that the probe tip penetrates until it finds the most coronal intact fibers of the connective tissue attachment.[38,72]

Probing depth is a dynamic parameter that may naturally change over time, even in healthy patients with no history of periodontitis, as a result of changes in the position of the gingival margin. Therefore probing depth changes may be unrelated to attachment loss. This is important to consider when evaluating differences in probing depth before and after treatment, because the reduction in probe penetration may be primarily related to a reduction in gingival inflammation rather than a gain in attachment.[37,40]

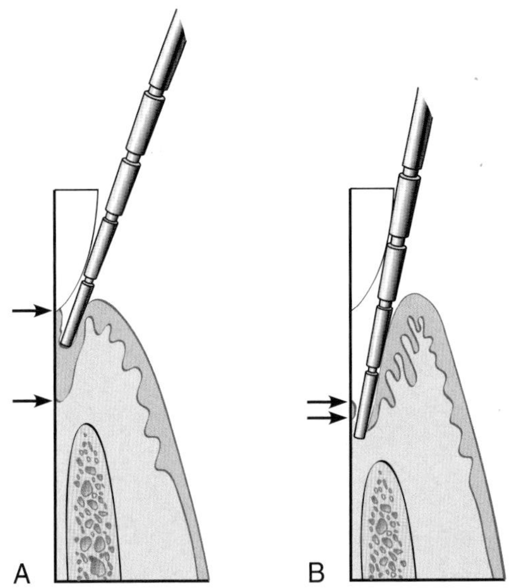

Fig. 38.15 (A) In a normal sulcus, the probe penetrates about one-third to half the length of the junctional epithelium *(between arrows)*. (B) In an inflamed periodontal pocket, the probe penetrates beyond the apical end of the junctional epithelium *(between arrows)*.

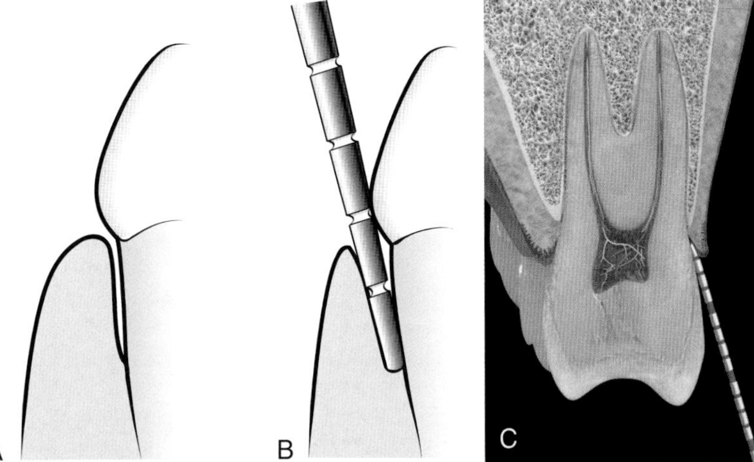

Fig. 38.14 (A) The biologic or histologic pocket depth is the distance between the gingival margin and the base of the gingival sulcular epithelium. (B) The probing or clinical pocket depth is the distance from the gingival margin to the bottom of the probeable crevice. (C) Graphical illustration showing periodontal probing. (© Periopixel.)

LEARNING BOX 38.7

Probing depth is a dynamic parameter that may change over time, even in the absence of attachment loss.

Bleeding on Probing

If the gingiva is inflamed, the insertion of a probe into the bottom of the pocket typically elicits a bleeding response. Non-inflamed sites rarely bleed, and if they do, it is often the result of an inadequate probing technique (e.g., excessive probing force). In most cases, bleeding on probing is an earlier sign of inflammation than gingival color changes (see Chapter 15).[45] However, gingival color changes may be identified without concomitant bleeding on probing.[24] Depending on the severity of inflammation, bleeding can vary from a tenuous red line along the gingival sulcus to profuse bleeding.[1] If periodontal treatment is successful and biofilm control is optimal, bleeding on probing will cease.[3]

To test for bleeding after probing, the probe is carefully introduced to the bottom of the pocket and gently moved laterally along the pocket wall. Sometimes bleeding appears immediately after the removal of the probe; other times it may be delayed. Therefore it is generally recommended that the examiner recheck for bleeding 30 to 60 seconds after probing.

As a single test, bleeding on probing is not a reliable predictor of progression of attachment loss; however, its absence is an excellent indicator of periodontal stability.[4] When bleeding is present in multiple sites that exhibit other signs of advanced periodontitis (e.g., probing depth >5 mm), bleeding on probing is a good indicator of attachment loss progression.[4,21]

LEARNING BOX 38.8

The absence of bleeding on probing is an excellent indicator of periodontal stability.

Pain on Probing

Pain is a cardinal sign of inflammation. However, gingival inflammation in gingivitis and periodontitis is generally not associated with pain. Probing of healthy sites does not typically induce pain, as long as the probing technique is adequate, while probing of sites presenting inflammation is more likely to produce pain. The level of pain is usually related to the severity and extent of gingival inflammation. Unless gingival inflammation is generalized and severe, patients do not normally report the same level of pain upon probing at every site. Although the clinician cannot directly measure pain on probing, for education purposes, it is useful to make the patient aware that pain usually indicates the presence of inflammation.

Probing Around Implants

Similar to the periodontium, the peri-implant tissues are susceptible to biofilm-induced inflammatory diseases. Hence, probing around implants is an integral component of the periodontal examination. It has been demonstrated that a conventional periodontal probe may be used under light force (e.g., 0.25 N) without damaging the peri-implant mucosal seal.[17] Peri-implant evaluation and probing of implants are further discussed in more detail in Chapter 74.

Probing in the Presence of Severe Disease

Recording probing depth measurements before, during, and after treatment is essential for effective diagnosis and monitoring of periodontal diseases and conditions, such as periodontitis. In the presence of severe gingival inflammation (see Figs. 38.5 and 38.12), accurate probing depth measurement may be difficult to obtain without anesthesia due to the pain and discomfort associated with the insertion of the periodontal probe into the inflamed periodontal pocket. Therefore when periodontal disease is overt and obvious clinically and radiographically, local anesthesia may facilitate the conduction of a thorough clinical periodontal examination, including probing depth assessments. Additionally, in cases presenting heavy subgingival calculus deposits, probing depth measurements may not be accurate until after completion of subgingival debridement. Clinicians should keep in mind that, in moderate and advanced periodontitis cases, a dramatic change in probing depths is normally observed after improvements in biofilm control and following scaling and root planing (Fig. 38.16). Obtaining accurate probing depths at the reevaluation following nonsurgical therapy holds more clinical relevance than obtaining accurate probing depths at the pretreatment periodontal examination, as the post-therapy measurements have more value in the context of clinical decision-making processes pertaining to recommendations for further treatment, whether it is corrective or supportive therapy.

LEARNING BOX 38.9

In the presence of severe periodontal disease, local anesthesia may facilitate the conduction of a thorough clinical periodontal examination.

Attachment Loss

Attachment loss is the apical migration of the dentogingival junction. Attachment loss may be induced by a variety of etiologies, such as inflammatory disease (e.g., periodontitis) or sustained trauma. The dentogingival junction is constituted by the junctional epithelium and the connective tissue attachment. The classic term to refer to the apicocoronal dimension of the dentogingival junction is the biologic width, which has been recently replaced with the term "supracrestal tissue attachment"[29] (Fig. 38.17).

The supracrestal tissue attachment averages 2.04 mm in humans.[20] In healthy conditions, without attachment loss, the connective tissue attachment of the dentogingival junction inserts into the root surface immediately apical to the cementoenamel junction. *Clinical attachment loss* refers to the *amount* of apical migration of the dentogingival junction that has occurred, using the cementoenamel junction as the reference point. If the cementoenamel junction is absent, another fiduciary mark can be used (e.g., restorative margin). Clinical attachment loss is typically measured using a calibrated probe as the distance from the cementoenamel junction to the bottom of the probeable crevice (i.e., attachment level). When the gingival margin is located coronal to the cementoenamel junction (on the anatomic crown), the clinical parameter "*clinical attachment loss*" is determined by subtracting the distance from the gingival margin to the cementoenamel junction from the probing depth. If both are the same, the actual clinical attachment loss is zero. When the gingival margin coincides with the cementoenamel junction, clinical attachment loss is equal to the probing depth. When the gingival margin is located apical to the cementoenamel junction, clinical attachment loss is greater than the probing depth. Therefore clinical attachment loss is the sum of gingival recession depth and probing depth. Refer to Fig. 38.18 to see how clinical attachment loss is determined in different clinical scenarios. Entering the probing depths and drawing the gingival margin on the periodontogram allows one to determine this important clinical landmark.[70]

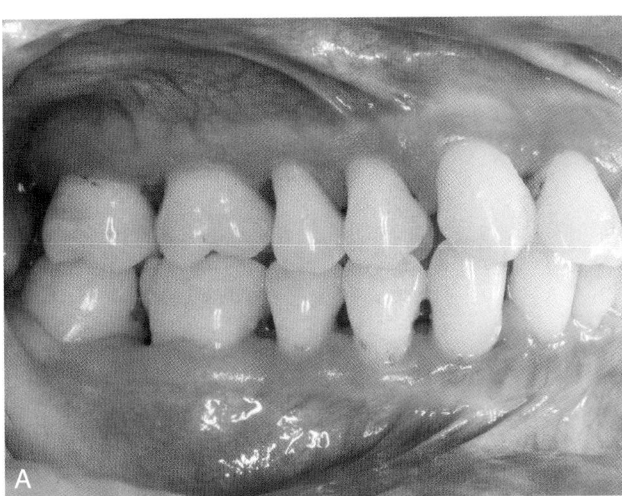

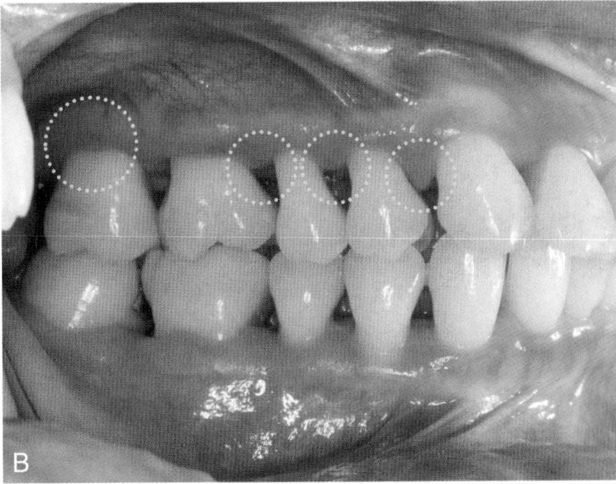

Fig. 38.16 Clinical presentation prior to scaling and root planing (A). Note the presence of supra- and subgingival calculus along the gingival margin. Following scaling and root planing, at the 6-week reevaluation (B), resolution of gingival inflammation resulted in dramatic gingival shrinkage or apical migration of the gingival margin *(circles)*. (Copyright Jonathan H. Do, DDS. All rights reserved.)

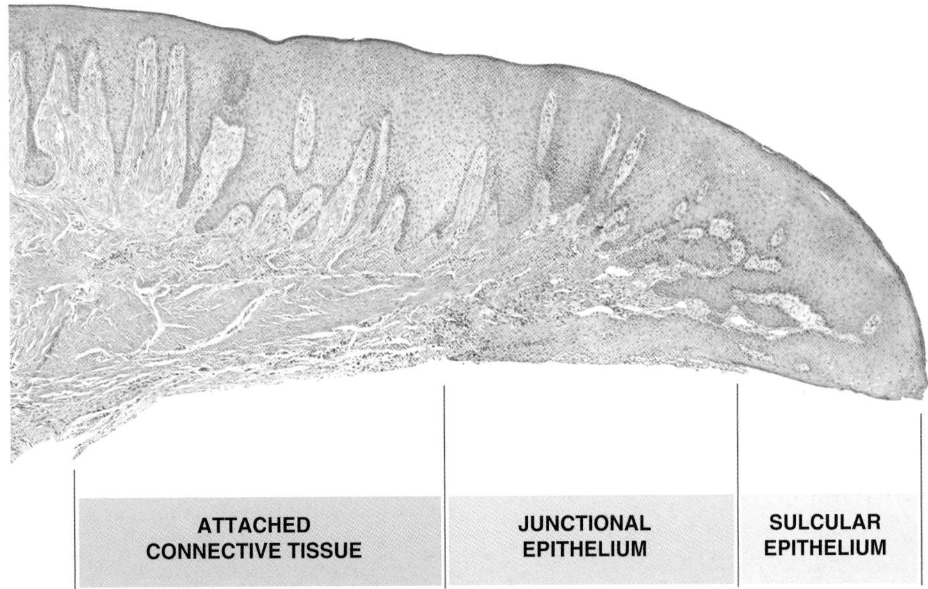

Fig 38.17 Histologic image of a human gingival sample depicting the apicocoronal dimension of the dentogingival junction showing the sulcular epithelium, the junctional epithelium, and the attached connective tissue. (Copyright Gustavo Avila-Ortiz, DDS, MS, PhD. All rights reserved.)

Clinical attachment loss is automatically calculated in many dental practice management software programs as the sum of probing depth and recession depth. This calculation is accurate only when both the probing and the recession depth are entered into the software correctly. However, when recession depth is not entered, many software programs assume the cementoenamel junction is at the level of the gingival margin and equate clinical attachment loss to probing depth. This is not necessarily correct, as many clinicians do not enter a value for recession depth when the cementoenamel junction is subgingival and not visible. As such, automatically calculated clinical attachment loss values must be scrutinized before they are used to establish a diagnosis.

Attachment Level

Attachment level refers to the most coronal location of the dentogingival junction on the tooth surface. For example, the attachment level of a tooth can be on the coronal third of the root or the apical third of the root. As aforementioned, clinical attachment loss measures the distance between the attachment level and a reference point, such as the cementoenamel junction or a restorative margin. Changes in attachment level can be the result of gain or loss of attachment, and they can provide valuable information to make clinical decisions.

LEARNING BOX 38.10

Clinical attachment loss measures *how much* apical migration of the dentogingival junction has occurred using the cementoenamel junction, or another fiduciary mark, as the reference point. **Clinical attachment level** refers to *where* the most coronal aspect of the dentogingival junction is located on the tooth surface.

Attached Gingiva

Establishing the relationship between the bottom of the gingival sulcus (or the periodontal pocket) and the mucogingival junction is a critical component of the periodontal examination, especially

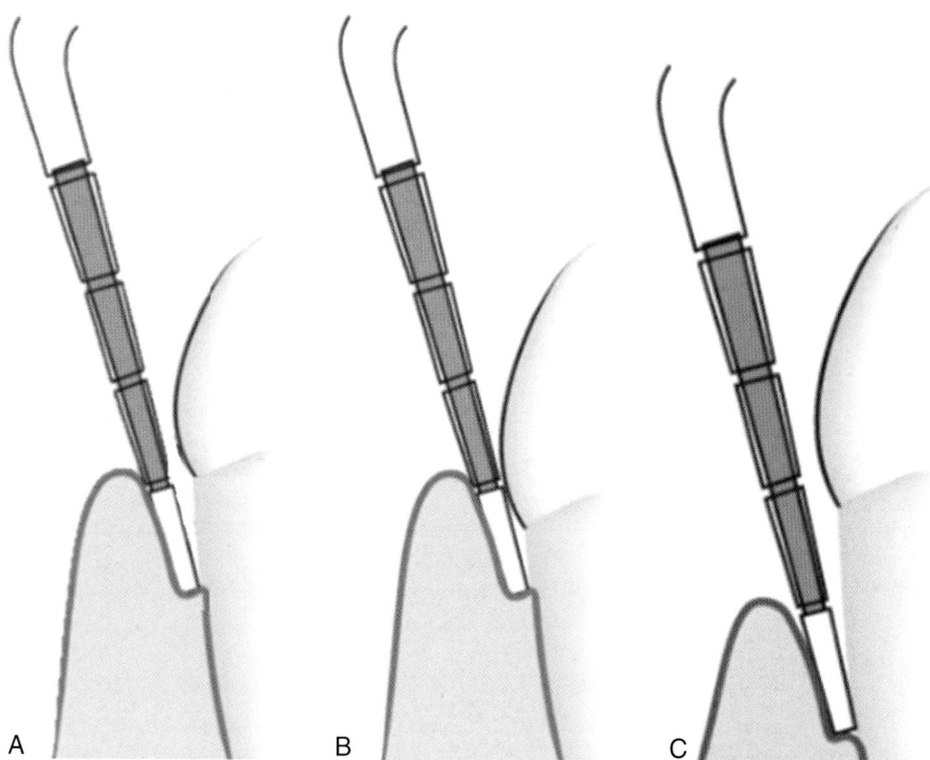

Fig. 38.18 Schematic illustration of three clinical scenarios where the probing depth is the same but with differing gingival margin locations with respect to the cementoenamel junction (CEJ), which result in different clinical attachment loss (CAL) measures. In scenario A, the gingival margin is at the level of the CEJ and, hence, the probing depth equals the CAL. In scenario B, the gingival margin is coronal to the CEJ, therefore CAL is calculated by subtracting the distance from the gingival margin to the CEJ from the probing depth. Scenario C presents a gingival recession defect. In this case, CAL is determined by adding the gingival recession measure (distance from the CEJ to the gingival margin) and the probing depth.

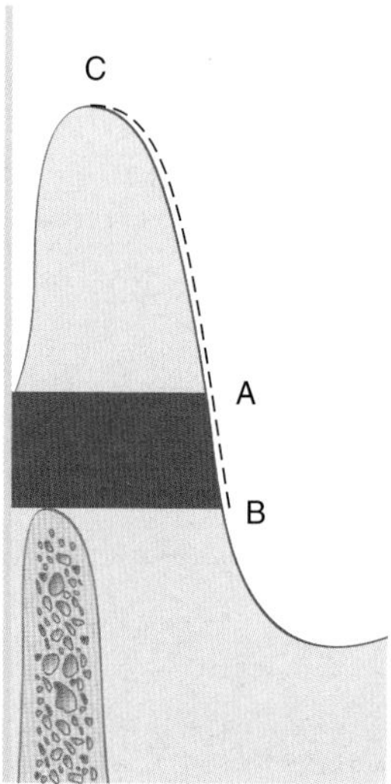

Fig. 38.19 The *shaded area* shows the attached gingiva, which extends between the projection on the external surface of the bottom of the gingival sulcus or periodontal pocket (A) and the mucogingival junction (B). The keratinized tissue (gingiva) extends from the mucogingival junction (B) to the gingival margin (C).

at sites presenting gingival recession defects and narrow gingival width (see Fig. 38.11). The width of the attached gingiva is the distance between the mucogingival junction and the bottom of the gingival sulcus (or the periodontal pocket). Attached gingiva width should not be confused with the gingival width, a dimension that also includes the marginal gingiva (Fig. 38.19).

The width of the attached gingiva is determined by subtracting the sulcus or pocket depth from the total gingival width (i.e., the distance from the gingival margin to the mucogingival junction). The amount of attached gingiva is generally considered to be insufficient when it presents a dimension of less than 1 mm, which sometimes correlates with movement of the free gingival margin when the lip or cheek are stretched. Other methods that are used to determine the amount of attached gingiva include pushing the apical alveolar mucosa coronally with a dull instrument or swabbing Schiller's potassium iodine solution over the mucosa, which stains keratin.

Periodontal Charting

Periodontograms provide a record of a comprehensive examination of the patient's periodontal condition and associated findings (Fig. 38.20A and B). These records are necessary to evaluate the initial status, the response to treatment, and for further comparison at recall visits. Electronic clinical records provide rapid and easy access to information and allow for the incorporation of digital clinical and radiographic images.[64] Computerized dental examination systems that make use of high-resolution graphics and voice-activated technology allow for easy retrieval and comparison of data.[11] See Chapter 37 for more information on recent advances in electronic health records.

Periodontal Pockets

As part of the periodontal examination, it is important to record the presence, distribution, and characteristics of periodontal pockets, including probing depth and attachment level.

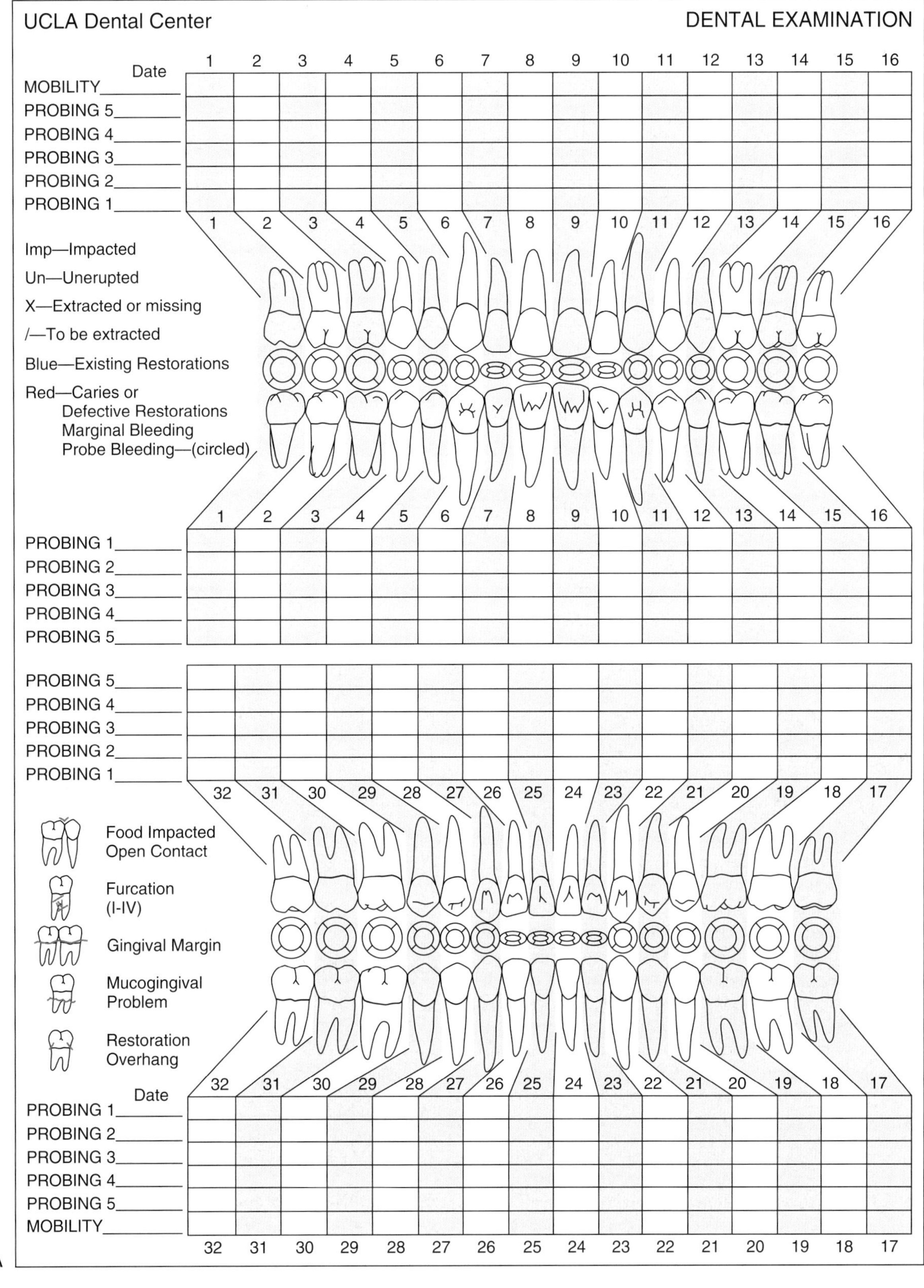

UCLA Dental Center

DENTAL EXAMINATION

Date

MOBILITY

PROBING 5

PROBING 4

PROBING 3

PROBING 2

PROBING 1

1 2 3 4 5 6 7 8 9 10 11 12 13 14 15 16

Imp—Impacted

Un—Unerupted

X—Extracted or missing

/—To be extracted

Blue—Existing Restorations

Red—Caries or
Defective Restorations
Marginal Bleeding
Probe Bleeding—(circled)

PROBING 1

PROBING 2

PROBING 3

PROBING 4

PROBING 5

PROBING 5

PROBING 4

PROBING 3

PROBING 2

PROBING 1

32 31 30 29 28 27 26 25 24 23 22 21 20 19 18 17

Food Impacted
Open Contact

Furcation
(I-IV)

Gingival Margin

Mucogingival
Problem

Restoration
Overhang

Date

PROBING 1

PROBING 2

PROBING 3

PROBING 4

PROBING 5

MOBILITY

A

Signs and Symptoms

Although probing is the only reliable method of detecting periodontal pockets, clinical signs such as color changes (i.e., a bluish-red marginal gingiva or a bluish-red vertical zone that extends from the gingival margin to the attached gingiva); a "rolled" edge separating the gingival margin from the tooth surface; or an enlarged, edematous gingiva may suggest their presence. Gingival bleeding and/or suppuration, and loose, extruded teeth may also denote the presence of a pocket.

Periodontal pockets are generally painless, but they may give rise to symptoms such as localized or sometimes radiating pain, or the sensation of pressure after eating that gradually diminishes. A foul taste, sensitivity to hot and cold, and toothache in the absence of caries are also sometimes reported by periodontitis patients.

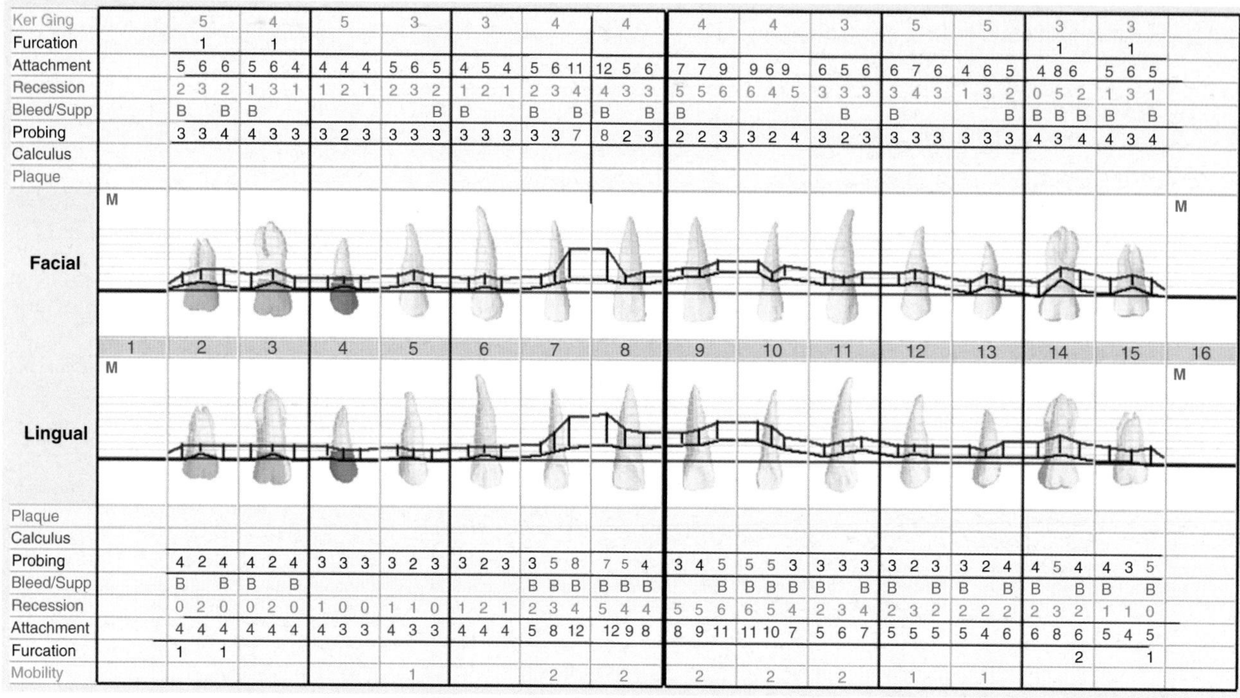

Fig. 38.20 (A) Periodontal chart (periodontogram) used at the University of California, Los Angeles. (B) Periodontal chart of maxillary teeth within an Electronic Health Record System

Detection of Periodontal Pockets

As previously mentioned, the only accurate method of detecting and measuring periodontal pockets is careful exploration with a periodontal probe. Pockets cannot be detected by radiographic examination. The periodontal pocket is essentially a soft tissue change. Radiographs can reveal areas of bone loss in which pockets may be suspected, but they do not show pocket presence or depth, and consequently, they are not valid to differentiate between the periodontal status before and after pocket elimination, other than monitoring bone levels.

Gutta-percha points or calibrated silver points[28] can be inserted in periodontal pockets prior to obtaining a radiograph to assist with the determination of the level of attachment. This approach can be used effectively for individual pockets or in clinical research, but its routine use throughout the mouth is impractical and unacceptable from a radiation protection standpoint. Again, clinical examination, including meticulous probing, is a direct and efficient way to assess the presence of periodontal pockets. See Chapter 39 for detailed information about the radiographic examination in the context of periodontal practice.

Determination of Disease Activity

A precise, site-specific determination of periodontitis activity may have a direct effect on diagnosis, prognosis, and therapy (e.g., treatment goals and strategy). Unfortunately, there are no accurate chairside methods currently available to determine the activity or inactivity of a periodontal lesion. In general, inactive (quiescent) lesions may show little or no bleeding on probing and minimal amounts of gingival crevicular fluid, while active lesions may bleed more readily with probing and exhibit large amounts of fluid and exudate. However, no differences between both active and non-active sites may be observed with regard to bleeding with probing, even in patients with aggressive periodontitis (i.e., a separate category in the previous disease classification to group periodontitis patients presenting a rapid progression pattern with a tendency to occur in relatively young patients).[31]

Assessment and comparison of clinical attachment level at different time points allows the examiner to determine whether attachment loss has occurred over time, which can be used as an indicator of disease progression. The automated Florida Probe provides a means of recording relative clinical attachment level changes over time. A later model of the probe has a modified sleeve with a prominent 0.125-mm edge to facilitate a "catch" of the cementoenamel junction. The width of this edge is considered small enough not to interfere with probing-depth measurements, thus providing concurrent assessments of clinical attachment level and pocket depth.[32,66] See Chapters 8, 9, 10 and 11 for descriptions of other methods used to determine disease activity that are still in a developmental stage.

Alveolar Bone Loss

Interproximal alveolar bone levels are primarily evaluated via radiographic examination. Probing can be helpful for estimating the following: (1) the approximate height and contour of the facial and lingual bone, which are obscured by the roots on conventional 2D radiographs, and (2) the architecture of the interdental bone. Transgingival probing (Figs. 38.21 and 38.22), which should be performed after anesthesia is achieved, can be used as a method of evaluation of the crestal bone architecture.[23,33,73]

Furcation Invasion

Attachment loss can result in *furcation invasion*, which is the pathologic resorption of inter-radicular bone within the furca of a multi-rooted tooth. Furcation invasion is detected by carefully probing the root surface for horizontal concavities where the roots start to diverge. As previously mentioned, specialized probes, such as the Nabers probe (Fig 38.23), may facilitate detection of furcation invasion. Several classifications of furcation invasion exist. The Glickman Classification[22] of furcation invasion is one of the most commonly used, and it is as follows:

- Grade I: pocket formation into the flute but intact inter-radicular bone.

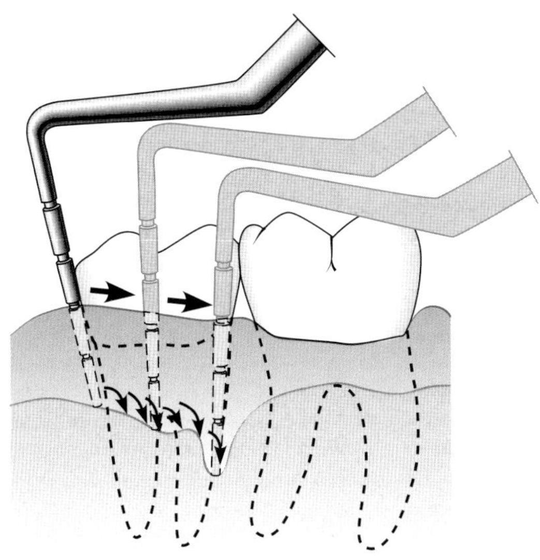

Fig. 38.21 Bone sounding: under local anesthesia, the probe is inserted down to the bone crest to explore the bone architecture.

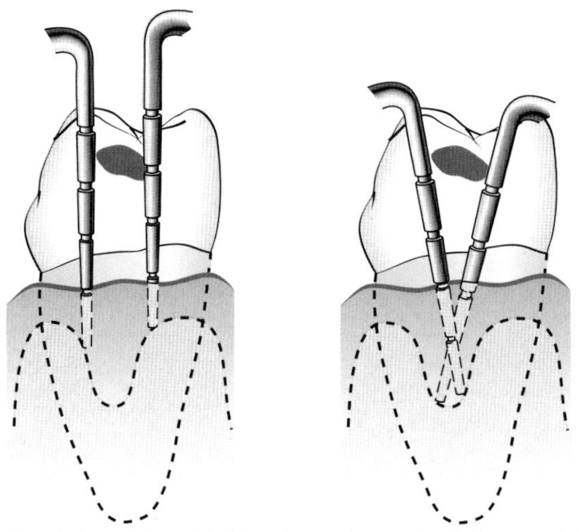

Fig. 38.22 A straight vertical insertion of the probe *(left)* may not detect interdental craters; oblique positioning of the probe *(right)* helps to reach the true depth of the crater.

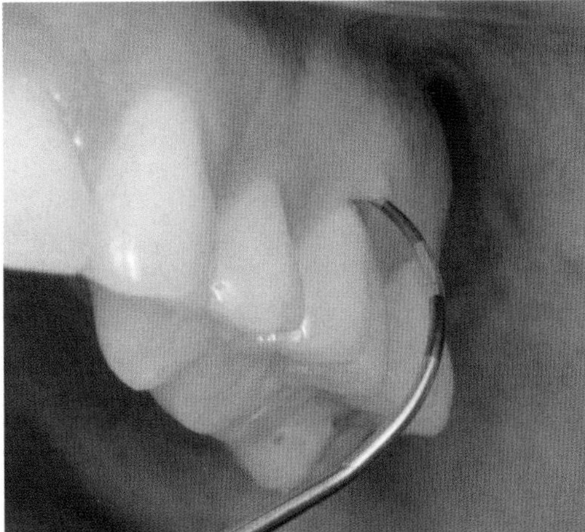

Fig. 38.23 Assessment of furcation involvement on the buccal aspect of the maxillary left first molar using a Nabers probe. Note the alternating colored bands in the probe, which are 3 mm in length.

- Grade II: loss of inter-radicular bone and pocket formation of varying depths into the furcation but not completely through to the opposite side of the tooth.
- Grade III: through-and-through lesion,
- Grade IV: same as grade III with gingival recession, rendering the furcation clinically visible.

Another popular classification scheme is the one proposed by Hamp, Nyman, and Lindhe in 1975 that categorizes furcation invasion into three degrees[26]:

- Degree I: horizontal loss of periodontal tissue supports less than 3 mm.
- Degree II: horizontal loss of periodontal tissue support exceeding 3 mm but not encompassing the total width of the furcation area.
- Degree III: horizontal "through and through" destruction of the periodontal tissue in the furcation.

Further information on furcation invasion and its treatment is available in Chapter 62.

Periodontal Abscess

A periodontal abscess is a localized accumulation of exudate within the gingival wall of a periodontal pocket (see Chapters 22 and 69). Periodontal abscesses may be acute or chronic.

The *acute periodontal abscess* appears as an ovoid elevation of the gingiva along the surface of the root. The gingiva usually appears edematous and red, with a smooth, shiny surface. The shape and consistency of the elevated area may vary; it may be domelike and relatively firm, or pointed and soft. In most cases, gentle digital pressure elicits exudate discharge through the gingival margin. An acute periodontal abscess is typically accompanied by symptoms such as throbbing, radiating pain, and tenderness to gingival palpation. Other symptoms may include sensitivity to tooth palpation or percussion; tooth mobility and lymphadenitis; and, less frequently, systemic effects such as fever, leukocytosis, and malaise. Occasionally, a patient may refer symptoms of an acute periodontal abscess without any notable clinical lesion or radiographic changes.

A *chronic periodontal abscess* usually presents a sinus tract that opens onto the gingival mucosa. There may be a history of intermittent exudation. The orifice of the sinus tract may appear as a difficult-to-detect pinpoint opening, which, when probed, reveals a sinus tract that leads deep into the periodontium. The sinus tract orifice may be covered by a small, pink, beadlike mass of granulomatous tissue. A chronic periodontal abscess is usually asymptomatic. However, the patient may report episodes of dull, gnawing pain; a slight elevation of the tooth; and a desire to bite down and grind the tooth. A chronic periodontal abscess may undergo acute exacerbation with all or some of the associated symptoms described previously. Fig. 38.24 is a clinical image that shows periodontal abscess on a mandibular molar tooth with furcation involvement.

Diagnosis of a periodontal abscess requires the correlation of the patient's medical and dental history with the clinical and radiographic findings. The suspected area should be probed carefully along the gingival margin in relation to each tooth surface to detect a channel from the marginal area to the deeper periodontal tissues. Continuity of the lesion with the gingival margin is clinical evidence that the abscess is periodontal.

An abscess is not necessarily located on the same surface of the root as the pocket from which it is formed. For example, a pocket on an interproximal surface may give rise to a periodontal abscess on the facial aspect of the tooth.

In children, a sinus orifice along the lateral aspect of a root is usually the result of a periapical infection of a deciduous tooth. In

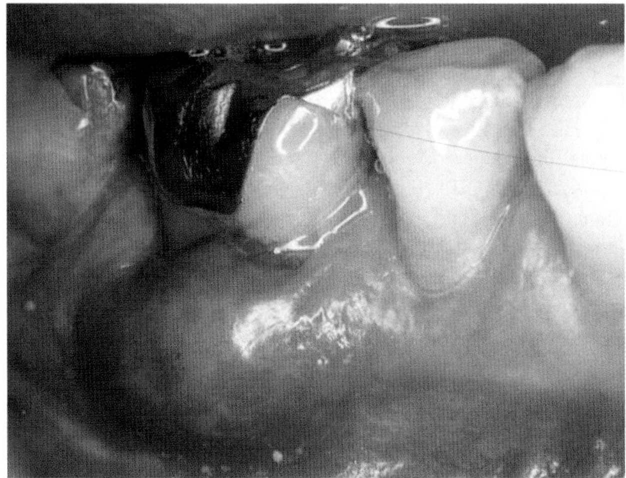

Fig. 38.24 Periodontal abscess associated with a furcation-involved mandibular molar.

the permanent dentition, such an orifice may be caused by a periodontal abscess or by apical involvement of endodontic origin and, therefore, a thorough examination is required to establish whether it is a purely periodontal, endodontic, or a combined lesion (see Chapter 49 for more information).

Periodontal Abscess and Gingival Abscess

The principal differences between the periodontal abscess and the gingival abscess are location and history (see Chapters 22 and 69). The gingival abscess is confined to the marginal gingiva, and it often occurs in previously disease-free areas. It is usually an acute inflammatory response to the presence of foreign material introduced into the gingiva. On the contrary, periodontal abscess involves supporting periodontal structures beyond the gingiva, and it generally occurs during the course of periodontitis or for other reasons (e.g., endodontic involvement, root fracture).

Periodontal Abscess and Periapical Abscess

Several characteristics can be used as guidelines when differentiating a periodontal abscess from a periapical abscess. If the tooth is non-vital, the lesion most likely has a periapical/endodontic origin. However, a previously non-vital tooth can have a deep periodontal pocket that may lead to the formation of a true periodontal abscess. Moreover, a deep periodontal pocket can extend to the apex and cause pulpal involvement and secondary necrosis.

A periapical abscess may spread along the root surface to the gingival margin. However, when the root apex and surface are involved with a single lesion that can be probed directly from the gingival margin, the lesion is more likely to have originated as a periodontal abscess.

Radiographic imaging can be helpful in differentiating between a periodontal and a periapical lesion (see Chapter 39). Early acute periodontal and periapical abscesses typically present with no radiographic changes. Ordinarily, a radiolucent area along the surface of the root suggests the presence of a periodontal abscess, whereas apical rarefaction suggests a periapical abscess. However, acute periodontal abscesses that show no radiographic changes may cause symptoms in teeth with long-standing, radiographically detectable periapical lesions that are not contributing to the patient's complaint. Clinical findings such as the presence of extensive caries, pocket formation, lack of tooth vitality, the existence of continuity between the gingival margin, and the abscess area often prove to be of greater diagnostic value than the radiographic appearance.

A draining sinus tract in the proximity of the gingival margin is suggestive of periodontal rather than periapical involvement, while a sinus tract from a periapical lesion is more likely to be located further apically. However, sinus location is not conclusive. In many instances, particularly in children, the sinus from a periapical lesion tends to drain coronally rather than at the apex (see Chapter 49). It is also important to note that abscesses are also associated with other dental conditions, such as vertical root fractures or cracked teeth. Refer to Chapter 49 for more information.

Examination of the Teeth and Implants

The teeth should be carefully examined for caries, poor restorations, developmental defects, anomalies of tooth form, wasting, hypersensitivity, and inadequate proximal contact relationships. The number, position, and stability of implants and their relationship to the adjacent natural dentition should also be examined.

Wasting Disease of the Teeth

Wasting is a generic term that refers to any gradual loss of tooth substance, which is characterized by the formation of smooth, polished surfaces. Depending on etiological factors and the process of development, tooth wasting can be classified as erosion, abrasion, attrition, and abfraction.[47,65] For more details, refer to the online version of this chapter.

Dental Stains

Dental stains are pigmented deposits on the surface of teeth that are not to be mistaken with calculus deposits. They should be carefully examined to determine their origin (see Chapter 24).

Hypersensitivity

Exposed root surfaces and sites presenting tooth wear may be hypersensitive to thermal changes or tactile stimulation. Patients often direct the clinician to the sensitive areas. These may be located by gentle exploration with an instrument (e.g., probe or explorer) or the direct application of cold air.

Proximal Contact Relations

Open contacts allow for food impaction, which can contribute to attachment loss. Open contacts may also be a result of inflammatory changes associated with periodontal diseases and conditions. The tightness of contacts should be checked by means of clinical observation and with dental floss. Abnormal contact relationships may also trigger occlusal changes, such as a shift in the median line between the central incisors with labial flaring of the maxillary canine, buccal or lingual displacement of the posterior teeth, and an uneven relationship of the marginal ridges. Teeth opposing an edentulous site may supra-erupt, thereby altering their proximal contacts.

Tooth Mobility

All teeth have a slight degree of physiologic mobility, which varies for different teeth and at different times of the day.[52,56] Tooth mobility is usually greatest when arising in the morning, and it progressively decreases through the day. The increased mobility in the morning is attributed to slight extrusion of the tooth as a result of limited occlusal contact during sleep. During the waking hours, mobility is reduced by chewing and swallowing forces, which "re-intrude" the teeth into the sockets. These 24-hour variations are less marked in persons with a healthy periodontium than in those with a history of attachment loss due to periodontitis or occlusal habits such as bruxism and clenching.

Single-rooted teeth typically exhibit greater mobility than multirooted teeth, with incisors having the most mobility. Mobility occurs

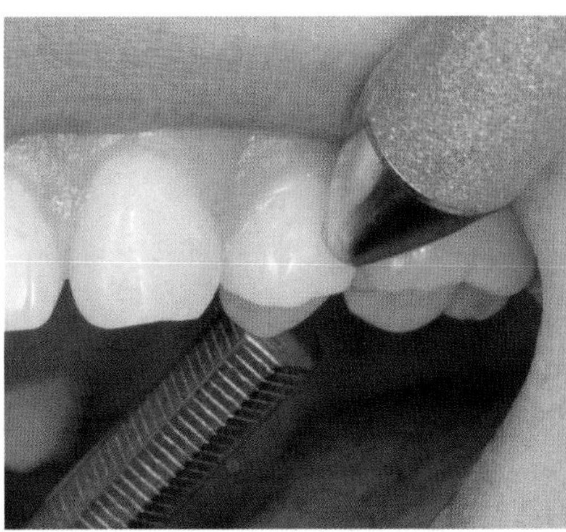

Fig. 38.25 Assessment of tooth mobility using two flat ends of rigid instruments (in this case mouth mirrors).

primarily in a horizontal direction, although some axial mobility can also be detected to a lesser degree.[54]

Tooth mobility occurs in the following two stages:

1. The initial or intra-socket stage: It occurs when the tooth moves within the confines of the periodontal ligament. This is associated with viscoelastic distortion of the principal fibers of the periodontal ligament and the redistribution of the periodontal fluids, inter-bundle content, and other interstitial fibers.[35] This initial movement occurs with forces exceeding about 100 lb, and it is on the order of 0.05 mm to 0.10 mm (50 μm to 100 μm).[48]
2. The secondary stage: This is a gradual process that entails elastic deformation of the alveolar bone in response to increased horizontal forces.[50] When a force of 500 g is applied to the crown, the resulting displacement is about 100 μm to 200 μm for incisors, 50 μm to 90 μm for canines, 8 μm to 10 μm for premolars, and 40 μm to 80 μm for molars.[48]

When a force such as that applied to teeth in occlusion is discontinued, the teeth return to their original position in two stages: the first is an immediate, spring-like elastic recoil; the second is a slow, asymptomatic recovery movement. Interestingly, the recovery movement is pulsating, and it is apparently associated with the normal pulsation of the periodontal vessels, which occurs in synchrony with the cardiac cycle.[49]

Many attempts have been made to develop mechanical or electronic devices for the precise measurement of tooth mobility.[49,53,55,68] Although standardization of grading mobility would be helpful for the diagnosis of some periodontal diseases and conditions and for the evaluation of treatment outcomes, these devices are not widely used. As a general rule, mobility is graded clinically by holding the tooth firmly between the handles of two rigid instruments (Fig. 38.25) or with one rigid instrument and one finger. An effort is then made to move the tooth in all directions. Abnormal mobility most often exhibits a faciolingual pattern. Tooth mobility is generally scored in daily practice according to the ease and extent of tooth movement according to the Miller Index, as follows:[46]

- Mobility no. 1: first distinguishable sign of movement greater than "normal."
- Mobility no. 2: movement of a tooth that allows the crown to move 1 mm from its normal position, in any direction.
- Mobility no. 3: Mobility that allows a tooth to move more than 1 mm, in any direction.

Physiologic mobility is generally defined as tooth movement up to 0.2 mm horizontally and 0.02 mm vertically. Mobility beyond the physiologic range is termed *abnormal* or *pathologic*. However, the periodontium is not *necessarily* diseased at the time of examination.

Increased mobility can be caused by one or more of the following factors:

1. The amount of mobility is related to the severity and distribution of bone loss at individual root surfaces and the shape and length of the roots as compared with that of the crown.[55] For the same amount of bone loss, a tooth with short, tapered roots is more likely to exhibit mobility than one with normal-size or bulbous roots. Post-orthodontic cases should be carefully evaluated for possible apical shortening of the root, which may lead to supra-physiologic mobility.
2. *Trauma from occlusion* (i.e., injury produced by excessive occlusal forces as a result of parafunctional habits, such as bruxism and clenching) is a common cause of tooth mobility. Mobility produced by trauma from occlusion occurs initially as a result of resorption of the inner cortical layer of bone (i.e., alveolar bone proper), which leads to reduced fiber support, and later, as an adaptation phenomenon that results in a widened periodontal ligament space. Notably, mobility may also be increased in response to hypofunction.
3. *Spread of inflammation* from the gingiva or the periapex into the periodontal ligament results in tissue changes that may increase tooth mobility. A good example of this is the spread of inflammation from an acute periapical abscess that increases tooth mobility in the absence of periodontitis.
4. *Periodontal surgery* temporarily increases tooth mobility immediately after the intervention and for a short period.[58–61] Mobility is a common but transient postoperative sequela, especially if a resective intervention to correct osseous deformities is performed (Chapter 62).
5. Tooth mobility can increase during *pregnancy,* and it is sometimes associated with the *menstrual cycle* or the use of *hormonal contraceptives.* This is unrelated to periodontitis, and it occurs presumably because of physicochemical changes in the periodontal tissues in response to fluctuations in hormone levels.
6. *Pathologic processes of the jaws* that destroy the alveolar bone or the roots of the teeth can also result in mobility. Osteomyelitis and tumors of the jaws belong in this category.

LEARNING BOX 38.11

The three main etiologic factors of tooth mobility are attachment loss, occlusal trauma, and periodontal inflammation.

Trauma From Occlusion

Trauma from occlusion refers to *tissue injury* produced by supra-physiologic occlusal forces (see Chapter 32). The threshold that defines a "supra-physiologic" force is different depending on multiple local and functional factors inherent to the site and the patient, respectively. The criterion that determines whether an occlusion is traumatic is whether it causes damage to the periodontal tissues. Therefore the diagnosis of trauma from occlusion is made considering the condition of the periodontal tissues, not the magnitude of the force *per se*. The periodontal findings are used as a guide to identify etiological occlusal relationships.

Periodontal findings that suggest the presence of trauma from occlusion include abnormal tooth mobility, particularly in teeth that show radiographic evidence of a widened periodontal space; vertical or angular bone destruction; and pathologic migration, especially of the anterior teeth.

Pathologic Tooth Migration

Alterations in tooth position should be carefully noted as part of the periodontal exam, particularly with a view toward identifying

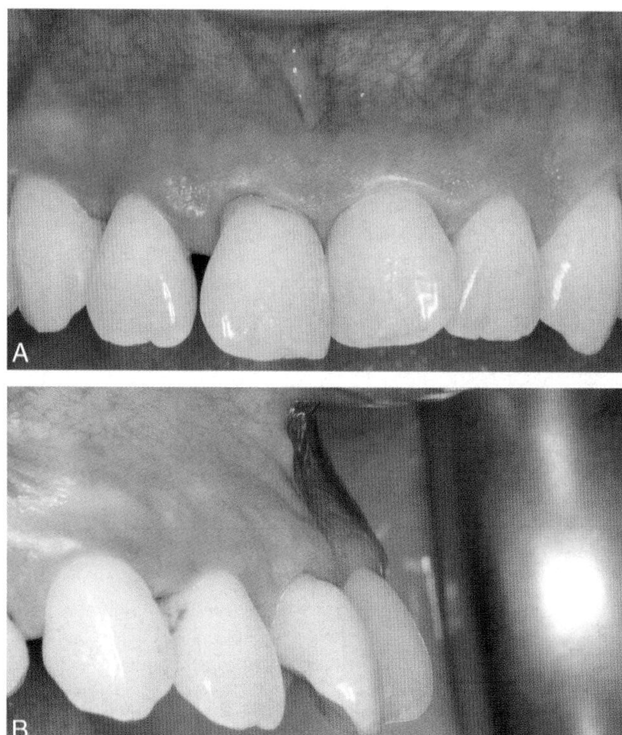

Fig. 38.26 Facial flaring and supraeruption of the right central incisor and spacing between the lateral and central incisors result from pathologic migration due to chronic periodontitis. Facial view (A) and side view (B) (Copyright Jonathan H. Do, DDS. All rights reserved.)

abnormal forces, a tongue-thrusting habit, or other habits that may be contributing etiologic factors (Fig. 38.26 see Chapter 32). Premature tooth contacts in the posterior region that deflect the mandible anteriorly contribute to the destruction of the periodontium of the maxillary anterior teeth and, secondarily, to pathologic migration (see also Chapter 32). The loss of posterior teeth can also lead to facial "flaring" of the anterior dentition. This is due to the increased trauma that the mandibular anterior dentition places against the palatal surface of the maxillary anterior dentition. Pathologic migration of the anterior teeth in young individuals may be a sign of periodontitis with a molar-incisor pattern (previously termed "localized aggressive or juvenile periodontitis").

Sensitivity to Percussion

Sensitivity to percussion may be indicative of acute inflammation of the periodontal ligament. Gentle tooth percussion at different angles with respect to the long axis often helps to localize the inflamed site.

Dentition with the Jaws Closed

Examination of the dentition with the jaws closed should be performed to detect conditions such as irregularly aligned teeth, supra-erupted teeth, improper proximal contacts, and areas of food impaction, all of which may favor microbial biofilm accumulation.

Excessive *overbite,* which is seen most often in the anterior region, may cause impingement of the teeth on the gingiva and food impaction, which may subsequently lead to gingival inflammation and periodontal pocket formation. The real significance of the detrimental effect of an excessive anterior overbite on gingival health is still controversial.[2]

In *open-bite* relationships, abnormal spacing exists between the maxillary and mandibular teeth. This condition is more common in the anterior region, although posterior open bite can be occasionally seen. Reduced mechanical cleansing by the passage of food may lead to the accumulation of plaque and debris, calculus formation, and tooth extrusion.

Crossbite is an inversion of the normal transversal relationship of the mandibular teeth with the maxillary teeth in which the maxillary teeth are lingual to the mandibular teeth. Crossbite may be anterior or posterior, and if posterior, it may be bilateral or unilateral. It may also affect multiple teeth or only a pair of antagonists. Crossbite may lead to food impaction, tooth migration, trauma from occlusion, and other periodontal disturbances.

Functional Occlusal Relationships

A meticulous examination of functional occlusal relationships is an important part of the diagnostic procedure. Dentitions that appear to be normal when the jaws are closed may actually present marked functional abnormalities. Systematic procedures for the detection and correction of functional abnormalities are presented in Chapters 34 and 35.

Radiographic Examination

The standard radiographic survey in a complete dentition normally consists of a minimum of 14 periapical and 4 posterior bitewing radiographs (Fig. 38.27). Panoramic radiographs are a simple and convenient method of obtaining a survey view of the dental arch and the surrounding structures (Fig. 38.28). They are helpful for the detection of developmental anomalies, pathologic lesions of the teeth and jaws, and fractures. Panoramic radiographs provide an overall radiographic picture of the distribution and severity of bone destruction in periodontitis cases, but *a complete intraoral series consisting of periapical and bitewing radiographs is required for a proper periodontal diagnosis and treatment planning.* In patients with severe bone loss, vertical rather than horizontal bitewings are the preferred radiographs to adequately capture the location of the crestal bone. Chapter 39 gives a detailed description of radiographic interpretation in periodontics.

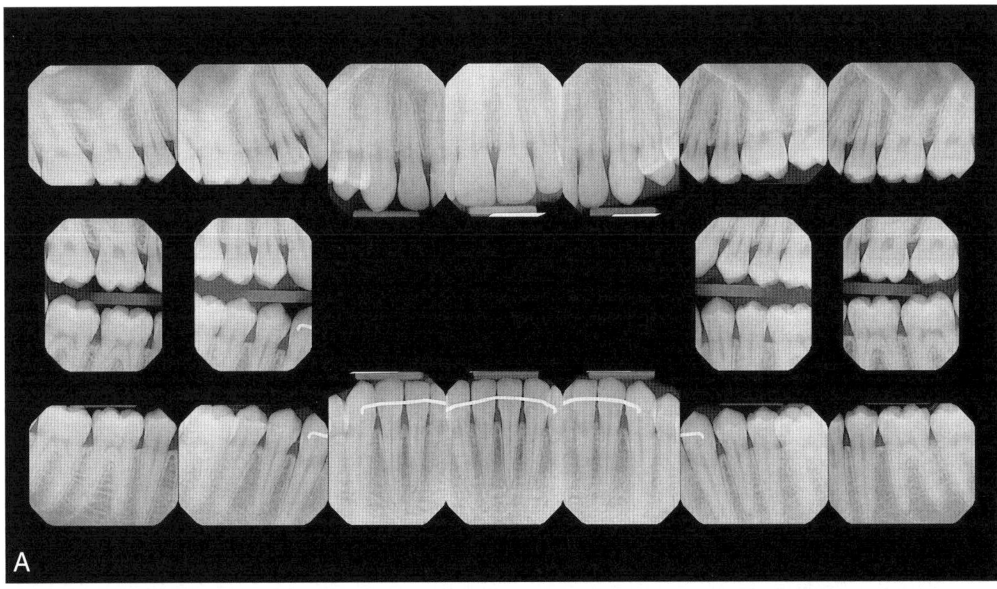

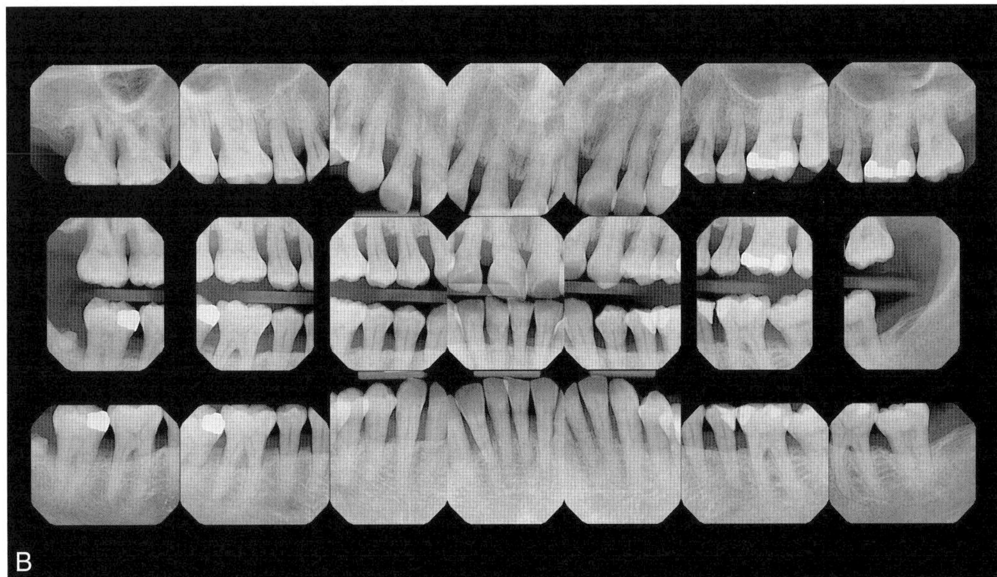

Fig. 38.27 A complete intraoral radiographic set is an essential adjunct to periodontal diagnoscomponent of the periodontal examinationis. (A) Intraoral radiographs of a patient with gingivitis. Note the radiopaque fixed lingual orthodontic retainer. (B) Intraoral radiographs of a patient with generalized moderate to severe chronic periodontitis. Vertical bitewing radiographs are useful to evaluate crestal bone loss. (Copyright Jonathan H. Do, DDS. All rights reserved.)

Laboratory Tests to Aid Clinical Diagnosis

When unusual gingival or periodontal findings that cannot be explained by local causes are detected, the possible contribution of systemic factors must be explored. The signs and symptoms of oral manifestations of systemic disease have to be clearly understood and analyzed, and their presence discussed with the patient's physician. See Chapter 25 for more information on this topic.

Laboratory tests may aid in the diagnosis of systemic diseases that contribute to periodontitis and other oral diseases; these tests may also be needed to make treatment decisions when dealing with medically compromised patients (see Chapter 67). Analyses of blood smears, blood cell counts, white blood cell differential counts, and erythrocyte sedimentation rates are used to evaluate the presence of blood dyscrasias and generalized infections. Determinations of platelet counts, coagulation time, bleeding time, clot retraction time, prothrombin time, and capillary fragility, as well as bone marrow studies, may be required to determine the presence of coagulation disorders. In a patient presenting with a suspicious oral lesion, biopsy of the abnormal tissue followed by histopathological evaluation is warranted.

Diagnosis and Classification of Periodontitis

Once the patient's medical and dental history has been obtained; clinical, radiographic, and other necessary examinations have been performed; and a diagnosis of periodontitis has been confirmed, the information acquired can be synthesized and utilized in a multidimensional staging and grading system to classify the periodontitis case. This system, which was devised in the context of the 2017 World Workshop on the Classification of Periodontal and Peri-implant Diseases and Conditions, takes the following factors into consideration: severity, treatment complexity, tooth loss due to periodontitis, rate of disease progression, and the presence of risk factors. The process of classifying a case of periodontitis is carried out according to the following key steps:

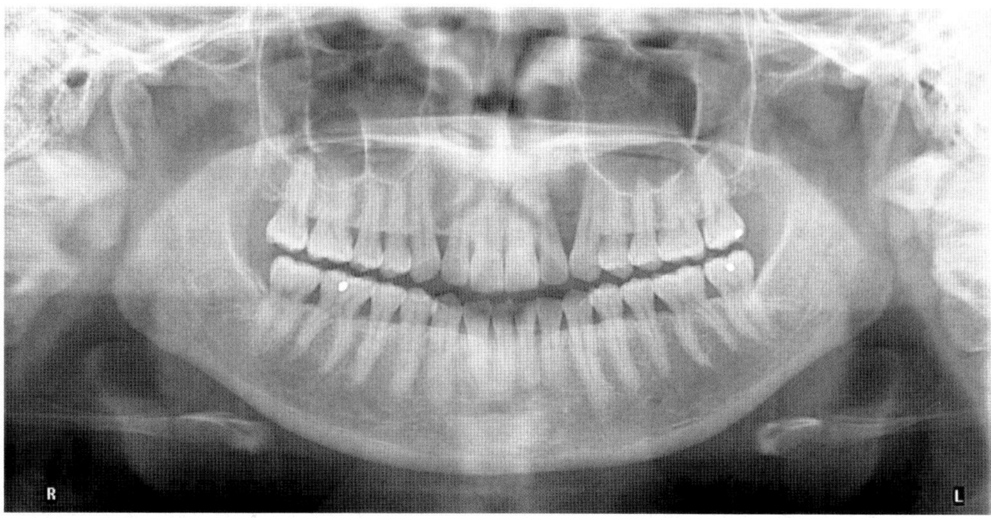

Fig. 38.28 Panoramic radiographs provides an overview of the dental arch and the surrounding structures.

Step 1: Confirm the Case of Periodontitis

A patient is considered to have periodontitis if one of the following two criteria is satisfied: Interdental clinical attachment loss is detectable at ≥2 non–adjacent teeth or buccal or oral clinical attachment loss ≥3 mm with pocketing greater than 3 mm is detectable at ≥2 teeth and the observed clinical attachment loss cannot be attributed to the following clinical scenarios: (a) trauma-induced gingival recession, (b) dental caries extending subgingivally, (c) clinical attachment loss on the distal aspect of second molar (associated with malposition or extraction of third molar), (d) endodontic pathology draining through periodontium, and (e) vertical root fracture[74].

Step 2: Establish the Stage and Extent

There are four stages (I through IV). Stage is determined based on the site with the most severe disease (attachment loss) and tooth loss. Stages I and II represent mild to moderate periodontitis without any tooth loss due to periodontitis. Stages III and IV represent severe periodontitis associated with (or potential for) tooth loss (≤4 in stage III and ≥5 teeth in stage IV). Table 38.2 presents the key features of each of the stages of periodontitis.

The extent should be described after the determination of the stage. Assessment of extent describes the percentage of teeth at the stage-defining severity level based on a 30% threshold.[34,67] Localized periodontitis is defined as periodontitis affecting ≤30% of teeth, while periodontitis affecting greater than 30% of teeth is considered generalized. If the periodontal attachment loss is completely or mostly confined to the first molars and incisors, the term molar-incisor pattern is used for the disease extent. Refer to Chapter 5 for more in-depth information on periodontal diagnoses.

Step 3: Establish the Grade

There are three grades (A, B, and C). Grade A denotes a slow rate of disease progression, while grades B and C denote a moderate and severe rate of disease progression, respectively. When direct evidence of radiographic or clinical disease progression over time is not available, indirect evidence in the form of % bone loss/age is used as the primary method to assign a grade. For grades A, B, and C, the corresponding % bone loss age measures are less than 0.25, 0.25 to 1.0. and greater than 1.0, respectively. Established periodontal risk factors such as smoking and its frequency and glycemic control status are both used as grade modifiers.

Assessment of Biofilm Control and Patient Education

Patients presenting for periodontal consultations typically expect to find out the problems they have and the treatments they need. By the end of the periodontal consultation, it may not be possible to determine a detailed prognosis and formulate a complete treatment plan, as a careful analysis of the information obtained, the acquisition of more diagnostic information, or consultation with other dental and medical professionals may be required. However, the patient can be educated on the problems identified in his or her mouth upon initial examination, the need for further diagnostics, and the etiologies and prevention of these problems. Clinical photographs, radiographs, and models may be useful to help the patient understand their current status of oral health. Upon completion of the periodontal examination, the patient may be presented with a preliminary treatment plan that may include emergency and palliative treatments as well as nonsurgical periodontal therapy as part of infection control therapy.

Although patient education and biofilm control are not the focus of this chapter, a preventive approach to oral health care demands behavior modification through effective patient education, which requires time, effort, and repetition. As such, every opportunity to educate and motivate patients should be seized in order to implement positive behavioral changes. Patients should be given personalized, site-specific oral hygiene instructions for biofilm control and to improve their oral health, including periodontal health. It is not uncommon for patients presenting with poor plaque control and the presence of disease to report brushing and flossing multiple times daily. For that reason, the effectiveness of the patient's biofilm control must be evaluated and monitored over time. If suboptimal plaque control is evident, the patient should be asked to demonstrate biofilm control (toothbrushing, flossing, etc.) in front of a mirror so that both the patient and the clinician can see their oral hygiene techniques. The patient should then be taught proper biofilm control techniques with a demonstration in their own mouth in front of a mirror. Detailed information on biofilm control strategies is presented in Chapter 50.

Ideally, unless emergency treatment is required, patients should be given at least 1 or 2 weeks to improve their oral hygiene, to control biofilm and reduce periodontal inflammation, and to appreciate how meticulous biofilm control can positively impact their oral health before any periodontal treatment is rendered.

TABLE 38.2 Salient Clinical and Radiographic Features of the Four Different Stages of Periodontitis According to the Classification Released in 2018.

Stage I	Stage II	Stages III and IV
• Incipient periodontitis 1–2 mm interdental CAL • Probing depths ≤4 mm • No tooth loss or planned for extraction due to periodontitis	• Progression beyond incipient periodontitis • 3–4 mm interdental CAL • Probing depths ≤5 mm • No tooth loss or planned to be removed due to periodontitis	• Tooth loss or planned for extraction due to periodontitis • ≥5 mm interdental CAL and probing depths ≥6 mm • Deep vertical bony defects • Deep furcation involvements • Extent of tooth loss and complexity of management distinguishes stage III from stage IV disease.
Radiographic Findings • Bone loss in the coronal third (<15% of the root)	• Bone loss in the coronal third (15%–33% of the root)	• Bone loss extending to middle third of root and beyond
A	B	C

CAL, Clinical attachment loss.

Conclusion

Periodontal examination begins with the acquisition of a thorough medical and dental history. Although, for didactic purposes, the sequence of periodontal examination presented in this chapter is divided into two parts (visual and tactile examination), in practice, both visual and tactile assessments overlap and occur simultaneously, as do the evaluations of the teeth and the periodontium. A proper periodontal examination should include an overall survey of biofilm and calculus, clinical signs of inflammation, and other obvious signs of disease to obtain insights into the patient's oral hygiene performance and disease status.

Once a detailed patient history has been obtained and a thorough clinical examination has been completed, the information collected is analyzed and synthesized to arrive at a diagnosis or a list of diagnoses. The periodontal examination is the basis from which the diagnosis, prognosis, and treatment plan are derived. Therefore a thorough and accurate periodontal examination is of the utmost importance to render optimal periodontal therapy.

LEARNING BOX 38.12

Examination and Information Gathering → Diagnosis → Prognosis ↔ Treatment

- Diagnosis requires gathering information from a thorough and careful examination.
- Prognosis is based on accurate diagnosis.
- Treatment decisions are based on prognosis.
- Treatment is provided to improve prognosis.
- Diagnosis and prognosis could change with treatment.

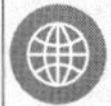
A Case Scenario is found on the companion website eBooks.Health.Elsevier.com.

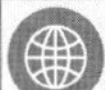
References for this chapter are found on the companion website eBooks.Health.Elsevier.com.

CHAPTER 39

Radiographic Aids in the Diagnosis of Periodontal Disease

Sanjay M. Mallya | Sotirios Tetradis

CHAPTER OUTLINE

Radiologic imaging provides essential information that contributes to diagnosis and management of patients with periodontal disease.[11,21,22] Objectives of imaging include assessment of the extent and pattern of osseous changes, identification of local causative factors, and an assessment of local anatomy. Radiographs illustrate the current status of calcified tissues—these imaging findings reflect the cumulative effects of inflammation on bone and teeth and do not always reflect current cellular activity in the periodontium. *Thus radiographs must be used as an adjunct to and not as a substitute for a clinical examination.* Radiologic evaluation provides information on the morphology of intrabony defects, the extent of furcation bone loss, and anatomic restrictions to root instrumentation—factors that contribute to treatment planning and outcome. In addition, radiographs provide longitudinal assessment of bone loss.

LEARNING BOX 39.1

Radiographic (periodontal) bone loss (RBL) reflects cumulative bone resorption from current and prior inflammation and must be interpreted in the context of the patient's periodontal history and current clinical presentation. Periodontal health cannot be determined by radiologic evaluation alone.

Imaging Modalities for Periodontal Assessment

Intraoral Imaging

Intraoral radiologic imaging with periapical and bite-wing projections serves as the primary imaging examination to assess periodontal disease.[1] Radiologic assessments include evaluation of the bone level, the destruction pattern, periodontal ligament (PDL) space width, and the radiodensity, trabecular pattern, and marginal contour of the interdental bone. Depiction of these details requires optimization of technique for radiographic projection and exposure. Standardized, reproducible techniques are important to obtain reliable radiographs for pretreatment and posttreatment comparisons.[4,27]

Prichard[23] established the following four criteria to determine adequate angulation of periapical radiographs (Fig. 39.1):

1. The radiograph should show the tips of molar cusps with little or none of the occlusal surface showing.
2. Enamel caps and pulp chambers should be distinct.
3. Interproximal spaces should be open.
4. Proximal contacts should not overlap unless teeth are anatomically misaligned.

For periapical radiographs, the long-cone paralleling technique accurately projects the alveolar bone level (Fig. 39.2). The bisecting angle technique typically elongates the projected image, making the bone margin appear closer to the crown; the facial bone level is distorted more than the lingual alveolar crest. Inappropriate horizontal angulation results in tooth overlap, changes the shape of the interdental bone image, alters the radiographic width of the PDL space and the appearance of the lamina dura, and may distort the extent of furcation involvement (see Fig. 39.2). Periapical radiographs frequently do not reveal the correct relationship between the alveolar bone and the cementoenamel junction (CEJ).[27] This is particularly true when a shallow palate or high floor of the mouth does not allow ideal placement of the receptor parallel to the tooth.

Bite-wing radiographs are a better approach to evaluate periodontal bone levels.[27] For a bite-wing projection, the image receptor is placed lingual to the crowns of the upper and lower teeth and parallel to the long axis of the crowns. The x-ray beam is directed through the contact areas of the teeth and perpendicular to the image receptor. Thus the bite-wing projection geometry permits evaluation of the relationship between the interproximal alveolar crest and the CEJ without distortion (Figs. 39.3 and 39.4).[27] When the periodontal bone loss is severe and the bone level cannot be visualized on horizontally positioned bite-wing radiographs, receptors may be placed vertically to encompass more root length (Fig. 39.5). More than two vertical bite-wing images may be necessary to cover all of the interproximal spaces in the area of interest.

A full mouth radiologic examination with periapical and bite-wing radiographs provides detailed evaluation of the periodontal bone and is the preferred examination[1] to assess the osseous impact of periodontal disease (Fig. 39.6).

LEARNING BOX 39.2

Bite-wing imaging is the preferred technique to depict interdental bone levels in the posterior dentition. In addition, vertical bite-wing radiographs are preferred when periodontal bone loss is severe.

Panoramic Imaging

Panoramic imaging (Fig. 39.7) encompasses regions of the jaw beyond the dentoalveolar region, including the basal body and rami of the mandible, the temporomandibular joints, the maxillary sinuses, and nasal cavity. Panoramic imaging is a low-radiation-dose procedure, is relatively quicker and easier than a full mouth intraoral survey, and is more comfortable for the patient.[24] However, panoramic image resolution is lower than that of intraoral radiographs, and assessments of root shape and resorption are more accurate on intraoral radiographs.

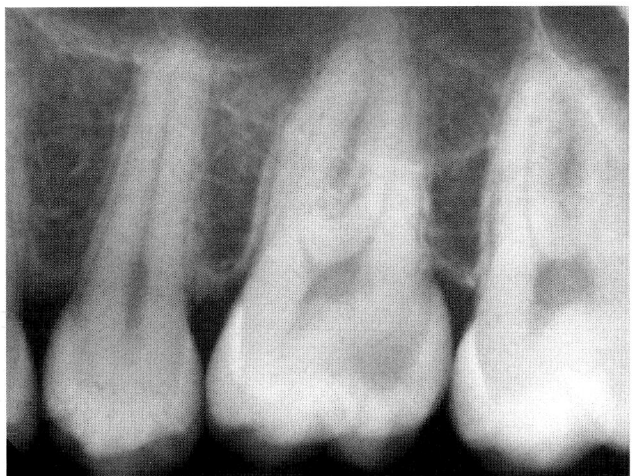

Fig. 39.1 Periapical radiograph of the posterior maxilla. Note that the cusps are superimposed and the enamel appears as a distinct cap separated from the pulp space. The approximal surfaces are separated, and the interdental bone is distinct.

LEARNING BOX 39.3

A full mouth intraoral radiographic survey (see Fig. 39.6) is the examination of choice for initial evaluation of patients with generalized periodontal disease or with a history of extensive dental restorations.[1]

Digital Radiologic Imaging

Globally, the use of digital technologies for intraoral and extraoral imaging has grown rapidly over the past two decades. Digital imaging provides several advantages over film-based imaging[20] and, importantly, also decreases patient radiation dose. In the United States, more than 80% of intraoral imaging is done using digital receptors.[12] Two technologies are used for digital intraoral imaging—solid-state detectors and photostimulable phosphors (PSPs). Solid-state sensor-based systems use complementary metal oxide semiconductor (CMOS) or charge-coupled device (CCD) chips to detect x-ray photons and record an image. These systems provide immediate image display after acquisition. PSP technology uses rare earth crystals to store energy and record a latent radiographic image. The stored energy is then released by stimulating the plate with an appropriate wavelength of light causing the crystal to emit light photons. Unlike CCD/CMOS receptors, PSP plates do not provide an instantaneous display of the radiographic image. Irrespective of acquisition method, digital images can be modulated, and most vendors provide software tools to adjust density and contrast, magnify images, and enhance edges to sharpen the image. Some software vendors have incorporated preprogrammed algorithms that can be applied to enhance digital images for specific diagnostic tasks (e.g., to enhance visualization of interproximal caries, periodontal bone [Fig. 39.8], and pulp canals). However, it is important to recognize that such image manipulations produce artifacts that may be misinterpreted as disease (see Fig. 39.8).[19]

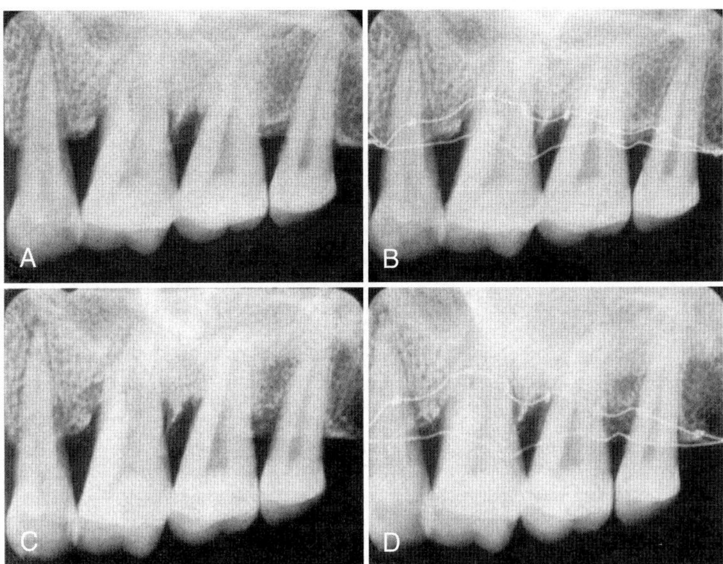

Fig. 39.2 Comparison of long-cone paralleling and bisection-of-the-angle techniques. (A) Long-cone paralleling technique, radiograph of dried specimen. (B) Long-cone paralleling technique, same specimen as shown in part A. Smooth wire is on the margin of the facial plate and knotted wire is on the lingual plate to show their relative positions. (C) Bisecting angle technique, same specimen as in parts A and B. (D) Bisecting angle technique, same specimen. Both bone margins are shifted toward the crown, the facial margin (smooth wire) more than the lingual margin (knotted wire), creating the illusion that the lingual bone margin has shifted apically. (*Courtesy Dr. Benjamin Patur, Hartford, Connecticut.*)

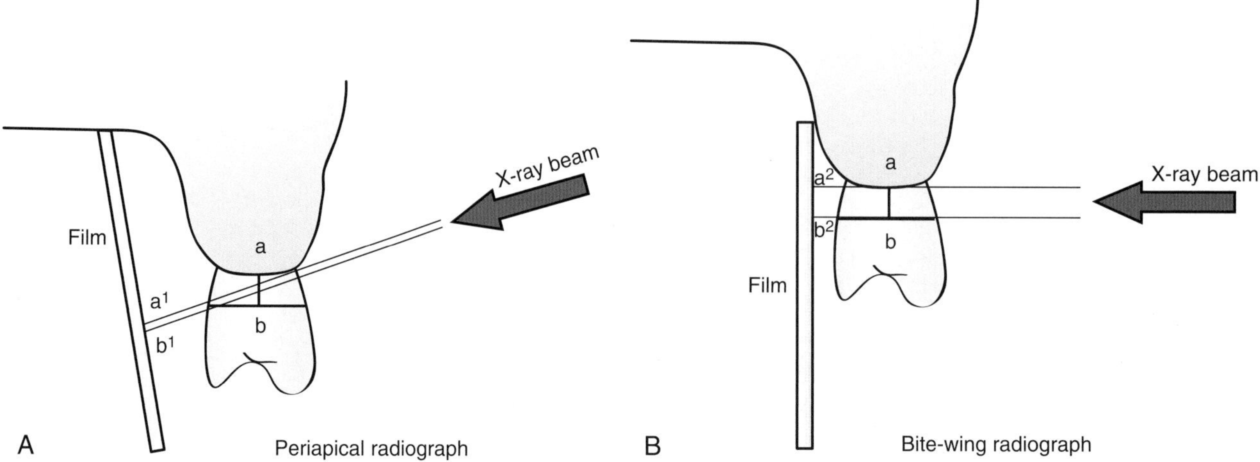

Fig. 39.3 Schematic diagram of periapical (A) and bite-wing (B) radiographs. Angulation of the x-ray beam and the receptor on the periapical radiograph distort the distance between the alveolar crest and the cementoenamel junction (CEJ) (compare a–b versus a^1–b^1). In contrast, the projection geometry of the bite-wing radiograph allows a more accurate depiction (a^2–b^2) of the distance between the alveolar crest and the CEJ (a–b).

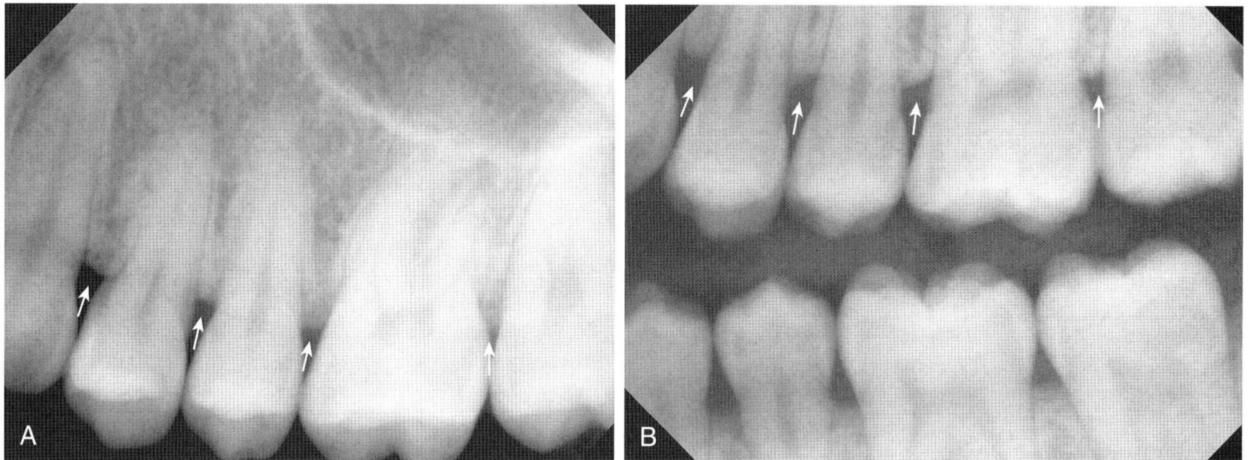

Fig. 39.4 Periapical (A) and bite-wing (B) radiographs from a full-mouth series of a patient with periodontitis. The periapical film clearly underestimates the amount of bone loss *(white arrows).* Because of appropriate projection geometry, the alveolar crest height is accurately depicted on the bite-wing radiograph *(white arrows).*

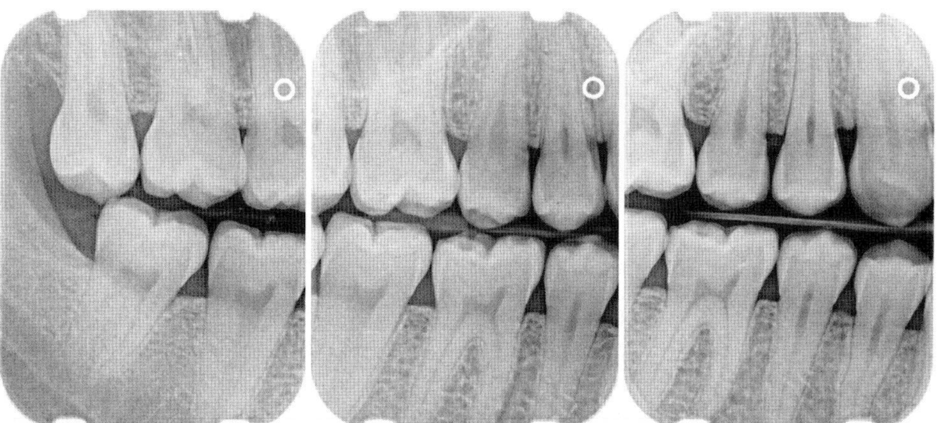

Fig. 39.5 Vertical bite-wing radiographs can be used to encompass a longer length of root and alveolar bone.

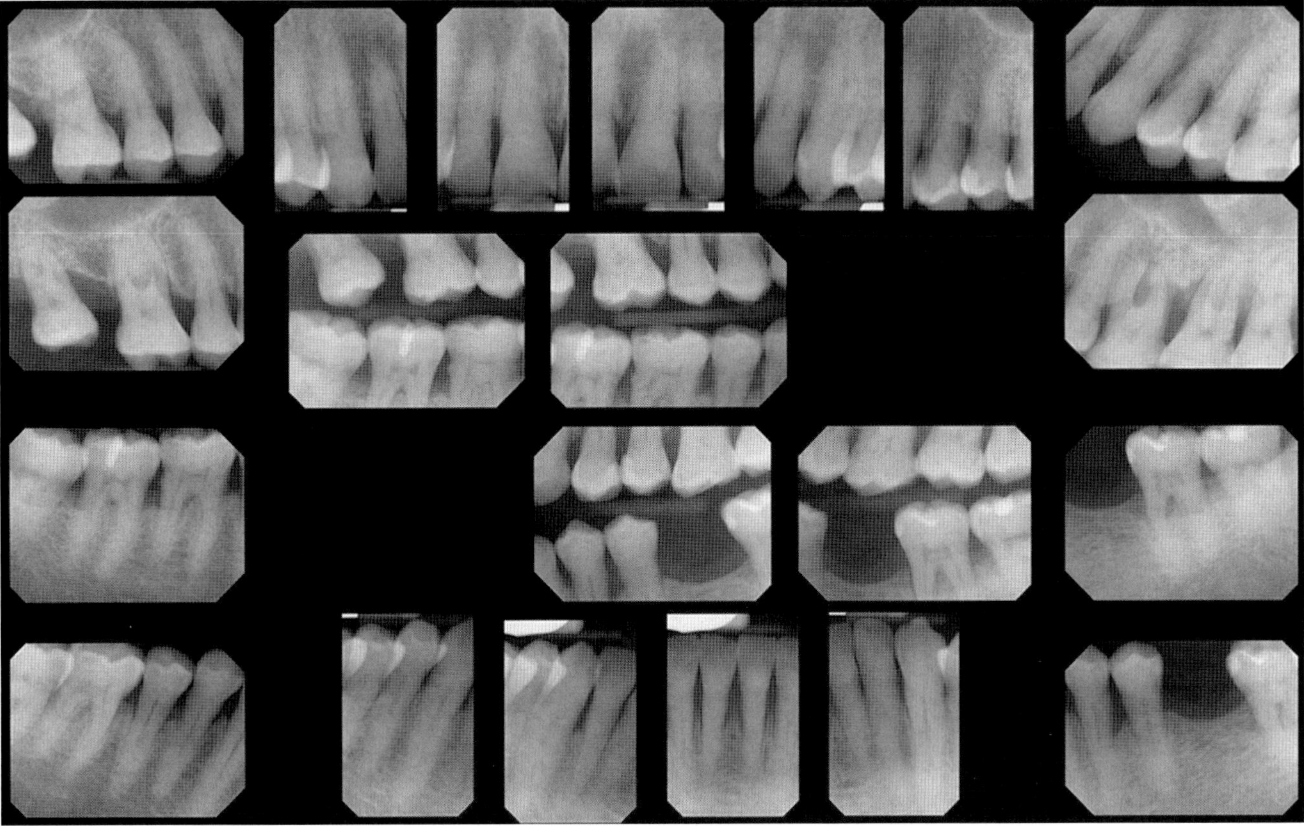

Fig. 39.6 Image display of a full-mouth radiographic series acquired using digital receptors. Specific features of the software program allow for image manipulation, measurements, and annotations.

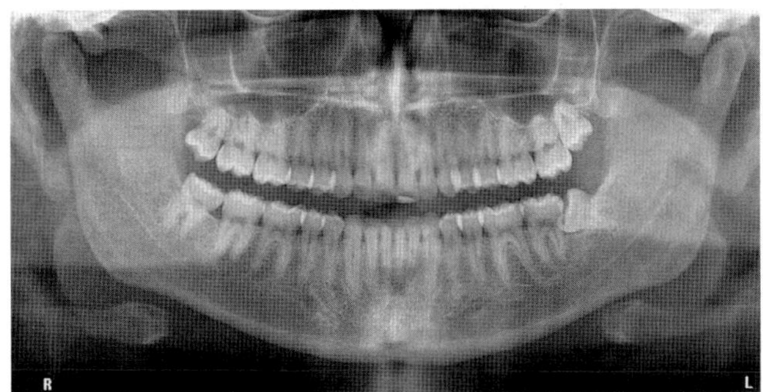

Fig. 39.7 Panoramic radiograph. Note the extended anatomic coverage relative to a full-mouth radiographic series.

Digital radiologic imaging offers additional conveniences for documentation of care. Providers can easily transmit images to other providers for consultation or transfer of care and to insurance companies and other payors. Digital radiologic images are typically stored with metadata that identifies the patient, exam date, and other information regarding the acquisition. Coupling this information along with the image pixel data allows an end user to accurately retrieve this information. The digital imaging and communication in medicine (DICOM) standard is an international standard that allows interoperability of this information, irrespective of the patient management software used by individual offices. This standard specifies how clinical and radiologic images are to be transmitted, stored, retrieved, archived, and displayed, allowing vendors to develop interoperable products for image display and archival.

More recently, artificial intelligence (AI) algorithms have been applied for image-based pattern recognition to highlight unusual patterns or areas of altered radiodensity. In dentomaxillofacial imaging, AI-based approaches have been developed to aid caries detection, score periodontal bone loss, and identify periapical lesions. Such products may facilitate radiologic review by presenting annotated images that are subsequently validated by the clinician (Fig. 39.9).

Cone-Beam Computed Tomography

Computed tomography (CT) is an advanced imaging technique that provides three-dimensional evaluation of the anatomy examined. In CT imaging, the x-ray source and detector revolve around the patient, acquiring projection images at hundreds of angles. Attenuation data from these projections are spatially reconstructed to provide a three-dimensional volumetric dataset that can be evaluated in multiple planes. CT imaging is dimensionally accurate and overcomes the limitations of image superimposition that are inherent to two-dimensional projection radiography. Maxillofacial cone-beam CT (CBCT) is a type of CT that uses an x-ray beam with a cone-shaped geometry to image the dentomaxillofacial hard tissues, including teeth and bones.[30,31] Depending on the extent of anatomy imaged, referred to as field of view (FOV), CBCT imaging protocols are categorized as:

- ***Limited*** FOV: Typically 3 to 5 cm and encompasses a dentoalveolar region with two to four teeth.
- ***Single arch*** FOV: Encompasses *one* dentoalveolar arch.
- ***Dentoalveolar*** FOV: Encompasses *both* dentoalveolar arches.
- ***Maxillofacial*** FOV: Encompasses the entire mandible and maxilla and part of the craniofacial skeleton extending cranially to the nasion.

In general, images acquired at a smaller FOV have a higher resolution. Imaging periodontal structures requires high resolution to detect the PDL space and the lamina dura, and thus limited, and single arch protocols are preferred to evaluate the teeth and periodontium in three dimensions.

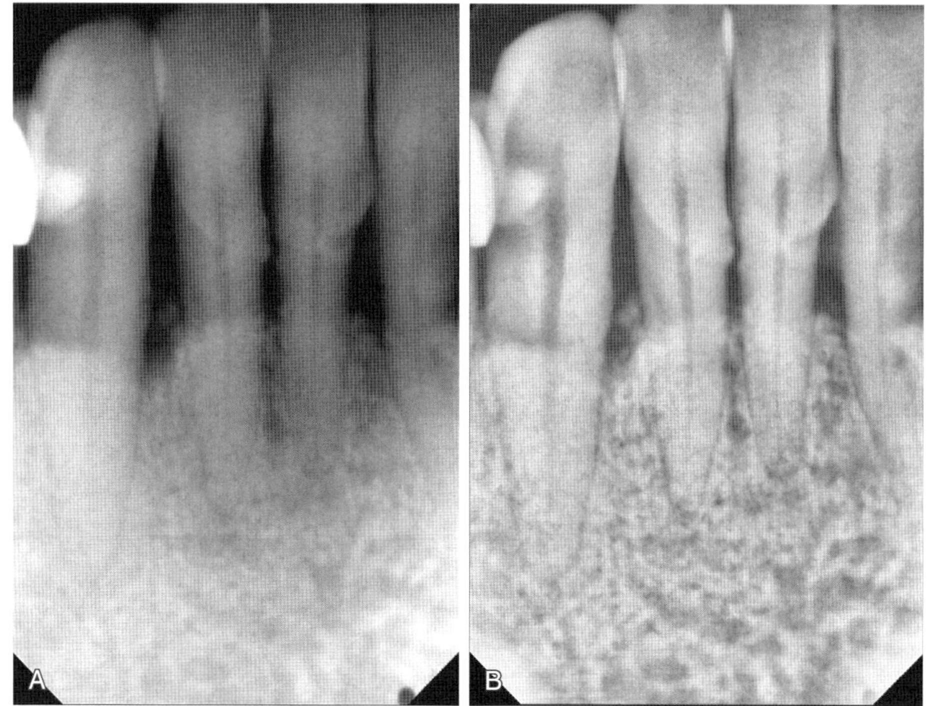

Fig. 39.8 (A) Periapical radiograph acquired with a digital complementary metal oxide semiconductor sensor. (B) Radiograph with a "perio" image enhancement filter applied to highlight the contrast of alveolar bone. Note the enhanced image highlights the contrast of calculus and the alveolar crest. Note artifactual radiolucent area adjacent to the restoration on the mandibular canine, which may be mistaken for caries.

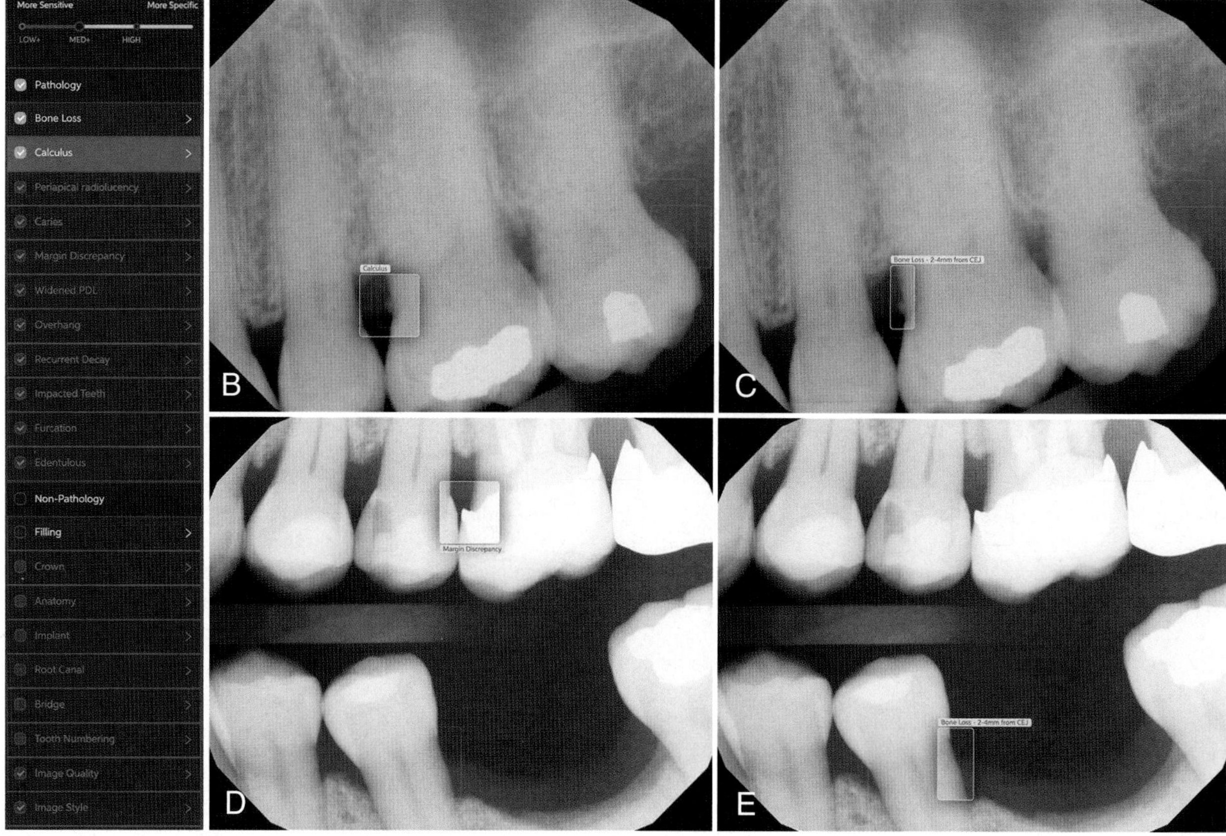

Fig. 39.9 Example of artificial intelligence–based assessments of relevance to periodontal evaluation. (A) Tool panel to select specific assessments. Note that the assessments parallel the assessments of morphology and disease that are performed during a systematic human radiologic evaluation of an intraoral radiograph. (B and C) Periapical radiograph with calculus deposits and bone loss highlighted by the program. (D and E) Bite-wing radiograph with an overhanging margin and periodontal bone loss highlighted by the program. (*Radiographs evaluated using "Second Opinion" [Pearl, West Hollywood, CA, USA], a computer vision platform for intraoral radiographic analysis. Images courtesy of Dr. Kyle Stanley.*)

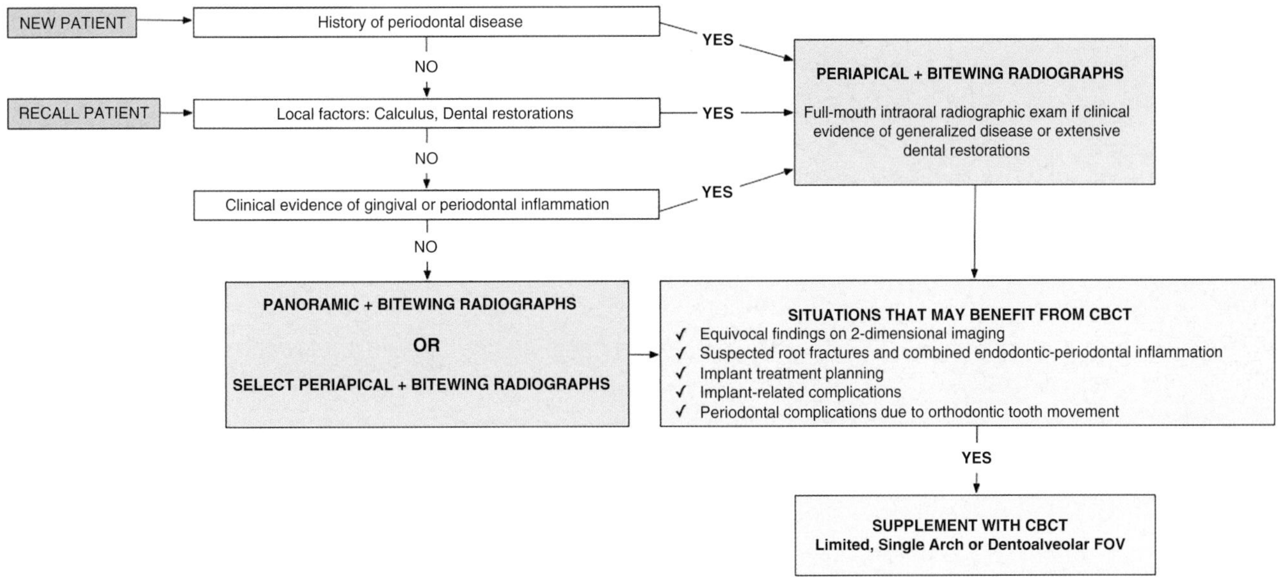

Fig 39.10 Flowchart to guide imaging evaluation of teeth and periodontal structures. The goal of this flowchart is to provide a broad guideline with respect to selection of radiographs in the management of periodontal conditions. The need and selection must be assessed on a case-by-case basis. Information collated from the recommendations, position statements, and best evidence reviews from the American Association of Endodontists,[7] the American Association of Oral and Maxillofacial Radiology,[7,33] the American Academy of Periodontology Best Evidence Reviews,[14,17,18,29] and the American Dental Association.[1]

Due to its inherent three-dimensional nature, CBCT provides significantly more information relative to intraoral and panoramic imaging. For example, interdental craters, an early sign of periodontal bone loss, is often masked on intraoral images but will be evident with multiplanar imaging. Specifically for periodontal management, two-dimensional imaging does not accurately depict the morphology of the periodontal defect—information that is important to determine disease severity and access to periodontal instrumentation, both important prognostic factors. Indeed, CBCT imaging is superior to intraoral imaging for identification of interdental craters, furcation involvement, and dehiscence and fenestration defects (see example in Fig. 39.17).[2,15,16] Despite these demonstrated advantages, an American Academy of Periodontology Best Evidence Review found limited evidence to justify CBCT imaging for routine diagnosis and treatment planning of moderate-to-severe (**stage II, III, or IV**) periodontitis.[14] Nevertheless, the review identified specific situations where CBCT imaging provides value beyond intraoral imaging. These include periodontal bone loss that has extended to the maxillary sinus or inferior alveolar canal, suspected endodontic and periodontal-endodontic lesions with equivocal findings on intraoral radiographs, to assess the periodontal impact of orthodontic tooth movement, and periodontal retreatment cases that fail to respond to localized therapy.[14,17,18,29]

LEARNING BOX 39.4

Intraoral radiographs provide adequate information for most periodontal diagnosis and treatment planning needs. In select situations, cone-beam computed tomography (CBCT) imaging provides useful information beyond that provided by conventional imaging and should be used to supplement conventional imaging in these cases (Fig. 39.10).

Selection of Appropriate Imaging

The decision to prescribe radiologic imaging is based on:

- The *diagnostic objectives* to be accomplished by imaging—the minimum essential information that is needed to diagnose and manage the patient,
- The *diagnostic efficacy* of the radiologic procedure—the ability of the radiologic technique to provide the required information,
- The *radiation-associated risks* of the procedure—to ensure that the benefits from the radiologic procedure far exceed the associated risk of radiation-induced cancer, the only risk of significance from maxillofacial radiologic imaging, and
- The *cost of imaging*—to ensure that the added benefits from imaging are provided at an appropriate cost.

Table 39.1 provides information on the radiation doses and associated risks from select radiologic examinations. Relative to most radiologic procedures used in health care, doses from dental radiologic examinations are low and are considered low risk. Thus the decisions to select an imaging technique are driven predominantly by its efficacy and cost. Fig. 39.10 provides guidance for imaging of the teeth and periodontal structures based on current evidence and recommended best practices. This imaging algorithm considers benefits, costs, and risks and is based on current evidence and follows the recommendations of the American Association of Endodontists,[7] the American Association of Oral and Maxillofacial Radiology,[7,33] the American Academy of Periodontology,[14,17,18,29] and the American Dental Association.[1]

Normal Interdental Bone

Standard radiologic assessments for periodontal disease use intraoral radiographs.[1] On these projections the facial and lingual bony plates are obscured by the relatively dense root structure (Fig. 39.11D). Thus evaluation of bone changes in periodontal disease is based predominantly on the appearance of the interdental bone. It is important to recognize normal appearances of the interdental bone—periodontal bone loss is categorized based on the extent and the pattern of resorption relative to this normal interdental bone level. Fig. 39.11 outlines a systematic approach to periodontal bone evaluation on intraoral radiographs.

The boundaries of the interdental bone are the cortical outlines of the tooth socket and the alveolar crest. The tooth socket appears as a thin, radiopaque line adjacent to the PDL and is referred to as

TABLE 39.1 Radiation Doses and Risks From Dentomaxillofacial Radiologic Imaging

Examination	Effective Dose (mSv)[a]	Equivalent Background Radiation[b]	Estimated Cancer Risk[c]	Relative Radiation Level[d]
4 Bite-wing radiographs	0.005	<1 day	1 in 4 million	☢☢
Air travel, Los Angeles to New York, 5 h	0.015	~1.5 days		
Panoramic, direct digital	0.02	~2 days	1 in a million	☢☢
Full mouth, digital sensor, rectangular collimation	0.03	~3 days	1 in 600,000	☢
Air travel, Los Angeles to Osaka, 15 h	0.045	~5 days		
CBCT, limited FOV	0.05	~6 days	1 in 400,000	☢
Full mouth, digital sensor, round collimation	0.1	~12 days	1 in 200,000	☢☢
CBCT, dentoalveolar				☢☢
Air travel, Los Angeles to Singapore, round trip, 33 h	0.1	~12 days		
CBCT, maxillofacial with cranium	0.15	~2 weeks	1 in 130,000	☢☢
Mammogram	0.4	~7 weeks	1 in 50,000	☢☢
MDCT, maxillofacial	0.8	~14 weeks	1 in 25,000	☢☢
MDCT, chest	7.0	~2 years	1 in 3000	☢☢☢

[a]Median effective doses of typical imaging protocols collated from multiple published studies.
[b]Equivalent background radiation is based on the average annual US background exposure of 3.1 mSv.
[c]Cancer risk estimated at 5.5%/Sv as per ICRP publication no. 103.
[d]Relative radiation levels. From American College of Radiology. *ACR Appropriateness Criteria.* Available at https://www.acr.org/-/media/ACR/Files/Appropriateness-Criteria/RadiationDoseAssessmentIntro.pdf.

CBCT, Cone-beam computed tomography; *FOV,* field of view; *MDCT,* multidetector computed tomography.
Adapted from Table 2 in Mallya SM. Effective and safe use of x-rays: understanding the risks for decision-making. *J Calif Dent Assoc.* 2021;49:301–309.[16]

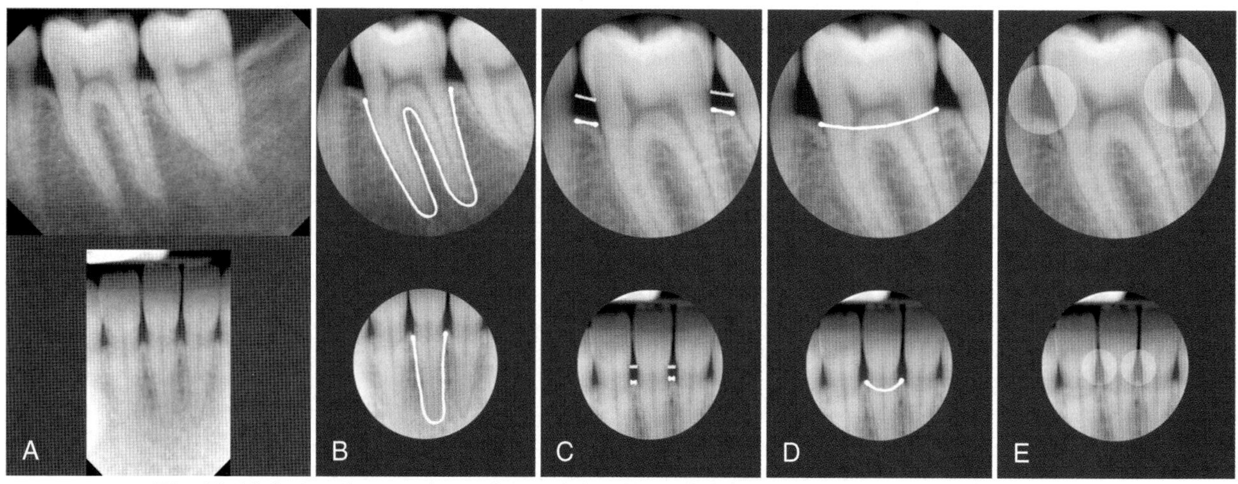

Fig. 39.11 Systematic approach to evaluate periodontal bone. (A) Periapical radiographs of the mandibular posterior region *(top)* and mandibular anterior region *(bottom).* (B) Evaluate the lamina dura *(white lines)* for continuity, in particular, in the furcation region. (C) Identify the line joining the adjacent cementoenamel junctions *(yellow line).* The interdental bone level (*white* line) is normally 1 to 2 mm below this line. (D) Trace the contour of the facial and lingual alveolar crest over the roots and examine their relation to the furcation. (E) Examine the embrasure spaces *(yellow highlight)* for evidence of calculus or overhanging restoration margins.

the *lamina dura* (see Fig. 39.11B).[3] The shape and position of the root and changes in the angulation of the x-ray beam produce considerable variations in the appearance of the lamina dura.[35] When the x-ray photons traverse a longer distance through the cortical bone, the lamina dura appears as a well-demarcated radiopaque line. When the x-ray photons intersect a shorter segment of the lamina dura, the resultant image is less distinct and thinner. Outlining the lamina dura identifies the margin of the interdental bone. In particular, evaluate the lamina dura in the furcation region to help identify early furcation involvement (see Fig. 39.11B).

Likewise, the cortical bone at the alveolar crest is also depicted as a thin radiopaque line between adjacent teeth. The width and shape of the interdental bone and the angle of the crest normally vary with the convexity of the proximal tooth surfaces and the relative levels of the cementoenamel junction (CEJ) of the approximating teeth. The dimension of the interdental bone is determined by the width of the proximal root surface and space between approximal teeth. In the posterior dentition, the crestal table of the interdental bone appears as a corticated line parallel to a line between the CEJs of the approximating teeth and approximately 1 to 2 mm below this line

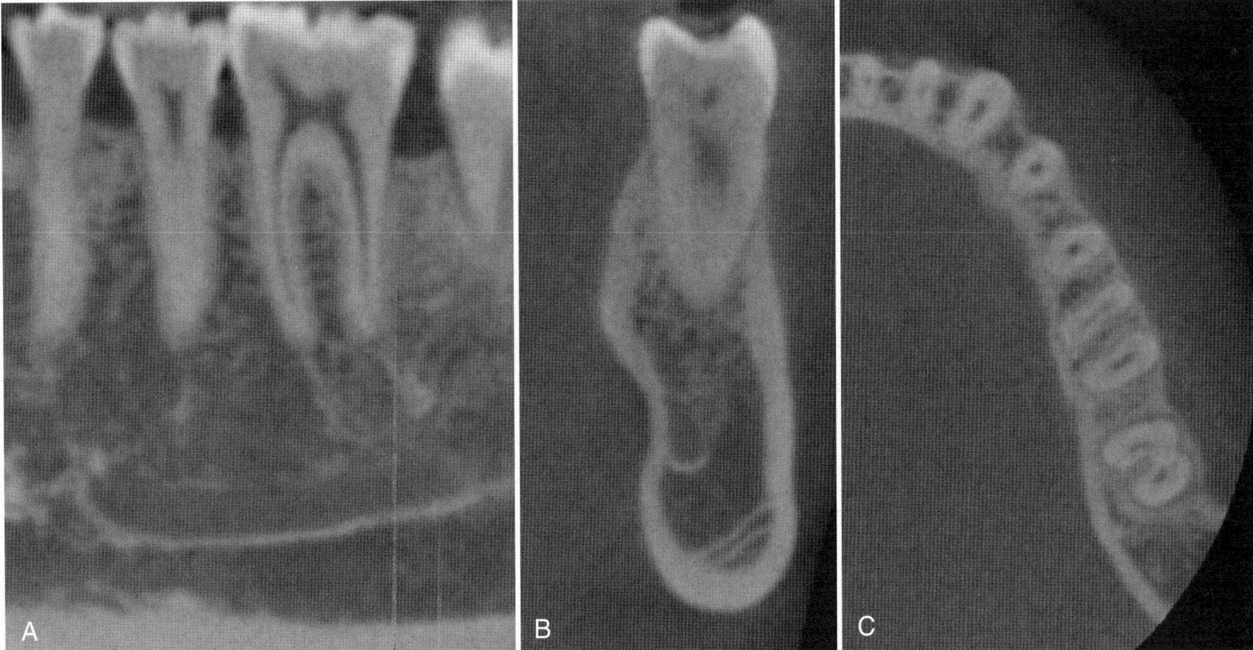

Fig. 39.12 Evaluation of periodontal bone on cone-beam computed tomography (CBCT) examinations. (A) Sagittal plane sections resemble the projection of a periapical radiograph and the lamina dura and periodontal ligament (PDL) space should be examined along the root length and in the furcation. (B) Coronal plane section shows the facial and lingual plates and the crest height on the root surface. (C) Axial section shows the PDL circumferentially around the root and continuity of the facial and lingual bone adjacent to the roots. Videos corresponding the CBCT sections presented in this figure are available on the Expert Consult version of the book.

(see Fig. 39.11C, top panel). When there is a difference in the level of the CEJs, as with tooth migration or tipping, the crest of the interdental bone appears inclined, relative to the crowns. In the anterior dentition, the interproximal spaces are narrower, and the interdental bone is triangular in shape (see Fig. 39.11C, bottom panel).

The dense root structure superimposes over and masks the facial and lingual plates of the tooth socket. On close examination, the crest of the facial and lingual plates can be identified as a faint radiopaque line across the root surface (see Fig. 39.11D). When the extent of loss of the buccal and lingual plates differs, two distinct bone levels may be apparent over the root surface.

In addition to evaluation of periodontal bone, radiographs also depict calculus deposits or faulty contours of restorations—local factors that increase risk for periodontal disease. Radiologic evaluation must include an assessment for the presence of these risk factors and their impact on the adjacent periodontal bone (see Fig. 39.11D).

The same systematic approach is also applied to the evaluation of periodontal bone support on CBCT examinations (Fig. 39.12). For evaluation of periodontal bone support, limited FOV scans depict the PDL space, lamina dura, and trabecular bone with high detail. The width of the PDL is approximately 0.2 mm, and imaging protocols with pixel dimensions less than 0.15 mm provide optimal evaluation of periodontal defects.[15] Unlike with conventional imaging, sectional imaging displays the lamina dura and PDL spaces on all the root surfaces, and these structures must be evaluated in the sagittal, coronal, and axial planes (see Fig. 39.12).

LEARNING BOX 39.5

A systematic approach to evaluation of radiographic images of teeth and periodontal bone on radiographs facilitates consistent detection and categorization of osseous changes. These changes must be interpreted in the context of clinical findings including probing depths, clinical attachment loss, and clinical manifestations of inflammation.

Radiographic Appearance of Periodontal Disease

Early destructive changes of bone that do not remove sufficient mineralized tissue cannot be captured on radiographs. Therefore radiographic manifestations suggest that the disease has progressed beyond its initial stages.[5] The earliest signs of periodontal disease must be detected clinically. Radiographic changes of periodontal inflammation follow the pathophysiology of periodontal tissue destruction and include the following:

1. *Fuzziness and disruption of lamina dura and crestal cortication* are the earliest radiographic changes of periodontitis (Fig. 39.13A–B) and results from bone resorption activated by extension of gingival inflammation into the periodontal bone. Depicting these early changes depends greatly on the radiographic technique and on anatomic variations (thickness and density of interdental bone, position of adjoining teeth). The presence of crestal lamina dura on radiographs is associated with periodontal stability,[25,26] but its absence is not associated with clinical inflammation, bleeding on probing, periodontal pockets, or loss of attachment.[9] Therefore the presence of an intact crestal lamina dura is considered an indicator of periodontal health, whereas its absence does not always imply periodontal disease.
2. Continued periodontal bone loss and widening of the periodontal space results in a *wedge-shaped radiolucency* at the mesial or distal aspect of the crest (see Fig. 39.13A–B). The apex of the area is pointed in the direction of the root.
3. Subsequently, the destructive process extends across the alveolar crest, reducing the height of the interdental bone. As increased osteoclastic activity results in increased bone resorption along the endosteal margins of the medullary spaces, the remaining interdental bone may appear partially eroded (see Fig. 39.13C).
4. The height of the interdental septum is progressively reduced by the extension of inflammation and the resorption of bone (see Fig. 39.13D).

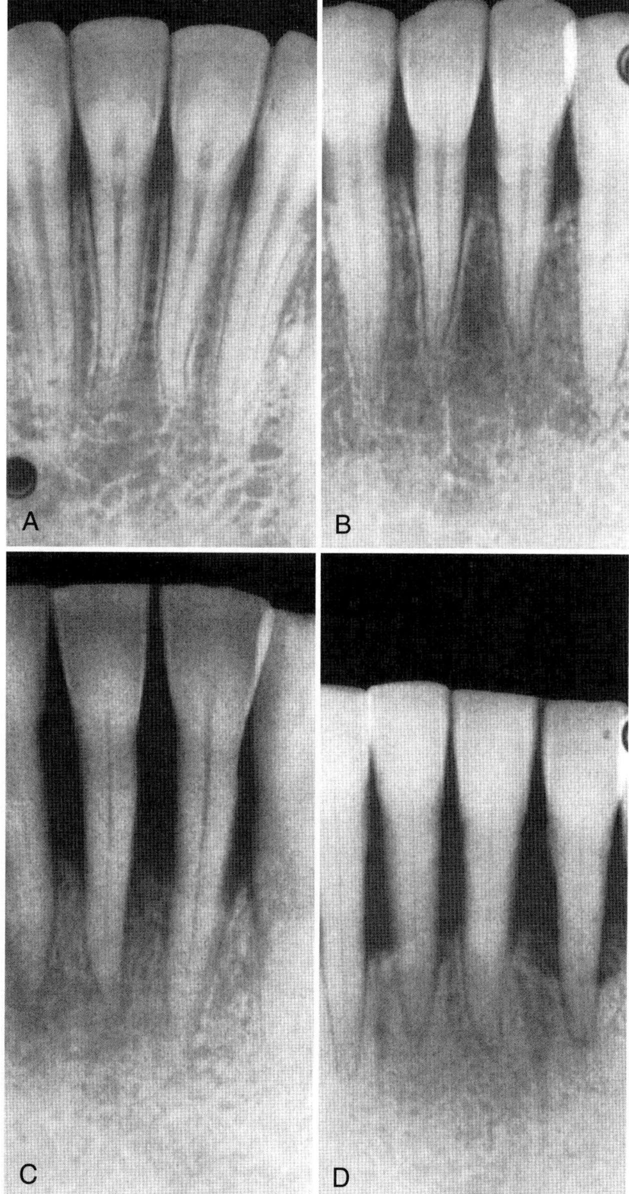

Fig. 39.13 Radiographic changes in periodontitis. (A) Normal appearance of interdental bone. (B) Fuzziness and a break in the continuity of the lamina dura at the crest of the bone distal to the central incisor *(left)*. There are wedge-shaped radiolucent areas at the crest of the other interdental bone. (C) Radiolucent projections from the crest into the interdental bone indicate extension of destructive processes. (D) Severe bone loss.

5. Frequently a radiopaque horizontal line can be observed across the roots of a tooth. This opaque line demarcates the portion of the root where the labial or lingual bony plate has been partially or completely destroyed from the remaining bone-supported portion (Fig. 39.14 and see Fig 39.11D).

LEARNING BOX 39.6

The earliest changes of periodontal disease often do not manifest on radiographs. Even when radiographic changes are evident, radiographic examination may underestimate the extent of bone loss. Thus determination of periodontal health should be based on clinical and radiologic findings.

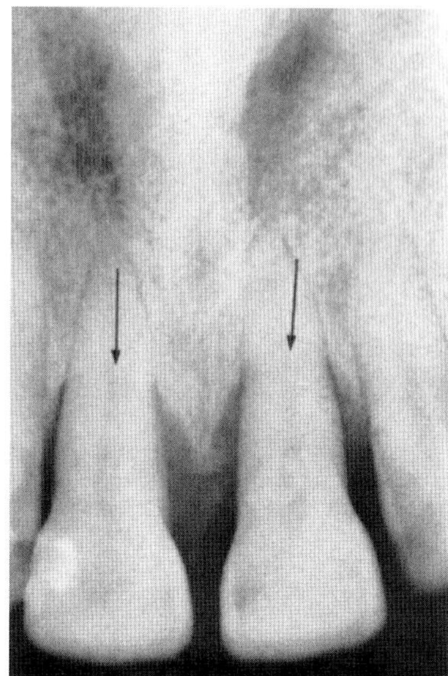

Fig. 39.14 Horizontal lines across the roots of the central incisors *(arrows)*. The area of the roots below the horizontal lines is partially or completely denuded of the facial and lingual bony plates.

Radiographic Bone Loss

Bone loss is the final manifestation of the periodontal inflammatory process. The radiographic image tends to underestimate the severity of bone loss. The difference between the alveolar crest height and the radiographic appearance ranges from 0 to 1.6 mm, mostly accounted for by x-ray angulation.[28] Radiologic assessment of bone loss must include both the amount of bone loss and the distribution and pattern of bone destruction.

Radiographs are an indirect method for determining the amount of bone loss in periodontal disease; they show the amount of remaining bone rather than the amount lost. The amount of bone lost is estimated to be the difference between the physiologic bone level and the height of the remaining bone. Several investigators have analyzed the distance from the CEJ to the alveolar crest—it is generally accepted that the alveolar crest is less than 2 mm from this reference line.[9,10,13,28] Current periodontal disease staging and grading relies on radiographic bone loss (RBL) at the site of greatest loss.[32] RBL is categorized based on the extent of bone loss along the root length (Fig. 39.15), with increasing bone loss associated with later stage disease. Refer to Chapter 5 for detailed description of staging and grading criteria of periodontitis. The distribution of bone loss is an important assessment. It identifies the locations of destructive local factors in different areas of the mouth and in relation to different surfaces of the same tooth.

Patterns of Bone Destruction

Periodontal bone loss changes the height and contour of the bone. The patterns of bone destruction are broadly categorized as horizontal bone loss and vertical or angular defects. Refer to Chapter 22 for details on bone loss patterns. In horizontal bone loss, the height of interdental bone is reduced with the crest perpendicular to the long axis of the adjacent teeth (Fig 39.16A). In contrast, vertical or angular defects are oblique troughlike bone loss adjacent to the root surface, with base of the defect located apically (see Fig 39.16B). The defects are classified as *one-*, *two-*, or *three*-wall defects, depending on the number of bony walls that surround the defect (see Fig 22.39). Contiguous defects that form a trough along more than one surface are called *circumferential* defects.

The internal morphology and depth of vertical defects are not apparent on two-dimensional radiographs. Furthermore, radiographs

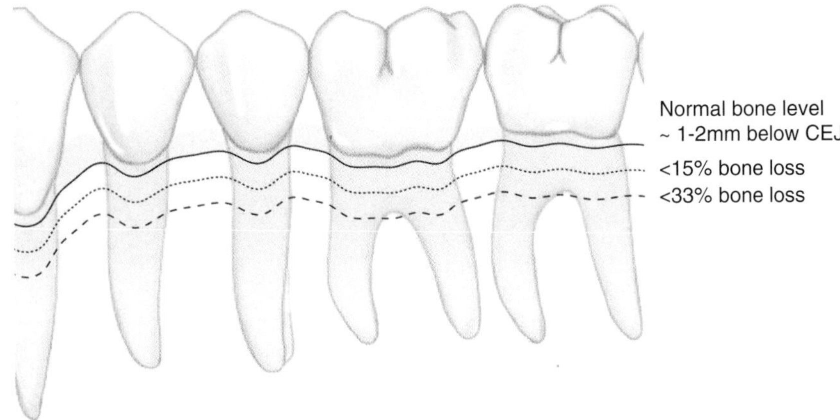

Fig. 39.15 Scoring radiographic bone loss for periodontal disease staging. Note that bone loss extending to and beyond the middle third of the root may involve the furcation of molar teeth. (*Modified from Mallya S, Lam E.* White and Pharoah's Oral Radiology. *8th ed. Mosby.*)

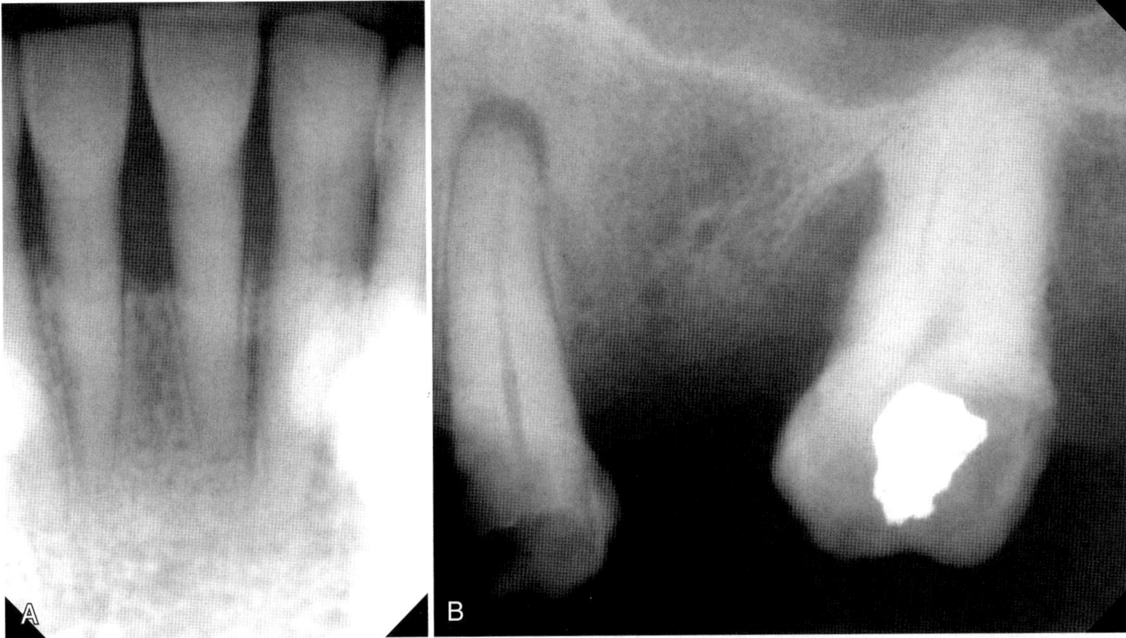

Fig. 39.16 (A) Horizontal bone loss. (B) Vertical or angular defect.

do not reveal the extent of involvement on the facial and lingual surfaces. Bone destruction of facial and lingual surfaces is masked by the dense root structure, and bone destruction on the mesial and distal root surfaces may be partially hidden by superimposed anatomy, such as a dense mylohyoid ridge (Fig. 39.17). In most cases, it can be assumed that bone loss seen interdentally continues in either the facial or lingual aspect, creating a troughlike lesion. Bone loss along the facial and lingual alveolar crest is apparent on CBCT examination, best visualized on cross-sectional images (Fig. 39.18).

Dense cortical facial and lingual plates of interdental bone obscure destruction of the intervening cancellous bone. Thus a deep, craterlike defect between the facial and lingual plates might not be depicted on conventional radiographs. To record destruction of the interproximal cancellous bone radiographically, the cortical bone must be involved. A reduction of only 0.5 to 1 mm in the thickness of the cortical plate is sufficient to permit radiographic visualization of the destruction of the inner cancellous trabeculae.

Interdental craters are a specific type of two-wall defect—they are concavities in the interdental bone between the facial and lingual plates. Interdental craters are common manifestations of periodontal destruction and constitute a third of osseous defects. They are more common in the mandible, especially in the posterior regions. Radiographically, interdental craters are recognized as irregular areas of reduced density on the alveolar bone crests. Craters are generally not sharply demarcated but gradually blend

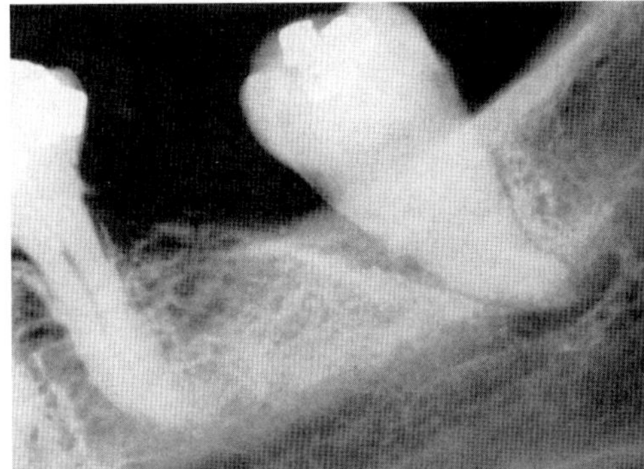

Fig. 39.17 Angular bone loss on mandibular molar partially obscured by a dense mylohyoid ridge.

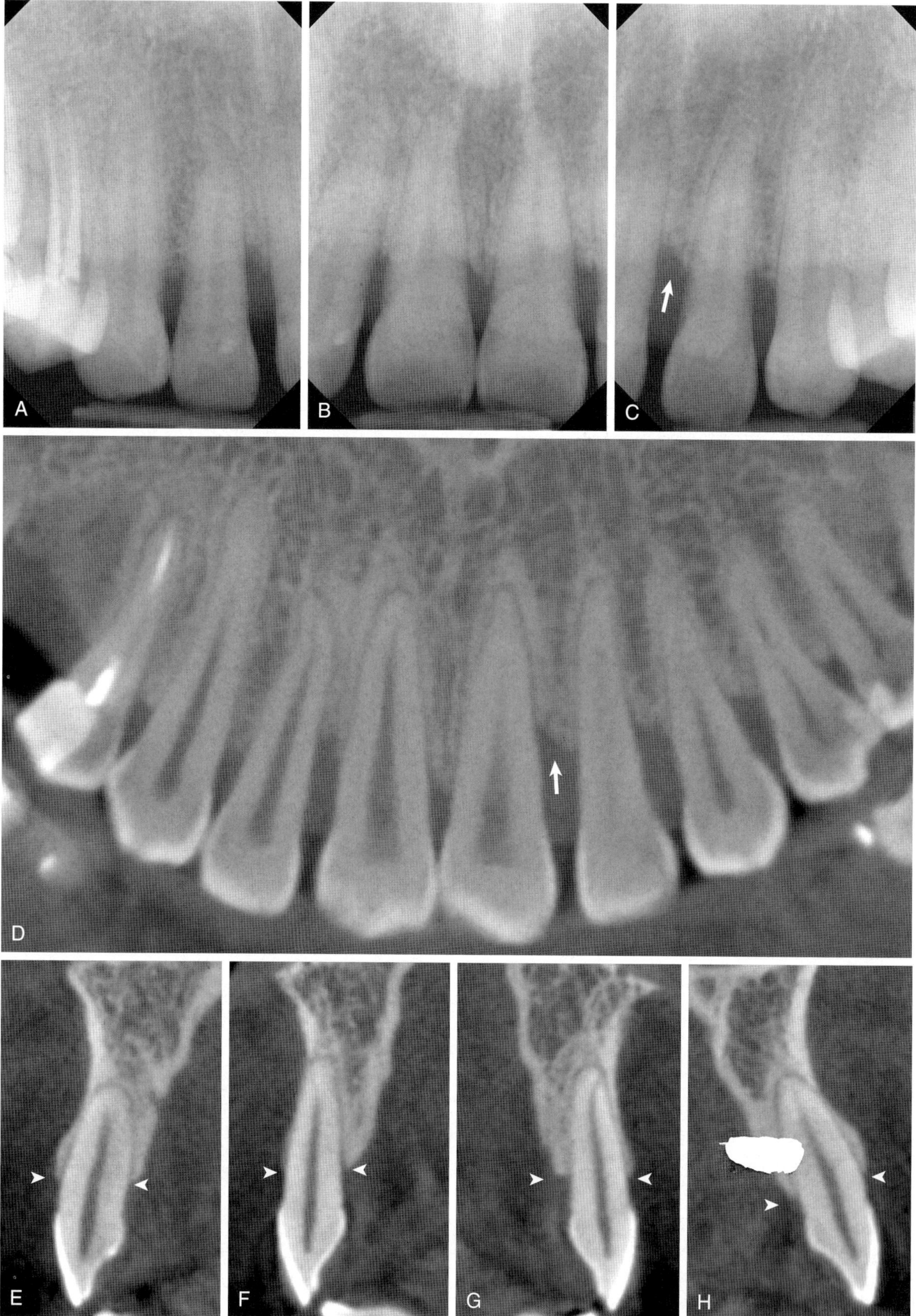

Fig. 39.18 Cone-beam computed tomography (CBCT) examination of the anterior maxilla. (A–C). Periapical radiographs show horizontal bone loss and a vertical defect between the left maxillary central incisor and the maxillary left lateral incisor *(arrow)*. (D). Panoramic reconstruction of a CBCT examination depicting the vertical periodontal defect noted in panel A *(arrow)*. (E–H). Cross-sections through the long axes of the maxillary incisors. The height of the crestal bone is evident *(arrow heads)*. Note that the facial bone adjacent to the maxillary right central incisor (panel F) is markedly thin.

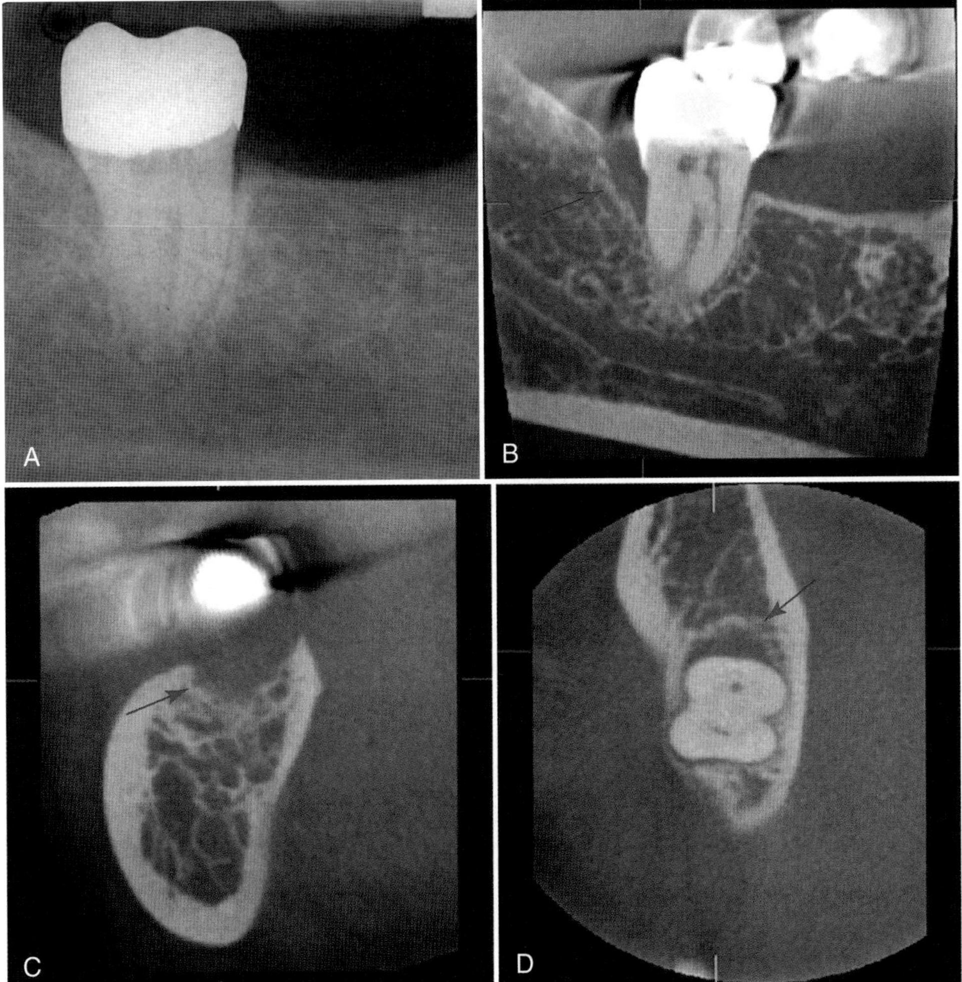

Fig. 39.19 Periapical radiograph (A) and sagittal (B), cross-sectional (C), and axial (D) cone-beam computed tomography (CBCT) sections of the mandibular right second molar. No periodontal defect is apparent on the periapical radiograph. However, CBCT images clearly illustrate a deep, vertical, three-wall defect on the distal surface of the mandibular right second molar *(red arrow)*.

with the rest of the bone. Conventional radiographs do not accurately depict the morphology or depth of interdental craters, which sometimes appear as vertical defects. CBCT imaging allows for better evaluation of the three-dimensional morphology of the defect (Fig. 39.19).

Interdental bone loss may continue facially or lingually to form a troughlike defect that could be difficult to interpret on radiographs. These lesions may terminate on the radicular surface or may communicate with the adjacent interdental area to form one continuous lesion (Fig 39.20).

Fig. 39.21 shows two adjacent interdental lesions connecting on the radicular surface to form one interconnecting osseous lesion. In addition to clinical probing to identify pocket depth, imaging with a radiopaque pointer, such as a gutta percha point, placed into the defect will demonstrate the extent of the bone loss.

Periodontal bone loss should be differentiated from normal anatomy or anatomic variants that can resemble disease. For example, nutrient canals in the alveolar bone can appear as linear and circular radiolucent areas (Fig 39.22). These canals can be seen more frequently in the anterior mandible, although they can be present throughout the alveolar ridge.

Finally, as emphasized earlier, radiographs can assess only the amount of existing periodontal bone to deduce the extent of prior bone loss. However, it is sometimes necessary to determine whether the reduced bone level is the result of periodontal disease that is no longer destructive (usually after treatment and proper maintenance)

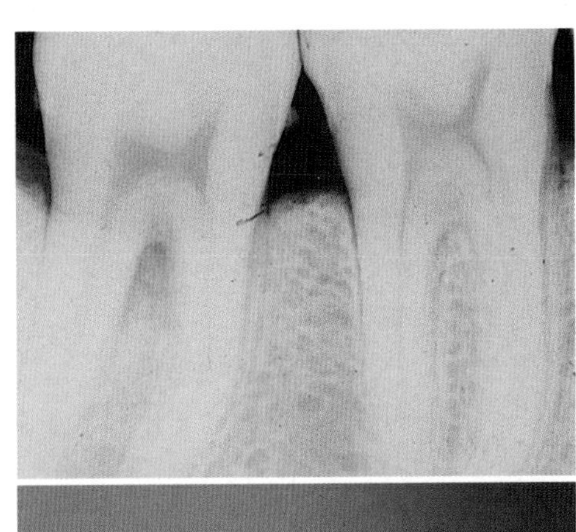

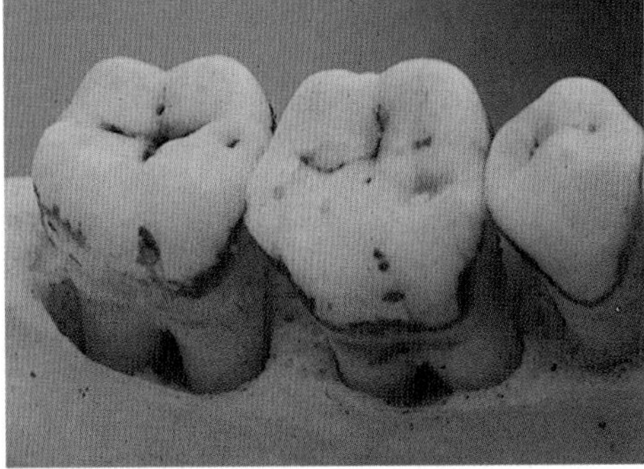

Fig. 39.20 Interdental lesion that extends to the facial or lingual surfaces in a troughlike manner.

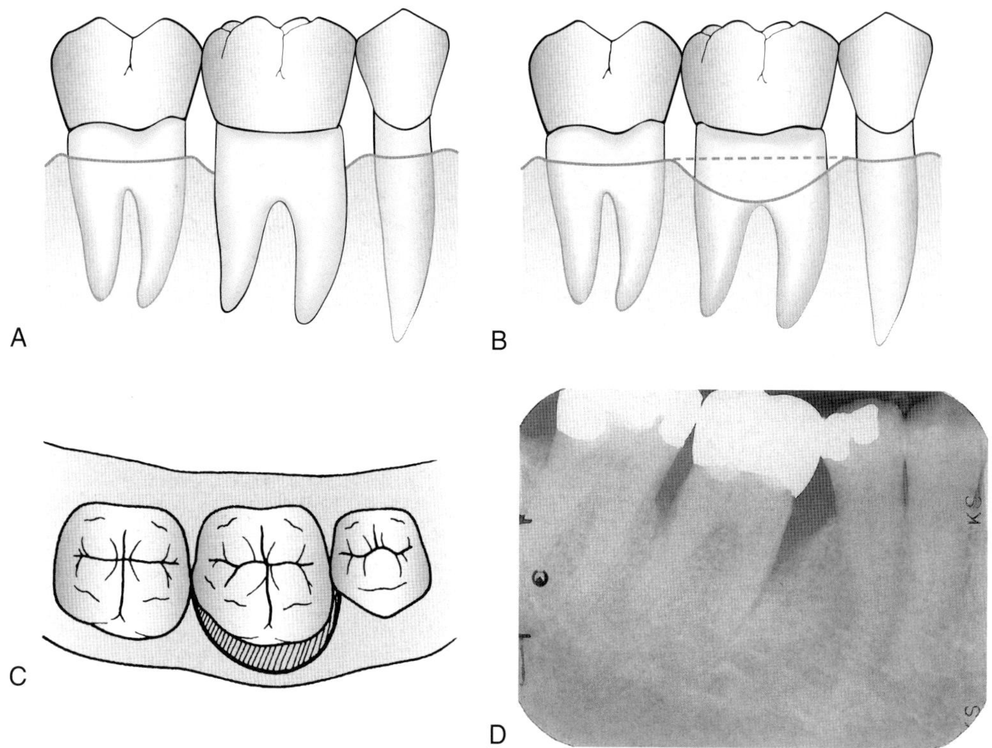

Fig. 39.21 (A) Interdental mesial and distal lesions. (B) Facial or lingual outlines of the actual lesion. (C) Occlusal view of the lesion. (D) Radiograph of mesial and facial lesions.

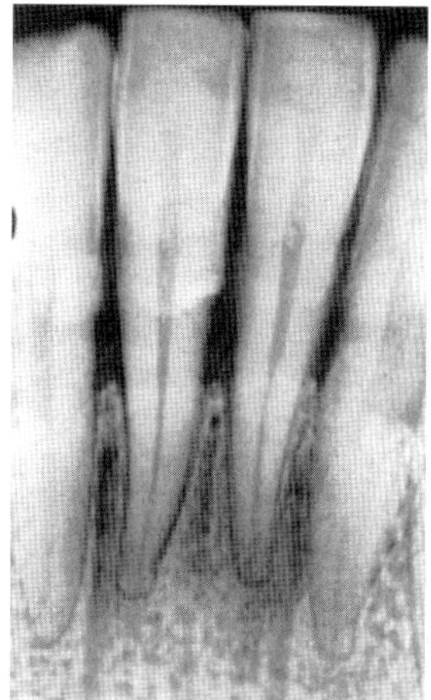

Fig. 39.22 Prominent nutrient canals in the mandible.

or whether active periodontal disease is present. Differentiation between treated versus active periodontal disease can only be achieved by clinical assessment.

Furcation Involvement

Definitive diagnosis of furcation involvement is made by clinical examination, which includes careful probing with a specially designed probe (e.g., Nabers). Radiographs are helpful, but root superimposition, caused by anatomic variations or improper technique, can obscure bone loss in the furcation. As a general rule, bone loss is greater than it appears in the radiograph. A tooth may present marked furcation involvement in one image (Fig. 39.23A) but appear to be uninvolved in another (see Fig. 39.23B). Radiographs should be taken at different angles to reduce the risk of missing furcation involvement.

A large, clearly defined radiolucency in the furcation area is easy to identify (see Fig. 39.23A), but less clearly defined radiographic

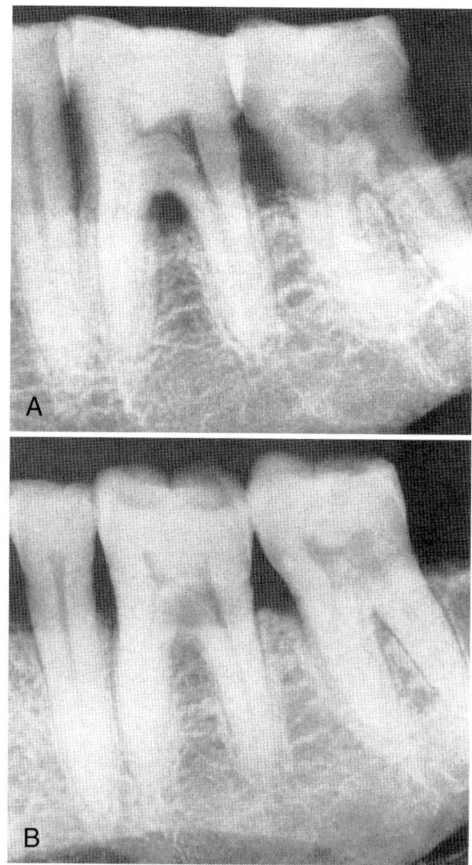

Fig. 39.23 (A) Furcation involvement indicated by triangular radiolucency in the bifurcation area of mandibular first molar. The second molar presents only a slight thickening of the periodontal space in the bifurcation area. (B) Radiograph of the same region as in A with different angulation. The triangular radiolucency in the bifurcation of the first molar is obliterated, and furcation involvement of the second molar is apparent.

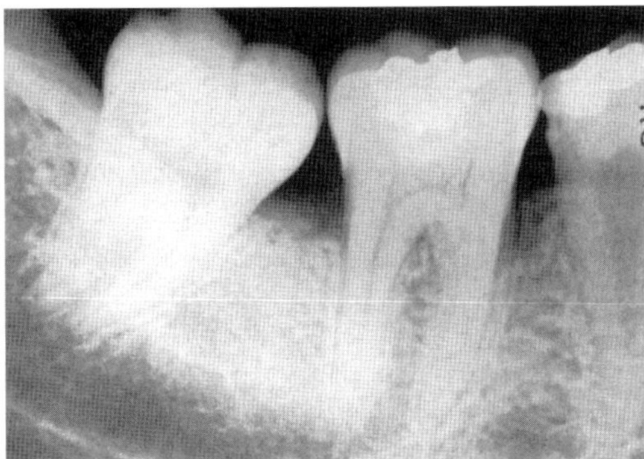

Fig. 39.24 Early furcation involvement suggested by fuzziness in the furcation of the mandibular first molar, particularly when associated with bone loss on the roots.

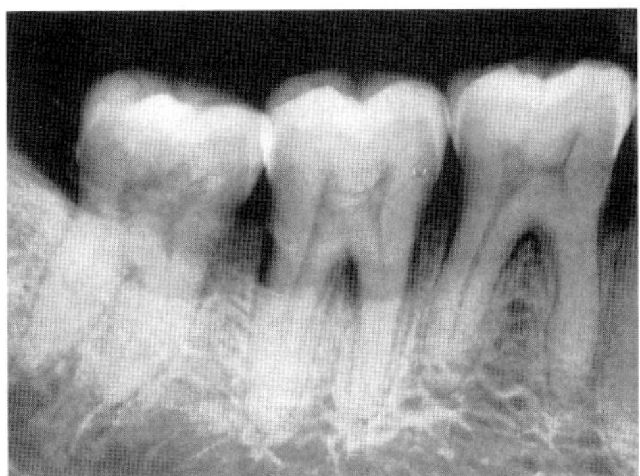

Fig. 39.25 Furcation involvement of mandibular first and second molars indicated by thickening of the periodontal space in the furcation area. The furcation of the third molar is also involved, but the thickening of the periodontal space is partially obscured by the external oblique line.

changes are often overlooked. To assist in the radiographic detection of furcation involvement, the following evaluation scheme is suggested:

1. The slightest radiographic change in the furcation area should be investigated clinically, especially if there is bone loss on adjacent roots (Fig. 39.24 and 39.27A).
2. Diminished radiodensity in the furcation area in which outlines of bony trabeculae are visible suggests furcation involvement (Fig. 39.25 and 39.27A).
3. Whenever there is marked bone loss in relation to a single molar root, it may be assumed that furcation is also involved (Fig. 39.26 and 39.27A).

Bone loss patterns and furcation involvement is often masked by superimposition of teeth and osseous structures on intraoral radiographs. The complexity of the bone loss extent and pattern is better depicted on CBCT images, especially for multirooted teeth (see Fig. 39.27).

Periodontal Abscess

The typical radiographic appearance of a periodontal abscess is a discrete area of radiolucency along the lateral aspect of the root (Figs. 39.28 and 39.29). However, the radiographic manifestation is often not characteristic (Fig. 39.30). This can be due to the following:

1. *The stage of the lesion.* The early stages of an acute periodontal abscess are extremely painful but present no radiographic changes.

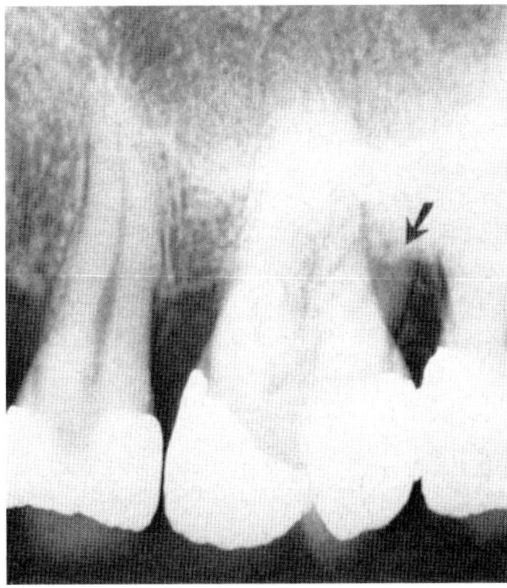

Fig. 39.26 Furcation involvement of the first molar partially obscured by the radiopaque lingual root. The horizontal line across the distobuccal root demarcates the apical portion *(arrow),* which is covered by bone, from the remainder of the root, where the bone has been destroyed.

2. *The extent of bone destruction and the morphologic changes of the bone.*
3. *The location of the* ***abscess****.* Lesions in the soft tissue wall of a periodontal pocket are less likely to produce radiographic changes than those deep in the supporting tissues. Abscesses on the facial or lingual surface are obscured by the radiopacity of the root; interproximal lesions are more likely to be visualized radiographically.

Therefore radiographs alone cannot provide a final diagnosis of a periodontal abscess but need to be accompanied by careful clinical examination.

Clinical Probing

Regenerative and resective flap designs and incisions require prior knowledge of the underlying osseous topography. Careful probing of these pocket areas ("bone sounding") after scaling and root instrumentation often requires local anesthesia and definitive radiographic evaluation of the osseous lesions. Radiographs taken with periodontal probes, gutta-percha points, or other indicators (e.g., Hirschfeld pointers) placed into the anesthetized pocket show the true extent of the bone lesion. As indicated previously, the attachment level on the radicular surface or interdental lesions with thick facial or lingual bone cannot be visualized in the radiograph. The use of radiopaque indicators is an efficient and necessary diagnostic aid (Fig. 39.31).

Localized Aggressive Periodontitis

Prior classifications of periodontal disease considered "aggressive periodontitis" as a separate entity distinct from other forms of periodontal inflammation. However, the distinction between these two entities has not been consistently applied. Currently, there is no evidence that these disease patterns are due to distinct pathophysiologic pathways, and the evidence to consider them as separate diseases is inconsistent.[8,32] In the 2018 disease classification, in addition to localized and generalized extent categories, "molar-incisor pattern" was added, which is now used to describe the previous disease category "localized aggressive periodontitis." As the name suggests, in this condition, the radiographic bone loss (mostly vertical) typically occurs in younger individuals and is restricted primarily to first molars and incisors.

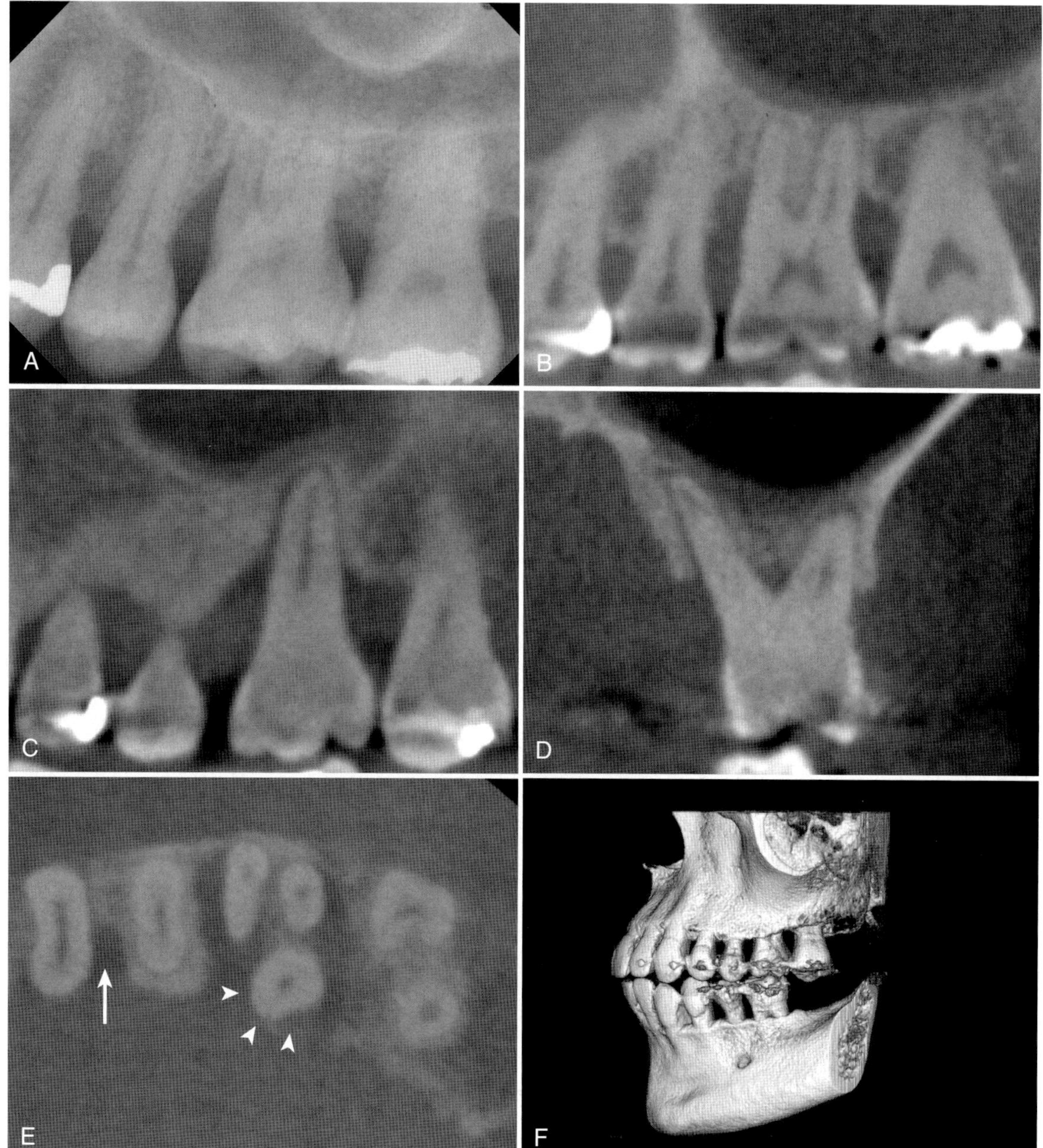

Fig. 39.27 (A). Periapical radiograph showing a vertical defect on the mesial and distal aspects of the maxillary first molar. The palatal root is superimposed over the furcation. (B) Sagittal section through the maxillary first molar buccal roots. Note clear depiction of extent of bone loss along the root length. (C) Sagittal section through the palatal root. Note that bone loss along this root is underestimated on the periapical radiograph. (D) Coronal section through the furcation of the maxillary first molar. Note bone loss between the palatal and mesiobuccal root that is not evident of the periapical radiograph in panel A. (E). Axial section at a level immediately apical to the furcation. Note bone loss along the mesiobuccal root extending to cause palatal dehiscence and merging with the circumferential bone loss around the palatal root *(arrow heads)*. Note palatal bone loss between the premolars *(arrows)* that is obscured on the periapical radiograph in panel A by the remnant interdental bone. (F) Volume-rendered cone-beam computed tomography (CBCT) image. Videos corresponding the CBCT sections presented in this figure are available on the Expert Consult version of the book.

Trauma From Occlusion

Trauma from occlusion can produce radiographically detectable changes in the thickness of the lamina dura, morphology of the alveolar crest, width of the PDL space, and density of the surrounding cancellous bone.

Traumatic lesions manifest more clearly in faciolingual aspects because mesiodistally the tooth has added stability provided by the contact areas with adjacent teeth. Therefore slight variations in the proximal surfaces may indicate greater changes in the facial and lingual aspects. *The radiographic changes listed next are not pathognomonic for trauma from occlusion and must be interpreted in combination with clinical findings,* particularly tooth mobility, presence of wear facets, pocket depth, and analysis of occlusal contacts and habits.

The *injury phase* of trauma from occlusion produces a loss of the lamina dura that may be noted in apices, furcations, and marginal areas. This loss of lamina dura results in widening of the PDL space (Fig. 39.32). The *repair phase* of trauma from occlusion results in an attempt to strengthen the periodontal structures to better support the increased loads. Radiographically, this is manifested by a widening of the PDL space, which may be generalized or localized.

Although microscopic measurements have determined normal variations in the PDL space width along the root surface, these are generally not detected radiographically. Thus, when seen on radiographs, variations in PDL space width suggest that the tooth is being subjected to increased forces. Successful attempts to reinforce the periodontal structures by widening the PDL space can be accompanied by increased width of the lamina dura and sometimes by condensation of the perialveolar cancellous bone.

More advanced traumatic lesions may result in deep angular bone loss, which, when combined with marginal inflammation, may lead to intrabony pocket formation. In terminal stages, these lesions extend around the root apex, producing a wide, radiolucent periapical image (cavernous lesions).

Root resorption may also result from excessive forces on the periodontium, particularly those caused by orthodontic appliances. Although trauma from occlusion produces many areas of root resorption, these areas are usually of a magnitude insufficient to be detected radiographically.

Conclusion

Intraoral radiographic examination with periapical and bite-wing radiographs should supplement a thorough history and clinical evaluation of manifestations of gingival and periodontal inflammation, including a detailed recording of probing depths and clinical attachment loss. Radiographic evaluation should be updated based on clinical need. Periapical radiographs often underestimate the amount of periodontal bone loss, and early periodontal disease

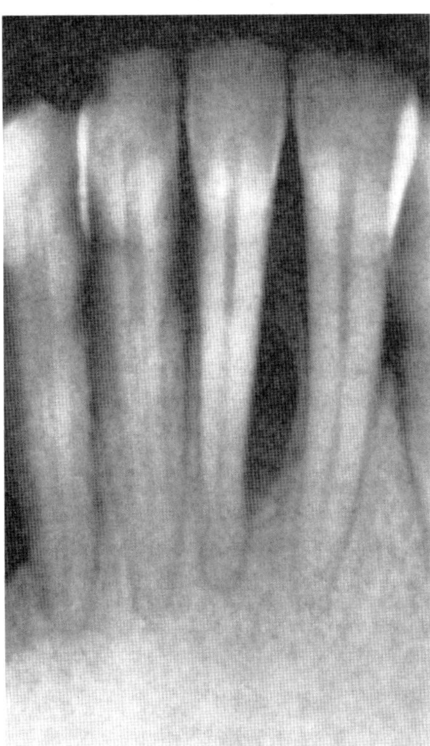

Fig. 39.28 Radiolucent area on lateral aspect of root with chronic periodontal abscess.

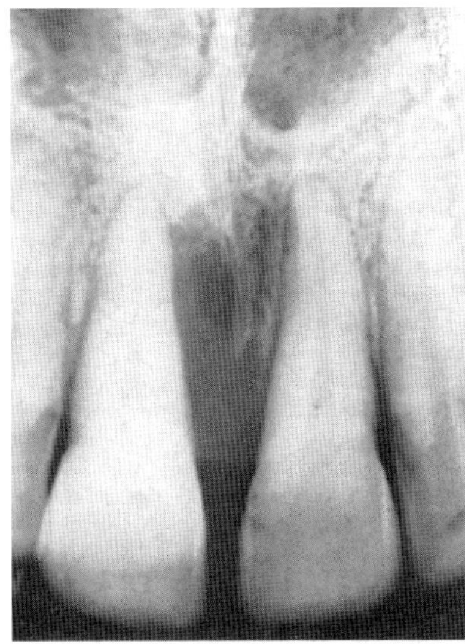

Fig. 39.29 Typical radiographic appearance of periodontal abscess on right central incisor.

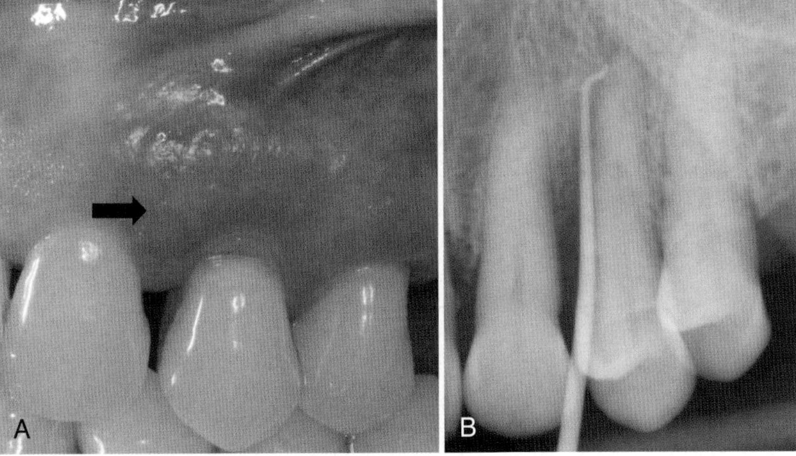

Fig. 39.30 Chronic periodontal abscess. (A) Periodontal abscess in the left maxillary first premolar area. (B) Extensive bone destruction on the mesial surface of the first premolar. Gutta-percha point traces to the root apex.

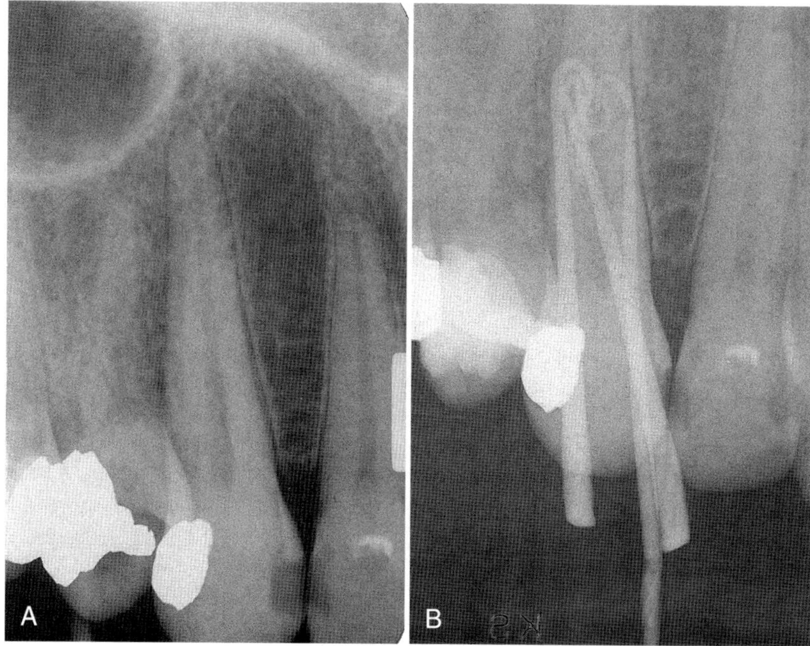

Fig. 39.31 (A) Radiograph of maxillary cuspid. This view does not show facial bone loss. (B) Radiograph of same maxillary cuspid as in part A, with gutta-percha points placed in the facial pocket to indicate bone loss.

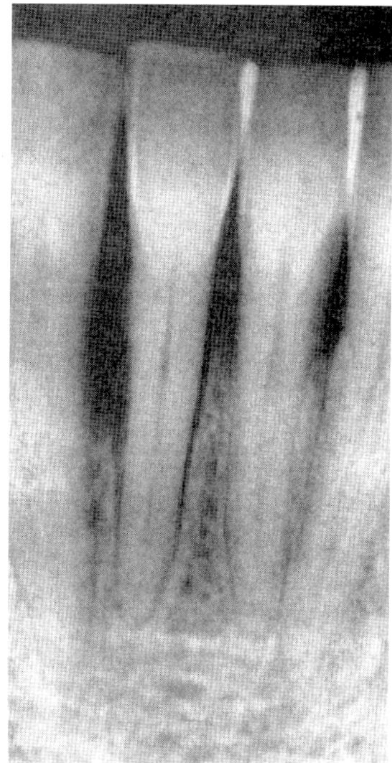

Fig. 39.32 Widened periodontal space caused by trauma from occlusion. Note the increased density of the surrounding bone caused by new bone formation in response to increased occlusal forces.

is usually not apparent on radiographs. Significant interdental bone loss can occur and on periapical radiographs may be masked by the radiodensity of the intact buccal and lingual or palatal bone plates. Despite these limitations, intraoral radiographs taken with a reproducible technique provide adequate information to diagnose and treat periodontal disease and periodically monitor outcomes. Three-dimensional imaging with CBCT provides additional value in select cases, either by providing better diagnostic accuracy or by providing morphological information of relevance to treatment planning.

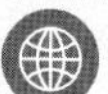 References for this chapter are found on the companion website eBooks.Health.Elsevier.com.

CHAPTER 40

Periodontal Risk Assessment[a]

Joel M. White | Satheesh Elangovan | Chun-Teh Lee

For online-only content on risk indicators, risk markers/ predictors, and clinical risk assessment for periodontal disease, please visit the companion website at eBooks.Health.Elsevier.com.

CHAPTER OUTLINE

Definitions

Risk assessment is defined by numerous components.[2,38] Disease risk is the probability that an individual will develop a specific disease in a given period. The risk of developing the disease will vary from individual to individual.

Risk factors may be environmental, behavioral, or biologic factors that, when present, increase the likelihood that an individual will develop the disease. Risk factors are identified through longitudinal studies of patients with the disease of interest. Exposure to a risk factor or factors may occur at a single point in time, over multiple separate points in time, or continuously. However, to be identified as a risk factor, the exposure must occur before disease onset. Interventions often can be identified and, when implemented, can help modify risk factors.

The term *risk determinant/background characteristic*, which is sometimes substituted for the term *risk factor*, should be reserved only for factors that cannot be modified. *Risk indicators* are *probable* or *putative* risk factors that have been identified in cross-sectional studies but not confirmed through longitudinal studies. *Risk predictors/markers,* although associated with increased risk for disease, do not cause the disease. These factors also are identified in cross-sectional and longitudinal studies. Box 40.1 lists elements of these categories of risk for periodontal disease.

CLINICAL CORRELATION

Lack of bleeding on probing does appear to serve as an excellent indicator of periodontal health, but the presence of bleeding on probing alone is not a good predictor of future attachment loss.

[a]Authors would like to thank Drs. Karen F. Novak and M. John Novak for their contributions to this chapter in the previous edition of this textbook.

Risk Factors for Periodontal Disease

Tobacco Smoking

Tobacco smoking is a well-established risk factor for periodontitis.[2,13] A direct relationship exists between smoking and the prevalence of periodontal disease (see Chapter 23). This association is independent of other factors such as oral hygiene or age.[23] Studies comparing the response to periodontal therapy in smokers, previous smokers, and nonsmokers have shown that smoking has a negative impact on the response to therapy. However, former smokers respond similarly to nonsmokers.[3] These studies demonstrate the therapeutic impact of smoking cessation on patients who smoke (see Chapter 23).

Diabetes

Diabetes is a clear risk factor for periodontitis.[2] Epidemiologic data demonstrate that the prevalence and severity of periodontitis are significantly higher in patients with type 1 or type 2 diabetes mellitus than in those without diabetes and that the level of diabetic control is an important variable in this relationship (see Chapter 25).

Pathogenic Bacteria and Biofilm Deposit

It is well documented that the accumulation of bacterial plaque at the gingival margin results in the development of gingivitis and that the gingivitis can be reversed with the implementation of oral hygiene measures.[32] These studies demonstrate a causal relationship between the accumulation of bacterial plaque and gingival inflammation. However, a causal relationship between *plaque accumulation* and *periodontitis* has been more difficult to establish. We come across clinical scenarios in which patients with severe loss of attachment have minimal levels of bacterial plaque on the affected teeth, indicating that the *quantity* of plaque is not of major importance in the disease process. However, although quantity may not indicate risk, there is evidence that the composition, or *quality,* of the complex plaque biofilm is important.

BOX 40.1 Categories of Risk Elements for Periodontal Disease

Risk Factors
Tobacco smoking
Diabetes
Pathogenic bacteria in dental biofilm deposit

Risk Determinants/Background Characteristics
Genetic factors
Age
Gender
Socioeconomic status
Stress

Risk Indicators
Human immunodeficiency virus (HIV)/acquired immunodeficiency syndrome (AIDS)
Osteoporosis
Infrequent dental visits

Risk Markers/Predictors
Previous history of periodontal disease
Bleeding on probing

In terms of the quality of plaque, three specific bacteria have been identified as etiologic agents for periodontitis: *Aggregatibacter actinomycetemcomitans* (formerly *Actinobacillus actinomycetemcomitans*), *Porphyromonas gingivalis,* and *Tannerella forsythia* (formerly *Bacteroides forsythus*).[15] To be considered periodontal pathogens, these bacteria have to fulfill a set of criteria (in relation to the disease in question): association, elimination, host response, virulence factor, animal studies, and risk assessment.[20] *P. gingivalis* and *T. forsythia* are often found in periodontitis, whereas *A. actinomycetemcomitans* is often associated with aggressive periodontitis (a separate disease category in the previous disease classification to group periodontitis patients with rapid progression pattern occurring in relatively younger patients). Additional evidence that these organisms are causal agents includes the following[20]:

1. Their elimination or suppression impacts the success of periodontal therapy (elimination).
2. There is elevated antibody in serum, saliva, or in periodontal tissue to these pathogens (host response).
3. Virulence factors (e.g., leukotoxin, endotoxin) are associated with these pathogens (virulence factor).
4. Inoculation of these bacteria into animal models induces periodontal disease (animal studies).
5. Cross-sectional and longitudinal studies support the delineation of these three bacteria as risk factors for periodontal disease (risk assessment).

Although not completely supported by these criteria for causation, moderate evidence also suggests that *Campylobacter rectus, Eubacterium nodatum, Fusobacterium nucleatum, Prevotella intermedia, Prevotella nigrescens, Peptostreptococcus micros, Streptococcus intermedius,* and *Treponema denticola* are etiologic factors in periodontitis.[15]

It is becoming clear from recent investigations that the plaque composition shifts from a more symbiotic microbial community to one that is more dysbiotic (an imbalance in the relative abundance of microbes leading to disease), composed primarily of anaerobes, as we go from periodontal health to periodontal disease. Certain pathogens (termed *keystone pathogens*) such as *P. gingivalis* play a major role in inducing such a shift, converting commensals into disease-provoking microbes (termed *pathobionts*).[21] Therefore the quantity of plaque present may not be as important as the quality of the plaque in determining the risk for periodontitis.

Anatomic factors, such as furcations, root concavities, developmental grooves, cervical enamel projections, enamel pearls, and bifurcation ridges, may predispose the periodontium to disease as a result of their potential to harbor bacterial plaque and present a challenge to the clinician during instrumentation. Similarly, the presence of subgingival and overhanging margins in restorations can result in increased plaque accumulation, increased inflammation, and increased bone loss. Although not clearly defined as risk factors for periodontitis, anatomic factors and restorative factors that influence plaque accumulation may play a role in disease susceptibility for specific teeth.[7]

The presence of calculus, which serves as a reservoir of bacterial plaque, has been suggested as a risk factor for periodontitis. Although the presence of some calculus in healthy individuals receiving routine dental care does not result in a significant loss of attachment, the presence of calculus in other groups of patients, such as those not receiving regular care and those with poorly controlled diabetes, can have a negative impact on periodontal health.[38]

Risk Determinants/Background Characteristics for Periodontal Disease

Genetic Factors

Evidence indicates that genetic differences between individuals may explain why some patients develop periodontal disease and others do not. Studies conducted on twins have shown that genetic factors influence clinical measures of gingivitis, probing pocket depth, attachment loss, and interproximal bone height.[35–37] The familial aggregation seen in localized and generalized aggressive periodontitis (periodontitis with rapid progression in relatively younger patients) also indicates genetic involvement in these diseases (see Chapter 9).

Kornman and colleagues[26] demonstrated that alterations (polymorphisms) in specific genes encoding inflammatory cytokines such as interleukin-1α (IL-1α) and interleukin-1β (IL-1β) were associated with severe periodontitis in nonsmoking subjects.[26] However, the results of other studies have shown a limited association between these altered genes and the presence of periodontitis. Overall, it appears that changes in the IL-1 genes may be only one of several genetic changes involved in the risk for periodontitis. Therefore, although an alteration in the IL-1 genes may be a valid marker for periodontitis in defined populations, its usefulness as a genetic marker in the general population may be limited.[25]

Immunologic alterations, such as neutrophil abnormalities,[22] monocytic hyperresponsiveness to lipopolysaccharide stimulation in patients with a molar-incisor pattern of periodontitis (formerly called localized aggressive periodontitis)[44] and alterations in the monocyte/macrophage receptors for the Fc portion of an antibody,[25,56] also appear to be under genetic control. In addition, genetics plays a role in regulating the titer of the protective immunoglobulin G2 (IgG2) antibody response to *A. actinomycetemcomitans* in patients with aggressive periodontitis.[19]

Age

Both the prevalence and severity of periodontal disease increase with age.[10,13,39] It is possible that degenerative changes related to aging may increase susceptibility to periodontitis. However, it is also possible that the attachment loss and bone loss seen in older individuals are the result of prolonged exposure to other risk factors over a person's life, creating a cumulative effect over time. In support of this theory, studies have shown minimal loss of attachment in aging subjects enrolled in preventive programs throughout their lives.[40,41] Therefore it is suggested that periodontal disease is not an inevitable consequence of the aging process and that aging alone does not increase disease susceptibility. However, it remains to be determined whether changes related to the aging process, such as medication intake, decreased immune function, and altered nutritional status, interact with other well-defined risk factors to increase susceptibility to periodontitis.

Evidence of loss of attachment may have more consequences in younger patients. The younger the patient, the longer the time for continuous exposure to causative factors since the disease starts early. In addition, aggressive periodontitis (periodontitis with rapid progression in relatively younger patients) in young individuals is often associated with unmodifiable risk factors, such as a genetic predisposition to disease.[13] Therefore young individuals with periodontal disease may be at greater risk for continued disease as they age.

Gender

Gender plays a role in periodontal disease.[2] Surveys conducted in the United States since 1960 demonstrate that men have more loss of attachment than women.[51,53,54] In addition, men have poorer oral hygiene than women, as evidenced by higher levels of plaque and calculus.[1,52,54] Therefore gender differences in the prevalence and severity of periodontitis appear to be related to preventive practices rather than any genetic factor.

Socioeconomic Status

Gingivitis and poor oral hygiene can be related to lower socioeconomic status (SES).[2,51,53] This most likely can be attributed to decreased dental awareness and decreased frequency of dental visits compared with more educated individuals with higher SES. Emerging evidence suggests low education attainment to be an important factor associated with periodontitis.[8,58]

Stress

The incidence of necrotizing ulcerative gingivitis increases during periods of emotional and physiologic stress, suggesting a link between the two.[14,46] Emotional stress may interfere with normal immune function[6,49] and may result in increased levels of circulating hormones, which can affect the periodontium.[43] Specifically, it is known that stress deregulates the immune system via the hypothalamic-pituitary-adrenal cortex axis or via the sympathetic-adrenal medullary axis.[9] The resulting increase in cortisol and epinephrine/norepinephrine, respectively, are shown to cause hyperglycemia, affect the immune system, and also affect the wound healing process.

Stressful life events, such as bereavement and divorce, appear to lead to a greater prevalence of periodontal disease,[17] and an apparent association exists between psychosocial factors and risk behaviors such as smoking, poor oral hygiene, and periodontitis.[12] Adult patients with periodontitis who are resistant to therapy are more stressed than those who respond to therapy.[5] Individuals with financial strain, distress, depression, or inadequate coping mechanisms have a more severe loss of attachment.[16] Although epidemiologic data on the relationship between stress and periodontal disease are limited, stress can be a putative risk factor for periodontitis.[13] Stress is listed as a risk determinant, but it is important to know that unlike other risk determinants listed above, it can be alleviated and hence its negative effect on periodontium can be minimized or negated.

CLINICAL CORRELATION

The ultimate goal of performing a periodontal risk assessment is to develop a more personalized treatment plan for a specific patient, taking into account the periodontal risk profile of that patient. Once an at-risk patient is identified and a diagnosis is made, the treatment plan may be modified accordingly.

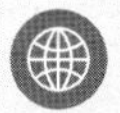

A Case Scenario is found on the companion website eBooks.Health.Elsevier.com.

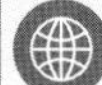

References for this chapter are found on the companion website eBooks.Health.Elsevier.com.

CHAPTER 41

Determination of Prognosis

Chun-Teh Lee | Jonathan H. Do | Henry H. Takei | Karen F. Novak | Satheesh Elangovan

CHAPTER OUTLINE

Definitions

A *prognosis* is a prediction of the probable course, duration, and outcome of a disease based on a general knowledge of the pathogenesis of the disease and the presence of prognostic factors for the disease. It is established after the diagnosis is made and before the treatment plan is established. The prognosis is based on specific information about the disease and the manner in which it can be treated, but it also can be influenced by the clinician's previous experience with treatment outcomes (successes and failures) as they relate to the particular case and the patient's medical and dental history. It is important to note that determination of prognosis is a dynamic process. As such, the prognosis initially assigned should be reevaluated after completion of all phases of therapy, including periodontal maintenance.

Prognosis is often confused with the term *risk*. Risk generally deals with the likelihood that an individual will develop a disease in a specified period (see Chapter 6). Risk factors are characteristics that put an individual at increased risk for developing a disease (see Chapter 6). In contrast, *prognosis* is the prediction of the course or outcome of a disease. *Prognostic factors* are characteristics that predict the outcome once the disease is present. Some characteristics can be both risk factors and prognostic factors. For example, patients with diabetes or patients who smoke are at higher risk for acquiring periodontal disease, and once they have it, they generally have a worse prognosis.

Types of Prognosis

Although some factors may be more important than others when assigning a prognosis based on the clinical evidence (Box 41.1),[32,33] it may benefit the clinician to consider each factor. Historically, prognosis classification schemes have been designed based on studies evaluating tooth mortality (tooth loss).[1,2,25,32,35] One scheme[25,32] assigns the following categories:

Good prognosis: Control of etiologic factors and adequate periodontal support ensure the tooth will be easy to maintain by the patient and clinician.

Fair prognosis: Approximately 25% attachment loss or grade I furcation invasion (location and depth allow proper maintenance with good patient compliance).

Poor prognosis: 50% attachment loss, grade II furcation invasion (location and depth make maintenance possible but difficult).

Questionable prognosis: Greater than 50% attachment loss, poor crown-to-root ratio, poor root form, grade II furcation invasion (location and depth make access difficult) or grade III furcation invasion; mobility no. 2 or no. 3; root proximity.

Hopeless prognosis: Inadequate attachment to maintain health, comfort, and function. Therefore, extraction is recommended.

It should be recognized that this classification was developed to assign prognosis to individual tooth, and good, fair, and hopeless prognostic categories in this classification system can be established with a reasonable degree of accuracy. However, poor and questionable prognoses are likely to change to other categories because they depend on a large number of factors that can interact in an unpredictable number of ways.[8,14,48] In the original study investigating this prognostication system, approximately 80% of the teeth that were initially assigned to questionable prognosis ended up with better prognosis, after 5 years of periodontal supportive therapy. It is important to know that prognosis is dynamic and bound to change over time. Therefore, the care provider should assess and update the prognosis of teeth on a consistent basis.[35]

In contrast to schemes based on tooth mortality, Kwok and Caton[25] proposed a scheme based on "the probability of obtaining stability of the periodontal supporting apparatus." This scheme is based on the probability of disease progression as related to local and systemic factors (see Box 41.1). Although some of these factors may affect disease progression more than others, consideration of each factor is important in assigning a prognosis. This scheme is as follows:

BOX 41.1 Factors to Consider When Determining a Prognosis

Overall Clinical Factors
Patient age
Disease severity
Biofilm control
Patient compliance

Systemic and Environmental Factors
Smoking
Systemic disease or condition
Genetic factors
Stress

Local Factors
Biofilm and calculus
Anatomic factors
- Short, tapered roots
- Cervical enamel projections
- Enamel pearls
- Bifurcation ridges
- Root concavities
- Developmental grooves
- Root proximity
- Furcation invasion

Tooth mobility
Caries
Tooth vitality
Root resorption

Prosthetic and Restorative Factors
Subgingival restorations
Tooth-supported prosthesis
Abutment selection

Favorable prognosis: Comprehensive periodontal treatment and maintenance will stabilize the status of the tooth. Future loss of periodontal support is unlikely.

Questionable prognosis: Local or systemic factors influencing the periodontal status of the tooth may or may not be controllable. If controlled, the periodontal status can be stabilized with comprehensive periodontal treatment. If not, future periodontal breakdown may occur.

Unfavorable prognosis: Local or systemic factors influencing the periodontal status cannot be controlled. Comprehensive periodontal treatment and maintenance are unlikely to prevent future periodontal breakdown.

Hopeless prognosis: The tooth must be extracted.

Because periodontal stability is assessed on a regular basis using clinical measures, it may be more practical in making treatment decisions and prognosis predictions than in trying to determine the likelihood that the tooth will be lost. However, since this prognostication system does not have specific criteria based on clinical parameters, the care provider should decide the importance and the status of each factor based on scientific evidence and clinical experience. Compared to other prognostication systems, this system described by Kwok and Caton is a somewhat straightforward system, but the inherent subjectivity cannot be completely eliminated.

In many of these cases, it may be advisable to establish a *provisional prognosis* until phase I therapy is completed and evaluated. The provisional prognosis allows the clinician to initiate treatment of teeth that have a doubtful outlook in the hope that a favorable response may tip the balance and allow teeth to be retained. Providing information on provisional prognosis to the patient can also help set treatment outcome expectations with the patient. The reevaluation phase in the treatment sequence allows the clinician to examine the tissue response to oral hygiene, subgingival root instrumentation (scaling and root planing), as well as to the possible use of adjunctive chemotherapeutic agents (see Chapters 53 and 54) where indicated. The patient's compliance with the proposed treatment plan also can be determined. The prognosis decided at the time of reevaluation will help guide the clinician in deciding on the need for surgical periodontal therapy and also selecting the proper interval for periodontal maintenance (supportive periodontal therapy).

LEARNING BOX 41.1

A prognosis based on whether periodontal stability can be achieved with periodontal therapy and maintenance is as follows: favorable—likely, questionable—maybe, unfavorable—unlikely, hopeless—impossible.

Overall Versus Individual Tooth Prognosis

Prognosis can be divided into overall prognosis and individual tooth prognosis. The *overall prognosis* is concerned with the dentition as a whole. Factors that may influence the overall prognosis include patient age, current severity of periodontal diseases and conditions, systemic diseases, smoking, the presence of biofilm, calculus, and other local factors, patient compliance, and prosthetic possibilities (see Box 41.1). The overall prognosis answers the following questions:

- Should treatment be undertaken?
- Is treatment likely to succeed?
- When prosthetic replacements are needed, are the remaining teeth able to support the added burden of the prosthesis?

The *individual tooth prognosis* is determined after the overall prognosis and is affected by it.[35] For example, in a patient with an overall unfavorable prognosis due to uncontrolled diabetes and existing generalized and severe periodontal disease, treating a tooth with a questionable prognosis can be more challenging as compared to treating a tooth with similar condition in a patient with an overall questionable prognosis. The factors that should be considered for overall prognosis that will have a direct effect on the prognosis of individual teeth are presented in Box 41.1.

Factors in Determination of Prognosis

Overall Clinical Factors

Patient Age

For two patients with comparable levels of remaining connective tissue attachment and alveolar bone, the prognosis is generally better for the older of the two. For the younger patient, the prognosis is not as good because of the shorter time frame in which the periodontal destruction has occurred; the younger patient may also have an aggressive pattern of disease progression because of systemic disease, smoking, or other factors. In addition, although the younger patient would ordinarily be expected to have a greater reparative capacity, the occurrence of so much destruction in a relatively short period would exceed any naturally occurring periodontal repair.

Disease Severity

Studies have demonstrated that a patient's history of previous periodontal disease may be indicative of their susceptibility to future periodontal breakdown. Therefore, the following variables should be carefully recorded because they are important in determining the patient's past history of periodontal disease: probing pocket depth, clinical attachment level, amount of bone loss, and type of bony defect. These factors are determined by clinical and radiographic evaluation (see Chapters 38 and 39).

Determining clinical attachment loss reveals the approximate extent of root surface that is devoid of periodontal ligament; the radiographic examination shows the amount of root surface still invested in bone. Probing pocket depth is less important than the level of attachment in determining the severity of tissue destruction because sometimes the pocket depth is not necessarily related to bone loss. In general, it is necessary to consider clinical attachment level, radiographic bone level and probing pocket depth together to assess disease severity which in turn affects prognosis. Lower attachment level, less remaining bone, and deeper pocket depth are associated with a worse prognosis.

Prognosis is adversely affected if the probing pocket depth is deep (≥5 mm). Compared to a site with a shallower probing pocket depth, it will be challenging to remove biofilm and calculus from a deeper pocket site. When the base of the pocket (level of attachment) is too deep and close to the root apex, the presence of apical disease as a result of endodontic involvement also worsens the prognosis. However, surprisingly, optimal repair of the attachment apparatus can sometimes be achieved by combining endodontic and periodontal therapy (see Chapter 49).

The prognosis also can be related to the height of remaining bone. Assuming bone destruction can be arrested, is there enough bone remaining to support the teeth? The answer is readily apparent in extreme cases—that is, when there is so little bone loss that tooth support is not in jeopardy (Fig. 41.1) or when bone loss is so severe that the remaining bone is obviously insufficient for proper tooth support (Fig. 41.2). Most patients, however, do not fit into these extreme categories. The height of remaining bone is usually somewhere in between, making bone level assessment alone insufficient for determining the overall prognosis.

The type of defect also must be determined. The prognosis for horizontal bone loss depends on the height of the existing bone because it is unlikely that clinically significant bone height regeneration will be induced by therapy. In the case of angular, intrabony defects, if the contour of the existing bone and the number of osseous walls are favorable (e.g., a narrow 3-wall defect), there is an excellent chance that therapy could regenerate bone to approximately the level of the existing alveolar crest.[45] The extent of bone loss around a tooth will also affect the prognosis. For example, a tooth with a circumferential bone loss may have worse prognosis than a tooth with bone loss limited to a localized area.

When greater bone loss has occurred on one surface of a tooth, the bone height on the less involved surfaces should be taken into consideration when determining the prognosis. Because of the greater height of bone in relation to other surfaces, the center of rotation of the tooth will be nearer the crown (Fig. 41.3). This results in a more favorable distribution of forces to the periodontium and less tooth mobility.[50]

In dealing with a tooth that has an unfavorable prognosis, the chances of successful treatment should be weighed against any benefits that would accrue to the adjacent teeth if the tooth under consideration was extracted. Strategic extraction of teeth was first proposed as a means of improving the overall prognosis of adjacent teeth or enhancing the prosthetic treatment plan.[9] It has now been expanded to include the extraction of teeth with an unfavorable prognosis to enhance the likelihood of partial restoration of the bone support of the adjacent teeth (Fig. 41.4A–D) or successful implant placement. With the growing evidence of the long-term success of dental implants, it is proposed that a "watch and wait" approach may allow an area to deteriorate to the point that placing an implant is no longer a viable option. This means that the practitioner should carefully weigh the potential success of one treatment option (extraction and implant placement) versus the other (periodontal therapy and maintenance) when dealing with a tooth with unfavorable prognosis.[20] Having said that, a patient's needs and expectations should be taken into account prior to performing any irreversible treatment such as tooth extraction.

LEARNING BOX 41.2

Strategic extraction of teeth with unfavorable prognosis may improve the prognosis of adjacent teeth, enhance the prosthetic treatment, and increase the success rate of implants replacing the strategically extracted teeth.

Biofilm Control

Bacterial biofilm is the primary etiologic factor associated with periodontal disease (see Chapter 10). Therefore, effective removal of biofilm on a daily basis by the patient is critical to the success of periodontal therapy and the overall prognosis.

Patient Compliance

The prognosis for patients with gingival and periodontal disease is critically dependent on the patient's attitude, desire to retain the natural teeth, and willingness and ability to effectively control biofilm. Without these, treatment cannot succeed. Patients should be educated on the etiology and prevention of dental caries and periodontal diseases, and they should be clearly informed of the important role they must play for treatment to succeed. Additionally, it is well known that patients' noncompliance with supportive periodontal therapy (periodontal maintenance) is significantly associated with periodontal disease progression and tooth loss.[26,41] Maintaining good oral hygiene and being compliant with the recommended professional periodontal maintenance visits are critical to maintaining better prognosis. If a patient is unwilling to perform adequate biofilm control and receive the timely periodic maintenance checkups and treatments that the dentist deems necessary, the dentist can refuse to accept the patient for treatment. The dentist should make it clear to the patient and in the patient record that further treatment is needed but will not be performed because of a lack of patient cooperation.

Systemic and Environmental Factors

Smoking

Epidemiologic evidence suggests that smoking may be the most important environmental risk factor impacting the development and progression of periodontal disease (see Chapter 23). Therefore, it should be made clear to patients that a direct relationship exists between smoking and the prevalence and incidence of periodontitis. In addition, patients should be informed that smoking affects not only the severity of periodontal destruction but also the healing potential of the periodontal tissues. As a result, patients who smoke do not respond as well to conventional periodontal therapy as patients who have never smoked.[42,44] There is a dose-response effect with the more the patient smokes, the more severe the tissue destruction and the poorer the treatment outcome. Therefore, the prognosis in patients who smoke and have slight to moderate (stage I or stage II) periodontitis is generally questionable. In smokers with severe periodontitis (stage III or stage IV), the prognosis may be unfavorable or hopeless.

However, it should be emphasized that smoking cessation can affect the treatment outcome and therefore the prognosis.[4,17] As such, for patients who stop smoking, the prognosis can improve to

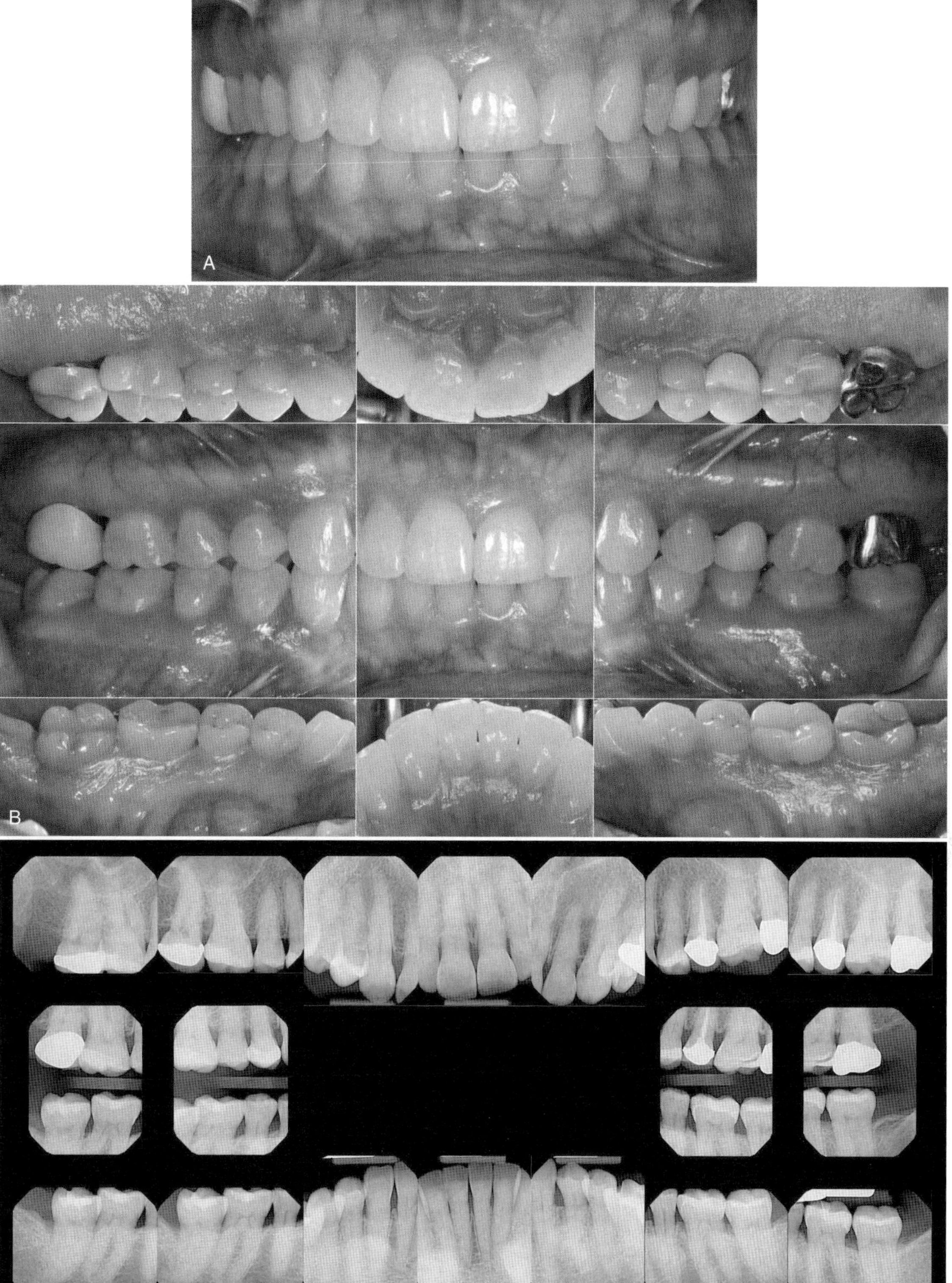

Fig. 41.1 Generalized stage I, grade B periodontitis in a healthy, nonsmoking 67-year-old female. Minimal clinical biofilm and gingival inflammation (A and B) and radiographic bone loss (C). Overall prognosis is favorable. (*Copyright Jonathan H. Do, DDS. All rights reserved.*)

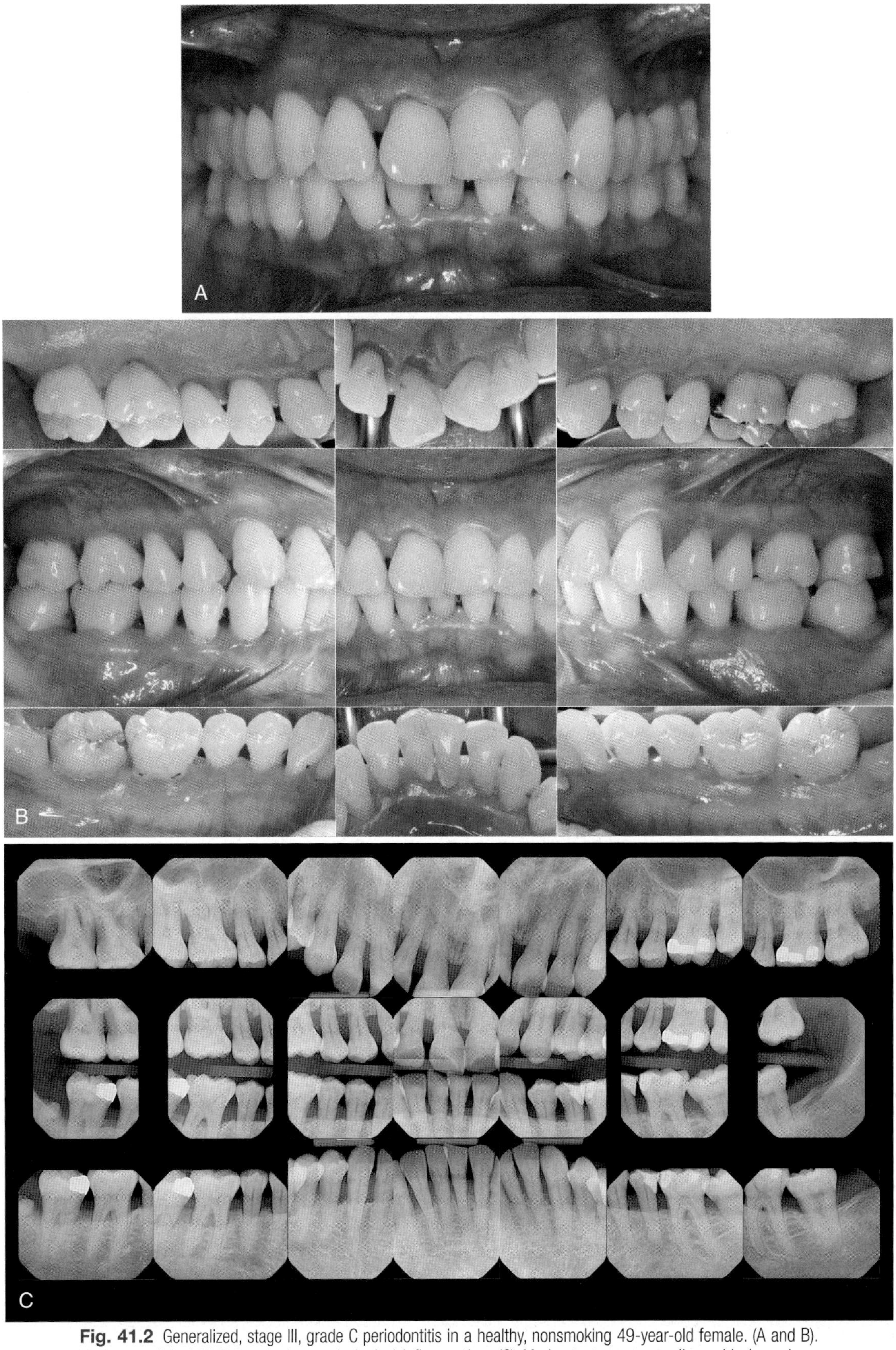

A

B

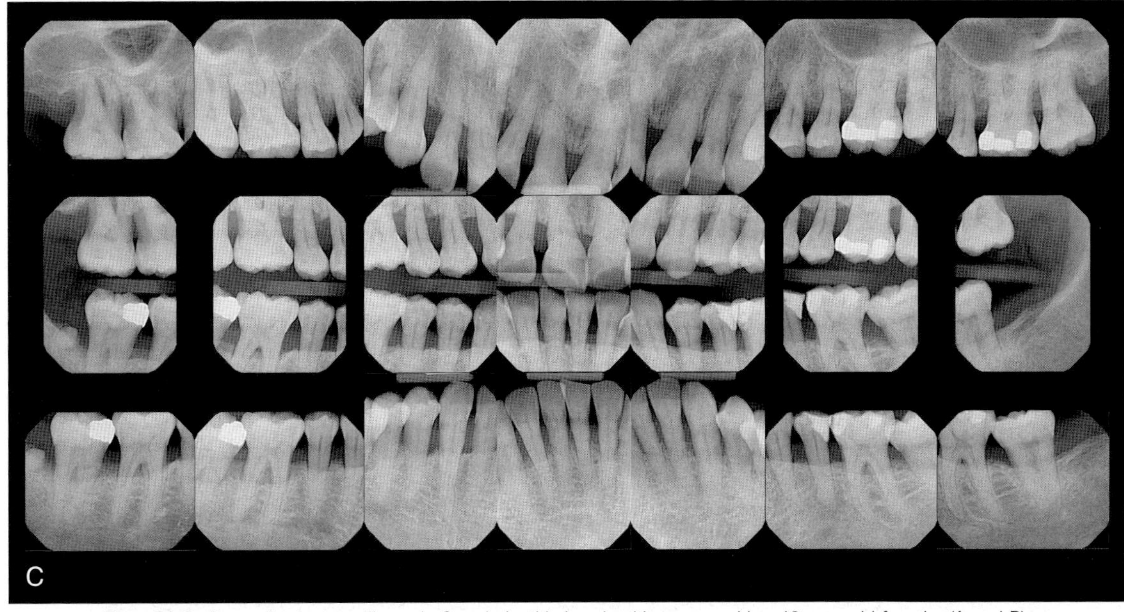

Fig. 41.2 Generalized, stage III, grade C periodontitis in a healthy, nonsmoking 49-year-old female. (A and B). Moderate clinical biofilm, calculus, and gingival inflammation. (C) Moderate to severe radiographic bone loss. Overall prognosis is questionable/unfavorable. (*Copyright Jonathan H. Do, DDS. All rights reserved.*)

favorable in those with slight to moderate periodontitis and to questionable in those with severe periodontitis.

Systemic Disease or Condition

The patient's systemic background affects the overall prognosis in several ways. For example, evidence from epidemiologic studies clearly demonstrates that the prevalence and severity of periodontitis are significantly higher in patients with poorly controlled diabetes than in those whose diabetes is well controlled or those who do not have diabetes (see Chapter 6). Therefore, patients at risk for diabetes should be identified as early as possible and informed of the relationship between periodontitis and diabetes. Similarly, patients diagnosed with diabetes must be informed of the impact of diabetic control on the development and progression of periodontitis. It follows that the prognosis in these cases depends on patient compliance relative to both medical and dental status. Patients with well-controlled diabetes and slight to moderate periodontitis who comply with their recommended periodontal treatment should generally have a favorable prognosis. Similarly, in patients with other systemic disorders that could affect disease progression, prognosis improves with correction of the systemic problem.

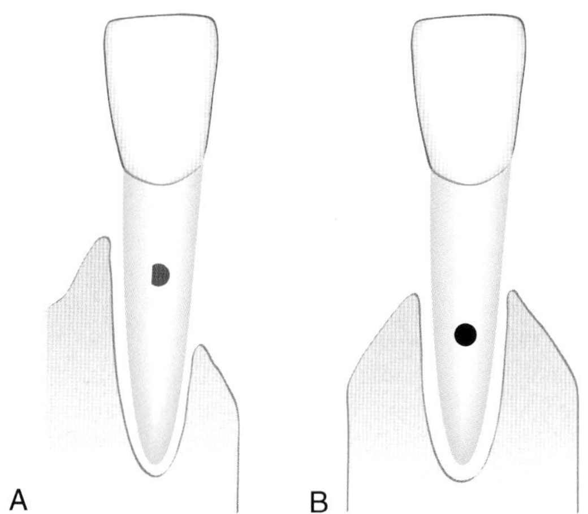

Fig. 41.3 Prognosis for tooth A is better than for tooth B, despite less bone on one of the surfaces of A. Because the center of rotation of tooth A is closer to the crown, the distribution of occlusal forces to the periodontium is more favorable than in B.

The prognosis is questionable when surgical periodontal treatment is required but cannot be provided because of the patient's systemic health (see Chapter 67). Incapacitating conditions that limit the patient's performance of oral procedures (e.g., Parkinson disease) also adversely affect the prognosis. Newer "automated" oral hygiene devices, such as electric toothbrushes, may be helpful for these patients and may improve their prognosis (see Chapter 50).

Genetic Factors

Periodontal diseases represent a complex interaction between a microbial challenge and the host's response to that challenge, both of which may be influenced by environmental factors such as smoking. In addition to these external factors, evidence also indicates that genetic factors may play an important role in determining the nature of the host response.[18] Evidence for this type of genetic influence exists for patients with periodontitis. Genetic polymorphisms in the interleukin-1 (IL-1) genes, resulting in increased production of IL-1β, have been associated with a significant increase in risk for severe and generalized periodontitis.[24,36] It has been demonstrated that knowledge of the patient's IL-1 genotype and smoking status can aid the clinician in assigning a prognosis.[34] Genetic factors also appear to influence serum immunoglobulin G2 (IgG2) antibody

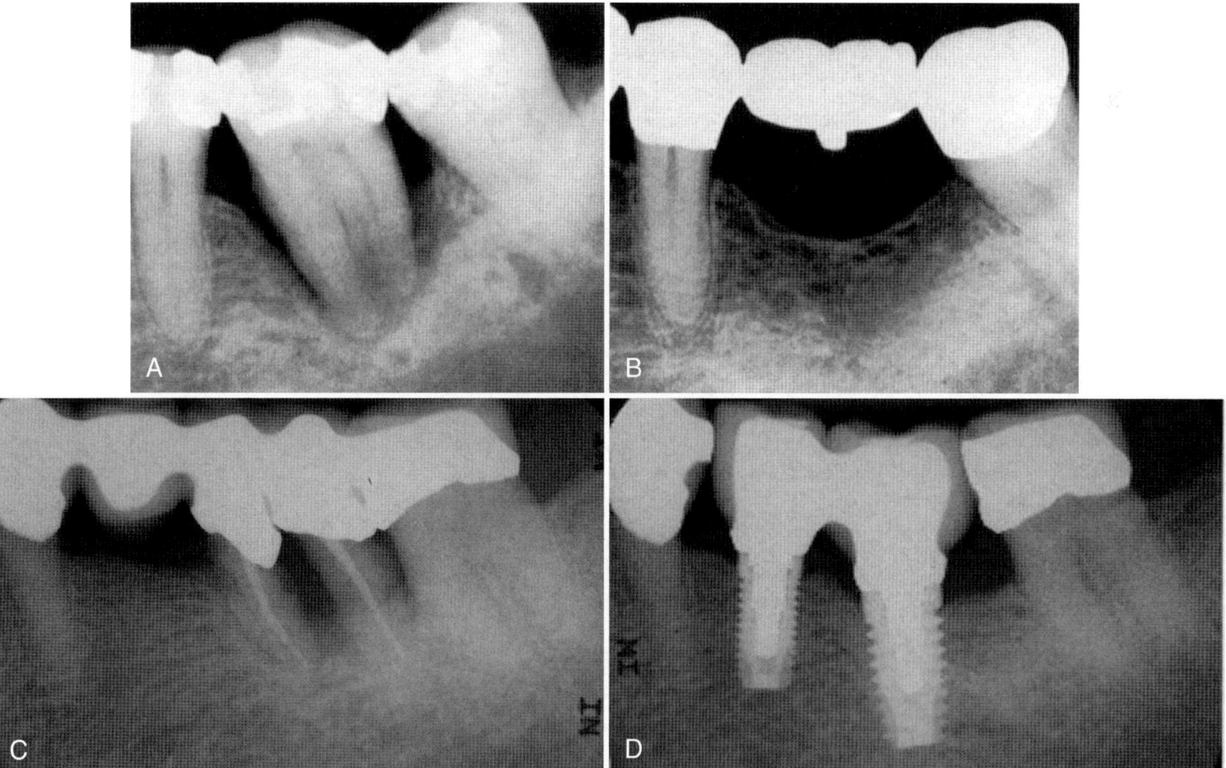

Fig. 41.4 Extraction of severely involved tooth to preserve bone on adjacent teeth. (A) Extensive bone destruction around the mandibular first molar. (B) Radiograph made years after extraction of the first molar and replacement by a prosthesis. Note the excellent bone support. (C) Extraction of periodontally involved bicuspid and molar. (D) Implant replacement of both teeth. (*Courtesy Dr. S. Angha, University of California, Los Angeles.*)

titers and the expression of FcγRII receptors on neutrophils, both of which may be significant in aggressive periodontitis (a separate disease category in the previous disease classification to group periodontitis with rapid progression pattern happening in relatively younger patients).[18] Other genetic disorders, such as leukocyte adhesion deficiency type 1, can influence neutrophil function, creating an additional risk factor for this aggressive pattern of periodontitis.[18] Finally, the familial aggregation that is characteristic of this periodontitis with rapid progression pattern (previously termed aggressive periodontitis) indicates that additional, as yet unidentified, genetic factors may be important in one's susceptibility to this form of disease.

The influence of genetic factors on prognosis is not simple. Although microbial and environmental factors can be altered through conventional periodontal therapy and patient education, genetic factors currently cannot be altered. However, detection of genetic variations linked to periodontal disease can potentially influence the prognosis in several ways. First, early detection of patients at risk because of genetic factors can lead to early implementation of preventive and treatment measures for these patients. Second, identification of genetic risk factors later in the disease or during the course of treatment can influence treatment recommendations, such as the use of adjunctive antibiotic therapy or increased frequency of maintenance visits. Third, identification of young individuals who have not been evaluated for periodontitis but who are recognized as being at risk because of the familial aggregation seen in periodontitis with rapid progression (previously termed aggressive periodontitis) pattern can lead to the development of early intervention strategies. In each of these cases, early diagnosis, intervention, and alterations in the treatment regimen may lead to an improved prognosis for the patient.

Stress

Physical and emotional stress, as well as substance abuse, may alter the patient's ability to respond to the periodontal treatment performed. These factors must be realistically faced when attempting to establish a prognosis.

Local Factors

Biofilm and Calculus

The microbial challenge presented by bacterial biofilm and calculus is the most important local factor in periodontal diseases. Therefore, in most cases, having a favorable prognosis depends on the ability of the patient and the clinician to remove these etiologic factors (see Chapters 10 and 24).

LEARNING BOX 41.3

Periodontal prognosis depends on the ability of the patient and clinician to effectively remove bacterial biofilm and resolve **inflammation**.

Anatomic Factors

Anatomic factors that may predispose the periodontium to disease and therefore affect the prognosis include short, tapered roots with large crowns, cervical enamel projections and enamel pearls, intermediate bifurcation ridges, root concavities, and developmental grooves. The clinician must also consider root proximity and the location and anatomy of furcations when assigning a prognosis.

Prognosis is less favorable for teeth with short, tapered roots and relatively large crowns. Because of the disproportionate crown-to-root ratio and the reduced root surface available for periodontal support,[21] the periodontium may be more susceptible to injury by occlusal forces.

Cervical enamel projections (CEPs) are flat, ectopic extensions of enamel that extend beyond the normal contours of the cementoenamel junction.[30] CEPs extend into the furcation of 28.6% of mandibular molars and 17% of maxillary molars.[30] CEPs are most likely to be found on buccal surfaces of mandibular second molars.[16,51] Enamel pearls are larger, round deposits of enamel that can be located in furcations or other areas on the root surface.[38] Enamel pearls are seen less frequently (1.1% to 5.7% of permanent molars; most prevalent in maxillary third molars[38]) than CEPs. An intermediate bifurcation ridge has been described in 73% of mandibular first molars, crossing from the mesial to the distal root at the midpoint of the furcation.[10] The presence of these enamel projections on the root surface interferes with the attachment apparatus and may prevent regenerative procedures from achieving their maximum potential. Therefore, their presence may have a negative effect on the prognosis for an individual tooth.

Subgingival root instrumentation ("scaling and root planing") is a fundamental procedure in periodontal therapy. Anatomic factors that decrease the efficiency of this procedure can have a negative impact on the prognosis. Therefore, the morphology of the tooth root is an important consideration when discussing prognosis. *Root concavities* exposed through loss of attachment can vary from shallow flutings to deep depressions. They appear more marked on maxillary first premolars, the mesiobuccal root of the maxillary first molar, both roots of mandibular first molars, and the mandibular incisors (Figs. 41.5 and 41.6).[5,6] Any tooth, however, can have a proximal concavity.[13] Although these concavities increase the attachment area and produce a root shape that may be more resistant to torquing forces, they also create areas that can be difficult for both the clinician and the patient to clean.

Other anatomic considerations that present accessibility problems are developmental grooves, root proximity, and furcation involvement. The presence of any of these can worsen the prognosis. *Developmental grooves,* which sometimes appear in the maxillary lateral incisors (palatogingival groove[52]; Fig. 41.7) or in the lower incisors, create an accessibility problem.[11,15] They initiate on enamel and can extend a significant distance on the root surface,

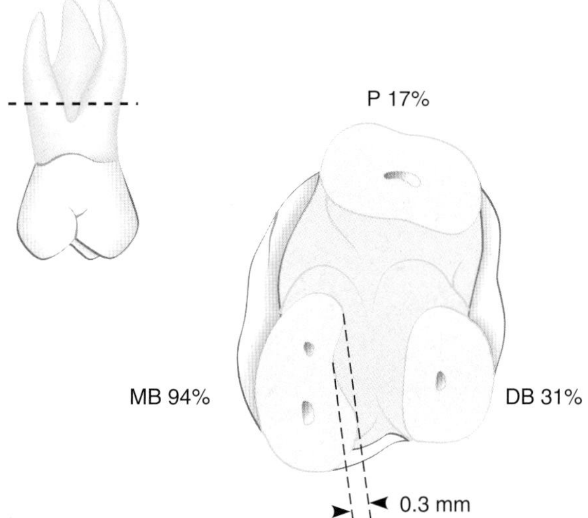

Fig. 41.5 Root concavities in maxillary first molars sectioned 2 mm apical to the furca. The furcal aspect of the root is concave in 94% of the mesiobuccal *(MB)* roots, 31% of the distobuccal *(DB)* roots, and 17% of the palatal *(P)* roots. The deepest concavity is found in the furcal aspects of the mesiobuccal roots (mean concavity, 0.3 mm). The furcal aspect of the buccal roots diverges toward the palate in 97% of teeth (mean divergence, 22 degrees). *(Redrawn from Bower RC. Furcation morphology relative to periodontal treatment. Furcation root surface anatomy.* J Periodontol. *1979;50:366.)*

providing a plaque-retentive area that is difficult to instrument. These palatogingival grooves are found on 5.6% of maxillary lateral incisors and 3.4% of maxillary central incisors.[23] Similarly, *root proximity* can result in interproximal areas that are difficult for the clinician and patient to access. Also, when periodontally involved, the narrow interproximal bone associated with the root proximity is susceptible to rapid bone loss. Finally, *access to the furcation area* is usually difficult to obtain. In 58% of maxillary and mandibular first molars, the furcation entrance diameter is narrower than the width of conventional periodontal curettes (Fig. 41.8).[6] Maxillary first premolars present the greatest difficulty, and therefore their prognosis is usually unfavorable when the lesion reaches the mesiodistal furcation which is averaged at 7 to 8 mm below the cementoenamel junction.[19] Maxillary molars also present some difficulty in access when interproximal furcation defects are present. The root trunk length of maxillary and mandibular molars is approximately 2.5 to 5 mm.[31] Therefore, attachment loss over 3 mm at these areas can be a sign of furcation involvement in molars and should be carefully assessed. Generally, furcation involvement is associated with a poorer prognosis due to difficult access for both the clinician and the patient to clean these sites. When buccal and lingual furcations of mandibular molars or buccal furcations of maxillary molars offer good access for oral hygiene measures, the prognosis is usually better.

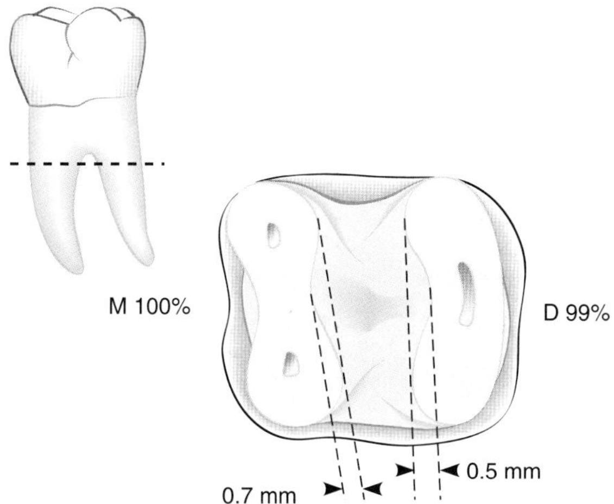

Fig. 41.6 Root concavities in mandibular first molars sectioned 2 mm apical to the furca. Concavity of the furcal aspect was found in 100% of mesial *(M)* roots and 99% of distal *(D)* roots. Deeper concavity was found in the mesial roots (mean concavity, 0.7 mm). (*Redrawn from Bower RC. Furcation morphology relative to periodontal treatment. Furcation root surface anatomy.* J Periodontol. *1979;50:366.*)

Tooth Mobility

The principal causes of tooth mobility are loss of alveolar bone, inflammatory changes in the periodontium, and trauma from occlusion. Tooth mobility caused by inflammation and trauma from occlusion may be correctable.[37] However, tooth mobility resulting from loss of alveolar bone is not likely to be corrected. The likelihood of restoring tooth stability is inversely proportional to the extent to which mobility is caused by the loss of supporting alveolar bone. A longitudinal study of the response to treatment of teeth with different degrees of mobility revealed that pockets on clinically mobile teeth do not respond as well to periodontal therapy as pockets on nonmobile teeth exhibiting the same initial disease severity.[12] Another study, however, in which ideal plaque control was attained, found similar healing in both hypermobile and firm teeth.[45] The stabilization of tooth mobility through the use of splinting may have a beneficial impact on the overall and individual tooth prognosis during treatment. However, it should be noted that splinting may potentially increase biofilm accumulation, resulting in inflammation. It is important to identify the cause of mobility, and assess patient's oral hygiene and compliance before splinting is considered.

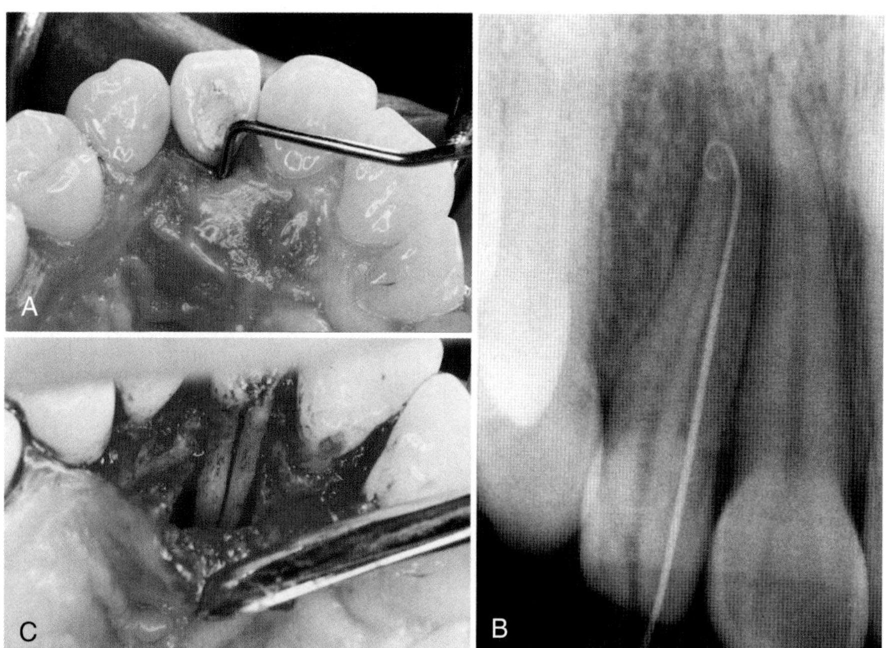

Fig. 41.7 Palatogingival groove. (A) Probe in place to indicate a deep pocket along the palatogingival groove. (B) Radiograph with a gutta-percha point placed in the pocket. (C) The area is surgically opened. Note the palatogingival groove along the entire palatal portion of the root. (*Courtesy Dr. Nadia Chugal, University of California, Los Angeles.*)

LEARNING BOX 41.4

Tooth mobility is often used to condemn a tooth to a prognosis of questionable, unfavorable, or hopeless depending on the degree of mobility and its etiology. It must be recognized that, depending on the cause, mobility may be correctable. Eliminating the cause of mobility can stabilize a tooth and improve its prognosis.

Caries, Tooth Vitality, and Root Resorption

For teeth mutilated by extensive caries, the feasibility of adequate restoration and endodontic therapy should be considered before undertaking periodontal treatment. Extensive idiopathic root resorption or root resorption resulting from orthodontic therapy or endodontic infection jeopardizes the stability of teeth and adversely affects the response to periodontal treatment. The periodontal prognosis of treated nonvital teeth does not differ from that of vital teeth. New attachment can occur to the cementum of both nonvital and vital teeth.

Restorative and Prosthetic Factors

Subgingival margins may contribute to increased biofilm accumulation, increased inflammation, and increased bone loss[3,39,47,49] when compared with supragingival margins. Furthermore, discrepancies in these margins (e.g., overhangs) can negatively impact the periodontium (see Chapter 24). The size of these discrepancies and duration of their presence are important factors in the amount of destruction that occurs. In general, a tooth with a discrepancy in its subgingival margins has a worse prognosis than a tooth with well-contoured supragingival margins. However, for esthetic reasons, it is common to keep the anterior crown margin at the level or below the gingival margin.

The overall prognosis requires a general consideration of bone levels (evaluated radiographically) and attachment levels (determined clinically) to establish whether enough teeth can be saved either to provide functional and esthetic dentition or to serve as abutments for a useful prosthetic replacement of the missing teeth.

At this point, the overall prognosis and individual tooth prognosis overlap because the prognosis for key individual teeth may affect the overall prognosis for prosthetic rehabilitation. For example, saving or losing a key tooth may determine whether other teeth are saved or extracted or whether the prosthesis is fixed or removable (see Fig. 41.4). When few teeth remain, the prosthodontic needs become more important, and sometimes periodontally treatable teeth may have to be extracted if they are not compatible with the design of the prosthesis.

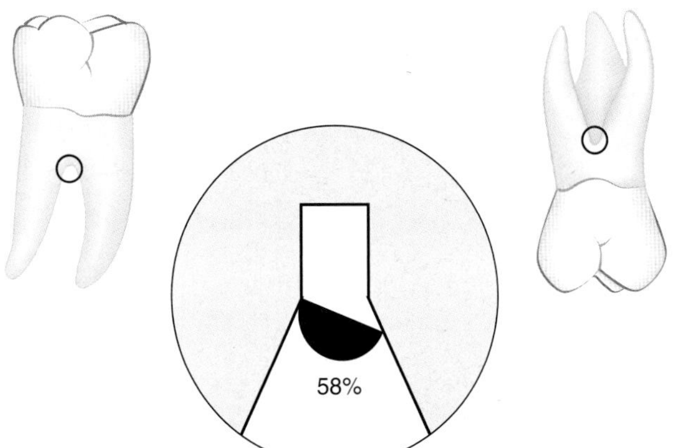

Fig. 41.8 The furcation entrance is narrower than a standard curette in 58% of first molars. (*Redrawn from Bower RC. Furcation morphology relative to periodontal treatment. Furcation root surface anatomy.* J Periodontol. *1979;50:366.*)

Teeth that serve as abutments are subjected to increased functional demands. Therefore, more rigid standards are required when evaluating the prognosis of teeth adjacent to edentulous areas. A tooth with a post that has undergone endodontic treatment is more likely to fracture when serving as a distal abutment supporting a distal removable partial denture. Additionally, special oral hygiene measures must be instituted in these areas.

In general, prognostication systems in periodontics were proposed to assign prognosis of a tooth based on its periodontal condition. However, clinically, it is important to consider restorability and the overall prosthetic plan when assigning individual or overall prognosis.

Prognosis of Specific Periodontal Diseases

Many of the criteria used in the diagnosis of periodontal diseases and conditions[7] (see Chapter 5) are also used in assigning prognosis (see Box 41.1). Factors such as patient age, severity of disease, genetic susceptibility, and presence of systemic disease are important criteria in the diagnosis of the condition and in developing a prognosis. This section discusses potential prognoses for the various periodontal diseases and conditions outlined in Chapter 5.

Prognosis for Patients With Gingival Disease

Dental Plaque-induced Gingivitis Associated With Biofilm Alone

Dental plaque-induced gingivitis is a reversible disease that occurs when bacterial biofilm accumulates at the gingival margin.[28,29] This disease can occur on a periodontium that has experienced no attachment loss or on a periodontium with nonprogressing attachment loss. In either case, the prognosis is good for patients with gingivitis associated with bacterial biofilm only, provided that all local irritants are removed, other local factors contributing to biofilm retention are eliminated, gingival contours conducive to the preservation of health are attained, and the patient cooperates by maintaining good oral hygiene.

Dental Plaque-Induced Gingivitis Mediated by Systemic or Local Risk Factors

Gingivitis is primarily induced by dental plaque but the inflammatory response to bacterial biofilm at the gingival margin can be influenced by systemic and local factors. Systemic factors include endocrine-related changes associated with puberty, menstruation, pregnancy, and diabetes; the presence of blood dyscrasias; smoking; and malnutrition. Local factors include dental plaque retention factors (e.g., prominent subgingival restoration margins) and hyposalivation (see Chapter 24).

In many cases, the frank signs of gingival inflammation that occur in these patients are seen in the presence of relatively small amounts of bacterial biofilm. Therefore, the long-term prognosis for these patients depends not only on control of bacterial biofilm but also on control or correction of these systemic and local factors.

Dental Plaque-Induced Gingivitis—Drug-Influenced Gingival Enlargement

The third group of conditions under dental plaque-induced gingivitis is drug-influenced gingival enlargement. This is often seen in patients taking antiepileptic medication such as phenytoin, immunosuppressants like cyclosporine, or calcium channel blockers like nifedipine. In drug-influenced gingival enlargement, the severity of the lesions is associated with inflammation, which is usually induced by bacterial biofilm. Inflammation may also be induced by repeated trauma (Fig. 41.9). Eliminating the source of inflammation,

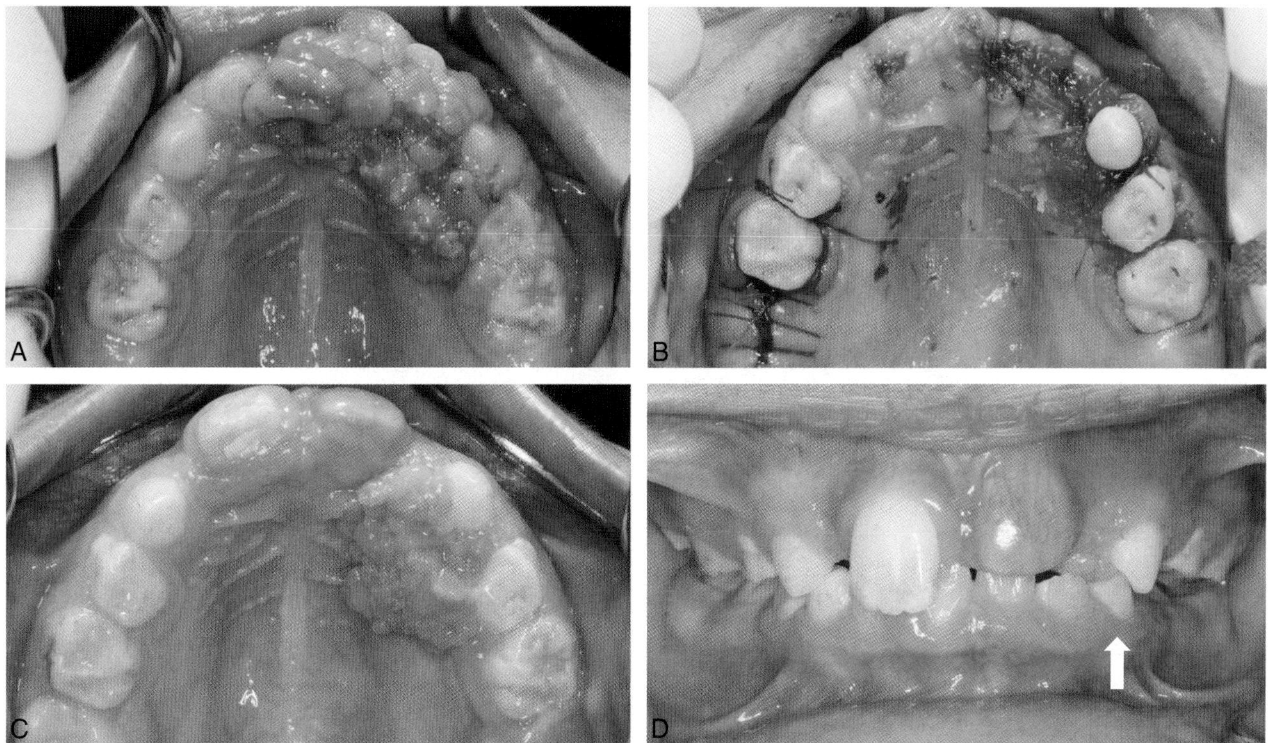

Fig. 41.9 (A) Gingival overgrowth in a 5-year-old male patient who was taking cyclosporine for the management of aplastic anemia. (B) The gingival overgrowth was resected surgically. (C) Recurrence of gingival overgrowth on the maxillary left quadrant at 1-year post-op due to trauma from the opposing mandibular teeth occluding on the maxillary left palatal tissue (D). (*Copyright Jonathan H. Do, DDS. All rights reserved.*)

either biofilm or trauma, can limit the severity of the gingival overgrowth. However, surgical intervention is usually necessary to correct the alterations in gingival contour. Continued use of the drug and persistence of inflammation usually result in recurrence of the enlargement, even after surgical intervention (see Chapter 19). Therefore, the long-term prognosis depends on whether the etiology of the inflammation can be completely eliminated, or the patient's systemic problem can be treated with an alternative medication that does not have gingival enlargement as a side effect.

Non-Dental Plaque Induced Gingival Diseases

Some gingival diseases are primarily induced genetic/developmental disorders (hereditary gingival fibromatosis), specific infections (bacterial, viral, or fungal origin), inflammatory and immune conditions (hypersensitivity reactions, autoimmune diseases of skin and mucous membranes, granulomatous inflammatory lesions), reactive processes (epulides), neoplasms, endocrine disorders, nutritional deficiency (vitamin C deficiency), metabolic diseases, or trauma. These gingival conditions will not be fully resolved by removal of dental plaque alone. However, uncontrolled plaque accumulation can worsen these conditions. Therefore, the long-term prognosis in these patients depends on the control of these contributing factors along with dental plaque control.

Prognosis for Patients With Periodontitis

Periodontitis

In general, there is a significant overlap in the prognostic factors for gingivitis and periodontitis. However, with the same prognostic factor(s), the prognosis for a periodontally affected tooth is worse than a tooth with gingival inflammation only.

Previously, periodontitis was further categorized into chronic periodontitis and aggressive periodontitis. Chronic periodontitis is a slowly progressive disease associated with well-known risk factors, such as biofilm and calculus.[27] Aggressive periodontitis is a rapidly progressive disease associated with abnormal host responses and featured bacterial species. However, since there is no strong evidence supporting the differences in etiology and pathophysiology between these two types of diseases, they are both categorized as periodontitis in the 2018 classification of periodontal diseases and conditions. In the 2018 classification, a staging and grading system was introduced to the periodontitis disease category and presented with the following components: generalized, localized or molar-incisor pattern (extent); stage I, II, III, or IV (severity and complexity); and grade A, B or C (progression rate). Refer to Chapter 5 for more information on staging and grading of periodontitis.

In cases in which the clinical attachment loss and bone loss are slight to moderate (stage I or II periodontitis) with slow or moderate progression rate (grade A or B), the prognosis is generally favorable, provided the inflammation can be controlled through good oral hygiene and the removal of local biofilm-retentive factors (see Fig. 41.1). In patients with more severe disease (stage III or IV) (see Fig. 41.2), as evidenced by bone loss extending to the middle third of root and beyond, furcation invasion, vertical defect and multiple tooth loss due to periodontitis, with rapid progression rate (grade C), the prognosis may be questionable or unfavorable, or even hopeless for some teeth.

When rapid progression rate is present and associated with systemic factors (e.g., uncontrolled diabetes) and smoking history, the host response might be altered and these patients usually do not respond well to conventional nonsurgical or surgical periodontal therapy. Therefore, the higher the stage and/or grade of periodontitis, the poorer the individual and overall prognoses will be.[43]

The overall prognosis in localized periodontitis is generally better than in generalized periodontitis since the disease is less extensive in the former category. When compared with localized periodontitis, the molar/incisor pattern of periodontitis that tends to occur in younger patients (previously known as localized aggressive periodontitis), is associated with rapid disease progression and therefore has worse overall prognosis (Fig. 41.10).

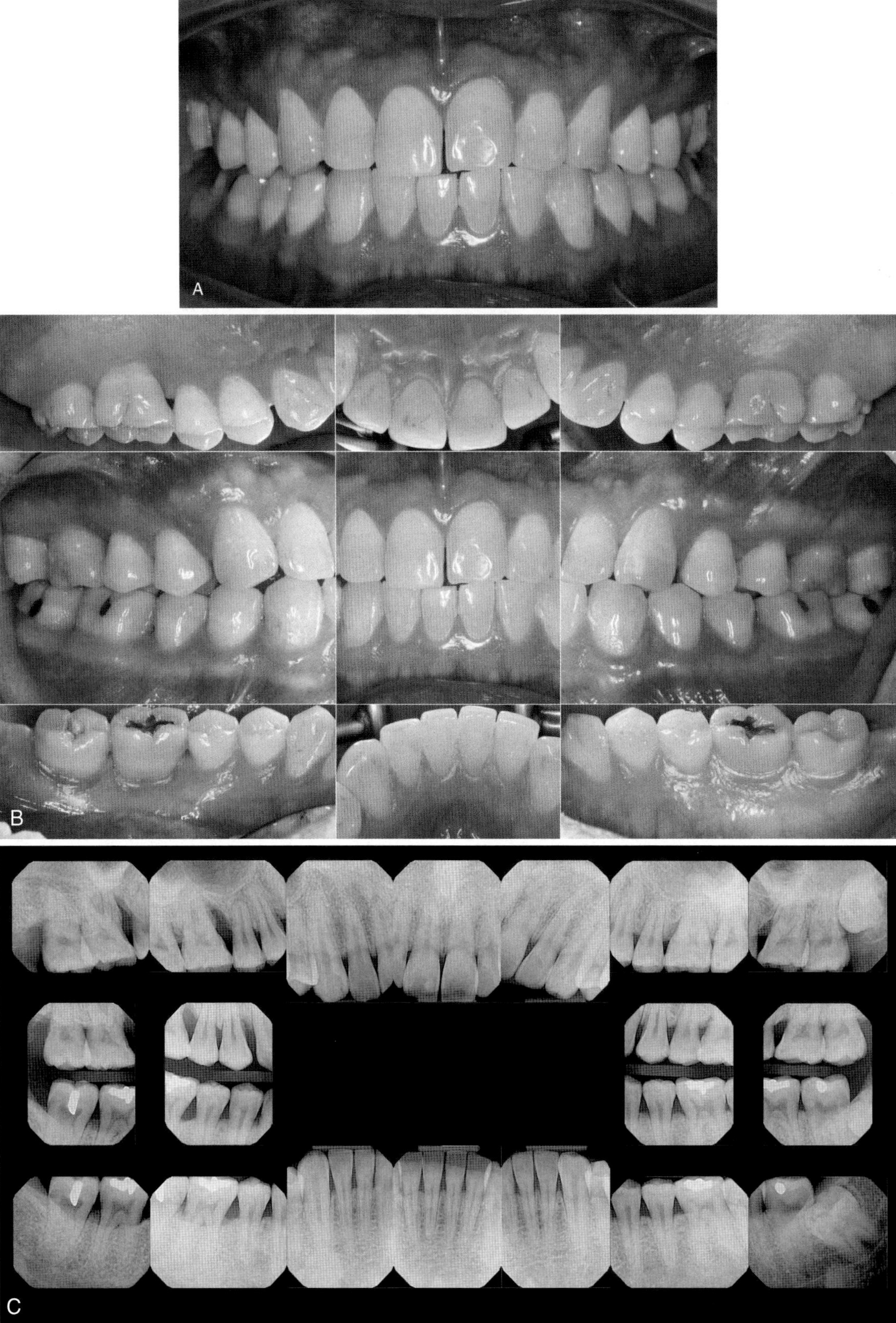

Fig. 41.10 Clinical photos (A and B) and full mouth radiographic series (C) of a patient who had molar-incisor pattern of periodontitis (used to be called "localized aggressive periodontitis"). The overall prognosis is favorable except for the maxillary right first molar (unfavorable), maxillary left first molar (questionable), and mandibular right first molar (questionable).

Periodontitis as a Manifestation of Systemic Diseases

Although the primary etiologic factor in periodontal diseases is bacterial plaque, systemic diseases that alter the ability of the host to respond to the microbial challenge may affect the progression of disease and therefore the prognosis for the case (see Chapters 5 and 25). For example, decreased numbers of circulating neutrophils (as in acquired neutropenia) may contribute to widespread destruction of the periodontium. Unless the neutropenia can be corrected, these patients can present with a questionable to unfavorable prognosis. Similarly, genetic disorders that alter the way the host responds to bacterial plaque (as in leukocyte adhesion deficiency syndrome) also can contribute to the development of periodontitis. Because these disorders generally manifest early in life, the destruction of periodontium can be severe and aggressive. The prognosis in these cases will be questionable or unfavorable.

Other systemic disorders do not affect the host's ability to combat infections but still affect the development of periodontitis. Examples include (1) hypophosphatasia, in which patients have decreased levels of circulating alkaline phosphatase, severe alveolar bone loss, and premature loss of deciduous and permanent teeth, and (2) Ehlers–Danlos syndrome, a connective tissue disorder in which patients may present with clinical characteristics of severe periodontitis. In both examples, the prognosis can be questionable or unfavorable.

Necrotizing Periodontal Disease

Necrotizing periodontal disease can be divided into necrotic diseases that affect the gingival tissues exclusively (necrotizing gingivitis [NG]); necrotic diseases that affect deeper tissues of the periodontium, resulting in a loss of connective tissue attachment and alveolar bone (necrotizing periodontitis [NP]); and necrotic diseases that affect gingiva, periodontium and mucosa in the oral cavity (necrotizing stomatitis [NS]).[40,46] In NG, the primary predisposing factor is bacterial plaque. However, this disease is usually complicated by the presence of secondary factors such as acute psychological stress, tobacco smoking, and poor nutrition, all of which can contribute to immunosuppression. The superimposition of these secondary factors on preexisting gingivitis can result in the painful, necrotic lesions characteristic of NG. With control of the bacterial plaque and the secondary factors, the prognosis for a patient with NG is favorable. Uncontrolled and repeated NG may progress to NP, negatively affecting the prognosis.

The clinical presentation of NP is similar to that of NG, except the necrosis extends from the gingiva into the periodontal ligament and alveolar bone. In systemically healthy patients, this progression may have resulted from multiple episodes of NG, or the necrotizing disease may occur at a site previously affected with periodontitis. In these patients, the prognosis depends on alleviating the biofilm and secondary factors associated with NG. However, many patients presenting with NP are immunocompromised by systemic conditions such as human immunodeficiency virus (HIV) infection. In these patients, the prognosis depends not only on reducing local and secondary factors but also on dealing with the systemic problem (see Chapter 27).

Determination and Reassessment of Prognosis

Determination of prognosis of a tooth or teeth requires a careful and thorough assessment of the presence of disease and its severity, extent, and progression rate. An accurate prognosis cannot be made without an accurate diagnosis. Once disease has been properly and accurately diagnosed, determining the prognosis can still be difficult, particularly for teeth with disease. Many factors can influence disease progression and the response to therapy, and the specific influence of any factor is unknown and likely different from one patient to another. In addition, each patient can respond differently at different times. Moreover, the outcome of therapy significantly depends on the treatment to be rendered, the quality of the treatment, the skills and knowledge of the treating clinician, and patient home care. For these reasons, determining an accurate prognosis can be challenging.

Prognosis of teeth with minimal disease is favorable and by far the easiest to assign with accuracy and precision. As disease develops and severity increases, prognosis becomes progressively harder to assign correctly and accurately, especially for teeth with moderate to advanced disease that have a questionable or unfavorable prognosis. Once disease progresses to a point that teeth are no longer functional or treatable, the prognosis is again easy to determine. These teeth are assigned a hopeless prognosis and the treatment is extraction. However, the treatability of a tooth can be easily skewed by the skills and expertise of the treating clinician, or lack thereof. It is also easier for a clinician to make a diagnosis, determine a prognosis, and create a treatment plan that aligns with his or her expertise. For example, a prosthodontist may assign mandibular incisors with moderate attachment loss and grade 2 mobility a hopeless prognosis and develop a treatment plan that involves replacement of these teeth with a removable partial denture or dental implants. However, a periodontist may assign these teeth a questionable prognosis if the patient is compliant. With the proper periodontal treatment and effective patient biofilm control, the health and function of these mandibular anterior teeth may be restored and maintained for many years.

It is not always possible to accurately determine the prognosis prior to initiating periodontal treatment. During the periodontal examination, due to the lack of anesthesia, it may not be possible to accurately and carefully probe a tooth to determine the true extent of bone loss and severity of disease. During subgingival root instrumentation ("scaling and root planing") under anesthesia, it is possible to probe to the depth of the periodontal pocket. However, the anatomy of the osseous defect may not be determined until a periodontal flap has been elevated and all the granulation tissue removed. Additionally, heavy subgingival calculus deposits before treatment may affect the accuracy of the examination, resulting in an imprecise diagnosis and prognosis. As such, the prognosis may change as more specific diagnostic information is discovered during the treatment phase.

Prognosis may also change with periodontal treatment or disease progression. During therapy, the patient's motivation and commitment, acknowledged as critical in all forms of periodontal therapy, can be determined, as well as the host response and the healing capacity of the patient.

A frank reduction in probing depth and inflammation after therapy indicates a favorable response to treatment and may suggest a better prognosis than previously assumed (Fig. 41.11). If the inflammatory changes cannot be controlled or reduced by therapy, the overall prognosis would be poorer. Adverse treatment outcomes usually indicate existence of uncontrolled or unidentified local and/or systemic factors. Therapy allows the clinician an opportunity to work with the patient and the patient's other care providers to control local, systemic, and environmental factors such as overhanging restorations, diabetes, and smoking, respectively, which may have a positive effect on prognosis, if adequately controlled.

The progression of periodontitis generally occurs in an episodic manner, with alternating periods of quiescence and shorter

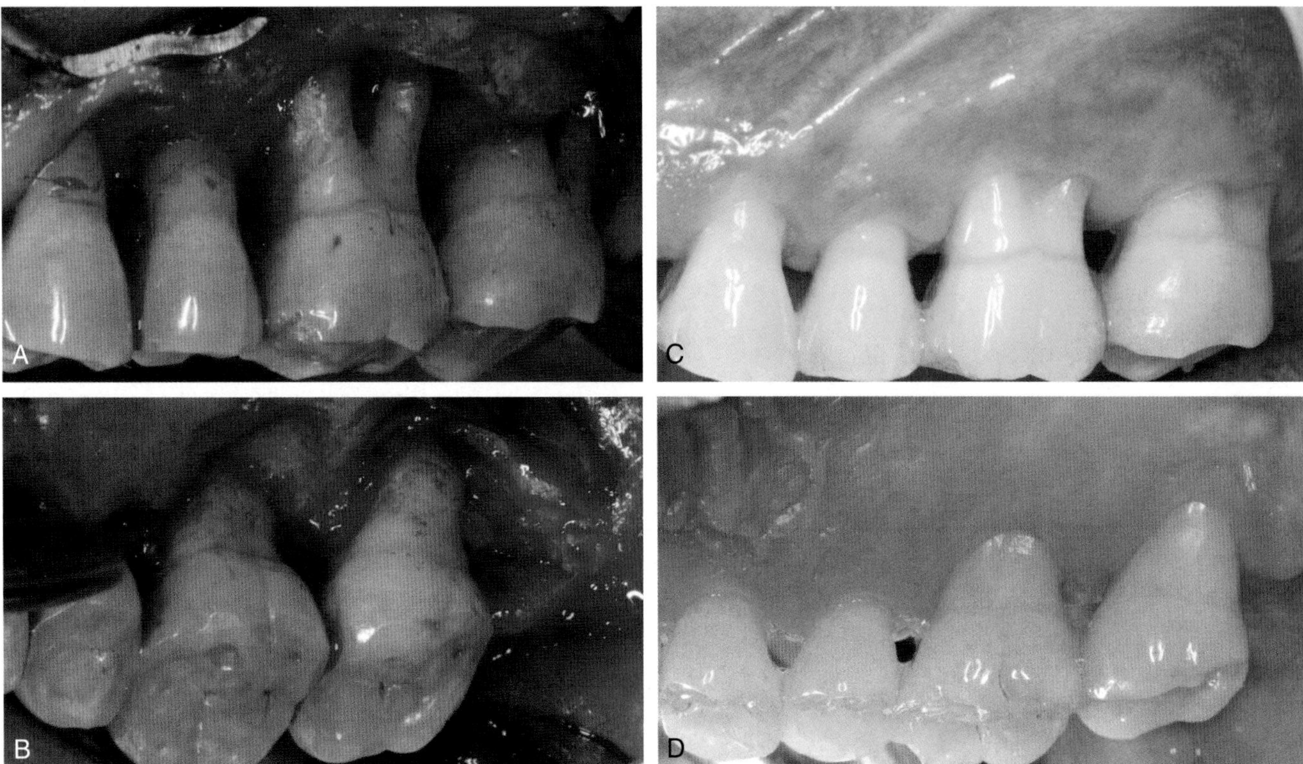

Fig. 41.11 Prognosis changes with treatment. The maxillary left first and second molars were initially assigned an unfavorable prognosis due to advanced bone loss and deep grade II furcation invasion (A, B). The clinician contemplated extraction of both teeth. However, both teeth were vital, stable, and did not require any restorative treatment, and the patient wanted to keep them and was willing to effectively control biofilm. Both teeth were treated with periodontal surgery. After 5 years, they remain healthy, functional with shallow probing pocket depths, and the prognosis improved to favorable (C, D). (*Copyright Jonathan H. Do, DDS. All rights reserved.*)

destructive stages (see Chapter 8). No methods are available at present to accurately determine whether a given lesion is in a stage of remission or exacerbation. Advanced lesions, if active, may progress rapidly to a hopeless stage, whereas similar lesions in a quiescent stage may be maintainable for long periods. Stable lesions in a patient in periodontal maintenance may also break down and advance due to changes in biofilm control, systemic health, or stress level. For these reasons, prognosis along with diagnosis must be carefully evaluated and reassessed throughout the course of treatment and over time during supportive maintenance therapy.

LEARNING BOX 41.5

Due to the dynamic nature of patients and periodontal disease, prognosis must be reevaluated during all phases of treatment.

Conclusion

The periodontal prognosis plays a pivotal role in therapy, as treatment decisions are made based on prognosis and to improve prognosis. Teeth with a hopeless prognosis are extracted, whereas teeth with more favorable prognoses are treated, with the intent of restoring health and stability and ultimately improving the prognosis. A hopeless prognosis is perhaps the easiest prognosis to assign, because hopeless teeth usually have overt and severe disease. The hopeless prognosis is also perhaps the easiest to be erroneously assigned, due to clinical bias or lack of training and expertise. Therefore, the hopeless prognosis must be assigned with caution, as the consequences are irreversible. It must also be recognized that patients and diseases are dynamic. As such, a prognosis will change and must be reevaluated over time. Depending on the controllability of local and systemic factors that affect the prognosis, the questionable or unfavorable prognostic categories can change and could go in either direction and therefore should be continually monitored.

LEARNING BOX 41.6

Examination and Information Gathering→ Diagnosis → Prognosis ↔ Treatment

- Diagnosis requires thorough and careful examination.
- Prognosis is based on accurate diagnosis.
- Treatment decisions are based on the prognosis.
- Treatment decisions are made to improve prognosis.
- Diagnosis (in select cases) and prognosis could change with treatment.

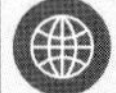
References for this chapter are found on the companion website eBooks.Health.Elsevier.com.

CHAPTER 42

Periodontal Treatment Plan

Satheesh Elangovan | Jonathan H. Do | Henry H. Takei | Fermin A. Carranza | Michael G. Newman

CHAPTER OUTLINE

A thorough and diligent "information gathering" process is an absolute prerequisite for the clinician to formulate a comprehensive treatment plan that takes into account not just local factors in the oral cavity but also the systemic health status of the patient and other critical treatment modifiers like psychosocial and behavioral factors. With the growing body of scientific evidence and validation of molecular markers of health and disease, the information-gathering process now expands to these domains as well in order to render preventive and/or therapeutic precision health care. In addition, digitalization of diagnostic information—be it periodontal charting, radiographs, or intraoral scans—allows for the effective integration of artificial intelligence and machine-learning capabilities that can aid the clinician in the decision-making process. In addition, three-dimensional imaging like cone-beam computed tomography (CBCT), with its seamless capability to connect to third-party software programs and the ability to link intraoral scanning images to CBCT images, has greatly expanded the diagnostic and treatment planning possibilities. The previous chapters in this section provide a more detailed information on the process of information gathering and how that information is utilized to diagnose periodontal diseases and conditions and to generate a personalized treatment plan for a patient. Fig 42.1 provides a broad overview of this process and how and where "arriving at diagnosis," "prognostication," and "formulating a treatment plan" fits in the broader scheme of things. Refer to Chapters 84 and 85 for more information on digital implant planning.

As shown in Fig. 42.1, after the periodontal diagnosis and prognosis have been established, the treatment is planned. The plan should encompass immediate, intermediate, and long-term goals.

The *immediate goals* are the elimination and resolution of infectious and inflammatory processes, respectively, that cause periodontal and other oral problems that may hinder the patient's general health. Basically, the immediate goals are to bring the oral cavity to a state of health. This may require patient education on infectious oral diseases and disease prevention, periodontal procedures, endodontics, caries control, extractions, and treatment of oral mucous membrane pathologies. Referral to other dental and medical specialties may be necessary at this stage of therapy.

From a periodontal viewpoint, the immediate goals are important, because they consist of the resolution of gingival inflammation and the correction of conditions that cause and perpetuate it. These include not only elimination of root surface accretions but also pocket reduction and the establishment of good gingival contours and mucogingival relationships conducive to periodontal health. Extraction of hopeless teeth, restoration of carious lesions, and correction of defective existing restorations may be necessary.

The *intermediate goals* are the reconstruction of a healthy dentition that not only fulfills all functional and aesthetic requirements but lasts many years. Restoration of health, function, aesthetics, and longevity involves endodontic, orthodontic, periodontal, and prosthodontic considerations as well as the age, health, and desires of the patient. The financial impact of restoring the dentition to health, function, aesthetics, and longevity requires careful consideration and understanding by the patient. The intermediate goals may be quickly achieved or require treatments over months or even years depending on the complexity of the case, the therapy involved, and the financial/compliance status of the patient.

The *long-term goal* is maintenance of health through prevention and professional supportive periodontal therapy. The long-term goal is set, and both the patient and the clinician work toward it from the very first visit. Once active disease has been controlled, all infectious and inflammatory processes have been addressed, and health has been attained, health should be maintainable for the rest of the patient's life. Maintenance of health requires patient education on disease prevention and oral hygiene at the onset of treatment and at repeated intervals, meticulous daily home care by the patient, and patient adherence to professional recall maintenance.

KEY FACT

Maintenance of health depends on disease prevention, meticulous daily patient home care, and patient adherence to professional recall maintenance at a regular interval.

The treatment plan is the blueprint for case management. It includes all procedures required for the establishment and maintenance of oral health and involves decisions regarding the following:

- Emergency treatment (pain, acute infections)
- Removal of nonfunctional and diseased teeth and possibly strategic extraction of healthy teeth to facilitate the prosthetic reconstruction of the patient
- Treatment of periodontal diseases (nonsurgical or surgical)
- Endodontic therapy (necessary and intentional)

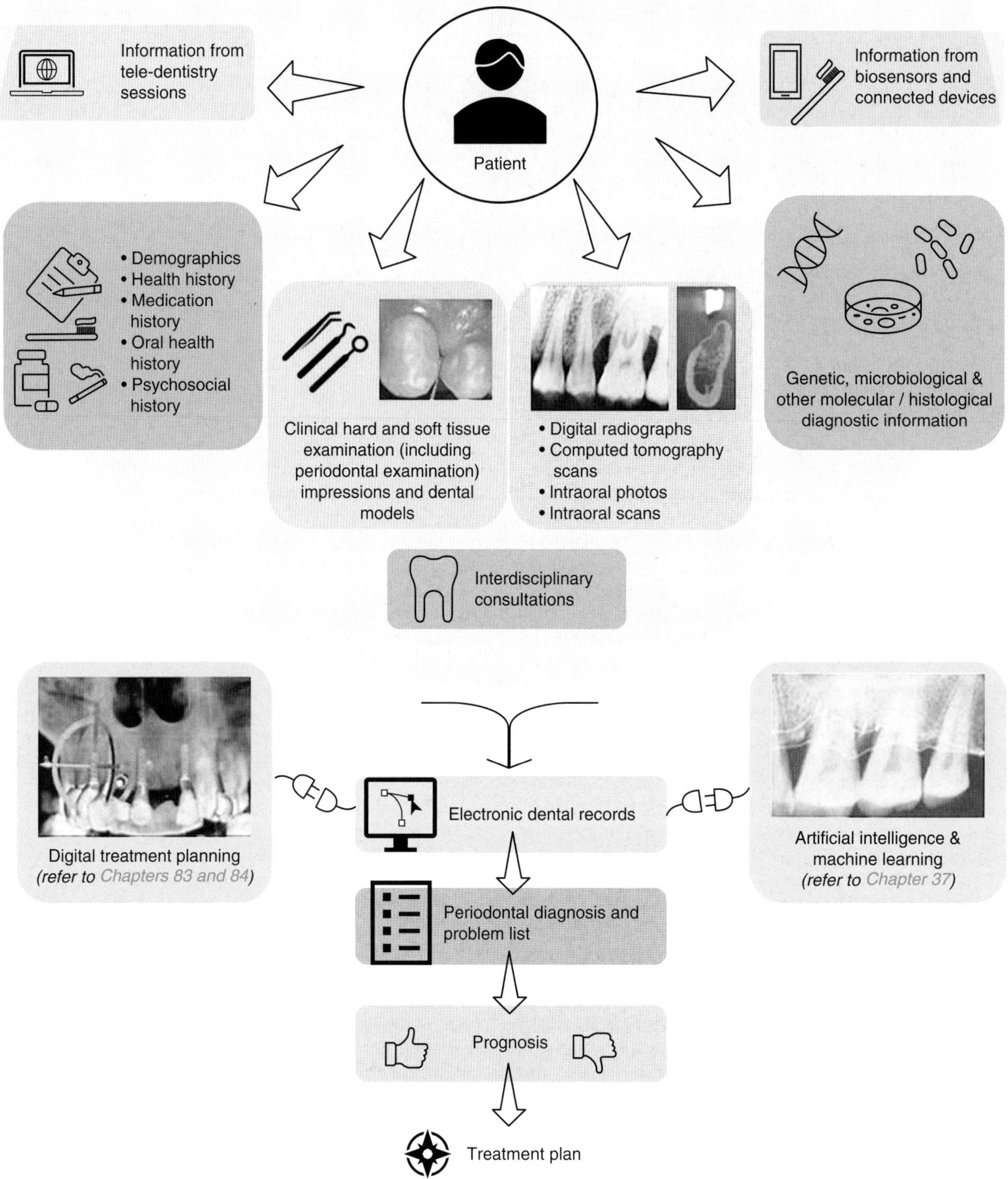

Fig. 42.1 Schematic illustrating the information-gathering process and how it leads to the formulation of a periodontal treatment plan in the era of precision dentistry.

- Caries removal and placement of temporary and final restorations
- Occlusal adjustment and orthodontic therapy
- Replacement of missing teeth with removable or tooth/implant-supported fixed dental prostheses
- Aesthetic demands
- Sequence of therapy

Treatment decisions are made with the diagnosis and prognosis of the individual teeth and the overall dentition in mind. The prognosis is usually established based on the diagnosis. Treatment decisions are made based on the prognosis and to improve the prognosis, and therefore prognosis will change with treatment. In the 2017 World Workshop, it was determined that once a stage of periodontitis is established, it cannot regress even with successful treatment outcomes—with the exception of successful regeneration of vertical defects and furcation with regenerative approaches changing the stage from III to possibly II.

Unforeseen developments during treatment may necessitate modification of the initial treatment plan. However, except for emergencies, no therapy should be initiated until a treatment plan has been established.

KEY FACT

Prognosis is established based on diagnosis. Treatment decisions are made based on prognosis and to improve prognosis.

Overall Treatment Plan

The aim of the treatment plan is to render comprehensive care—that is, the coordination of all the immediate, intermediate, and long-term goals for the purpose of creating a well-functioning dentition in a healthy periodontal environment. The periodontal treatment encompasses different areas of therapeutic objectives for each patient according to his or her needs. It is based on the diagnosis, prognosis, disease severity, risk factors, and other factors outlined in previous chapters.

Extracting or Preserving a Tooth

Periodontal treatment requires long-range planning. Its value to the patient is measured in years of healthy functioning of the entire dentition and not by the number of teeth retained at the time of treatment. Treatment is directed to establishing and maintaining the health of the periodontium throughout the mouth rather than attempting spectacular efforts to "tighten loose teeth."

Implant replacement of missing teeth has become a predictable course of therapy. Therefore, attempts to save questionable teeth may jeopardize adjacent teeth and may lead to the loss of bone needed for implant therapy. Teeth on the borderline of a hopeless prognosis do not contribute to the overall usefulness of the dentition. Such teeth become sources of recurrent problems for the patient and detract from the value of the greater service rendered by the establishment of periodontal health in the remainder of the oral cavity.

Removal, retention, or temporary (interim) retention of one or more teeth is an important part of the overall treatment plan. A tooth should be extracted under the following conditions:

- It is so mobile that function becomes painful or if it poses an aspiration (tooth reaching the lungs) risk.
- It can cause acute abscesses during therapy.
- There is no use for it in the overall treatment plan.

In some cases, a tooth can be retained temporarily, postponing the decision to extract until after treatment is completed. A tooth in this category can be retained under the following conditions:

- It maintains posterior stops; the tooth can be removed after treatment when it can be replaced by an implant or another type of prosthesis.
- It maintains posterior stops and may be functional after implant placement in adjacent areas. When the implant is restored, these teeth can be extracted.
- In the anterior aesthetic zone, a tooth can be retained during periodontal therapy and removed when treatment is completed and a permanent restorative procedure can be performed. The retention of this tooth should not jeopardize the adjacent teeth. This approach avoids the need for temporary appliances in the aesthetic zone during therapy.
- Extraction of hopeless teeth can be delayed during the nonsurgical periodontal therapy and can be performed during periodontal surgery of the adjacent teeth. This approach reduces the number of appointments needed for surgery in the same area.

In addition to the proper function of the dentition, aesthetic considerations play an important role in the formulation of the treatment plan. Different patients value aesthetics differently according to their age, gender, profession, social status, and life experiences. The clinician should carefully evaluate and consider a final aesthetic outcome of treatment that will be acceptable to the patient without jeopardizing the basic need of attaining health.

With the predictable use of implants, questionable teeth should be carefully evaluated as to whether their removal and replacement with an implant may be a better and more satisfactory course of therapy.

In complex cases, interdisciplinary consultation with other specialty areas is necessary before a final plan can be made. The opinions of orthodontists and prosthodontists are especially important for the final decision in these patients.

Occlusal evaluation and therapy may be necessary during treatment, which may necessitate planning for occlusal adjustment (see Chapters 34 and 35), orthodontics (see Chapter 48), and splinting. The correction of bruxism and other occlusal habits may also be necessary.

Systemic conditions should be carefully evaluated, because they may require special precautions during the course of periodontal treatment. The tissue response to treatment procedures may be affected, or the preservation of periodontal health may be threatened after treatment is completed. The patient's physician should always be consulted when the patient presents with medical and systemic problems that may affect the periodontal therapy.

Supportive periodontal therapy is also of paramount importance for maintenance of treatment outcomes. Such care entails all procedures for maintaining periodontal health after it has been attained. It consists of instruction in oral hygiene and recall therapy at regular intervals, according to the patient's needs. Please refer to Chapter 70 for detailed information on supportive periodontal therapy.

Sequence of Therapy

The periodontal treatment sequence is presented in Box 42.1, and a nonsurgical periodontal treatment decision tree is presented in Fig. 42.2. Periodontal therapy is an inseparable part of dental therapy, and all treatments must be well coordinated.

Although the phases of treatment are numbered, the recommended sequence does not follow the numbers (Fig. 42.3). Phase I, or the *nonsurgical phase,* is directed to the elimination of the etiologic factors of dental, gingival, and periodontal diseases. When successfully performed, this phase controls and stops the progression of dental and periodontal disease.

Immediately after completion of Phase I therapy, the patient should be placed on the *maintenance phase* (Phase IV) to preserve the results obtained and prevent any further deterioration and recurrence of disease. While on the maintenance phase with its periodic evaluation based on need, the patient enters into the *surgical phase* (phase II) and the *restorative phase* (phase III) of treatment (Fig. 42.4). These phases include periodontal surgery to treat and improve the condition of the periodontal and surrounding tissues. This may include reconstruction of gingival and bone defects for function and aesthetics, placement of implants, and restorative therapy.

KEY FACT

Immediately after the completion of phase I therapy, the patient should be placed on the maintenance phase.

Explaining the Treatment Plan to the Patient

The following discussion includes suggestions for explaining the treatment plan to the patient.

BOX 42.1 Periodontal Treatment Sequence

Periodontal Evaluation

Comprehensive periodontal examination
Diagnosis, prognosis, and risk assessment
Patient education

- Clinical findings and disease status
- Disease pathogenesis and prevention
- Personalized oral hygiene instruction

Reduction of systemic and environmental risk factors

- Physician consultation
- Smoking cessation

Periodontal treatment plan

- Oral hygiene assessment and education

Nonsurgical Therapy

Oral hygiene assessment and education[a]
Infection control

- Nonsurgical periodontal therapy
- Supragingival scaling and subgingival root instrumentation ("scaling and root planing")
- Extraction of hopeless teeth

Reduction of local risk factors

- Removal or reshaping of overhangs and over-contoured restorations
- Restoration of carious lesions
- Restoration of open contacts

Periodontal Reevaluation

Inquiry of new concerns or problems
Inquiry of changes in patient's medical and oral health status
Oral hygiene assessment and education[a]
Comprehensive periodontal examination
Assessment of outcome of nonsurgical therapy
Determination of required additional nonsurgical and adjunctive therapy

Surgical Therapy

Adjunct to nonsurgical therapy
Should only occur once patient demonstrates proficient biofilm control
Objectives:

- Primary: Access for root instrumentation
- Secondary: Pocket reduction through soft tissue resection, osseous resection, or periodontal regeneration

Periodontal pocket reduction surgery

- Resective
- Regenerative

Extraction of hopeless teeth
Periodontal plastic surgery

- Mucogingival surgery
- Aesthetic crown lengthening

Preprosthetic surgery

- Prosthetic crown lengthening
- Implant site preparation and implant placement

Periodontal Maintenance Therapy

Inquiry of new concerns or problems
Inquiry of changes in patient's medical and oral health status
Oral hygiene assessment and education[a]
Comprehensive periodontal examination
Professional maintenance care

- Supragingival and subgingival biofilm and calculus removal
- Selective subgingival root instrumentation ("scaling and root planing")

Assessment of recall interval and plan for next visit

[a]Patient oral hygiene is critical to the overall short-term and long-term treatment outcome. Therefore, oral hygiene must be repeatedly assessed and reinforced.

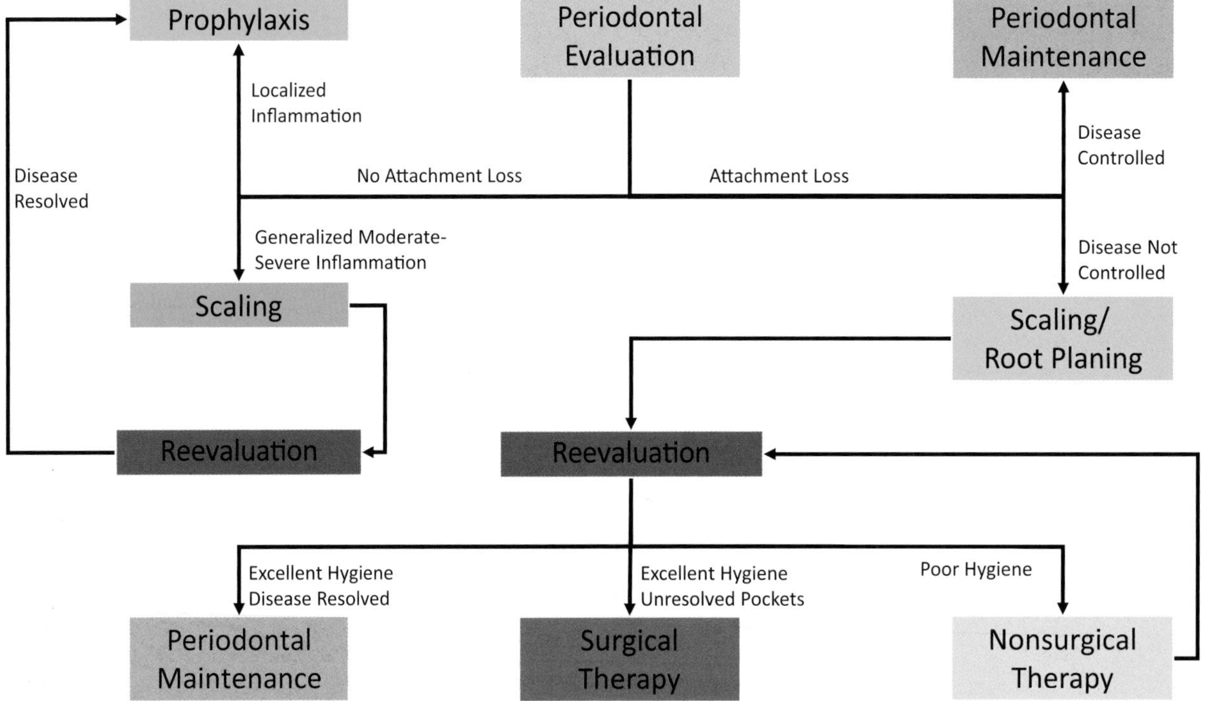

Fig. 42.2 Periodontal treatment decision tree.

Be specific. Tell your patient, "You have gingivitis" or "You have periodontitis," then explain exactly what the condition is.

Avoid vague statements. Do not use statements such as, "You have trouble with your gums" or "Something should be done about your gums." The patient may not understand the significance of such statements and may disregard them.

Begin your discussion on a positive note. Talk about the teeth that can be retained and the long-term service they can be expected to render. Do not begin your discussion with the statement "The following teeth have to be extracted." This creates a negative impression, which adds to the erroneous attitude of hopelessness the patient may already have regarding his or her mouth. Make it clear that every effort will be made to retain as many teeth as possible, but do not dwell on the patient's loose teeth. Emphasize that the important purpose of the treatment is to prevent the other teeth from becoming as severely diseased as the loose teeth.

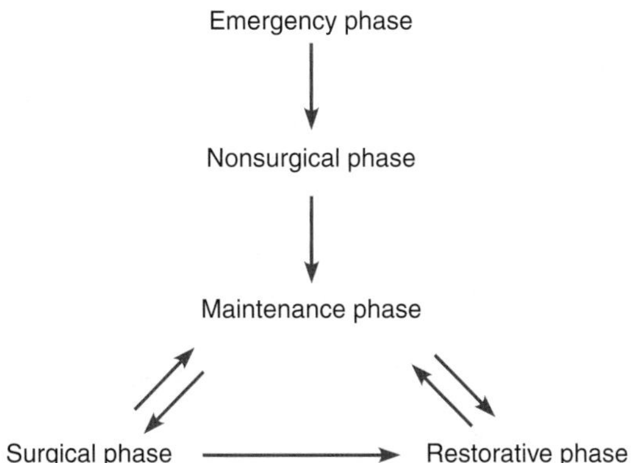

Fig. 42.3 Preferred sequence of therapy.

Present the entire treatment plan as one unit. Avoid creating the impression that treatment consists of separate procedures, some—or all—of which may be selected by the patient. Make it clear that dental restorations and prostheses contribute as much to the health of the gingiva as the elimination of inflammation and periodontal pockets. Do not speak in terms of "having the gums treated and then taking care of the necessary restorations later" as if these were unrelated treatments.

Patients often seek guidance from the dentist with questions such as the following:

- "Are my teeth worth treating?"
- "Would you have them treated if you had my problem?"
- "Why don't I just go along the way I am until the teeth really bother me and then have them all extracted?"

Explain that "doing nothing" or holding on to hopelessly diseased teeth as long as possible is inadvisable for the following reasons:

1. Periodontal disease with inflammation as a bridge is associated with several medical conditions such as stroke, cardiovascular disease, pulmonary disease, and diabetes, as well as the possibility for premature, low-birth-weight babies in women of childbearing age.
2. It is not feasible to place restorations or fixed bridges on teeth with untreated periodontal disease, because the usefulness of the restoration would be limited by the uncertain condition of the supporting structures.
3. Failure to eliminate periodontal disease not only results in the loss of teeth already severely involved, but also shortens the life span of other teeth. With proper treatment, these teeth can serve as the foundation for a healthy and functioning dentition.

Therefore, the dentist should make it clear to the patient that if the periodontal condition is treatable, the best results are obtained by prompt treatment. If the condition is not treatable, the teeth should be extracted.

It is the dentist's responsibility to advise the patient of the importance of periodontal treatment. However, if treatment is to be successful, the patient must be sufficiently interested in retaining his or her natural teeth and to maintain the necessary oral hygiene. Individuals who are not particularly perturbed by the thought of

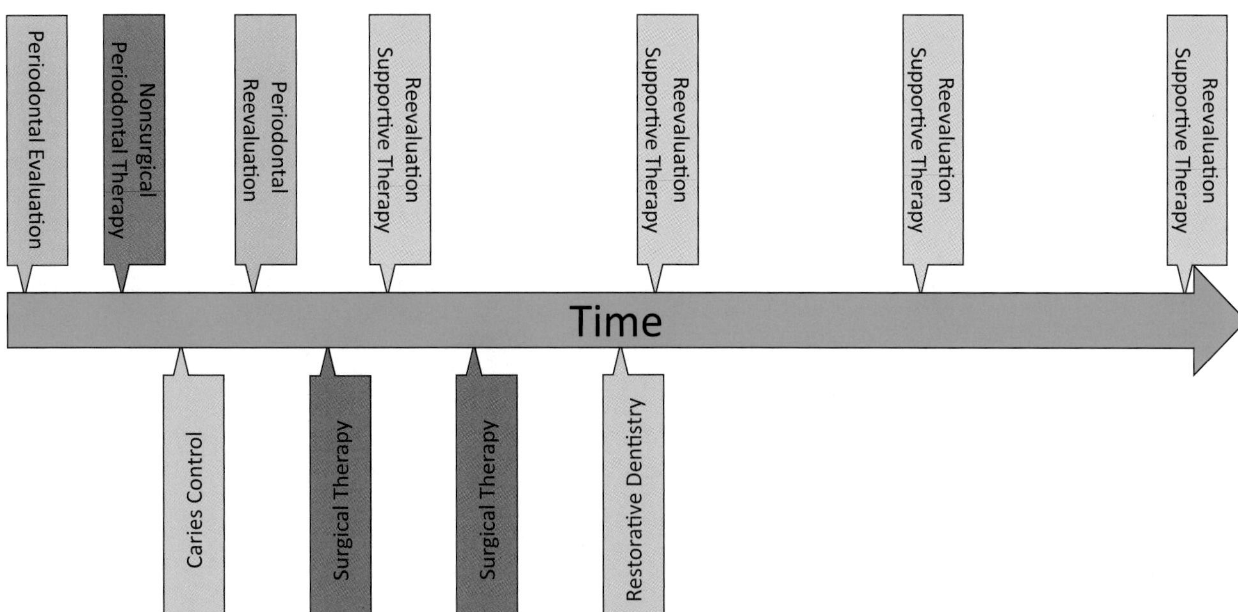

Fig. 42.4 Sample treatment timeline. Following nonsurgical periodontal therapy, the patient is placed on periodontal maintenance at regular intervals. Surgical and restorative treatments are scheduled between periodontal recalls.

losing their teeth are generally not good candidates for periodontal treatment.

Conclusion

The ultimate goal for every patient is to bring his or her mouth to a state of health and maintain it long term. This begins with educating the patient on the problems in his or her mouth and the etiologies, treatment, and prevention of these problems. A properly formulated treatment plan is paramount to achieving this goal. A treatment plan is a plan for therapy formulated only after a thorough examination has been completed, the diagnosis and prognosis have been determined, and the needs and desires of the patient have been taken into consideration. It must be recognized that as the diagnosis (in select cases) and prognosis will change with treatment, therapeutic needs may also change. As such, the treatment plan must be changed accordingly.

KEY FACT

Examination and Information Gathering → Diagnosis → Prognosis ↔ Treatment

- Diagnosis requires thorough and careful examination.
- Prognosis is based on accurate diagnosis.
- Treatment decisions are based on the prognosis.
- Treatment decisions are made to improve the prognosis.
- Diagnosis (in select cases) and prognosis could change with treatment.

CHAPTER **43**

Nonsurgical Phase of Periodontal Therapy

Satheesh Elangovan | Henry H. Takei

CHAPTER OUTLINE

Nonsurgical (phase I) or cause-related therapy[10] is the first in the chronologic sequence of procedures that constitute periodontal treatment. The objective of phase I therapy is to alter or eliminate the microbial etiology and factors that contribute to gingival and periodontal diseases to the greatest extent possible, thereby halting the progression of disease and returning the dentition to a state of health and comfort.[5] Phase I therapy is referred to by a number of names, including *initial therapy,*[5,10] *nonsurgical periodontal therapy,*[18] and *cause-related therapy.*[10] All terms refer to the procedures performed to treat gingival and periodontal infections up to and including tissue reevaluation, which is the point at which the course of ongoing care is determined.

Rationale

The evidence-based American Association of Periodontology practice guidelines[5] defined phase I therapy as the initiation of a comprehensive daily plaque or biofilm control regimen, management of periodontal-systemic interrelationships as needed, and thorough removal of supragingival and subgingival bacterial plaque or biofilm and calculus. Other components of this phase include the use of chemotherapeutic agents as necessary and correction of local factors[1–4,6] such as elimination of defective restorations and treatment of carious lesions.[7,9,15,16,20] These procedures are a required part of periodontal therapy, regardless of the extent of disease present. In many cases, only phase I therapy is required to restore periodontal health, or it constitutes the preparatory phase for surgical therapy. Figs. 43.1 and 43.2 show the results of phase I therapy in two patients with periodontitis. Cause-related phase I periodontal therapy has been succinctly stated as the approach *aimed at removal of pathogenic biofilms, toxins, and calculus, and the reestablishment of a biologically acceptable root surface.*[10]

Phase I therapy is a critical aspect of periodontal treatment. Data from clinical research indicate that the long-term success of periodontal surgical treatment is dependent on maintaining the plaque or biofilm control results achieved with phase I therapy. In fact, patients who do not have adequate plaque or biofilm control will continue to lose attachment regardless of what surgical procedures are performed and therefore are not good candidates for phase II or surgical therapy.[12] In addition, phase I therapy provides an opportunity for the dentist to evaluate tissue response and provide reinforcement about home care, both of which are crucial to the overall success of treatment.

Based on the knowledge that microbial plaque or biofilm is the major etiologic agent in gingival inflammation, one specific aim of phase I therapy for every patient is *effective daily plaque or biofilm removal* at home. These home care procedures can be complex and time-consuming and often require modifying long-standing habits. Good oral hygiene is more easily accomplished if the tooth surfaces are free of calculus deposits and other irregularities so that they are easily accessible. Management of all contributing local factors is required in phase I therapy. The following list of elements makes up phase I therapy:

1. Patient education and oral hygiene instruction
2. Complete removal of supragingival calculus (see Chapters 51 and 52)
3. Correction or replacement of poorly fitting restorations and other prosthetic devices (see Chapter 45)
4. Restoration or temporization of carious lesions
5. Orthodontic tooth movement (see Chapter 48)
6. Treatment of food impaction areas
7. Treatment of occlusal trauma (see Chapter 34)
8. Extraction of hopeless teeth
9. Possible use of antimicrobial agents, including necessary plaque or biofilm sampling and sensitivity testing (see Chapters 53 and 54)

Treatment Sessions

After careful analysis and diagnosis of the specific periodontal condition present, the clinician must develop a treatment plan that includes all required procedures to treat the periodontal condition and an estimate of the number of appointments necessary to complete phase I therapy. In most cases, patients require several treatment sessions for complete debridement of the tooth surfaces. All

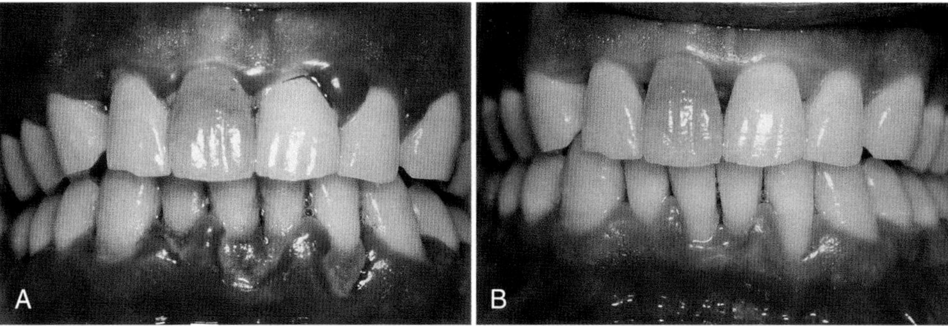

Fig. 43.1 Results of phase I therapy, severe chronic periodontitis. (A) A 45-year-old patient with deep probe depths, bone loss, severe swelling, and redness of the gingival tissues. (B) Results 3 weeks after the completion of phase I therapy. Note that the gingival tissue has returned to a normal contour, with redness and swelling dramatically reduced.

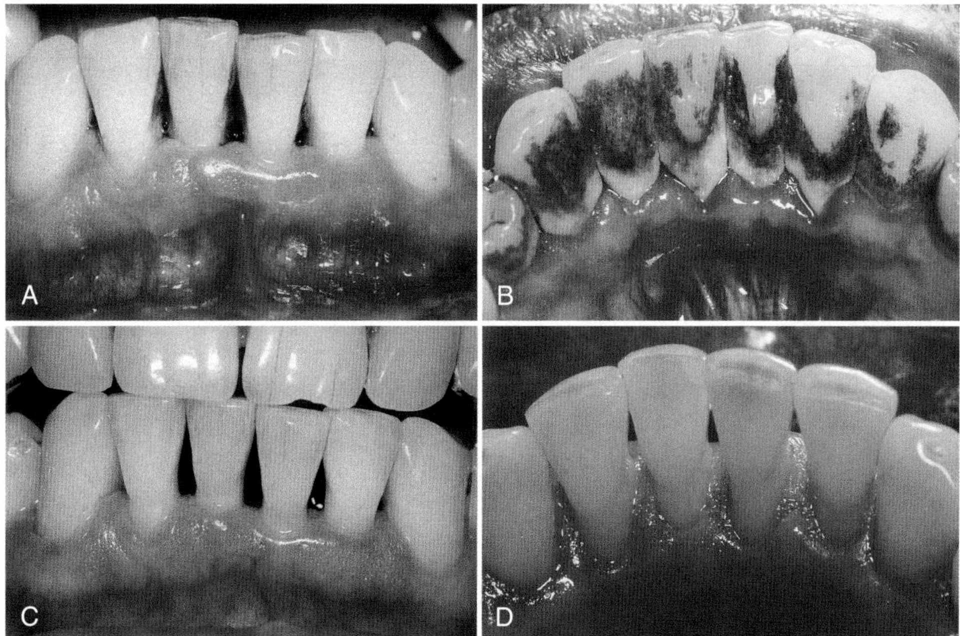

Fig. 43.2 Results of phase I therapy, moderate chronic periodontitis. (A) A 52-year-old patient with moderate attachment loss and probe depths in the 4- to 6-mm range. Note that the gingiva appears pink because it is fibrotic. Inflammation is present in the periodontal pockets but disguised by the fibrotic tissue. Bleeding occurs on probing. (B) Lingual view of the patient with more visible inflammation and heavy calculus deposits. (C and D) At 18 months after phase I therapy the same areas show significant improvement in gingival health. The patient returned for regular maintenance visits at 4-month intervals.

the following conditions must be considered when determining the phase I treatment plan:[18]

- General health and tolerance of treatment
- Number of teeth present
- Amount of subgingival calculus
- Probing pocket depths
- Attachment loss
- Furcation involvement
- Alignment of teeth
- Margins of restorations
- Developmental anomalies
- Physical barriers to access the dentition (e.g., limited opening or tendency to gag)
- Patient cooperation and sensitivity to therapy (requiring use of anesthesia or analgesia)
- Presence of dental implants in the oral cavity (requiring special tips and instruments)

Sequence of Procedures

Step 1: Plaque or Biofilm Control Instruction

Plaque or biofilm control is an essential component of successful periodontal therapy, and instruction should begin at the first treatment appointment. Before oral hygiene instruction, the patient must understand the reason that he or she must actively participate in therapy. The explanation of the etiology of the disease must be presented to the patient. Once the patient understands the nature of periodontal disease and the etiology, it will be easier to teach the hygiene that he or she must practice. The patient must be instructed on the correct technique to remove the plaque or biofilm; this means focusing on applying the bristles at the gingival third of the clinical crowns, where the tooth meets the gingival margin. This technique is sometimes referred to as *targeted oral hygiene* (H. Takei, Personal communication, 2009) and is synonymous with the Bass technique. Instructions are also initiated for interdental cleaning with dental floss and interdental brushes. The use of the multiple appointment approach to phase I therapy is favored by many clinicians because it permits the use of numerous appointments to evaluate, reinforce, and improve the patient's oral hygiene skills (see Chapter 50, which details plaque and biofilm control options).

Step 2: Removal of Supragingival and Subgingival Plaque or Biofilm and Calculus

Removal of calculus is accomplished using scalers, curettes, ultrasonic instrumentation, or combinations of these devices during one or more appointments. Evidence suggests that the treatment results for periodontitis are similar for all instruments, which could be hand instrumentation or other mechanical instruments, such as ultrasonic scalers.[12,13] Most clinicians advocate the combination of hand instruments (scalers, curettes) and ultrasonic devices. In addition to calculus and plaque or biofilm removal, cementum exposed to the pocket environment should be removed. At one time it was thought that the removal of all cementum was necessary to attain a smooth, glassy, hard surface. The rationale was that cementum became necrotic from penetration of endotoxins from the microbial biofilm and would interfere with healing. Current studies have indicated that endotoxins do not penetrate into the cementum as deeply as once believed and complete removal of the cementum may not always be necessary, but removal of the plaque or biofilm and calculus is absolutely necessary. In a clinical situation, it is difficult to know whether the removal of some or all of the cementum is achieved.

Laser treatment has also been advocated for periodontal therapy by some clinicians.[8] However, some reviews suggest that further well-designed studies are needed to confirm the outcomes. In addition, gingival curettage, the systematic removal of the soft tissue lining of the pockets, has not been shown to improve the results of treatment. Thorough plaque or biofilm removal and excellent root therapy result in conversion of the soft, edematous, inflamed gingival tissue to a healthier state without removing this tissue by using intentional soft tissue curettage. Therefore, curettage of the soft tissue pocket wall in phase I therapy is no longer advocated.

Photodynamic therapy has also been presented as an adjunct to scaling and root planing. This therapy uses light at specific wavelengths to "target microorganisms treated with a photosensitizer." Studies have not found this intervention to be useful as an alternative to scaling and root planing to improve treatment outcomes. Further research is necessary to ascertain the efficacy of this treatment.[12]

KEY FACT

Current studies have indicated that endotoxins do not penetrate into the cementum as deeply as once believed, and complete removal of the cementum may not always be necessary, but removal of the plaque or biofilm and calculus is absolutely necessary.

Another interesting approach to calculus removal and debridement is full-mouth disinfection. In this technique, full-mouth treatment is performed during one session or multiple sessions within a few days. Disinfectants are used after therapy with the intention of preventing reinfection of treated sites from untreated sites.[14,17,19,22] This treatment approach is used during phase I therapy by some clinicians, but the results have not been shown to be superior to those of any other phase I therapeutic approaches.[11,12,21]

Multiple approaches are used to plan and perform nonsurgical phase I therapy. Decisions on how to proceed should be discussed and agreed on by the patient and the dentist based on the extent and severity of disease present and the patient's tolerance to the therapy.[11] Staged therapy has the advantage of evaluating and reinforcing the oral hygiene status of the patient, but the one- or two-appointment approach can be more efficient in reducing the number of office visits the patient is required to attend.

Step 3: Recontouring Defective Restorations and Crowns

Corrections of restorative defects, which are plaque- or biofilm-retentive areas, may be accomplished by smoothing the rough surfaces and removing overhangs from the faulty restorations with burs or hand instruments, or complete replacement of the failing restorations may be necessary. All these steps are important to remove the local risk factors that perpetuate the inflammatory process. These procedures can be completed concurrently with other phase I procedures.

Step 4: Management of Carious Lesions

Removal of the carious lesions and placement of either temporary or permanent restorations are indicated in phase I therapy because of the infectious nature of the carious process. Healing of the periodontal tissues is maximized by removing the reservoir of bacteria in these lesions so that they cannot repopulate the microbial plaque.

Step 5: Tissue Reevaluation

After scaling, root planing, and other phase I procedures, the periodontal tissues require approximately 4 weeks to heal. This time allows the connective tissues to heal, and accurate probe depths can be measured. Patients will also have the opportunity to improve their home care skills to reduce gingival inflammation and adopt new habits that will ensure the success of treatment. At the reevaluation appointment, periodontal tissues are probed, and all related anatomic conditions are carefully evaluated to determine whether further treatment, including periodontal surgery, is indicated. Additional improvement from periodontal surgical procedures can be expected only if phase I therapy results in gingival tissues that are free of overt inflammation, and the patient has adopted effective daily plaque or biofilm control procedures.

Results

Subgingival root instrumentation ("scaling and root planning") have been studied extensively to evaluate their effects on periodontal disease. Many studies have indicated that this treatment is both effective and reliable. Studies ranging from 1 month to 2 years in length demonstrated up to 80% reduction in bleeding on probing and mean probing depth reductions of 2 to 3 mm. Other studies demonstrated that the percentage of periodontal pockets of 4 mm or deeper was reduced by more than 50% and in many cases up to 80%.[9] Figs. 43.1 and 43.2 show examples of the effectiveness of phase I therapy.

In addition, deeper probing depths present the dentist with greatly increased instrumentation challenges due to the complexity of root anatomy and difficulty accessing the root surfaces. Badersten and colleagues[7] reported in the 1980s that residual calculus remained on 44% of the surfaces in deeper pockets. Other studies have confirmed these findings, including studies comparing the use of hand instruments with that of powered scaling instruments.[12]

Additional individual treatments, such as caries control and correction of poorly fitting restorations, clearly help the healing gained by good plaque or biofilm control and debridement by making tooth surfaces accessible to hygiene procedures. Fig. 43.3 demonstrates the

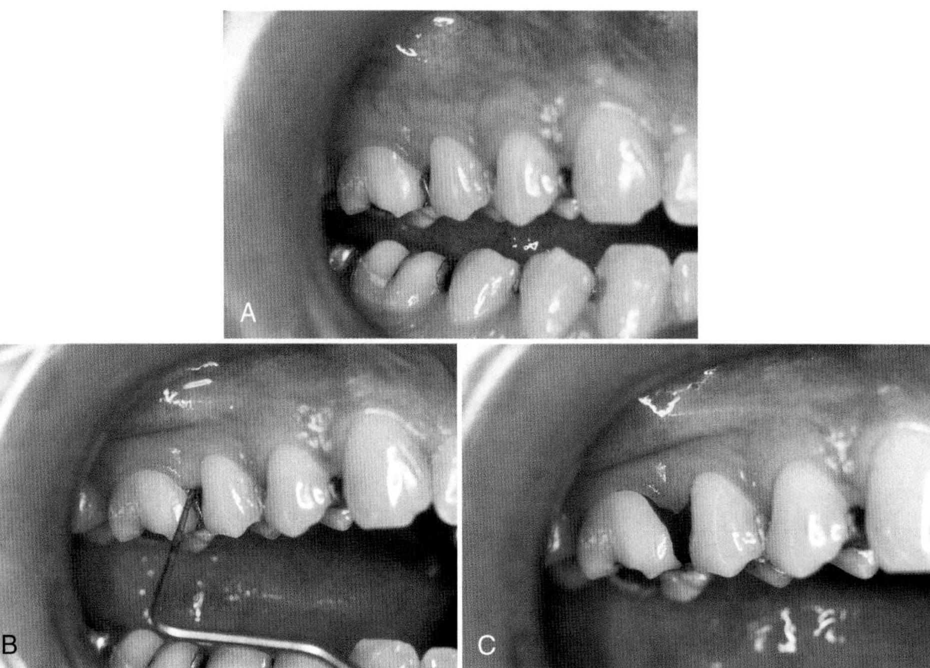

Fig. 43.3 Effects of overhanging amalgam margin on interproximal gingiva of maxillary first molar in otherwise healthy mouth. (A) Clinical appearance of rough, irregular, and overcontoured amalgam. (B) Gentle probing of interproximal pocket. (C) Extensive bleeding elicited by gentle probing indicating severe inflammation in the area.

effects of an overhanging amalgam restoration on gingival inflammation in an otherwise healthy periodontium. Maximal healing from phase I treatment is not possible when local conditions retain biofilm and provide reservoirs for repopulation of periodontal pathogens.

Healing

Healing of the gingival epithelium consists of the formation of a long junctional epithelium rather than new connective tissue attachment to the root surfaces. This long junctional epithelium occurs about 1 week after therapy. Gradual reductions in inflammatory cell population, crevicular fluid flow, and repair of connective tissue result in decreased clinical signs of inflammation, including less redness and swelling. One or two millimeters of recession is often apparent as the result of tissue shrinkage.[9] Connective tissue fibers are disrupted and lysed by the disease process and also by the inflammatory reaction to treatment. These tissues require 4 or more weeks to reorganize and heal, and many cases may require several weeks for complete healing.

Transient root sensitivity frequently accompanies the healing process. Although evidence suggests that relatively few teeth in a few patients become highly sensitive, this problem can be disconcerting to patients. The extent of the sensitivity can be diminished with good plaque or biofilm removal, but this may take several weeks to months.[23] Patients should also be warned and educated before the therapy is undertaken regarding the potential outcomes of several changes, such as the teeth appearing longer due to shrinkage of the periodontal tissues and root sensitivity. Knowledge of these changes before therapy will prevent the possibility of the patient complaining if they should occur. Unexpected and possible uncomfortable consequences of treatment may result in the patient's distrust and loss of motivation to continue therapy.

Decision to Refer for Specialist Treatment

It is fortunate that many periodontally involved cases do not require any further therapy beyond phase I therapy. Therefore, these patients can be seen by general dentists for routine maintenance therapy. However, advanced or complicated cases benefit from specialist care. Heitz-Mayfield and Lang[12] demonstrated that surgical treatment in deep pockets—those greater than 6 mm—gained 0.6 mm more probing depth reduction and 0.2 mm more clinical attachment gain than did deep pockets treated with scaling and root planing alone. This study also confirmed that in pockets of 4- to 6-mm probing depth, scaling and root planing resulted in 0.4 mm more attachment gain than surgical procedures, and shallow pockets of 1 to 3 mm had 0.5 mm less attachment loss compared with surgical results.[12] It is critical to be skilled in determining which patients would benefit from specialist care and deciding when a patient should be referred.

The concept of the *critical probing depth* of 5.4 mm has been advanced to assist in making the determination to proceed to surgical intervention. This is the measurement above which surgical therapy will result in clinical attachment gain and below which it will result in clinical attachment loss. This determination was made based on statistical analysis of surgical outcome data.[12] A similar *5-mm standard* has been commonly used as a guideline for identifying candidates for surgical referral based on the understanding that the typical root length is about 13 mm, and the crest of the alveolar bone is at a level approximately 2 mm apical to the bottom of the pocket. When there is 5 mm of clinical attachment loss, the crest of bone is about 7 mm apical to the cemento-enamel junction, and therefore only about half of the bony support for the tooth remains. Periodontal surgery can help improve the health and support for teeth in these cases through pocket reduction and regeneration procedures. Fig. 43.4 depicts the relationship of clinical attachment loss to tooth support.

In addition to the 5-mm probing depth criterion, other factors must be considered in the decision to refer to a periodontal specialist:

1. *Extent and severity of the disease process.* The amount of bone loss, even in localized areas, suggests the need for specialized surgical techniques.
2. *Root length.* Short-rooted teeth are jeopardized to a greater extent by the 5-mm clinical attachment loss criterion than teeth with long roots.

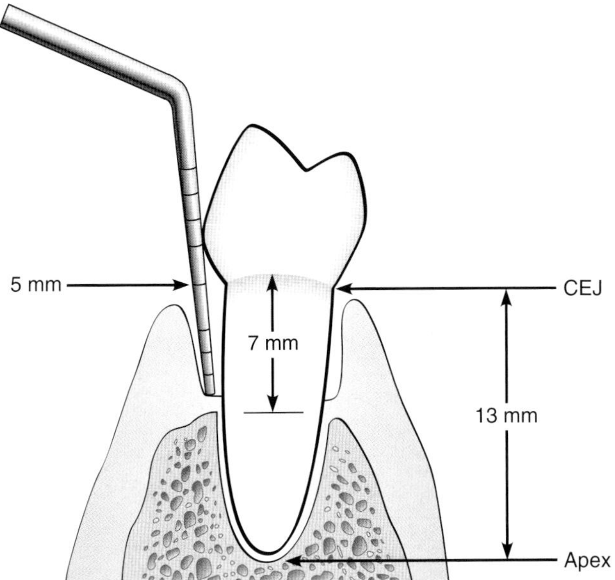

Fig. 43.4 The 5-mm standard for referral to a periodontist is based on root length, probing depth, and clinical attachment loss. The standard serves as a reasonable guideline to analyze the case for referral for specialist care. *CEJ,* Cementoenamel junction. (Redrawn with permission from Armitage G, ed. *Periodontal Maintenance Therapy.* Berkeley, CA: Praxis; 1974.)

3. *Hypermobility.* Excessive tooth mobility suggests that contributing factors may be responsible for the mobility. The extent of mobility could mean that the prognosis for the tooth may be unfavorable to poor.
4. *Difficulty of scaling and root planing.* The presence of deep pockets and furcations makes instrumentation difficult, but the results can often be improved with surgical access.
5. *Restorability and importance of particular teeth for reconstruction.* Long-term prognosis of each tooth is important when considering extensive restorative work.
6. *Age of the patient.* Younger patients with extensive attachment loss are more likely to have aggressive forms of disease that require advanced therapy.
7. *Lack of resolution of inflammation after thorough plaque or biofilm removal and excellent scaling and root planing.* If inflammation and progressive deepening of the pocket continue, further therapy will be necessary. Such cases require an understanding of the etiology to determine the best course of treatment.
8. *Rapid progression of disease.* In cases with rapid disease progression (grade C periodontitis), proper referral to a periodontist in a timely fashion is required for effective management.
9. *Defects that can be regenerated.* Vertical defects with multiple walls and early furcation defects in molars (see Chapters 22 and 63) have better prognosis with regeneration approaches when they are treated early.

Every patient is unique, and the decision process for each patient is complex and difficult. The considerations presented in this chapter should provide guidance for understanding the significance of phase I therapy and making referral decisions. For detailed information on factors dictating periodontal referral, refer to Chapter 47.

Conclusion

The major goal of phase I therapy is to control the factors responsible for periodontal inflammation; this involves educating the patient in the removal of bacterial plaque or biofilm. Phase I therapy also includes scaling, root planing, and other therapies such as caries control, replacement of defective restorations, occlusal therapy, orthodontic tooth movement, and cessation of confounding habits such as tobacco use. Comprehensive reevaluation after phase I therapy is essential to determine treatment options and establish a prognosis. Many patients can attain periodontal disease control with phase I therapy alone and do not require further surgical intervention. For patients who require surgical intervention, phase I therapy is an advantageous element of treatment in that it permits tissue healing, thus improving the surgical management and healing response of the tissues.

Periodontal surgical intervention should be considered for patients with deep pocket depths and those with 5 mm or more of attachment loss after phase I therapy. Periodontal specialists can best provide treatment to preserve the teeth for patients with advanced disease. Moreover, patients who do not demonstrate the ability to control plaque or biofilm on a daily basis effectively are poor candidates for surgery and should be closely monitored on a recall maintenance program unless conditions change.

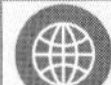
References for this chapter are found on the companion website eBooks.Health.Elsevier.com.

CHAPTER 44

Clinical Practice Guideline for Treatment of Periodontitis

Srinivas Myneni | Seyed Hossein Bassir

CHAPTER OUTLINE

Introduction

A clinical practice guideline (CPG) is a framework based on the highest level of available evidence, assisting the clinician in the decision-making process to support best practices. CPG development typically begins with defining the clinical problem, assembling a team of experts, conducting a systematic review or reviews on the given topic and finally, translating the findings of the reviews into clinical recommendations. In the context of clinical management of periodontal disease, only a handful of evidence-based CPGs have been developed over the years. In 2015, based on the best available evidence at that time, a CPG was developed specifically focusing on the nonsurgical management chronic periodontitis (this form of periodontitis is not a separate category in the 2018 classification). This CPG highlighted that the available evidence was in favor of subgingival root instrumentation (in the form of scaling and root planing) and the use of systemic antimicrobial dose doxycycline for nonsurgical management of periodontitis.[15]

In 2020, a CPG was developed focusing on the clinical management of patients with stage I to III periodontitis. This is the first comprehensive guideline in periodontology providing guidance and clinical recommendations on all aspects of periodontal therapy from behavioral changes to nonsurgical and surgical periodontal therapy.[13] With the implementation and global adoption of the 2018 disease classification, this recent CPG provides a good framework in establishing an individualized, dynamic, stepwise treatment plan for the treatment of periodontitis, based on a patient's stage, grade, risk factors and response to therapy. In this chapter, an overview of this CPG is provided focusing primarily on interventions with highest grade of recommendation, followed by case scenarios to depict how this CPG can be applied in the management of different stages of periodontitis, based on individual patient needs. The guideline proposes a stepwise approach (total of four steps) in the treatment of periodontitis that is presented in the following section. For more information on the specific interventions and the associated grade of recommendation and strength of consensus, please refer to the original publication.[13]

Steps in the Management of Periodontitis (Fig. 44.1)

Step 1: Behavior and Risk Factors Modification (See Chapters 25, 50, 51, and 52)

The aim of the first step of therapy is to encourage behavioral changes in the patient, including improvement in biofilm control, and lifestyle and behavioral changes which may modify existing risk factors for periodontitis. Interventions during the first step in therapy include:

- Supragingival biofilm control
- Improvement in oral hygiene instruction
- Professional mechanical plaque removal (PMPR)
- Control of known risk factors for periodontitis
  - Smoking cessation
  - Glycemic control of diabetic patients.

Supragingival Biofilm Control and Oral Hygiene Instruction (See Chapter 50)

Supragingival biofilm control is an essential intervention when discussing the treatment of periodontitis as it allows the patient to control the oral biofilm, which is the known etiological factor, for the development of gingival and periodontal diseases. Supragingival biofilm control is completed through a combination of mechanical removal (e.g., toothbrushing, interdental cleaning) and chemical removal (e.g., use of antiseptic or antimicrobial agents) of the oral biofilm from the dentition. Supragingival biofilm control is accomplished through proper oral hygiene instruction and patient motivation. Oral hygiene instruction (OHI) establishes the habits to control the oral biofilm and gingival inflammation needed to achieve the desired endpoints of periodontal therapy. Supragingival biofilm control and OHI are therefore essential interventions that should be encouraged and reassessed at all steps in periodontal therapy, including supportive periodontal care.[21]

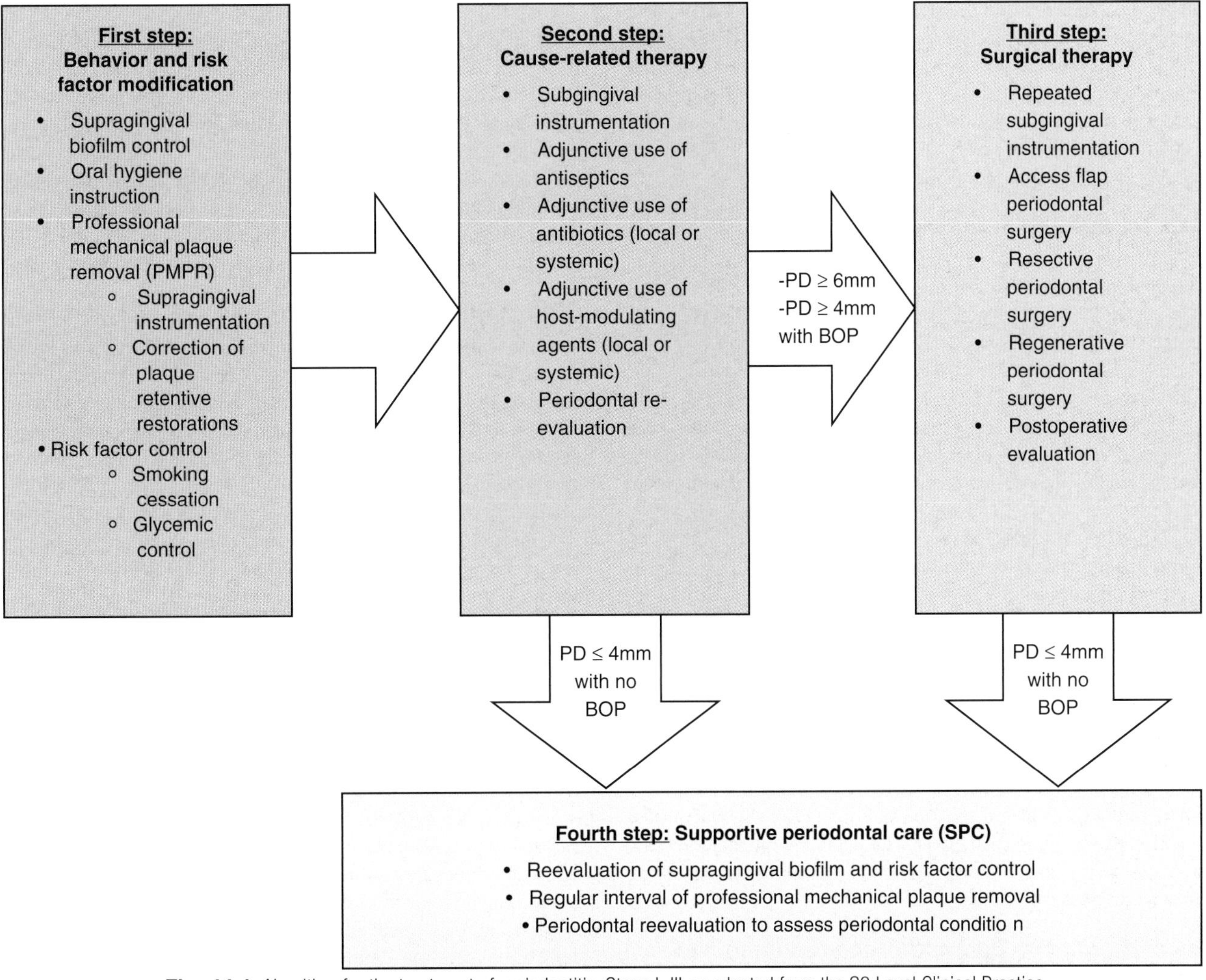

Fig. 44.1 Algorithm for the treatment of periodontitis: Stage I–III as adapted from the S3 Level Clinical Practice Guidelines *(CPG)* for treatment of Stage I–III Periodontitis. The intention of this algorithm is to provide a broad overview of treatment phases in periodontics. Clinician should take into consideration the available clinical and radiographic findings along with presenting risk factors and patient expectations before finalizing a treatment plan. (Based on Sanz, M, Herrera D, Kebschull M, et al. Treatment of stage I–III periodontitis—The EFP S3 level clinical practice guideline. *J Clin Periodontol.* 2020;47:4–60. https://doi.org/10.1111/jcpe.13290.)

Professional Mechanical Plaque Removal (See Chapters 51 and 52)

PMPR is the removal of supragingival biofilm and supragingival calculus by a dental professional. PMPR is a critical intervention for the treatment and prevention of progression of periodontal diseases, as it removes oral biofilm, a key etiological factor for plaque-induced gingival and periodontal diseases.[2] Supragingival instrumentation has been shown to induce a beneficial change in the subgingival microbiota, causing a shift from the pathogenic red complex bacteria.[22] PMPR also includes identifying and correcting plaque retentive factors within the dentition, including anatomical grooves, and restorative margins. The current body of evidence supports that plaque retentive factors, such as restorative overhangs, can increase the risk of gingival inflammation and can lead to disease progression in patients with periodontitis.[1]

Control of Known Risk Factors of Periodontitis (See Chapters 23, 24, and 25)

The last component in the first step of periodontal therapy is intervention to control known risk factors to the etiology and pathogenesis of periodontitis: smoking and diabetes.[9] Risk factor control is a critical intervention when formulating a patient's plan for periodontal therapy because smoking and/or glycemic control will directly impact the success of periodontal treatment.

Smoking cessation allows for improved treatment outcomes following nonsurgical and surgical periodontal therapy. Smoking cessation may include a combination of the following interventions: (1) patient education and counseling, (2) referral for advanced counseling programs, and (3) use of pharmacotherapeutic agents (e.g., nicotine replacements).[11]

In diabetic patients, uncontrolled diabetics will exhibit more advanced disease progression and a reduced response to nonsurgical and surgical periodontal treatment as compared to a well-controlled diabetic patient. Before initiating periodontal therapy, it is therefore important for patients to have glycemic control. Interventions include (1) patient education, (2) dietary counseling, (3) regular check of blood glucose levels and hemoglobin A1c (HBA1c%), and (4) referral to an endocrinologist to achieve glycemic control in patients who are uncontrolled diabetics.[11]

The first step of periodontal therapy is indicated in all periodontitis patients, regardless of stage. Although step 1 is not effective enough to treat the periodontal condition alone, it provides foundational knowledge of the disease, as well as education on management (oral hygiene practices, control of risk factors), which can be used to increase compliance and achieve the desired endpoints of periodontal therapy. Patients should be reassessed to ensure that a patient has effective biofilm control, is compliant and continues to control known risk factors throughout all phases of treatment, including supportive periodontal care.[1]

Step 2: Cause-Related Therapy

The onset and progression of periodontitis is driven by a dysbiosis of the oral biofilm and the inflammatory response in a susceptible host, leading to clinical signs of periodontitis, specifically, gingival inflammation, bleeding on probing (BOP) and alveolar bone loss and clinical attachment loss (CAL). The aim of the second step of therapy, cause-related therapy, is to control the etiology of periodontitis, leading to a reduction in gingival inflammation, probing depth (PD) and an improvement in biofilm and calculus control in the patient. This is accomplished by the physical removal of the subgingival biofilm and subgingival calculus through the following interventions:

- Subgingival instrumentation
- Use of adjunctive chemotherapeutic agents
- Use of host modulating agents
- Use of adjunctive antimicrobial agents (local or systemic)

*Subgingival Instrumentation (See **Chapters 51 and 52**)*

Subgingival instrumentation (like scaling and root planing) is completed to reduce the subgingival biofilm, calculus accumulation, and infected cementum, therefore leading to a reduction in inflammation, probing depths within the dentition. Subgingival instrumentation can be performed either with hand instrumentation (e.g., curettes, scalers) or with the use of power-driven instruments (e.g., ultrasonic or piezoelectric).[17]

*Use of Adjunctive Chemotherapeutic Agents (See **Chapters 51 and 52**)*

Antiseptic mouthrinses, such as chlorhexidine, have shown to have slight therapeutic advantage when used as an adjunctive therapy to subgingival instrumentation.[4]

*Use of Host Modulating Agents (See **Chapter 55**)*

Current evidence supporting the use of host modulating agents (local or systemic) as an adjunct to subgingival instrumentation is limited.[5]

*Use of Adjunctive Antimicrobial Agents (Local or Systemic) (See **Chapters 53 and 54**)*

Current evidence on the use of antimicrobial agents on a local or systemic level as an adjunct to subgingival instrumentation is inconclusive with mixed results. As described by Herrera et al.[6] there is some evidence supporting the use of certain sustained-release locally delivered antibiotics as an adjunct to mechanical treatment. Atridox, Ligosan, and Arrestin were shown to provide a significant reduction in probing depth when used as an adjunct to subgingival debridement in short-term outcomes.[6]

The current body of evidence for the use of systemic antimicrobials only supports the use of specific antimicrobials (amoxicillin and metronidazole) for specific patient categories (stage III or stage IV in a molar incisor pattern or generalized disease in a young patient). In select cases where the combination of amoxicillin and metronidazole were utilized, there was a significant reduction in probing depth when used as an adjunct to mechanical therapy with significant pocket closure, reduction in BOP, and CAL gain at 6 and 12 months.[18]

The second step of periodontal therapy is indicated for the treatment of periodontitis patients—stage I–III. Following gingival healing (4 to 6 weeks post therapy), patients should undergo a periodontal re-evaluation to assess response to therapy and to determine their individual additional treatment needs. Periodontal stability is defined as probing depths ≤4 mm with an absence of bleeding on probing. Patients who have healed following the second step of periodontal therapy should be placed on a supportive periodontal care regimen (fourth step of periodontal therapy). Patients who have residual deep probing depths (≥6 mm) or probing depths ≥4 mm with bleeding on probing may require additional periodontal therapy and should progress to the third step of periodontal therapy.[13]

Step 3: Surgical Therapy

Prior to initiating the third step of periodontal therapy, patients should demonstrate proper supragingival and subgingival biofilm control as well as improved OH and risk factor control following the first and second step of therapy. The third step of periodontal therapy is indicated for the treatment of sites which did not respond appropriately to the second step of periodontal therapy, resulting in persistent pocketing (PD ≥ 6 mm) and/or inflammation (PD > 4 mm with bleeding on probing). The aim of phase 3 therapy is (1) access to the root surfaces for effective subgingival instrumentation (2) access to alveolar defects for regenerative or resective treatment through the following interventions:

- Repeating Subgingival Instrumentation
- Access Flap Periodontal Surgery
- Resective Periodontal Surgery
- Regenerative Periodontal Surgery

*Access Flap Periodontal Surgery (See **Chapter 60**)*

In the presence of deep pockets (≥6 mm), flap surgery is recommended to provide better access for proper subgingival instrumentation and removal of subgingival calculus and infected cementum. Access flap periodontal surgery is performed with the goal of further instrumentation without addressing alveolar defects (e.g., infrabony defects or furcation defects). Access flaps include (1) open flap debridement, (2) flaps with para-marginal incisions (modified Widman flaps), and (3) papilla preservation flaps.[14]

*Resective Periodontal Surgery (See **Chapter 62**)*

The aim of resective periodontal surgery is to (1) gain access for subgingival instrumentation and (2) to correct the architecture of the hard and/or soft tissue to allow for elimination or reduction of pocketing, post-treatment. In stage III periodontitis patients, resective periodontal surgery has been more effective at achieving desired endpoints of therapy as compared to access flap periodontal surgery. Resective periodontal surgery demonstrates a greater reduction in probing depths with greater gingival recession present as compared to more conservative access flaps.[10]

*Regenerative Periodontal Surgery (See **Chapter 63**)*

The aim of regenerative periodontal surgery is to reestablish the periodontal attachment apparatus (alveolar bone, periodontal ligament, and cementum) when an intrabony or furcation defect 3 mm or deeper is present. In the presence of intrabony defects, regenerative therapy leads to an increased CAL gain and reduction in probing depths as compared to open flap debridement.[8] Teeth treated with regenerative therapies demonstrate improved tooth retention rates when maintained with regular periodontal supportive care.[16] In addition to intrabony defects, regenerative periodontal therapies are also used in the treatment of furcation defects. Regenerative approaches for the treatment of class 2 furcation defects in mandibular molars is superior to open flap debridement in probing depth reduction and gain in CAL.[7]

Following the third step in periodontal therapy are the goals to achieve periodontal stability (PD ≤ 4 mm with no BOP) and for the patient to be placed on supportive periodontal care. Not all teeth may achieve the desired endpoints of therapy with the third step of periodontal therapy; teeth with severe stage III disease should be properly evaluated and reevaluated following each step in therapy. In some cases, extraction may be recommended at any step in treatment when a tooth is given a hopeless prognosis.

Step 4: Supportive Periodontal Care (See Chapters 70 and 71)

Following a successful second step of therapy or third step in therapy, a patient can enter the fourth step of periodontal care: supportive periodontal care (SPC). The aim of the fourth step in periodontal therapy is preventing further disease progression and maintaining a patient's periodontal health. The fourth step combines the first and second step therapies through the following interventions:

- Reinforcement of proper biofilm control through oral hygiene and modification if necessary
- Assessment and modification of risk factors for periodontitis (smoking cessation, evaluation of glycemic control for diabetes)
- Professional supragingival and subgingival biofilm and calculus control
- Re-evaluation of periodontal tissue at regular maintenance intervals to prevent disease progression, and to diagnose/treat sites if repocketing occurs

SPC intervals should be tailored to an individual's specific needs, compliance, and response to therapy. SPC interval is most commonly set to 3 months.[12,19,20] In addition to establishing an SPC interval, it is also important to continue educating and motivating patients of the importance of regular maintenance visits. Costa et al.[3] showed that patients with irregular compliance demonstrated greater tooth loss and disease progression as compared to patients with regular SPC visits.[3]

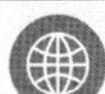
Case Scenarios are found on the companion website eBooks.Health.Elsevier.com.

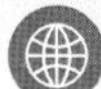
References for this chapter are found on the companion website eBooks.Health.Elsevier.com.

CHAPTER 45

Restorative Interrelationships

Frank M. Spear | Todd R. Schoenbaum | Julie Mitchell | Joseph P. Cooney

For expanded discussions on margin placement, supracrestal attached tissue, and esthetic tissue management as well as online-only content on special restorative considerations, please visit the companion website at eBooks.Health.Elsevier.com.

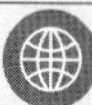
Videos for this chapter can be viewed on the companion website at eBooks.Health.Elsevier.com.

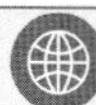
Animation (slide show) has been added by the editors as a supplement to the chapter and can be found on the companion website eBooks.Health.Elsevier.com. It was produced by My Dental Hub as a patient education tool and covers the basic elements in a conceptual manner. It is not intended to be a procedural guide for dental professionals.

CHAPTER OUTLINE

The relationship between periodontal health and the restoration of teeth is intimate and inseparable. For restorations to survive long term, the periodontium must remain healthy so that the teeth are maintained. For the periodontium to remain healthy, restorations must be critically managed from design to maintenance so that they are in harmony with their surrounding periodontal tissues. To maintain or enhance the patient's esthetic appearance, the tooth–tissue interface must present a healthy natural appearance, with gingival tissues framing the restored teeth in a harmonious manner. Once this harmony is achieved, the restoration must allow for regular hygiene maintenance procedures and the patient must be able to perform adequate plaque control. This chapter reviews the key areas of restorative management necessary to optimize periodontal health, with a focus on the esthetics and function of restorations.

Biologic Considerations

Supracrestal Tissue Attachment (formerly, Biologic Width) as a Restorative Consideration

One of the most important aspects of understanding the periodontal–restorative relationship is the location of the restorative margin to the adjacent gingival tissue. Restorative clinicians must understand the role of "biologic width" (now termed as supracrestal tissue attachment or supracrestal attached tissue) in preserving healthy gingival tissues and controlling the gingival form around restorations.

A clinician is presented with three options for margin placement: supragingival, equigingival (even with the tissue), and subgingival (or intracrevicular).[102] The *supragingival margin* has the least impact on the periodontium. Classically, this margin location has been applied in unesthetic areas because of the marked contrast in color and opacity of traditional restorative materials against the tooth. With the advent of more translucent restorative materials, adhesive dentistry, and resin cements, the ability to place supragingival margins in esthetic areas is now a reality (Figs. 45.1 and 45.2). Therefore whenever possible, these restorations should be chosen not only for their esthetic advantages but also for their favorable periodontal impact (Fig. 45.3).

The use of *equigingival margins* traditionally was not desirable because they were thought to retain more plaque than supragingival or subgingival margins and therefore resulted in greater gingival inflammation. There was also the concern that any minor gingival recession would create an unsightly margin display. These concerns are not valid today, not only because the restoration margins can be esthetically blended with the tooth, but also because restorations can be finished easily to provide a smooth, polished interface at the gingival margin. From a periodontal viewpoint, both supragingival and equigingival margins are well tolerated.

The greatest biologic risk occurs when placing *subgingival margins*.[66] These margins are not as accessible as supragingival or

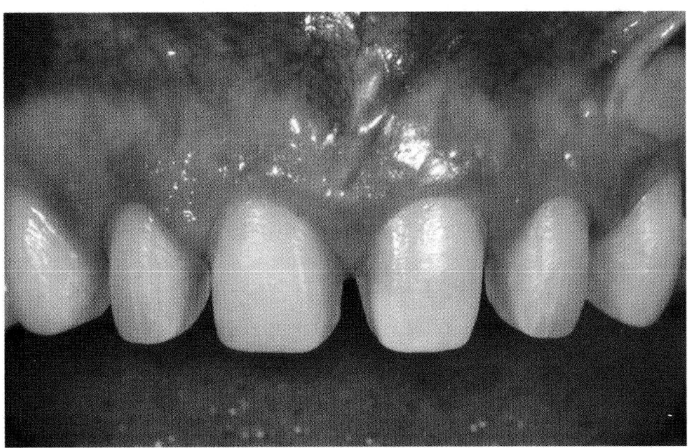

Fig. 45.1 With the advent of adhesive dentistry and ultrathin ceramic veneers, it now is possible to prepare restorations equigingival without visible margins. The preparations for six porcelain veneers with the margins placed at the level of tissue are shown.

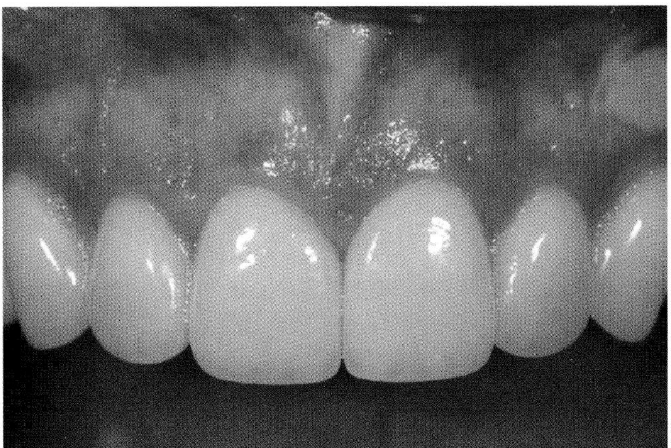

Fig. 45.2 The completed veneers from Fig. 45.1. Note the invisible gingival finish line, even though the margin has not been carried below tissue.

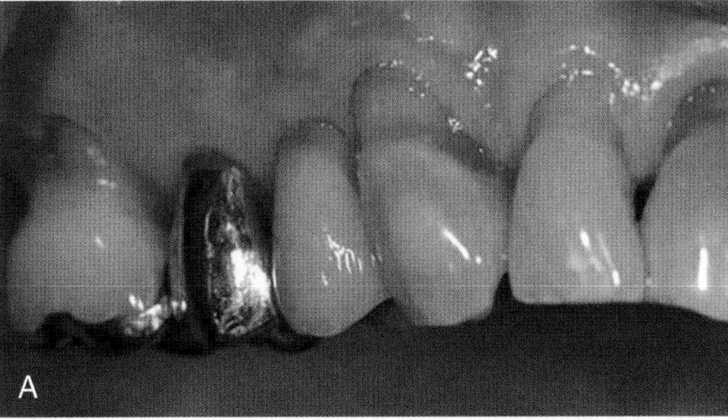

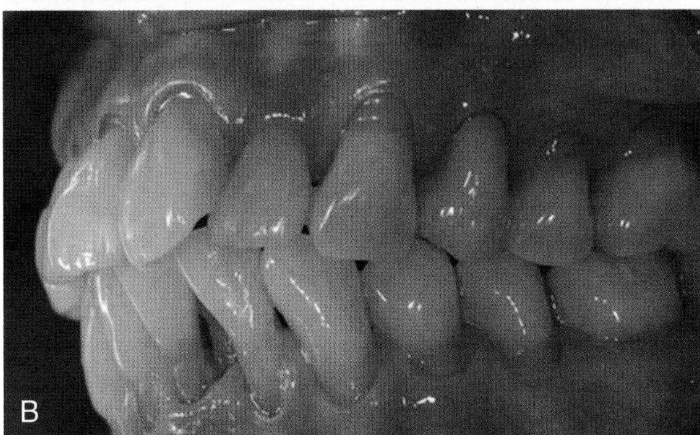

Fig. 45.3 Supragingival margin placement on tooth #4 restored with gold crown and tooth #5 restored with lithium disilicate (A) and on tooth #5 restored with lithium disilicate (B) that blends nicely with the anterior teeth and will allow for optimal hygiene and periodontal maintenance procedures.

equigingival margins for finishing procedures. In addition, if the margin is placed too far below the gingival tissue crest, it could violate the gingival attachment apparatus.

As described in Chapter 4, the dimension of space that the healthy gingival tissues occupy between the base of the sulcus and the underlying alveolar bone is composed of the junctional epithelial attachment and the connective tissue attachment. The combined attachment width has long been called *biologic width,* though it was updated in 2018 to the term supracrestal tissue attachment.[46] Most authors credit Gargiulo, Wentz, and Orban's 1961 study[31] on cadavers with the initial research establishing the dimensions of space required by the gingival tissues. They found that, in the average human, the connective tissue attachment occupies 1.07 mm of space above the crest of the alveolar bone and that the junctional epithelial attachment below the base of the gingival sulcus occupies another 0.97 mm of space above the connective tissue attachment. The combination of these two measurements, averaging approximately 1 mm each, constitutes the supracrestal attached tissue (Fig. 45.4). Clinically, this information is applied to diagnose supracrestal attached tissue violations when the restoration margin is placed 2 mm or less away from the alveolar bone and the gingival tissues are inflamed with no other etiologic factors evident.

Restorative considerations frequently dictate the placement of restoration margins beneath the gingival tissue crest. Restorations may need to be extended gingivally (1) to create adequate resistance and retentive form in the preparation, (2) to make significant

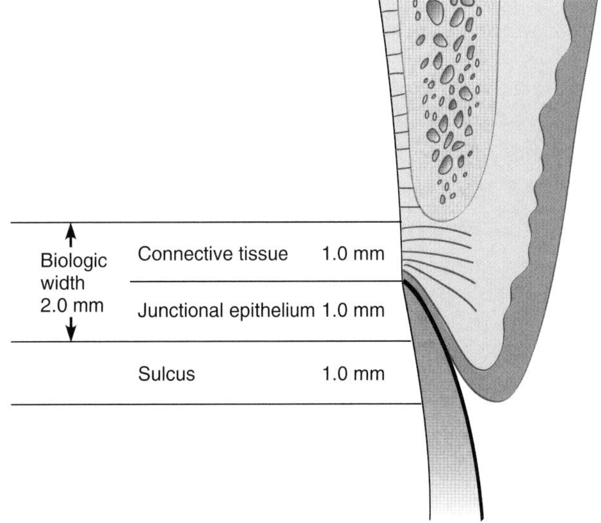

Fig. 45.4 Average human supracrestal attached tissue: connective tissue attachment 1 mm in height; junctional epithelial attachment 1 mm in height; sulcus depth of approximately 1 mm. The combined connective tissue attachment and junctional epithelial attachment, or supracrestal attached tissue, equals 2 mm.

contour alterations because of caries or other tooth deficiencies, (3) to mask the tooth–restoration interface by locating it subgingivally, or (4) to lengthen the tooth for esthetic reasons. When the restoration margin is placed too far below the gingival tissue crest, it impinges on the gingival attachment apparatus and creates a violation of supracrestal attached tissue.[75] Two different responses can be observed from the involved gingival tissues (Fig. 45.5). The earlier of these is marginal tissue inflammation characterized by increased gingival indices.[38]

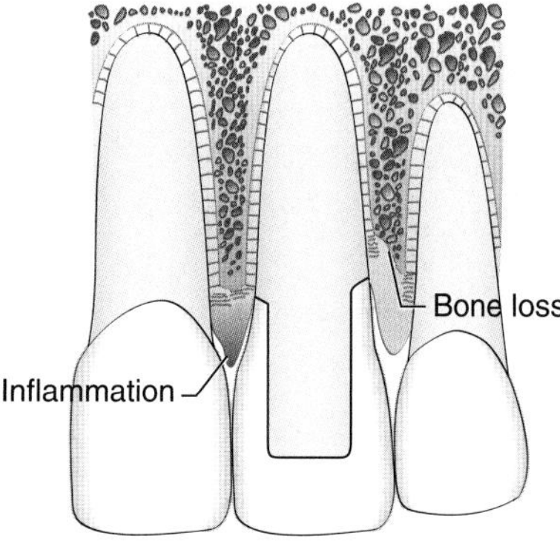

Fig. 45.5 Ramifications of a supracrestal attached tissue violation if a restorative margin is placed within the zone of the attachment. On the mesial surface of the left central incisor, bone has not been lost, but gingival inflammation occurs. On the distal surface of the left central incisor, bone loss has occurred, and a normal supracrestal attached tissue has been reestablished.

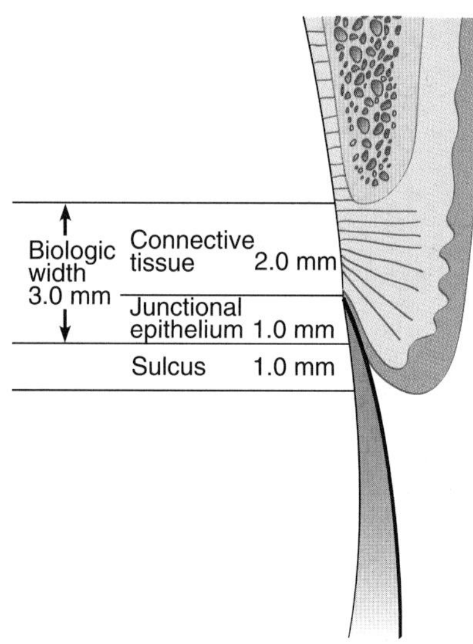

Fig. 45.6 Possible variations exist in supracrestal attached tissue. Connective tissue attachments and junctional epithelial attachments may be variable. In this example, the connective tissue attachment is 2 mm in height, the junctional epithelial attachment 1 mm in height, and the sulcus depth 1 mm, for a combined total tissue height above bone of 4 mm. However, the supracrestal attached tissue is 3 mm. This is just one variation that can occur from the average depicted in Fig. 45.4.

The other possibility is that bone loss of an unpredictable nature and gingival tissue recession occurs as the body attempts to recreate room between the alveolar bone and the margin to allow space for tissue reattachment. This is more likely to occur in areas in which the alveolar bone surrounding the tooth is very thin in width. Trauma from restorative procedures, particularly placement of retraction cord or rotary instrumentation during tooth preparation, can play a major role in causing this fragile tissue to recede. Other important factors that may impact the likelihood of recession is periodontal phenotype: this includes gingival (thickness and width) and the underlying alveolar bone characteristics.[63] It has been found that highly scalloped, thin gingiva is more prone to recession than a flat periodontium with thick fibrous tissue.[73]

KEY FACT

Thin gingiva and highly scalloped papilla are more highly prone to recession after normal restorative procedures.

The more common finding with deep margin placement is that the bone level appears to remain unchanged, but gingival inflammation develops and persists. To restore gingival tissue health, it is necessary to establish space clinically between the alveolar bone and the margin. This can be accomplished either by surgery to alter the bone level or by orthodontic extrusion to move the restoration margin farther away from the bone level. It is important to note that the adverse periodontal responses noted with subgingival restorative margins of indirect restorations [bleeding on probing (BOP), increased gingival index (GI), and plaque index (PI)] were observed predominantly in cross-sectional studies.[8,9,25,27,33,84,86,89,104] Longitudinal assessments show that periodontal health can be maintained in patients with intracrevicular indirect restorations, provided patients are motivated and instructed to perform optimal oral hygiene and remain in supportive periodontal therapy.[18,20,25,39,47,70,80] With respect to direct restorations, it is clear that the type of restoration has an effect on its interactions with periodontal tissues. Increased GI, BOP, probing depths (PD), and clinical attachment loss (CAL) were observed with subgingival amalgam restorations, while the periodontal tissue response was compatible with subgingival adhesive restorations (like composite and glass ionomer).[25] Based on animal studies, it is clear that when restorative margins are placed at the level of the bone crest, the bone loss occurs to allow for the reestablishment of supracrestal tissue attachment.[75,76,99] Bone loss is usually accompanied by inflammatory changes in the gingiva but studies show that the type of restorative material has an influence on the degree of gingival inflammation.[25,90]

Supracrestal Attached Tissue Evaluation

Radiographic interpretation can identify interproximal violations of supracrestal attached tissue. However, with the more common locations on the mesiofacial and distofacial line angles of teeth, radiographs are not diagnostic because of tooth superimposition. If a patient experiences tissue discomfort when the restoration margin levels are being assessed with a periodontal probe, it is a good indication that the margin extends into the attachment and that a supracrestal attached tissue violation has occurred.

A more positive assessment can be made clinically by measuring the distance between the bone and the restoration margin using a sterile periodontal probe. The probe is pushed through the anesthetized attachment tissues from the sulcus to the underlying bone. If this distance is less than 2 mm at one or more locations, a diagnosis of supracrestal attached tissue violation can be confirmed. This assessment is completed circumferentially around the tooth to evaluate the extent of the problem. However, supracrestal attached tissue violations can occur in some patients in whom the margins are located more than 2 mm above the alveolar bone level.[38] In 1994 Vacek and colleagues[103] also investigated the supracrestal attached tissue phenomenon. Although their average width finding of 2 mm was the same as that previously presented by Gargiulo and associates,[31] they also reported a range of different supracrestal attached tissues that were patient specific. They reported supracrestal attached tissues as narrow as 0.75 mm in some individuals, whereas others had supracrestal attached tissues as tall as 4.3 mm (Fig. 45.6).

This information dictates that specific supracrestal attached tissue assessment should be performed for each patient to determine if the patient needs additional supracrestal attached tissue, in excess of 2 mm, for restorations to be in harmony with the gingival tissues. The biologic, or attachment, width can be identified for the individual patient by probing to the bone level (referred to as "sounding to bone") and subtracting the sulcus depth from the resulting measurement. This measurement must be done on teeth with healthy gingival tissues and should be repeated on more than one tooth to ensure an accurate assessment. The technique allows the variations in sulcus depths found in individual patients to be assessed and factored into the diagnostic evaluation. The information obtained is then used for definitive diagnosis of supracrestal attached tissue violations, the extent of correction needed, and the parameters for placement of future restorations.

Margin Placement Guidelines

Given the materials and adhesives available today, it is the standard of care to keep margins of restorative work supragingival (without any esthetic compromise) unless the defective tooth structure extends below the gingival crest or esthetics require preparation subgingivally (Fig. 45.7). This is particularly true when patients have thin biotype/phenotype, in the interest of avoiding the need for gingival displacement. When intracrevicular margins are deemed necessary, it is recommended that the patient's existing sulcular depth be used as a guideline in assessing the supracrestal attached tissue requirement for that patient. The base of the sulcus can be viewed as the top of the attachment, and therefore the clinician accounts for variations in attachment height by ensuring that the margin is placed in the sulcus and not in the attachment.[6,59,60,85] The variations in sulcular probing depth are then used to predict how deep the margin can safely be placed below the gingival crest. With shallow PD (1 to 1.5 mm), extending the preparation more than 0.5 mm subgingivally risks violating the attachment. This assumes that the periodontal probe will penetrate into the junctional epithelial attachment in healthy gingiva an average of 0.5 mm. Deeper sulcular PD provide more freedom in locating restoration margins farther below the gingival crest, which can be advantageous when trying to change the esthetics of a tooth (e.g., closing an open gingival embrasure or "black triangle" or redistributing space to create a more pleasing esthetic). Locating the restorative margin deep subgingivally should be done with care, as it increases the difficulty in making an accurate impression, finishing the restoration margins, removing excess resin cement, and increases the likelihood of inflammation.

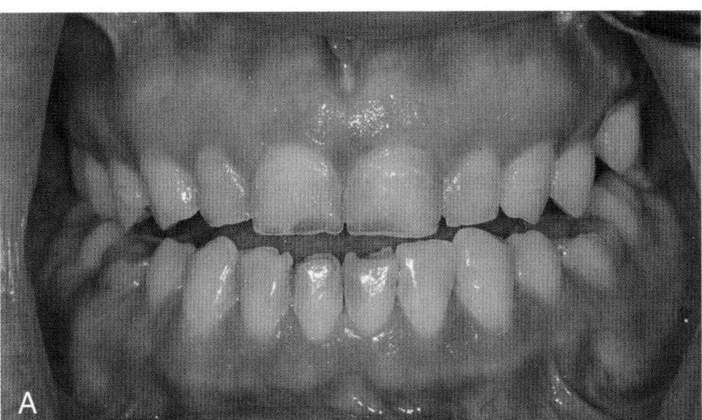

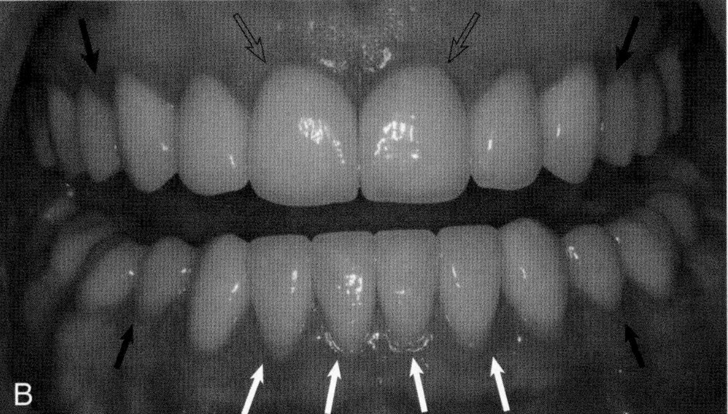

Fig. 45.7 Part (A) demonstrates the patient's initial condition. Clinical photo of a completed (B) full-mouth reconstruction demonstrates supragingival *(white arrows)*, equigingival *(empty arrows)*, and subgingival/intracrevicular *(black arrows)* margin placement in different areas of the dentition. With proper case and material selection, all may be compatible with periodontal health.

KEY FACT

Technical difficulties related to impression making and cementation of indirect restorations may be avoided using techniques referred to as "deep margin elevation" or "cervical margin relocation" in cases where loss of tooth structure dictates intracrevicular margins. However, these techniques have not been shown to be beneficial to gingival health as measured by indices.[28,48]

Provisional Restorations

Three critical areas must be effectively managed to produce a favorable biologic response to provisional restorations.[5,108] The marginal fit, crown contour, and surface finish of the interim restorations must be appropriate to maintain the health and position of the gingival tissues during the interval until the final restorations are delivered. Provisional restorations that are poorly adapted at the margins, that are overcontoured or undercontoured, and that have rough or porous surfaces can cause inflammation, overgrowth, or recession of gingival tissues. The outcome can be unpredictable, and unfavorable changes in the tissue architecture can compromise the success of the final restoration. It should be kept in mind that the presence of inflamed, edematous tissue or hemorrhage may compromise final cementation, particularly when using adhesives and resin cement. It is recommended that gingival displacement techniques be used if necessary during cementation of final restorations to achieve a dry and clean field.

Marginal Fit

Marginal fit has clearly been implicated in producing an inflammatory response in the periodontium. It has been shown that the level of gingival inflammation can increase corresponding with the level of marginal opening.[27] Margins that are significantly open (several tenths of a millimeter) are capable of harboring large numbers of bacteria and may be responsible for the inflammatory response seen. However, the quality of marginal finish and the margin location relative to the attachment are much more critical to the periodontium than marginal fit (Fig. 45.8).[50,66,72,91]

Restoration Contour

Restoration contour has been described as extremely important to the maintenance of periodontal health and is also critical in achieving a pleasing esthetic and allowing for hygiene access.[43,109] A concept that is related to crown contour is emergence profile (EP), which dictates the circumferential apical third of the restoration. Ideal contour and EP provide access for hygiene, has the fullness to create the desired gingival form, and has a pleasing visual tooth contour in esthetic areas. Evidence from human and animal studies clearly demonstrates a relationship between overcontouring and gingival inflammation, whereas undercontouring produces no adverse periodontal effect.[74,78] The most frequent cause of overcontoured restorations is inadequate tooth preparation by the dentist, which forces the technician to produce a bulky restoration to provide room for the restorative material. In areas of the mouth in which esthetic considerations are not critical, a flatter contour is always acceptable. In spite of the observed benefits of a flat contour or EP, a recent review concluded that human longitudinal evidence on the effect of EP on periodontal parameters is limited.[25]

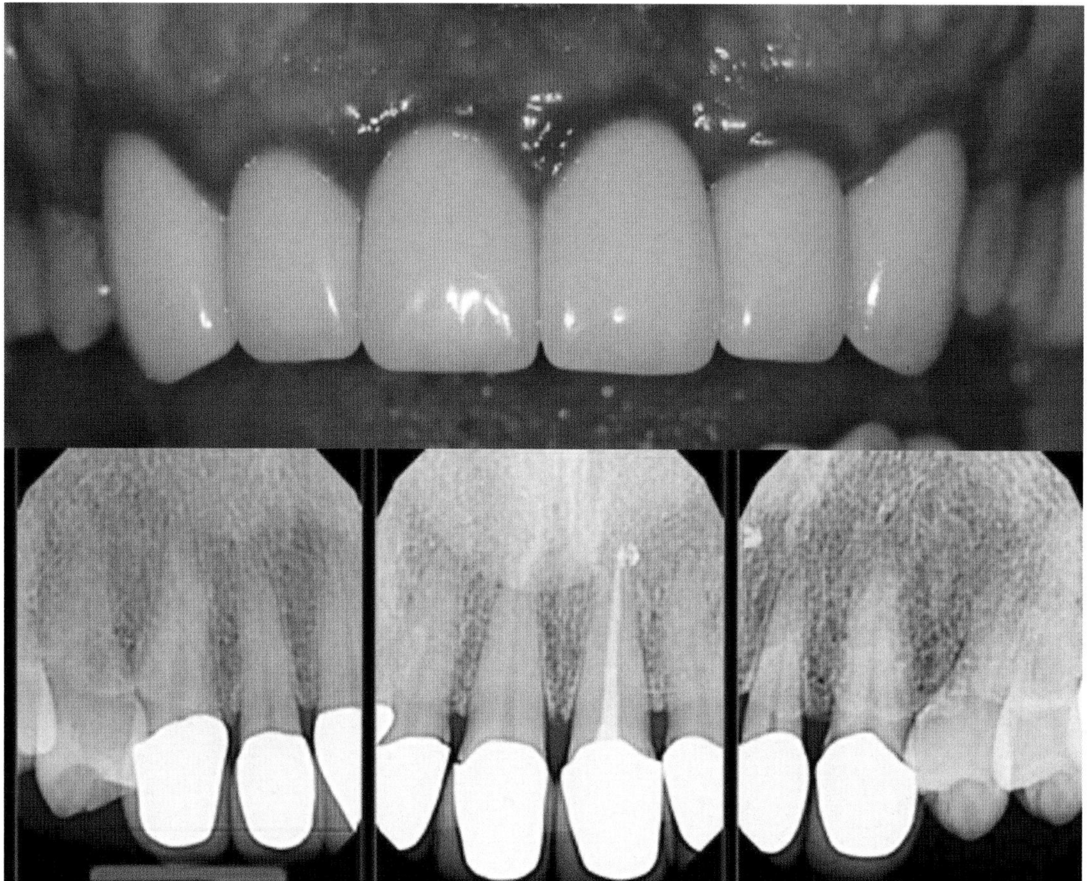

Fig. 45.8 These crowns have been in place for 15 years and their margins do not appear to violate the supracrestal attached tissue. This case exemplifies chronic gingival inflammation brought on by a combination of rough margins, poor marginal fit, and possible hypersensitivity response.

Subgingival Debris

Leaving debris below the tissue during restorative procedures can create an adverse periodontal response. Often, the patient presents with discomfort or tenderness around the recently prepared or recently restored tooth. The cause can be retraction cord, impression material, provisional material, or either temporary or permanent cement.[83] The diagnosis of debris as the cause of gingival inflammation can be confirmed by examining the sulcus surrounding the restoration with an explorer, removing any foreign bodies and performing curettage of the area, and then monitoring the tissue response. It may be necessary to provide tissue anesthesia for patient comfort during the procedure.

Dental Materials

Materials selection is of utmost importance in achieving restorative/periodontal harmony for both direct and indirect restorations. Importantly, tissues respond more to the differences in surface roughness of the material than they do to the composition of the material.[3,98] The rougher the surface of the restoration subgingivally, the greater the plaque accumulation and gingival inflammation. Class II restorations, particularly amalgam, with intracrevicular margins have been implicated in the development of increased gingival bleeding and dental calculus.[1,19,37] Class V restorations of both composite and resin-modified glass ionomers, for treatment of both caries and non-carious cervical lesions (NCCLs), have been demonstrated in clinical research to be compatible with periodontal health under optimal hygiene conditions.[11,90] This is particularly true when application of the composite or glass ionomer is performed impeccably as finishing methods can increase surface roughness. It should be kept in mind that it is difficult if not impossible to highly polish an intracrevicular direct restoration for a restorative clinician without surgical access.

For indirect restorations, inflammatory gingival responses have been reported related to the use of nonprecious alloys in dental restorations.[79] Typically, the responses have occurred to alloys containing nickel, although the frequency of these occurrences is controversial.[77] Hypersensitivity responses to precious alloys are extremely rare, and these alloys provide an easy solution to the problems encountered with the nonprecious alloys. When considering modern options for indirect restorations, lithium disilicate, zirconia, highly polished gold, and highly polished resin can all be placed with the expectation of periodontal harmony as long as a smooth surface is established. Clinical research has demonstrated significantly lower plaque accumulation intraorally on yttria-stabilized zirconia materials when compared to feldspathic glass-ceramic and lithium disilicate.[13] Additionally, there are extensive publications on surface properties of ceramics and other restorative materials in vitro and in vivo as they relate to bacterial adhesion and biofilm formation. However, clinical applicability of these results has not been established.[24,54]

Esthetic Tissue Management

Managing Interproximal Embrasures

Current restorative and periodontal therapy must consider a good esthetic result, especially in the esthetic zone. As discussed in Chapters 59 and 65, the interproximal papilla is an important part in creating this esthetic result. The interproximal embrasure created by restorations and the form of the interdental papilla have a unique and intimate relationship.[93,94] The ideal interproximal embrasure should house the gingival papilla without impinging on it and should also extend the interproximal tooth contact to the top of the papilla so that no excess space exists to trap food and to be esthetically displeasing.

Papillary height is established by the level of the bone, the supracrestal attached tissue, and the form of the gingival embrasure. Changes in the shape of the embrasure can impact the height and form of the papilla. The tip of the papilla behaves differently than the free gingival margin on the facial aspect of the tooth. Whereas the free gingival margin averages 3 mm above the underlying facial bone, the tip of the papilla averages 4.5 to 5 mm above the interproximal bone (Fig. 45.9). This means that if the papilla is farther above the bone than the facial tissue but has the same supracrestal attached tissue, the interproximal area will have a sulcus 1 to 1.5 mm deeper than that found on the facial surface.

CLINICAL CORRELATION

If you create restorations with no more than 5 mm from the contact to the bone, open gingival embrasures can be avoided. The downside to this approach is that the teeth will look square and blocky. However, some patients can support a 7-mm papilla. Well-made provisional restorations allow accurate determination of an individual's actual papilla length.

Van der Veldon[106] completely removed healthy papillae to the bone level and found that they routinely regenerated 4 to 4.5 mm

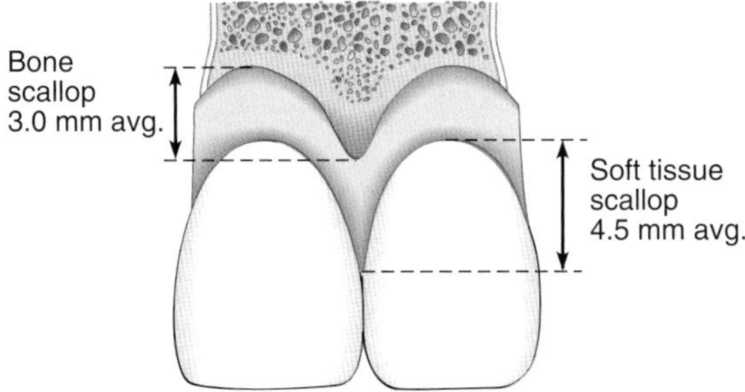

Fig. 45.9 Comparison of the behavior of the interproximal papilla relative to bone and the free gingival margin relative to bone in the average human. There is a 3-mm scallop from the facial bone to the interproximal bone. However, on average, a 4.5- to 5-mm gingival scallop exists between the facial tissue height and the interproximal papilla height. This extra scallop of 1.5 to 2 mm of gingiva compared with bone is the result of the extra soft-tissue height above the attachment interproximally.

of total tissue above bone, with an average sulcus depth of 2 to 2.5 mm. The height above bone that the papilla strives to maintain was indirectly confirmed by Tarnow and coworkers,[100] who studied the relationship of the papilla between the interproximal contact and the underlying bone. When the distance from the interproximal bone to the interproximal contact of the teeth measured 5 mm or less, 98% of these sites had complete papilla fill. When the distance was 6 mm, only 56% of the sites had complete papilla fill. When the distance was 7 mm, only 27% of the sites had complete papilla fill (Fig. 45.10).

Because there is individual variability to the required supracrestal attached tissue, this information relative to the papilla is applied by locating the lowest point of the interproximal contact in relation to the top of the epithelial attachment. The ideal contact should be 2 to 3 mm coronal to the attachment, which coincides with the depth of the average interproximal sulcus. In assessing the soft tissues to determine margin location, it is imperative that they be healthy and mature. Performing the analysis on inflamed or immature tissues will result in supragingival margins when the tissues heal. If the papillary sulcus measures greater than 3 mm, there is some risk of recession with restorative procedures. Critical adjustments to margin and soft tissue positions should be ultimately diagnosed with the use of well-designed and adapted provisional restorations. This will allow for treatment to be accurately designed based on the individual's unique supracrestal attached tissue.

Intimately tied to the notion of contact placement is gingival embrasure form. If the embrasure extending apically from the contact is of ideal width, the papilla assumes a pointed form, has a sulcus of 2.5 to 3 mm, and is healthy. With an embrasure that is too wide, the papilla flattens out, assumes a blunted shape, and has a shallow sulcus. If the embrasure is too narrow, the papilla may grow out to the facial and lingual, form a col, and become inflamed. This information is applied when evaluating an individual papilla with an open embrasure. The papilla in question is compared with the adjacent papillae. If the papillae are all on the same level, and if the other areas do not have open embrasures, the problem is one of gingival embrasure form. If the papilla in the area of concern is apical to the adjacent papillae, however, the clinician should evaluate the interproximal bone levels. If the bone under that papilla is apical to the adjacent bone levels, the problem is caused by bone loss. If the bone is at the same level, the open embrasure is caused by the embrasure form of the teeth and not a periodontal problem with the papilla. The papillae in the anterior maxilla average 4 mm long and are the same heights at the mesial and distal sides of the tooth. Ultimately, deficient papillae and open gingival embrasures are most predictably corrected with restorations to close the space (Fig. 45.11).

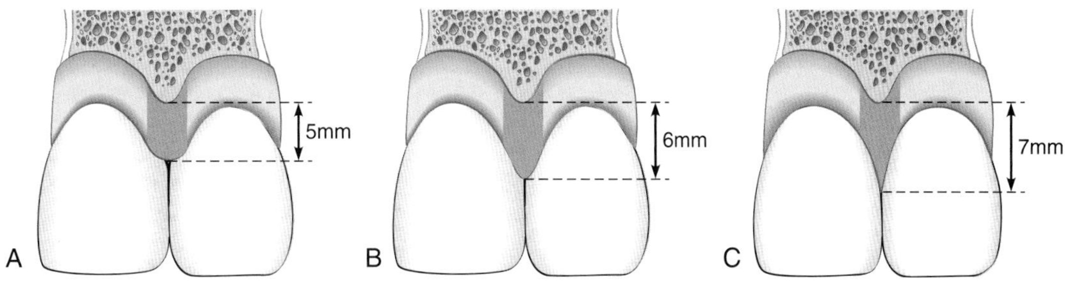

Fig. 45.10 The probability of complete fill of gingival embrasure by papilla. (A) With 5 mm from crest of bone to the apical contact point, there is a 98% chance of complete fill of the space. (B) At 6 mm from crest to contact, the chance of filled embrasure drops to 56%. (C) At 7 mm from crest to contact, the chance of complete fill drops to 27%.

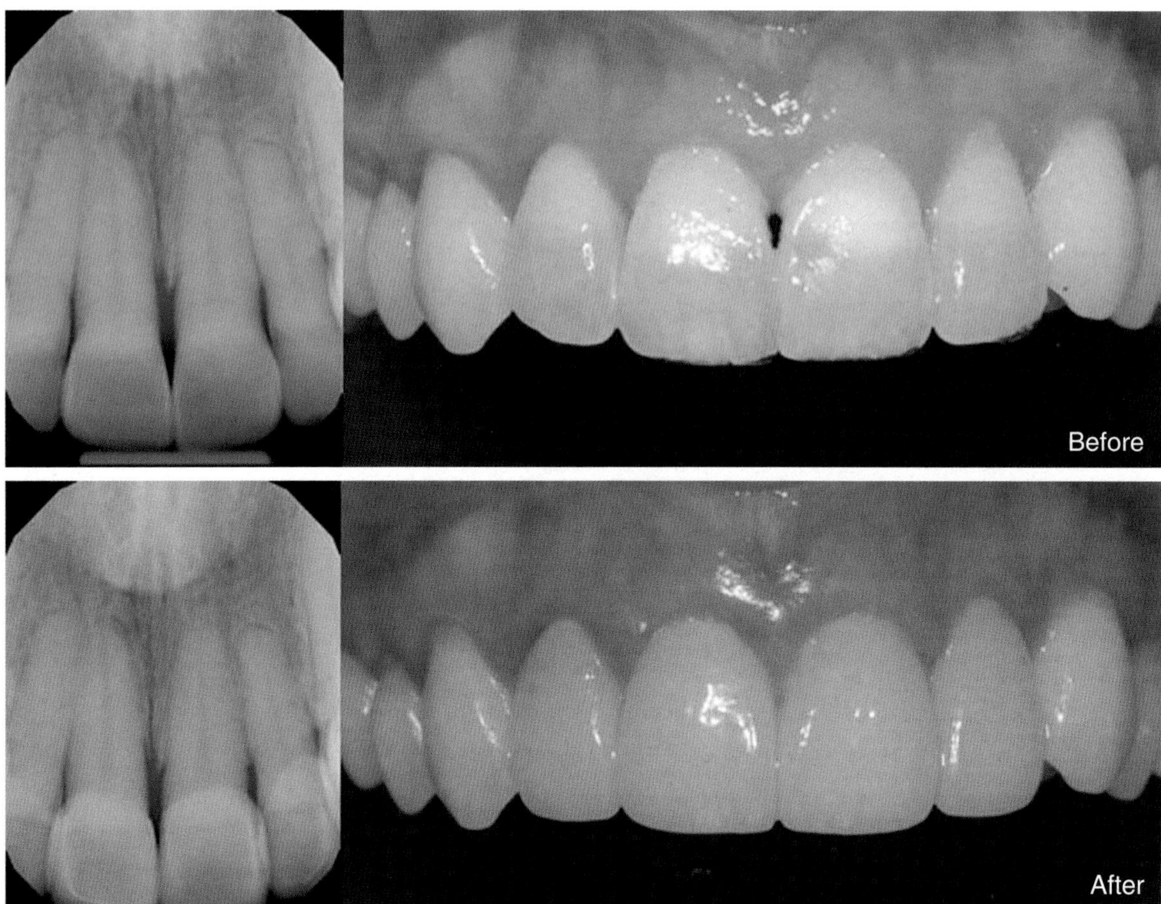

Fig. 45.11 An example of a patient in which papilla closure was achieved before and after veneer placement in a deep embrasure. Note the bone height in corresponding radiographs as it relates to the contact point and change in embrasure volume.

Occlusal Considerations in Restorative Therapy

KEY FACT

A mutually protective occlusion is created when nearly all the teeth touch at the same time in a normal closing arc, but when the mandible moves, all contacts are on the anterior teeth.

Chapter 35 presents details on the biology of occlusion and related clinical evaluation procedures. The importance of occlusal trauma as a factor in periodontal disease and its role in orofacial pain have been deemphasized in numerous papers.[14,26,57,58,69,71,82,97,105] However, the role that occlusion plays in restorative dentistry has been reemphasized. The increased use of dental implants and nonmetallic restorations has resulted in increased concern over force management. Some of these materials are more sensitive to occlusal trauma, and resulting fracture, than are metal restorations. Consequently, for the clinician who wants a high degree of predictability, understanding occlusion is critical. The clinician must know how to create an occlusion, with the following guidelines as a goal:

1. There should be even, simultaneous contacts on nearly all teeth in maximal intercuspal position (MIP). This distributes the force of closure over all the teeth instead of the few teeth that may touch first.
2. When the mandible moves from maximum intercuspal position (MIP), some form of canine or anterior guidance is desirable, with no posterior tooth contacts. This mutually protective occlusion reduces the ability and force of the muscles of mastication, while it more evenly distributes the forces. It has been shown that, as a result of the class III lever action, the anterior teeth receive approximately one-ninth the force of a second molar.[41,92]
3. The anterior guidance needs to be in harmony with the patient's envelope of function. The harmony of this relationship is demonstrated by a lack of fremitus and mobility on the anterior teeth, by the ability of the patient to speak clearly and comfortably, and by the patient's general sense of comfort with the overbite, overjet, and guidance created during chewing and when holding the head upright.
4. The occlusion should be created at an occlusal vertical dimension (OVD) that is stable for the patient. It is generally accepted that the patient's existing vertical dimension is at equilibrium between the eruptive forces of the teeth and the repetitive contracted length of the elevator muscles. It has been demonstrated that vertical dimension can be altered with no sense of pain from muscles and joints.[14,16,36,51] However, if this alteration lengthens the pterygomasseteric sling beyond its ability to adapt, the patient will not maintain the vertical change and will close the OVD back down by intruding the teeth.[17,56,62,64,65]
5. When managing a pathologic occlusion or when restoring a complete occlusion, the clinician needs to work with a repeatable condylar reference position. Centric relation, defined as the

most anterior superior condylar position, provides such a starting point.[34] Centric relation has been shown to be reproducible over multiple appointments, allowing the clinician to create the occlusion indirectly on an articulator and return it to the same reference position in the mouth.[23,61,68,107] It is the only position that has been shown to shut off lateral pterygoid muscle contraction.[32] Because it is a border position, any mandibular movement will result in the condyle moving inferiorly. Therefore, centric relation is the most predictable position from which an interference-free occlusion can be created.

To manage the occlusion as previously described, the clinician must be able to make accurate casts, use a facebow, create centric relation and protrusive records so that the information can be transferred to a suitable articulator. Although the details of these procedures are beyond the scope of this chapter, they are a routine part of any restorative treatment plan and must be mastered for the clinician to achieve predictable, long-term restorative success. The reader is referred to Chapter 35 for a more comprehensive overview of occlusal evaluation and therapy.

Special Restorative Considerations

Splinting

Splinting therapy may be applied with bonded external appliances, intracoronal appliances, or indirect cast restorations to connect multiple teeth, with the goal of improving tooth stability. Unstable teeth may be caused by a lack of periodontal support from bone loss, a lack of support from tooth loss, or the need to splint abutment teeth to support pontics. Indications for splinting are (1) mobility of teeth that is increasing or that impairs patient comfort, (2) migration of teeth, and (3) prosthetics in which multiple abutments are necessary.

Before considering splinting, the clinician must identify the etiology of the instability.[4] Excessive occlusal forces from parafunction or deflective tooth contacts are frequent causes of excessive mobility. Whenever the occlusion is the cause, occlusal therapy is always performed first. The mobility is then evaluated over time to determine if it resolves before splinting is considered. In addition, any inflammation of the periodontal supporting apparatus must be controlled before making a decision on splinting because inflammation can produce mobility in the presence of normal occlusal forces and normal periodontal support. When the teeth are splinted, all the teeth in the splint share the occlusal load to some extent.[29] The rigidity of the splint and the number of teeth used determine how the forces are distributed.

The most common indication to splint mobile teeth is to improve patient comfort and to provide better control of the occlusion. If the anterior teeth are mobile, adequate crown length on the teeth being splinted is critical so that the interproximal connectors do not impinge on the interdental papilla. Also, adequate space must exist between the connector and the papilla for access with dental floss anteriorly and with an interproximal brush on posterior teeth.

Anterior Esthetic Surgery

The importance of gingiva in relation to anterior esthetics has been well documented.[15,49,88,96] Various methods for altering gingival levels have been described, including gingivectomy, apically positioned flaps with osseous recontouring, and the use of orthodontic therapy to position the gingival tissue level apically or coronally by intruding or extruding the teeth (Video 45.1 ).[7,21,55,101]

Whenever an alteration in gingival levels is contemplated, the expected outcome must be communicated to the patient to determine if the planned surgery is acceptable. A wide variety of computer design and virtual imaging programs can be used to provide the patient with a visual plan for the final esthetic result.[30,110] Digital design can be converted into three-dimensional (3D)-printed waxup, or a conventional stone model waxup may be used to confirm the desired final outcome. However, this design process may not allow the dentist or patient to include the dynamics of lip movement in the evaluation of the proposed changes.

When the surgery will involve many or all of the anterior teeth and will result in moving gingiva several millimeters, to the extent that a flap will be raised and bony levels altered, an esthetic template guide is desirable. Before constructing the guide, treatment planning is completed as described above to determine the desired incisal edge position and the desired gingival level of the tissues. This will establish the amount of tooth display at rest and at full smile. For a patient who is undergoing both periodontal and restorative esthetic procedures to change the architecture of the smile, this step is critical.

Once the conventional or digital waxup is completed and accepted by the patient, a mock-up procedure using composite or acrylic resin may be performed using direct putty technique to evaluate intraorally the desired incisal edge position. From there, the gingival positions are confirmed and an esthetic template guide can be made on the patient's initial cast to be used at the time of surgery. This guide can be made of either clear thermoplastic material or the same composite or acrylic used for the mock-up.

When the patient approves the gingival levels established with the guide, the desired gingival correction can be completed using the esthetic guide as a surgical template. In addition to locating the initial incisions at the correct level, the guide can also be employed after flap reflection to aid in the bony recontouring to ensure adequate supracrestal attached tissue and sulcus depth at the new gingival position. The surgeon replaces the flap at closure to the gingival level established with the guide. Employing an esthetic template in this manner optimizes the predictability of the surgical therapy and establishes the ideal tissue framework to complete the esthetic restorations (Figs. 45.12–45.19). It is also common practice to place provisionals at the time of suturing/surgery to guide healing and maintain tissue levels. Absolute care and attention to detail must be paid to ensure highly polished, closed margins on provisionals.

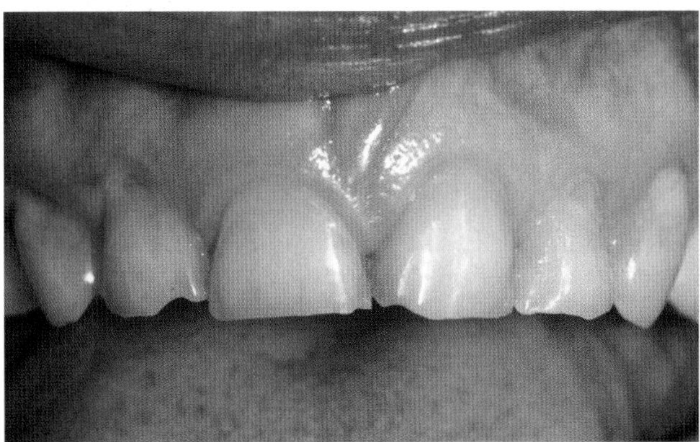

Fig. 45.12 This patient is unhappy with the appearance of her maxillary teeth and the discrepancies of tissue height and tooth form (see Figs. 45.13–45.19).

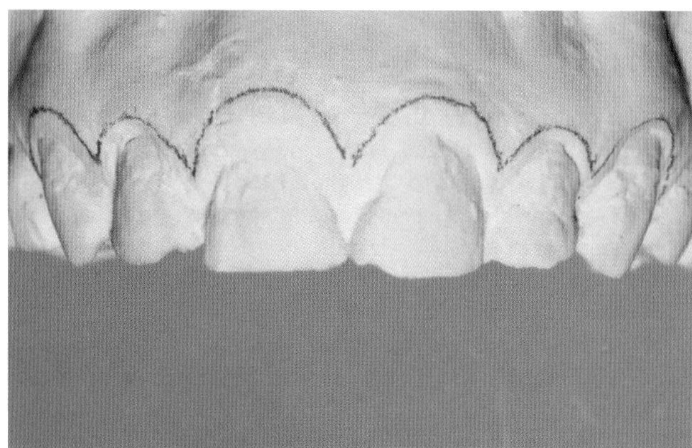

Fig. 45.13 To create a surgical guide for the patient in Fig. 45.12, a stone cast is modified by drawing the desired soft-tissue profile with a red wax pencil.

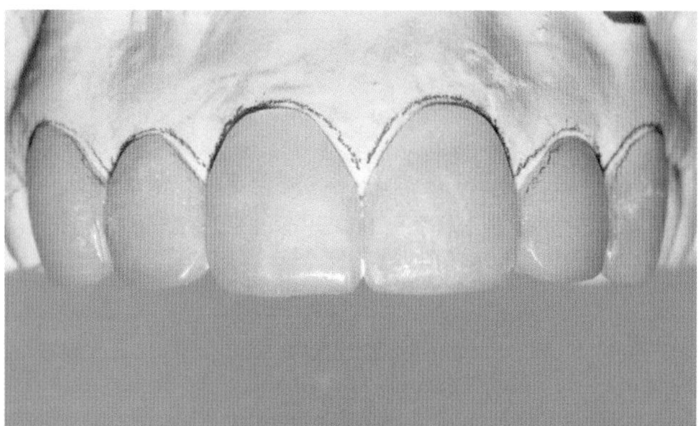

Fig. 45.14 A composite-resin surgical guide is fabricated on this stone cast, extending to the line drawn. This guide can be taken to the mouth for try-in and verification by the patient (see Fig. 45.12).

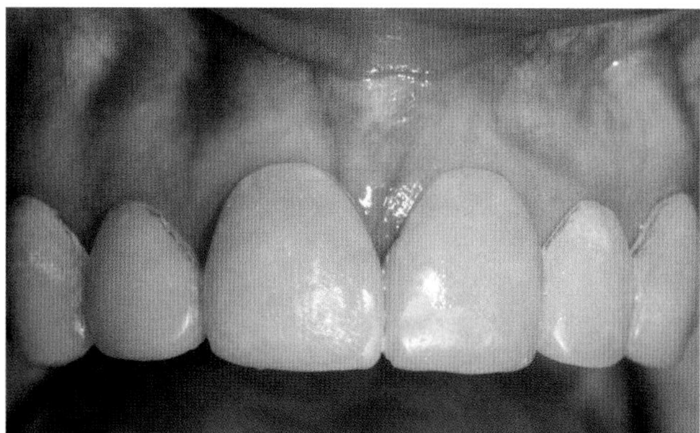

Fig. 45.15 Photograph taken the day the surgical guide was tried-in. The patient in Fig. 45.12 approved the new length of the maxillary anterior teeth and the form created by altering the soft-tissue profile.

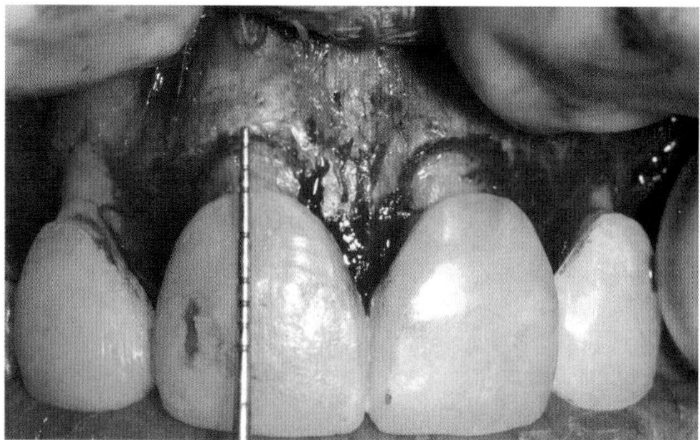

Fig. 45.16 By placing the surgical guide during the surgery, it is possible to recognize where the bone needs to be placed. The surgical guide represents the desired final free gingival margin position and can be used as a reference for osseous recontouring. This patient had an average supracrestal attached tissue of 2 mm (see Fig. 45.12). Allowing an additional 1 mm for sulcus depth, the desired distance between the bone and the free gingival margin will be 3 mm. With this knowledge, the periodontist can use the guide and remove bone until it is 3 mm from the position of the guide on each tooth.

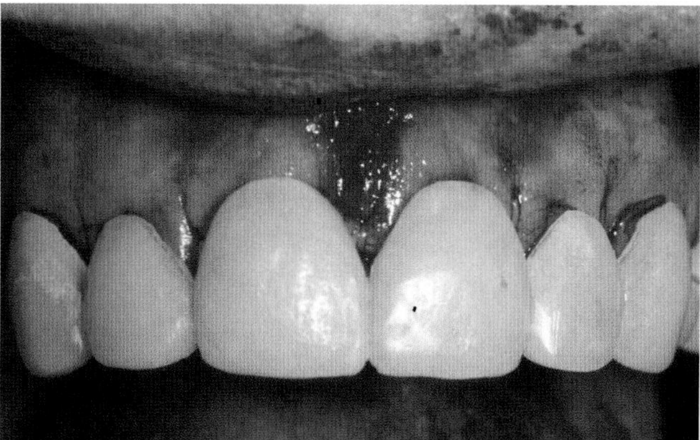

Fig. 45.17 Surgical guide is also useful during suturing. Because the guide represents the desired free gingival margin position, it is possible to suture to the level of the guide, knowing that the surgery has now recreated supracrestal attached tissue and a 1-mm sulcus. This shortens the amount of time necessary for healing and eliminates the need to wait for tissue rebound before restorative dentistry.

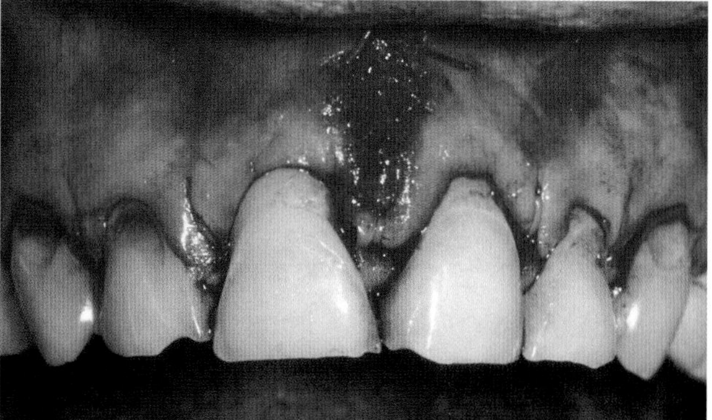

Fig. 45.18 Soft-tissue profile as seen the day of surgery with the guide removed. Note that in this patient, the interproximal papillae were not changed because the interproximal papillary form and height were deemed acceptable (see Figs. 45.12–45.17).

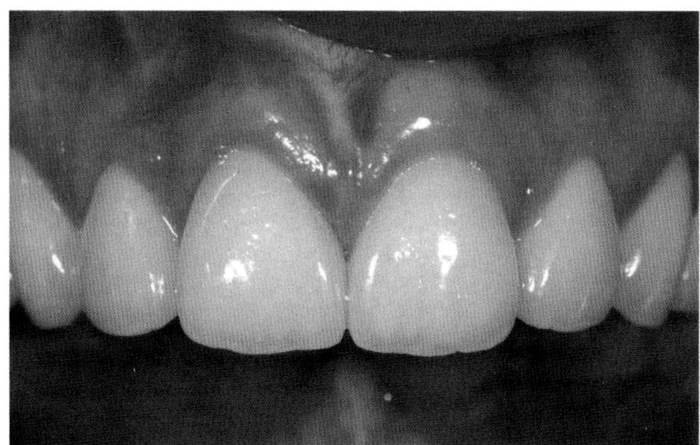

Fig. 45.19 Photograph taken 4 years after placement of the final restoration of the patient in Fig. 45.12. Note the excellent soft-tissue health and the attainment of the desired free gingival margin and papillary form.

Embrasures of sufficient height for papilla healing are to be meticulously cut with a diamond disc

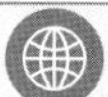

Case Scenarios are found on the companion website eBooks.Health.Elsevier.com.

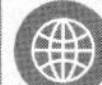

References for this chapter are found on the companion website eBooks.Health.Elsevier.com.

CHAPTER 46

Multidisciplinary Versus Interdisciplinary Approaches to Dental and Periodontal Problems

Dennis P. Tarnow | Mitchell J. Bloom

CHAPTER OUTLINE

Traditionally, periodontal treatment has been delivered using an interdisciplinary model of therapy with general dentists and specialists each providing their respective aspects of care to the same patients according to a comprehensive plan of therapy (Figs. 46.1–46.22). Conversely, a multidisciplinary approach is centered on a single provider delivering care across a range of dentistry disciplines. This practitioner can be a general dentist or a specialist, as traditional modes of practice have evolved and, in some aspects, look quite different from the classic model. The interdisciplinary system has worked well because the patient benefits from the best mix of talent from a "team" of dentists. Regardless of whether an interdisciplinary or multidisciplinary approach is utilized, it is critical for primary providers to have a thorough understanding of the signs, symptoms, local and systemic risk factors, and pathophysiology of disease processes as they relate to periodontal and dental implant therapy. Additionally, they must possess a strong working knowledge of the range of treatment options available along with their respective indications, contraindications, benefits, and liabilities to effectively formulate a proper treatment plan. At this point the dentist can then decide whether he or she has the requisite knowledge, expertise, and experience to meet the patient's needs to proceed in a multidisciplinary fashion or should refer the patient to a specialist for care at a more advanced level.

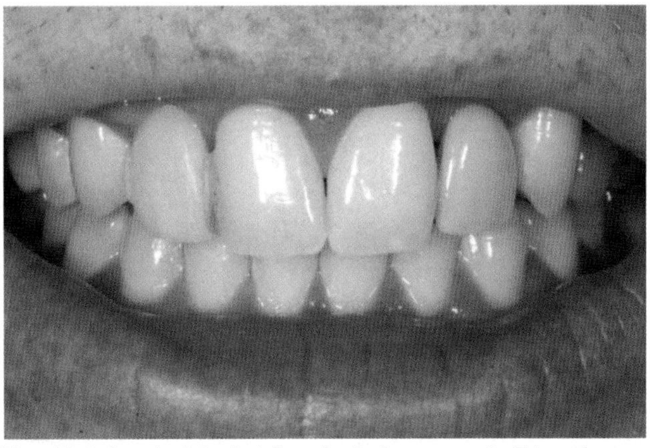

Fig. 46.1 Complex interdisciplinary implant care scenario. Extraoral preoperative condition. Aesthetic compromise is evident in this challenging treatment scenario where there is significant gingival display.

Many of the early innovators in the field of implant dentistry were general practitioners. Subsequently, their early accomplishments were built on using rigid and narrowly defined surgical and prosthetic protocols whose effectiveness and predictability were supported by well-documented long-term research studies put forth by Dr. P. I. Brånemark. His namesake implant design, when used precisely as directed with respect to case type and patient selection, strict surgical protocols, specialized armamentarium, and a narrow range of treatment options, made it possible for clinicians to achieve highly predictable treatment outcomes. The initial offering of training in the Brånemark method was limited only to specialist prosthodontists and oral surgeons—the former group focusing on the restorative aspect of care and the latter group on the surgical phase of therapy. However, as implant dentistry continued to evolve, periodontists became increasingly more active in the field, ultimately sharing the same role and stature as their oral surgeon colleagues in this arena. The same was true for many general practitioners with respect to their prosthodontist colleagues in terms of delivering implant restorative care.

The range of indications for the use of dental implants expanded beyond the limited mandibular full arch case type Brånemark initially taught to include partial edentulism, single teeth, and even orthodontic and maxillofacial applications. Regenerative techniques have been developed as well to address hard- and soft-tissue deficiencies that, for many patients, had previously deemed them unsuitable candidates for dental implant therapy. Autogenous intraoral block grafting, guided bone regeneration, maxillary sinus grafting, transposition of the inferior alveolar nerve, ridge splitting, distraction osteogenesis, and biologics are among the many strategies that have emerged to overcome limitations for less-than-optimal sites.

Early implant designs and materials were subject to limitations and even prone to problems. Those with machined surfaces suffered from a significantly higher failure rate in sites with poor-quality bone, whereas those with rough surfaces, coupled with other design flaws, were prone to late failure resulting from inflammatory peri-implant disease or prosthetic complications. With all of

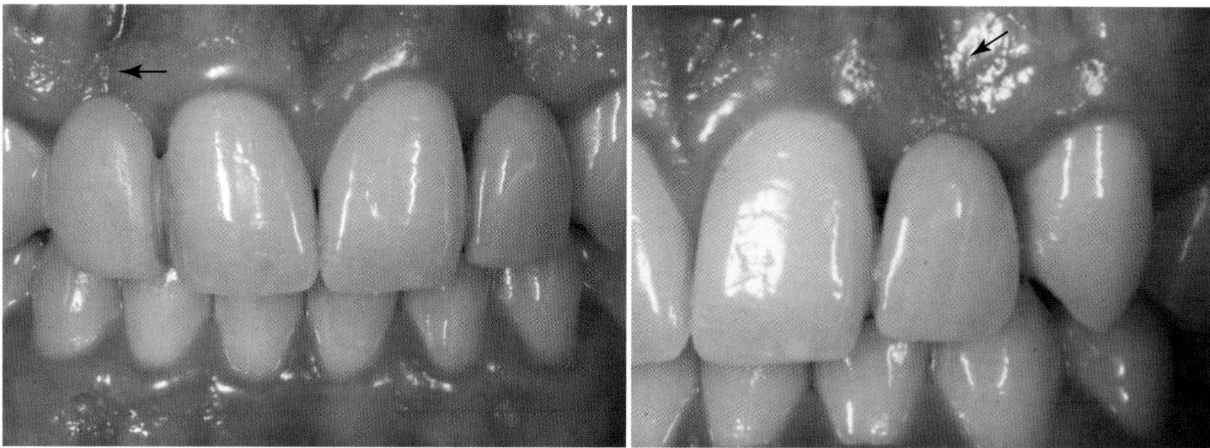

Fig. 46.2 Intraoral preoperative condition. A concave soft-tissue profile that contributes to a dark shadow and aesthetic compromise is evident bilaterally *(arrows).*

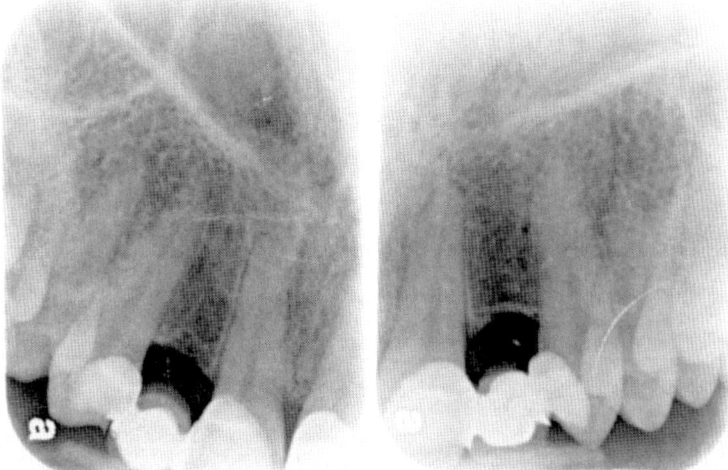

Fig. 46.3 Preoperative radiographs. The roots of adjacent teeth do not converge to interfere with proper orientation of the positions of the planned dental implants. However, there is limited space between the adjacent tooth roots.

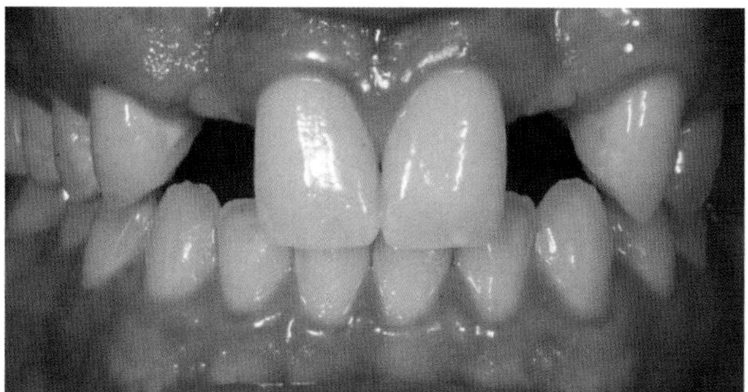

Fig. 46.4 Intraoral preoperative clinical view. Soft-tissue contours as seen with the existing restorations removed.

these variables in play and emerging so rapidly during the formative years, implant dentistry was relegated largely to the specialty care arena. Through innovative implant designs, advances in material science, opportunities for simplified surgical techniques, digital planning and manufacturing technologies, systematic treatment protocols, and better data to appreciate success and risk factors, predictable outcomes have become readily achievable. The widespread emergence and acceptance of implant dentistry and the fact that it is both a surgical and prosthetic modality puts it at the center of many of the trends transforming traditional practice models.

Periodontology, like other specialties, has evolved to embrace a more global view of patient care. It is suggested that in addition to learning all of the standard periodontal procedures of the past, the contemporary periodontist should also be able to *restore* simple implant cases such as those located outside of the aesthetic zone (Figs. 46.23–46.32). Periodontists will continue to be trained to manage hard and soft tissues and perform all of the latest periodontal plastic surgical procedures to preserve and reconstruct pleasing gingival architecture in the aesthetic zone to the highest level of sophistication and complexity. However, as the definition of what is deemed a successful outcome continues to evolve and the bar for the definition is raised, the surgeon must remain acutely aware of the restorative aspects of care and abreast of related advances. In other words, it has become essential that periodontists not limit their knowledge and care to the treatment of periodontal disease alone.

Surgical specialists (i.e., periodontists) who are trained according to a multidisciplinary approach will provide even greater benefit to their patients from this evolved philosophy. Consider the case for immediate dental implant placement along with simultaneous fabrication and insertion of a provisional restoration at the time of tooth extraction. This treatment is a series of steps that integrates both

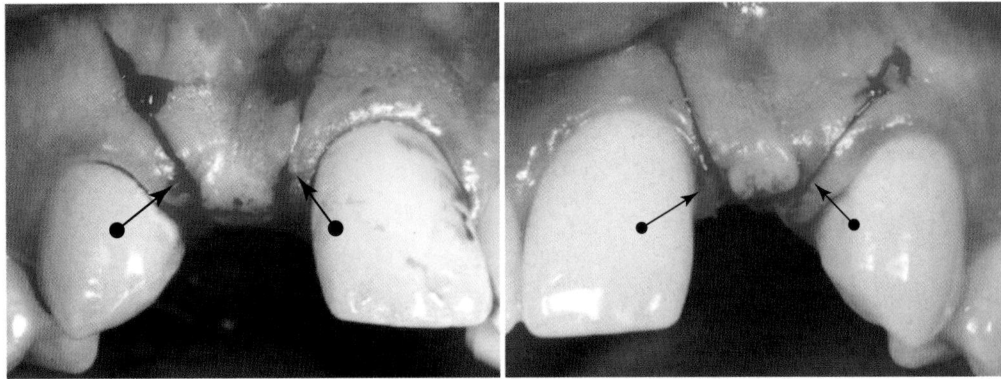

Fig. 46.5 Implant surgery. Initial incisions using a papilla-sparing technique to minimize disturbing the healthy supracrestal attachment on the surfaces of the adjacent teeth.

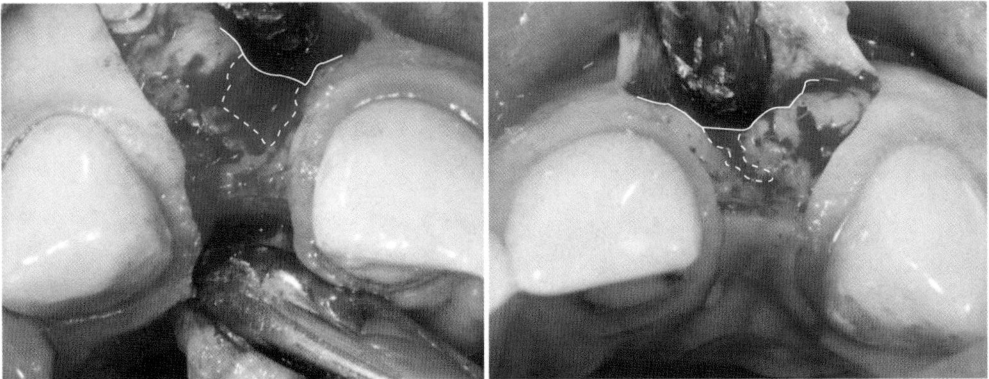

Fig. 46.6 Intraoperative clinical view. Edentulous right and left treatment areas both show concave bony defects labially.

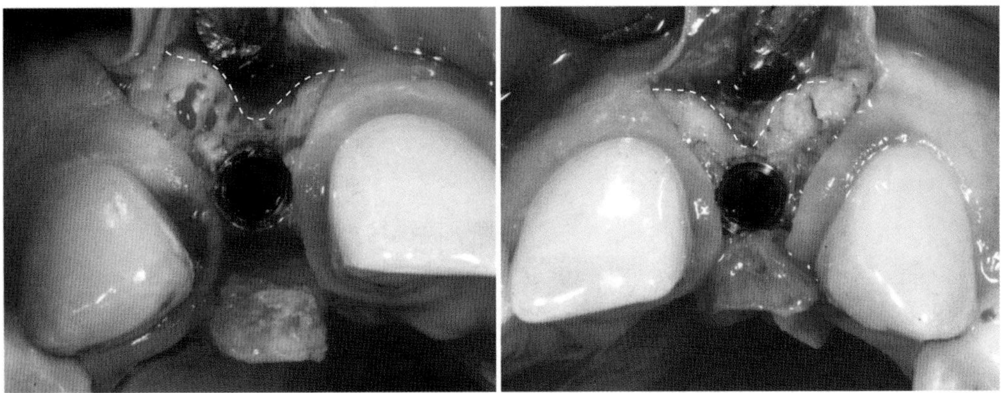

Fig. 46.7 Intraoperative clinical view. Implants placed in a prosthetically guided orientation that is palatal to the buccal depression.

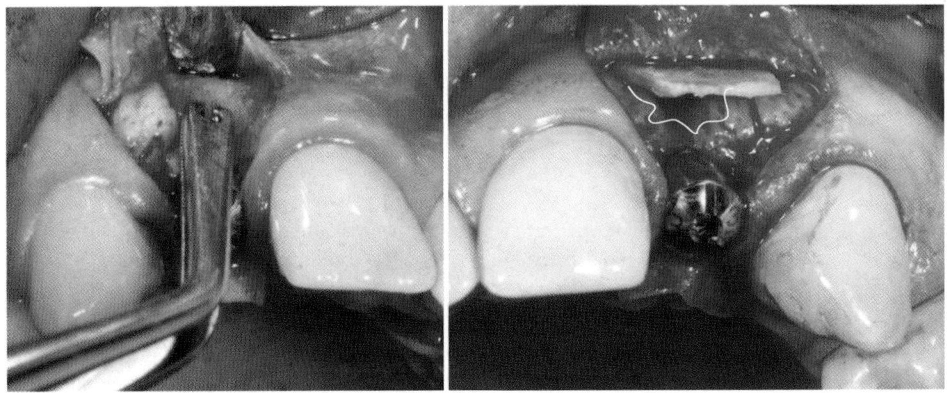

Fig. 46.8 Intraoperative clinical view. Correction of bony defects using guided bone regeneration technique. Resorbable barrier membranes are shown in position after being trimmed to a suitable shape and fitted in place.

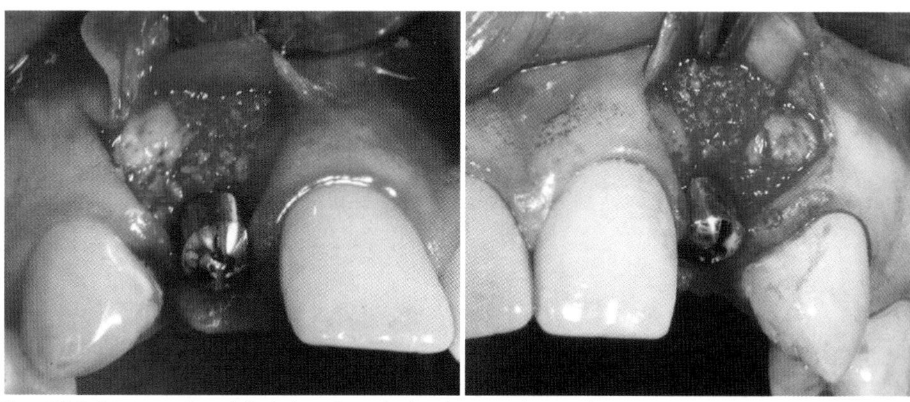

Fig. 46.9 Intraoperative clinical view. A particulate bone graft material is placed and shaped to fill the bony depression under the previously fitted membrane.

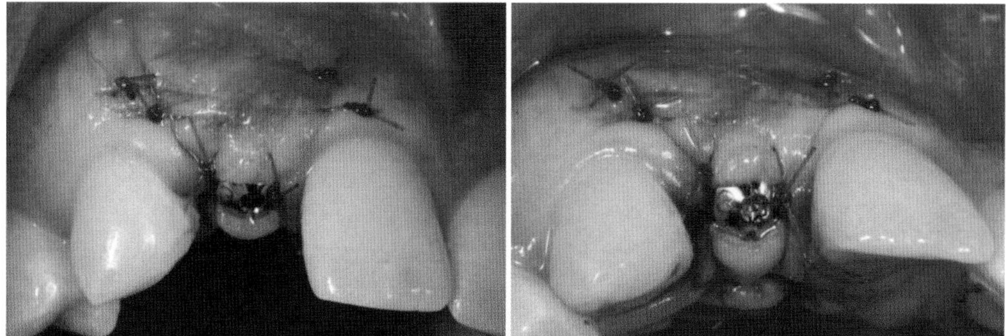

Fig. 46.10 Implant healing abutments, which act to facilitate coronal and labial positioning of the soft-tissue flap, were previously placed. This will work in conjunction with the augmentation procedure to correct the preoperative soft-tissue concavity.

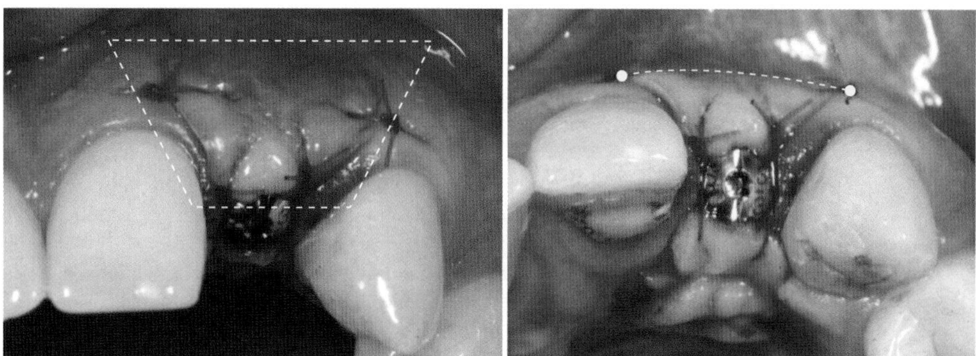

Fig. 46.11 Convex ridge shape after augmentation is shown after completion of the surgical procedure.

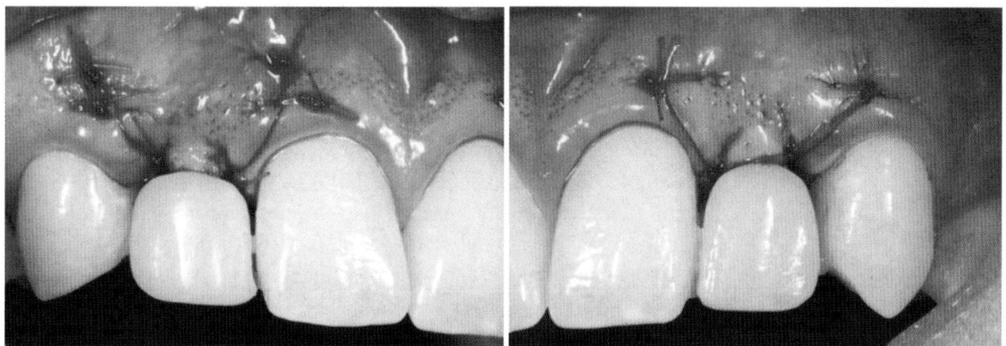

Fig. 46.12 The gingival third of the provisional restoration has been reduced so it does not impinge on the surgical site. The vertical position of the soft-tissue height on completion of the surgery is favorable as compared with that of the adjacent natural teeth.

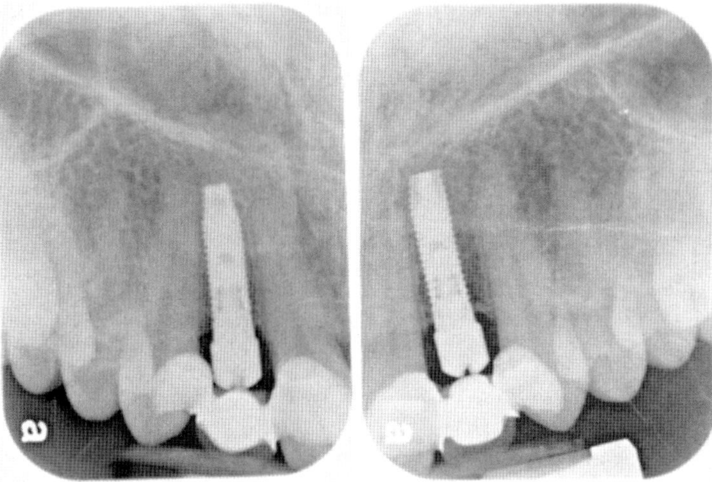

Fig. 46.13 Postoperative radiograph. The dental implants are in good position. Given the amount of available space between the adjacent tooth roots, a narrow-diameter implant was selected as part of the treatment plan to yield a biologically and prosthetically favorable result.

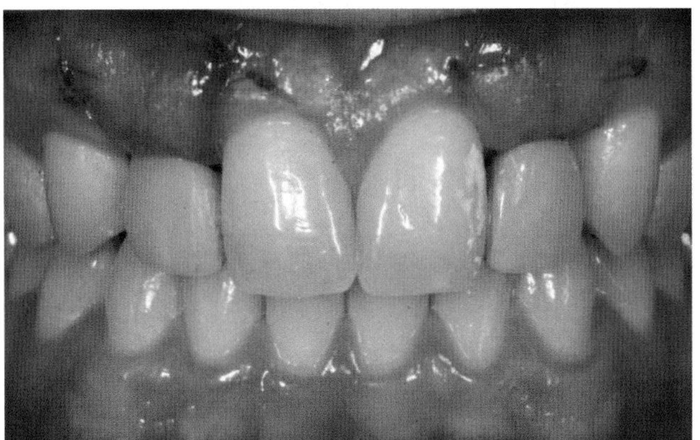

Fig. 46.14 Postoperative clinical view at 1 week after surgery. The soft tissue is healing well. Note the favorable soft-tissue response where the papillae were not disturbed using a conservative incision design.

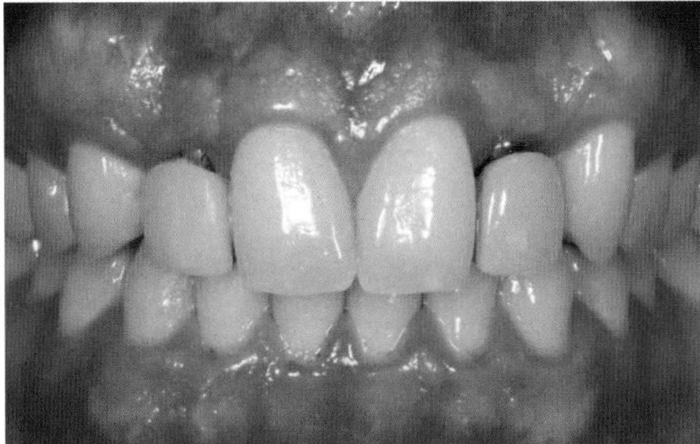

Fig. 46.15 Postoperative clinical view 3 months after surgery. The soft tissues have healed favorably with maintenance of the free gingival margin position situated to yield a prosthetic clinical crown of appropriate length.

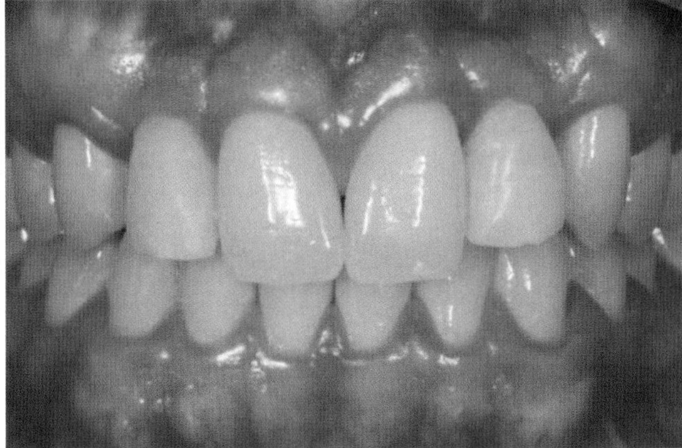

Fig. 46.16 Screw-retained single provisional crowns inserted and connected to the dental implants to begin nonsurgical sculpting of the peri-implant soft tissue.

surgical and restorative areas of dentistry. As such, suitable depth of knowledge in all phases is needed to allow for proper diagnosis, case selection, and clinical delivery of care for predictable outcomes and to yield the wide range of benefits this treatment offers to both the patient and the doctor. Even when the role of implant surgeons is limited to the surgical phase of therapy, achieving the best and most predictable outcomes requires that they possess a thorough understanding of the realities and intricacies related to the fabrication and delivery of the planned prosthesis. This "restorative" knowledge and experience will help them to place implants in as close to ideal orientation in all three spatial dimensions and to avoid such common errors as excessive implant angulation by understanding the restorative challenges that may otherwise result. Additionally, the well-versed periodontist will be better able to communicate effectively with restorative colleagues and may even serve as a resource to guide and educate those who might have less familiarity with the subject matter when an interdisciplinary approach is utilized.

Another significant factor in the delivery of care and who might provide it is the rapid evolution in the development of digital dentistry. Its widespread introduction into clinical practice holds limitless potential for diagnosis, manufacturing, and chairside delivery of care. Digital technologies also expand communication and collaboration between the members of the clinical and laboratory dental team—whether in the same office, across town, or in another country—at every phase of therapy.

What was once thought impossible, such as digital intraoral impressions and scanning that seamlessly integrates with the manufacturing of orthodontic aligners, printing or milling prostheses, and guided dental implant surgery, are just a few of what is already available in contemporary practice. Also, as artificial intelligence

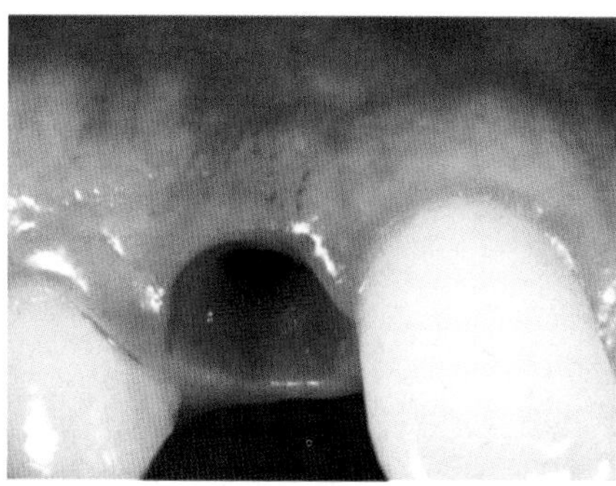
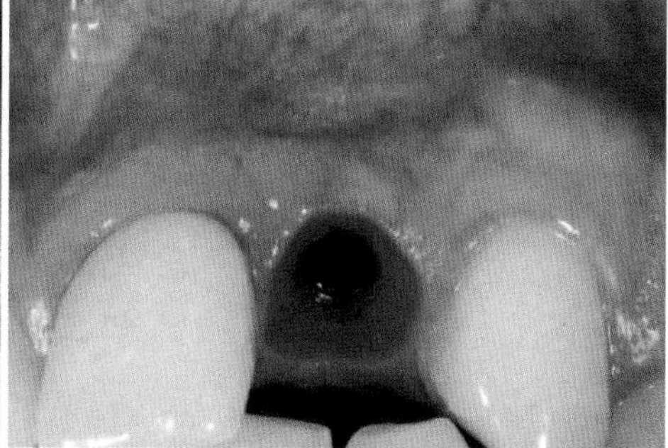

Fig. 46.17 The peri-implant soft tissue is sculpted three-dimensionally to represent the cross-section of the natural tooth being replaced to create a more natural appearance in the final restoration than possible with prefabricated round healing abutments.

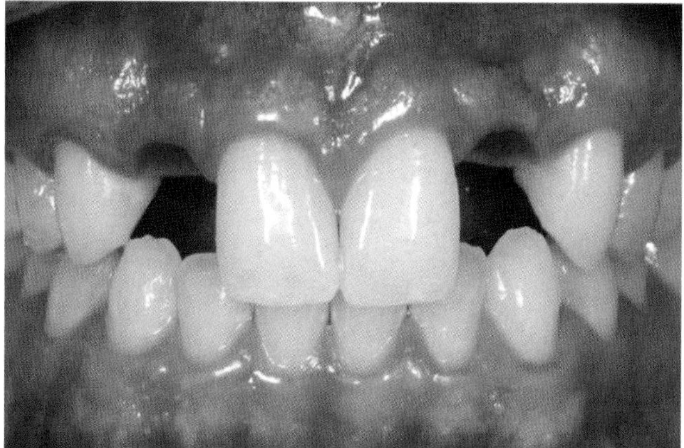

Fig. 46.18 Peri-implant soft tissue after nonsurgical sculpting. Notice the early stages of papillae reforming in the spaces between the natural teeth and dental implants.

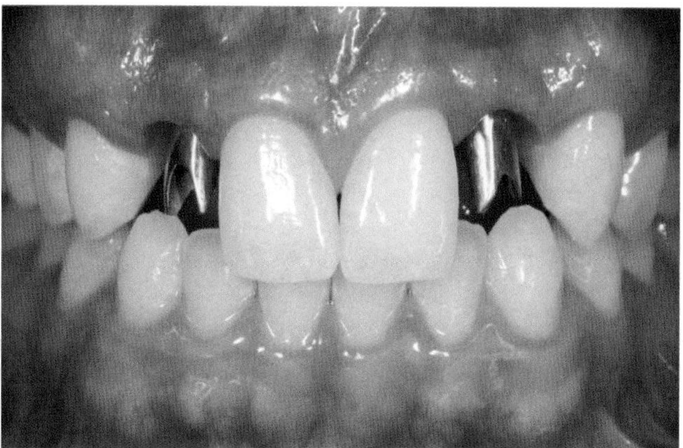

Fig. 46.19 Custom abutments in place on the dental implants. Gold plating of the custom abutments was done to impart a hue to the peri-implant sulcus and soft tissue to optimize the aesthetic outcome.

evolves parallel with material science and digital manufacturing, we can expect enhanced patient care outcomes in the form of improvement in accuracy, reduced treatment times, and even less-invasive surgical interventions. However, the caveat here is to always remain mindful of the fact that digital technologies only follow the commands that humans program and direct them to do.

This fact remains a central tenet in deciding between when a multidisciplinary approach will suffice or if an interdisciplinary approach is indicated to meet the unique needs of each individual patient who entrusts us with their care.

KEY FACT

Like any other instrument, digital technology is not a replacement for sound knowledge, training, and expertise that are essential to oversee, verify, and troubleshoot every step of treatment.

Educational Trends Toward Multidisciplinary Specialist Education in Implant Treatment

For the multidisciplinary model of practice to be able to deliver care at the level presently available through the interdisciplinary model, the provider (general practitioner or specialist) needs to be comprehensively trained with a broader scope and depth of expertise than typical contemporary norms often deliver. This is reflected in the many changes and opportunities in continuing and postgraduate training, particularly those centered on the surgical aspects of dental implant therapy.

Continuing education offerings span a broad range. Some are limited to didactic teaching with laboratory simulation, whereas others take the form of clinical fellowship-style programs that encompass a patient care component lasting a year or longer. As such, some general practitioners and traditionally trained prosthodontists who have sought out advanced postgraduate training might add some aspects of surgical care (commensurate with the scope and level of their respective training) to the range of services they personally provide. Conversely, members of the surgical specialties (e.g., periodontists and oral surgeons) would have received a level of training that would enable them to recommend, guide, and, if necessary, provide a range of restorative treatments. Indeed, rigidly defined accreditation standards for some postgraduate specialties have already been revised and reflect this trend toward encouraging multidisciplinary training. With recent changes in accreditation standards, implant provisionalization is now an integral component of periodontology training programs in the United States. Also, traditional nonsurgical restorative training programs now include basic implant surgical training in their curricula. Advanced education specialty programs in prosthodontics, among other topics, now include an increased allocation of time in their didactic and clinical curricula for the area of diagnosis as well as training to the level of competency with respect to simple single-tooth implants in healed ridges of favorable dimension and in sites outside the aesthetic zone.

The Future

It has already become the accepted norm that not all surgery will be done by a periodontist or oral surgeon, nor is it likely that all restorative work will be done by a general dentist or prosthodontist.

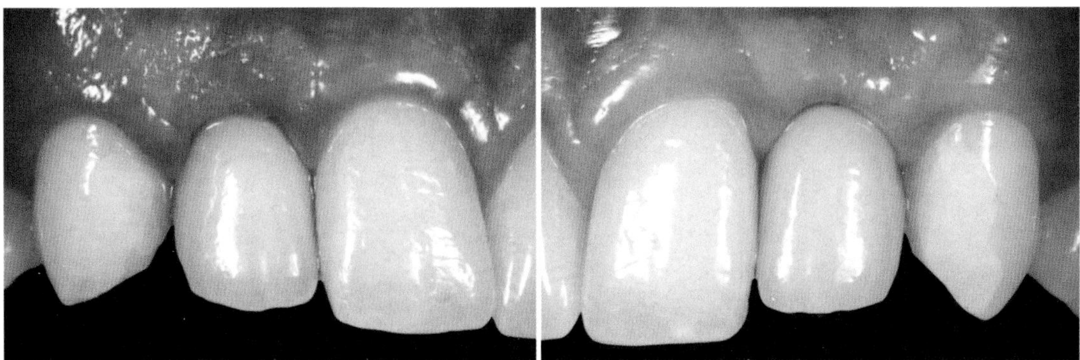

Fig. 46.20 Final crowns are seen here on the date of insertion. The crown contours dictate the gingival contours.

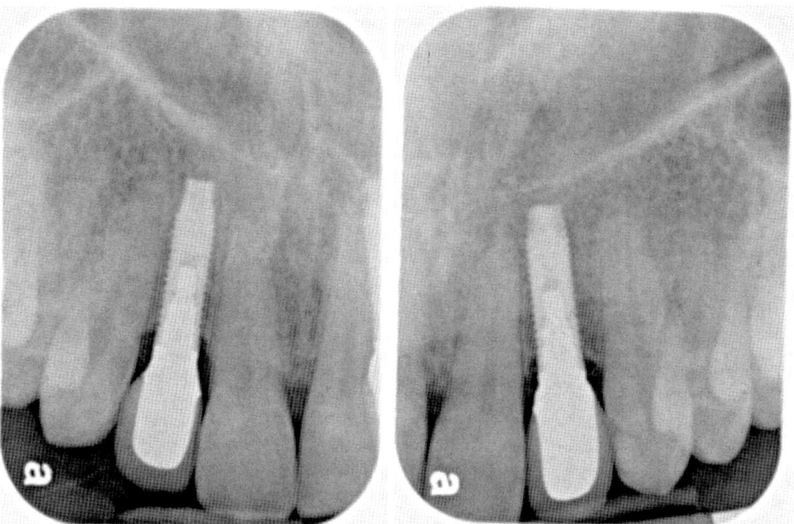

Fig. 46.21 Radiograph following final crown insertion. Note the customized emergence profile of the prosthetic components on the dental implants.

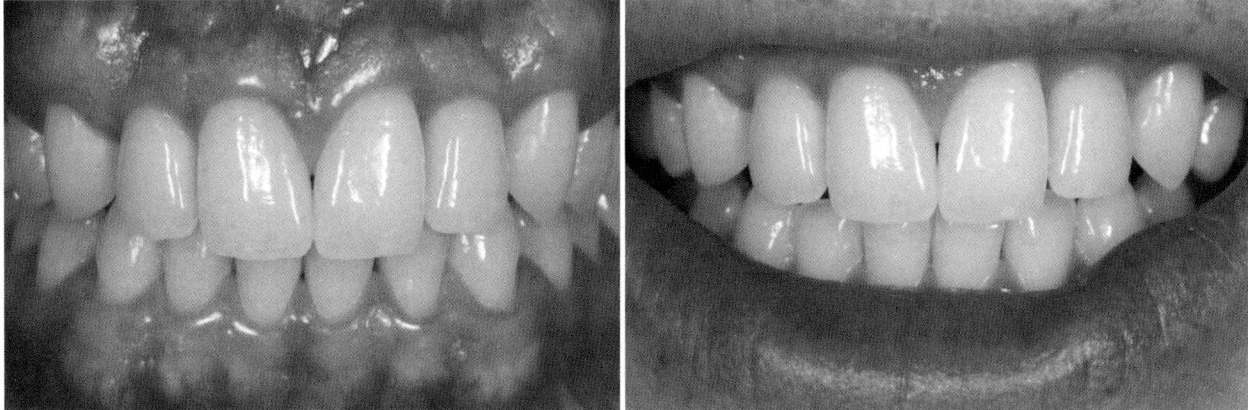

Fig. 46.22 Final aesthetic outcome from both an intraoral and extraoral perspective.

Instead, simple cases that require surgery and restoration will probably be performed entirely by either a well-trained general dentist or a specialist. In fact, many periodontists have already begun working with their restorative colleagues by making the final impression or index of the implant at the time of surgery and forwarding it to them. In such a scenario, the restorative dentist may now only need to insert the final restoration when it comes back from the laboratory, thus expediting treatment and enhancing the experience for both the patient and the doctor. Although it is conceivable that simple implant cases will more likely be treated in a multidisciplinary fashion, an interdisciplinary approach will still exist and be utilized for patients who require advanced treatments, particularly when there is a deficiency of soft and/or hard tissues.

Periodontists of the future will have a multidisciplinary approach to patient care. They will continue to provide all of the specialty services that "classically" trained periodontists have done for decades, but they will also be well suited to better support their restorative colleagues.

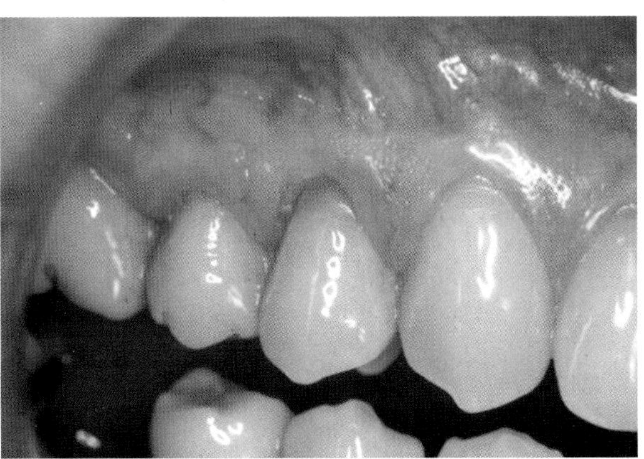

Fig. 46.23 Multidisciplinary simple implant care scenario: favorable soft-tissue parameters combined with a low smile line. Preoperative view of the maxillary right first premolar. With the exception of a small degree of gingival recession, all other aspects of the surrounding periodontium are intact.

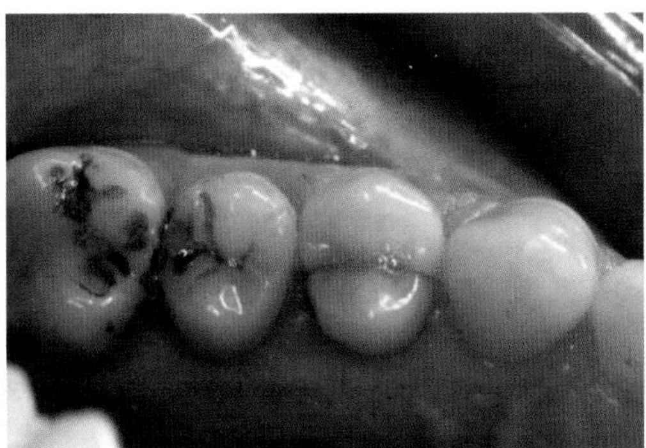

Fig. 46.24 A fracture extending in a mesiodistal orientation is evident on the occlusal surface of the maxillary first premolar.

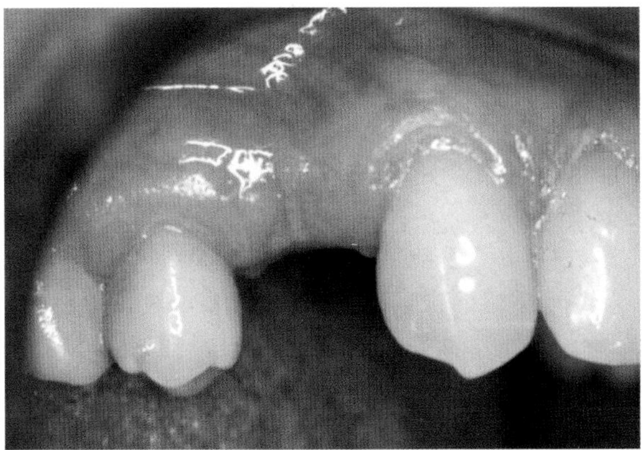

Fig. 46.25 Healed ridge 3 months after tooth extraction. Note the wide zone of keratinized tissue present and favorable maintenance of the height of the adjacent interdental papillae.

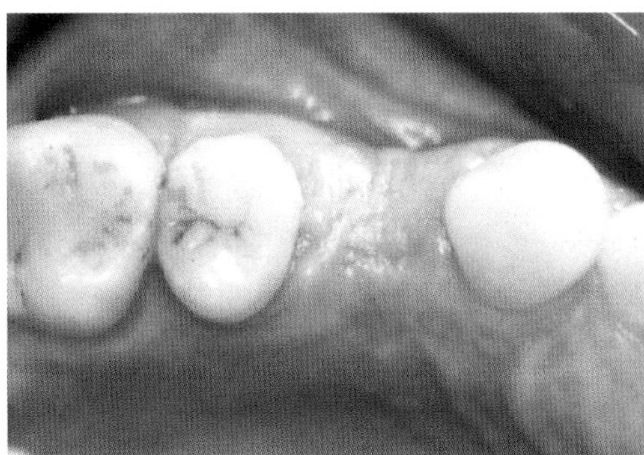

Fig. 46.26 The healed ridge demonstrates favorable buccolingual dimension and soft-tissue quality. Based on preoperative clinical and radiographic evaluation, placement of a dental implant in an uncomplicated fashion can be expected.

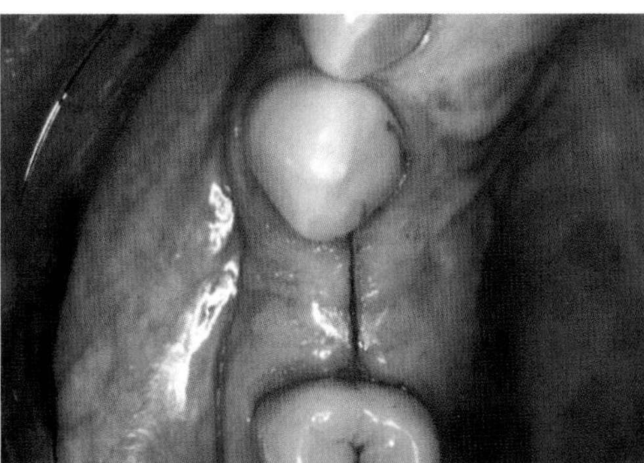

Fig. 46.27 Surgical access for placement of the dental implant using a horizontal incision that extends intrasulcularly to the nearest buccal and palatal line angles of the adjacent teeth.

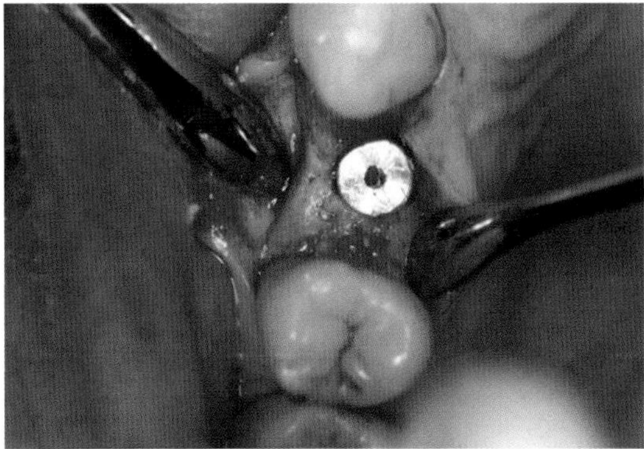

Fig. 46.28 The endosseous implant is properly positioned to facilitate an optimal prosthetic outcome in the final restoration.

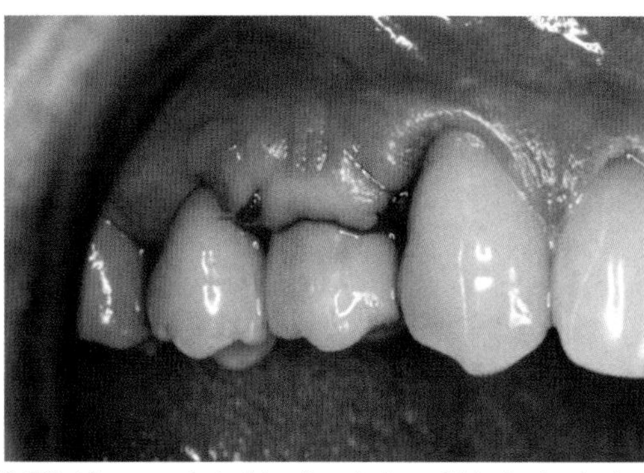

Fig. 46.29 After a period of healing during which the implant was submerged, stage II surgery to expose it was accomplished. In this scenario, a fixed provisional restoration was secured to the implant to serve as a matrix and begin sculpting the resultant soft-tissue profile in lieu of using a conventional nonanatomic round healing abutment. Note the position of the flap margin on the prosthetic crown. It is located occlusal to the expected cementoenamel junction (CEJ) location to compensate for expected soft-tissue healing and remodeling and yield a favorable aesthetic outcome.

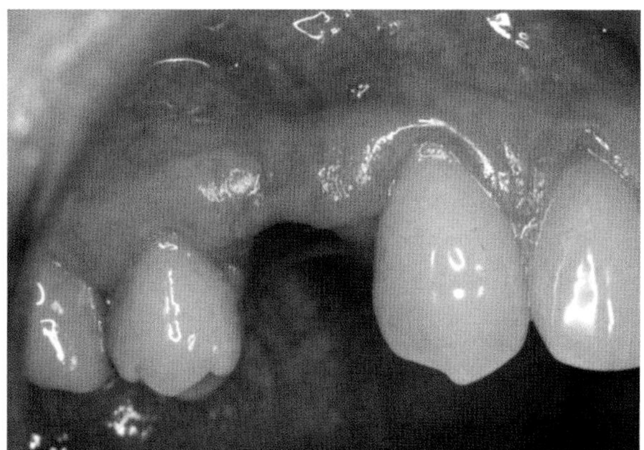

Fig. 46.30 The healed peri-implant sulcus demonstrates the three-dimensionally generated result achieved using a provisional crown for soft-tissue sculpting. Note the recreation of the interdental papilla, the result of a favorable relationship between the interproximal bone height of the adjacent teeth and reestablishment of contact areas between the natural teeth and the provisional restoration.

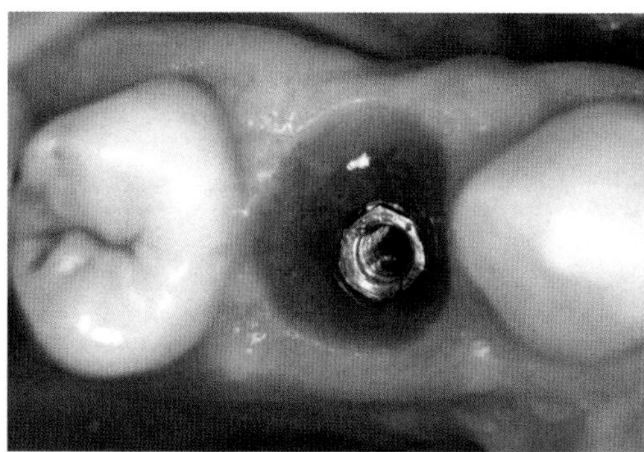

Fig. 46.31 Occlusal view of the anatomic peri-implant sulcus formed by the contours of the provisional restoration subgingivally.

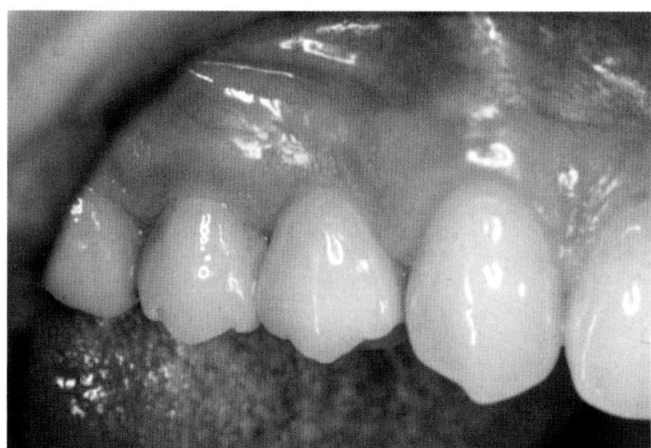

Fig. 46.32 Final implant-supported restoration in place.

CHAPTER 47

Periodontal Referral

Sukirth M. Ganesan | Megumi A. Williamson

CHAPTER OUTLINE

Introduction

Patient referral is a broad term that also includes patient referral to physicians by a periodontist for a medical consultation prior to or during periodontal therapy. In this chapter, the focus is primarily on patient referral to periodontists by another dental provider (general dentists or other dental specialists). Appropriate referrals are an essential component of comprehensive patient management. According to General Guidelines for Referring Dental Patients by the American Dental Association,[1] referral may be requested for a variety of reasons. Broadly, the reasons for referral can be divided into (1) provider-related factors and (2) patient-related factors.

Some provider-related factors include:

1. Dentist's level of training and experience
2. Dentist area of interest (specialization) and clinical expertise
3. Special equipment and instrument availability in the office
4. Staff capabilities and training
5. Desire to share responsibility for patient care
6. Patient volume and availability of appointments

Patient-related factors include both disease associated, and other patient associated reasons, such as:

1. Behavioral concerns of the patient
2. Patient's preference due to logistical reasons such as geographical proximity of the specialist
3. Medical complications
4. Extensiveness and complexity of the clinical condition

Management of periodontal disease is not a one-time process, and most periodontal patients require lifelong disease management. Hence, the most integral part of referral is clear communication between the referring dentist and periodontist to establishing an appropriate periodic recall and maintenance appointment after the completion of periodontal therapy to ensure early detection and timely management of disease recurrence.

Current State of Periodontal Referral

A study on periodontal referral patterns between 1980 and 2000 showed that the referred patients exhibited decreased smoking frequency; however, they presented with a greater loss of teeth and more severe disease, and required a higher number of extractions.[4] In another study cohort, close to 30% of patients referred to a periodontal practice required two or more extractions because of the severity of disease.[5] Additionally, more than 70% of the referred patients were diagnosed with severe periodontal disease, and the average number of cleanings that these patients received in their general dental practitioners' offices was less than the standard of care. The study demonstrated a lack of (a) timely diagnosis of periodontal disease and (b) appropriate treatment, and/or timely referral for treatment.

The results were corroborated by another group that reported that at least 13% of the general dentists made no referral to a periodontal office in the last month, and 69% made between one to five referrals in the last month.[15] With at least one-half of the American adults suffering from at least some form of periodontal disease and approximately 9% suffering from severe periodontal disease,[6–8] the referral numbers reported in the study are disproportionately low. Several factors have been listed as potential causes for poor periodontal referral patterns, including socioeconomic status and insurance coverage of patients, patient's apprehension, and lack of access to care. However the most alarming finding is the lack of appropriate diagnostic skills, thus resulting in a delay in or absence of appropriate referral for periodontal therapy. Lack of periodontal diagnostic skills was discussed in 2002 in a study that identified that only 6% of training hours in the US dental curriculum were spent on periodontal training.[15]

Therefore this chapter's primary goals are to provide clinical guidelines for referral based on the extent and severity of periodontal disease condition as described in the 2018 periodontal disease classification criteria.

Patient Referral Based on Periodontist and General Dentist Involvement in Treatment

The guidelines for managing patients with periodontal diseases published by the American Academy of Periodontology in 2006[14] classified patients into three levels based on the involvement of the periodontist and the general dentist in the patient care.

Level 3 patients: These are patients who should be treated by a periodontist. Examples of level 3 patients include patients diagnosed with severe chronic periodontitis ("stage III or IV periodontitis"), furcation involvement, vertical/angular bony defect(s), aggressive periodontitis ("periodontitis with molar-incisor pattern"), periodontal abscess and other acute periodontal conditions, significant root surface exposure and/or progressive gingival recession, peri-implant diseases, and any patients with periodontal diseases, regardless of severity, whom the referring dentist prefers not to treat because of lack of expertise and/or support in the office.

Level 2 patients: These are patients who would likely benefit from co-management by the referring dentist and the periodontist. Level 2 patients have local or systemic risk factors or indicators of periodontal disease progression and include the following: early onset of periodontal diseases, persistent gingival inflammation characterized by redness of the tissue, bleeding on probing (BOP) or suppuration, probing depth 5 mm or greater, vertical bone defects, radiographic evidence of progressive bone loss, progressive tooth mobility, progressive attachment loss, anatomic gingival deformities, exposed root surfaces, and a deteriorating risk profile.

Level 1 patients: These patients may benefit from co-management by the referring dentist and the periodontist. Level 1 patients include any patient with systemic conditions such as diabetes, pregnancy, cardiovascular disease, or chronic respiratory disease, presenting with periodontal inflammation/infection. Additionally, patients who undergo cancer therapy, cardiovascular surgery, joint-replacement surgery, or organ transplantation may benefit from co-management.

Table 47.1 lists the recommendation of co-management levels based on the 2018 periodontal disease classification scheme.

Patient Referral Based on Periodontal Condition

Periodontal Health, Gingival Diseases and Conditions

In general, (a) non-periodontitis patients with clinically healthy gingiva characterized by less than 10% BOP and ≤3 mm probing depth[3] or (b) dental biofilm-induced gingivitis characterized by ≥10% BOP and ≤3 mm probing depth[3] can be managed by general dentists. Patients with non-dental biofilm-induced gingival diseases should be referred to appropriate health care providers as they are frequently oral manifestations of systemic diseases. Gingival health on a reduced periodontium is a clinical diagnosis given to patients with a history of periodontitis, but was successfully treated and currently presents with healthy gingival tissue, characterized by less than 10% BOP and ≤4 mm probing depth.[3] In these patients, as the susceptibility to periodontitis still remains, these patients should be co-managed with a periodontist and can be considered as level 2 or level 1 patients (depending on the risk profile).

Periodontitis Patients

Necrotizing periodontal diseases are characterized by three typical clinical features: papilla necrosis, bleeding, and pain and associated with compromised host immune response.[16] When identified, these patients should be immediately referred to and treated by a periodontist (level 3) and appropriate health care provider (if needed) to manage the underlying systemic conditions.

For periodontitis patients, stage I and II periodontitis patients can be treated and managed by general dentists. However, patients with stage III or IV periodontitis presents with more severe disease that requires more complex procedures. Examples of clinical indicators that will put the patients under stage III or IV include clinical attachment loss ≥5 mm, deep probing depth (≥6 mm), vertical bone loss (≥3 mm), furcation involvement (class II or III), moderate ridge defects, and need of complex rehabilitation. Therefore, when identified, stage III and IV periodontitis patients should be referred to and treated by a periodontist (level 3). Since the host susceptibility does not change even after the successful treatment in these patients, successfully treated stage III and IV patients should be co-managed by the referring dentist and the periodontist (level 2 or 1). For detailed information on the staging and grading scheme of periodontitis, refer to Chapter 5.

Patients with any known risk factors such as cigarette smoking and diabetes would likely or may benefit from co-management by the referring dentist and the periodontist (level 2 or 1). Patients diagnosed with periodontitis as a manifestation of systemic diseases should be treated by a periodontist if the disease severity falls under stage III and IV and will likely benefit from co-management, if periodontitis is less severe (stage I or II) or successfully treated. In addition, on a need basis, these patients should be managed by appropriate health care professionals. Fig. 47.1 shows a decision-making algorithm that can be used as a guide by general dentists to make appropriate periodontal referrals.

Patients With Other Conditions Affecting the Periodontium

When a patient presents with systemic conditions that may affect the periodontium, the patient should be treated by the appropriate health care provider first. If periodontitis is confirmed, the patient may benefit from co-management by the referring dentist and periodontist. Periodontal abscesses are destructive lesions in the periodontium, characterized by localized accumulation of pus within the gingival wall of the periodontal pocket or sulcus.[11,12] Periodontal abscesses are frequently seen in preexisting periodontal pocket and can be acute or chronic in nature. Acute periodontal abscess accompanies pain and is a common dental emergency that requires immediate management by periodontist due to its destructive nature. In some cases, periodontal abscesses are associated with systemic dissemination. When periodontal abscess is identified, the patient should be immediately referred to a periodontist for timely management (level 3).

Patients with Endodontic-Periodontal Lesions or Signs of Occlusal Trauma

Endodontic-periodontal lesion is a pathological communication between the pulpal and periodontal tissues on the same tooth.[12] Acute form of this type of lesion is a common dental emergency. When a given tooth presents with isolated deep probing depth with signs of pulpal involvement, the tooth likely has an endodontic-periodontal lesion. When an endodontic-periodontal lesion is identified, the patient should be referred to a periodontist (level 3). In many of these conditions, patients will be co-managed by a periodontist and an endodontist. Traumatic occlusal force leads to injury of the periodontal attachment apparatus. Signs of occlusal trauma include progressive tooth mobility, fremitus, occlusal discrepancies, wear facets, pathologic tooth migration, tooth fracture, thermal sensitivity, root resorption, cemental tear, and widening of periodontal ligament space observed on a radiograph.[9] As traumatic occlusal force may accelerate the progression of existing periodontitis and complicate the treatment course, patients with traumatic occlusal forces with signs of occlusal trauma should be referred to a periodontist for management (level 3).

TABLE 47.1 Recommendation of Co-Management Levels Based on AAP/EFP 2018 Classification Scheme

RECOMMENDATION / CLASSIFICATION				**Patients who should be treated by a periodontist (Level 3)**	**Patients who would likely benefit from co-management by the referring dentist and the periodontist (Level 2)**	**Patients who may benefit from co-management by the referring dentist and the periodontist (Level 1)**
Periodontal health, gingival diseases and conditions	Periodontal health and gingival health	Periodontal health		N/A	N/A	N/A
		Gingival health on a reduced periodontium in non-periodontitis patient		N/A	N/A	N/A
		Gingival health on a reduced periodontium (stable periodontitis patient)			✓	
	Gingivitis, dental biofilm-induced	Associated with dental biofilm alone	Gingivitis in non-periodontitis patient	N/A	N/A	N/A
			Gingivitis on a reduced periodontium in stable periodontitis patient		✓	
		Mediated by systemic or local risk factors			✓	
		Drug-induced		✓		
	Gingival diseases: non-dental biofilm-induced			✓	✓	
Periodontitis	Necrotizing periodontal diseases			✓		
	Stage I periodontitis					✓, depending on the grade (risk factors/modifiers)
	Stage II					✓, depending on the grade (risk factors/modifiers)
	Stage III			✓		
	Stage IV			✓		
	Periodontitis as a manifestation of systemic diseases			✓ (If it is stage III & IV)	✓ (If it is stage I & II)	
Other conditions affecting periodontium	Systemic diseases or conditions affecting the periodontal supporting tissue			✓	✓	
	Periodontal abscesses and endodontic-periodontal lesions			✓		
	Mucogingival deformities and conditions			✓ (if it is progressing)		
	Traumatic occlusal forces			✓		
	Tooth- and prosthesis-related factors					
Peri-implant diseases	Peri-implant health					✓ (annual check if the implant was placed by the periodontist)
	Peri-implant mucositis			✓		
	Peri-implantitis			✓		
	Peri-implant soft and hard tissue deficiencies			✓		

✓ denotes recommended management levels, and *N/A* indicates that those patients may not need referral to periodontists. This is a broad guideline and referral decisions should be made on a case-by-case basis.

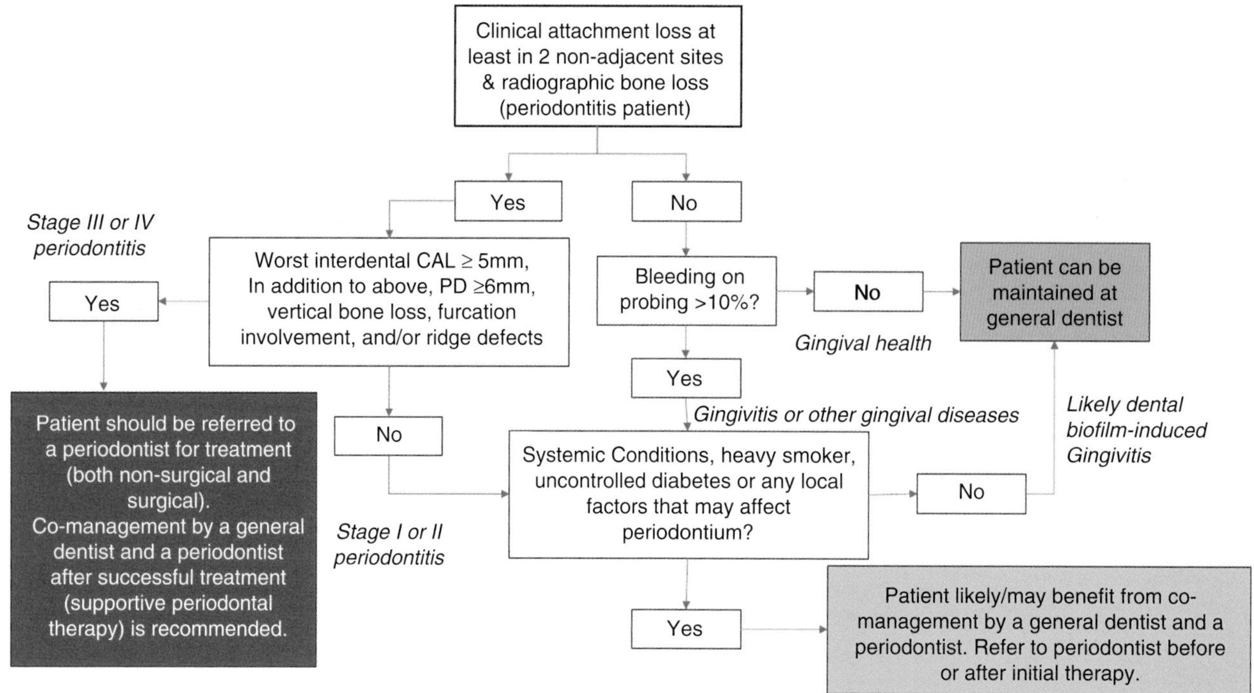

Fig. 47.1 Referral flowchart for patients presenting with periodontal conditions. Note this is just a broad guideline and referral decisions should be made on a case-by-case basis.

Patients With Mucogingival Deformities and Conditions around Natural Dentition

Mucogingival deformities and conditions around natural dentition includes gingival recession and lack of keratinized gingiva. If gingival recession is progressive or causing esthetic concerns, the patient should be referred to a periodontist for evaluation and appropriate treatment. In many patients, lack of keratinized tissue is not an immediate indication for treatment. However, it may affect proper oral hygiene habits and contribute to localized chronic inflammation. Therefore, when above conditions are identified, referral to a periodontist (level 3) should be made for an evaluation and treatment. Thin periodontal phenotype increases risk for gingival recession, especially with buccal movement of the tooth during orthodontic treatment.[13] It is recommended to make a referral to a periodontist (level 3) for evaluation and treatment as needed, prior to initiation of orthodontic therapy, when the patient presents with existing gingival recession, lack of keratinized gingiva, or thin periodontal phenotype.

Patients With Dental Prosthesis and Tooth-Related Factors

Dental prosthesis and tooth-related factors can negatively affect periodontium. Dental prosthesis–related factors include restoration margins placed within the supracrestal attached tissues, clinical procedures related to the fabrication of indirect restorations, and hypersensitivity/toxicity to dental materials (Chapter 45). Localized tooth-related factors include tooth anatomic factors, root fractures, cervical root resorption, root proximity, and altered passive eruption.[13] When such conditions are suspected, the patient should be referred to a periodontist for further evaluation and treatment as needed.

Peri-implant Diseases and Conditions

Patients With Peri-implant Health

Peri-implant health is characterized by absence of erythema, BOP, swelling, suppuration, and absence of bone loss beyond crestal bone level changes resulting from initial bone remodeling.[2] Therefore it is necessary to probe around implant to be able to detect these inflammatory signs and take periodic radiographs to compare crestal bone changes around implant. Patients with peri-implant health may still benefit from co-management by the general dentist and periodontist for a periodic evaluation on the implant so that any peri-implant changes can be detected early and managed appropriately (level 1). Peri-implant health can be observed around an implant with a reduced bone support. In such case, patients should be seen more frequently by a periodontist as the susceptibility to peri-implant diseases is higher in these patients (level 2).

Patients With Peri-implant Mucositis

Peri-implant mucositis is characterized by clinical signs of inflammation such as BOP, erythema, swelling, and/or suppuration but absence of bone loss beyond crestal bone level changes resulting from the initial bone remodeling.[2] Other clinical signs that can aid in diagnosis include increased probing depth compared to the previous examinations. Therefore it is necessary to probe around implants and take periodic radiographs for early detection of those signs and radiographic changes. When peri-implant mucositis is identified, the patient should be referred to and treated by a periodontist (level 3).

Patients With Peri-implantitis

Peri-implantitis is characterized by clinical signs of inflammation in the peri-implant mucosa and subsequent progressive loss of supporting bone.[2] If the previous examination data are not available, diagnosis of peri-implantitis can be made with the following clinical and radiographic signs: presence of inflammation, probing depth of ≥6 mm, and bone levels ≥3 mm apical of the most coronal portion of the intraosseous part of the implant.[2] When these signs are identified around implants, the patient should be referred to and treated by a periodontist (level 3).

Referral form

Patient details

First name	Middle name	Last name
D.O.B	Age	Gender
Address (street)	City	Zip
Phone number	Phone type	Email

Insurance information ______________________

Referring dentist details

First name	Last name	
Practice address (street)	City	Zip
Dentist email	Phone number	Fax number

Reason for referral/previous treatment/comments

Radiographs

- Accompanying patient
- Please take new radiographs
- Email: gohawksperio@iowa.com
- Needs/evaluate for CBCT

Periodontal concerns

- Emergency treatment teeth # ______________
- Comprehensive periodontal examination
- Limited periodontal evaluation teeth #/area ______________
- Extraction teeth # ______________
- Crown lengthening (C/L) teeth # ______________
    - Restorability of teeth requiring C/L ______________
- Recession or mucogingival problem teeth #/area ______________
- Frenum attachment area ______________
- Exposure of impacted teeth # ______________
- Biopsy area ______________
- Other ______________

Esthetic concerns

- Esthetic crown lengthening teeth #/area ______________
- Gingival augmentation teeth #/area ______________

Dental implant therapy

- Implant site development. teeth #/area ______________
- Dental implant
    - Preferred system ______________
    - Surgical/radiographic stent (please circle an option)
        - Periodontist Referring dentist
    - Restorative abutment (please circle an option)
        - Periodontist Referring dentist

Follow-up care

- Scaling and root planing (root instrumentation)(please circle an option)
    - Periodontist Referring dentist
- Maintenance and hygiene (please circle an option)
    - Periodontist Referring dentist Alternate intervals ______________

Fig. 47.2 A sample periodontal referral form.

Patient With Peri-implant Soft and Hard Tissue Deficiencies

Peri-implant soft tissue deficiencies, in the form of recession of peri-implant mucosa, are associated with malpositioning of implants, lack of buccal bone, thin soft tissue, lack of keratinized tissue, status of attachment of adjacent teeth affecting the papilla height, surgical trauma, and migration of teeth and lifelong skeletal changes.[10] Crestal bone loss due to peri-implantitis also causes soft tissue deficiencies around implants. Soft tissue deficiencies around implants affect esthetics of implants as well as long-term implant health. When soft tissue deficiencies are identified and/or patient expresses esthetic concerns, referral to periodontist should be made for an evaluation and treatment (level 3). Hard tissue deficiencies around implant can be associated with defects in healthy situations such as bony undercuts, malpositioning of implants, peri-implantitis, mechanical overload, thin soft tissue around implants, and systemic diseases.[10] When hard tissue defects are causing esthetic problems or results from peri-implantitis, the patient should be referred to a periodontist for management of these defects.

Referral Process

Once the level of management/co-management is identified, and when the need for a referral to a periodontist is determined, for effective communication of patient needs between clinics, completing a periodontal referral form is advised. The purpose of the referral form is to provide efficient, clear, and precise communication between the primary provider and the specialist office. Any relevant medical and dental condition and a detailed explanation of the current problem and reason (s) for the referral need to be furnished. For example, if a functional crown lengthening is requested, the primary provider must confirm the restorability of the tooth. Similarly, for the dental implant procedures, enough information should be furnished related to the fabrication of guides, provisionalization, and the type of implant that the primary provider has expertise in restoring. Fig. 47.2 is a model periodontal referral form.

A closed-loop tracking for referral completion followed by patient feedback/follow-up is essential to confirm that appropriate treatment has been rendered and ensure the highest patient satisfaction. This will also ensure continuity of care. Once the treatment is complete, the periodontist should communicate with the referring dentist and provide the following information:

1. Nature of treatment/surgery rendered
2. Timeline of healing and when the patient will need a referring dentist's appointment.

Conclusions

An appropriate periodontal referral starts with accurate diagnosis of periodontal conditions. Periodontal referral can be challenging due to the dynamic nature of the process, and this chapter provides some guidance on this important process in the overall scheme of patient management. For many periodontal conditions, making timely referral to a periodontist is vital for its successful management and resolution.

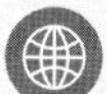
References for this chapter are found on the companion website eBooks.Health.Elsevier.com.

CHAPTER 48

Orthodontics in Periodontal Therapy

Frank Celenza | Vincent G. Kokich† | Conchita Martin

For discussions of preorthodontic osseous surgery, orthodontic treatment of osseous defects, the orthodontic treatment of gingival discrepancies, and implant interactions in orthodontics and aligners please go to the companion website at eBooks.Health.Elsevier.com.

CHAPTER OUTLINE

Orthodontic appliances have become smaller, less noticeable, and easier to maintain during orthodontic therapy. Also, the use of temporary anchorage devices (TADs) has facilitated the mechanics in complex cases. Many adults are taking advantage of the opportunity to have their teeth aligned to improve the esthetics of their smile. Underlying gingival or osseous periodontal defects often can be improved during orthodontic therapy if the orthodontist is aware of the situation and designs the appropriate tooth movement. In addition, implants have become a major part of the treatment plan for many adults with missing teeth. If adjacent teeth have drifted into edentulous spaces, orthodontic therapy is often helpful to provide the ideal amount of space for implants and subsequent restorations. This chapter shows the ways in which adjunctive orthodontic therapy can enhance the periodontal health and restorability of teeth, reviews how orthodontic therapy can be implemented in adults with periodontally affected dentitions, and presents the role of implant dentistry in both periodontics and orthodontics.

Benefits of Orthodontic Therapy

Orthodontic therapy can provide several benefits to adult periodontal patients. The following eight factors should be considered:

1. Aligning crowded or malpositioned maxillary or mandibular anterior teeth permits adult patients better access to clean all surfaces of their teeth. This could be a tremendous advantage for patients who are susceptible to periodontal disease or do not have the dexterity to maintain oral hygiene.
2. Vertical orthodontic tooth repositioning can improve certain types of osseous defects in periodontal patients. Often, moving the tooth eliminates the need for resective osseous surgery.
3. Horizontal orthodontic tooth movement undertaken immediately after tooth extraction can counteract the resultant physiologic alveolar ridge contraction, and thus develop an appropriately sized alveolar ridge.
4. Orthodontic treatment can improve the esthetic relationship of the maxillary gingival margins before restorative dentistry. Aligning the gingival margins orthodontically avoids gingival recontouring, which could also entail bone removal and exposure of the roots of the teeth (Fig. 48.1).
5. Orthodontic therapy also benefits the patient with a severe fracture of a maxillary anterior tooth that requires forced eruption to permit adequate restoration of the root. Erupting the root allows the crown preparation to have sufficient resistance form and retention for the final restoration.
6. Orthodontic treatment allows open gingival embrasures to be corrected to regain lost papillae. If open gingival embrasures are located in the maxillary anterior region, this can present an esthetic problem. In most patients, these areas can be corrected with a combination of orthodontic root movement, tooth reshaping, and restoration.
7. Orthodontic treatment could improve adjacent tooth positioning before implant placement or tooth replacement. This is especially true for the patient who has been missing teeth for several years and has drifting and tipping of the adjacent dentition.
8. A common tooth malalignment problem that results in periodontal pockets is the mesially tipped molar. Orthodontic uprighting of tipped molars corrects the deep gingival contours and eliminates or reduces the mesial periodontal pocket (Fig. 48.2).

†Deceased.

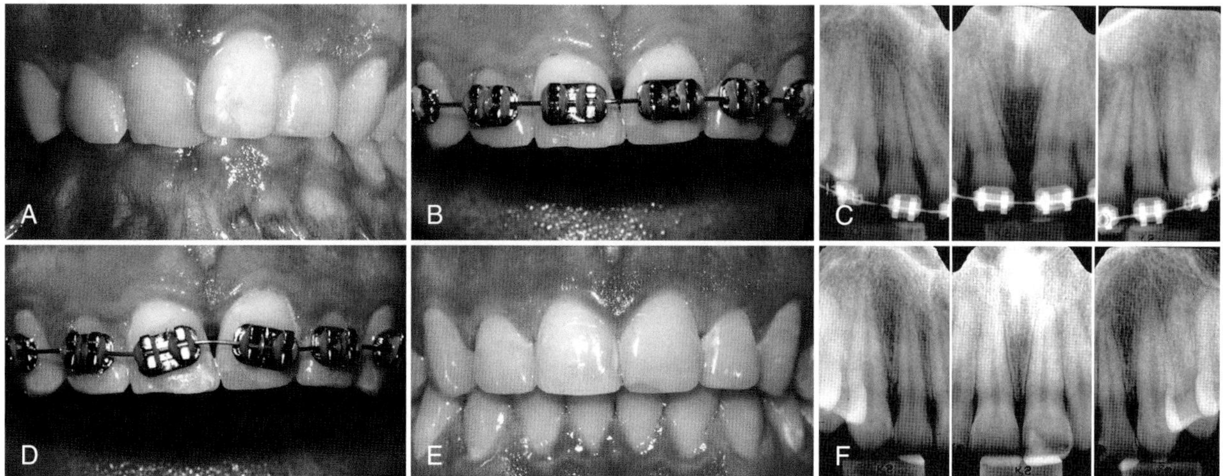

Fig. 48.1 This patient initially had overlapped maxillary central incisors (A), and, after initial orthodontic alignment of the teeth, an open gingival embrasure appeared between the centrals (B). Radiography showed that the open embrasure was caused by divergence of the central incisor roots (C). To correct the problem, the central incisor brackets were repositioned (D), and the roots were moved together. This required restoration of the incisal edges after orthodontic therapy (E) because these teeth had worn unevenly before therapy. As the roots were paralleled (F), the tooth contact moved gingivally and the papilla moved incisally, resulting in elimination of the open gingival embrasure.

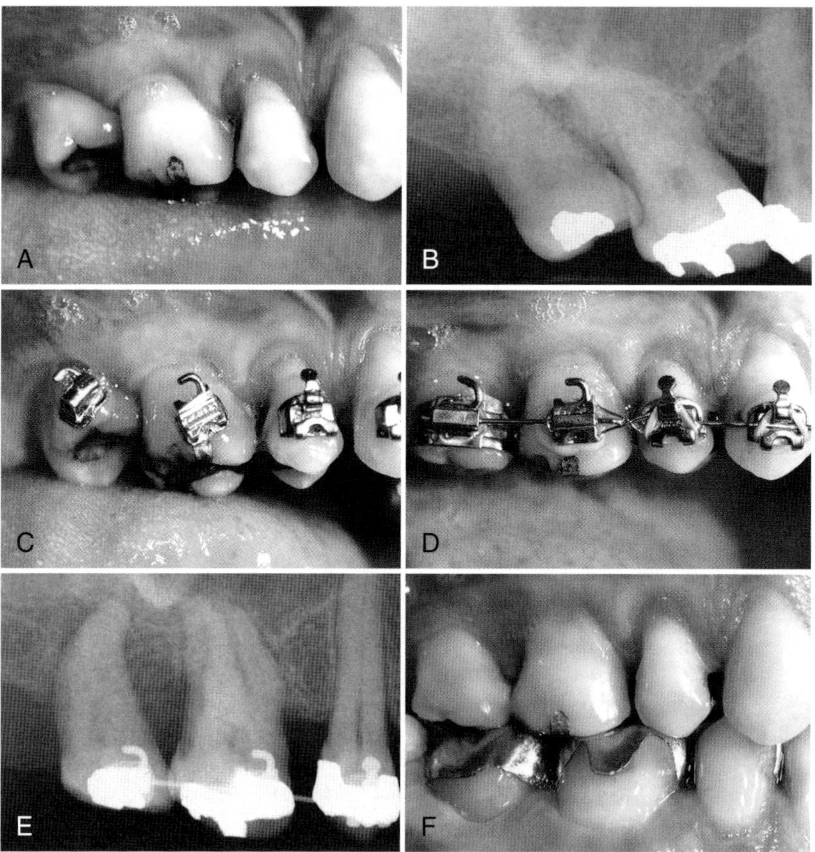

Fig. 48.2 Before orthodontic treatment, this patient had significant mesial tipping of the maxillary right first and second molars, causing marginal ridge discrepancies and deep periodontal pockets (A). The tipping produced root proximity between the molars as well as a disruption of the normal gingival anatomy (B). To eliminate the root proximity, the brackets were placed perpendicular to the long axes of the teeth (C). This method of bracket placement facilitated root alignment and elimination of the root proximity, as well as leveling of the marginal ridge discrepancies (D through F).

LEARNING BOX 48.1

Orthodontic therapy can contribute in many ways to help patients with periodontal problems. In selected cases, vertical orthodontic tooth repositioning can improve certain types of osseous defects to eliminate the need for resective periodontal surgery. Many patients have crowded, malaligned, and malpositioned maxillary or mandibular anterior teeth, presenting a difficult biofilm control problem. Aligning the crowded teeth orthodontically will help patients maintain improved biofilm control. The incorporation of orthodontic therapy in the treatment of these clinical periodontal problems is a great aid to the clinician and the patient.

Effects of Orthodontic Therapy on the Periodontium

Although the effects of orthodontic forces on the periodontium have been studied extensively, there are contradictory findings in the scientific literature on the impact of orthodontic therapy on periodontal health. A systematic review about the effect of orthodontic treatment on periodontal outcomes concluded that orthodontic treatment with fixed appliances has little to no clinically relevant effect on periodontal clinical attachment levels.[72]

In some patients with poor oral hygiene, the fixed orthodontic appliances may promote gingival enlargement, which further enhances plaque accumulation. In these situations, subgingival instrumentation is indicated to resolve the inflammation, and reinstatement of efficient oral hygiene practices are mandatory. Sometimes the marginal tissues do not revert to their appropriate position with only subgingival instrumentation, and surgical removal of the excessive gingival tissue is needed.[41,82] Orthodontic tooth movements *per se* do not cause periodontal attachment loss and/or gingival recession.

Orthodontic Therapy in Severe Periodontitis Patients

In the 2018 classification of periodontal and peri-implant diseases, stage IV periodontitis defines the clinical situation where severe periodontitis is accompanied by extensive tooth loss and the sequelae of tooth drifting and altered masticatory function. This stage of periodontitis will usually need not only the appropriate treatment of the periodontal condition but also a multidisciplinary rehabilitation, including orthodontic therapy.[73]

A recent systematic review concluded that in stable, treated stage IV periodontitis patients, orthodontic therapy had no significant impact on periodontal outcomes. In those studies in which periodontal outcomes were reported before periodontal therapy, combined periodontal and orthodontic therapy had a significant benefit on clinical attachment level, probing pocket depth, and radiographic bone level.[60] In fact, many clinical studies have clearly shown that with adequate plaque control, orthodontic treatment in patients with a reduced but healthy periodontium achieves the orthodontic objectives without aggravating their periodontal condition, and the risk of periodontal recurrence in these patients had not increased during orthodontic therapy.[76] When periodontal inflammation is not fully controlled during orthodontic treatment, however, these inflammatory processes may accelerate the progression of periodontal destruction, leading to further loss of attachment.

The timing of initiating orthodontic treatment after periodontal therapy in periodontitis patients is still controversial. Three main time points were found in the literature: less than 2 weeks, 1 to 2 months, or more than 3 months after periodontal surgeries. The best results were observed when the active force was applied 2 months after the patients were periodontally controlled. There was even a randomized controlled trial that compared the application of orthodontic forces before or after periodontal therapy and found no difference in attachment levels.[97] Although there is no consensus on the best moment to apply orthodontic forces in periodontitis patients, it is mandatory to start orthodontic therapy once periodontal health has been optimally restored.

Orthodontics, Implants and Periodontal Interactions

Whereas the interrelationships between the disciplines of orthodontics and implantology might not seem close to the casual observer, in fact they are quite intimate. In addition, the integration of periodontics with orthodontics and implants presents an even more interesting and important combination. Although the conventional orthodontic patient might be quite different in nature from the periodontal patient, there are many useful and interesting interactions between the disciplines that can and should be harnessed for the best treatment outcomes. This is especially true in current treatment planning in which implants are used as anchors to move teeth.

The conventional orthodontic patient might be characterized as an adolescent or young adult, usually with a healthy, although not always complete, dentition. This patient most often does not present with a significant medical or dental history. Conversely, the periodontal patient often does present with a significant and contributory medical history and a long list of dental problems, which often includes restorative considerations. Further, the periodontium will be compromised and in need of treatment, usually preparatory to orthodontic intervention. Also, there will often be tooth replacement considerations to be sequenced into the therapy. It is in this situation that implant therapy may be part of the treatment scenario. How, then, are these two divergent patient types to be managed by combining treatment modalities from these three disciplines?

This section delineates some of the interrelationships that can be utilized for better therapeutic outcomes. When the clinician gains an appreciation for the periodontal apparatus that supports a tooth and applies an understanding of the physiology of tooth movement, one can utilize the body's reparative and remodeling capacities to effect periodontal alterations as a result of tooth movement. Further, as implant modalities are called upon, a greater demand for accurate tooth position arises. Moreover, as more adult patients are seeking orthodontic and implant treatment, an understanding of the need for and methods of ensuring periodontal health before and during orthodontic and implant care becomes paramount. Consequently, the intimate relationships among these three distinct dental disciplines become apparent in both the treatment planning and treatment execution phases of therapy. We can truly address this topic as *interdisciplinary dentistry*.

Implant Interactions in Orthodontics

Planning Phase

As implant dentistry has impacted virtually all realms of the profession and clinical practice, so too has implantology interacted with orthodontics. As with the other clinical disciplines of dentistry, these potential interactions must be considered prior to the onset of treatment, in the treatment planning stages, because the appropriate sequencing and timing of various steps is important for maximizing the benefits of their coordination.

More specifically, including implants in orthodontic therapy can have two fundamentally different goals, and the clinician needs to clarify the intent, which in turn will dictate the treatment sequence. There are two basic circumstances in which implants (of various configurations) should be considered.

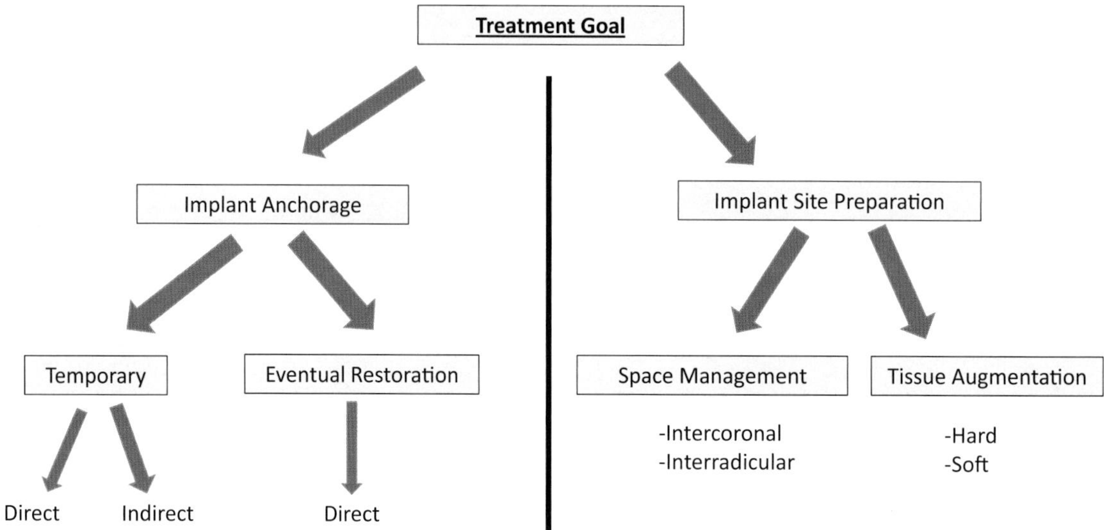

Fig. 48.3 Flowchart for treatment plan.

First, are implants being included in the actual orthodontic mechanotherapy (e.g., used for anchorage purposes)? If so, these types of devices need to be sequenced early in treatment, so as to best utilize them in facilitating the orthodontic movement. Implants used solely for providing orthodontic anchorage will be subsequently explanted when their intended function is completed, and consequently they are referred to as TADs (Fig. 48.3).

Second, are implants under consideration for the replacement of missing or lost teeth? In this more conventional role, implant placement is usually sequenced much later, if not at the conclusion of orthodontic movement. In fact, the orthodontic mechanotherapy treatment in this instance is preparatory to the implant therapy, and it is now employed as a means of implant site development.

It is also feasible that an implant scheme can be devised in which the fixture serves both functions: to provide anchorage for orthodontic mechanotherapy and to be subsequently used as a means of dental replacement.

LEARNING BOX 48.2

Implants can be used to facilitate orthodontic mechanotherapy by providing anchorage, and orthodontic treatment can facilitate implant therapy by providing site development. The sequence of therapy is determined by which of these roles are being harnessed. When an implant is utilized to provide a source of orthodontic anchorage, it should be placed and loaded early in the orthodontic treatment. When orthodontics is being employed for site development, the implant placement will follow the orthodontic treatment.

Conclusion

There are many benefits to integrating orthodontics and periodontics in the management of adult patients with underlying periodontal defects. The key to treating these patients is communication and proper diagnosis before orthodontic therapy, as well as continued dialog during treatment. Not all periodontal problems are treated in the same way. This section provides a framework for the integration of orthodontics to solve periodontal problems. Significant and fascinating interplays exist between the practices of orthodontics and periodontics, which also include implantology. Reciprocal relationships can be harnessed through proper sequencing of treatments to enhance outcomes. Utilization of various implants can facilitate orthodontic mechanotherapy, streamline treatment, eliminate compliance dependency, improve predictability, and even introduce new treatment options. Conversely, orthodontic preparation prior to implant placement can yield a more favorable environment through orthodontically induced site development in which both hard and soft tissue can be augmented and remodeled. Further, spatial management of implant sites and neighboring tooth positions is often essential to ideal implant location.

Periodontal treatment preparatory to orthodontic treatment is often required to eliminate inflammation and bolster the investing tooth structures, thereby permitting successful tooth movement without further loss of attachment. Likewise, orthodontic modalities can be employed to remodel the hard and soft tissues of the periodontium to benefit various situations, such as defect eradication.

Consequently, there are many instances in which interdisciplinary interactions can facilitate treatment, and these interactions can be considered bidirectional. Thus implant utilization can sometimes enhance orthodontic outcomes, while other times orthodontic treatment should be employed to enhance implant outcomes. Just as applicable are the bidirectional possibilities between orthodontics and periodontics. This chapter has illustrated these concepts and has stressed the importance of proper sequencing of therapy to maximize these possibilities.

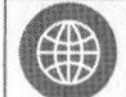
Case Scenarios are found on the companion website eBooks.Health.Elsevier.com.

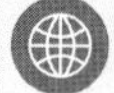
References can be found on the companion Expert Consult website at eBooks.Health.Elsevier.com.

CHAPTER 49

Endo-Perio Lesions: Pathogenesis, Diagnosis, and Treatment Considerations

Mo K. Kang | Shebli Mehrazarin | Kenneth C. Trabert

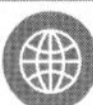 Videos for this chapter can be viewed on the companion website at eBooks.Health.Elsevier.com.

CHAPTER OUTLINE

Anatomic Considerations of the Pulpal and Periodontal Continuum

Periodontium and pulpal spaces represent the two primary modes of dental infection from oral bacteria. These two spaces are separated by a hard shell of dentin but may communicate through various portals, such as root canal foramen, dentinal tubules, and even crack lines, through which bacteria and microbial irritants may trigger inflammatory responses in surrounding tissues. At the clinical level, compound dentoalveolar infections involving both periodontium and pulpal spaces are common and present challenges for diagnosis and treatment. Conversations occur daily between periodontists, endodontists, and general practitioners to try and ascertain whether a lesion surrounding one or more teeth is of a periodontal or endodontic origin or is possibly a truly combined lesion that impacts both compartments and will require endodontic as well as subsequent periodontal treatment. The complex lesions presenting the characteristics of both endodontic and periodontic infections are referred to as endo-periodontal lesions (EPLs), and these lesions may present challenges in terms of proper diagnosis and treatment planning. In this chapter, we will discuss the proper diagnosis of these various conditions and offer treatment modalities to ensure the retention of teeth that might otherwise be extracted.

Persistent infection in the pulp tissue leads to secondary infection and breakdown of tissues in the periodontium. Conversely, severe periodontal disease may initiate or exacerbate inflammatory changes in the pulp tissue. This mutuality of infection between pulp and periodontium is mediated through anatomical routes, allowing for communication between the two spaces. The main and obvious route of communication is the apical foramen. Advanced pulpitis will lead to pulp necrosis, which often is accompanied by inflammatory bone resorption at the root apex, as found in cases of apical periodontitis or an apical abscess (Fig. 49.1). This is also known as *retrograde periodontitis* because it represents the periodontal tissue breakdown from an apical to a coronal direction and is the opposite of orthograde periodontitis, which results from a sulcular infection. This is typically identified as a periapical radiolucency (PARL) (Fig. 49.2). Retrograde periodontitis is the most common example of pulpal diseases leading to secondary periodontal breakdown. The presence of patent apical foramen may also lead to inflammatory changes in the pulp, secondary to severe periodontitis in cases where the periodontal defect reaches the apical foramen.

Alternatively, lateral or accessory canals may be the route of periodontal/pulpal communications. The prevalence of accessory root canals in various human teeth and their contribution to the complexity of the root canal system have been well established. Accessory canals are found along the length of the root canals, albeit to varying frequencies depending on their location. Using the "clearing technique" for transparent root canal visualization, prior studies showed that 59.5% of maxillary second premolars possess lateral canals; 78.2% of those are located in the apical regions of the root canals.[1] Notably, accessory canals were also found in both midroot and cervical regions, albeit with reduced frequencies at 16.2% and 4.0%, respectively. A subsequent study showed that 28.4% of permanent molars exhibit patent accessory canals in furcation regions,[2] suggesting that these accessory canals allow a pulpal and periodontal communication to exist. Root canal therapies fail frequently in maxillary molars because of unidentified second mesiobuccal canals. These canals are found in a surprisingly high percentage (80.8%) of teeth.[3] Clearly, accessory canals can lead to asymptomatic apical periodontitis resulting from chronic pulpal diseases. This can be readily detected in periapical radiographs (Fig. 49.3), and the periodontal lesions usually heal after the successful completion of endodontic therapy. Questions also arise as to whether pulpitis develops from periodontal infections through accessory root canals. Kirkham (1975) reported that only 2% of teeth possessed accessory

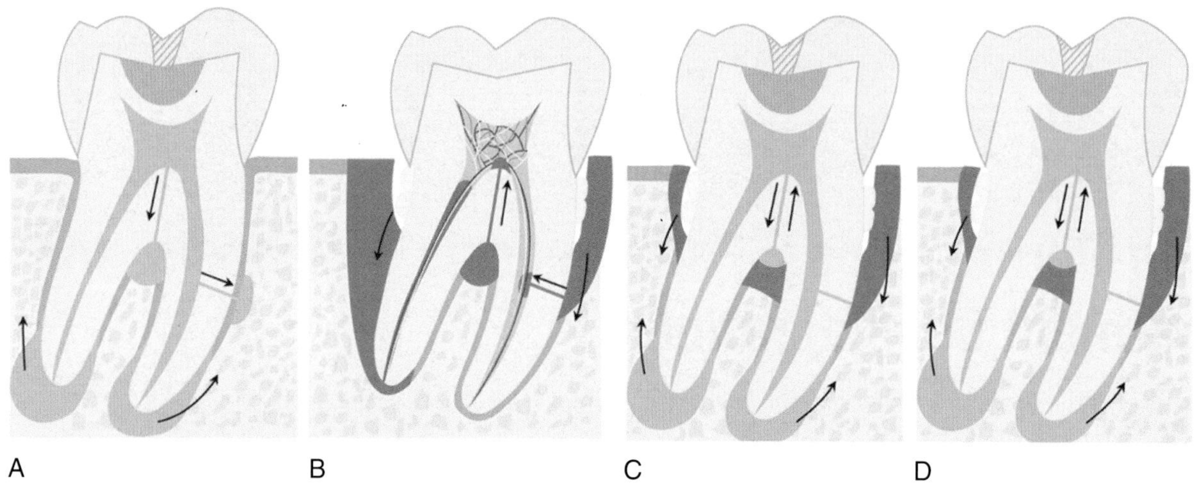

Fig. 49.1 Classification of endo-periodontal lesions (EPLs). (A) Primary pulpal infection can lead to chronic periradicular periodontitis by which a periapical radiolucency (PARL) can develop and migrate cervically. Mandibular molars can also have accessory canals in lateral orientation or in the furcation area. These accessory canals can allow migration of the primary pulpal infection and cause secondary breakdown of the periodontium at their respected loci. (B) Primary periodontal infection can lead to extensive breakdown of alveolar crest bone that migrates from the cervical area to the apex. In these lesions, one would find generalized bone loss around a single tooth or often might involve multiple adjacent teeth. Because of the pulpal-periodontal continuum through main root canal foramen or through accessory canals, extensive periodontal infection can cause irritation in the pulp tissues. (C) Both primary pulpal and primary periodontal infection can occur simultaneously in an "independent" EPL, exhibiting the characteristics of both. (D) Primary pulpal and primary periodontal infections can occur extensively in this "combined" EPL.

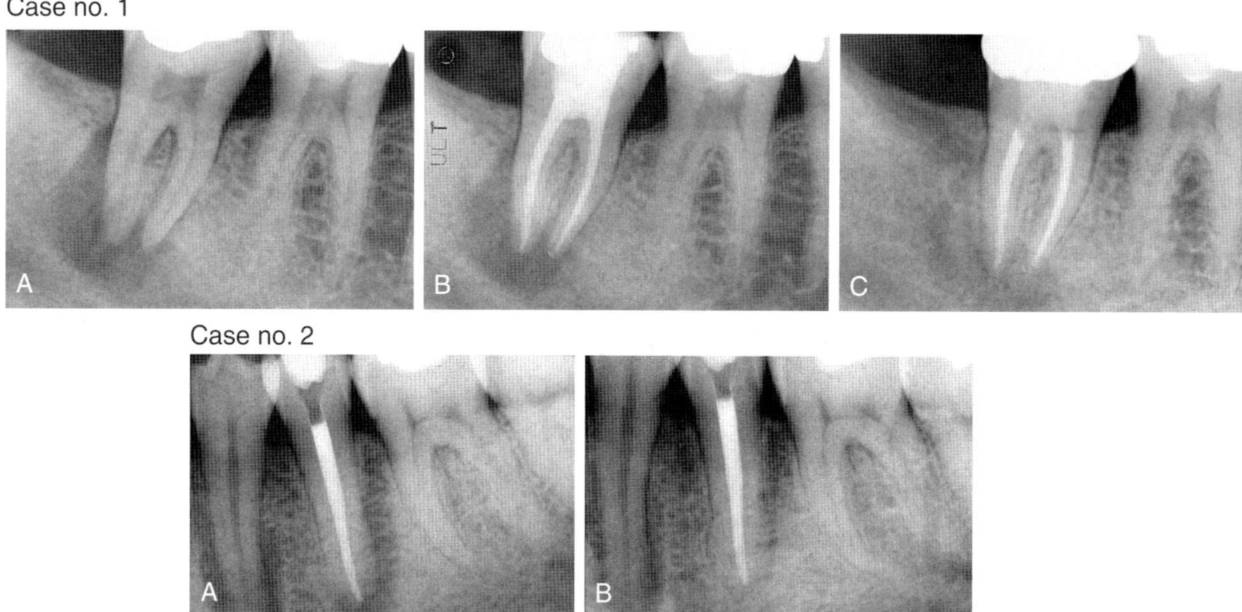

Fig. 49.2 Retrograde periodontitis. *Case 1:* (A) Large periapical lesion extending around the periapex of tooth #31. No visible fractures were detected on the mesial or distal marginal ridges. The tooth tested nonvital. A sinus tract was visible on the buccal gingiva. (B) Endodontic therapy was completed in two visits, and the canals were obturated. (C) Healing of the periradicular bone is evident at 6 months, and a crown providing complete coverage has been placed. *Case 2:* (A) Tooth number 20 presented with broad peri-raiduclar lesion extending from the apex to the distal root surface, resembling a J-shaped lesion. Conventional RCT was completed. (B) Healing of periradicular bone lesion after 6 months recall. *(Case 1, Courtesy Dr. Thomas Rauth.)*

canals within the periodontal pockets among those extracted due to severe periodontal disease.[4] Thus, the likelihood that primary periodontal infections will reach the dental pulp through accessory canals is highly remote.

The third route of communication between the periodontium and the pulp is through the dentinal tubules. Dentinal tubules maintain a tapered structure along the length from the pulpo-dentinal complex (PDC) to the dentinoenamel junction (DEJ) with a diameter of 2.5 μm at PDC and 0.9 μm at the DEJ.[5] It is therefore conceivable that dentinal permeability changes at different locations along the root surface according to the size and density of the dentinal tubules. Bacterial colonization in the tubules from infected root canals has been well documented.[6] Also, bacterial invasion into dentinal tubules from the periodontal pocket has been demonstrated,[7] suggesting that dentinal tubules may allow pulpal irritation from chronic periodontal infections. Also, periodontal

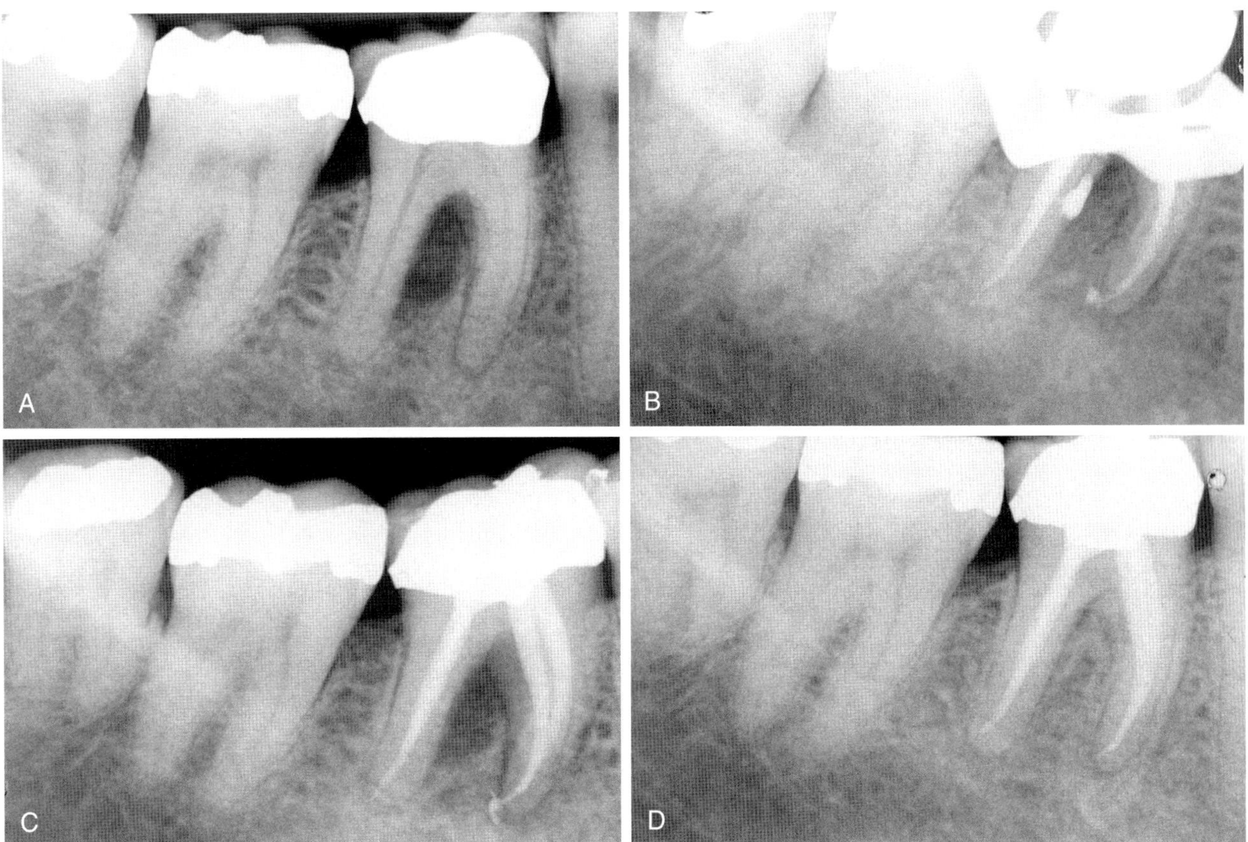

Fig. 49.3 Lateral canal-led periodontal defect from a primary endodontic infection. (A) Bone loss is present in the furcation with sinus tract present on the buccal mucosa. Tooth #30 tested nonvital. (B) During condensation, a large amount of sealer was expressed through a large lateral canal in the distal root. (C) Sealer was removed after obturation by curettage of the furcation and irrigation with anesthetic solution through the sinus tract. (D) Healing at 12 months demonstrates complete repair of periradicular bone. *(Courtesy Dr. Thomas Rauth.)*

pathogens penetrating the dentinal tubules may be the source of persistent periodontal infection.[7]

Dentin permeability through dentinal tubules is a clinically important issue. The permeability may be measured through hydraulic conductance described earlier.[8] Subsequently, investigators have studied the effects of various agents and stresses on dentin permeability. Subgingival root instrumentation in the form of root planing, as part of routine periodontal therapy, for example, is shown to decrease dentin permeability and result in the formation of a smear layer that is acid-labile.[9] However, dentin permeability may increase on the removal of the smear layer, resulting in tubular penetration of oral pathogens and subsequent pulpal irritation. Further study is necessary to delineate the role of dentinal tubules in causing secondary infection in pulpal or periodontal tissues. Clinicians need to be cognizant of the fact that patent dentinal tubules can provide effective irritant conduits between these two otherwise distinct tissues.

In addition to the above routes of anatomical communication between pulpal and periodontal tissues, there are instances in which communication is established between the pulp and periodontium by

iatrogenic defects such as vertical root fractures (VRFs) (Video 49.1) and tooth perforations. Both of these situations represent non-anatomic communication between the pulp and periodontium and result in the spread of infection from one compartment to the other. Based on the etiology of the EPLs, the lesion may behave differently in terms of symptomology, clinical presentation, and responses to the treatments. Recognizing this important distinction in EPLs, Herrera et al. proposed a new classification of EPLs into those without root damage or with root damage.[10] EPLs without root damage primarily arise from bacterial infections in pulp and/or periodontal tissues, while those with root damage may arise from vertical tooth defect, perforation defect, or resorptive defects Among these iatrogenic factors, EPLs linked with vertical tooth defect is very common, especially in mandibular second molars and maxillary first molars. It is important to recognize that the vertical tooth defects can be either coronal tooth crack or VRF, both of which are very different pathologies with vastly different treatment outcomes. This will be further discussed later in the chapter.

Factors Initiating Pulpal and Apical Diseases

Pulpal and apical diseases are initiated by numerous external factors that may include microorganisms, trauma, excessive heat, restorative procedures, restorative agents, and malocclusion. These insults lead to inflammatory changes in the pulp, starting from reversible or irreversible pulpitis and ultimately progressing to pulpal necrosis and subsequent breakdown of the periodontium. Dental caries is a prominent cause of pulpal disease, and bacterial infection is the primary form of microbial insult to the pulp. A systematic review of literature from 1966 to 2000 showed causative effects of mutans streptococci and the lactobacilli for human dental caries, whereas others like sanguinis streptococci, *Streptococcus salivarius*, or enterococci could not be associated with the disease.[11] Recent understanding of the caries process has adopted the importance of the homeostatic balance in biofilm, which describes the microbial ecosystem on tooth surfaces rather than the virulence of individual bacterial species.[12] Regardless, pulpal infection is polymicrobial and often starts from incipient caries causing localized pulpal inflammation or pulpitis.

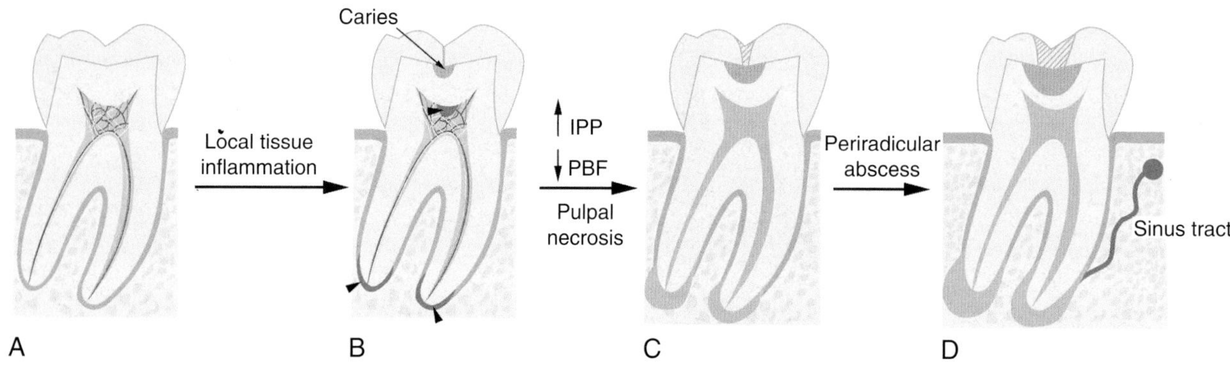

Fig. 49.4 Progression of the pulpal and periradicular pathosis. (A) Normal tooth without any pulpal pathosis is richly vascularized and innervated. (B) With microbial challenges, such as caries, local tissue inflammation can occur in the pulp adjacent to the site of carious lesions as well as in the apical regions *(arrowheads).* (C) Pulpal inflammation can lead to reduction in pulpal blood flow *(PBF)* caused by an increase in intrapulpal pressure *(IPP),* causing pulpal necrosis (shown in *gray*). (D) Pulpal necrosis, if left untreated, can lead to the chronic inflammation of periradicular tissues and abscess formation, leading to a draining sinus tract.

Local invasion of the cariogenic bacteria or a shift in the bacterial content of biofilm can lead to inflammatory changes in the dental pulp. This frequently happens in the absence of caries extension into the pulp chamber. Bacterial by-products relevant to pulpitis include lactic acid, ammonia, urea, lipopolysaccharide (LPS), and lipoteichoic acid (LTA). It is notable that the dental pulp is capable of managing numerous microbial insults because of its extensive intrapulpal lymphatic system. However, an overwhelming pulpal inflammatory response may be induced through various mechanisms and numerous microbial challenges. LPS and LTA bind to toll-like receptors (TLRs) that are present on the surface of some immune cells in the pulp and induce the release of inflammatory mediators such as prostaglandins, cytokines, and chemokines.[13] In particular, tumor necrosis factor-alpha (TNF-α), interleukin-1 (IL-1), IL-8, IL-12, and chemokines CCL2 and CXCL2 are well described for their role in pulpitis.[14] IL-1 is known to be released from macrophages after stimulation with LPS and is responsible for bone resorption leading to apical periodontitis.[15] During acute pulpitis, the inflammatory mediators trigger vasodilation, transient increase of pulpal blood flow (PBF), inflammatory cell infiltration, increased intrapulpal pressure, and finally, ischemic necrosis of the pulp (Fig. 49.4).

In an acute apical abscess, anaerobic bacteria are predominant over aerobic strains and anaerobes, and microaerophiles were predominant in 82% of the cases studied.[16] The most prevalent isolated bacteria are *Fusobacterium nucleatum, Parvimonas micra,* and *Porphyromonas endodontalis.*[17] Depending on the virulence of the organisms and host resistance, a lesion that has been chronic may exacerbate and become an acute apical abscess. The presence of spirochetes is also well documented in apical and periodontal abscesses and has been studied by various identification techniques.[18] Spirochetes most often isolated in root canal infections are *Treponema denticola* and *Treponema maltophilium.*[19,20] When comparing chronic and acute apical abscesses, Baumgartner found that there was a significantly higher incidence of spirochetes in acute abscesses or cellulitis than in asymptomatic infected root canals. *Treponema socranskii* was the most frequently encountered species.[21]

Thermomechanical irritants can induce altered pulpal circulation and pulp tissue damage. Earlier studies demonstrated that thermal changes caused by dental procedures, such as tooth preparation, led to a marked diminution of PBF and plasma extravasation, resulting in an inflammatory response.[22,23] Extreme heat caused by dry tooth preparation triggers vascular stasis and hemorrhage in the subodontoblastic vascular plexus.[24] It was noted that even a small increase in pulpal temperature (5°C to 6°C) is capable of inducing necrotic changes in the pulp.[25] Pulpal necrosis will eventually lead to apical periodontitis. Likewise, chemical irritants impose measurable changes in the pulp status. A recent study showed the cytotoxicity of dental resin material (2-hydroxyethyl methacrylate [HEMA]) on pulp stromal cells through induction of apoptotic cell death.[26] Etching the dentin surface with high phosphoric acid content resulted in deleterious effects on dental pulp.[27] Also, bonding resins used as pulp capping materials led to acute pulpitis and varying degrees of necrosis in human teeth.[28] Root canal overfills with gutta-percha and sealers invariably cause severe inflammatory reactions in the apical tissues, even though patients may be completely asymptomatic.[29] Thus, dental materials often contain chemical irritants that affect both the pulpal and periodontal tissues, and one must be cognizant of the potential iatrogenic endodontic pathosis associated with their misuse.

Classification of Pulpal and Periapical Diseases

The diagnosis of endodontic lesions that may often have a periodontal component can be confusing. The diagnostic terminology used in various dental schools and textbooks further compounds the confusion for students and practitioners alike. In an attempt to simplify and unify a standardized diagnostic terminology, the American Association of Endodontists published the glossary of endodontic diagnosis terminology in 2009.[30] These endodontic diagnostic terminologies are summarized in Tables 49.1 and 49.2.

In order to make a proper endodontic diagnosis, the clinician must evaluate the symptoms of the patient, the radiographic and clinical findings, and the presence, absence, and location of any swelling or drainage. Given all of these variables, it is easy to understand why a lack of clarity exists, and mistakes are made as to whether the lesion is primarily endodontic, periodontal, or a truly combined lesion.

The classification of diseases of the dental pulp depends on the extent of pulpal injury and its ability to repair. Many factors influence whether a tooth will be classified as normal, develop reversible pulpitis, irreversible pulpitis, or will become necrotic.

Previous studies have found little correlation between the histology of pulpal disease and the symptoms that the patient experienced before treatment.[31,32] A review of the diagnosis of pulpal pain by IB Bender (2000) found that 80% of patients who give a previous history of odontogenic pain manifested histopathologic evidence of pulpitis and partial necrosis in the dental pulp.[33] Bender also concluded that a clinician is able to determine the degree of pulp

TABLE 49.1 Classification of Pulpal Diseases[a]

Pulpal State	Symptom	Vitality	Response to Cold
Normal pulp	Asymptomatic	Vital	Within normal limits
Reversible pulpitis	Sensitive to pressure or temperature[b]	Vital	Hypersensitive to cold
Symptomatic irreversible pulpitis[c]	Spontaneous, throbbing pain	Vital	Hypersensitive to cold and lingering response
Asymptomatic irreversible pulpitis[d]	None	Vital	Within normal limits
Pulp necrosis[e]	Asymptomatic[e]	Nonvital	No response
Previously treated	Variable	Nonvital	No response
Previous initiated therapy	Variable	Variable	Variable

[a]Different pulpal conditions cannot be discerned by periapical radiographs. Symptoms and responses to cold explained herein are the general findings, but exceptions can occur.
[b]Patients' response to pressure may be due to hyperocclusion in reversible pulpitis cases. In the absence of such factors, patients' complaints mainly revolve around thermal sensitivity.
[c]Symptomatic irreversible pulpitis may be symptomatic and painful as described or may be asymptomatic and nonpainful.
[d]Asymptomatic irreversible pulpitis is based on presence of pulpal inflammation, e.g., extensive caries, hyperemia, or traumatic injuries, in the absence of patients' subjective symptoms.
[e]Necrotic pulp may cause acute exacerbation of symptoms, including spontaneous throbbing pain. However, such sensitivity results from periradicular inflammation.
This diagnostic terminology is based on the recommendations of the AAE Consensus Conference, as shown in the *Journal of Endodontics*. 2009, 35:1634.

TABLE 49.2 Classification of Periapical Diseases[a]

Periradicular State	Symptom	Pulpal Status	Percussion Response	Palpation Response	PARL	Sinus Tract
Normal periapex	None	Varies[b]	None	None	Not present	Not present
Symptomatic apical periodontitis[c]	Painful	Inflamed	Painful	Varies[d]	Not present	Not present
Asymptomatic apical periodontitis	None	Nonvital	None	None	Present	Not present
Acute apical abscess[c]	Painful	Inflamed	Painful	Painful	Varies[e]	Not present
Chronic apical abscess	None	Nonvital	None	None	Present	Present
Condensing osteitis	None/pain	Inflamed	None	None	Radiopaque	Not present

[a]Symptom and other descriptions of the individual periradicular pathosis are the general findings to which deviations can occur.
[b]Normal periapex can be associated with either normal, inflamed, or necrotic pulp.
[c]Difference between acute periradicular periodontitis and acute periradicular abscess is that the former is confined to the involved tooth and the latter is more generalized and frequently presents with gross swelling in the affected periradicular tissues.
[d]Palpation in acute periradicular periodontitis may elicit tenderness after progression of the disease through the cortical plate.
[e]PARL may be present in advanced acute periradicular abscess.
PARL, Periapical radiolucency.
This diagnostic terminology is based on the recommendations of the AAE Consensus Conference, as shown in *Journal of Endodontics*. 2009, 35:1634.

histopathosis by asking the patient about their previous pain history and symptoms related to the involved tooth.[33] There still remains controversy, however, as to the degree of correlation between pulpal symptoms and the histopathology of the pulpal tissues and additional studies are needed to confirm the correlation between the two.

Apical pathoses of endodontic origin are inflammatory processes occurring in periradicular tissues surrounding root apices. They result from various microbial agents that originate from the root canal infection and create a series of inflammatory and immunologic responses. These agents exit through the apical foramen, lateral canals, or dentinal tubules.[4,34] It is an infectious process caused by a large number of microbial species, unlike classic infectious diseases occurring elsewhere in the body that may consist of only one or two specific organisms. These species reside in ecologically balanced communities discussed previously and constitute the *biofilm.*[35] The different characteristics of pulpal and periodontal lesions are summarized in Table 49.3.

Biologic Effects of Endodontic Infection on Periodontal Tissues

The effects of the pulpal disease on the surrounding periodontal tissues are widely accepted by clinicians and researchers and have been studied for more than 50 years. Early inflammatory changes in the pulp exert very little effect on the periodontium. Even a pulp that is significantly inflamed may have little or no effect on the surrounding periodontal tissues. It is believed that this initial pulpal inflammatory response is an attempt to prevent the spread of infection to the apical tissues.

When the pulp becomes necrotic, however, it produces a significant inflammatory response involving extremely complex inflammatory and immune reactions. This response can traverse the apical foramen, the furcation, lateral canals, dentinal tubules, or areas of trapped necrotic tissue along the surface of the root that extends

TABLE 49.3 Different Characteristics of the Lesions of Endodontic and Periodontic Infection[a]

	Primary Pulpal	Primary Periodontal	Independent Endo-Perio	Combined Endo-Perio
Patient symptom	Varies[b]	Mild discomfort	Varies[b]	Varies[b]
Coronal integrity	Compromised	Intact	Compromised	Compromised
Radiographic lesions	PARL	Crestal bone loss	Separate PARL and crestal lesions	Continuous bony lesions from alveolar crest to apex
Vitality	Nonvital	Vital	Nonvital	Nonvital
Periodontal probing	Narrow probing to apex[c]	Generalized bone loss	Generalized bone loss	Generalized bone loss with narrow probing to apex

[a]These are generalized summaries, and deviations can occur.
[b]Patient symptom for pulpal lesions may vary, depending on the type of pathosis. Chronic lesions can be completely asymptomatic, whereas acute symptoms without any radiographic lesions can trigger pain.
[c]Primary pulpal lesions may not present with any periodontal defect. Narrow probing in pulpal lesions may indicate sinus tract through sulcus.
PARL, Periapical radiolucency.

past the periodontal ligament (PDL) and into the surrounding apical tissues.[36] This initial inflammatory response of the pulp and subsequent necrosis that permeates through the numerous spaces of the canal system includes various bacterial strains, spirochetes, fungi, yeasts, and viruses.[37] The nature and extent of the periodontal destruction that follows depend on the virulence of the pathogens in the root canal system, the chronicity of the disease, and the defense mechanisms of the host.[38]

In a classic study by Kakehashi et al., the infected pulps of germ-free rats remained vital, whereas the infected pulps of normal rats that were left open to the oral environment developed pulpal necrosis with subsequent inflammation and formation of periapical lesions.[39] This was the first experimental evidence to demonstrate microbial infection as the etiology of pulpal and periapical pathoses. Likewise, bacterial infection plays a pivotal role in endo-perio lesions, in the form of bacterial biofilm, which is composed of a 15% cellular component and a matrix material that comprises the remaining 85%. The formation of biofilm communities is under the control of complex chemical signals that both regulate and guide the formation of the slime-enclosed colonies and water channels.[40] Proteolytic bacteria predominate in early root canal infections and then change over time to a flora that contains a greater number of anaerobes.[41,42]

Several nonliving irritants have also been implicated in the inflammatory process as well. These include foreign bodies, epithelial rests, cholesterol crystals, Russell bodies, Rushton hyaline bodies, and Charcot-Leyden crystals. These irritants have not only been implicated in the inflammatory process, but may also be responsible for the lack of healing of apical lesions in teeth that have received appropriate endodontic treatment.[43] If the growth of the epithelial cells is stimulated by any of these living or nonliving pathogens, then the integrity of the periodontal tissues may be affected as well.

As the degree of pulpal inflammation becomes more extensive, a greater amount of destruction of the periodontal tissues ensues. Extension of the infection through the PDL space, tooth socket and surrounding bone occurs, and the patient begins to experience a localized or diffuse swelling that may result in cellulitis that invades the various facial spaces. Most often, however, the infection erupts through the labial, buccal, or lingual mucosa and results in a draining sinus tract. In cases where the path of least resistance to the infectious process is along the attached gingiva, the infection may dissect the PDL space and result in the formation of a deep but narrow periodontal pocket. This pocket usually extends to the main site of the infection, for example, root apex, when probed or traced with a gutta-percha point. Confusion often results among both general dentists and specialists as to whether the probing defect is the result of an endodontic or periodontal infection, or from VRF. Generally, a narrow probing defect combined with a nonvital pulpal response indicates that the problem is usually of endodontic origin rather than of periodontal lesion. Also, a probing defect associated with VRF generally extends to the level of the crack as opposed to the root apex. VRF is generally detected during access into the pulp chamber under high-power magnification or by using transillumination. If VRF is not detected, it should be ruled out as the potential cause of the narrow probing defect.

In a few situations, adjacent teeth, their root surfaces, or furcation areas may also probe deeply. Care must be taken to thoroughly test all maxillary and mandibular teeth to correctly assess whether the problem is endodontic or periodontal. Once the correct diagnosis is made, only then should the treatment plan be formulated and discussed with the patient. When endodontic infection is the main cause of the swelling or breakdown of the periodontium, successful endodontic treatment usually results in the healing of both the periapical and periodontal tissues. There are times, however, when trauma to the tooth, severe loss of adjacent periodontal tissues, continued tooth mobility, and occlusal trauma do not provide an environment that allows for apical healing to occur. In these cases, splinting is sometimes necessary to help stabilize the tooth and allow for potential repair of the apical tissues (Fig. 49.5).

If an endodontic infection is left untreated, the progression of periodontal disease continues. Untreated and unresolved infections of endodontic origin can sustain the growth of various endodontic pathogens that may lead to an increased pocket formation, bone loss, calculus deposition, osteoclastic activity, and subsequent bone and tooth resorption. They may additionally impair wound healing and aggravate the development and progression of the periodontal disease state.[44]

The ability of the periodontium to regenerate and heal the lost attachment apparatus in the context of endodontically treated tooth and the cement layer is no longer present.[45] A study by Sanders et al. demonstrated a 60% osseous regeneration rate in teeth that had not undergone endodontic treatment compared with a regeneration rate of only 33% in teeth that had endodontic treatment completed.[46] One study compared the loss of attached gingiva and found that there was a 0.2 mm greater loss of attached tissue in the presence of teeth with a root canal infection and a PARL.[47] These same investigators in a later study found a three times greater loss of marginal proximal bone utilizing radiographic measurements in teeth with endodontic infections compared to those without endodontic infections or subsiding endodontic involvement.[48] Other investigators, however,

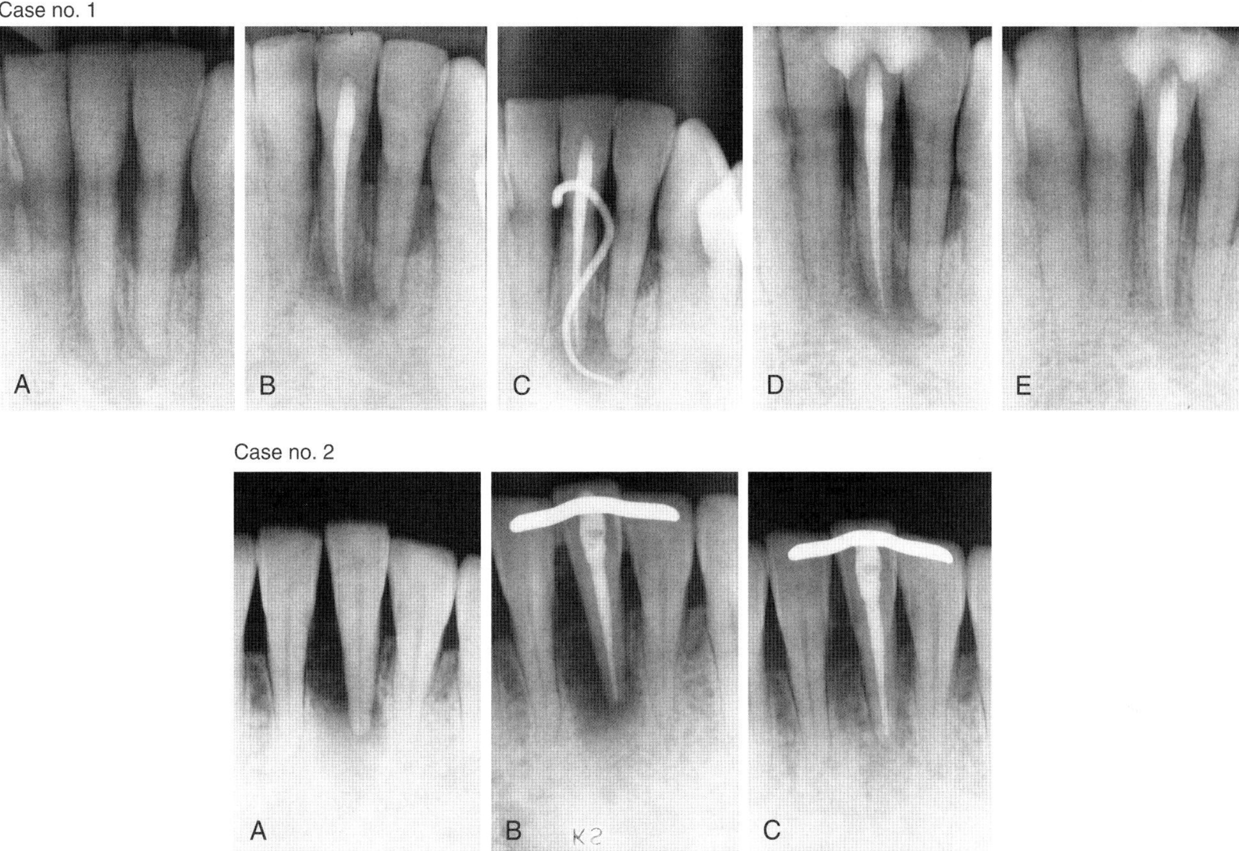

Fig. 49.5 *Case 1.* (A) Previous trauma of tooth #25 with complaints of pain to biting and chewing. The tooth tested nonvital and tooth #26 probed 6 mm on the lingual. (B) Postoperative radiograph after obturation of the canal. Treatment was completed in two appointments with the interappointment placement of calcium hydroxide. (C) Four months later the tooth was mobile, and there was a sinus tract present. (D) The occlusion was adjusted, and composite resin was bonded to the mesial and distal surfaces to stabilize both tooth #25 and #26. (E) Healing of the periradicular lesion is apparent after 13 months and tooth #26 probed only 4 mm. *Case 2.* (A) Previously traumatized tooth #25. The tooth was Class III mobile and tested nonvital to both CO_2 and electric pulp testing. (B) After obturation of the tooth with gutta percha, a cast gold splint was bonded to the lingual surface to stabilize the tooth. (C) 13-month recall demonstrates repair of the periradicular bone and no mobility as a result of the placement of stabilization and splint. *(Case 1, Courtesy Dr. Thomas Rauth.)*

have reported that all periodontal tissues have the ability to regenerate, regardless of whether the tooth is vital, partially treated and medicated, partially filled, or whether an endodontic treatment has been successfully completed.[49] Additional studies need to be completed to better understand the relationship between the presence of endodontic infection and the increased loss of marginal bone and attached tissue in patients prone to periodontal disease.

It is evident that endodontium and periodontium are closely related in structural, functional, and pathogenic perspectives and that microorganisms and nonliving irritants play an important role in the disease progression of both structures. Proper diagnosis of EPLs, therefore, is critically important and will dictate the appropriate course of treatment.

Biologic Effects of Periodontal Infection on the Dental Pulp

Effects of periodontal disease on the dental pulp appear to be more controversial compared to the effects of pulpal disease on the periodontium.[50,51] Not all studies agree about the effect of periodontal disease on the pulp. Even though inflammation and localized pulpal necrosis have been observed next to lateral canals exposed to periodontal diseases,[36,51,52] other studies have not confirmed a correlation between periodontal disease and changes within the pulp.[53–55] Langeland et al. indicated that when pathologic changes do occur in the pulp as a result of advanced periodontal disease, the pulp does not usually undergo degenerative changes as long as the main canal has not been involved.[31] If the vasculature of the pulp remains vital, no inflammatory reaction occurs, and there are no symptoms of pulpal pathosis. An animal study conducted by Bergenholtz found that 70% of animal specimens showed no pathologic changes even when 30% to 40% of the periodontal attachment was lost.[56] The remainder showed only minor inflammatory changes, formation of reparative dentin, or resorptive defects where the root had been exposed.

Researchers and clinicians, however, have observed the spread of advanced periodontal lesions that extend to the apical foramen and result in pulpal necrosis. This retrograde infection may proliferate through large accessory canals on the lateral surfaces of the tooth, canals positioned closer to the apical foramen, and the area where the main canal exits the tooth apex.[52] Kobayashi et al.[57] compared the microflora from root canals and periodontal pockets of caries-free teeth that were necrotic and tested nonvital with an electric pulp tester. The aerobic/anaerobic ratio in the periodontal pocket was 0.23 compared to 0.0022 in the root canal. Although there were far fewer bacteria in the root canal, both areas demonstrated similar bacterial strains. The authors concluded that the similarity of strains in both areas suggested that the periodontal pocket may be the source of bacteria found in infections within the root canal system.[58]

Protection and preservation of the cementum and dentin surrounding the tooth also play important roles in preserving the health of the pulp and preventing the ingress of periodontal pathogens. The presence of an intact layer of cementum is important in protecting the pulp from dental plaque and other periodontal pathogens that migrate along the root surface during the development of advanced periodontal disease. Excessive root planing and curettage (that are not recommended anymore) remove the cementum and dentin from the root surface and encourage narrowing of the pulp canals. This process is thought to be reparative rather than inflammatory.[50,59] Several studies also suggest that periodontal disease is degenerative to pulpal tissues resulting in continued calcification, fibrosis, collagen resorption, and inflammation.[31,60.]

Dentin thickness also contributes to the protection of the pulp. Stanley stated that if a 2-mm thickness of dentin remains between the pulp and irritating stimulus, there is little chance of pulpal damage.[61] Weine summarized the precautions that can be taken during the course of periodontal therapy: (1) avoid using irritating chemicals on the root surface, (2) minimize the use of ultrasonic scalers when there is less than 2 mm of remaining dentin, and (3) allow minor pulpal irritations to subside before completing additional procedures.[62] When these precautions are not followed, and the microvasculature of the pulp is damaged during periodontal procedures that involve deep curettage or periodontal surgical efforts to save the tooth, necrosis may result.[63]

The healing success and failure rates after endodontic microsurgery were studied in teeth that had lesions of only endodontic origin compared to those teeth that had lesions of a combined endodontic-periodontal origin. Lesions only of endodontic origin had a successful outcome of 95.2%, whereas those teeth with combined lesions had a successful outcome of only 77.5%. This suggests that bone and tissue healing are negatively affected after endodontic surgery with lesions of combined origin.[64]

It appears, therefore, that both the pulp and periodontal compartments influence each other. Periodontal disease, however, seems to have less of an influence on the pulpal tissues compared to the influence of pulpal disease on the periodontium. Clearly, advanced periodontal disease has some biological effect on the pulpal state (Fig. 49.6). Unless the microvasculature of the pulp is compromised during aggressive periodontal procedures or excessively deep curettage severs the apical vessels, most periodontal interventions result in only a localized pulpal response and dentin hypersensitivity.[65]

Endo-Perio Lesions With Vertical Tooth Defects

Vertical tooth defects are very common. A previous study showed that approximately 10% of all patients seen with pulpitis symptoms demonstrate a tooth crack.[66] When the vertical tooth defect involves the radicular dentin and invades the periodontal space, it can be the conduit between the pulp and periodontal tissues and lead to EPL. Vertical tooth defects can be either coronal tooth crack or VRF. There are several clear differences between coronal tooth crack and VRF. First, the location is different. A coronal tooth crack initiates within the coronal dentin and migrates apically, while VRF affects primarily radicular dentin. Secondly, the orientation of the defect is different. The tooth crack extends mesiodistally. It is most frequently found at the distal marginal ridge of mandibular second molars, followed by the mesial marginal ridge of maxillar first molars.[67] These coronal cracks would then migrate mesiodistally and apically. On the contrary, VRF is almost always found at the buccolingual root surfaces, often initiated from the radicular dentin.[68] Finally, the prognosis is different. An earlier study reported 2-year survival of endodontically treated teeth with a coronal crack at 85%.[69] One of the most important factors that influence the prognosis of a cracked tooth after endodontic therapy is the probing defect at the location of the crack.[67] The 2-year survival of teeth with more than 6 mm probing defect was 74.1%, while those with less than 6 mm probing defect were 94.8%.[67] On the other hand, teeth with VRF exhibit a very poor prognosis and account for a significant portion of endodontically treated teeth that are extracted.[70] Therefore, it is critically important for clinicians to recognize EPLs with vertical tooth defects and identify whether it is coronal tooth crack or VRF.

The differences in the clinical characteristics of EPLs linked to coronal tooth crack and VRF are illustrated in the two cases shown in Fig. 49.7. Case 1, representing symptomatic teeth, #18 and #19 presented with a buccal fistula on #18 and was diagnosed with pulpal necrosis, chronic apical periodontitis (#18), and symptomatic apical periodontitis (#19). Both #18 and #19 exhibited no other coronal defects than a crack at the distal marginal ridges but showed large periradicular bone loss (see in the pre-op

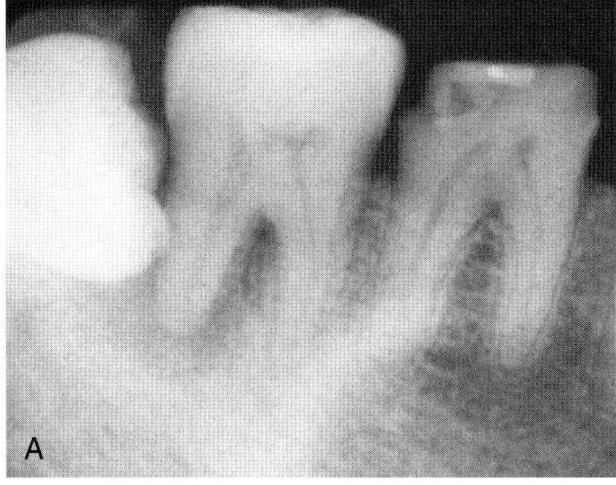

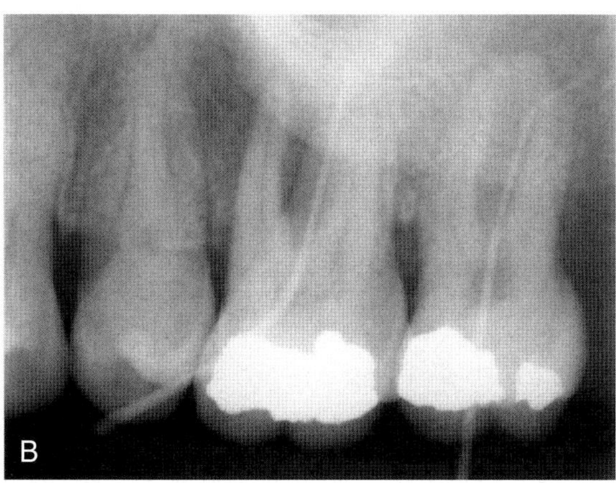

Fig. 49.6 Primary periodontal defects causing periradicular bony lesions and pulpal irritation. (A) Primary periodontal lesion is evident on the distal of tooth #31. The defect was probed to a depth of 7 mm, and the tooth tested vital to both thermal and electrical pulp testing. The defect was most likely the result of the impacted third molar and formation of a chronic periodontal abscess. (B) Primary periodontal lesions both probing 12 mm into the furcation. Teeth #14 and #15 tested vital to thermal and electrical testing. The patient's chief complaint was discomfort to cold, thus exemplifying pulpitis secondary to the primary periodontal infection. *(B, Courtesy Dr. Gregory Kolber.)*

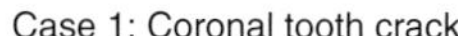

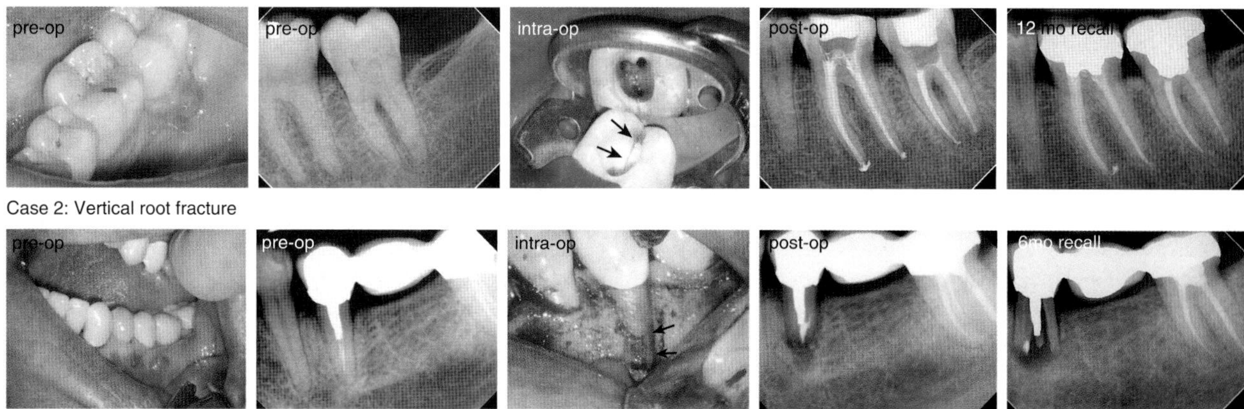

Fig. 49.7 *Case 1.* EPL with coronal tooth crack. #18 and #19 were diagnosed with pulpal necrosis and chronic apical abscess (#18) and symptomatic apical periodontitis (#19). Conventional RCT was performed on both #18 and #19. Intraoperatively, a coronal tooth crack was detected at the distal marginal ridge. RCT was completed successfully on #18 and #19. Patient came back for 12-month recall with final restoration, resolution of the symptoms, and radiographic healing of periradicular osseous lesions. *Case 2.* EPL with VRF. Patient came in with symptomatic tooth #20 and buccal fistula and no detectable radiographic lesion. Apical surgery was performed with full thickness mucogingival flap, which exposed bony dehiscence over the buccal root surface of #20 and buccolingual fracture line that starts from the midroot and migrated apically. Upon 6-month recall, patient presented with completely failed tooth with root fragments split open.

radiograph). These teeth were endodontically treated successfully, and upon 12-month recall, showed complete healing of the osseous lesions and resolution of the patient's symptoms. On the contrary, case 2 presented with symptomatic tooth #20 and buccal fistula, which served as an anterior abutment for a 3-unit bridge with the cast post. Radiographically, no apical bone loss was detected. However, during explorative apical surgery, bony dehiscence was detected directly over the buccal surface of the apical root segment of tooth #20. Interestingly, VRF was detected on the buccal root surface from the midroot to the root apex. Although apicectomy was completed, when the patient came back for a 6-month recall, the tooth completely failed with the root split open. These two seemingly similar EPLs with vertical tooth defects demonstrate completely different ways in which coronal tooth crack or VRF behave in terms of location of the defect, orientation of the defect, and the outcome of the treatment.

Effect of Endodontic Pathosis on Development of Retrograde Peri-implantitis

The management and resolution of adjacent endodontic and periapical infection is an important consideration when treatment planning the placement of a dental implant. The persistence of endodontic bacteria and inflammatory cells commonly facilitates the development of retrograde peri-implantitis, or the development of a radiographically evident periapical lesion at the apex of an osseointegrated implant accompanied by swelling, pain, tenderness, and sinus tract formation.[71,72] Although retrograde peri-implantitis can occur as a result of overloading or premature loading on the implant or contamination of the external surface of the implant upon placement, the presence of pre-existing periapical inflammation, endodontic bacteria, or inflammatory cells at, near, or adjacent to the site of implant placement has also been shown to play an important role in its development.[73,74] Understanding the role that persistent periapical infection plays in the development of retrograde peri-implantitis and the treatment options that exist in cases of refractory periapical periodontitis is critical to long-term periodontal and implant success.

There exist two scenarios by which the interaction between the implant and adjacent tooth may lead to retrograde peri-implantitis. Under circumstances where complications arise during implant placement, such as overheating of bone during the preparation of the implant space, placement of the implant too close to the adjacent tooth, or the altering of the blood supply of the adjacent tooth during implant surgery, the implant placement itself may result in devitalization of the adjacent tooth and subsequent development of peri-implantitis.[75] More common, however, is the presence of existing or recurrent periapical pathology from an endodontically treated tooth resulting in contamination of the adjacently placed implant, which may also lead to peri-implantitis development.[75,76]

Root canal therapy is critical for the resolution of intraradicular and periapical infection. Although there may be radiographic evidence of periapical lesion healing upon endodontic treatment, periapical inflammation may continue to persist and only be detectable histologically.[77–79] Brisman et al.[80] demonstrated several cases in which implants placed adjacent to asymptomatic, endodontically treated teeth exhibiting no clinical or radiographic signs of periapical pathology resulted in peri-implantitis development, which resolved with surgical intervention.[80] The presence of persistent or refractory periapical inflammation adjacent to the implant may increase the risk of developing retrograde peri-implantitis.

Certain treatment considerations should be made when planning implant placement adjacent to an endodontically involved tooth. First and foremost, conventional root canal therapy (RCT) should be performed to resolve underlying symptomatic or radiographic endodontic and periapical pathology, and endodontic retreatment should be performed to address the failure of endodontic therapy.[81,82] Delaying the placement of an implant after completion of endodontic treatment on an adjacent tooth or increasing the distance between the implant and the adjacent endodontically treated tooth may reduce the likelihood of peri-implantitis development.[76] The use of non-machined surfaced implants may also decrease the chances of implant failure, as machined surfaced implants placed adjacent to or at the site of previous endodontic infection are more likely to result in the development of retrograde peri-implantitis.[73]

Under circumstances where endodontic infection results in the development of peri-implantitis, surgical debridement, disinfection of the implant surface, and resolution of the endodontic pathosis are critical to the continued success of the implant.[83] Implant stability is also an important consideration when planning for the treatment of retrograde peri-implantitis. Affected implants exhibiting poor stability require removal of the implant, debridement of granulation tissue within the implant socket, and either placement of the bone graft and subsequent implant placement, or immediate placement of a longer or wide implant after the debridement.[83,84,85] Stable implants exhibiting radiographic evidence of periapical pathosis may be surgically debrided and the implant surface disinfected using chlorhexidine or tetracycline while ensuring that the implant surface is not damaged and that systemic antibiotics are administered upon successful debridement.[71,86] Brisman et al.[80] demonstrated a case in which an implant placed at the site of the mandibular incisor succumbed to retrograde peri-implantitis and fistula that, upon removal of the implant, was found to lead to the adjacent mandibular canine, which had been endodontically treated several years prior. Subsequent apicoectomy of the adjacent tooth and placement of a new implant prevented further implant apical inflammation and failure.[80] Thus, management of both endodontic and implant periapical pathology is critical to the resolution of retrograde peri-implantitis and the long-term prognosis of the implant.

Interactions Between Extraradicular Infection and the Periodontium

Although the failure of endodontic therapy and persistence of periapical pathology is typically the result of persistent or secondary infection arising from incomplete obturation or the presence of abnormal root canal anatomy, there are instances when extraradicular infection is to blame. This bacterial infection occurs periapically along the external surface of the root apex and can lead to or exacerbate acute periapical abscess development.[87–89] Extraradicular infection can occur either as a result of, or independent of, intraradicular infection,[90] and unhealed periapical lesions resulting from extraradicular lesions have been found to harbor bacteria belonging to *Actinomyces*, *Propionibacterium*, *Treponema*, *Porphyromonas*, *Prevotella,* and *Fusobacterium* bacterial species.[87,91]

Among the causes of extraradicular infection, the formation of acute apical abscesses resulting secondary to intraradicular infection is the most common and can be resolved nonsurgically by endodontic therapy. Unlike periapical abscess formation, extraradicular infection can less commonly occur as a result of periapical actinomycosis, or the asymptomatic development of a granulomatous infection facilitated by gram-positive bacteria that belong to *Actinomyces* and *Propionibacterium* species.[90,91] Among these, *Actinomyces israelii* and *Propionibacterium propionicus* have been predominately found in actinomycosis lesions.[90,92,93] Whereas periapical abscesses are resolved by conventional RCT, periapical actinomycosis does not respond to endodontic therapy and requires apical surgery.[90] Periapical actinomycosis may develop when infected intraradicular tissue or debris are moved past the apex during instrumentation, intraradicular bacteria are moved into the periapical lesion, or when an apical abscess persists, resulting in extraradicular infection that requires surgical intervention.[90,93]

Though intraradicular infection is the predominant source of extraradicular infection, there exist far less common external factors that propagate extraradicular pathosis. One such source is the accumulation of calculus on the external surface of the root apex, which is associated with failed periapical lesion healing, persistent sinus tract formation, and refractory apical periodontitis. Several case reports have identified the presence of calculus along the root apex upon removal by apicoectomy and have found the presence of persistent sinus tract and periapical pathology to resolve upon their removal.[94–96] The formation of calculus around the root apex is thought to be the result of accumulation and calcification of plaque from the external oral environment and periodontium by means of the open, persistent sinus tract present in these cases.[95]

In addition to calculus, bacterial biofilms held together by extracellular polysaccharides have also been found along the external surface of the root tip.[97] *Actinomyces naeslundii*, *Actinomyces meyeri*, *P. propionicum*, *Clostridium botulinum*, *P. micra*, *Bacteroides ureolyticus*, *Tannerella forsythensis*, *F. nucleatum*, *and Porphyromonas gingivalis* have been identified within bacterial biofilms found around the root apex that led to extraradicular infection and refractory apical periodontitis.[88,98] Although the origin of these biofilms is unclear, it is possible that they may originate from leaking exudate from the junctional epithelium due to periodontal inflammation.[97] Extraradicular bacteria have proven difficult to eliminate by means of systemic antibiotic administration, and in cases where bacterial biofilms are found, this may be due to the presence of bacteria within the extracellular polysaccharide, which facilitates their survival and proliferation.[97,99,100] Although extraradicular infection is not common,[101] its implications in endodontic failure and management of refractory periapical periodontitis are evident. Whereas conventional RCT successfully treats intraradicular infection, the presence of microorganisms beyond the apical foramen often makes extraradicular periapical infections difficult to resolve without surgical intervention.[90,95]

Differential Diagnosis of Endodontic and Periodontic Infection

Acute infection of both the periodontium and the pulp must be differentiated from one another for clinicians to be able to establish a correct diagnosis with reasonable certainty and initiate appropriate therapy. A thorough understanding of both disease processes and the correct interpretation of clinical and radiographic findings will aid the dentist in establishing a diagnosis that results in the rapid relief of acute and painful conditions.

When the pulpal and periodontal abscesses are separate from one another, most clinicians feel that the diagnosis is usually easier. There are instances, however, when each primary disease may have similar clinical characteristics and make the diagnosis more difficult. In other situations, there may be no demarcation between the two areas of pathosis that both clinically and radiographically appear as one large and continuous lesion with extreme pain and swelling. When this occurs, the clinician must avoid classifying these continuous lesions as truly combined lesions. One must rely on all available clinical testing methods to help clarify the correct clinical diagnosis prior to beginning treatment.[45]

Making the accurate differentiation between pulpal and periodontal lesions can be challenging. If the lesion originates from a pulpal infection and yet was treated by extensive periodontal therapy, it will not resolve. Conversely, performing endodontic therapy on a tooth that has an extensive periodontal defect and a vital pulp will result in the persistence of the periodontal infection. Thus, identifying the primary cause of infection is a critical determinant of treatment outcome. Perhaps the most important consideration when making such a distinction is to base the diagnosis on multiple findings. These include patients' symptoms, coronal integrity, shape and size of the radiographic lesions, periodontal probing, and tooth vitality. It is possible that one or more of these findings suggest a pulpal or periodontal infection, whereas others point to the contrary. For instance, a tooth may exhibit extensive failing restorations, recurring decay, and radiographic lesions, suggesting probable pulpal involvement. However, the tooth may test completely vital and lack any evidence of irreversible pulpitis upon thermal testing. Under these circumstances, one would rule out the primary pulpal infection and examine the patient for periodontal involvement. Thus, making the distinction between pulpal or periodontal infection requires collectively dissecting the multiple findings and synthesizing the most probable diagnosis (see Table 49.3).

Patients' Subjective Symptoms

Patients suffering from the acute phase of pulpal infection present with the symptoms that are generally absent in chronic periodontal infection. During the initial stage of pulpitis, patients may complain about sensitivity and pain exacerbated by certain stimuli, including temperature changes, pressure, and/or biting. If the symptoms result from reversible pulpitis, they will usually resolve spontaneously with time as the result of various mechanisms such as the closure of dentinal tubules, clearance of microbial irritants and toxins, and reparative dentin formation. Persistent inflammation leads to symptomatic irreversible pulpitis, which is often associated with sharp and spontaneous pain, although asymptomatic irreversible pulpitis may also occur as described previously. Acute pain to thermal stimuli may subside after several days as the pulp becomes necrotic, and the bacteria and their by-products migrate down the complex canal system. As the infection extends to and then past the apical foramen or a lateral root canal, the tooth becomes particularly sensitive to bite pressure and percussion. After several days, the necrotic tooth may develop either an acute apical abscess which results in the elevation of the tooth from the dentoalveolar complex. Patients frequently report that the tooth feels "high" on occlusion. However, patients with irreversible pulpitis or a necrotic pulp may be asymptomatic. Thus, making the diagnosis of primary pulpal infection must be based on multiple objective findings, such as the patients' responses to percussion, palpation, biting, periodontal probing, and vitality testing, as well as a thorough evaluation of the patients' subjective symptoms.

In apical and periodontal abscesses, the extent of pain may vary. Generally, an acute apical abscess causes extreme pain to pressure, bite, percussion, and, at times, palpation if the infection has penetrated the cortical bone. Periodontal abscesses are thought to cause less pain because there is little or no elevation of the periosteum. Edema and swelling are characteristics that may be shared by both conditions. The swelling and edema with a periodontal abscess are generally confined to the cervical portion of the tooth. An apical abscess is usually more sensitive to palpation around the tooth apex if the infection has penetrated through the bony cortical plate. Redness and a smooth appearance of the marginal gingival tissues are more common with abscesses of periodontal origin, whereas redness can be detected more apically if a pulpal abscess has started to swell and elevate surrounding tissues. Objective findings in periodontal abscesses include bleeding on probing, suppuration, increased pocket depth, increased tooth mobility, and occasionally, lymphadenopathy.[102] Abscesses of endodontic origin usually probe normally but may also display increased mobility, depending on the amount of bone loss. Patients may describe the tooth as feeling longer or higher than the adjacent teeth.[103]

Suppuration and drainage from periradicular and periodontal abscesses may also differ. Periodontal abscesses are associated with severe periodontal destruction. In a study investigating the incidence of anaerobes in periodontal abscesses, approximately 66% were determined to have a suppurative exudate that was evident during probing. In the same study, 100% of the patients had bleeding during probing, more than 75% had severe edema, redness, and swelling, and 78% of the patients had some degree of mobility. Only a few of the patients suffered from lymphadenopathy. Over 60% of the patients had not received previous periodontal therapy, and nearly 70% of the teeth were molars. The average measured pocket depth was 7.28 mm.[102] In another study that cultured facultative anaerobic bacteria, the teeth most affected were maxillary and mandibular anteriors and mandibular molars. One of the typical features of this study, as in the previous one, was the fact that most of the teeth had been previously untreated.[104] Other aspects of periodontal therapy that correlate highly with the development of acute periodontal abscess formation are (1) patients undergoing current periodontal treatment,[105] (2) incomplete removal of calculus,[106] (3) a history of a previous abscess at the same site,[107] and (4) the previous use of antibiotics for dental or non-dental reasons.[108]

Drainage from apical abscesses usually comes from one of two sites. The most prevalent area of drainage is a sinus tract that develops when the area of swelling breaks through the mucoperiosteum and exits the mucosal tissue either near or at some distance from the site of the infection. Additionally, the path of least resistance may be along the PDL, and the infection may dissect the ligament along the surface of the root and exit the tooth at the height of the epithelial attachment. This results in a periodontal defect that probes along a narrow path to the apex of the root, as previously discussed. Both the sinus tract and narrow sulcular lesions can usually be traced to the infected tooth or offending root using a gutta-percha point.

Coronal Integrity

Periodontal infection without pulpal involvement may present with intact crown structure and absence of coronal defects. On the other hand, endodontic infection is almost always associated with loss of coronal integrity, such as caries, failing restorations, extensive restorations, and the existence of cracks or fractures that extend to the pulpal tissues. However, this does not mean that all periodontal infections are devoid of coronal defects nor that all endodontic lesions exhibit loss of coronal integrity. When pulp tissue is severed by trauma, for example, one might expect to find a necrotic pulp in the absence of coronal defects. If left untreated, such lesions originating from primary pulpal infection lead to the breakdown of the periodontium as in asymptomatic apical periodontitis or apical abscess. Of course, primary periodontal lesions can develop in teeth with coronal defects. Furthermore, combined EPLs would present with periodontal infection and extensive coronal destruction. However, careful examination of the coronal status either during the intraoral or radiographic examination can provide supportive information in deciding whether the lesion originates from an endodontic or periodontal infection.

Radiographic Appearance

Periapical radiographs can provide distinguishing information on whether the lesion is of pulpal or periodontal origin. Although radiographic findings are objective data, *interpretation* of radiographs can be highly subjective, depending on who is reading the radiograph. Thus, it is important to *understand* and focus on specific entities on a radiograph. These should include the coronal status, crestal bone height and shape, presence of an apical or lateral radiolucency, bony trabeculation, the integrity of the lamina dura, and careful evaluation of the obturation of the root canal if present. Coronal status, as revealed on a radiograph, can also help in the differential diagnosis, as described previously. Also, apical lesions originating from a primary pulpal infection lead to retrograde periodontitis that migrates from the root apex in a cervical direction. On the contrary, periodontal infections will lead to the loss of crestal bone from the cervical area of the tooth in an apical direction. Thus, radiographic lesions appear different in endodontically treated teeth compared to periodontal lesions, and the shape of the bony lesions can help distinguish between the two. For example, radiographic lesions representing severe periodontitis will appear wider at the cervical end than the apical portion of the lesion. Apical or lateral radiolucencies may also result from differences in trabeculation patterns not associated with pulpal infection. For this reason, it is critical to consider the integrity of the lamina dura. A break in the lamina dura, accompanied by an apical or lateral radiolucency, is usually indicative of a chronic or acute pulpal infection. If the tooth had been endodontically treated, assessment of the previous obturation qualities (i.e., voids, short fills or overfills, missed canals, etc.) is also important. These radiographic features will provide very useful and often distinguishing information in making the differential diagnosis between pulpal and periodontal lesions more accurate.

Vitality

Testing of tooth vitality often becomes one of the most important tests that can differentiate between periodontal and endodontic infections. Teeth with periodontal infection usually test vital to thermal testing unless the acute condition is a combined lesion in which both endodontic and periodontal compartments have become diseased. Teeth with both endodontic infection and periodontal abscess usually test nonvital. Exceptions to this are extremely calcified canals, extensively restored teeth, or multirooted teeth where canals may be partly necrotic as a result of either pulpal or periodontal disease. Other canals may still retain vital tissue that responds to thermal or electric pulp testing. Thermal testing is usually the most reliable way of determining pulpal health or disease. Patients with symptomatic irreversible pulpitis often report a lingering painful response to a thermal stimulus. In later stages of pulpitis, heat exacerbates the symptom more than the cold, and the application of cold may even cause short-term pain relief.[109] Although thermal testing can be informative as to the status of the pulp, a patient's response to thermal stimuli may be confused with hypersensitivity resulting from exposed dentin and patent dentinal tubules in the absence of pulpitis.[110] Therefore, thermal testing must be combined with other diagnostic criteria, as discussed previously, to distinguish between the lesions originating from pulpal or periodontal infection.

Treatment Considerations of Endo-Perio Lesions (EPL)

In managing the lesions of pulpal or periodontal origin, making an accurate diagnosis as to the source of infection is a critical determinant of the treatment outcome. *Primary* pulpal pathoses combined with *secondary* periodontal defects would be completely resolved by conventional RCT alone. Fig. 49.3 shows a chronic pulpal infection associated with a necrotic pulp that led to a periodontal defect via the apical foramen. This is a classic example of primary pulpal infection causing a secondary periodontal defect. In this case, RCT alone led to complete resolution of the chronic apical periodontitis involving the furcal defect. In fact, this type of lesion and the healing pattern is observed in almost all secondary periodontal defects resulting from root canal infection.

Lesions originating from pulpal infections require endodontic therapy and would not resolve from periodontal treatment alone. This is exemplified in Fig. 49.8, a preoperative radiograph of an "independent" EPL showing an apical radiolucency spanning the entire length of the distal root of tooth #19 and moderate bone loss at the mesial aspect. Upon completion of RCT, the periodontal breakdown around the distal root completely resolved, whereas the mesial bony defect remained unchanged. Case 2 shows a "combined" EPL involving extensive apical defects around the apices of tooth #19 and a periodontal defect in the bifurcation. After successful endodontic therapy alone, the apical lesions and the furcation defect have resolved, but incomplete healing is noted in the coronal aspect of the furcation. This finding presumes that the unhealed defect originates from primary periodontal infection.

Therefore, EPLs require both endodontic and periodontal therapies for complete healing to occur. This is true whether the EPLs are independent or combined. One important consideration is the sequence of therapies: Which of the two should be performed first? As discussed earlier, endodontic lesions are often associated with more pronounced symptoms than periodontal lesions. More importantly, in combined EPLs, some periodontal defects will resolve on completion of the endodontic treatment, whereas the opposite would not be the case. After resolution of the secondary periodontal defect stemming from a primary pulpal infection, the residual periodontal disease may be more accurately and predictably managed. These considerations indicate that combined EPLs are best treated by first performing the necessary endodontic treatment followed by periodontal therapy.

When patients present with an abscess, the periodontal and apical abscesses are managed differently. Previous studies have suggested that the treatment of the patient with an acute periodontal abscess should be performed in two stages. In the first stage, the management of the acute lesion is performed. In the second stage, a more comprehensive treatment of the original and any residual lesions are accomplished. The management of the acute periodontal abscess involves establishing drainage via the periodontal pocket and subgingival scaling and root planing.

Curettage of the epithelium lining, the pocket, and surrounding connective tissue is then accomplished followed by compression of the pocket wall. If the swelling is large and fluctuant, flap surgery or incision and drainage (IND) may be necessary to relieve the pressure. In cases in which the bone loss is too extensive and the prognosis for the tooth is hopeless, extraction may be required.[111]

The rationale for the use of antibiotics should be considered in acute periodontal abscesses.[112] The use of systemic antibiotics may be indicated when patients have elevated temperatures, cellulitis, or systemic disease and are immunocompromised.[111] In a study by Jaramillo,[112] some periodontal pathogens showed resistance to tetracycline, metronidazole, and amoxicillin but not azithromycin. In the management of acute apical abscesses, the abscess should be drained by IND and/or root canal debridement. Depending on the maturity of the abscess, IND may not establish draining exudate from the periapical tissues. However, it is highly recommended to initiate RCT to debride the root canal infection and eliminate the source of infection. IND procedure is efficient and yet relieves the pressure that has accumulated under the subperiosteal tissues, resulting in a fluctuant, swollen, and painful lesion. Pulpectomy removes the infected pulp tissues and microorganisms within the canal system, and calcium hydroxide is placed into each of the canals. Its use has proved to be a suitable intracanal medicament because of its stability and bactericidal effect in a limited space.[113] There is quite substantial evidence that systemic antibiotic therapy may not be beneficial for patients with acute apical abscesses unless the patient presents with systemic complications, such as fever, lymphadenopathy, cellulitis, or in an immunocompromised patient.[114–116]

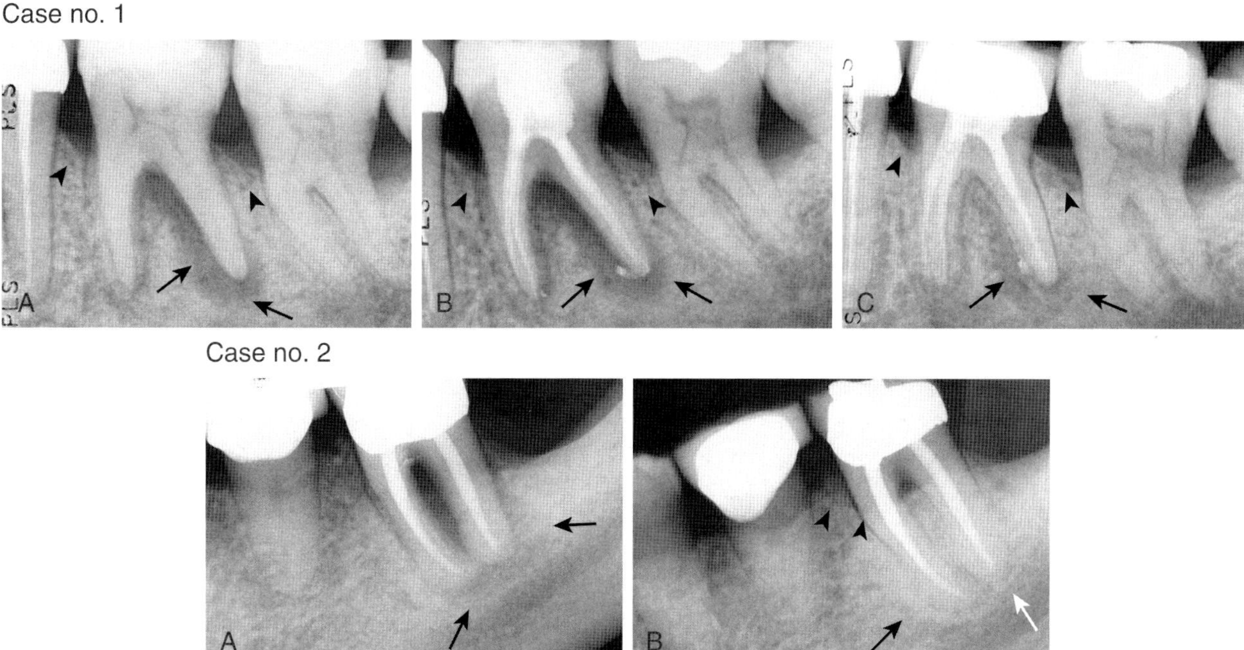

Fig. 49.8 *Case 1.* "Independent" endo-periodontal lesion (EPL). (A) "Truly separate" EPL. Vertical periodontal bone loss can be seen at the mesial surface of both teeth #18 and #19. A large endodontic lesion extends around the apex and into the bifurcation. An apical and furcal defect is evident radiographically. (B) Final condensation film 2 weeks after initiating treatment. (C) Nearly complete healing of the endodontic lesion at 6 months and restoration of the tooth with a porcelain-fused-to-metal (PFM) crown. The areas of vertical bone loss from the periodontal lesions are still present. *Case 2.* "Combined" EPL. (A) Nonvital tooth with a narrow 9-mm probing defect in the bifurcation of tooth #19 and a large periapical lesion. Normal probing depths were found on the remaining tooth surfaces. (B) Nine-month healing demonstrates significant bone repair in the furcation and periapical areas. A small amount of bone loss in the furcation still remains because of a persistent periodontal defect. *(Case 1, Courtesy Dr. Thomas Rauth.)*

Penicillin V or amoxicillin are still the antibiotics of choice against the majority of bacteria isolated from acute endodontic infections. If penicillin V therapy is ineffective, the combination of penicillin V with metronidazole or amoxicillin–clavulanate potassium is recommended. The use of clindamycin is another excellent alternative.[16] The management of pain associated with acute apical periodontitis is well controlled by prescribing systemic nonsteroidal antiinflammatory drugs (NSAIDs) with or without the additional use of Tylenol. Narcotics are usually unnecessary unless an acute flare-up occurs.[115] The correct diagnosis of periodontal and apical abscesses is the most critical step in the resolution of the disease process. Failure to properly diagnose and treat these often encountered conditions results in the progression of the disease, continued loss of bone and periodontal attachment apparatus, and a poor prognosis and possible loss of the tooth.

Summary

Bacterial-induced inflammations of the pulpal and periodontal tissues often occur together. Endodontic lesions are more likely to spread to surrounding periodontal tissues with subsequent bone and tissue destruction compared to the less frequent involvement of periodontal infections on the pulpal tissues resulting in retrograde pulpitis.

The etiology and diagnosis of dental abscesses are based on patient history and clinical and radiographic findings. Pulpal pathosis often results in significant pain to thermal stimuli, tissue swelling, or may be totally asymptomatic. A radiographic evaluation may demonstrate a circumscribed periapical lesion when the tooth tests necrotic and the origin of the lesion is pulpal. Vitality testing can detect changes in sensation caused by pulpal inflammation and necrosis. If there is evidence of pulpal disease and the possibility of associated periodontal bone loss, the endodontic treatment should be completed first, and then the patient should be reevaluated. In many cases, apparent periodontal pathology, including bone loss, suppuration, and pocket depth, resolves if there has been a pulpal lesion that has been successfully treated endodontically.

Residual periodontal problems can be treated after the completion of successful endodontic treatment, and in many cases, successful regeneration of periodontal defects is possible in endodontically treated teeth.

The importance of knowledge of these two disciplines is necessary for a successful treatment outcome for the patient.

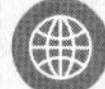 References for this chapter are found on the companion website eBooks.Health.Elsevier.com.

CHAPTER 50

Plaque Biofilm Control for the Periodontal Patient[a]

Carol A. Jahn | Deborah Mancinelli-Lyle

For online-only content on oral irrigation, caries control, chemical plaque biofilm control with oral rinses, disclosing agents, frequency of plaque biofilm removal, and patient motivation and education, please visit the companion website at eBooks.Health.Elsevier.com.

CHAPTER OUTLINE

Microbial plaque biofilm accumulation is an important etiological factor for periodontal disease.[19] Thorough biofilm removal via daily self-care that includes toothbrushing and interdental cleaning is an effective way of treating and preventing gingivitis and is essential to the long-term success of all periodontal and dental treatment.[19] In 1965, Löe et al. conducted the classic study demonstrating the relationship between microbial plaque biofilm accumulation and the development of experimental gingivitis in humans.[59] Subjects with healthy gingiva in the study ceased all daily self-care resulting in the development of gingivitis in every person within 7 to 21 days. During this time, the composition of the biofilm bacteria shifted with more virulent gram-negative organisms predominating. Importantly, these changes were shown to be reversible within 7 days once daily self-care was resumed.[59] In concordance, a systematic review by Needleman et al. concluded that daily self-care combined with regular professional care helps reduce plaque and gingival bleeding/inflammation and even concluded that thorough self-care can achieve a benefit similar to repeated professional maintenance.[60] A 2020 Clinical Practice Guideline affirms regular the importance of maintenance visits along with individually tailored self-care instructions including interdental cleaning for optimal periodontal health.[72] It is well-established that the periodontal disease typically starts interdentally. It has been demonstrated in healthy subjects that plaque biofilm formation begins on the interproximal surfaces, where the toothbrush does not reach. Masses of biofilm first develop in the molar and premolar areas, followed by the proximal surfaces of the anterior teeth and the facial surfaces of the molars and premolars. Lingual surfaces accumulate the least amount of biofilm. Patients consistently leave more plaque biofilm on the posterior teeth than the anterior teeth, with interproximal surfaces retaining the highest amounts of biofilm.[88] Additionally, periodontal patients may have increased susceptibility to future disease progression[89] due to complex defects in gingival architecture and long exposed root surfaces to clean, which compounds the difficulty of practicing thorough hygiene.

CLINICIAN'S CORNER

Effective daily plaque biofilm control practices result in improved periodontal and gingival health. Cessation of plaque control practices for 7–21 days results in:

- Accumulation of thick plaque on tooth surfaces
- Reddened gingiva that bleeds easily
- Shift to more virulent gram-negative flora
- Changes that are completely reversed in about 7 days when plaque control practices are resumed

[a]The authors would like to thank Drs. Dorothy A. Perrry, Henry Takei, and Jonathan H. Do for their contribution to this chapter in the 13th edition. The authors would also like to thank Lauren Hutchison (Colgate Palmolive Piscataway, NJ) for the inputs provided regarding connected tooth brush and arginine dentifrice.

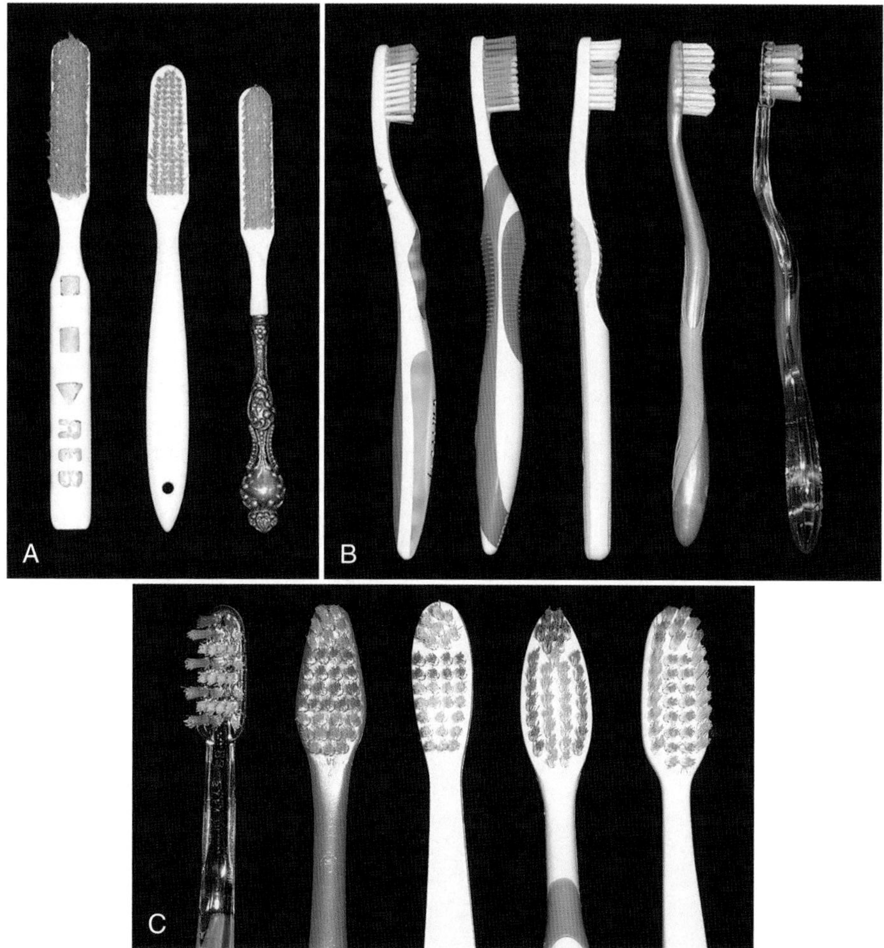

Fig. 50.1 Manual toothbrushes. (A) Various types of toothbrushes are available; note the variations in brush head and handle design. (B and C) Brush heads, showing various bristle configurations.

Effective daily plaque biofilm control is essential to optimal periodontal health. Fundamental elements of biofilm control include toothbrushing (manual or powered) and interdental cleaning (floss, floss holders, interdental brushes, water flosser, toothpicks, and other devices). Mouthrinsing may provide supplemental biofilm control.

Toothbrushes

It is well-established that toothbrushes are the most commonly used, and often only used, tool for daily plaque biofilm removal. Toothbrushing efficacy is dependent on several variables, including toothbrush design, individual skill, and frequency and duration of brushing.[36] The majority of toothbrushes on the market are manual and require the user to master a brushing technique to effectively clean the exposed tooth surface. Toothbrushes vary in size and design, as well as in length, stiffness, and configuration of the bristles (natural) or filaments (synthetic) (Fig. 50.1A–C). Handle design may be straight, contoured, or angled and also differ in width and curvature.

Electrically powered toothbrushes are widely available on the global retail market. There are basic mechanisms of action for electric toothbrushes such as oscillating-rotating (Fig. 50.2A and B) or sonic vibrations (Figs. 50.3 and 50.4A and B) of the brush head with different features and benefits including timers, pressure sensor, and artificial intelligence-empowered systems.

Brushing Frequency, Duration, and Force

The general rule is to instruct patients to brush for 2 minutes twice a day. Most individuals overestimate the amount of time they brush reporting times of 2 minutes or more.[79] In reality, the best estimates for manual brushing range from 30 to 60 seconds.[10,96] There is a belief that increased brushing time results in better plaque biofilm removal. This is hard to quantify due to heterogeneity of brushing methods and self-reported frequency. Brushing performed by dental professionals found that 2 minutes of brushing showed the best efficacy for both manual and powered toothbrushes.[96]

Resolution of experimental gingivitis required brushing once a day or every other day, but gingivitis persisted in subjects who brushed every third or fifth day.[15] This outcome shows that the maturity of the plaque biofilm may be more important for the onset of gingival inflammation than the amount. The quality of brushing may be more important than the frequency of brushing within reason.[14,36] A consideration is to judge efficacy based on the patient's clinical signs of disease where once a day with a manual toothbrush may be optimal for one individual but more frequent brushing may be needed for another individual.

Research on brushing force has mostly focused on gingival abrasion and recession. Studies that evaluated plaque biofilm removal to force found increased pressure corresponded to an increase in plaque biofilm removal.[97,98] However, there is a point of diminishing return where excess pressure resulted in reduced efficacy. Lower force with a powered toothbrush has shown better results than a higher force.[94] Toothbrushes with mechanisms that provide feedback on brushing force may benefit individuals who tend to brush vigorously and present with poor oral hygiene or soft and hard tissue lesions (Fig. 50.5).

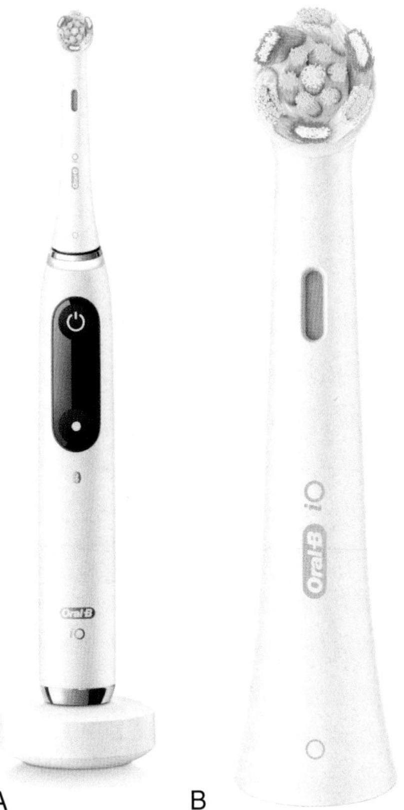

Fig. 50.2 (A) Oscillating power brush. (B) Oscillating power brush head. (Courtesy of Oral B/Procter & Gamble, Inc.)

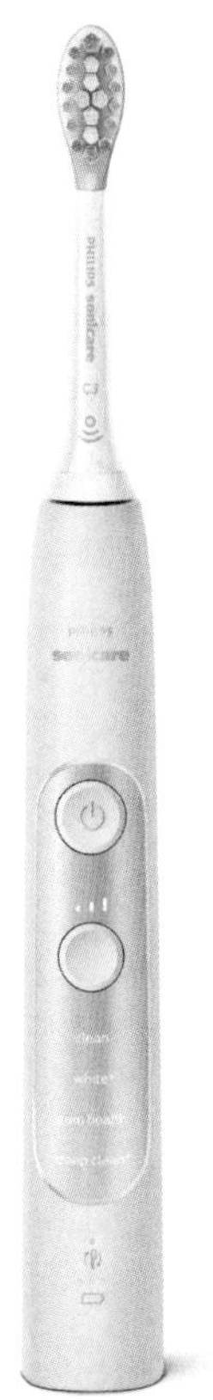

Fig. 50.3 Sonic power toothbrush. (Courtesy of Philips Sonicare.)

Toothbrush Design

Early toothbrushes used hog hair (bristles) embedded in a wooden handle, whereas today most bristles or filaments are made of nylon or polyester. The ends of the filaments are rounded by machine to minimize trauma to the gingival tissue and exposed cementum or dentin. Toothbrush filaments are grouped in tufts that are embedded into the brush head and usually arranged in rows or groupings. The features of the ideal toothbrush include:[30]

- Handle size that is appropriate to age and dexterity
- Head size that is appropriate to the size of the individual patient's requirement
- Use of end-rounded nylon or polyester filaments not larger than 0.23 mm (0.009 inch) in diameter
- Use of a soft filament configuration as defined by the acceptable international industry standards (ISO)
- Filament patterns that enhance plaque removal in the proximal spaces and along the gumline

Soft-bristled brushes have gained wide acceptance. Softer bristles are more flexible, and they clean slightly below the gingival margin when used with a sulcular brushing technique.

Electrically powered toothbrushes designed to mimic back-and-forth brushing techniques were invented in 1939. Subsequent models featured circular or elliptical motions, and some had combinations of motions. Currently, powered toothbrushes have either oscillating and rotating motions, or use low-frequency acoustic energy to enhance cleaning ability. Powered toothbrushes rely primarily on mechanical contact between the bristles and the teeth to remove plaque biofilm. The addition of low-frequency acoustic energy generates dynamic fluid movement and provides cleaning slightly away from the bristle tips.[35]

Most clinicians recommend that toothbrushes be replaced every 3 to 4 months. The filaments or bristles do not retain their shape over time and lose the ability to remove plaque effectively.[76] Toothbrush wear is different for each individual because of the varied techniques, pressure, and filaments.

Toothbrush Efficacy

A conventional flat-trim filament toothbrush has been compared to newer designs with multilevel and angled filaments designed to fit to the curvature of the teeth to improve access along the gingival margin and mesial and distal line angles. A meta review reported a reduction in plaque scores of approximately 42% (range 30% to 53% depending on index), demonstrating ineffective manual brushing technique.[94] A single brushing exercise is often used to demonstrate plaque biofilm removal or superiority between different designs. Superiority of one filament design over another has not been included in a meta-analysis. Separately, the flat-trim design showed a 24% to 27% reduction in plaque biofilm, multi-level design a 33% to 54% reduction, and crisscross design a 39% to 61% reduction.[84] However, research does not indicate significant changes in gingivitis scores or bleeding indices, which are the more important measures of improved gingival health.

When recommending a particular toothbrush, ease of use and preference by the patient are important considerations. The effectiveness of and potential injury from different types of brushes depend to a great degree on how the brushes are used.

Electrically powered toothbrushes have either oscillating and rotating motions or use low-frequency acoustic energy to enhance cleaning ability. Typically, comparison studies of powered toothbrushes, manual toothbrushes, and other powered devices demonstrate slightly improved plaque biofilm removal for the device of interest in short-term clinical trials. A Cochrane review reported that mechanical brushes with oscillating and rotating motions reduced microbial plaque biofilm 11% better and demonstrated 6% greater reduction in gingival bleeding than manual brushing.[102] These improvements were maintained over 3 months. Although long-term benefits have not been established, this particular style

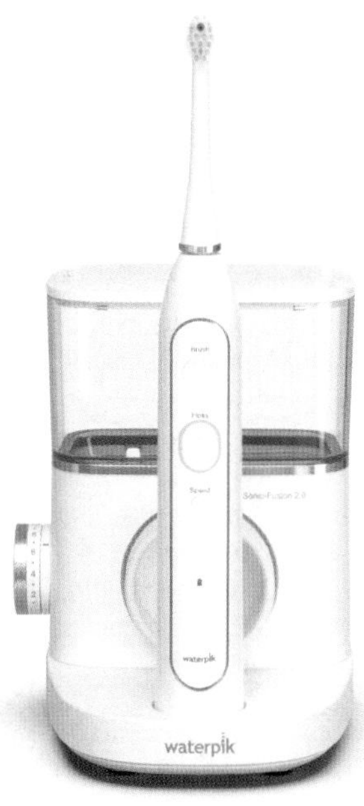

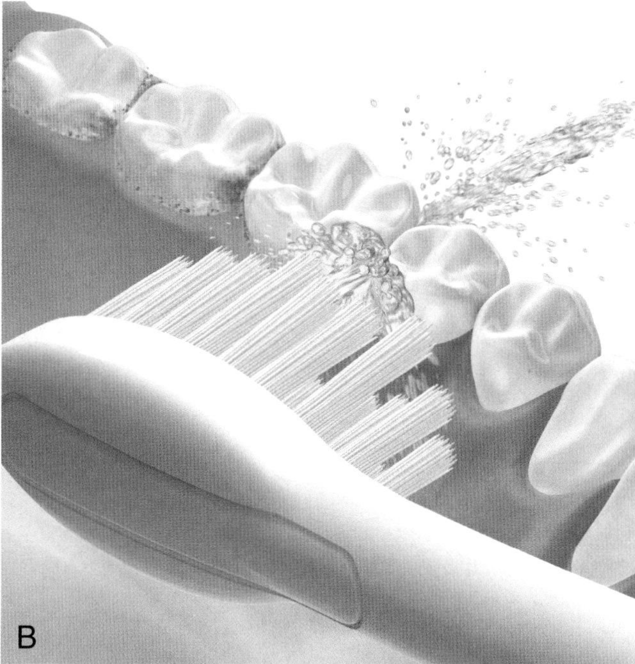

Fig 50.4 (A) Combination sonic toothbrush with built-in water flosser. (B) Brush head in action. (Courtesy of Philips Sonicare.)

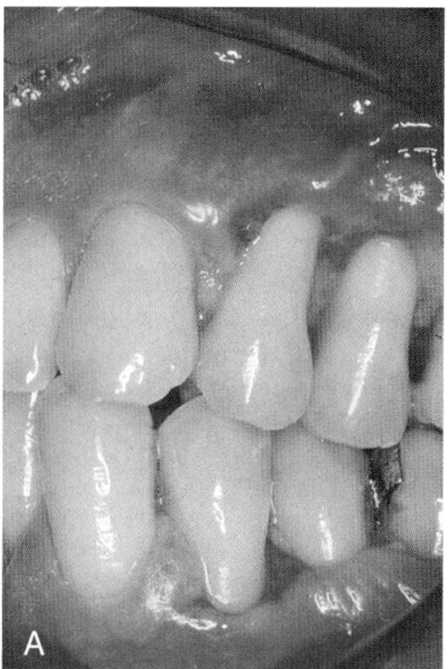

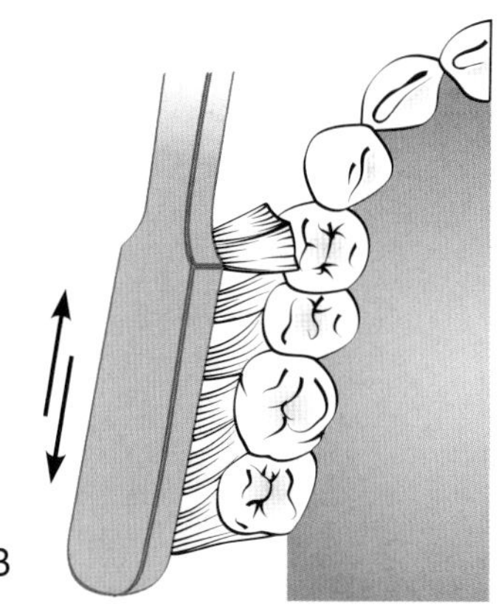

Fig. 50.5 Vigorous toothbrushing can result in trauma to the gingiva and wearing away of the tooth surfaces, especially root surfaces, and can contribute to gingival recession.

of mechanical brush resulted in better microbial plaque biofilm and gingivitis reduction in a number of well-controlled studies.

Powered toothbrushes have been shown to improve oral health for the following special situations: (1) children and adolescents; (2) people with physical or mental disabilities; (3) hospitalized patients, including older adults who require the assistance of caregivers for hygiene; and (4) patients with fixed orthodontic appliances.[48]

Connected Brush

An evolution of the powered brush is the connected brush. Connected brushes are connected to an application via wireless technology. They are most often powered brushes but may be manual. Information about brushing is combined with big data analytics and artificial intelligence to enhance the patient experience and give feedback on how the patient is brushing. Toothbrush smartphone apps can help assist in behavior change through sending reminders to brush. Connected brushes have the ability to improve both brushing and duration of brushing.[20] Connected brushes may be well suited for patients who need assistance in better brushing practices.

KEY FACT

When recommending toothbrushes, keep these general recommendations in mind:

- Soft nylon bristle toothbrushes clean effectively when used properly.
- Toothbrushes become worn due to wear and should be replaced about every 3–4 months.
- If patients perceive a benefit from a particular design of toothbrush, they should use it as long as it is effective for their needs.
- Patients who want to use powered toothbrushes should be encouraged to do so.

Toothbrushing Methods

Patients who lack manual dexterity, children, and caregivers may particularly benefit from using powered toothbrushes.

Many methods for brushing the teeth have been long-established. They are described and promoted as being efficient and effective. These methods can be categorized primarily according to the pattern of motion when brushing and are primarily of historic interest, as follows:

- *Roll:* Roll or modified Stillman technique
- *Vibratory:* Stillman, Charters, and Bass techniques
- *Circular:* Fones technique
- *Vertical:* Leonard technique
- *Horizontal:* Scrub technique

Patients with periodontal disease are most frequently taught a sulcular brushing technique using a vibratory motion to improve access to the gingival margin areas. It is important for patients to understand that plaque biofilm removal at the dentogingival junction is necessary to prevent caries as well as periodontal disease. The method most often recommended is the *Bass technique* because it emphasizes the placement of the bristles angled toward the gingival margin. This method places a focus at the gingival margin, an area that is often missed. It also provides slight access subgingivally depending on the filament design. A controlled vibrating motion is used to dislodge microbial plaque biofilm and avoid trauma. The brush is systematically placed on all the teeth in both arches (Fig. 50.6A and B).

Bass Technique

1. Place the head of a soft brush parallel to the occlusal plane, with the brush head covering three to four teeth. This hygiene procedure begins at the most distal tooth in the arch and systematically proceeds mesially.
2. Place the bristles at the gingival margin, pointing at a 45-degree angle to the long axis of the teeth (Fig. 50.7A and B).
3. Exert gentle vibratory pressure using short, back-and-forth motions without dislodging the tips of the bristles. This motion forces the bristle ends into the gingival sulcus area as well as partly into the interproximal embrasures. The pressure should be firm enough to blanch the gingiva.

Brushing With Powered Toothbrushes

The patient should follow the manufacturer's instructions for use of a powered toothbrush (Fig. 50.8).

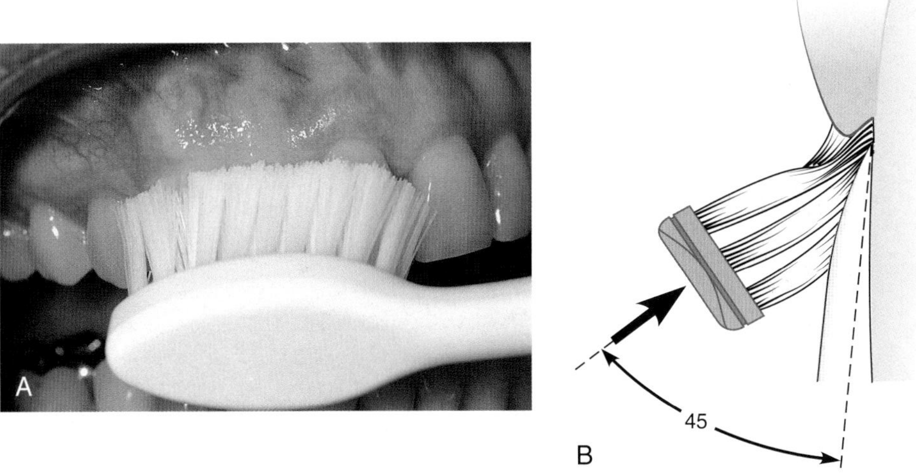

Fig. 50.6 Bass method. (A) Proper positioning of the brush in the mouth aims the bristle tips toward the gingival margin. (B) Diagram shows the ideal placement, which permits slight subgingival penetration of the bristle tips.

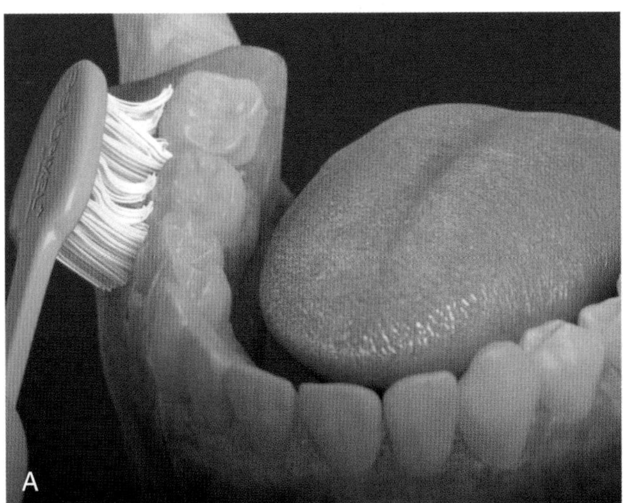

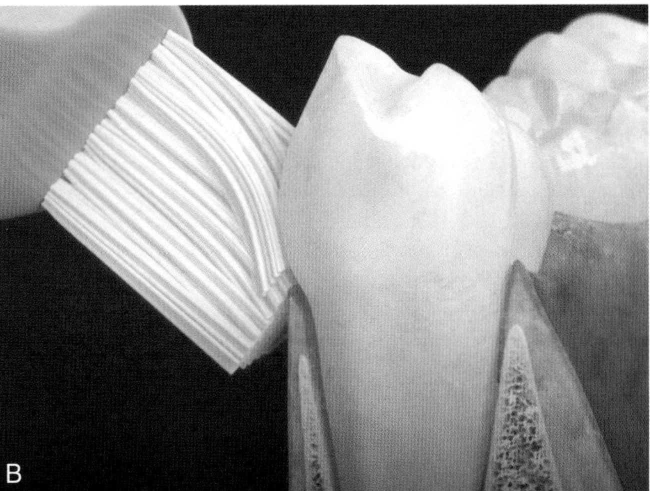

Fig. 50.7 Bass method. (A) Proper positioning of the brush in the mouth aims the bristle tips toward the gingival margin. (B) Illustration showing 45 degrees angulation between bristles of the brush and long axis of a tooth. (Courtesy of Periopixel.)

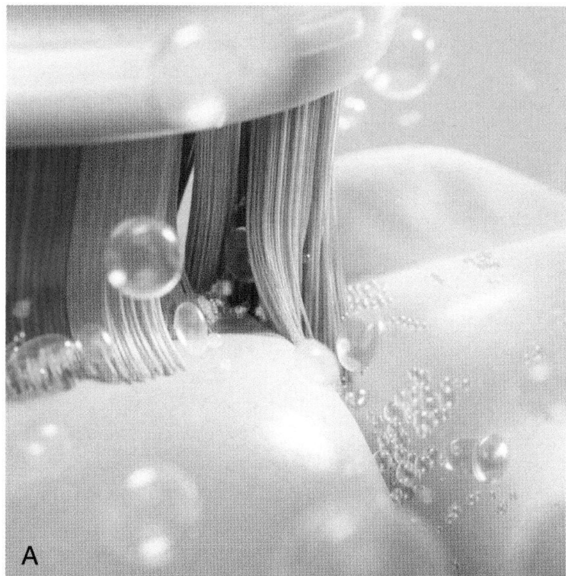

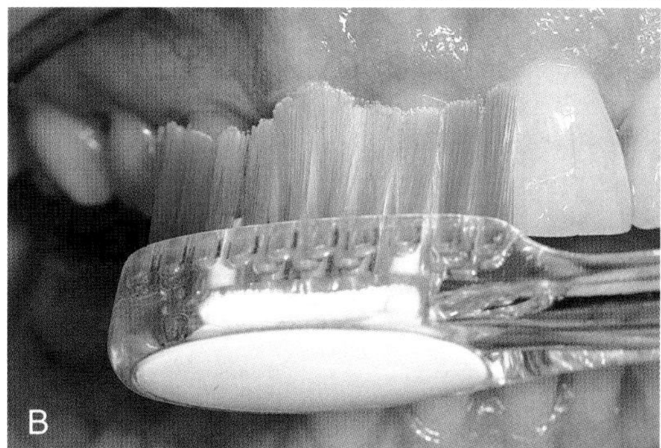

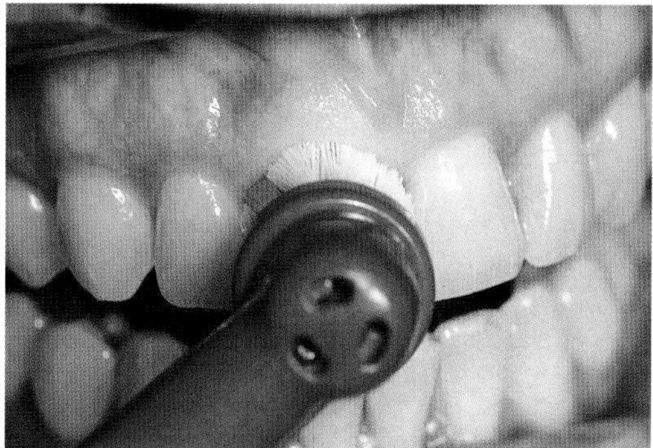

Fig. 50.8 Positioning the powered toothbrush head and bristle tips so that they reach the gingival margin is critical to achieving the most effective cleaning results. (A) Sonic brush head placement needed. (B) Straight and round head placement. (Courtesy of Philips Sonicare.)

Interdental Cleaning Devices

Daily interdental plaque biofilm removal is crucial for preventing gingivitis and maintaining periodontal health. Toothbrushing, including power brushing, is most effective for facial and lingual surfaces but fails to fully cleanse the interdental area.[101] This is true for all patients, even for periodontal patients with wide-open embrasures.

Periodontal disease can lead to loss of alveolar bone and supporting tissue.[78] This may result in large, open interproximal spaces and exposed root surfaces with anatomic concavities and furcations. These defects also occur after resective periodontal surgery. The best example of an anatomic root concavity is the mesial root surface of the maxillary first bicuspid. With attachment loss, the concavity located on this mesial surface is exposed where plaque biofilm will accumulate. In addition, dental floss does not reach these concave surfaces (Fig. 50.9).

Many devices are available for interproximal cleaning. What product is recommended should be based on the size of the interdental spaces, presence of furcations, root surface concavities, tooth alignment, and the presence of orthodontic appliances or other fixed prostheses. Importantly, patient preference along with the ability to effectively use the product at a level that produces results is critical. Common aids for interdental hygiene are interdental brushes, water flossers, toothpicks, dental floss, dental floss holders, rubber tips, and wooden or plastic tips.

Dental floss has been considered the gold standard of interdental cleaning, yet evidence does not support this.[51,77,78,83]

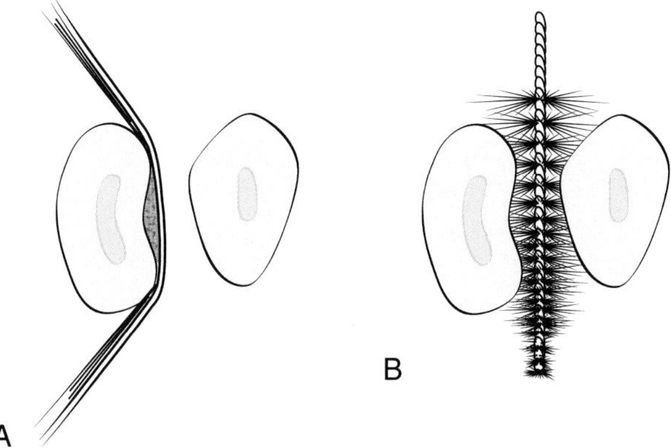

Fig. 50.9 Cleaning of concave or irregular proximal tooth surfaces. (A) Dental floss may be less effective than (B) an interdental brush on long root surfaces with concavities.

Moreover, compliance with dental floss is low at around 32%.[32] A 2020 Clinical Practice Guideline noted that dental floss should not be the first choice for interdental cleaning for people with periodontitis.[78] Kotsakis et al. conducted a network meta-analysis of interproximal oral hygiene methods for the reduction of inflammation and found interdental brushes and water flossers ranked high for reducing gingival bleeding while toothpicks and floss ranked last.[51]

KEY FACT

When recommending interdental aids:

- Flossing is often the first recommendation, but research has found other devices may be more effective for interdental plaque biofilm removal
- Interdental brushes and water flossers have been found to be most effective followed by dental floss and toothpicks.

The right product for the right patient needs to be a combination the physical need (embrasure size), manual dexterity, and interest in the product.

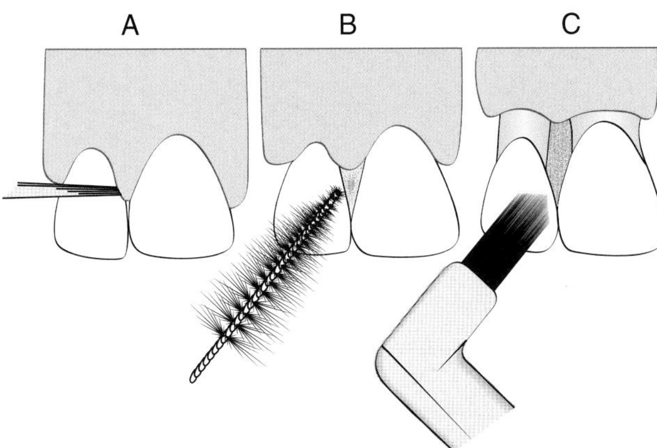

Fig. 50.10 Interproximal embrasure spaces vary greatly in patients with periodontal disease. (A) In general, embrasures with no gingival recession may be adequately cleaned using dental floss. (B) Larger spaces with exposed root surfaces require the use of an interproximal brush. (C) Single-tufted brushes clean efficiently in interproximal spaces with no papillae.

Interdental Brushes

Interdental brushes have been shown to be an effective tool in areas where the papilla does not completely fill the interdental space, or there are concave root surfaces.[51,69,77,78,83,101] The 2020 Clinical Practice Guidelines on the treatment of stage I-III periodontitis found evidence that interdental brushes provided significantly better cleaning in periodontal maintenance patients versus dental floss.[78] Other systematic reviews have concurred the finding that interdental brushes enhance the removal of plaque[19,78,84,102] and treat gingivitis better[19,77,101] over brushing alone, and are a preferred choice for interproximal cleaning for periodontal maintenance patients.[19,51,78,83]

Interdental brushes come in a variety of shapes and sizes to accommodate different embrasure sizes (Figs. 50.11A and B). Fig. 50.10 provides a representation of the size and anatomy of three types of embrasures and the interdental cleaning instrument most often recommended for each. Slot et al. concluded that the cylindrical shape was more effective at removing plaque than the conical shape.[83] As a general rule, the larger the spaces, the larger the brush size needed to clean thoroughly. Care must be taken to match the size of the brush to the opening or soft tissue trauma may result.

Technique

An interdental brush is inserted through the interproximal spaces and moved back and forth between the teeth with short strokes. The diameter of the brush should be slightly larger than the gingival embrasures to be cleaned. This size permits the bristles to exert pressure on both proximal tooth surfaces by working their way into concavities on the roots. The brush bristles must also reach the interdental gingival margin (Fig. 50.12A and B).

Single-tufted brushes provide access to furcation areas, or isolated areas of deep recession, and are effective on the lingual surfaces of mandibular molars and premolars. These areas are often missed when using a toothbrush and floss.

Water Flosser (Oral Irrigation)

See also Chapter 52.

Water flossers (oral irrigators) work via a combination of pulsation and pressure. Pulsation creates a decompression phase that allows the water or solution to penetrate subgingivally followed by a compression phase that expels bacteria and debris from the pocket (Fig. 50.13).[12,13,79] Physiologically, pulsation, along with pressure and water velocity, creates shear hydraulic forces that are capable of removing up to 99.9% of bacterial biofilm from treated areas.[39] Research on water flossing demonstrates its safety and effectiveness.[25,43] Evaluated outcomes included removal of plaque biofilm,[33–41] reductions in calculus,[42] gingivitis,[33–36,38,40,41,43–46] bleeding upon probing,[4,9,21,28,37,42,61,62,75,80] probing depth,[28,33,34,42,75] periodontal pathogens,[21,25,68] and inflammatory mediators.[4,28]

The most common agent used and demonstrated effective in a water flosser is plain water. The use of an antimicrobial agent, such as diluted chlorhexidine, may enhance reductions in gingivitis and bleeding.[21,33]

Evidence indicates that using a water flosser can lead to oral health improvements over what has been traditionally seen with string floss[9,41,43,62,75,80] or interdental brushes.[40,60] Barnes et al. found that a water flosser added to either manual or sonic toothbrushing was significantly more effective than dental floss for removing plaque and reducing bleeding and gingivitis.[9] Studies comparing water flossing to interdental brushes have found that water flossing was 56% more effective at reducing bleeding[40] and 18% more effective at removing plaque biofilm.[60]

The water flosser has been found safe and effective for those with special needs such as implants,[62] orthodontics,[17,80] and diabetes.[4] There is a well-established body of evidence demonstrating that water flossing improves the oral health for those in periodontal maintenance.[4,28,37,68] Studies have found that water flossing with water reduced bleeding upon probing (BOP) by 50% over a 6-month time frame[34] and was more effective at reducing BOP than rinsing with 0.12% chlorhexidine mouthrinse.[33]

Water flossing is the most common device recommended for self-care with implants (Fig. 50.14).[105] It has been demonstrated safe and effective around implants. Magnuson found water flossing with water at medium pressure with a tip specifically designed for use with implants was twice as effective at reducing bleeding around implants than string floss.[62] Despite strong evidence to the contrary, many myths abound regarding the safety of water flossing including appropriate pressure settings, penetration of bacteria into the pocket, and concerns about bacteremia. A 6-week study demonstrated that the water flosser can be safely used at any setting including 100 psi.[43] Water flossing has been shown to safely reduce bacteria up to 6-mm depth.[25] The rate of bacteremia from water flossing has been shown to range from 7%[74] in those with gingivitis to 50%[31] in people with periodontitis. In comparison, the rate of bacteremia from dental flossing has been shown to be around 40% in those with periodontitis[54]

Technique

1. The most widely used water flosser tip is a plastic nozzle with a 90-degree bend at the tip (Fig 50.15). Modifications to this tip include one with a tuft of bristles and one with three filaments.
2. Patients should be instructed to aim these tips at a 90-degree angle across the proximal papilla, hold it there for 3 to 5 seconds, trace along the gingival margin to the next proximal space, and

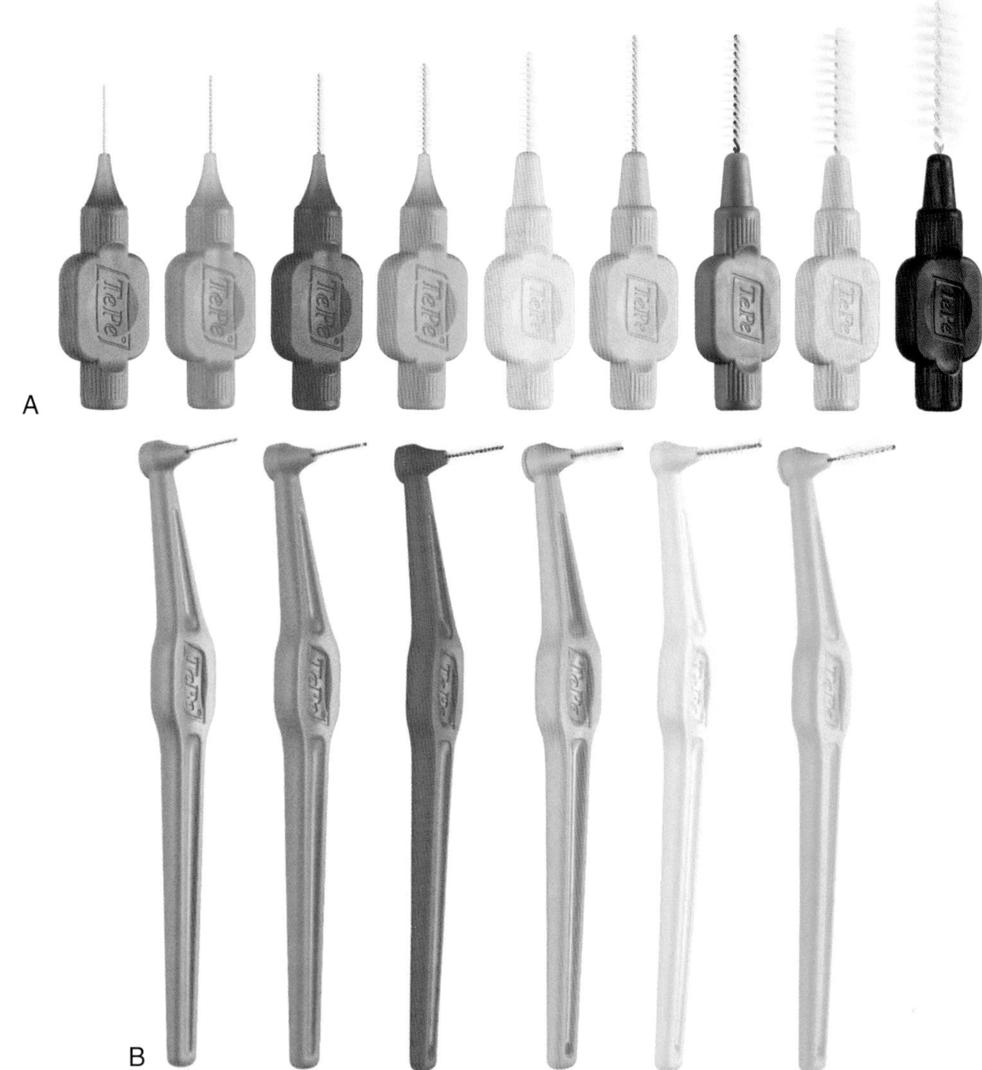

Fig. 50.11 (A) Different sizes of interdental brushes. (B) Handles of interproximal brushes. (Courtesy of TePe.)

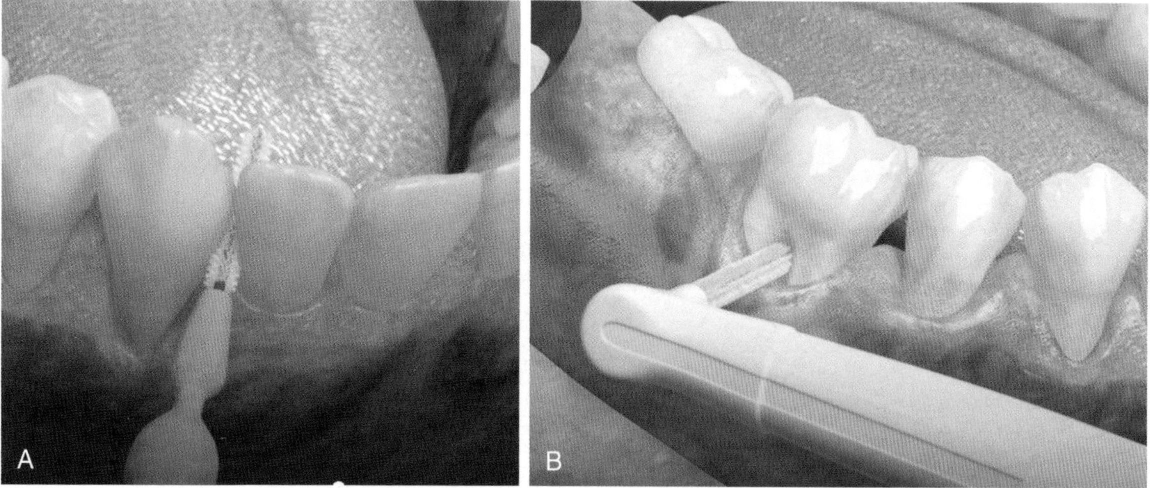

Fig 50.12 (A) Placement of an interdental brush interproximally. (B) Placement of an interdental brush into a furcation. (Courtesy of Periopixel.)

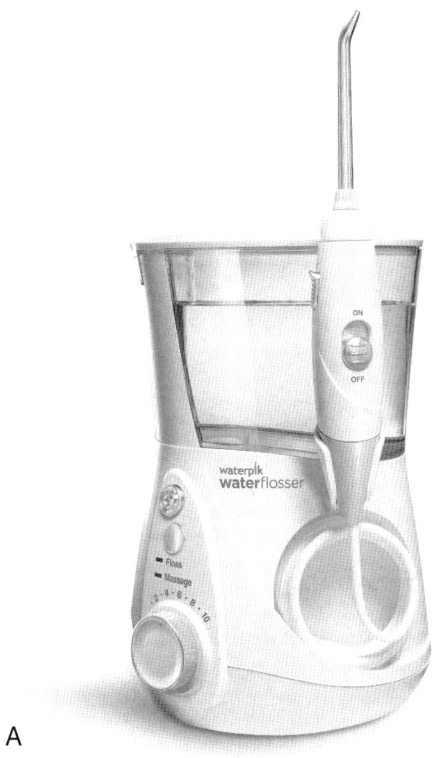

A

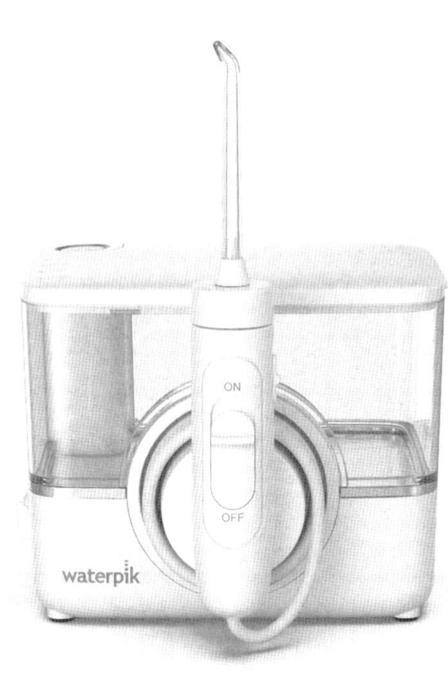

B

Fig. 50.13 (A and B) A water flosser device has been found to be highly effective in plaque biofilm removal. (Courtesy of Water Pik, Inc.)

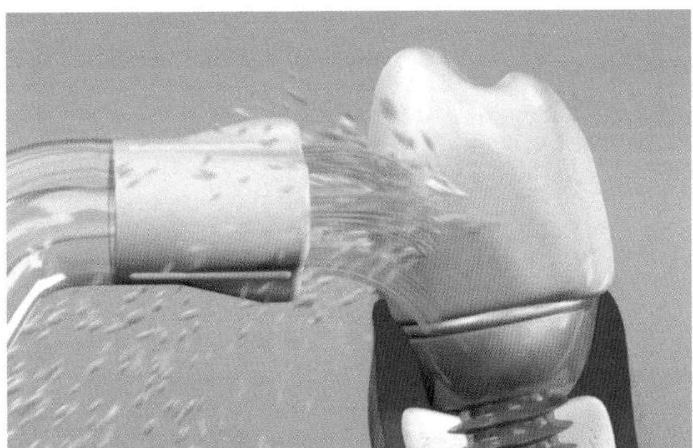

Fig. 50.14 Placement of the water flosser tip around an implant. (Courtesy of Water Pik, Inc.)

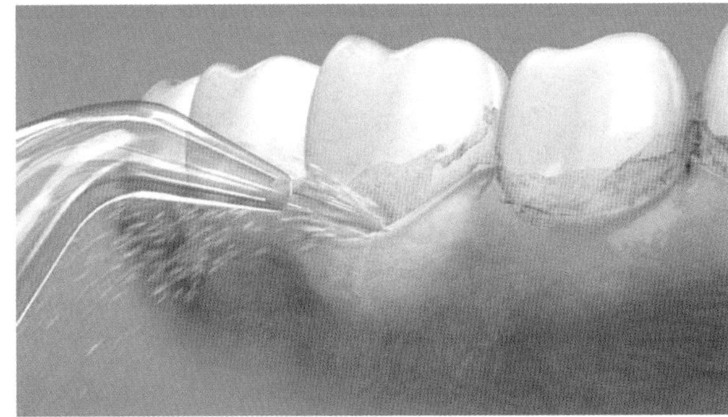

Fig. 50.15 Use of the jet tip. (Courtesy of Water Pik, Inc.)

repeat throughout the mouth both from the buccal and lingual surfaces

3. When using a tip with tuft of bristles or fine filaments, the ends of the bristles or filaments can be placed along the gingival margin to enhance plaque removal.
4. All patients should start at low pressure and increase the pressure as comfortable to at least the medium as tissue health improves. Patient comfort should be the guide for pressure setting.
5. A soft rubber tip may be used as an adjunct to any of the above tips to deliver a medication deep into the pocket. This tip is designed to deliver at a low-pressure setting regarding of the setting of the unit. Its purpose is to deliver a medication into a deep pocket, furcation, or other difficult to access area.
6. This tip should be place slightly subgingivally into the pocket and held for a few seconds (Fig.50.16). Research indicates that this tip can deliver an agent up to 70% of the depth of a 6-mm pocket.[16]

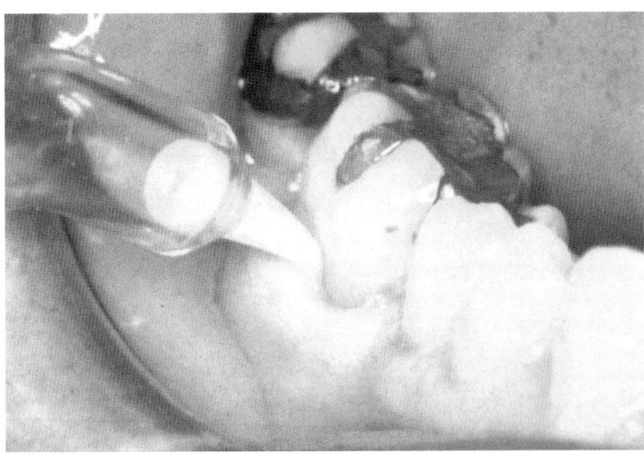

Fig. 50.16 Soft rubber tip for medicament delivery for water flossing. (Courtesy of Water Pik, Inc.)

CLINICIAN'S CORNER

Oral irrigation has been found to be a safe and effective tool for plaque biofilm removal.

- The water flosser can be safely used at any setting including 100 psi
- The rate of bacteremia from water flossing is similar to dental flossing
- The water flosser is the most recommended self-care device for dental implants.

Dental Floss

Dental floss was invented by Dr. Levi Spear Parmly in 1815 as a way to help his patients clean between their teeth. It is well-established that dental floss has become the most widely recommended tool for removing biofilm from proximal tooth surfaces. Most dental professionals have long considered it to be the best tool for interdental care. However, dental floss has largely escaped the scientific rigor that is required of many products today. Over the last decade, several researchers have explored the efficacy of floss. To the surprise and dismay of many, data indicate that dental floss often does not improve oral health beyond that of toothbrushing.[11,19,51,69,83] Dental floss has been commonly believed to be effective in controlling interproximal decay; however, no studies have been conducted on adults to evaluate this, and studies on children have provided mixed results.[49] Having said that, it is important to note that there are many reasons (including ethical ones and lack of funding) for not being able to conduct large randomized controlled trials to assess the effectiveness of dental flossing. So, longitudinal observational studies will be the next best option to explore flossing effectiveness. Using longitudinal data, researchers have shown that older adults (over 65 years of age) who flossed maintained overall oral health better and lost fewer teeth.[65]

Dental floss is technique-sensitive and requires a high level of skill to achieve an optimal oral health outcome. It is a challenging skill to master, and this is likely a driving factor in weak evidence findings.[11,69] Lang et al. found that only about 22% of individuals could use dental floss correctly.[54] Moreover, data indicate that the utilization of floss is low with about 32% of individuals reporting daily flossing.[32] A survey by the American Academy of Periodontology found people are dishonest with their dentist about how often they floss and would rather perform unpleasant tasks such as sitting in traffic or cleaning their toilet versus daily flossing.[6]

Based on emerging evidence, a routine recommendation of dental floss for all patients is becoming outdated.[11,19,49,69,78,101] Berchier et al. and Hujoel et al. concluded that dental professionals should determine on an individual basis whether high-quality flossing is an achievable goal.[11,49] While floss is a skill that can be taught, it requires that the patient have an interest in flossing. Data on repeated educational attempts to influence patients to floss are inconsistent.[11] Flossing is best for those who have the interest, motivation, skill, and an intact periodontium.

Floss is made from nylon filaments or plastic monofilaments; comes in waxed, unwaxed, thick, thin, and flavored varieties. Some prefer monofilament floss made of nonstick material because they are slick and do not fray. Clinical research has demonstrated no significant differences in the ability of the various types of floss to remove dental plaque biofilm.[23,52] Waxed dental floss was once thought to leave a waxy film on proximal surfaces, thus contributing to biofilm accumulation and gingivitis. This has been proven incorrect.[72] Factors influencing the choice of dental floss include the tightness of tooth contacts, the roughness of proximal surfaces, and the patient's preference and not the superiority of any one product.

CLINICIAN'S CORNER

Dental flossing requires a high level of skill to achieve good oral health. Many patients lack the manual dexterity or the desire to improve the skill. Therefore when recommending dental floss, it's imperative to make a carefully considered decision regarding the patients' level of skill to be able to floss effectively. A floss holder may be beneficial.

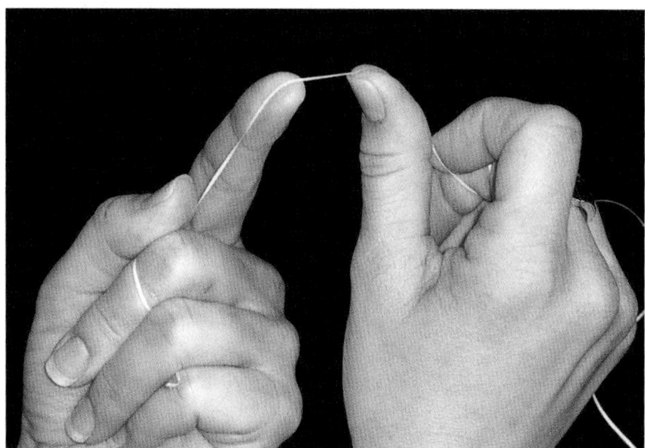

Fig. 50.17 Dental floss should be held securely in the fingers or tied in a loop.

Technique for the Use of Dental Floss

The floss must contact the proximal surface from line angle to line angle to clean effectively. It must also clean the entire proximal surface, including accessible subgingival areas. Flossing technique requires the following:

1. Start with a piece of floss long enough to grasp securely; 12 to 18 inches is usually sufficient. It may be wrapped around the middle fingers, or the ends may be tied together in a loop.
2. Stretch the floss tightly between the thumb and forefinger (Fig. 50.17) or between both forefingers, and pass it gently through each contact area with a firm back-and-forth motion. Do not snap the floss past the contact area, because this may injure the interdental gingiva. In fact, zealous snapping of floss through contact areas creates proximal grooves in the gingiva.
3. Once the floss is apical to the contact area between the teeth, wrap the floss around the proximal surface of one tooth and slip it under the marginal gingiva. Move the floss firmly along the tooth up to the contact area and gently down into the sulcus again, repeating this up-and-down stroke two or three times (Fig. 50.18A and B). Then move the floss across the interdental gingiva, and repeat the procedure on the proximal surface of the adjacent tooth.
4. Continue through the whole dentition, including the distal surface of the last tooth in each quadrant. When the working portion of the floss shreds or becomes contaminated, move the floss to a fresh portion.

Flossing can be facilitated by using a *floss holder* (Fig. 50.19A–C). Floss holders are helpful for patients lacking manual dexterity and for caregivers assisting patients in cleaning their teeth. A floss holder should be rigid enough to keep the floss taut when penetrating tight contact areas, and it should be simple to string the floss onto the holder. The disadvantage of these floss holders is that using them tends to be time-consuming because they must be rethreaded frequently when the floss shreds.

Disposable single-use floss holders with prethreaded floss are also available. Short-term clinical studies suggested that plaque biofilm reduction and improvement in gingivitis scores are similar for patients using disposable floss devices and patients who hold the floss with their fingers.[18,85]

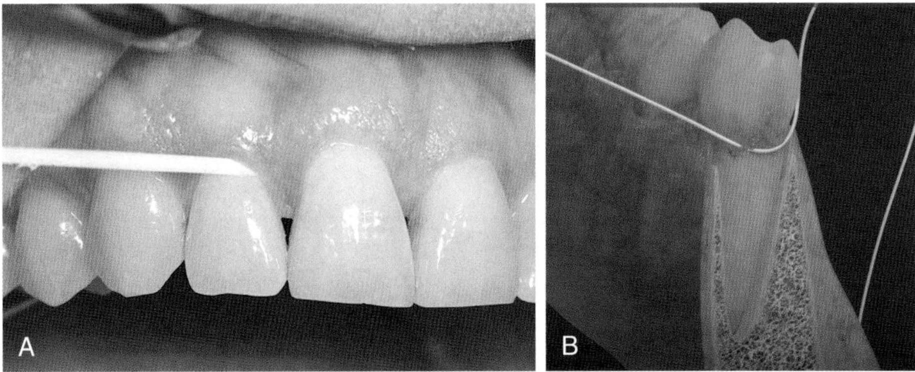

Fig. 50.18 Dental floss technique. The floss is slipped between the contact areas of the teeth (in this case, teeth #7 and #8) and wrapped around the proximal surface, and removes plaque by using several up-and-down strokes (A). The process must be repeated for the distal surface of tooth #8. Schematic showing the interdental location of dental floss below the contact point (B). (Courtesy of Periopixel.)

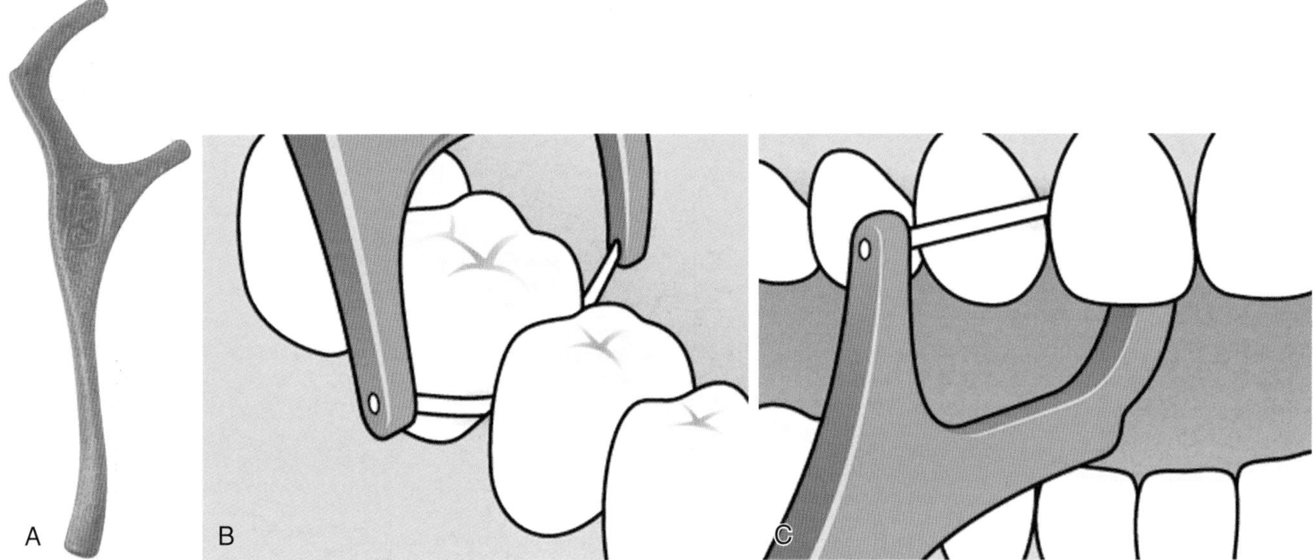

Fig. 50.19 Single-use floss holder (A) and placement of the floss holder (B and C). (Courtesy of TePe.)

Other Interdental Cleaning Devices: Rubber Tips, Wooden Toothpicks, and Tufted Brushes

Other interdental cleaning devices are available for removing microbial plaque biofilm from between the teeth. Rubber tips with angled shanks, tapered wooden toothpicks that are round or triangular in cross-section, and single-tufted brushes may be helpful in attaining interdental hygiene. Moreover, patients may prefer these devices as they can be easier to use than dental floss.

Wooden toothpicks are used either with or without a handle (Fig. 50.20). Access is easier from the buccal surfaces for tips without handles but is limited primarily to the anterior and bicuspid areas. Wooden toothpicks on handles improve access to all areas and have been shown to be as effective as dental floss in reducing plaque biofilm and bleeding scores in subjects with gingivitis.[55]

Triangular wooden tips are typically larger than toothpicks and need a sufficient interdental space to be used effectively. A systematic review by Sälzer et al. found that wooden sticks did not remove plaque better than toothbrushing but were effective at reducing bleeding.[77] A 2009 review by Ng et al. had similar findings.[69]

Rubber tip stimulators are conical and are mounted on handles or the ends of toothbrushes. They have been often recommended for plaque removal, but they have rarely been clinically evaluated. One study found the rubber tip stimulator removed more plaque than toothbrushing alone but did not reduce gingivitis.[66] Some have recommended a rubber tip for gingival massage; however, no evidence indicates that massaging the gingiva is essential or necessary to attain gingival health.

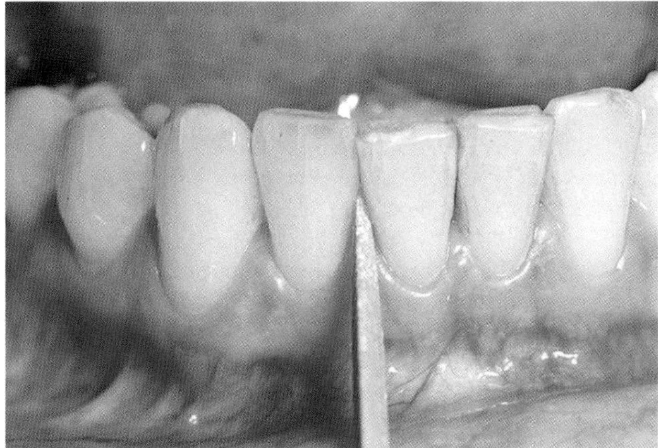

Fig. 50.20 A triangular wooden tip,

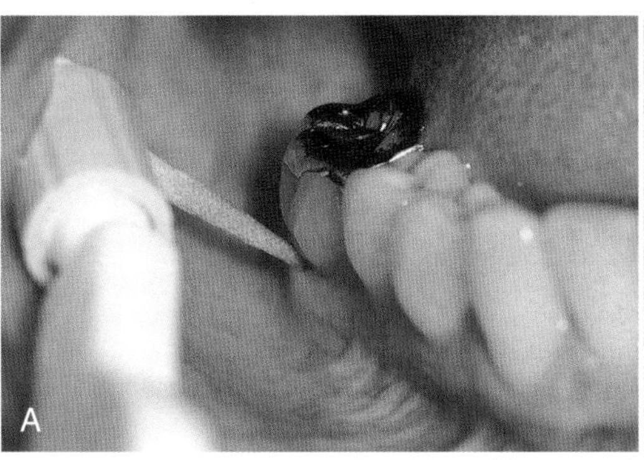
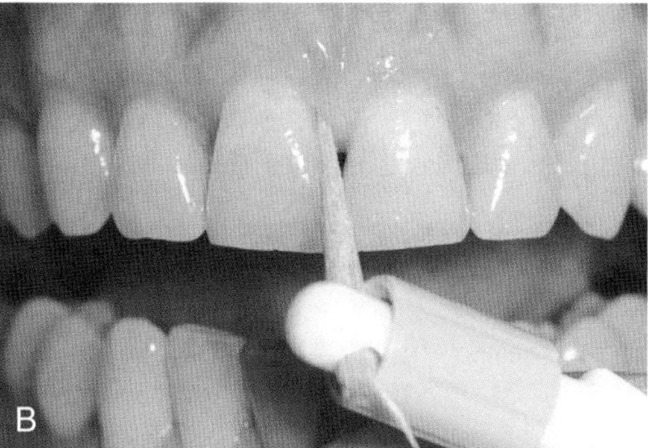

Fig. 50.21 Placement of wooden toothpicks (A and B).

Technique

Toothpicks are common devices and readily available in most homes. They can be used around all surfaces of the teeth when attached to commercially available handles. Once mounted on the handle, the toothpick is broken off so that it is only 5 or 6 mm long. The tip of the toothpick is used to trace along the gingival margin and into the proximal areas from both the facial and lingual surface of each tooth (Fig. 50.21A and B).

Soft triangular wooden picks or plastic picks are placed in the interdental space with the base of the triangle resting on the gingiva and the sides in contact with the proximal tooth surfaces. The pick is then moved in and out of the embrasure several times to remove the biofilm. The disadvantage of triangular wooden or plastic tips is that they do not reach into the posterior areas or on the lingual surfaces.

KEY FACT

Periodontal patients often have to clean large interdental spaces, so it is extremely important to find an interdental device that is easy to manipulate and that the patient will use regularly.

- Patients may need to try several of the many devices available before finding one that satisfies their needs.
- In general, the largest brush or device that fits into a space will clean most efficiently (see Fig. 50.9).

Dentifrices

Dentifrice is a term used to describe toothpastes or gels that are used in combination with toothbrushing to help clean and polish teeth and deliver fluoride.[90] It is well-established that a fluoride dentifrice helps with caries control. These medicaments, as with any drug, should be recommended and prescribed according to the needs of the individual patient. Patients like the fresh feeling that comes from a dentifrice and are also attracted to products that improve cosmetics. There is growing interest in natural products such as aloe vera, but the evidence base supporting the use of these products is currently lacking valid studies to determine their efficacy.[22,90]

In general, dentifrices have not been shown to enhance plaque removal.[90,91] Valkenburg et al. found that on average, 49.2% of plaque was removed when brushing without a dentifrice compared to 50.3% with a dentifrice.[91] When a dentifrice with triclosan or stannous fluoride (SnF) was compared with a sodium fluoride dentifrice, findings demonstrated that both SnF and triclosan enhanced plaque removal.[92] When a triclosan and an SnF dentifrice were compared, SnF fluoride was significantly better for the reduction of gingival bleeding while triclosan was more effective at removing plaque.[90]

Historically, sodium fluoride (NaF) has been the primary added fluoride ingredient in dentifrice. To earn the American Dental Association (ADA) Seal of Acceptance, a dentifrice must contain fluoride. More recently, SnF has become popular due to its antimicrobial properties. One issue with SnF has been staining. Newer formulations contain the agent, hexametaphosphate, which reduces staining.[90] For several years, triclosan was a popular ingredient. Recently, concerns over their environmental and health effects have resulted in the restricted use of the agent in both Europe and the USA.[90] Tartar control pastes may contain pyrophosphates or zinc compounds. These agents have been found to help reduce supragingival calculus.[90] Baking soda is a long-time common toothpaste ingredient. A systematic review indicated that a baking soda toothpaste helped to reduce bleeding.[93] Periodontal patients may also prefer a paste that reduces hypersensitivity. NaF can do this to some extent. Products with arginine, calcium sodium phophosilicate, or SnF and strontium have been shown to be clinically effective in treating dentinal hypersensitivity.[99]

KEY FACT

Considering dentifrices, keep in mind that:

- Dentifrices typically do not enhance plaque removal
- Products containing fluoride and antimicrobial agents provide additional benefits for controlling caries and inflammation
- Patients who form significant amounts of supragingival calculus benefit from the use of a calculus control dentifrice
- Sensitivity toothpastes may also be needed for select periodontal patients

Arginine

More recently, dentifrices containing the amino acid arginine, often in combination with fluoride, have become available. Arginine has been shown to help disrupt biofilm architecture,[46,64] making biofilm less adhesive/sticky.[81] Arginine has also been shown to have an impact on the composition of the oral microbiome where evidence indicates it actively promotes caries-fighting bacteria and impairs caries-causing bacteria.[20,46] Clinical research studies with arginine have indicated that dentifrices containing arginine with fluoride as well as arginine alone inhibit the development of dental caries.[1,2,57,103,104] Large-scale clinical studies with arginine-containing dentifrices are currently underway.

Two concerns about dentifrices are allergic reactions/sensitivity and abrasiveness. Patients may sometimes react to certain agents in toothpaste. More common is a sensitivity to sodium lauryl sulfate (SLS). This agent has been shown to irritate the oral mucosa and has been linked to the development of aphthous ulcers in some people.[90] Abrasiveness is another concern. The abrasive quality of dentifrices affects enamel slightly and is a much greater concern for patients with exposed root surfaces. Dentin is abraded 25 times faster and cementum even faster, 35 times the rate of enamel.[87] The ADA, along with governmental agencies and other stakeholders, has developed a standardized scale called the Relative Dentin

Abrasivity (RDA) to quantify the abrasivity of toothpastes. All dentifrices are assigned a standard RDA value of 100. Any toothpaste at or below 2.5 times the reference value or 250 is considered safe and effective. To earn the ADA Seal of Acceptance, a toothpaste must demonstrate an RDA of 250 or less.[7]

KEY FACTS

Periodontal patients should be aware of caries, and the use of fluoride products minimizes the risk for caries.

- All periodontal patients should be encouraged to use a fluoride-containing toothpaste daily.
- Patients at high risk for root caries should use higher-concentration fluoride toothpaste or gel.
- Other considerations in caries control, such as diet and reduced salivary flow, should be evaluated, and modifications should be made where possible.

Root Caries

Periodontal patients may be at risk for root caries. Exposed root surfaces, older age, tobacco use, and poor oral hygiene are risk factors for root caries.[106] Because the root surface has fewer inorganic minerals in comparison with enamel, demineralization can proceed quickly.[3]

Good oral hygiene and fluoride are essential in helping arrest and prevent root caries. To arrest a cavitated root carious lesion or arrest or reverse a noncavitated root caries lesion, an expert panel from the American Dental Association recommended prioritizing treating lesions with 5000 parts per million fluoride NaF toothpaste or gel once per day. This was found to provide a three times greater chance of arrest or reversal than no treatment.[82] Others have found silver diamine fluoride (SDF) effective for arresting cavitated root caries. SDF will turn the carious lesion black, so patients must be informed that esthetics may be compromised.[27]

KEY FACT

Strategies that will assist you in educating and motivating your patients include:

- Listen to your patient and recommend products based on their needs, lifestyle, and preferences.
- Provide encouragement and positive reinforcement including directing them to online videos and smart phone applications.
- Demonstrate how devices work, and allow practice time.
- Provide or dispense products to patients to enhance value and convenience.
- Show and reinforce improvements at subsequent appointments, even if changes are modest.

Conclusion

Effective control of the plaque biofilm is the foundation of good oral health especially periodontal health. Toothbrushing combined with an interdental aid is essential for everyone. Power toothbrushes can be helpful for those who struggle to effectively remove plaque with a manual toothbrush. For interdental aids, current research indicates that interdental brushes and water flossers may be more effective than dental floss or toothpicks. Some people, depending upon their level of dexterity, may need an adjunctive rinse to help control plaque. Because some may have exposed root surfaces, caries control via an over-the-counter or prescription paste may be necessary. The best tool is the one that meets the patient's needs, abilities, lifestyle, and preferences.

A Case Scenario is found on the companion website eBooks.Health.Elsevier.com.

Suggested Readings

1. Araujo MWB, Charles CA, Weinstein RB, et al. Meta-analysis of an essential oil-containing mouthrinse on gingivitis and plaque. *J Am Dent Assoc*. 2015;146:610–622. PubMed PMID: 26227646. PMID: .
2. Barnes CM, Russell CM, Reinhardt RA, et al. Comparison of irrigation to floss as an adjunct to toothbrushing: effect on bleeding, gingivitis, and supragingival plaque. *J Clin Dent*. 2005;16:71–77. PubMed PMID: 10476890. PMID: .
3. Chapple ILC, Van der Weijden F, Doerfer C, et al. Primary prevention of periodontitis: managing gingivitis. *J Clin Periodontol*. 2015;42(suppl. 16):S71–S76. PubMed PMID: 25639826. PMID: .
4. Chen Y, Wong RW, McGrath C, et al. Natural compounds containing mouthrinses in the management of dental plaque and gingivitis: a systematic review. *Clin Oral Investig*. 2014;18:1–16. PubMed PMID: 23860901. PMID: .
5. Fleming EB, Nguyen D, Afful J, et al. Prevalence of daily flossing among adults by selected risk factors for periodontal disease – United States, 2011-2014. *J Periodontol*. 2017;89:933–939. PubMed PMID: 29644699. PMID: .
6. Genovesi AM, Lorenzi C, Lyle DM, et al. Periodontal maintenance following scaling and root planing, comparing minocycline treatment to daily oral irrigation with water. *Minerva Stomatol*. 2013;62(suppl 1):1–9. PubMed PMID: 24423731. PMID: .
7. Gobat N, Bogle V, Lane C. The challenge of behavior change. In: Ramseier CA, Suvan JE, eds. *Health Behavior Change in the Dental Practice*. Ames, IA: Wiley-Blackwell; 2010:13–34.
8. Gorur A, Lyle DM, Schaudinn C. Biofilm removal with a dental water jet. *Compend Contin Educ Dent*. 2009;30:1–6. PubMed PMID: 19385349. speciall . PMID:.
9. Haps S, Slot DE, Berchier CE, et al. The effect of cetylpyridinium chloride-containing mouth rinses as adjuncts to toothbrushing on plaque and parameters of gingival inflammation: a systematic review. *Int J Dent Hygiene*. 2008;6:290–303. PubMed PMID: 19138180. PMID: .
10. Hujoel PP, Cunha-Cruz J, Banting DW, et al. Dental flossing and interproximal caries: a systematic review. *J Dent Res*. 2006. PubMed PMID: 16567548. 85298-305. PMID: .
11. Kotsakis GA, Lian Q, Ioannou AL, et al. A network meta-analysis of interproximal oral hygiene methods in the reduction of clinical indices of inflammation. *J Periodontol*. 2018;89:558–570. PubMed PMID: 29520910. PMID: .
12. Ng E, Lim LP. An overview of different interdental cleaning aids and their effectiveness. *Dent J*. 2019;7:56. PubMed PMID: 31159354. PMID: .
13. Sälzer S, Slot DE, Van Der weijden FA, et al. Efficacy of inter-dental mechanical plaque control in managing gingivitis- a meta-review. *J Clin Periodnotol*. 2015;42(suppl. 16):S92–S105. PubMed PMID: 25581718. PMID: .
14. Sanz M, Herrer D, Kebschull M, et al. Treatment of stage I-III periodontitis-the EFP S3 level clinical practice guideline. *J Clin Periodontol*. 2020;47(suppl 22):4–60. PubMed PMID: 32383274. PMID: .
15. Slayton RL, Urquhart O, Araujo WB, et al. Evidence-based clinical practice guideline on nonrestorative treatments for carious lesions: a report from the American Dental Association. *J Am Dent Assoc*. 2018;149:837–849. PubMed PMID: 30261951. PMID: .
16. Toothpastes: Relative Dentin Abrasivity (RDA). American Dental Association, www.ada.org/en/member-center/oral-health-topics/toothpastes Accessed July 19, 2021.
17. Valkenburg C, Van der Weijden FA, Slot DE. Plaque control and reduction of gingivitis: the evidence for dentifrices. *Periodontology*. 2000;79:221–232. PubMed PMID: 30892760. 2019 . PMID:.
18. Van der Weijden GA, Hioe KPA. Systematic review of the effectiveness of self-performed mechanical plaque removal in adults with gingivitis using a manual toothbrush. *J Clin Periodontol*. 2005;32:214–228. PubMed PMID: 16128840. PMID: .

19. Van Strydonck DA, Slot D, Van der Velden U, et al. Effective of a chlorhexidine mouthrinse on plaque, gingival inflammation and staining in gingivitis patients: a systematic review. *J Clin Periodontol.* 2012;39:1042–1055. PubMed PMID: 22957711. PMID: .
20. Worthington HV, MacDonald L, Poklepovic PT, et al. Home use of interdental cleaning devices, in addition to toothbrushing, for preventing and controlling periodontal diseases and dental caries. *Cochrane Database Syst Rev.* 2019;(4). PubMed PMID: 30968949. PMID: .

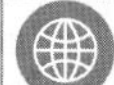
References for this chapter are found on the companion website eBooks.Health.Elsevier.com.

CHAPTER 51

Scaling and Root Instrumentation (Root Planing)[a]

Anna M. Pattison | Gordon L. Pattison

 For online-only content on general principles of instrumentation, principles of scaling and root instrumentation, and instrument sharpening, please visit the companion website at eBooks.Health.Elsevier.com.

CHAPTER OUTLINE

Periodontal instruments are designed for specific purposes, such as calculus removal, biofilm removal, and subgingival root instrumentation (root planing). On first investigation, the variety of instruments available for similar purposes appears confusing. With experience, however, clinicians select a relatively small set that fulfills all requirements.

LEARNING BOX 51.1

Special Note on Terminology

In this chapter and in the entire book, we utilized the term *root instrumentation* to encompass both *root planing* and *root debridement*. It is important to note that in the United States, treatment codes (D4341 and D4342) submitted for insurance purposes utilize the term root planing.

Classification of Periodontal Instruments

Periodontal instruments are classified according to the purposes they serve, as follows:

1. *Periodontal probes* are used to locate, measure, and mark pockets, as well as determine their course on individual tooth surfaces.
2. *Explorers* are used to locate calculus deposits and caries.
3. *Scaling, root instrumentation (root planing), and curettage instruments* are used for the removal of biofilm and calcified deposits from the crown and root of a tooth, removal of altered cementum from the subgingival root surface, and debridement of the soft tissue lining the pocket. Scaling and curettage instruments are classified as follows:
   - *Sickle scalers* are heavy instruments used to remove supragingival calculus.
   - *Curettes* are fine instruments used for subgingival scaling, root instrumentation (root planing), and removal of the soft tissue lining the pocket. The removal of the soft tissue wall of the pocket or curettage is seldom performed these days.
   - *Hoe and file scalers* are used to remove tenacious subgingival calculus and altered cementum. Their use is limited compared with that of curettes.
   - *Implant instruments* are plastic or titanium scalers and curettes designed for use on implants and implant restorations.
   - *Ultrasonic and sonic instruments* are used for scaling and cleansing tooth surfaces and curetting the soft tissue wall of the periodontal pocket.[1–3]
4. *Periodontal endoscopes* are used for deep visualization into subgingival pockets and furcations, thereby allowing the detection of deposits.
5. *Cleansing and polishing instruments*, such as rubber cups, brushes, and dental tape, are used to clean and polish tooth surfaces. Air-powder abrasive systems are also available for

[a]Material in this chapter was derived from Pattison A, Pattison G, Matsuda S: Periodontal instrumentation, ed 3, New York, 2018, Pearson Education.

Systematic and subgingival cleaning and polishing of tooth, root, and implant surfaces.

The wearing and cutting qualities of some types of steel used in periodontal instruments have been tested,[4–6] but specifications vary among manufacturers.[6] Stainless steel is used most often in instrument manufacturing. High-carbon content steel instruments are available and are considered by some clinicians to be superior. Newer advanced proprietary manufacturing processes for heat treating and cryogenically tempering stainless steel are producing blades that are sharper and longer lasting than ever before. In addition, other processes produce stainless steel instruments with titanium nitride or other surface coatings that are not embedded or diffused into the base material. Their cutting edges are sharp when new, but these coatings wear down during normal use and cannot be resharpened. Each group of instruments has characteristic features; individual therapists often develop variations with which they operate most effectively. Small, miniaturized instruments are recommended to fit into periodontal pockets without injuring the soft tissues.[7–10]

The parts of each instrument are referred to as the working end, shank, and handle (Fig. 51.1).

Periodontal Probes

Periodontal probes are used to measure the depth of pockets and to determine their configuration. The typical probe is a tapered, rodlike instrument calibrated in millimeters, with a blunt, rounded tip (Fig. 51.2). Several other designs with various millimeter calibrations are available (Fig. 51.3). The World Health Organization probe has millimeter markings and a small, round ball at the tip (see Fig. 51.3E). Ideally, these probes are thin, and the shank is angled to allow easy insertion into the pocket. Furcation areas can best be evaluated with the curved, blunt Nabers probe (Fig. 51.4).

LEARNING BOX 51.2

Periodontal probes are used to measure the depth of pockets and to determine their configuration.

When measuring a pocket, the probe is inserted with firm, gentle pressure to the bottom of the pocket. The shank should be aligned with the long axis of the tooth surface to be probed. Several measurements are made ("walking the probe") to capture the level of attachment along the surface of the tooth.

Explorers

Explorers are used to locate subgingival deposits and carious areas and to check the smoothness of the root surfaces after root instrumentation (root planing). Explorers are designed with different shapes and angles, with various uses (Fig. 51.5), as well as limitations (Fig. 51.6). The periodontal probe can also be useful in the detection of subgingival deposits (see Fig. 51.6D).

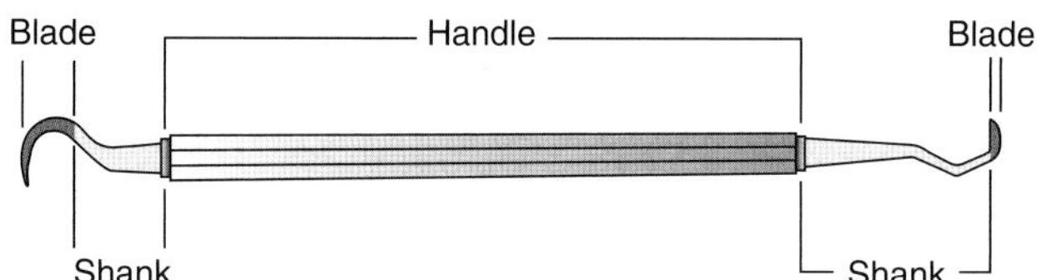

Fig. 51.1 Parts of a typical periodontal instrument.

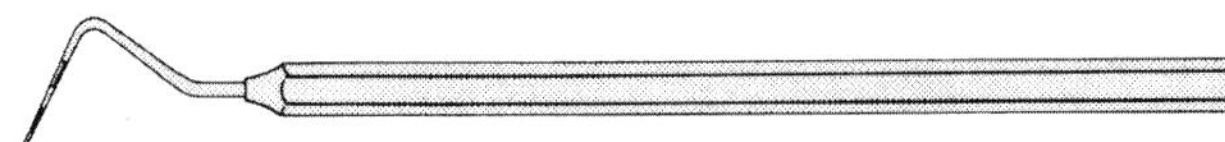

Fig. 51.2 Periodontal probe is composed of the handle, shank, and calibrated working end.

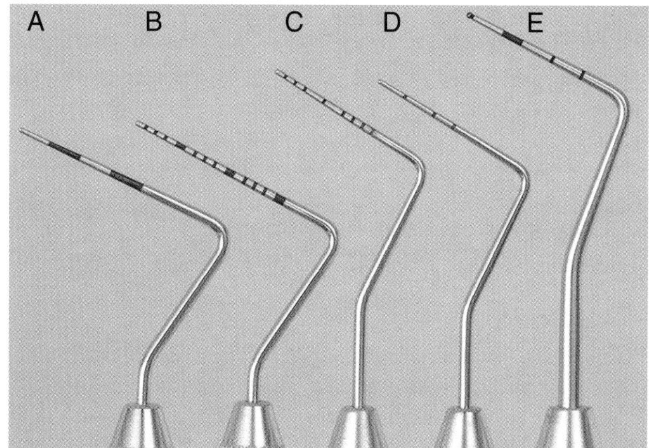

Fig. 51.3 Types of periodontal probes. (A) Marquis color-coded probe. Calibrations are in 3-mm sections. (B) University of North Carolina 15 probe, a 15-mm long probe marked at each millimeter and color-coded at the 5th, 10th, and 15th millimeters. (C) University of Michigan "0" probe, with Williams markings (at 1, 2, 3, 5, 7, 8, 9, and 10 mm). (D) Michigan "0" probe with markings at 3, 6, and 8 mm. (E) World Health Organization probe, which has a 0.5-mm ball at the tip and markings at 3.5, 8.5, and 11.5 mm and color coding from 3.5 to 5.5 mm.

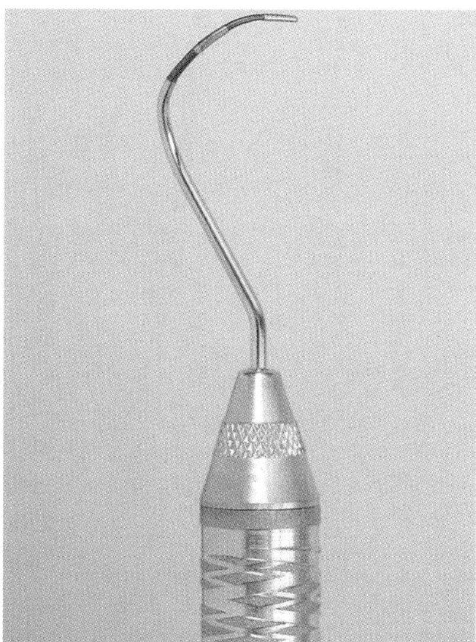

Fig. 51.4 Curved #2 Nabers probe for detection of furcation areas, with color-coded markings at 3, 6, 9, and 12 mm.

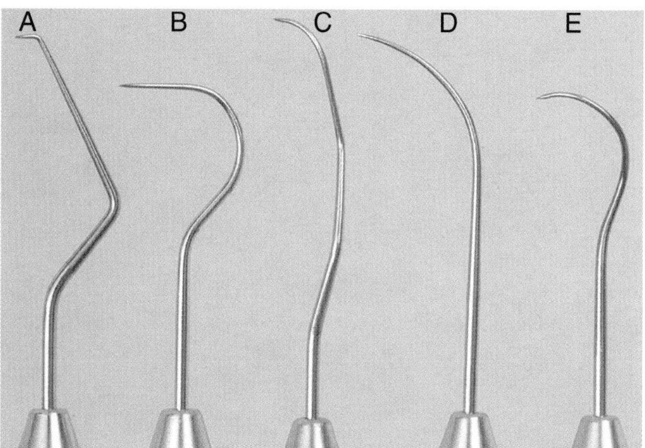

Fig. 51.5 Five typical explorers. (A) #17; (B) #23; (C) EXD 11-12; (D) #3; (E) #3CH pigtail.

LEARNING BOX 51.3

Explorers are used to locate subgingival deposits and carious areas and to check the smoothness of the root surfaces after root instrumentation (root planing).

Scaling and Curettage Instruments

Scaling and curettage instruments are illustrated in Fig. 51.7.

Sickle Scalers

Sickle scalers have a flat surface and two cutting edges that converge in a sharply pointed tip. The shape of the instrument makes the tip strong so that it will not break off during use (Fig. 51.8). The sickle scaler is used primarily to remove supragingival calculus (Fig. 51.9). Because of the design of this instrument, it is difficult to insert a large sickle blade under the gingiva without damaging the surrounding gingival tissues (Fig. 51.10). Small, curved sickle scaler blades such as the 204SD can be inserted under ledges of calculus several millimeters below the gingiva. Sickle scalers are used with a pull stroke.

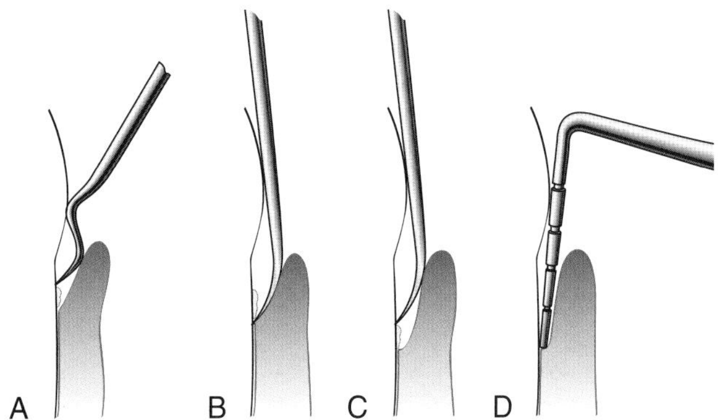

Fig. 51.6 Insertion of two types of explorers and a periodontal probe in a pocket for calculus detection. (A) The limitations of the pigtail explorer in a deep pocket. (B) Insertion of the #3 explorer. (C) Limitations of the #3 explorer. (D) Insertion of the periodontal probe.

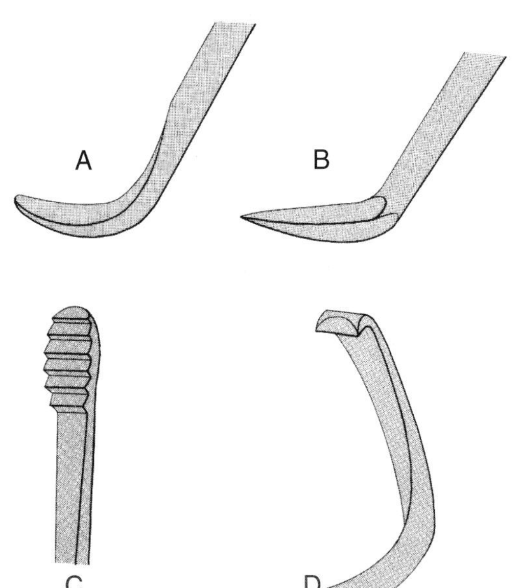

Fig. 51.7 The four basic scaling instruments. (A) Curette; (B) sickle; (C) file; (D) hoe.

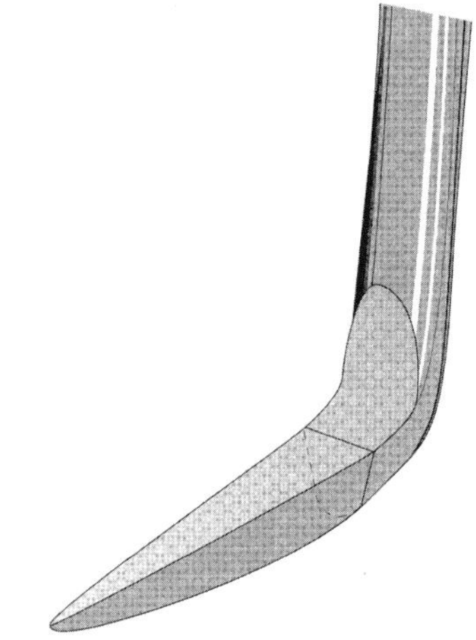

Fig. 51.8 Basic characteristics of a sickle scaler: triangular shape, double-cutting edge, and pointed tip.

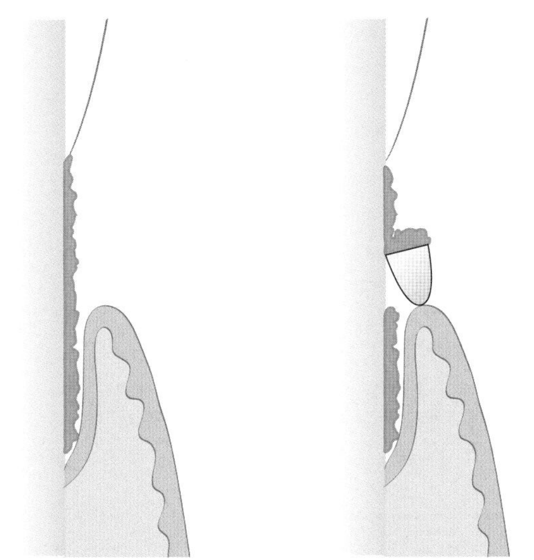

Fig. 51.9 Use of a sickle scaler for removal of supragingival calculus.

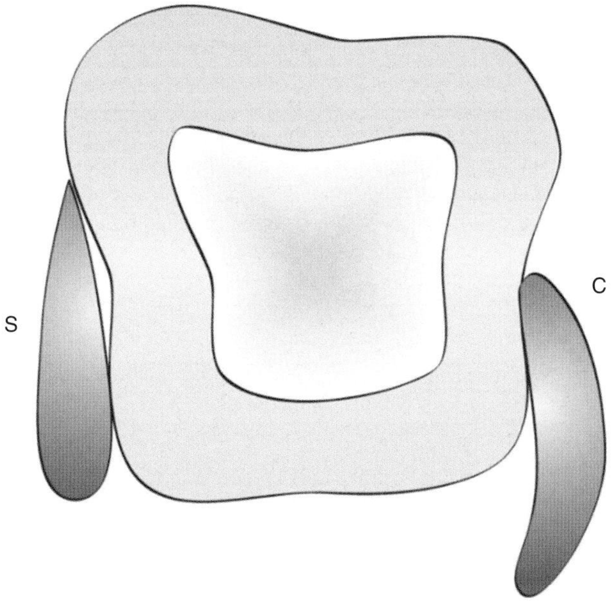

Fig. 51.10 Subgingival adaptation around the root is better with the curette than with the sickle. *C*, Curette; *S*, sickle.

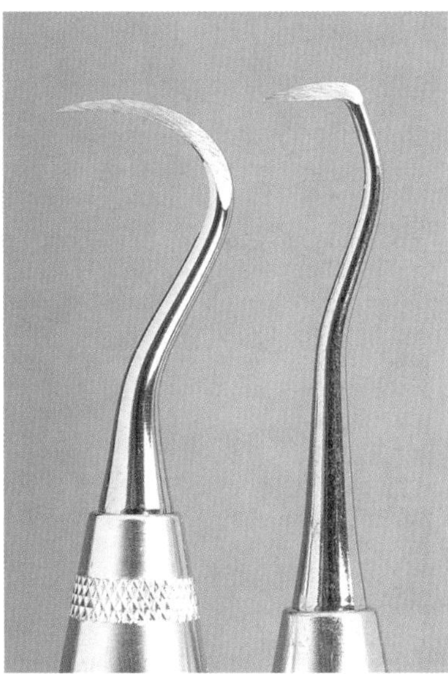

Fig. 51.11 Both ends of a U15/30 scaler.

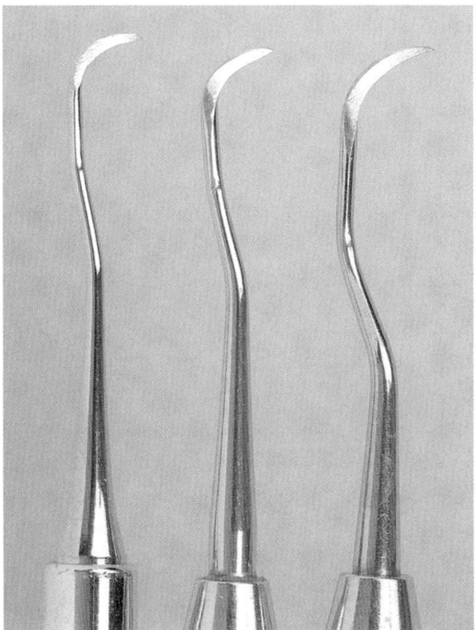

Fig. 51.12 Three different sizes of 204 sickle scalers.

Sickle scalers of the same basic design can be obtained with different blade sizes and shank types to adapt to specific uses. The U15/30 (Fig. 51.11), Ball, and Indiana University sickle scalers are large. Jaquette sickle scalers #1, #2, and #3 have medium-size blades. Curved 204 posterior sickle scalers are available with large, medium, or small blades (Fig. 51.12). The Montana Jack sickle scaler and the Nevi 2, Nevi 3, and Nevi 4 curved posterior sickle scalers are all thin enough to be inserted several millimeters subgingivally for removal of light to moderate ledges of calculus. The selection of these instruments should be based on the area to be scaled. Sickle scalers with straight shanks are designed for use on anterior teeth and premolars. Sickle scalers with contra-angled shanks adapt to posterior teeth.

Curettes

The curette is the instrument of choice for the removal of deep subgingival calculus, root instrumentation (root planing) of altered cementum, and removal of the soft tissue lining the periodontal pocket (Fig. 51.13). Each working end has a cutting edge on both sides of the blade and a rounded toe. Curettes are finer than sickle scalers and do not have any sharp points or corners other than the cutting edges of the blade (Fig. 51.14). Therefore, curettes can be adapted for and provide good access to deep pockets, with minimal soft tissue trauma (see Fig. 51.10). In cross section, the blade appears semicircular with a convex base. The lateral border of the convex base forms a cutting edge with the face of the semicircular blade. Cutting edges are present on both sides of the blade. Both single- and double-end curettes may be obtained, depending on the preference of the operator.

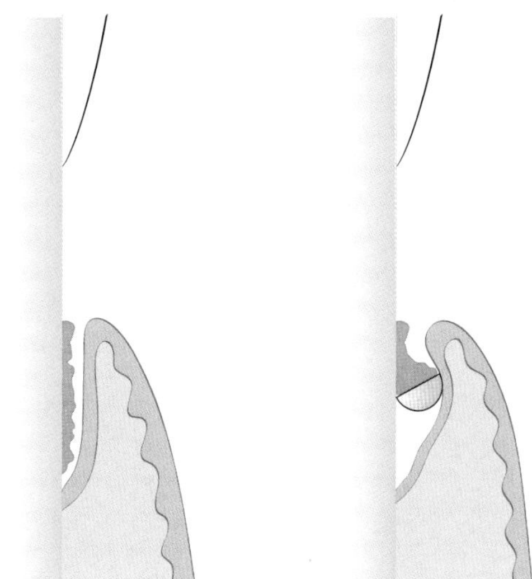

Fig. 51.13 The curette is the instrument of choice for subgingival scaling and root instrumentation (root planing).

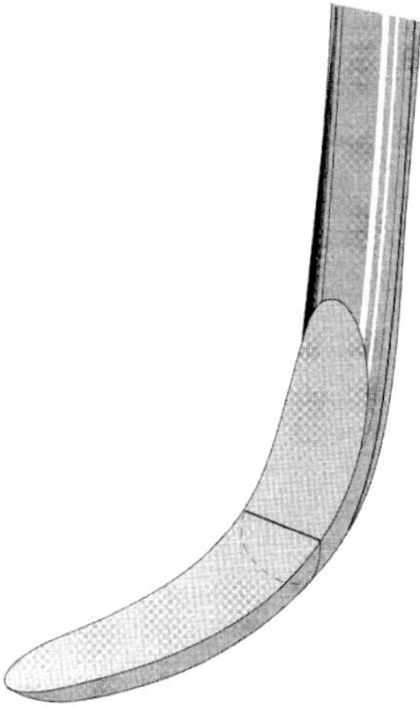

Fig. 51.14 Basic characteristics of a curette: spoon-shaped blade and rounded tip.

LEARNING BOX 51.4

The curette is the instrument of choice for the removal of deep subgingival calculus, root instrumentation (root planing) of altered cementum, and removal of the soft tissue lining the periodontal pocket ("curettage").

As shown in Fig. 51.10, the curved blade and rounded toe of the curette allow the blade to adapt better to the root surface, unlike the straight design and pointed end of a sickle scaler, which can cause tissue laceration and trauma. The two basic types of curettes are universal and area specific.

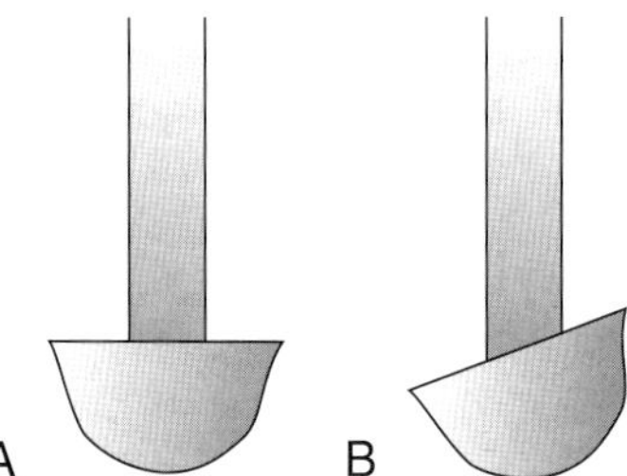

Fig. 51.15 Principal types of curettes as seen from the toe of the instrument. (A) Universal curette. (B) Gracey curette. Note the offset blade angulation of the Gracey curette.

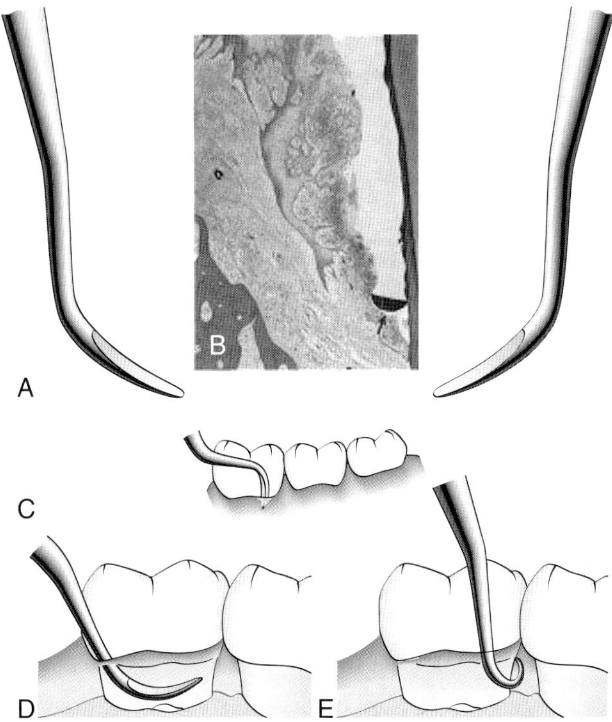

Fig. 51.16 (A) Double-ended curette for the removal of subgingival calculus. (B) Cross section of the curette blade *(arrow)* against the cemental wall of a deep periodontal pocket. (C) Curette inserted in a pocket with the tip directed apically. (D) Curette in position at the base of a periodontal pocket on the facial surface of a mandibular molar. (E) Curette in position at the base of a pocket on the mesial surface of the mandibular molar.

Universal Curettes

Universal curettes have cutting edges that may be inserted in most areas of the dentition by altering and adapting the finger rest, fulcrum, and hand position of the operator. The blade size and the angle and length of the shank may vary, but the face of the blade of every universal curette is at a 90-degree angle (perpendicular) to the lower shank when seen in cross section from the tip (Fig. 51.15A). The blade of the universal curette is curved in one direction from the head of the blade toward the toe. Barnhart curettes #1-2 and #5-6 and Columbia curettes #13-14, #2R-2L, and #4R-4L (Figs. 51.16 and 51.17A) are examples of universal curettes. Other popular universal curettes are the Younger-Good #7-8, and the McCall's #17-18 (see Fig. 51.17B).

LEARNING BOX 51.5

Universal curettes have cutting edges that may be inserted in most areas of the dentition by altering and adapting the finger rest, fulcrum, and hand position of the operator.

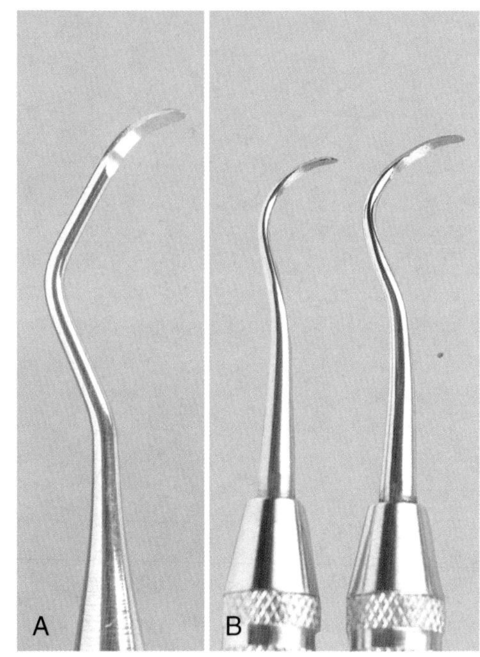

Fig. 51.17 (A) Columbia #4R-4L universal curette. (B) Younger-Good #7-8 and McCall's #17-18 universal curettes.

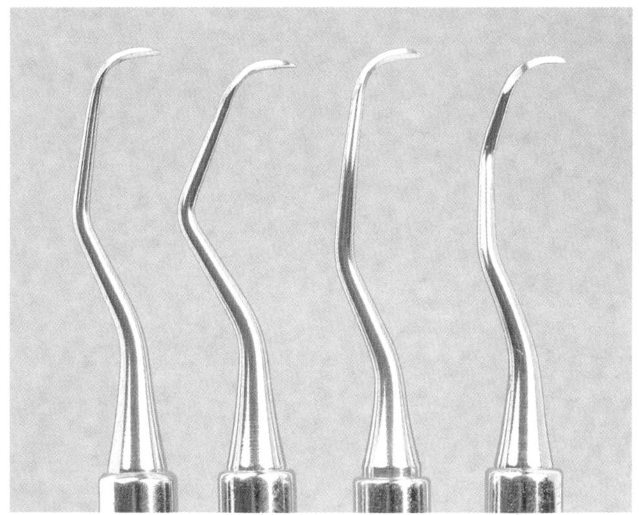

Fig. 51.18 Reduced Set of Gracey Curettes. *Left to right,* #5-6, #7-8, #11-12, and #13-14.

Area-Specific Curettes

Gracey Curettes. Gracey curettes are representative of the area-specific curettes, a set of several instruments designed and angled to adapt to specific anatomic areas of the dentition (Fig. 51.18). These curettes and their modifications are the best instruments for subgingival scaling and root instrumentation (root planing) because they provide the best adaptation to complex root anatomy.

LEARNING BOX 51.6

Gracey curettes are representative of the area-specific curettes, a set of several instruments designed and angled to adapt to specific anatomic areas of the dentition.

Double-ended Gracey curettes are paired in the following manner:
Gracey #1-2 and #3-4: Anterior teeth
Gracey #5-6: Anterior teeth and premolars

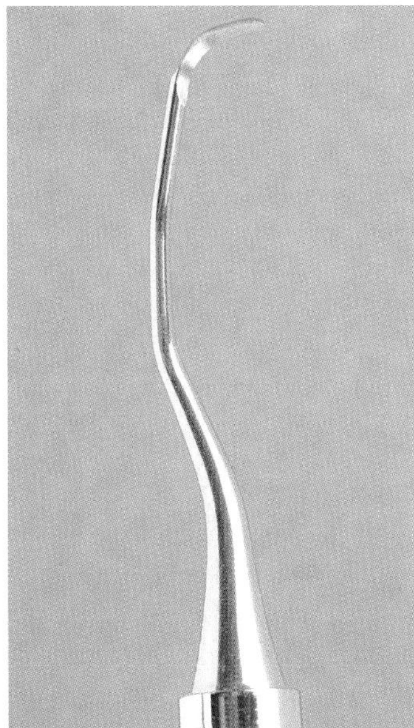

Fig. 51.19 Gracey #11-12 curette. For mesial surfaces.

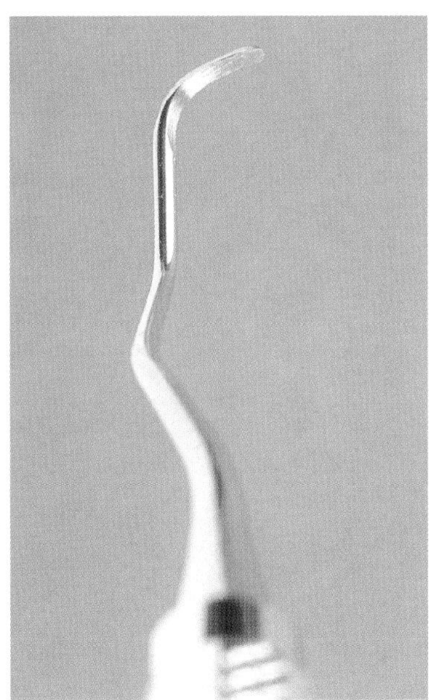

Fig. 51.20 Gracey #13-14 curette. For distal surfaces.

Gracey #7-8 and #9-10: Posterior teeth, facial and lingual
Gracey #11-12: Posterior teeth, mesial (Fig. 51.19)
Gracey #13-14: Posterior teeth, distal (Fig. 51.20)

Single-ended Gracey curettes can also be obtained; a set comprises 14 instruments. Although these curettes are designed to be used in specific areas, an experienced operator can adapt each instrument for use in several different areas by altering the position of his or her hand and the position of the patient.

Gracey curettes also differ from universal curettes in that the blade is not at a 90-degree angle to the lower shank. The term *offset blade* is used to describe Gracey curettes because they are angled approximately 70 degrees from the lower shank (see Fig. 51.15B). This unique angulation allows the blade to be inserted in the precise position necessary for subgingival scaling and root instrumentation (root planing), provided the lower shank is parallel to the long axis of the tooth surface being scaled.

LEARNING BOX 51.7

Gracey curettes also differ from universal curettes in that the blade is not at a 90-degree angle to the lower shank.

Area-specific curettes also have curved blades. Whereas the blade of the universal curette is curved in one direction (Fig. 51.21A), the Gracey blade is curved from shank to toe and also appears to be curved along the side of the cutting edge (see Fig. 51.21B). Table 51.1 lists some of the major differences between Gracey (area-specific) curettes and universal curettes.

Gracey curettes are available with either a "rigid" or "finishing" type of shank. The rigid Gracey has a larger, stronger, and less flexible shank and blade than the standard finishing Gracey. The rigid shank allows the removal of moderate to heavy calculus without using a separate set of heavy scalers, such as sickles and hoes. Although some clinicians prefer the enhanced tactile sensitivity that the flexible shank of the finishing Gracey provides, both types of Gracey curettes are suitable for root instrumentation (root planing).

More recent additions to the Gracey curette set have been #15-16 and #17-18. The Gracey #15-16 is a modification of the standard #11-12 and is designed for the mesial surfaces of posterior teeth (Fig. 51.22). It consists of a Gracey #11-12 blade combined with the more

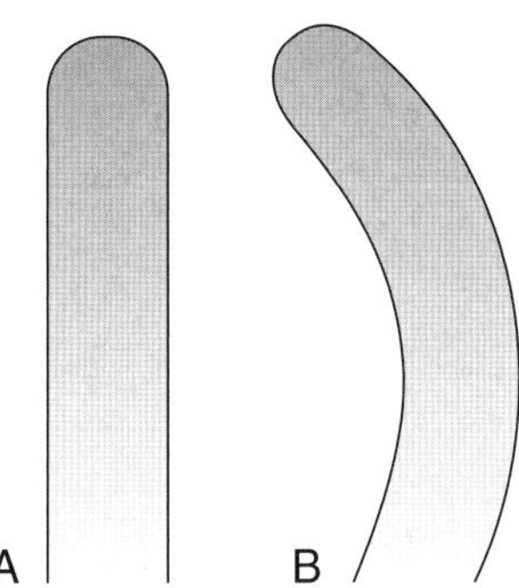

Fig. 51.21 (A) Universal curette as seen with the face of the blade parallel to the floor. Note that the blade is straight. (B) Gracey curette as seen with the face of the blade parallel to the floor. Only the outer convex cutting edge is used.

TABLE 51.1 Comparison of Area-Specific (Gracey) and Universal Curettes

	Gracey Curette	Universal Curette
Area of use	Set of many curettes designed for specific areas and surfaces	One curette designed for all areas and surfaces
Cutting Edge		
Use	One cutting edge used; work with outer edge only	Both cutting edges used; work with either outer or inner edge
Curvature	Blade curves from the shank toward the toe and also appears to curve to the side	Blade curves only from the shank toward the toe, not to the side
Blade angle	Offset blade; face of blade beveled at 60 degrees to shank	Blade not offset; face of blade beveled at 90 degrees to shank

Modified from Pattison G, Pattison A. *Periodontal Instrumentation.* 2nd ed. Norwalk, CT: Appleton & Lange; 1992.

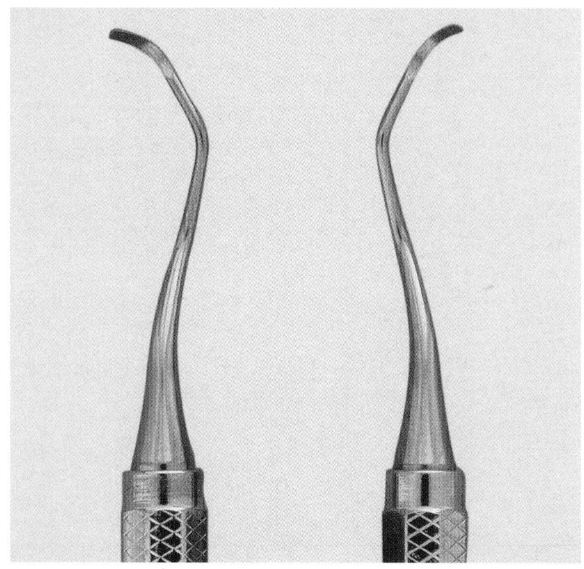

Fig. 51.22 Gracey #15-16. New Gracey curette, designed for mesioposterior surfaces, combines a Gracey #11-12 blade with a Gracey #13-14 shank. (Copyright A. Pattison.)

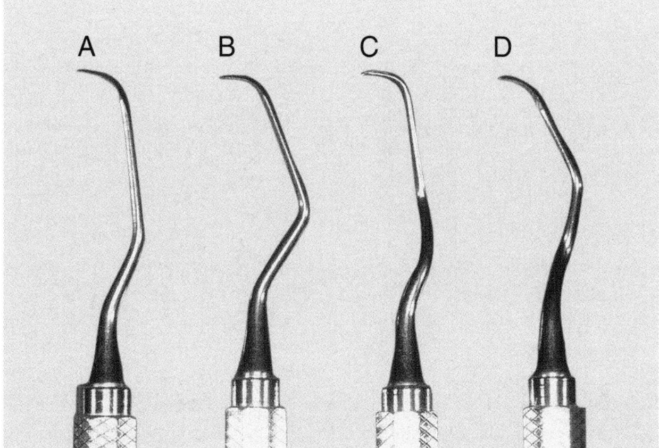

Fig. 51.23 After Five curettes. Note the extra 3 mm in the terminal shank of After Five curettes compared with standard Gracey curettes. (A) #5-6; (B) #7-8; (C) #11-12; (D) #13-14. (Copyright A. Pattison.)

acutely angled #13-14 shank. When the clinician is using an intraoral finger rest, it is often difficult to position the lower shank of the Gracey #11-12 so that it is parallel to the mesial surfaces of the posterior teeth, especially on the mandibular molars. The newer shank angulation of the Gracey #15-16 allows better adaptation to posterior mesial surfaces from a front position with intraoral rests. If alternative fulcrums, such as extraoral or opposite-arch rests, are used, the Gracey #11-12 works well and the #15-16 is not essential. The Gracey #17-18 is a modification of the #13-14. It has a terminal shank elongated by 3 mm and a more accentuated angulation of the shank to provide complete occlusal clearance and better access to all posterior distal surfaces. The horizontal handle position minimizes interference from opposing arches and allows a more relaxed hand position when scaling distal surfaces. In addition, the blade is 1 mm shorter to allow better adaptation of the blade to distal tooth surfaces.

Extended-Shank Curettes. Extended-shank curettes, such as *After Five* curettes (Hu-Friedy, Chicago, IL), are modifications of the standard Gracey curette design. The terminal shank is 3 mm longer, allowing extension into deeper periodontal pockets of 5 mm or more (Figs. 51.23 and 51.24). Other features of After Five curettes include a thinned blade for smoother subgingival insertion and reduced tissue distention and a large-diameter, tapered shank. All standard Gracey numbers except for the #9-10 (i.e., #1-2, #3-4, #5-6, #7-8, #11-12, or #13-14) are available in the After Five series. After Five curettes are available in finishing or rigid designs. For heavy or tenacious calculus removal, rigid After Five curettes should be used. For light scaling or deplaquing in a periodontal maintenance patient, the thinner finishing After Five curettes will insert subgingivally more easily.

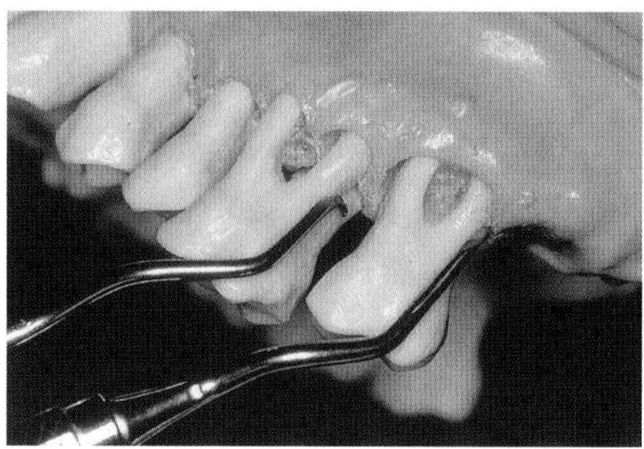

Fig. 51.24 Comparison of After Five curette with standard Gracey curette. Rigid Gracey #13-14 adapted to the distal surface of the first molar and rigid After Five #13-14 adapted to the distal surface of the second molar. Notice the extralong shank of the After Five curette, which allows deeper insertion and better access. (Copyright A. Pattison.)

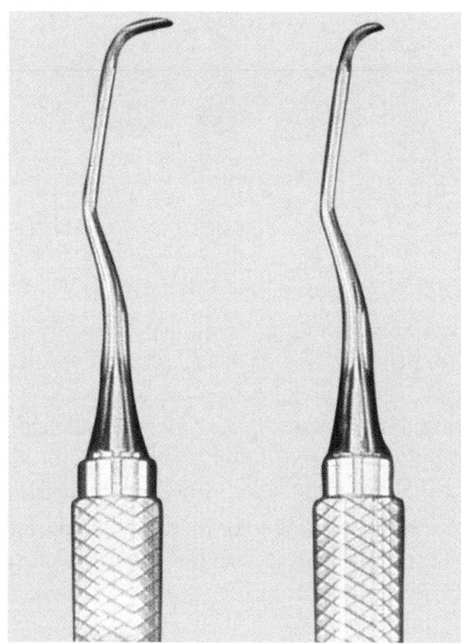

Fig. 51.25 Comparison of After Five curette and Mini Five curette. The shorter Mini Five blade (half the length) allows increased access and reduced tissue trauma.

LEARNING BOX 51.8

Extended-shank curettes, such as After Five curettes (Hu-Friedy, Chicago, IL), are modifications of the standard Gracey curette design.

Mini-Bladed Curettes. Mini-bladed curettes, such as Hu-Friedy *Mini Five* curettes, are modifications of the After Five curettes. Mini Five curettes feature blades that are half the length of After Five or standard Gracey curettes (Fig. 51.25). The shorter blade allows easier insertion and adaptation in deep, narrow pockets; furcations; developmental grooves; line angles; and deep, tight facial, lingual, or palatal pockets. In any area where root morphology or tight tissue prevents full insertion of the standard Gracey or After Five blade, Mini Five curettes can be used with vertical strokes, with reduced tissue distention and no tissue trauma (Fig. 51.26).

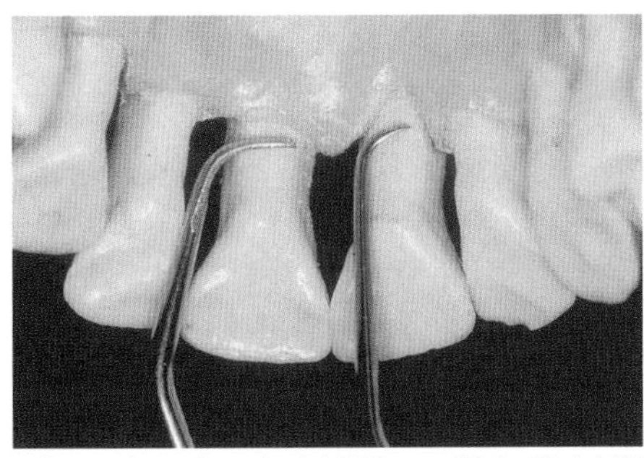

Fig. 51.26 Comparison of standard rigid Gracey #5-6 with rigid Mini Five #5-6 on the palatal surfaces of the maxillary central incisors. Mini Five curette can be inserted into the base of these tight anterior pockets and used with a straight vertical stroke. The standard Gracey or After Five curette usually cannot be inserted vertically in this area because the blade is too long. (Copyright A. Pattison.)

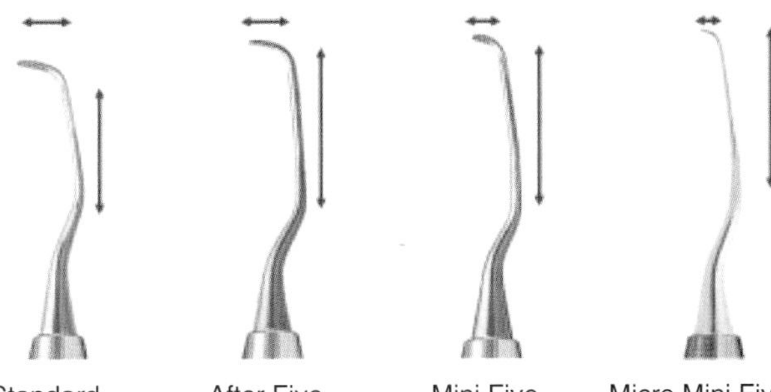

Fig. 51.28 Comparison of Gracey curette designs. *Left to right,* Standard #1-2, After Five #1-2, Mini Five #1-2, Micro Mini Five #1-2. (Courtesy Hu-Friedy, Chicago, IL.)

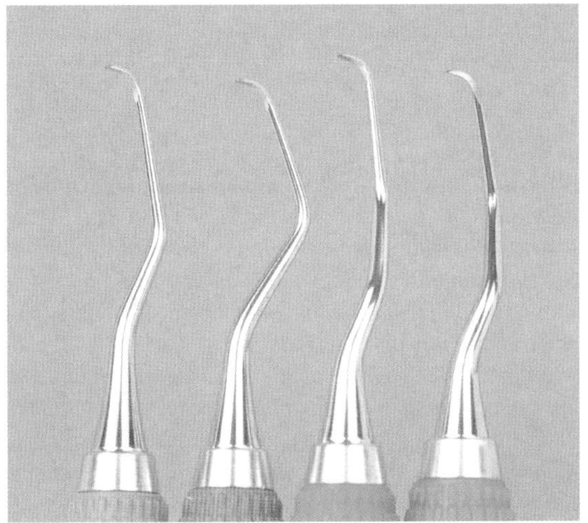

Fig. 51.27 Micro Mini Five Gracey curettes. *Left to right,* #1-2, #7-8, #11-12, #13-14. (Copyright A. Pattison.)

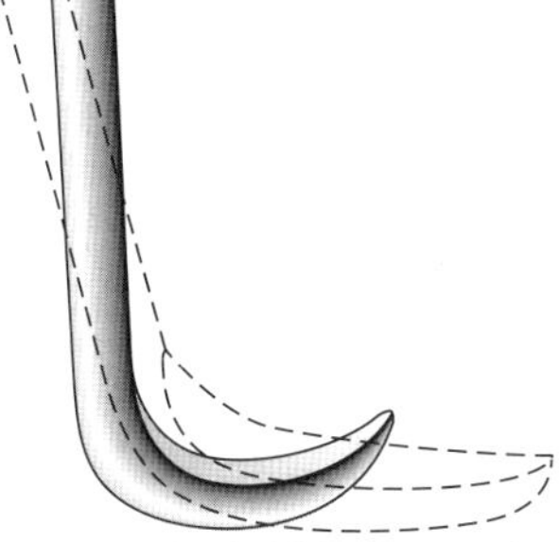

Fig. 51.29 Gracey curvette blade. This diagram shows the 50% shorter blade of the Gracey Curvette superimposed on the standard Gracey curette blade *(dotted lines).* Notice the upward curvature of the Curvette blade and blade tip. (Redrawn from Pattison G, Pattison A. *Periodontal Instrumentation,* 2nd ed. Norwalk, CT: Appleton & Lange; 1992.)

LEARNING BOX 51.9

Mini Five curettes (Hu-Friedy, Chicago, IL) feature blades that are half the length of After Five or standard Gracey curettes. The shorter blade allows easier insertion and adaptation in deep, narrow pockets; furcations; developmental grooves; line angles; and deep, tight facial, lingual, or palatal pockets.

In the past, the only solution in most of these areas of difficult access was to use Gracey curettes with a toe-down horizontal stroke. Mini Five curettes, along with other short-bladed instruments recently introduced, opened a new chapter in the history of root instrumentation by allowing access to areas that previously were extremely difficult or impossible to reach with standard instruments. Mini Five curettes are available in both finishing and rigid designs. Rigid Mini Five curettes are recommended for calculus removal. The more flexible shanked finishing Mini Five curettes are appropriate for light scaling and deplaquing in periodontal maintenance patients with tight pockets. As with the After Five series, Mini Five curettes are available in all standard Gracey numbers, except the #9-10.

The recently introduced *Micro Mini Five* Gracey curettes (Hu-Friedy) have blades that are 20% thinner and smaller than the Mini Five curettes (Figs. 51.27 and 51.28). These are the smallest of all curettes, and they provide exceptional access and adaptation to tight, deep, or narrow pockets; narrow furcations; developmental depressions; line angles; and deep pockets on facial, lingual, or palatal surfaces. In areas where root morphology or tight, thin tissue prevents easy insertion of other mini-bladed curettes, Micro Mini Five curettes can be used with vertical strokes without causing tissue distention or tissue trauma.

LEARNING BOX 51.10

Micro Mini Five Gracey curettes (Hu-Friedy, Chicago, IL) have blades that are 20% thinner and smaller than the Mini Five curettes These are the smallest of all curettes, and they provide exceptional access and adaptation to tight, deep, or narrow pockets; narrow furcations; developmental depressions; line angles; and deep pockets on facial, lingual, or palatal surfaces.

Gracey Curvettes comprise another set of four mini-bladed curettes; the Sub-0 and #1-2 are used for anterior teeth and premolars, the #11-12 is used for posterior mesial surfaces, and the #13-14 is used for posterior distal surfaces. The blade length of these instruments is 50% shorter than that of the conventional Gracey curette, and the blade is curved slightly upward (Fig. 51.29). This curvature allows Gracey Curvettes to adapt more closely to the tooth surface than any other curettes, especially on the anterior teeth and on line angles (Fig. 51.30). However, this curvature also carries the risk of gouging or "grooving" into the root surfaces on the proximal surfaces of the posterior teeth when #11-12 or #13-14 is used. Additional features that represent improvements on the standard Gracey curettes are a precision-balanced blade tip in direct

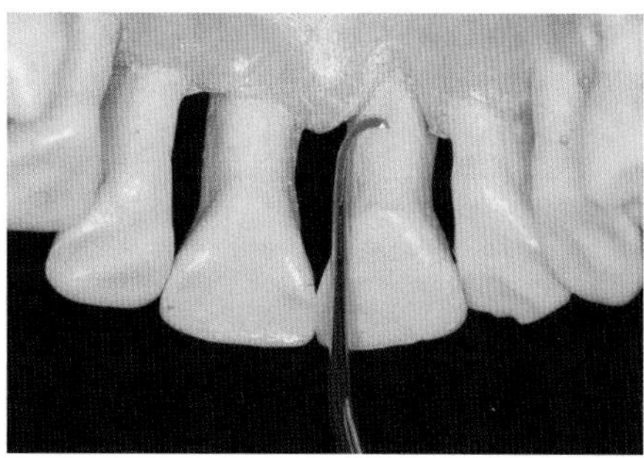

Fig. 51.30 Gracey curvette sub-0 on the palatal surface of a maxillary central incisor. The long shank and short, curved, blunted tip make this a superior instrument for deep anterior pockets. This curette provides excellent blade adaptation to the narrow root curvatures of the maxillary and mandibular anterior teeth. (Copyright A. Pattison.)

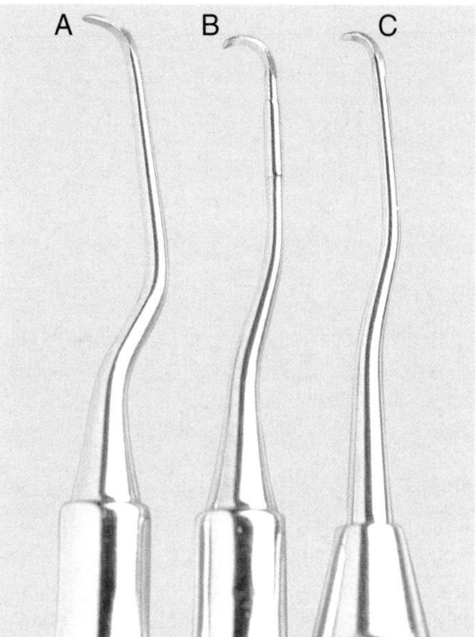

Fig. 51.31 Comparison of three different mini-bladed instruments designed for use on the maxillary and mandibular anterior teeth. (A) Hu-Friedy Mini Five #5-6; (B) Hu-Friedy Curvette Sub-0; (C) Hartzell Sub-0. (Copyright A. Pattison.)

alignment with the handle, a blade tip perpendicular to the handle, and a shank closer to parallel with the handle.

For many years, the *Morse scaler,* a miniature sickle, was the only mini-bladed instrument available. However, mini-bladed curettes have largely replaced this instrument (Fig. 51.31).

Periodontal Maintenance Curettes. The most recent Gracey curette innovation is a category called periodontal maintenance Gracey curettes, introduced in November 2015. These instruments are specifically designed for patients with tight tissue, recession, and residual pocket depth following initial periodontal therapy or periodontal surgery. They can also be used on maintenance patients with healthier tight tissue without attachment loss or recession. In both cases, patients require a small, thin blade to allow subgingival insertion with ease (Fig. 51.32).

LEARNING BOX 51.11

The most recent Gracey curette innovation is a category called periodontal maintenance Gracey curettes, introduced in November 2015. These instruments are specifically designed for patients with tight tissue, recession, and residual pocket depth following initial periodontal therapy or periodontal surgery.

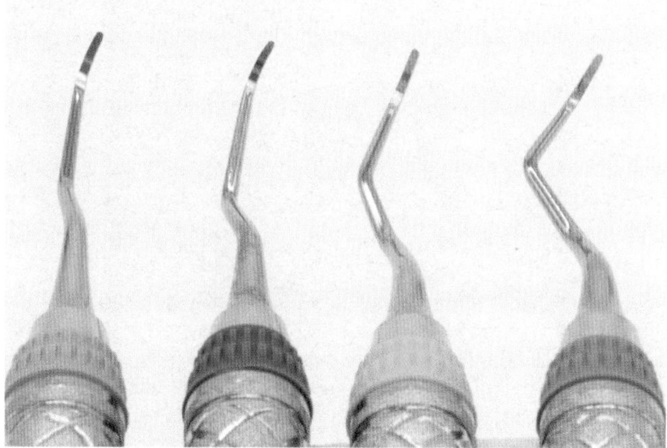

Fig. 51.32 Periodontal maintenance Gracey curettes (Hu-Friedy) shorter, thinner three-quarter–sized Gracey curettes with modified rigid shanks. *Left to right,* Pattison Gracey Lite #1-2, Pattison Gracey Lite #7-8, Pattison Gracey Lite #11-12, Pattison Gracey Lite #13-14. (Copyright A. Pattison.)

This newer blade is 1 mm shorter and 20% thinner, and the face of the blade is offset from the terminal shank at 60 degrees as opposed to all other Gracey designs, which are offset at 70 degrees. This slight modification to the blade-to-shank angle and the thinner, narrow blade allows easier insertion and better access to root surfaces with tight tissue and loss of attachment. Working angulation can be achieved without as much tissue distention, thus increasing patient comfort. The three-quarter blade length of this new type of Gracey curette is between the blade lengths of the standard and mini-bladed Gracey curettes. The shorter blade adapts more easily to root anatomy and furcation areas and helps to prevent spanning across root depressions.

The shank length is 2 mm longer than that of the standard Gracey curette, but 1 mm shorter than that of the extended shank Gracey curette. This length enables better access to molar areas with attachment loss but still allows ease of use in the anterior areas where a very long shank is not necessary. The shank angle of the new Gracey #11-12 is between the regular Gracey #11-12 and the Gracey #15-16, and the shank angle of the new Gracey #13-14 is between the regular Gracey #13-14 and the Gracey #17-18. These shank angle modifications were developed to enhance access to the mesial and distal surfaces of the posterior teeth.

The shanks of these newer instruments are rigid so they can withstand firm pressure when the removal of residual burnished calculus is necessary. However, they are not designed for moderate or heavy calculus removal. The clinician must be mindful that the instrument blade is at a slightly more closed angle than the traditional Gracey curette, so if more substantial or tenacious calculus is encountered, the clinician must slightly open the blade angulation, or switch to a rigid standard Gracey curette, or use a different manual or ultrasonic instrument.

Langer and Mini-Langer Curettes. Langer and Mini Langer curettes comprise a set of three curettes combining the shank design of standard Gracey #5-6, #11-12, and #13-14 curettes with a universal blade honed at 90 degrees rather than the offset blade of the Gracey curette. This marriage of the Gracey and universal curette designs allows the advantages of the area-specific shank to be combined with the versatility of the universal curette blade. The Langer #5-6 curette adapts to the mesial and distal surfaces of anterior teeth; the Langer #1-2 curette (Gracey #11-12 shank) adapts to the mesial and distal surfaces of mandibular posterior teeth; the Langer #3-4 curette (Gracey #13-14 shank) adapts to the mesial and distal surfaces of maxillary posterior teeth (Fig. 51.33). These instruments can be adapted to both

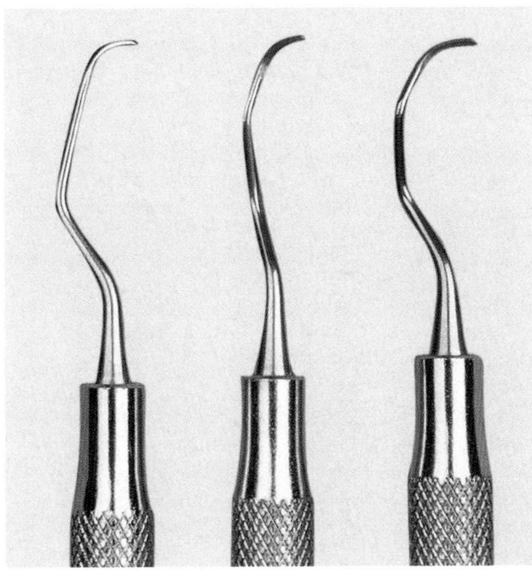

Fig. 51.33 Langer curettes combine Gracey-type shanks with universal curette blades. *Left to right,* #5-6, #1-2, and #3-4. (Copyright A. Pattison.)

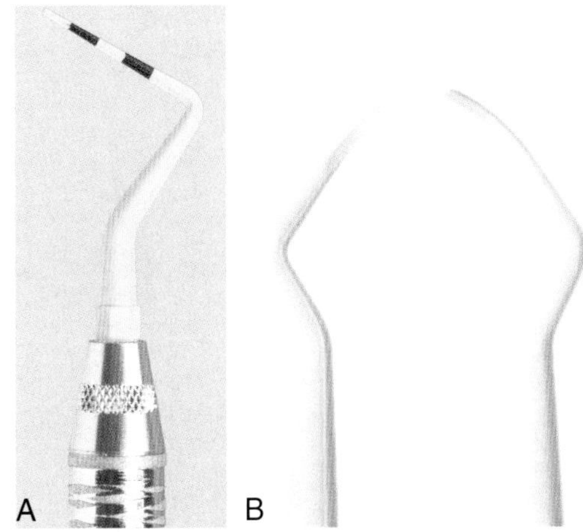

Fig. 51.35 (A) Plastic probe: Colorvue. (B) New Implacare II Barnhart #5-6 cone socket plastic curette tips that screw into an autoclavable stainless steel handle. (Courtesy Hu-Friedy, Chicago, IL.)

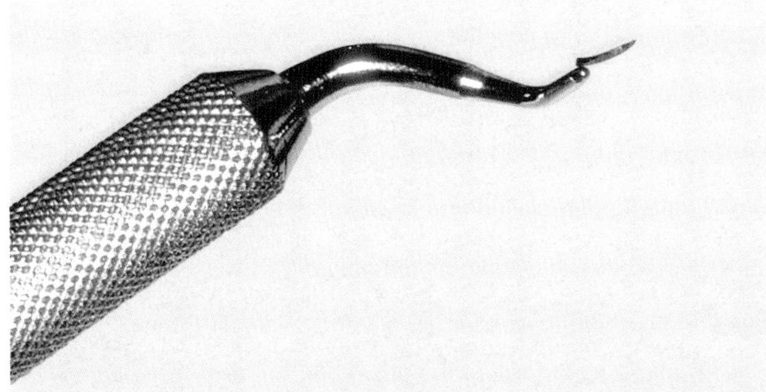

Fig. 51.34 Broken instrument tip attached to the magnetic tip of a Schwartz periotriever (Daness Dental Distributors, Nyack, NY). (From Pattison G, Pattison A. *Periodontal Instrumentation.* 2nd ed. Norwalk, CT: Appleton & Lange; 1992.)

mesial and distal tooth surfaces without changing instruments. The standard Langer curette shanks are heavier than a finishing Gracey but less rigid than the rigid Gracey. Langer curettes are also available with either rigid or finishing shanks and can be obtained in extended-shank (After Five) and mini-bladed (Mini Five) versions.

Schwartz Periotrievers

Schwartz Periotrievers comprise a set of two double-ended, highly magnetized instruments designed for retrieval of a broken instrument tip from the periodontal pocket (Fig. 51.34). They are indispensable when the clinician has broken a curette tip in a furcation or deep pocket.[11]

Plastic and Titanium Instruments for Implants

Several companies are manufacturing plastic and titanium instruments for use on titanium and other implant abutment materials. It is important that plastic or titanium instruments be used to avoid scarring and permanent damage to implants (Figs. 51.35–51.37).[12–17]

Mini-bladed titanium implant instruments are now available in both universal and Gracey curette designs (see Fig. 51.37B). Although most standard titanium implant instrument blades are large, the newer mini-bladed titanium curettes insert more easily under tight tissue and adapt more easily around implants and implant restorations. They may be used for implant maintenance with careful, light-pressured strokes for biofilm and light calculus removal.

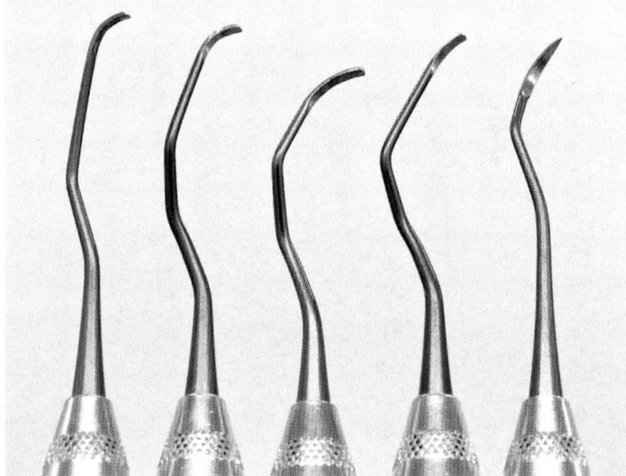

Fig. 51.36 New mini-titanium implant scalers (Hu-Friedy, Chicago). *Left to right,* Mini Five Gracey #1-2, Mini Five Gracey #11-12, Langer #1-2, Mini Five Gracey #13-14, 204SD Sickle Scaler.

Moderate- or heavy-pressured strokes should be avoided to prevent scratching or roughening of implant surfaces. These instruments are not intended for the removal of heavy calculus or cement. Such deposits are often found in cases of peri-implantitis with moderate to advanced bone loss and exposure of implant threads. Removal of tenacious deposits requires other forms of instrumentation and surgical treatment of the implant. (See Chapter 86 for information on treatment of peri-implantitis.)

LEARNING BOX 51.12

Several companies are manufacturing plastic and titanium instruments for use on titanium and other implant abutment materials. It is important that plastic or titanium instruments be used to avoid scarring and permanent damage to implants

Hoe Scalers

Hoe scalers are used for scaling of ledges or rings of calculus (Fig. 51.38). The blade is bent at a 99-degree angle, and the cutting edge is formed by the junction of the flattened terminal surface with the inner aspect of the blade. The cutting edge is beveled at 45 degrees.

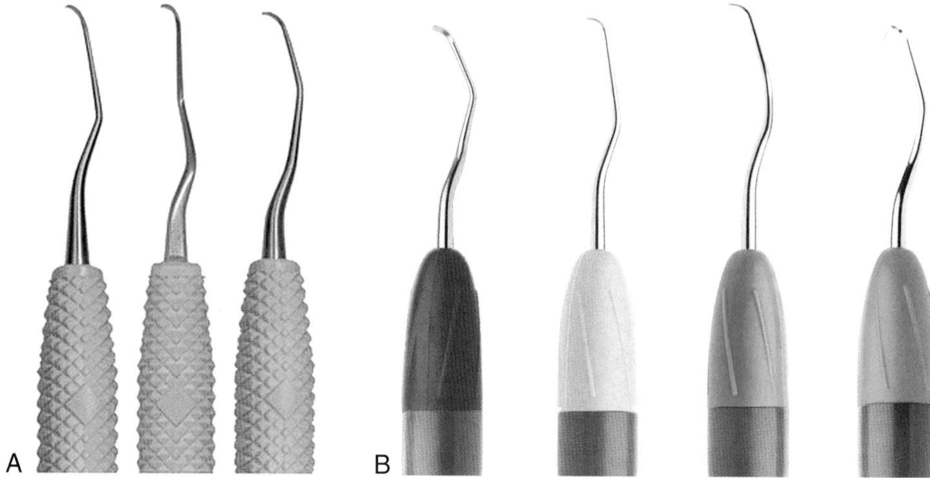

Fig. 51.37 (A) Micro mini-titanium implant curettes (Paradise Dental Technologies, Missoula, MT). *Left to right,* Gracey #1-2 Micro Mini, Gracey #11-12 Micro Mini, Gracey #13-14 Micro Mini. (B) Mini-bladed titanium implant curettes (LM Instruments, Parainen, Finland): Mini universal curette, Mini Gracey #1-2, Mini Gracey #13-14, Mini Gracey #11-12.

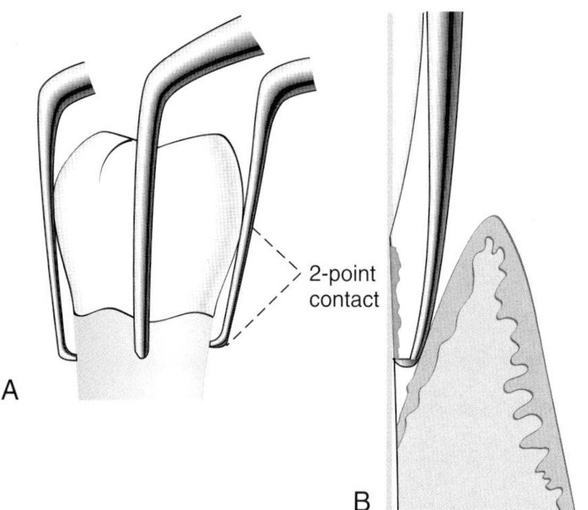

Fig. 51.38 (A) Hoe scalers designed for different tooth surfaces, showing "two-point" contact. (B) Hoe scaler in a periodontal pocket. The back of the blade is rounded for easier access. The instrument contacts the tooth at two points for stability.

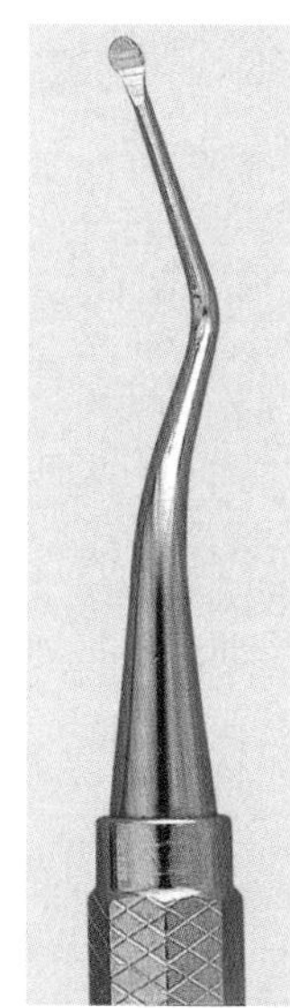

Fig. 51.39 Hirshfeld file.

The blade is slightly bowed so that it can maintain contact at two points on a convex surface. The back of the blade is rounded, and the blade has been reduced to minimal thickness to permit access to the roots without interference from the adjacent tissues.

Hoe scalers are used in the following manner:

1. The blade is inserted into the base of the periodontal pocket so that it makes two-point contact with the tooth (see Fig. 51.38). This stabilizes the instrument and prevents nicking of the root.
2. The instrument is activated with a firm pull stroke toward the crown, with every effort made to preserve the two-point contact with the tooth.

McCall's #3, #4, #5, #6, #7, and #8 comprise a set of six hoe scalers designed to provide access to all tooth surfaces. Each instrument has a different angle between the shank and the handle.

Files

Files have a series of blades on a base (Fig. 51.39). Their primary function is to fracture or crush large deposits of tenacious calculus or burnished sheets of calculus. Files can easily gouge and roughen root surfaces when they are used improperly. Therefore they are not suitable for fine scaling and root instrumentation (root planing). Mini-bladed curettes are currently preferred for fine scaling in areas where files were once used. Files are sometimes used for removing overhanging margins of dental restorations.

LEARNING BOX 51.13

Files have a series of blades on a base. Their primary function is to fracture or crush large deposits of tenacious calculus or burnished sheets of calculus.

Quétin Furcation Curettes

Quétin furcation curettes are actually hoes with a shallow, half-moon radius that fits into the roof or floor of the furcation. The curvature of the tip also fits into developmental depressions on the inner aspect of the roots. The shanks are slightly curved for better access, and the tips are available in two widths (Fig. 51.40). The BL1 *(buccal-lingual)* and MD1 *(mesial-distal)* instruments are small and fine, with a 0.9-mm blade width. The BL2 and MD2 instruments are larger and wider, with a 1.3-mm blade width.

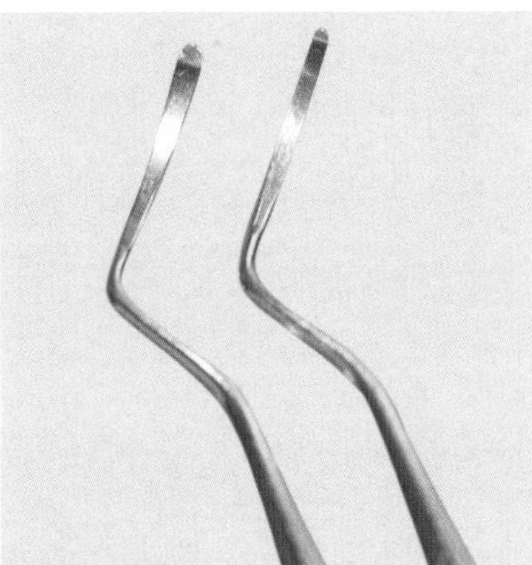

Fig. 51.40 Quétin furcation curettes: BL2 (larger) and BL1 (smaller). (Copyright A. Pattison.)

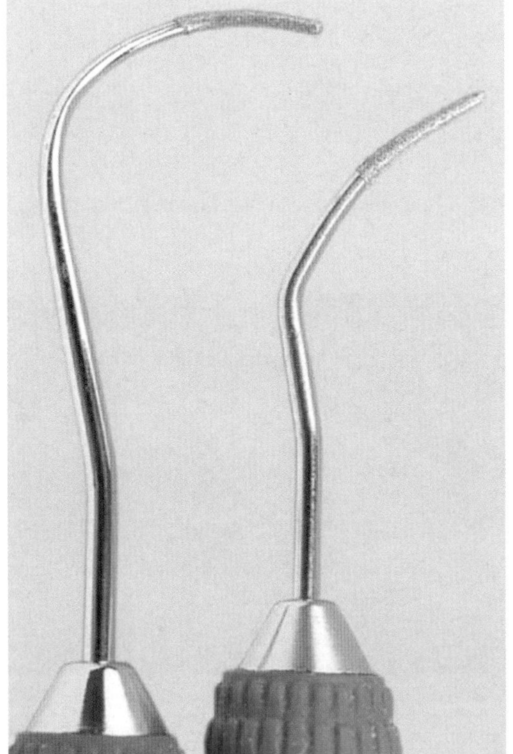

Fig. 51.41 Diamond files. SDCN 7, SDCM/D 7. (Hu-Friedy, Chicago.) (Copyright A. Pattison.)

These instruments remove burnished calculus from recessed areas of the furcation where curettes, even mini-bladed curettes, are often too large to gain access. Using mini-bladed Gracey curettes and Gracey Curvettes on the ceiling or floor of the furcation may unintentionally create gouges and grooves. The Quétin instruments, however, are well suited for this area and lessen the likelihood of root damage.

Diamond-Coated Files

Diamond-coated files are unique instruments used for the final finishing of root surfaces. These files do not have cutting edges; instead, they are coated with very fine-grit diamond (Fig. 51.41). The most useful diamond files are the buccal-lingual instruments, which are used in furcations and also adapt well to many other root surfaces.

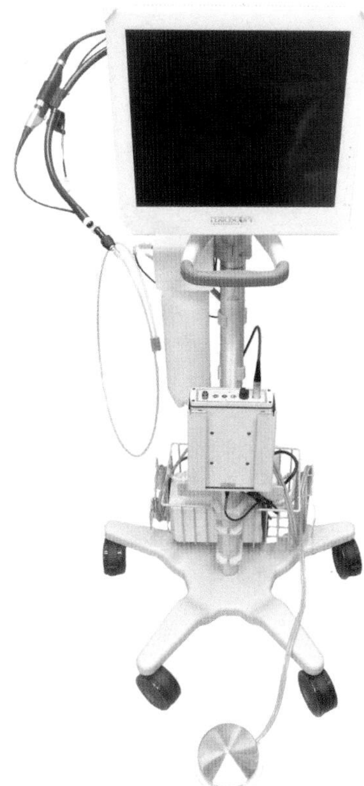

Fig. 51.42 Perioscopy system, dental endoscope. (Courtesy Perioscopy, Inc., Zest Dental Solutions, Carlsbad, CA.)

New diamond files are sharply abrasive and should be used with light, even pressure against the root surface to avoid gouging or grooving. When viewing the root surface with the dental endoscope after all tactilely detectable deposits are gone, one can observe small embedded remnants of calculus in the root surface. Diamond files are used similar to an emery board to remove these minute remnants of calculus from the root, to create a surface that is free of all visible accretions. Diamond files can produce a smooth, even, clean, and highly polished root surface.

Diamond files must be used carefully because they can cause overinstrumentation of the root surface. They will remove too much root structure if they are used with excessive force, are poorly adapted to root morphology, or are used too long in one place.

Diamond files are particularly effective when used with the dental endoscope, which reveals residual deposits and directs the clinician to the exact area for instrumentation.

Ultrasonic and Sonic Instruments

Ultrasonic instruments may be used for removing biofilm, scaling, curetting, and removing stains (see Chapter 52).

Dental Endoscope

The dental endoscope is used subgingivally in the diagnosis and treatment of periodontal disease (Fig. 51.42). The device consists of a 0.99-mm-diameter reusable fiberoptic endoscope over which a disposable sterile sheath is placed. The fiberoptic endoscope fits onto periodontal probes that have been designed to accept it (Fig. 51.43). The sheath delivers water irrigation that flushes the pocket while the endoscope is being used, thereby keeping the field clear. The fiberoptic endoscope attaches to a medical-grade charge-coupled device (CCD) video camera and a light source that produces an image on a flat-panel monitor for viewing during subgingival exploration and instrumentation. This device allows clear

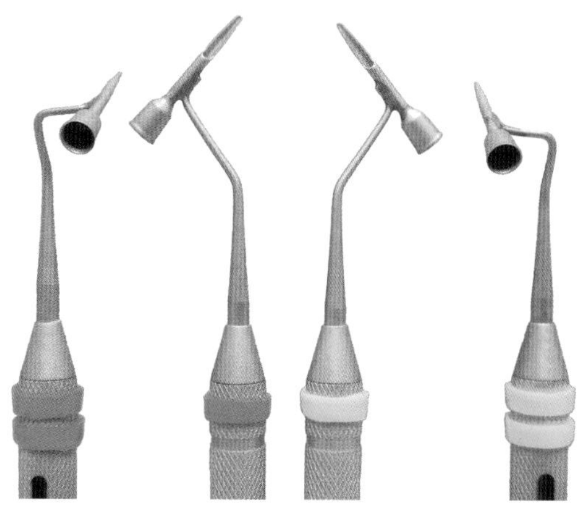

Fig. 51.43 Viewing periodontal explorers (left/right/full viewing) for the perioscopy system. (Courtesy Perioscopy, Inc., Zest Dental Solutions, Carlsbad, CA.)

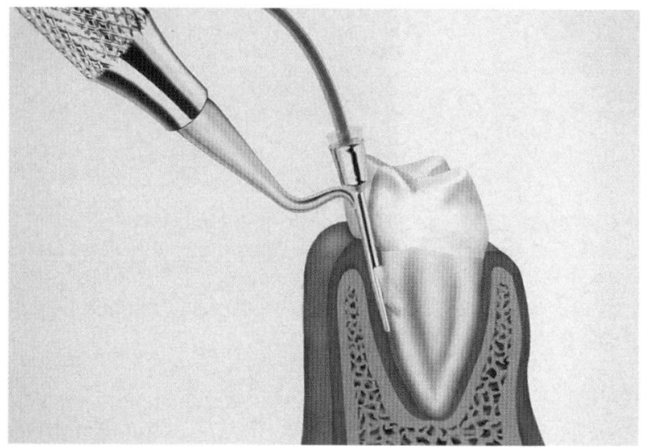

Fig. 51.44 Perioscopic instrumentation permits deep subgingival visualization in pockets and furcations. (Courtesy Perioscopy, Inc., Zest Dental Solutions, Carlsbad, CA.)

visualization deep into subgingival pockets and furcations (Fig. 51.44). It permits operators to detect the presence and location of subgingival deposits and guides them in the thorough removal of these deposits. Magnification ranges from 24 to 48 times, enabling visualization of even minute deposits of plaque and calculus. Using this device, operators can achieve levels of root debridement and cleanliness that are much more difficult or impossible to produce without it.[18–24] The dental endoscope can also be used to evaluate subgingival areas for caries, defective restorations, root fractures, and resorption.

LEARNING BOX 51.14

Using this device, clinicians can achieve levels of root debridement and cleanliness that are much more difficult or impossible to produce without it. The dental endoscope can also be used to evaluate subgingival areas for caries, defective restorations, root fractures, and resorption.

Cleansing and Polishing Instruments

Rubber Cups

Rubber cups consist of a rubber shell with or without webbed configurations in the hollow interior (Fig. 51.45). They are used in the handpiece with a prophylaxis angle. The handpiece, prophylaxis angle, and rubber cup must be sterilized after each patient use, or a disposable plastic prophylaxis angle and rubber cup may be used and then discarded (Fig. 51.46). Recently, an innovative anti-splatter prophylaxis angle has been introduced. A small plastic flange positioned against the side of the rubber cup prevents splatter by removing excess saliva and polishing paste from the spinning cup (Fig. 51.46A) (Lotus DPA, Diamond Bar, CA).

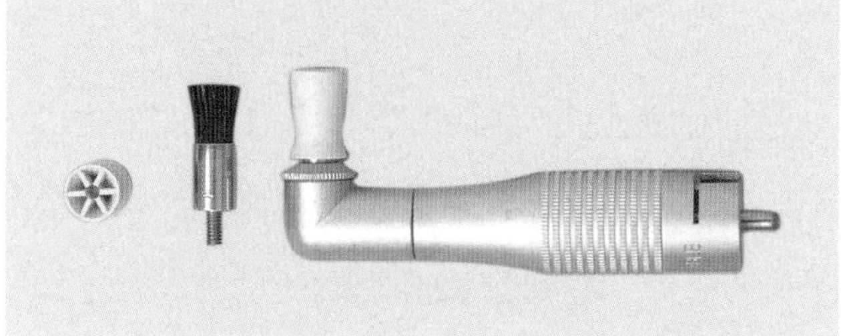

Fig. 51.45 Metal prophylaxis angle with rubber cup and brush.

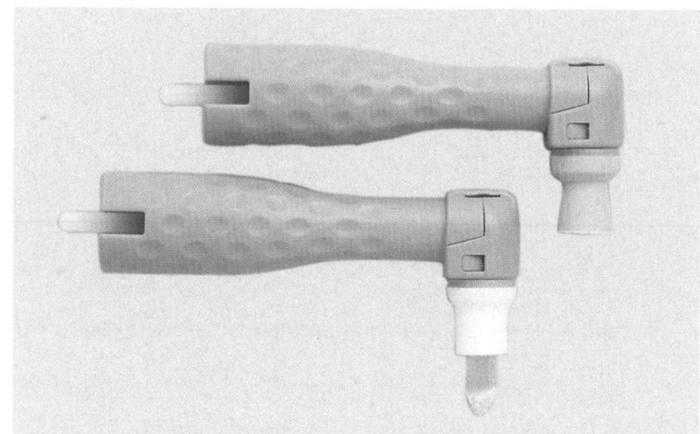

Fig. 51.46 Disposable plastic prophylaxis angle with rubber cup and with brush.

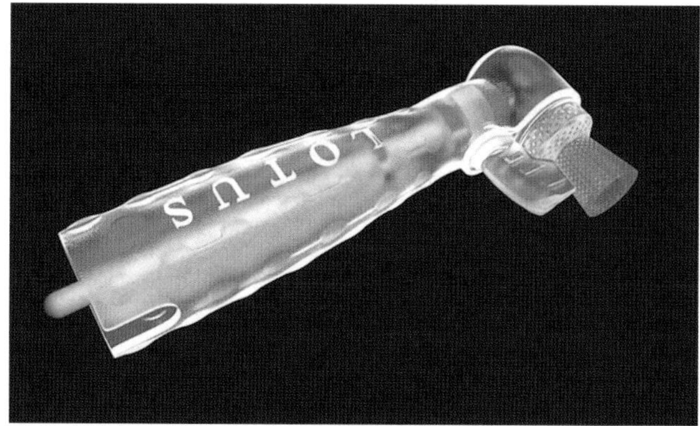

Fig. 51.46a Lotus anti-splatter prophylaxis angle. Dimples on the outside of the cup retain the slurry then the splatter guard removes the accumulated excess saliva and paste during each cup rotation. (Courtesy Lotus DPA, Diamond Bar, CA.)

A good cleansing and polishing paste that contains fluoride should be used and kept moist to minimize frictional heat as the cup revolves. Polishing pastes are available in fine, medium, or coarse grit and are packaged in small, convenient, single-use containers. Aggressive use of the rubber cup with any abrasive may remove the layer of cementum, which is thin in the cervical area.

Bristle Brushes

Bristle brushes are available in wheel and cup shapes (see Fig. 51.45). The brush is used in the prophylaxis angle with a polishing paste. Because the bristles are stiff, use of the brush should be confined to the crown to avoid injuring the cementum and the gingiva.

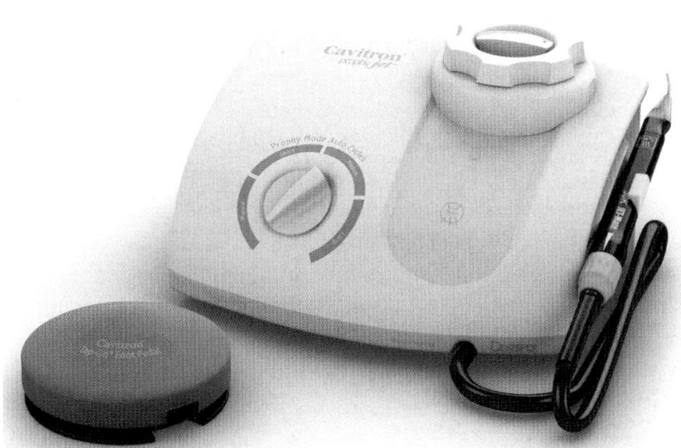

Fig. 51.47 Cavitron ProphyJet Air-powder polishing device. (Courtesy Dentsply International, York, PA.)

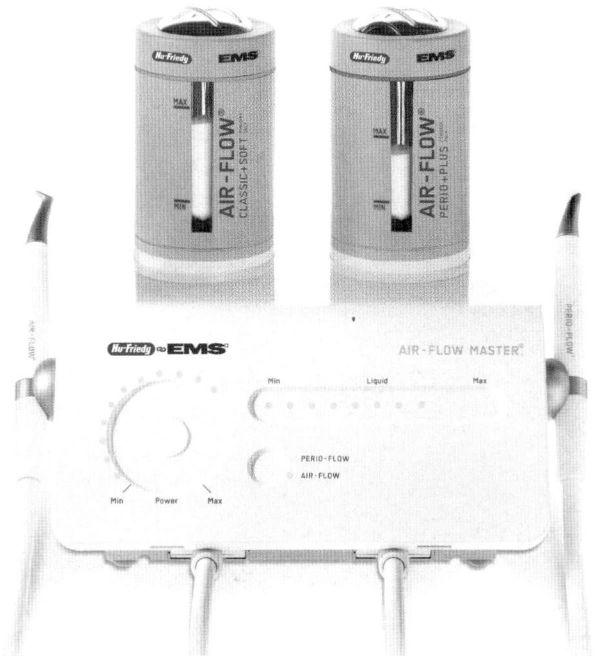

Fig. 51.48 Hu-Friedy EMS Air Flow Master air polishing device with perio and standard handpieces and tips for both supragingival and subgingival air polishing. (Courtesy Hu-Friedy, Chicago, IL.)

Dental Tape

Dental tape with polishing paste is used for polishing proximal surfaces that are inaccessible to other polishing instruments. The tape is passed interproximally while being kept at a right angle to the long axis of the tooth and is activated with a firm labiolingual motion. Particular care is taken to avoid injury to the gingiva. The area should be cleansed with warm water to remove all remnants of paste.

Air-Powder Polishing

The first specially designed handpiece to deliver an air-powered slurry of warm water and sodium bicarbonate for polishing was introduced in the early 1980s. This device, called the *Prophy-Jet* (Dentsply International, York, PA), is very effective for removing extrinsic stains and soft deposits (Fig. 51.47). The slurry removes stains rapidly and efficiently by mechanical abrasion and provides warm water for rinsing and lavage. The flow rate of the abrasive cleansing power can be adjusted to increase the amount of powder for heavier stain removal. Currently, many manufacturers produce improved air-powder polishing systems with both supragingival and subgingival tips that use various powder formulas (Fig. 51.48).

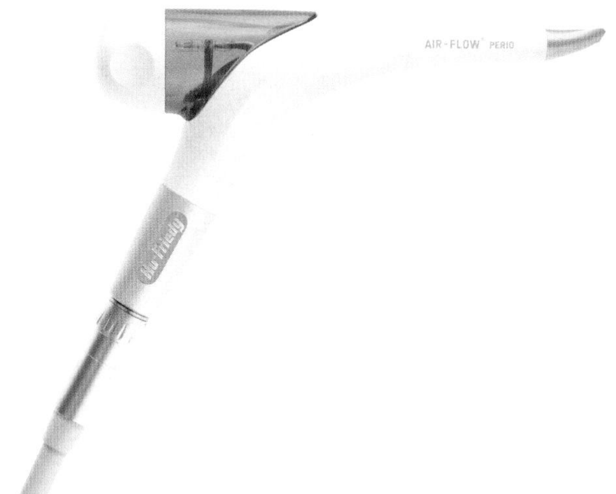

Fig. 51.49 Hu-Friedy EMS Air Flow Perio Handy smaller air polishing device with subgingival air polishing tip for glycine or erythritol powder polishing. (Courtesy Hu-Friedy, Chicago, IL.)

The results of studies on the abrasive effect of air-powder polishing devices using sodium bicarbonate and aluminum trihydroxide on cementum and dentin show that significant tooth substance can be lost.[25–28] Damage to gingival tissue is transient and insignificant clinically, but amalgam restorations, composite resins, cements, and other nonmetallic materials can be roughened.[29–33] Polishing powders containing glycine or erythritol rather than sodium bicarbonate are commonly used for subgingival biofilm removal from root surfaces and implants.[34,35]

Both supragingival and subgingival air polishing with glycine or erythritol powder are safe and very effective for the removal of biofilm from titanium implant surfaces and restorative materials (Fig. 51.49).[36–38]

LEARNING BOX 51.15

Both supragingival and subgingival air polishing with glycine or erythritol powder are safe and very effective for the removal of biofilm from titanium implant surfaces and restorative materials.

No soft tissue abrasion occurs, and at probing depths of 1 mm to greater than 5 mm, the use of glycine or erythritol powder in an air-polishing device with a subgingival nozzle (Fig. 51.50) is more effective for subgingival biofilm removal than the use of either manual or ultrasonic instruments.[39–50]

LEARNING BOX 51.16

The use of glycine or erythritol powder in an air-polishing device with a subgingival nozzle is more effective for subgingival biofilm removal than the use of either manual or ultrasonic instruments.

Patients with a medical history of respiratory illness or hemodialysis are not candidates for the use of the air-powder polishing device.[51,52] Powder containing sodium bicarbonate should not be used on patients with a history of hypertension, sodium-restricted diet, or medication use affecting electrolyte balance.[53]

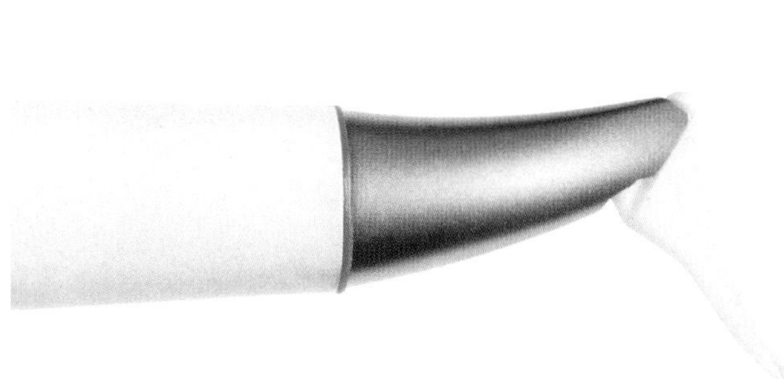

Fig. 51.50 Hu-Friedy EMS Perio Flow Tip disposable plastic tip with millimeter markings for subgingival air polishing of implants or deep pockets with glycine or erythritol powder. (Courtesy Hu-Friedy, Chicago IL.)

Aerosol-Generating Devices and Communicable Diseases

Aerosol-generating devices (AGDs) such as air polishers and ultrasonic scalers create a large amount of contaminated aerosol.[54–56] Patients with diseases that can be transmitted by aerosols should not be treated in the dental office or clinic. However, since any patient could be an asymptomatic or prodromal carrier of coronavirus disease 2019 (COVID-19), tuberculosis, or other communicable blood-borne or airborne disease, air polishers should only be used with proper aerosol control measures.[57] Aerosols linger in the air for 30 minutes up to several hours in the entire operatory and in areas of the dental office outside the operatory.[58–61] Unprotected patients are more susceptible to infection by aerosols than dental personnel who wear protective barriers such as face shields, respirators, masks, gloves, eyewear, and disposable clinical clothing.[62–64] High volume evacuation,[57] preprocedural rinsing with antimicrobial mouth wash,[65] flushing of the handpiece and water lines or a self-contained sterile water source, disinfection of environmental surfaces, adequate ventilation and air filtration units with high-efficiency particulate air (HEPA) filters are all important measures to minimize the hazards of microbial aerosols.[66–69]

Summary

Various periodontal instruments and devices are specifically designed for examination of the periodontium, removal of calculus and biofilm from tooth and implant surfaces, and root instrumentation (root planing).

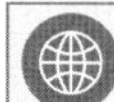

Important information on techniques for the use and sharpening of these instruments is described in detail in the online continuation of this chapter.

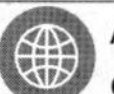

A Case Scenario is found on the companion website eBooks.Health.Elsevier.com.

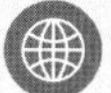

References for this chapter are found on the companion website eBooks.Health.Elsevier.com.

CHAPTER 52

Sonic and Ultrasonic Instrumentation and Irrigation

Carol A. Jahn

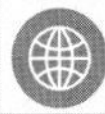
Videos for this chapter can be viewed on the companion website at eBooks.Health.Elsevier.com.

CHAPTER OUTLINE

Scaling and subgingivalroot instrumentation (like "root planing") is considered the initial nonsurgical treatment of choice for periodontitis. Ultrasonic and sonic power scalers have transformed the role of power-driven oscillating instruments and made them essential in periodontal therapy. For post care at home, the pulsating water flosser (oral irrigator) has been clinically proven to help patients stabilize and maintain periodontal health by removing biofilm and reducing inflammation.

Power-Driven Instruments: Overview

Power-driven instruments are everyday mainstays in periodontal therapy and maintenance. They may be used alone or more commonly in combination with hand instruments. Evidence indicates that power-driven instruments provide clinical outcomes similar to those derived from hand instruments alone,[2,14,32,49,50,53,63,68,70.64] or a combination of hand and power-driven instruments.[14,50,53] There is some evidence that power instrumentation has the potential to make scaling less demanding and more time efficient.[2,53] Potential hazards from using power-driven devices include rough root surfaces/defects,[36,38,39,51] production of bioaerosols,[37,46,67] and interference with cardiovascular implantable electronic devices.[16,45,66]

CLINICIAN'S CORNER

Power-driven instruments are essential tools for the nonsurgical treatment of periodontal disease and periodontal maintenance. They can be used alone or in combination with hand instruments. They have the potential to make scaling more time efficient and less physically demanding; however regardless of instrument type, thorough root debridement takes time and perseverance.

Mechanism of Action of Power Scalers

Various physical factors play a role in the mechanism of action of power scalers. These factors include frequency, stroke, and water flow. In addition to rate of flow, the physiologic effects of water may contribute to the efficacy of power instruments (Fig. 52.1).

Water contributes to three physiologic effects that play a role in the efficacy. These are acoustic streaming, acoustic turbulence, and cavitation. Acoustic steaming is unidirectional fluid flow caused by ultrasound waves. Acoustic turbulence is created when the movement of the tip causes the coolant to accelerate, producing an intensified swirling effect. This turbulence continues until cavitation occurs. Cavitation is the formation of bubbles in water caused by the high turbulence. The bubbles implode and produce shock waves in the liquid, thus creating further shock waves throughout the water.[35,68] In vitro, the combination of acoustic streaming, acoustic turbulence, and cavitation has been shown to disrupt biofilm.[21,52,65,69]

Type and Benefit of Power Instruments

Sonic units work at a frequency of 2000 to 6500 cycles per second and use a high- or low-speed air source from the dental unit. Water is delivered via the same tubing used to deliver water to a dental handpiece. Sonic scaler tips are large in diameter and universal in design. A sonic scaler tip travels in an elliptical or orbital stroke pattern. This stroke pattern allows the instrument to be adapted to all tooth surfaces. Box 52.1 outlines the advantages and disadvantages of mechanized instruments compared with manual instruments.

Magnetostrictive ultrasonic devices work in a frequency range of 18,000 to 50,000 cycles per second (Figs. 52.2 and 52.3). Metal stacks that change dimension when electrical energy is applied

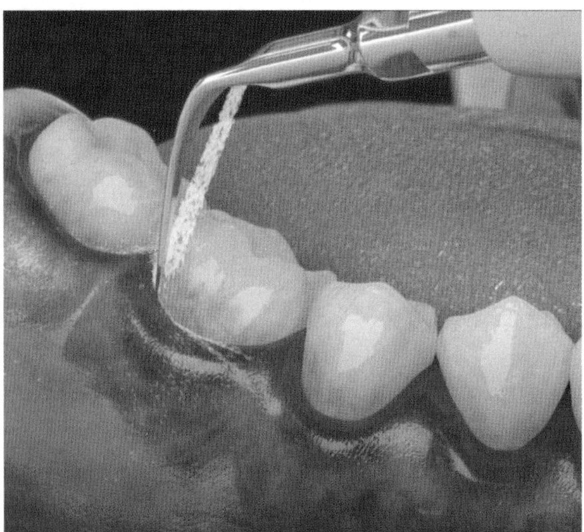

Fig. 52.1 Graphical illustration of an activated power scaler tip. (Courtesy Periopixel.)

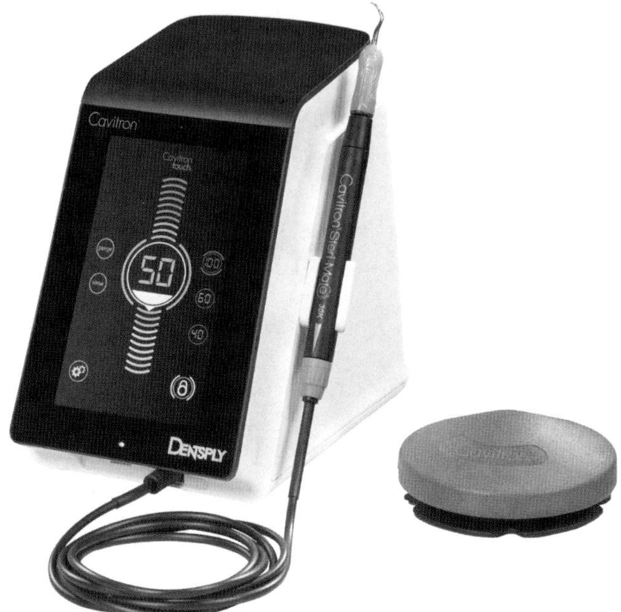

Fig. 52.2 Magnetostrictive ultrasonic device. (Courtesy Dentsply Sirona, York, PA.)

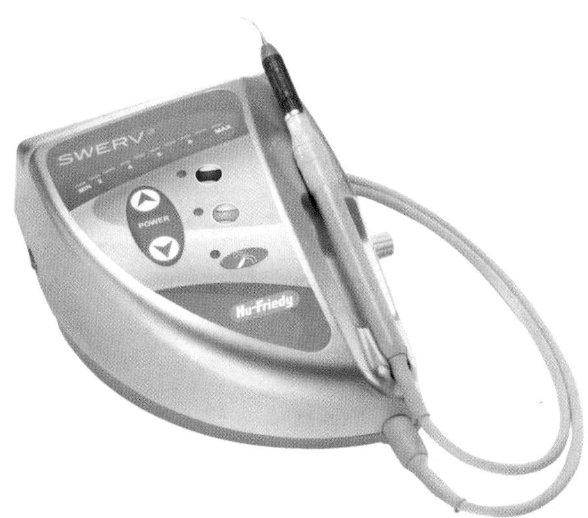

Fig. 52.3 Magnetostrictive ultrasonic device. (Courtesy Hu-Friedy, Chicago, IL.)

BOX 52.1 Advantages and Disadvantages of Mechanized Instruments Compared With Manual Instruments

Advantages

Increased efficiency
- Multiple surfaces of tip are capable of removing deposits
- No need to sharpen
- Less chance for repetitive stress injuries
- Large handpiece size
- Reduced lateral pressure
- Less tissue distention
- Water
- Lavage
- Irrigation
- Acoustic microstreaming

Disadvantages

More precautions and limitations
- Client comfort (water spraying)
- Bioaerosol production
- Temporary hearing shifts
- Noise
- Less tactile sensation
- Reduced visibility

From Darby ML, Walsh MM. *Dental Hygiene.* 3rd ed. St. Louis: Saunders; 2010.

power the magnetostrictive technology. Vibrations travel from the metal stack to a connecting body that causes the vibration of the working tip. Tips move in an elliptical or orbital stroke pattern. This gives the tip four active working surfaces (Fig. 52.4).

Piezoelectric ultrasonic units work in a frequency range of 18,000 to 50,000 cycles per second (Fig. 52.5). Ceramic disks located in the handpiece power the piezoelectric technology and change in dimension as electric energy is applied. Piezoelectric tips move primarily in a linear pattern, giving the tip two active surfaces (Fig. 52.6). Various insert tip designs and shapes are available for use.

Efficiency

Modified tip designs allow for improved access in many areas, including furcations. Newer, slimmer designs operate effectively at lower power settings, thus improving patients' comfort. Flat-edged tips (rectangular in cross section) or bladed designs seem to engage deposits and remove them more efficiently than conical (in cross section) tips.

Tip Designs

Some tips are designed to remove heavy gingival calculus or debride periodontal pockets definitively. Large-diameter tips are created with a universal design and are indicated for the removal of large, tenacious deposits. A medium to medium-high power setting is generally recommended. Thinner-diameter tips may be site specific in design and *in vitro* have been shown to be beneficial for use in removing biofilm.[52] The right and left contra-angled instruments allow for greater access and adaptation to root morphology. These inserts are designed to work on a low-power setting. A deactivated tip can be used for exploration. The amount of water delivered for lavage can be controlled through the

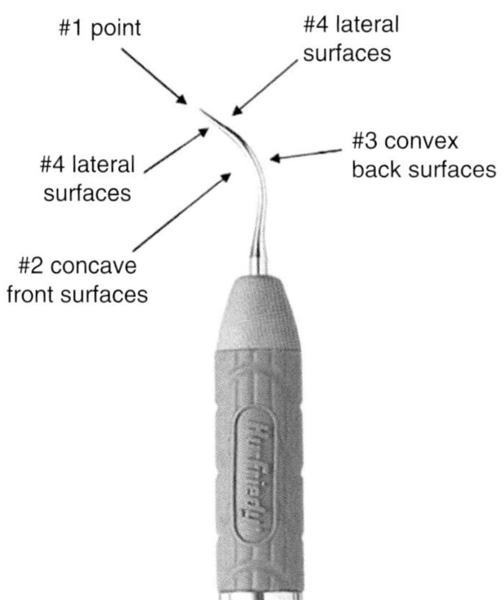

Fig. 52.4 Working sides of a magnetostrictive tip. (Courtesy Hu-Friedy, Chicago, IL.)

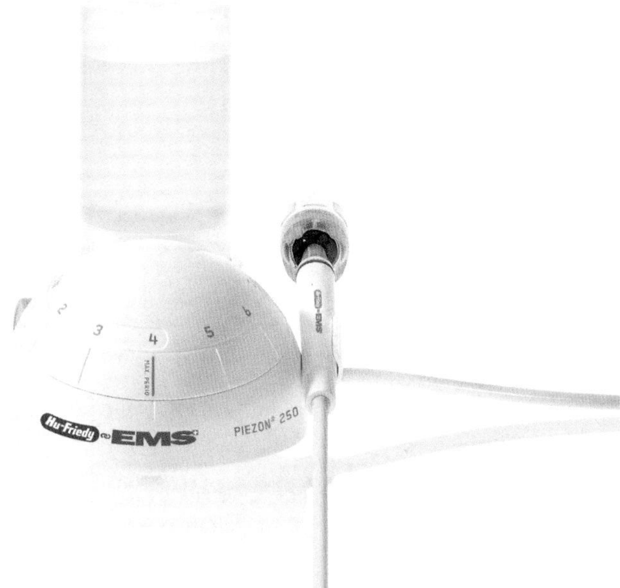

Fig. 52.5 Piezoelectric ultrasonic device. (Courtesy Hu-Friedy, Chicago, IL.)

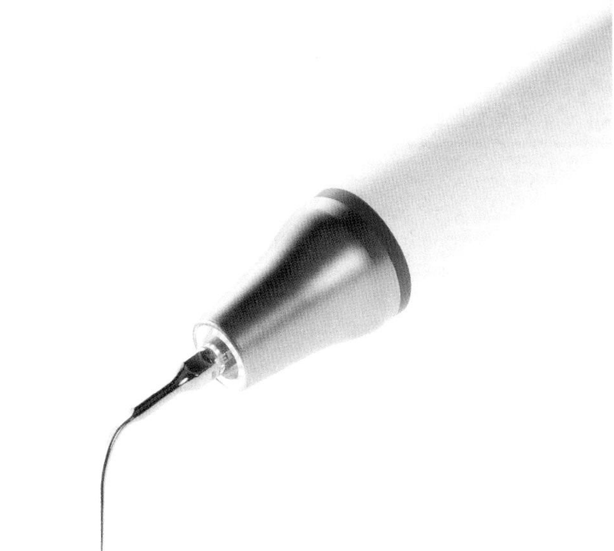

Fig. 52.6 Working sides of a piezoelectric tip. (Courtesy Hu-Friedy, Chicago, IL.)

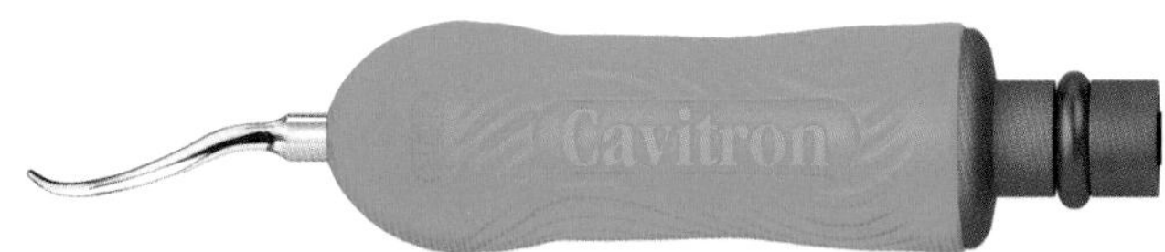

Fig. 52.7 Site-specific designed insert. (Courtesy Dentsply Sirona, York, PA.)

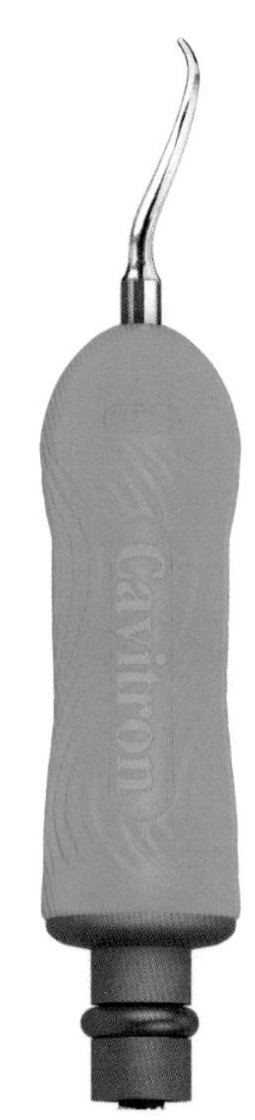

Fig. 52.8 Site-specific designed insert. (Courtesy Dentsply Sirona, York, PA.)

selection of either traditional flow or focused-tip delivery flow. Contra-angled designs and larger ergonomic grips enhance comfort and ergonomics (Figs. 52.7 and 52.8).

Clinical Outcomes of Power-Driven Instruments

Numerous clinical outcomes have been evaluated from the use of power-driven instruments. Reviews of the literature have found the effectiveness of subgingival debridement using ultrasonic or sonic scalers to be similar to that achieved with or in combination with manual instruments.[2,14,32,50,53,63,70]

Power-driven instruments remove calculus through mechanical action.[38,60] In vitro studies have found that power scalers may be effective at removing biofilm on root surfaces.[21,52,65,69] Ultrasonic instruments, through high-speed action, produce cavitational activity and acoustic microstreaming that some believe may help enhance the disruption of bacteria in subgingival biofilm even when the tip is not in contact with the root surface.[21,52,69]

KEY FACT

Power-driven instruments are not just for heavy calculus removal. Depending on tip design and size, they are beneficial for supragingival calculus removal, subgingival debridement, and general biofilm removal.

The primary expected clinical outcomes from scaling and subgingival root instrumentation ("root planing") is a reduction in bleeding and probing depth and a gain in clinical attachment.[62] Comparing power scalers with manual instruments, both types demonstrate similar outcomes for reductions in bleeding on probing and probing depth and gains in clinical attachment.[2,14,32,50,53,63,70] Power scalers also appear to provide similar microbiological[14,32] and immunological[14] outcomes as manual scaling. Because the opening of a furcation is narrower than with conventional hand instruments, power scalers may be recommended as a means to improve access when scaling this type of defect.[3]

Special Considerations

Power-driven instruments must be used with some caution. Roots may be rougher post scaling than with hand instruments. Due to aerosol production, proper infection control procedures including high volume evacuation (HVE) need to be implemented. Power-driven instruments may be contraindicated for people with cardiac vascular implantable electronic devices.

Root Surface Roughness

The data are mixed on whether power-driven instruments cause more root surface roughness than hand instruments.[36,38,39,51,61] Although it could be assumed that using the device at a higher power may cause more roughness, this is not been proven.[38] It is also not known how much root surface roughness affects the healing process.[40] Power-driven instruments may increase the roughness of resin or glass ionomer restorative materials; therefore repolishing post scaling is recommended.[17]

Aerosol Production

Power-driven devices produce bioaerosols and splatter, which can contaminate the operator and remain in the air for up to 30 minutes,[67] thus creating the potential for the spread of contagious respiratory diseases.[37] Recent data indicate that it is the irrigant in the power scaler that is the potential source of disease transmission.[46] Following the Centers for Disease Control and Prevention (CDC) recommended infection prevention and control practices can help minimize bioaerosol risks to patients and providers.[31] This includes appropriate personal protective equipment (PPE) such as gowns, surgical caps, surgical grade mask, and face shields. Data have shown that preprocedural rinsing and high-speed evacuation are the most efficient ways to reduce bioaerosols.[46,47]

KEY FACT

Infectious bioaerosols from power-driven devices can remain in the air for up to 30 min. A well-fitting surgical grade mask is recommended. A face shield may be required. To help minimize bioaerosols, preprocedural rinsing and high-speed evacuation have been shown to be effective.

Cardiovascular Implantable Electronic Devices

The use of ultrasonics on patients with cardiovascular implantable electronic devices such as cardiac pacemakers and cardioverter-defibrillators has been a cause of concern.[16,45,66] Newer models of pacemakers often have bipolar titanium insulation that is believed to make ultrasonic and sonic instruments generally safe for use. In support of this, in vivo studies have found that ultrasonics did not interfere with pacemaker or defibrillators' pacing or sensing functions.[16,45] Conversely, an in vitro study found that ultrasonic scalers interfered with the activity of dual-system pacemakers.[54] A best practice is to consult with the physician regarding any precautions or warnings from the manufacturer of the product. Box 52.2 outlines the indications, precautions, and contraindications of using mechanized instrumentation.

BOX 52.2 Indications, Precautions, and Contraindications for Use of Mechanized Instruments

Indications

- Supragingival debridement of dental calculus and extrinsic stains
- Subgingival debridement of calculus, oral biofilm, root surface constituents, and periodontal pathogens
- Removal of orthodontic cement
- Gingival and periodontal conditions and diseases
- Surgical interventions
- Margination (reduces amalgam overhangs)

Precautions

- Unshielded pacemakers
- Infectious diseases: human immunodeficiency virus, hepatitis, tuberculosis (active stages), active herpetic lesions, contagious respiratory infections like SARS, COVID or influenza
- Demineralized tooth surface
- Exposed dentin (especially associated with sensitivity)
- Restorative materials (porcelain, amalgam, gold, composite)
- Titanium implant abutments unless using special insert (e.g., Quixonic SofTip Prophy Tips)
- Children (primary teeth)
- Immunosuppression from disease or chemotherapy
- Uncontrolled diabetes mellitus

Contraindications

- Chronic pulmonary disease: asthma, emphysema, cystic fibrosis, pneumonia
- Cardiovascular disease with secondary pulmonary disease
- Swallowing difficulty (dysphagia)

From Darby ML, Walsh MM. *Dental Hygiene.* 3rd ed. St. Louis: Saunders; 2010.

Principles of Instrumentation

Ultrasonic technique is different from instrumentation with hand scalers. A pen grasp is used with an ultrasonic scaler, along with an extraoral fulcrum (Fig. 52.9). The purpose of the extraoral fulcrum is to allow the operator to maintain a light grasp and have easier access physically and visually to the oral cavity. Alternate cross-arch or opposite-arch fulcrums are acceptable alternatives.

CLINICIAN'S CORNER

Instrumentation with the ultrasonic device is different from hand instrumentation. A pen grasp with light pressure is preferred, as is using an extraoral fulcrum. Deposits are removed coronally to apically. For deposits in the embrasure area, a horizontal or transverse stroke is recommended.

Light pressure is needed with a power instrument. The tip is traveling at a set frequency in a set stroke pattern. Increased clinician pressure on the tip causes decreased clinical efficacy.

Sonic or ultrasonic instrumentation requires removal from the coronal to the apical portion of the deposit. This stroke pattern allows the

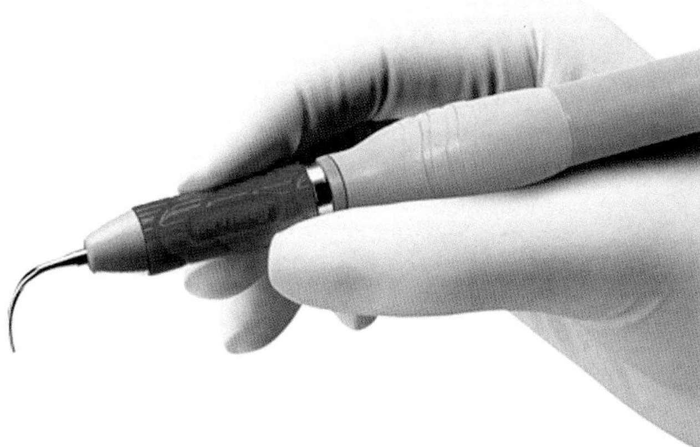

Fig. 52.9 Pen grasp of tip. (Courtesy Hu-Friedy, Chicago, IL.)

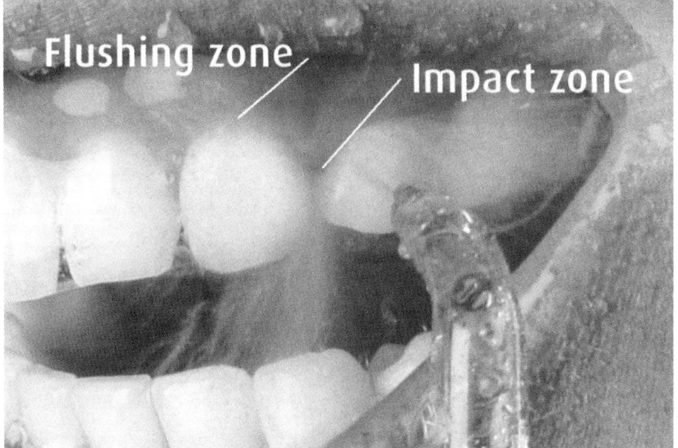

Fig. 52.10 Pulsation creates two zones of hydrokinetic activity: the impact zone and the flushing zone. (Courtesy Water Pik, Inc., Fort Collins, CO.)

insert to work at its optimal stroke pattern and frequency for quick, effective deposit removal. For coronal deposits located in the embrasure area, a horizontal or transverse tip orientation is recommended. A deplaquing stroke should be used when the focus is removal of biofilm and soft debris for the resolution of gingival inflammation. This stroke entails accessing every square millimeter of the tooth surface during ultrasonic deplaquing as a result of the limited lateral dispersion of the lavage subgingivally (Videos 52.1 and 52.2).

Home and Self-Applied Irrigation

The oral irrigator (also called a dental water jet or water flosser) was introduced in 1962. Contrary to myth and misunderstanding, long-standing replication of research results show that water flossing safely and effectively reduces inflammation and bleeding on probing.[33,34] Evidence also indicates that the oral irrigator effectively removes biofilm[23,24] and it is as effective as dental floss when added to toothbrushing.[4,44,56,59]

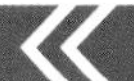

FLASH BACK

The oral irrigator has had many different names throughout the years. It has been referred to as a water jet or dental water jet. Today, the more common name is water flosser. The term is supported by clinical evidence and has been shown to be useful in helping patients understand the benefit of the device.

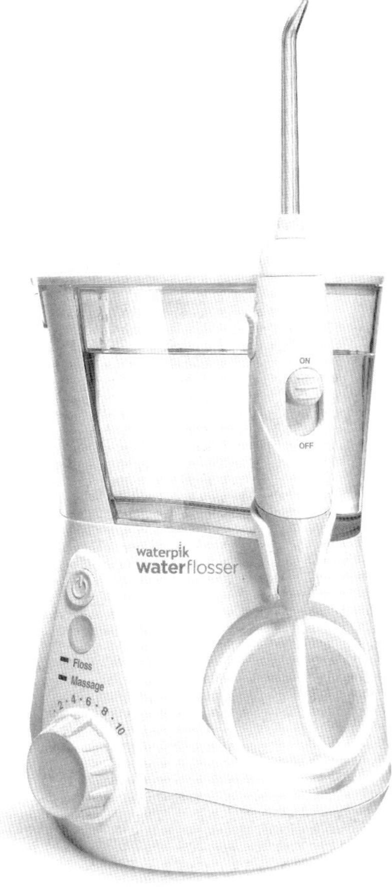

Fig. 52.11 A dental water jet with 1200 ppm and a pressure setting that ranges from 10 to 100 psi. (Courtesy Water Pik, Inc., Fort Collins, CO.)

Mechanism of Action of Irrigation

The mechanism of action of irrigation is through pulsation and pressure.[6,7,57] Pulsation creates a decompression phase that allows the water or solution to penetrate subgingivally. It is followed by a compression phase that expels bacteria and debris from the pocket (Fig. 52.10). Physiologically, pulsation, along with pressure and water velocity, creates shear hydraulic forces that are capable of removing bacterial biofilm from treated areas.[23] Clinical efficacy of home irrigation has been found for units that pulsate from 1200 to 1400 pulses per minute set at a minimum of 60 psi.[33] The oral irrigator is safe to use at higher pressure settings.[29] Many types of oral irrigators are commercially available; however, research data from one product brand cannot be extrapolated to other brands, because different brands may have different pressure settings and pulsation rates (Figs. 52.11 and 52.12). A best practice is to determine if the product carries the American Dental Association (ADA) Seal of Acceptance, which indicates that the product has been evaluated for safety and efficacy.

KEY FACT

Pulsation and pressure create a compression-decompression phase that allows for both penetration of the agent into the sulcus or pocket and expelling of bacteria and debris. Unlike simple rinsing, pulsation, pressure, and water velocity create shear hydraulic forces capable of removing biofilm.

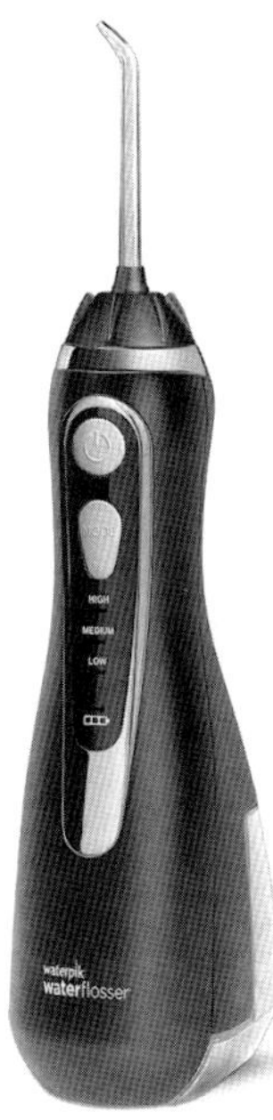

Fig. 52.12 A cordless dental water jet, which also has 1200 ppm. (Courtesy Water Pik, Inc., Fort Collins, CO.)

A variety of tips can be used with an oral irrigator. The traditional jet tip is placed supragingivally (slightly above the gingival margin) at a 90-degree angle. Data indicate this results in an average pocket penetration of 50% (Fig. 52.13).[15] A soft, site-specific subgingival tip (Pik Pocket subgingival irrigation tip, Water Pik, Inc., Fort Collins, CO) (Fig. 52.14) is placed slightly subgingivally and it penetrates to about 90% of the depth of pockets that are 6 mm or less and 64% of pockets that are 7 mm or greater[8] (Videos 52.3 and 52.4).

Tips that are placed supragingivally are recommended for full-mouth irrigation or cleansing. These tips include a traditional jet tip along with jet tips of this configuration that have been enhanced with bristles or filaments to assist in biofilm removal (Figs. 52.15 and 52.16).[56,59] The subgingival tip is recommended after full-mouth cleaning for localized irrigation of a specific site that is difficult to access, such as a deep pocket, a furcation, an implant, or a crown and bridge. A new tip with a candy cane design is available to help patients clean under implant-retained dentures (Fig. 52.17).

Safety

Oral irrigation is supported by a large body of scientific evidence and has been used by people since the 1960s.[34] Clinical studies on oral irrigation evaluate for adverse events, and none have been reported. Despite the scientific evidence, myths about trauma to soft tissue, penetration of bacteria into the pocket, increased pocket depth, and rates of bacteremia still exist.

CLINICIAN'S CORNER

It is well-established that oral irrigation is both safe and effective. Concerns and anecdotes about trauma to soft tissue, penetration of bacteria into the pocket, and increased pocket depth are not supported by clinical evidence. The device has been recommended by dental professionals and used by the general population since the 1960s.

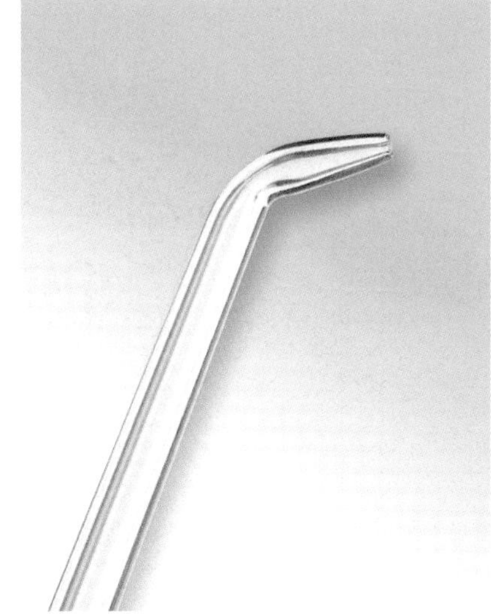

Fig. 52.13 Jet tip. (Courtesy Water Pik, Inc., Fort Collins, CO.)

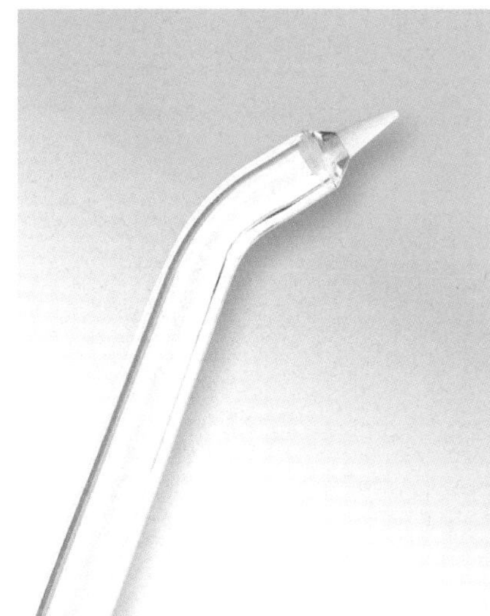

Fig. 52.14 Site-specific tip. (Courtesy Water Pik, Inc., Fort Collins, CO.)

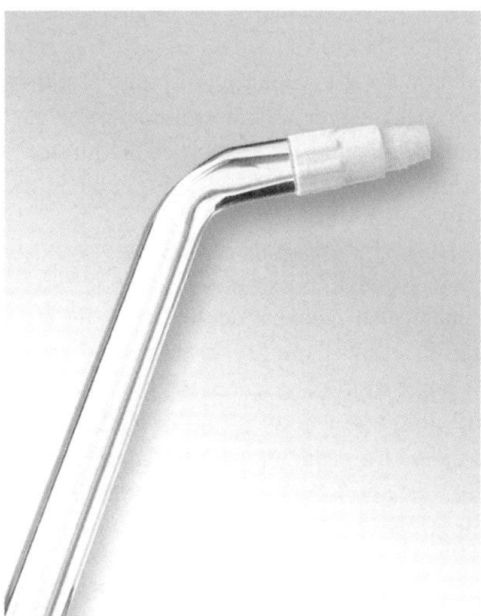

Fig. 52.15 Tip with soft tapered bristles. (Courtesy Water Pik, Inc., Fort Collins, CO.)

The water flosser has been shown to be safe and effective on gingival and epithelial tissue at multiple pressure settings including 100 psi. In a 6-week, 3-arm study that measured probing pocket depth (PPD) and clinical attachment levels (CAL), individuals used a manual toothbrush and water flosser and were compared to subjects using a manual toothbrush and floss or manual toothbrushing only. Those in the water flosser group increased the pressure settings during the first 2 weeks followed by 2 weeks use at 90 psi and 2 weeks

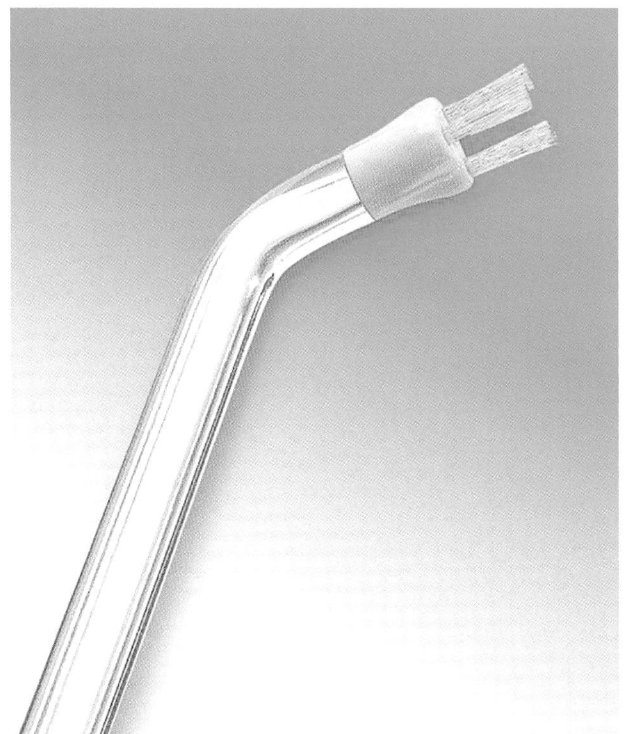

Fig. 52.16 Tip with soft filaments. (Courtesy Water Pik, Inc., Fort Collins, CO.)

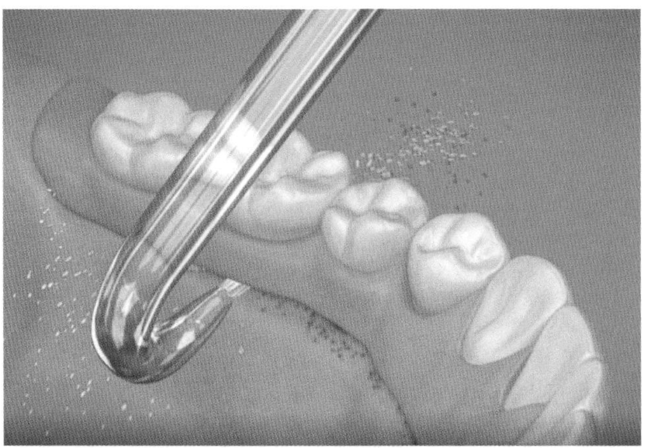

Fig. 52.17 Tip designed for an implant-retained denture. (Courtesy Water Pik, Inc., Fort Collins CO.)

use at 100 psi. The results demonstrated that manual brushing and water flossing reduced PPD and maintained CAL, and these results exceeded those seen in the other two groups.[29]

Trauma to tissue and penetration of bacteria were evaluated in a study that used scanning electron microscopy (SEM) to assess the differences between irrigated and nonirrigated untreated periodontal pockets. Examination with SEM showed no observable differences between the irrigated and nonirrigated pocket tissue with regard to physical features and appearance of the epithelium. Irrigated pockets had significantly fewer bacteria up to 6 mm, compared with nonirrigated pockets. The investigators concluded that oral irrigation induces a qualitative change on subgingival plaque and is not injurious to soft tissue.[11]

One long-held assumption is that using an oral irrigator will result in a higher incidence of bacteremia compared with flossing. Studies contradict this. Data have shown that the incidence of bacteremia can range from 7% in people with gingivitis[55] to 50% in those with periodontitis.[18] Other investigators have found similar results, with one study finding no incidence of bacteremia[64] post irrigation and another study noting a rate of 27%.[5] In comparison, the incidence of bacteremia from string flossing has been shown to be 40% in people with periodontitis and 41% in periodontally healthy individuals.[12]

Clinical Outcomes of Irrigation

Table 52.1 highlights the body of evidence on the oral irrigator. Evaluated outcomes include removal of plaque biofilm and reductions in calculus, gingivitis, bleeding on probing, probing depth, periodontal pathogens, and inflammatory mediators.[1,4,9,10,13,19,20,22,24-28,41,43,44,48,49,56,58,59] Oral irrigation has been studied and found to be safe and effective for those with additional needs such as implants,[44] orthodontics,[9,59] and diabetes.[1]

Emerging evidence indicates that using an oral irrigator can lead to oral health improvements over what has been traditionally seen with string floss[4,24,44,56,59] or interdental brushes.[25,42] Barnes et al. found that an oral irrigator added to either manual or sonic toothbrushing was significantly more effective than dental floss for removing plaque and reducing bleeding and gingivitis.[4] Studies comparing water flossing to interdental brushes have found that water flossing was 56% more effective at reducing bleeding[25] and 18% more effective at removing plaque biofilm.[42]

The oral irrigator has been demonstrated to remove biofilm.[1,4,13,23–25,27,28,42,43] The combination of pulsation, pressure, and water velocity creates shear hydraulic forces that can significantly remove biofilm. Researchers who assessed the action of the oral irrigator with SEM found that a 3-second application at medium pressure removed 99.9% of biofilm from treated areas (Figs. 52.18 and 52.19).[23]

CLINICIAN'S CORNER

Over 80 studies have been conducted on the oral irrigator. Consistent clinical outcomes demonstrate reductions in biofilm, periodontal pathogens, bleeding on probing, gingivitis, and probing depth. The device has been tested on people in periodontal maintenance and in those with gingivitis, orthodontic appliances, implants, and diabetes.

Oral irrigation is beneficial regardless of the type of toothbrush used. Oral irrigation added to manual toothbrushing was 2.4 times more effective at removing plaque biofilm, 3.1 times more effective at reducing bleeding, and 2.7 times more effective at reducing gingivitis than manual brushing alone.[28]

Patients who added an oral irrigator to an oscillating brush routine were 33% more effective at removing plaque biofilm, 37% more effective at reducing bleeding, and 35% more effective at reducing gingivitis versus those who only used the oscillating brush.[43] A recent entry to the water flosser market features a sonic toothbrush with a built-in water flossing (Fig. 52.20). This allows patients to brush and water floss with one device. When used for 2 minutes of power brushing followed by 1 minute of water flossing, this device was up to twice as effective as traditional brushing and flossing for reducing plaque biofilm, gingival bleeding, and inflammation.[30]

The most common agent used and demonstrated effective in a water flosser is plain water. The use of an antimicrobial agent, such as diluted chlorhexidine, may enhance reductions in gingivitis and bleeding.[10,20]

TABLE 52.1 Reduction of Inflammation and Plaque Biofilm

Study	Duration	*N*	Agent Used	Bleeding Reduction (%)	Gingivitis Reduction (%)	Plaque Biofilm Reduction (%)
Al-Mubarek et al.[1]	3 months	50	Water	43.8	66.9	64.9
Barnes et al.[4]	4 weeks	105	Water	36.2–59.2	10.8–15.1	8.8–17.3
Burch et al.[9]	2 months	47	Water	57.1–76.6	NR	52–55.7
Chaves et al.[10]	6 months	105	CHX (0.04%)	54	26	35
			Water	50	26	16
Cutler et al.[13]	2 weeks	52	Water	56	50	40
Flemmig et al.[19]	6 months	175	CHX (0.06%)	35.4	42.5	53.2
			Water	24	23.1	0.1
Flemmig et al.[20]	6 months	60	Acetylsalicylic acid 3%		8.9	55.6
			Water	50	29.2	0
Genovesi et al.[22]	30 days	30	Water	81%	NR	45%
			Minocycline hydrochloride, 1 mg per pocket in-office/1 time	75%	NR	61%
Lobene et al.[41]	5 months	155	Water	NR	52.9	7.9
Magnuson et al.[44]	30 days	44 implants	Water	82%	NR	NR
Newman et al.[48]	6 months	155	Water	22.8	17.8	6.1
			Water and zinc sulfate (0.57%)	8.8	6.5	9.2
Rosema et al.[56]	30 days	104	Water	17%	NR	9.0
Sharma et al.[59]	4 weeks	128	Water	84.5	NR	38.9

CHX, Chlorhexidine; *NR*, not reported.

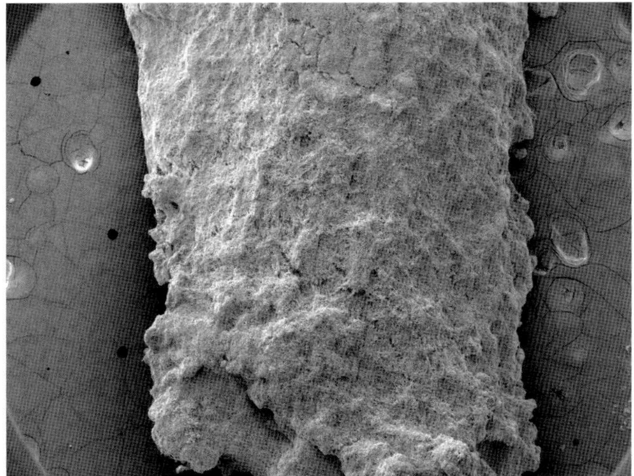

Fig. 52.18 Control tooth with no irrigation. (Courtesy Water Pik, Inc., Fort Collins, CO.)

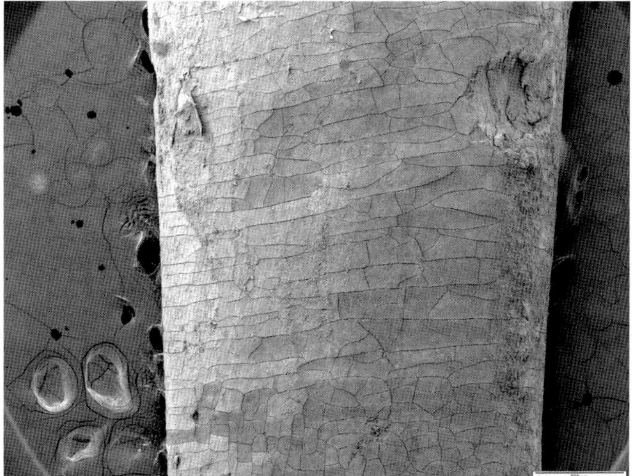

Fig. 52.19 Tooth after a 3-s pulsating lavage with a jet tip at medium pressure. (Courtesy Water Pik, Inc., Fort Collins, CO.)

Individuals With Special Considerations

Some clinical trials have focused on groups with special oral or medical health needs. Both children and adults undergoing orthodontic therapy have shown significant benefits from using a dental water jet (Video 52.5).[9,59] A newer small brush tip that cleans and irrigates simultaneously has been shown to remove 3.76 times more plaque than brushing and flossing with a floss threader.[59] For individuals with implants, a modified jet tip with filaments has been found to be both safe and effective (Video 52.6). Patients who used the oral irrigator at 60 psi with warm water had twice the reduction in bleeding around implants compared with patients who used floss. No adverse events were reported.[44] The oral irrigator has also been found to improve periodontal health in people with type 1 or 2 diabetes.[1] For patients who prefer natural products, subjects who used the oral irrigator for 30 days post scaling and root planing effectively reduced the clinical parameters of periodontitis and periodontal bacteria similar to scaling and root planing followed by the placement of 1 mg of minocycline hydrochloride. Any differences between the two therapies were not statistically significant.[22].

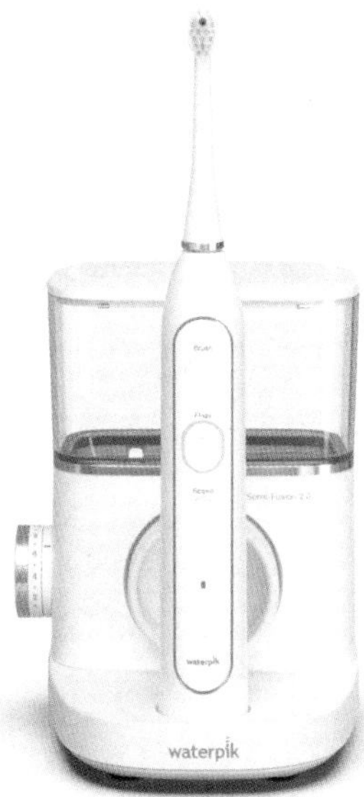

Fig. 52.20 Sonic toothbrush with built-in water flosser. (Courtesy Water Pik, Inc., Fort Collins, CO.)

Action of a Tip With Filaments Cleaning Around an Implant

Video 52.7 shows the action of the site-specific tip in a periodontal pocket.

Conclusion

Power scalers have emerged from being adjuncts for removing heavy supragingival calculus to a tool that may be used for all aspects of scaling: biofilm removal, supragingival scaling, and subgingival scaling. The clinical outcomes achieved are similar to those seen with hand instrumentation. The advantages gained from using power instruments are potentially greater access subgingivally and in furcation areas and increased efficiency in time needed for scaling.

Oral irrigation is safe and effective for a wide variety of patients, including those in periodontal maintenance; those with gingivitis, orthodontic appliances, implants, or diabetes; and those who are noncompliant with floss. Clinical outcomes include reductions of plaque, calculus, gingivitis, bleeding on probing, probing depth, periodontal pathogens, and inflammatory mediators.

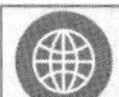 A Case Scenario is found on the companion website eBooks.Health.Elsevier.com

Suggested Readings

Al-Mubarek S, Ciancio S, Aljada A, et al. Comparative evaluation of adjunctive oral irrigation in diabetes. *J Clin Periodontol.* 2002;29:295–300. PMID: 11966926.

Arabaci T, Cicek Y, Canakci CF. Sonic and ultrasonic scalers in periodontal treatment: a review. *Int J Dent Hyg.* 2007;5:2–12. PMID: 17250573.

Barnes CM, Russell CM, Reinhardt RA, et al. Comparison of irrigation to floss as an adjunct to toothbrushing: effect on bleeding, gingivitis, and supragingival plaque. *J Clin Dent.* 2005;16:71–77. PMID:10476890.

Cobb CM, Rodgers RL, Killoy WF. Ultrastructural examination of human periodontal pockets following the use of an oral irrigation device in vivo. *J Periodontol.* 1988;59:155–163. PMID: 3162980.

Cutler CW, Stanford TW, Cederberg A, et al. Clinical benefits of oral irrigation for periodontitis are related to reduction of pro-inflammatory cytokine levels and plaque. *J Clin Periodontol.* 2000;27:134–143. PMID: 10703660.

Del Peloso Ribeiro E, Bittencourt S, Sallum EA, et al. Periodontal debridement as a therapeutic approach for severe chronic periodontitis: a clinical, microbiological and immunological study. *J Clin Periodontol.* 2008;35:789–798. PMID: 18647203.

Genovesi AM, Lorenzi C, Lyle DM, et al. Periodontal maintenance following scaling and root planing, comparing minocycline treatment to daily oral irrigation with water. *Minerva Stomatol.* 2013;62(suppl 1):1–9. PMID: 24423731.

Gorur A, Lyle DM, Schaudinn C. Biofilm removal with a dental water jet. *Compend Contin Educ Dent.* 2009;30(special1):1–6. PMID: 19385349.

Goyal CR, Qaqish JG, Schuller R, et al. Evaluation of the safety of a water flosser on gingival and epithelial tissue at different pressure settings. *Compend Cont Dent Educ.* 2018;39(suppl 2):8–13.

Goyal CR, Qaqish JG, Schuller R, et al. Comparison of a novel sonic toothbrush with a traditional sonic toothbrush and manual brushing and flossing on plaque, gingival bleeding, and inflammation. *Compend Cont Dent Educ.* 2018;39(suppl 2):14–22.

Ioannou I, Dimitriadis N, Papadimitriou K, et al. Hand instrumentation versus ultrasonic debridement in the treatment of chronic periodontitis: a randomized clinical and microbiological trial. *J Clin Periodontol.* 2009;36:132–141. PMID: 19207889.

Jolkovsky DL, Lyle DM. Safety of a water flosser: a literature review. *Compend Contin Educ Dent.* 2015;36:146–149. PMID: 25822642.

Kumar P, Das SJ, Sonowal ST, et al. Comparison of root surface roughness produced by hand instruments and ultrasonic scalers: an in vitro study. *J Clin Diagn Res.* 2015;9:56–60. PMID: 26675445.

Kumar PS, Subramanian K. Demystifying the mist: sources of microbial bioload in dental aerosols. *J Periodontol.* 2020;91:1113–1122. PMID: 32662070.

Magnuson B, Harsono M, Stark PC, et al. Comparison of the effect of two interdental cleaning devices around implants on the reduction of bleeding: a 30-day randomized clinical trial. *Compend Contin Educ Dent.* 2013;34(special 8):2–7. PMID: 24568169.

Puglisi R, Santos A, Pujol A, et al. Clinical comparison of instrumentation systems for periodontal debridement: a randomized clinical trial. *Int J Dent Hyg.* 2021. May online head of print. PMID: 34018671.

Suvan J, Leira Y, Sancho FMM. Subgingival instrumentation for treatment of periodontitis. A systematic review. *J Clin Periodontol.* 2020;47:155–175. PMID: 31889320.

Tom J. Management of patients with cardiovascular implantable electronic devices in dental, oral, and maxillofacial surgery. *Anesth Prog.* 2016;63:95–104. PMID: 27269668.

Veena HR, Mahantesha S, Joseph PA, et al. Dissemination of aerosol and splatter during ultrasonic scaling: a pilot study. *J Infec Public Health.* 2015;8:260–265. PMID: 25564419.

Walmsley AD, Laird WR, Williams AR. Dental plaque removal by cavitational activity during ultrasonic scaling. *J Clin Periodontol.* 1988;15:539–543. PMID: 2848873.

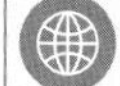 References for this chapter are found on the companion website eBooks.Health.Elsevier.com.

CHAPTER 53

Chemotherapy: Use of Systemic Antibiotics[a]

Sukirth M. Ganesan | Angelo Mariotti | Yvonne L. Hernandez-Kapila

CHAPTER OUTLINE

Learning Objectives

- Evaluate the rationale for use of anti-infective agents as adjuncts to periodontal therapy.
- List the clinical indications for use of anti-infective agents.
- Evaluate the pharmacology of anti-infective agents indicated as adjuncts to periodontal therapy.

It has been well established that the various periodontal diseases are caused by bacterial infection. Bacteria begin reattaching to tooth surfaces soon after the teeth have been cleaned and start to form a biofilm. Over time, this supragingival plaque biofilm becomes more complex, which leads to a succession of bacteria that are more pathogenic. Bacteria grow in an apical direction and become subgingival. Eventually, as bone is destroyed, a periodontal pocket is formed. In a periodontal pocket, the bacteria form a highly structured and complex biofilm. As this process continues, the bacterial biofilm extends so far subgingivally that the patient cannot reach it during oral hygiene efforts. In addition, this complex biofilm may now offer some protection from the host's immunologic mechanisms in the periodontal pocket as well as from antibiotics used for treatment. It has been suggested that an antibiotic strength that is 500 times greater than the usual therapeutic dose may be needed to be effective against bacteria that have become arranged in biofilms.[30]

Systemic Administration of Antibiotics
Tetracyclines
Metronidazole
Penicillins
Cephalosporins
Clindamycin
Ciprofloxacin
Macrolides

It is therefore logical to treat periodontal pockets by mechanically removing local factors (including the calculus that harbors bacteria) and by disrupting the subgingival plaque biofilm itself. Mechanical removal includes manual instrumentation (e.g., scaling and root planing/subgingival root instrumentation) and machine-driven instrumentation (e.g., ultrasonic scalers). *Systemic* antibiotic therapy (oral antibiotics) has been shown to reduce the number of periodontal pathogens and improve clinical outcomes in various forms of periodontal diseases when used in conjunction with the mechanical instrumentation.[22] This chapter reviews the indications and protocols for optimizing the use of systemically administered antibiotics during the treatment of periodontal diseases.

KEY FACT

Bacteriostatic Versus Bactericidal Antibiotics

Pharmacologic agents that prevent the growth of bacteria are bacteriostatic antibiotics, whereas pharmacologic agents that actually kill the bacteria are bactericidal antibiotics. Examples of bacteriostatic antibiotics include tetracycline and clindamycin, whereas penicillin and metronidazole are good examples of bactericidal antibiotics.

Definitions

An antibiotic is a naturally occurring, semisynthetic, or synthetic type of chemotherapeutic agent that destroys or inhibits the growth of select microorganisms, generally at low concentrations. An antiseptic is a chemical antimicrobial agent that can be applied topically or subgingivally to mucous membranes, wounds, or intact dermal surfaces to destroy microorganisms and inhibit their reproduction or metabolism. In dentistry, antiseptics are widely used as the active ingredient in antiplaque and antigingivitis oral rinses and dentifrices. Disinfectants (a subcategory of antiseptics) are antimicrobial agents that are generally applied to inanimate surfaces to destroy microorganisms.[14]

When antibiotics are administered orally, they reach all surfaces and fluids, including the gingival crevicular fluid (GCF). The purpose of a *systemic administration* of antibiotics is to reduce the number of bacteria present in the diseased periodontal pocket; this is often a necessary adjunct for controlling bacterial infection because bacteria can invade periodontal tissues, thereby making mechanical therapy alone sometimes ineffective.[3,12,13,25,51]

[a]Authors would like to thank Dr. Sebastian G. Ciancio (deceased) for his contribution to this chapter in the previous editions of this book.

Systemic Administration of Antibiotics

Background and Rationale

The treatment of periodontal diseases is based on their infectious nature (Table 53.1). Ideally, the causative microorganisms should be identified, and the most effective agent should be selected with the use of antibiotic-sensitivity testing. Although this appears simple, the difficulty lies primarily in identifying the specific etiologic microorganisms rather than the microorganisms that are simply associated with various periodontal disorders.[13]

An ideal antibiotic for use in the prevention and treatment of periodontal disease should be specific for periodontal pathogens, allogenic, nontoxic, substantive, not in general use for the treatment of other diseases, and inexpensive.[26] Currently, however, an ideal antibiotic for the treatment of periodontal disease does not exist.[36] Although oral bacteria are susceptible to many antibiotics, no single antibiotic at the concentrations achieved in body fluids inhibits all putative periodontal pathogens.[64] Indeed, a combination of antibiotics may be necessary to eliminate all putative pathogens from some periodontal pockets (Table 53.2).[49]

As always, the clinician, in concert with the patient, must make the final decision regarding any treatment. Thus, the treatment of an individual patient must be based on the patient's clinical status, the nature of the colonizing bacteria, the ability of the agent to reach the site of infection, and the risks and benefits associated with the proposed treatment plan. The clinician is responsible for choosing the correct antimicrobial agent. Some adverse reactions include allergic or anaphylactic reactions, superinfections of opportunistic bacteria, development of resistant bacteria, interactions with other medications, upset stomach, nausea, and vomiting.[4] Most adverse reactions take the form of gastrointestinal upset.[36] Other concerns include the cost of the medication and the patient's willingness and ability to comply with the proposed therapy.

No consensus exists regarding the magnitude of risk for the development of bacterial resistance. The common and indiscriminate use of antibiotics worldwide has contributed to increasing numbers of resistant bacterial strains since the late 1990s, and this trend is likely to continue given the widespread use of antibiotics.[11,19,65] The overuse, misuse, and widespread prophylactic application of anti-infective drugs are some of the factors that have led to the emergence of resistant microorganisms. Increasing levels of resistance of subgingival microflora to antibiotics have been correlated with the increased use of antibiotics in individual countries.[11,61] At least one Antibiotic Resistance Gene (ARG) has been identified in a majority of the population in a cross-sectional study, and the disease sites exhibited a further increase in prevalence of these ARGs.[2] However, researchers have noted that the subgingival microflora tends to revert to similar proportions of antibiotic-resistant isolates 3 months after therapy.[21,32]

Tetracyclines

Tetracyclines have been widely used for the treatment of periodontal diseases. They have been frequently used to treat refractory periodontitis, including *localized* aggressive periodontitis (LAP), currently termed as periodontitis with molar-incisor pattern in 2018 classification[35,66] (see Table 53.1). Tetracyclines have the ability to concentrate in the periodontal tissues and inhibit the growth of *Aggregatibacter actinomycetemcomitans*. In addition, tetracyclines exert an anticollagenase effect that can inhibit tissue destruction and may help with bone regeneration.[10,41,63]

Pharmacology

The tetracyclines are a group of antibiotics that are produced naturally from certain species of *Streptomyces* or derived semisynthetically. These antibiotics are bacteriostatic and are effective against rapidly multiplying bacteria. They generally are more effective against gram-positive bacteria than against gram-negative bacteria. Tetracyclines are effective for the treatment of periodontal diseases in part because their concentration in the gingival crevice is 2 to 10 times that found in serum.[1,5,28] This allows a high drug concentration to be delivered into the periodontal pockets. In addition, several studies have demonstrated that tetracyclines at a low GCF concentration (i.e., 2 μg/mL to 4 μg/mL) are very effective against many periodontal pathogens.[6,7]

Clinical Use

Tetracyclines have been investigated as adjuncts for the treatment of LAP.[35,54] *A. actinomycetemcomitans* is a microorganism that is frequently associated with LAP, and it invades tissue. Therefore, the mechanical removal of calculus and plaque from root surfaces may

TABLE 53.1 Antibiotics Used to Treat Periodontal Diseases

Category	Agent	Major Features
Penicillin[a]	Amoxicillin	Extended spectrum of antimicrobial activity; excellent oral absorption; used systemically
	Augmentin[b]	Effective against penicillinase-producing microorganisms; used systemically
Tetracyclines	Minocycline	Effective against a broad spectrum of microorganisms; used systemically and applied locally (subgingivally)
	Doxycycline	
	Tetracycline	Effective against a broad spectrum of microorganisms; used systemically and applied locally (subgingivally)
		Chemotherapeutically used in subantimicrobial doses for host modulation (Periostat)
		Effective against a broad spectrum of microorganisms
Quinolone	Ciprofloxacin	Effective against gram-negative rods; promotes health-associated microflora
Macrolide	Azithromycin	Concentrates at sites of inflammation; used systemically
Lincomycin derivative	Clindamycin	Used in penicillin-allergic patients; effective against anaerobic bacteria; used systemically
Nitroimidazole[c]	Metronidazole	Effective against anaerobic bacteria; used systemically and applied locally (subgingivally) as gel

[a]Indications: localized aggressive periodontitis, generalized aggressive periodontitis, medically related periodontitis, and refractory periodontitis.
[b]Amoxicillin and clavulanate potassium.
[c]Indications: localized aggressive periodontitis, generalized aggressive periodontitis, medically related periodontitis, refractory periodontitis, and necrotizing ulcerative periodontitis.

not eliminate this bacterium from the periodontal tissues. Systemic tetracycline can eliminate tissue bacteria and has been shown to arrest bone loss and suppress *A. actinomycetemcomitans* levels in conjunction with scaling and root planing.[53] This combination therapy allows for the mechanical removal of root surface deposits and the elimination of pathogenic bacteria from within the tissues.[56] Increased posttreatment bone levels have been noted with the use of this method (Figs. 53.1–53.4).

As a result of increased resistance to tetracyclines, metronidazole or amoxicillin in combination with metronidazole has been found to be more effective for the treatment of aggressive periodontitis (currently classified as Generalized Stage III or IV Grade C Periodontitis or Localized Stage III/IV Grade C Periodontitis with molar-incisor pattern) in children and young adults. Some investigators think that metronidazole in combination with amoxicillin–clavulanic acid is the preferable antibiotic.[62]

TABLE 53.2 Common Antibiotic Regimens Used to Treat Periodontal Diseases[a]

	Regimen	Dosage/Duration
Single Agent		
Amoxicillin	500 mg	Three times daily for 8 days
Azithromycin	500 mg	Once daily for 4 to 7 days
Ciprofloxacin	500 mg	Twice daily for 8 days
Clindamycin	300 mg	Three times daily for 10 days
Doxycycline or minocycline	100–200 mg	Once daily for 21 days
Metronidazole	500 mg	Three times daily for 8 days
Combination Therapy		
Metronidazole + amoxicillin	250 mg of each	Three times daily for 8 days
Metronidazole + ciprofloxacin	500 mg of each	Twice daily for 8 days

[a]These regimens are prescribed after a review of the patient's medical history, periodontal diagnosis, and antimicrobial testing. Clinicians must consult pharmacology references such as *Mosby's GenRx*[45] or the manufacturer's guidelines for warnings, contraindications, and precautions.

Data from Jorgensen MG, Slots J. Practical antimicrobial periodontal therapy. *Compend Contin Educ Dent.* 2000;21:111.

Long-term use of low antibacterial doses of tetracyclines has been advocated in the past. One long-term study of patients taking low doses of tetracycline (i.e., 250 mg/day for 2 to 7 years) demonstrated the persistence of deep pockets that did not bleed after probing. These sites contained high proportions of tetracycline-resistant gram-negative rods *(Fusobacterium nucleatum)*. After the antibiotic was discontinued, the flora was characteristic of sites with disease.[36] A recent cross-sectional study identified a higher prevalence of tetracycline resistance bacteria, tetracycline resistance genes *(tet)*, and multi-drug resistance genes in their study cohort. Therefore, it is not advisable to prescribe a long-term regimen of tetracyclines because of the possible development of resistant bacterial strains.[38] Although tetracyclines were often used in the past as anti-infective agents, especially for LAP and other types of aggressive periodontitis, they are now frequently replaced by more effective combination antibiotics.[36]

Specific Agents

Tetracycline, minocycline, and doxycycline are semisynthetic members of the tetracycline group that have been used in periodontal therapy.

Tetracycline

Treatment with tetracycline hydrochloride requires the administration of 250 mg four times daily. It is inexpensive, but compliance may be reduced by the need to take the medication so frequently. Side effects include gastrointestinal disturbances, photosensitivity, hypersensitivity, increased blood urea nitrogen levels, blood dyscrasias, dizziness, and headache. In addition, tooth discoloration occurs when this drug is administered to children who are 12 years old or younger.

Tetracycline and Tooth Discoloration

Tetracycline has the ability to chelate with calcium and therefore gets deposited in mineralized tissues such as bone or teeth during the mineralization process, resulting in yellow to brown discoloration of teeth.

Minocycline

Minocycline is effective against a broad spectrum of microorganisms. In patients with adult periodontitis, it suppresses spirochetes and

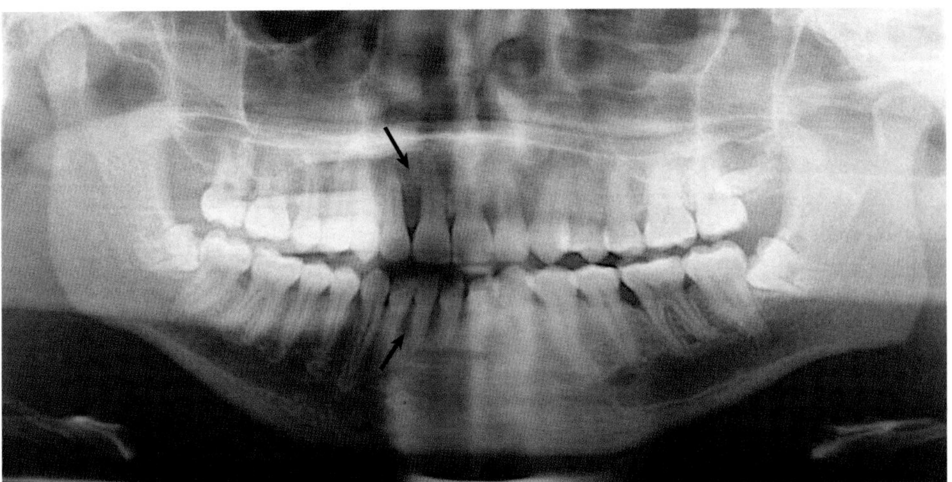

Fig. 53.1 Panoramic image of 17-year-old African American male exhibiting signs of localized aggressive periodontitis. (Photo courtesy Dr. Sasi Sunkari.)

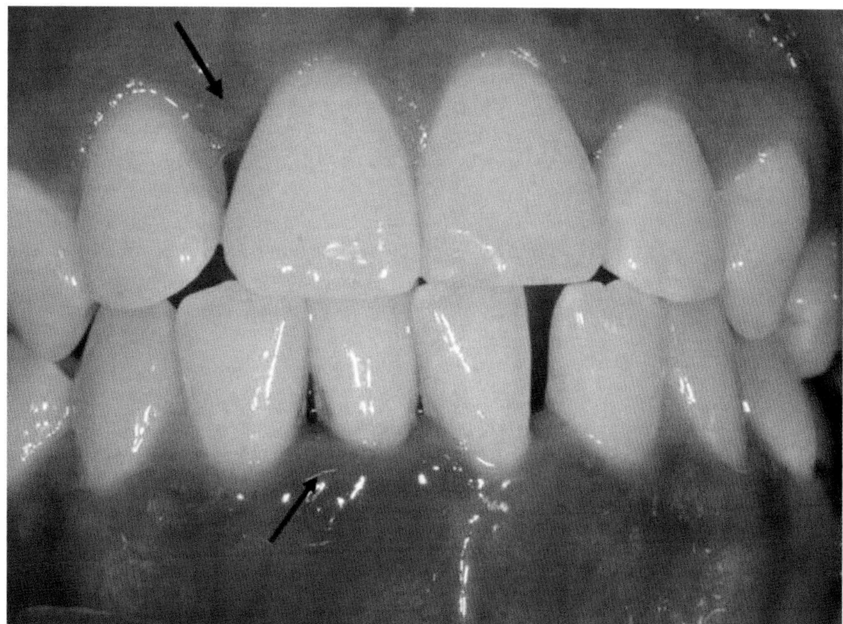

Fig. 53.2 Image of anterior dentition in 17-year-old African American male with localized aggressive periodontitis. (Photo courtesy Dr. Sasi Sunkari.)

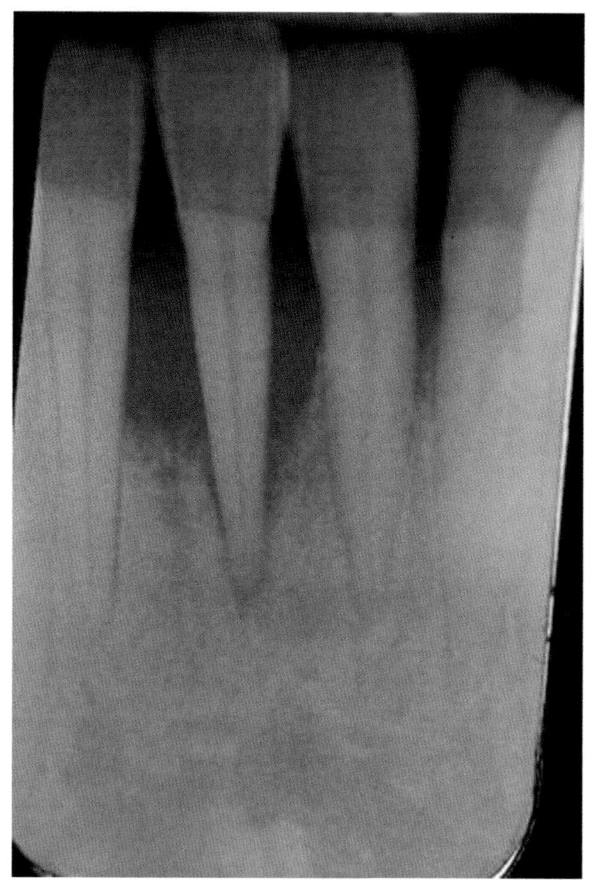

Fig. 53.3 Preoperative radiograph of anterior mandible in localized aggressive periodontitis patient. (Photo courtesy Dr. Sasi Sunkari.)

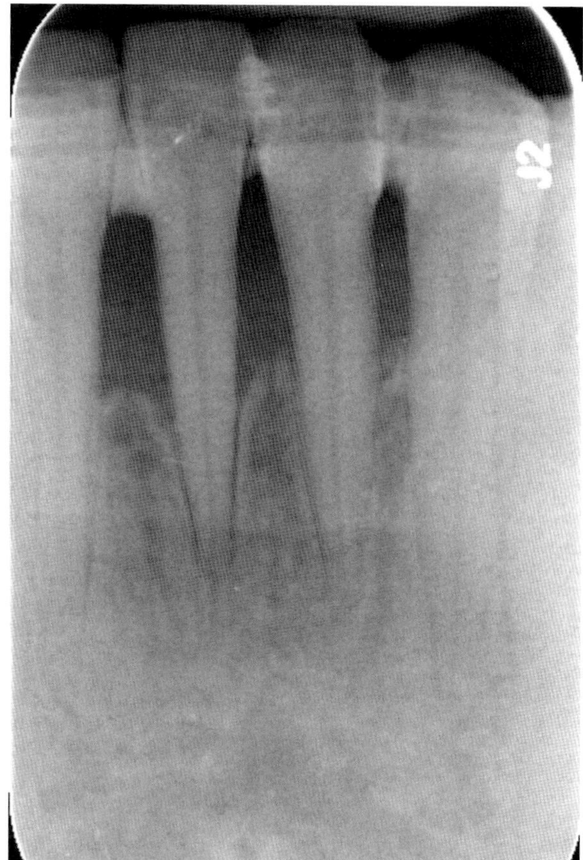

Fig. 53.4 Postoperative radiograph of anterior mandible in localized aggressive periodontitis patient treated with a combination of antibiotic therapy, scaling and root planing, and surgical intervention. (Photo courtesy Dr. Sasi Sunkari.)

motile rods as effectively as scaling and root planing, with suppression evident up to 3 months after therapy. Minocycline can be given twice daily, thereby facilitating compliance as compared with tetracycline. Although it is associated with less phototoxicity and renal toxicity than tetracycline, minocycline may cause reversible vertigo. Minocycline administered at a dose of 200 mg/day for 1 week results in a reduction of total bacterial counts, complete elimination of spirochetes for up to 2 months, and improvement of all clinical parameters.[14,15]

Side effects are similar to those of tetracycline; however, there is an increased incidence of vertigo. It is the only tetracycline that can permanently discolor erupted teeth and gingival tissue when administered orally.

Doxycycline

Doxycycline has the same spectrum of activity as minocycline and can be equally effective.[13] Because doxycycline can be given only once daily, patients may be more compliant. Compliance is also improved because its absorption from the gastrointestinal tract is only slightly altered by calcium, metal ions, or antacids, as is absorption of other tetracyclines. Side effects are similar to those of tetracycline hydrochloride; however, it is the most photosensitizing agent in the tetracycline category.

The recommended dosage when doxycycline is used as an anti-infective agent is 100 mg twice daily the first day, which is then reduced to 100 mg daily. To reduce gastrointestinal upset, 50 mg can be taken twice daily after the initial dose. When given as a subantimicrobial dose (to inhibit collagenase), 20 mg of doxycycline twice daily is recommended.[10,17]

Metronidazole

Pharmacology

Metronidazole is a nitroimidazole compound that was developed in France to treat protozoal infections. It is bactericidal to anaerobic organisms and is thought to disrupt bacterial DNA synthesis in conditions with a low reduction potential. Metronidazole is not the drug of choice for treating *A. actinomycetemcomitans* infections. However, metronidazole is effective against *A. actinomycetemcomitans* when used in combination with other antibiotics.[49,50] Metronidazole is also effective against anaerobes such as *Porphyromonas gingivalis* and *Prevotella intermedia*.[29]

Clinical Use

Metronidazole has been used clinically to treat acute necrotizing ulcerative gingivitis, chronic periodontitis, and aggressive periodontitis. It has been used as monotherapy and also in combination with root planing and surgery or with other antibiotics. Metronidazole has been used successfully to treat necrotizing ulcerative gingivitis.[43]

Studies in humans have demonstrated the efficacy of metronidazole for the treatment of periodontitis.[42] A single dose of metronidazole (250 mg orally) appears in both serum and GCF in sufficient quantities to inhibit a wide range of suspected periodontal pathogens. When it is administered systemically (i.e., 750 mg/day to 1000 mg/day for 2 weeks), metronidazole reduces the growth of anaerobic flora, including spirochetes, and it decreases the clinical and histopathologic signs of periodontitis.[42] The most common regimen is 250 mg 3 times daily for 7 days.[43] Currently, the critical level of spirochetes that is needed to diagnose an anaerobic infection, the appropriate time to give metronidazole, and the ideal dosage or duration of therapy are unknown.[29] As monotherapy (i.e., with no concurrent root planing), metronidazole is inferior and at best only equivalent to root planing. Therefore, if it is used, metronidazole should not be administered as monotherapy.

Soder and colleagues[55] demonstrated that metronidazole was more effective than placebo for the management of sites that were unresponsive to root planing. Nevertheless, many patients still had sites that bled with probing despite metronidazole therapy. The existence of refractory periodontitis as a diagnostic consideration indicates that some patients do not respond to conventional therapy, which may include root planing, surgery, or both.

Studies have suggested that when it is combined with amoxicillin or amoxicillin–clavulanate potassium (Augmentin), metronidazole may be of value for the management of patients with LAP or refractory periodontitis. This is discussed in more detail later in this chapter.

Side Effects

Metronidazole has an Antabuse effect when alcohol is ingested. The response is generally proportional to the amount ingested and can result in severe cramps, nausea, and vomiting. Products that contain alcohol should be avoided during therapy and for at least 1 day after therapy is discontinued. Metronidazole also inhibits warfarin metabolism. Patients who are undergoing anticoagulant therapy should avoid metronidazole because it prolongs prothrombin time.[43] It also should be avoided in patients who are taking lithium. This drug produces a metallic taste in the mouth, which may affect compliance.

Penicillins

Pharmacology

Penicillins are the drugs of choice for the treatment of many serious infections in humans and are the most widely used antibiotics. Penicillins are natural and semisynthetic derivatives of broth cultures of the *Penicillium* mold. They inhibit bacterial cell wall production and therefore are bactericidal.

Clinical Use

Penicillins other than amoxicillin and amoxicillin–clavulanate potassium (Augmentin) have not been shown to increase periodontal attachment levels, and their use in periodontal therapy does not appear to be justified.

Side Effects

Penicillins may induce allergic reactions and bacterial resistance.

 **KEY FACT**

Penicillin Allergy

Up to 10% of patients may be allergic to penicillin. Reactions to ingestion of penicillin or its derivatives, such as amoxicillin, in allergic patients can range from skin rash to life-threatening anaphylaxis.

Amoxicillin

Amoxicillin is a semisynthetic penicillin with an extended anti-infective spectrum that includes gram-positive and gram-negative bacteria. It demonstrates excellent absorption after oral administration. Amoxicillin is susceptible to penicillinase, which is a β-lactamase produced by certain bacteria that breaks the penicillin ring structure and thus renders penicillins ineffective.

Amoxicillin may be useful for the management of patients with severe form of periodontitis (previously classified as localized/generalized aggressive periodontitis). The recommended dosage is 500 mg 3 times daily for 8 days.[36,37]

Amoxicillin–Clavulanate Potassium

The combination of amoxicillin with clavulanate potassium makes this anti-infective agent resistant to penicillinase enzymes produced by some bacteria. Amoxicillin with clavulanate (Augmentin) may be useful for the management of patients with LAP or refractory periodontitis.[47] Bueno and colleagues[9] reported that Augmentin arrested alveolar bone loss in patients with periodontal disease that was refractory to treatment with other antibiotics, including tetracycline, metronidazole, and clindamycin.

Cephalosporins

Pharmacology

The family of β-lactams known as cephalosporins is similar in action and structure to penicillins. These drugs are frequently used in medicine, and they are resistant to a number of β-lactamases that are normally active against penicillin.

Clinical Use

Cephalosporins are generally not used to treat dental-related infections. Penicillins are superior to cephalosporins with regard to their range of action against periodontal pathogenic bacteria.

Side Effects

Patients who are allergic to penicillins must be considered to be allergic to all β-lactam products. More specifically, up to 10% of patients who have an allergy to penicillin may also have an adverse reaction to cephalosporins. Rashes, urticaria, fever, and gastrointestinal upset have all been associated with cephalosporins.[65]

Clindamycin

Pharmacology

Clindamycin is effective against anaerobic bacteria and has a strong affinity for osseous tissue.[60] It is effective for situations in which the patient is allergic to penicillin.

Clinical Use

Clindamycin has demonstrated efficacy in patients with periodontitis that are refractory to tetracycline therapy. Walker and colleagues[65] showed that clindamycin helped stabilize refractory patients; the dosage used was 150 mg 4 times daily for 10 days. Jorgensen and Slots[37] recommend a regimen of 300 mg twice daily for 8 days.

Side Effects

Clindamycin has been associated with pseudomembranous colitis, but the incidence is higher with cephalosporins and ampicillin. When needed, however, clindamycin can be used with caution, but it is not indicated for patients with a history of colitis. Diarrhea or cramping that develops during clindamycin therapy may be indicative of colitis, and it should be discontinued. If symptoms persist, the patient should be referred to an internist.

Ciprofloxacin

Pharmacology

Ciprofloxacin is a quinolone that is active against gram-negative rods, including all facultative and some anaerobic putative periodontal pathogens.[45]

Clinical Use

Because it demonstrates a minimal effect on *Streptococcus* species, which are associated with periodontal health, ciprofloxacin therapy may facilitate the establishment of a microflora that is associated with periodontal health. At present, ciprofloxacin is the only antibiotic in periodontal therapy to which all strains of *A. actinomycetemcomitans* are susceptible. It has also been used in combination with metronidazole.[49]

Side Effects

Nausea, headache, metallic taste in the mouth, and abdominal discomfort have been associated with ciprofloxacin. Quinolones inhibit the metabolism of theophylline, and caffeine and concurrent administration can produce toxicity. Quinolones have also been reported to enhance the effects of warfarin and other anticoagulants.[65]

Macrolides

Pharmacology

Macrolide antibiotics contain a many-membered lactone ring to which one or more deoxy sugars are attached. They inhibit protein synthesis by binding to the 50S ribosomal subunits of sensitive microorganisms. Macrolides can be bacteriostatic or bactericidal depending on the concentration of the drug and the nature of the microorganism. The macrolide antibiotics used for periodontal treatment include erythromycin, spiramycin, and azithromycin.

Clinical Use

Erythromycin does not concentrate in GCF and is not effective against most putative periodontal pathogens. For these reasons, erythromycin is not recommended as an adjunct to periodontal therapy.

Spiramycin is active against gram-positive organisms; it is excreted in high concentrations in saliva. It is used as an adjunct to periodontal treatment in Canada and Europe but is not available in the United States. Spiramycin has a minimal effect on attachment levels.

Azithromycin is a member of the azalide class of macrolides. It is effective against anaerobes and gram-negative bacilli. After an oral dosage of 500 mg 4 times daily for 3 days, significant levels of azithromycin can be detected in most tissues for 7 to 10 days.[8,34] The concentration of azithromycin in tissue specimens from periodontal lesions is significantly higher than that of normal gingiva.[44] It has been proposed that azithromycin penetrates fibroblasts and phagocytes in concentrations that are 100 to 200 times greater than that of the extracellular compartment. Azithromycin is actively transported to sites of inflammation by phagocytes, where it is released directly into the sites of inflammation as the phagocytes rupture during phagocytosis.[27] Therapeutic use requires a single dose of 250 mg/day for 5 days after an initial loading dose of 500 mg.[65]

Data have suggested that azithromycin may be an effective adjunctive therapy for increasing attachment levels in patients with aggressive periodontitis[31] as well as for reducing the degree of gingival enlargement.[16] These data must be carefully considered because they were derived from small subject populations. Currently, the literature presents conflicting reports regarding the efficacy of this antibiotic as an adjunct to periodontal therapy. One study concluded that adjunctive azithromycin provides no additional benefit over nonsurgical periodontal treatment for the parameters investigated in patients with severe generalized chronic periodontitis. Furthermore, an additional study reported that there was an increase in cardiovascular deaths among patients who received azithromycin; this increase was most pronounced among patients with a high baseline risk of cardiovascular disease. As a result of this study, the U.S. Food and Drug Administration issued a warning that the drug can alter the electrical activity of the heart, which may lead to a potentially fatal heart rhythm known as *prolonged QT interval.* This rhythm causes the timing of the heart's contractions to become irregular. The warning stated that physicians should use caution when giving the antibiotic to patients who are known to have this condition or who are at risk for cardiovascular problems.

To ascertain the efficacy of azithromycin for the management of periodontal diseases, future studies will need to increase the number of subjects, improve diagnostic methods and tools, and determine the appropriate dose, duration, and frequency of azithromycin therapy.

Serial and Combination Antibiotic Therapy

Rationale

Because periodontal infections may contain a wide variety of bacteria, no single antibiotic is effective against all putative pathogens. Indeed, differences exist in the microbial flora associated with the various periodontal disease syndromes.[66] These "mixed" infections can include a variety of aerobic, microaerophilic, and anaerobic bacteria, which may be both gram-negative and gram-positive. In these cases, it may be necessary to use more than one antibiotic, either serially or in combination.[50] Before combinations of antibiotics are used, however, the periodontal pathogens being treated should be identified and antibiotic-susceptibility testing performed.[67]

Clinical Use

Antibiotics that are bacteriostatic (e.g., tetracycline) generally require rapidly dividing microorganisms to be effective. They do not function well if a bactericidal antibiotic (e.g., amoxicillin) is given concurrently. *When both types of drugs are required, they are best given serially rather than in combination.*

Rams and Slots[50] reviewed combination therapy involving the use of systemic metronidazole along with amoxicillin, amoxicillin–clavulanate (Augmentin), or ciprofloxacin. The metronidazole–amoxicillin and metronidazole–Augmentin combinations provided excellent elimination of many organisms in adults with LAP who had been treated unsuccessfully with tetracyclines and mechanical debridement. These drugs have an additive effect that involves the suppression of *A. actinomycetemcomitans*. Tinoco and colleagues[59] found metronidazole and amoxicillin to be clinically effective for the treatment of LAP, although 50% of patients who were treated with this regimen harbored *A. actinomycetemcomitans* 1 year later. The metronidazole–ciprofloxacin combination is effective against *A. actinomycetemcomitans;* metronidazole targets obligate anaerobes, and ciprofloxacin targets facultative anaerobes. This is a powerful combination against mixed infections. Studies of this drug combination for the treatment of refractory periodontitis have documented marked clinical improvement. This combination may provide a therapeutic benefit by reducing or eliminating pathogenic organisms and a prophylactic benefit by giving rise to a predominantly streptococcal microflora.[49]

Systemic antibiotic therapy in combination with mechanical therapy appears to be valuable for the treatment of recalcitrant periodontal infections and LAP infections that involve *A. actinomycetemcomitans*. Antibiotic treatment should be reserved for specific subsets of periodontal patients who do not respond to conventional therapy. The selection of specific agents should be guided by the results of cultures and sensitivity tests for subgingival plaque microorganisms. A handful of randomized clinical trials and meta-analyses demonstrated that the combination of amoxicillin and metronidazole showed superior clinical outcomes with a significant decrease in probing pocket depths, frequency of occurrence of deeper pockets, clinical attachment level (CAL) gain, and reduction in bleeding on probing (BOP) when compared to metronidazole and azithromycin combination. Although no meta-analyses were able to be performed, the amoxicillin and metronidazole combination was also associated with a higher number of side effects.[2,58,53]

Pharmacologic Implications

Principles of antibiotic therapy for the proper selection of an antibiotic minimally require identification of the causative organism, determination of the antibiotic sensitivity, and an effective method of administration.[33] The use of antibiotics to treat gingival diseases is contraindicated, because this is a local infection that can be easily treated with scaling and appropriate home care by the patient.[57] With regard to destructive periodontal diseases, there are limited data to support the use of systemic antibiotic treatment. Although bacterial infections of the periodontium are considered to be important to initiation of the disease, currently no one microbe or group of microbes has been demonstrated to be the cause of these diseases. It is therefore not surprising that systemic antibiotics have had only a modest effect on the management of periodontal diseases. Systemic antibiotics for the treatment of periodontal diseases have been

TABLE 53.3 Therapeutic Uses of Systemic Antimicrobial Agents for Various Periodontal Diseases

Disease	Systemic Antimicrobial Agents	Adjunct or Stand-Alone Therapy
Gingival diseases	Antibiotic use not recommended	Not applicable
Necrotizing gingivitis	Antibiotic use not recommended unless there are systemic complications (e.g., fever, swollen lymph nodes)	As an adjunct when necessary
Generalized Stage III Grade B Periodontitis	Limited benefit; antibiotic use not recommended	Not applicable
Aggressive periodontitis (AAP 1999 classification) Currently classified as Generalized Stage III or IV Grade C Periodontitis or Localized Stage III/IV Grade C Periodontitis with molar-incisor pattern	Antibiotic use recommended; for greatest benefit, therapeutic levels of antibiotics should be achieved by the time scaling and root planing are completed (all debridement should be completed within a week); the optimal antibiotic type, dose, frequency, and duration have not been identified	As an adjunct
Necrotizing periodontitis	Antibiotic use dependent on the systemic condition of the patient	As an adjunct when necessary
Periodontitis as a manifestation of systemic disease	Antibiotic use dependent on the systemic condition of the patient	As an adjunct when necessary
Periodontal abscess	Antibiotic use not recommended	As an adjunct when necessary

"As an adjunct when necessary" refers to presence of associated systemic conditions/complications.

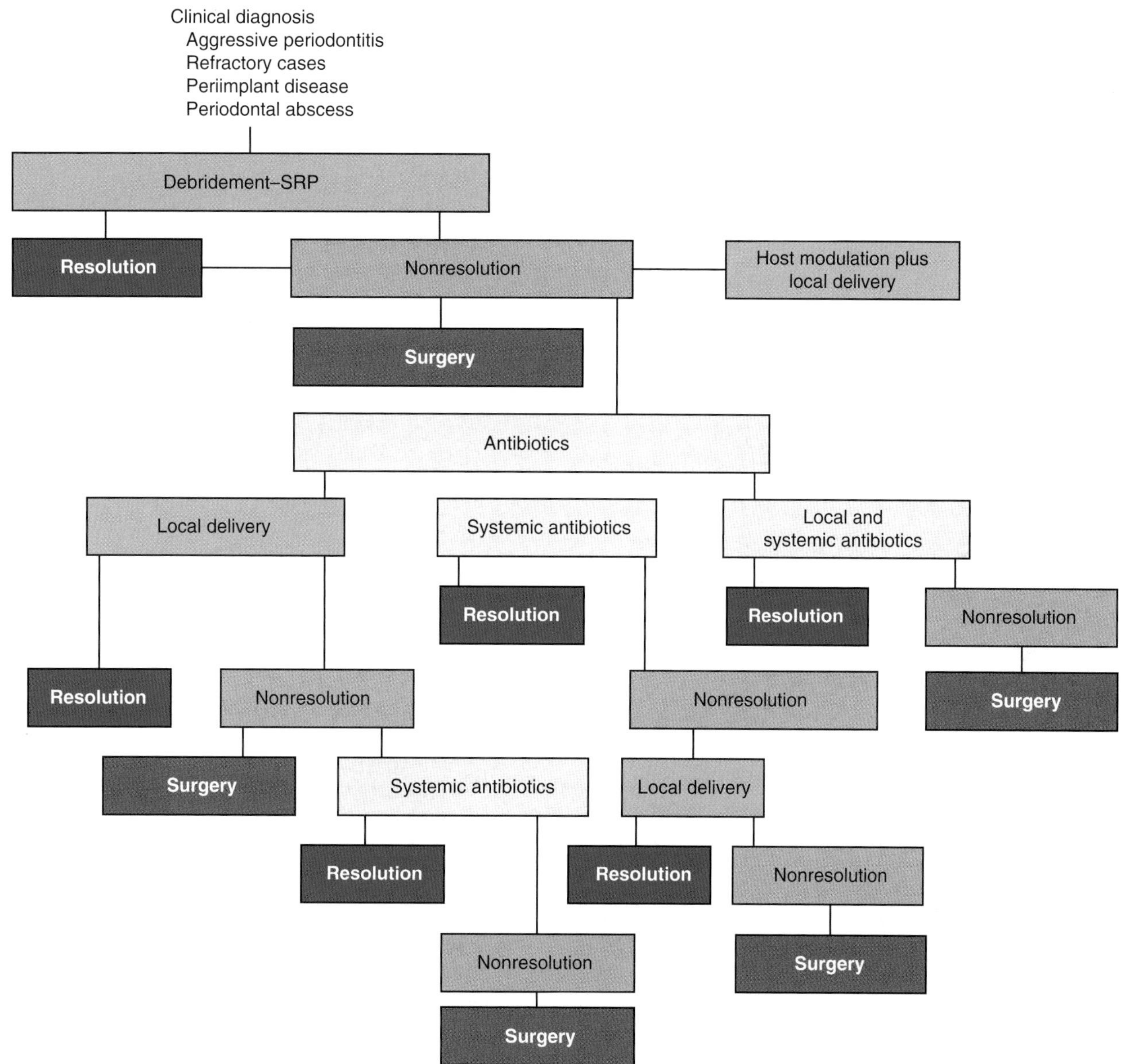

Fig. 53.5 A decision tree for the selection of antibiotic therap. *SRP*, Scaling and root planing.

indicated primarily for adjunctive use in the treatment of aggressive periodontal diseases (Table 53.3).[30,32]

Guidelines for the use of antibiotics in periodontal therapy include the following:

1. The clinical diagnosis and situation dictate the need for possible antibiotic therapy as an adjunct for controlling active periodontal disease (Fig. 53.5).
2. Disease activity as measured by continuing attachment loss, purulent exudate, and bleeding on probing[39,40] may be an indication for periodontal intervention and possible microbial analysis through plaque sampling.
3. When they are used to treat periodontal disease, antibiotics are selected on the basis of the patient's medical and dental status, current medications,[36] and the results of microbial analysis, if it is performed.
4. Microbiologic plaque sampling may be performed according to the instructions of the reference laboratory. The samples are usually taken at the beginning of an appointment before instrumentation of the pocket. Supragingival plaque is removed, and an endodontic paper point is inserted subgingivally into the deepest pockets to absorb bacteria in the loosely associated plaque. This endodontic point is placed in reduced transfer fluid or a sterile transfer tube and sent to the laboratory. The laboratory will then send the referring dentist a report that includes the pathogens that are present and any appropriate antibiotic regimen. At this time, there are scant data to suggest that microbial identification from a plaque sample can be used to clinically improve the periodontal condition of the patient.
5. Meta-analyses of randomized clinical trials and quasi-experimental studies have shown that systemic antibiotics can improve attachment levels when they are used as adjuncts to root instrumentation. The same benefits could not be demonstrated when antibiotics were used as a stand-alone therapy.[32]
6. When systemic antibiotics were used as adjuncts to scaling and root planing, improvements were observed in the attachment levels of patients with chronic and aggressive periodontitis, although patients with aggressive periodontitis experienced greater benefits.[32] The mean attachment level change depended on the antibiotic used and ranged from 0.09 mm to 1.10 mm.[32] The more severe the disease and the deeper the pocket, the better the response to antibiotic therapy.[58]

7. The identification of which antibiotics were most effective for the treatment of destructive periodontal diseases was limited by the insufficient sizes of the samples found in the randomized clinical trials used as part of a systematic review.[32] One of the recent systematic reviews and meta-analysis demonstrated that the amoxicillin and metronidazole combination has the most significant impact on clinical outcomes, including pocket reduction, BOP reduction, and CAL gain.[58]
8. Debridement of root surfaces, optimal oral hygiene, and frequent periodontal maintenance therapy are important parts of comprehensive periodontal therapy. As mentioned previously, an antibiotic strength that is 500 times greater than the systemic therapeutic dose may be required to be effective against bacteria that have been arranged into biofilm. It is therefore important to disrupt the biofilm physically so that the antibiotic agents can have access to the periodontal pathogens.[30]
9. Although there are adequate data to suggest that systemic antibiotics can be of benefit for the treatment of destructive periodontal diseases, there are limited data available to identify which antibiotics are suitable for which infection; the optimum dosage, frequency, and duration of antibiotic therapy; when the regimen should be introduced during the treatment schedule; the long-term outcomes of antibiotic use; the potential hazards of these agents (e.g., antibiotic resistance, changes in oral microflora);[32] and the economic ramifications of this type of pharmacologic intervention.

The selection of an antibiotic must be made on the basis of factors other than the empirical decisions made by the clinician. Unfortunately, there is no one best choice of antibiotic at present (i.e., there is no "silver bullet"). Therefore, the clinician must integrate the history of the patient's disease, the clinical signs and symptoms, and the results of radiographic examinations and possibly microbiologic sampling to determine the course of periodontal therapy. The clinician must obtain a thorough medical history, including current medications and the possible adverse effects of combining these medicines, before prescribing any antibiotic therapy. The clinician must make the final decision with the patient. Risks and benefits concerning antibiotics as adjuncts to periodontal therapy should be discussed with the patient before antibiotics are used.

Alternatives to systemic antibiotics:

Prevalence of side effects associated with systemic antibiotics and the emerging antibiotic-resistant organisms and genes warrant a dire need for antibiotic alternatives in the future. Several novel preventive and therapeutic strategies, such as probiotics, prebiotics, and secreted bacterial products—such as bacteriocins—are being investigated as alternatives for antibiotics. Emerging evidence demonstrates their ability to suppress the periodontal pathogens and/or change the environment to be unfavorable for pathogens while protecting the commensal bacterial species. Future research is warranted to investigate the clinical application of these findings and identify a suitable target for delivering these alternatives.[24,46,48,52] (Refer to Chapter 10 for a detailed description of probiotics, prebiotics, bacteriocins.)

Conclusion

Manual instrumentation (scaling and root planing) alone is effective for reducing pocket depths, gaining increases in periodontal attachment levels, and decreasing inflammation levels (i.e., bleeding on probing). When systemic antibiotics are used as adjuncts to root instrumentation, the evidence indicates that some systemic antibiotics (e.g., metronidazole, tetracycline) provide additional improvements in attachment levels (0.35 mm for metronidazole; 0.40 mm for tetracycline) depending on the severity and form of the disease.[32] The use of anti-infective chemotherapeutic treatment adjuncts does not result in significant adverse effects for patients.

The decision regarding when to use systemic antimicrobials should be made on the basis of the clinician's consideration of the clinical findings, the patient's medical and dental history,[18,20] the patient's preferences, and the potential benefits of adjunctive therapy with these agents.

CHAPTER HIGHLIGHTS

- The *systemic administration* of antibiotics may be a necessary adjunct for controlling bacterial infection because bacteria can invade periodontal tissues, thereby making mechanical therapy alone sometimes ineffective.
- Although oral bacteria are susceptible to many antibiotics, no single antibiotic at the concentrations achieved in body fluids inhibits all putative periodontal pathogens.
- The protocol for use of antibiotic agents depends on the mechanism of action, the patient's health status and history, and the clinical presentation.

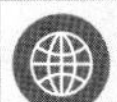
A Case Scenario is found on the companion website eBooks.Health.Elsevier.com.

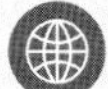
References for this chapter are found on the companion website eBooks.Health.Elsevier.com.

CHAPTER 54

Locally Delivered, Controlled-Release Antimicrobials

Richard D. Finkelman  | Hector L. Sarmiento | Alan M. Polson

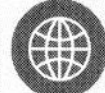 For online-only information regarding cost-effectiveness of locally delivered antimicrobials, clinical studies of non-U.S. agents, ongoing and future research considerations, and case reports, please visit the companion website at eBooks.Health.Elsevier.com.

CHAPTER OUTLINE

Background and Objectives

Periodontitis is a bacterial infection. The focus of most nonsurgical periodontal therapy, including mechanical therapy such as subgingival root instrumentation (like scaling and root planing [SRP]), is to combat infection. Chemical antibacterial strategies include systemic drug delivery, oral rinses or toothpastes, and irrigating devices, but none of these therapies have provided significant clinical benefit in reducing the signs of chronic periodontitis.

In the past few decades, a new strategy has emerged. Several controlled-release delivery systems have been developed to deposit antimicrobials directly into the periodontal pocket and maintain effective concentrations of drug for an extended period. After extensive study, these agents have been declared safe and effective for the treatment of chronic adult periodontitis. In some cases, they are used as monotherapy and, in other cases, they are administered adjunctively with SRP, which is generally considered by the professional community to be the best approach.

Evidence-based practice, which provides dental treatment based on research, produces optimal care for the greatest number of patients.[117,118] Locally delivered, controlled-release antimicrobials may have the most robust data of any periodontal therapy to support their clinical use. This chapter considers the available clinical data that support the use of these agents for the treatment of periodontitis and provides evidence-based guidance for their use. In this discussion, locally delivered, controlled-release antimicrobials are considered as a drug class rather than individually.

Because appropriate comparative trials have not been performed, there are insufficient data on which to base comparisons of agents or consider differential indications for use. The indications for use of each product are described in their respective full prescribing information. Some commentary is provided regarding these agents and available research for potentially new indications that have not been evaluated by the U.S. Food and Drug Administration (FDA) (Box 54.1).

U.S. Locally Delivered, Controlled-Release Antimicrobials

Three locally delivered, controlled-release antimicrobial products are available for dental use in the United States (Table 54.1): a chlorhexidine-containing chip (PerioChip), a doxycycline gel (Atridox), and minocycline microspheres (Arestin). A fourth product, an ethylene or vinyl acetate copolymer fiber containing the antibiotic tetracycline (Actisite as a 12.7-mg, 9-inch filament), was the first product introduced into the U.S. market in the early 1990s and was the prototypic system. The tetracycline fiber is no longer commercially available in the United States, and its clinical use is not further considered, but it is included because data generated from clinical studies of the product are pertinent to a discussion of the general effects of locally delivered, controlled-release antimicrobials.

Chlorhexidine Chip

The chlorhexidine chip is a small chip (4.0 × 5.0 × 0.35 mm) that contains 2.5 mg of the active ingredient chlorhexidine gluconate in a resorbable, biodegradable matrix of hydrolyzed gelatin that is cross-linked with glutaraldehyde and packaged in individual foil containers (Fig. 54.1A). The chip is stored at 20°C to 25°C (68°F to 77°F), with excursions permitted to 15°C to 30°C (59°F to 86°F). The chlorhexidine chip is placed into the pocket directly from the foil container using a forceps (see Fig. 54.1B).

The chlorhexidine chip is indicated as an adjunct to SRP procedures for the reduction of pocket depth in adults with periodontitis, and it can be used as part of a periodontal maintenance program, which includes good oral hygiene and SRP.[133] After placement in the pocket, the chip has been reported to release chlorhexidine into the gingival crevicular fluid (GCF) over 7 to 10 days.[166] Chlorhexidine is active against a broad range of microbes. It disrupts the cell membrane and causes precipitation of the cytoplasm, resulting in cell death. No adverse alterations in the oral microbial

BOX 54.1 Adjunctive Therapy

- Adjunctive therapy makes subgingival root instrumentation (SRP) more effective.
- Because most pockets are quiescent, mean changes are modest when all pockets are included.
- Significantly more patients show large pocket depth reductions with adjunctive therapy.
- Clinical responses are evident only after time and with clinical pocket measurements.
- The greatest clinical benefit is likely to result when adjunctive agents are routinely included as part of SRP procedures and in a long-term periodontal maintenance program.

TABLE 54.1 Locally Delivered, Controlled-Release Antimicrobials Developed and FDA Approved for Dental Use in the United States

Product	Antimicrobial Agent
Actisite[a]	Tetracycline
PerioChip	Chlorhexidine
Arestin	Minocycline
Atridox	Doxycycline

[a]No longer commercially available in the United States.

flora or overgrowth of opportunistic microorganisms have been observed.[133] The chip is biodegradable and does not require removal, but dental floss should be avoided for 10 days to avoid dislodging it.

Doxycycline Gel

Doxycycline gel is a subgingival, controlled-release delivery product composed of a two-syringe mixing system (Fig. 54.2A). Syringe A contains 450 mg of a bioabsorbable polymeric formulation of 36.7% poly(D,L,-lactide) dissolved in 63.3% *N*-methyl-2-pyrrolidone. Syringe B contains 50 mg of doxycycline hyclate, equivalent to 42.5 mg of doxycycline. The two syringes are stored at 2°C to 30°C (36°F to 86°F). When mixed, the product is a viscous liquid of 500 mg, which contains 50 mg (10%) of doxycycline hyclate.

Doxycycline gel is indicated for the treatment of chronic adult periodontitis for a gain in clinical attachment, reduction in probing depth, and reduction of bleeding on probing.[15] Doxycycline, a broad-spectrum semisynthetic tetracycline, is bacteriostatic, inhibiting bacterial protein biosynthesis by interfering with transfer RNA (tRNA) and messenger RNA (mRNA) at the ribosome. No overgrowth of opportunistic organisms was observed after use of the doxycycline gel.[15]

The gel has been reported to release doxycycline in the GCF over 7 days.[174] The doxycycline gel is biodegradable and does not require removal. If not used immediately, the mixed contents in syringe A can be stored in an airtight container at room temperature for a maximum of 3 days. The doxycycline gel is used by injecting the mixed contents of the two syringes directly into the pocket (see

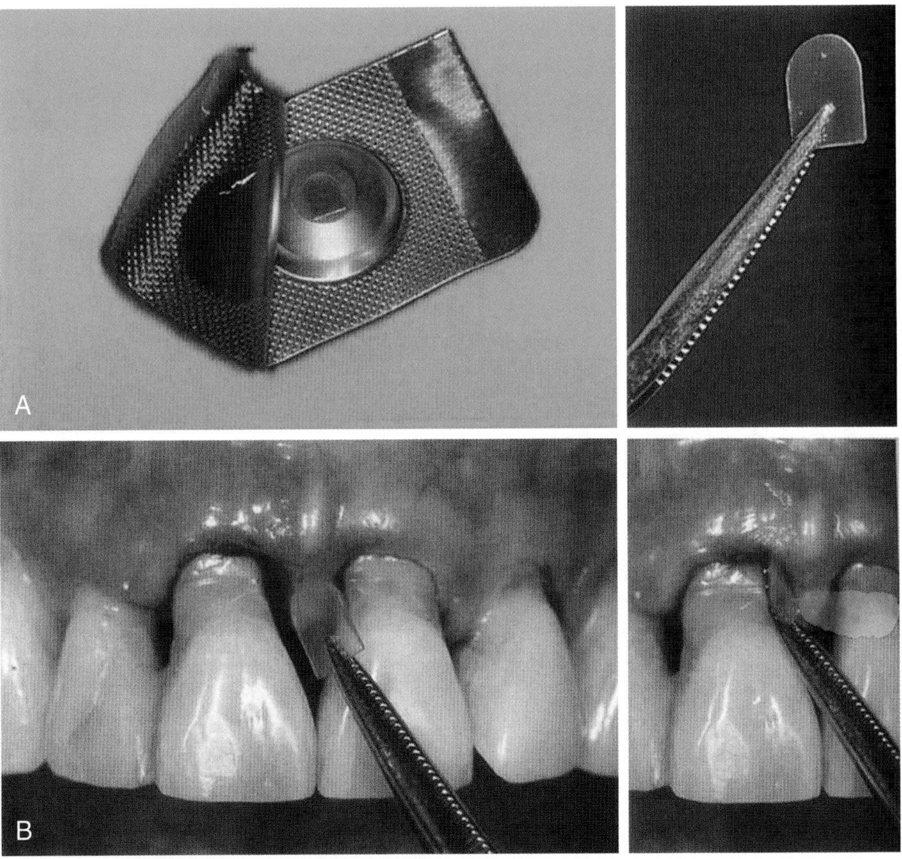

Fig. 54.1 Chlorhexidine Gluconate Chip (PerioChip). (A) The chip is packaged in a foil packet *(left)*. The chip is removed from the foil container with a suitable forceps *(right)*. (B) The chip is inserted into the pocket, curved end first *(left)*. After insertion, the chip is pressed apically to the base of the pocket *(right)*. (Reprinted from Wolf HF, Hassell TM. *Color Atlas of Dental Hygiene: Periodontology.* 1st ed. Stuttgart, Germany: Thieme; 2006, with permission.)

Fig. 54.2B). The pocket contents are then covered with a periodontal dressing or a cyanoacrylate dental adhesive.

Minocycline Microspheres

The minocycline microspheres product is a subgingival, controlled-release delivery system containing the antibiotic minocycline hydrochloride incorporated into a bioresorbable (glycolide-co-D,L-lactide) polymer in unit-dose cartridges (Fig. 54.3). Each cartridge delivers minocycline hydrochloride equivalent to 1 mg of minocycline free base. Minocycline microspheres are indicated as an adjunct to SRP for the reduction of pocket depth in patients with adult periodontitis and as part of a periodontal maintenance program, which includes good oral hygiene and SRP.[14]

Minocycline belongs to the tetracycline class of antibiotics and has a broad spectrum of activity. Its bacteriostatic, antimicrobial activity results from the inhibition of protein biosynthesis. No overgrowth of opportunistic microorganisms was reported from clinical studies. No changes in the number of minocycline-resistant bacteria,

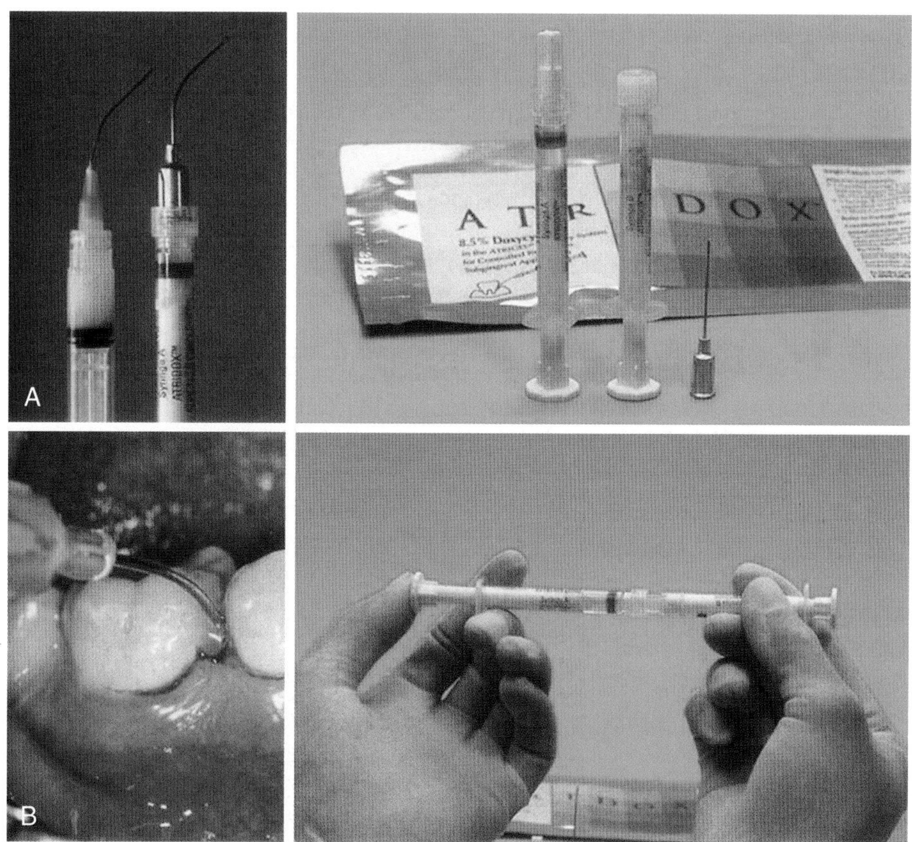

Fig. 54.2 Doxycycline Hyclate Gel (Atridox). (A) Doxycycline gel is packaged as a two-syringe mixing system *(right)*. After mixing the gel, a cannula is attached for injection *(left)*. (B) The two syringes are coupled, and the liquid contents of syringe A are injected into the powder within syringe B; the contents are mixed within the two syringes for 100 cycles (1 cycle/s) and then left within syringe A *(right)*. The mixed solution is injected into the pocket through the cannula attached to syringe A until the pocket is completely filled *(left)*. The pocket contents are covered with a periodontal dressing or a cyanoacrylate dental adhesive. (Reprinted from Wolf HF, Hassell TM. *Color Atlas of Dental Hygiene: Periodontology.* 1st ed. Stuttgart, Germany: Thieme; 2006, with permission.)

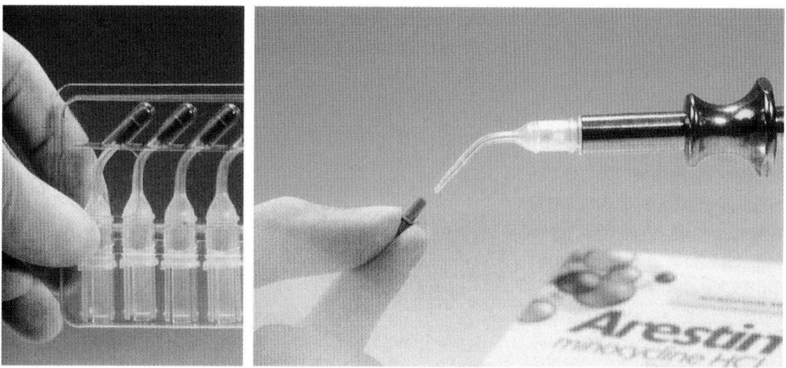

Fig. 54.3 Minocycline Hydrochloride Microspheres (Arestin). Minocycline microspheres are packaged into unit-dose cartridges *(left)*. Microspheres are used by injecting the cartridge contents directly with a syringe into the periodontal pocket *(right)*. (Reprinted from Wolf HF, Hassell TM. *Color Atlas of Dental Hygiene: Periodontology.* 1st ed. Stuttgart, Germany: Thieme; 2006, with permission.)

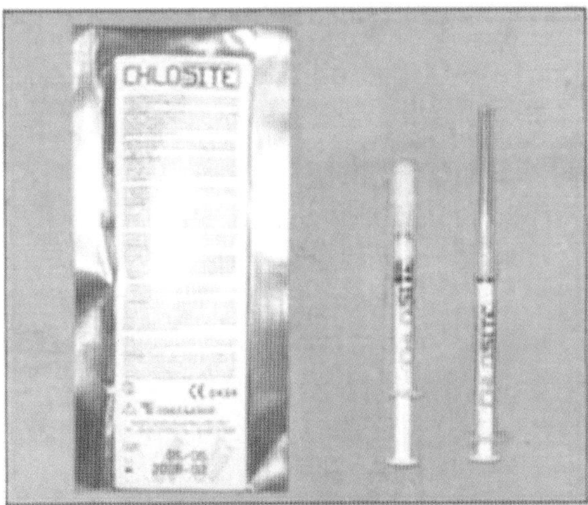

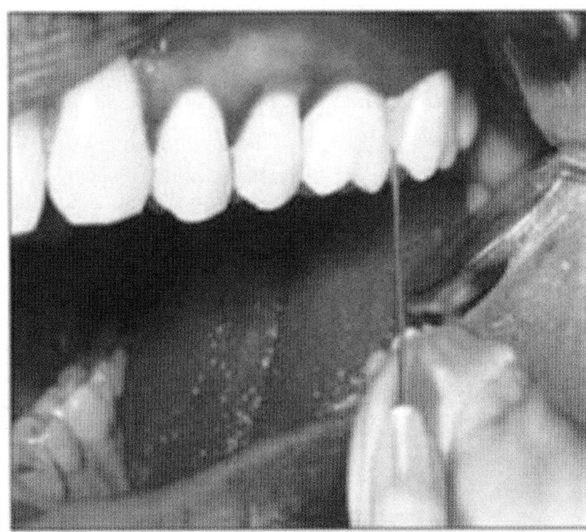

Fig. 54.4 Chlo-Site gel packaging is shown *(left)*. The xanthan gel with chlorhexidine is inserted into the periodontal pocket *(right)*. (Reprinted from Gill JS. Nonsurgical management of chronic periodontitis with two local drug delivery agents—a comparative study. *J Clin Exp Dent.* 2011;3:e424–e429.)

Candida albicans or *Staphylococcus aureus*, in the gastrointestinal tract were detected at the end of a 56-day study, although there was a slight increase in the numbers of minocycline-resistant bacteria in periodontal pocket plaque samples after 9 months.[14] The clinical significance of the changes is unknown.

Patients should avoid hard or sticky foods at the treated teeth for 1 week and interproximal cleaning devices for about 10 days. The minocycline microspheres formulation is biodegradable and does not require removal. The cartridges are stored at 20°C to 25°C (68°F to 77°F), with excursions permitted to 15°C to 30°C (59°F to 86°F). Excessive heat should be avoided. The minocycline microspheres are used by injecting the contents of a unit-dose cartridge into the pocket. Neither a periodontal dressing nor an adhesive is needed.

Complete details on the use of locally delivered, controlled-release antimicrobials and their safety profiles are available in the full prescribing information for each product.[14,15,133] The reader is also referred to a companion website for online video demonstrations of the administration of each of these three agents.

Non-U.S. Locally Delivered, Controlled-Release Antimicrobials

After approval by the FDA of locally delivered, controlled-release antimicrobials for clinical use in the United States, several products were approved for use in other countries. These products typically use antimicrobial agents that were discussed earlier for U.S. products.

Chlorhexidine-Based Products

PerioCol-CG

PerioCol-CG is a small, 10-mg chip (4 × 5 × 0.25 to 0.32 mm) designed as a collagen matrix into which chlorhexidine gluconate (2.5 mg) is incorporated from a 20% chlorhexidine solution that is its active ingredient. The chip is designed for insertion into the periodontal pocket and resorbs after 30 days, but its coronal edge degrades within 10 days.[12,32] It releases chlorhexidine in vitro at a rate of approximately 40% to 45% in the first 24 hours, followed by a linear release for 7 to 8 days, and it has a shelf life of 2 years.[12,65]

Chlo-Site

Chlo-Site is a xanthan gel, consisting of a saccharide polymer as a three-dimensional mesh containing 1.5% chlorhexidine in 0.5 mL of gel, which is injected into the periodontal pocket (Fig. 54.4). The gel product is sterilized by gamma radiation at 2.5 Mrad and is individually packed for delivery in 0.25-mL prefilled syringes fitted with a blunt side-exit needle.[10,32,42]

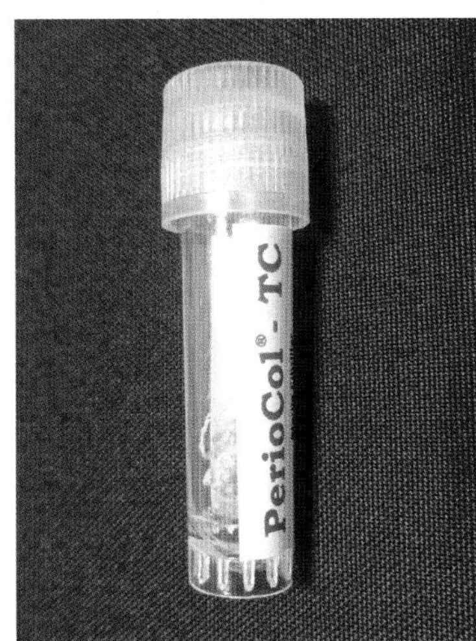

Fig. 54.5 PerioCol-TC fibers are packaged in an individual vial. (Courtesy Eucare Pharmaceuticals, Ltd., Chennai, India. http://www.eucare.in/dental-regeneration-concepts.html.)

The gel contains two types of chlorhexidine: a slow-release chlorhexidine digluconate (0.5%) and a rapid-release chlorhexidine dihydrochloride (1.0%).[10] The gel is retained within the pocket and is not easily dislodged by the GCF or saliva. The gel disappears from the pocket in 10 to 30 days and is reported to achieve a chlorhexidine concentration in GCF of more than 100 µg/mL for an average of 6 to 9 days and to maintain an effective concentration for at least 15 days.[32,66]

Tetracycline-Based Products

PerioCol-TC

As reported by the manufacturer,[46] each PerioCol-TC vial contains fish type I collagen (approximately 25 mg) impregnated with approximately 2.0 mg of tetracycline hydrochloride, which is sterilized by gamma radiation (Fig. 54.5). PerioCol-TC releases tetracycline in vitro for 8 to 10 days. A periodontal dressing should be placed to avoid dislodging the fibers.

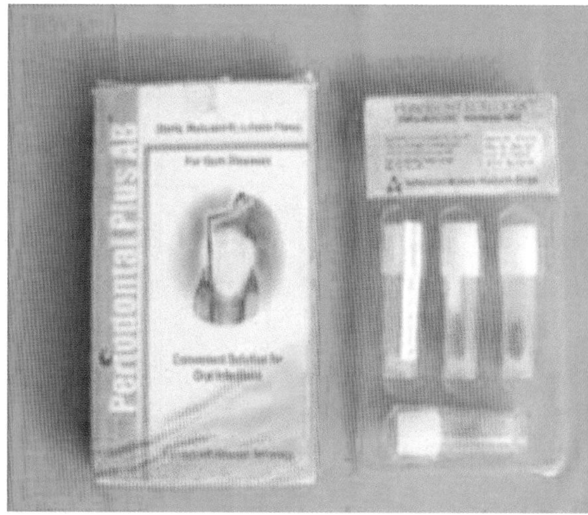

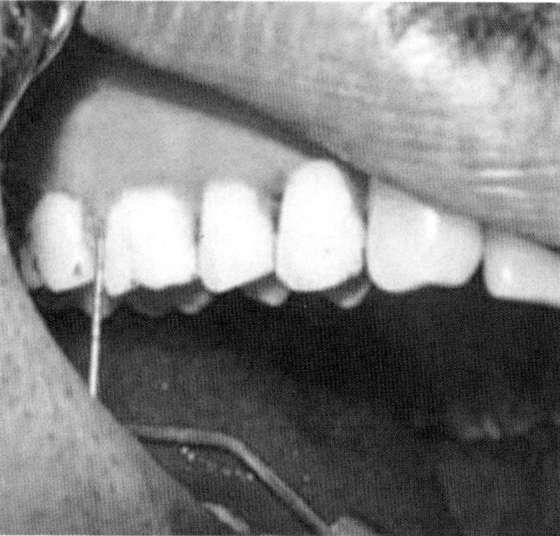

Fig. 54.6 Periodontal Plus AB packaging *(left)*. Fibers are Inserted into the periodontal pocket *(right)*. (Reprinted from Gill JS. Nonsurgical management of chronic periodontitis with two local drug delivery agents—a comparative study. *J Clin Exp Dent.* 2011;3:e424–e429.)

PerioCol-TC is indicated for the treatment of adult periodontitis as an adjunct to SRP for pockets more than 5 mm deep, and it can be administered every 3 months. The fibers are moistened with saline and placed into the periodontal pocket to the depth of the pocket base; they are biodegradable and do not have to be removed. PerioCol-TC is stored in a dry place between 5°C (41°F) and 25°C (77°F) and has a shelf life of 2 years with proper storage.

Periodontal Plus AB

Periodontal Plus AB is a bioresorbable tetracycline fiber. It is 25 mg of pure fibrillar collagen evenly impregnated with approximately 2 mg of tetracycline hydrochloride (Fig. 54.6).[158] The fibers are packaged as a strip containing four individually packed and separable sterile product packs. The fiber biodegrades in the periodontal pocket within 7 days.[32] The fiber should be retained with a periodontal dressing or covered with a dental adhesive for 10 days.

Doxycycline-Based Products

Ligosan Slow Release

Ligosan Slow Release is a 14% (w/w), resorbable doxycycline gel for periodontal application provided in a laminate pouch and stored under refrigeration. It contains 1, 2, 4, 8, 10, or 16 single-application cylinder cartridges, each containing 260 mg of Ligosan Slow Release (Fig. 54.7).[98]

The product is used by inserting the cartridge into the caulking gun, opening the spray nozzle, and then discharging the gel to the bottom of the pocket. The doxycycline release profile was studied in 20 patients.[98] The maximal value in the GCF within the first 5 hours (i.e., at 15 minutes) was 19.97 ± 5.58 mg /mL; after 3 days, the concentration was 577.1 ± 127.3 μg/mL. Concentrations in the GCF remained above 16 μg/mL for at least 12 days. Mechanical hygiene in the area should be avoided for 7 days.

Rationale for Local Delivery and Controlled Release

Periodontitis is a multifactorial disease (Fig. 54.8). The first requirement is a susceptible host, largely due to genetics, and not modifiable. Another nonmodifiable risk factor is age. Disease risks that may be modifiable include pathogenic oral plaque microorganisms and behavioral or environmental factors such as tobacco use. Mediating the pathogenesis are host-derived elements, including immune and inflammatory responses that can affect soft and hard tissue metabolism and feed back on the pathogenic flora.

From the most basic perspective, periodontal diseases are bacterial infections; the requirement for bacteria to initiate the periodontal lesion is well recognized. The antibacterial effect of SRP or other mechanical therapy generally results from a reduction of the bacterial load or an alteration of the composition of the bacterial flora at the periodontal site, but the antibacterial effect of mechanical treatment alone is insufficient, providing the rationale for chemically augmenting the mechanical therapy.

Many strategies have been used to deliver antimicrobial agents to the periodontal pocket at effective doses to reduce the bacterial microflora, including systemic administration or local administration by local irrigation of fluid formulations or placement of various gels or ointments. None of these strategies have proved as effective as controlled-release antimicrobials.

A drawback of antimicrobials delivered to the pocket but not in controlled-release formulations results from the dynamics of the GCF. The GCF fills the periodontal pocket space, but the copious flow out of the pocket continuously moves GCF contents to the oral cavity.[56,62] The flow rate can be markedly enhanced in the setting of inflammation. Antimicrobials delivered to the pocket are quickly washed out of the pocket by the GCF, rapidly reducing the concentration of drug locally to subantimicrobial levels (Figs. 54.9 and 54.10). GCF drug concentrations may need to be elevated above usual levels because microorganisms in the pocket can exist within a protective biofilm structure in the periodontal ecosystem.[35,169] (For reviews of periodontal microbiology and biofilms, see Palmer,[127] Teughels et al.,[177] or Kuboniwa and Lamont.[95]) Bacterial biofilms can be highly resistant to penetration by fluids,[45] emphasizing the critical need for high GCF concentrations of active antimicrobials, which are achievable only with locally delivered, controlled-release agents (see Pharmacokinetics) but not possible with locally delivered antimicrobials not in controlled-release formulations or by systemic routes. Drisko[43] suggested that the high antimicrobial concentrations in the GCF as a result of local delivery could help to reach infected sites within the root or tissue.

Drug concentrations of systemically delivered antimicrobials in the GCF are orders of magnitude less than those achievable with controlled-release local delivery, and they cannot provide equivalent therapy.[159,174] Drugs that are transferred from the plasma compartment to the GCF in the periodontal pocket are quickly washed

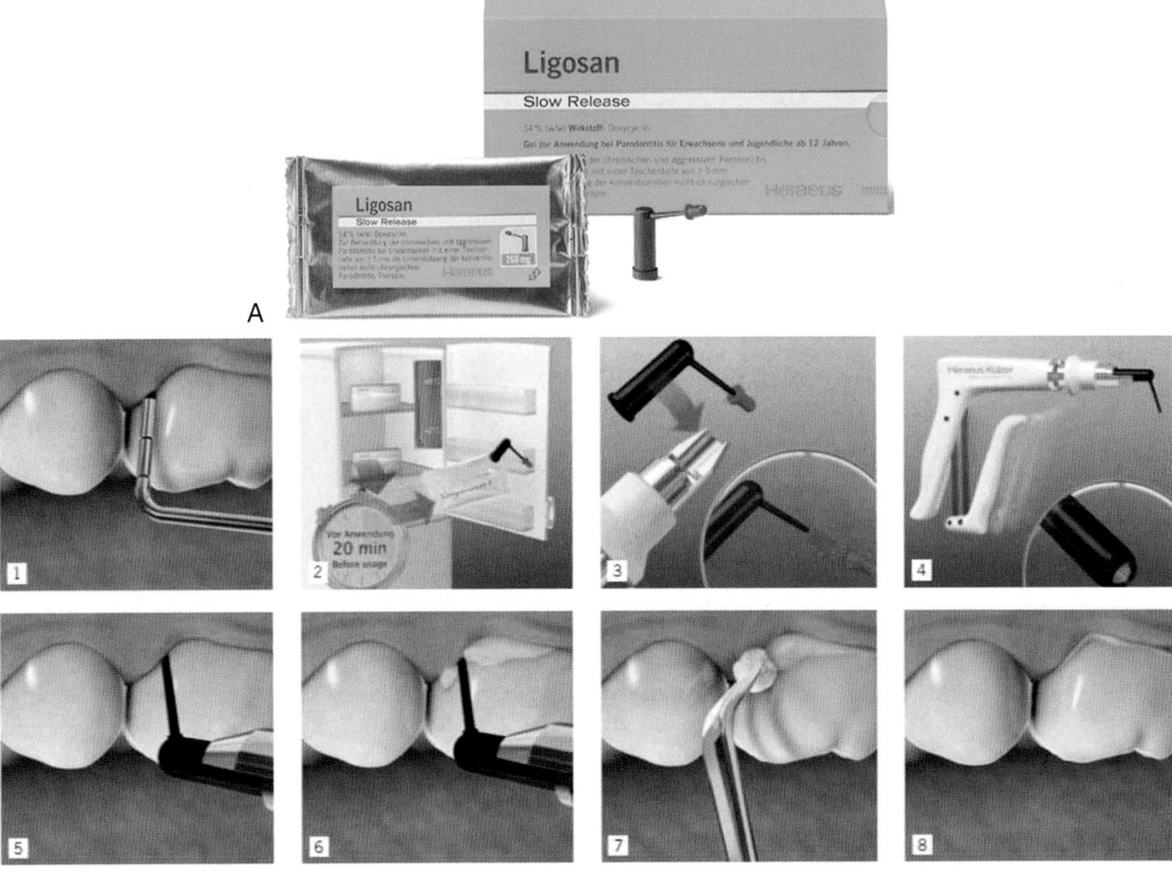

Fig. 54.7 (A) Ligosan Slow Release; box, laminate pouch and caulking gun tip. (B) Steps 1 through 8 in the placement procedure. (From http://www.zm-online.de/markt/heraeus-kulzer/produkte/Ligosan-Slow-Release-in-Einer-Packung_69583.html; http://heraeus-kulzer.de/media/webmedia_local/downloads_new/ligosan_4/Ligosan_Produktinformation_DE.pdf.)

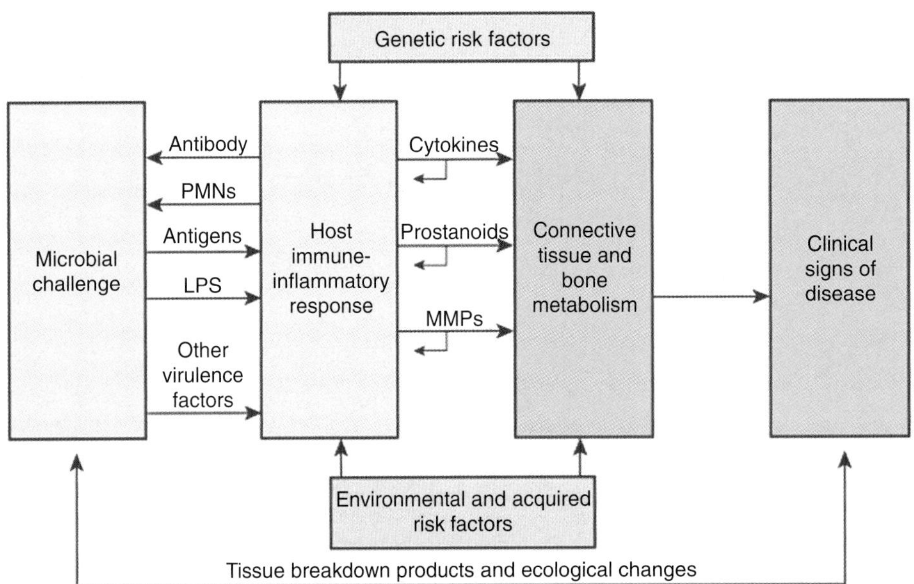

Fig. 54.8 Schematic representation of the pathogenesis of periodontal diseases and possible avenues for prevention or treatment. Through several **virulence** factors such as **antigens** or lipopolysaccharides *(LPS)*, pathogenic microorganisms stimulate a host immune-inflammatory response. Immune elements, including **polymorphonuclear leukocytes** (PMNLs) and antibodies, can inhibit the offending microorganisms, and various **cytokines**, prostanoids, or **enzymes** can affect connective tissue and bone metabolism, ultimately resulting in the clinical signs of periodontitis initiation and progression. Genetic factors or environmental/acquired factors can separately affect disease risk. Potential avenues for intervention include subgingival root instrumentation (scaling and root planing) and use of **antimicrobial agents** to inhibit pocket microorganisms (i.e., affecting the microbial challenge), nonsteroidal or other antiinflammatory agents to inhibit cytokines or prostanoids (i.e., affecting the host immune-inflammatory response), antiresorptive agents (e.g., bisphosphonates) to inhibit osteoclastic bone resorption, and host-modulation therapy (e.g., low-dose oral doxycycline) to inhibit matrix-metalloproteinase *(MMP)* activity (i.e., affecting connective tissue and bone metabolism). (Modified from Page RC, Kornman KS. The pathogenesis of human periodontitis: an introduction. *Periodontol 2000.* 1997;14:9–11.)

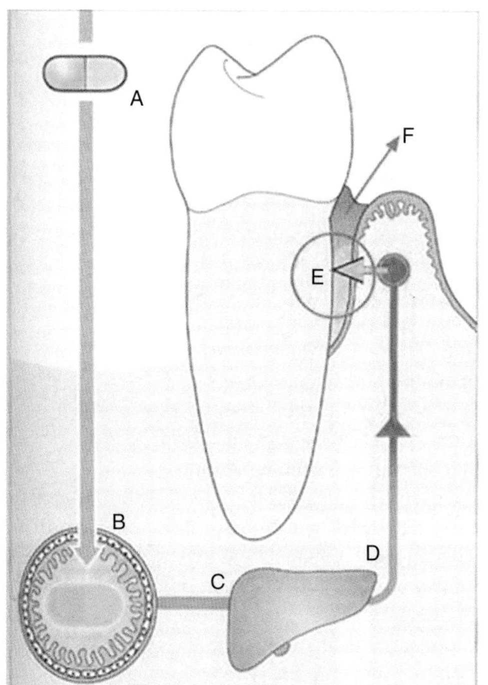

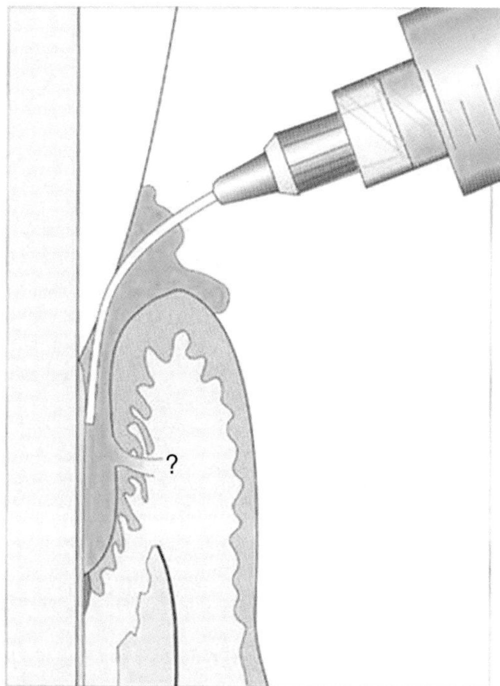

Fig. 54.9 Schematic representation of the inability to achieve therapeutically sufficient concentrations in the periodontal pocket for sufficient time with antimicrobials delivered systemically or locally but not in controlled-release formulations. *Left,* Orally administered drug *(A)* is absorbed in the gastrointestinal tract *(B)*, transported by the portal pathway to the liver *(C)*, and enters the circulatory system *(D)*, from which drug exits the vasculature into the periodontal pocket *(E)*. Drug is quickly eliminated from the pocket into the oral cavity by the copious flow of gingival crevicular fluid (GCF) *(F)*. Locally administered drugs not in controlled-release formulations suffer from the same limitation. *Right,* Locally delivered, controlled-release antimicrobial is administered into the periodontal pocket, where it remains until it degrades, continuously releasing drug into the GCF over time. Antimicrobial drug may be active against plaque bacteria that have invaded the surrounding periodontal tissues. (Reprinted from Wolf HF, Hassell TM. *Color Atlas of Dental Hygiene: Periodontology.* 1st ed. Stuttgart, Germany: Thieme; 2006, with permission.)

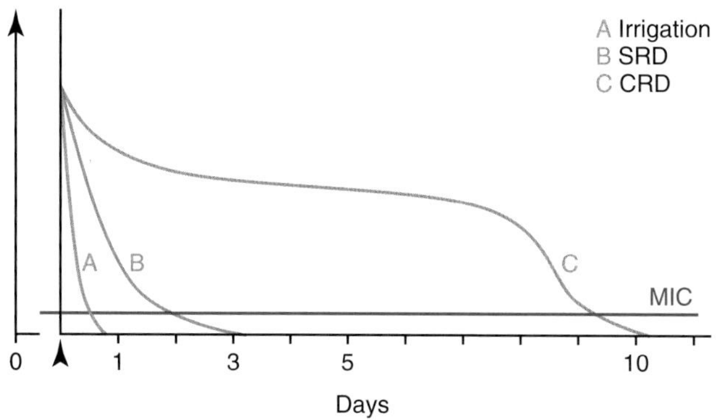

Fig. 54.10 Graph shows the release profile of locally delivered, sustained-release or controlled-release antimicrobials by irrigation. Drug concentration in the gingival crevicular fluid (GCF) is diminished rapidly after irrigation *(A)*. Drug concentration can be extended for several days with drug administered in a modified, sustained-release formulation *(B)*. Drug concentration in the GCF can be maintained at therapeutically relevant concentrations for up to 10 days with controlled-release formulations *(C)*. Area under the curve but above the minimal inhibitory concentration *(MIC)* line represents drug concentration in the gingival crevicular fluid greater than MIC values. The MIC for subgingival plaque bacteria may be substantially greater than typically reported bacterial MIC values because of the potentially protective effect of a subgingival biofilm formation. *CRD*, Controlled-release delivery; *SRD*, sustained-release delivery; *arrowhead*, administration of locally delivered agent. (Adapted from Wolf HF, Hassell TM. *Color Atlas of Dental Hygiene: Periodontology.* 1st ed. Stuttgart, Germany: Thieme; 2006, with permission.)

away by the GCF flow (see Fig. 54.9). It was previously thought that systemically delivered tetracyclines markedly concentrated drugs in the GCF compared with plasma,[60,132] but the hypothesis was not supported by later studies.[159,174] Some investigators have suggested that systemic therapies, rather than locally delivered agents, should be considered when there are multiple pocket sites for the sake of convenience and to save costs,[61,153] but if high concentrations of an antimicrobial drug are desired in the periodontal pockets, systemic delivery is not the appropriate therapy. Other benefits of locally delivered, controlled-release antimicrobials include decreased systemic, off-target effects and a decreased risk for promoting microbial resistance.

Pharmacokinetics

The pharmacokinetic principles of controlled-release local delivery are illustrated in Fig. 54.10. Drugs delivered locally to the periodontal pocket but not in a controlled-release formulation (e.g., by irrigation) are washed out of the pocket by the GCF flow, quickly reducing the concentration of drugs in the GCF.[56] Locally delivered, controlled-release antimicrobials have been designed to maintain high and clinically relevant concentrations of drugs in the GCF for extended periods. The pharmacokinetics of the chlorhexidine chip, doxycycline gel, and minocycline microspheres have been studied in clinical trials.

CLINICAL CORRELATION

Controlled-release agents maintain clinically effective intrapocket concentrations of antimicrobial for an extended period of time.

Chlorhexidine Chip

The release profile of the chlorhexidine chip was evaluated in a single-center, 10-day clinical trial in 19 patients with chronic adult periodontitis.[166] Each patient received a single chip administered into each of four pocket sites, and concentrations of chlorhexidine were determined in GCF, plasma, and urine at various times after dosing. Peak GCF concentrations were achieved 2 hours after dosing (2007 ± 422 μg/mL), with GCF concentrations maintained between approximately 1300 and 1900 μg/mL to 4 days after dosing. Mean chlorhexidine concentrations then steadily decreased to 57 ± 13 μg/mL at 9 days. Chlorhexidine was below detectable limits in plasma and urine at all time points. For perspective, Wilson and colleagues[189] reported that chlorhexidine (125 μg/mL) killed 99.9% of cultivable bacteria from plaque samples from patients with chronic periodontitis within 15 minutes.

Doxycycline Gel

The release profile of the doxycycline gel was evaluated in a single-center, 28-day clinical trial in 32 patients with adult periodontitis and compared with oral doxycycline.[174] All patients assigned to receive local delivery had doxycycline gel administered to all pocket sites with probing depths of 5 mm or more that bled on probing. Drug was retained after placement with a noneugenol (NE) periodontal dressing (n = 13) or 2-octyl cyanoacrylate (2-O) (n = 13). Mean GCF concentrations peaked 2 hours after dosing (1473 ± 328 μg/mL for NE; 1986 ± 445 μg/mL for 2-O). At day 7, mean concentrations were 309 ± 127 μg/mL (NE) and 148 ± 49 μg/mL (2-O). Mean salivary concentrations peaked at 2 hours (4.05 ± 1.24 μg/mL for NE; 8.78 ± 1.48 μg/mL for 2-O) and were 2 μg/mL or less at 24 hours. Serum concentrations after local administration remained at 0.1 μg/mL or less.

For oral doxycycline (200 mg on day 0 and then 100 mg/day for 7 days; n = 6), GCF concentrations peaked at 12 hours after dosing (2.53 ± 1.56 μg/mL), and serum concentrations ranged from 0.91 to 2.26 μg/mL for the 8 days of data collection. Salivary concentrations never exceeded 0.11 μg/mL.

Minocycline Microspheres

The release profile of minocycline microspheres was studied in 18 patients with moderate to advanced chronic periodontitis.[13,14] Minocycline microspheres (mean dose, 46.2 mg; 25 to 112 unit doses) were administered to eligible periodontal pocket sites with a 5 mm or more probing depth (i.e., minimum of 30 sites on at least eight teeth; 1 mg/treatment site) after SRP. Serum and saliva samples were collected before dosing and at various times after dosing to 14 days. The mean dose-normalized saliva area under the curve and maximal concentration (C_{max}) were approximately 125 and 1000 times that of serum parameters, respectively. In saliva, the minocycline C_{max} was 254.0 ± 139.3 mg/mL at 0.75 ± 0.56 hours after dosing, with a half-life of 44.7 ± 19.2 hours.[13] In serum, the mean minocycline concentrations peaked at 4.8 ± 1.8 hours after dosing (C_{max}: 216.4 ± 122.9 μg/mL) and were undetectable by 7 days. Minocycline concentrations in saliva and GCF were sufficient (>1 μg/mL) to kill bacteria associated with periodontal disease in vitro.[13] These concentrations were evident for up to 14 days without significant systemic exposure.[13]

For information regarding the magnitude of effect of locally delivered, controlled-release antimicrobials, please refer to the online version of this chapter (eBooks.Health.Elsevier.com).

CLINICAL CORRELATION

Potential Indications

Additional dental indications for locally delivered, controlled-release antimicrobials have not been evaluated by the FDA. Examples include combination adjunctive therapy and adjuncts for surgical therapy or peri-implantitis. Preliminary data for these indications are available and discussed in the following sections.

Combination Adjunctive Therapy

Many local and systemic adjunctive therapies are available with supportive data on their use in patients. None is labeled for use in combination therapy. It seems likely, however, that some practitioners may already be providing off-label combination adjunctive therapy for their patients, even though appropriate data do not exist.

Locally delivered, controlled-release antimicrobials enhance the clinical efficacy of SRP. Similarly, adjunctive systemic therapy with low-dose (20-mg) doxycycline, given orally twice daily as a host-modulating agent (later reported as a once-daily, modified-release formulation[144]) also can enhance the clinical efficacy of SRP.[27,33,143] Reddy and colleague[149] and Ryan and Golub[156] have reviewed matrix metalloproteinase modulation as a treatment strategy. The question is whether a combination of local antimicrobial and host-modulating adjunctive therapies can provide greater clinical benefit than either adjunctive agent used alone.

In a 6-month clinical trial, combination adjunctive therapies resulted in significantly greater improvements in probing depth and clinical attachment compared with SRP alone.[121] More sites showed a probing depth reduction of 2.0 mm or more, and fewer sites had a residual probing depth 5.0 mm or more.[121] A single case report from this trial was published.[135] Because the appropriate control groups (i.e., SRP plus single adjunctive therapy) were not included in the trial, definitive conclusions regarding increased benefit from combination versus single adjunctive therapy cannot be made. The potential for combined adjunctive therapy to enhance clinical benefit is promising and warrants additional research.

The focus of this chapter is locally delivered, controlled-release antimicrobials. Data support the efficacy of locally delivered, controlled-release antimicrobials,[67] supporting the conclusion that SRP plus adjunctive therapy could be considered a new standard for nonsurgical periodontal therapy. Available data also support the adjunctive efficacy of systemic, low-dose oral doxycycline[27,33,79,144] to an extent that is numerically similar to that reported for locally delivered, controlled-release antimicrobials. Because appropriate comparative data are not available, comparisons of these therapies is not appropriate, and no conclusion can be reached regarding the most efficacious approach for adjunctive therapy, local or systemic adjunctive therapy or with single or combined agents.

In addition to the possibility of combination adjunctive therapy with a locally delivered agent and host modulatory therapy with low-dose oral doxycycline, Goodson and coworkers[59] reported outcomes from a randomized trial enrolling 231 patients that considered SRP alone and various combinations of SRP, systemic antimicrobials, and surgery using a 2 × 2 × 2 factorial design. Patients were followed for 24 months. Maximal reductions in probing depth and gains in attachment level were observed at 6 months, which were maintained at 24 months in all treatment groups. At 24 months, gains in attachment were increased by systemic antimicrobials (0.50 mm), and probing depth reductions were further augmented by systemic antimicrobials (0.51 mm) and surgical treatment (0.36 mm). Both types of improvements were reduced by smoking.

Surgical Therapy

Pocket sites that do not seem to respond adequately to nonsurgical therapy and evidence residual probing depth with inflammation are often treated with follow-up surgical therapy. A question is whether locally delivered, controlled-release antimicrobials could augment surgical results. This hypothesis was tested in a pilot study by Hellström and coworkers[73] with minocycline microspheres at all pocket sites of 5 mm or more. Sixty patients with at least one nonmolar pocket site with a probing depth of 6 mm or more in each of two quadrants were treated with (1) microspheres at baseline and immediately after each of two surgical procedures at weeks 2 and

3 and again at week 5 or (2) standard surgical therapy. The mean probing depth was reduced in both treatment groups, but the reduction was significantly greater in the test group than in controls at 25 weeks (2.51 ± 0.10 mm vs. 2.18 ± 0.10 mm, $P = .027$). In contrast, the probing depth reduction after SRP with a limited surgical approach using adjunctive minocycline microspheres was not significantly different compared with SRP in a smaller pilot trial.[196]

A specialized periodontal surgical procedure, regenerative surgery, has become a standard procedure in periodontal practice. It had been suggested verbally as early as 1993 (Killoy WJ, personal communication, 2002) and in print in 1998[89,90] that adjunctive locally delivered, controlled-release antimicrobials might improve outcomes after regenerative periodontal surgery. In a pilot trial, the adjunctive use of the chlorhexidine chip with regenerative surgery resulted in more than a 100% greater mean improvement from baseline in bone height and mass 9 months after surgical treatment compared with SRP alone and surgery.[150] Both groups had also received prophylactic systemic antimicrobial treatment before surgery, but the addition of a locally administered antimicrobial resulted in a significant benefit compared with the control arm.

Other reports support the lack of efficacy of systemic antimicrobials[112] and the benefit of locally delivered antimicrobials[195] as adjunctive treatments in the regenerative setting. A microbiologic rationale for the use of locally delivered antimicrobials (i.e., tetracycline fiber) in the regenerative setting was also supported by Sbordone and colleagues.[161] Aichelmann-Reidy and Reynolds[5] suggested that regenerative surgical procedures should include an adjunctive, locally delivered, controlled-release antimicrobial agent to provide a more consistent clinical benefit.

These preliminary reports suggested that the adjunctive use of locally delivered, controlled-release antimicrobials can improve clinical outcomes after periodontal surgery in regenerative and nonregenerative settings. These hypotheses require testing in prospective, adequate, and well-controlled trials. None of the three available agents is approved as an adjunct to surgery.

Peri-Implantitis

Similar to periodontitis, peri-implantitis is an inflammatory disease process that is initiated by local microorganisms and affects the tissues surrounding an implant. An opportunity exists to treat diseased implant sites chemically by targeting the local microflora. There is a potential rationale for the use of locally delivered, controlled-release antimicrobials for the treatment of peri-implantitis. Although the treatment of peri-implantitis is an off-label use, it seems likely that some clinicians have tried local delivery in this setting.

Renvert and coworkers[151] studied 32 patients with at least one implant site with a probing depth of 4 mm or more plus bleeding or exudate on probing. Patients were treated with debridement followed by minocycline microspheres (17 patients, 57 implants) or a chlorhexidine gel formulation (15 patients, 38 implants). Treatments were repeated at 30 and 90 days. Follow-up examinations were performed at 10 days and 1, 3, 6, 9, and 12 months. There were significant reductions in probing depth compared with chlorhexidine at 1, 3, and 6 months and marked reductions in indicator microorganisms in both treatment groups. The study authors concluded that adjunctive minocycline microspheres could be of value in treating peri-implant lesions.

Buchter and colleagues[25] studied 28 patients with a total of 48 peri-implant defects. Two to 18 weeks before baseline measurements, patients had been treated for peri-implantitis (including scaling with a plastic instrument). Patients then continued to receive this treatment alone or with the additional adjunctive use of the doxycycline gel. At 18 weeks, the test group evidenced a significant reduction in mean probing depth and a significant gain in mean attachment levels compared with controls.

Schar and associates[162] and Bassetti coworkers[19] studied 40 patients with peri-implantitis who had probing depths of 4 to 6 mm and less than 2 mm of radiographic bone loss that was treated with mechanical debridement and air polishing and adjunctively with local minocycline microspheres or photodynamic therapy for 12 months. A significant decrease in probing depth from baseline values was observed in photodynamic sites up to 9 months and in minocycline sites up to 12 months. Decreases in *Porphyromonas gingivalis* and *Tannerella forsythia* concentrations and in GCF levels of IL-1β were seen in both groups. There were no significant differences between groups, and no conclusions can be drawn about either therapy compared with mechanical therapy alone because an appropriate control group was not included. Finally, in a recent publication, Wang and colleagues[184] estimated that at least 25% of implants suffer from peri-implantitis, characterized by distinct immune profiles; common pathogens in the microenvironment around diseased implants were recently reported by de Melo and colleagues[39] in a systematic review.

Labels for the available locally delivered, controlled-release antimicrobials do not include an indication for peri-implantitis. Their potential treating peri-implantitis, however, is an exciting possibility, and one that warrants additional research. There seems a clear need for additional antimicrobial support for the treatment of peri-implantitis. Phase III trials are needed to test the hypothesis that locally delivered, controlled-release antimicrobials offer clinical benefit as part of a treatment regimen to manage peri-implantitis.

Tobacco Smoking

Smoking is a well-known risk factor for the development or progression of periodontitis, and it can limit the effectiveness of periodontal therapy.[21,76,81,142] The adjunctive use of locally delivered, controlled-release antimicrobials can enhance the efficacy of SRP in smokers. In a 3-month trial, SRP plus adjunctive doxycycline gel resulted in significantly greater probing depth reduction and clinical attachment gain compared with SRP alone about equally in smokers and nonsmokers.[179] This result was consistent with subset analyses of current smokers, former smokers, and nonsmokers from two 9-month, multicenter trials of doxycycline gel[157] and of microspheres smokers versus nonsmokers in studies of minocycline microsphers.[188] Subset analyses of therapy with minocycline microspheres showed that results for smokers were consistent with overall trial results.[124,131]

Consistent results also were seen in a later clinical trial of minocycline microspheres.[64] Beneficial periodontal microbiologic alterations in adjunctively treated sites compared with SRP alone were reported for doxycycline gel and minocycline microspheres (Fig. 54.11).[64,104,163] A 2-year trial of doxycycline gel with a small number of patients provided further evidence of clinical efficacy.[103]

In a pilot trial to test the use of adjunctive minocycline microspheres in a surgical setting, clinical improvement was seen similarly in smokers and nonsmokers.[73] Adjunctive therapy may lessen the adverse impact of smoking on the periodontium and improve treatment outcomes for patients who smoke. A systematic review of the doxycycline gel and minocycline microspheres found that available data are insufficient to conclude that adjunctive therapy significantly enhances SRP specifically in smokers, and it recommended additional clinical trials (i.e., adequate and well-controlled trials) to assess outcomes for smokers.[9]

Adverse Effects and Cautions for Use

A complete listing of cautions for use and possible adverse effects as listed on the FDA labels for these locally delivered, controlled-release antimicrobials is beyond the scope of this chapter, but

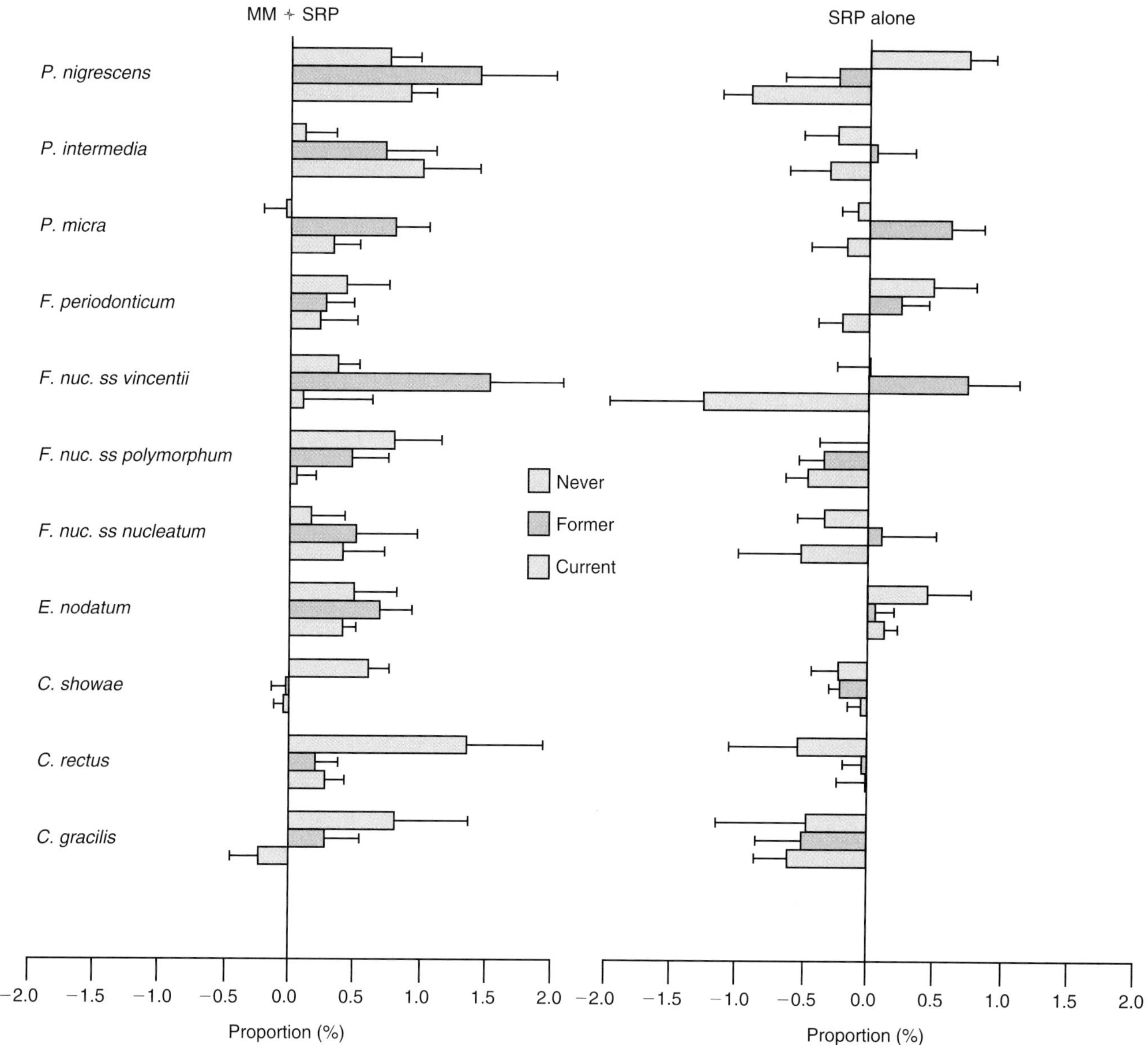

Fig. 54.11 Microbiologic effects are shown after the adjunctive administration of minocycline microspheres in smokers and nonsmokers. Therapy causes changes in the proportion of orange complex bacteria. Positive changes represent antibacterial effects as reductions in proportions. Negative changes represent proportional increases or proliferation of bacterial groups. *F. nuc.*, *Fusobacterium nucleatum; MM,* minocycline microspheres; *SRP,* scaling and root planing. (Reprinted from Grossi SG, Goodson JM, Gunsolley JC, et al. Mechanical therapy with adjunctive minocycline microspheres reduces red-complex bacteria in smokers. *J Periodontol.* 2007;78:1741, with permission from the American Academy of Periodontology.)

complete details about the use of these products and their safety profiles are available in the full prescribing information.[14,15,133]

Clinicians are cautioned about adverse effects of this class of drugs:

- Potential for hypersensitivity reactions (i.e., not to be used in patients with a known sensitivity to any ingredient)
- Potential for the overgrowth of nonsusceptible microorganisms, including fungi
- Use in pregnancy
- Potential for discoloration during tooth development (i.e., tetracyclines only)
- Use in an acutely abscessed periodontal pocket or in extremely severe periodontal defects with little remaining periodontium

Use of local mechanical oral hygiene procedures (e.g., toothbrushing, interdental cleaning devices) for approximately 7 to 10 days after administration.

The most frequently reported adverse reactions reported in the clinical trials without mention of causality include headache, infection (including upper respiratory tract infection), flu syndrome, pain, tooth disorder and toothache, and various oral signs or symptoms. Toothache was the only adverse reaction that was significantly higher ($P = .042$) in the chlorhexidine chip group compared with placebo.[133]

For information regarding cost-effectiveness of locally delivered antimicrobials, clinical studies of non-U.S. agents and ongoing and future research considerations, please refer to the online version of this chapter (eBooks.Health.Elsevier.com).

Conclusions

The evidence is very strong that adjunctive, locally delivered, controlled-release antimicrobials make SRP significantly more effective and have a known safety profile. SRP without adjunctive treatment in appropriately eligible sites (i.e., probing depth ≥5.0 mm) may be less than maximally effective. It is not appropriate to determine therapy based solely on clinical judgment. The practitioner should evaluate the evidence and suggest a treatment that has the greatest probability for success based on current data.

Spielman and Wolff[170] commented on the unfortunate tendency for many dentists to base treatment on personal experience rather than reported evidence. They stated that optimal care is evidence based. As an example of the suboptimal care that can result from the lack of incorporation of the best available evidence into clinical practice, O'Donnell and colleagues[122] reported on the underutilization of pit-and-fissure sealants in dental practice despite published American Dental Association (ADA) recommendations.[20] Available data support the adjunctive use of locally delivered, controlled-release antimicrobials, which provides significant additional clinical benefit.

SRP procedures have been considered the nonsurgical standard of care.[24] The evidence supports the idea that adjunctive locally delivered, controlled-release antimicrobials make SRP more effective[67] and have a known safety profile. Based on available data, when these agents are used routinely as adjuncts to SRP as indicated as part of initial periodontal treatment or maintenance therapy, clinicians can expect a significantly greater mean reduction in probing depth and usually maintenance or gain in attachment level in comparison with SRP alone. SRP plus adjunctive therapy, used in a manner that is consistent with the approved full prescribing information, could be considered a new standard for nonsurgical periodontal therapy for the management of periodontitis.[47]

Acknowledgment

The authors thank Laurel K. Graham from the University of Pennsylvania library for excellent library services to provide the literature search to support this chapter.

CLINICAL CORRELATION

SRP plus adjunctive therapy could potentially be considered a new standard for nonsurgical periodontal therapy.

A number of pilot trials have suggested additional indications for adjunctive locally delivered, controlled-release antimicrobials. More research is necessary to test these hypotheses before further clinical comments can be made.

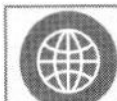

Case Scenarios are found on the companion website eBooks.Health.Elsevier.com.

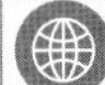

References can be found on the companion Expert Consult website at eBooks.Health.Elsevier.com.

CHAPTER 55

Host Modulation

Maria Emanuel Ryan  | *Ying Gu*

CHAPTER OUTLINE

Introduction

Host modulation is a term that has been incorporated into our dental jargon, but it has not been well defined. *Host* can be defined as "the organism from which a parasite obtains its nourishment," or in the transplantation of tissue, "the individual who receives the graft." *Modulation* is defined as "the alteration of function or status of something in response to a stimulus or an altered chemical or physical environment" (*Taber's Medical Dictionary,* 2004). In diseases of the periodontium that are initiated by bacteria, the "host" clearly is the individual who harbors these pathogens; however, it was not clear for many years whether it was possible to modulate the host response to these pathogens and other stimuli, leading to the breakdown of the attachment apparatus. Host modulation with chemotherapeutic agents or drugs is the latest adjunctive therapeutic option for the management of periodontal diseases. The concept of host modulation is fairly new to the field of dentistry but is universally understood by most physicians who routinely apply the principles of host modulation to the management of a number of chronic progressive disorders such as arthritis and osteoporosis. The concept of host modulation was first introduced to dentistry by Williams[118] and Golub et al.[42] and then expanded on by many other scholars in the dental profession. In 1990, Williams concluded, "there are compelling data from studies in animals and human trials indicating that pharmacologic agents, that modulate the host responses believed to be involved in the pathogenesis of periodontal destruction, may be efficacious in slowing the progression of periodontitis."[118] In 1992, Golub and colleagues discussed "host modulation with tetracyclines and their chemically modified analogues."[42] The future that these authors described has arrived, and to better understand this new era in disease management, we must first look at the pathogenesis of periodontitis.

Many clinicians previously believed that periodontal disease was an inevitable consequence of aging and was uniformly distributed in the population. They thought that disease severity was directly correlated with plaque levels (i.e., the worse the oral hygiene, the worse the periodontal disease) and that disease progression occurred in a continuous, linear manner throughout life. Now, as a result of better epidemiologic data, there has been a paradigm shift in how clinicians and scientists view the prevalence and progression of this common disease. It has been well established that periodontal disease is not a natural consequence of aging and disease severity is not necessarily correlated with plaque levels. Theories about the pathogenesis of periodontitis have evolved from a purely plaque-associated disease to the more recent hypotheses that place considerable emphasis on the host's response to the bacteria.[13] The first Surgeon General's report on "Oral Health in America," published in 2000, recognized the importance of dental health in the overall general health and well-being of a patient.[108] Recent research findings indicate possible associations between chronic oral infections, such as periodontitis, and systemic disorders, such as diabetes, cardiovascular and lung diseases, stroke, osteoporosis, and rheumatoid arthritis. The Surgeon General's report assesses these emerging associations and explores factors that may underlie oral-systemic disease connections. Along with these findings and the emergence of the discipline of periodontal medicine, there have been many developments in therapeutic approaches to the management of periodontitis. The development of the chemotherapeutic approach known as "host modulation" required a thorough understanding of the host response and the impact of a variety of risk factors.

Anecdotally, many dentists have identified patients with abundant plaque and calculus deposits, which may manifest itself as gingivitis with shallow pocketing. By contrast, other patients, despite

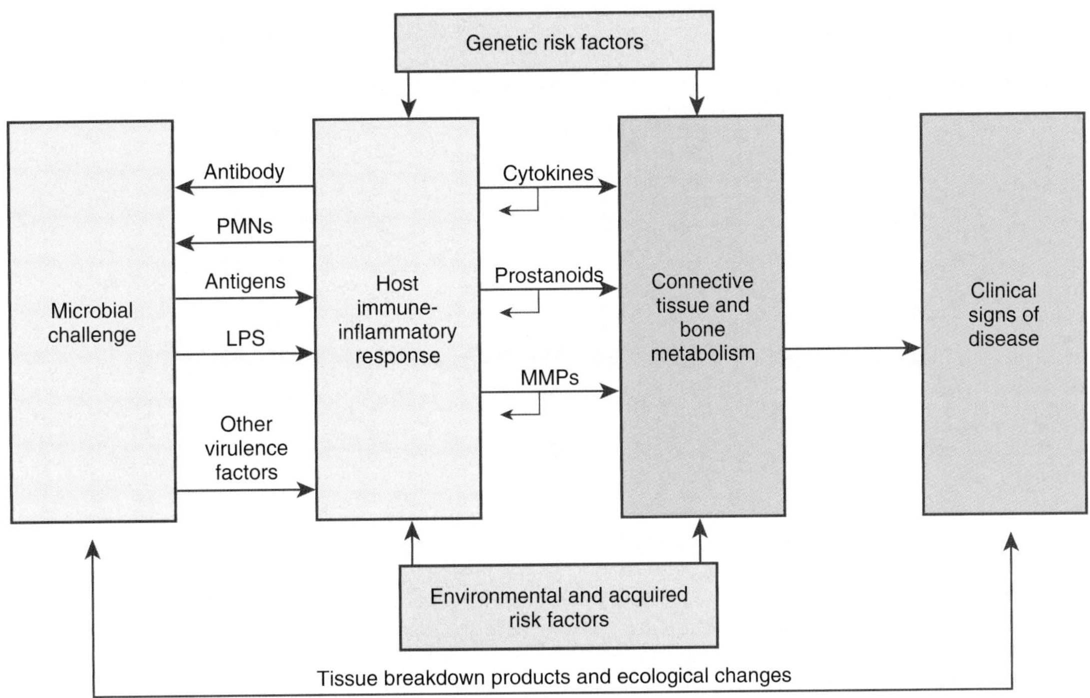

Fig. 55.1 Schematic illustration of the pathogenesis of periodontitis. The microbial challenge presented by subgingival plaque bacteria results in an upregulated host immune-inflammatory response in the periodontal tissues that is characterized by the excessive production of inflammatory cytokines (e.g., interleukins, tumor necrosis factor), prostanoids (e.g., prostaglandin E_2), and enzymes, including the matrix metalloproteinases *(MMPs).* These proinflammatory mediators are responsible for the majority of periodontal breakdown that occurs, leading to the clinical signs and symptoms of periodontitis. The process is modified by environmental (e.g., tobacco use) and acquired risk factors (e.g., systemic diseases) and genetic susceptibility. *PMNs,* Polymorphonuclear leukocytes; *LPS,* lipopolysaccharide. (Modified from Kornman KS. *Clin Infect Dis.* 1999;28:520.)

maintaining a high standard of plaque control, succumb to aggressive forms of periodontitis, with deep pocketing, tooth mobility, and early tooth loss. The former group of patients is *periodontal disease resistant,* whereas the latter group is *periodontal disease susceptible.* Clearly, the response of the periodontal tissues to plaque is different in these two types of patients, and certain patients undergo advanced periodontal breakdown even though they achieve a high standard of oral hygiene. Previous observations led researchers to realize that the *host response* to the bacterial challenge presented by subgingival plaque is perhaps the *most* important determinant of disease severity, rate of progression, and even response to therapy. Although plaque bacteria are capable of causing direct damage to the periodontal tissues (e.g., by release of H_2S, butyric acid, and other enzymes and mediators), it is now recognized that the great majority of the destructive events occurring in the periodontal tissues result from the activation of destructive processes that occur as part of the host immune-inflammatory response to plaque bacteria. The host response is essentially protective by intent but, paradoxically, can also result in significant tissue damage, including breakdown of connective tissue fibers in the periodontal ligament (PDL) and resorption of alveolar bone.

In 1985, research began to focus on bacterial-host interactions.[70] It has been recognized that although bacterial pathogens initiate the periodontal inflammation, the host response to these pathogens is equally, if not more, important in mediating connective tissue breakdown, including bone loss. It has become clear that the host-derived enzymes known as the *matrix metalloproteinases* (MMPs), as well as changes in osteoclast activity driven by cytokines and prostanoids, cause most of the tissue destruction in the periodontium.[80] This shift in paradigms, with a focus on the host response, led to the development of *host modulatory therapies* to improve therapeutic outcomes, slow the progression of disease, and allow for more predictable management of patients with periodontitis. This therapeutic strategy not only may be relevant to individuals at greater risk for periodontal disease but also may be important in the management of those at risk for a number of related systemic conditions. To better understand the host factors that clinicians are attempting to modulate, we need a more detailed assessment of the role of the host response in periodontal pathogenesis (Fig. 55.1). After the accumulation of subgingival plaque bacteria, a variety of microbial substances, including chemotactic factors such as *lipopolysaccharide* (LPS), microbial peptides, and other bacterial antigens, diffuse across the junctional epithelium into the gingival connective tissues. The periodontium is anatomically unique in that the junctional epithelium ends on the tooth surface, which is nonliving tissue; there is no other such discontinuous lining over the entire surface of the body. The dentogingival junction indicates a priori vulnerability to bacterial attack. Epithelial and connective tissue cells are thus stimulated to produce inflammatory mediators that result in an inflammatory response in the tissues. The gingival vasculature dilates (vasodilation) and becomes increasingly permeable to fluid and cells. Fluid accumulates in the tissues, and defense cells migrate from the circulation toward the source of the chemotactic stimulus (bacteria and their products) in the gingival crevice. Neutrophils, or polymorphonuclear leukocytes (PMNs), predominate in the early stages of gingival inflammation to phagocytose and kill plaque bacteria. Bacterial killing by PMNs involves both intracellular mechanisms (after phagocytosis of bacteria within membrane-bound

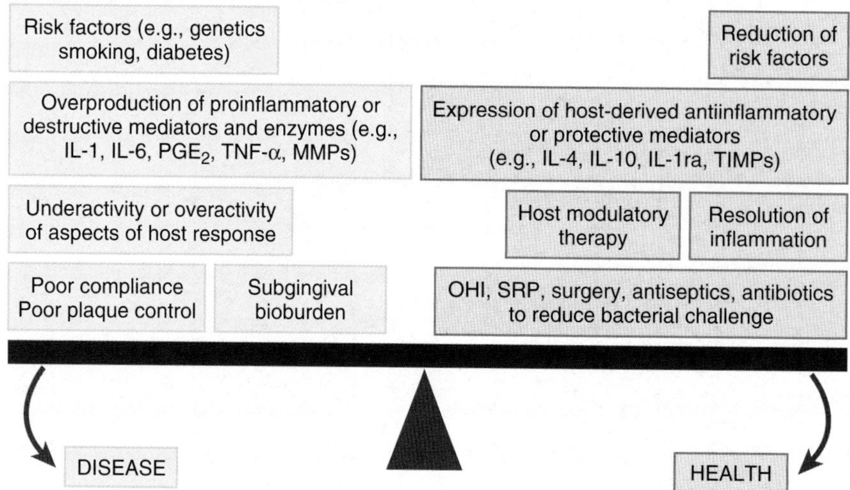

Fig. 55.2 The periodontal balance. The balance between periodontal breakdown ("disease") and periodontal stability ("health") is tipped toward disease by risk factors, excessive production of inflammatory cytokines and enzymes (e.g., *IL-1* and *IL-6,* interleukin-1 and -6; *PGE_2,* prostaglandin E_2; *TNF-α,* tumor necrosis factor alpha; *MMPs,* matrix metalloproteinases), underactivity or overactivity of aspects of the immune-inflammatory host response, poor compliance, and a pathogenic microflora. The balance can be tipped toward health by risk factor modification, upregulation, and restoration of balance between naturally occurring inhibitors of inflammation (e.g., *IL-4* and *IL-10,* interleukins-4 and -10; *IL-1ra,* interleukin-1 receptor antagonist; *TIMPs,* tissue inhibitors of metalloproteinases), host modulatory therapy, and antibacterial treatments such as *OHI* (oral hygiene instructions), *SRP* (scaling and root planing), surgery, antiseptics, and antibiotics.

structures inside the cell) and extracellular mechanisms (by release of PMN enzymes and oxygen radicals outside the cell). As bacterial products enter the circulation, committed lymphocytes return to the site of infection, and B lymphocytes are transformed into plasma cells, which produce antibodies against specific bacterial antigens. Antibodies are released in the gingival tissues and, in the presence of complement, facilitate and enhance PMN phagocytosis and bacterial killing.

Thus a host immune-inflammatory response is established in the gingival tissues, and the clinical signs of gingivitis develop as the tissues become more edematous and erythematous. This response is essentially protective in intent, to combat the bacterial infection and prevent the ingress of bacteria into the tissues. In persons who are not susceptible to periodontitis *(disease resistant),* these primary defense mechanisms control the infection, and chronic inflammation (i.e., chronic gingivitis) may persist indefinitely. In *disease-susceptible* individuals, however, inflammatory events extend apically and laterally to involve deeper connective tissues and alveolar bone. There is proliferation of the junctional epithelium, which becomes increasingly permeable and ulcerated, thus accelerating the ingress of bacterial products and the inflammation worsens. Further defense cells are recruited to the area, including macrophages and lymphocytes. Large numbers of PMNs migrate into the tissues, secreting excessive quantities of destructive enzymes and inflammatory mediators indiscriminately into the tissues. These enzymes include the MMPs, such as collagenase and gelatinase, which break down collagen fibers in the gingival and periodontal tissues. The infiltrating inflammatory and immune cells are accommodated by the breakdown of structural components of the periodontium. MMPs are a primary target for host modulation. Pharmacologic agents or chemotherapeutics can be administered to suppress excessive levels of MMPs.

Macrophages are recruited to the area and are activated (by binding to LPS) to produce prostaglandins (e.g., prostaglandin E_2 [PGE_2]), interleukins (e.g., IL-1α, IL-1β, IL-6), tumor necrosis factor alpha (TNF-α), and MMPs. The cytokines (interleukins and TNF-α) and prostanoids are additional targets for host modulatory therapeutics. Interleukins and TNF-α bind to fibroblasts, which are stimulated to produce additional quantities of PGE_2, interleukins, TNF-α, and MMPs in positive-feedback cycles. The concentration of these enzymes and inflammatory mediators becomes pathologically high in the periodontal tissues. Host modulatory therapy (HMT) can be used to interrupt these positive-feedback loops and ultimately reduce the excessive levels of cytokines, prostanoids, and enzymes resulting in tissue destruction. MMPs break down collagen fibers, disrupting the normal anatomy of the gingival tissues and ultimately resulting in destruction of the periodontal ligament. The inflammation extends apically, and osteoclasts are stimulated to resorb alveolar bone by the high levels of prostaglandins, interleukins, and TNF-α in the tissues. The osteoclasts themselves are targets for host modulation. Drugs can be administered to downregulate osteoclastic activity and ultimately to inhibit bone resorption by these cells.

The elevations in the proinflammatory or destructive mediators in response to bacterial challenge are counterbalanced by elevations in anti-inflammatory or protective mediators such as the cytokines IL-4 and IL-10, as well as other mediators, such as IL-1ra (receptor antagonist), and tissue inhibitors of metalloproteinases (TIMPs) (Fig. 55.2). Under conditions of health, the anti-inflammatory or protective mediators serve to control tissue destruction. If there are adequate levels of these anti-inflammatory or protective mediators to keep the host response to the bacterial challenge in check, the individual will be disease resistant. If an imbalance occurs, with excessive levels of the proinflammatory or destructive mediators present in the host tissues, tissue destruction will ensue in the susceptible host. Another potential target for host modulation could entail the use of pharmacologic agents that either mimic or result in elevations of endogenous anti-inflammatory or protective mediators.

Thus plaque bacteria initiate the disease, and bacterial antigens that cross the junctional epithelium drive the inflammatory process. Therefore bacteria are essential for periodontitis to occur, but they are insufficient by themselves to cause disease. For periodontitis to

BOX 55.1 Risk Factors for Periodontal Disease

- Heredity: family history, PST test
- Smoking: frequency, current history, past history
- Diabetes: duration, control
- Obesity
- Stress: reported by patient
- Medications: calcium channel blockers, Dilantin, cyclosporin, drugs known to cause dry mouth
- Nutrition
- Poor oral hygiene: plaque and calculus
- Faulty dentistry: overhangs, subgingival margins
- Hormonal variations: *pregnancy* (increased estradiol and progesterone), *menopause* (decreased estrogen, osteoporosis)
- Immunocompromise: HIV, neutropenia
- Connective tissue diseases
- Previous history of periodontitis

PST, Periodontal screening test; *HIV*, human immunodeficiency virus.

BOX 55.2 Risk Reduction Strategies

- Heredity: HMT chemotherapeutics
- Smoking: cessation, HMT chemotherapeutics
- Diabetes: improved control, work with physician; HMT chemotherapeutics
- Obesity: weight loss
- Stress: management, HMT chemotherapeutics
- Medications: change medications, work with physician; HMT chemotherapeutics
- Nutrition: supplements
- Poor oral hygiene: improved oral hygiene, HMT chemotherapeutics
- Faulty dentistry: corrective dentistry
- Hormonal variations: consult with physician, HMT chemotherapeutics
- Immunocompromise: consult with physician, HMT chemotherapeutics
- Connective tissue diseases: consult with physician, HMT chemotherapeutics

HMT, Host modulatory therapy.

develop, a susceptible host is also required. The majority of periodontal breakdown (bone loss, attachment loss) is caused by host-derived destructive enzymes (MMPs) and inflammatory mediators (prostaglandins, interleukins) that are released during the cascade of destructive events that occur as part of the inflammatory response (see Fig. 55.1).[83] Paradoxically, the inflammatory response, which is essentially protective in design, is responsible for much of the breakdown of the soft and hard periodontal tissues. Periodontal disease is characterized by high concentrations of MMPs, cytokines, and prostanoids in the periodontal tissues, whereas periodontal health is characterized by the opposite.[82] The purpose of HMT is to restore the balance of proinflammatory or destructive mediators and anti-inflammatory or protective mediators to that seen in healthy individuals. Pocket formation that occurs as coronal junctional epithelium is broken down and restored at a more apical location. Plaque bacteria then migrate apically along the root surface deeper into the pocket, where the physical conditions favor the proliferation of gram-negative anaerobic species. Bacterial products continue to challenge the host, and the host continues its frustrated response against these bacteria and their products. Inflammation extends further and further apically, more bone is resorbed, and PDL is broken down. The pocket deepens, and the associated attachment and bone loss result in clinical and radiographic signs of periodontitis. Intervention is required to prevent eventual tooth loss and other sequelae of the disease.

The nature of the host response to the presence of plaque is modified by genetic factors (helping to explain why aggressive periodontitis tends to have a familial aggregation) and systemic and environmental factors (e.g., smoking, diabetes, stress). These risk factors may lead to the imbalance between the proinflammatory and anti-inflammatory mediators seen in susceptible individuals (see Fig. 55.2). Risk factors can affect the onset, rate of progression, and severity of periodontal disease, as well as response to therapy (Box 55.1).[31,48,100] Risk assessment is extremely important as we now recognize that some of these risk factors can be modified to reduce a patient's susceptibility to periodontitis. Risk reduction strategies may include smoking cessation, improved control of diabetes, nutritional supplementation, improved oral hygiene, changes in medication, stress management, weight loss, and more frequent dental visits (Box 55.2). The use of chemotherapeutic agents or drugs specifically designed to treat periodontal diseases is emerging as an aid as a risk reduction strategy. Intervention in periodontal disease can now include HMT as one of the available adjunctive treatment options. The term *adjunctive* is meant to imply "in addition to conventional therapies" or "in addition to other established therapies." For the management of periodontal diseases, conventional approaches were initially mechanical in nature, that is, surgery as well as scaling and root planing (SRP). Initially, adjunctive therapies were solely antimicrobial, such as the use of antiseptics and antibiotics (local and/or systemic). New adjunctive approaches involve modulation of the host response. Researchers are also investigating HMTs, which aim to modify or reduce destructive aspects of the host response so that the immune-inflammatory response to plaque is less damaging to the periodontal tissues. Removal of plaque by SRP targets one aspect of the pathogenic process by reducing the bacterial burden and, therefore, the antigenic challenge that drives the inflammatory response in the host tissues. However, the bacterial challenge is never completely eliminated after SRP, as recolonization by bacterial species occurs. HMTs offer the potential for downregulating destructive aspects and upregulating protective aspects of the host response so that, in combination with conventional treatments to reduce the bacterial burden, the balance between health (resolution of inflammation and wound healing) and disease progression (continued proinflammatory events) is tipped in the direction of a healing response.

HMT is a *means of treating the host side of the host-bacteria interaction*. The host response is responsible for most of the tissue breakdown that occurs, leading to the clinical signs of periodontitis (i.e., loss of connective tissue attachment and bone). HMTs offer the opportunity to modulate or reduce this destruction by treating aspects of the chronic inflammatory response. HMTs do not "switch off" normal defense mechanisms or inflammation; instead, they ameliorate excessive or pathologically elevated inflammatory processes to enhance the opportunities for wound healing and periodontal stability.

HMT can be used to reduce excessive levels of enzymes, cytokines, and prostanoids and should not reduce levels below constitutive levels. HMTs can also modulate osteoclast and osteoblast function (Fig. 55.3) but should not impact normal tissue turnover. HMT is key to addressing many of the risk factors that have adverse effects on the host response that are either not easily managed (e.g., smoking, diabetes) or cannot be changed (e.g., genetic susceptibility). In addition, host modulatory agents might be used to increase the levels of a person's own protective or anti-inflammatory mediators. Use of systemic HMTs for the treatment of a patient's periodontal condition may also provide benefits for other inflammatory

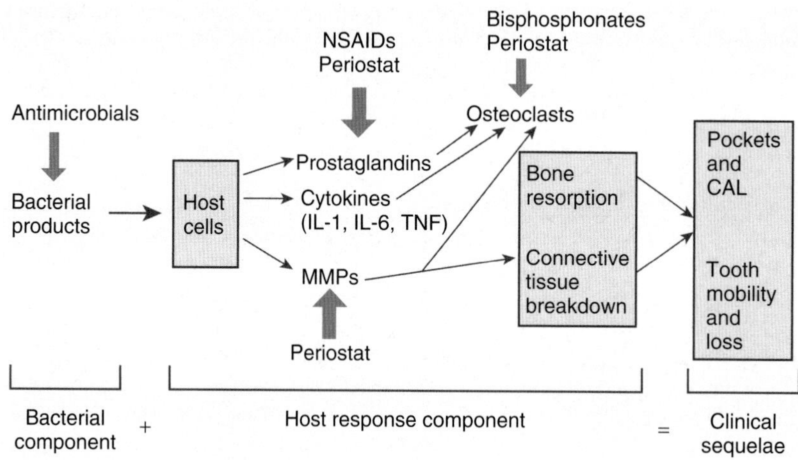

Fig. 55.3 Potential adjunctive therapeutic approaches. Possible adjunctive therapies and points of intervention in the treatment of periodontitis are presented related to the pathologic cascade of events. *CAL*, Clinical attachment loss; *IL-1 and IL-6*, interleukin-1 and -6; *MMPs*, matrix metalloproteinases; *NSAID*, nonsteroidal anti-inflammatory drug; *TNF-α*, tumor necrosis factor alpha.

disorders such as arthritis, cardiovascular disease (CVD), dermatologic conditions, diabetes, rheumatoid arthritis, and osteoporosis. Also, patients who are currently taking host modulatory agents, such as nonsteroidal anti inflammatory drugs (NSAIDs), bisphosphonates, or tetracyclines, as well as newer agents targeting specific cytokines for the management of medical conditions, may be experiencing periodontal benefits from these systemic medications prescribed for the management of other chronic inflammatory conditions.

A variety of different drug classes have been evaluated as host modulation agents, including the NSAIDs, bisphosphonates, tetracyclines, enamel matrix proteins, growth factors, bone morphogenetic proteins, and more recently the Probiotics, omega-3 polyunsaturated fatty acids (PUFAs), and resolvins. This section discusses chemotherapeutics developed as HMTs researched as adjuncts to treat periodontitis to date, the use of HMTs in clinical practice, and what the future might hold for HMTs.

Systemically Administered Agents

Nonsteroidal Anti-Inflammatory Drugs

NSAIDs inhibit the formation of prostaglandins, including PGE_2, which are produced by neutrophils, macrophages, fibroblasts, and gingival epithelial cells in response to the presence of LPS, a component of the cell wall of gram-negative bacteria. PGE_2 has been extensively studied in periodontal disease because it upregulates bone resorption by osteoclasts.[43,56,81] Levels of PGE_2 have been shown to be elevated in patients with periodontal disease compared with healthy patients.[45,81] PGE_2 also inhibits fibroblast function and has inhibitory and modulatory effects on the immune response.[46]

NSAIDs inhibit prostaglandins and therefore reduce tissue inflammation. They are used to treat pain, acute inflammation, and a variety of chronic inflammatory conditions. NSAIDs include the salicylates (e.g., aspirin), indomethacin, and the propionic acid derivatives (e.g., ibuprofen, flurbiprofen, and naproxen). The ability of NSAIDs to block PGE_2 production, thereby reducing inflammation and inhibiting osteoclast activity in the periodontal tissues, has been investigated in patients with periodontitis. Short-term administration of NSAIDs showed a reduction of GCF MMP-8 levels, but no statistically significant differences were observed in CAL levels.[12] Studies have also suggested that low-dose aspirin as an adjunct periodontal therapy may be beneficial in reducing periodontal attachment loss.[27,29] In addition, studies have shown that systemic NSAIDs, such as indomethacin,[120] flurbiprofen,[119] and naproxen[55] administered daily for up to 3 years, significantly slowed the rate of alveolar bone loss compared with placebo. However, NSAIDs have some serious disadvantages when considered for use as HMT for periodontitis. Daily administration for extended periods is necessary for periodontal benefits to become apparent, and NSAIDs are associated with significant side effects, including gastrointestinal problems, hemorrhage (from decreased platelet aggregation), and renal and hepatic impairment. Furthermore, research shows that the periodontal benefits of taking long-term NSAIDs are lost when patients stop taking the drugs, with a return to or even an acceleration of the rate of bone loss seen before NSAID therapy, often referred to as a "rebound effect."[121] For these reasons, the long-term use of NSAIDs as an adjunctive treatment for periodontitis has never really developed beyond research studies.

It was previously anticipated that selective cyclooxygenase-2 (COX-2) inhibitors may offer promise as adjunctive treatments in the management of periodontitis. The enzyme cyclooxygenase, which converts arachidonic acid to prostaglandins, exists in two functionally distinct isoforms, COX-1 and COX-2. COX-1 is constitutively expressed and has antithrombogenic and cytoprotective functions. Therefore, inhibition of COX-1 by nonselective NSAIDs causes side effects such as gastrointestinal ulceration and impaired hemostasis. COX-2 is induced after stimulation by various cytokines, growth factors, and LPS and results in the production of elevated quantities of prostaglandins. Inhibition of COX-2 by selective COX-2 inhibitors results in a reduction of inflammation. Researchers considered that the use of selective COX-2 inhibitors offered the prospect of reducing periodontal inflammation without the side effects typically observed after long-term (nonselective) NSAID therapy, and preliminary studies identified that selective COX-2 inhibitors slowed alveolar bone loss in animal models[6,54] and modified prostaglandin production in human periodontal tissues.[112] However, the selective COX-2 inhibitors were later identified to be associated with significant and life-threatening adverse effects (i.e., myocardial infarction), resulting in some drugs being withdrawn from the market. In summary, NSAIDs (including the selective COX-2 specific inhibitors) are presently not indicated as adjunctive HMTs in the treatment of periodontal disease.

Bisphosphonates

The bisphosphonates are bone-seeking agents that inhibit bone resorption by disrupting osteoclast activity. Their precise mechanism of action is unclear, but research has shown that bisphosphonates interfere with osteoblast metabolism and secretion of lysosomal enzymes.[117] More recent evidence has suggested that bisphosphonates also possess anticollagenase properties.[76] The ability of bisphosphonates to modulate osteoclast activity clearly indicates that they may be useful in the treatment of periodontitis. Research has demonstrated that in naturally occurring periodontitis in beagle dogs, treatment with the bisphosphonate, alendronate, significantly increased bone density compared with placebo.[94] In animal models of experimentally induced periodontitis, bisphosphonates reduced alveolar bone resorption.[102,117] In human studies, these agents resulted in enhanced alveolar bone status and density.[9,22,96]

Some bisphosphonates have the unwanted effects of inhibiting bone calcification and inducing changes in white blood cell counts. Also, there have been recent reports of avascular necrosis of the jaws following bisphosphonate therapy, with the resultant risk of bone necrosis following dental extractions.[14] The recent reports of bisphosphonate-related osteonecrosis of the jaw (BRON/ONJ), although primarily associated with intravenous administration of bisphosphonates rather than oral administration, have impeded the development of bisphosphonates as an HMT to manage periodontitis. As with NSAIDs, at present there are no bisphosphonate drugs that are approved and indicated for treatment of periodontal diseases.

Sub-Antimicrobial-Dose Doxycycline

Sub-antimicrobial-dose doxycycline (SDD) is a 20-mg dose of doxycycline (Periostat) that is approved and indicated as an adjunct to SRP in the treatment of chronic periodontitis. It is taken twice daily for 3 months, up to a maximum of 9 months of continuous dosing. The 20-mg dose exerts its therapeutic effect by enzyme, cytokine, and osteoclast inhibition rather than by any antibiotic effect. Research studies have found no detectable antimicrobial effect on the oral flora or the bacterial flora in other regions of the body and have identified clinical benefit when used as an adjunct to SRP. At present, SDD (Periostat) is the only systemically administered HMT specifically indicated for the treatment of chronic periodontitis that is approved by the US Food and Drug Administration (FDA) and accepted by the American Dental Association (ADA). Studies conducted by Preshaw et al.,[91] utilizing this same modified-release SDD versus placebo in 266 subjects with periodontitis as an adjunct to SRP resulted in significantly greater clinical benefits than SRP alone in the treatment of periodontitis. A review paper on the nonsurgical treatment of chronic periodontitis by means of sub gingival root instrumentation in the form of SRP with or without adjuncts showed that clinical improvements with SRP alone resulted in a mean gain of 0.5 mm in clinical attachment levels (CAL), while adjunctive therapy with sub-antimicrobial dose doxycycline resulted in an additional 0.35-mm gain in CAL above and beyond that seen with mechanical therapy alone, representing a 70% improvement in CAL.[103] In addition, a modified-release SDD was more recently approved by the FDA (Oracea) for the treatment of the common skin disorder rosacea and is routinely prescribed within the dermatology community. It will be interesting to see what the long-term benefits to oral health will be for rosacea patients being prescribed this time-released formulation of SDD. There has also been considerable off-label use of this new modified-release SDD for the treatment of periodontal diseases based on the understanding that once-a-day administration can increase the level of compliance as compared to twice-a-day oral administration. In fact, Preshaw et al. demonstrated that this modified-release SDD resulted in significantly improved clinical benefits in the treatment of periodontitis.[91]

Locally Administered Agents

Nonsteroidal Anti-Inflammatory Drugs

Topical NSAIDs have shown benefit in the treatment of periodontitis. One study of 55 patients with chronic periodontitis who received topical ketorolac mouthrinse reported that gingival crevicular fluid (GCF) levels of PGE_2 were reduced by approximately half over 6 months and that bone loss was halted.[58] In addition, locally administered ketoprofen has been investigated. To date, topically administered NSAIDs have not been approved as local HMTs for the management of periodontitis.

Enamel Matrix Proteins, Growth Factors, and Bone Morphogenetic Proteins

A number of local HMTs have been investigated for potential use as adjuncts to surgical procedures, not only to improve wound healing but also to stimulate regeneration of lost bone, periodontal ligament, and cementum, restoring the complete periodontal attachment apparatus. These have included enamel matrix proteins, bone morphogenetic proteins (BMP-2, BMP-7), growth factors (platelet-derived growth factor, insulin-like growth factor), and tetracyclines. The locally applied HMTs currently approved by the FDA for adjunctive use during surgery are enamel matrix proteins (Emdogain), recombinant human platelet-derived growth factor-BB (GEM 21S), and BMP-2 (INFUSE), which are covered in much greater detail in other chapters. The initial local host modulatory agent approved by the FDA for adjunctive use during surgery to assist with clinical attachment gain and wound healing was Emdogain. This has been followed by platelet-derived growth factor combined with a resorbable synthetic bone matrix (GEM 21S) to assist in regenerative procedures approved by the FDA, as well as rhBMP-2 (INFUSE) soaked on to an absorbable collagen sponge to assist with ridge and sinus augmentation. The technology behind GEM 21 has also been approved and marketed for use in wound healing, particularly in patients with diabetes, and INFUSE has been used for quite some time for the healing of fractures by the orthopedic community. However, adverse events associated with the administration of BMPs have been reported, including: osteolysis, seroma/hematoma, infection, arachnoiditis, dysphagia, increased neurological deficits, and cancer.[26] The remainder of this chapter focuses on the clinical utility of host modulation for nonsurgical procedures in clinical practice and the use of SDD (Periostat) in clinical practice.

Host Modulation and Comprehensive Periodontal Management

The term *periodontal management* suggests a much broader concept of periodontal care than the term *periodontal treatment.* This concept is extremely important considering the chronic nature of the disease. Disease management includes thorough medical and dental history and examination (clinical charting and radiographs), assessment of risk factors, diagnosis, development of a treatment strategy, initial and definitive treatment planning, review of treatment outcomes and reevaluation, long-term supportive periodontal therapy (maintenance care), and assessment of prognosis. In addition, as new data continue to emerge regarding biochemical assessments of disease activity (measuring levels of proinflammatory mediators, bone and connective tissue breakdown products in the GCF, saliva, and tissues of the oral cavity), new diagnostic and prognostic tests may become part of our established protocols

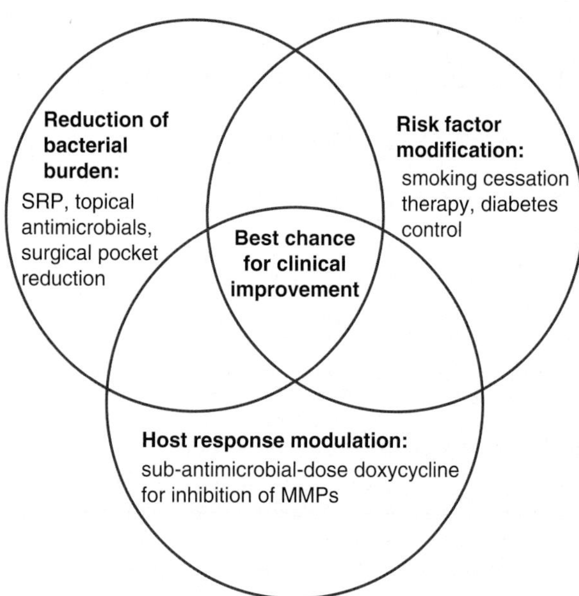

Fig. 55.4 Complementary treatment strategies in periodontitis. The best chance for clinical improvement may come from implementing complementary treatment strategies that target different aspects of the periodontal balance. Reduction of the bacterial burden by scaling and root planing *(SRP)* is the cornerstone of treatment and can be augmented by the use of topical antimicrobials and surgical pocket therapy. In addition to this antibacterial treatment approach, the host response can be treated by the use of host modulatory therapy, such as sub-antimicrobial-dose doxycycline, for the inhibition of matrix metalloproteinases *(MMPs)*. Risk factor assessment and modification must form a key part of any periodontal treatment strategy, including smoking cessation counseling. These different but complementary treatment strategies can be used together as part of a comprehensive management approach.

for comprehensive periodontal disease management in the future. However, controlling the bacteria that cause periodontal infections remains a central focus of effective periodontal treatment. Understanding the importance of the host response and the impact of risk factors now allows clinicians to provide complementary treatment strategies simultaneously for their patients (Fig. 55.4).

Those patients most likely requiring the use of HMT include those with risk factors that are either nonmodifiable or not easily modified. If the decision is made to use HMT, this must be discussed with the patient and the rationale for treatment thoroughly explained. This takes time at the chairside, but it is time well spent; patients become increasingly interested in their periodontal status and are more likely to develop ownership of their management, thereby enhancing compliance with all aspects of care, including plaque control, risk reduction, and treatment protocols. Compliance with HMT is greatly facilitated if the rationale for prescribing is clearly explained. The need for compliance with the prescribed drug regimen is important because with SDD, for example, a tablet must be taken twice daily (once in the morning and once in the evening) and should not be taken with calcium supplements. Compliance may be improved by the administration of a modified-release SDD capsule taken only once a day. It should be emphasized to the patient that the use of HMT is not a substitute for excellent plaque control (just as it is not a substitute for excellent debridement and root surface instrumentation by the treating clinician). To achieve the best results, patients must be interested and well informed about their condition so that compliance is maximized. Furthermore, patients must also be convinced that comprehensive and frequent recall appointments are absolutely necessary in the maintenance phase of this chronic and often progressive disease, which can be very well controlled with adequate follow-up.

In addition to patient motivation, oral hygiene instruction, and SRP to reduce the bacterial challenge, a key treatment strategy when managing periodontitis patients is *risk factor modification.* The harmful effects of smoking on the periodontal tissues are well documented,[61] and successful smoking cessation therapy will likely be a major benefit to patients with periodontitis. Smoking cessation counseling can be undertaken in the dental office (if staff are appropriately trained) or through collaboration with the patient's physician or specialized clinics. Given the evidence that smokers have worse periodontal disease than nonsmokers[104,122] and that the magnitude and predictability of clinical improvements after treatment are significantly reduced in smokers,[1,87] smoking cessation counseling should form a major part of treatment for smokers with periodontitis. Patients with poorly controlled diabetes are also at an increased risk for periodontitis,[71] and periodontal therapy may have an impact on diabetic control.[46] Collaboration with medical colleagues when treating patients with diabetes and periodontitis is warranted to ascertain the degree of diabetic control.[30] Other possible risk factors for the development of periodontitis include nonmodifiable factors such as genetics, gender, and race. As the relevance of different risk factors is established through epidemiologic research, clinicians must remain aware of their responsibilities for informing and attempting to change patients' behaviors in relation to modifiable risks.

The management of patients with periodontitis can therefore involve the following complementary treatment strategies:

- Patient education and motivation, including oral hygiene instruction; use of powered toothbrushes and connected technologies, interproximal cleaners (floss, interdental brushes), antiseptics in rinses, toothpastes with actives, and irrigation; and explanation of the rationale for any adjunctive treatments.
- Reduction of the bacterial burden by high-quality SRP.
- Site-specific antibacterial treatment with local delivery systems or systemic antimicrobial therapy in select cases.
- Host response modulation by HMT.
- Risk factor modification and risk reduction strategies.
- Periodontal surgery with or without HMT.

It is the responsibility of the dentist to customize the treatment plan for each individual patient by selecting and providing appropriate treatments, taking into consideration individual risk, following discussion and informed decision-making by the patient. Good communication and showing an interest in the patient's condition are essential to maximize compliance and modify risk factors. The best chance for clinical improvement may come from a combination of targeted treatment approaches for each patient (see Fig. 55.4). In fact, Novak et al. published very striking improvements in probing depth reductions and CAL gains in a 6-month, randomized, multicenter, examiner-blinded, placebo-controlled study, which showed that combination therapy of HMT (SDD) plus a locally delivered antimicrobial (doxycycline hyclate gel) and SRP provided optimal improvements in clinical parameters when compared to SRP alone in the treatment of moderate-to-severe periodontitis.[78]

Sub-Antimicrobial-Dose Doxycycline

As previously discussed, SDD is currently the only FDA-approved, systemically administered HMT indicated specifically in the treatment of periodontitis. SDD is used as an adjunct to SRP and must not be used as a stand-alone therapy (monotherapy). Because SDD,

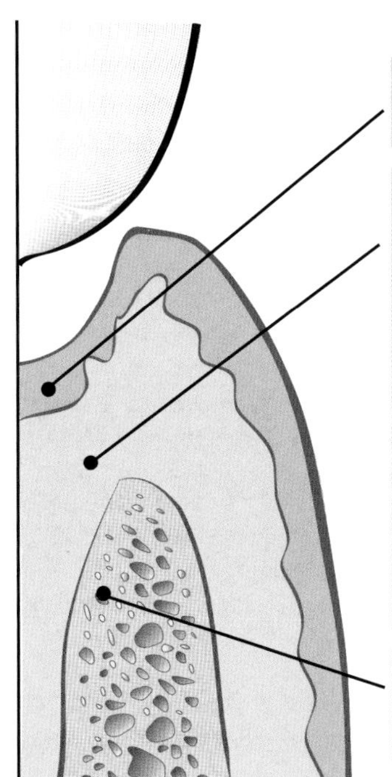

Fig. 55.5 Schematic of periodontal pocket indicating the pleiotropic mechanisms by which doxycycline inhibits connective tissue breakdown. Downregulation of destructive events occurring in the periodontal tissues by doxycycline results from modulation of a variety of different proinflammatory pathways. Tetracyclines inhibit connective tissue breakdown by multiple non-antimicrobial mechanisms. Rights were not granted to include this figure in electronic media. Please refer to the printed book. (From Golub LM, Lee HM, Ryan ME, et al. *Adv Dent Res.* 1998;12:12.)

previously called "low-dose doxycycline" (LDD) and currently marketed as Periostat, is based on a sub-antimicrobial dosage of doxycycline, a member of the tetracycline family of compounds, the use of tetracyclines for the management of periodontal diseases must be put into perspective.

In regard to the incorporation of a medical pharmacologic approach into the management of a disease in the dental practice setting, no class of drugs has had more of an impact on periodontal therapy than the tetracyclines. They have been used in conjunction with SRP, the "gold standard" of nonsurgical therapy, as well as with both resective and regenerative surgical procedures. The tetracyclines have been used locally and systemically as antimicrobial agents and, more recently, systemically as a host modulation agent (SDD). The tetracyclines have been prescribed not only to address chronic periodontitis but also to manage specific and often more aggressive types of periodontitis. Most recently, the tetracyclines have been advocated for the management of patients with systemic diseases such as diabetes, rheumatoid arthritis, and rosacea (Oracea); doxycycline has led to improvements in both the periodontal health of compromised diabetic patients and long-term markers of glycemic control (e.g., glycated hemoglobin).[47] As an adjunct to mechanical therapies, the goal of tetracycline therapy has been to enhance reattachment or even to stimulate new attachment of the supporting apparatus and osseous formation.

This section concentrates on the use of these pleiotropic compounds for modulation of the host response in the treatment of periodontitis.

Mechanisms of Action

In addition to its antibiotic properties, doxycycline (as well as the other members of the tetracycline family) has the ability to downregulate MMPs, a family of zinc-dependent enzymes that are capable of degrading extracellular matrix molecules, including collagen.[7,98] MMPs are secreted by the major cell types in the periodontal tissues (fibroblasts, keratinocytes, macrophages, PMNs, endothelial cells) and play a key role in periodontitis. Excessive quantities of MMPs are released in inflamed periodontal tissues, resulting in the breakdown of the connective tissue matrix. The predominant MMPs in periodontitis, particularly MMP-8 and MMP-9, are derived from PMNs[40] and are extremely effective in degrading type I collagen, the most abundant collagen type in gingiva and periodontal ligament.[69] Levels of PMN-type MMPs have been shown to increase with severity of periodontal disease and decrease after therapy.[33,40] The release of large quantities of MMPs in the periodontium leads to significant anatomic disruption and breakdown of the connective tissues, contributing to the clinical signs of periodontitis.

The rationale for using SDD as an HMT in the treatment of periodontitis is that doxycycline downregulates the activity of MMPs by a variety of synergistic mechanisms, including reductions in cytokine levels, and stimulates osteoblastic activity and new bone formation by upregulating collagen production (Fig. 55.5).

Clinical Research Data on Distinct Patient Populations

Tetracyclines work well as host modulation agents because of their pleiotropic effects on multiple components of the host response (see Fig. 55.3). The only enzyme (MMP) inhibitors that have been approved for clinical use and tested for the treatment of periodontitis are members of the tetracycline family of compounds. In early studies investigating the use of different commercially available tetracyclines, Golub et al.[41] reported that the semisynthetic compound (e.g., doxycycline) was more effective than the parent compound tetracycline in reducing excessive collagenase activity in the GCF of chronic periodontitis patients. Because doxycycline was found to be a more effective inhibitor of collagenase than either minocycline or tetracycline[12,34] and because of its safety profile, pharmacokinetic properties, and ready systemic absorption, recent clinical trials have focused on this compound. In an effort to eliminate the side effects of long-term tetracycline therapy, especially the emergence of tetracycline-resistant organisms, SDD capsules were prepared and tested.[40] Each capsule contained 20 mg of doxycycline versus the commercially available 50 and 100 mg, antimicrobially effective, capsules or tablets. Multiple clinical studies using subantimicrobial doses of doxycycline have shown no difference in the composition or resistance level of the oral flora.[106,116] More recent studies also demonstrate no appreciable differences in either fecal or vaginal microflora samples.[114] In addition, these studies have shown no overgrowth of opportunistic pathogens, such as *Candida,* in the oral cavity, gastrointestinal system, or genitourinary system.

With regard to MMP inhibition, Golub et al.[33] reported that a 2-week regimen of SDD reduced collagenase in GCF and in the adjacent gingival tissues surgically excised for therapeutic purposes. Subsequent studies using SDD therapy as adjunctive to routine scaling and prophylaxis indicated continued reductions in the excessive levels of collagenase in the GCF after 1 month of treatment. After cessation of SDD administration, however, there was a rapid rebound of collagenase activity to placebo levels, suggesting that a 1-month treatment regimen with this host modulation agent was insufficient to produce a long-term benefit.[3] In contrast, during the same study, a 3-month regimen produced a prolonged drug effect without a rebound in collagenase levels to baseline during the no-treatment phase of the study. The mean levels of GCF collagenase were significantly reduced (47.3% from baseline levels) in the SDD group versus the placebo group, who received scaling and prophylaxis alone (29.1% reduction from baseline levels). Accompanying these reductions in collagenase levels were gains in the relative attachment levels in the SDD group.[3,39] As discussed earlier, a recent review paper revealed that adjunctive therapy with SRP and SDD can result in a 70% improvement in CAL.[103] Continuous drug therapy over several months appears to be necessary for maintaining collagenase levels near normal over prolonged periods. It is reasonable to speculate that levels of MMPs will eventually increase again in the more susceptible patients after drug cessation, and those individuals having the most risk factors and the greatest microbial challenge will require more frequent HMT than other patients.

General Patient Populations

Data from clinical trials of SDD are summarized in Table 55.1. In addition, a series of double-blind, placebo-controlled studies of 3, 6, and 9 months' duration all showed clinical efficacy based on reductions in probing depth and gains in clinical attachment as well as biochemical efficacy, based on the inhibition of collagenase activity and protection of serum α_1-antitrypsin (a naturally occurring protective mediator) from collagenase attack in the periodontal pocket.[18,34,64] Golub et al.[36] showed that a 2-month regimen of SDD significantly decreased both the level of bone-type collagen breakdown products (C-terminal telopeptide of type I collagen (ICTP); carboxy terminal peptide, a pyridinoline-containing cross-linked peptide of type I collagen) and MMP-8 and MMP-13 enzyme levels (neutrophil and bone-type collagenase) in chronic periodontitis subjects (Fig. 55.6).

The Phase III, 9-month, randomized, double-blind, placebo-controlled trial conducted at five dental centers demonstrated the clinical efficacy and safety of SDD versus placebo as an adjunct to SRP. The benefits of HMT as an adjunct to mechanical therapy were seen again, with statistically significant reductions in probing depths and gains in CALs, as well as the prevention of disease progression.[15] When SDD administration was discontinued after 9 months of continuous therapy, the incremental improvements demonstrated in the SDD group were maintained for at least 3 months. There was no rebound effect in either the pocket depth reductions or the CAL gains; in fact, there appeared to be slight continued improvement in both these clinical parameters, presumably because of the enhanced clinical status of the patients who had benefited from adjunctive SDD, and possibly also because of the known persistence or substantivity of doxycycline in the bone and soft tissue of the periodontium. The clinical relevance of such findings confirms the utility of an MMP inhibitor in the management of chronic periodontitis.

High-Risk Patients: Smokers

The harmful effects of cigarette smoking and the reduced response to periodontal treatment in smokers compared with nonsmokers are well established.[61] A recent meta-analysis of randomized clinical trials of SDD used as an adjunct to SRP revealed a benefit when using SDD in smokers with periodontitis (see Table 55.1).[77,88] A hierarchical treatment response was observed, such that nonsmokers who received SDD demonstrated the best clinical improvements and smokers who received placebo had the poorest treatment response. The responses of the smokers who received SDD and the nonsmokers who received placebo were intermediate between the two extremes and were broadly identical. This suggests that even patients traditionally considered resistant to periodontal treatment (i.e., smokers) can benefit from SDD, with a treatment response similar to that expected when treating a nonsmoker by SRP alone.

Special Patient Populations

More recent Phase IV (i.e., post-licensing) clinical studies have revealed success using SDD in particular populations of susceptible individuals. Much interest has focused on genetic susceptibility to periodontal disease, particularly whether a specific variation in the genes that regulate the cytokine IL-1 confers increased susceptibility to disease. This polymorphism is known as the *periodontitis-associated genotype* (PAG), the presence of which can be characterized using a screening test, the PST genetic susceptibility test. Investigation of patients who possess this gene polymorphism has been driven by the assumption that local phenotypic differences exist in chronic periodontitis associated with this genotype (e.g., that PAG-positive patients produce more IL-1 cytokines for a given bacterial challenge, resulting in increased tissue damage and more extensive periodontal disease). IL-1β levels in shallow periodontal pockets have been reported to be higher in patients with this genotype than in those without.[25] The studies that have investigated associations between PAG and periodontal disease status have thus far generated conflicting data (as reviewed by Taylor et al.).[105] A reasonable assumption currently is that there are genetic associations between polymorphisms in the IL-1 gene cluster and periodontal disease but that unambiguous results are not yet apparent because of the heterogeneity of the disease and/or the variable design of the reported studies. Cullinan et al. concluded that the IL-1 genotype is a contributory but nonessential risk factor for periodontal disease progression.[19] Despite the controversy surrounding the acceptance of this genotype as a risk factor, insurance companies have utilized testing as a determinant of covered treatment.[10]

A 5-month preliminary investigation by Ryan et al.[99] was designed to evaluate the impact of treatment on IL-1β and MMP levels in PST-positive (PAG) patients who presented with elevated levels of these biochemical markers in their GCF. These patients were initially treated with SRP, resulting in no change in the levels of these biochemical markers after 1 month. Al-Shammari et al.[2] reported similar findings, with no changes in GCF levels of IL-1β and ICTP before and after SRP in patients who had not been genotyped. When the genotype-positive patients received SDD and these biochemical markers were monitored at 2 and 4 months, a significant decrease (50% to 61%) in the IL-1β and MMP-9 levels was noted after treatment with SDD. Correspondingly, gains in clinical

TABLE 55.1 Summary of Data Reported in Clinical Trials of Sub-Antimicrobial-Dose Doxycycline[90]

			MEAN CAL CHANGE (mm)		MEAN PD REDUCTION (mm)		% SITES WITH CAL GAIN[c]		% SITES WITH PD REDUCTION[b]	
Study (Year)	**Duration**	**Study Groups (*N*)**	**4–6 mm Pockets**	**7+ mm Pockets**	**4–6 mm Pockets**	**7+ mm Pockets**	**≥2 mm**	**≥3 mm**	**≥2 mm**	**≥3 mm**
Caton et al. (2000)[15]	Study: 9 months (drug: 9 months)	SRP + SDD (90)	1.03[a]	1.55[a]	0.95[b]	1.68[b]	46	22	47[a]	22[a]
		SRP + placebo (93)	0.86	1.17	0.69	1.20	38	16	35	13
Novak et al. (2002)[79]	Study:9 months (drug: 6 months)	SRP + SDD (10)	1.00	1.78	1.20	3.02	29	15	48	26
		SRP + placebo (10)	0.56	1.24	0.97	1.42	21	11	21	6
Emingil et al. (2004)[23]	Study: 12 months (drug: 3 months)	SRP + SDD (10)	0.21 (all sites)	1.59[a] (all sites)						
		SRP + placebo (10)	0.05 (all sites)	1.32 (all sites)						
Preshaw et al. (2004)[89]	Study: 9 months (drug: 9 months)	SRP + SDD (107)	1.27[b]	2.09[a]	1.29[b]	2.31[b]	58[a]	33[b]	62[b]	37[b]
		SRP + placebo (102)	0.94	1.60	0.96	1.77	44	20	45	21
Lee et al. (2004)[65]	Study: 9 months (drug: 9 months	SRP + SDD (240)	1.56[a] (all sites)	1.63[a] (all sites)						
		SRP + placebo (17)	0.80 (all sites)	1.19 (all sites)						
Choi et al. (2004)[16]	Study: 4 months (drug: 4 months)	SRP + SDD (15)	2.2[a] (test sites)	1.6[a] (test sites)						
		SRP + placebo (17)	0.6 (test sites)	1.1 (test sites)						
Gurkan et al. (2005)[51]	Study: 6 months (drug: 3 months)	SRP + SDD (13)	1.12	2.15	1.80	3.38				
		SRP + placebo (13)	0.78	1.76	1.46	2.57				
Preshaw et al. (2005)[e,88]	Study: 9 months (drug: 9 months)	SRP + SDD[#] (116)	1.23[a]	1.89[b]	1.22[b]	2.16[a]	59[b]	33[b]	63[d]	37
		SRP + placebo[#] (135)	0.96	1.43	0.88	1.53	43	19	44	18
		SRP + SDD[##] (81)	1.03	1.71	1.01	1.80	44	21	45[b]	20
		SRP + placebo[##] (60)	0.85	1.58	0.80	1.62	37	15	31	13
Mohammad et al. (2005)[75]	Study: 9 months (drug: 9 months)	SRP + SDD (12)	2.14[d]	3.18[a]	1.57[d]	3.22[d]				
		SRP + placebo (12)	0.02	0.25	0.63	0.98				
Górska and Nedzi-Góra (2006)[44]	Study: 3 months (drug: 3 months)	SRP + SDD (33)	0.33[a] (all sites)	0.29[a] (all sites)						
		SRP + placebo (33)	0.04 (all sites)	0.08 (all sites)						
Needleman et al. (2007)[77]	Study: 6 months (drug: 3 months)	SRP + SDD[##] (18)	0.65 (all sites)	1.40 (all sites)						
		SRP + placebo[##] (16)	0.40 (all sites)	0.98 (all sites)						

[a] $P < .05$ compared with placebo.
[b] $P < .01$ compared with placebo.
[c] Percentage of sites with CAL gain and PD reduction ≥2 mm and ≥3 mm calculated for all sites that had 6+ mm probing depths at baseline.
[d] $P < .001$ compared with placebo.
[e] Same study population as Preshaw et al. (2004),[89] stratified by smoking status: *#*, nonsmokers, *##*, smokers.
N, Number of subjects; *CAL*, clinical attachment level, CAL change can be positive (CAL gain) or negative (CAL loss); *PD*, probing depth; *SRP*, scaling and root planing.

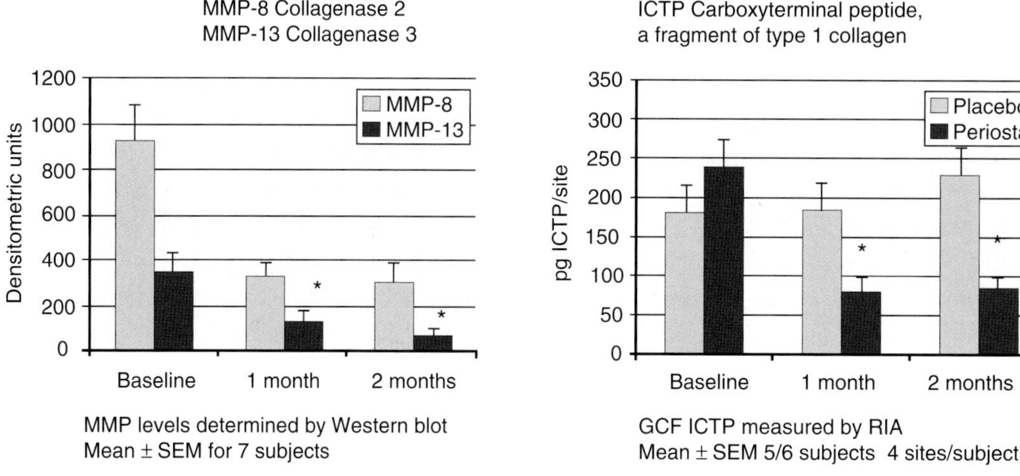

Fig. 55.6 Effect of sub-antimicrobial-dose doxycycline (SDD) on gingival crevicular fluid *(GCF)* collagenase *(MMP-8, MMP-13)* and ICTP. A 2-month regimen of SDD significantly decreased levels of matrix metalloproteinases (MMP-8 and MMP-13, neutrophil and bone-type collagenases, respectively) and ICTP compared with placebo in GCF samples of adult periodontitis patients. Decreased levels of GCF bone-type collagen breakdown products (ICTP, pyridinoline-containing cross-linked peptide of type I collagen) in the SDD group versus the placebo group provide biochemical evidence of a reduction in bone resorption. *RIA*, Radioimmunoassay. A matrix metalloproteinase inhibitor reduces bone-type collagen degradation fragments and specific collagenases in gingival crevicular fluid during adult periodontitis, (From Golub LM, Lee HM, Greenwald RA, et al. *Inflamm Res.* 1997;46:310.)

attachment and reduced probing depths were also observed. The study concluded that a sub-antimicrobial dose of doxycycline may provide PST-positive patients with a therapeutic strategy that specifically addresses their exaggerated host response.

Another study was conducted in susceptible patients with severe generalized periodontitis using host modulation (SDD) as an adjunct to repeated subgingival debridement.[79] Seventy percent of the patients who completed this 9-month double-blind, placebo-controlled study were smokers. SDD as an adjunct to mechanical therapy versus mechanical therapy alone resulted in significantly greater mean probing depth reductions in pockets of 7 mm or greater at baseline as early as 1 month after therapy (2.52 mm vs. 1.25 mm, respectively). These improvements in the SDD group compared with the group receiving mechanical therapy only were maintained during the 5.25 months of therapy (2.85 mm vs. 1.48 mm, respectively) and even at 3 months after stopping drug therapy (3.02 mm vs. 1.41 mm), demonstrating that no rebound effect occurred. Because of the beneficial effects of HMT in susceptible patients, multicenter studies are using SDD in other susceptible populations, including diabetic, osteoporotic, and institutionalized geriatric patients, as well as smokers.

Since periodontitis is associated with many systemic diseases (e.g., osteoporosis, diabetes, and CVD), researchers have investigated the effect of SDD on these systemic conditions. Payne et al.[84] conducted a 2-year randomized, double-blind, placebo-controlled trial in osteopenic women at two dental centers demonstrating that SDD can effectively reduce the levels of localized and systemic inflammatory mediators in osteopenic patients in addition to improving on the clinical measurements of periodontitis[37]; SDD significantly reduced the progression of periodontal attachment loss[95] and the severity of gingival inflammation and alveolar bone loss in postmenopausal osteopenic women.[85] Golub et al.[37] reported that collagenase activity in the GCF of these osteopenic women was significantly reduced by SDD treatment. ICTP showed a similar pattern of change during SDD treatment with GCF collagenase activity and ICTP levels positively correlated at all time periods ($P < .001$). MMP-8 accounted for approximately 80% of total collagenase in the GCF, with much lower levels of MMP-1 and -13. SDD dramatically reduced the elevated MMP-8 levels by 60%. This 2-year study also demonstrated that long-term continuous use of SDD did not produce antibiotic side effects,[115] confirming what had been reported previously in studies of continuous use of up to 12 months. Previously reported studies have demonstrated a relationship between serum high-sensitivity C-reactive protein (hsCRP) concentration and biochemical bone turnover markers in healthy pre- and post-menopausal women.[59] These findings suggest that low-grade systemic inflammation may be a common linking factor between the development of atherosclerosis and an increased bone turnover rate. Payne et al.[82] demonstrated that the two-year SDD regimen described above in post-menopausal women significantly reduced serum inflammatory biomarkers (hs-CRP and MMP-9) and, among women more than five years post-menopausal, increased the HDL cholesterol level. These preliminary findings suggest that SDD may play a role in managing the care of patients at risk for developing coronary artery disease. Other studies have shown that SDD reduces systemic inflammatory biomarkers in CVD patients[11] and SDD decreases glycosylated hemoglobin level (HbA1c) in patients who are taking normally prescribed hypoglycemic agents.[24] The impact of SDD therapy on periodontitis may be amplified by the concurrent use of other HMTs used to manage other inflammatory diseases.

Suggested Uses and Other Considerations

Until relatively recently, treatment options for periodontal disease have focused solely on reducing the bacterial challenge through nonsurgical therapy, surgery, and systemic or local antimicrobial therapy. The development of SDD as an HMT, driven by research into the pathogenesis of periodontal disease, is a great example of how translational research can lead to new treatments. By better understanding the biochemical processes that are important in periodontal disease, a pharmacologic principle (doxycycline downregulates MMP activity) has been used in the development of a new drug treatment. Data presented from research studies show the clinical benefits of adjunctive SDD, and the science behind SDD has been transferred into clinical practice. In other words, dentists now have the opportunity to use SDD for patient care, with the aim being to enhance the treatment response to conventional therapy.

Candidate Patients

When deciding whether to use SDD as an adjunct to SRP, first consider the patient's motivation toward periodontal care, the medical history, and the patient's willingness to take a systemic drug treatment. SDD is contraindicated in any patient with a history of allergy or hypersensitivity to tetracyclines. It should not be given to pregnant or lactating women or children less than 12 years old (because of the potential for discoloration of the developing dentition). Doxycycline may reduce the efficacy of oral contraceptives, and, therefore, alternative forms of birth control should be discussed, if necessary. There is a risk of increased sensitivity to sunlight (manifested by an exaggerated sunburn) seen with higher doses of doxycycline, although this has not been reported in the clinical trials using the sub-antimicrobial dose.

The rationale for using SDD must be clearly explained to the patient. By discussing the etiology of periodontal disease, the available treatment options, and the anticipated outcomes, patients become more interested in their periodontal management, are more likely to comply with treatment, and take more responsibility for managing their disease. Therefore the anticipated compliance and likely commitment to treatment must also be gauged when considering SDD. Patients who show little enthusiasm for complying with the treatment plan or with oral hygiene practices are less likely to be good candidates for systemic drug therapy.

Treatable Periodontal Conditions

SDD is indicated in the management of chronic periodontitis, and studies to date have focused on chronic and aggressive forms of periodontitis.[15,23,79,89] SDD should not be used in conditions such as gingivitis and periodontal abscess or when an antibiotic is indicated. SDD can be used in patients with aggressive periodontitis who are being treated nonsurgically. Furthermore, emerging studies have supported the efficacy of SDD as an adjunct to periodontal surgery.[28] SDD may also be of benefit in cases that are refractory to treatment, as well as in patients with risk factors such as smoking, diabetes, osteoporosis/osteopenia, and genetic susceptibility, in whom the treatment response might be limited.

Side Effects

Doxycycline at antibiotic doses (≥100 mg) is associated with adverse effects, including photosensitivity, hypersensitivity reactions, nausea, vomiting, and esophageal irritation. However, in the clinical trials of SDD (20-mg dose), it was reported that the drug was well tolerated and the profile of unwanted effects was virtually identical in the SDD and placebo groups.[15,23,79,89] The types of adverse events did not differ significantly between treatment groups, and the typical side effects of the tetracycline class were not observed, indicating that the appearance of adverse events is dose related.[15,89] Furthermore, there was no evidence of adverse events that could be attributed to antimicrobial effects of treatment and no evidence of developing antibiotic resistance of the microflora after 2 years of continuous use.[15,106,107,115,116] Therefore the drug appears to be well tolerated, with a very low incidence of adverse effects.

Sequencing Prescription With Periodontal Treatment

SDD is indicated as an adjunct to mechanical periodontal therapy and should not be used as a stand-alone or monotherapy. SDD should be prescribed to coincide with the first round of SRP and is prescribed for 3 months, up to a maximum of 9 to 24 months of continuous dosing depending on the patient's risk. Modification of any risk factors, such as smoking, nutrition, stress, contributing medications, faulty restorations, poor oral hygiene, and poor diabetic control, should also be addressed at this time. A patient's refusal or inability to modify contributing risk factors is an important consideration for treatment planning and evaluation of therapeutic responses.

After initial periodontal treatment, the patient is enrolled in an intensive periodontal maintenance program. This involves regular monitoring of probing depths, reinforcement of oral hygiene, and re-motivation of the patient, with further SRP to disrupt the plaque biofilm and remove re-forming calculus deposits. The 3-month prescription of SDD fits in well with the typical maintenance recall interval of 3 months, which in turn is based on the duration reported for recolonization of treated periodontal pockets.[67]

Thus SDD therapy is commenced at the start of initial periodontal therapy and continues for 3 months until the first reevaluation or maintenance appointment. At maintenance appointments, the need for further prescription of SDD can be assessed. For patients demonstrating a good treatment response with significant reductions in probing depths, further SDD may not be necessary. Periodontal maintenance care must continue, with an emphasis on plaque control, monitoring, and prophylaxis. In other patients, the treatment response after completion of initial therapy may be less favorable. Sites with persisting or progressing pockets may require additional instrumentation, and the prescription of SDD may be extended for an additional 3 months. SDD may be combined with the use of locally applied antimicrobials and surgical procedures. Remember that periodontitis is a chronic disease, and the treatment (whether SDD is used or not) is long-term. The patient must be regularly reevaluated to determine disease stability or progression and the need for additional active therapy.

Therefore patients may cycle between phases of "active" treatment (SRP + SDD) and long-term periodontal maintenance. The success of the maintenance phase of treatment will be affected by many factors, including the following:

- Compliance with the maintenance regimen.
- Compliance with oral hygiene instruction.
- Presence of risk factors, such as smoking, poorly controlled diabetes, or stress.
- Extent (i.e., number) and severity (i.e., depth) of residual deep pockets.

Maintenance therapy is more likely to be successful in patients with good compliance, good oral hygiene, minimal or no systemic risk factors, and minimal residual deep pocketing. The patient who enters the maintenance program may have periodontal stability for months or years. However, plaque control may deteriorate, the patient may develop or acquire new risk factors, and disease progression (i.e., further loss of attachment) may become apparent, indicating that a further course of treatment is required. A further course of SRP will then be undertaken together with adjunctive SDD to restore periodontal stability.

Combining With Periodontal Surgery or Local Delivery Systems

Most clinical research to date has focused on using SDD as an adjunct to nonsurgical periodontal treatment. However, when SDD was used as an adjunct to access flap surgery in 24 patients, clinical evaluation revealed better probing depth reductions in surgically treated sites greater than 6 mm compared with surgically treated sites in patients given placebo.[28] Furthermore, the SDD group demonstrated greater reductions in ICTP (carboxy-terminal peptide, a breakdown product of collagen) than the placebo group, indicating that collagenolytic activity was reduced in the patients taking SDD.

SDD treatment can also be combined with the local delivery of antibiotics into the periodontal pocket through sustained-delivery systems. The two treatment approaches target different aspects of the pathogenic process: local delivery systems deliver antimicrobial concentrations of an antibacterial agent directly into the site of the pocket, whereas SDD is a systemic host response modulator. Thus combining these two complementary treatment strategies is another example of how antibacterial therapy (SRP + local antibiotics) can be combined with HMT (SDD) to maximize the clinical benefit for patients. Preliminary results from a 6-month, 180-patient clinical trial designed to evaluate the safety and efficacy of SDD combined with a locally applied antimicrobial (Atridox) and SRP versus SRP alone demonstrated that patients receiving the combination of treatments experienced more than a 2-mm improvement in mean attachment gains and probing depth reductions ($P < .0001$) compared with SRP alone.[78]

Monitoring Benefits of Therapy

To improve the ability of dentists to make appropriate treatment decisions for patients undergoing periodontal therapy, it would be extremely useful if they had access to the types of diagnostic tests available to their medical colleagues. Such tests might be used, for example, to distinguish between active and inactive lesions. Studies have shown that SRP alone, although effective for improving clinical parameters such as probing depths, may not be sufficient to reduce excessive levels of many underlying destructive mediators, particularly in more susceptible patients. It would be valuable, therefore, if it were possible to monitor the levels of such inflammatory mediators as treatment progresses. SDD results in the downregulation of MMP activity in inflamed periodontal tissues.[33,36] Therefore in theory, MMP levels could be monitored before, during, and after SRP plus SDD treatment. Published data support a concomitant reduction in MMP levels in GCF[16,23] and improvements in clinical parameters when combining SDD and SRP.[23] Although chairside tests for MMPs have been developed,[68] they are not in widespread use because of concerns about their specificity or sensitivity.

In the absence of new chairside tests or a centralized diagnostic facility for monitoring the inflammatory status of the tissues, dentists must rely on clinical periodontal monitoring to assess the outcomes of treatment. In addition to the reductions in probing depths and gains in attachment that may be observed after SRP plus SDD, the quality of the periodontal tissues also tends to improve after treatment with SDD, with significant reductions in gingival indices and bleeding on probing. More sensitive radiographic techniques, assessments of bone density, and bone height changes used solely in clinical trials in the past may be possible in clinical practice in the future. Until such diagnostic techniques are made widely available, however, clinicians must rely on clinical judgment to determine the most appropriate course of therapy.

Emerging Host Modulatory Therapies

Recently, a variety of HMTs have been studied as adjunctive treatments for periodontitis.

Chemically Modified Tetracyclines

A promising group of potential HMTs is the *chemically modified tetracyclines* (CMTs). These nonantibiotic tetracycline analogs are tetracycline molecules that have been modified to remove all antibiotic properties but which retain host modulatory and anticollagenolytic effects. The CMTs are also designed to be more potent inhibitors of proinflammatory mediators and can increase levels of anti-inflammatory mediators such as IL-10. Because they have no antimicrobial properties, the clinician would be able to increase the dose for more susceptible patients with more risk factors and who might be more difficult to manage without experiencing the side effects seen with antibiotics. CMTs, such as CMT-3 and CMT-8 (both of which lack antibiotic activity but retain anti-MMP activity), have been shown to inhibit osteoclastic bone resorption and promote bone formation,[101] enhance wound healing,[86] and inhibit proteinases produced by periodontal pathogens.[45] CMTs also are being studied for other effects, such as inhibition of tumor cell invasion[66] and attenuation of intimal thickening after arterial injury.[57] CMTs will likely emerge as drugs that have beneficial effects in a variety of disease states because of their host modulation capabilities.

Anti-Cytokine Therapy

Anti-cytokine therapy utilizes monoclonal antibodies against cytokines or cytokine receptor antagonists to reduce destructive inflammatory processes associated with a variety of conditions. Novel *anticytokine drugs* have been developed for the management of rheumatoid arthritis, a disease with a pathobiology similar to that of periodontitis.[74] Cytokines such as TNF-α have been targeted by Infliximab (monoclonal antibody to TNF-α) and Etanercept (a TNF-α receptor antagonist), which have been shown to be effective in treating rheumatoid arthritis.[113] Recent studies have demonstrated that these two anti-TNF-α drugs also significantly improve clinical parameters such as probing depth (PD), CAL, and Bleeding on probing BOP in patients with periodontitis ([4]). IL-6 is another important cytokine that plays a major role in periodontal disease. Tocilizumab is a recombinant mAb against IL-6 shown to significantly reduce PD with gains in CAL after 6 months of treatment in patients with periodontitis and rheumatoid arthritis.[62] Since these disease-modifying anti-rheumatic drugs (DMARDs) are associated with significant unwanted side effects, additional studies are necessary to determine new therapeutic regimens that may be efficacious against periodontal disease yet may ameliorate the untoward effects of these drugs.

Anti-cytokine therapy could offer potential benefits given the importance of inflammatory cytokines, such as TNF-α and IL-6, in periodontal pathogenesis. In addition, drugs designed to increase the levels of anti-inflammatory or protective mediators, such as IL-1ra, can perform similar functions. Evidence is emerging to support the benefits of combining HMTs that target different aspects of the disease process. For example, the combination of SDD with bisphosphonates has also demonstrated synergy in animal models of bone loss.[63]

Probiotics

Studies have revealed that probiotics can be beneficial in the management of periodontitis. From animal studies to human clinical trials, Lactobacillus-based probiotics demonstrated potential therapeutic effects on reduction of gingival index (GI) and PD, with gains in CAL compared with a placebo control when administered as an adjunctive treatment to SRP.[4,52] The underlying mechanisms are not completely understood, as probiotics seem to modulate both the periodontal pathogens and host inflammatory responses. Probiotics have been used to reduce the levels of gram-negative bacteria, temporarily shifting the oral microbial environment to a more healthy microbiome. With regards to host modulation, it is proposed that probiotics can modulate T-regulatory cell activity to inhibit inflammation and periodontal bone loss, and may play a role in the inhibition of nitric oxide synthesis. It is clear that more extensive studies of probiotics demonstrating safety and efficacy are needed before this approach can be available clinically.

Omega-3 Polyunsaturated Fatty Acids and Resolvins

As the concept of host modulation has become more widely accepted, we have seen much research looking toward the development of additional HMTs. Some have focused on the efficacy of available nutritional supplements such as fish oils. Studies have indicated that n-3 polyunsaturated fatty acids (n-3 PUFAs; fish oil), as an adjunct to oral hygiene instructions, can significantly lower GCF IL-8, IL-6, and PGE_2 levels compared to placebo controls.[20] Other studies have found that a combination therapy with n-3 PUFA and low-dose aspirin as an adjunct to regenerative procedures utilizing decalcified freeze-dried bone allografts results in greater mean probing depth reductions ($P < .001$) and gains in clinical attachment ($P < .05$) accompanied by a trend for modulation of the cytokine profile of IL-1β and IL-10 in GCF compared to placebo-controlled regenerative therapy.[21] More recent researches confirmed that PUFAs have therapeutic effects on treating various chronic inflammatory diseases such as CVD, diabetes, and COVID.[4]

Recent research has indicated that there is an active biochemical resolution phase involved in inflammation. It is recognized that it is a key component of the normal inflammatory process. Failure of this resolution pathway can cause prolonged chronic inflammation, delayed wound healing, and can play a role in the pathogenesis of many medical conditions, including periodontal diseases.[109] Specialized pro-resolving mediators (SPMs) are a family of agents including lipoxins, resolvins (Resolvin Ds and Es), and protectins, which are derived from PUFAs. They play a fundamental role in promoting restoration of normal cellular function and resolution of inflammation. Studies have shown that during the resolution phase, SPMs can inhibit inflammatory cell infiltration, promote phagocytosis to remove dead cells and foreign objects, and ultimately restore tissue homeostasis.[111]

Restoration of the resolution pathway by the introduction of resolving molecules may provide new potential therapeutic methods for the management of inflammatory periodontitis.[8] In rabbit animal models of periodontitis, topical application of Resolvin E1 has been shown to protect bone loss mediated by osteoclasts.[53] In a rat model of periodontitis Resolvin E1 was shown to reverse periodontal bone loss and inflammatory gene expression with reductions in osteoclast density reported.[110] A small-scale human clinical study with localized aggressive periodontitis showed that Resolvin E1 can restore impaired macrophage cell function.[92] To date, resolvins have demonstrated great potential as an HMT drug candidate to resolve inflammation and reduce the severity of periodontal diseases in animal models with promising results in small human clinical studies. More research involving larger-scale clinical trials is needed to validate these findings.

Metalloproteinases Inhibitors

New collagenase (MMP) inhibitors known as poly-enolic zinc-binding compounds (PEZBINs) for periodontitis have also been investigated. These new inhibitors are based on the natural product curcumin, which contains a calcium and zinc binding β-diketone moiety that is similar to that found in tetracyclines. The anti-inflammatory properties of curcumin have been demonstrated not only in periodontal disease but also in CVDs, cancer, arthritis, and diabetes.[123] A novel group of chemically modified curcumins (CMC) with increased bioavailability and improved anti-inflammatory activity has been tested. In vitro and in vivo findings demonstrate that these potential new host modulatory agents can decrease pathologically elevated MMP levels in the plasma and gingiva of animal models of periodontitis.[38] Recently, one of the lead compounds has demonstrated a significant effect on reducing alveolar bone loss in experimental periodontitis models. More research is being conducted to evaluate this new group of compounds as an HMT not only in periodontal diseases but also in other systemic chronic inflammatory conditions such as arthritis and diabetes. In an experimental diabetic rat model, CMC has shown a resolving-like activity to restore the impaired macrophage cell function, increase Rev D1 levels, resolve the chronic inflammation and attenuate the alveolar bone loss (publication pending).

Other approaches recently reported indicate the therapeutic potential of a novel semi-synthetic glycosamino glycan ether (SAGE) or sulfated polysaccharide to suppress inflammatory mediators in high-risk individuals, such as those with diabetes and smokers, based on their ability to reduce the impact of advanced glycation end products (AGEs), thereby resulting in reductions of pro-inflammatory mediators of disease.[49] In vitro and in vivo studies found that systemic administration of SAGE significantly reduced local and systemic inflammation by modulating the production of cytokines and MMPs. Periodontal bone loss was significantly attenuated in the diabetic rats with Pg-infection.[49,50] In a recent dog study with naturally occurring periodontitis, SAGE has significantly reduced pro-inflammatory cytokines and MMPs, improved clinical parameters of periodontitis, and decreased alveolar bone loss in beagle dogs.[93]

Other Emerging Host Modulation Therapies

Recent innovations in stem cell research have presented possibilities for the application of stem cells in the development of novel strategies for HMT. These new approaches offer interesting alternatives to existing therapies. Studies have demonstrated that human periodontal stem cells can modulate neutrophil function and reduce excessive inflammation.[17] In addition, bone marrow-derived mesenchymal stem cells have shown great potential for periodontal regeneration in animal models.[60] Additional studies will be needed to characterize dental stem cells and evaluate the therapeutic efficacy of stem cell-based periodontal therapy.

As more innovative potential HMT therapeutics emerge, different categories of agents are being investigated, including complement inhibitors, Homeostatic proteins with epidermal growth factor-like and dicoidin-like domains, nuclear metabolic receptor agonists such as liver X receptors, immune cell inhibitors targeting T-helper 17 cells, and immunization against periodontal pathogens. We can speculate that more enhanced and innovative HMT strategies may achieve desired periodontal outcomes.

Host Modulation Factors in Systemic Disorders

In susceptible patients demonstrating an excessive local inflammatory response to the bacterial stimuli leading to periodontal disease, another consideration involves the loss of epithelial integrity in the periodontal pocket. This tissue response allows for bacterial penetration into the inflamed tissues and eventual entry of the bacteria into the systemic circulation. Patients with untreated periodontitis have an increased risk of transient bacteremias. Bacteremia and associated endotoxemia may incite the overproduction of destructive proinflammatory mediators at distant sites in the periodontitis patient. Therefore patients with periodontitis may be at greater risk for developing a number of systemic conditions associated with a similar overactive host response to external stimuli, such as CVD and diabetic complications. Elevated levels of cytokines, prostanoids, and enzymes are evident in all these conditions.

In the era of periodontal medicine, systemic host modulatory approaches need to be considered. As mentioned, host modulators used to manage periodontal disease, such as an MMP, cytokine and prostanoid inhibitors, may have additional beneficial effects on systemic diseases that have been linked to periodontal disease, such as CVD and diabetes. In CVD, preliminary studies have indicated that individuals with periodontal disease are almost twice as likely to have a fatal heart attack and three times as likely to have a stroke.[5]

MMPs and cytokines have been found to play a major role in weakening the plaques formed by CVD, leading to rupture and eventual thrombosis and infarction.[32] In fact, Golub et al.[35] suggested that tetracyclines could reduce the incidence of acute myocardial infarction[73] by blocking collagenase and stabilizing the collagen cap on the atheroscleromatous arterial plaques. In diabetes, the same MMPs and cytokines involved in the development of periodontitis, the sixth long-term complication of diabetes[72] also play a role in the development of other well-known complications of diabetes such as nephropathy, angiopathy, retinopathy, and wound-healing problems.[97] Modulation of these proinflammatory mediators in patients with diabetes may impede the development of multiple long-term complications. An inhibitor of MMPs, cytokines, and prostanoids used in the treatment of periodontitis may have an indirect effect on these disease processes if a patient's risk for developing these disorders is increased by the presence of untreated periodontitis. HMT may also directly aid in the treatment and prevention of CVD and diabetic complications.

Summary

Periodontal pathogens and destructive host responses are involved in the initiation and progression of periodontitis. Therefore the successful long-term management of this disease may require a treatment strategy that integrates therapies that address both etiologic components. Evidence for the role of MMPs, cytokines, and other mediators in the pathogenesis of periodontal disease distinguishes them as viable targets for a chemotherapeutic approach. The introduction of novel, adjunctive therapies such as host modulation to enhance the efficacy of existing mechanical procedures can contribute favorably to an integrated approach for the long-term, clinical management of periodontitis.

HMTs are an emerging treatment concept in the management of periodontitis. The use of HMT as an adjunct may be particularly useful in susceptible, high-risk patients in whom a prolonged and excessive host response to the presence of bacteria promotes the activity of MMPs and osteoclasts. SDD is the only systemically administered HMT currently approved and indicated as an adjunct to SRP for treating periodontitis. Clinical trials have demonstrated a clear treatment benefit when using SDD versus SRP alone. SDD should be used as part of a comprehensive treatment strategy that includes antibacterial treatments (SRP, plaque control, oral hygiene instruction, local antimicrobials, and periodontal surgery), host response modulation (SDD), and assessment and management of periodontal risk factors. In the future, a range of HMTs targeting different aspects of the destructive cascade of breakdown events in the periodontal tissues are likely to be developed as adjunctive treatments for periodontitis. The further development of these agents will permit dentists to treat specific aspects of the underlying biochemical basis for periodontal disease. The goal is to maximize and make more predictable the treatment response by reducing inflammation and inhibiting destructive processes in the tissues, which will result in enhanced periodontal stability after conventional periodontal treatments such as SRP and surgery. The dentist is now in the exciting position of being able to combine established treatment strategies with new systemic and local drug treatments for this common, chronic disease.

The findings discussed with regard to the use of HMT to better manage chronic periodontal disease may have applications to other chronic systemic diseases such as arthritis, diabetes, osteoporosis, and CVD. In addition, studies utilizing locally applied antimicrobials as part of an intensive periodontal therapy (IPT) regimen have shown very promising results. Future studies may demonstrate that in addition to our current standard therapies, IPT with adjunctive antibiotics and/or host modulation for the management of periodontal disease may have profound positive effects on the overall health status of high-risk patients. The proper management of local infection and inflammation (periodontitis) will have a significant impact on the general, overall health of the population.

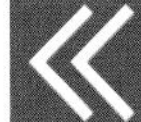

CLINICAL IMPLICATIONS

- HMT is an emerging treatment option in the management of periodontitis.
- A promising group of potential HMTs is the chemically modified tetracyclines (CMTs).
- FDA-approved agent for host modulation treatment of periodontal disease is sub-antimicrobial dose doxycycline (SDD) 20 mg/day.
- SDD is the only systemically administered HMT currently approved and indicated as an adjunct to SRP for treating periodontitis.
- Clinical trials have demonstrated a clear treatment benefit when using SDD versus SRP alone.

FLASH BACK

The downregulation of the destructive elements of the host immune response has the potential to add to the spectrum of treatment choices in the future; however, other agents, such as systemic nonsteroidal anti-inflammatory drugs (NSAIDs) such as ibuprofen, can cause significant side effects with long-term use and are not advised. Antiosteoporotic agents, such as bisphosphonates, have minimal effect on periodontal bone loss and carry other risks, such as localized bone necrosis.

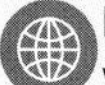

KEY FACT

A range of HMTs targeting different aspects of the destructive cascade of breakdown events in the periodontal tissues are likely to be developed as adjunctive treatments for periodontitis. The further development of these agents provides clinicians with the option to treat specific aspects of the underlying biochemical basis for periodontal disease. The goal is to enhance the response to therapy and achieve periodontal stability.

References for this chapter are found on the companion website eBooks.Health.Elsevier.com.

CHAPTER 56

Surgical Phase of Periodontal Therapy

Satheesh Elangovan | Henry H. Takei

CHAPTER OUTLINE

Therapy for periodontal disease, which encompasses many techniques and procedures, depends on the disease status and objective of the final outcome. Early problems can be corrected with successful nonsurgical (phase I) therapy, consisting of biofilm removal by the patient on a daily basis, scaling, and root instrumentation when necessary.

Many moderate to advanced cases cannot be resolved without surgically gaining access to the root surface for root instrumentation and reducing or eliminating pocket depth to help the patient remove biofilm. The surgical phase of periodontal therapy is also referred to as phase II therapy. This chapter provides an overview of the surgical techniques used for the following purposes:

- Controlling or eliminating periodontal disease
- Correcting anatomic conditions that favor periodontal disease, impair esthetics, or impede placement of prosthetic appliances
- Placing implants to replace lost teeth and improving the environment for their placement and function

Many cases are successfully treated and maintained by phase I therapy. The chapters in Part 2, Section 2, will discuss the in-depth techniques and concepts used to treat periodontal diseases that require a surgical approach to reduce or eliminate pockets and obtain access to the root surface to remove accretions.

Objectives of the Surgical Phase

The surgical phase of periodontal therapy has the following objectives:

1. To improve the prognosis for teeth and their replacements
2. To improve esthetics

Surgical techniques are used for pocket therapy and for correction of related morphologic problems (i.e., mucogingival defects). In many cases, therapies are combined to provide one surgical intervention that fulfills both objectives but there will be scenarios in which attaining both objectives is not feasible.

Surgical techniques can do the following:(1) increase access to the root surface, allowing the clinician to remove all irritants; (2) reduce or eliminate pocket depth, making it possible for the patient to maintain the root surfaces free of biofilm; and (3) reshape soft and hard tissues to attain a harmonious topography. Resective or regenerative surgery or both is used to reduce pocket depth (Box 56.1; see Chapters 61 to 64).

The second objective of phase II therapy is to correct anatomic defects that favor plaque or biofilm accumulation and pocket recurrence or impair esthetics. The aim of correcting anatomic problems is to alter defects of the gingival and mucosal tissues that predispose these areas to disease. Three types of techniques are performed on noninflamed tissues and in the absence of periodontal pockets (see Box 56.1):

- *Plastic surgery techniques* are used to create or widen the attached keratinized gingiva by placing soft tissue grafts of various types.
- *Esthetic surgery techniques* are used to cover denuded root surfaces resulting from recession and to re-create lost papillae.
- *Preprosthetic techniques* are used to modify the periodontal and neighboring tissues to receive prosthetic replacements. They include crown lengthening, ridge augmentation, and vestibular deepening.

Fig. 56.1 provides a three-tiered classification of the surgical procedures used in periodontics: pocket reduction surgery, periodontal plastic surgery, and preprosthetic surgery. Pocket reduction surgery consists of resective and/or regenerative procedures; periodontal plastic surgery includes esthetic and gingival augmentation (anatomic) procedures. Crown lengthening, ridge augmentation, and implant procedures are listed under preprosthetic surgery. Plastic and esthetic surgery techniques are explored in depth in Chapter 65 and preprosthetic techniques are discussed in Chapter 66.

Periodontal surgical procedures also are available for the placement of dental implants. They include implant placement techniques

BOX 56.1 Periodontal Surgery

Pocket Reduction Surgery

- Resective (e.g., gingivectomy, apically displaced flap, undisplaced flap with or without osseous resection)
- Regenerative (e.g., flaps with grafts, membranes)

Correction of Anatomic or Morphologic Defects

- Plastic surgery techniques used to widen attached gingiva (e.g., free gingival grafts)
- Esthetic surgery (e.g., root coverage, recreation of gingival papillae)
- Preprosthetic techniques (e.g., crown lengthening, ridge augmentation, vestibular deepening)
- Placement of dental implants, including techniques for site development for implants (e.g., guided bone regeneration, sinus grafts)

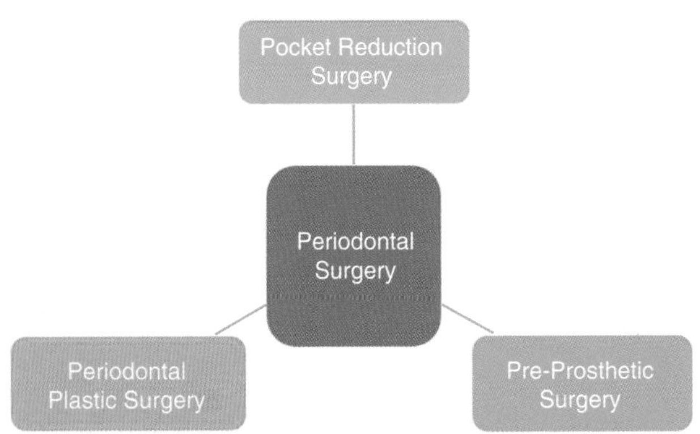

Fig. 56.1 Classification of periodontal surgery. The surgical procedures accomplished in periodontics are organized as pocket reduction surgery, periodontal plastic surgery, and preprosthetic surgery.

and a variety of surgical procedures to modify neighboring tissues for the placement of implants. Bone augmentation of the sinus floor or for a narrow edentulous ridge is an example (see Box 56.1). These topics are discussed in Chapters 78, 79, and 80.

Surgical Pocket Therapy

Surgical pocket therapy can be used to gain access to the diseased root surface to ensure the removal of calculus located subgingivally before surgery and to eliminate or reduce the depth of the periodontal pocket.

Successful periodontal therapy completely eliminates calculus, plaque, or biofilm and diseased cementum from the tooth surface. Numerous investigations have shown that the difficulty of this task increases as the pocket becomes deeper.[2,5] The irregularities and concavities on the root surface also increase, which adds to the difficulty of instrumenting the root surfaces.[11,15]

Furcations also create problems for scaling and subgingival root instrumentation in these areas[4] (see Chapters 50 through 52). Most of these problems can be rectified by resecting or displacing the soft tissue wall of the pocket, which increases the visibility and accessibility of the root surface.[3] The surgical flap technique allows the clinician to overcome these problems of access to the root surface.

Pocket elimination is another important consideration. It consists of reducing the depth of the periodontal pocket to that of a physiologic sulcus to enable cleaning by the patient. By proper case selection, resective and/or regenerative techniques can be used to accomplish this goal. A pocket makes it impossible for the patient to remove biofilm, which is part of the vicious cycle depicted in Fig. 56.2.

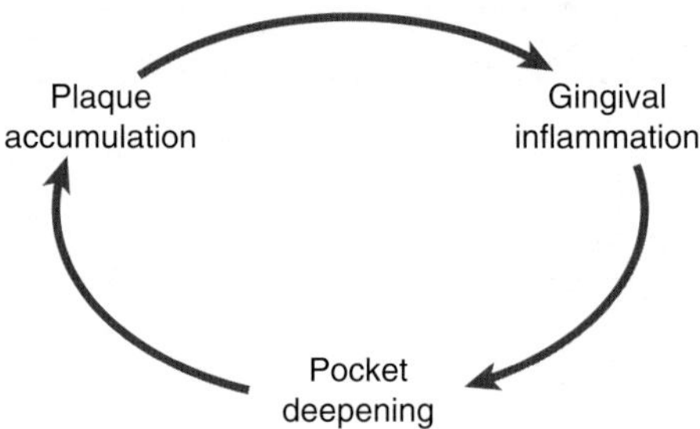

Fig. 56.2 Accumulation of plaque leads to gingival inflammation and pocket deepening, which increases the area of plaque accumulation.

Results of Pocket Therapy

A periodontal pocket can be in an active state or a period of inactivity or quiescence. In an active pocket, underlying bone is being lost (Fig. 56.3, *top left*). It often is diagnosed clinically by bleeding that occurs spontaneously or in response to probing. After phase I therapy, the inflammatory changes in the pocket wall subside, rendering the pocket inactive and reducing its depth (see Fig. 56.3, *top center*). The extent of this reduction depends on the depth before treatment and the degree to which the depth is the result of the edematous and inflammatory component of the pocket wall (i.e., pseudopocket).

Whether the pocket remains inactive depends on the depth, the individual characteristics of the plaque or biofilm components, and the host response. Recurrence of the initial activity is likely.

Inactive pockets sometimes heal with a long junctional epithelium (see Fig. 56.3, *top right*). This condition can be unstable, and the chance of recurrence and re-formation of the original pocket remains because the epithelial union with the tooth is weak. However, one study in monkeys showed that the long junctional epithelial union could be as resistant to biofilm infection as a true connective tissue attachment.[9]

Several studies reported that inactive pockets could be maintained for long periods with little loss of attachment by means of frequent therapy[6,10,12] and by excellent plaque or biofilm removal by the patient on a daily basis. A more reliable and stable result is obtained by transforming the pocket into a healthy sulcus. The bottom of the healthy sulcus can be located where the bottom of the pocket was located or coronal to it. In the first case (see Fig. 56.3, *bottom left*), there is no gain of attachment, and the area of the root that was previously the tooth wall of the pocket becomes exposed. Rather than causing recession, periodontal treatment uncovers the recession previously caused by disease.

The healthy sulcus can be located coronal to the bottom of the preexisting pocket (see Fig. 56.3, *bottom center* and *right*). This is conducive to a restored marginal periodontium; the result is a sulcus of normal depth with a gain of attachment. The creation of a healthy sulcus and a restored periodontium entails total restoration of the status that existed before periodontal disease began, which is the ideal result of treatment. The bone regeneration diagram in Fig. 56.3 (*bottom center* and *right)* is for illustrative purpose only because bone regeneration without an osseous wall is seldom achieved (see Chapter 22).

Pocket Elimination Versus Pocket Maintenance

Pocket elimination (i.e., depth reduction to gingival sulcus levels) has traditionally been considered a type of periodontal therapy. It was considered vital because of the need to improve access to root surfaces for the therapist during treatment and for the patient

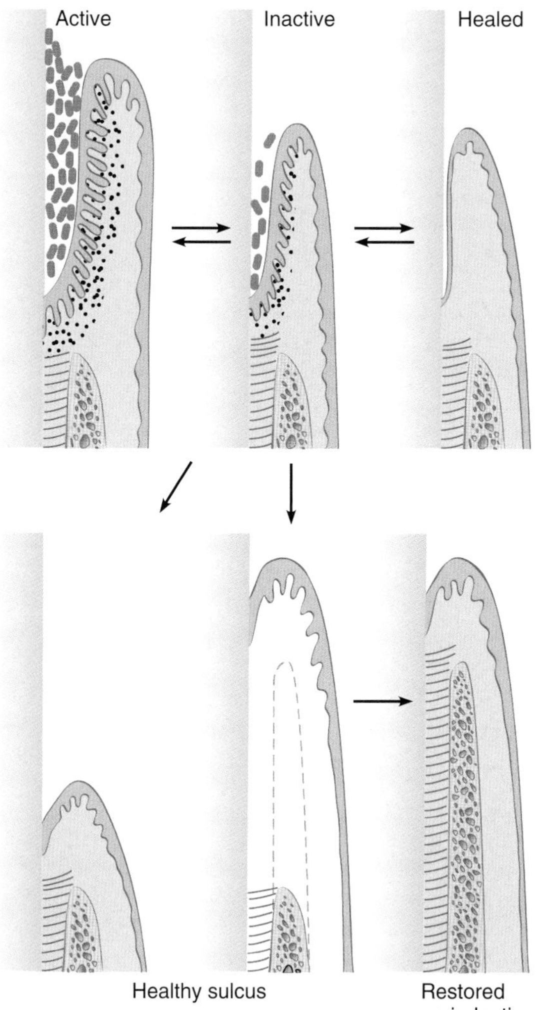

Fig. 56.3 Possible results of pocket therapy are shown. An active pocket can become inactive and heal by means of a long junctional epithelium. Surgical pocket therapy can result in a healthy sulcus, with or without gain of attachment. Improved gingival attachment promotes restoration of bone height, with re-formation of periodontal ligament fibers and layers of cementum.

after healing. Prevailing opinion considers that deep pockets after therapy represent a greater risk of disease progression than shallow sites. Individual probing depths are not good predictors of future clinical attachment loss. Conversely, the absence of deep pockets in treated patients is an excellent predictor of a stable periodontium.[5]

Longitudinal studies of different therapeutic modalities over the past 30 years have produced conflicting results,[7,16] probably because of problems created by the split-mouth design. After surgical therapy, pockets that rebound to a shallow or moderate depth can be maintained in a healthy state and without radiographic evidence of advancing bone loss by maintenance visits consisting of scaling and root instrumentation, with oral hygiene reinforcement performed at regular intervals of 3 months or less.

The findings emphasize the importance of the maintenance phase and close monitoring of the level of attachment and pocket depth, along with the other clinical variables (e.g., bleeding, exudation, tooth mobility). *Transformation of the initial deep, active pocket into a shallower, inactive, maintainable pocket requires some form of definitive pocket therapy and constant supervision thereafter.*

Pocket depth is an extremely useful and widely used clinical parameter, but it must be evaluated together with the level of attachment and degree of bleeding, exudation, and pain. The most important variable for evaluating whether a pocket is progressing is the *level of attachment,* which is measured in millimeters from the cementoenamel junction. Apical displacement of the level of attachment places the tooth in jeopardy, not the increase in pocket depth, which may be caused by coronal displacement of the gingival margin (as in gingival inflammation or gingival overgrowth).

Pocket depth remains an important clinical variable in making decisions about treatment. Lindhe and colleagues[8] compared the effect of root planing alone or using a modified Widman flap with the resultant level of attachment and in relation to initial pocket depth. They reported that scaling and root planing procedures induced loss of attachment if performed in pockets shallower than 2.9 mm, whereas gain of attachment occurred in deeper pockets. The modified Widman flap induced loss of attachment if performed in pockets shallower than 4.2 mm but resulted in a greater gain of attachment than root planing in pockets deeper than 4.2 mm. The loss is a true loss of connective tissue attachment, whereas the gain can be considered a false gain because of the reduced penetrability of connective tissues apical to the bottom of the pocket after treatment.[9,17]

Probing depths established about 6 months after active therapy and healing can be maintained, remain unchanged, or be reduced even further during a maintenance period involving careful reevaluation, plaque or biofilm removal, and root therapy as necessary every 3 months.[8]

Ramfjord[12] and Rosling[13] and their colleagues reported that a certain pocket depth recurs regardless of the surgical technique used for pocket therapy. *Maintaining this depth without any further loss of attachment becomes the goal.*

Reevaluation After Phase I Therapy

Longitudinal studies found that all patients should be treated initially with subgingival root instrumentation (scaling and root planing) and plaque or biofilm control and that a final decision on the need for periodontal surgery should be made only after a thorough evaluation of the effects of phase I therapy.[5] Assessment typically is made no less than 1 to 3 months and sometimes as much as 9 months after the completion of phase I therapy.[1] Reevaluation of the periodontal condition includes repeat probing of the entire mouth. Calculus, root caries, defective restorations, and signs of persistent inflammation should also be evaluated.

Critical Zones in Pocket Surgery

Criteria for the selection of a surgical technique for pocket therapy are based on clinical findings in the soft tissue pocket wall, tooth surface, underlying bone, and attached gingiva.

Zone 1: Soft Tissue Pocket Wall

The clinician should determine the morphologic features, thickness, and topography of the soft tissue pocket wall and persistence of inflammatory changes in the wall.

Zone 2: Tooth Surface

The clinician should identify the deposits on and alterations of the cementum surface and determine the accessibility of the root surface to instrumentation. Phase I therapy should have solved many or all of the problems on the tooth surface. Evaluation of the results of phase I therapy can determine the need for further therapy and the method to be used.

Zone 3: Underlying Bone

The clinician should establish the shape and height of the alveolar bone next to the pocket wall through careful probing and clinical and radiographic examinations. The number of osseous walls—one, two, or three—helps determine whether resective or regenerative therapy can be used (see Chapter 22). Bony craters, horizontal or angular bone losses, and other bone deformities also are important criteria in selection of the treatment technique.

Zone 4: Attached Gingiva

The clinician should consider the presence or absence of an adequate band of keratinized attached gingiva when selecting the pocket treatment method. Diagnostic techniques for mucogingival problems are described in Chapter 65. An inadequate attached gingiva can be caused by a high frenum attachment, marked gingival recession, or a deep pocket that reaches the level of the mucogingival junction. All these conditions should be explored and their influence on pocket therapy considered.

Indications for Periodontal Surgery

The following findings can indicate the need for a surgical phase of therapy:

1. Areas with irregular bony contours, deep craters, and other defects usually require a surgical approach.
2. Pockets around teeth where access to the root surface for complete removal of root irritants is not possible by nonsurgical means are an indication for surgery. These occur frequently around molars and premolars.
3. Furcation involvement of grade II or III may require a surgical approach to ensure the removal of irritants around root surfaces. If root resection or hemisection is necessary, surgical intervention will be needed.
4. Intrabony pockets distal to the last molars, which in many cases are complicated by mucogingival problems, often require surgery.
5. Areas with furcation involvements and intrabony defects that can be predictably treated by regenerative approaches require surgical intervention (see Chapter 63).
6. Persistent inflammation at sites with moderate to deep pockets that were treated nonsurgically in the past may require a surgical approach. These are usually areas where all the subgingival calculus could not be removed.
7. Cases with shallow pockets and good hygiene but bleeding on probing can be caused by mucogingival problems in areas where there is no keratinized tissue. Trauma to these areas can cause bleeding.

Methods of Pocket Therapy

The methods for pocket therapy can be classified as follows:

1. *New attachment techniques* offer the ideal result because they eliminate pocket depth by reuniting the attachment apparatus with the tooth at a position coronal to the bottom of the preexisting pocket. New attachment involves regeneration of bone, connective tissue, periodontal ligament, and cementum.
2. *Removal of the pocket wall* is the most common method. The wall of the pocket consists of soft tissue and can include bone in the case of intrabony pockets. It can be removed by the following methods:
    - Retraction or shrinkage, where plaque or biofilm removal by the patient and subgingival root instrumentation (scaling and root planing) resolve the inflammatory process, can occur. The gingival tissue shrinks, reducing the pocket depth.
    - Surgical removal of the pocket is done by gingivectomy or the undisplaced flap technique.
    - Apical displacement of the flap is performed with an apically positioned flap.
3. *Removal of the tooth side of the pocket*, which is accomplished by tooth extraction or by partial tooth extraction in the case of furcation involvement (i.e., hemisection or root resection).

The techniques, what they accomplish, and the factors governing their selection are discussed in Chapters 60 through 64.

Criteria for Selection of the Method of Surgical Therapy

Scientific criteria to establish indications for the use of each technique are difficult to determine. Criteria are based on longitudinal studies that follow a significant number of cases over a number of years, standardization of multiple factors, and long-term clinical experience. Selection of a technique for treating a particular periodontal lesion is based on the following considerations:

1. Characteristics of the pocket—depth, relation to bone, and configuration
2. Accessibility to instrumentation, including furcation involvement
3. Existence of mucogingival problems
4. Response to phase I therapy
5. Patient cooperation, including the ability to perform effective oral hygiene and quit smoking (smoking cessation)
6. Age and general health (e.g., diabetic status) of the patient
7. Overall diagnosis of the case—various types of gingival enlargement and different stages and grades of periodontitis
8. Esthetic considerations and patient expectations
9. Previous periodontal treatments

Each variable is analyzed in relation to the pocket therapy techniques available. A specific technique is then selected. The one most likely to solve the problem successfully, with the fewest undesirable effects, should be selected. Clinicians who adhere to one technique to solve all problems are not taking advantage of the wide repertoire of techniques that are at their disposal.

Approaches to Specific Pocket Problems

Therapy for Gingival Pockets

Gingival pockets do not have an osseous component (i.e., no attachment loss) and usually have edematous or fibrotic gingival tissue. Two factors are taken into consideration: the character of the pocket wall and accessibility of the pocket.

The pocket wall can be edematous or fibrotic. *Edematous tissue* shrinks after the elimination of local factors, reducing or totally eliminating pocket depth. Subgingival root instrumentation in the form of scaling and root planing is the technique of choice for these cases.

Pockets with a *fibrotic wall* are not appreciably reduced in depth after subgingival root instrumentation. These pockets are eliminated or reduced by surgical therapy. In the past, gingivectomy was frequently used to reduce these pockets. This solved the problem, but in cases of marked gingival enlargement (e.g., severe phenytoin-related enlargement), treatment could leave a large, open wound, and the patient had to endure a painful and prolonged healing process. Currently, a modified flap technique is used, and fewer postoperative problems are associated with primary closure of the wound (see Chapter 19). Some clinicians have advocated the use of laser therapy to manage gingival enlargement (see Chapters 19 and 64).

Therapy for Stage I Periodontitis (Incipient Disease)

In patients with slight or incipient periodontitis with minimal attachment and bone loss, the pocket depths are shallow or a moderate depth. In these patients, the conservative approach of good oral hygiene and subgingival root instrumentation (scaling and root planing), when necessary, usually suffices to control the disease. Incipient periodontitis that recurs in previously treated sites with good hygiene may require a thorough analysis of the recurrence, which may be caused by remnants of calculus that were missed during previous treatment or other factors such as open margins of a restoration located subgingivally. Occasionally, a surgical approach may be required to correct these problems.

Therapy for Stages II to IV Periodontitis (Moderate to Severe Disease) in the Anterior Sector

Because the maxillary anterior teeth are important esthetically, techniques that cause the least amount of visual root exposure should be considered. However, each patient has different expectations regarding the final result of therapy. The clinician must explain that the therapy may be a compromise between complete pocket elimination and achieving an esthetic result that is acceptable to the patient. The patient must be educated before therapy on the possibility of some degree of gingival recession and some loss of the interdental papilla (see Chapter 61 and 66).

The anterior dentition has two advantages for using a conservative (nonsurgical) approach: (1) the teeth are all single rooted and easily accessible for subgingival root instrumentation (scaling and root planing); and (2) patient compliance and thoroughness in plaque or biofilm control may be easier to attain. *Nonsurgical therapy is therefore the technique of choice for the maxillary anterior dentition.*

In some situations, surgical therapy may be necessary to improve accessibility for root instrumentation or regenerative therapy may be possible. Chapters 60 through 64 discuss the surgical aspects in detail. The papilla preservation flap or modified papilla preservation flap can be used for both purposes and offers a better postoperative result, with less recession and reduced soft tissue crater formation interproximally.[14]

When the interdental space is minimal, papilla preservation techniques may not be feasible. Instead, a technique that splits the papilla and retains as much of the papilla as possible is the appropriate surgical technique.

When the esthetic outcome is not the primary consideration and a flap procedure is necessary for root surface access, the *modified Widman flap* can be selected. This technique uses an internal bevel incision about 1 to 2 mm from the gingival margin without thinning the flap. This procedure may result in minor recession of the surrounding gingival tissue.

In cases with advanced osseous involvement, bone contouring may be needed, despite the resultant root exposure. The technique of choice is the *apically displaced flap with osseous bone contouring*. The clinician must educate the patient before therapy about the possibility of esthetic compromises due to the expected recession of gingival tissue.

Therapy for Stages II to IV Periodontitis (Moderate to Severe Disease) in Posterior Areas

Treatment for the maxillary and mandibular premolars and molars does not entail esthetic problems but frequently involves difficult access for root therapy. Bone defects occur more often in the posterior area than the anterior, with many areas having deep infrabony lesions and anatomic root problems with concavities, such as the mesial surface of the maxillary first premolar. A difficult problem encountered in the posterior area is the furcation lesion. Because this area can pose insurmountable problems for instrumentation unless a flap is reflected, surgery is frequently indicated.

Surgery is used in the posterior area for enhanced access to the root surface or for definitive pocket reduction requiring osseous surgery. Access can be obtained by an undisplaced or apically displaced flap (see Chapter 60).

Most patients with stage II to stage IV periodontitis have developed osseous defects that require some degree of bone remodeling or reconstruction. For osseous defects amenable to reconstruction, the *papilla preservation flap* or *modified papilla preservation flap* is the technique of choice because it better protects the interproximal areas where defects frequently occur. Second and third choices are the *sulcular flap* and *modified Widman flap,* maintaining as much of the papilla as possible.

For osseous defects with no possibility of reconstructive therapy, such as interdental craters, the technique of choice is an undisplaced or apically displaced flap with osseous contouring. All surgical flap procedures are discussed in Chapters 60 through 63. It is important to note that in spite of the disease being present only in the posterior sextant, if severe and presenting with tooth loss or posterior bite collapse (stage IV), it can negatively affect the esthetics of the anterior dentition and warrants an interdisciplinary form of care.

Surgical Techniques for Correction of Morphologic Defects

The rationales and objectives for techniques performed to correct morphologic defects (i.e., mucogingival, esthetic, and preprosthetic) are described in Chapters 64 through 66.

Surgical Techniques for Implant Placement and Related Problems

The rationales and objectives for techniques performed for implant placement and related problems are described in Chapters 78 through 86.

Conclusions

Many steps are required to achieve and maintain a healthy periodontal status. After completion of phase I therapy, which consists of patient education, biofilm control, and thorough root therapy, the involved periodontal areas are reevaluated. The necessity of phase II therapy, which is the surgical phase of treatment, depends on the success of the initial phase and the severity of the periodontal condition. Periodontal surgery, which includes plastic, esthetic, resective, and regenerative procedures, becomes necessary when access for root therapy is required or correction of anatomic or morphologic defects is necessary. Placement of dental implants can be part of this therapy.

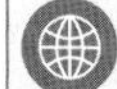
References for this chapter are found on the companion website eBooks.Health.Elsevier.com.

CHAPTER 57

Surgical Training and Technology

Carilynne Yarascavitch

CHAPTER OUTLINE

Introduction

Digital technologies are transforming how clinicians train for and perform surgical procedures. Health professions education, which includes dental education, has been markedly improved by an expanded pedagogic repertoire that cultivates expertise through the attainment of individual competencies. The traditional Halstedian apprenticeship (training) model,[28] sometimes colloquially referred to as "see one, do one, teach one," is now an anomaly rather than an educational best practice. In this era of rapid change, what type of understanding does a clinical expert require to be able to acquire, transform, and apply information to practice their skills at the highest level of competence? This chapter will briefly review the advances in cognitive and educational science that help us understand how surgical skill is acquired and maintained.

Knowledge Acquisition

The Science of Learning

All learning requires memory. Therefore, the way in which information is learned and retained so that it can be conveniently retrieved for future application is of interest to clinicians who need to first establish and then maintain expert knowledge. Discoveries in the field of psychology and cognitive science provide useful strategies for maximizing learning opportunities. Although many mysteries remain regarding memory science, scientists have identified some general memory principles with applications for learning through decades of research. Understanding broad principles of the science of memory can help future and current clinicians acquire and retain the knowledge required for expert performance. Four guiding principles of memory are as follows: (1) deep processing, (2) transfer-appropriate processing, (3) desirable difficulties, and (4) metacognition for learning.[39]

Deep (elaborative) processing involves a learning focus on the meaning of the material. In contrast, unsophisticated attempts at learning tend to be superficial and focus on processing information in the way the information is presented (i.e., lists, illustrations). This has limited benefit for memory. Deliberate elaboration on what information means in relationship to other information or prior learning and understanding benefits retention. Deep processing suggests that even simple associations, such a rhyming, can have excellent benefits for retention and that greater context during learning strengthens later performance.

Transfer-appropriate processing emphasizes that successful recall of information requires attention to the congruence between encoding (learning phase) and retrieval (remembering phase) conditions. Retrieval is more successful when the processes during retrieval are similar to the processes during encoding. This theory suggests that information should be practiced in the way it will be used to enhance memory cues. For example, students who are expected to perform in an oral examination should practice material verbally "out loud," rather than in quiet study.

Desirable difficulty suggests that long-term memory is enhanced by processing challenge rather than ease. This phenomenon is often counterintuitive to students, who tend to erroneously view fluency (ease of processing) and the resulting confidence as deep understanding. By contrast, discomfort with material due to variability and complexity in the initial conditions of processing (e.g., testing oneself on material rather than repeated re-reading) often leads to better understanding and improved memory. However, it is important that the challenge is not excessive, because an extremely poor initial performance has neither short- nor long-term benefit for memory. Challenge during the initial acquisition of information that makes learning more effortful has benefits for the ability to retrieve information later and is the desirable difficulty that benefits long-term retention.

Metacognition for learning refers to an ability to understand one's own cognitive processes. This principle asserts that learning is aided by an ability to place attention on one's own thoughts about learning and monitor one's own progress. Students who can monitor their own learning processes can make good decisions about the "what and how" of information that is essential to successful performance—what to learn and how it should be learned.

These broad principles of deep processing, transfer appropriate learning, desirable difficulty, and metacognition can be practically applied by guiding specific strategies and techniques that contribute to successful learning and memory. Putnam and Roediger have described seven tools for learning[39] that are relevant to surgical education (Box 57.1).

BOX 57.1 Seven Tools for Learning

1. Retrieval practice
2. Spaced practice
3. Interleaving
4. Elaborative interrogation
5. Self-explanation
6. Mnemonics
7. Self-regulated learning

Adapted from Putnam AL, Roediger III HL. Education and memory: Seven ways the science of memory can improve classroom learning. https://doi.org/10.1002/9781119170174.epcn106.

CASE STUDY A

Students in a periodontology program are studying for their board examination to obtain certification for specialty practice. To prepare for the oral examination, they thought about complex clinical patient encounters in residency and created relevant questions that could be asked during oral examination. They rehearsed their answers to these questions out loud. When they thought that their answer seemed unsupported, they reviewed major texts and publications to solidify their knowledge and then rehearsed the answers out loud again.

What guiding principles are these students using to enhance their learning?

Seven Tools for Learning

All students understand that repetition enhances memory. However, students are incorrect in assuming that more time on task inherently leads to improved performance. The so-called testing effect, also known as *retrieval practice*, refers to the long-term memory benefit gained from the effect of repeated retrieval of information. Studies have shown that the direct effect of repeated retrieval is distinct and in addition to the indirect effects of exposure to and organization of the material through repeated study.[42] For example, a student using flash cards benefits more from using the cards to practice answering questions and subsequently revealing the answers (self-testing) than from using the flash cards as a concise summary for re-reading (self-studying).

The effectiveness of the testing effect can be enhanced by another older, even more well-known robust learning phenomenon, called the "spacing effect". Also known as *spaced practice*, the spacing effect shows that time between learning sessions (distributed practice) is more effective for long-term retention than when learning occurs in a single session (massed practice). Even when the time available to study is the same, performance is improved by dividing this time between two spaced learning sessions (between-session spacing). For example, a student using flash cards benefits more from 30 minutes of study over 2 days than by 1 hour of study in a single day. This effect can also be observed within a learning session (within-session spacing). For example, the same student using flash cards would benefit from rotation of the cards several times within a session, rather than focusing on each card in turn. Students should be careful to consider that too much space between sessions can be counterproductive to memory and that the optimal gap for spacing is poorly defined.

KEY FACT

Studies have shown that re-reading notes or textbook material is the primary and most often used learning strategy.[27] However, repeated re-reading is a poor strategy compared to repeated re-testing. Re-testing, also known as retrieval practice, enhances learning and leads to greater long-term retention. This phenomenon, known as the testing effect, shows that the act of retrieving information from memory has a robust positive effect on learning.

Interleaving is a closely related but distinct concept from spaced practice that shows variability in the type of practice (mixed practice) benefits learning the most. Mixed practice is useful for both conceptual and motor learning. Mixed practice confers benefit from creating contrast between examples, which can help later to discriminate between categories and tasks. This is counterintuitive to students, who often practice information in categories as a way of promoting organization of knowledge. However, interleaving suggests that there is greater benefit to long-term memory by mixing different types of information presentations and practice during learning sessions. For example, practicing multiple types of suture ties in a different order in one session would confer a greater benefit than focusing on one type of suture tie practice at a time.

Students may be surprised to find that actively questioning their efforts can have positive effects on learning and memory. Two tools that function this way are elaborative interrogation and self-explanation. In elaborative interrogation, students are encouraged to pause to answer "why" questions when processing information. For example, a student might ask, "Why do I need to know this?" Interestingly, this pause in processing for reflection on the learning itself has demonstrated benefits in later recall of information. Elaborative interrogation has the greatest benefit when a student already has some knowledge on the topic of interest. When background knowledge is low, it may exert its effects through increased attention, arousal, or effort. However, when background knowledge is high, "why" questions foster deep processing by connecting new knowledge to previous knowledge. This suggests that elaborative interrogation may be a particularly useful learning technique for expert clinicians.

A related concept to elaborate interrogation is *self-explanation*. The self-explanation effect is the ability of think-aloud explanations during tasks to benefit recall, comprehension, and problem solving. Examples of self-explanation prompts are questions such as the following:

- "What is new to me?"
- "What does this mean?"
- "What don't I understand?"

Self-explanation may be more complex without mentorship because it requires a higher level of metacognition from the student. Novice students may require that an instructor make specific prompts to encourage self-explanation, whereas expert students may already possess enabling abilities. Self-explanation is more time-consuming than other learning tools, and the research remains unclear regarding how the accuracy or quality of the self-explanation affects learning. Although more research is needed, the apparent ability to improve knowledge transfer from familiar to novel tasks is a high reward aspect of self-explanation.

A common memory device used by health care students is the use of mnemonics, which refers to word association strategies. Although the term *mnemonic* refers generally to any strategy to improve memory, it more commonly applies to word associations that aid memory through visual imagery and are either multiple-use (e.g., key word method, journey method, or "memory palace") or single-use mnemonics (e.g., acronyms, acrostics). Research on this subject is mixed, and the magnitude of the benefit to learning is unclear compared to other learning tools. Suggested best practices for the use of mnemonics include choosing a simple learning objective, using information that is easily adaptable to the objective, and using other strategies such as retrieval practice and spaced rehearsal to reinforce recall.

Although learning tools that improve recall are important, the ability to *self-regulate* learning is a key concept in developing expert performance. Self-regulation is a broad and complex area of study. One of the challenges of self-regulation is that judgments of learning are often incorrect. For example, if asked how well a student will perform an upcoming task, the response may have a high degree of error due to differing biases. Often, students are not assessing the strength of their memory for factual or procedural information, but instead are evaluating other cues such as subject difficulty. These inaccuracies persist in judgments about how to prepare for tasks. Students sometimes make poor choices in the preparation for tasks, known as the "labor-in-vain effect," by choosing learning strategies with little memory benefit, such as re-reading rather than self-testing material. There is also evidence that students may "triage" knowledge when under time pressures—choosing to study items of moderate difficulty that they think they can master, sometimes ignoring the most difficult items. This can be a disadvantage if the difficult task is also a necessary one. From a more positive position, it is reassuring to know that self-regulation is universally improved by almost any type of feedback, such as standards, checklists, videos, peers, and experts[7]. Therefore, students and clinicians aiming to improve self-regulation should actively seek feedback from a variety of sources.

CASE STUDY B

A dentist who aspired to complete an online continuing education program failed the multiple-choice final assessment and will not receive certification points for the time and is disappointed with the test performance, given that he/she worked very hard to learn the material. The dentist was highly motivated by the high stakes of the testing and re-read all the assigned material at least three times to make condensed notes on flash cards. The flash cards were then each read repeatedly until the dentist felt confident that she/he knew the material in one 3-hour practice session the night before the test.

What advice would you give to this dentist to improve the test performance?

Technical Skills

Technical skill training is a foundation of surgical training. Technical skills refer to the cognitive and psychomotor abilities necessary to carry out a task to a prescribed standard. In health care, the idealized surgical goal is an error-free performance of a psychomotor task. In dentistry, it is obvious that good hand-eye coordination and manual dexterity are essential abilities for surgical performance. However, there are also cognitive features beyond motor skills such as perception, attention, and decision-making that contribute to success. Individuals able to carry out surgical tasks to the highest level demonstrate expert performance because they are proficient in meeting the surgical goals.[37] Reznick and MacRae[40] have provided three stages of skill acquisition, adapted from the Fitts-Posner Three-Stage Theory of Motor Skill Acquisition.[20] The stages and reflected goals are as follows: (1) cognition (understanding the task); (2) integration (comprehend and perform mechanics of the task); and (3) automation (perform the task with speed, efficiency, and precision). Consequently, in this process, a novice will first perform a task in erratic distinct steps, then become more fluid with fewer interruptions, and finally develop a continuous, fluid, and adaptive task performance.

Technical Skills Assessments

Manual skills can be assessed in a variety of formats and can be subjective or objective. Based on the objective structured clinical examination (OSCE) model, the Objective Standardized Assessment of Technical Skills (OSATS) has helped create objective standards for otherwise historically subjective evaluations of surgical performance.[41] Widely adopted in surgical education in medicine, these assessments typically consist of series of stations where a candidate performs a task under observation, with scoring according to strict dimensions of performance. Although there is a strong tradition in dentistry of rigorous technical skills evaluation, historically these rely on assessment of the final product rather than on elements of the process.[30] Structured assessments for surgical skills remain relatively uncommon[21] although in the past decade there has been significant renewed interest[8] (Fig. 57.1). Objective measurement of technical skills can also be accomplished by tracking movement and kinetics using motion tracking systems.[37] This can provide information about surgical efficiency through measurement of economy of movement.[44] Subjective and objective assessments of technical skill are supported by the vast use of simulation-based education, which is well known to have benefits for students.[12]

Simulation in Surgical Education

The benefits of the use of simulation in surgical education are many and function primarily to transform inherently high-stakes procedures into low-stakes encounters, with the ability for repetition and feedback. Some studies have shown transfer validity; students who receive simulation training compared to those who have received no simulation training demonstrate improved outcomes, including in subsequent supervised patient procedures.[23] Simulation refers to any artificial (contrived) situation that attempts to recreate (mimic) a real-life situation. Simulation training for surgical education can use a variety of models to support training.[44] Simulation can be "wet" or "dry", with the former referring to tissue-based models (Fig. 57.2) and the latter to bench-top artificial material models (Fig. 57.3). Wet-labs typically use animal tissues and can be described as in-vivo (living anesthetized animals) and ex-vivo (animal tissue or human cadaver). Wet-labs can be particularly helpful for recreating conditions of tissue-handling to closely mimic patient conditions in delicate tasks such as tissue grafting and suturing (Fig. 57.4). Dry-labs use artificial materials and can incorporate digital elements such as augmented reality or be entirely virtual. While dry-labs may not be able to replicate the human body with high fidelity, they are excellent for providing context for procedural rehearsal, often at a lower cost[34] (Fig. 57.5).

Simulation-Based Learning Opportunities

Simulation creates the opportunity for mastery learning. Mastery learning refers to learning that occurs in a competency-based framework in which the learning objectives for a skill are translated into a series of leveled tasks that are scaffolded according to progressive difficulty.[37] A key feature of mastery learning is that the student is not permitted to progress to the next level of learning until they have met the previous minimum standard for the learning objective, which is evaluated by rigorous formative assessments. Simulation in a mastery learning framework benefits the students as it provides structured opportunities for practice and feedback, which improve skill retention.

Practice

It is often assumed that "practice makes perfect". However, practice must occur in a specific context to promote expertise. Many clinicians might assert that their increased time in clinical practice inevitably leads to better care; unfortunately a consistent finding is that increased professional experience with familiar tasks does not improve performance.[14] Simulation is uniquely helpful to surgical skill acquisition and maintenance as it can provide essentially unlimited access to repetitive practice.

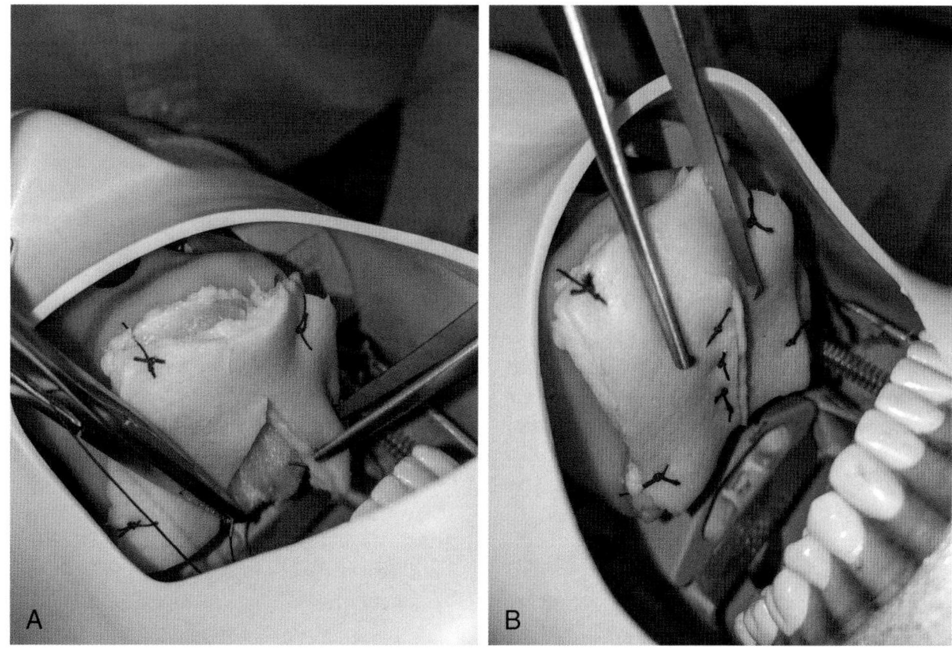

Fig. 57.1 (A) Objective Standardized Assessment of Technical Skills (OSATS) station for cleft palate closure—simple suture placement in muscle. A layer of pig belly muscle and skin is dissected to create a cleft and placed in a pediatric dentiform to replicate the space constriction of the oral cavity. (B) OSATS station for cleft palate closure, completed skill. The task goal is to perform three simple sutures in the muscle and a horizontal mattress suture in the mucosa. (Adapted from Caminiti MF, Driesman V, DeMontbrun S. The Oral and Maxillofacial Objective Structured Assessment of Technical Skills (OMOSATS) examination: a pilot study. *Int J Oral Maxillofac Surg.* 2021;50(2):277-284.)

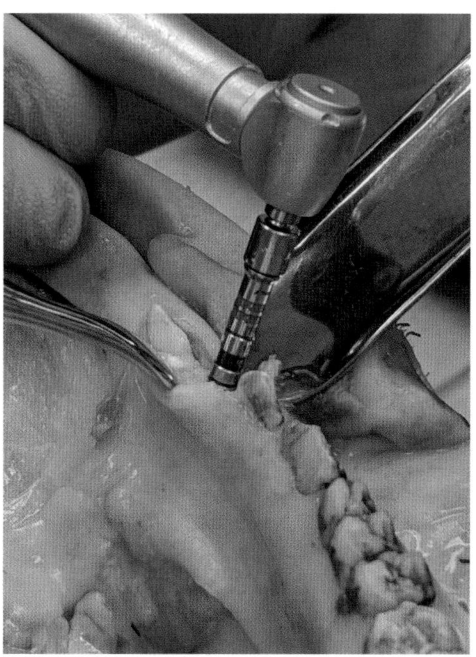

Fig. 57.2 Wet-lab simulation placing implants in the edentulous area of a pig mandible. (Adapted from Caminiti MF, Driesman V, DeMontbrun S. The Oral and Maxillofacial Objective Structured Assessment of Technical Skills (OMOSATS) examination: a pilot study. *Int J Oral Maxillofac Surg.* 2021;50(2):277-284.)

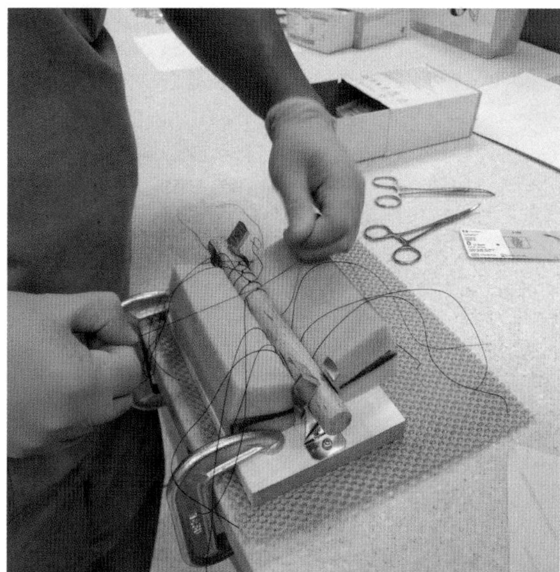

Fig. 57.3 Dry-lab simulation using a benchtop model for hand-tying of sutures. (Adapted from Caminiti MF, Driesman V, DeMontbrun S. The Oral and Maxillofacial Objective Structured Assessment of Technical Skills (OMOSATS) examination: a pilot study. *Int J Oral Maxillofac Surg.* 2021;50(2):277-284.)

Deliberate practice is one type of practice to develop expertise that was original based on mastery in music instrumental performance. Deliberate practice occurs when a solitary student is given explicit goals for performance by an instructor who provides informative feedback and remedial training. In deliberate practice, the training is individualized: (1) the instructor is able to assess the areas that require improvement, (2) communicate these goals to the students, (3) assist the students to obtain the goal by assisting with immediate feedback, and (4) provide opportunity for repeated attempts until the desired goal is reached.[15] While this kind of individualized learning has benefit, it can be logistically complex to incorporate individualized instructor observation and feedback for all students in any training environment. Fortunately, other forms of practice which can promote expertise have been described. *Purposeful practice* is described as when a solitary student engage in practice with the goal of improving performance, without constant access to individualized evaluation and guidance by an instructor. *Structured practice*, in comparison, is a group activity that is guided by an instructor where activities are not tailored to individual skill levels.[16] *Naïve practice*, in contrast to deliberate, purposeful, and structured practice, does not have a specific performance goal, and might be better thought of as engagement with a task or subject. Deliberate or purposeful practice is more strongly associated with performance than naïve practice[16]. These findings can be applied to continuing education in dentistry and suggests that clinicians of all levels should seek individualized coaching for better skill development.

Feedback

Feedback is an essential element of the learning process and is the most frequently cited design feature in simulation.[22] Influential factors in motor skill learning and performance that enhance effectiveness and efficiency of learning have been described[50] (Table 57.1). While theoretically supported, the evidence for the precise role of feedback in procedural skill training is limited. A meta-analysis of feedback in procedural skill training[22] provides insights into the specific features of feedback that benefit students. These authors found that diverse sources of feedback (instructor, peer or other) are superior to any single source of feedback. Notably their review

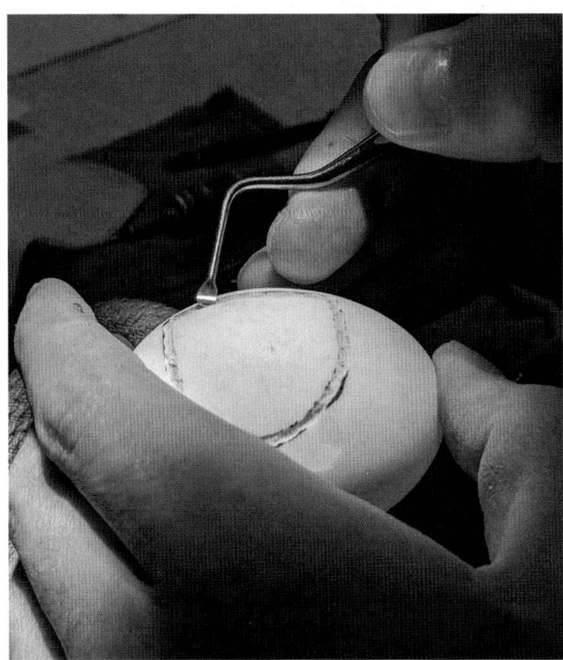

Fig. 57.4 Simulation of sinus lift creation using an animal tissue model. A duck egg provides tactile feedback for drilling and lifting of the shell, without perforation of the membrane. (Modified from Caminiti MF, Driesman V, DeMontbrun S. (2021). The Oral and Maxillofacial Objective Structured Assessment of Technical Skills (OMOSATS) examination: a pilot study. *Int J Oral Maxillofac Surg* 2021;50(2):277-284.)

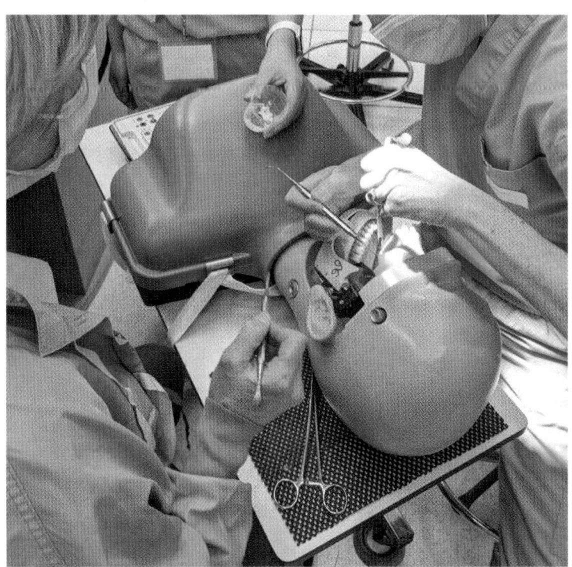

Fig. 57.5 Simulation of sinus lift and dental implant placement using a dentiform artificial tissue model in a mannequin. (Adapted from Caminiti MF, Driesman V, DeMontbrun S. The Oral and Maxillofacial Objective Structured Assessment of Technical Skills (OMOSATS) examination: a pilot study. *Int J Oral Maxillofac Surg.* 2021;50(2):277-284.)

TABLE 57.1 Influential Factors in Motor Skill Learning and Performance

Factor	Definition	Influence
Observational practice	Performer's observation of the physical practice of others, including dyad (paired) practice	Observing others' performance enhances learning; more benefit is derived from practice in pairs compared to practice alone.
Focus of attention	Performer's focus, either internal (directed at the body movements) or external (directed at the result of the movement)	External focus facilitates automaticity and promotes movement efficiency.
Feedback	Information provided to the performer about their process or result	Sociocomparative (normative) feedback to the performer that their performance is better than average benefits learning.
Self-controlled practice	Performer controls the timing of demonstration and feedback.	Self-controlled practice is more effective than externally-controlled practice (i.e., instructor pace).

Adapted from Wulf G, Shea C, Lewthwaite R. Motor skill learning and performance: a review of influential factors. *Med Educ.* 2010;44(1):75–84.

provided support for feedback at the end of a practice attempt (terminal feedback) rather than feedback during teach attempt (concurrent feedback). The underlying mechanism for this observation is based on the "guidance hypothesis", which suggests novice students may develop an over-reliance on feedback from an instructor.[43] However, this effect depends on the level of task difficulty and the experience of the students. Novice students and low-difficulty tasks benefit most from conditions of terminal feedback. Cognitive load theory is another framework to explain motor skill acquisition in novice students, and suggests that students attempting new skills may experience "information overload" with concurrent feedback during tasks.[48] Researchers in motor learning recommend that high complexity motor skills should be rehearsed in a full sequence before receiving individualized feedback.[6]

KEY FACT

The relationship between practice and feedback is critical for optimal motor skill learning. Research suggests that novice students should rehearse high complexity motor skill tasks as a complete sequence before receiving feedback on performance.[6]

Skill Retention

Skill decay is a threat to good surgical outcomes as skills that are not practiced often can result in a loss of performance. Skill decay refers to the partial or full loss of previously trained or acquired knowledge and skill following a period of nonpractice or nonuse.[4] Controlled simulation encounters can afford the ability to practice skills to mastery, but also assist in maintaining skills at a high level. Studies examining skill retention note that immediate outcomes of surgical skill assessment are often positive. However, when assessments are delayed to longer intervals, the duration of retention of skills varies.[23] Studies show that skills can be retained without further practice between three and six months. An understanding of the precise interval of skill decay is impaired to some degree by methodological choices since assessment intervals vary in research. Studies to date suggest that cognitive and psychomotor skill decay across various learning contexts begins as early as 90 days, and is almost always observed beyond one year, reinforcing the anecdotal experience of "use it or lose it".[38] This is relevant to students, in that reinforcement of skills on a routine basis appears necessary to maintain high skill levels. For clinicians, this reinforces the need for retraining, especially for procedures that are performed infrequently.

CASE STUDY C

A surgical trainee is new to suture tying and is asked to perform a horizonal mattress suture on a benchtop simulated tissue model. They are being coached by an instructor who is providing in-the-moment feedback, interrupting them during their suture tying to provide corrective instruction that focuses on the movement of the hands and instruments. At the end of the session time, the surgical trainee feels frustrated. They complain, "I still don't think I can tie this suture correctly".

What feedback features might have improved this student's experience and learning?

Nontechnical Skills

Traditionally, manual technical skills have dominated the discourse in surgical expertise. However, there is growing acknowledgment that effective care requires more than psychomotor performance.[1] *Nontechnical skills* (NTS) encompass a broad group of ideas that informs the application of knowledge in practice. Interest of non-technical aspects of performance in health care developed following the understanding that causal factors in patient harm are most often due to failures that fall outside of a traditional surgical psychomotor skill set.[19] For example, failures in communication amongst team members can result in diagnostic or therapeutic errors that impact patient outcomes. As such, the highest levels of surgical performance can only be achieved through attention to non-technical aspects of surgical skill. The training of non-technical skills relates primarily to cognitive, social, and affective skill domains that impact surgical performance.[51]

Cognitive Skills

The cognitive skills that impact surgical performance have been described in several typologies. Some important areas of cognitive skill that are relevant at the individual level in surgery include areas of mental readiness, cognitive flexibility, decision-making, and situational awareness.[9,51] Mental readiness refers to a state of readiness to carry out a task and is related to concepts of self-confidence and mental resilience. Mental readiness can be promoted by mental rehearsal, which is considered the act of performing a motor task in one's "mind's eye" rather than physical enactment. Cognitive flexibility can be thought of as the ability of a surgeon to adapt to novel situations by generating new hypotheses between performance and outcome, which replace the automated, learned, or previously successful behaviors that are less appropriate to the surgical context. Decision-making is sometimes referred to as "surgical judgment", but such a broad term is not helpful unless it can be more precisely defined. To that end, decision-making has been specifically broken down into elements of (1) considering options, (2) selecting and communicating an option, and (3) implementing and reviewing decisions.[13] Finally, situational awareness is a person's understanding of what is happening in a current state of circumstances[17]. Preparatory knowledge of the characteristics of information can facilitate perception of information. In other words, the anecdotal experience that you "can't see what you don't know" is relevant to situation awareness. Short-term memory processes such as working memory also play an important role, as it allows a clinician to hold previous information while assessing and classifying new information. Situation awareness can be considered a skill whereby a clinician is able to maintain a broad view of the circumstance and accommodate new information.

Social Skills

Surgical practice most often requires a team to accomplish task goals, and therefore can be viewed as an interpersonal activity. There are strong relationships between teamwork failures and technical errors.[24] These errors are mostly the result of poor underlying skills in leadership and communication. The need to assess nontechnical skill performance and its contribution to surgical outcomes has led to operationalization of many "soft" or subjective skills. For example, leadership has been conceptualized as three behaviors of (1) setting and maintaining standards, (2) supporting others, and (3) coping with pressure.[52] Effective communication has many elements, and has been analyzed from the perspectives of information flow (communication from sender to receiver), purpose (intention of communication as it relates to the task), relevance (relevant or irrelevant to task goal), mode (verbal or nonverbal), and response accuracy (correctness)[10]. This type of nomenclature allows for discourse analysis to identify communication breakdown (failure) that can be important for reflection on frank errors or "near misses" that may lead to adverse events.

One study of team communication noted communication failures were common and that these occurrences can be categorized into failures of occasion, content, purpose, and audience.[33] Occasion failures occur most frequently and are problems in a situation or context of the communication of event. For example, initiating a question about antibiotic prophylaxis for infective endocarditis after a surgical procedure is already underway, is a problem as it should have been addressed prior to the procedure start. Content failures are concerns with insufficient or inaccurate transfer of information. For example, a surgeon might request a particular instrument and be told by an assistant that the instrument is not in the room, yet the surgery continues without comment. This leaves a gap in understanding whether the instrument is needed to complete the surgery, whether the surgery is compromised without it, and what the next step is that should be taken. Purpose failures occur when the purpose is unclear, not achieved, or inappropriate. Communication modes that do not benefit the team, such as confrontational exchanges that add nothing positive to execution of task goals and are an example of a purpose failure. Audience failures are gaps in communication because the receiver is either not present or not engaged in the procedure. For example, making a request to a dental assistant for a missing instrument that remains unanswered because the assistant is busy charting patient information; this is an audience failure as the assistant's focus is on a different task goal. Notably, communication failures can affect system processes, such as loss of efficiency, resource waste, time delays, and result in patient inconvenience and procedural errors.[33] Such harms are relevant to dental practice and reinforce that attention to social skills is necessary for optimal performance.

KEY FACT

Communication is a critical non-technical skill in surgical care. In health care, communication errors account for most patient adverse events. Studies suggest that communication issues can account for up to 50% of adverse events[5] and that adverse events from poor communication are twice as likely as those from poor clinical skill.[49] Attention to communication is therefore one of the simplest and most cost-effective ways to improve clinical patient care and safety[11].

Affective Skills

New attention has been directed at affective (emotional) skills that can impact performance. Surgeons face challenges in their training and practice that can cause stress, which is understood to affect performance in a variety of ways[3,32]. Investigations in acute stress suggest deficits in attention, memory, decision-making, and team performance. Chronic stress can lead to mental illness such as anxiety, depression, and burnout. Consequently there is a developing interest in emotional regulation to optimize performance, promote wellness, and support professional longevity[2].

Mental skills training (MST) refers to a set of psychological techniques used to promote adaptive emotional regulation[2]. Techniques are described as somatic or cognitive, depending on the nature of the intervention. Somatic, or body-based interventions, focus on the use of mindfulness for situational awareness of both internal and external stimuli, emotional response regulation to manage situational feelings, and metacognition to be able to intentionally retrieve and apply these learned techniques. Cognitive interventions can be preparatory in nature with the use of mental rehearsal, pre-performance mental routines, and goal setting, or in-the-moment with the use of mental imagery and refocusing strategies.

Another area of interest relevant to emotional resiliency is the concept of cognitive flow. Cognitive flow is the idea of "being in the zone". It is a state of positive well-being wherein an individual has both high focus and control, and is associated with enhanced performance and satisfaction[35]. The cognitive flow experience is defined by a series of elements. The flow experience requires clear goals and immediate task feedback. In the flow experience, there is total concentration on a task, such that time can be transformed and experienced as faster or slower than real time, and a loss of self-conscious rumination, such as failure to notice hunger or thirst. There is also a positive feeling of a balance between an obtainable challenge and the high skill required to execute the task. This results in a sense of control over the task, which is accompanied by a feeling of effortless and intrinsic reward. Coaching to promote flow appears to have benefit in health care settings, including increased work engagement and job satisfaction[35].

While the science on MST in high-stakes domains such as sport and music performance are well-established, studies of the effectiveness of MST in health care performance are few resulting in limited available evidence to support its routine incorporation into surgical practice. Similarly, the concept of cognitive flow is not well adapted in health care. However, it is likely that some principles are universal and may translate well into surgical domains, and trainees and clinicians should be aware of their potential benefits.

CASE STUDY D

A periodontist is placing a challenging maxillary anterior tissue graft for an anxious young adult under intravenous moderate sedation. The team includes a dental assistant and a registered nurse. The nurse notices thirty minutes into the procedure that the patient is squirming in the chair and says, "Should I give more, doctor?" but receives no reply. The periodontist notices the patient appears alert and is coughing intermittently, and asks, "Can someone help me out?" To help the periodontist who is placing the graft, the dental assistant picks up the high-volume excavator tip to clear a small amount of saliva and accidentally suctions the graft tissue into the high-volume suction.

What types of communication failures occurred in this scenario?

The Surgeon in the Digital Era

Surgical education continues to be transformed by the evolving digital environment. Twenty-first century clinicians must not only consider their nontechnical and technical skill sets, but their digital fluency as another major competence in future patient care. There are many well-established digital tools for learning. E-learning through online or virtual learning platforms creates new opportunities for learning, including unprecedented 24/7 access to structured content for students to adopt at their own pace. Serious games are another frontier in digital learning, adopting immersive learning in a virtual environment similar to recreational digital gaming, which potentially offer similar outcomes to traditional learning but with increased student engagement and satisfaction[46]. As technology evolves digital simulation is most likely to transform dental education for its potential to meet the significant challenges of replicating spatial environments for skill acquisition[36]. Indeed, the use of artificial intelligence is already being explored in various aspects of training to characterize and support surgical skills[31].

Practice in the Digital Era

The digital transformation of workflow is now well-established in dentistry. Digital workflow encompasses computer-aided data gathering, design, and manufacturing. Examples of these kinds of technology included a myriad of devices from digital radiography[45] to computer-aided design (CAD) and computer-aided manufacturing (CAM; Fig. 57.6). Critical changes already in motion shaping surgical practice is the adoption of robot-assisted surgery and precision-guided surgery. Robot-assisted surgery is a type of computer-integrated surgery (CIS) that involves digital systems designed to carry out surgical procedures and can include both planning phases and surgical practices.[47] Robotic assistance that uses remote manually controlled tools can be further defined by the level of autonomy, such as preprogrammed sequences versus teleoperation or cooperative control.

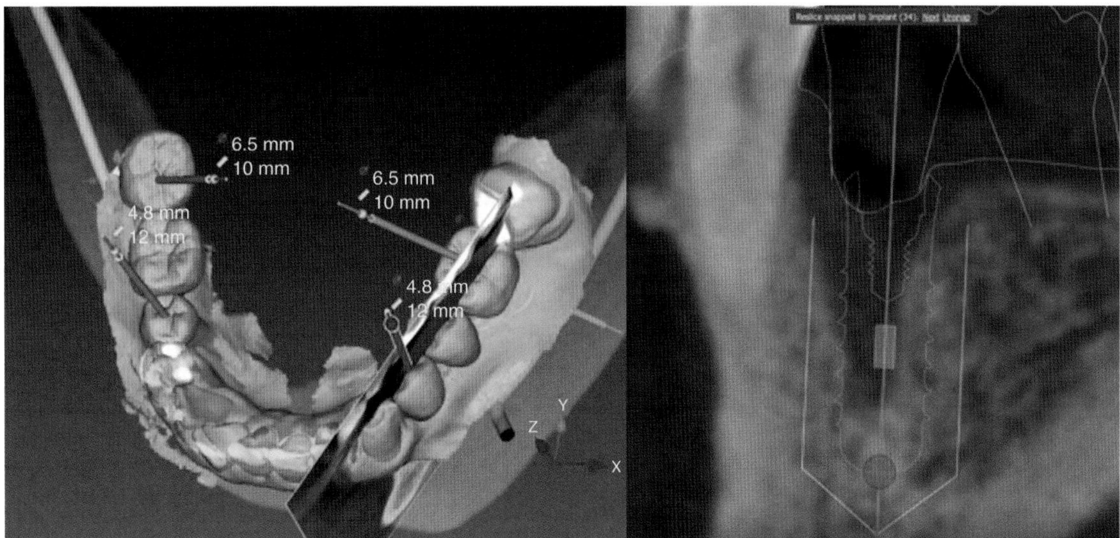

Fig. 57.6 Digital imaging in digital workflow for implant placement. A cone-beam computed tomography (CBCT)-based 3D interactive environment of a partially edentulous patient with fused optical scan and virtual tooth setup. Modern implant software allows for the addition of virtual teeth in partially edentulous jaws based on the aligned digital impression of the respective jaw and opposing tooth. (From Vandenberghe B. The crucial role of imaging in digital dentistry. *Dent Mater.* 2020;36(5):581-591.)

BOX 57.2 Top Trends in Digital Workflow

1. Electronic health records, virtual records
2. Telehealth care, virtual care
3. Rapid prototyping
4. Virtual and augmented reality
5. Artificial intelligence
6. Machine learning

Adapted from Joda T, Bornstein MM, Jung RE, et al. Recent trends and future direction of dental research in the digital era. *Int J Environ Res Public Health.* 2020;17(6):1987.

Precision-guided surgery, which uses digital imaging for planning and intraoperative three-dimensional (3D) localization has the potential to provide unprecedented patient-specific modelling and care, with the possibility of better therapeutic outcomes. Top trends and innovations in digital workflow (Box 57.2) have been described as follows: (1) electronic health records (EHRs) and virtual records; (2) telehealth care and virtual care; (3) rapid prototyping (RP); (4) virtual reality and augmented reality (VR/AR); (5) artificial intelligence (AI); and (6) machine learning (ML)[25].

EHRs are a transformative technology—the electronic data capture creates a new ease of availability of information that can be shared within and across systems.[25] The EHR also allows patients and caregivers greater access to personal health care information. Structured assessments and systematic collection of information, including individual biomarkers, allow health care opportunities in diagnosis and therapy that can be patient- or population- specific. The use of a comprehensive EHR facilitates other digital technologies, such as RP, VR/AR, and AI/ML.

Teledentistry is the remote provision of dental care without physical personal contact.[29] Consultation by means of telecommunication rather than an in-person visit is essentially synonymous with "virtual care," which is emerging as a broad term to describe consultations in which patients are remote from their care provider. The advantages of virtual care visits include improved access for special care patients who may have reduced mobility due to physical limitations, the need for behavioral supports, or complex living and travel arrangements. Patient travel and time costs can be reduced for all patients, but especially rural patients, because virtual care is often delivered within or near the patient's home. Live video streaming is a common modality. However, future potential for virtual care can be expanded by complimentary technologies such as EHR access, including digital radiography, which when combined can transform screening, consultation, and follow-up care appointments.

Rapid prototyping is the construction of 3D models using 3D printers to create product components or finished components.[26] Current use is limited by the availability of materials suitable for intraoral applications, but applications of this technology for dental models or implant surgical guides are obvious. Fabrication of biologically compatible and even biologic materials to replace lost tooth structure is an exciting possibility of RP that has yet to be realized.

Virtual and augmented reality are both types of interactive technologies that use computer animation to create immersive virtual environments. Virtual reality can use any combination of visual, auditory, and haptic sensations to replicate the real-world environment within a computer-based system. Augmented reality provides virtual content to augment rather than replace the real world, with a common form being visual superimposition of images or information. VR/AR software applications can be used as patient or interdisciplinary communication tools for 3D treatment planning, surgical rehearsal, and image projection for dynamic computer (precision)-guided surgery. VR/AR has vast potential for dental education.[25] Complex clinical procedures can be rehearsed fully in virtual simulation without any patient risk prior to real-world practice. VR/AR simulations can be used for both skill development and maintenance and can include validated recertification of competencies. Promising research in the application of VR suggests that it can enhance dental manual skill acquisition, even after brief interventions, and may also enhance theoretical knowledge.[36] A review of published studies suggest that the most interest in the use of augmented reality is in the field of maxillofacial surgery, followed by restorative dentistry, implantology, and endodontics[18].

Artificial intelligence and ML are helpful elements for any task that is aided by the gathering, analysis, and evaluation of what is referred to as "big data." AI is the use of computer algorithms to mimic human decision-making and problem-solving capabilities. ML is an application of AI, where the algorithm is generated or "learned" from data patterns without explicit programming. Diagnostic accuracy in digital imaging is an area that can benefit from AI/ML, where training with large datasets may allow for recognition of patterns that are prone to human error due to fatigue or high workload. AI can permit automated localization of anatomic features such as required for cephalometry, cyst or tumor identification, and periodontal or periapical disease classification. In this way, ML may be able to identify pathology, predict disease, recommend therapy, or forecast prognosis. Future digital workflow frontiers are likely to develop the use of AI and ML.

Conclusion

The future of surgical education is one that seamlessly leverages digital technologies to benefit learning and practice. Cognitive and educational science aid in the implementation of technology by presenting frameworks and evidence-based principles that help ensure that learning is effective and efficient. The science of memory guides knowledge acquisition, with important implications for the acquisition of technical and nontechnical skills. Surgical training and technology benefit from the use of simulation to provide learning opportunities. In this age of digital transformation, the clinical expert must be aware of technologic innovation in training and practice to provide patient care at the highest levels of competence.

CASE STUDY ANSWERS

Case Study A. This periodontology student was using techniques known to enhance memory. Considering previous patient care experiences and creating questions for self-studying use deep processing, and oral rehearsal for oral assessment considers transfer-appropriate processing. Furthermore, this student was using metacognition to self-monitor progress and seek out missing knowledge.

Case Study B. This dentist relied on a learning strategy of re-reading, which has little demonstrated benefit for learning. Performance may have been improved by use of the testing effect. The flash cards, rather than being condensed notes, could have supplied a question or topic prompt on one side, with an answer or content on the other. This would have allowed the dentist to practice recalling the information, rather than relying on simple re-exposure. In addition, the dentist could have used the spacing effect. For example, he or she could have practiced for 1 hour over 3 days, rather than 3 hours the night before, and rotated each flash card several times in each session.

Case Study C. This surgical student is a novice student. For a complex task, she or he would benefit most from terminal feedback that occurs at the end of the complete motor task, which is the full sequence of suturing movements. The instructor should have held back on comments until the motor task sequence of suture tying was complete and then provided corrective notes. The instructor should also have directed focus to the result of the movement, such as location of entry or exit points of the needle, rather than step-by-step naming of physical movements of the hand and instruments, because an external focus of attention has greater benefits to learning.

Case Study D. The failure of the periodontist to hear the nurse request more sedation for the patient is an audience failure. The periodontist was likely engaged in the clinical work and therefore was less attentive to the sedation requirements. When the periodontist also notices that the patient is alert, there is a purpose failure. The periodontist wants more sedative drug given, but because this communication is not directed specifically to the nurse, the dental assistant believes that the comment is directed to them and takes an unwanted action, resulting in an adverse event. The lack of direction in the periodontists' request for help might also be considered a content failure because of the insufficient transfer of information leaving a gap in understanding.

Suggested Readings

Agha RA, Fowler AJ, Sevdalis N. The role of non-technical skills in surgery. *Ann Med Surg*. 2015;4(4):422–427.

Arora S, Sevdalis N, Nestel D, et al. The impact of stress on surgical performance: a systematic review of the literature. *Surgery*. 2010;147(3):318–330.

Cha JS, Yu D. Objective measures of surgeon nontechnical skills in surgery: a scoping review. *Hum Factors*. 2021. https://doi.org/10.1177/0018720821995319.

Cook DA, Hatala R, Brydges R, et al. Technology-enhanced simulation for health professions education: a systematic review and meta-analysis. *J Am Med Assoc*. 2011;306(9):978–988.

Ericsson KA, Harwell KW. Deliberate practice and proposed limits on the effects of practice on the acquisition of expert performance: why the original definition matters and recommendations for future research. *Front Psychol*. 2019;10:1–19. https://doi.org/10.3389/fp-syg.2019.02396. https://www.ncbi.nlm.nih.gov/pmc/articles/PMC6824411/pdf/fpsyg-10-02396.pdf.

Farronato M, Maspero C, Lanteri V, et al. Current state of the art in the use of augmented reality in dentistry: a systematic review of the literature. *BMC Oral Health*. 2019;19(1):1–15.

Hatala R, Cook DA, Zendejas B, et al. Feedback for simulation-based procedural skills training: a meta-analysis and critical narrative synthesis. *Adv Health Sci Educ*. 2014;19(2):251–272.

Higgins M, Madan C, Patel R. Development and decay of procedural skills in surgery: a systematic review of the effectiveness of simulation-based medical education interventions. *Surgeon*. 2021;19(4):e67–e77.

Hull L, Arora S, Aggarwal R, et al. The impact of nontechnical skills on technical performance in surgery: a systematic review. *J Am College Surg*. 2012;214(2):214–230.

Joda T, Bornstein MM, Jung RE, et al. Recent trends and future direction of dental research in the digital era. *Int J Environ Res Public Health*. 2020;17(6):1–8. https://doi.org/10.3390/ijerph17061987.

Kirubarajan A, Young D, Khan S, et al. Artificial intelligence and surgical education: a systematic scoping review of interventions. *J Surg Educ*. 2021. https://doi.org/10.1016/j.surg.2021.09.012.

LeBlanc VR. The effects of acute stress on performance: implications for health professions education. *Acad Med*. 2009;84(10):S25–S33.

Lingard L, Espin S, Whyte S, et al. Communication failures in the operating room: an observational classification of recurrent types and effects. *BMJ Qual Saf*. 2004;13(5):330–334.

Lu J, Cuff RF, Mansour MA. Simulation in surgical education. *Am J Surg*. 2021;221(3):509–514.

Moussa R, Alghazaly A, Althagafi N, et al. Effectiveness of virtual reality and interactive simulators on dental education outcomes: systematic review. *Eur J Dentist*. 2021. https://doi.org/10.1055/s-0041-1731837.

Norman GR, Grierson LE, Sherbino J, et al. Expertise in medicine and surgery. In: Ericsson KA, Hoffman RR, Kozbelt A, Williams AM, eds. *The Cambridge Handbook of Expertise and Expert Performance*. 2nd ed. Cambridge University Press; 2018.

Putnam AL, Roediger III HL. Education and memory: seven ways the science of memory can improve classroom learning. *Stevens' Handbook of Experimental Psychology and Cognitive Neuroscience*. 2018;1:1–45.

Reznick RK, MacRae H. Teaching surgical skills—changes in the wind. *N Engl J Med*. 2006;355(25):2664–2669.

Wulf G, Shea C, Lewthwaite R. Motor skill learning and performance: a review of influential factors. *Med Educ*. 2010;44(1):75–84.

Yule S, Flin R, Paterson-Brown S, Maran N. Non-technical skills for surgeons in the operating room: a review of the literature. *Surgery*. 2006;139(2):140–149.

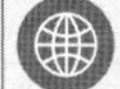

References for this chapter are found on the companion website eBooks.Health.Elsevier.com.

CHAPTER 58

Sedation in Periodontics and Implant Surgery

Robert L. Merin 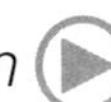 | Perry R. Klokkevold

 For online-only content on mild sedation, anxiolysis, and moderate conscious sedation, please visit the companion website at eBooks.Health.Elsevier.com.

CHAPTER OUTLINE

Periodontal and implant surgery should be performed painlessly and with minimal or no apprehension. The patient should be assured at the initial consultation. The most reliable means of providing painless surgery is effective administration of local anesthesia. However, patients who are apprehensive may require treatment under minimal or moderate sedation. The use of sedation can help make patients more comfortable during periodontal and implant surgery, especially when the procedure is expected to continue for 2 hours or more. Routes of administration for sedation agents include inhalation, oral, sublingual, nasal, intramuscular, and intravenous.[7,9,17,21,38,47] The specific agents and modality of administration are based on the desired level of sedation, anticipated length of the procedure, overall condition of the patient, and training of the clinician and staff. This chapter reviews the rationale, definitions, techniques, and guidelines for the use of minimal to moderate conscious sedation in the dental office for periodontal and implant surgical procedures.

Rationale for Sedation During Periodontal and Implant Surgical Procedures

Many patients delay or avoid having needed dental treatment because of fear and anxiety. This avoidance behavior often results in compromised health and quality of life. In a study of 174 patients referred for dental implant therapy, only 40.8% proceeded with therapy, and 24% listed dental fear as the reason for refusing to accept treatment.[42,52] Those who proceeded with therapy had low anxiety ratings as measured by the Modified Dental Anxiety Scale.[42]

Anxiety about dental therapy has not changed significantly during the past 50 years; publications report that about 30% to 50% of patients are at least somewhat fearful of dental procedures.[6,20,22–23,52,77,87] Evidence suggests that genetic variations are associated with anxiety related to dental care, which could help explain the consistent avoidance patterns, despite improved treatment methods.[11] According to a national survey of the Canadian population, more than 68% of patients would prefer to have sedation or general anesthesia for periodontal surgery[12] (Fig. 58.1). Anxiety reduction that includes moderate sedation is an important part of delivering advanced periodontal services.[1,68,82]

Because dental anxiety results in avoidance behavior and is associated with more dental and periodontal problems,[27,56,87] it is likely that disproportionate numbers of patients referred to periodontal specialists have dental anxiety. Patients may develop a high degree of fear and avoid treatment they have not received.[54] There appears to be a close relationship between anxiety and postoperative pain, and preoperative anxiety can be a predictor of postoperative pain.[30,33,55] High levels of anxiety (i.e., stress) can affect wound healing after periodontal treatment[46,50,85] (see Chapter 25). Sedation techniques have been effective in reducing physiologic markers of stress.[63,74] For these reasons, it is important for clinicians who provide advanced periodontal and implant therapy to be knowledgeable and skilled in providing sedation to reduce anxiety in their patients.

American Dental Association Policy Statement and Guidelines for Conscious Sedation

The American Dental Association (ADA) has released three documents related to the use of sedation and general anesthesia in dentistry—the ADA Policy Statement on the Use of Sedation and General Anesthesia by Dentists,[4] the ADA Guidelines for the Use of Sedation and General Anesthesia by Dentists,[3] and the ADA Guidelines for Teaching Pain Control and Sedation to Dentists and Dental Students.[2] The policy statement and guidelines provide educational and practice standards for anxiety control in dental practice. The ADA Committee on Anesthesiology, consisting of

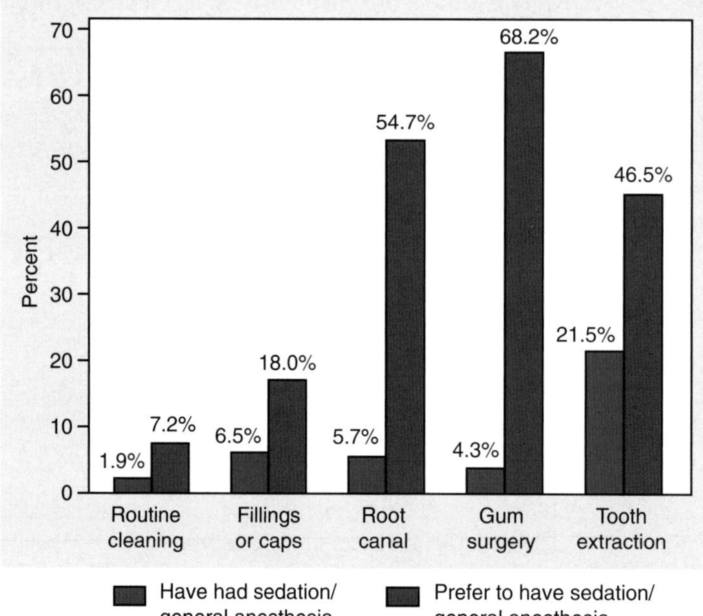

Fig. 58.1 Patient preferences for sedation or general anesthesia by dental procedure. (From Chanpong B, Haas DA, Locker D: Need and demand for sedation or general anesthesia in dentistry: a national survey of the Canadian population, *Anesth Prog* 2005;52:3–11.)

representatives from dental organizations involved with sedation and anesthesia, produced these documents after reviewing the relevant scientific evidence, expert opinions, and comments by all communities of interest. The following sections describe the important elements of these documents as they relate to treating anxious periodontal patients.

American Dental Association Policy Statement on the Use of Sedation and General Anesthesia by Dentists

The dental profession's continued ability to control anxiety and pain effectively depends on a strong educational foundation in the discipline. Training to competency in minimal and moderate sedation techniques may be acquired at the predoctoral, postgraduate, graduate, or continuing education level. Dentists who wish to use minimal or moderate sedation are expected to successfully complete formal training, which is structured in accordance with the ADA Guidelines for Teaching Pain Control and Sedation for Dentists and Dental Students.

The knowledge and skills required for the administration of deep sedation and general anesthesia are beyond the scope of predoctoral and continuing education. Only dentists who have completed an advanced education program accredited by the Commission on Dental Accreditation (CODA) that provides training in deep sedation and general anesthesia are considered educationally qualified to use these modalities in practice.

Use of Sedation and General Anesthesia by Dentists

The ADA guidelines refer to the effects of sedation on the central nervous system and do not depend on the route of administration. The purpose of the guidelines is to assist dentists in the delivery of safe and effective sedation and anesthesia. The ADA adopted the American Society of Anesthesiologists (ASA) definitions for levels of sedation (Fig. 58.2) and expanded and commented on them as they relate to treating adult dental patients.[5]

For children, the ADA supports the use of the American Academy of Pediatric Dentistry (AAPD) series of Guidelines for Monitoring and Management of Pediatric Patients During and After Sedation for Diagnostic and Therapeutic Procedures.[18]

Definitions and Levels of Sedation

Pediatric Sedation

The definition of *child* is not discussed in the ADA guidelines but has been defined in other sources. The end of childhood can be defined by age, size, and development.[18,19,28,70] With normal size and development, an individual becomes an adolescent between the ages of 11 and 13 years.[28]

Sedation is often administered to children to control behavior, which often requires deeper levels of sedation. Children can become moderately sedated despite an intended level of minimal sedation. Except in extraordinary situations, the use of preoperative sedatives for children must be avoided because of the risk of unobserved respiratory obstruction during transport by untrained individuals. The management of conscious sedation in children is beyond the scope of this chapter but is addressed by the American Academy of Pediatrics/American Academy of Pediatric Dentists (APA/AAPD) Guidelines for Monitoring and Management of Pediatric Patients During and After Sedation for Diagnostic and Therapeutic Procedures.[18]

Adult Sedation

Minimal Sedation

Minimal sedation is defined as a minimally depressed level of consciousness produced by a pharmacologic method that retains the patient's ability to independently and continuously maintain an airway and respond normally to tactile stimulation and verbal commands. Although cognitive function and coordination can be modestly impaired, respiratory and cardiovascular functions are unaffected. Minimal sedation can be achieved by the administration of a drug (singly or in divided doses) by the enteral route to achieve the desired clinical effect, not to exceed the maximum recommended dose as printed in U.S. Food and Drug Administration (FDA)–approved labeling for unmonitored home use. The administration of enteral drugs exceeding the FDA-recommended

CONTINUUM OF DEPTH OF SEDATION: DEFINITION OF GENERAL ANESTHESIA AND LEVELS OF SEDATION/ANALGESIA*
Committee of Origin: Quality Management and Departmental Administration (Approved by the ASA House of Delegates on October 13, 1999, and amended on October 23, 2019)

	Minimal Sedation Anxiolysis	Moderate Sedation/Analgesia ("Conscious Sedation")	Deep Sedation/Analgesia	General Anesthesia
Responsiveness	Normal response to verbal stimulation	Purposeful† response to verbal and tactile stimulation	Purposeful† response following repeated and painful stimulation	Unarousable even with painful stimulus
Airway	Unaffected	No intervention required	Intervention may be required	Intervention often required
Spontaneous ventilation	Unaffected	Adequate	May be inadequate	Frequently inadequate
Cardiovascular function	Unaffected	Usually maintained	Usually maintained	May be impaired

Minimal Sedation (Anxiolysis) is a drug-induced state during which patients respond normally to verbal commands. Although cognitive function and coordination may be impaired, ventilatory and cardiovascular functions are unaffected.

Moderate Sedation/Analgesia ("Conscious Sedation") is a drug-induced depression of consciousness during which patients respond purposefully† to verbal commands, either alone and accompanied by light tactile stimulation. No interventions are required to maintain a patent airway, and spontaneous ventilation is adequate. Cardiovascular function is usually maintained.

Deep Sedation/Analgesia is a drug-induced depression of consciousness during which patients cannot be easily aroused but respond purposefully† following repeated and painful stimulation. The ability to independently maintain ventilatory function may be impaired. Patients may require assistance in maintaining a patent airway, and spontaneous ventilation may be inadequate. Cardiovascular function is usually maintained.

General Anesthesia is a drug-induced loss of consciousness during which patients are not arousable, even by painful stimulation. The ability to independently maintain ventilatory function is often impaired. Patients often require assistance in maintaining a patent airway, and positive pressure ventilation may be required because of depressed spontaneous ventilation or drug-induced depression of neuromuscular function. Cardiovascular function may be impaired.

Because sedation is a continuum, it is not always possible to predict how an individual patient will respond. Hence, practitioners intending to produce a given level of sedation should be able to rescue†† patients whose level of sedation becomes deeper than initially intended. Individuals administering Moderate Sedation/Analgesia ("Conscious Sedation") should be able to rescue†† patients who enter a state of Deep Sedation/Analgesia, while those administering Deep Sedation/Analgesia should be able to rescue†† patients who enter a state of General Anesthesia.

*Monitored anesthesia care ("MAC") does not describe the continuum of depth of sedation, rather it describes "a specific anesthesia service in which an anesthesiologist has been requested to participate in the care of a patient undergoing a diagnostic or therapeutic procedure." Indications for monitored anesthesia care include "the need for deeper levels of analgesia and sedation than can be provided by moderate sedation (including potential conversion to a general or regional anesthetic."

†Reflex withdrawal from a painful stimulus is NOT considered a purposeful response.

††Rescue of a patient from a deeper level of sedation than intended is an intervention by a practitioner proficient in airway management and advanced life support. The qualified practitioner corrects adverse physiologic consequences of the deeper-than-intended level of sedation (such as hypoventilation, hypoxia, or hypotension) and returns the patient to the originally intended level of sedation.

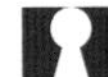

Fig. 58.2 Continuum of depth of sedation—definitions of general anesthesia and levels of sedation or analgesia. The information was approved by the American Society of Anesthesiologists House of Delegates on October 13, 1999, and was last amended on October 15, 2014. (From the American Society of Anesthesiologists: Continuum of depth of sedation: definition of general anesthesia and levels of sedation/analgesia, 2014. https://www.asahq.org/standards-and-guidelines/continuum-of-depth-of-sedation-definition-of-general-anesthesia-and-levels-of-sedationanalgesia.)

dose during an appointment is considered moderate sedation, and the moderate sedation guidelines apply.

Inhalation sedation with nitrous oxide and oxygen (N_2O/O_2) can be used in combination with a single enteral drug for minimal sedation. When used in combination with one or more sedative agents, N_2O/O_2 can produce sedation that is minimal, moderate, or deep and, in some cases, can produce general anesthesia. If more than one enteral drug is administered to achieve the desired sedation effect, with or without the concomitant use of N_2O, the guidelines for moderate sedation apply.

Maximum Recommended Dose

The *maximum recommended dose* is the maximum FDA-recommended dose of a drug as printed in FDA-approved labeling for unmonitored home use.

KEY FACT

Minimal sedation is a drug-induced minimally depressed level of consciousness. The ability to independently and continuously maintain an airway and respond to tactile stimulation and verbal commands is maintained. Respiratory and cardiovascular functions are unaffected.

Moderate Sedation

Moderate sedation is a drug-induced depression of consciousness during which patients respond purposefully to verbal commands, alone or accompanied by light tactile stimulation. No interventions are required to maintain a patent airway, and spontaneous ventilations are adequate. Cardiovascular function is usually maintained.

In accord with this definition, the drugs and techniques used should carry a margin of safety wide enough to render unintended loss of consciousness unlikely. Repeated dosing of an agent before the effects of previous dosing can be fully appreciated may result in greater alteration of the state of consciousness than intended by the dentist. A patient whose only response is reflex withdrawal from a painful stimulus is not considered to be in a state of moderate sedation.

Titration

Titration is the administration of incremental doses of an intravenous or inhalation drug until a desired effect is reached. Knowledge about each drug's time of onset, peak response, and duration of action is essential to avoid oversedation. The concept of titration to effect is critical for patient safety and, when the intent is moderate sedation, the clinician must know whether the previous dose has taken full effect before administering an additional drug increment.

KEY FACT

Moderate sedation is a drug-induced depression of consciousness. Patients respond purposefully to verbal commands, possibly requiring light tactile stimulation. A patent airway is maintained, and spontaneous ventilation is adequate. Cardiovascular function is usually maintained.

Deep Sedation

Deep sedation is drug-induced depression of consciousness during which patients cannot be easily aroused but respond purposefully to repeated or painful stimulation. The ability to maintain respiratory function independently can be impaired. Patients may require assistance in maintaining a patent airway, and spontaneous ventilation may be inadequate. Cardiovascular function is usually maintained.

KEY FACT

Deep sedation is a drug-induced depression of consciousness. Patients may not be easily aroused but respond purposefully to repeated or painful stimulation. Respiratory function may be impaired, and assistance may be necessary to maintain a patent airway. Spontaneous ventilation may be inadequate. Cardiovascular function is usually maintained.

General Anesthesia

General anesthesia is drug-induced loss of consciousness during which patients are not aroused, even by painful stimulation. The ability to maintain respiratory function independently is often impaired. Patients often require assistance in maintaining a patent airway, and positive-pressure ventilation may be required because of depressed spontaneous ventilation or drug-induced depression of neuromuscular function. Cardiovascular function can be impaired.

Clinical Guidelines for Minimal and Moderate Sedation

The following clinical guidelines apply to minimal and moderate sedation[3]: (1) patient evaluation; (2) preoperative preparation; (3) personnel and equipment; (4) monitoring and documentation; and (5) recovery and discharge. Differences between guidelines for minimal and moderate sedation are indicated.

Patient History and Evaluation

The patient's health status is assessed before any sedation procedure. Evaluation includes determination of the ASA physical status (Table 58.1). For healthy or medically stable individuals (i.e., ASA 1 or 2), a review of the medical history and medication use may be adequate. For patients with significant medical considerations (i.e., ASA 3 or 4), a consultation with the primary care physician or consulting medical specialist is indicated. The

TABLE 58.1 American Society of Anesthesiologists Physical Status Classification System

ASA Class	Definition	Examples
1	A normal healthy patient	No disease, nonsmoking, no or minimal alcohol use
2	A patient with mild systemic disease	Mild conditions or diseases without substantive functional limitations, such as current tobacco use, social drinking, pregnancy, obesity (BMI = 30–40), well-controlled DM or HTN, mild lung disease
3	A patient with severe systemic disease	Substantive functional limitations; one or more moderate to severe diseases, such as poorly controlled DM or HTN, COPD, morbid obesity (BMI ≥ 40), active hepatitis, alcohol dependence or abuse, implanted pacemaker, moderate reduction of ejection fraction, ESRD undergoing regularly scheduled dialysis, premature infant (PCA < 60 wk), history (>3 mo) of MI, CVA, TIA, or CAD/stents
4	A patient with severe systemic disease that is a constant threat to life	Recent (<3 mo) MI, CVA, TIA, or CAD/stents; ongoing cardiac ischemia or severe valve dysfunction; severe reduction of ejection fraction; sepsis, DIC, or ARD or ESRD not undergoing regularly scheduled dialysis
5	A moribund patient who is not expected to survive without the operation	Ruptured abdominal or thoracic aneurysm, massive trauma, intracranial bleed with mass effect, ischemic bowel in the setting of significant cardiac pathology or multiple organ or system dysfunction
6	A declared brain-dead patient whose organs are being removed for donation purposes	

ARD, Acute renal disease; *BMI*, body mass index; *CAD*, coronary artery disease; *COPD*, chronic obstructive pulmonary disease; *CVA*, cardiovascular accident; *DIC*, disseminated intravascular coagulation; *DM*, diabetes mellitus; *ESRD*, end-stage renal disease; *HTN*, hypertension; *MI*, myocardial infarction; *PCA*, postconceptional age; *TIA*, transient ischemic attack.
Modified from American Society of Anesthesiologists: ASA physical status classification system, 2014. https://www.asahq.org/resources/clinical-information/asa-physical-status-classification-system.

evaluation must include a focused physical examination, including baseline vital signs and a focused examination of alertness, respiratory function, airway, and appearance, as well as a specific evaluation of identified medical conditions (Box 58.1 and Fig. 58.3). Assessment of body mass index (BMI) should be considered for patients undergoing moderate sedation. Konicki and colleagues[51] evaluated point-of-care pregnancy testing prior to outpatient oral surgery for women of childbearing age. Prior to oral surgery, they tested 176 women between the ages of 12 and 50 years and found five positive subjects (2.8%). They suggested that pregnancy tests (which may cost less than $2 each) allow providers and patients to make fully informed decisions prior to elective surgical and anesthesia treatment.

Preoperative Preparation

The patient, or a parent, guardian, or caregiver if the patient is a minor, must be informed about the planned procedure that will occur while under sedation, including benefits, risks, and instructions for sedation (Fig. 58.4). Informed consent for the proposed procedure and sedation must be obtained.

Determination of an adequate oxygen supply and the equipment necessary to deliver oxygen under positive pressure must be completed. Baseline vital signs, including weight, height, blood pressure, pulse rate, and respiration rate, must be obtained. For moderate-sedation patients, blood oxygen saturation must be obtained by pulse oximetry. Body temperature should be measured when clinically indicated. Preoperative verbal or written instructions must be given to the patient, parent, escort, legal guardian, or caregiver.

BOX 58.1 Preoperative Physical Evaluation

1. Blood pressure and pulse
2. Oxygen saturation and respiration; ability to breathe deeply and cough
3. Mallampati airway classification and neck flexibility
4. Appearance and skin color
5. Alertness
6. Exercise tolerance and ambulation
7. Height, weight, body mass index

For moderate sedation, this includes preoperative fasting instructions based on the ASA summary of fasting and pharmacologic recommendations.

Preoperative dietary restrictions are based on the sedation technique prescribed (Boxes 58.2 and 58.3). For moderate sedation, NPO (nothing by mouth) status should be confirmed.

Personnel and Equipment

At least one person trained in basic life support (BLS) for health care providers must be present in addition to the dentist. Monitoring equipment includes a sphygmomanometer, positive-pressure oxygen delivery system, suction and, if inhalation sedation is used, a fail-safe and scavenging system. In the case of moderate sedation, a pulse oximeter, equipment for monitoring end-tidal carbon dioxide (CO_2), a precordial or pretracheal stethoscope, equipment for intravenous or intraosseous access, and reversal agents for drugs used must be available (Table 58.2).

A positive-pressure oxygen delivery system suitable for the patient being treated must be immediately available. Documentation of compliance with the manufacturer's recommended maintenance of monitors, anesthesia delivery systems, and other anesthesia-related equipment should be maintained. A preprocedural check of equipment and a preoperative review of the patient's records and physical status are performed immediately before each administration of sedation (Box 58.4). When inhalation equipment is used, it must have a fail-safe system that is appropriately checked and calibrated. The equipment must also have a functioning device that prohibits the delivery of less than 30% oxygen or an appropriately calibrated and functioning in-line oxygen analyzer with an audible alarm. An appropriate scavenging system must be available if gases other than oxygen or air are used.

For moderate sedation, the equipment necessary to establish intravascular or intraosseous access should be available until the patient meets the discharge criteria. This includes a catheter or butterfly needle, an intravenous drip line, a solution bag (i.e., saline or dextrose), a tourniquet, and appropriate antiseptic or dermal disinfectant (Fig. 58.5). For moderate sedation, the equipment necessary for monitoring end-tidal CO_2 and auscultation of breath sounds must be immediately available.

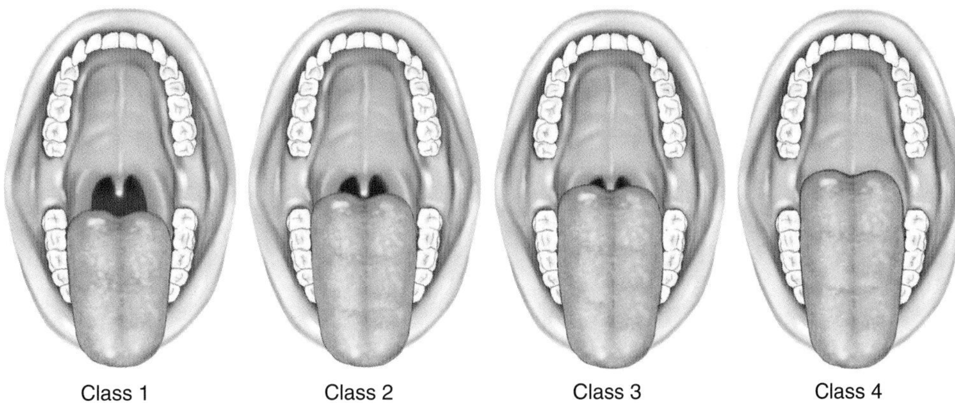

Class 1: soft palate, fauces, uvula, pillars
Class 2: soft palate, fauces, portion of uvula
Class 3: soft palate, base of uvula
Class 4: hard palate only

Fig. 58.3 Mallampati classifications used to predict difficult tracheal intubations. (Modified from Mallampati SR, Gatt SP, Gugino LD, et al: A clinical sign to predict difficult tracheal intubation: a prospective study. *Can Anaesth Soc J.* 1985;32:429–434.)

An explanation of IV conscious sedation, its purpose, benefits, possible risks, and complications as well as alternative methods of anesthesia has been discussed with you at your consultation, and we obtained your verbal consent to undergo treatment planned for you. Please read this document, which repeats issues we discussed, and provide the appropriate signatures. Please ask us to clarify anything that you do not understand.

PRESEDATION INFORMATION

1. The premedication you will receive by vein is NOT sodium pentothal. Its purpose is not to put you to sleep but to relax and sedate you. In addition, local anesthetics will be administered in your mouth.
2. You must have a responsible adult bring you to the office and drive you home, and you must remain in the company of a responsible adult until you are fully alert. Make arrangements for the person driving you home to come to the waiting room.
3. You should not have any solid food for 6 hours before your appointment. You can have clear liquids up to 2 hours before your appointment. Examples of clear liquids are apple juice, lemonade, Jell-O, or decaffeinated coffee without cream or cream substitutes.
4. Please wear short sleeves or sleeves that may be raised above the elbows.
5. No alcoholic beverages for 12 hours before sedation.
6. Possible risks and side effects: I have been informed and understand that occasionally there are complications associated with IV conscious sedation including, but not limited to, pain, phlebitis (inflammation of the vein), infection, swelling, bleeding, numbness, discoloration, nausea, vomiting, allergic reaction, depressed breathing, and, in extremely rare instances, intraarterial injection with damage to the part of the body supplied by the artery.
7. I have read and understand the presedation instructions and have also read the enclosed postsedation instructions.

Patient's Signature Date

Fig. 58.4 Consent form for and explanation of intravenous conscious sedation.

BOX 58.2 Mild Sedation: Protocol for the Use of Adult Oral Sedative Premedication for Anxious or Fearful Dental Patients

1. The dentist determines the extent of dental treatment, evaluates the patient's medical history, researches potential drug interactions, consults with the patient's physician, if appropriate, and obtains informed consent.
2. The patient must have a responsible adult companion for travel to and from the dental office. The patient must be escorted by this companion to and from the parking lot to prevent stumbling.
3. The patient should take the prescribed medication according to directions and is instructed to have a light meal such as toast and a beverage without caffeine.
4. A patient who has received an oral sedative is monitored visually and never left alone.
5. After treatment is complete, postoperative directions are given to the patient and a responsible adult, and the patient is released into the care of his or her companion for travel home. The companion is informed that the patient may have psychomotor and cognitive impairment for the rest of the day.

From Merin RL: Adult oral sedation in California: what can a dentist do without a special permit or certificate from the Dental Board of California? *J Calif Dent Assoc.* 2006;34:959–968.

BOX 58.3 Mild Sedation: Suggested Patient Pretreatment Instructions

1. The sedative ____________________ (name of medication) is being prescribed to help reduce your anxiety before and during your dental procedure.
2. The medication may make you sleepy and impair your thinking and coordination. You must have a responsible adult companion for travel to and from the dental office.
3. You must be escorted by this companion to and from the parking lot to prevent stumbling.
4. You should take the prescribed medication according to directions. You can have a light meal (no fat) such as toast without butter or margarine and a beverage without caffeine. No grapefruit juice is allowed.
5. After the treatment is complete, a responsible adult must escort you out of the office and take you home. Because the sedative effects may linger for the rest of the day, you should not plan to do anything, and it is advisable to have a responsible adult stay until you are able to take care of yourself.

From Merin RL: Adult oral sedation in California: what can a dentist do without a special permit or certificate from the Dental Board of California? *J Calif Dent Assoc.* 2006;34:959–968.

Monitoring

For minimal sedation, a dentist or, at the dentist's direction, an appropriately trained individual, must remain in the operating room during active dental treatment to monitor the patient continuously until he or she meets the criteria for discharge to the recovery area. The appropriately trained individual must be familiar with monitoring techniques and equipment.

In the case of moderate sedation, a dentist administering moderate sedation must remain in the room to monitor the patient continuously until he or she meets the criteria for recovery. When active treatment concludes and the patient recovers to a minimally sedated level, a qualified auxiliary may be directed by the dentist to remain with the patient and continue to monitor him or her as explained in the guidelines until discharged from the facility. The dentist must not leave the facility until the patient meets the criteria for discharge and is discharged to go home with a responsible adult (Box 58.5).

TABLE 58.2 Equipment Required for Mild or Moderate Sedation

Mild or Moderate Sedation	Moderate Sedation
Sphygmomanometer	Pulse oximeter
Positive-pressure oxygen delivery system	Equipment for establishing intravenous access
Suction equipment	Reversal agents for drugs used
Inhalation equipment with a fail-safe system and scavenging system	End-tidal CO_2 monitor (i.e., capnography)

BOX 58.4 Safety Checklist for Office-Based Sedation

Check Before Patient Is Brought to the Procedure Room

1. Ensure functional monitors:
   Pulse oximeter
   Capnograph
   Blood pressure monitor
   Printer
   Bluetooth pretracheal stethoscope
   Electrocardiograph if required
2. Oxygen source and delivery
3. Dinitrogen dioxide (N_2O) scavenger and fail-safe system
4. Suction functioning
5. Emergency equipment and medications
   Positive-pressure oxygen delivery system
   Airway adjuncts
   Laryngeal suction device
   Reversal agents
   Emergency medications
6. Fire hazard precautions with oxygen if laser, electrosurgery, flame sources, or burs and drills are used
7. Necessary instruments and devices for procedure

Preoperative Encounter with the Patient

1. Sedation record available
2. Correct patient chart
3. Recent radiographs
4. Correct procedure listed
5. Informed consent signed
6. Review of medical history, including allergies, adverse drug reactions, and changes in health
7. Medications taken
8. American Society of Anesthesiologists (ASA) score, Mallampati classification
9. NPO status (no oral intake)
10. Name of responsible adult escort
11. Preoperative vital signs

KEY FACT

For moderate sedation, a dentist administering moderate sedation must remain in the operating room to monitor the patient continuously until he or she meets the criteria for recovery. When the patient recovers to a minimally sedated level, a qualified auxiliary person may be directed by the dentist to remain and monitor the patient until he or she meets the criteria for discharge. The dentist must not leave the facility until the patient meets the criteria for discharge and is discharged to home with a responsible adult.

Vital signs, level of sedation, and oxygen perfusion must be continuously monitored throughout the conscious sedation procedure. There are many methods of monitoring.

Circulation

For minimal sedation, blood pressure and heart rate should be evaluated preoperatively, postoperatively, and intraoperatively, as necessary. For moderate sedation, the dentist must continually evaluate blood pressure and heart rate unless invalidated by the nature of the patient, procedure, or equipment, and this information is noted in the time-oriented anesthesia record. Continuous electrocardiographic monitoring should be considered for patients with significant cardiovascular disease. All-in-one monitors with printers can efficiently perform these functions.

Consciousness

The level of consciousness or sedation (e.g., responsiveness to verbal command) must be continually assessed. In 1990, Chernik and colleagues[14] developed the Observer's Assessment of Alertness/Sedation Scale (Table 58.3), which has been used in many studies to evaluate the degree of alertness of patients undergoing sedation. The method developed by Dr. Katherine Wilson and coworkers in 2011 at the Newcastle University School of Dental Sciences (Table 58.4) is also an efficient method for assessing the level of sedation.[88]

Ventilation and Oxygenation

For minimal sedation, the dentist or appropriately trained individual must observe chest movements and verify respirations. Oxygen saturation by pulse oximetry may be clinically useful and should be considered. For moderate sedation, the dentist must observe chest movements continuously, and oxygen saturation must be evaluated continuously by pulse oximetry. Ventilation or breathing can also be assessed by monitoring end-tidal CO_2 (i.e., capnography). Ventilation should be monitored by continual observation of qualitative signs, including auscultation of breath sounds with a precordial or pretracheal stethoscope.

The color of the mucosa, skin, and/or blood must be evaluated continuously to assess oxygenation. Oxygen saturation by pulse oximetry is clinically useful and should be considered for minimal sedation. For moderate sedation, oxygen saturation must be continuously evaluated by pulse oximetry. Approximately 98% to 99% of the total oxygen content in arterial blood is bound to hemoglobin in red blood cells. The pulse oximeter measures the degree to which hemoglobin is saturated with oxygen (Spo_2). The remaining 1% to 2% of oxygen is dissolved in plasma and produces a gas pressure referred to as arterial oxygen tension (Pao_2). The Pao_2 level is what determines how much oxygen is entering the body tissues and is referred to as *oxygenation*. Normally, the Spo_2 level is at 98% to 99% and sustains a Pao_2 level of about 95%. Normal oxygenation is defined as a Pao_2 of 80 to 100 mm Hg. There is a nonlinear relationship between Spo_2 and Pao_2. Spo_2 readings of 95% and higher maintain Pao_2 at or above 80 mm Hg and prevent hypoxemia (Table 58.5).

Capnography

Adequate ventilation and respiration can be monitored by assessing end-tidal CO_2 using capnography. This method monitors CO_2 concentrations in exhaled respiratory gases. A capnography monitor provides a graphic representation of the partial pressure of CO_2 and is more effective than other clinical assessments of ventilation.[53,71,78] A report of a randomized controlled clinical trial of patients undergoing moderate sedation demonstrated that capnography improved patient monitoring, with earlier detection of respiratory compromise prompting intervention to minimize hypoxemia compared with other care methods.[53] A systematic review by Askar and colleagues[8] concluded that training dental providers on the use of capnography monitoring would help reduce adverse events during intravenous sedation.

CLINICAL CORRELATION

A capnography monitor provides a measure of exhaled CO_2 that is more effective than pulse oximetry. It provides an immediate alarm for life-threatening breathing problems during moderate sedation. Pulse oximeters, which have been the standard of care, take much longer to register respiratory distress because oxygen levels in the blood can remain normal for several minutes after a patient stops breathing. Capnography provides earlier detection.

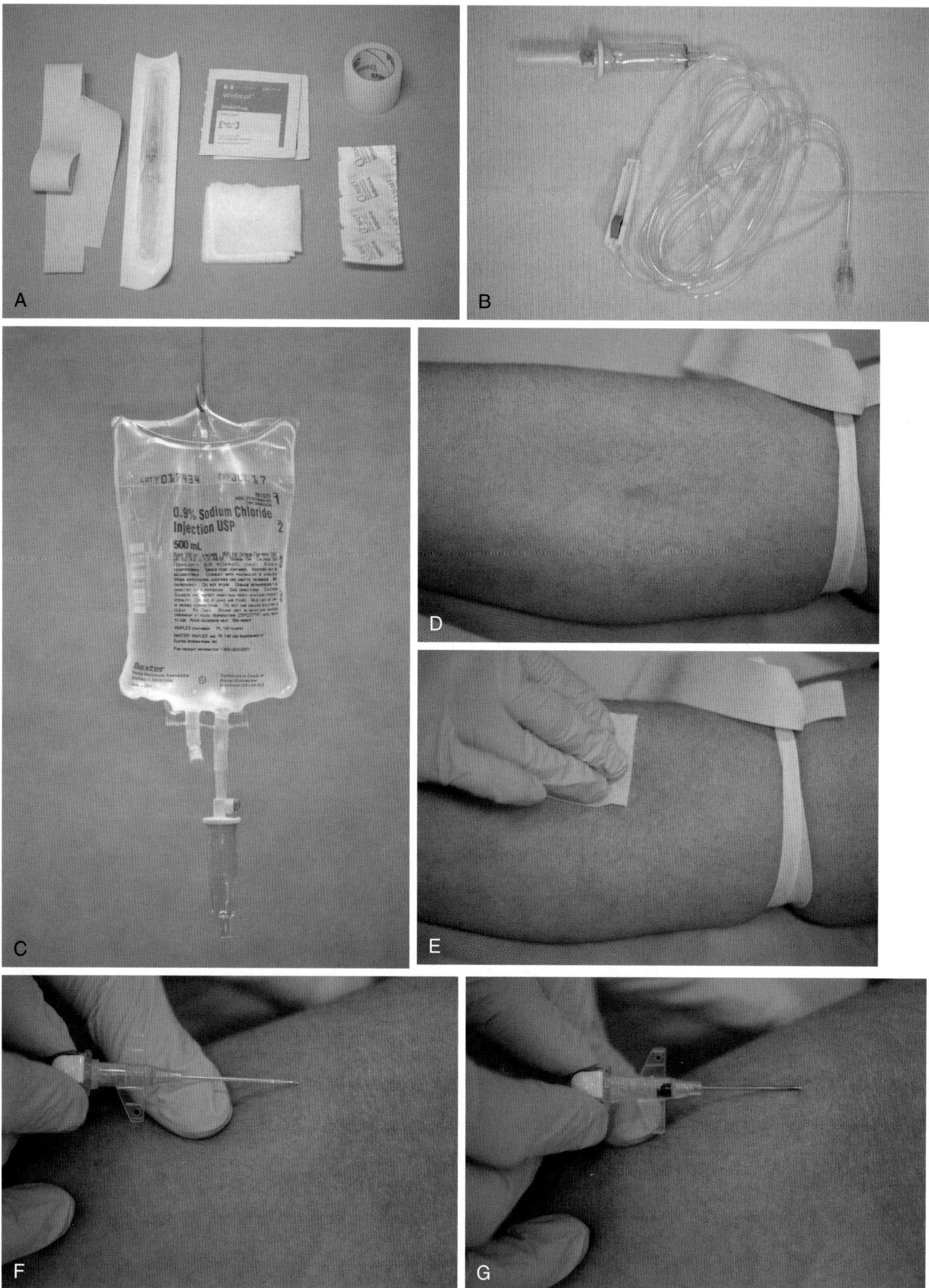

Fig. 58.5 Equipment and supplies needed for the administration of moderate intravenous (IV) sedation. (A) A tourniquet, indwelling catheter, appropriate antiseptic or dermal disinfectant wipes, tape, and adhesive bandage. (B) An IV line with drip chamber and administration ports. (C) Saline solution. (D) A tourniquet is placed proximal to the antecubital fossa, and veins are visualized and palpated. (E) The skin is prepared with an antiseptic wipe. (F) The indwelling catheter is directed toward a vein, with the bevel of the needle facing up. (G) The needle with catheter is advanced into the vein (notice the blood flashback).

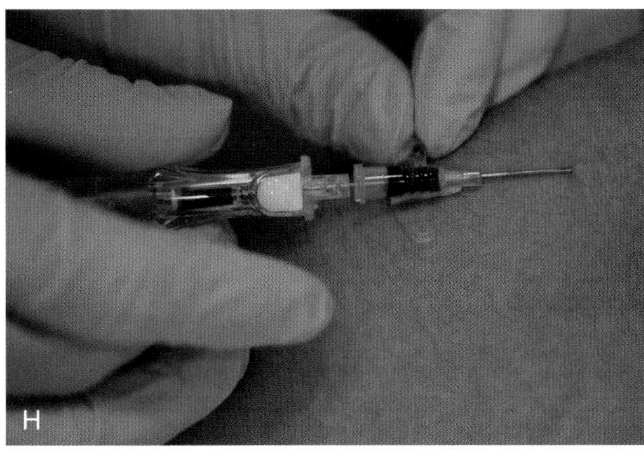
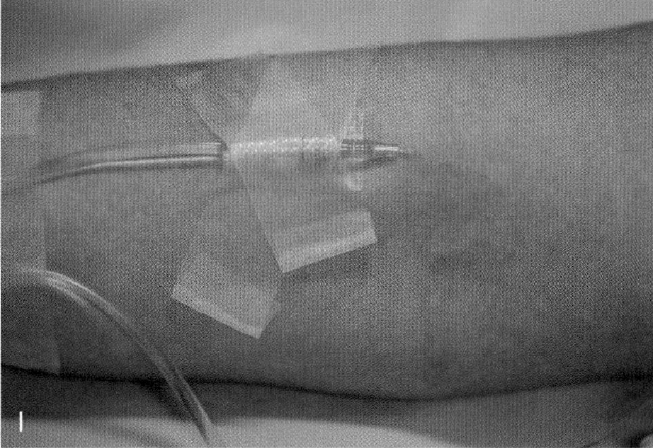

Fig. 58.5, cont'd (H) The catheter is advanced, and the needle is removed. (I) The IV line is connected, the tourniquet is removed, and the IV line is opened to check fluid flow and then secured with tape.

BOX 58.5 Discharge Criteria

1. Alertness: patient able to answer three simple questions
   Who is driving you home?
   Where are you?
   What day is it?
2. Breathing
   Normal oxygen saturation on room air
   Able to breathe deeply and cough
3. Circulation
   Systolic blood pressure within 20% of baseline
4. Ambulation
   Able to walk with minimal assistance
5. Color
   Normal skin color and appearance

TABLE 58.3 Observer's Assessment of the Alertness/Sedation Scale

Category	Observation	Score[a]
Responsiveness	Responds readily to name spoken in normal tone	5
	Lethargic response to name spoken in normal tone	4
	Responds only after name is called loudly and/or repeatedly	3
	Responds only after mild prodding or shaking	2
	Does not respond to mild prodding or shaking	1
Speech	Normal	5
	Mild slowing or thickening	4
	Slurring or prominent slowing	3
	Few recognizable words	2
Facial expression	Normal	5
	Mild relaxation	4
	Marked relaxation (slack jaw)	3
Eyes	Clear, no ptosis	5
	Glazed or mild ptosis (less than half of the eye)	4
	Glazed and marked ptosis (half of the eye or more)	3

[a]This score is used to evaluate the level of sedation.
Modified from Chernik DA, Gillings D, Laine H, et al: Validity and reliability of the Observer's Assessment of Alertness/Sedation Scale: study with intravenous midazolam, *J Clin Psychopharmacol.* 1990;10:244–251.

TABLE 58.4 Description of Levels of Sedation

Level of Sedation	Description
1	Awake and anxious
2	Awake not anxious
3	Partial ptosis and/or slurred speech
4	Eyes closed, responds to speech
5	Eyes closed, responds to mild stimulation (shaking or earlobe pull)
6	Unresponsive to mild stimulation

Adapted from Wilson KE, Thorpe RJ, McCabe JF, et al: Complications associated with intravenous sedation in anxious dental patients. *Prim Dent Care.* 2011;18:161–166.

TABLE 58.5 Arterial Oxyhemoglobin Saturation and Oxygen Tension Values for Monitoring Tissue Oxygenation

Oximeter Arterial Oxyhemoglobin Saturation (Spo_2)	Arterial Oxygen Tension (Pao_2) (mm Hg)	Interpretation
95%–99%	80–100	Normal oxygenation
90%	60	Alarm goes off; patient is hypoxemic
80%	45–50	Severe hypoxemia

Documentation

An appropriate, time-oriented anesthetic record (Fig. 58.6) must be maintained with the names of all administered drugs (including local anesthetics), along with dosages, times administered, and routes of administration. Physiologic parameters, including heart rate, respiratory rate, blood pressure, and level of consciousness, must be recorded. For moderate sedation, oxygen saturation (i.e., pulse oximetry) must be monitored and recorded continually. The anesthesia record should also include BMI, Mallampati classification, and capnography information.

Recovery and Discharge

Oxygen and suction equipment must be immediately available in the treatment room and the recovery room (if a separate recovery area is used). The qualified dentist or appropriately trained clinical staff must continually monitor the patient's blood pressure, heart

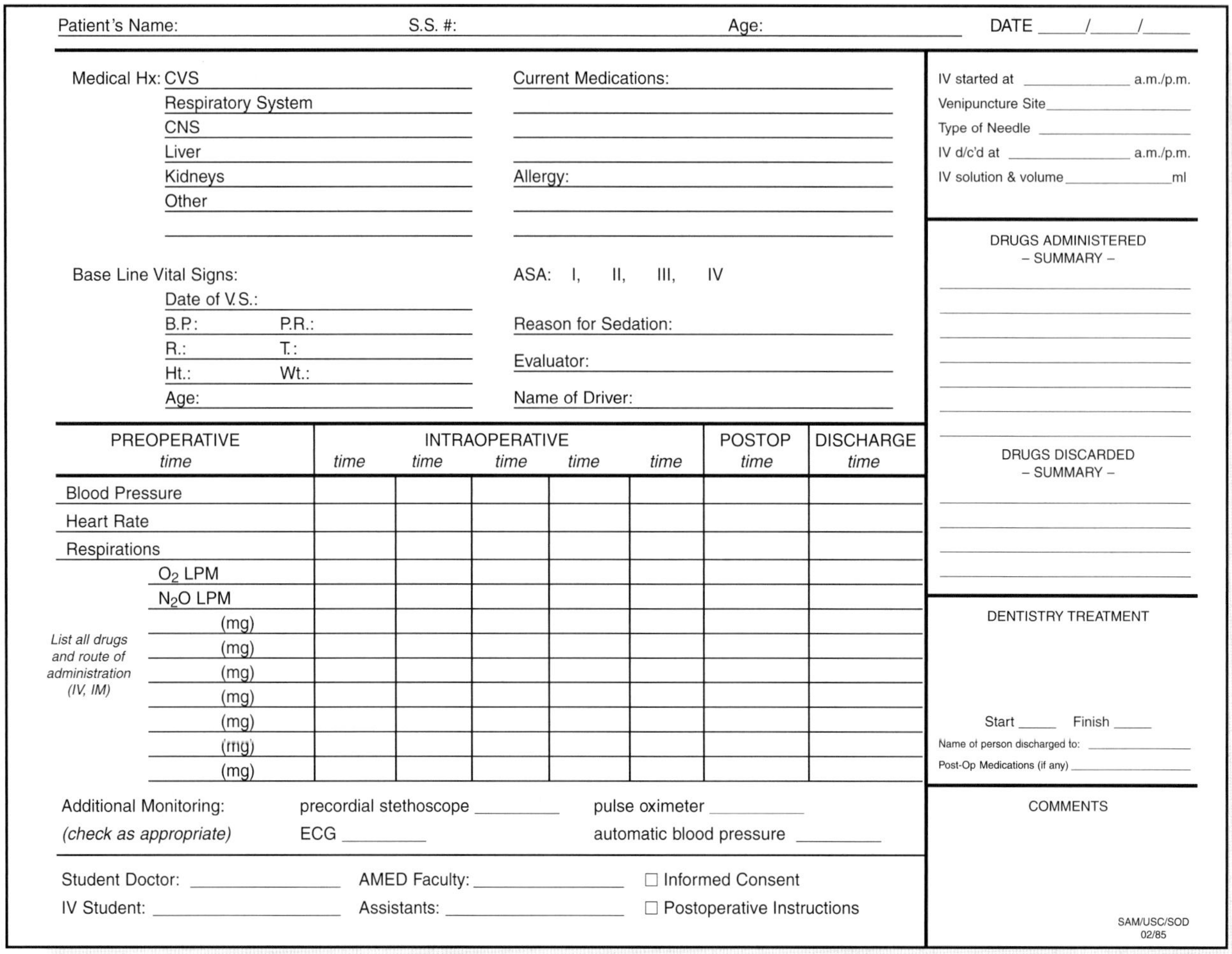

Patient's Name: S.S. #: Age: DATE ___/___/___

Medical Hx: CVS
Respiratory System
CNS
Liver
Kidneys
Other

Current Medications:

Allergy:

IV started at ______ a.m./p.m.
Venipuncture Site ______
Type of Needle ______
IV d/c'd at ______ a.m./p.m.
IV solution & volume ______ ml

DRUGS ADMINISTERED
– SUMMARY –

Base Line Vital Signs:
Date of V.S.:
B.P.: P.R.:
R.: T.:
Ht.: Wt.:
Age:

ASA: I, II, III, IV

Reason for Sedation:

Evaluator:

Name of Driver:

PREOPERATIVE time	INTRAOPERATIVE time	time	time	time	time	POSTOP time	DISCHARGE time
Blood Pressure							
Heart Rate							
Respirations							
O_2 LPM							
N_2O LPM							
List all drugs and route of administration (IV, IM) (mg)							
(mg)							
(mg)							
(mg)							
(mg)							
(mg)							
(mg)							

DRUGS DISCARDED
– SUMMARY –

DENTISTRY TREATMENT

Start ____ Finish ____
Name of person discharged to: ______
Post-Op Medications (if any) ______

Additional Monitoring: precordial stethoscope ______ pulse oximeter ______
(check as appropriate) ECG ______ automatic blood pressure ______

COMMENTS

Student Doctor: ______ AMED Faculty: ______ ☐ Informed Consent
IV Student: ______ Assistants: ______ ☐ Postoperative Instructions

SAM/USC/SOD
02/85

Fig. 58.6 Example of a moderate sedation record. (From Malamed SF: *Sedation: a guide to patient management,* ed 5. St. Louis, 2010, Elsevier.)

rate, and respiration. In cases of moderate sedation, oxygen saturation and level of consciousness must be evaluated continuously. The qualified dentist must determine and document that the levels of consciousness, oxygenation, ventilation, and circulation are satisfactory before discharge (see Box 58.5). Postoperative verbal and written instruction must be given to the patient and a responsible adult (e.g., parent, escort, guardian, or caregiver).

If a reversal agent is administered before discharge criteria have been met, the patient must be monitored until recovery is ensured. A potential problem when using reversal agents is the possibility that the duration of action of the reversal agent can be shorter than the sedative agent used, and the patient can become sedated again. It is critical for the clinician to understand and appreciate the duration of action of all sedative and reversal agents used.

Sedation Failures

When performing outpatient mild or moderate sedation, the clinician must realize that sedation will not be 100% effective for all patients. A certain percentage of patients will not respond appropriately to minimal or moderate sedation protocols (Table 58.6). If a patient is not responding to the sedation procedure, it is extremely

TABLE 58.6 Sedation Failure in Dentistry by Route of Administration

Technique	Expected Failure Rate (%)
Oral (child, older)	40–50
Oral (child, younger)	50–65
Oral (adult)	20–50
Inhalation	15–20
Oral + inhalation	5–10
Intravenous	4.3–5
Oral + intravenous	2–3
Deep sedation/general anesthesia	1.6

Data from Malamed SF: Sedation and safety: 36 years of perspective *Alpha Omegan.* 2006;99:70–74; Senel FC, Buchanan JM Jr, Senel AC, et al: Evaluation of sedation failure in the outpatient oral and maxillofacial surgery clinic. *J Oral Maxillofac Surg.* 2007;65:645–650; Skehan SJ, Malone DE, Buckley N, et al: Sedation and analgesia in adult patients: evaluation of a staged-dose system based on body weight for use in abdominal interventional radiology. *Radiology.* 2000;216:653–659; Wilson KE, Thorpe RJ, McCabe JF, Girdler NM: Complications associated with intravenous midazolam sedation in anxious dental patients. *Prim Dent Care.* 2011:18:161–166.

hazardous to go beyond dose limits or to attempt putting the patient into a deeper level of sedation. It is best to abort the procedure and reschedule the appointment for another day, with a different technique or with a dental anesthesiologist.

Emergency Preparedness

Because sedation and general anesthesia are on a continuum of drug-induced depression of consciousness to loss of consciousness, it is not always possible to predict how an individual patient will respond. Practitioners intending to produce a given level of sedation should be able to diagnose and manage the physiologic consequences for patients whose level of sedation becomes deeper than initially intended (i.e., rescue). For all levels of sedation, the practitioner must have the training, skills, drugs, and equipment to identify and manage such an occurrence until assistance arrives (i.e., emergency medical service) or the patient returns to the intended level of sedation without airway or cardiovascular complications. The qualified dentist is responsible for sedation management, adequacy of the facility, competence of the staff, diagnosis and treatment of emergencies related to the administration of sedation, and providing and maintaining the equipment and protocols for patient rescue.

If a patient enters a deeper level of sedation than the dentist is qualified to provide, the dentist must stop the procedure and focus attention on the patient until his or her condition returns to the intended level of sedation. This can involve monitoring the patient, providing airway management and support, administering reversal agents, or activating emergency medical services.

Conclusions

As periodontal procedures become more complex, there is an increased need for the use of conscious sedation techniques for patients with fear and anxiety. The ADA guidelines and policy are outlined in documents that need to be followed. Minimal sedation with N_2O inhalation techniques must be used with appropriate patient monitoring. The practitioner should have a minimum of 14 hours of instruction, including a clinical component.

After appropriate recovery, patients usually can be allowed to function normally and do not need another adult to monitor them. Minimal sedation using oral agents, such as triazolam in one dose, should not exceed the MRD for home use but, after recovery, these patients cannot drive and need another adult to supervise them. Moderate to deep sedation should be performed only by practitioners with appropriate postdoctoral training in an accredited advanced education program, which carries additional responsibilities for patient monitoring, restrictions on food and liquid intake, recovery, and additional trained support staff. The qualified dentist is responsible for sedative management, adequacy of the facility and staff, diagnosis and treatment of emergencies related to the administration of minimal or moderate sedation, and providing the equipment, drugs, and protocol for patient rescue.

Patients with systemic problems should undergo preoperative evaluation from a physician, and older patients frequently need downward adjustments of normal dosage. Children require special care from trained practitioners, and preoperative sedation in children younger than 12 years of age should be carried out by specialists in pediatric anesthesia. Patients with significant systemic problems are best treated in a hospital environment rather than in an outpatient surgical center.

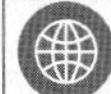
A Case Scenario is found on the companion website eBooks.Health.Elsevier.com.

Suggested Readings

American Academy of Periodontology: Statement on the use of moderate sedation by periodontists. *J Periodontol*. 2013;84:435.

American Dental Association. *Guidelines for the Use of Sedation and General Anesthesia by Dentists.* Adopted by the ADA House of Delegates; 2016. www.ada.org/~/media/ADA/Advocacy/Files/anesthesia_use_guidelines.

American Dental Association. *Guidelines for Teaching Pain Control and Sedation to Dentists and Dental Students*. Adopted by the ADA House of Delegates; 2016. www.ada.org/~/media/ADA/Member%20Center/Files/anxiety_guidelines.

American Society of Anesthesiologists. *Continuum of Depth of Sedation: Definition of General Anesthesia and Levels of Sedation/Analgesia*; 2019. http://www.asahq.org/quality-and-practice-management/standards-guidelines-and-related-resources/continuum-of-depth-of-sedation-definition-of-general-anesthesia-and-levels-of-sedation-analgesia.

Araújo JO, Bergamaschi CC, Lopes LC, et al. Effectiveness and safety of oral sedation in adult patients undergoing dental procedures: a systematic review. *BMJ Open*. 2021;11:1–10.

Askar H, Misch J, Chen Z, et al. Capnography monitoring in procedural intravenous sedation: a systematic review and meta-analysis. *Clin Oral Investig*. 2020;24:3761–3770.

Chen Q, Wang L, Ge L, et al. The anxiolytic effect of midazolam in third molar extraction: a systematic review. *PLoS One*. 2015;10:e0121410.

Lin C-S, Wu S-Y, Yi C-A. Association between anxiety and pain in dental treatment: a systematic review and meta-analysis. *J Dent Res*. 2017;96:153–162.

Malamed SF. *Sedation: a Guide to Patient Management*. 5th ed. St. Louis: Elsevier; 2009.

Venchard GR, Thomson PJ, Boys R. Improved sedation for oral surgery by combining nitrous oxide and intravenous midazolam: a randomized, controlled trial. *Int J Oral Maxillofac Surg*. 2006;35:522–527.

Yagiela JA. Recent developments in local anesthesia and oral sedation. *Compend Contin Educ Dent*. 2004;25:697–706, quiz 708.

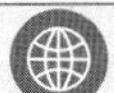
References for this chapter are found on the companion website eBooks.Health.Elsevier.com.

CHAPTER 59

Periodontal and Peri-Implant Surgical Anatomy

Perry R. Klokkevold | Joseph M. Miller | Fermin A. Carranza

CHAPTER OUTLINE

A sound knowledge of the anatomy of the periodontium and the surrounding hard and soft tissue structures is essential to determine the scope and possibilities of periodontal and implant surgical procedures and to minimize their risks. The spatial relationship of bones, muscles, blood vessels, and nerves, as well as the anatomic spaces located in the vicinity of the periodontal or implant surgical field, are particularly important. Only those features with periodontal and implant surgery relevance are mentioned in this chapter; the reader is referred to oral and head and neck anatomy books for a more detailed and comprehensive description of these structures.[4,5]

Mandible

The mandible is a horseshoe-shaped bone connected to the skull by the temporomandibular joints, stylomandibular and sphenomandibular ligaments, and the muscles of mastication (temporalis, masseter, medial and lateral pterygoids). It presents several landmarks of great surgical importance for both periodontal and implant surgical procedures.

The *mandibular canal,* which is occupied by the inferior alveolar nerve and vessels, begins at the mandibular foramen on the medial surface of the mandibular ramus and curves inferiorly and anteriorly until it becomes horizontal below the apices of the molars (Fig. 59.1). The distance from the canal to the apices of the teeth is shortest in the third molar area. A significant percentage of mandibular canals (up to 27%) were found to bifurcate in a systematic review and meta-analysis of 15 studies of anatomic variation using samples of more than 300 individuals from different geographic regions.[11] Trifid mandibular canals have also been documented. The mandibular canal status may have clinical significance in anesthesia failure, mandibular third molar extraction, implantation, and other surgical procedures.[18] In the premolar area, the mandibular canal divides in two branches, with one exiting the mandible and the other continuing anteriorly—the *incisive canal,* which continues horizontally to the midline, and the *mental canal,* which turns superiorly and opens in the mental foramen.

The *mental foramen,* from which the mental nerve and vessels emerge, is located on the buccal surface of the mandible below the apices of the premolars, sometimes closer to the second premolar and usually halfway between the inferior border of the mandible and the alveolar margin (Fig. 59.2). It is often but not always visible on conventional radiographs. The opening of the mental foramen, which may be oval or round, typically faces superiorly and distally, with its posterior-superior border slanting gradually to the bone surface. An "anterior loop" of the mental foramen has been described, with the use of cadaver dissection, as a reverse turn and looping back of the mental nerve within the body of the mandible before its exit out of the mental foramen; the estimated length of the anterior loop ranges from 0.5 to 5.0 mm.[9] A more recent evaluation of the anterior loop of the mental nerve involving the use of cone beam scans and cadaveric dissection reported this loop extension to range from 0.0 to 9.0 mm.[24,25] The anterior loop of the mental nerve has a high prevalence (88%), symmetric occurrence, and mean length of 4.13 ± 1.08 mm.[19] As it emerges, the *mental nerve* divides into three branches. One branch of the nerve turns anteriorly and inferiorly to supply the skin of the chin. The other two branches course anteriorly and superiorly to supply the skin and mucous membranes of the lower lip and the mucosa of the labial alveolar surface.

Surgical trauma (e.g., pressure, manipulation, postsurgical swelling) to the mental nerve can produce paresthesia of the lip, which recovers slowly. Partial or complete cutting of the nerve can result in permanent paresthesia, dysesthesia, or both. Familiarity with the location and appearance of the mental nerve reduces the likelihood of injury (Fig. 59.3).

KEY FACT

Surgical trauma, including pressure, manipulation, and postsurgical swelling of the mental nerve tissues, may result in transient paresthesia of the lip. Partial or complete nerve cutting of the mental nerve may result in permanent paresthesia, dysesthesia, or both.

In partially or totally edentulous jaws, the disappearance of the alveolar portion of the mandible brings the mandibular canal and mental foramen closer to the superior border (Figs. 59.4 and 59.5). When these patients are evaluated for the placement of implants, the distance between the canal and superior surface of the bone, as well as the location of the mental foramen, must be carefully determined to avoid surgical injury to the nerve (see Chapter 73).

The anterior extension of the inferior alveolar nerve or incisive nerve has been measured with the use of conventional radiography, computed tomography (CT) scans, cadaver dissections, and cone beam scans.[3,10,24,25] This nerve, which is less evident on conventional radiographs and often unnoticed, extends beyond the anterior loop of the mental foramen in a horizontal direction toward the midline. The length of the incisive canal has been reported to be up to 21.45 mm from the mesial aspect of the mental foramen and to terminate just 4 mm from the midline.[3]

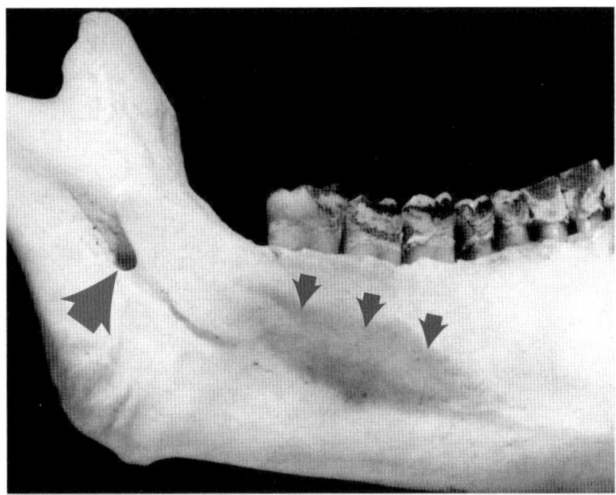

Fig. 59.1 Mandible, lingual surface view. Note the lingual or mandibular foramen *(blue arrow),* where the inferior alveolar nerve enters the mandibular canal, and the mylohyoid ridge *(red arrows).*

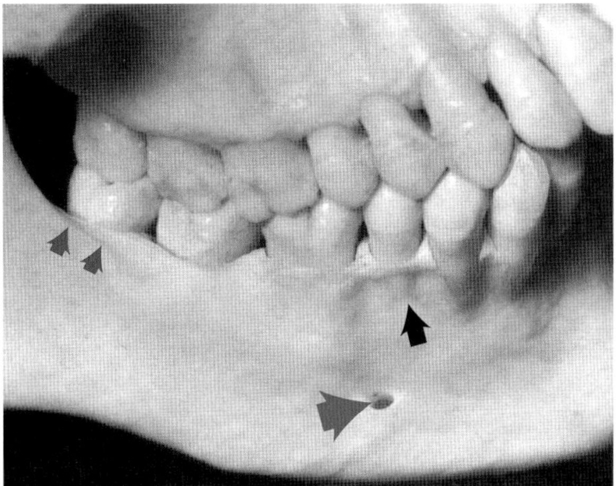

Fig. 59.2 Mandible, facial surface view. Note the location of the mental foramen *(blue arrow),* which is slightly distal and apical to the apex of the second premolar, and the shelflike area in the region of the molars *(red arrows),* which is created by the external oblique ridge. Note also the fenestration that is present in the second premolar *(black arrow).*

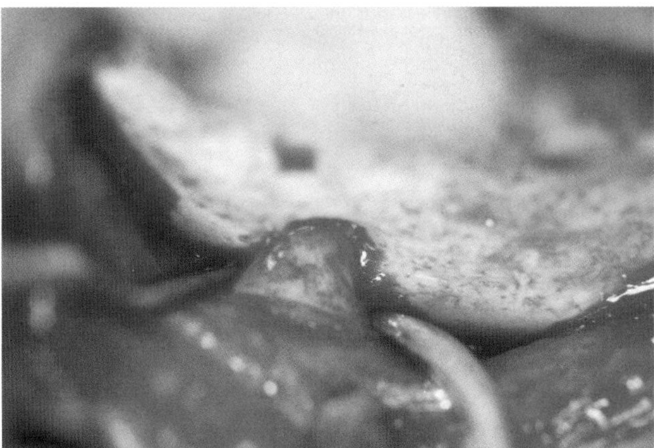

Fig. 59.3 Surgical view of the mental nerve emerging from the foramen in the premolar area.

The *lingual nerve,* along with the inferior alveolar nerve, is a branch of the posterior division of the mandibular nerve. It descends along the mandibular ramus medial and anterior to the inferior alveolar nerve. The lingual nerve lies close to the surface of the oral mucosa in the third molar area and goes deeper as it travels anteriorly (Fig. 59.6). It can be damaged during anesthetic injections and during oral surgery procedures (e.g., third molar extractions).[14] Less often, the lingual nerve may be injured when a periodontal partial-thickness flap is raised in the third molar region or when releasing incisions are made in the area.

The *alveolar process,* which provides the supporting bone to the teeth, has a narrower distal curvature than the body of the mandible (Fig. 59.7), thus creating a flat surface in the posterior area between the teeth and anterior border of the ramus. This results in the formation of the *external oblique ridge,* which runs inferiorly and anteriorly to the region of the second or first molar (Fig. 59.8) to create a shelflike bony area. Resective osseous therapy may be difficult or impossible in this area because of the amount of bone that must be removed distally toward the ramus to achieve resection of a periodontal osseous defect on the distal aspect of the mandibular second or third molar.

Distal to the third molar, the external oblique ridge circumscribes the *retromolar triangle* (see Fig. 59.8). This region is occupied by glandular and adipose tissue and covered by unattached, nonkeratinized mucosa. If sufficient space exists distal to the last molar, a band of attached gingiva may be present; only in such a case can a distal flap procedure be performed effectively (see Chapter 56).

The medial side of the body of the mandible is traversed obliquely by the *mylohyoid ridge,* which starts close to the alveolar margin in the third molar area and continues anteriorly in an apical direction, thereby increasing its distance from the osseous margin as it travels anteriorly (Fig. 59.9). The *mylohyoid muscle* inserts along this ridge and separates the *sublingual space,* which is located superiorly or more anteriorly and superiorly, from the submandibular space, which is located inferiorly or more posteriorly and inferiorly.

Maxilla

The maxilla is a paired bone that is hollowed out by the maxillary sinuses and the nasal cavity. The maxilla has the following four processes:

- The *alveolar process* contains the sockets for and supports the maxillary teeth.
- The *palatine process* extends horizontally from the alveolar process to meet its counterpart from the opposite maxilla at the midline intermaxillary suture, and it extends posteriorly with the horizontal plate of the palatine bone to form the hard palate.
- The *zygomatic process* extends laterally from the area above the first molar and determines the depth of the posterior vestibular fornix on the lateral aspect of the maxilla.
- The *frontal process* extends in an ascending direction and articulates with the frontal bone at the frontomaxillary suture.

The terminal branches of the nasopalatine nerve and vessels pass through the incisive canal, which opens in the midline anterior area of the palate (Fig. 59.10). The mucosa overlying the incisive canal presents a slight protuberance called the *incisive papilla.* Vessels that emerge through the incisive canal are of small caliber, and their surgical interference is of little consequence.

The *greater palatine foramen* opens 3 to 4 mm anterior to the posterior border of the hard palate (Fig. 59.11). The greater palatine nerve and vessels emerge through this foramen and run anteriorly in the submucosa of the palate, between the palatal and alveolar processes (Fig. 59.12). Palatal flaps and donor sites for gingival and connective tissue grafts should be carefully performed and selected to avoid invading these areas because profuse hemorrhage may ensue, particularly if vessels are damaged at the greater palatine foramen. Vertical incisions in the molar region should be avoided.

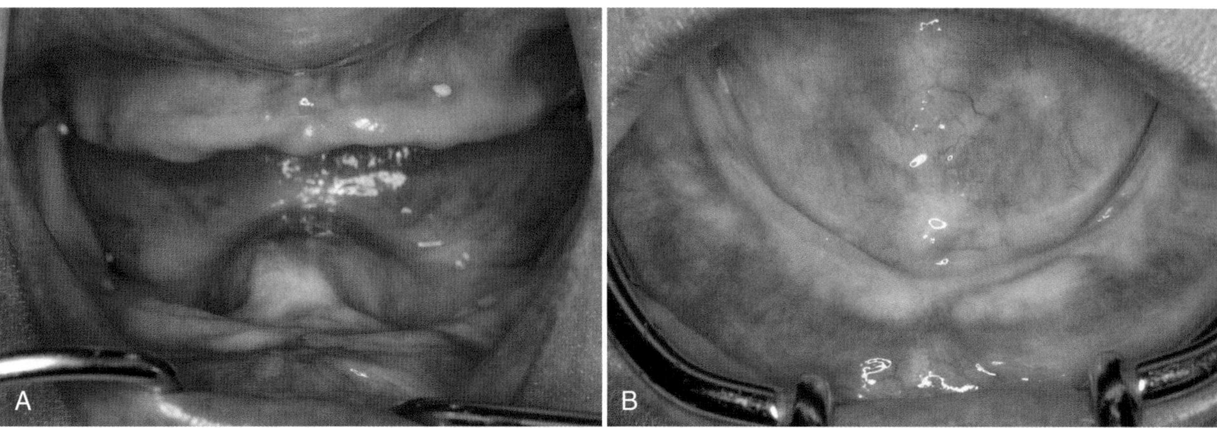

Fig. 59.4 Loss of the alveolar ridge in an edentulous patient brings the mental foramen and mandibular canal closer to the surface, which may lead to discomfort for the patient. (A) Anterior view demonstrating a severe loss of vertical alveolar ridge height. (B) Occlusal view of the same patient demonstrating a loss of vestibular depth with alveolar bone loss.

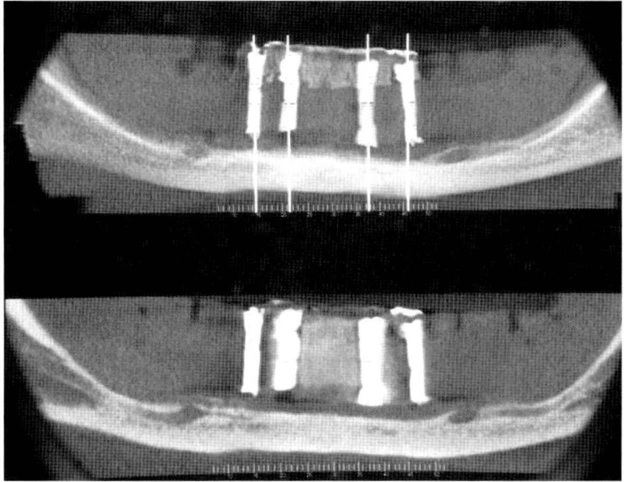

Fig. 59.5 Panoramic radiograph of an edentulous patient with a loss of alveolar bone height. This results in the mental foramen exiting the jaw at the superior aspect of the remaining bone (ridge crest), which is the denture-bearing surface. Pressure from the complete removable denture over this area causes pain.

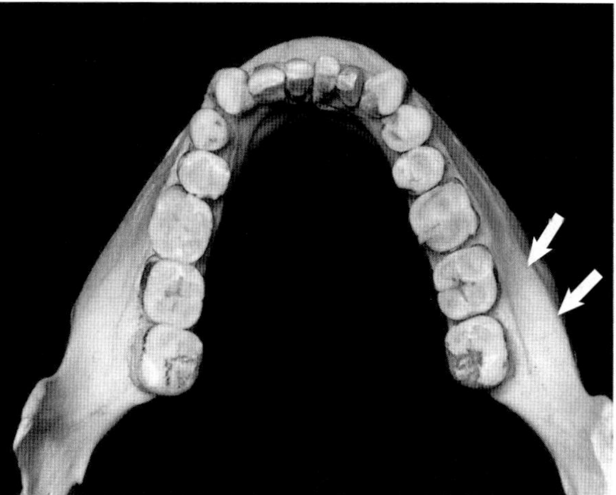

Fig. 59.7 Occlusal view of the mandible. Note the shelf that is created in the facial molar areas by the external oblique ridge. *Arrows* show the attachment of the buccinator muscle.

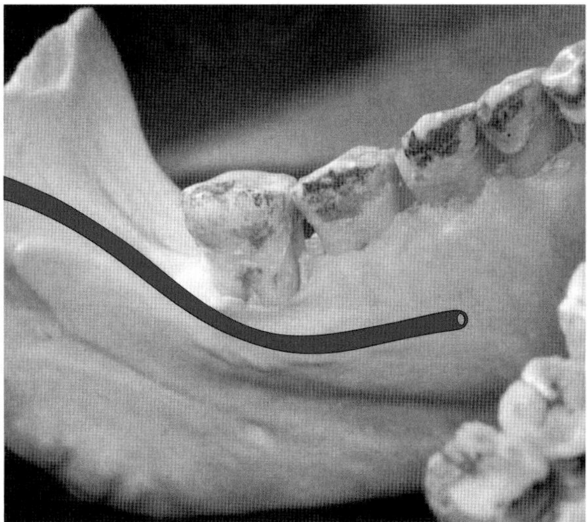

Fig. 59.6 Lingual view of the mandible showing the pathway of the lingual nerve *(red)*, which courses near the gingiva in the third molar area and then continues forward, running deeper and medially toward the tongue.

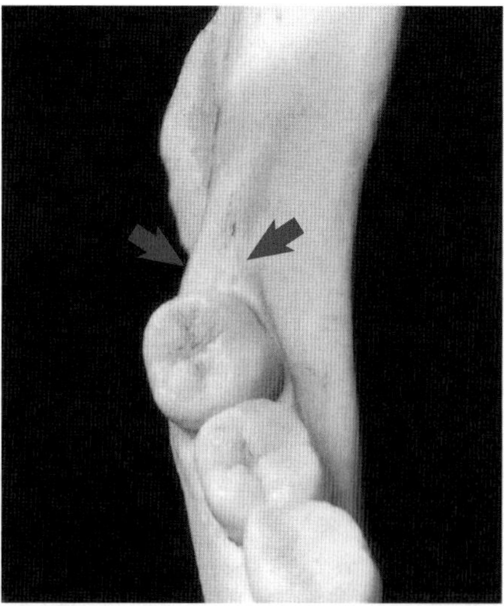

Fig. 59.8 Mandible; occlusal view of the ramus and molars. Note the retromolar triangle area distal to the third molar *(arrows)*.

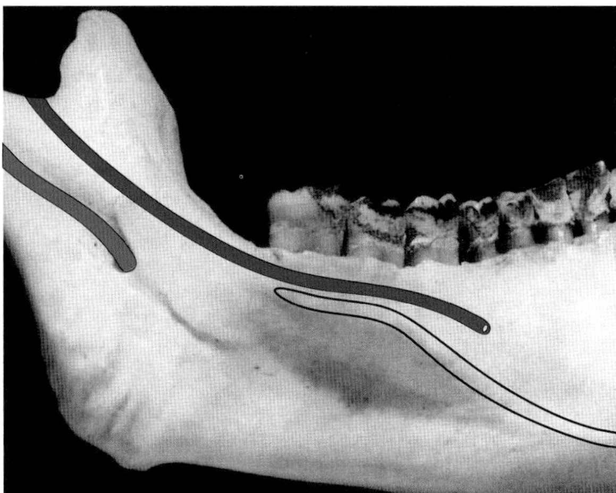

Fig. 59.9 Lingual view of the mandible showing the inferior alveolar nerve entering the mandibular canal *(blue)*, the lingual nerve traversing near the lingual surface of the third molar *(red)*, and the attachment of the mylohyoid muscle inferiorly *(outline)*.

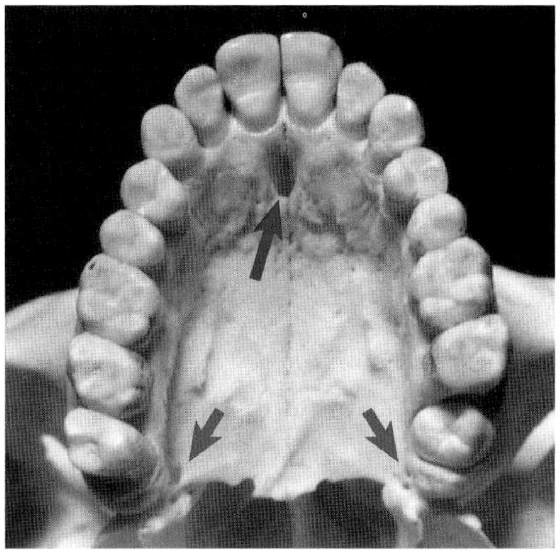

Fig. 59.10 Occlusal view of the maxilla and palatine bone. Note the opening of the incisive canal *(red arrow)* and the greater palatine foramina *(blue arrows)*.

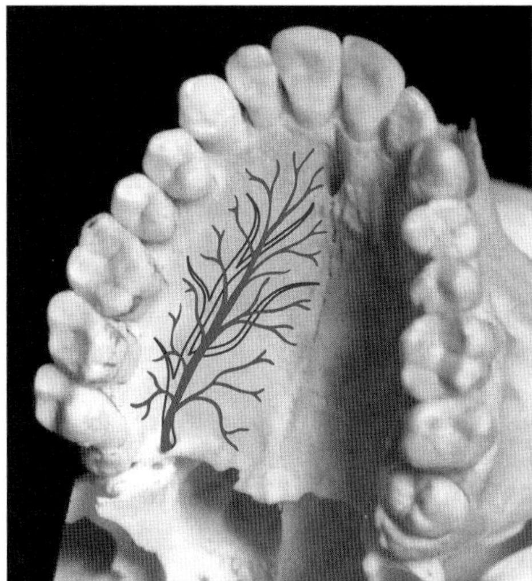

Fig. 59.11 Occlusal lateral view of the palate showing nerves *(red)* and vessels *(blue)* emerging from the greater palatine foramen and continuing anteriorly on the palate.

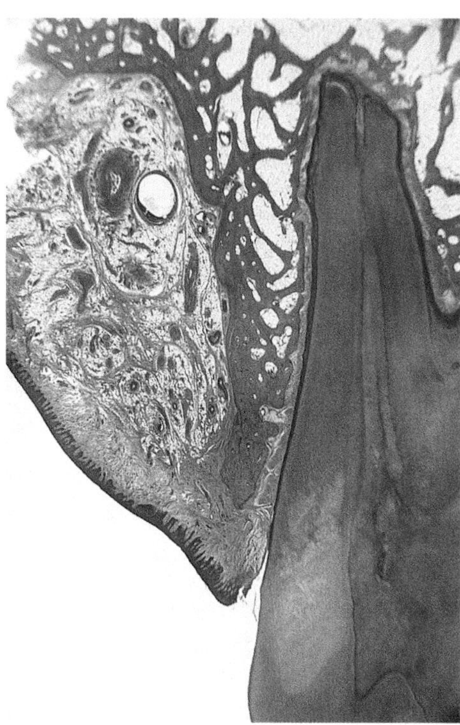

Fig. 59.12 Histologic frontal section of a human palate at the level of the first molar showing the location of the vessels and the nerve surrounded by adipose and glandular tissue. Hematoxylin and eosin stained tissues; 2× magnification.

The mucous membrane that covers the hard palate is firmly attached to the underlying bone. The submucosal layer of the palate posterior to the first molars contains the *palatal glands,* which are more compact in the soft palate and extend anteriorly, thereby filling the gap between the mucosal connective tissue and periosteum and protecting the underlying vessels and nerves (see Fig. 59.22, later).

The area distal to the last molar, called the *maxillary tuberosity,* consists of the posterior-inferior angle of the infratemporal surface of the maxilla. Medially it articulates with the pyramidal process of the palatine bone. It is covered by dense, fibrous connective tissue, and it contains the terminal branches of the lesser (middle and posterior) palatine nerves. Excision of the area for distal flap surgery may reach medially to the tensor veli palatini muscle. The tensor veli palatini muscle originates from the scaphoid fossa and spine of the sphenoid bone and ends by forming a tendon that winds around the pterygoid hamulus; it then expands medially to form the palatine aponeurosis, which then inserts onto the posterior border of the hard palate.

The body of the maxilla is occupied by the *maxillary sinus,* which is the largest of the paranasal sinuses. It is an air-filled cavity located in the posterior maxilla, superior to the teeth. The lateral wall of the nasal cavity borders the sinus medially; it is bordered superiorly by the floor of the orbit and laterally by the lateral wall of the maxilla, alveolar process, and zygomatic arch (Fig. 59.13). It is pyramidal, with its apex in the zygomatic arch and its base at the lateral wall of the nasal cavity. The size of the maxillary sinus varies from one individual to another (depending on the individual and his or her age) and from very small and narrow to quite large and expansive.

The maxillary sinus is frequently subdivided (incompletely) into recesses by one or more septa. Maxillary sinus septa vary in size and location. Clinical and radiographic examinations suggest that septa are frequently present (≤39% of sinuses).[7,13,27] CT and cone-beam computed tomography (CBCT) scans are the preferred methods for detecting septa because panoramic radiographs are not reliable (i.e.,

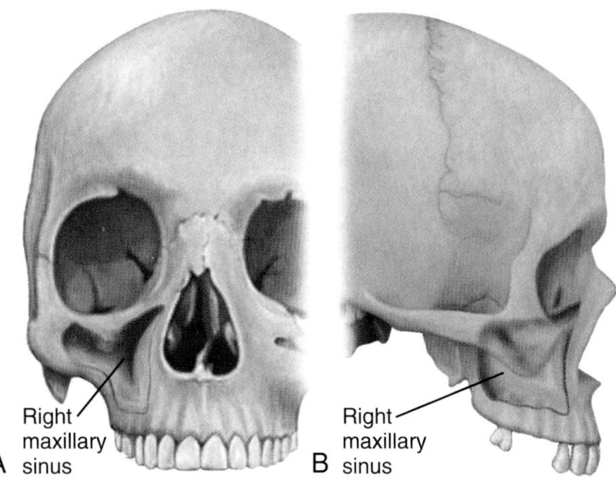

Fig. 59.13 Location and anatomy of the maxillary sinus. (A) Frontal view. (B) Lateral view.

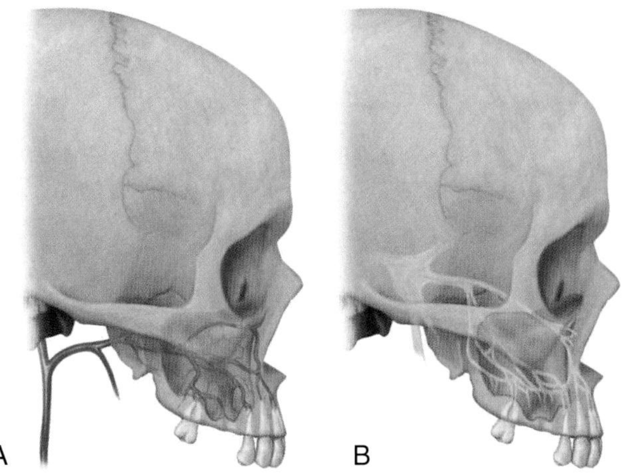

Fig. 59.14 Blood supply and innervation of the maxillary sinus. (A) Arterial blood supply. (B) Innervation of the maxillary sinus.

26.5% false diagnosis of the presence or absence of septa).[13,15] Septa are found in the anterior (24%), middle (41%), and posterior (35%) aspects of the maxillary sinus, with the most common location being between the second premolar and first molar.[12,27] The height of septa varies as well, ranging from 0 to 20.6 mm.[27] Only 0.5% of septa form a complete separation of the sinus cavity into separate chambers.[16]

The entire maxillary sinus is lined with a thin mucosal membrane called the Schneiderian membrane. This specialized structure of the respiratory mucous membrane, with its motile cilia and rich blood supply, is well adapted to purifying, moistening, and warming air to protect the lungs. The entrance to the maxillary sinus, through the orifice or maxillary duct, is located at the superior medial aspect of the sinus cavity. The orifice is relatively small, measuring only 3 to 6 mm in length and diameter. An accessory opening is occasionally found inferior and posterior to the main opening. The maxillary sinus drains into the middle meatus of the nasal cavity through the maxillary duct or ostium, which passes secretions medially to the semilunar hiatus. Normal amounts of secretion are moved from the sinus by the spiral pattern of the beating cilia that surround the orifice. If the maxillary sinus becomes infected or chronically inflamed, swelling of the mucosa around the orifice impairs drainage. The floor of the maxillary sinus extends inferiorly below the level of the nasal cavity into the alveolar process.

The roots of the maxillary first and second molars are often in close proximity to the floor of the sinus. Less frequently, the roots of the premolars and third molars may be observed in close proximity to the floor of the sinus. It has been suggested that the maxillary sinus expands or pneumatizes with age. It becomes more pneumatized down around the roots of the maxillary teeth, sometimes resulting in exposure of the roots through the bony floor into the sinus, with only the thin mucosal membrane covering the root surface. The ability to perform periodontal osseous surgery in the posterior maxilla may be limited when the sinuses are severely pneumatized. Extraction of teeth with roots exposed into the maxillary sinus (i.e., without bone to maintain integrity of the maxillary sinus floor) can result in an oroantral communication. A recent (2019) retrospective analysis using CBCT to assess maxillary sinus pneumatization has refuted the idea that it expands with age.[20] Following CBCT evaluation of 50 dentate and 50 edentulous maxillae, the authors concluded that edentulism did not have an impact on maxillary sinus dimension, suggesting that there is no ongoing pneumatization in the sinus after tooth loss. Males had larger sinuses than females.

Blood supply to the maxillary sinus arises from the superior alveolar (anterior, middle, and posterior) branches of the maxillary artery (Fig. 59.14A).[26] The maxillary artery, which is a large terminal branch of the external carotid artery, gives off many branches to supply the maxillary sinus, including the infraorbital artery, which travels superiorly and anteriorly and gives off the anterior superior alveolar artery.[8] Branches of the greater palatine artery contribute to a lesser extent. Venous blood drains via the pterygoid plexus. Much of the vasculature travels through channels in the bony walls of the maxillary sinus, with many branches anastomosing with the highly vascularized Schneiderian membrane. Innervation of the maxillary sinus is supplied by the superior alveolar nerves (anterior, middle, and posterior) and branches of the maxillary nerve (see Fig. 59.14B).

Knowledge of the arterial blood supply is particularly important when considering a lateral window approach to sinus floor elevation and bone augmentation. Solar and colleagues[21] found an intraosseous branch of the posterior superior alveolar artery anastomosing with the infraorbital artery in 100% of their human cadaver specimens (134 sinuses, all male cadavers). On average, the vessel was located 18.9 mm from the alveolar crest. By studying 50 CT scans from 625 patients (both male and female) who were undergoing sinus bone augmentation, Elian and colleagues[6] found that the vessel was radiographically evident in 52.9% of sinuses. The vessel was located an average of 16.4 mm from the alveolar crest, a slightly shorter distance but consistent with the previous study. Human cadaver dissection and CT scan evaluations of the vessels running through the lateral wall of the maxillary sinus have revealed that intraosseous vessels are present in the lower two thirds of the anterolateral wall in approximately 10.5% of cases (Fig. 59.15).[8] In 57.1% of those cases (≈6% of all sinuses), the vessel diameter ranged in size from 1 to 2.5 mm. The location of the artery in relation to the position of the lateral window for sinus augmentation presents a risk for bleeding complications in 10% to 20% of cases.[6,8]

The floor of the maxillary sinus is frequently separated from the apices and roots of the maxillary posterior teeth by a thin bony plate (Fig. 59.16). In edentulous posterior areas, the maxillary sinus bony wall may only be a thin plate that is in intimate contact with the alveolar mucosa (Fig. 59.17). Adequate determination of the extension of the maxillary sinus into the surgical site is important to avoid creating an oroantral communication, particularly in relation to osseous reduction in periodontal surgery, surgical procedures for bone augmentation, or the placement of implants in edentulous areas. Determining the amount of available bone in the anterior area, inferior to the floor of the nasal cavity, is also critical for the placement of implants (see Chapter 73).

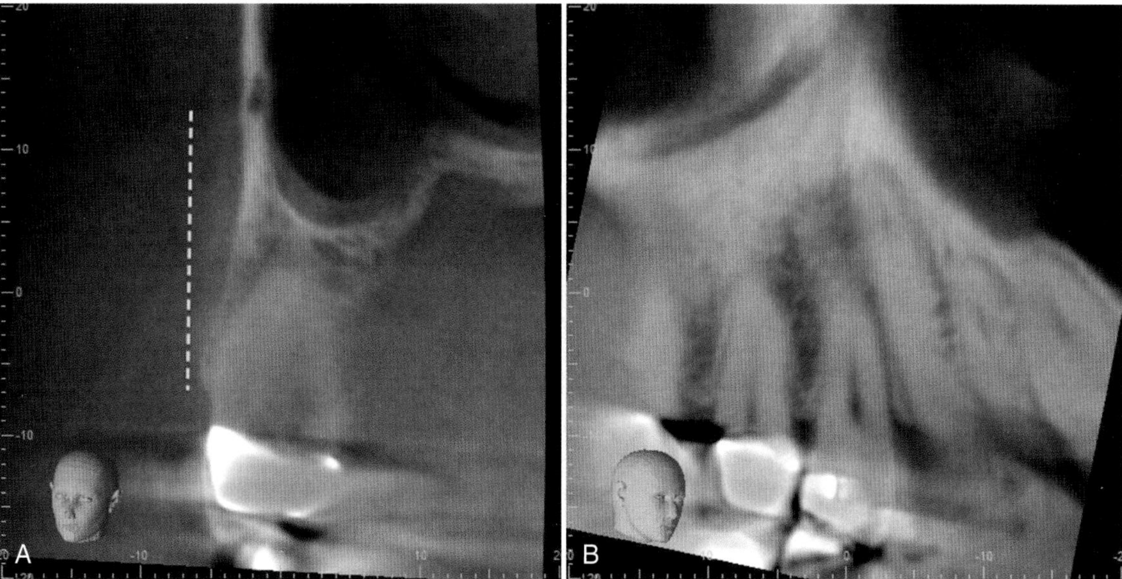

Fig. 59.15 (A) Cross-sectional image from a cone-beam computed tomography scan of the maxillary sinus demonstrating the presence of an intraosseous vessel in the lateral wall approximately 20 mm from the alveolar crest. (B) Sagittal section through the maxillary sinus in the same patient demonstrating an intraosseous vessel extending along the maxillary sinus. The diameter of the intraosseous canal is 2 mm.

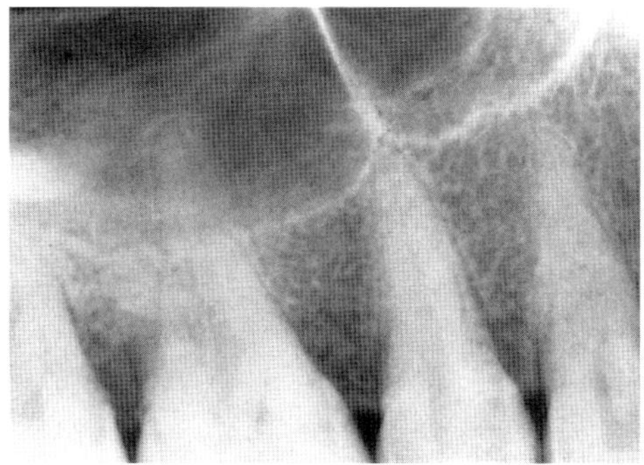

Fig. 59.16 Radiograph of the maxillary molars and premolars, with the maxillary sinus apparently near the apices. A radiopaque structure suggestive of a maxillary sinus septum is observed superior to the apex of the maxillary second premolar.

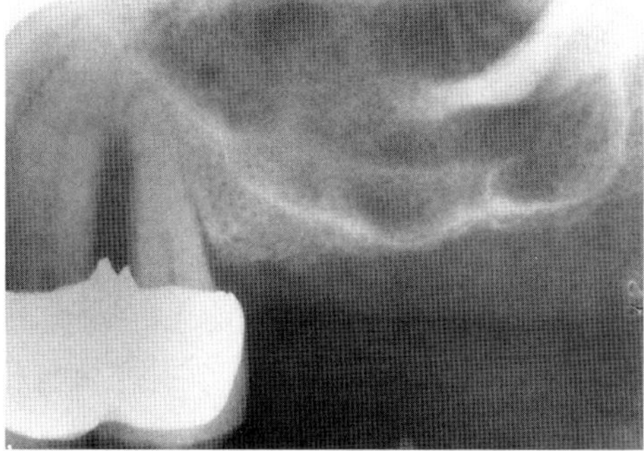

Fig. 59.17 Radiograph of an edentulous molar maxillary area demonstrating severe pneumatization of the maxillary sinus. Only a thin layer of cortical bone separates the sinus from the oral cavity.

Exostoses

Both the maxilla and mandible may have exostoses or tori, which are considered to be within the normal range of anatomic variation. Sometimes these structures may hinder the daily biofilm removal by the patient and may have to be removed to improve the prognosis of adjacent teeth. Additional indications for the removal of exostoses include the inability to wear removable prostheses comfortably over these areas. The most common location of a mandibular torus is in the lingual area of the canines and premolars, superior to the mylohyoid muscle (Fig. 59.18). Mandibular tori can also be found on the buccal and labial surfaces of the mandibular teeth. Maxillary tori are usually located in the midline of the hard palate (Fig. 59.19). Smaller tori may be seen over the palatal roots of the maxillary molars, in the area inferior to the greater palatine foramen (see Fig. 59.19), or on the buccal and labial surfaces of the maxillary teeth (Fig. 59.20).

Muscles

Several muscles may be encountered when performing periodontal and implant placement flap surgery, particularly during mucogingival surgery and bone augmentation procedures. These are the mentalis, incisivus labii inferioris, depressor labii inferioris, depressor anguli oris (triangularis), incisivus labii superioris, and buccinator muscles. Their bony attachments are shown in Fig. 59.21. These muscles provide mobility to the lips and cheeks.

Anatomic Spaces

Several anatomic spaces or *compartments* are found close to the operative field of periodontal and implant surgery sites. These spaces contain loose connective tissue, but they can be easily distended by hemorrhage, inflammatory fluid, and infection.

Surgical invasion of these areas may result in dangerous hemorrhage (intraoperative) or infections (postoperative) and should be carefully avoided. Some of these spaces are briefly described in the following paragraphs. For more information, the reader is referred to other sources.[2,10,22,23]

The *canine fossa* contains varying amounts of connective tissue and fat. It is bounded superiorly by the levator (quadratus) labii superioris muscle, anteriorly by the orbicularis oris, and posteriorly by the buccinator. Infection of this area results in swelling of the upper lip, which obliterates the nasolabial fold, and possibly the upper and lower eyelids, resulting in closure of the eye.

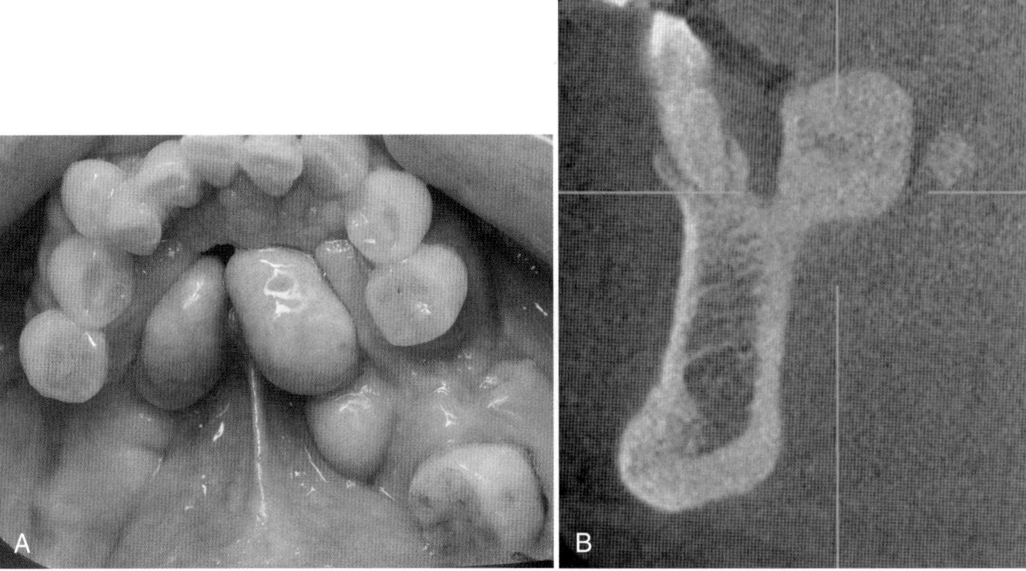

Fig. 59.18 (A) Clinical photograph of large mandibular tori on the lingual aspect of both the right and left mandibles. (B) Cross-sectional image of a mandibular torus in the premolar area in the same patient.

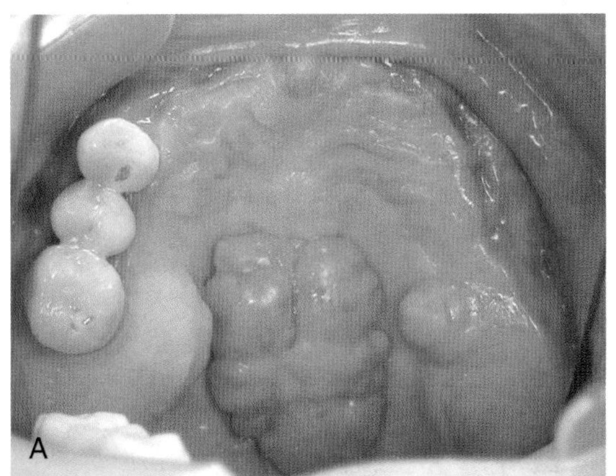

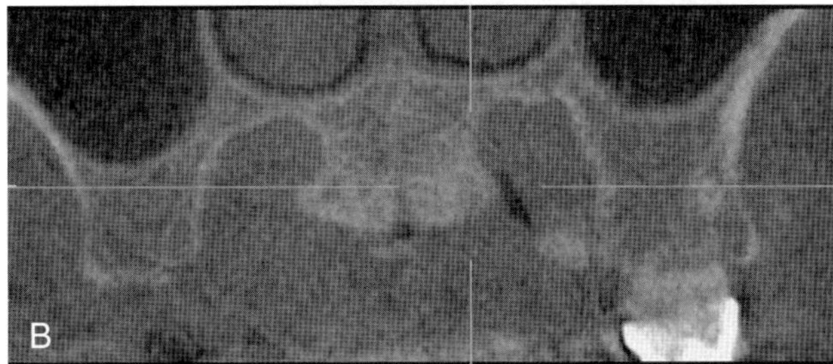

Fig. 59.19 (A) Clinical photograph of a large palatal torus located in the midline of the palate. Note also the large tori on the palatal aspects of the maxillary alveolar ridge. (B) Cross-sectional image of the maxillary midline torus in the same patient. Note also the torus located on the palatal aspect of the alveolar ridge.

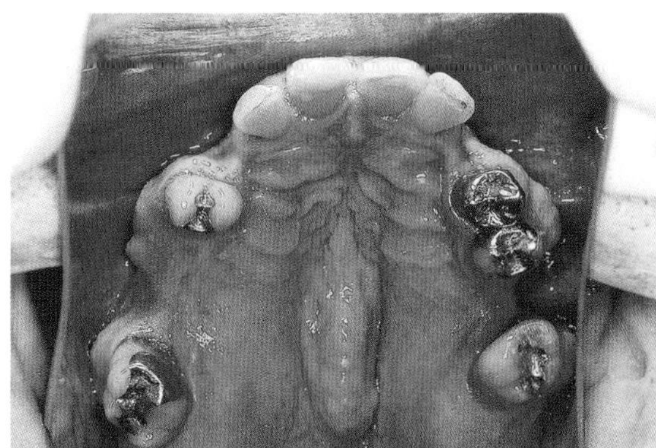

Fig. 59.20 Clinical photograph of large buccal exostosis in the maxillary arch. The patient also has a large midline palatal torus.

The *buccal space* is located between the buccinator and masseter muscles. Infection of this area results in swelling of the cheek that may extend to the temporal or the submandibular spaces, with which the buccal space communicates.

The *mental* or *mentalis space* is located in the region of the mental symphysis, where the mentalis muscle, depressor labii inferioris, and depressor anguli oris are attached. Infection of this area results in large swelling of the chin, which extends inferiorly.

The *masticator space* contains the masseter muscle, pterygoid muscles, tendon of insertion of the temporalis muscle, mandibular ramus, and posterior part of the body of the mandible. Infection of this area results in swelling of the face, severe trismus, and pain. If the abscess occupies the deepest part of this compartment, facial swelling may not be obvious, but the patient may complain of pain and trismus. Patients may also complain of difficulty and discomfort when moving the tongue and swallowing.

The *sublingual space* is located below the oral mucosa in the anterior part of the floor of the mouth. It contains the sublingual gland and its excretory ducts and the submandibular (Wharton) duct. The sublingual space is traversed by the lingual nerve and vessels and by the hypoglossal nerve (Fig. 59.22). Its boundaries are the geniohyoid and genioglossus muscles medially, the lingual surface of the mandible inferiorly, and the mylohyoid muscle laterally and anteriorly (Fig. 59.23). Infection of this area raises the floor of the mouth and displaces the tongue, which results in pain and difficulty in swallowing, but little facial swelling.

The *submental space* is found between the mylohyoid muscle superiorly and the platysma inferiorly. It is bounded laterally by the mandible and posteriorly by the hyoid bone. It is traversed by the anterior belly of the digastric muscle. Infections of this area arise from the region of the mandibular anterior teeth and result in swelling of the submental region; infections become more dangerous as they proceed posteriorly.

The *submandibular space* is found external to the sublingual space, inferior to the mylohyoid and hyoglossus muscles (see Figs. 59.22 and 59.23). This space contains the deep part of the submandibular gland, the superficial part of which extends partially superior to the mylohyoid muscle, thereby communicating with the sublingual space and numerous lymph nodes. Infections of this area originate in the molar or premolar area and result in swelling that obliterates the submandibular line and in pain with swallowing. Ludwig angina is a severe form of infection of the submandibular space that may extend to the sublingual and submental spaces. It results in the hardening of the floor of the mouth and may lead to asphyxiation from edema of the neck and glottis. Although the bacteriology of these infections has not been completely determined, they are presumed to be mixed infections with an important anaerobic component.[1,17]

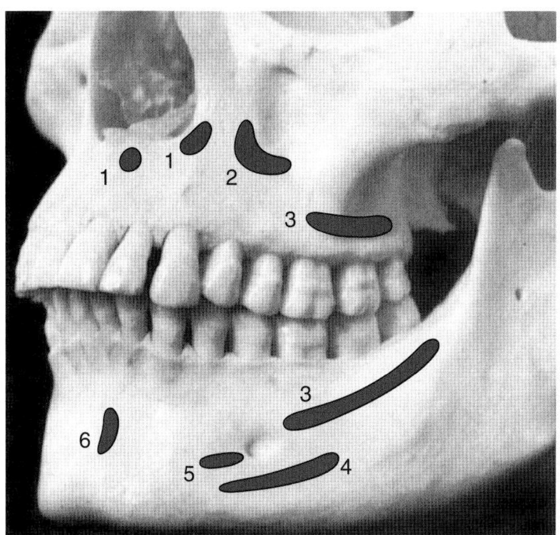

Fig. 59.21 Muscle attachments that may be encountered in mucogingival surgery. *1,* Nasalis; *2,* levator anguli oris; *3,* buccinator; *4,* depressor anguli oris; *5,* depressor labii inferioris; *6,* mentalis.

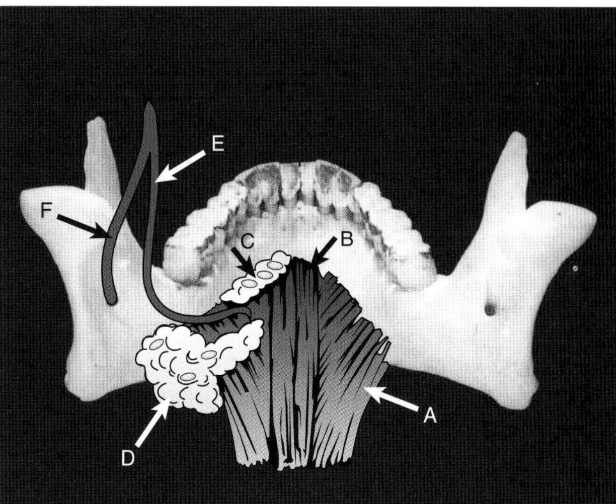

Fig. 59.23 Posterior view of the mandible showing the attachment of the mylohyoid muscles (A), geniohyoid muscles (B), sublingual gland (C), submandibular gland, which extends inferior to and also to some extent superior to the mylohyoid muscle (D), lingual nerve (E), and inferior alveolar nerve (F).

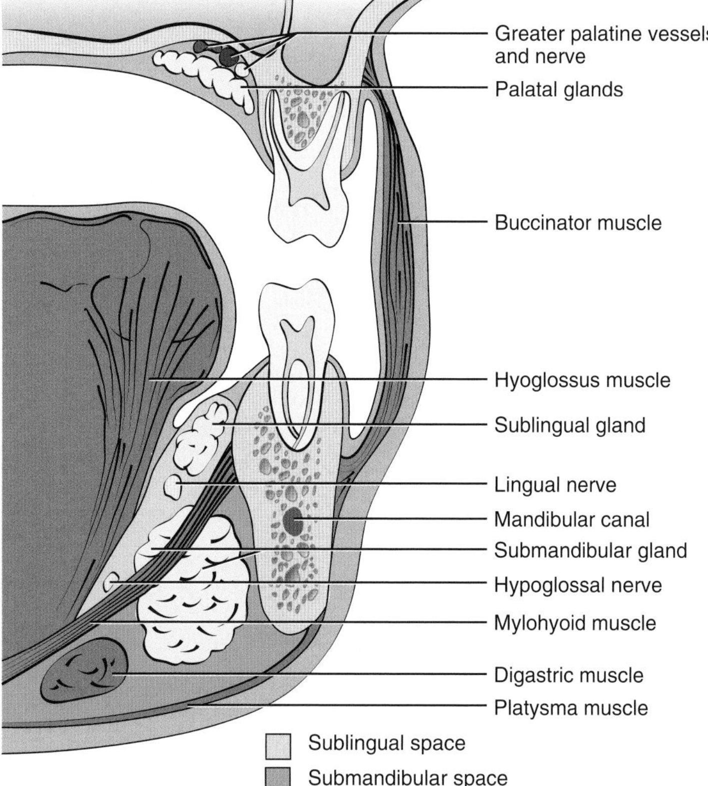

Fig. 59.22 Diagram of a frontal section of the human head at the level of the first molars depicting the most important structures in relation to periodontal surgery. Note the location of the sublingual space, submandibular space, and greater palatine nerve and vessels.

FLASH BACK

Ludwig angina is a life-threatening fascial space infection involving the submandibular, sublingual, and submental spaces. It is characterized by extraoral swelling and edema of the lower face and neck, with intraoral swelling that raises the floor of the mouth and tongue. If not treated urgently, it can lead to airway obstruction requiring tracheostomy. Infection can spread to other fascial spaces of the head and neck, including the retrosternal space.

Conclusions

Having a thorough understanding of the anatomic structures of the periodontium and the surrounding hard and soft tissues, including innervation and vasculature, is essential for periodontal and implant surgical procedures. Knowledge of anatomy and function is important for proper execution of surgical procedures, as well as to minimize the risk of injury and complications. The spatial relationship of bones, muscles, blood vessels, and nerves, as well as the anatomic spaces located in the vicinity of the periodontal or implant surgical field, are particularly important. This chapter describes anatomic features that are significant to clinicians performing periodontal and implant surgical therapy.

Case Scenarios are found on the companion website eBooks.Health.Elsevier.com.

Suggested Readings

De Andrade E, Otomo-Corgel J, Pucher J, et al. The intraosseous course of the mandibular incisive nerve in the mandibular symphysis. *Int J Periodontics Restorative Dent*. 2001;21:591–597.

Elian N, Wallace S, Cho SC, et al. Distribution of the maxillary artery as it relates to sinus floor augmentation. *Int J Oral Maxillofac Implants*. 2005;20:784. –787.

Ella B, Noble Rda C, Lauverjat Y, et al. Septa within the sinus: effect on elevation of the sinus floor. *Br J Oral Maxillofac Surg*. 2008;46:464–467.

Ella B, Sedarat C, Noble Rda C, et al. Vascular connections of the lateral wall of the sinus: surgical effect in sinus augmentation. *Int J Oral Maxillofac Implants*. 2008;23:1047–1052.

Greenstein G, Tarnow D. The mental foramen and nerve: clinical and anatomical factors related to dental implant placement: a literature review. *J Periodontol*. 2006;77:1933–1943.

Haas LF, Dutra K, Porporatti AL, et al. Anatomical variations of mandibular canal detected by panoramic radiography and CT: a systematic review and meta-analysis. *Dentomaxillofac Radiol*. 2016;45:20150310.

Kiesselbach JE, Chamberlain JG. Clinical and anatomic observations on the relationship of the lingual nerve to the mandibular third molar region. *J Oral Maxillofac Surg*. 1984;42:565–567.

Ngeow WC, Chai WL. The clinical anatomy of accessory mandibular canal in dentistry. *Clin Anat*. 2020;33:1214–1227.

Schriber M, Bornstein MM, Suter VGA. Is the pneumatisation of the maxillary sinus following tooth loss a reality? A retrospective analysis using cone beam computed tomography and a customised software program. *Clin Oral Investig.* 2019;23(3):1349–1358. https://doi.org/10.1007/s00784-018-2552-5. Epub 2018 Jul 17. PMID: 30014166.

Spilka CJ. Pathways of dental infections. *J Oral Surg*. 1966;24:111–124.

Topazian RG, Morton H, Goldberg MH, et al. *Oral and maxillofacial Infections*. London: Saunders; 2002.

Uchida Y, Noguchi N, Goto M, et al. Measurement of anterior loop length for the mandibular canal and diameter of the mandibular incisive canal to avoid nerve damage when installing **endosseous** implants in the interforaminal region: a second attempt introducing cone beam computed tomography. *J Oral Maxillofac Surg*. 2009;67:744–750.

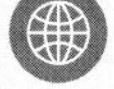

References for this chapter are found on the companion website eBooks.Health.Elsevier.com.

CHAPTER 60

General Principles of Periodontal Surgery

Perry R. Klokkevold | Henry H. Takei | Fermin A. Carranza

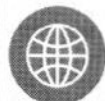 For online-only content on the treatment of root sensitivity and hospital periodontal surgery, please visit the companion website at eBooks.Health.Elsevier.com.

CHAPTER OUTLINE

All periodontal surgical procedures must be carefully planned and executed. Clinicians must be knowledgeable and prepared for the surgical procedure as well as any untoward outcomes. Likewise, they need to prepare the patient medically, psychologically, and practically for all aspects of the surgical intervention. This chapter reviews general considerations that are common to all periodontal surgical procedures, including preparation of the patient, surgical instruments, intraoperative and postsurgical considerations, and management. Finally, although periodontal surgical procedures are usually performed in the dental office, an online section of this chapter briefly discusses situations that may require hospitalization and treatment using general anesthesia in the operating room.

Presurgical Patient Preparation

Reevaluation After Phase I Therapy

Most patients with periodontitis will have an initial or preparatory phase of therapy, which consists of patient education and thorough root instrumentation (scaling and root planing) to debride and remove all root surface accretions, endotoxins, or other irritants responsible for the periodontal inflammation. When these procedures are executed well and combined with good daily biofilm control, the results will: (1) eliminate some pockets entirely; (2) render the periodontal tissues firm and consistent, thereby facilitating the ability to perform more accurate and less invasive surgery; and (3) acquaint the patient with the office, the clinician, and the assistants, thereby reducing the patient's apprehension and fear.

LEARNING BOX 60.1

Phase I therapy and reevaluation are important to reduce periodontal inflammation, improve periodontal condition, and minimize the need for periodontal surgery. When thorough root instrumentation is performed by the clinician and excellent daily biofilm removal is completed by the patient, some cases will not require surgical therapy, or if it is necessary, the extent of required surgical intervention can be minimized.

The reevaluation phase consists of reprobing and reexamining all of the pertinent findings that previously indicated the need for surgery. The persistence of findings, such as deep pocket depth, confirms the indication for surgery. The number of surgical procedures, the anticipated outcome, and the postoperative care necessary should be determined and explained to the patient before scheduling treatment. Once the important information regarding the surgery is discussed, a final decision is made that incorporates any necessary adjustments to the original plan.

Premedication

For patients who are not medically compromised, the value of administering antibiotics for periodontal surgery has not been clearly demonstrated.[36] Given the very low incidence of infection after periodontal surgery, there does not seem to be justification for the prophylactic use of antibiotics in healthy patients.[38,41] Some older studies reported reduced postoperative complications, including reduced pain and swelling, when antibiotics are given before periodontal surgery and continued for 4 to 7 days after surgery.[5,13,24,39]

The prophylactic use of antibiotics in patients who are otherwise healthy has been advocated for bone-grafting procedures and purported to enhance the results. Although the rationale for such use appears logical, published research to support it is scant. A systematic review of the literature assessing randomized controlled clinical trials (RCTs) and systematic reviews and meta-analyses that reported results of preventive antibiotic therapy for bone augmentation procedures in oral implantology found only one systematic review and four RCTs that met the inclusion criteria.[47] The conclusion from this systematic review of bone augmentation for oral implantology recommended the prescription of 2 or 3 g of amoxicillin 1 hour prior to surgery to reduce early failure of one-stage implants and to decrease bacterial loads in grafted bone. A survey of prescribing practices, among periodontists in California, for periodontal surgery confirmed there is a greater tendency for clinicians to prescribe antibiotics when bone grafts are used as opposed to when periodontal surgery is performed without the addition of bone grafts.[18] In any case, the risks inherent in the administration of antibiotics should be evaluated together with the potential benefits.

Additional presurgical medications that may be administered include a nonsteroidal antiinflammatory drug such as ibuprofen (e.g., Motrin) 1 hour before the procedure, and rinsing with an antimicrobial mouthrinse such as 0.12% chlorhexidine gluconate (e.g., Peridex or PerioGard).[48]

Precautions to be taken with medically compromised patients are discussed in Chapter 67.

Smoking

The deleterious effect of smoking on the healing of periodontal wounds has been amply documented (see Chapter 23).[23,42,53] Patients should be clearly informed about the adverse effect of smoking and advised to quit completely or to stop smoking for a minimum of 3 to 4 weeks after the procedure. For patients who are unwilling to follow this advice, an alternative treatment plan that does not include complex procedures (e.g., regenerative, mucogingival, esthetic) should be considered.

Informed Consent

Obtaining informed consent from the patient for surgical treatment is essential. The patient should be informed at the initial visit regarding the diagnosis, prognosis, and recommended treatment options that include explanations about expected outcomes. The pros and cons of each approach should be discussed prior to scheduling the surgery, and the patient should be encouraged to ask questions. On the day of surgery, the patient should again be reminded about the procedure to be performed, including the risks and expected outcomes. Patients should be given the opportunity to ask any additional questions, and, once their questions are answered, they should indicate their agreement to undergo the procedure by signing the informed consent.

Emergency Equipment

The clinician, all assistants, and office personnel should be trained to handle all possible medical emergencies that could arise. Each member of the team needs to know their role should an emergency situation present. Drugs and equipment for medical emergencies should be routinely checked for expiration and readily available at all times.

Syncope, which is a transient loss of consciousness caused by a reduction in cerebral blood flow, is the most common emergency. It is often precipitated by fear and anxiety. The syncope event is usually preceded by a feeling of weakness, and then the patient experiences pallor, sweating, coldness of the extremities, dizziness, and a slowing of the pulse. The patient should be placed in a supine position with the legs elevated; tight clothes should be loosened, and a wide-open airway should be ensured. Oxygen administration should be started. Unconsciousness may persist for a few minutes. A previous history of syncope during dental appointments should be explored before the treatment is started. If the patient has had other experiences with syncope, every effort should be made to minimize the patient's fear and anxiety. The use of oral sedatives should be considered as well.

It is important to be prepared for any medical emergency. The reader is referred to Chapter 58 and other texts for details and a complete analysis of this important topic.[3,32,33]

Infection Control

Preventing the transmission of infections to the dental team or to other patients is a critical precaution that must be a part of every appointment in the dental office, especially with the threat of life-threatening infections, which are transmitted through body fluids. In the dental setting, blood-borne viruses including hepatitis B virus (HBV), hepatitis C virus (HCV), and human immunodeficiency virus (HIV), along with respiratory pathogens, present the highest risks of cross-infection.[21] Universal precautions, the use of personal protective equipment (PPE), and barrier techniques must be incorporated into the surgical protocol for every procedure. These include the use of disposable sterile gloves, gowns, caps, surgical masks, and protective eyewear. All surfaces that may be contaminated with blood or saliva but that cannot be sterilized (e.g., light handles, chairs) must be covered with sterile aluminum foil or plastic wrap. Aerosol-producing devices (e.g., ultrasonic scalers) should not be used on patients with suspected infections, and their use should be kept to a minimum in all other patients. This is especially true for preventing the spread of contagious infections, such as the SARS-Co-V2 coronavirus, which is an airborne pathogen and a concern for dental offices, but adhering to safe infection prevention practices, including screening patients for symptoms should mitigate the risk.

At the conclusion of each procedure, all instruments, handpieces, and burs must be properly cleansed of biologic debris in ultrasonic cleaners, dried, packaged, and sterilized. Excised tissues and contaminated gauze must be disposed as biohazard waste, and sharps (i.e., needles and blades) need to be carefully removed and disposed in special sharps containers.

Surgical Instruments

Periodontal surgery is accomplished with a set of instruments designed for incision, flap reflection, debridement, recontouring, root instrumentation, and suturing; Fig. 60.1 shows a typical surgical cassette. Periodontal surgical instruments are classified as follows: (1) incisional and excisional instruments, (2) periosteal elevators, (3) surgical curettes and sickles, (4) surgical chisels, (5) tissue forceps, (6) scissors, and (7) needle holders.

Incisional and Excisional Instruments

Periodontal Knives (Gingivectomy Knives)

The Kirkland knife is representative of the knives that are typically used for gingivectomy. These knives can be obtained as either double-ended or single-ended instruments. The entire periphery of these kidney-shaped knives is the cutting edge (Fig. 60.2A).

Interdental Knives

The Orban knife #1 and #2 (see Fig. 60.2B), and the Merrifield knife #1 through #4 are examples of knives that can be used for interdental areas. These spear-shaped knives have cutting edges on both sides of the blade, and they are designed with either double-ended or single-ended blades.

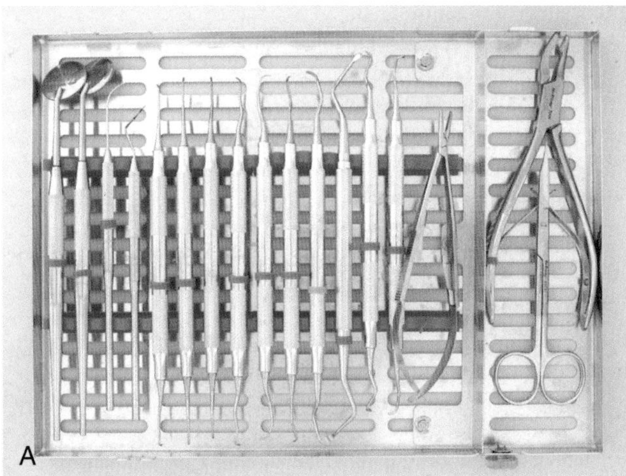

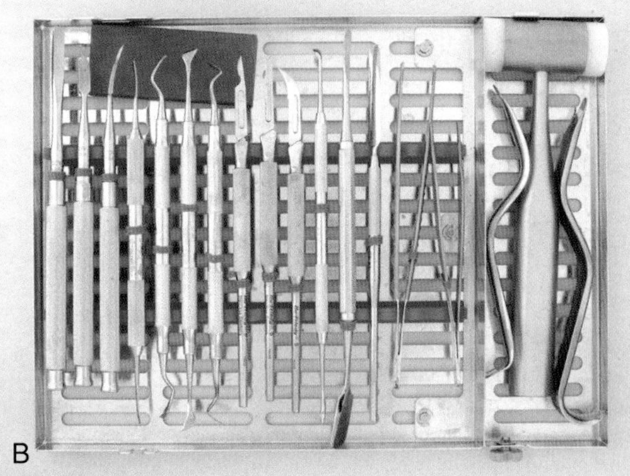

Fig. 60.1 A typical series of periodontal surgical instruments, divided into two cassettes. (A) *From left,* Mirrors, explorer, probe, series of curettes, needle holder, rongeurs, and scissors. (B) *From left,* Series of chisels, Kirkland knife, Orban knife, scalpel handles with surgical blades (#15C, #15, and #12D), periosteal elevators, spatula, tissue forceps, cheek retractors, and mallet; also shown is a sharpening stone. (A, Courtesy Hu-Friedy, Chicago, IL. B, Courtesy G. Hartzell & Son, Concord, CA.)

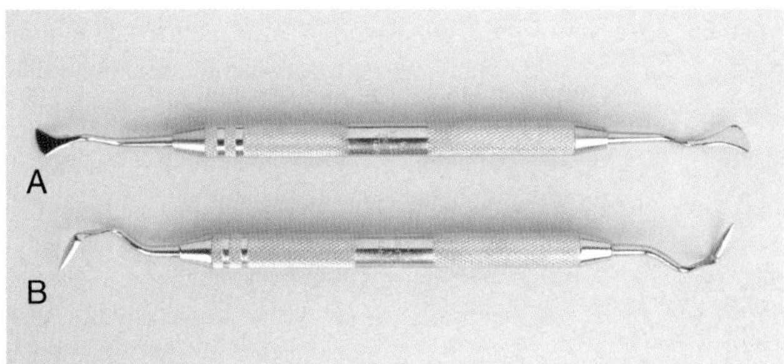

Fig. 60.2 Gingivectomy knives. (A) Kirkland knife. (B) Orban interdental knife.

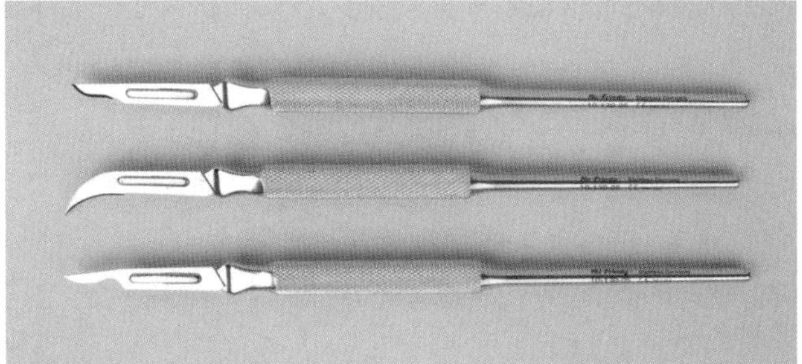

Fig. 60.3 Surgical blades. *Top to bottom,* #15, #12D, and #15C. These blades are disposable.

Surgical Blades

A variety of scalpel blades with different shapes and sizes are available for use in periodontal surgery. The most common blades are #12D, #15, and #15C (Fig. 60.3). The #12D blade is a curved, beak-shaped blade with cutting edges on both sides that allow the operator to engage narrow, restricted areas with both pushing and pulling cutting motions. The #15 blade is used for thinning the flaps and is also used for general purposes. The #15C blade, which is a narrower version of the #15 blade, is useful for making the initial, scalloping-type incision. The slim design of this blade allows for incising into the narrow interdental portion of the flap. All of these blades are disposable and must be discarded after one patient use. The contact of blades with the bone, teeth, or dense tissues during procedures will dull the edge and may require changing the blade. Currently, there are an enormous variety of mini and micro scalpel blades available in different shapes and sizes for use in microsurgical techniques. See Chapter 68.

Electrosurgery (Radiosurgery)

The terms electrosurgery and radiosurgery[49] are currently used to identify surgical techniques performed on soft tissue with the use of controlled, high-frequency electrical (radio) currents in the range of 1.5 to 7.5 million cycles per second (megahertz). Three classes of active electrodes are available: single-wire electrodes for incising or excising; loop electrodes for planing tissue; and heavier, bulkier electrodes for coagulation procedures.[17,35]

The four basic types of electrosurgical techniques are electrosection, electrocoagulation, electrofulguration, and electrodesiccation. Electrosection, which is also referred to as electrotomy or acusection, is used for incisions, excisions, and tissue planing. Incisions and excisions are performed with single-wire active electrodes that can be bent or adapted to accomplish any type of cutting procedure. Electrocoagulation provides a wide range of coagulation and hemorrhage control by using the electrocoagulation current. Electrocoagulation can prevent bleeding or hemorrhage at the initial entry into soft tissue, but it cannot stop bleeding once it is present. All forms of hemorrhage must be stopped first by some form of direct pressure (e.g., compress, hemostat). After bleeding has momentarily stopped, the final sealing of the capillaries or large vessels can be accomplished with a short application of the electrocoagulation current. The active electrodes that are used for coagulation are much bulkier than the fine tungsten wire used for electrosection. Electrosection and electrocoagulation are the procedures that are most often used in all areas of dentistry. Two monoterminal techniques, electrofulguration and electrodesiccation, are not used in dentistry.

The most important basic rule of the use of electrosurgery is *always keep the tip moving*. The prolonged or repeated application of current to tissue induces heat accumulation and undesired tissue destruction, whereas interrupted application at intervals adequate for tissue cooling (5 to 10 seconds) reduces or eliminates heat buildup. Electrosurgery is not intended to destroy tissue; it is a controllable means of sculpturing or modifying oral soft tissue with little discomfort and hemorrhage for the patient. Electrosurgery is contraindicated for patients who have incompatible or poorly shielded cardiac pacemakers.

Lasers

Lasers are used in periodontal therapy for surgical procedures such as gingivectomy, flap surgery, and crown lengthening. They are also used for nonsurgical procedures such as depigmentation, nonsurgical periodontal therapy, decontamination and antimicrobial therapy, and biomodulation. However, their use and effectiveness remain controversial, and the evidence to support the advantages of laser therapy is limited at this time.[9,34]

A variety of lasers have been used in periodontics, including diode, Nd:YAG, Er:YAG, Er,Cr,YSGG, and CO_2. See Chapter 64 for a description of laser types. Selection of the laser type is based on the wavelength and the amount of energy transmitted to the tissue during a procedure. Photothermal energy is measured in watts (W = joules/second) and hertz (Hz = cycles/second). The energy beam can be delivered in a continuous or pulsed manner. A continuous laser transmits more energy than a pulsed laser because there are momentary breaks or cooling periods in the latter. When comparing lasers and laser therapy outcomes, it is imperative to consider the type of laser, the wavelength, and the amount of energy delivered to tissues including watts, hertz, and total time of exposure. Care must be taken to avoid delivering excessive thermal energy to the tissues. The amount of energy delivered is critical to the desired outcome. Although the optimal energy delivered to tissues can be advantageous, excessive energy may be adverse. Consider the results of a study comparing incision wound healing made with a scalpel versus Nd:YAG laser at two different power settings. Healing was best following the incision with the laser applied at 1.75 W, 20 Hz, and worst when the energy was increased to 3 W, 20 Hz. The scalpel incision healed better than the laser incision at the higher energy setting.[43]

The selective absorption by water makes erbium lasers (Er:YAG, Er,Cr:YSGG) effective for both soft and hard tissue procedures. Among the various lasers used in periodontics, it is generally accepted that erbium lasers can be used effectively for nonsurgical and surgical periodontal treatments without producing major side effects or complications. Erbium laser ablation wounds heal rapidly due to very little thermal effects, shallow penetration depth, minimal tissue damage, and a low inflammatory response.[4]

Periosteal Elevators

Periosteal elevators are used to reflect and move the flap after the incision has been made. The Woodson and Prichard elevators are well-designed periosteal instruments for flap elevation (Fig. 60.4).

Surgical Curettes and Sickles

Larger and heavier curettes and sickles are often needed during surgery for the removal of granulation tissue, fibrous interdental tissues, and tenacious subgingival deposits. The Prichard surgical curette (Fig. 60.5) and the Kirkland surgical instruments are heavy curettes, whereas the Ball scaler (#B2 and #B3) is a popular heavy sickle. The wider, heavier blades of these instruments are suitable for surgical procedures that require reflection of firmly bound fibrous tissues and the removal of granulation tissue and tenacious calculus.

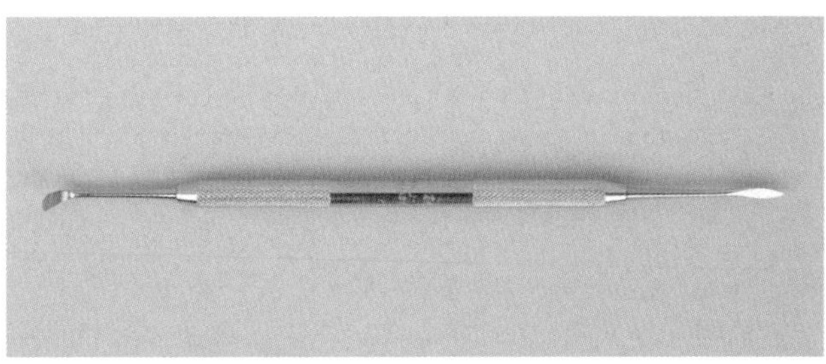

Fig. 60.4 Woodson periosteal elevator.

Surgical Chisels

The back-action chisel (Fig. 60.6) is used with a pulling motion, whereas the straight chisel (e.g., Wedelstaedt, Ochsenbein #1 and #2) is used with a pushing motion. The Ochsenbein chisel (Fig. 60.7) is a useful chisel with a semicircular indentation on both sides of the shank that allows the instrument to engage around the tooth and into the interdental area. The Rhodes chisel is another popular back-action chisel that has an edge that is offset from the shank. These are particularly useful for removing and recontouring bone with a pull stroke.

Tissue Forceps

The tissue forceps is used to hold the flap during reflection, suturing, or other flap manipulation. This instrument is also used to position and displace the flap after it has been reflected. They are available in a variety of lengths, angles, and sizes. The tips can be serrated or flat and available with or without teeth. The DeBakey tissue forceps is an efficient instrument for the atraumatic grasping and manipulating of flaps (Fig. 60.8).

Scissors

Scissors and nippers are used in periodontal surgery to remove tabs of tissue during gingivectomy, to trim the margins of flaps, to enlarge incisions in periodontal abscesses, and to remove muscle attachments in mucogingival surgery. They are also used to cut sutures during wound closure. Many types are available, and individual

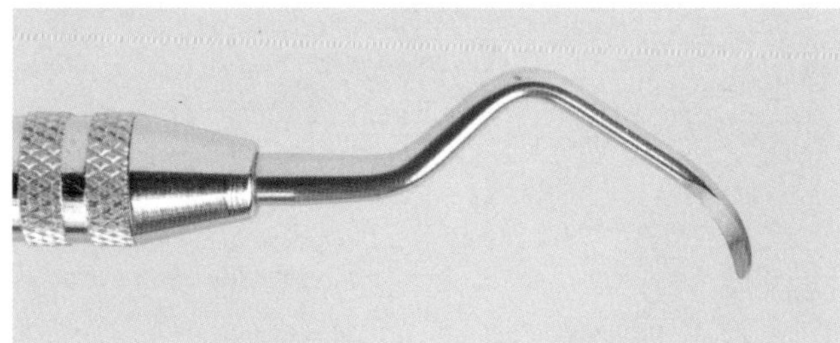

Fig. 60.5 A Prichard surgical curette. The curettes that are used in surgery have wider blades than those that are used for conventional scaling and root planing.

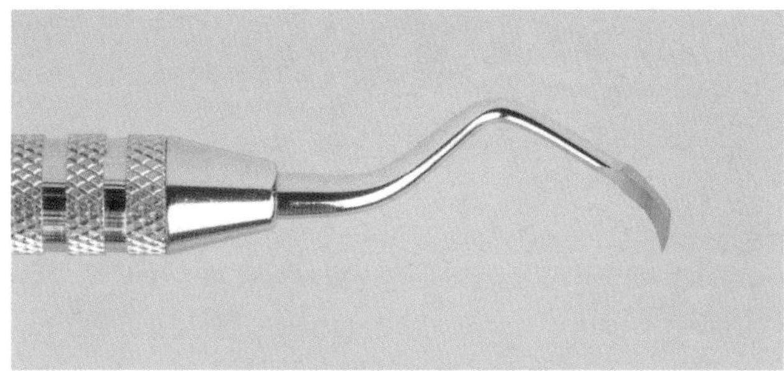

Fig. 60.6 Back-action chisel.

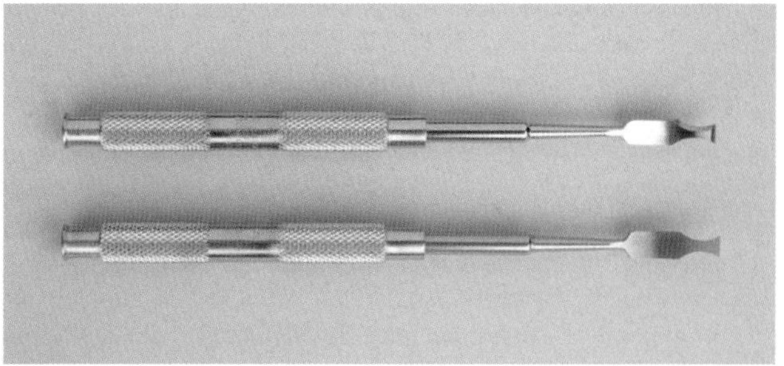

Fig. 60.7 Ochsenbein chisels are paired, with their cutting edges in opposite directions.

preference determines the choice. The Goldman–Fox #16 scissors have a curved, beveled blade with serrations (Fig. 60.9).

Needle Holders

Needle holders are used to suture the flap at the desired position after the surgical procedure has been completed. In addition to the regular types of needle holders (Fig. 60.10A), the Castroviejo needle holder is used for delicate, precise techniques that require quick and easy grasp and release of the suture needle (see Fig. 60.10B).

Intraoperative Surgical Considerations

Sedation and Anesthesia

Pain control during periodontal surgery is very important. Most procedures should be painless. The patient should be assured of this at the beginning and throughout the procedure. The most reliable means of providing painless surgery is the effective administration of local anesthesia. The area to be treated should be thoroughly anesthetized by means of regional block and local infiltration. Injections directly into the interdental papillae may also be helpful.

Apprehensive and neurotic patients may require special management with antianxiety or sedative-hypnotic agents. Modalities for the administration of these agents include inhalation, oral, intramuscular, and intravenous routes. The specific agents and the modality of administration are based on the desired level of sedation, the anticipated length of the procedure, and the overall condition of the patient. Specifically, the patient's medical history and physical and emotional status should be considered when determining the need for sedation, as well as the specific agents and techniques to be used. See Chapter 58 for a detailed description of conscious sedation methods.

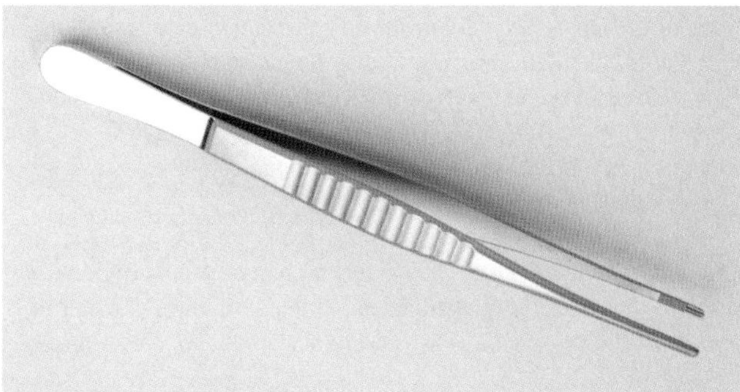

Fig. 60.8 DeBakey tissue forceps.

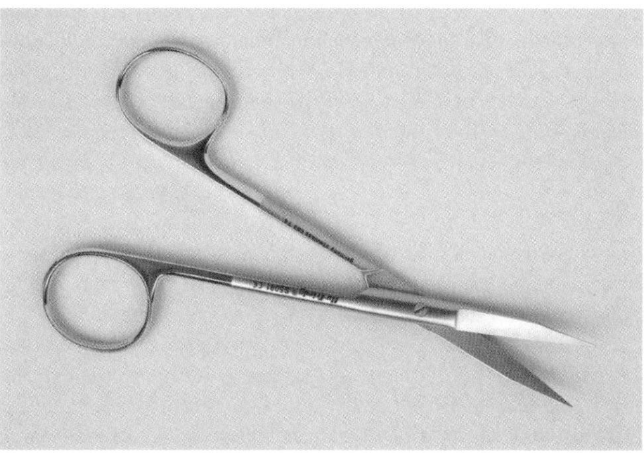

Fig. 60.9 Goldman-Fox scissors.

Tissue Management

It is important to manage tissues well during surgery to optimize healing and minimize postoperative discomfort. There are some specific guidelines to follow including operating gently, ensuring that instruments are sharp and monitoring the patient at all times.

1. *Operate gently and carefully.* In addition to being most considerate to the patient, this is also the most effective way to operate. Tissue manipulation should be precise, deliberate, and gentle. It is essential to be thorough, but traumatic instrumentation and aggressive tissue manipulation must be avoided because it produces excessive tissue injury, causes postoperative discomfort, and delays healing.
2. *Be certain that the instruments are sharp.* Instruments must be sharp to be effective; a successful treatment outcome will be more likely when using sharp instruments. Dull instruments inflict unnecessary trauma as a result of inefficient cutting and excessive forces applied to compensate for their ineffectiveness. A sterile sharpening stone should be available on the operating table at all times. Sharpening instruments during a procedure is essential and may be necessary.
3. *Observe the patient at all times.* It is important to pay careful attention to the patient's reactions. Facial expressions, pallor, and perspiration are distinct signs that may indicate when a patient is experiencing pain, anxiety, or fear. The clinician's responsiveness to these signs can be the difference between success and failure.

Root Instrumentation

Although root instrumentation (scaling and root planing) may have been performed previously as part of the initial phase I therapy, all exposed root surfaces should be carefully inspected, explored, and instrumented as needed during the surgical procedure. In particular, areas of difficult

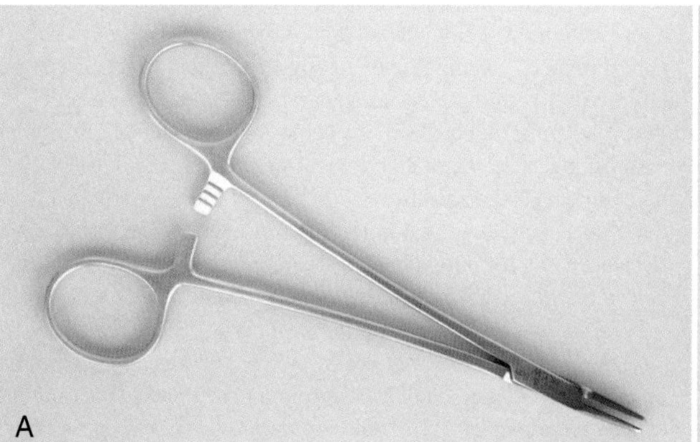

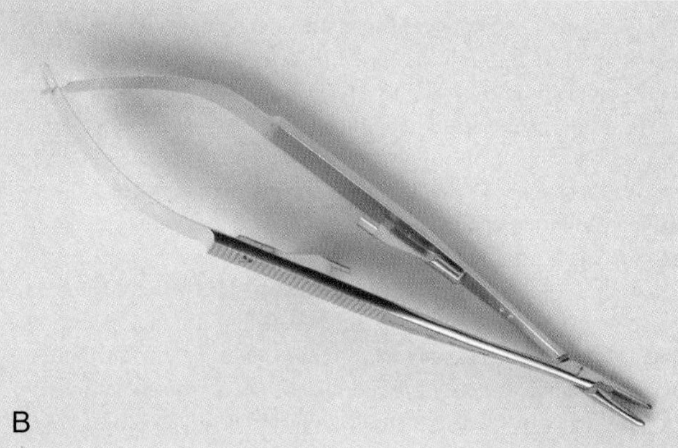

Fig. 60.10 (A) Conventional needle holder. (B) Castroviejo needle holder.

access (e.g., furcations, deep infrabony pockets) often have rough areas or residual calculus that was inaccessible or undetected during the preparatory sessions. The assistant who is retracting the tissues and using the aspirator should also check for the presence of calculus and the smoothness of each surface from a different angle.

LEARNING BOX 60.2

The most important objective of periodontal pocket reduction surgery is to gain access to the root surface for root instrumentation (scaling and root planing). The exposure obtained to the subgingival root surfaces when the flap is reflected allows not only access for visualization and root instrumentation but also the opportunity to reduce and recontour osseous defects.

Hemostasis

Hemostasis is an important aspect of periodontal surgery because good intraoperative control of bleeding permits accurate visualization of the extent of disease, the pattern of bone destruction, and the anatomy and condition of the root surfaces. It provides the operator with a clear view of the surgical site, which is essential for wound debridement and root instrumentation. In addition, good hemostasis also prevents excessive loss of blood into the mouth, oropharynx, and stomach.

Periodontal surgery can produce profuse bleeding, especially during the initial incisions and flap reflection. Once the flap is reflected and granulation tissue is removed, bleeding stops or will be considerably reduced. Control of the typical intraoperative bleeding can be managed with aspiration. Continuous suctioning of the surgical site with an aspirator is indispensable when performing periodontal surgery. The application of pressure to the surgical wound with moist gauze can be a helpful adjunct to control site-specific bleeding. Intraoperative bleeding that is not controlled with these simple methods may indicate a more serious problem and require additional control measures. High blood pressure is a condition that will often cause excessive bleeding during surgery. Blood pressure measurements should be taken for all patients prior to surgery, and procedures should be rescheduled if it is not in the normal range.

Excessive hemorrhaging after initial incisions and flap reflection may be caused by the laceration of venules, arterioles, or larger vessels. Fortunately, the laceration of medium or large vessels is rare because incisions near highly vascular anatomic areas (e.g., the posterior mandible [the lingual and inferior alveolar arteries], the posterior midpalatal regions [the greater palatine arteries]) are avoided by incision and flap procedures. Proper design of the flaps that takes these areas into consideration will help avoid these accidents (see Chapter 59). However, even when all anatomic precautions are taken, it is possible to cause bleeding from medium or large vessels due to anatomic variations that occur resulting in inadvertent laceration. If a medium or large vessel is lacerated, a suture around the bleeding end may be necessary to control the hemorrhage. Pressure should be applied through the tissue to determine the location that will stop blood flow from the severed vessel. A suture can then be passed through the tissue at that point and tied to restrict blood flow. Excessive bleeding from a surgical wound may also result from incisions across a capillary plexus. Minor areas of persistent bleeding from capillaries can usually be stopped by applying cold pressure to the site with moist gauze for several minutes.

The use of a local anesthetic with a vasoconstrictor (epinephrine) may also be useful for controlling minor bleeding from the periodontal flap. Both of these methods act through vasoconstriction, thereby reducing the flow of blood through incised small vessels and capillaries. This action is relatively short lived, and it should not be relied on for long-term postoperative hemostasis. It is important to avoid the use of vasoconstrictors to control bleeding just before sending a patient home. If a more serious bleeding problem exists or if a firm blood clot is not established, bleeding is likely to recur when the vasoconstrictor has metabolized and the patient is no longer in the office.

LEARNING BOX 60.3

Along with the usual procedures to help control hemorrhage during surgery (pressure; irrigation with cold, sterile water; removal of granulation tissue) the use of local anesthesia with epinephrine is helpful. It is important to remember that this action is effective for a short duration and should not be used toward the end of the surgical procedure to control bleeding. When the patient is dismissed from the appointment and the effect of the vasoconstriction is no longer present, bleeding may recur at home.

For a slow, constant blood flow and for oozing, hemostasis may be achieved with hemostatic agents. Absorbable gelatin sponge (Gelfoam), oxidized cellulose (Oxycel), oxidized regenerated cellulose (Surgicel Absorbable Hemostat), microfibrillar collagen hemostat (Avitene), collagen bovine/glycosaminoglycans (CollaCote, CollaTape, CollaPlug), and chitosan-based dressings (HemCon Dental Dressing Pro) are useful hemostatic agents for the control of bleeding in capillaries, small blood vessels, and deep wounds (Table 60.1).

Absorbable gelatin sponge is a porous matrix prepared from pork skin that helps to stabilize a normal blood clot. The sponge can be cut to the desired dimensions and either sutured in place or positioned within the wound (e.g., an extraction socket). It is absorbed in 4 to 6 weeks.

Oxidized cellulose is a chemically modified form of surgical gauze that forms an artificial clot. The material is friable, and it can be difficult to keep it in place. It is absorbed in 1 to 6 weeks.

Oxidized regenerated cellulose is prepared from cellulose via a reaction with alkali to form a chemically pure and uniform structure of oxidized cellulose. The material is prepared in a cloth or thin gauze form that can be cut to the desired size and sutured or layered on the bleeding surface. It can be used as a surface dressing because it does not impair epithelialization, and it is bactericidal against many gram-negative and gram-positive microorganisms that are both aerobic and anaerobic. Caution should be used if wounds are infected or have an increased potential to becoming infected (e.g., immunocompromised patients) because, although they have a bactericidal effect, the absorbable hemostatic agents can serve as a nidus for infection.

Microfibrillar collagen hemostat is type I collagen derived from bovine skin. It is commonly dispensed in a flour form but also comes in a nonwoven sponge form. It binds tightly to blood surfaces and causes the aggregation of platelets, thus working even when the field is not dry. In addition to its blood binding properties as a collagen product, it also activates platelets.

Collagen bovine/glycosaminoglycans is an absorbable collagen hemostat composed of purified and lyophilized bovine dermal collagen. It reduces bleeding when ligation and other conventional methods are ineffective or impractical.

Chitosan-based dressing is a hemostatic product that is capable of establishing hemostasis independent of the normal platelet aggregation and coagulation pathways.[25,26,40] The chitosan product has a positive molecular charge that attracts negatively charged red blood cells to create a clot forming a seal to stop bleeding. This product may have advantages for individuals on antiplatelet or anticoagulant medications.

Thrombin is a drug that is capable of hastening the process of blood clotting. It is intended for topical use only, and it is applied as a liquid or powder. Thrombin should never be injected into tissues because it can cause serious or even fatal intravascular coagulation. In addition, because thrombin is a bovine-derived material, caution should be used for any patient with a known allergic reaction to bovine products.

TABLE 60.1 Absorbable Hemostatic Agents

Generic (Brand)	Directions	Adverse Effects	Precautions
Absorbable gelatin sponge (Gelfoam)	May be cut into various sizes and applied to bleeding surfaces	May form nidus for infection or abscess	Should not be overpacked into extraction site or wound—may interfere with healing
Oxidized cellulose (Oxycel)	Most effective when applied to wound dry as opposed to moistened	May cause foreign body reaction	Extremely friable and difficult to place; should not be used adjacent to bone—impairs bone regeneration; should not be used as a surface dressing—inhibits epithelialization
Oxidized regenerated cellulose (Surgicel Absorbable Hemostat)	May be cut to various shapes and positioned over bleeding sites; thick or excessive amounts should not be used	Encapsulation, cyst formation, and foreign body reaction possible	Should not be placed in deep wounds—may physically interfere with wound healing and bone formation
Microfibrillar collagen hemostat (Avitene)	May be cut to shape and applied to bleeding surface	May potentiate abscess formation, hematoma, and wound dehiscence; possible allergic reaction or foreign body reaction	May interfere with wound healing; placement in extraction sockets has been associated with increased pain
Collagen hemostat/ glycosaminoglycans (CollaCote, CollaTape, CollaPlug)	May be cut to shape and applied to bleeding surface	May become infected	Do not use on infected or contaminated wounds
Chitosan-based dressing (HemCon Dental Dressing Pro)	May be trimmed to fit; most effective in presence of blood to wet surface	Contains chitosan from shellfish.	Sutures may be used but not always required since dressing sticks to wound. Do not place into wound with primary closure.
Thrombin (Thrombostat)	May be applied topically to bleeding surface	Allergic reaction can occur in patients with known sensitivity to bovine materials	Must not be injected into tissues or vasculature—can cause severe (and possibly fatal) clotting

Finally, it is imperative to recognize that excessive bleeding may be caused by systemic disorders, including (but not limited to) platelet deficiencies, coagulation defects, medications, and hypertension. As a precaution, all surgical patients should be asked about any current medications that may contribute to bleeding, any family history of bleeding disorders, and hypertension. All patients, regardless of health history, should have their blood pressure evaluated before surgery, and anyone who is diagnosed with hypertension must be advised to see a physician and improve control before surgery. Patients with known or suspected bleeding deficiencies or disorders must be carefully evaluated before any surgical procedure. A consultation with the patient's physician is recommended, and laboratory tests should be performed to assess the risk of bleeding. It may be necessary to refer the patient to a hematologist for a comprehensive workup and to coordinate the surgical plan for managing hemostasis.

LEARNING BOX 60.4

Thrombin is a very effective drug to help coagulate blood and is applied topically. This drug should never be injected into tissues because it can cause serious or even fatal intravascular coagulation. In addition, thrombin is a bovine-derived drug, so caution should be used for patients with a known allergy to bovine products.

Postsurgical Management

Periodontal Dressings (Periodontal Packs)

At completion of the periodontal surgical procedure, clinicians may elect to cover the area with a periodontal dressing. In general, dressings have no curative properties but assist healing by protecting the tissue rather than providing "healing factors." The dressing minimizes the likelihood of postoperative infection, facilitates healing by preventing surface trauma during mastication, and protects the patient from pain induced by contact of the wound with food or with the tongue during mastication. For a complete literature review on this subject, see the article by Sachs and colleagues.[46] In a study comparing the postoperative pain experienced by patients with and without periodontal dressings, Checchi and Trombelli reported no significant difference between treatment groups with respect to frequency of analgesic use.[11] Most patients stated a psychological feeling of protection with the periodontal dressing.

Zinc Oxide–Eugenol Dressing

Dressings that are based on the reaction of zinc oxide and eugenol include the Wonder Pak, which was developed by Ward[56] in 1923, and several other dressings that use modified forms of Ward's original formula. The addition of accelerators, such as zinc acetate gives the material better working time.

Zinc oxide–eugenol dressings are supplied as a liquid and a powder that are mixed before use. Eugenol in this type of dressing may induce an allergic reaction that produces reddening of the area and burning pain in some patients.

Noneugenol Dressing

The reaction between a metallic oxide and fatty acids is the basis for Coe-Pak, which is the most widely used periodontal dressing in the United States. This is supplied in two tubes, the contents of which are mixed immediately before use until a uniform color is obtained. One tube contains zinc oxide, an oil (for plasticity), a gum (for cohesiveness), and lorothidol (a fungicide).

The other tube contains liquid coconut fatty acids that have been thickened with colophony resin (or rosin) and chlorothymol (a bacteriostatic agent).[46,50] This dressing does not contain asbestos or eugenol, thereby avoiding the problems associated with these substances.

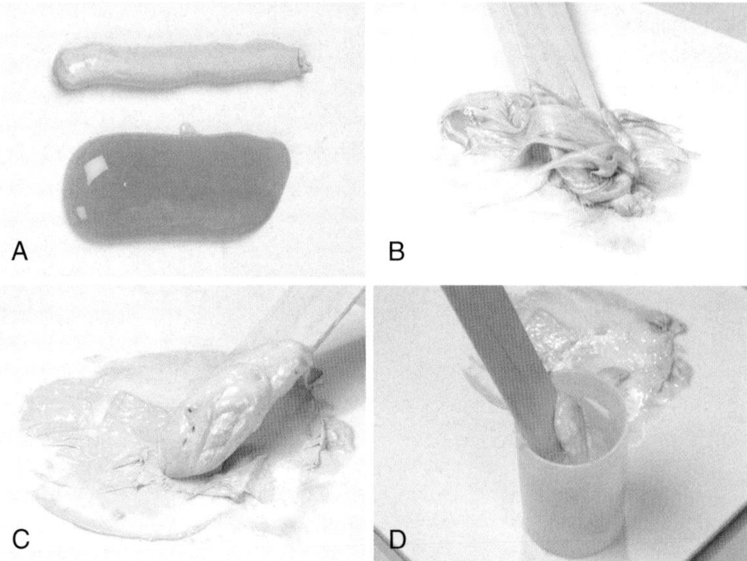

Fig. 60.11 Preparing the surgical pack (Coe-Pak). (A) Equal lengths of the two pastes are placed on a paper pad. (B) The pastes are mixed with a wooden tongue depressor for 2 or 3 minutes until (C) the paste loses its tackiness. (D) The mixed paste is placed in a paper cup of water at room temperature. With lubricated fingers, it is then rolled into cylinders and placed on the surgical wound.

Other noneugenol dressings include cyanoacrylates[8,22,29] and tissue conditioners (methacrylate gels).[2] However, these products are not in common use.

Retention of Dressing

Periodontal dressings are usually kept in place mechanically by interlocking the dressing in interdental spaces and joining the lingual and facial portions of the dressing. In isolated teeth or when several teeth in an arch are missing, retention of the dressing may be difficult. Numerous reinforcements, splints, and stents for this purpose have been described.[19,20,57] The placement of dental floss tied loosely around the teeth enhances retention of the dressing.

Antibacterial Properties of Dressing

Improved healing and patient comfort with less odor and foul taste[8] have been obtained by incorporating antibiotics into the dressing. Bacitracin,[7] oxytetracycline (Terramycin),[14] neomycin, and nitrofurazone have been used. Care must be taken when any antibiotic products are used because they may produce hypersensitivity reactions. The emergence of resistant organisms and opportunistic infections has also been reported.[45] The incorporation of tetracycline powder into the Coe-Pak is generally recommended, particularly when long and traumatic surgical procedures are performed.

Allergy

Contact allergies to eugenol and rosin have been reported.[44]

Preparation and Application of Dressing

Zinc oxide dressings are mixed with eugenol or noneugenol liquids on a wax paper pad with a spatula or a wooden tongue depressor. The powder is gradually incorporated with the liquid until a thick paste is formed.

Coe-Pak is prepared by mixing equal lengths of paste from tubes that contain the accelerator and the base until the resulting paste is a uniform color (Fig. 60.11A–C). A capsule of tetracycline powder can be added at this time. The dressing is then placed in a cup of water at room temperature (see Fig. 60.11D). After 2 to 3 minutes, the paste loses its tackiness, and it can be handled and molded. The mixed dressing remains workable for 15 to 20 minutes. The working time can be shortened by adding a small amount of zinc oxide to the accelerator (pink paste) before spatulating.

The dressing is then rolled into two strips that are approximately the length of the treated area. The end of one strip is bent into a hook shape and fitted around the distal surface of the last tooth to approach that tooth from the distal surface (Fig. 60.12A). The remainder of the strip is brought forward along the facial surface to the midline and gently pressed into place along the gingival margin and interproximally. The second strip is applied from the lingual surface. It is joined to the dressing at the distal surface of the last tooth and then brought forward along the gingival margin to the midline and gently pressed (see Fig. 60.12B). The strips are joined interproximally by applying gentle pressure on the facial and lingual surfaces of the dressing (see Fig. 60.12C). For isolated teeth separated by edentulous spaces, the dressing should be made continuous from tooth to tooth to cover the edentulous areas (Fig. 60.13).

When split-thickness flaps have been performed, the area should be covered with a sterile tinfoil to protect the wound and sutures before the dressing is placed.

The dressing should cover the gingiva, but overextension onto uninvolved mucosa should be avoided. *Excess dressing irritates the mucobuccal fold and the floor of the mouth, and it interferes with the tongue.* Overextension also jeopardizes retention of the dressing because the excess tends to break off and loosens the dressing from the operated area. *Dressing that covers occlusal surfaces or otherwise interferes with the occlusion should be removed before the patient is dismissed* (Fig. 60.14). Failure to do this causes discomfort and jeopardizes retention of the dressing.

The operator should ask the patient to move the tongue forcibly out and to each side, and the cheek and lips should be displaced in all directions to mold the dressing while it is still soft. After the dressing has set, it should be trimmed to eliminate all excess.

As a general rule, the dressing is kept on for 1 week after surgery. This guideline is based on the usual timetable of healing and clinical experience. It is not a rigid requirement; the period may be extended, or the area may be redressed for an additional week.

Portions of the dressing may not remain during the week, but this should not present a problem. If the dressing is lost from the operated area and the patient is uncomfortable, it is usually best to redress the

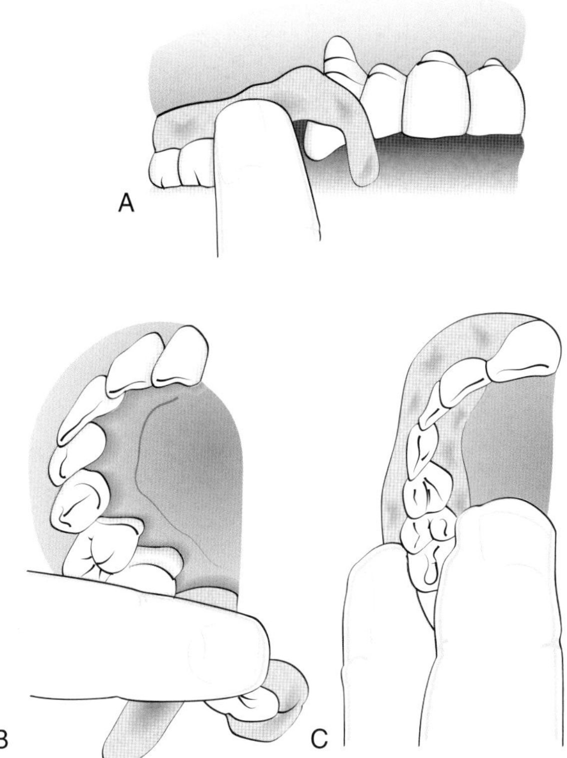

Fig. 60.12 Inserting the periodontal pack. (A) A strip of pack is hooked around the last molar and pressed into place anteriorly. (B) The lingual pack is joined to the facial strip at the distal surface of the last molar and fitted into place anteriorly. (C) Gentle pressure on the facial and lingual surfaces joins the pack interproximally.

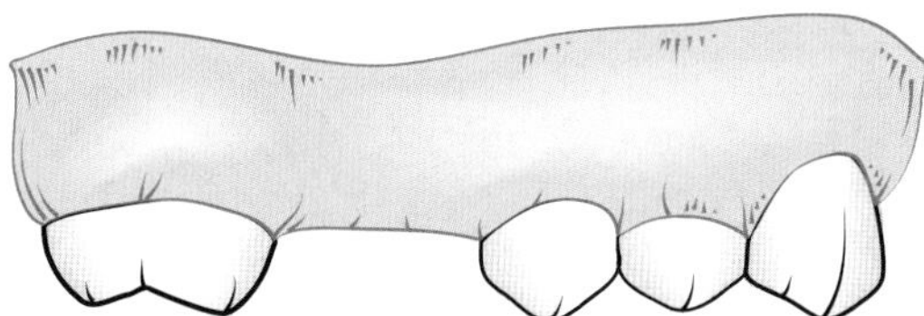

Fig. 60.13 Continuous pack covers the edentulous space.

area. The clinician should remove the remaining dressing, irrigate the area with warm water, and apply a topical anesthetic before replacing the dressing, which is then retained for another week. The excess dressing should be trimmed away with care taken to ensure that the new margin is not rough before the patient is dismissed.

Postoperative Instructions

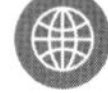

After the dressing is placed, postoperative instructions (eBox 60.1, online) are given verbally and in writing before the patient is dismissed from the chair.

First Postoperative Week

When the therapy is properly performed, periodontal surgery should present minimal postoperative problems. If biofilm control is compromised, patients can be instructed to rinse with 0.12% chlorhexidine gluconate (Peridex, PerioGard) immediately after the surgical procedure and twice daily thereafter until normal biofilm control can be resumed.[37,48,55] The following complications may arise during the first postoperative week, although they are the exception rather than the rule:

1. *Persistent bleeding after surgery.* The dressing is removed, and local anesthesia may be needed before the bleeding areas are located. The bleeding is stopped with pressure, or if necessary, the area may have to be anesthetized and resutured. After the bleeding has been stopped, the area is again redressed.
2. *Sensitivity to percussion.* Extension of inflammation into the periodontal ligament may cause sensitivity to percussion. The patient should be questioned regarding the progress of the symptoms. Gradual diminishing discomfort is a favorable sign. The dressing should be removed and the surgical area checked for localized areas of infection or irritation. The area should be irrigated or incised to provide drainage if areas of localized exudate are present. Particles of calculus that may have been overlooked should be removed. Adjusting the occlusion can be helpful. Sensitivity to percussion may also be caused by excess dressing, which interferes with the occlusion. Removal of the excess usually corrects the condition.
3. *Swelling.* During the first 2 postoperative days, some patients may report a soft, painless swelling of the cheek in the surgical area. Lymph node enlargement may occur, and the temperature may be slightly elevated. The area of operation itself is usually symptom free. This type of involvement results from a localized inflammatory reaction to the surgical procedure. It generally subsides by the fourth postoperative day without necessitating the removal of the dressing. If swelling persists, enlarges, or is associated with increased pain, amoxicillin (500 mg) should be taken every 8 hours for 1 week and moist heat can be applied intermittently to the area. The patient should be monitored closely until resolved.
4. *Feeling of weakness.* Occasionally, patients report having experienced a "washed-out," weakened feeling for about 24 hours after surgery. This represents a systemic reaction to transient bacteremia induced by the procedure. This reaction can be mitigated by premedication with amoxicillin (500 mg) every 8 hours. This protocol should be started 24 hours before the next procedure and continued for 5 days postoperatively.

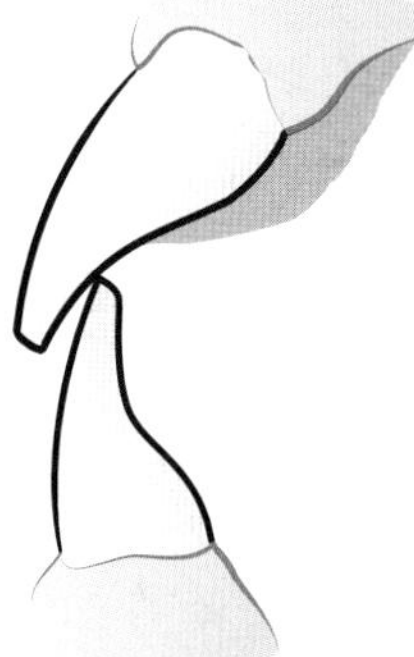

Fig. 60.14 Periodontal pack should not interfere with the occlusion.

Postoperative Visit and Removal of the Dressing

When the patient returns in 1 week, the periodontal dressing is removed by inserting a curette along the margin and exerting gentle lateral pressure. Pieces of the dressing retained interproximally and particles adhering to the tooth surfaces are also removed with curettes. Particles of dressing and debris may be enmeshed in the surgical surfaces and should be carefully removed with cotton pliers. The entire area is irrigated with peroxide or saline to remove the superficial debris.

Findings at the Time of Dressing Removal

Typical findings when the dressing is removed include the following:

- If g*ingivectomy* has been performed, the incised surface is covered with a friable meshwork of new epithelium. This tissue should not be disturbed. If calculus has not been completely removed, red, beadlike protuberances of granulation tissue will persist. The granulation tissue must be removed with a curette to expose the calculus so the root can be planed. Granulation tissue will recur if the residual calculus is not completely removed.

- After a *flap operation*, the areas that correspond to the incisions are epithelialized, but they may bleed readily if irritated. These areas should not be disturbed nor probed.
- The facial and lingual mucosa may be covered with a grayish-yellow or white granular layer of debris that has entered under the dressing. This is easily removed with a moist cotton pellet or swab. The root surfaces may be sensitive to touch or to thermal change. The patient should be advised that these changes will diminish with time (4 to 6 weeks). The dentition that was beneath the dressing may be stained in a brownish-yellow color that can be removed by polishing at a later date.
- *Fragments of calculus delay healing.* Each root surface should be carefully rechecked visually to be certain that no calculus was missed during surgery. The grooves on proximal root surfaces and furcations are areas where calculus is likely to have been overlooked or missed.

Redressing

After the dressing is removed, it is usually not necessary to replace it. However, redressing for an additional week is advised for the following types of patients: (1) those with a low pain threshold who are particularly uncomfortable when the dressing is removed; (2) those with unusually sensitive root surfaces after surgery; or (3) those with an open wound where the flap edges have necrosed. Clinical judgment helps when deciding whether to redress the area or to leave the initial dressing for a longer period.

LEARNING BOX 60.5

Periodontal dressings have no curative properties but assist healing by protecting the tissue rather than providing "healing factors." The dressing facilitates healing by preventing surface trauma during mastication and protects the patient from pain induced by contact of the wound with food debris or with the tongue during mastication.

Tooth Mobility

Tooth mobility usually increases immediately after surgery.[10] This is caused by edema in the periodontal ligament space from the inflammation that occurs following surgery. The mobility diminishes to the pretreatment level by the fourth week.[31] The patient should be reassured before surgery that the increased tooth mobility after surgery is temporary.

Mouth Care Between Procedures

Care of the mouth by the patient between the treatments as well as after the surgery is extremely important.[58] Biofilm control should begin after the dressing is removed. The patient has had instructions on oral hygiene before surgical therapy but must be instructed again after surgical therapy. Biofilm removal after surgery is different from that of presurgical hygiene because the areas are still healing and uncomfortable. There may also be spaces that did not exist previously.

Vigorous brushing is not feasible during the first week after the dressing is removed. However, the patient should be informed that biofilm and food accumulation impair healing and they should be advised to try to keep the area as clean as possible with the gentle use of an extra soft toothbrush and light water irrigation. Rinsing with a chlorhexidine mouthwash or applying such a rinse topically with cotton-tipped applicators may be indicated for the first few postoperative weeks, especially for those who are not effective or too timid to try. Return to normal brushing is introduced when the healing of the tissues permits, and the overall hygiene regimen is increased as healing progresses. Patients should be told that (1) keeping the area clean will aid in optimal healing; (2) some gingival bleeding will occur when the wounded areas are gently cleaned; (3) this bleeding is normal and will subside as healing progresses; and (4) the bleeding should not deter them from performing their oral hygiene regimen.

Management of Postoperative Pain

Periodontal surgery that follows the basic principles outlined here should produce only minimal pain and discomfort.[51] A study of 304 consecutive periodontal surgical interventions revealed that 51.3% of the patients reported minimal or no postoperative pain, and only 4.6% reported severe pain. Of these, only 20.1% took five or more doses of analgesic.[12] This is consistent with the finding of another study that reports a 4.1% incidence of severe pain following periodontal flap surgery.[6] The previous study indicated that mucogingival surgery was 3.5 times more likely to cause pain than osseous surgery and 6 times more likely than plastic soft tissue surgery. For the few patients who may experience severe pain, analgesia becomes an important part of patient management.[36]

As indicated earlier, a common source of postoperative pain is overextension of the periodontal dressing onto the soft tissue apical to the mucogingival junction, on a frenum, or beyond the vestibule. Overextended dressings cause localized areas of edema that are usually noticed 1 to 2 days after surgery. The removal of excess dressing is followed by resolution in about 24 hours.

Extensive and excessively prolonged exposure of bone with poor irrigation during surgery induces greater pain. For most healthy patients, a preoperative dose of ibuprofen (600 to 800 mg) followed by one tablet every 8 hours for 24 to 48 hours is very effective for reducing discomfort after periodontal surgery. Alternatively, a preoperative dose of acetaminophen (500 to 1000 mg) may be taken followed by one tablet every 6 hours for 24 to 48 hours. Patients are advised to continue taking ibuprofen or acetaminophen thereafter, if needed. If pain persists, a narcotic such as acetaminophen plus codeine (Tylenol #3) can be prescribed. Caution should be used when prescribing or dispensing ibuprofen to patients with hypertension that is controlled by medications because it can interfere with the effectiveness of the medication. Ibuprofen should be avoided for patients with impaired kidney function. Patients experiencing severe postoperative pain should be seen on an emergency basis. The area should be anesthetized by infiltration, and the dressing should be removed to allow for the examination of the area in pain. Postoperative pain related to infection is accompanied by signs of infection (e.g., increased erythema, exudate, swelling), localized lymphadenopathy, and a slight elevation in temperature.[38] This type of pain should be treated with systemic antibiotics and analgesics.

Dentin (Root) Hypersensitivity

Dentin or root hypersensitivity is a relatively common problem in dental and periodontal practices. It may occur spontaneously when the root becomes exposed as a result of gingival recession or pocket formation, or it may appear after root instrumentation (scaling and root planing) or periodontal surgical procedures. This type of sensitivity is manifested as pain that is induced by thermal changes (cold or hot temperature), by citrus fruits or sweets, or by contact with a toothbrush or a dental instrument.

Root sensitivity occurs more frequently in the cervical area of the root, where the cementum is extremely thin. Root instrumentation procedures remove this thin cementum, thereby inducing the hypersensitivity.

The transmission of stimuli from the surface of the dentin to the nerve endings located in the dental pulp or in the pulpal region of the dentin could result from the odontoblastic process or from a hydrodynamic mechanism (i.e., the displacement of dentinal fluid in the dentinal tubules). The latter process seems more likely and has been widely accepted as the mechanism,[30] which would also explain the importance of burnishing desensitizing agents to obturate the dentinal tubule.

An important factor for reducing or eliminating hypersensitivity is adequate biofilm control. The problem is that hypersensitivity often prevents the patient from performing biofilm control, and therefore a vicious cycle of escalating hypersensitivity, avoidance, and biofilm accumulation ensues.

The patient should be informed about the possibility of root hypersensitivity *before* treatment. A patient who is educated about any potential adverse issues before surgery will be more understanding and less likely to complain because he or she is aware and expects the sensitivity may occur. The following information on how to cope with the problem should also be given to the patient:

1. Dentin hypersensitivity appears as a result of dentin exposure, which is inevitable if calculus, biofilm, and endotoxins are removed via root instrumentation.
2. Dentin hypersensitivity slowly disappears in a few weeks.
3. Biofilm control is an important factor in reducing dentin hypersensitivity.
4. Desensitizing agents do not produce immediate relief and must be used for at least 2 weeks to produce results.

Desensitizing Agents

Numerous desensitizing agents have been proposed to control dentin hypersensitivity. Clinical evaluation of these agents is difficult for the following reasons: (1) measuring and comparing pain among patients with different thresholds are difficult, (2) the time required for hypersensitivity resolution is different for each patient, and (3) each desensitizing agent acts differently both in terms of time and the level of relief it offers.

Desensitizing agents can be applied by the patient at home or by the dentist or hygienist in the dental office. The most likely mechanism of action is the reduction of the diameter of the dentinal tubules or blockage to limit the displacement of fluid. According to Trowbridge and Silver,[54] this can be attained in the following ways: (1) by the formation of a smear layer produced by burnishing the exposed surface, (2) via the topical application of agents that form insoluble precipitates within the tubules, or (3) with the impregnation or sealing of tubules with plastic resins.

The most common agents used by the patient for oral hygiene are dentifrices. Although many dentifrice products contain stannous fluoride, which can help to decrease dentin hypersensitivity, additional active ingredients for desensitization are strontium chloride, potassium nitrate, sodium citrate, and arginine. The American Dental Association has approved several dentifrices for desensitizing purposes (Table 60.2).[1] Fluoride rinsing solutions and gels can also be used after the usual biofilm control procedures.[52]

Patients should be aware that several factors must be considered during the treatment of dentin hypersensitivity, including the history and severity of the problem, as well as the physical findings of the tooth or teeth involved. A proper diagnosis is required before any treatment can be initiated so that pathologic causes of pain, such as dental caries, chipped or cracked tooth, fractured or leaking restoration, trauma from occlusion, and other pulpal problems can be ruled out before attempting to treat the dentin hypersensitivity.[30] Desensitizing agents act through the precipitation of crystalline salts on the dentin surface that block dentinal tubules. Patients must be aware that their use will not prove to be effective unless they are used continuously for at least 2 weeks or longer. Consistent use over time may be necessary to control dentin hypersensitivity.

Table 60.3 lists various products used for the desensitization of dentin hypersensitivity. These products and treatments aim to decrease hypersensitivity by blocking dentinal tubules with either a crystalline salt precipitation or an applied coating (varnish or bonding agent) on the root surface.[1,44]

TABLE 60.2 Common ADA Approved Dentifrices for Desensitization

Toothpaste	Active Ingredient(s)	Company
Sensodyne Original	Strontium chloride	GlaxoSmithKline Consumer Healthcare
Sensodyne Sensitivity and Gum	Stannous fluoride (0.454%) Sodium fluoride (0.072%)	GlaxoSmithKline Consumer Healthcare
Crest Pro-Health Gum and Sensitivity	Stannous fluoride (0.454%)	Proctor & Gamble Co.
Colgate Sensitive Prevent and Repair	Potassium nitrate (5.0%) Sodium fluoride (0.24%)	Colgate-Palmolive Co.
Colgate Sensitive Pro-Relief	Arginine (8.0%) Sodium fluoride (0.24%)	Colgate-Palmolive Co.

Note: This table is not intended to be an exhaustive or comprehensive list of dentrifrices for desensitization.
ADA, American Dental Association.

Several agents have been used to precipitate crystalline salts on the dentin surface in an attempt to occlude the dentinal tubules. *Fluoride solutions* and *pastes* historically have been the agents of choice. In addition to their antisensitivity properties, fluoride agents have the advantage of anticaries activity, which is particularly important for patients with a tendency to develop root caries. Certain agents, such as chlorhexidine, decrease the ability of fluoride to bind with calcium on the root surfaces. Thus it is important to advise patients not to rinse or eat for 1 hour after applying a fluoride-based desensitizing treatment.

Another method of treating hypersensitive dentin is the use of varnishes or bonding agents to occlude dentinal tubules. Newer restorative materials, such as glass-ionomer cements and the dentin bonding agents, are under investigation. These materials are considered for use when the tooth requires recontouring or when difficult cases do not respond to other treatments. Resin primers alone could be promising, but the effects are not permanent, and further investigations are ongoing.[15] Despite some success with decreasing dentin hypersensitivity, these "dental office" treatments have not been predictable in resolving hypersensitivity, and the success that is achieved is often short lived. The crystalline salts, varnishes, and other sealants can be washed away over time, and the hypersensitivity may return. Repeated therapy will be necessary to help alleviate the hypersensitivity for these patients.

More recently, attempts have been made to improve the success and longevity of these treatments with the use of lasers. Low-level laser "melting" of the dentin surface appears to seal dentinal tubules without damage to the pulp.[16,28] In a combined treatment modality, the neodymium:yttrium-aluminum-garnet (Nd:YAG) laser has been used to congeal fluoride varnish on root surfaces. This in vitro study demonstrated that the laser-treated fluoride varnish resisted removal by electric toothbrushing, with 90% of tubules remaining blocked. In the control subjects (i.e., those who did not undergo laser treatment), the fluoride varnish was almost completely brushed away.[27] Despite these convincing preliminary results, further research is needed before laser treatment can be considered an effective and predictable means of desensitization (see Chapter 64).

TABLE 60.3 Desensitizing Products

Name	Active Ingredient(s)	Usage/Instructions
Desensitizing Agents		
Sensitive Pro-Relief Desensitizing Paste with Pro-Argin	Arginine 8%, calcium carbonate, sodium Monofluorophosphate	**Office**: Place paste in rotary cup; apply to area and polish at low to moderate speed for 3 s and repeat. **Home**: Patients advised to use paste as directed.
Bis-Block, Sensodyne Sealant, SuperSeal	Oxalate products	**Office**: Dry dentin surface; dispense 10–12 drops; apply with cotton pellet 1 min to area with light pressure; do not burnish; may require multiple 1 min applications. Expectorate after use.
Sultan Sodium Fluoride Paste	Sodium fluoride 33.50%	**Office**: Burnish onto sensitive area using orangewood stick for 1 min; followed by rinsing; sequential 1-min treatments may be required.
Many brands of over-the-counter toothpaste	Potassium nitrate, sodium fluoride	**Home**: Apply 1-inch toothpaste onto soft-bristled toothbrush; brush thoroughly at least 1 min twice a day or as recommended.
Gel-Kam Dentin Block	Sodium fluoride, stannous fluoride	**Office**: Dry dentin surface; dispense 10–12 drops; apply with cotton pellet for 1 min to area with light pressure; do not burnish; may require multiple 1-min applications. Expectorate after use.
Sealants/Adhesives/Resins/Bonding Agents		
Dentin Protect, Ivoclar Vivadent, Prime & Bond, Scotch Bond	Barrier dental sealant	**Office**: Apply chairside according to manufacturer's recommendations.
GC Tooth Mousse, MI Paste, Recaldent	Casein derivatives	**Office**: Apply chairside according to manufacturer's recommendations.
Seal & Protect, Vitrebond-Lite	Light-cured adhesives	**Office**: Apply chairside according to manufacturer's recommendations.
All-Bond DS, MicroPrime, Gluma Desensitizer, Glu/Sense, Hema Seal G	Methacrylate polymer	**Office**: Apply chairside according to manufacturer's recommendations.
Varnishes		
Cervitec Plus	Chlorhexidine dental varnish	**Office**: After isolating the area and drying, apply topically to all tooth surfaces and instruct patient to avoid eating for 3 h, and brushing teeth for 24 h, according to manufacturer's recommendations.
Cavity Shield, Durafluor, Duraphat, Fluoline, Fluor Protector, PreviDent Clear, Waterpik UltraThin	Sodium fluoride solutions	**Office**: Apply chairside according to manufacturer's recommendations.

Note: This table is not intended to be exhaustive or comprehensive. Clinicians are advised to read manufacturer's instructions and warnings.
Excerpted from *ADA/PDR Guide to Dental Therapeutics,* 5th ed. Chicago, IL.: American Dental Association; Physicians Desk Reference Inc.; 2009.

LEARNING BOX 60.6

Root sensitivity occurs more frequently in the cervical area of the root, where the cementum is extremely thin. Scaling and root planing procedures can remove this thin cementum, thereby inducing the hypersensitivity.

 Periodontal Surgery in the Hospital

For most patients, periodontal surgical procedures are managed well in the dental office with local anesthesia only or with some form of sedation. If multiple surgeries are indicated, they are typically performed by quadrant or sextant at biweekly or longer intervals. However, certain patients and procedures warrant treatment in the hospital operating room with general anesthesia. These include patients who are not well enough to undergo treatment in a dental office and procedures that are more extensive and difficult for patients to endure. Readers are referred to the online material for a discussion of indications and procedures in a hospital setting.

Conclusions

The majority of periodontal surgical procedures can be carried out with effective use of local anesthesia. Clinicians have the obligation to ensure a patient-centered approach that includes oral, intravenous, and inhalational sedation in their spectrum of available services for their patients.

The efficient, precise, and minimally traumatic management of tissues is necessary to achieve the most predictable and comfortable result and outcome for the patient. Most patients need oral analgesic support, and they should be given the necessary pain-relieving medications so that an effective level of analgesia is present during the immediate postsurgical period. The use of longer-acting local anesthetic agents (e.g., bupivacaine) and protective periodontal dressings also helps to reduce postsurgical pain.

During the immediate postsurgical weeks, biofilm control and healing can be facilitated with the use of antimicrobial mouthrinses such as chlorhexidine. Postsurgical root sensitivity is well controlled by ensuring that biofilm control is optimal, and occasionally desensitizing agents will be needed.

A Case Scenario is found on the companion website eBooks.Health.Elsevier.com.

Suggested Reading

ADA/PDR Guide to Dental Therapeutics. 5th ed. Chicago, IL: American Dental Association; Physicians Desk Reference Inc.; 2009.

Askar H, Di Gianfilippo R, Ravida A, Tattan M, Majzoub J, Wang HL. Incidence and severity of postoperative complications following oral, periodontal, and implant surgeries: a retrospective study. *J Periodontol.* 2019;90(11):1270–1278.

Checchi L, Trombelli L. Postoperative pain and discomfort with and without periodontal dressing in conjunction with 0.2% chlorhexidine mouthwash after apically positioned flap procedure. *J Periodontol.* 1993;64(12):1238–1242.

Hai JH, Lee C, Kapila YL, Chaffee BW, Armitage GC. Antibiotic prescribing practices in periodontal surgeries with and without bone grafting. *J Periodontol.* 2020;91(4):508–515.

Jakubovics N, Greenwood M, Meechan JG. General medicine and surgery for dental practitioners: part 4. Infections and infection control. *Br Dent J.* 2014;217(2):73–77.

Liu XX, Tenenbaum HC, Wilder RS, Quock R, Hewlett ER, Ren YF. Pathogenesis, diagnosis and management of dentin hypersensitivity: an evidence-based overview for dental practitioners. *BMC Oral Health.* 2020;20(1):220.

Malamed SF. *Medical Emergencies in the Dental Office.* 7th ed. St. Louis: Mosby; 2014.

Mills MP, Rosen PS, Chambrone L, Greenwell H, Kao RT, Klokkevold PR, et al. American Academy of Periodontology best evidence consensus statement on the efficacy of laser therapy used alone or as an adjunct to non-surgical and surgical treatment of periodontitis and peri-implant diseases. *J Periodontol.* 2018;89(7):737–742.

Pack PD, Haber J. The incidence of clinical infection after periodontal surgery. A retrospective study. *J Periodontol.* 1983;54(7):441–443.

Pippi R, Santoro M, Cafolla A. The effectiveness of a new method using an extra-alveolar hemostatic agent after dental extractions in older patients on oral anticoagulation treatment: an intrapatient study. *Oral Surg Oral Med Oral Pathol Oral Radiol.* 2015;120(1):15–21.

Powell CA, Mealey BL, Deas DE, McDonnell HT, Moritz AJ. Post-surgical infections: prevalence associated with various periodontal surgical procedures. *J Periodontol.* 2005;76(3):329–333.

Preber H, Bergstrom J. Effect of cigarette smoking on periodontal healing following surgical therapy. *J Clin Periodontol.* 1990;17:324.

Salgado-Peralvo AO, Mateos-Moreno MV, Velasco-Ortega E, Peña-Cardelles JF, Kewalramani N. Preventive antibiotic therapy in bone augmentation procedures in oral implantology: A systematic review. *J Stomatol Oral Maxillofac Surg.* 2022;123(1):74-80.

Trowbridge HO, Silver DR. A review of current approaches to in-office management of tooth hypersensitivity. *Dent Clin North Am.* 1990;34:583.

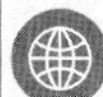
References for this chapter are found on the companion website eBooks.Health.Elsevier.com.

CHAPTER 61

Periodontal Surgical Therapy

Michael G. Newman | Jonathan H. Do | Henry H. Takei | Michael Whang | Kitetsu Shin

 For online-only content on periodontal surgery fundamentals and specific techniques, please visit the companion website at eBooks.Health.Elsevier.com.

 Animations have been added by the editors as a supplement to the chapter. They are produced by PerioPixel as patient education tools and cover the basic elements in a conceptual manner. They are not intended to be procedural guides for dental professionals.

CHAPTER OUTLINE

Periodontal surgical therapy has a long history and evolution. It started with subgingival curettage and pocket elimination with gingivectomy. Understanding of healing, development of sophisticated periodontal flap techniques, and esthetic demands have made gingival curettage obsolete and have relegated gingivectomy to limited cases of gingival enlargement or instances where flap surgery is not possible.

Periodontal flap surgery is the most widely used surgical procedure for periodontal pocket therapy. Periodontal flaps are advantageous and versatile in providing not only access for root instrumentation but also access for osseous surgery and periodontal regeneration. Flap surgery also allows for primary closure, which enhances wound healing and minimizes patients' discomfort.

Rationale for Periodontal Access Surgery

In patients with furcation invasion and infrabony defects, it may be difficult and even impossible to resolve periodontal inflammation completely because residual pockets remain after nonsurgical treatment. Periodontal access surgery is necessary to definitively treat, create anatomies that are maintainable long-term by both the patient and the clinician, and, when feasible, reconstruct lost periodontal structures.

Periodontal access surgery refers to various surgical procedures that permit the clinician to debride adequately and, if necessary, modify the underlying infrabony pockets by either osseous surgical or regenerative procedures. Periodontal access surgery is an adjunct to nonsurgical periodontal therapy and should occur only once the patient has demonstrated effective biofilm control.

Periodontal access surgery enhances access for root instrumentation and allows for the reduction of periodontal pockets and the correction of osseous defects. However, periodontal access surgery in patients with periodontitis frequently results in gingival recession and loss of interdental papillae because the disease process destroys the underlying tissues.

In the anterior maxilla, where esthetics is of high priority, recession and loss of interdental papillae can present major esthetic problems that are both difficult and unpredictable to treat surgically. Fortunately, the anterior location of these teeth and their single-rooted and convex root surface anatomies facilitate nonsurgical root instrumentation. When specialized instruments such as mini Gracey curettes and Vision Curvettes are used in conjunction with illumination and magnification, access to these periodontal pockets is enhanced, and nonsurgical periodontal therapy can be very efficacious.

In the posterior sextants, access for definitive root instrumentation is much more restricted due to multiple anatomic factors, especially around multirooted teeth. Wide proximal surfaces, root grooves and concavities, furcations, angulation and proximity of roots, depth of the periodontal pocket, the cheek, the tongue, and the opposing dentition can all contribute to hinder the removal of subgingival biofilm and calculus on these teeth. Fortunately, gingival recession and loss of interdental papillae in the posterior regions generally do not present esthetic problems for most patients. Many patients and clinicians are willing to accept recession and the associated transient root sensitivity and food impaction in exchange for periodontal health. In many patients, periodontal access surgery is a treatment modality that is essential and frequently used in the treatment of periodontal disease in the non-esthetic area.

There are two main modalities of periodontal access surgery, gingivectomy and periodontal flap surgery, which provide access for root instrumentation. Pocket reduction is achieved by resection of the suprabony soft tissue pocket by gingivectomy, whereas with periodontal flap surgery, a pocket reduction is achieved via soft tissue resection, osseous resection, or periodontal regeneration.

LEARNING BOX 61.1

For the clinician, the objectives of periodontal access surgery are to facilitate root instrumentation and permit soft and hard tissue resection or periodontal regeneration.

For the patient, surgical intervention will enhance the ability for home care and long-term professional, supportive maintenance

Fundamentals of Periodontal Surgery

Incisions

Periodontal surgery involves using horizontal (mesial-distal) and vertical (occlusal-apical) incisions. The #15 or #15C surgical blade is often used to make these incisions.

Horizontal Incisions

Horizontal incisions are directed along the gingiva in a mesial or distal direction. Flaps can be reflected with only horizontal incision if sufficient access can be obtained in this way and if the flap's apical, lateral, or coronal displacement is not anticipated. If vertical incisions are not made, the flap is called an *envelope flap*.

Straight and Scalloped Incisions

A horizontal incision that follows the scalloped morphology of the gingival architecture is called a scalloped incision, as opposed to a straight incision, which follows a straight line (Fig. 61.1). The scalloped incision is advantageous in preserving the interdental architecture in gingivectomy and in creating surgical papillae and preserving soft tissue over the interdental areas to allow coverage of the interdental bone in flap surgery.

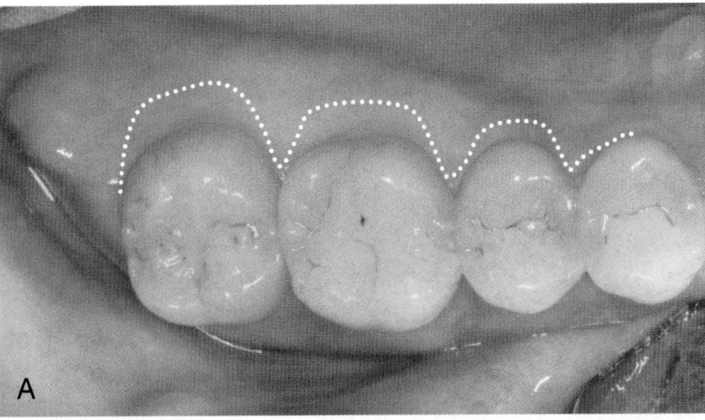

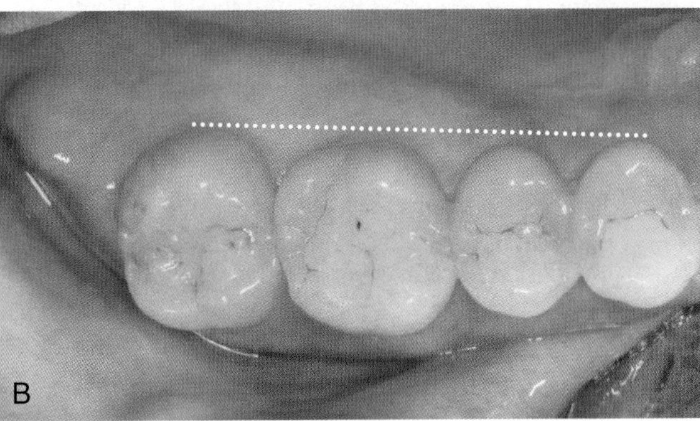

Fig. 61.1 (A) Scalloped incision. (B) Straight incision.

Historical Reference. Historically, horizontal incisions were used in gingivectomy and flap surgery to eliminate the interdental tissue, where periodontal disease and periodontal pockets frequently occur. The *interdental denudation procedure* used horizontal internal bevel incisions to remove the gingival papillae and to denude the interdental spaces.[2,3,24,28] This technique completely eliminates the inflamed interdental tissue. Healing is by secondary intention and results in excellent gingival contour and shallow probing depths. However, the initial healing is slow and uncomfortable due to exposure and necrosis of the interdental bone. For this reason, the interdental denudation procedure has very limited clinical application.

The use of scalloped incisions in flap surgery allows the interdental bone to be covered once the flap is coapted. Coaptation is the process of firmly placing the flap back onto the bone and teeth. This enhances patients' comfort and allows for faster closure of the wound.

When scalloping the incision, the scallop is from the mesial line angle to the distal line angle to maximize the width of the surgical papillae and to allow tight adaptation of the flap to the roots once the flap is coapted. In interdental areas, the incision is maintained close or in the sulcus to maximize coverage of the interdental bone. The scallop incision should take into account root anatomy to optimize primary closure. For example, the mesial-distal palatal dimension of a maxillary molar decreases from the cementoenamel junction down to the palatal root as the tooth transitions from a root trunk to a single root. An aggressive scallop may leave bone around the palatal root of a maxillary molar exposed.

External Bevel and Internal Bevel Incisions

The external bevel incision starts at the surface of the gingiva apical to the periodontal pocket and is directed coronally toward the tooth apical to the bottom of the periodontal pocket. The external bevel incision, or simply bevel incision, is used primarily in gingivectomy, and it can be made with a scalpel or a knife. The internal bevel incision, also called the reverse bevel incision and inverse bevel incision, is the opposite of the external bevel incision (Fig. 61.2). The internal bevel incision[27] starts at the surface of the gingiva and is directed apically to the bone crest. It is the incision from which the flap is reflected to expose the underlying bone and root. The internal bevel incision accomplishes three important objectives: (1) it removes the pocket lining; (2) it conserves the relatively uninvolved outer surface of the gingiva, which, if apically positioned, becomes attached gingiva; and (3) it produces a sharp, thin flap margin for adaptation to the bone–tooth junction. The internal bevel incision is basic to most periodontal flap procedures. Both bevel and internal bevel incisions can be straight or scalloped.

Crevicular, Crestal, and Submarginal Incisions

The crevicular incision is also called intercrevicular incision, intracrevicular incision, sulcular incision, intrasulcular incision, and intersulcular incision. It starts in the gingival crevice and is directed apically through the junctional epithelium and connective tissue attachment and down to the bone (Fig. 61.3).

- The crestal incision is also called the marginal incision. It starts at the surface of the gingiva at the gingival margin and is directed apically down through the epithelium and connective tissue to the bone. Both the crevicular and crestal incisions are internal bevel incisions. The submarginal incision starts at the surface of the gingiva apical to the gingival margin and can be an external

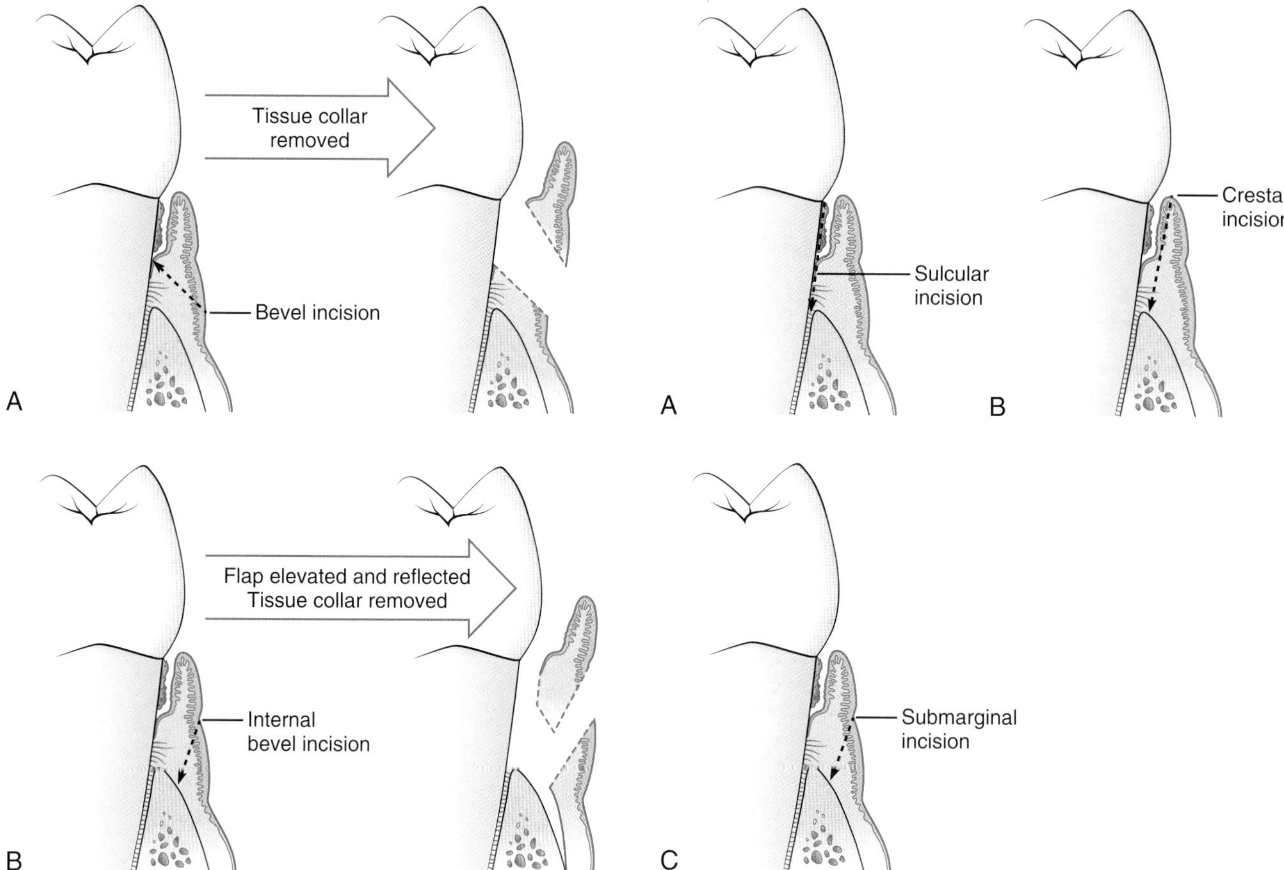

Fig. 61.2 (A) Bevel incision. (B) Internal bevel incision.

Fig. 61.3 (A) Sulcular incision. (B) Crestal incision. (C) Submarginal incision.

or internal bevel. In flap surgery, the submarginal incision is an internal bevel incision, whereas in gingivectomy, it is an external one.

- The use of a crevicular, marginal, or submarginal internal bevel incision in periodontal flap surgery depends on the objectives of the surgery and the anatomy of the area. The crevicular incision is frequently used in regenerative periodontal surgery to retain all gingival tissue to maximize blood supply and to obtain primary wound closure. The crevicular incision is also the incision of choice when the recession is not desired. The anterior maxilla is an area where recession and loss of interdental papillae can compromise esthetics.

When flap surgery is required in the anterior maxilla, the crevicular incision is recommended. In resective periodontal surgery, the marginal and submarginal scalloped incisions are frequently used to create flaps with thin margins and to leave a collar of tissue around the tooth that contains the epithelium of the pocket lining and the adjacent granulomatous tissue. This collar of tissue is discarded after flap elevation. The marginal incision maximizes the remaining keratinized tissue, whereas the submarginal scalloped incision allows for more aggressive soft tissue resection and reduction of the periodontal pocket.

LEARNING BOX 61.2

When the submarginal scalloped incision is used, *how submarginal should be incision be?* The placement of the submarginal incision always depends on: (1) the transgingival interdental probing depth, (2) the **mucogingival junction**, and (3) the depth of the palatal vault.

The transgingival interdental probing depth is used to provide a guide for the placement of the submarginal scalloped incision. The transgingival probing depth is the distance from the gingival margin down to the bone. It is measured by inserting the probe into the gingival crevice through the attachment apparatus and down to the bone.

Transgingival probing is also called *bone sounding*. The submarginal scalloped incision is placed a distance of one-half to two-thirds the transgingival interdental probing depth away from the tooth surface (Fig. 61.4). For example, if the mesial and distal interdental probing depths are 6 mm, then the submarginal scalloped incision will be placed 3 mm apical to the gingival margin at the midbuccal and midlingual surface of the tooth.

LEARNING BOX 61.3

Why is the transgingival interdental probing depth used as a guide for the placement of the submarginal scalloped incision in resective periodontal surgery? Periodontal disease occurs most commonly in the interdental areas due to inadequate biofilm removal below the interdental proximal contact. Interdental attachment and bone loss result in reverse/negative bony architecture. To reestablish positive architecture, the radicular bone is resected apical to the interdental bone, whereas the interdental bone is maintained. Therefore, the transgingival interdental probing depth is used as the guide for submarginal incision placement.

Although the presence of keratinized tissue is not required for periodontal health, its presence facilitates oral hygiene. Therefore, the submarginal scalloped incision will be placed depending on

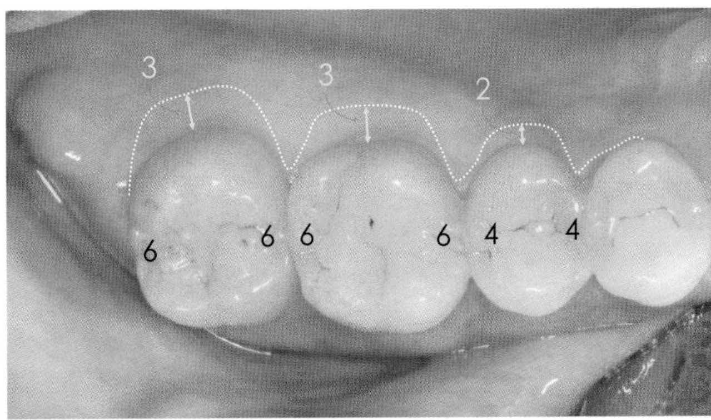

Fig. 61.4 The submarginal scalloped incision is placed at a distance of one-half to two-thirds the transgingival interdental probing depth away from the tooth surface. Numbers shown in black represent the interdental probing depths. Numbers shown in yellow represent the distance from the tooth where the submarginal scalloped incision should be placed.

the mucogingival junction to preserve ≥3 mm of keratinized tissue. If the width of keratinized tissue is narrow, the submarginal scalloped incision will be placed closer to the gingival margin. A marginal incision would be used in lieu of a submarginal incision if the width of the keratinized tissue is less than 3 mm. If the width of the keratinized tissue is broad, then the submarginal scalloped incision will be placed based on the transgingival interdental probing depth (Fig. 61.5).

On the *palatal maxilla*, where the lack of keratinized tissue is not a concern, placement of the submarginal scalloped incision must take into consideration the depth of the palatal vault (Fig. 61.6). A high palatal vault will allow the submarginal incision to be placed based on one-half to two-thirds the transgingival interdental probing depth. In shallow palates, the more submarginal an incision, the closer it will be to the midline and the farther away it will be from the tooth surface. A submarginal incision placed in a shallow palatal vault based on the transgingival probing depth may result in a palatal flap that is too short to provide complete coverage of the alveolar bone and primary closure once it is coapted. Therefore, the flatter the palatal vault, the closer the submarginal incision must be to the gingival margin. If the palatal flap is too long when it is coapted, it can always be trimmed and rescalloped.

In areas where a mucogingival junction is present, such as the buccal or facial maxilla and the buccal or facial and lingual mandible, resection of soft tissue with the submarginal scalloped internal bevel incision is not the only way to obtain pocket reduction. A marginal incision can be used to maximize remaining keratinized tissue, and reduction of soft tissue height can be achieved by apically repositioning the flap margin to the level of the alveolar crest. The only area in the mouth where the submarginal incision must be used to reduce soft tissue height is the palate, where it is not possible to reposition the soft tissue apically due to the absence of a mucogingival junction.

LEARNING BOX 61.4

Reduction of soft tissue height may be achieved using the submarginal scalloped incision or a combination of a marginal scalloped incision and an apically displaced flap.

Vertical Incisions

Vertical or oblique releasing incisions can be used on one or both ends of the horizontal incision, depending on the design and purpose of the flap. Vertical incisions at both ends may be necessary if the

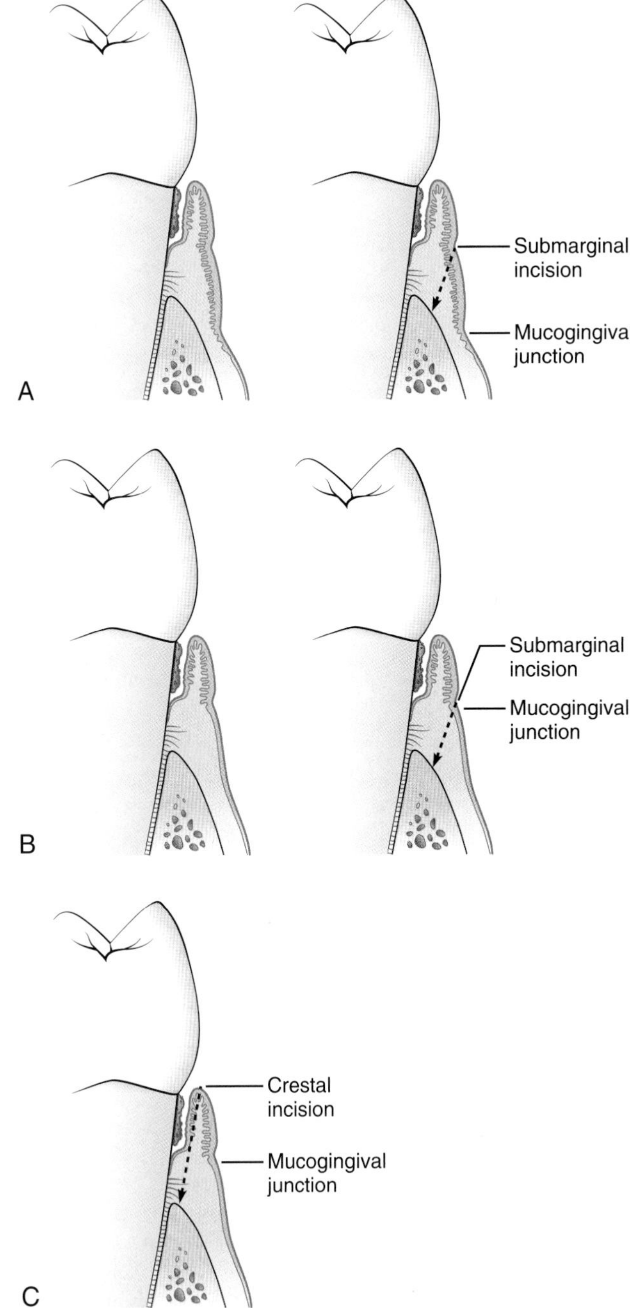

Fig. 61.5 (A) When keratinized tissue is abundant, a submarginal incision may be used. (B) When keratinized tissue is limited, a submarginal incision eliminates keratinized tissue that must be retained. (C) A crestal incision maximizes the retained keratinized tissue.

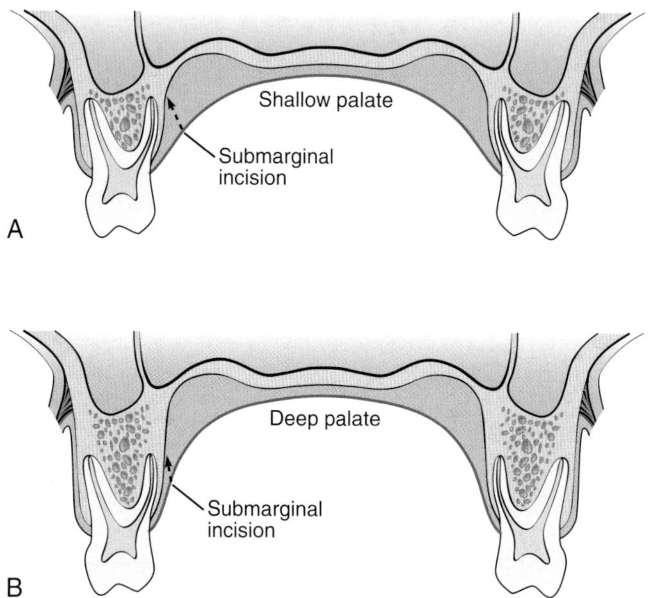

Fig. 61.6 (A) In a shallow palate, the more submarginal an incision, the closer it will be to the midline and the farther away it will be from the tooth surface. (B) In a high palate, a submarginal incision remains close to the tooth and allows for primary closure of the flap.

flap is to be apically displaced. Several factors need to be considered when making vertical incisions:

- Vertical incisions must extend beyond the mucogingival junction to reach the alveolar mucosa, allowing the release of the flap to be displaced.
- In general, vertical incisions in the lingual and palatal areas should be avoided.
- Facial vertical incisions should not be made in the center of an interdental papilla or over the radicular surface of a tooth.
- Incisions should be made at the line angles of a tooth either to include the papilla in the flap or to avoid it completely.
- The vertical incision should also be designed to avoid long (coronal-apical) and narrow (mesial-distal) flaps, and flaps with the base narrower than the margin, because this could jeopardize the blood supply to the flap (Fig. 61.7).

Papilla Management

The papilla may be thinned, preserved, or split beneath the contact point. Management of the papilla depends on the dimension of the interdental space, esthetics, and the secondary objective of the surgery, which could be resective or regenerative. In resective surgery, the scalloped incision creates surgical papillae to cover the interdental bone. The surgical papilla may or may not include the original papilla, depending on the submarginal placement of the scalloped incision. The surgical papilla is thinned to create the same thickness as the remainder of the flap to allow intimate adaptation of the papilla and the flap with the bone once the flap is coapted. In regenerative therapy and in esthetic cases, the *papilla preservation technique* (Fig. 61.8),[34] which retains the entire papilla, is favored when the interdental space is adequate to allow the intact papilla to be reflected with the facial or lingual-palatal flap. When the interdental space is narrow, and the reflection of an intact papilla is not possible, the interdental papilla is split beneath the contact point of the two approximating teeth to allow for the reflection of the buccal and lingual flaps. The papilla is not thinned in these cases to minimize tissue shrinkage.

Flap Elevation

A periodontal flap may be elevated in full thickness or partial thickness (Fig. 61.9). In a *full-thickness flap,* all of the soft tissue, including the periosteum, is reflected to expose the underlying bone. This complete exposure of and access to the underlying bone is indicated when resective or regenerative osseous surgery is contemplated. This type of flap is also called the mucoperiosteal flap. Elevation of a full-thickness flap requires the internal bevel incision to penetrate the periosteum, the last tissue overlying the bone. Once the periosteum has been completely incised along the length of the flap, a full-thickness flap is reflected by elevating the periosteum off the bone via blunt dissection. A periosteal elevator or curette is used to separate the periosteum from the bone by moving it mesially, distally, and apically on the bone until the desired reflection is accomplished, usually a millimeter apical to the mucogingival junction. Elevation of the periosteum off the bone should be performed with ease, and it can even be done with gauze. Difficulty in elevating a full-thickness flap is usually due to incomplete and noncontiguous incision of connective tissue and periosteum along the length of the flap.

The *partial-thickness flap* includes only the epithelium and a layer of the underlying connective tissue. The bone remains covered by a layer of connective tissue that includes the periosteum. This type of flap is also called the *split-thickness flap.* The partial-thickness flap is indicated when the flap is to be positioned apically or when exposure of bone is not desired. Elevation of a partial-thickness flap is completed by sharp dissection with a surgical scalpel (#15). When the tissue is thin, a flap may be elevated at full thickness slightly past the mucogingival junction and at partial thickness apical to the mucogingival junction. The combination of full-thickness and partial-thickness flaps reduces the risk of flap perforation at the mucogingival junction, where the tissue is often the thinnest. This also allows for access to the bone around the teeth and preserves tissue over the bone apical to the mucogingival junction, which can be used to help stabilize the flap should it be apically displaced.

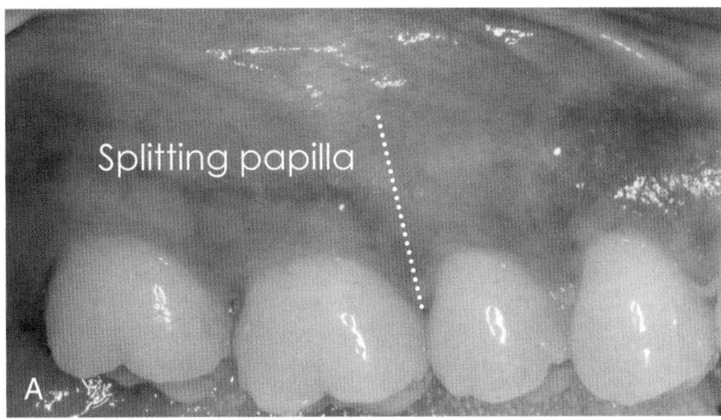

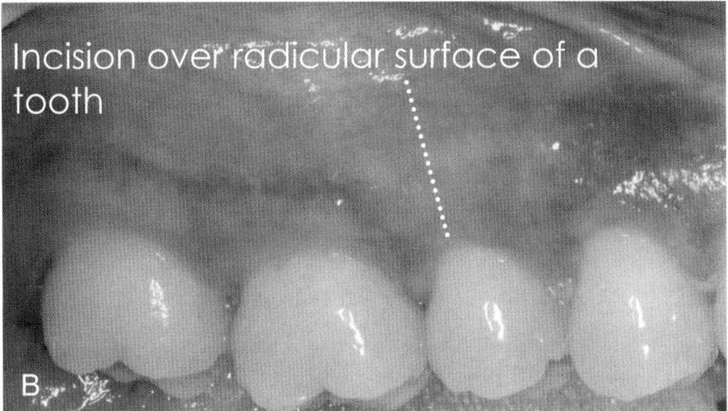

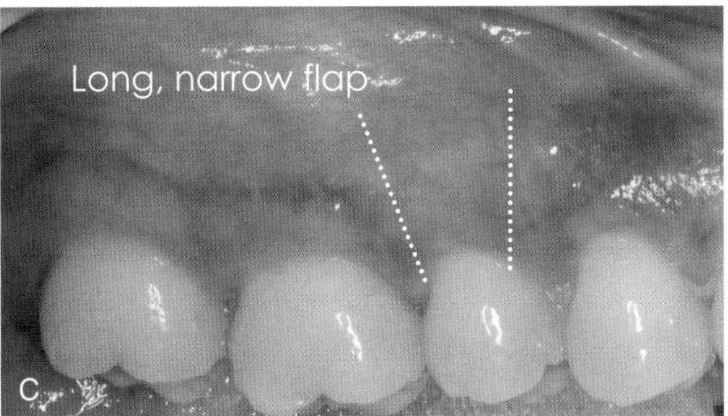

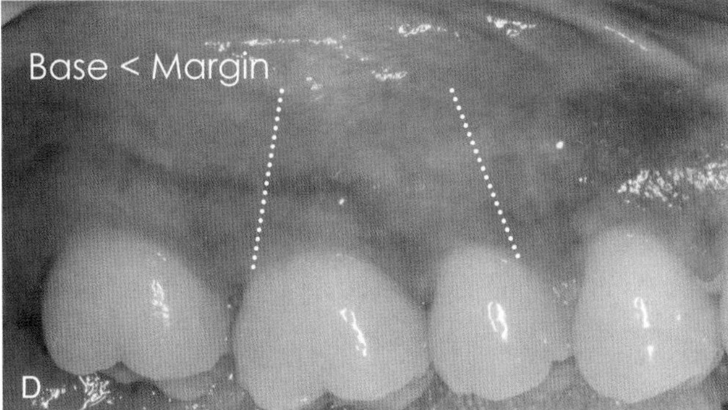

Fig. 61.7 Vertical incisions should not (A) split a papilla or (B) be placed over a root prominence. When two vertical incisions are used, (C) the length of the flap should not be longer than the width of the flap, and (D) the base of the flap should not be narrower than the margin of the flap.

Conflicting data surround the advisability of uncovering the bone when this is not actually needed. When bone is stripped of its periosteum, a loss of marginal bone occurs, and this loss is prevented when the periosteum is left on the bone.[6] Although this is usually clinically insignificant,[13] the difference may be significant in some cases. The partial-thickness flap may be necessary when the crestal bone margin is thin or when dehiscences or fenestrations are present.

An apically displaced flap may be stabilized by suturing it to the intact periosteum.

LEARNING BOX 61.5

When the tissue is thin, a flap may be elevated at full thickness slightly past the mucogingival junction and at partial thickness apical to reduce flap perforation at the mucogingival junction and use the advantages of each flap.

Flap Coaptation

For flap coaptation after surgery, flaps are classified as either (1) *nondisplaced flaps,* when the flap is placed and sutured in its original position, or (2) *displaced flaps,* which are placed apically, coronally, or laterally to their original position (Fig. 61.10). Both full-thickness and partial-thickness flaps can be displaced. For a full-thickness flap to be displaced, the attached gingiva must be completely separated from the underlying bone, and the flap must be elevated apical to the mucogingival junction, thereby enabling mobility of the flap. Flap mobility may also require the use of vertical incisions and the release of the periosteum, especially for full-thickness flaps. Although the periosteum is only a few cells thick, it is not elastic. The periosteum may be folded over itself to allow apical displacement of the flap. However, it does not stretch, and coronal flap displacement requires the periosteum to be incised along the length of the flap. Palatal flaps cannot be displaced due to the absence of a mucogingival junction and mobile elastic tissue.

Apically displaced flaps have the important advantage of preserving the outer portion of the pocket wall and transforming it into attached gingiva. Therefore, these flaps accomplish the double objective of eliminating the pocket and increasing the width of the attached gingiva. The apically displaced flap also allows for a pocket reduction in instances where keratinized tissue is limited, and the internal bevel incision must be made close to or at the gingival margin.

At locations where keratinized tissue is abundant and pocket reduction is desired, such as the palate, a nondisplaced flap is created with a submarginal scalloped incision to eliminate marginal tissue.

Flap Closure and Sutures

After all of the necessary procedures are completed, the area is reexamined and cleansed, and the flap is placed in the desired position. The flap should remain in this position without tension. It is convenient to keep the flap in place with light pressure via the use of a piece of gauze to allow the blood clot to form. The purpose of suturing is to maintain the flap in the desired position until healing has progressed to the point at which sutures are no longer needed.

Many types of sutures, suture needles, and materials are available.[8,19] Suture materials may be either *non-resorbable* or *resorbable,* and they may be further categorized as *braided* or *monofilament* (eBox 61.1). Resorbable sutures have gained popularity because they enhance patients' comfort and eliminate suture removal appointments. The most common resorbable sutures used today are plain and chromic gut sutures. Both are monofilaments, and both are processed from purified collagen of either sheep or cattle intestines. The chromic suture is a plain gut suture that has been processed with chromic salts to make it resistant to enzymatic resorption, thereby increasing the resorption time. Synthetic resorbable sutures are also often used.

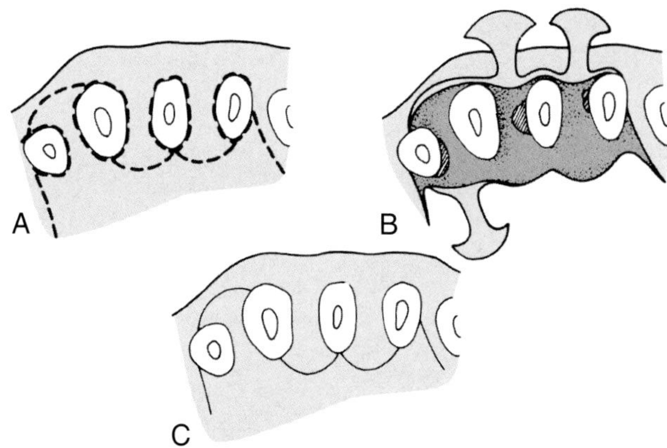

Fig. 61.8 Flap design for a papilla preservation flap. (A) Incisions for this type of flap are depicted by interrupted lines. The preserved papilla can be incorporated into the facial or the lingual–palatal flap. (B) The reflected flap exposes the underlying bone. Several osseous defects are seen. (C) The flap has been returned to its original position, where it covers all of the interdental spaces.

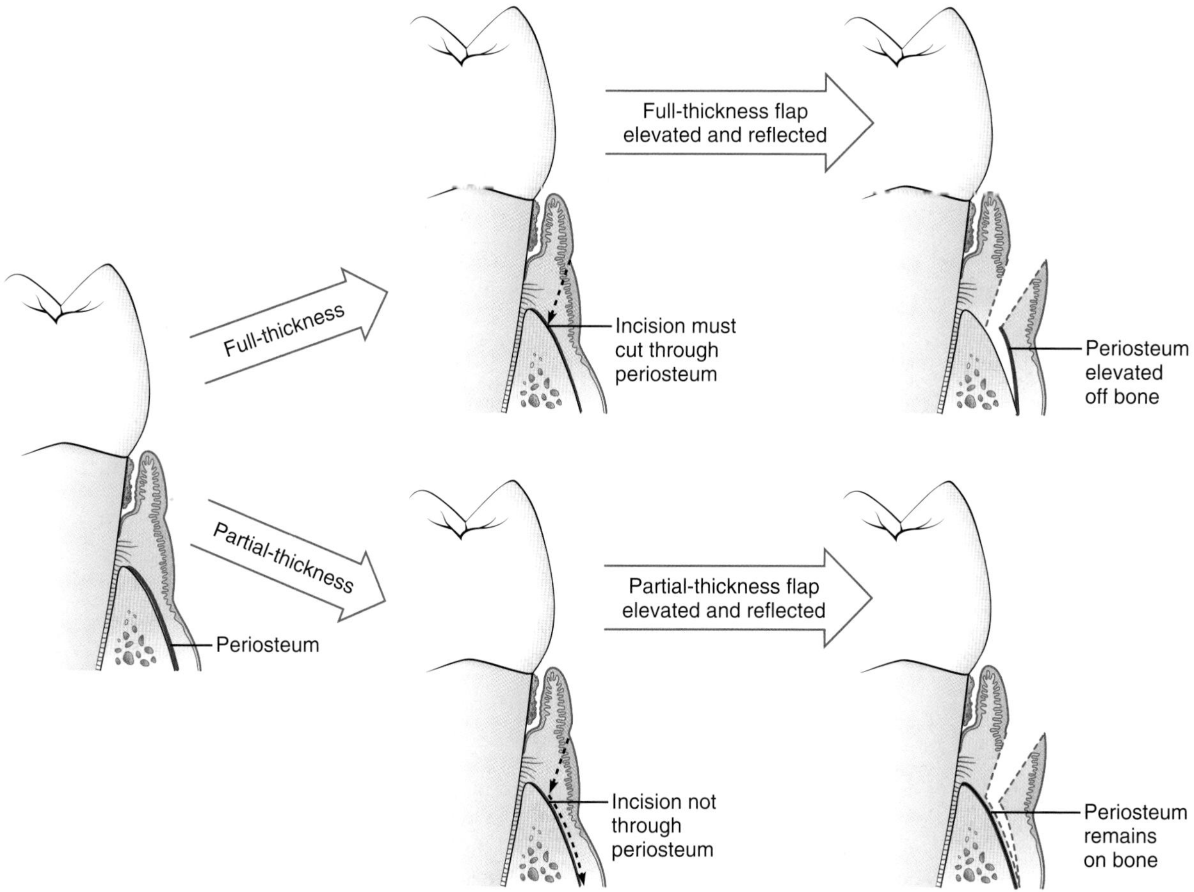

Fig. 61.9 In full-thickness flap elevation, the periosteum is elevated off the bone by blunt dissection. In partial-thickness flap elevation, the flap is split by sharp dissection to leave the periosteum and connective tissue intact over the bone.

The monofilament type of suture alleviates the "wicking effect" of braided sutures that may allow bacteria from the oral cavity to be drawn through the suture to the deeper areas of the wound. The braided silk suture was the most common non-resorbable suture used in the past because of its ease of use and low cost. The expanded polytetrafluoroethylene, synthetic, monofilament suture, is an excellent non-resorbable suture that is widely used today.

Periodontal Surgical Techniques

Periodontal surgery limited to the gingival tissues only without the use of periodontal flaps can be classified as *gingival curettage* and *gingivectomy.* The current understanding of disease etiology and therapy limits the use of *gingival curettage,* but its place in surgical therapy is still warranted for limited situations. Gingivectomy may be used in some cases of gingival enlargement (see Chapter 19).

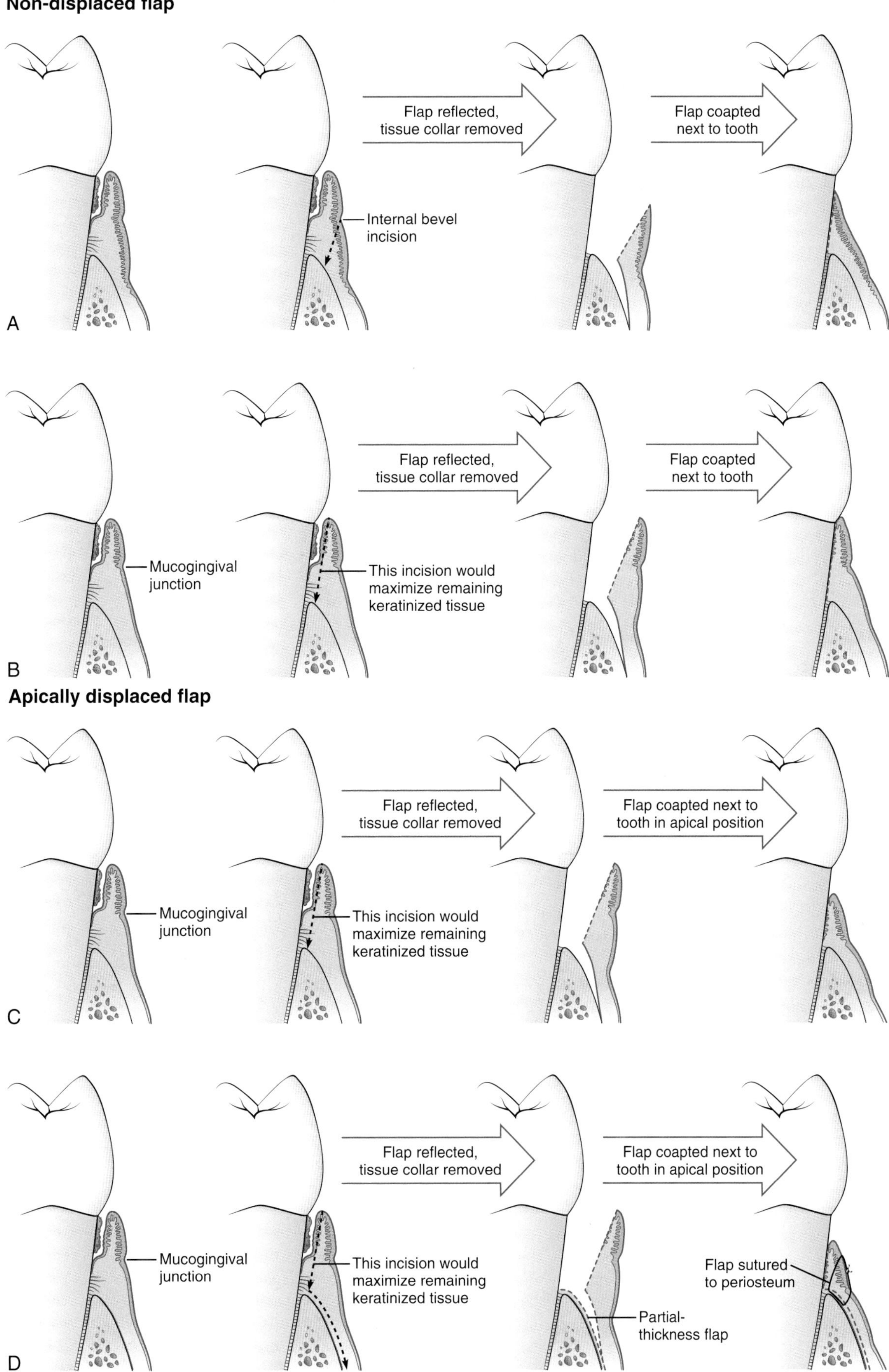

Fig. 61.10 (A) In the presence of abundant keratinized tissue, a reduction in soft tissue height is obtained with a submarginal scalloped incision. (B) A marginal incision is used to maximize the remaining keratinized tissue. A nondisplaced flap results in thick, soft tissue height. This is desirable in an esthetic area where recession needs to be minimized. (C) A marginal incision, to maximize keratinized tissue, is combined with an apically displaced flap to reduce soft tissue height. (D) A partial-thickness flap is used to allow the stabilization of an apically positioned flap with a periosteal suture.

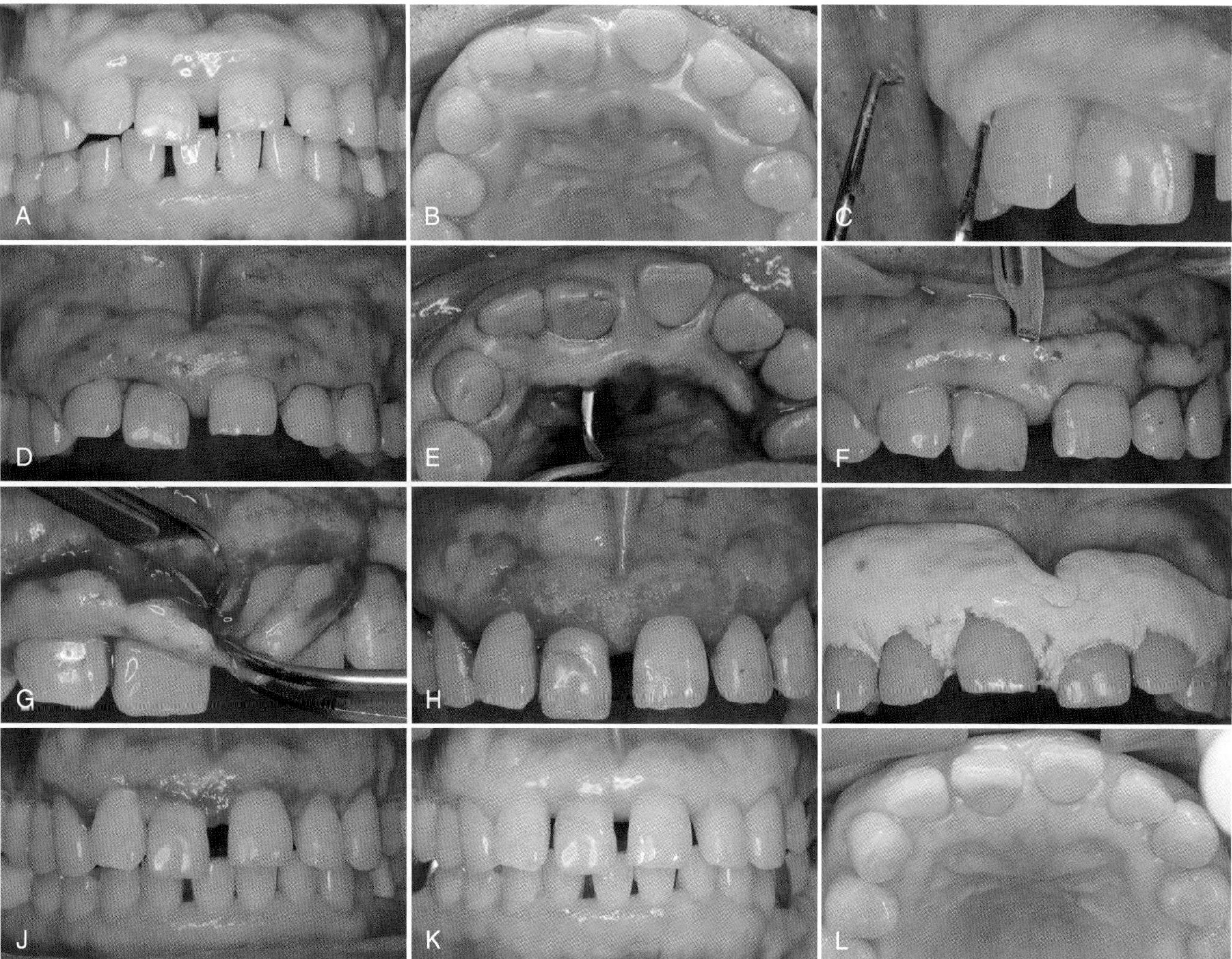

Fig. 61.11 Results obtained by treating a suprabony pocket with gingivectomy. (A and B) Preoperative facial and palatal views. (C) Marking of the depth of the suprabony pocket. (D) The bottoms of the pockets are indicated by pinpoint markings. (E) A beveled palatal incision with an Orban knife. (F) A facial beveled incision with a Bard-Parker #15 blade extends apical to the perforations made by the pocket marker. Note that the beveled incision can also be made with a Kirkland knife. (G) The interdental incision and excision of the pocket wall with a Bard-Parker #12 blade. (H) A completed gingivectomy. (I) The surgical site is covered with periodontal dressing. (J) One week after healing. (K and L) Results 22 months after the operation. (Courtesy Dr. Kitetsu Shin, Saitama, Japan.)

Periodontal flap surgery is one of the most frequently employed procedures, particularly for moderate and deep pockets in the posterior areas. Periodontal flap surgery provides access for root instrumentation and pocket reduction via gingival resection, osseous resection, and periodontal regeneration.

Gingival Surgery

Gingivoplasty

Gingivoplasty is *recontouring the gingiva* in the absence of pockets.[11] It may be accomplished with a periodontal knife, a scalpel, or rotary coarse diamond stones.[23]

Gingivectomy

The word *gingivectomy* means "excision of the gingiva." By removing the pocket wall, gingivectomy provides visibility and accessibility for complete calculus removal and thorough root planing. This creates a favorable environment for gingival healing and restoration of a physiologic gingival contour.

Although gingivectomy was widely performed in the past, an improved understanding of healing and the development of sophisticated flap techniques have relegated it to a lesser role in periodontal surgery. However, it remains an effective form of treatment when indicated (Fig. 61.11).

Gingivectomy may be performed for the following indications:[10]

1. Elimination of suprabony pockets if the pocket wall is fibrous and firm
2. Elimination of gingival enlargements

Contraindications to gingivectomy include the following:

1. Access to bone required
2. Narrow zone of keratinized tissue
3. Esthetics
4. Patients with a high postoperative risk of bleeding

The step-by-step technique for gingivectomy is as follows:

Step 1: The periodontal pocket is mapped out on the external gingival surface by inserting a probe into the bottom of the pocket and puncturing the external surface of the gingiva at a depth of probe penetration (see Figs. 61.11C and D; Figs. 61.12 and 61.13).

Step 2: Periodontal knives (e.g., Kirkland) are used for incisions on the facial and lingual surfaces. Orban periodontal knives are used for interdental incisions (see Fig. 61.11E–G). Bard-Parker blades (#12 and #15) and scissors are used as auxiliary instruments.

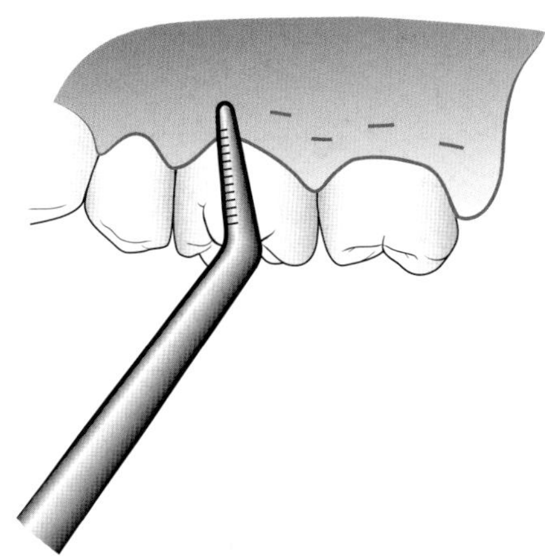

Fig. 61.12 The pocket marker makes pinpoint perforations that indicate pocket depth.

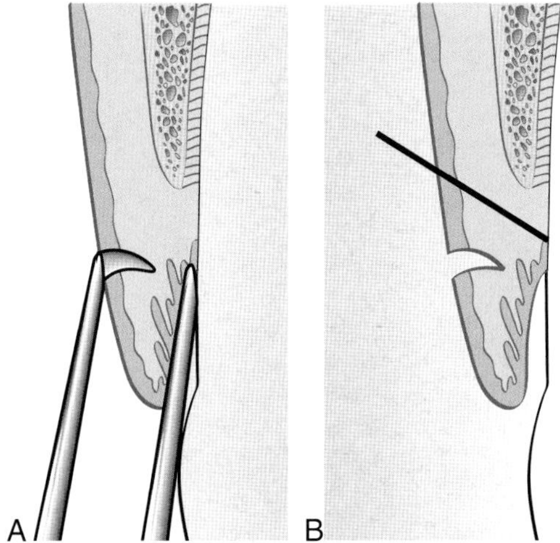

Fig. 61.13 Marking the depth of a suprabony pocket. (A) A pocket marker in position. (B) The beveled incision extends apical to the perforation made by the pocket marker.

The external bevel incision is started apical to the points marking the course of the pockets,[29,35] and it is directed coronally to a point between the base of the pocket and the crest of the bone. It should be as close as possible to the bone without exposing it to remove the soft tissue coronal to the bone. Exposure of bone is undesirable. If this occurs, healing usually presents minimal complications if the area is adequately covered by the surgical dressing.

Either interrupted or continuous incisions may be used. The incision should be beveled at approximately 45 degrees to the tooth surface, and it should re-create the normal festooned pattern of the gingiva. Failure to bevel the incision will leave a broad, fibrous plateau that will delay the development of a physiologic contour.

Step 3: Remove the excised pocket wall, irrigate the area, and examine the root surface.

Step 4: Scale and root plane.

Step 5: Cover the area with a surgical dressing (see Fig. 61.11I and Chapter 59).

Healing After Gingivectomy

The *initial response* after gingivectomy is the formation of a protective surface blood clot. The underlying tissue becomes acutely inflamed with necrosis. The clot is then replaced by granulation tissue. In 24 hours, an increase occurs in new connective tissue cells, which are mainly angioblasts beneath the surface layer of inflammation and necrotic tissue. By the third day, numerous young fibroblasts are located in the area.[26] The highly vascular granulation tissue grows coronally, creating a new free gingival margin and sulcus.[22] Capillaries derived from the blood vessels of the periodontal ligament migrate into the granulation tissue, and within 2 weeks they connect with the gingival vessels.[36]

After 12 to 24 hours, epithelial cells at the margins of the wound begin to migrate over the granulation tissue, thereby separating it from the contaminated surface layer of the clot. Epithelial activity at the margins reaches a peak after 24 to 36 hours.[9]

The new epithelial cells arise from the basal and deeper spinous layers of the epithelial wound edge and migrate over the wound over a fibrin layer that is later resorbed and replaced by a connective tissue bed.[14] The epithelial cells advance by a tumbling action, with the cells becoming fixed to the substrate by hemidesmosomes and a new basement lamina.[12,15]

After 5 to 14 days, surface epithelialization is generally complete (see Fig. 61.11J). During the first 4 weeks after gingivectomy, keratinization is less than it was before surgery. Complete epithelial repair takes about 1 month.[33] Vasodilation and vascularity begin to decrease after the fourth day of healing, and they appear to be almost normal by the 16th day.[20] Complete repair of the connective tissue takes about 7 weeks.[33]

The flow of gingival fluid in humans is initially increased after gingivectomy, and it diminishes as healing progresses.[1,31] Maximal flow is reached after 1 week, which coincides with the time of maximal inflammation.

Although the tissue changes that occur during postgingivectomy healing are the same in all individuals, the time required for complete healing varies considerably among sites and individuals. In patients with physiologic gingival melanosis, the pigmentation is diminished in the healed gingiva.

Flap Surgery

Periodontal flaps are used in surgical periodontal therapy to accomplish the following:

1. Access for root instrumentation
2. Gingival resection
3. Osseous resection
4. Periodontal regeneration

To fulfill these purposes, five different flap techniques are used: (1) the modified Widman flap,[27] (2) the undisplaced flap, (3) the apically displaced flap, (4) the papilla preservation flap,[7,34] and (5) the distal terminal molar flap.

The modified Widman flap facilitates root instrumentation. It does not attempt to reduce the pocket depth but eliminates the pocket lining. The objectives of the undisplaced and apically displaced flaps include root surface access and the reduction of probing depth. The choice of which procedure to use depends on two important anatomic landmarks: the transgingival probing depth and the location of the mucogingival junction. These landmarks establish the presence and width of the attached gingiva, which are the basis for the decision. The papilla preservation flap is used when possible in regenerative and esthetic cases to minimize recession and loss of interdental papillae. The distal terminal molar flap is used for treating pockets and osseous defects on the distal surface of the terminal maxillary and mandibular molars.

Modified Widman Flap

The original Widman[37] flap used two vertical releasing incisions connected by a submarginal scalloped internal bevel incision to demarcate the area of surgery. A full-thickness flap was reflected, and the marginal collar of tissue was removed to provide access for

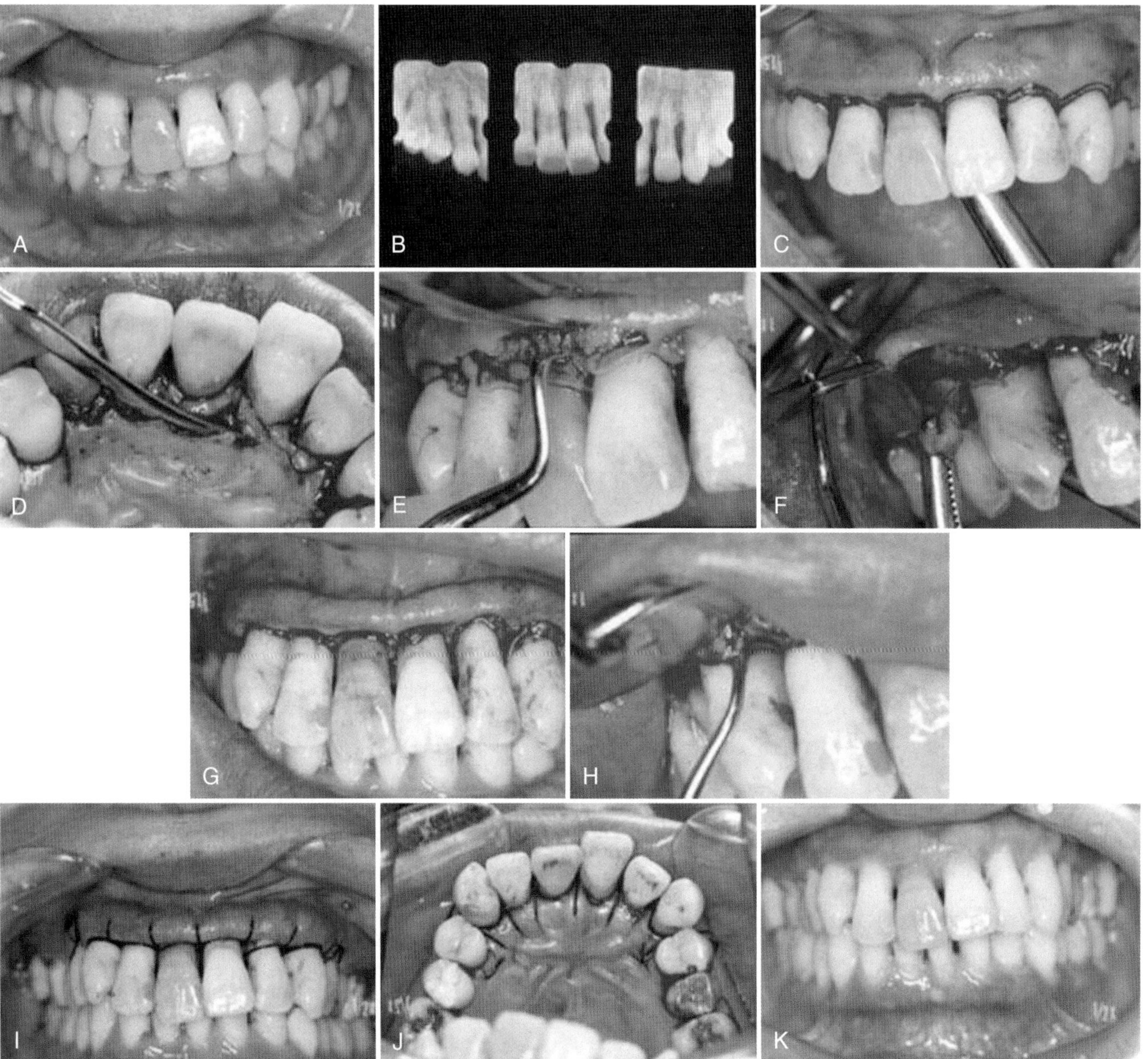

Fig. 61.14 Modified Widman flap technique. (A) Facial view before surgery. The probing of pockets revealed interproximal depths that ranged from 4 to 8 mm and facial and palatal depths of 2 to 5 mm. (B) Radiographic survey of the area. Note the generalized horizontal bone loss. (C) Facial internal bevel incision. (D) Palatal incision. (E) Elevation of the flap, which left a wedge of tissue attached to its base. (F) Removal of tissue. (G) Tissue removed and ready for scaling and root planing. (H) Scaling and root planing of exposed root surfaces. (I) Continuous, independent sling suture of facial portion of the surgery. (J) Continuous, independent sling suture of palatal portion of the surgery. (K) Postsurgical result. (Courtesy Dr. Kitetsu Shin, Saitama, Japan.)

root instrumentation and osseous recontouring. In 1974, Ramfjord and Nissle[27] published the "modified Widman flap" (Fig. 61.14), which used only horizontal incisions. This technique offers the possibility of establishing an intimate postoperative adaptation of healthy collagenous connective tissue to tooth surfaces,[4,17,25,27] and it provides access for adequate instrumentation of the root surfaces and immediate closure of the area.

The step-by-step technique for the modified Widman flap is as follows:

Step 1: The first incision (Fig. 61.15A) parallel to the long axis of the tooth is a scalloped internal bevel incision to the alveolar crest starting 0.5 to 1 mm away from the gingival margin (see Fig. 61.14C). The papillae are dissected and thinned to have a thickness similar to that of the remaining flaps.

Step 2: Full-thickness flaps are reflected 2 to 3 mm away from the alveolar crest (see Fig. 61.14D).

Step 3: The second crevicular incision (see Fig. 61.15B) is made in the gingival crevice to detach the attachment apparatus from the root.

Step 4: The interdental tissue and the gingival collar are detached from the bone with a third incision (see Fig. 61.15C; see also Fig. 61.14E and F).

Step 5: The gingival collar and granulation tissue are removed with curettes. The root surfaces are scaled and planed (see Fig. 61.14G and H). Residual periodontal fibers attached to the tooth surface should not be disturbed.

Step 6: Bone architecture is not corrected unless it prevents intimate flap adaptation. Every effort is made to adapt the facial and lingual interdental tissue so that no interdental bone remains exposed during suturing. The flaps may be thinned to allow for close adaptation of the gingiva around the entire circumference of the tooth.

Step 7: The flaps are stabilized with sutures (see Fig. 61.14I and J) and covered with a surgical dressing.

Ramfjord[25] performed an extensive longitudinal study that compared the modified Widman procedure with the curettage technique and the pocket elimination (gingivectomy and osseous surgery) methods. Patients were assigned randomly to one of the techniques, and results were analyzed yearly for up to 7 years after therapy. The researchers reported similar results for each of the three methods tested. Pocket depth was initially similar for all methods, but it was maintained at shallower levels with the modified Widman flap; the attachment level remained higher with the modified Widman flap.

Undisplaced Flap

Currently, the undisplaced flap may be the most frequently performed type of periodontal surgery. For the undisplaced flap, the submarginal scalloped internal bevel incision is initiated at a distance from the tooth, roughly one-half to two-thirds of the interdental transgingival probing depth. This incision can be accomplished only if sufficient attached gingiva remains apical to the incision. Therefore, the two anatomic landmarks, the transgingival interdental probing depth, and the mucogingival junction must be considered to evaluate the amount of attached gingiva that will remain after surgery. The internal bevel incision should be scalloped to create surgical papillae, which are essential to covering the interdental bone (see Fig. 61.4). If the tissue is too thick, the flap margin should be thinned with the initial incision. Proper placement of the flap margin at the alveolar crest during closure is important to prevent either recurrence of the pocket or exposure of bone.

The step-by-step technique for the undisplaced flap is as follows:

Step 1: The periodontal probe is inserted into the gingival crevice and penetrates the junctional epithelium and connective tissue down to the bone.

Step 2: The mucogingival junction is assessed to determine the amount of keratinized tissue.

Step 3: The initial placement of the submarginal scalloped internal bevel incision is based on the transgingival interdental probing depth and the mucogingival junction (Fig. 61.16). The incision is made parallel to the long axis of the tooth and directed down to the alveolar bone. The angulation of the incision may be altered depending on the thickness of the gingiva, as well as the initial placement of the submarginal scalloped incision, to produce a thin flap margin. The thicker the tissue, the more apically the incision will end (see Fig. 61.16). A short mesial vertical incision may be employed to allow flap release on the palate or to avoid extension of the horizontal incision into the esthetic area.

Step 4: Full-thickness flaps are reflected 1 mm apical to the mucogingival junction.

Step 5: The crevicular is made in the gingival crevice to detach the attachment apparatus from the root.

Step 6: The gingival collar and granulation tissue are removed with curettes. The root surfaces are scaled and planed.

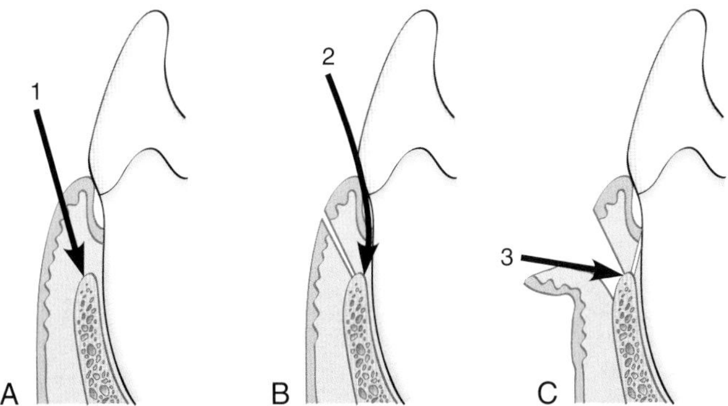

Fig. 61.15 The three incisions necessary for flap surgery. (A) First (internal bevel) incision; (B) second (crevicular) incision; and (C) third (interdental) incision.

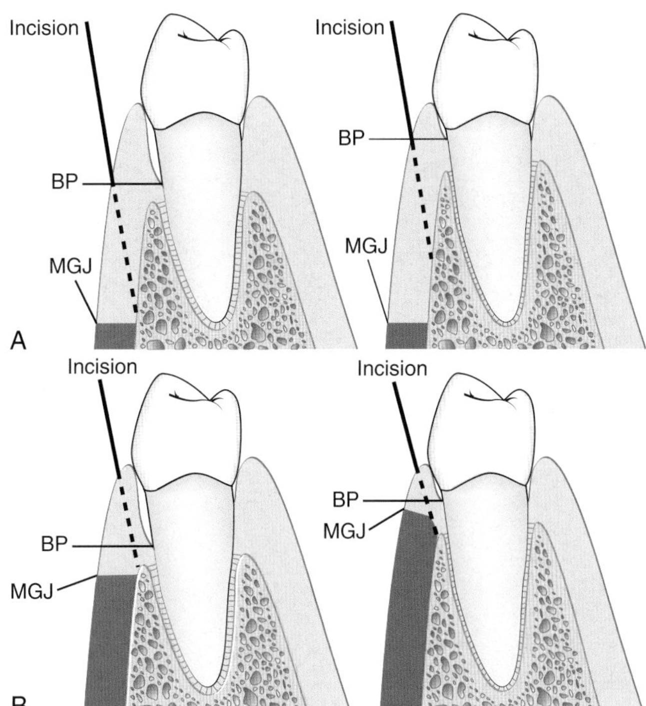

Fig. 61.16 (A and B) The location of two different areas where the internal bevel incision is made in an undisplaced flap. The incision is made at the level of the pocket to discard the tissue coronal to the pocket if the remaining attached gingiva is sufficient. *BP,* Bottom of pocket; *MGJ,* mucogingival junction.

Step 7: Osseous recontouring is performed to eliminate defects and reestablish positive architecture.

Step 8: The flaps are coapted on the alveolar crest, with the flap margin well adapted to the roots. The flaps may be trimmed and rescalloped if necessary.

Step 9: The flaps are stabilized with sutures and covered with a surgical dressing.

Apically Displaced Flap

The apically displaced flap is selected for cases that present with a minimal amount (<3 mm) of attached gingiva. For this reason, the internal bevel incision should be made as close to the tooth as possible (i.e., 0.5 to 1.0 mm). No need exists to determine where the bottom of the pocket is in relation to the incision for the apically displaced flap as one would for the undisplaced flap. The flap is placed at the tooth–bone junction by apically displacing the flap. Its final position is not determined by the placement of the first incision.

With some variants, the apically displaced flap can be used for pocket eradication, widening the zone of attached gingiva, or both. Depending on the purpose, the apically displaced flap can be a full-thickness flap or a split-thickness flap. The split-thickness flap requires more precision and finesse, as well as a gingiva that is thick enough to split. The split-thickness flap can be more precisely positioned and sutured in an apical position with the use of a periosteal suturing technique.

The step-by-step technique for the apically displaced flap is as follows:

Step 1: A marginal scalloped internal bevel incision parallel to the long axis of the tooth is made down to the crest of the bone (Fig. 61.17).

Step 2: If used, vertical incisions are made extending beyond the mucogingival junction. It is important that the vertical incisions—and therefore the flap elevation—reach past the mucogingival junction to provide adequate mobility to the flap for its apical displacement.

Step 3: The flap is reflected in full thickness or partial thickness, depending on the thickness of the gingiva and the objective of the surgery.

Step 4: Crevicular and interdental incisions are made, and the marginal collar of tissue is removed.

Step 5: After degranulation, scaling and root planing, and osseous surgery if needed, the flap is displaced apically.

Step 6: If a full-thickness flap is reflected, an independent sling suture positions the flap margin at the alveolar crest, and a surgical dressing can prevent its coronal movement. If a partial-thickness flap was reflected, it could be apically displaced with an independent sling suture, and further stabilized with periosteal sutures. A periodontal dressing can prevent its coronal movement.

After 1 week, dressings and sutures are removed. The area is usually repacked for another week, after which the patient is to brush gently along the gingival margin with a soft brush and interdentally with interdental brushes.

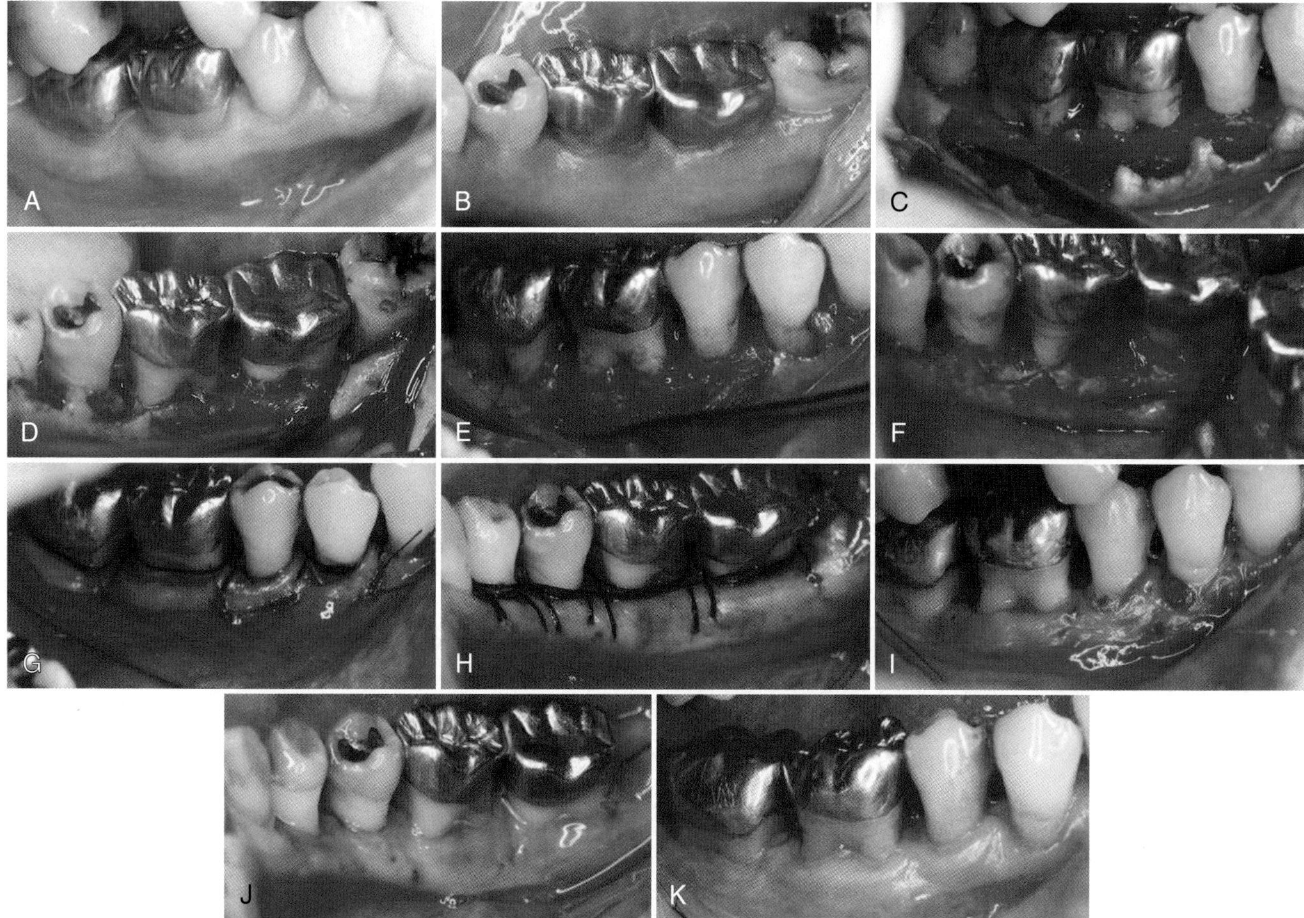

Fig. 61.17 An apically displaced flap. (A and B) Facial and lingual preoperative views. (C and D) The facial and lingual flaps have been elevated. (E and F) After debridement of the areas. (G and H) The sutures are in place. (I and J) Healing after 1 week. (K) Healing after 2 months. Note the preservation of the attached gingiva is displaced to a more apical position. (Courtesy Dr. Thomas Han, Los Angeles, CA.)

Distal Terminal Molar Flap

The treatment of periodontal pockets on the distal surface of terminal molars is often complicated by the presence of bulbous fibrous tissue over the maxillary tuberosity or prominent retromolar pads in the mandible. Some of these osseous lesions may result from incomplete repair after the extraction of impacted third molars (Fig. 61.18).

Access to these distal areas may be obtained by a single horizontal incision, two converging horizontal incisions, or two parallel incisions extending distally from the distal surface of the terminal molar to the mucogingival junction distal to the tuberosity or the retromolar pad. The distal horizontal incision is connected with the crevicular incision on the distal surface of the terminal molar, which merges mesially with the buccal and lingual or palatal scalloped incisions. If the secondary objective of surgery is regenerative or the buccolingual width of the distal keratinized tissue is limited, a single horizontal incision in keratinized tissue is used. If the secondary objective of surgery is resective and adequate keratinized tissue is present buccolingually, two distal horizontal incisions are placed in keratinized tissue. The two horizontal incisions technique were described by Robinson[30] and Braden[4] and modified by several other investigators. These techniques are called the *distal wedge* and the *modified distal wedge*.

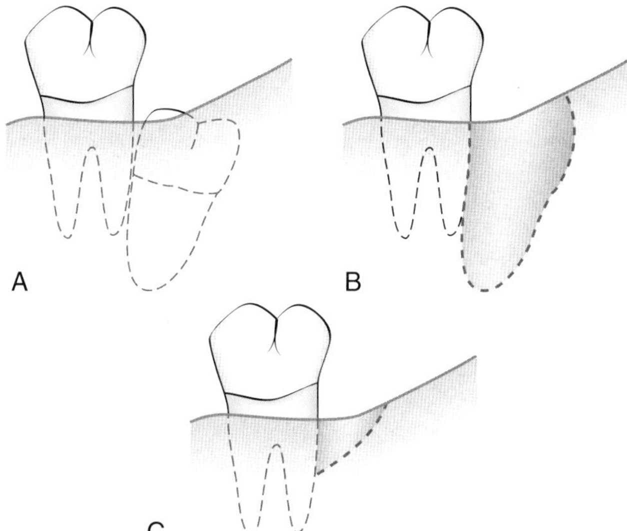

Fig. 61.18 (A) Impaction of a third molar distal to a second molar with little or no interdental bone between the two teeth. (B) Removal of the third molar creates a pocket with little or no bone distal to the second molar. (C) This often leads to a vertical osseous defect distal to the second molar.

The distal wedge technique employs two horizontal incisions that begin at the distal surface of the terminal molar and *converge* distally at the mucogingival junction distal to the tuberosity or the retromolar pad. The modified distal wedge technique employs two *parallel* horizontal incisions that extend distally from the distal surface of the terminal molar and are connected by a transverse incision distal to the mucogingival junction distal to the tuberosity or retromolar pad. The buccolingual distance between the two horizontal incisions in both techniques depends on the transgingival probing depth and the amount of fibrous tissue involved. When the flaps are thinned, and the tissue between the two incisions is removed, the two flap edges must approximate each other at a new apical position without overlapping (Fig. 61.19). Generally, the distance between the two parallel incisions is roughly one-half to two-thirds the distal transgingival probing depth and should never be farther apart than the distance between the buccal and lingual line angles of the tooth.

To ensure primary closure of the distal flaps, especially in the tuberosity, it is advantageous to use one horizontal incision or two horizontal incisions that are closer together rather than farther apart. Flaps that overlap when they are coapted can be easily trimmed by placing one flap over the other, grabbing the superficial flap with a hemostat, and cutting away the overlapped tissue with a sharp scalpel or scissors.

In regenerative therapy, the distal flaps are not thinned; they are reflected in full thickness. Whereas in resective therapy, before the flaps are completely reflected, they are undermined and thinned with a #15 blade. It is easier to thin the flap before it is completely reflected and mobile. The flaps are then reflected in full thickness.

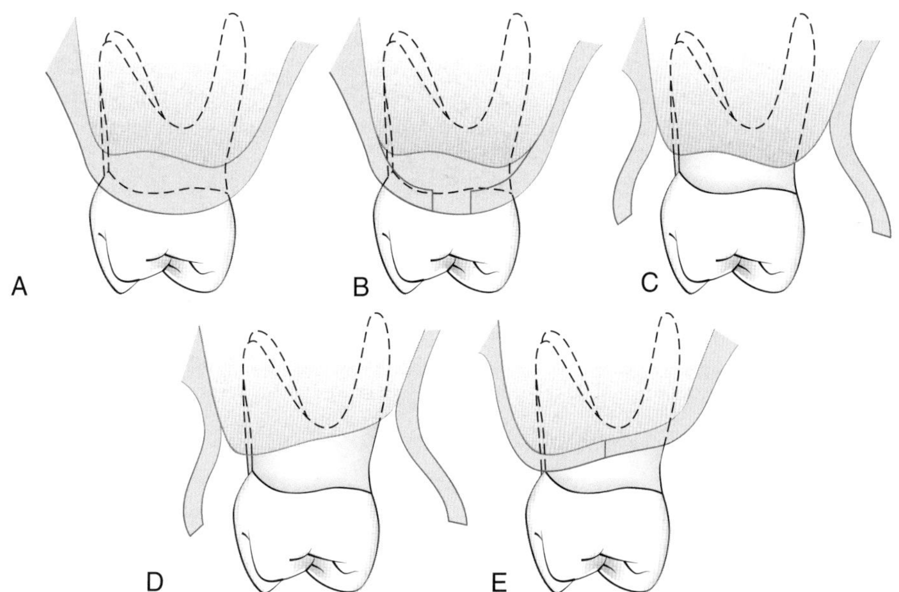

Fig. 61.19 (A) Coronal view from behind a maxillary second molar with an osseous defect. (B) Distal terminal flap surgery employs two horizontal incisions; both buccal and lingual flaps are thinned. (C) Buccal and lingual flaps are elevated, and the "wedge" of tissue is removed. (D) The bone is sloped to the palatal side to eliminate the osseous defect. (E) The flaps are coapted on the bone in the apical position.

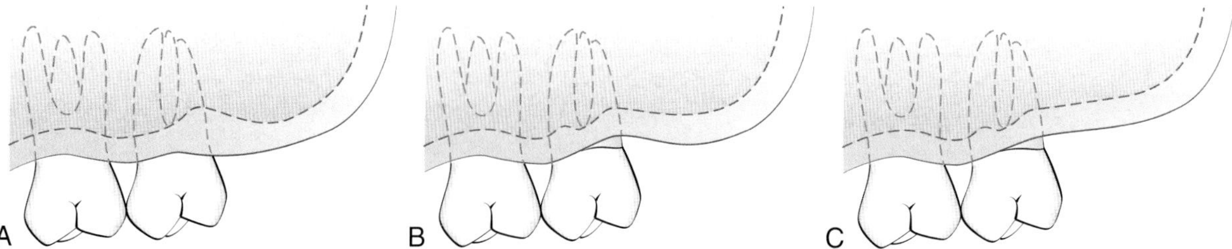

Fig. 61.20 (A) Sagittal view of a distal defect on a maxillary second molar. (B) Treatment with distal wedge results in an acute angle between the tuberosity and the distal surface of the second molar. (C) Treatment with modified distal wedge results in a wider angle between the tuberosity and the distal surface of the second molar that is more accessible for hygiene.

Maxillary Molars

The treatment of distal pockets in the maxilla is usually less challenging than that in the mandible. The tuberosity presents a greater amount of fibrous attached gingiva than does the retromolar pad. The use of the distal wedge with two converging incisions causes the tissue next to the tooth to be displaced more apically than the tissue away from the tooth. Consequently, healing of a distal wedge in the maxilla results in an acute angle between the distal tooth surface and the tuberosity that is biofilm retentive and difficult to clean (Fig. 61.20B). In contrast, the use of the modified distal wedge with two parallel distal incisions allows the soft tissue along the whole length of the distal flap to be evenly displaced apically (see Fig. 61.20C). This is advantageous in the maxilla in maintaining a wide angle between the tooth and the tuberosity that is much easier to clean. Therefore, the modified distal wedge is preferred in the maxilla. The two parallel incisions are usually made at the midline of the tuberosity where the tissue is the thickest or slightly to the palatal side to maximize buccal keratinized tissue and to provide easier access for flap closure (Fig. 61.21).

LEARNING BOX 61.6

The two parallel distal horizontal incisions in the maxillary tuberosity are advantageous in allowing the soft tissue along the whole length of the distal flap to be evenly displaced. This results in a wide angle between the tooth and the tuberosity that is much easier to clean.

Mandibular Molars

Incisions in the distal mandible differ from those in the tuberosity due to differences in the anatomy of the area. The retromolar pad usually has limited attached gingiva and vestibular depth. The attached gingiva, if present, may not be found directly distal to the molar. The greatest amount may be distolingual or distobuccal, and it may not be over the bony crest. The ascending ramus of the mandible may also create a short or completely eliminate the horizontal area distal to the terminal molar (Fig. 61.22). The shorter this area, the more difficult it is to treat any deep distal lesion around the terminal molar. The anatomy of the posterior mandible is further discussed in Chapter 59.

The mandibular retromolar tissue ascends distally to merge with the ascending ramus. This anatomy favors the distal wedge technique in the mandible, although parallel distal incisions and a single horizontal incision may be used. The two distal incisions should follow the area with the greatest amount of attached gingiva and must be made over bone (Fig. 61.23). Therefore, the incisions could be directed distally or distobuccally, depending on which area has more attached gingiva. Incisions directing distolingually should be avoided due to the potential presence of the lingual nerve.

Papilla Preservation Flap

In current regenerative therapy, bone grafts, membranes, or a combination of these are used with or without other biologics (see Chapter 63). The flap design should maximize the amount of gingival tissue and papilla retained to cover the material placed in the osseous defect. In the esthetic area, when surgery is necessary, flap design must minimize recession and loss of interdental papillae. As such, the crevicular incision is the incision of choice for the anterior esthetic area and regenerative therapy. The interdental papilla is retained with the papilla preservation technique when the interdental space is adequate for reflection of the intact papilla; otherwise, it is split beneath the contact point of the two approximating teeth. The flap is elevated in full thickness without thinning of the flap or the papilla.

The step-by-step technique for the papilla preservation flap (see Fig. 61.8; Fig. 61.24) is as follows:

Step 1: A crevicular incision is made around each tooth, with no incisions across the interdental papilla.

Step 2: The preserved papilla can be incorporated into the facial-buccal flap (original papilla preservation technique[34]) or lingual-palatal flap (modified papilla preservation technique[7]). If the preserved papilla is reflected with the facial-buccal flap, the semilunar incision at the base of the papilla is on the lingual-palatal side of the interdental space. If the preserved papilla is reflected with the lingual-palatal flap, the semilunar incision at the base of the papilla is on the facial-buccal side of the interdental space. This semilunar incision dips apically from the line angles of the tooth so that the incision is at least 5 mm from the crest of the papilla.

Step 3: The papilla is then elevated with an Orban knife or curettes and is reflected intact with the flap.

Step 4: The flap is reflected without thinning the tissue.

Healing After Flap Surgery

Time sequence for healing:

- *Immediately after suturing (≤24 hours),* a connection between the flap and the tooth or bone surface is established by a blood clot consisting of a fibrin reticulum with many polymorphonuclear leukocytes, erythrocytes, debris of injured cells, and capillaries at the edge of the wound.[5] Bacteria and an exudate or transudate also result from tissue injury.
- *One to 3 days after flap surgery,* the space between the flap and the tooth or bone is thinner. Epithelial cells migrate over the border of the flap, and they usually contact the tooth at this time. When the flap is closely adapted to the alveolar process, the inflammatory response is minimal.[5]

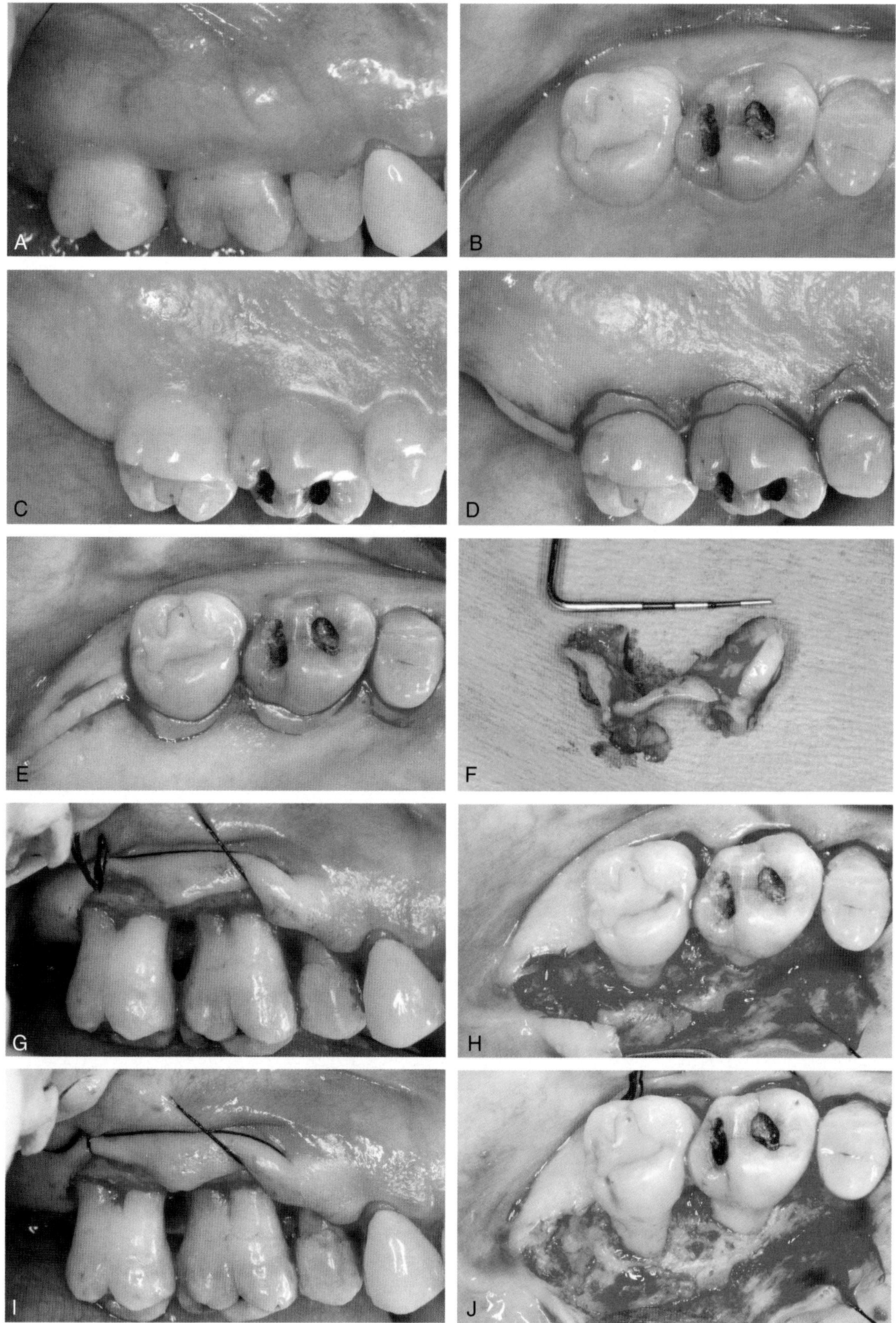

Fig. 61.21 (A–C) Presurgical views. (D and E) Palatal submarginal scalloped incisions and parallel distal horizontal incisions. (F) Distal "wedge" of tissue removed. (G) Buccal and (H) palatal bone before osseous recontouring. (I) Buccal and (J) palatal bone after osseous recontouring.

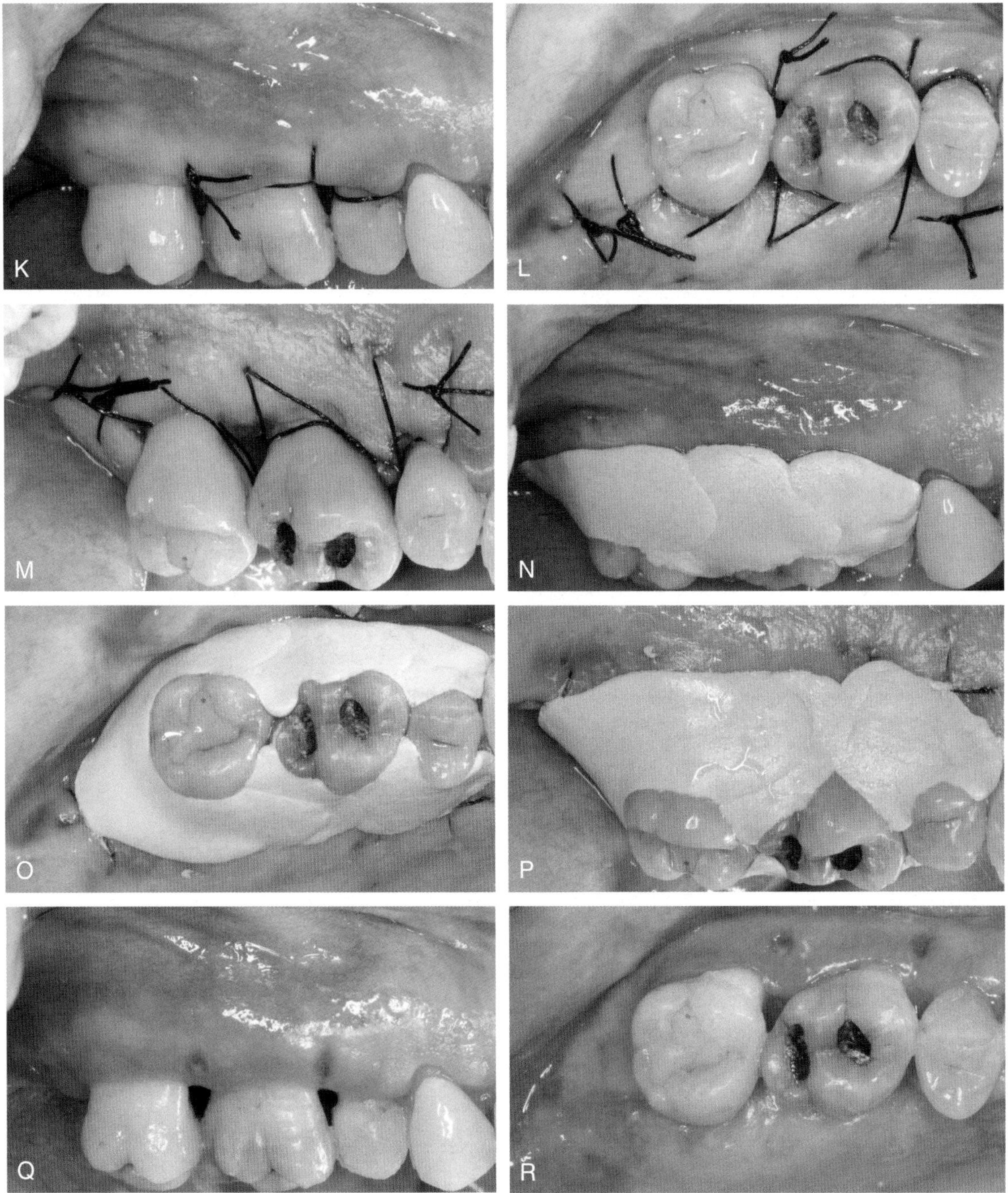

Fig. 61.21, cont'd (K) to (M) Primary closure of flaps with 4-0 silk sutures. (N –P) Placement of surgical dressing. (Q–S) Postoperative healing at 2 weeks.

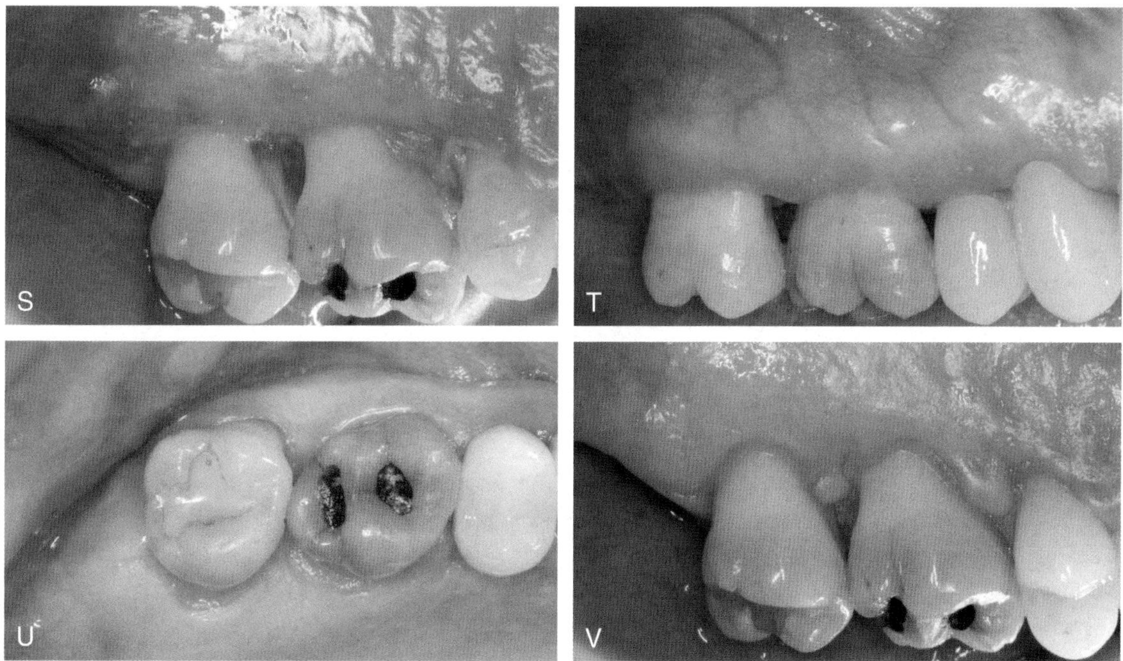

Fig. 61.21, cont'd (T –V) Postoperative healing at 8 months. (Copyright Jonathan H. Do, DDS. All rights reserved.)

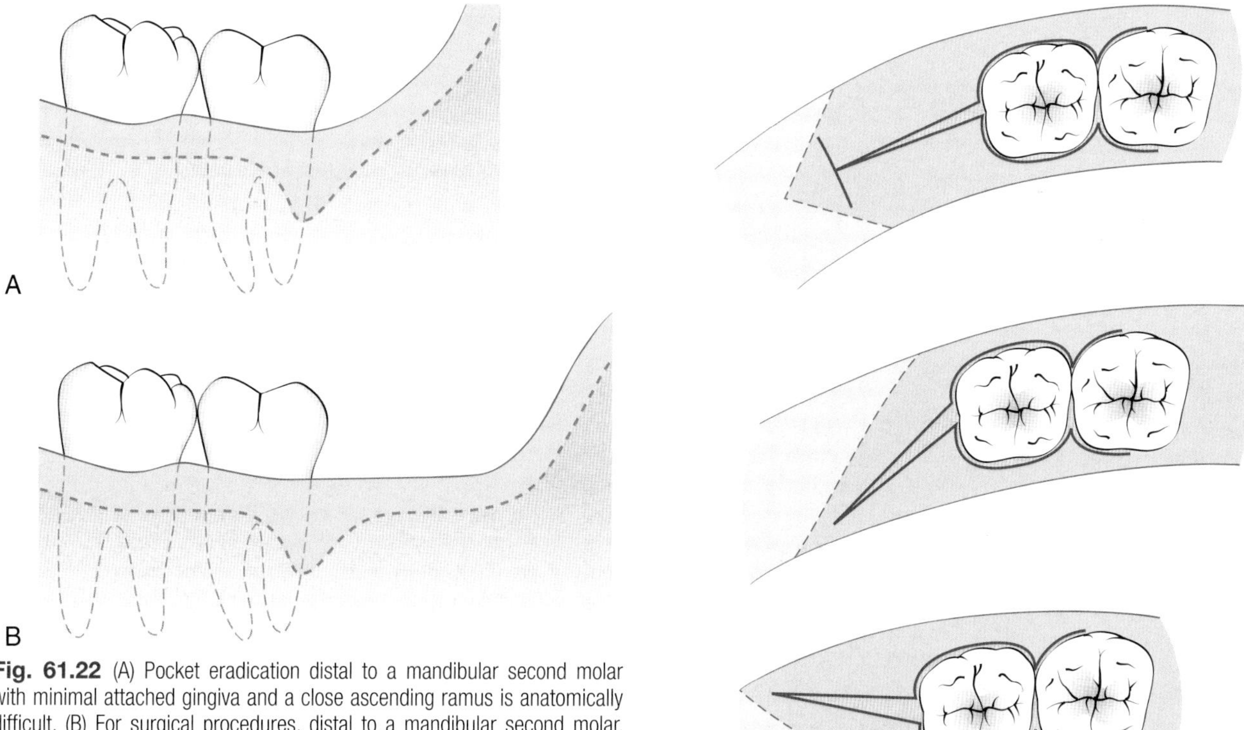

Fig. 61.22 (A) Pocket eradication distal to a mandibular second molar with minimal attached gingiva and a close ascending ramus is anatomically difficult. (B) For surgical procedures, distal to a mandibular second molar, abundant attached gingiva, and distal space are ideal.

Fig. 61.23 Incision designs for surgical procedures distal to the mandibular second molar. The incision should follow the areas of the greatest attached gingiva and underlying bone.

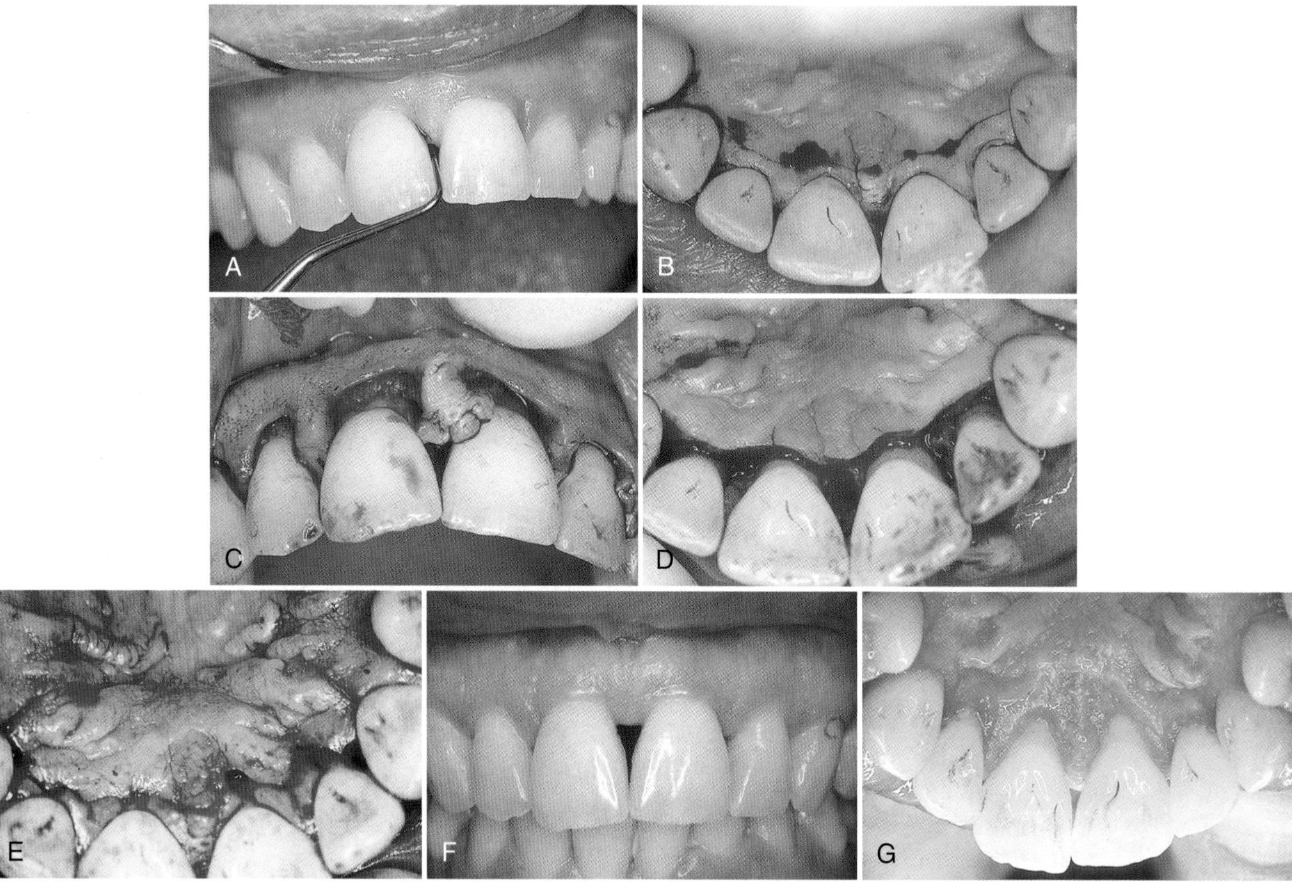

Fig. 61.24 Papilla preservation flap. (A) Facial view after sulcular incisions have been made. (B) Straight-line incision in the palatal area about 3 mm from the gingival margins. This incision is then connected to the margins with vertical incisions at the midpart of each tooth. (C) Papillae are reflected with the facial flap. (D) Lingual view after the reflection of the flap. (E) Lingual view after the flap is brought back to its original position. It is then sutured with independent sutures. (F) Facial view after healing. (G) Palatal view after healing. (Courtesy Dr. Thomas Han, Los Angeles, CA.)

- *One week after surgery,* an epithelial attachment to the root has been established by means of hemidesmosomes and a basal lamina. The blood clot is replaced by granulation tissue derived from the gingival connective tissue, the bone marrow, and the periodontal ligament.
- *Two weeks after surgery,* collagen fibers begin to appear parallel to the tooth surface.[5] Union of the flap to the tooth is still weak because of the presence of immature collagen fibers, although the clinical aspect may be almost normal.
- *One month after surgery,* a fully epithelialized gingival crevice with a well-defined epithelial attachment is present. A functional arrangement of the supracrestal fibers is beginning.

Full-thickness flaps denude the bone, resulting in superficial bone necrosis after 1 to 3 days. Osteoclastic resorption follows and peaks at 4 to 6 days, then declines thereafter.[32] This results in a loss of bone of about 1 mm^3; the bone loss is greater if the bone is thin.[38,39]

Osteoplasty with the use of diamond burs results in areas of bone necrosis with a reduction in bone height, which is later remodeled by new bone formation. The final shape of the crest is determined more by osseous remodeling than by surgical reshaping.[16] Therefore, osseous surgery around the crestal areas must be carefully managed.

This may not be the case when osseous remodeling does not include excessive thinning of the radicular bone.[18] Bone repair reaches its peak after 3 to 4 weeks.[39]

A loss of bone occurs during the initial healing stages both in the radicular bone and in the interdental bone areas. However, in the interdental areas, which have cancellous bone, the subsequent repair stage results in total restitution without any loss of bone; in radicular bone (particularly if it is thin and unsupported by cancellous bone), bone repair results in the loss of marginal bone.[39]

Conclusion

Short- and long-term success of periodontal access surgery is dependent on biofilm control and long-term maintenance. The patient must understand the etiology of periodontal disease and its prevention. Surgery in the absence of effective biofilm control and maintenance will result in failure and the recurrence of disease.

Periodontal access surgery is an adjunct to nonsurgical periodontal therapy and should be performed only after the patient has demonstrated effective biofilm control. The primary objective for the clinician is access for root instrumentation. The secondary objective of periodontal access surgery is pocket reduction through soft tissue resection, osseous resection, or periodontal regeneration.

The clinician must also take esthetics into consideration; in some areas, such as the anterior maxilla, periodontal disease should be treated nonsurgically, and periodontal access surgery is rendered only when absolutely necessary. Papilla preservation techniques are useful in regenerative therapy, as well as in minimizing recession and loss of interdental papilla in the esthetic area.

Although the submarginal scalloped incision is useful in reducing periodontal pockets, it must be used with caution. Placement of a submarginal scalloped incision without regard for the mucogingival junction and the width of keratinized tissue may result in a mucogingival problem. The only area in the mouth where the submarginal scalloped incision is necessary is the palatal maxilla. In places where a mucogingival junction is present, marginal incisions and apically displaced flaps may be used in lieu of submarginal scalloped incisions to maximize remaining keratinized tissue and reduce soft tissue height. The palatal maxilla is unique in that all the tissue is keratinized, attached, and immobile. Pocket reduction must be obtained by tissue resection. The precise placement of the submarginal scalloped incision on the palatal maxilla is essential for intimate adaptation, coaptation of the flap, and primary closure.

Although the "distal wedge" procedure is popular and widely practiced, it is perhaps one of the most difficult procedures to execute well due to the location of the surgical site, as well as the challenges presented by the anatomy of the mandibular retromolar pad and the maxillary tuberosity. *The distal wedge procedure is not simply removing a "wedge of tissue" distal to the terminal molar to reduce or eliminate a pocket.* Well-executed distal terminal molar flap surgery requires the flaps to approximate intimately to allow for primary closure and in an apical position to achieve pocket reduction. Execution of distal terminal molar flap surgery requires understanding of the anatomy and behavior of the tissue, as well as surgical experience.

References for this chapter are found on the companion website eBooks.Health.Elsevier.com.

CHAPTER 62

Pocket Reduction Therapy—Resective Approach

Beatriz Bezerra

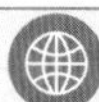 For online-only content on osseous resection technique, flap placement and closure, specific osseous reshaping situations, root resection, hemisection, and postoperative maintenance, please visit the companion website at eBooks.Health.Elsevier.com.

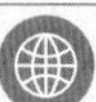 Animations have been added by the editors as a supplement to the chapter. They are produced by PerioPixel as patient education tools and cover the basic elements in a conceptual manner. They are not intended to be procedural guides for dental professionals.

CHAPTER OUTLINE

Periodontal disease results in a loss of connective tissue attachment in association with uneven destruction of the alveolar bone. The destruction of periodontal tissues progresses in the apical direction and is influenced by several factors, including local anatomy and the inflammatory response. In the posterior teeth, this progression can lead to exposure of the furcation area, which presents an additional anatomical challenge. Bone loss resulting from the progression of periodontitis is often a combination of horizontal or vertical bone loss, and this pattern is normally a result of the local osseous anatomy (i.e., the thickness of cortical bone affects the manner in which bone loss progresses).

With these varying presentations of bone loss, it is important to carefully consider the most appropriate ways to recontour the bony housing to provide a more physiological bone pattern. This allows the soft tissues to properly heal, leading to a reduction in probing depths and improved access for patients to perform proper plaque control.

Resective therapy has been used in the treatment of osseous defects as well as in the management of furcation defects for many years. The goal of resective surgery is to reshape the bone and tooth/root structure to achieve proper contours that will result, many times, in bone levels slightly more apical than preexisting levels.

In this chapter, we discuss the surgical management of periodontal disease via resective surgery. The anatomical features of furcation areas are briefly discussed as they relate to the proper management of these defects via a resective approach.

Rationale

The primary goal of resective surgery is to eliminate periodontal pockets and create shallow gingival sulci that allow for proper maintenance by the patient and the dental professional. This is the most predictable surgical technique for pocket elimination.[13,48] However, because of its nature, this surgical technique is performed at the expense of bony tissue and attachment levels.[4]

The conversion of deep periodontal pockets to shallow gingival sulci allows the patient to properly maintain periodontal health by daily plaque removal by means of oral hygiene measures. Similarly, the ability of a dental professional to successfully scale shallow pockets allows for the maintenance of periodontal health. Studies have demonstrated that the deeper the pocket, the more difficult it is to properly scale and completely remove all plaque and calculus.[50,58] On the same note, proper debridement of furcation areas is impaired by the reduced size of the furcation entrance in relation to the size of periodontal instruments,[5] the presence of ridges,[12] and concavities.[5,16] These local anatomical features render furcation sites difficult to effectively reach with an instrument. Therefore, the successful elimination of pockets and furcation defects via resective surgery followed by an effective periodontal maintenance therapy will lead to greater longitudinal stability of the surgical results.

 **KEY FACT**

Bone determines the form of the gingiva as well as the residual pocket depth.

 **KEY FACT**

Instrumentation of furcation areas is difficult because instruments often are wider than the furcation entrance.

Local Anatomy

Bone Defect Morphology

The patterns of bone loss associated with periodontal disease can lead to variations in local bone morphology. For a review of the different bony defects, the reader is encouraged to review Chapter 22 of this book.

Osseous craters, also known as *two-wall defects*, are the most common bony defect resulting from periodontal bone loss,[34,35,41] representing one-third of all bony defects identified in the maxilla and two-thirds of all defects observed in the mandible.[35]

Furcation

Furcation is defined as the anatomical area of a multirooted tooth where the roots diverge.[19] This area presents with a complex anatomic morphology that affects proper debridement by routine periodontal instrumentation.[5]

To properly diagnose a furcation involvement one must carefully probe the area to the determine the presence and extent of attachment loss. This assessment is made with a specific periodontal probe called a *Nabers probe* (Fig. 62.1). The Nabers probe allows for the measurement of horizontal attachment loss, which should be an integral part of a thorough periodontal examination.

Radiographic evaluation may not be reliable for the assessment of early furcation involvement, but it does provide valuable information for treatment planning.[9,23] Information furnished by well-made radiographs include the following: root trunk length, root length, root form, root separation, position of interproximal bone in relation to furcation entrance, anatomy of the furcation, and cervical enamel projections.

Root trunk length: This is the distance between the cementoenamel junction (CEJ) and the furcation entrance. This is an important anatomic factor because variations in length can place a tooth at greater risk for furcation involvement (Fig. 62.2A–C). It can also affect the outcomes of therapy. The shorter the root trunk, the less attachment needs to be lost before the furcation is involved. This allows for early intervention and may facilitate some surgical procedures. Conversely, teeth with long root trunks or fused roots may not be appropriate candidates for treatment once the furcation is affected.

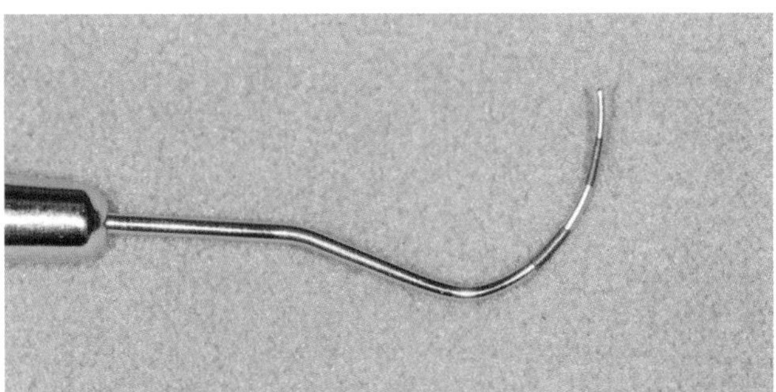

Fig. 62.1 The Nabers probe, which is designed to probe into a furcation.

Root length: Root length goes hand in hand with root trunk length. Teeth with long root trunks and short roots are more likely to present with a hopeless prognosis once furcation involvement is detected.[16,17] Teeth with long roots and short to moderate root trunks are more readily treated because there is still sufficient attachment remaining to meet the functional demands.

Root form: Concavities are often observed on the root surfaces associated with furcation area. Bower[5] noted that mandibular first molars presented with concavities on both mesial and distal roots, where the mesial root concavity was deeper. Maxillary first molars present with concavities on the furcal side of the roots in 94% of mesial–buccal roots, 31% of disto-buccal roots, and 17% of palatal roots.[5] As bone loss progresses into the furcation area, these concavities act as niches for plaque accumulation, and proper debridement of these areas is impaired because of the non-flat anatomy. Maxillary first premolars present with a mesial concavity that can place these teeth at greater risk for attachment loss due to inadequate access for proper root debridement.

Root separation: The wider the separation between roots, the more treatment options are available for the management of furcation involvements (Fig. 62.3A–D). Fused and closely approximated roots are observed in 33% of teeth, with 42% of these being maxillary molars and 24% occurring in mandibular molars.[26]

Cervical enamel projections (CEPs): CEPs are extensions of the cervical enamel margin toward or into the root furcation area (Fig. 62.4). Their prevalence ranges from 8.6% to 28.6%, with mandibular molars having the highest prevalence. Their presence has been highly correlated with furcation involvement; one study demonstrated that 63% of furcation involved teeth presented with CEPs.[27] The extent of CEPs was classified by Masters and Hoskins[36] on the basis of their extension toward the furcation area (Box 62.1). CEPs should be removed to facilitate maintenance.

Classification of Furcation Defects

The extent and severity of furcation defects need to be assessed to properly propose the most predictable treatment approach. Several classification systems have been developed, and they provide information on the horizontal as well as vertical extent of the involvement.

The classification system proposed by Glickman[18] (1953) has been widely used; it provides information on the horizontal component to attachment loss and is divided into four grades (Box 62.2

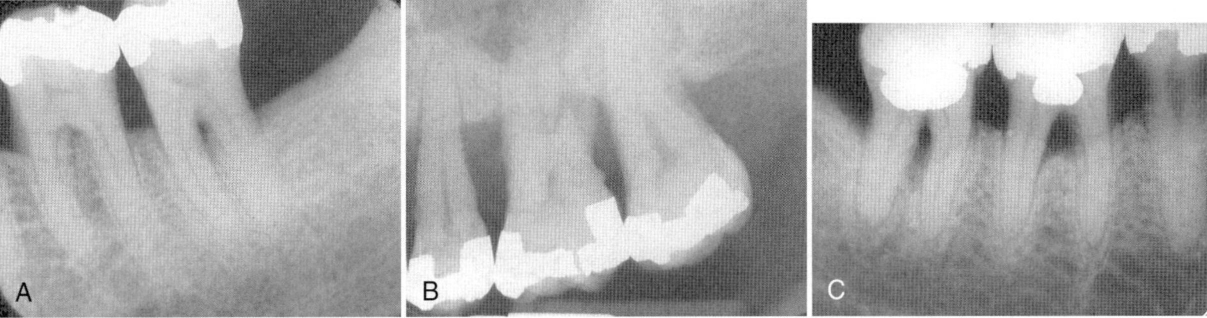

Fig. 62.2 Different degrees of furcation involvement in radiographs. (A) A grade I furcation on the mandibular first molar and a grade III furcation on the mandibular second molar. The root approximation on the second molar may be sufficient to impede accurate probing of this defect. (B) Multiple furcation defects on a maxillary first molar. Grade I buccal furcation involvement and grade II mesiopalatal and distopalatal furcations are present. Deep developmental grooves on the maxillary second molar simulate furcation involvement in this molar with fused roots. (C) Grades III and IV furcations on mandibular molars.

and Fig. 62.5). Hamp[22] proposed a classification in which furcation involvement is measured in millimeters to determine the extent of horizontal involvement. Tarnow and Fletcher[54] further elaborated on the classification system by proposing a subclassification that measures the vertical depth from the roof of the furcation apically.

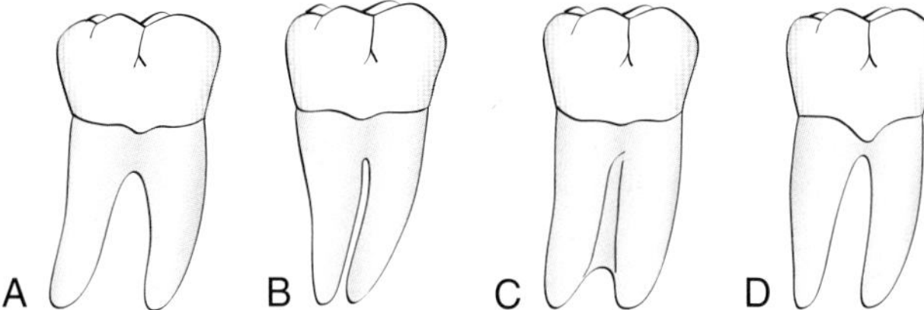

Fig. 62.3 Different anatomic features that may be important in the prognosis and treatment of furcation involvement. (A) Widely separated roots. (B) Roots are separated but close. (C) Fused roots separated only in their apical portion. (D) Presence of enamel projection that may be conducive to early furcation involvement.

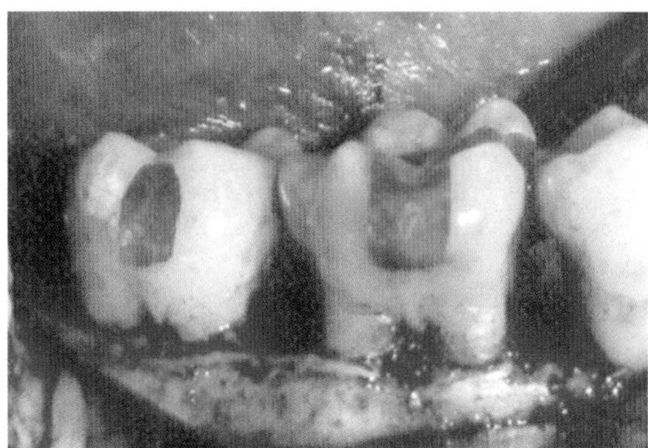

Fig. 62.4 Furcation involvement by grade III cervical enamel projections.

Understanding the configuration of the furcation defect, both vertically and horizontally, can facilitate treatment planning.

Normal Alveolar Bone Morphology

To successfully achieve pocket elimination by means of osseous resection, an understanding of the morphology of a healthy bony periodontium is of utmost importance (Fig. 62.6). Normal bony architecture can be characterized as follows:

1. The interproximal bone is located coronal to the buccal and lingual/palatal bone.

BOX 62.1 Classification of Cervical Enamel Projections

Grade I: The enamel projection extends from the cementoenamel junction to the tooth toward the furcation entrance

Grade II: The enamel projection approaches the entrance to the furcation. It does not enter the furcation, and therefore no horizontal component is present.

Grade III: The enamel projection extends horizontally into the furcation

From Masters DH, Hoskins SW. Projection of cervical enamel into molar furcations. *J Periodontol.* 1964;35:49.

BOX 62.2 Glickman's Furcation Classification

Grade I: Incipient involvement. Pocket formation into the flute, but intact interradicular bone.

Grade II: Loss of interdental bone and pocket formation, but not extending through to the opposite side.

Grade III: Through-and-through lesion.

Grade IV: Through-and-through lesion with gingival recession, leading to a clearly visible furcation area.

From Glickman I. *Clinical Periodontology.* Philadelphia: Saunders; 1953.

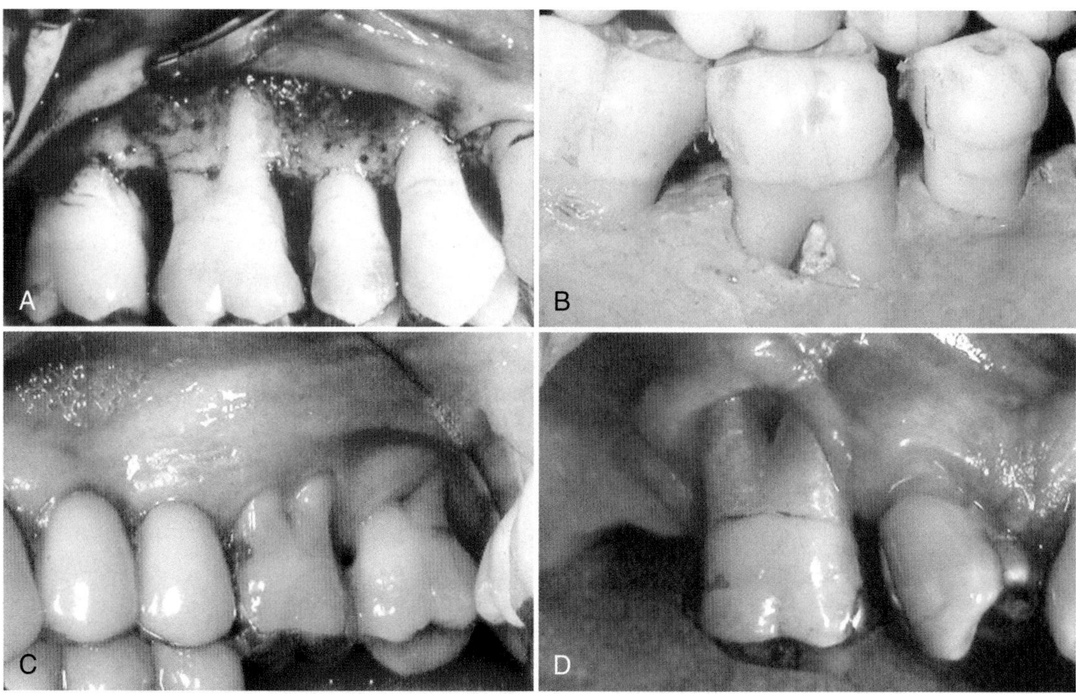

Fig. 62.5 Glickman's classification of furcation involvement. (A) Grade I furcation involvement. Although a space is visible at the entrance to the furcation, no horizontal component of the furcation is evident on probing. (B) Grade II furcation in a dried skull. Note both the horizontal and the vertical components of this cul-de-sac. (C) Grade III furcations on maxillary molars. Probing confirms that the buccal furcation connects with the distal furcation of both these molars, yet the furcation is filled with soft tissue. (D) Grade IV furcation. The soft tissues have receded sufficiently to allow direct vision into the furcation of this maxillary molar.

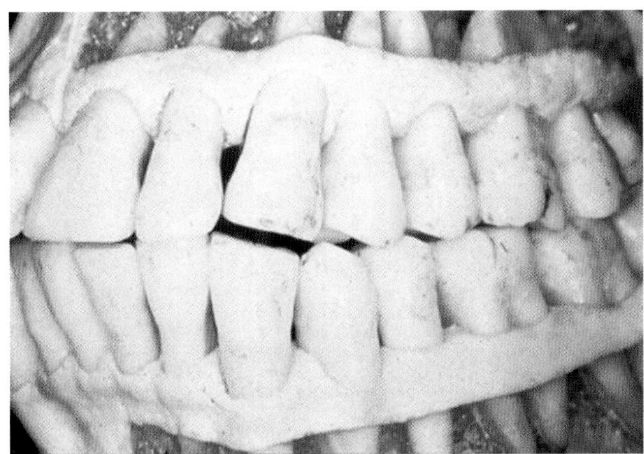

Fig. 62.6 Photograph of a healthy bony periodontium in a skull. Although a slight amount of attachment may have been lost, this skull demonstrates the characteristics of normal form.

2. On molars, the furcation area presents with bone located coronal to the buccal and lingual/palatal radicular bone.
3. The bony contours follow the contours of the CEJ.
4. The shape of interdental bone is determined by the relative position of the CEJs of adjacent teeth.[51] In the molar regions it is predominantly flat, and in the anterior region (mesial to second premolars) it has a more pyramidal shape.[46]
5. The "scalloping" observed on the buccal and lingual/palatal surfaces is associated with the tooth and root form, where incisors and bicuspids present with a more pronounced scalloping than molars.

Even though these are general observations, it is important to be aware that variations can occur from patient to patient and the morphology may be normal and healthy.

Terminology

Osseous resective surgery is accomplished via two methods of bone removal: osteoplasty and ostectomy.[19] *Osteoplasty* consists of reshaping the alveolar process to achieve a more physiological form without removing supporting bone (bone directly involved in the attachment of the tooth). *Ostectomy* refers to the excision of tooth-supporting bone to correct or reduce deformities caused by periodontal disease. One or both types of resections may be necessary to achieve the desired results. In the management of furcation defects, reshaping of a portion of the tooth may be necessary to eliminate local anatomical factors (i.e., CEPs, bifurcation ridges, reshaping of furcation areas); this is referred to as *odontoplasty*.

Another important concept to understand is the morphological description of bony contours after osseous resection. *Positive architecture* and *negative architecture* are the terms used to describe the relative position of the interdental bone in relation to the radicular bone (Fig. 62.7). The term *positive* refers to a case in which the interdental bone is located coronal to the radicular bone, whereas *negative* refers to the interdental bone being more apical than the radicular bone. One will also come across the term *flat architecture*, which means the interdental and radicular bones are reduced to the same height. Therefore, when the osseous form is considered to be *ideal*, this means that the bone at interdental areas is located coronal to the buccal and lingual surfaces.

Examination and Treatment Planning

A thorough examination of patients presenting with signs and symptoms of periodontitis allows the clinician to identify the areas that can benefit from resective surgery.

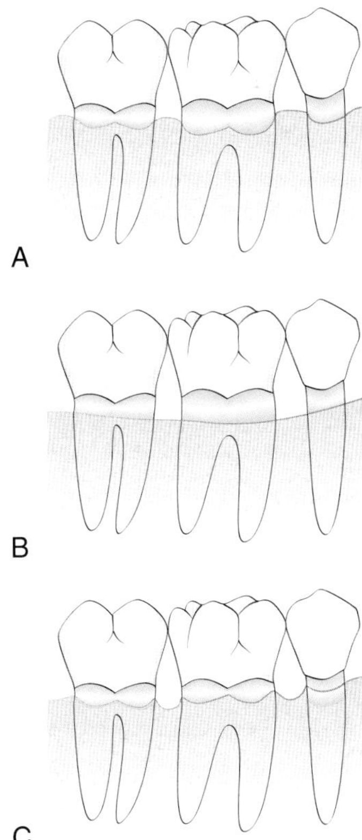

Fig. 62.7 Diagram of types of bony architecture. (A) Positive bony architecture. (B) Flat bony architecture. (C) Reversed, or negative, bony form.

Periodontal probing provides the clinician with important information regarding the (1) depth of the pocket, (2) location of the base of the pocket relative to the mucogingival junction and attachment level on adjacent teeth, (3) number of bony walls, and (4) presence of furcation defects. *Transgingival probing*, also known as *bone sounding*, performed using local anesthesia, can confirm the extent and configuration of the intrabony component of the pocket and of the furcation involvement.[11,39]

Intraoral radiographs are an adjunct tool that provides useful information on the extent of the interproximal bone loss, the presence of vertical bony defects, caries, root trunk length, root proximities, and other anatomical features. Intraoral radiographs, however, cannot accurately document the number of bony walls and the presence or extent of bone lesions on the facial or lingual walls. Even though cone-beam computed tomography images allow for the three-dimensional assessment of these changes, limited evidence supporting its use for the diagnosis of intrabony and furcation defects is available.[30]

The ultimate goal of periodontal treatment is to achieve periodontal health. The means by which this goal is achieved includes the use of nonsurgical and surgical procedures. When the clinician is designing a plan for the treatment of periodontal disease, they should also consider the overall dental picture of the patient, because the periodontal treatment should facilitate the performance of other dental procedures.

After completion of Phase 1 periodontal therapy (see Chapter 42 for phases of periodontal therapy), the patient's periodontal condition is reassessed. The resolution of inflammation, with reduction in swelling, may result in the return of normal depths and configuration of some pockets. However, other areas may still present with persistent pocketing and bleeding on probing. These signs may be an indication that residual plaque and calculus are present, because achieving complete debridement of root surfaces in deep

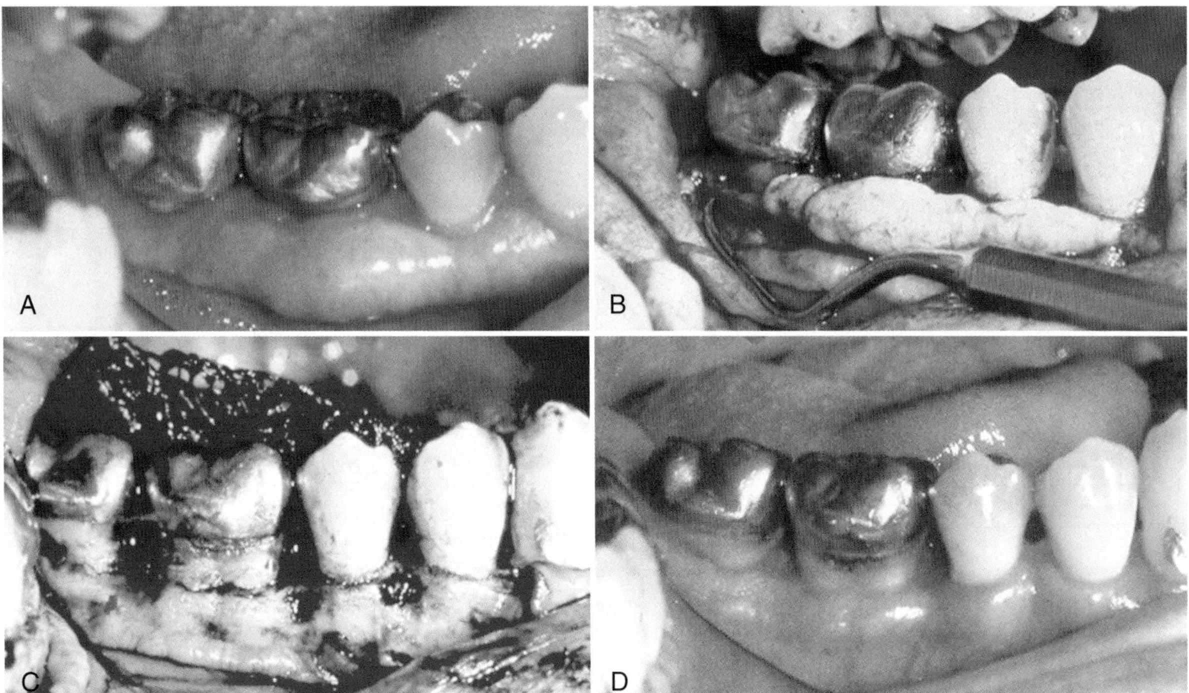

Fig. 62.8 Reduction of bony ledges and exposure of caries by osteoplasty. (A) Buccal preoperative photograph showing two crowns, exostoses, and caries. (B) Flap reflected to reveal caries on both molars at the restoration margins, interdental cratering, and a facial exostosis. (C) After osseous surgery; the bulk of the bony removal was by osteoplasty, with minor ostectomy between the two molars. The caries are now exposed, and the crowns are lengthened for restoration. (D) Postoperative photograph at 6 weeks. Plaque control is deficient, but the teeth should be readily restorable at this time. (Courtesy Dr. Joseph Schwartz, Portland, OR.)

pockets has proven difficult.[50] This can also be an indication of the patient's inability or unwillingness to properly perform adequate oral hygiene. If patients present with inadequate oral hygiene, they are not good candidates for surgical therapy. On the other hand, if plaque control is adequate and residual pocket depths of 5 mm or more are present, patients with these conditions may be candidates for periodontal surgery.[33]

Resective osseous surgery is also used to facilitate certain restorative and prosthetic dental procedures.[8,47] Dental caries can be exposed for restoration, fractured roots of abutment teeth can be exposed for removal, and bony exostoses and ridge deformities can be altered in contour to improve the performance of removable or fixed prostheses (Fig. 62.8). Severely decayed teeth, or teeth with short anatomic crowns, can be lengthened by resection or by a combination of orthodontic tooth extrusion and osseous resection. Such procedures allow the therapist to expose more tooth for restoration, prevent an invasion of the biologic width of attachment, and create a periodontal attachment of normal dimension.[8,15,37] Resection can also provide a means of producing optimal crown length for cosmetic purposes.[38]

CLINICAL CORRELATION

Some teeth cannot be restored without the assistance of resective osseous surgery.

Selection of Treatment Technique

The extent of osseous resection depends on the relationship between the depth and configuration of the bony defects with root morphology and the adjacent teeth. Because of the resective nature of osseous surgery, this is best applied to cases with early to moderate bone loss (2 to 3 mm) with moderate-length root trunks[7] presenting with bony defects of one or two walls. In cases in which advanced attachment loss is present with deep intrabony defects, significant osseous reduction is required to achieve positive architecture and will compromise the prognosis of the tooth.

Osteoplasty is used to treat buccal and lingual bony ledges or tori, shallow lingual or buccal intrabony defects, thick interproximal areas, and incipient furcation involvements that do not require removal of supporting bone.[14,42,43,49] Ostectomy is applied in the treatment of shallow to medium (1 to 4-mm deep) intrabony defects and correction of osseous topography.[20,44]

The performance of resective surgery should not compromise esthetics or increase tooth mobility; therefore, it presents with certain limitations, such as exposure of furcation areas, especially interproximal furcations in maxillary molars. If production of positive architecture would lead to the creation of other periodontal problems, compromised osseous reshaping should be considered. In these situations, partial defect elimination is accomplished, and residual pockets, although less deep than they were initially, are expected. When compromised osseous reshaping leads to a negative architecture it is important to remove peaks of bone that remain at the line angles of the teeth (*widow's peaks*). If these peaks are not removed, soft tissue will reattach, resulting in recurrence of deep interproximal pockets.

In the management of furcation defects, osseous resection may be indicated for the management of class II defects presenting with a shallow horizontal component without significant vertical bone loss. Osteoplasty and ostectomy, in association with odontoplasty to modify the furcation anatomy, usually result in favorable outcomes. Furcation defects presenting with deep two- or three-wall components may be suitable for regenerative procedures. Chapter 63 addresses regenerative therapies. When furcation involvement is extensive (class III to IV), root resections and tunneling procedures may be used. The surgical management of furcation defects has yielded good long-term results, with surgical resective modalities (root resections and hemisections) showing a survival rate ranging from 62% to 100% with an observation period of 5 to 13 years.[28]

KEY FACT

Osseous resective surgery should never compromise the prognosis of the tooth.

Conclusion

Resective surgery has been demonstrated to be an effective therapy in eliminating bony defects and furcation involvements. The clinician, however, must be aware of the limitations of this procedure. The recontouring of the tissues should not be accomplished at the expense of supporting bone. When the surgery is properly performed, the amount of bone removed is minimal, and osteoplasty allows for proper flap adaptation. The advantages of this surgical modality include a predictable amount of pocket reduction that can enhance oral hygiene and periodic maintenance. It also preserves the width of the attached tissue while removing granulomatous tissue and providing access for debridement of the radicular surfaces. In addition, resective techniques allow the recontouring of bony abnormalities, including hemiseptal defects, tori, ledges, and furcation defects. Some of the significant benefits include proper assessment for restorative procedures (e.g., crown lengthening) and assessment of restorative overhangs and tooth abnormalities (e.g., enamel projections, enamel pearls, perforations, fractures). Consequently, resective therapy can be an important technique in the armamentarium necessary to provide a maintainable periodontium for periodontal patients.

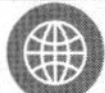

References for this chapter are found on the companion website eBooks.Health.Elsevier.com.

CHAPTER 63

Periodontal Regeneration

Richard T. Kao | Daniel R. Clark | Henry H. Takei | Guo-Hao Lin

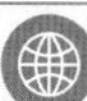

For online-only content on analysis of periodontal of wound healing, non-graft-associated procedures, analysis of laser associated periodontal wound healing, autologous bone grafts, guided tissue regeneration membranes, miscellaneous biologics for periodontal regeneration, scaffold or supporting matrices, and therapeutic considerations, please visit the companion website at eBooks.Health.Elsevier.com.

CHAPTER OUTLINE

Intrabony and furcation defects are sequelae of periodontal disease. Ideally, these defects are managed in a timely fashion through periodontal regeneration. In the past, the results of regenerative therapy were inconsistent and unpredictable. The current status of regenerative therapy has dramatically changed and improved due to research and a better understanding of the biology of the tissues that comprise the periodontal attachment. Various surgical approaches, including bone replacement grafts, guided tissue regeneration (GTR), and a better understanding of biologic mediators and tissue engineering have improved the predictability of regeneration. This chapter reviews the current strategies and clinical decision-making for optimizing regenerative success.

When the periodontium is damaged by inflammation or as a result of surgical treatment, the defect heals either through periodontal regeneration or repair.[9,84,136,164,240] In periodontal regeneration, healing occurs through the reconstitution of a new periodontium, which involves the formation of alveolar bone, functionally aligned periodontal ligament, and new cementum. Alternatively, repair due to healing by replacement with epithelial and/or connective tissue that matures into various nonfunctional types of scar tissue is termed *new attachment* (Fig. 63.1). Histologically, patterns of repair include long junctional epithelium, ankylosis, and/or new attachment (see Chapter 4). Although the stability of periodontal repair is not clear, the ideal goal of periodontal surgical therapy is periodontal regeneration.

Today, several highly reproducible regenerative approaches are used, as evidenced by clinical attachment gain, decreased pocket probing depth, radiographic evidence consistent with bone fill, and overall improvements in periodontal health.[3,9,131,223] These clinical improvements can be maintained over long periods (often greater than 10 years).[53,134,271]

Assessment of Periodontal Wound Healing versus Regeneration

It is sometimes difficult in clinical and experimental situations to determine whether regeneration or new attachment has occurred and the extent to which it has occurred. Although various types of evidence of reconstruction exist, the *proof of principle* for the type of healing is determined by histologic studies. Once defined, the evidence found subsequently by clinical, radiographic, and surgical reentry findings is implied.[37,38,157] All these methods have advantages and shortcomings that should be well understood and considered in individual cases when critically evaluating the literature.

LEARNING BOX 63.1

It is sometimes difficult in clinical and experimental situations to determine whether regeneration or new attachment has occurred and the extent to which it has occurred. Although various types of evidence of reconstruction exist, the *proof of principle* for the type of healing is determined by histologic studies. Once defined, the evidence found subsequently by clinical, radiographic, and surgical reentry findings is implied.[37,38,157] These methods have advantages and shortcomings that should be well understood and considered in individual cases and when critically evaluating the literature. A supplemental and detailed discussion regarding analysis of periodontal wound healing is detailed in the next online section in the eBook.

Regenerative-Associated Procedures

There are several procedures historically associated with the management of the junctional and pocket epithelium and root surface conditioning. The removal of junctional and pocket epithelium to encourage connective tissue attachment or soft tissue curettage is not clinically effective. It is the root planing procedure or removal of plaque/calculus and endotoxin affected cementum that is critical for regeneration. Another area of focus has been on root biomodification for periodontal regeneration. Research interests in root conditioning with citric acid, tetracycline, ethylenediaminetetraacetic acid (EDTA), and fibronectin have proven to be ineffective.[160]

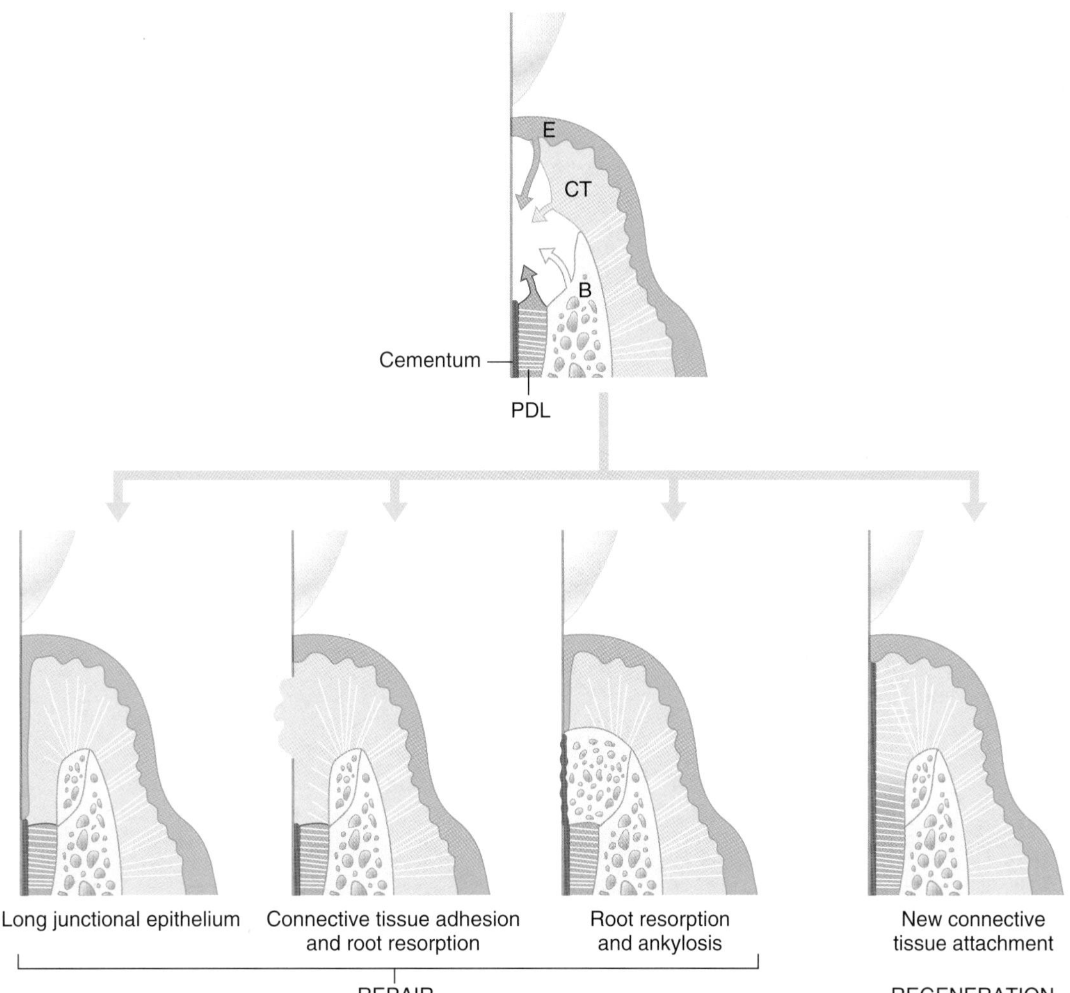

Fig. 63.1 Possible healing patterns for a periodontal wound. These patterns are dependent on the four possible cell types that predominate the wound site. The downgrowth of epithelial cells *(E)* results in a long junctional epithelium. The proliferation of connective tissue *(CT)* may result in connective tissue adhesion with or without root resorption. With the predominance of bone cells *(B)*, root resorption and/or ankylosis will occur. With the ingress of periodontal ligament *(PDL)* and perivascular cells from the bone, a regenerated periodontium develops. (From Rose LF, Meaney BL, Genco RJ, et al. *Periodontics: Medicine, Surgery, and Implants.* St. Louis: Mosby; 2004.)

Laser-Assisted New Attachment Procedure

The role of lasers in periodontal therapy remains controversial (see Chapter 64). Nevertheless, the use of neodymium:yttrium-aluminum-garnet (Nd:YAG) to perform surgical laser-assisted new attachment procedure (LANAP) has been reported for the management of chronic periodontitis,[133,181] and it can potentially result in new attachment and periodontal regeneration (see Chapter 64).[194,307] The LANAP procedure is based on the excisional new attachment procedure (ENAP) and many of the classical nongrafting procedures that promote connective tissue attachment and limited periodontal regeneration. The clinical and biologic basis for this technique is reviewed in online material, *Analysis of laser-associated periodontal wound healing.*

Many questions remain about LANAP. The first refers to the exact mechanism and parameters by which healing via new attachment occurs consistently. Also, the extent of regeneration has not been defined, nor has this approach been compared with other established regenerative therapies. This comparison, along with other randomized controlled trials, will be needed for a meta-analysis to determine whether LANAP is equivalent or superior to other conventional therapy. As with all periodontal therapy, the long-term stability and clinical parameters for regeneration also needs to be explored.

Regenerative Surgical Approaches

Regenerative techniques can be subdivided into three major therapeutic approaches: graft-associated, non–bone graft–associated, and biologic-based regeneration (Table 63.1). In clinical practice, it is common for clinicians to combine these various approaches in clinical management of intrabony defects.

Graft Materials and Procedures

Numerous therapeutic grafting modalities for restoring periodontal osseous defects have been investigated. Periodontal reconstruction can be attained without the use of bone grafts in meticulously treated three-wall defects (intrabony defects) and in periodontal and endodontic abscesses.[33,113,132,214] New attachment is more likely to occur when the destructive process has occurred rapidly, such as after treatment of pockets complicated by acute periodontal abscesses and after treatment of acute necrotizing ulcerative lesions.[190] Previously, the use of graft materials was thought to provide a regenerative inductive effect, but it is now thought to primarily provide a scaffold for healing.

The following classifications of bone graft materials are important. Grafts are categorized either by their origin or function during

TABLE 63.1 Comparative Analysis of Regenerative Approaches

Graft Material	CAL Gain (mm)	Bony Defect Fill (% or mm)	Histological Assessment	Comments[a]
Debridement	0.3–1.3mm	1.05–2.71 (ND in most studies)		
Autologous Extraoral (iliac crest)[78,243,245] Intraoral autologous[56,79,114,228,229]	3.3–4.2 mm • 2.60 mm in 0-wall • 3.75 mm in 1-wall • 4.16 mm in 2-walls 2.88–3.44 mm	— 73%	33 of 39 defects showed evidence of regeneration 0.7 mm of regeneration	Only evidence of regeneration in 0-wall defect. Only one controlled study with 2.98 mm of bone gain vs. 0.66 mm with debridement.
Allograft FDBA[171,236,239,263] DFDBA vs. OFD[167,169,170] Comparative studies • FDBA vs. FDBA + autologous graft[239]	2.0 mm 2.3–2.9 mm vs. 0.3–1.3 mm —	60%–80% pf 1401 defects w ≥50% fill 65% vs. 11% 63%–67% w ≥50% fill 78%–80% w ≥50% fill	--- 1.21 mm of regeneration —	Only controlled study using paired defects shows no difference between FDBA vs. debridement —
Xenograft[131] NBM	2.2–3.7 mm	1.3 mm		
GTR[131] OFD GTR-NR GTR-R GTR-R + DFDBA	1.39 3.0–3.3 2.39–3.5 3.8	1.25 1.5–2.1 1.5–2.7 4.7	Regeneration Regeneration Regeneration	
EMD[131] OFD EMD EMD + DFDBA EMD + NBM EMD + BG EMD + β-TCP EMD + NBM + PRP	1.7 2.2 3.0 (vs. 3.2 for EMD) 3.4 (vs. 2.9 for EMD) 5.2 (vs. 4.1 for EMD) 3.0 (vs. 3.1 for EMD) 4.9 (vs. 3.9 for EMD)	0–2.71 2.6 -4.29 3.7 (vs. 2.6 for EMD) 4.0 (vs. 3.1 for EMD) 2.8 (vs. 2.2 for EMD) ND ND	Regeneration Regeneration Regeneration ND ND ND	NS w comparison $P < .001$ vs. OFD $P < .001$ vs. EMD $P < .05$ $P < .05$
rhPDGF-BB + β-TCP[131] β-TCP rhPDGF + β-TCP	3.44 4.31	1.81 3.32	Regeneration	$P < .001$ vs. β-TCP

Synopsis of representative data cited and from data synopsis from Kao, Nares, and Reynold's review.[131] Note that variabilities in outcomes are often due to inclusion criteria for defects accepted for respective study.

[a]Regeneration results with grafting materials, GTR, and biologics.

BG, bone graft; *BG,* Bioglass; *DFDBA,* demineralized freeze-dried bone allograft; *EMD,* enamel matrix derivative; *FDBA,* freeze-dried bone allograft; *GTR,* guided tissue regeneration; *HA,* hydroxyapatite; *NBM,* natural bone mineral; *ND,* not done; *NR,* nonresorbable; *OFD,* open flap debridement; *PHA,* porous hydroxyapatite; *R,* resorbable; *Regeneration,* histological evidence(s); *β-TCP,* beta tricalcium phosphate.

healing. Categorization by origin includes the following: (1) *autografts* are bone obtained from the same individual; (2) allografts are bone obtained from a different individual of the same species; and (3) *xenografts* are bone from a different species. Bone graft materials are also evaluated based on their osteogenic, osteoinductive, or osteoconductive potential. (1) *Osteogenesis* refers to the formation or development of new bone by cells contained in the graft. (2) *Osteoinduction* is a chemical process by which molecules contained in the graft (e.g., bone morphogenetic proteins) convert the neighboring cells into osteoblasts, which in turn form bone. (3) *Osteoconduction* is a physical effect by which the matrix of the graft forms a scaffold that favors outside cells to penetrate the graft and form new bone.

Periodontal defects as sites for transplantation differ from osseous cavities surrounded by bony walls. Saliva and bacteria may easily penetrate along the root surface, and epithelial cells may proliferate into the defect, thus resulting in contamination and possible exfoliation of the grafts. Therefore, the principles established to govern transplantation of bone or other materials into closed osseous cavities are not fully applicable to transplantation of bone into periodontal defects.[67]

Schallhorn defined the considerations that govern the selection of a material as follows: biologic acceptability, predictability, clinical feasibility, minimal operative hazards, minimal postoperative sequelae, and patients' acceptance.[245] It is difficult to find a material with all these characteristics, and, to date, no ideal material or technique exists.

Graft materials have been developed and tried in many forms. To familiarize the reader with various types of graft material, as defined by either the technique or the material used, a brief discussion of each is provided.

All grafting techniques require presurgical scaling, occlusal adjustment as needed, and exposure of the defect with a full-thickness flap. The flap technique best suited for grafting purposes is the *papilla preservation flap* because it provides complete coverage of the interdental area after suturing (see Chapter 60). The use of antibiotics after the procedure is generally recommended.

Autogenous Bone Grafts

Historically, extraoral sites for bone harvesting have been from the iliac crest, but this approach is seldom performed due to medical and legal concerns. Intraoral autograft donor sites can be effective, especially when donor sites adjacent to the defects are available. Due to the morbidity of the secondary harvest site and the limited material that can be harvested, the autograft is not popular. The consequence is that the allograft is the clinical graft material of choice. Despite the popularity of using allograft, the material functions primarily as a scaffolding or osteoconductive agent with a minimal amount of osteogenic content. Historical development of the use of autografts from intraoral sites suggests that we should consider using an autograft when possible. (See online material, *Autologous bone graft of historical interest.)*

Bone Allografts

Obtaining donor material for autograft purposes necessitates inflicting surgical trauma on another part of the patient's body. Obviously, it would be to the patient's and provider's advantage if a suitable substitute could be used for grafting purposes that would offer similar potential for repair and not require the additional surgical removal of donor material from the patient. However, both allografts and xenografts are foreign to the patient and therefore have the potential to provoke an immune response. Attempts have been made to suppress the antigenic potential of allografts and xenografts by radiation, freezing, and chemical treatment.[27]

Bone allografts are commercially available from tissue banks. They are obtained from cortical bone within 12 hours of death of the donor, defatted, cut in pieces, washed in absolute alcohol, and deep-frozen. The material may then be demineralized, subsequently ground and sieved to a particle size of 250 to 750 μm, and freeze-dried. Finally, it is vacuum-sealed in glass vials.

Numerous steps are also taken to eliminate viral infectivity. These include exclusion of donors from known high-risk groups and various tests on the cadaver tissues to exclude individuals with any type of infection or malignant disease. The material is then treated with chemical agents or strong acids to inactivate the virus, if still present. The risk of human immunodeficiency virus (HIV) infection has been calculated as 1 in 1 to 8 million and is therefore characterized as highly uncommon.[173]

Freeze-Dried Bone Allograft

Several clinical studies by Mellonig, Bowers, and coworkers reported bone fill exceeding 50% in 67% of the defects grafted with freeze-dried bone allograft (FDBA) and in 78% of the defects grafted with FDBA in combination with autogenous bone.[24,171,189,239,263] FDBA, however, is considered an osteoconductive material, whereas demineralized freeze-dried bone allograft (DFDBA) is considered an osteoinductive graft. Laboratory studies have found that DFDBA has a higher osteogenic potential than FDBA and is therefore preferred.[167,169,170]

Demineralized Freeze-Dried Bone Allograft

Experiments by Urist established the osteogenic potential of DFDBA.[289–292] Demineralization in cold, diluted hydrochloric acid exposes the components of the bone matrix, which are closely associated with collagen fibrils and have been termed *bone morphogenetic proteins* (BMPs).[41,292]

In 1975, Libin and colleagues reported three patients with 4 to 10 mm of bone regeneration in periodontal osseous defects.[152] Subsequent clinical studies were done with cancellous DFDBA and cortical DFDBA.[204,212,215] DFDBA resulted in more desirable results (2.4 mm vs. 1.38 mm of bone fill).

Bowers and associates, in a histologic study in humans, showed new attachment and periodontal regeneration in defects grafted with DFDBA.[25] Mellonig and colleagues tested DFDBA against autogenous materials in the calvaria of guinea pigs and showed it to have similar osteogenic potential.[169,170,172]

These studies provide strong evidence that DFDBA in periodontal defects results in significant probing depth reduction, attachment level gain, and osseous regeneration. The combination of DFDBA and GTR has also proved to be very successful.[246] However, limitations of the use of DFDBA include the possible, although remote, potential of disease transfer from the cadaver.

A bone-inductive protein isolated from the extracellular matrix of human bones, termed *osteogenin* or *BMP-3,* has been tested in human periodontal defects and seems to enhance osseous regeneration.[26] This bone-inductive protein is discussed later in this chapter.

Xenografts

Bone products from other species have a long history of use in periodontal therapy. A few of these xenograft products are mentioned here for historical purposes but the only one used consistently by clinicians is an anorganic, bovine-derived bone marketed under the brand name Bio-Oss (Geistlich Pharma), which has been successfully used both for periodontal defects and in implant surgery. It is an osteoconductive, porous bone mineral matrix from bovine cancellous or cortical bone. The organic components of the bone are removed, but the trabecular architecture and porosity are retained.[31,165] The physical features permit clot stabilization and revascularization to allow for migration of osteoblasts, leading to osteogenesis. Bio-Oss is biocompatible with the adjacent tissues, and it elicits no systemic immune response.

Several studies have reported successful bone regeneration and new attachment with Bio-Oss in periodontal defects, as well as regeneration around implants and sinus grafting.[31,168]

Periodontally, Bio-Oss has been used as a graft material covered with a resorbable membrane (Geistlich Bio-Gide, Geistlich Pharma). The membrane prevents the migration of fibroblasts and connective tissues into the pores and between the granules of the graft. Histologic studies of this technique have shown significant osseous regeneration and cementum formation.

Yukna and associates have used Bio-Oss in combination with a cell-binding polypeptide (P-15) that is a synthetic analogue of a 15-amino acid sequence of type I collagen marketed as PepGen P-15 (Dentsply Sirona, York, PA).[308] This combination seems to enhance the bone regenerative results of the matrix alone in periodontal defects.

Calf bone (Boplant), treated by detergent extraction, sterilized, and freeze-dried, has been used for the treatment of osseous defects.[8,242] Kiel bone is calf or ox bone denatured with 20% hydrogen peroxide, dried with acetone, and sterilized with ethylene oxide. Anorganic bone is ox bone from which the organic material has been extracted by means of ethylenediamine; it is then sterilized by autoclaving.[166] These materials have been tried and discarded for various reasons.

Non–Graft-Associated Reconstructive Procedures

The following sections discuss the rationale and techniques that must be considered for a successful outcome in achieving new attachment or periodontal bone regeneration in response to non–graft-associated reconstructive surgical therapy. This approach is used in Europe and Asia where human bone graft is not available due to regulatory restraints.

The primary regenerative approach utilized in clinical practice is based on the concept of bioexclusion as proposed by Melcher and referred to as GTR. This technique utilizes a "barrier" membrane to obtain bioexclusion of a healing space, which is supported by a blood clot that subsequently becomes the healing environment for cells that will form the histological components of new cementum, periodontal ligament, and bone. The available membranes are detailed in the online material, *Analysis of Laser-Associated Periodontal Wound Healing*.

More recent evidence suggests that the LANAP may also result in new attachment and regeneration, but further clinical trials are needed to test its efficacy and parameters for success. The efficacy of laser for periodontal regeneration is discussed in detail in Chapter 64.

Lastly, there are several procedures of historical interest which provide insight for enhancing healing or result in regeneration in narrow intrabony defects, including: (1) the removal of the junctional and pocket epithelium; (2) the prevention of their migration into the healing area after therapy; (3) clot stabilization, wound protection, and space creation; and (4) biomodification of the root surfaces (see online material). Although these procedures are not used individually as reconstructive approaches, some of these strategies are currently incorporated into reconstructive surgery as adjuncts for other currently used regenerative techniques.

Guided Tissue Regeneration

GTR is a clinical application of bioexclusion whereby epithelial migration is prevented from dominating the wound site and the space is maintained for clot stabilization. Derived from the classic studies of Nyman, Lindhe, Karring, and Gottlow, this method assumes that periodontal ligament and perivascular cells have the potential for regeneration of the attachment apparatus of the tooth.[46,67,88–90,176,198,199,275] GTR consists of placing barriers of different types (membranes) to cover the bone and periodontal ligament, thus temporarily separating them from the gingival epithelium and connective tissue. Excluding the epithelium and the gingival connective tissue from the root surface during the postsurgical healing phase not only prevents epithelial migration into the wound, but also favors repopulation of the area by cells from the periodontal ligament and the bone (see Chapter 4).[39] In the United States, GTR is often performed with some type of bone graft as a scaffolding agent, so it is a combined therapy. As indicated earlier, in Europe and in other parts of the world, because of regulatory and religious constraints, human graft materials are not available, so it is performed as a traditional GTR procedure and may be occasionally used in conjunction with other graft materials as combined therapy.

Initial animal experiments using Millipore filters (Millipore Sigma, Burlington, MA) and Teflon membranes resulted in regeneration of cementum and alveolar bone and a functional periodontal ligament.[33,34,39] Clinical case reports indicate that GTR results in a gain in attachment level.[15,16] Histologic studies in humans provided evidence of periodontal reconstruction in most cases, even with horizontal bone loss.[89,275,276]

The use of PTFE membranes has been tested in controlled clinical studies in mandibular molar furcations and has shown statistically significant decreases in pocket depths and improvement in attachment levels after 6 months, but bone level measurements have been inconclusive.[151,210] A study of maxillary molar furcations did not result in significant gain in attachment or bone levels.[175]

With the regenerative success associated with the use of nonresorbable membrane, the advantages and disadvantages of this approach became apparent. Notably, problems such as membrane exposure, which resulted in no or limited regeneration, and the need for a secondary procedure for surgical removal, resulted in the development of biodegradable membranes.[262] Today in clinical practice, most GTR procedures use biodegradable membranes, whereas the nonresorbable membranes, especially those with titanium reinforcement struts, are used for regeneration of large intrabony defects and implant site development. Nevertheless, the historical research using nonresorbable membranes and the development of various types of biodegradable membranes are valuable. (See online material, *GTR membranes.*)

LEARNING BOX 63.2

Due to the osteoconductive nature and slow resorption rate of anorganic, bovine-derived bone graft, it acts as a bioexclusive graft material in that it excludes epithelial mesenchymal cell migration into the regeneration site. The slow resorption rate is also advantageous for grafting in implant surgical sites since it may be corrective for soft tissue defects, and it remains fairly stable. However, the use of this material in implant placement sites must be cautioned because over-compaction of this material may result in such low volume of native bone that it will not provide an adequate level of osseointegration for implant stability.

Periodontal Regeneration Utilizing Biologics

A new approach for regeneration that departs from the use of grafting materials and/or bioexclusion with GTR membranes is the use of biologics. This category of regenerative approach is based on a tissue engineering concept of enhancing regeneration by augmenting the defect site with signaling molecules, scaffolds, and/or cells (Fig. 63.2). This appears to result in periodontal regeneration in a relatively more rapid pace of regeneration as well as faster response. This category consists of the use of enamel matrix derivative (EMD), recombinant human platelet-derived growth factor-BB (rhPDGF), osteogenic allograft, platelet rich plasma (PRP), and platelet rich fibrin (PRF). Other biologics, such as recombinant human bone morphogenetic protein (rhBMP) and recombinant fibroblast growth factor -2 (rhFGF), have undergone clinical trials but have not been FDA approved for clinical use, and are discussed in the online material, *GTR membranes.*

Enamel Matrix Derivative

EMD has been available as a biologic periodontal regenerative material for 20 years.[110,111] The biologic properties of EMD have been summarized recently.[135] Several studies have provided human histologic evidence of intrabony regeneration associated with EMD therapy.[110,111,252,309] EMD is present on root surfaces for ≥4 weeks after application, and early signs of periodontal wound regeneration can be observed after 2 to 6 weeks.[255] Signs of clinical improvement are present as early as 6 months after treatment (Fig. 63.3).[95,96,123,147,148,249,294]

Studies have evaluated the efficacy of EMD versus open flap debridement, with the majority confirming that debridement followed by EMD application resulted in substantial improvements in clinical measurements and bone fill in the management of intrabony defects. They also found that neither postoperative antibiotics nor EDTA root conditioning improved the clinical outcome of EMD therapy.[256,259] In comparing EMD versus GTR, intrabony defect correction was comparable except in situations with deep, noncontained intrabony defects.[267] In these defects, GTR with titanium reinforcement was superior. The latter results suggest that, in situations in which defect configuration is broad or lacking in wall containment, a supported barrier membrane may be critical to the success of EMD-associated regeneration. Additionally, no added clinical advantage was observed when EMD was combined with GTR.[177,256]

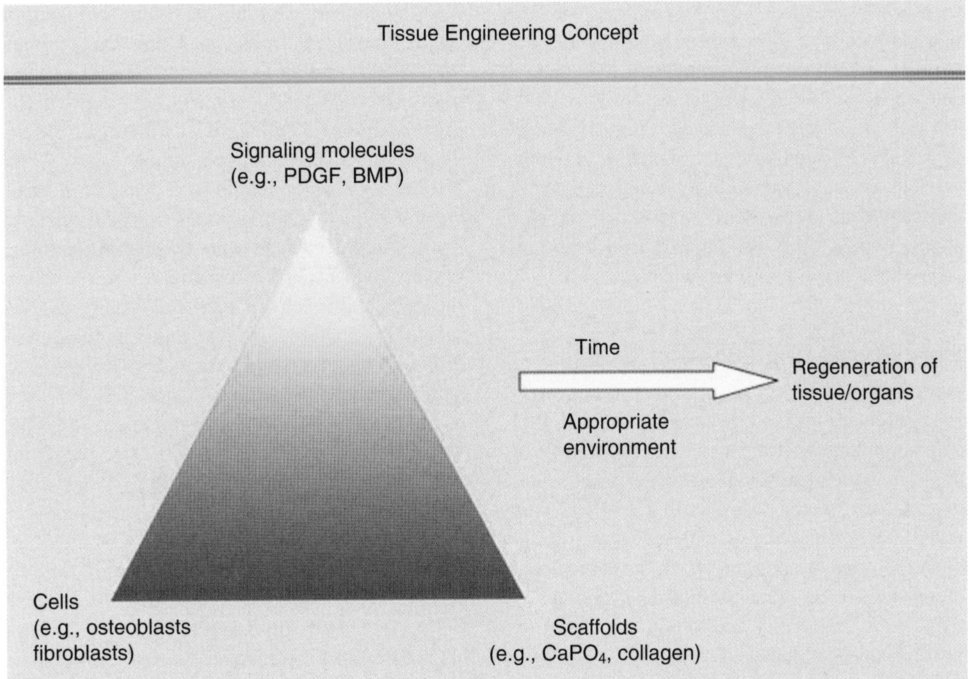

Fig. 63.2 Tissue engineering is the manipulation of one or more of the three elements: signaling molecules, scaffolds, or cells. *BMP,* Bone morphogenetic protein; *$CaPO_4$,* calcium phosphate; *PDGF,* platelet-derived growth factor. (Courtesy Dr. Samuel Lynch.)

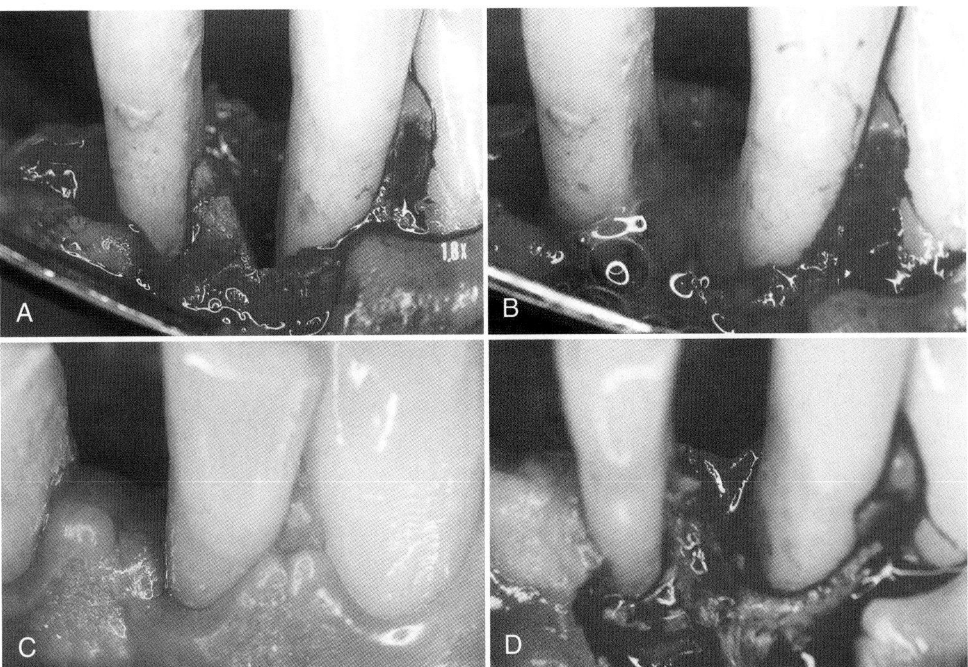

Fig. 63.3 (A) Deep vertical bone loss distal to the lower left central incisor. (B) Area flapped, root prepared, and defect filled with enamel matrix protein (Emdogain, Straumann, Andover, MA). (C) Postoperative photograph 6 months later. (D) Reentry surgery showing extensive bone fill. (Courtesy Dr. Marco Orsini, Aquila, Italy.)

There are several studies in which EMD has been used in combined therapy. Histologic evidence of periodontal regeneration has been demonstrated when EMD is used in combination with autogenous bone,[95] allografts,[96,115,231] a bovine-derived natural bone mineral (NBM),[249,254,257,258,294] bioactive glass,[115,123,143,253] NBM + PRP,[62] or biphasic calcium phosphate.[23,260] The majority of the studies indicated no added benefits in either clinical and radiographic gains when EMD is used with the addition of graft materials.[260]

EMD remains a very intriguing biologic mediator. As we better understand the mechanism of action of the potpourri of proteins and growth factors, this may strengthen the biologic rationale for clinical use of this material. The concern remains whether commercial batches of EMD will be consistent and provide comparable clinical results in all cases. Perhaps the message is that the achievement of maximum regenerative response will require a mixture of biologic mediators. With further characterization of EMD, we may better develop a synergistic blend that will provide an optimal result.

In summary, EMD is a semi-purified protein preparation from developing porcine teeth that contains a mixture of low-molecular-weight proteins. Although there were initial concerns about the poorly characterized nature of this preparation, recent reports suggest that the mixture may work synergistically on multiple levels to enhance periodontal regeneration.[130] When applied to root surfaces, the proteins are absorbed into the hydroxyapatite and collagen fibers of the root surface, in which they induce cementum formation followed by periodontal regeneration. Clinical use of EMD can generally be characterized as safe, with excellent clinical healing and limited complications. EMD alone, or in combination with graft materials, provides clinical outcome and long-term clinical stability comparable with GTR. Although characterization of the EMD preparation remains incomplete, the challenge, as with allografts, is to provide a consistent batch of EMD, so the regenerative response is predictable.

Recombinant Human Platelet-Derived Growth Factor-BB for Periodontal Regeneration

Platelet-derived growth factor (PDGF) is one of the earliest growth factors studied for its effect on wound healing because it is a potent mitogenic and chemotactic factor for mesenchymal cells in cell culture. Histologic evidence of periodontal regeneration was first reported in experimental defects in beagle dogs.[155,156] During the development of PDGF for clinical use, rhPDGF was used in conjunction with allogenic bone to correct Class II furcations and interproximal intrabony defects on hopeless teeth.[32,191] Histologic evidence of successful periodontal regeneration in the furcation lesion with excellent fill has been noted.

A human clinical trial was conducted using rhPDGF and recombinant human insulin-like growth factor 1 (rhIGF-1).[118] Using a split-mouth design, defects were treated with either a low dose (50 μg/mL) or high dose (150 μg/mL) of rhPDGF–rhIGF-1. After 9 months, the high-dose rhPDGF–rhIGF-1 induced 2.08 mm of new bone and 43.2% defect fill, compared with 0.75-mm vertical bone height and 18.5% bone fill in controls. Low-dose rhPDGF–rhIGF-1 results were statistically similar to those of the controls. Additionally, this study demonstrated that no adverse immunologic or clinical reaction resulted from use of these agents. A primate study examined the regenerative effects of PDGF–IGF-1 individually and in combination.[155] PDGF alone was found to be as effective as the PDGF–IGF-1 combination in producing new attachment after 3 months. No significant effect was found when IGF was used alone. This study suggests that IGF may not be important at the dose level tested.

Subsequently, the effectiveness of 0.3 mg/mL of rhPDGF in combination with beta tricalcium phosphate (β-TCP) to improve attachment level gain, bone level, and bone volume significantly compared with β-TCP alone was demonstrated after 6 months in a multicenter clinical trial.[192] A subset of these patients was followed for 24 months, and a representative case series was reported to be stable, with increases in radiographic bone fill compared with the end results after 6 months (Fig. 63.4).[164] A review of these cases indicates that the results were

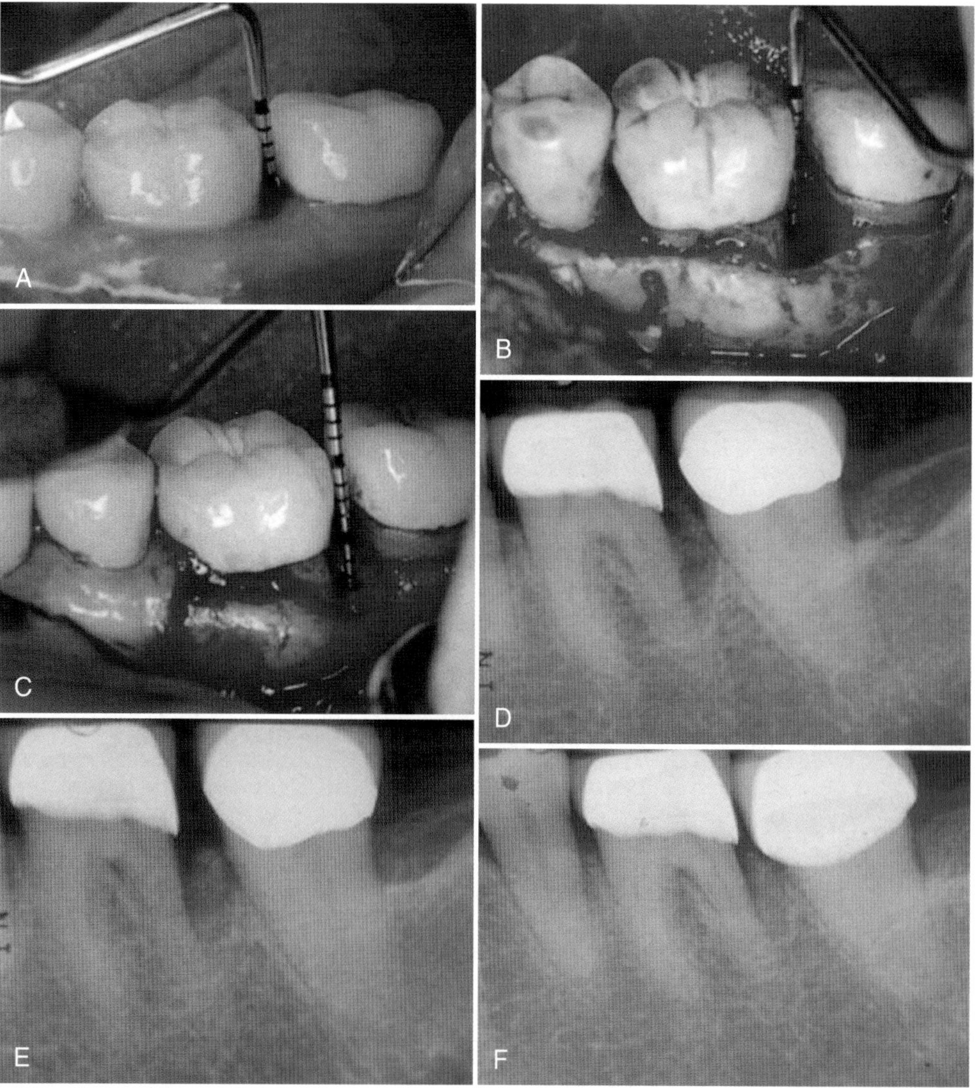

Fig. 63.4 A sample case of a patient treated in the pivotal trial. (A–C) The pretreatment situation preoperatively, at surgical debridement, and at postsurgical reentry. (D–F) The radiographic appearance after 12, 24, and 60 months. Surgical reentry after 12 months indicates good bone fill of the circumferential intrabony defect (C). The clinical pocket depth was 3 mm after 5 years.

stable after 3 and 5 years.[129,193] Another case series suggests that rhPDGF with freeze-dried bone allograft can be combined to achieve excellent results in severe periodontal intrabony defects.[329] These findings were confirmed by another randomized controlled trial.[122]

The combination of rhPDGF with a β-TCP carrier is now commercially available (GEM 21S, Osteohealth, Shirley, NY). These preliminary studies using rhPDGF-TCP suggest that it is easy to use, requires no barrier membranes, and has results comparable or superior to those of other regenerative graft materials. The potential for using rhPDGF for regeneration of furcation defects and implant site preparation still needs to be evaluated. Additionally, considerable clinical interest has been expressed in combining rhPDGF-BB with other bone replacement grafts, particularly bone allografts and xenografts.

Cell Therapy

Cell therapy has been used in periodontal surgery (Osteocel Plus, NuVasive, San Diego, CA). Stem cells have the potential to improve current bone regeneration. These cells can expedite cell recruitment, act as target cells for growth factor delivery, and promote early extracellular matrix formation. All of these cellular activities increase the bioactivity of the graft. The concentration of multipotential stromal cells (MSCs) in a commercially available cellular bone allograft was compared with fresh age-matched iliac crest bone and bone marrow aspirate.[11] Without cultivation or expansion, this allograft contains cells with cell surface markers called *cluster differentiation (CD) markers* that are found with immunotyping of osteoprogenitor cells and osteoblasts. These cells displayed an "osteoinductive" molecular signature and the presence of $CD45^+$, $CD271^+$, $CD73^+$, $CD90^+$, and $CD105^+$ MSC surface markers that were more than 100-fold of what are found in iliac crest bone. In comparison with bone marrow, MSC numbers enzymatically released from 1 g of cellular allograft were equivalent to approximately 45 mL of bone marrow aspirate. This MSC cellular allograft bone represents unique, nonimmunogenic material rich in MSCs, osteoblasts, and osteocytes. This osteoinductive cellular graft represents an attractive alternative to autograft bone by eliminating a secondary surgical harvest site and morbidity risk.

This stem cell preparation with bone scaffold has been used for implant site preparation by increasing alveolar ridge volume and sinus grafting.[86,163,271] Additionally, this cellular allograft has been used successfully in regenerative treatment of periodontal defects in both a single-rooted tooth and a multirooted tooth.[162] In the single-rooted case, a significant reduction in probing depth was obtained with radiologic evidence of approximately 4 mm of vertical bone fill at 6 months following grafting. In the multirooted case, clinical evidence showed decreased probing depths and radiographic bone improvement at 6 months. A cone-beam computed tomography scan taken at 14 months demonstrated three-dimensional bone fill. A similar result was presented in a case report, where this allograft cellular bone matrix was used in the successful treatment of a severe periodontal defect.[142] These case reports indicate a potential resolution of periodontal defects using cellular allograft material.

Use of Platelet-Rich Plasma/Platelet-Rich Fibrin for Periodontal Regeneration

PRP and PRF are autologous blood concentrate products that have been utilized in a variety of regenerative surgical applications.[58,59,178] While both products have unique preparation methods, both rely on concentrating the platelets of whole blood to produce a product that delivers the polypeptide growth factors associated with normal wound healing in a highly concentrated form to the surgical site.

The platelet-associated growth factors released from PRF and PRP include PDGF, VEGF, TGF-β, PDGEF, IGF-1, and bFGF (eTable 63.1).[59,106,238] These growth factors have been shown to contribute to periodontal regeneration and were released in significantly higher concentrations from the PRF and PRP products compared to whole blood.[58,59,248] In vitro studies have demonstrated that PRF and PRP can promote periodontal regeneration through the enhancement of cellular proliferation and differentiation of key progenitor cell populations.[277] In addition, the clinical benefits of PRF and PRP in periodontal regeneration in humans have been well studied. Across multiple randomized controlled trials, the addition of PRF was effective for the treatment of intrabony defects and Class II furcation defects compared to open flap debridement alone, resulting in decreased PPD and increased CAL.[178,280] The data have been inconclusive in terms of the benefit of adding PRF to bone graft material for the treatment of intrabony defects and Class II furcation defects.[1,264,280] The addition of PRP to intrabony and furcation defects has demonstrated more heterogenous results with minimal to no clinical benefit demonstrated when comparing its effectiveness to open flap debridement.[117,230] Proof of true periodontal regeneration using PRF or PRP via histological studies in humans is still lacking.

LEARNING BOX 63.3

Note that the use of biologic agents such as enamel matrix derivative (EMD) and platelet-derived growth factor (PDGF) is a relatively recent concept for periodontal regeneration. The process can proceed even with the short biologic half-life of these materials, so that the agents are often not present in the later stages of development. Readers should appreciate that these stimulated cells can somehow organize themselves to differentiate and, in a timely fashion, become three distinct histologic structures: new bone, cementum, and periodontal ligament. In addition, it is amazing that these three histologic structures "intertwine" with each other and stimulate regeneration using a different mechanism from the bioexclusion principle, as demonstrated with the use of guided tissue regeneration membranes. Finally, randomized controlled studies indicate that the addition of guided tissue regeneration membranes confers no advantage. All these factors indicate that the use of biologic agents can stimulate stem cells to be recruited to the intrabony or furcation defect site, proliferate, and differentiate into a newly regenerated periodontal apparatus. It is also interesting that this occurs in very rapid fashion, faster than the migration of epithelial and mesenchymal cells.

Combined Techniques

Periodontal new attachment and bone reconstruction have been challenges for clinicians throughout the history of periodontal therapy. To take advantage of the different bone graft materials and biologic mediators, clinicians have combined these graft materials with the use of membranes in an attempt to find a predictable technique to regenerate bone.

Several clinicians have proposed a combination of the techniques previously described in an attempt to enhance their results.[11,100,160,177] A classic paper published by Schallhorn and McClain[246] in 1988 described a combination technique using graft material, root conditioning with citric acid, and coverage with a nonresorbable membrane (the only available one at the time). More recently, with the advent of osteopromotive agents, such as the EMD (Emdogain, Straumann, Andover, MA) and osteoconductive bovine-derived anorganic bone (Bio-Oss) graft materials, other combination techniques have been advocated.[158] The combined use of these products, along with autogenous bone with resorbable membrane coverage, has resulted in an increased percentage of cases with successful new attachment and periodontal reconstruction. Many of these combination techniques were reviewed in previous sections of this chapter. Whereas the use of combination techniques may be appealing, it is important for clinicians to remember that these added materials often escalate the cost of the procedure and should be balanced with the quality and the long-term stability of the clinical results.

Regenerative Supportive Graft Materials

Many of the commercial regenerative materials are provided along with osteoconducive materials, such as tricalcium phosphate, collagen, and calcium that function as carriers, supportive matrix, or support bioexclusive properties. Many of these are FDA-approved carriers but clinicians have been known to discard these carriers in favor of DFDBA/FDBA. Though these materials do not provide osteogenic properties, it is important for clinicians to be aware of how and when these materials are clinically applied. More details are provided in the online material, *Miscellaneous biologics used for periodontal regeneration.*

Factors That Influence Therapeutic Success

Factors that adversely affect periodontal regeneration were reviewed at the 2013 AAP Regeneration Workshop.[84] Some of the therapeutic factors that have been implicated or shown to influence periodontal regenerative therapy adversely include (1) the selection of the appropriate surgical technique, accurate assessment of the periodontal defect, and the clinician's clinical experience (Fig. 63.5); (2) the importance of the tooth in the overall restorative treatment plan; and (3) the patient's personal preference for regenerative options.

Periodontal regeneration of intrabony defects can be predictable. There are several determinants which will influence the extent / ease for achieving defect fill.[195] Systematic reviews suggest that deeper defect areas are associated with more radiographic fill. Generally, regeneration of intrabony defects is predictable for defects that are ≥3 to 4 mm and narrow, as compared to wide/crater-type defects. An increased number of bony walls (3 walls greater than 2 walls greater than 1 wall) result in better defect fill while circumferential defects can be comparable to results obtained with 2-wall defects or better, depending on the defect width. There is a low level of evidence that suggests that the narrower the defect angle, the better the bone fill. Ideally, radiographic bone defects with less than 37° increase the likelihood for bone fill. The more of these criteria that are fulfilled, the greater the likelihood of bone fill. It should be noted that the extent of defect fill is not consistent nor completely predictable. There is 75% variability in terms of improvement in clinical attachment level and radiographic bone fill, assuming no membrane exposure, complete graft containment, number of walls, and defect angles.[284] Due to the high variability, it is not reasonable to define to the patient how much regeneration can be achieved. What is notable is that if membranes are used and become exposed, there is a significant negative effect on GBR around dental implants but only a minimal effect on GTR around natural teeth.[159]

Clinical Guidelines to Guide Clinicians in Their Patient Management

Clinical guidelines for the management of patients with periodontal disease are depicted in Fig. 63.5.[131] The ideal management of periodontal defects consists of early diagnosis and appropriately addressing the defect (see Fig. 63.5A). When defects are detected early, before the formation of intrabony and furcation lesions, a

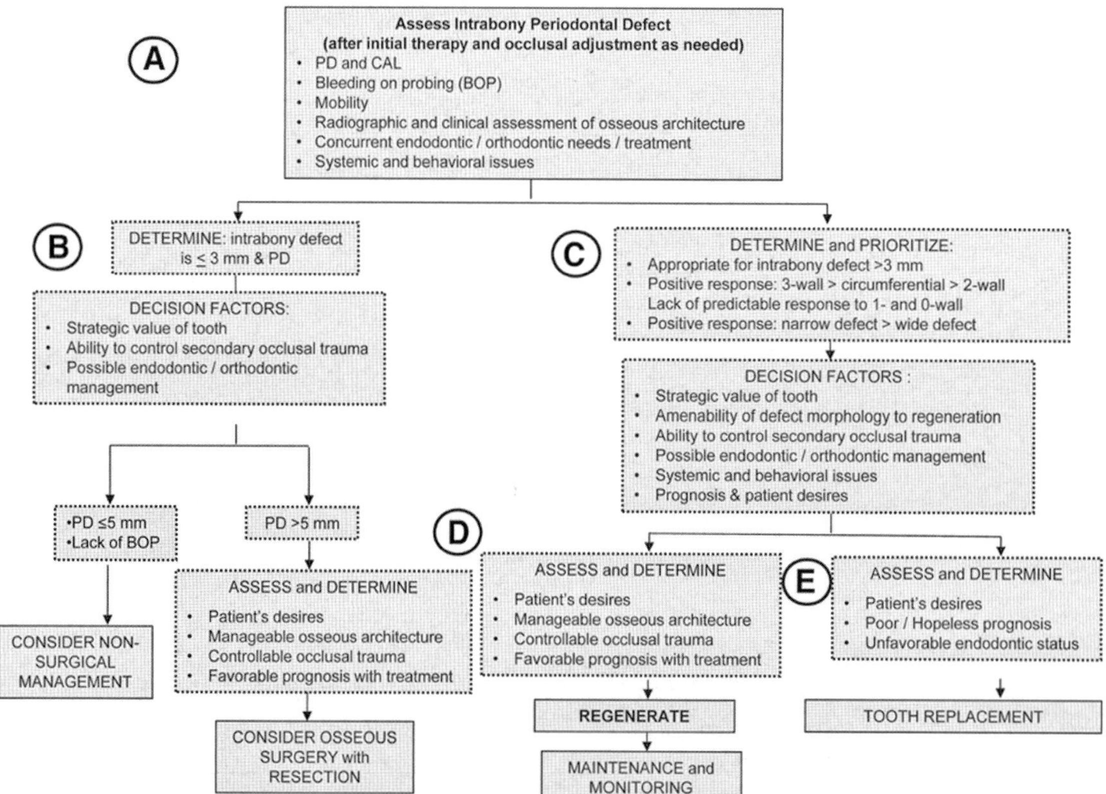

Fig. 63.5 Clinical decision tree for the management of advanced periodontal defects. *A* to *E* are explained in the text in the section titled "Clinical Guidelines to Guide Clinicians in Their Patient Management." *CAL*, Clinical attachment level; *PD*, periodontal defect. (From American Academy of Periodontology. *J Periodontol.* 2015;86[suppl]:S77.)

predictable outcome can be obtained with scaling, root planing, and conventional osseous surgery (see Fig. 63.5B). Even early narrow intrabony (less than 3 mm) and furcation defects can be blended in with the adjacent osseous contour. When the intrabony and furcation defects are greater than 3 mm, periodontal regeneration should be considered (see Fig. 63.5C). Assessment of defect morphology and the patient's clinical and systemic-behavioral determinants is critical for regenerative success. Consideration of these issues, in addition to the patient's desires, will define the selection of the regenerative approach used (see Fig. 63.5D). Long-term stability is possible, but the individual outcome is influenced by patient-related considerations, such as smoking and compliance with periodontal maintenance and monitoring. Should patient-related or clinical determinants be unfavorable for periodontal regeneration, a different, more appropriate, therapy must be selected in place of regeneration. Alternative therapeutic options include long-term maintenance or the removal of the tooth and replacement with a prosthesis, such as a dental implant or another form of prosthesis (see Fig. 63.5E).[128]

Before regenerative therapy, it is important to perform an endodontic assessment. This is to eliminate the possibility that the defect is the result of an endodontic-periodontal lesion. Should this be the case, endodontic treatment may resolve that portion of the defect due to the endodontic lesion. If a residual defect still persists, periodontal therapy should be initiated.

A common misconception is that regenerative therapy ends with a postoperative assessment a few months after treatment. Most therapeutic approaches have maximal healing results after 12 months. As such, postoperative monitoring should occur for at least 12 months after therapy. Additionally, these regenerated areas should be monitored at every recall visit because poor hygiene, uncorrectable tooth anatomy, and undiagnosed endodontic problems will cause these areas to relapse. Should failures due to these causes be determined, it may be prudent to consider strategic extraction.[128]

The **endpoint** for active periodontal therapy should comprise a stable periodontal attachment level, absence of inflammation or bleeding, and a periodontal anatomic environment that is conducive for the patient and the clinician to maintain excellent oral hygiene. A successful long-term periodontal outcome is also dependent on a patient who will be compliant with the maintenance visits. (See online material, *Therapeutic Considerations.*)

Future Directions for Periodontal Regeneration

In wound healing, the natural healing process usually results in tissue scarring or repair. By using tissue engineering, the wound healing process is manipulated so that tissue regeneration occurs.[87,165] This manipulation usually involves one or more of three key elements: (1) the signaling molecules, (2) scaffold or supporting matrices, and (3) cells (see Fig. 63.2). The cellular responses to these biologic mediators in vitro have been studied and are summarized in eTable 63.2. Some of these biologic mediators are commercially available (recombinant human bone morphogenetic protein [rhBMP], rhPDGF, EMD). The potential of tissue engineering in periodontal regeneration has been reviewed.[154,226]

Conclusion

Since the 1980s, the periodontal literature has been filled with numerous reports related to periodontal regeneration. This therapeutic goal, although ideal, is difficult to achieve. Various graft materials and regenerative strategies are now available; however, they all have limitations. The surgical procedure can be technically demanding, and when success is achieved, maintenance of positive results is highly dependent on patients' oral hygiene habits and compliance with periodontal maintenance. Despite these difficulties, periodontal regeneration is a clinical possibility that can be offered to patients. The clinician must carefully evaluate the various regenerative and reparative approaches and decide which technique may result in the best clinical outcome. With the advent of new regenerative approaches, such as biologic modifiers, including EMD and growth factors, we must critically evaluate how they may improve our ability to regenerate periodontal defects.

Treatment planning in periodontics has also changed dramatically because of the acceptance of dental implants as viable long-term options for replacing missing teeth. With the increased predictability of implants, questions arise regarding when to treat severe periodontal defects with regenerative procedures and when to perform strategic extraction in preparation for implant placement. Sometimes, the best management of a periodontal defect may be extraction in lieu of periodontal regeneration or when regenerative efforts have been unsuccessful. Extraction would minimize further bone loss and provide the maximum volume of bone at the future implant healing site. This paradigm shift has complicated our views about regeneration. Conversely, the increasing complications associated with dental implants, such as mechanical failures and peri-implantitis, makes regeneration attractive. In this debate, the patient should be brought into the decision-making process. The medical and dental history of the patient should be considered along with the decision-making for preserving the dentition through regeneration versus strategic extraction with the replacement with implant-supported dentition. As both dental implant and regenerative approaches improve, the clinician must consider the options and aid the patient in this decision-making process.

Periodontal regeneration continues to be one of the primary therapeutic approaches toward the management of periodontal defects. Although evidence suggests that present regenerative techniques can lead to periodontal regeneration, the use of GTR and biologic modifiers can enhance these results. The crucial challenge for the clinician is to assess critically whether a periodontal defect can be corrected with a regenerative approach, or whether it would be better managed with osseous resection for a slight periodontal defect and with strategic extraction for an advanced diseased state. In this assessment, the clinician should attempt to differentiate between techniques that have been studied in depth and with acceptable results and those that are still experimental and promising. Research articles must be critically evaluated for adequacy of controls, selection of cases, methods of evaluation, and long-term postoperative results. In addition, the clinician should remember that we treat patients based on clinical success and not statistical success. A resulting clinical attachment gain of half a millimeter may be a statistical success, but it is meaningless for the patients we treat and manage over the long term.

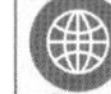
References for this chapter are found on the companion website eBooks.Health.Elsevier.com.

CHAPTER 64

Lasers in Periodontal and Peri-Implant Therapy

Richard T. Kao | Guo-Hao Lin | Stephen John | Perry R. Klokkevold | Charles M. Cobb

For online-only content on specific laser types, photodynamic therapy and low-level laser therapy, and literature on the use of lasers in the treatment of periodontitis, please visit the companion website at eBooks.Health.Elsevier.com.

CHAPTER OUTLINE

A variety of techniques and technologies have been proposed to replace traditional instrumentation used in periodontal therapy. Most such technology, including lasers, was developed to replace curettes, scalpels, and other types of instruments commonly used in invasive periodontal procedures. Despite the marketing efforts, studies confirmed that dental lasers are an adjunctive tool in the treatment of periodontal disease and are not intended to replace conventional therapies. As with any instrument, it is prudent for the therapist to identify clinical indications that are patient centric. In periodontics, lasers have potential application in three areas: (1) surgical procedures, such as gingivectomy and osseous crown lengthening, (2) scaling and root planing, and (3) the management of pathological changes resulting from periodontal disease. However, many questions remain and well-designed research studies are needed to evaluate the application of lasers in the treatment of periodontal and peri-implant diseases.

As with the introduction of most new technologies, advocates of laser therapy for periodontal and peri-implant diseases hope it will be able to replace or enhance traditional therapies. Determining whether a new technology should be incorporated into practice requires evidence from clinical studies to demonstrate equivalence or superiority to accepted therapies. Superiority is usually defined as greater than 20% of the effect of the established treatment. If the new treatment is no greater than or less than 20% of the effect of the established treatment, then the two groups are considered equivalent.[71] Additionally, the sample size required to statistically test superiority versus equivalence is generally much greater than what has been tested in clinical trials evaluating lasers currently. The limited number of longitudinal clinical trials and cohort studies for each laser type, along with the fact that different exposure settings and various protocols have been used in these studies, makes justification to implement this new technology for periodontal applications challenging. Published studies to date have too small a sample size and too heterogeneous methodology to make definitive conclusions, other than lasers are equivalent, at best, to conventional therapies. Nonetheless, if a new therapy is found to be equivalent, albeit not superior to a conventional therapy, utilization of the new technology may still be warranted for reasons such as safety, cost, or ease of use.[71] Systematic reviews and meta-analyses of available clinical trials have attempted to define whether lasers provide additional clinical benefits for periodontal applications.[166,167,169,171] Despite the large number of reports, there is a minimal number of randomized controlled clinical trials on which meta-analyses are based, so concluding any clinical benefit of lasers is speculative. This chapter describes some of the clinical applications of lasers for periodontal therapy and discusses the currently available literature.

Laser Physics and Biologic Interactions

Laser is an acronym for "*L*ight *A*mplification by *S*timulated *E*mission of *R*adiation." Lasers function by stimulating the emission of light energy from a given medium in a collimated, focused monochromatic ray of light. The energy beam reacts with a target tissue by being absorbed, reflected, or scattered, depending on wavelength and absorption characteristics (Fig. 64.1). If the light is well absorbed by the target tissue, the energy virtually explodes the cell and destroys the extracellular matrix in a process called *ablation.*[106] The efficiency of ablation is related to the wavelength and the affinity of the target tissue. If the wavelength is not well absorbed, there is scattering, and a thermal reaction occurs with carbonization, charring, and melting. Laser beams may also be reflected or bounced off the target (e.g., reflected off a metal surface) without interaction.

Argon lasers have wavelengths in the ultraviolet and visible light range and, as a consequence, they are primarily limited to dental applications involving composite resin placement, enamel and dentin bonding, preventive therapies, and endodontic procedures.[69,91,102,141] Reported periodontal applications for other laser types include soft tissue incision, ablation, depigmentation,

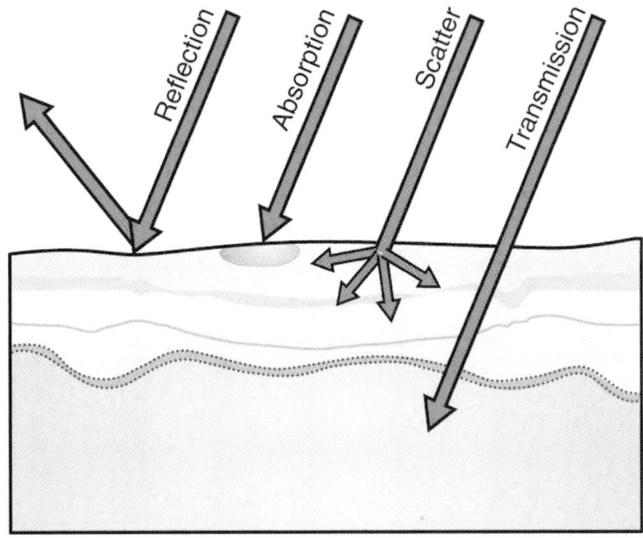

Fig. 64.1 Four potential laser-tissue interactions. The laser beam may be reflected, absorbed, scattered, or transmitted. (From Convissar RA. *Principles and Practice of Laser Dentistry.* 2nd ed. St. Louis: Mosby; 2016.)

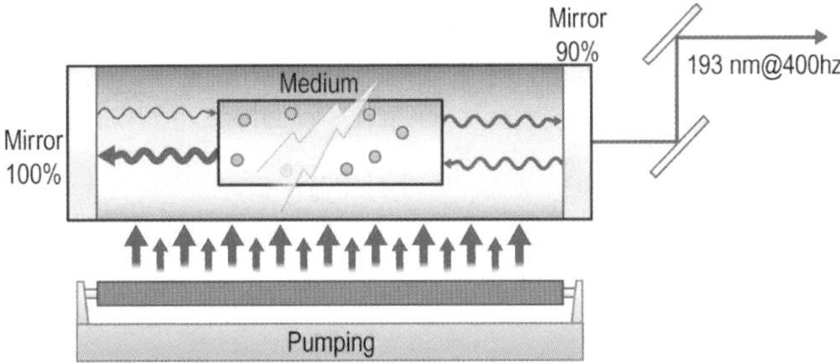

Fig. 64.2 Diagrammatic presentation of the main components of a laser device. Lasers require a medium, an optical chamber or laser tube, and an externally applied energy source to create an emitted monochromatic energy beam. (From Spaeth GL, Danesh-Meyer H, Goldberg I, et al. *Ophthalmic Surgery: Principles and Practice.* 4th ed. Edinburgh: Saunders; 2012.)

subgingival curettage, scaling of root surfaces, calculus removal, bacterial killing, osteoplasty, and ostectomy.

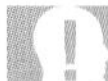

CLINICAL CORRELATION

Laser energy delivered to target tissues will vary depending on laser type (wavelength), settings (power), and exposure (time). Comparing the results of multiple studies is speculative, unless the same laser is used with identical settings and exposure time.

Production of a laser requires a medium, an optical chamber or laser tube, and an externally applied energy source to create an emitted monochromatic energy beam (Fig. 64.2). When energy is applied to the medium, electrons are "excited" to a higher energy orbit. When they return to the normal orbit, a photon (particle of light) is emitted. Because the photons are all the same wavelength, the laser beam is "coherent." The medium, which can be a gas, a solid, or a semiconductor, determines the laser wavelength. Lasers are named in relationship to the active element(s) that, when stimulated, generate the energy beam. The range of lasers used in dentistry consists of diodes (Gallium, Arsenic or Gallium, Aluminum, Arsenic), Nd:YAG, Er:YAG, Er,Cr:YSGG, CO_2, and argon. Clinicians must understand and appreciate not only how this energy is affecting the target tissues but also how it affects the adjacent tissues as well.

KEY FACT

Lasers function by stimulating the emission of light energy from a given medium in a collimated, focused monochromatic ray of light. The energy beam reacts with a target tissue by being absorbed, reflected, or scattered, depending on wavelength and absorption characteristics.

Each laser has a unique wavelength spectrum resulting in specific absorption characteristics that must be understood and appreciated as wavelength is the primary determinant for achieving a desired clinical outcome (Figs. 64.3 and 64.4). When applied to the various periodontal tissues, such as the gingiva, periodontal ligament, cementum, dentin, and bone, the biologic interactions will be unique for that wavelength. Tissues are composite structures of inorganic and organic elements with various constituents. Gingiva is composed of fibrous connective tissue, extracellular matrix components, layers of epithelial cells with melanin pigment, and 70% water. Bone is composed of 67% inorganic minerals (calcium hydroxyapatite) and 33% organic elements (collagen, noncollagenous proteins, cells, and water). Other factors to consider are the textures, compositions, and densities of these structures. For example, the varying percentages of mineralized structures, blood vessels, and fluid found in cortical bone versus cancellous bone will result in the laser energy beam encountering differing fluctuations in absorption and scattering, regardless of the wavelength. By contrast,

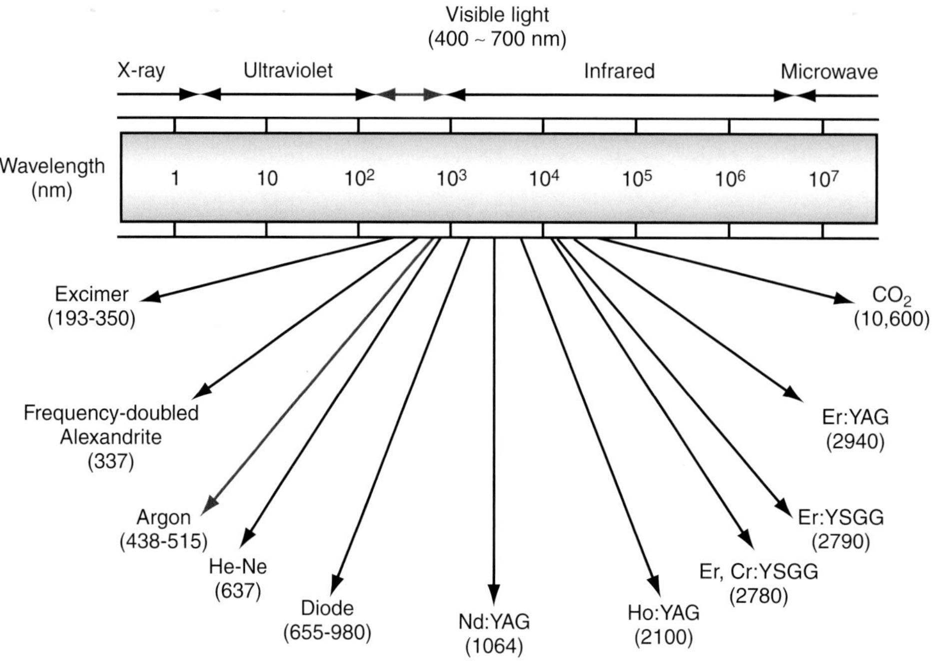

Fig. 64.3 Laser wavelengths. Each laser has a unique wavelength spectrum resulting in specific absorption characteristics. The wavelength of most of the lasers used in dentistry/periodontics is in the red and near-infrared spectrum.

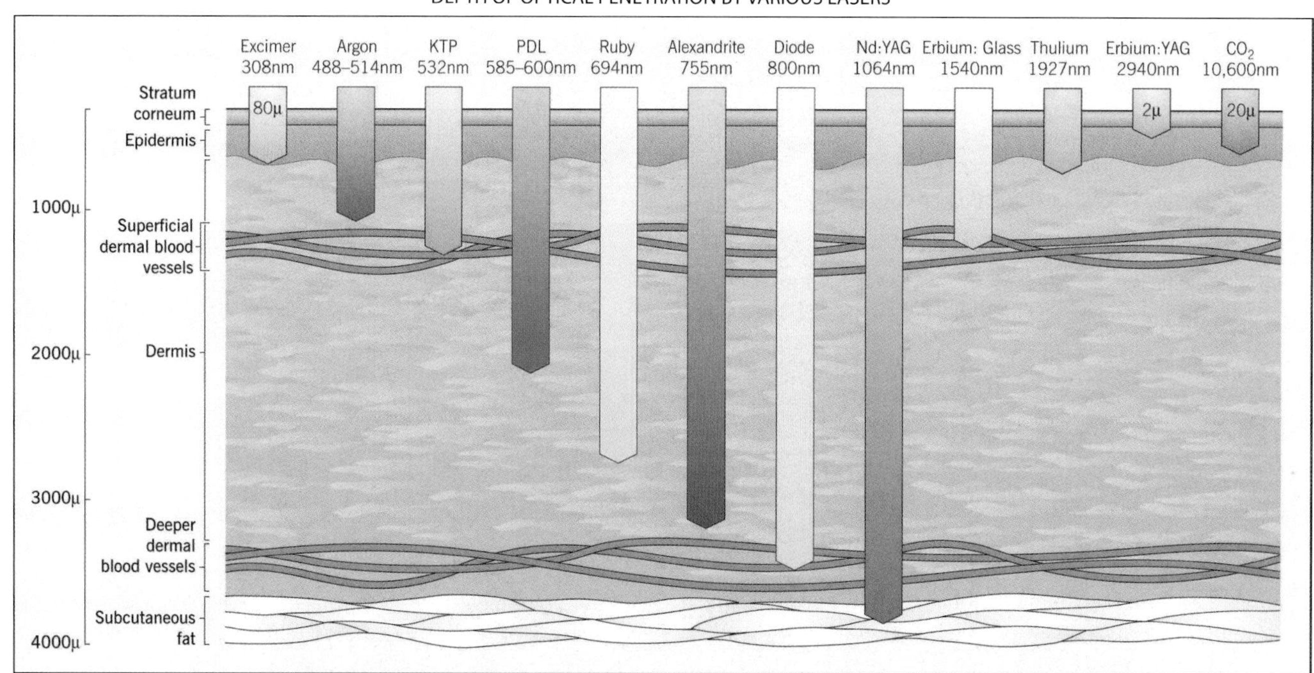

Fig. 64.4 Depth of optical penetration by various lasers. Tissue penetration is a function of laser wavelength and absorption characteristics. It should be noted that the treatment depth can greatly exceed the optical penetration depth for ablative lasers. On the face, the fat can be present at depth of 2–3 mm. For example, the depth of optical penetration for CO_2 lasers is only ~20 microns, but fractional CO_2 lasers can vaporize nearly full-thickness microchannels through the dermis. *KTP*, potassium titanyl phosphate; *Nd*, neodymium; *PDL*, pulsed dye laser; *YAG*, yttrium aluminum garnet. (From Bolognia JL, Jorizzo JL, Schaffer JV. *Dermatology*, Two-Volume Set. 3rd ed. Philadelphia: Saunders; 2012.)

blood contains 55% plasma (water containing salts and proteins) and 45% cells, such as red blood cells with hemoglobin, white blood cells, and platelets. The composition of the target tissue is relevant to a specific clinical application. Thus, when considering the use of lasers for a given clinical application, it is important to appreciate not only the type of laser being used and the target tissue but also the composition of that tissue. Recent advances in new wavelengths, delivery units, and power maximums refocused the use of lasers for soft tissue as well as hard tissue procedures (Table 64.1).[61,102] So when considering clinical application, it is important to ask: Is the

TABLE 64.1 Types of Lasers Currently Used in Dentistry

Laser Medium	Wavelength (nm)	Dental Uses
Argon	488–514	Tooth bleaching and advanced curing lights
Diode	655–980	Gingivectomy/gingivoplasty, oral medicine uses (aphthous ulcer therapy, biopsies, dentinal desensitizing), second-stage implant exposure, periodontal curettage (advocated but not evidence based)
Neodymium:yttrium-aluminum-garnet (Nd:YAG)	1064	Gingivectomy/gingivoplasty, oral medicine uses (aphthous ulcer therapy, biopsies, dentinal desensitizing), second-stage implant exposure, periodontal curettage (advocated but not evidence based)
Erbium, chromium:yttrium-scandium-gallium-garnet (Er,Cr:YSGG)	2780	Gingivectomy/gingivoplasty, oral medicine uses (aphthous ulcer therapy, biopsies, dentinal desensitizing), second-stage implant exposure, periodontal curettage (advocated but not evidence based), hard tissue cutting (dentin and osseous)
Erbium:yttrium-aluminum-garnet (Er:YAG)	2940	Gingivectomy/gingivoplasty, oral medicine uses (aphthous ulcer therapy, biopsies, dentinal desensitizing), second-stage implant exposure, periodontal curettage (advocated but not evidence based), hard tissue cutting (dentin and osseous)
Carbon dioxide (CO_2)	10,600	Gingivectomy/gingivoplasty, second-stage implant exposure, periodontal curettage (advocated but not evidence based)

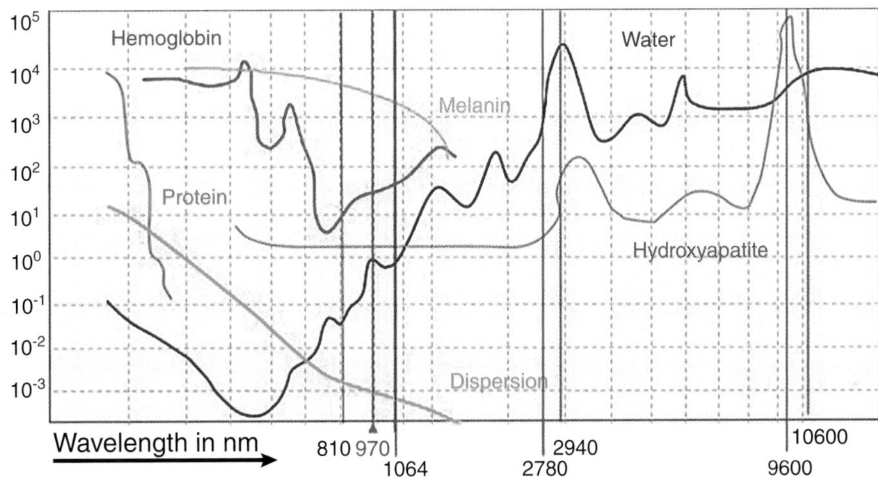

Fig. 64.5 Laser absorption coefficient of various tissue constituents as a function of wavelength.

specific laser wavelength appropriate for achieving the desired clinical outcome without adverse tissue interaction?

The affinity of a laser wavelength for the target tissue (absorption coefficient) is critical to its effectiveness for the procedure (Fig. 64.5). The light from the relatively short wavelengths of the diode (655 to 980 nm) and Nd:YAG (1064 nm) is well absorbed by pigment and is better suited for soft tissue procedures than for hard tissue procedures. The CO_2 laser has two different wavelengths, 9300 nm and 10,600 nm. The longer wavelength (10,600 nm) has an affinity for water and is best suited for soft tissue procedures. The shorter wavelength (9300 nm) has a high absorption affinity for hydroxyapatite that allows for efficient vaporization of tooth and bone structure, critical during the cutting of hard tissue. Its water absorption is much lower than an Erbium laser, so hydroxyapatite absorption and vaporization predominate during the cutting of enamel, dentin, and bone. Hard tissue ablation with the 9300 nm CO_2 laser is a photothermal event, not photoacoustic. As a result, higher temperatures are generated and much higher pulse rates are needed to cut. Diode and Nd:YAG wavelengths are not absorbed by hydroxyapatite and thus are not effective for hard tissues, such as cementum, dentin, and bone. The wavelengths of Er:YAG (2940 nm) and Er,Cr:YSGG (2780 nm) lasers have a positive affinity for both water and hydroxyapatite. The specificity for hydroxyapatite allows erbium lasers to cut hard tissues, including bone, dentin, and enamel,[10,26,28,29,31,32,37,64,65,81] and their additional absorption by water also makes them effective for soft tissue procedures.

Selection of the type of laser is also based on the amount of energy transmitted to the target tissue during a procedure, as determined by watts (W = joules/second) and hertz (Hz = cycles/second of a pulsed laser). The energy beam can have two types of waveforms: gated and/or pulsed energy beam. A continuous wave energy beam transmits more energy at the target surface than a pulsed energy beam, which has momentary breaks or cooling periods as compared to the former. Hertz (Hz) is the unit of measurement of the cycles/second of a pulsed laser. When comparing outcomes of different laser therapies, it is imperative when comparing protocols for laser treatment of periodontal and peri-implant disease that wavelength of laser, watts, hertz, and total time in contact with target tissues be assessed.

The benefits of using a laser can be compromised if the energy is excessive. Transmission of excessive thermal energy to target and adjacent tissues can result in cellular damage. Although the optimal energy delivered to tissues can be advantageous, excessive energy may completely negate the potential benefits. This effect is illustrated by a study comparing the wound healing of incisions made with a scalpel with the incisions made by two different power settings of an Nd:YAG laser. Healing was best following the incision applied with the laser, using settings of 1.75 W, 20 Hz., but delayed when the energy was increased to 3 W, 20 Hz. Healing of the scalpel incision was better than that for the laser incision at the higher energy setting.[145] The study demonstrates that differences in energy level delivered to tissues using the same laser can have significantly different results. It also shows the dilemma faced when attempting to compare the results of one study to another unless both studies use the same laser with the same energy settings and the same quantity of energy delivered. Unfortunately, the literature is inundated with reports of various applications using different lasers, varied settings, and a wide range of protocols.

KEY FACT

The type of tissue (e.g., hard versus soft tissue) as well as the composition of target tissue is important when applying laser therapy. For example, the varying percentages of mineralized structures, blood vessels, and fluid found in cortical bone versus cancellous bone will result in the laser energy beam encountering differing fluctuations in absorption and scattering, regardless of the wavelength.

Advantages and Disadvantages of Laser Therapy

There are many advantages to using a laser in dental surgical procedures: (1) decreased bleeding due to sealing of small vessels and lymphatics; (2) decreased swelling and edema; (3) reduced bacteremia due to sterilization of the wound surface during cutting; (4) decreased pain and discomfort; and (5) increased patient acceptance. Other purported advantages are less invasive surgery to gain access and minimal wound contraction and scarring. Many of these advantages are obvious but several need to be verified through further research. There are clearly many favorable reports of laser use in periodontal and peri-implant therapy, but further studies are necessary to establish which laser therapy protocols are most appropriate and effective.

The primary disadvantage of laser therapy is the potential for unintended tissue damage, as lasers can easily generate excessive temperatures. The exposure of bone to temperatures greater than 47°C (116.6°F) can induce cellular damage and osseous resorption.[61] Extreme temperature levels of greater than 60°C (140°F) result in tissue necrosis.[102]

Overexposure of laser energy has been the basis for complications, reports of tissue damage, and destruction of the periodontium. New, inexperienced operators as well as more seasoned, "cutting-edge" clinicians may encounter disastrous results from their initial treatments (Fig. 64.6). To avoid these negative outcomes, knowledge of the laser mechanics and manufacturer's recommended treatment protocol, and acquiring appropriate training and technique are essential to minimize tissue damage.

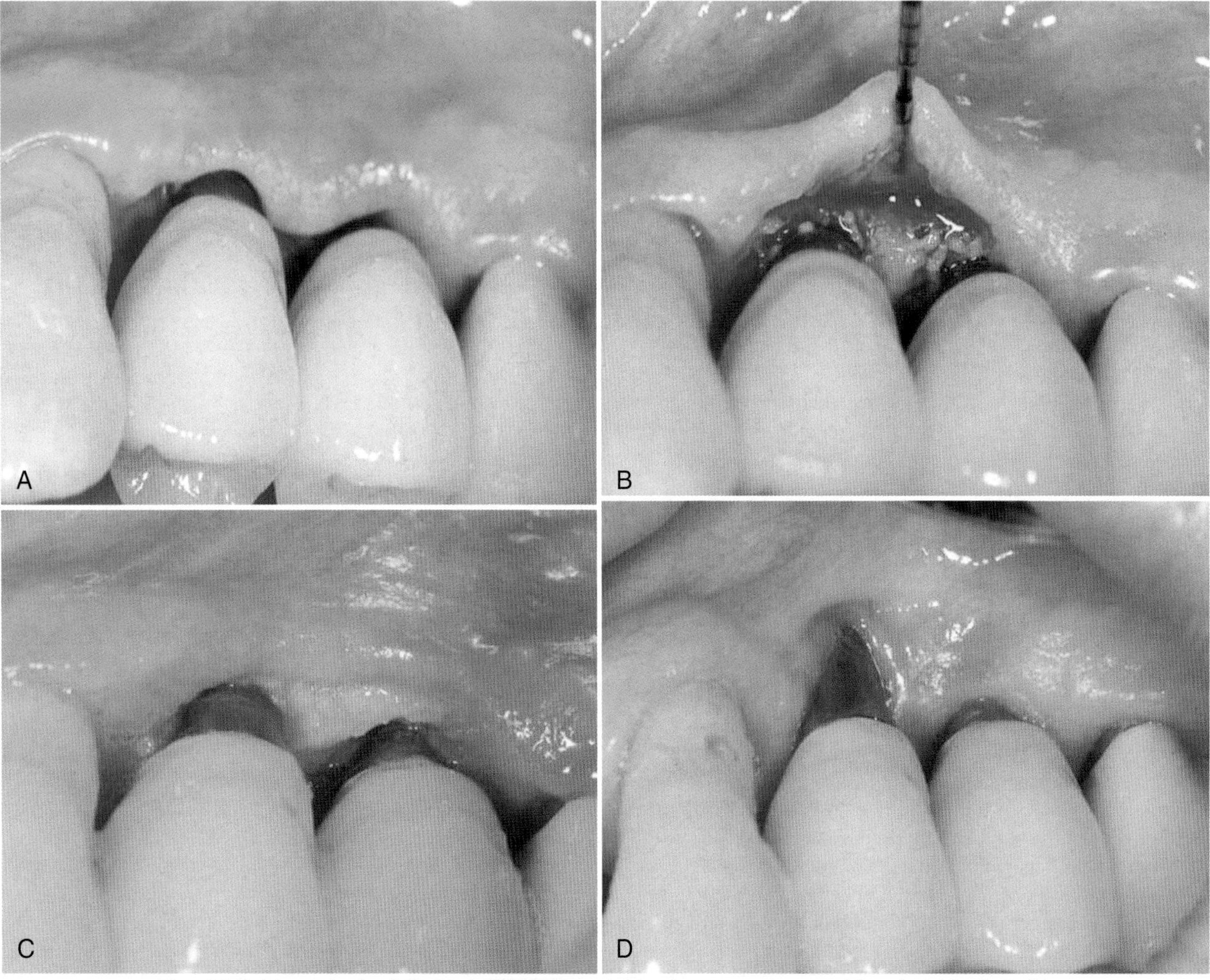

Fig. 64.6 Interproximal soft tissue cratering with underlying bone necrosis around two dental implants following laser treatment of peri-implantitis using inappropriate energy density and duration of exposure. Photos in sequence: (A–B) One-month post laser treatment. (C) Sequestration of necrotic interproximal and facial bone at 2 months post treatment. (D) Healing at 3 months post treatment. (Courtesy Dr. Charles Cobb, University of Missouri, Kansas City.)

Once mastery of the information has been achieved, it is critical to identify the desired laser application and the fashion in which it will be used. To avoid negative results and collateral damage to adjacent tissue requires a thorough knowledge of laser mechanics and the specific protocol technique. It cannot be emphasized enough that the commitment to incorporate the use of a laser obligates the practitioner to a commitment to the required training and continuous updating of requisite skill trainings.

In conclusion, the evidence for laser therapy is, at best, equivalent to conventional therapy. Given the significant investment, it behooves the clinician to be clear as to the additional clinical and patient management benefits that would justify the purchase and the incorporation of a laser in clinical practice.

Use of Common Types of Lasers in Periodontics

Lasers have been used in dentistry since 1989. The U.S. Food and Drug Administration must approve all lasers sold in the United States that are intended for medical and/or dental applications. At this stage, the American Academy of Periodontology (AAP) has reported there is not sufficient evidence in support of lasers, either as a monotherapy or as an adjunct, as being superior to traditional treatments for periodontal diseases.[49,114,125] The dental insurance industry usually determines reimbursement based on the actual treatment and not on the method or equipment used to achieve clinical outcome. As the readers review the attributes and skills required for the mastery of each laser type, the commitment to this technology requires an assessment of financial/time commitment, as well as treatment efficacy. Nevertheless, laser use for periodontal and soft tissue management has been promoted by thought leaders and commercial enterprise. Whether to have familiarity with the topic or to actually incorporate this tool into practice, it is important to have an understanding of the various laser types used in dentistry and their respective dental applications.

Laser applications can be basically divided into those with soft tissue applications and those with both soft and hard tissue applications. Appropriate soft tissue applications may include gingivectomy and/or gingivoplasty, management of aberrant soft tissue (such as gingival overgrowth, pericoronitis, and frena), and esthetic crown lengthening. Further, CO_2, Er,Cr:YSGG diode, and Nd:YAG lasers have been used for esthetic depigmentation. Hard tissue applications include caries detection, tooth preparation, tooth whitening, and decreasing dentinal hypersensitivities. Miscellaneous laser uses include optical coherence tomography (which has been used primarily as a research tool for caries and soft tissue research), photobiomodulation management of recurrent aphthous ulcers, temporomandibular joint treatment, airway management, and nerve regeneration. While these applications are interesting, the focus of this chapter is limited to laser use in periodontal and peri-implant applications. The lasers used and their clinical periodontal and soft tissue applications are listed in Table 64.1. Specific laser characteristics and applications can be found online.

> **Laser Applications in Periodontics**
>
> Currently, lasers are used in periodontal therapy for (1) microbial reduction within the pocket, (2) soft tissue management, such as frenectomy, gingival bleaching, gingivectomy, and gingivoplasty, (3) biopsy, (4) conservative management of the periodontal pocket, (5) photobiomodulation; and for water-affinity lasers, (6) decontamination of implant surfaces, and (7) osseous resection for osteoplasty, ostectomy, and crown lengthening procedures.

Esthetic and Soft Tissue Surgical Applications

Several types of laser wavelengths have been used for soft tissue surgical procedures.[11,72,73] Appropriate use of lasers has been well documented[23,67,88,113] for procedures, such as frenectomy, gingivectomy/gingivoplasty, reshaping of drug-induced gingival overgrowth, exposure of short crowns associated with altered passive/delayed eruption, and management of excess mucosal tissue, such as pericoronitis on the distal of mandibular second molars. Some of the positive aspects of laser therapy are good visibility during the surgical procedure as a result of coagulation, hemostasis, and minimal tissue damage adjacent to the laser wound. Additionally, laser therapy can offer greater precision and may be easier than using a scalpel in some restricted anatomical sites.

Esthetic applications for gingivectomy and gingivoplasty procedures allow delicate tissue reshaping. Also, the laser is effective for removing pigmentation from the gingival tissues, which can significantly improve the esthetics of highly pigmented areas. The CO_2, diode, Nd:YAG, Er:YAG, and Er,Cr:YSGG lasers have been used for depigmentation.[18,56,62,97,119]

Nonsurgical Periodontal Therapy

One of the more prevalent and controversial applications of lasers in periodontics is their use in nonsurgical treatment of moderate to advanced chronic periodontitis. Lasers have been used as a monotherapy or as an adjunct to scaling and root planing. The purported benefits of lasers for nonsurgical periodontal therapy include concurrent subgingival curettage, less invasive access for scaling and root planing and calculus removal, as well as detoxification and killing of subgingival periodontal microbial pathogens.[72,160,172,195] Lasers of various wavelengths have been shown to effectively kill periodontal pathogens.[37,74]

In vitro studies of bactericidal properties of lasers may not be clinically relevant as bacteria in a periodontal pocket do not exist as a suspension or monolayer, as they do in the laboratory. Clinically, subgingival periodontal pathogenic bacteria exist within a protective biofilm that has thickness and a significant extracellular polymeric matrix. Further, there are issues of clinical access, restorations, root anatomy, and the tortuous anatomy of infrabony pockets. Consequently, it is difficult for conventional periodontal therapies to completely eliminate subgingival microbes. Additionally, the microbial ecology is such that recolonization rapidly occurs. Thus, laser therapy may provide the benefit of reducing subgingival bacterial loads.

Currently, there is a clinical trend for advocating the use of diode/Nd:YAG lasers during supportive periodontal therapy. These clinical sessions are usually short in duration. The safe use of a laser and the completeness of debridement is questionable if time is an issue. It is not clear if the therapeutic objective is for the curettage effect or the suppression of the subgingival bacterial load. Incomplete debridement can potentially be more problematic than to use the traditional mechanical debridement. Additionally, the cost-benefit for adequate training for dental auxiliaries on the safe use of dental laser and the risk for iatrogenic periodontal tissue damage makes this therapeutic approach questionable.

Several questions to be considered when determining the effectiveness of using lasers for nonsurgical periodontal therapy are listed in Box 64.1.

BOX 64.1 Questions to Consider When Evaluating the Effectiveness of Laser Therapy

1. Do the in vivo studies demonstrate a reduction in pathogenic bacteria as compared with conventional therapy (e.g., scaling and root planing [SRP])?
2. Are positive microbial changes sustained, or do the periodontal pathogens return and recolonize the sites?
3. Are there any differences in clinical parameters following laser-assisted versus conventional therapy SRP? When evaluating nonsurgical periodontal therapy, gain in clinical attachment level (CAL) represents the gold standard. Pocket depth (PD) and levels of subgingival microbes are important because they correlate with changes in CAL.[47,152]
4. Are there changes in the root surface condition based on in vitro or in vivo studies?

The targeted elimination of subgingival bacteria has been demonstrated when a diode laser is used in concert with a photosensitizer. This combination of laser with photoactive dye is called PDT. Additionally, it has been proposed that use of a low-energy laser may have biomodulation properties that reduce inflammation and pain and improve healing and is referred to as LLLT. Currently, PDT and LLLT are more of experimental interest and have thus far not achieved wide clinical application. A synopsis of our understanding of these laser approaches is reviewed online.

CLINICAL CORRELATION

Laser therapy used to treat moderate to advanced chronic periodontitis is one of the more prevalent applications of this technology. The purported benefits of lasers for nonsurgical periodontal therapy include less invasive access for scaling and root planing, calculus removal, and the detoxification and killing of subgingival periodontal pathogens. Laser therapy may reach difficult-to-access areas more effectively than conventional therapy.

Crown Lengthening Procedure

The laser is an adjunct instrument in surgical therapy. The clinician must evaluate the best instrument to achieve their end result. The decision to use the laser in surgical therapy is based on the clinician's expertise and comfort level. This is best demonstrated with the crown lengthening procedure. Diode, Nd:YAG, CO_2, Er:YAG and Er,Cr:YSGG lasers are acceptable for soft tissue removal and/or recontouring, while the preferred lasers for osseous resection and/or osteoplasty are the Er:YAG, CO_2 and Er,Cr:YSGG. The Er,Cr:YSGG laser can safely cut bone without burning or altering the calcium-to-phosphate ratio of the irradiated bone.[93,189] The open crown lengthening approach provides optimal visual access with minimal bleeding. Additionally, the laser can be used for all steps of the crown lengthening procedure, which reduces the use of additional instruments and instrument transfer.

The use of lasers for flapless crown lengthening with osseous contouring remains controversial. Since both erbium lasers (e.g., Er:YAG and Er,Cr:YSGG) have an affinity for water and hydroxyapatite, it has been advocated that they may be used for clinical crown lengthening without gingival flap reflection.[64,65,93,175,187,189,192,193] No controlled longitudinal or cohort studies support the use of lasers for clinical crown lengthening using the closed-flap technique.

Decision-making for the use of lasers in crown lengthening in an open or closed approach is based on osseous biotypes and the skill level of the clinician.[94,101] In the closed approach, the Er,Cr:YSGG or Er:YAG laser is only feasible in medium biotype cases with an osseous crest that is at least 1 mm in thickness and in situations requiring only 1 to 2 mm of osseous removal (Fig 64.7). In this technique, bone sounding with a probe is used after the external gingivectomy to determine the thickness of the osseous biotype and the amount of bone required to be removed. In a pilot study to evaluate the use of Er:YAG laser for crown lengthening in a closed flap approach, the surgical objectives of a stable post-crown lengthening results were accomplished.[108] However, examination of the treated root surfaces indicated the flapless approach resulted in osseous troughs, insufficient /ragged bone removal, and root surface pitting. Some of these root defects were not correctable with root planing and can potentially serve as reservoirs for future plaque and calculus accumulation. A closed crown lengthening requires a high degree of competency.

Lasers in the Management of Periodontitis

The role of laser therapy in the management of periodontitis remains controversial. To date, the diode, Nd:YAG, and Er:YAG lasers have been advocated to use in managing the disease. Diodes may offer improved access for debridement, but microbial recolonization may result in recurrence of the periodontal defect. Much of the clinical focus has been with the use of Nd:YAG and Er:YAG lasers.

The Er,Cr:YSGG laser has been used for management of periodontitis in both a "closed" (no flap reflection) and an "open" (flap reflection) surgical approach. As with any surgery, the ability to see and treat with minimal intervention is the ideal approach. The "open" and "closed" approaches are very similar in their steps to achieve the optimal biologic environment for the potential of regeneration. The "closed" approach can be done if full visualization of the defect cannot be achieved and /or if reflection of the soft tissue may result in the compromised stability of the tooth.

Outcome Analysis of Laser Use Versus Conventional Therapies (Scaling and Root Planing) for Periodontitis

Traditional nonsurgical treatment of periodontitis (SRP) is remarkably effective in terms of reducing probing depths, bleeding on probing, and subgingival bacterial loads.[45,46] However, there is a caveat—the potential of recurrent disease in a relatively short period of time due to bacterial recolonization, incomplete removal of calculus, and the patient's lack of compliance with oral hygiene procedures. This caveat, therefore, dictates the need for continual maintenance therapy at regular intervals. Thus, lasers were introduced into the traditional nonsurgical treatment of periodontal disease as an alternative to SRP or as an adjunct to SRP[14,82,161] because of the purported inadequacies of traditional scaling and root planing. Yet, as applied to nonsurgical treatment of periodontal diseases, lasers also have inadequacies.[171,172,174]

The primary reason for the persistent uncertainty regarding the efficacy of lasers in both periodontal and peri-implant therapy is the lack of convincing evidence for achieving a consistent and clinically significant benefit. The American Academy of Periodontology Best Evidence Consensus (AAP BEC) statements[114,144] concluded that the number of well-designed clinical studies is limited, and the collective body of evidence was insufficient to support recommending developing clinical practice guidelines. Furthermore, the AAP BEC statement reported that only a slightly greater additive benefit should be expected following adjunctive use of lasers with traditional nonsurgical periodontal therapy. Based on current evidence, the use of lasers cannot justifiably replace conventional treatment. A summary of 73 systematic reviews of the literature, spanning 25 years (1996 to 2021), is presented in eTable 64.1 (see online material) and provides an evaluation of the body of evidence.

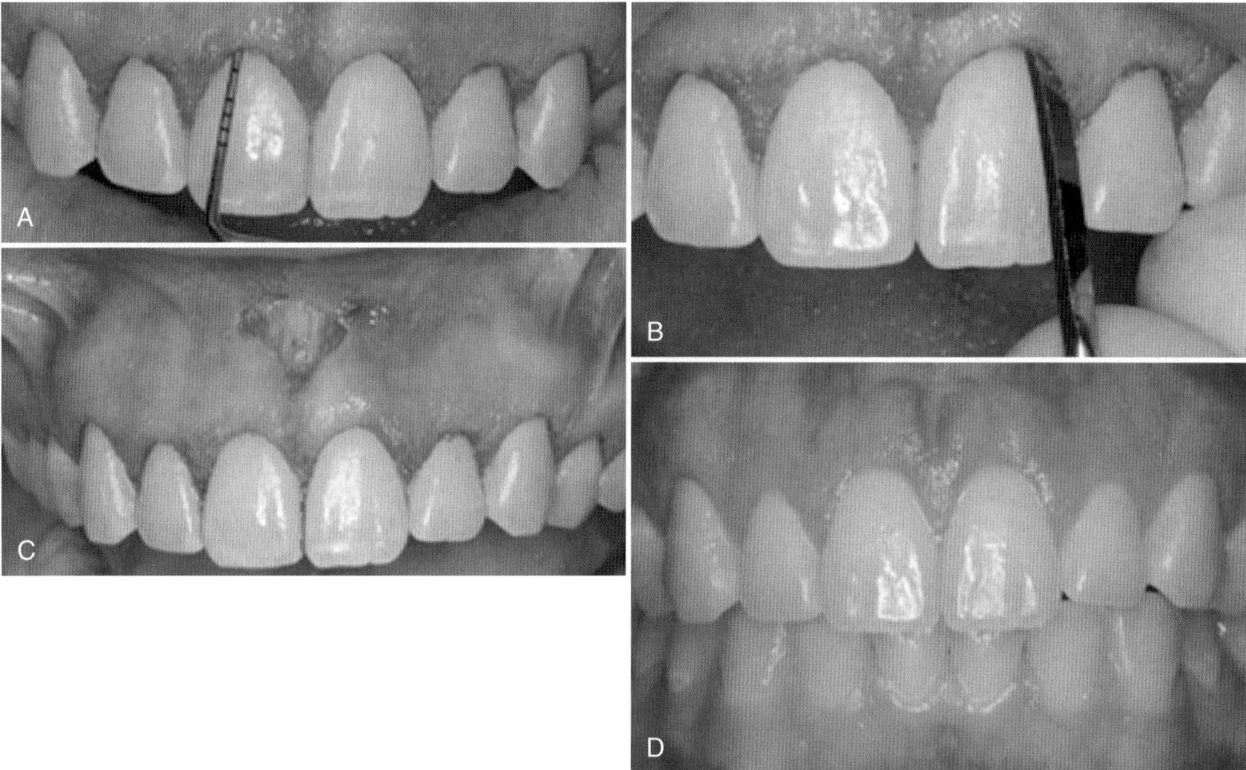

Fig. 64.7 Crown-lengthening procedure performed using a closed approach with a laser. (A) Periodontal sounding after the initial gingivectomy, which indicated the need for osseous contouring to achieve biologic width. (B) The osseous contouring was done via intrasulcular access. Sounding confirms 3 mm from the gingival to osseous crest. Final small fragments of bone are checked and removed with a small chisel. (C) Final surgical photograph shows minimal bleeding with no need for sutures. A frenectomy was also completed at the time of surgery. (D) Smile at 3 months postsurgery. (Case courtesy Dr. Bobby Butler, Seattle, WA.)

Lasers in the Management of Peri-implantitis

Interest has increased in the use of Nd-YAG lasers to manage peri-implantitis due to anecdotal reports of stabilization or reversal of radiographic changes associated with bone loss in peri-implantitis cases (eFig. 64.3). This clinical observation, although interesting, is an inconsistent finding and there appears to be no biological basis for when and why this phenomenon happens.

Several implant decontamination methods have been proposed for treating peri-implantitis. The mechanical methods refer to the use of plastic and/or metal inserts to debride the implant surface.[163] The application of chemicals, such as normal saline, root conditioners, disinfectants, and antibiotics have also been suggested to decontaminate the implant surface.[133] However, a complete implant decontamination using the aforementioned devices has been proven unsuccessful due to the limited access to implant microstructures, presence of resistant bacterial strains, ineffective drug dosages, and inadequate bactericidal effect.[70] As a result, adjunct use of lasers to detoxify the diseased implant surface was then proposed, aiming to optimize the treatment outcomes for peri-implantitis.[15,99]

Nevertheless, inconsistent results have been reported when lasers were used as an adjunct method for implant surface detoxification.[54,146,162] A recent systematic review reported that laser therapy provided similar outcomes as other surface detoxification methods for probing depth reduction, attachment level gain, and radiographic bone fill.[105] The authors reported that this heterogeneity in treatment outcomes after the use of lasers for peri-implant diseases could be attributed to several factors. Specifically, a wide range of lasers with varying settings (i.e., wavelength, power, waveform, pulse duration, energy/pulse, density of the energy, duration of the exposure, angulation of the energy towards the targeted tissue, peak power of the pulse, and the properties of the tissue)[47] have been used, so it is difficult to analyze their impact on treatment outcome. In addition, the frequency of laser use can also influence the treatment outcomes. Evidence suggested that the repeated application of lasers could have a positive impact on regeneration in peri-implant defects.[105,112]

Several clinical studies[54,145,162] have advocated laser use for surface decontamination methods as an adjunct to regenerative approaches when treating peri-implantitis surgically. In a case series study,[146] a CO_2 laser was used in combination with either autografts or xenografts to achieve a significant reduction in pocket depth around the implants with peri-implantitis. In contrast, Deppe et al.[54] concluded that no treatment outcome differences were found with or without the adjunct use of a CO_2 laser over a five-year period. Schwarz et al.[162] also failed to show the benefit of an adjunct Er:YAG laser in treating peri-implantitis. On the contrary, a recent clinical trial[188] reported a positive trend for PD reduction and CAL gain in the short term when treating narrow peri-implant infrabony defects with an Er:YAG laser. Due to the conflicting results, the American Academy of Periodontology best evidence review[99] recently reported that there is insufficient evidence to support the beneficial effect of adjunctive laser intervention on improving clinical parameters when treating peri-implantitis. Therefore, future clinical trials with a long-term follow-up are still needed to warrant the adjunctive use of lasers in peri-implantitis treatment.[36,99]

Conclusion

The use of laser therapy has many potential advantages, including better visualization of cutting, patient acceptance, wound detoxification, less invasive surgical access, and minimal wound contraction with less scarring.[23,79,113] Although these laser applications hold promise, many require more well-designed, controlled clinical trials to validate their effectiveness.[80]

The literature has numerous positive findings for the use of lasers in the management of periodontal and peri-implant disease; however, this literature is largely dominated by case reports and case series. There are relatively few well-designed randomized controlled clinical trials that are adequately powered in terms of the study population. Further confounding the issue is the variety of laser types at different wavelengths, the diversity of laser parameters, and variations in protocols in the different studies. The lack of consistency among studies has meant that no one laser type, parameter, and protocol has been adequately assessed to provide predictable parameters of use. Therefore, laser use for the treatment of periodontal or peri-implant disease continues to suffer from inconsistent results, controversy, and a lack of answers to important questions.

As in all professions, research and technological advances constantly provide better instrumentation, medications, and clinical techniques that allow clinicians to offer better and more predictable patient therapy. Lasers may become an integral part of periodontal therapy but, at the present time, further research, primarily focused on the parameters for clinical efficacy and the biologic basis of laser therapy, is required. Clinicians considering incorporating laser therapy should be familiar with what is known, understand the appropriate parameter for use, and receive adequate training to master their choice of laser.

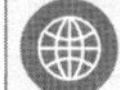
References for this chapter are found on the companion website eBooks.Health.Elsevier.com.

CHAPTER 65

Periodontal Plastic and Esthetic Surgery

Henry H. Takei | E. Todd Scheyer | Robert R. Azzi | Edward P. Allen | Thomas J. Han

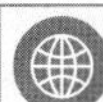
For online-only content on techniques to increase attached gingiva, gingival augmentation coronal to recession, tissue engineering, and techniques used to deepen the vestibule, remove the frenum, and improve esthetics, please visit the companion website at eBooks.Health.Elsevier.com.

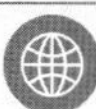
Videos for this chapter can be viewed on the companion website at eBooks.Health.Elsevier.com.

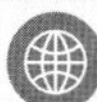
Animations have been added by the editors as a supplement to the chapter. They are produced by PerioPixel as patient education tools and cover the basic elements in a conceptual manner. They are not intended to be procedural guides for dental professionals.

CHAPTER OUTLINE

Terminology

The term *mucogingival surgery* was initially introduced in the literature by Friedman[39] to describe surgical procedures for the correction of relationships between the gingiva and oral mucous membranes, with special reference to three problem areas: attached gingiva, shallow vestibules, and a frenum interfering with the marginal gingiva. With the advancement of periodontal surgical techniques, the scope of nonpocket surgical procedures has increased and now encompasses a multitude of areas that were not addressed in the past. Recognizing this, the 1996 World Workshop in Clinical Periodontics renamed mucogingival surgery as *periodontal plastic surgery*,[3] a term originally proposed by Miller in 1993 and broadened to include the following areas[3,4]:

- Periodontal-prosthetic corrections
- Crown lengthening
- Ridge augmentation
- Esthetic surgical corrections
- Coverage of the denuded root surface
- Reconstruction of papillae
- Esthetic surgical correction around implants
- Surgical exposure of unerupted teeth for orthodontics

Periodontal plastic surgery is defined as the surgical procedures performed to correct or eliminate anatomic, developmental, or traumatic deformities of the gingiva or alveolar mucosa.[3,4] Mucogingival therapy is a broader term that includes nonsurgical procedures such as papilla reconstruction by means of orthodontic or restorative therapy. Periodontal plastic surgery includes only the surgical procedures of mucogingival therapy (Video 65.1).

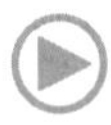

The periodontal plastic surgical techniques included in the traditional definition of mucogingival surgery are as follows: (1) widening of attached gingiva; (2) deepening of shallow vestibules; and (3) resection of the aberrant frena. Esthetic surgical therapy for natural dentition and tissue engineering (i.e., biologic mediators) also are addressed in this chapter. Other aspects of periodontal plastic surgery, such as periodontal-prosthetic surgery, esthetic surgery around implants, and surgical exposure of teeth for orthodontic therapy, are covered in Chapters 56, 60, 66, 68, and 78.

A classification system for periodontal surgery is shown in Fig. 65.1. It indicates the category of periodontal plastic surgery in surgical procedures that are used in periodontal therapy.

Objectives

Five objectives of periodontal plastic surgery are addressed in this chapter:

1. Problems associated with attached gingiva

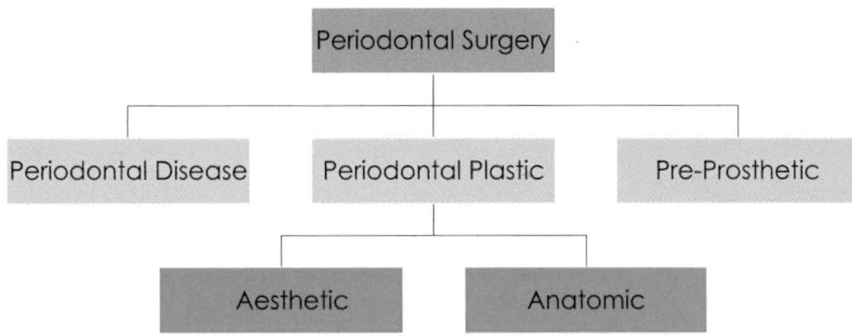

Fig. 65.1 Classification of periodontal surgery.

2. Problems associated with a shallow vestibule
3. Problems associated with an aberrant frenum
4. Esthetic surgical therapy
5. Tissue engineering

Problems Associated with Attached Gingiva

The ultimate goal of mucogingival surgical procedures is the creation or widening of attached gingiva around teeth and implants.[3] The width of the attached gingiva varies in different individuals and on different teeth of the same individual (see Chapter 4). Attached gingiva is not synonymous with keratinized gingiva because the latter also includes the free gingival margin. The width of the attached gingiva is determined by subtracting the depth of the sulcus or pocket from the distance between the crest of the gingival margin and mucogingival junction.

The original rationale for mucogingival surgery was predicated on the assumption that a minimal width of attached gingiva was required to maintain optimal gingival health. However, several studies have challenged the view that a wide attached gingiva is more protective against the accumulation of biofilm than a narrow or nonexistent zone. No minimal width of attached gingiva has been established as a standard necessary for gingival health. People who practice good, atraumatic oral hygiene can maintain excellent gingival health with almost no attached gingiva.

However, individuals whose oral hygiene practices are less than optimal can be helped by the presence of keratinized gingiva and vestibular depth. Vestibular depth provides space for easier placement of the toothbrush and prevents brushing on mucosal tissue. To improve esthetics, the objective is the coverage of the denuded root surface. The maxillary anterior area, especially the facial aspect of the canine, often has extensive gingival recession. In these cases, the covering of the denuded root surface widens the zone of attached gingiva and creates an improved esthetic result. Recession and the resultant denuded root surface have special esthetic concerns for individuals with a high smile line. A wider zone of attached gingiva is also needed around teeth that serve as abutments for fixed or removable partial dentures and in the ridge areas bearing a denture. Teeth with subgingival restorations and narrow zones of keratinized gingiva have higher gingival inflammation scores than teeth with similar restorations and wide zones of attached gingiva.[99,100] In these cases, techniques for widening the attached gingiva are considered preprosthetic periodontal surgical procedures. Chapter 68 discusses this subject in detail.

Widening the attached gingiva accomplishes four objectives:

1. Enhances plaque removal around the gingival margin
2. Improves esthetics
3. Reduces inflammation around restored teeth
4. Allows the gingival margin to bind better around teeth and implants with attached gingiva

Problems Associated With a Shallow Vestibule

Another objective of periodontal plastic surgery is the creation of vestibular depth when it is lacking. Gingival recession displaces the gingival margin apically, reducing vestibular depth, which is measured from the gingival margin to the bottom of the vestibule. With minimal vestibular depth, proper hygiene procedures are jeopardized. The sulcular brushing technique (Bass technique) requires placement of the toothbrush at the gingival margin, which may not be possible with reduced vestibular depth.

Minimal attached gingiva with adequate vestibular depth may not require surgical correction if proper atraumatic hygiene is practiced with a soft brush. Minimal amounts of keratinized attached gingiva with no vestibular depth benefit from mucogingival correction. Adequate vestibular depth is also necessary for the proper placement of removable prostheses.

LEARNING BOX 65.1

Gingival recession can be a functional and esthetic problem, and the biofilm is an oral hygiene problem because recession of the gingival margin reduces the vestibular depth. The proper position of the toothbrush (Bass technique) at the gingival margin becomes difficult or impossible without the space created by the vestibular depth.

Problems Associated with an Aberrant Frenum

An important objective of periodontal plastic surgery is correction of frenal or muscle attachments that may extend coronally to the mucogingival junction. If adequate keratinized, attached gingiva exists coronally to the frenum, it may not be necessary to remove the frenum. A frenum that encroaches on the margin of the gingiva can interfere with biofilm removal, and the tension on the frenum tends to open the sulcus. In these cases, surgical removal of the frenum is indicated.

Esthetic Surgical Therapy

Recession of the facial gingival margin alters the proper gingival symmetry and results in an esthetic problem. The interdental papilla is also important to satisfy the esthetic goals of the patient. A missing papilla creates a space that many call a *black hole*. Regeneration of the lost or reduced papilla is one of the most difficult goals in esthetic periodontal plastic surgery.

Another area of concern is an excessive amount of gingiva in the visible area. This condition is often called a *gummy smile,* and it can be corrected surgically by crown lengthening. Correction of these anatomic defects has become an important part of periodontal plastic surgery.

Tissue Engineering

The future of periodontal plastic surgery will encompass the use of tissue-engineered products at the recipient site to reduce donor site morbidity. Results of numerous experimental and clinical studies support the clinician's use of a minimally invasive approach to periodontal plastic surgery.

Cause of Marginal Tissue Recession

The most common cause of gingival recession and the loss of attached gingiva is abrasive and traumatic toothbrushing habits. The bone and soft tissue anatomy of the facial, radicular surface of the dentition is usually thin, especially around the anterior area. Teeth positioned facially may have an even thinner bone and gingiva. In many cases, the areas have a complete absence of bone beneath the thin overlying gingival tissue. This defect in the bone is called a *dehiscence.* This anatomic status combined with external trauma from overzealous brushing can lead to the loss of gingival tissue. Recession of the gingival tissue and bone exposes the cemental surface of the root, which results in abrasion and ditching of the cemental surface apical to the cementoenamel junction (CEJ). The cementum is softer than enamel and is destroyed before the enamel surface of the crown.

LEARNING BOX 65.2

Selection and daily use of the proper type of toothbrush are important. Daily use of a hard, improperly designed toothbrush is a poor instrument for biofilm removal and a principal cause of gingival recession.

Another cause of gingival recession is periodontal disease and chronic marginal inflammation. The loss of attachment caused by the inflammation is followed by the loss of bone and gingiva. Advanced periodontal involvement in areas of minimally attached gingiva results in the base of the pocket extending close or apical to the mucogingival junction. Periodontal therapy for these areas results in gingival recession caused by the loss of gingiva and bone.

Frenal and muscle attachments that encroach on the marginal gingiva can distend the gingival sulcus, which creates an environment for biofilm accumulation. This condition increases the rate of periodontal recession and contributes to the recurrence of recession, even after treatment (Fig. 65.2). These problems are more common on facial surfaces, but they may also occur on the lingual surface.[11]

Orthodontic tooth movement through a thin buccal osseous plate may lead to a dehiscence beneath a thin gingiva. This situation can also lead to the recession of the gingival margin[46,120] (Fig. 65.3).

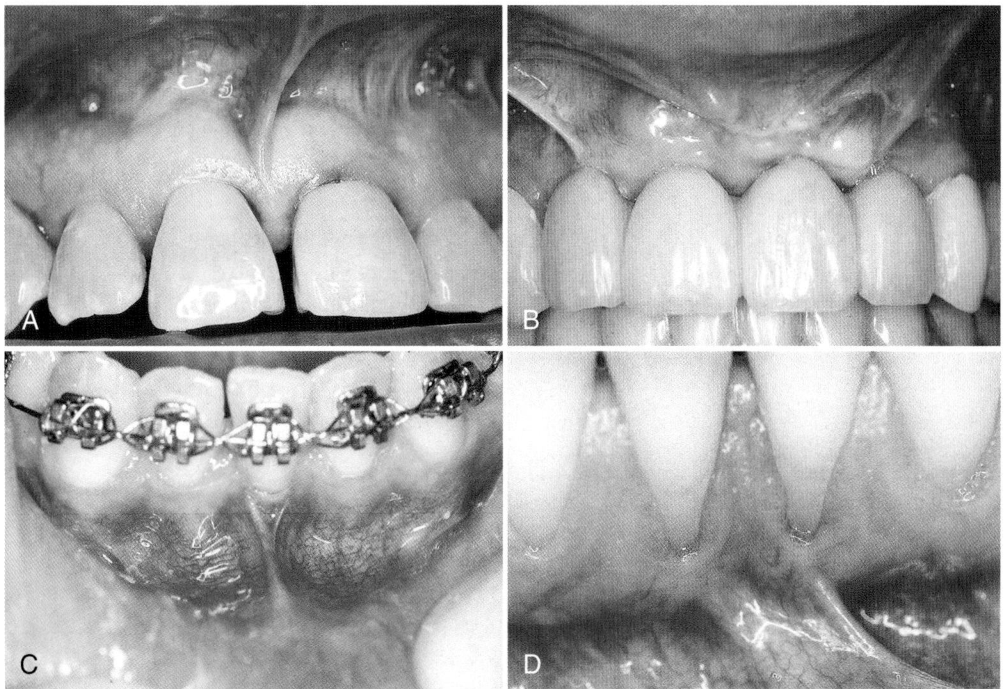

Fig. 65.2 High frenum attachments. (A) Frenum between the maxillary central incisors. (B) Frenum attached to the facial surface of the maxillary lateral incisors. (C) Frenum attached to the facial surface of a mandibular incisor. (D) Frenum attached to the facial surface of an incisor.

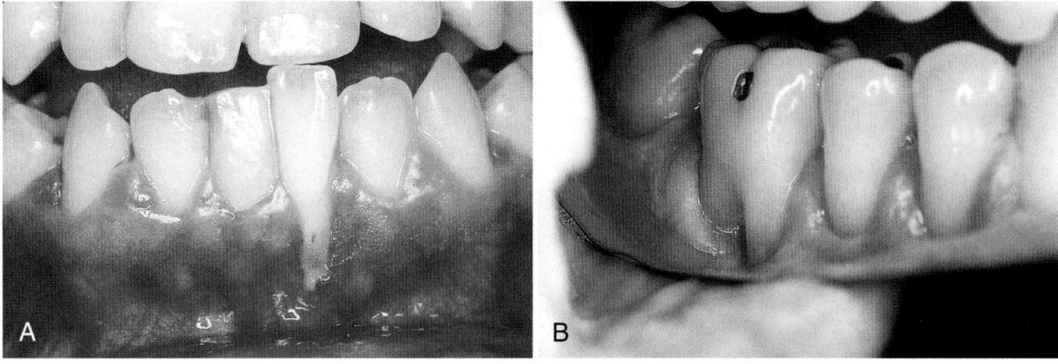

Fig. 65.3 (A) Gingival recession and extreme inflammation around a lower central incisor. (B) Advanced recession of the mesial root of a first lower molar.

Factors That Affect Surgical Outcome

Irregularity of Teeth

Abnormal tooth alignment is an important cause of gingival deformities that require corrective surgery and an important factor in determining the outcome of treatment. Location of the gingival margin, width of the attached gingiva, and alveolar bone height and thickness are affected by tooth alignment. On teeth that are tilted or rotated labially, the labial bony plate is thinner and located further apically than on the adjacent teeth. The gingival margin is recessed apically to follow the bone, which leads to the exposure of the root.[120] On the lingual surface of these teeth, the gingiva is bulbous and the bone margins are closer to the CEJ. The level of gingival attachment on the root surfaces and width of the attached gingiva after mucogingival surgery are affected as much by tooth alignment as by variations in treatment procedures.

Orthodontic correction is indicated when mucogingival surgery is performed on malposed teeth in an attempt to widen the attached gingiva or restore the gingiva over denuded roots. If orthodontic treatment is not feasible, the prominent tooth should be reduced to within the borders of the alveolar bone, with special care taken to avoid pulp injury.

Roots covered with thin bony plates pose a hazard in mucogingival surgery. Even the most minimally invasive flap, such as the partial-thickness flap, creates the risk of bone resorption on the periosteal surface.[49] Resorption in amounts that ordinarily are not significant may cause loss of bone height when the bone plate is thin or tapered at the crest.

LEARNING BOX 65.3

A facially malpositioned tooth and traumatic toothbrushing with a hard-bristled toothbrush are important factors in gingival recession.

Mucogingival Line

Normally, the mucogingival line (i.e., junction) in the incisor and canine areas is located approximately 3 mm apical to the crest of the alveolar bone on the radicular surfaces and 5 mm interdentally.[101] In periodontal disease and on malposed, disease-free teeth, the bone margin is located further apically and may extend beyond the mucogingival line. The distance between the mucogingival line and CEJ before and after periodontal surgery is not necessarily constant. After inflammation is eliminated, the tissue tends to contract and draw the mucogingival line in the direction of the crown.[31]

Criteria for Selection of Techniques

Numerous techniques are used for solving the mucogingival problems outlined in this chapter. Proper selection of a technique must be based on the predictability of success, which is based on specific criteria.

The following criteria are used for the selection of mucogingival techniques:

1. Surgical site free of biofilm, calculus, and inflammation
2. Adequate blood supply to the donor tissue
3. Anatomy of the recipient and donor sites
4. Stability of the grafted tissue to the recipient site
5. Minimal trauma to the surgical site

Surgical Site Free of Biofilm, Calculus, and Inflammation

Periodontal plastic surgical procedures should be undertaken in a biofilm-free and inflammation-free environment to enable the clinician to manage firm gingival tissue. Meticulous precise incisions and flap reflection cannot be achieved when tissue is inflamed and edematous. Thorough scaling and root planing and meticulous biofilm removal by the patient must be accomplished before any surgical procedure.

Adequate Blood Supply

To obtain the maximal amount of blood supply to the donor tissue, gingival augmentation apical to the area of recession provides a better blood supply than coronal augmentation because the recipient site is entirely periosteal tissue. Root coverage procedures involve a portion of the recipient site (i.e., denuded root surface) without blood supply. If esthetics is not a factor, gingival augmentation apical to the recession may be more predictable. A pedicle-displaced flap has a better blood supply than a free graft, with the base of the flap intact. If the anatomy is favorable, the pedicle flap or any of its variants may be the best procedure for root coverage.

The Langer SECTG procedure and the pouch and tunnel techniques use a split flap with the connective tissue sandwiched between the flaps. This flap design maximizes the blood supply to the donor tissue. If large areas require root coverage, these sandwich-type recipient sites provide the best flap design for blood supply.

Anatomy of the Recipient and Donor Sites

The presence or absence of vestibular depth is an important anatomic criterion at the recipient site for gingival augmentation. If gingival augmentation is indicated apical to the area of recession, there must be adequate vestibular depth apical to the recessed gingival margin to provide space for a free or pedicle graft. If a vestibule is necessary, only a free graft can accomplish this objective apical to the recession.

Mucogingival techniques, such as free gingival grafts and free connective tissue grafts, can be used to create vestibular depth and widen the zone of attached gingiva. Other techniques require vestibular depth to be present before the surgery, including pedicle grafts (lateral and coronal), the Langer SECTG, and pouch and tunnel procedures.

Availability of donor tissue is another anatomic factor that must be considered. Pedicle displacement of tissue necessitates an adjacent donor site that has gingival thickness and width. Palatal tissue thickness is also necessary for the connective tissue donor autograft. Gingival thickness is required at the recipient site for techniques using a split-thickness, sandwich-type flap or the pouch and tunnel techniques.

Stability of the Grafted Tissue to the Recipient Site

Good communication of the blood vessels from the grafted donor tissue to the recipient site requires a stable environment. This necessitates sutures that stabilize the donor tissue firmly against the recipient site. The least number of sutures and maximal stability should be achieved.

Minimal Trauma to the Surgical Site

As with all surgical procedures, periodontal plastic surgery is based on the meticulous, delicate, and precise management of oral tissues. Unnecessary tissue trauma caused by poor incisions, flap perforations, tears, or traumatic and excessive placement of sutures can lead to tissue necrosis. The proper selection of instruments, needles, and sutures is mandatory to minimize tissue trauma. Sharp contoured blades (see eFig. 65.16), smaller diameter needles, and resorbable monofilament sutures are important factors in achieving atraumatic surgery.

Conclusions

Periodontal plastic surgery refers to soft tissue relationships and manipulations. In all these procedures, blood supply is the most significant concern and must be the underlying consideration for all decisions regarding the individual surgical procedure. A major complicating factor is the avascular root surface, and many modifications to existing techniques are used to overcome this. Diffusion of fluids is short term and of limited benefit as tissue size increases. The formation of a circulation through anastomosis and angiogenesis is crucial to the survival of these therapeutic procedures.

Formation of vascularity is based on growth molecules, such as vascular endothelial growth factor (VEGF), and on cellular migration, proliferation, and differentiation. As tissue engineering techniques improve, the success and predictability of mucogingival surgery should dramatically increase. However, all advancements must have adequate circulation and blood supply as their basis.

New techniques are being developed and are slowly being incorporated into periodontal practice. The practitioner should be aware that new methods sometimes are published without adequate clinical research to ensure the predictability of the results and the extent to which the techniques may benefit the patient. Critical analysis of recently presented techniques should guide the evolution toward better clinical methods.

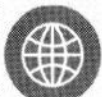
A Case Scenario is found on the companion website eBooks.Health.Elsevier.com.

Suggested Readings

Barootchi S, Tavelli L, Di Gianfilippo R, et al. Long-term assessment of root coverage stability using connective tissue graft with or without an epithelial collar for gingival recession treatment. A 12–year follow–up from a randomized clinical trial. *J Clin Periodontol*. 2019;46(11): 1124–1133.

Dai A, Huang JP, Ding PH, Chen LL. Long–term stability of root coverage procedures for single gingival recessions: a systematic review and meta–analysis. *J Clin Periodontol*. 2019;46(5):572–585.

Huang JP, Liu JM, Wu YM, Chen LL, Ding PH. Efficacy of xenogeneic collagen matrix in the treatment of gingival recessions: a systematic review and meta–analysis. *Oral Diseases*. 2019;25(4):996–1008.

Tavelli Lorenzo, et al. Biologics–based regenerative technologies for periodontal soft tissue engineering. *J Periodontol*. 2020;91(2):147–154.

Tonetti MS, Cortellini P, Pellegrini G, et al. Xenogenic collagen matrix or autologous connective tissue graft as adjunct to coronally advanced flaps for coverage of multiple adjacent gingival recession: randomized trial assessing non–inferiority in root coverage and superiority in oral health–related quality of life. *J Clin Periodontol*. 2018;45(1):78–88.

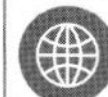
References for this chapter are found on the companion website eBooks.Health.Elsevier.com.

CHAPTER 66

Preparation of the Periodontium for Restorative Dentistry

Philip R. Melnick | Henry H. Takei

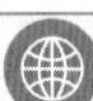 For online-only content on preprosthetic surgery, please visit the companion website at eBooks.Health.Elsevier.com.

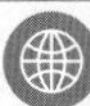 Videos for this chapter can be viewed on the companion website at eBooks.Health.Elsevier.com.

 An animation (slide show) has been added by the editors as a supplement to the chapter. It was produced by My Dental Hub as a patient education tool and covers the basic elements in a conceptual manner. It is not intended to be a procedural guide for dental professionals.

CHAPTER OUTLINE

Periodontal health is the *sine qua non* of successful, patient centric, interdisciplinary, comprehensive dentistry.[46] To achieve the long-term therapeutic targets of comfort, good function, treatment predictability, longevity, and ease of restorative and maintenance care, active periodontal infection must be treated and controlled before the performance of restorative, esthetic, and implant dentistry. In addition, the residual effects of periodontal disease or anatomic aberrations inconsistent with realizing and maintaining long-term stability must be addressed. This phase of treatment includes therapies performed in anticipation of esthetic or implant dentistry, such as surgical crown lengthening, covering denuded roots, alveolar ridge preservation or augmentation, and implant site development (Video 66.1).

Rationale for Therapy

The many reasons for establishing periodontal health before performing restorative dentistry include the following[29]:

1. Periodontal treatment is undertaken to establish stable gingival margins before tooth preparation. Noninflamed healthy tissues are less likely to change (e.g., recede) as a result of subgingival restorative treatment or postrestoration periodontal care or lapses in patient plaque control efforts.[51,52] In addition, tissues that do not bleed during restorative manipulation allow for a more predictable restorative and esthetic result.[43,44]
2. Many periodontal procedures are designed to provide for adequate tooth length for retention, access for tooth preparation, impression making, tooth preparation, and finishing of restorative margins in anticipation of restorative dentistry.[43,81] Failure to complete these procedures before restorative care adds to the complexity of treatment and introduces unnecessary risk for failure.[43]
3. Periodontal therapy should antecede restorative care because the resolution of inflammation may result in the repositioning of teeth[76] and/or soft tissue and mucosal changes.[41,82] Failure to anticipate these changes may interfere with prosthetic designs planned or carried out before periodontal treatment.
4. Traumatic forces placed on teeth with ongoimay increase tooth mobility, discomfort, and possibly the rate of periodontal attachment loss.[20] Restorations constructed on teeth free of periodontal inflammation, synchronous with a functionally appropriate occlusion, are more compatible with long-term periodontal stability, comfort, and patient satisfaction (see Chapters 32 and 35).
5. The quality, quantity, and topography of the periodontium may play essential roles as structural defense factors in maintaining periodontal health.[94] Orthodontic tooth movement and restorations completed without the benefit of the necessary periodontal therapies can result in adverse changes that complicate reconstructive efforts and maintenance of long-term health.[18,19,40,70,94]
6. Successful esthetic and implant procedures may be difficult or impossible in the absence of the necessary periodontal procedures.[36,58,66]

LEARNING BOX 66.1

Periodontal treatment is undertaken to establish stable gingival margins, at the desired level and morphology, before tooth preparation. Noninflamed healthy tissues are less likely to change (e.g., recede) as a result of subgingival restorative treatment or postrestoration periodontal care. In addition, tissues that do not bleed during restorative manipulation improve the ease of predictable reconstructive therapies and offer a superior esthetic result.

Sequence of Treatment

Treatment sequencing should be based on logical and evidence-based methodologies and grounded in the periodontal health status and psychological and esthetic concerns of the patient. Because periodontal and restorative therapies are situational and specific to each patient, every treatment plan must be adaptable to change, depending on the variables encountered during treatment. For example, teeth initially determined to be salvageable may be judged "hopeless," thus altering the preconceived treatment scheme.[41,82]

Generally, the preparation of the periodontium for restorative dentistry can be divided into two phases: (1) control of periodontal inflammation with nonsurgical and surgical approaches; and (2) preprosthetic periodontal surgery (Box 66.1).

Control of Active Disease

The initial step in preparing the periodontium for restorative dentistry is to address the active disease state. Any inflammatory condition of the supporting tissues must be eliminated or controlled with some combination of patient self-performed biofilm removal, scaling, root planing and, if necessary, periodontal surgery (see Chapters 43, 50, 51, 52, and 56).

In addition to removing the primary etiologic agents, biofilm, and root surface accretions, secondary local factors, such as plaque-retentive overhanging margins and untreated caries, must also be addressed.[18,19,27,32]

Emergency Treatment

The purpose of emergency treatment is to alleviate symptoms and stabilize acute infection. To the patient, the control of acute pain is often their primary reason for seeking dental care.[50] Treatment may include endodontic as well as periodontal conditions (see Chapters 49 and 69). This aspect of therapy must be addressed appropriately before any other treatments are instituted.

Extraction of Hopeless Teeth

The retention of untreated hopeless teeth often results in bone loss around the adjacent teeth.[55] Removing teeth with poor and/or hopeless prognoses if implant dentistry or other replacement options offer a more predictable alternative to attempting periodontal therapy should be considered. The extraction of hopeless teeth often includes preplanned temporization with fixed or removable prosthetics.

BOX 66.1 Sequence of Treatment in Preparing Periodontium for Restorative Dentistry

Control of Active Disease

- Emergency treatment
- Extraction of hopeless teeth
- Oral hygiene instructions
- Scaling and root planing
- Reevaluation
- Periodontal surgery
- Adjunctive orthodontic therapy

Preprosthetic Surgery

- Management of mucogingival problems
- Preservation of ridge morphology after tooth extraction
- Crown-lengthening procedures
- Alveolar ridge reconstruction

Oral Hygiene Measures

As indicated earlier, oral hygiene measures, when effectively applied, will reduce plaque biofilm and gingival inflammation[53,74,85] (see Chapters 43, 50, 51, and 52). Self-performed biofilm control measures alone are often inadequate for the resolution of subgingival infection and inflammation, particularly in pockets ≥5 mm. Beyond the inaccessibility of deep pockets to tenacious dental deposits, lack of patient dexterity, tooth position, and dental anatomy may further complicate removal. Furthermore, routine oral hygiene devices have been shown to be inefficient in reaching the base of deep periodontal pockets[74,91] (see Chapter 50).

Scaling and Root Planing

Scaling and root planing, combined with oral hygiene measures, have been shown to reduce gingival inflammation and the rate of the progression of periodontitis significantly[6,7,54] (see Chapters 50, 51, and 52). This finding even applies to patients with deep periodontal pockets[8,28,62] (Fig. 66.1).

LEARNING BOX 66.2

Pathologic periodontal conditions must be resolved before contemplating restorative dentistry.

Reevaluation

Four to 8 weeks after periodontal therapy, the gingival tissues are evaluated to determine oral hygiene adequacy, soft tissue response, and residual pocket depth[79] (see Chapter 43). This permits sufficient time for healing, reduction in inflammation and pocket depths, and gain in clinical attachment levels. Unfortunately, in deeper pockets (>5 mm), plaque biofilm and calculus removal are often incomplete,[2,90] increasing the chances of future periodontal breakdown[13,83] (Fig. 66.2). In such a situation, periodontal surgery to remove calculus and biofilm deposits and reduce periodontal pockets must be considered before proceeding with definitive restorative care.[25]

Periodontal Surgery

Periodontal surgery may be required for some patients (see Chapter 56). Indications for surgery include treating active periodontal disease, residual disease after nonsurgical therapy,[24,64] patients with future restorative, prosthetic, or dental implant needs, and orthodontic treatment.[94] This would include surgical crown lengthening for functional and esthetic purposes, alveolar ridge preservation, edentulous ridge augmentation[3,36,58,66], and mucogingival surgery.

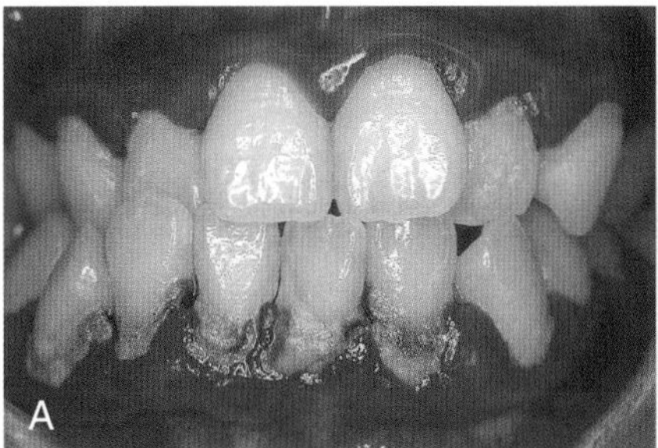

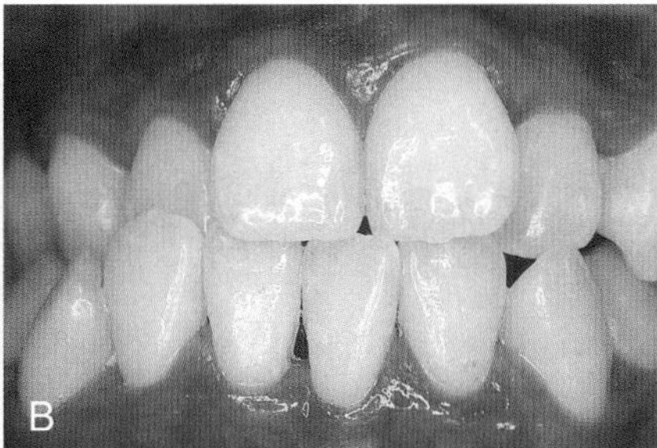

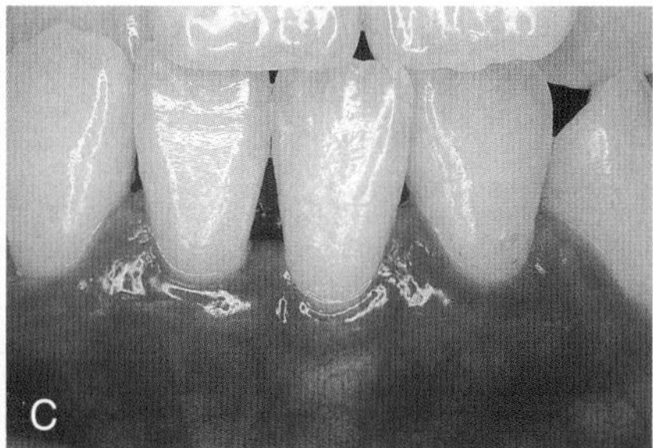

Fig. 66.1 (A–C) Root planing has resolved the gingival inflammation of this patient.

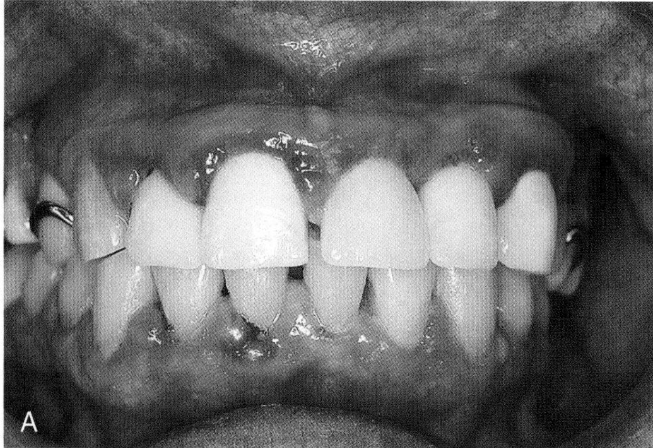

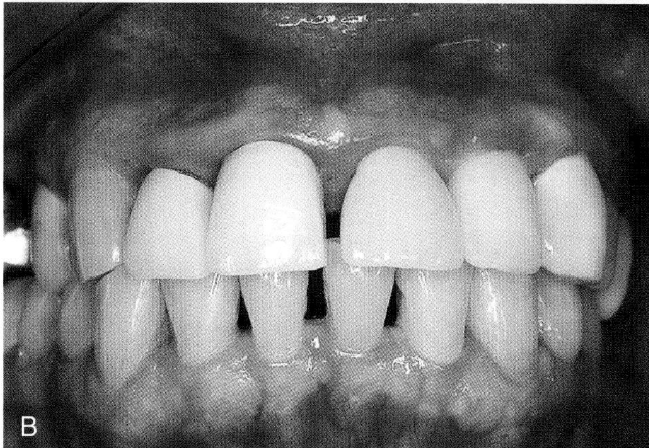

Fig. 66.2 (A) Before treatment. (B) After 4 weeks, oral hygiene instructions, scaling, and root planing have improved this patient's periodontal status. However, inflammation associated with pockets deeper than 5 mm suggests a need for periodontal surgery.

Adjunctive Orthodontic Therapy

Orthodontic treatment has been shown to be a useful adjunct to periodontal therapy[11,30,31,45,60] and, by extension, restorative, prosthetic, and implant dentistry (see Chapter 48). Orthodontic therapy should be undertaken only after active periodontal disease has been controlled.[21] If nonsurgical treatment is sufficient to establish and maintain periodontal health, definitive periodontal pocket therapy (e.g., surgery) may be postponed until after the completion of orthodontic tooth movement. This approach affords the advantage of the positive bone changes that orthodontic therapy can provide. However, deep pockets and furcation invasions often require surgical access for root instrumentation in advance of orthodontic tooth movement. Failure to control active periodontitis can result in acute exacerbations and bone loss during tooth movement.[22,35] As long as the periodontium is periodontally healthy, teeth with preexisting bone loss may be moved orthodontically without incurring additional attachment loss.[67,68] Soft tissue–grafting procedures are often indicated in anticipation of orthodontic therapy and restorative dentistry to reduce the possibility of gingival margin recession.[60,94]

LEARNING BOX 66.3

Periodontal surgery is performed for the treatment of active periodontal disease, as well as for preprosthetic preparation of the periodontium. Some procedures are intended to treat active disease successfully, and others are aimed at preparing the mouth for restorative or prosthetic care.

Patients undergoing orthodontic, restorative, or esthetic treatment must have a comprehensive clinical and radiographic periodontal examination and risk assessment.[14,39,40]

The Role of the Periodontal Phenotype

A patient's periodontal phenotype may play an essential role in the success of restorative dentistry and, by extension, complementary therapies, such as orthodontics and implant dentistry.[14,18,39,40]

An organism's *phenotype* is its observable characteristics influenced both by its genotype and its environment.[33,34,39] The *periodontal phenotype* has been defined as the combination of gingival phenotype (three–dimensional gingival volume—e.g., gingival thickness, keratinized tissue width) and thickness of the buccal bone plate (bone morphotype). The periodontal phenotype may change over time, depending on environmental factors and clinical intervention.[33,34,39] The dimensions of these structures may vary and can differ from patient to patient and from tooth to tooth in the same patient.[33,34,39]

The *gingival thickness* may be estimated by detecting a periodontal probe showing through the gingival tissue after insertion into the gingival sulcus: (1) probe visible, thin (≤1 mm), (2) probe not visible, thick (>1 mm).[39,56] The *keratinized tissue width* is measured from the gingival margin to the mucogingival junction. (KK) Cone-beam computed tomography (CBCT) can estimate *bone thickness*; however, the risk of radiation exposure versus the benefit of acquiring this data should be considered.[39]

Periodontal Phenotype and Restorative Dentistry

Patients with a thin periodontal phenotype, including those with minimal or no attached gingiva, can be maintained in periodontal health.[33,34,38] However, the risk of inflammation and recession increases when oral hygiene is suboptimal and thin periodontal tissues are subjected to restorative dentistry.[14,38] This would include routine occurrences such as trauma from gingival retraction, placement of intracrevicular restorative margins, and restorations with large restorative overhangs.[14,18,19,38]

In patients with a thin periodontal phenotype and no gingival recession, treating clinicians should correct potential harmful environmental influences and concentrate on prevention and monitoring.[38,39] However, in situations of an extremely thin phenotype, current gingival recession, minimal (≤2 mm), or no attached gingiva, an appropriate surgical gingival augmentation procedure should be considered in anticipation of potentially traumatic procedures and intracrevicular restorative dentistry.[33,34,38,39]

Periodontal Phenotype and Orthodontics

With appropriate oral hygiene, healthy gingiva of any dimension is considered sufficient to maintain periodontal health. However, during orthodontic tooth movement, the three-dimensional adequacy of periodontal hard and soft tissues is critical to preventing gingival recession. Tooth movement within the alveolar envelope, irrespective of gingival thickness or quality, is considered a lower risk of a future recession. If, however, the tooth is moved outside the alveolar process, resulting in a bony dehiscence, there is an increased potential for gingival recession. In that event, the gingival thickness is more likely to be a critical factor in preventing future gingival recession. Therefore, sites showing thin periodontal tissues (<2 mm) are potential candidates for periodontal surgical soft tissue augmentation (grafting) and fastidious preventive measures in advance of orthodontic treatment and in preparation for future restorative dentistry.[33,34,92,93]

Surgical Modification of Periodontal Phenotype

A thick periodontal phenotype is more resistant to gingival inflammation and recession. Conversely, sites with a thin periodontal phenotype are more suspectable to gingival recession when subjected to plaque-associated inflammation, restorative procedures, and orthodontic tooth movement.[38,39,40,77] Thus, the clinician needs to identify the deficiencies in patient-performed oral hygiene and periodontal phenotype and plan the most appropriate therapies, including surgical techniques, best suited to enhance the quality of soft tissue to support periodontal health and stability[38,39,77] (see Chapter 65).

Autogenous free gingival grafts to increase the dimension of attached gingiva and bilaminar tissue grafts to enhance gingival thickness are considered the gold standard for gingival augmentation[40] (see Chapter 65).

The gingival tissues will normally regenerate to their full dimension after correctly performed osseous surgery, including crown lengthening. This takes on special significance when planning for restorative dentistry. The healing period after surgical crown lengthening can vary and may be affected by several factors, including the patient's periodontal phenotype. Whereas a thin phenotype may regrow and mature sufficiently within 6 to 12 weeks to allow for the restorative process, a thick phenotype may take as long as 6 to 12 months to regenerate completely.[10,69] Consequently, tooth preparation and restoration in advance of healed and stable gingival tissues can invite placement of the restorative margin within the supracrestal attachment zone.

Conclusion

As described in this and other sections of this text, the therapeutic goals of patient comfort, function, esthetics, predictability, longevity, and ease of restorative and maintenance care are attainable only through thorough examination, insightful diagnosis. and a carefully constructed interdisciplinary plan. The dialectic interaction between periodontal therapy and successful restorative dentistry only serves to underscore this premise.

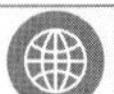
Case Scenarios are found on the companion website eBooks.Health.Elsevier.com.

References for this chapter are found on the companion website eBooks.Health.Elsevier.com.

CHAPTER 67

Periodontal Treatment of Medically Complex Patients

Perry R. Klokkevold | Brian L. Mealey  *| Joan Otomo-Corgel*

Content on thyroid and parathyroid disorders, adrenal insufficiency, thrombocytopenic purpuras, nonthrombocytopenic purpuras, blood dyscrasias, renal diseases, liver diseases, and pulmonary diseases can be accessed on the companion website at eBooks.Health.Elsevier.com.

CHAPTER OUTLINE

Many patients seeking dental care have significant medical conditions that can alter the course of their oral disease and the therapy provided. This is especially true for older patients who are more likely to have underlying disease(s). The therapeutic responsibility of the clinician includes identification of the patient's medical problems to formulate a proper treatment plan. A thorough medical history is paramount.[89] If significant findings are unveiled, consultation with or referral of the patient to an appropriate physician is indicated. This ensures correct management and provides medicolegal coverage for the clinician.

This chapter covers common medical conditions that clinicians will encounter when managing patients with periodontal disease. The review of each topic area can be supplemented by consulting other references for more detailed coverage of specific disorders. Understanding these conditions enables the clinician to appropriately treat the total patient, rather than focusing solely on their periodontal needs.

Cardiovascular Diseases

Cardiovascular diseases are the most prevalent category of systemic disease in the United States and many other countries, and they are more common with increasing age.[119] Health histories should be closely scrutinized for cardiovascular problems, including hypertension, angina pectoris, atrial fibrillation, myocardial infarction (MI), cardiac bypass surgery, cerebrovascular accident (CVA), congestive heart failure (CHF), infective endocarditis (IE), and implanted cardiac pacemakers or automatic cardioverter-defibrillators.

In most cases, the patient's physician should be consulted, especially if stressful or prolonged treatment is anticipated. Short appointments and a calm, relaxing environment help minimize stress and maintain hemodynamic stability.

Hypertension

Hypertension, the most common cardiovascular disease, affects more than 100 million American adults, many of whom are undiagnosed.[7] In 2017, the American Heart Association, the American College of Cardiology, and nine other health professional organizations revised the 2003 high blood pressure guidelines, lowering the definition of high blood pressure from 140/90 to 130/80 mm Hg. Nearly half (46%) of the U.S. adult population has high blood pressure based on the new definitions (Table 67.1).

The new guidelines were developed following the Systolic Blood Pressure Intervention Trial (SPRINT), which included more than 9000 adults aged 50 years old and older with at least one risk factor and a systolic blood pressure of 130 mm Hg or higher. The results demonstrated that a systolic blood pressure of 120 mm Hg or less reduced the chances of heart attack, heart failure, or stroke over a three-year period. The new guidelines eliminate the category of prehypertension, categorizing these patients as elevated (systolic 120 to 129 and diastolic <80) or stage 1 hypertension (systolic 130 to 139 or diastolic 80 to 89).[129]

TABLE 67.1 Blood Pressure Categories

Category	Systolic (mm Hg)		Diastolic (mm Hg)
Normal	<120	and	<80
Elevated	120–129	and	<80
Stage 1 Hypertension	130–139	or	80–89
Stage 2 Hypertension	≥140	or	≥90
Hypertensive Crisis	>180	and/or	>120

Hypertension is not diagnosed from a single elevated blood pressure (BP) recording. Rather, the diagnosis is based on the average value of two or more BP readings taken at two or more appointments. Both the systolic and diastolic pressure readings are considered in the diagnosis.

Hypertension is divided into primary and secondary types. *Primary* (i.e., essential) *hypertension* occurs when no underlying pathologic abnormality can be found to explain the disease. Approximately 90% to 95% of hypertensive patients have primary hypertension. The remaining 5% to 10% have *secondary hypertension,* in which an underlying cause can be found and is often treated. Conditions responsible for secondary hypertension include renal disease, endocrinologic changes, and neurogenic disorders.

In early hypertension, the patient may be asymptomatic. If not identified, diagnosed, and treated, hypertension can persist and increase in severity, leading eventually to coronary artery disease, angina, MI, CHF, CVA, or kidney failure.[65] Patients with hypertension enter dental practices every day. Hypertension is more common among the older populations who are frequently seen in periodontal practices, and the prevalence of patients with hypertension will certainly increase with the new, lower threshold guidelines. Prior evidence from the Framingham Heart Study revealed that people with normal BP at age 55 still have a 90% risk of becoming hypertensive later in life.[120]

The dental office can play a vital role in the detection of hypertension and maintenance care of the patient with hypertensive disease. The first dental office visit should include two BP readings spaced at least 10 minutes apart, which are averaged and used as a baseline. Before the clinician refers a patient to a physician because of elevated BP, readings should be taken at a minimum of two appointments, unless the measurements are extremely high (i.e., systolic pressure > 180 mm Hg or diastolic pressure > 120 mm Hg).

The periodontal recall maintenance visit is an ideal time for hypertension detection and monitoring. Only about one in four (24%) adults with hypertension in the United States have their condition under control.[22] Lack of compliance with antihypertensive therapy is the primary reason for this failure. Dentists can help patients achieve greater success in managing hypertension by taking BP readings at each periodontal recall maintenance visit and informing them about the readings.

Periodontal or other dental procedures should not be performed until accurate BP measurements and a thorough medical history have been taken to identify patients with significant hypertensive disease. The time of day should be recorded because BP varies significantly throughout the day.[82] Patient position and arm used to record blood pressure should also be recorded (e.g., right arm, seated).

Dental treatment for hypertensive patients is safe as long as stress is minimized.[65,71] If a patient is receiving antihypertensive therapy, consultation with the physician may be warranted regarding the current medical status, medications, periodontal treatment plan, and patient care. Many physicians are not knowledgeable about the details of dental or periodontal procedures. It is important for the dentist to inform the physician regarding the estimated degree of stress, length of the procedures, and complexity of the individualized treatment plan. Morning dental appointments were once suggested for hypertensive patients, but evidence indicates that BP usually increases around awakening and peaks at midmorning.[14,82,108] Because lower BP levels occur in the afternoon, afternoon dental appointments may be preferable.

No routine periodontal treatment should be given to a patient who is hypertensive and not under medical management. For patients with systolic BP greater than 180 mm Hg or diastolic BP greater than 120 mm Hg, treatment should be limited to emergency care only until hypertension is controlled. Immediate referral to manage hypertension should be considered. Analgesics are prescribed for pain and antibiotics for infection. Acute infections may require surgical incision and drainage, but the surgical field should be limited because excessive bleeding can occur with elevated BP.

When treating hypertensive patients, the clinician should not use a local anesthetic containing an epinephrine concentration greater than 1:100,000 or a vasopressor to control local bleeding. Local anesthesia without epinephrine can be used for short procedures (<30 minutes). In a patient with hypertensive disease, however, it is important to minimize pain by providing profound local anesthesia to avoid an increase in endogenous epinephrine secretion.[65,71]

The benefits of the small doses of epinephrine used in dentistry far outweigh the potential for hemodynamic compromise. The smallest possible dose of epinephrine should be used, and aspiration before injection of local anesthetics is critical. Intraligamentary (i.e., periodontal ligament) injection is usually contraindicated because hemodynamic changes are similar to an intravascular injection.[107] If the hypertensive patient exhibits anxiety, the use of conscious sedation in conjunction with periodontal procedures may be warranted (see Chapter 58).[117]

Although there is success with nonpharmacologic methods to control hypertension including diet, exercise, weight control, and limiting alcohol, most people require one or more medications to achieve blood pressure control.[2] There are several categories of antihypertensive medications (Table 67.2). See online material for a brief description of the various classes of medications used to control hypertension.

Clinicians need to be familiar with antihypertensive medications and recognize their side effects and potential drug interactions. *Postural hypotension* is common and can be minimized by slow positional changes of the dental chair.[65] *Depression* is a side effect of some antihypertensive medications that many patients are unaware of. Nausea, sedation, oral dryness, lichenoid drug reactions, and gingival enlargement are associated with certain classes of antihypertensive agents.[71]

! CLINICAL CORRELATION

Hypertension, the most common cardiovascular disease, affects more than 100 million American adults, many of whom are undiagnosed. Three of every four (76%) adults with hypertension do not control their blood pressure well enough. The dental office can play a vital role in the detection of undiagnosed hypertension and the compliance of patients being treated for hypertension. Blood pressure should be taken at the initial visit and at each periodontal recall maintenance visit.

TABLE 67.2 Classes of Medication Available in the U.S. to Treat Hypertension

Medication Categories	Common Examples
Alpha-Adrenergic Blockers	Doxazosin (Cardura) Prazosin (Minipress) Terazosin (Hytrin)
Central Alpha-Adrenergic (Alpha 2) Agonists	Clonidine (Catapres) Guanfacine (Tenex) Methyldopa (Aldomet)
Direct Vasodilators	Hydralazine (Apresoline) Minoxidil (Loniten)
Peripheral Adrenergic Inhibitors	Guanadrel (Hylorel) Reserpine (Serpasil)
Beta-Adrenergic Blockers	Atenolol (Tenormin) Bisoprolol (Zebeta) Metoprolol (Toprol XL) Propranolol (Inderal) Timolol (Blocadren)
Beta-Adrenergic Blockers with Intrinsic Sympathomimetic Activity	Acebutolol (Sectral) Pindolol (Visken)
Beta-Adrenergic Blockers with Alpha-Blocking Properties	Carvedilol (Coreg) Labetalol (Normodyne, Trandate)
Beta-Adrenergic Blockers with Nitric-Oxide Mediated Vasodilating Activity	Nebivolol (Bystolic)
Calcium-Channel Blockers - Dihydropyridines	Amlodipine (Norvasc, Lotrel) Isradipine (DynaCirc) Nicardipine (Cardene SR) Nifedipine (Adalat CC, Procardia XL)
Calcium-Channel Blockers - Nondihydropyridines	Diltiazem (Cardizem CD, Cardizem SR, Dilacor XR, Tiazac) Verapamil (Calan SR, Covera HS, Isoptin SR, Verelan)
Diuretics—Thiazide/Thiazide-Like	Chlorthalidone (Hygroton, Thalitone, Chlorthalidone) Chlorothiazide (Diuril) Hydrochlorothiazide (Dyazide, Maxzide)
Diuretics—Loop	Bumetanide (Bumex) Ethacrynic acid (Edecrin) Furosemide (Lasix) Torsemide (Demadex)
Diuretics—Potassium-Sparing	Amiloride (Midamor) Triamterene (Dyrenium)
Diuretics—Aldosterone Antagonists	Eplerenone (Inspra) Spironolactone (Aldactone)
Renin-Angiotensin System Inhibitors Angiotensin-Converting Enzyme (ACE) Inhibitors	Enalapril (Vasotec) Captopril (Capoten) Fosinopril (Monopril) Lisinopril (Prinivil, Zestril)
Renin-Angiotensin System Inhibitors Angiotensin II Receptor Blockers (ARB)	Candesartan (Atacand) Irbesartan (Avapro) Losartan (Cozaar) Valsartan (Diovan)
Renin-Angiotensin System Inhibitors Direct Renin Inhibitor	Aliskiren (Tekturna)

Excerpt from American Dental Association: Oral Health Topics—Hypertension. https://www.ada.org/en/member-center/oral-health-topics/hypertension. Last updated July 29, 2020.

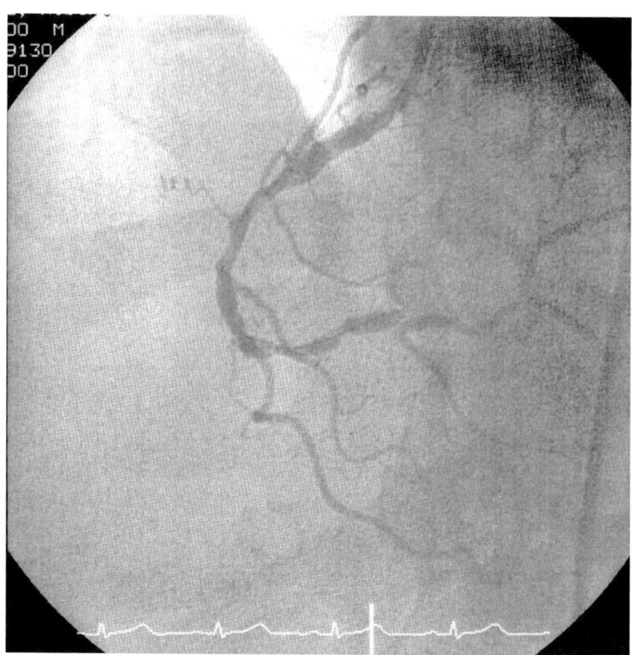

Fig. 67.1 As seen on a coronary angiogram, atherosclerosis can result in narrowing of the coronary arteries, producing signs and symptoms of ischemic heart disease.

Ischemic Heart Diseases

Ischemic heart disease (Fig. 67.1) includes disorders such as angina pectoris and MI. Angina pectoris occurs when myocardial oxygen demand exceeds supply, resulting in temporary myocardial ischemia.[46] Patients with a history of unstable angina pectoris (i.e., angina that occurs irregularly or on multiple occasions without predisposing factors) should be treated only for emergencies and then in consultation with their physician. Patients with stable angina (i.e., angina that occurs infrequently, is associated with exertion or stress, and is easily controlled with medication and rest) can undergo elective dental procedures. Because stress can induce an acute anginal attack, stress reduction is important. Profound local anesthesia is vital, and conscious sedation may be indicated for anxious patients (see Chapter 58).[117] Supplemental oxygen delivered by nasal cannula can also help prevent intraoperative anginal attacks.

Patients who manage acute anginal attacks with nitroglycerin should be instructed to bring their medication to dental appointments. Nitroglycerin should also be kept in the office medical emergency kit. For particularly stressful procedures, the patient may take a nitroglycerin tablet preoperatively to prevent angina, although this usually is not necessary. The patient's nitroglycerin should be readily accessible on the dental tray in case it is needed during treatment. Because the shelf life of nitroglycerin is relatively short, the expiration date of the patient's nitroglyce[illegible]t of the nitroglycerin in the office's medical emergency kit should be regularly checked and updated.

Patients with angina may be taking longer-acting forms of nitroglycerin (e.g., tablet, patch), β-blockers, or calcium channel blockers (also used for treating hypertension) for prevention of angina. Restrictions on the use of local anesthetics containing epinephrine are similar to those for the patient with hypertension. Intraosseous injection with epinephrine-containing local anesthetics using special systems (e.g., Stabident, Fairfax Dental) should be done cautiously in patients with ischemic heart disease because it results in transient increases in heart rate and myocardial oxygen demand.[86]

If the patient becomes fatigued or uncomfortable or has a sudden change in heart rhythm or rate during a periodontal procedure, the procedure should be discontinued as soon as possible. Box 67.1

BOX 67.1 Emergency Treatment Protocol for Patients Who Experience Angina in the Dental Chair

1. Discontinue the periodontal procedure.
2. Administer 1 tablet (0.3–0.6 mg) of nitroglycerin sublingually.
3. Reassure the patient, and loosen restrictive garments.
4. Administer oxygen with the patient in a reclined position.
5. If the signs and symptoms cease within 3 min, complete the periodontal procedure if possible, making sure that the patient is comfortable. Terminate the procedure at the earliest convenient time.
6. If the anginal signs and symptoms do not resolve with this treatment within 5 min, administer another dose of nitroglycerin, monitor the patient's vital signs, call the patient's physician, and be ready to accompany the patient to the emergency department.
7. A third nitroglycerin tablet can be given 5 min after the second. Chest pain that is not relieved by three tablets of nitroglycerin indicates likely MI. The patient should be transported to the nearest emergency medical facility immediately.

outlines the emergency medical treatment protocol for a patient who has an anginal episode in the dental chair.

Nitroglycerin lingual spray formulations have been popular in hospital pharmacies because of the increased shelf life compared with nitroglycerin tablets.[81] The lingual spray can provide greater and more rapid vasodilation with a longer duration of action.[32,93] The convenience and advantages of a nitroglycerin lingual spray are appealing, but the accuracy of dose delivery has been questioned and warrants additional studies before the spray can be recommended to replace the known tablet regimen.[81]

MI is the other category of ischemic heart disease encountered with patients in dental practice. Dental treatment is usually deferred for at least 6 months after MI because the peak mortality rate occurs during this time.[37] After 6 months, MI patients can usually be treated using techniques similar to those for stable angina patients.

Cardiac (aortocoronary) bypass, femoral artery bypass, angioplasty, arterial stent insertion, and endarterectomy have become common surgical procedures in patients with ischemic heart disease. If one of these procedures was recently performed, the physician should be consulted before elective dental therapy to determine the degree of heart damage or arterial occlusive disease, the stability of the patient's condition, and the potential for infective endocarditis or graft rejection. Prophylactic antibiotics are not usually necessary for cardiac bypass patients unless recommended by the cardiologist.

Congestive Heart Failure

CHF is a condition in which the pump function of the heart is unable to supply sufficient amounts of oxygenated blood to meet the body's needs.[37] CHF usually begins with left ventricular failure caused by a disproportion between the hemodynamic load and the capacity to handle that load. CHF can be caused by a chronic increase in workload (as in hypertension or aortic, mitral, pulmonary, or tricuspid valvular disease), direct damage to the myocardium (as in MI or rheumatic fever), or an increase in the body's oxygen requirements (as in anemia, thyrotoxicosis, or pregnancy).

Patients with poorly controlled or untreated CHF are not candidates for elective dental procedures. These individuals are at risk for sudden death, usually from ventricular arrhythmias.[36] For patients with treated CHF, the clinician should consult with the physician regarding the severity of CHF, underlying cause, and current medical management. Medical management of CHF can include the use of calcium channel blockers, direct vasodilators, diuretics, angiotensin-converting enzyme (ACE) inhibitors, α-receptor blockers, or cardiotonic agents such as digoxin.[34,53] Each medication has potential side effects that can affect periodontal therapy. Because of orthopnea (i.e., inability to breathe unless in an upright position) in some CHF patients, the dental chair should be adjusted to a comfortable level for the patient rather than placed in a supine position. Short appointments, stress reduction, profound local anesthesia, possibly conscious sedation, and use of supplemental oxygen should be considered.[37,65]

Cardiac Pacemakers and Implantable Cardioverter-Defibrillators

Cardiac arrhythmias are most often treated with medications, but some are also treated with implantable pacemakers or automatic cardioverter-defibrillators.[36,65,88] Pacemakers are usually implanted in the chest wall and enter the heart via transvenous catheter. Automatic cardioverter-defibrillators are more often implanted subcutaneously near the umbilicus and have electrodes passing into the heart via transvenous catheter or directly attached to the epicardium. Consultation with the patient's physician allows determination of the underlying cardiac status, the type of pacemaker or automatic cardioverter-defibrillator, and any precautionary measures to be taken.

Older pacemakers were unipolar and could be disrupted by dental equipment that generated electromagnetic fields, such as ultrasonic and electrocautery units. Newer units are bipolar and are usually not affected by dental equipment. Automatic cardioverter-defibrillators activate without warning when certain arrhythmias occur. This can endanger the patient during dental treatment because activation often causes sudden patient movement. Stabilization of the operating field during periodontal treatment with bite blocks or other devices can prevent trauma or injury from unexpected movements.

Infective Endocarditis

Infective endocarditis (IE) is a disease in which microorganisms colonize damaged endocardium or heart valves.[40] Although the incidence of IE is low, it is a serious disease with a poor prognosis despite modern therapy. The term *infective endocarditis* is preferred to the previous term *bacterial endocarditis* because the disease can also be caused by fungi or viruses. The organisms most often encountered in IE are α-hemolytic streptococci (e.g., *Streptococcus viridans*). However, non-streptococcal organisms, often found in the periodontal pocket, have been increasingly implicated, including *Eikenella corrodens, Aggregatibacter actinomycetemcomitans, Capnocytophaga,* and *Lactobacillus* species.[11]

IE has been divided into acute and subacute forms. The acute form involves virulent organisms, usually non-hemolytic streptococci and strains of staphylococci, which invade normal cardiac tissue, produce septic emboli, and cause infections that run a rapid, usually fatal course. The subacute form results from colony formation on damaged endocardium or heart valves by low-grade pathogenic organisms. The classic example is rheumatic carditis from rheumatic fever.

Following the earlier American Heart Association (AHA) publication on prevention of IE in 1997,[28] many questioned the efficacy of antimicrobial prophylaxis to prevent IE in patients who undergo dental or other procedures.[33,111] Members of the Rheumatic Fever, Endocarditis, and Kawasaki Disease Committee of the AHA Council on Cardiovascular Disease in the Young and a national and international group of experts on IE extensively reviewed data published on the prevention of IE. The committee concluded that only an extremely small number of IE cases might be prevented by antibiotic prophylaxis for dental procedures (even if such therapy was 100% effective). Consequently, the guidelines were changed and published in a 2007 report.[130,131] The new guidelines advise that

IE prophylaxis should be recommended only for cardiac conditions with the highest risk of adverse outcome from IE (Box 67.2). For these patients, antibiotic prophylaxis continues to be recommended for all dental procedures that involve manipulation of the gingival or periapical tissues, or perforation of the oral mucosa. Antibiotic prophylaxis is *not* indicated for individuals on the basis of an increased lifetime risk of contracting IE. A recent (2021) scientific statement from the American Heart Association, following review of currently available evidence, confirmed there are no changes to the 2007 viridans group streptococcal (VGS) IE prevention guidelines.[132]

The practice of periodontics is intimately concerned with the prevention of IE. However, bacteremia may occur even in the absence of dental procedures, especially in individuals with poor oral hygiene and significant periodontal inflammation. IE is much more likely to result from frequent exposure to random bacteremias associated with daily activities than to be caused by bacteremia associated with a dental procedure.[131] Prevention of periodontal inflammation is paramount. The AHA states that patients who are at risk for IE should "establish and maintain the best possible oral health to reduce potential sources of bacterial seeding." To provide adequate preventive measures for IE, the clinician's major concern should be to reduce the microbial biofilm in the oral cavity to minimize soft tissue inflammation and bacteremia.

BOX 67.2 Cardiac Conditions Associated With the Highest Risk of Adverse Outcome from Infective Endocarditis for Which Prophylaxis With Dental Procedures Is Recommended[a]

Previous history of infective endocarditis

Prosthetic cardiac valves or prosthetic material used for cardiac valve repair

Congenital heart disease (CHD), with the following conditions:

- Unrepaired cyanotic CHD, including palliative shunts and conduits
- Completely repaired congenital heart defect with prosthetic material or device, whether placed by surgery or catheter intervention, during the first 6 months after the procedure
- Repaired CHD with residual defects at or adjacent to the site of a prosthetic patch or prosthetic device (which inhibits endothelialization)

Cardiac transplantation recipients who develop cardiac valvulopathy.

[a]American Heart Association recommendations.[132]

From Wilson W, Taubert KA, Gewitz M, et al. Prevention of infective endocarditis: guidelines from the American Heart Association Rheumatic Fever, Endocarditis, and Kawasaki Disease Committee, Council on Cardiovascular Disease in the Young, and the Council on Clinical Cardiology, Council on Cardiovascular Surgery and Anesthesia, and the Quality of Care and Outcomes Research Interdisciplinary Working Group. *Circulation.* 2007;116:1736–1754.

KEY FACT

The updated American Heart Association (AHA) guidelines on the prevention of infective endocarditis (IE) were published in a 2007 report. The guidelines recommend that prophylaxis should be provided only for cardiac conditions with the highest risk of adverse outcomes from IE (see Box 67.2).

Preventive measures to reduce the risk of IE (for those with cardiac conditions with the highest risk of adverse outcomes) consist of the following:

1. *Define the susceptible patient.* A careful medical history can disclose a susceptible patient. Health questioning should cover the history in all categories of risk. If any doubt exists, the patient's physician should be consulted.
2. *Provide oral hygiene instruction.* Oral hygiene should be practiced with methods that improve gingival health. In patients with significant gingival inflammation, oral hygiene should initially be limited to gentle procedures (i.e., oral rinses and gentle toothbrushing with a soft brush) to minimize bleeding. As gingival health improves, more definitive oral hygiene procedures can be initiated. Oral irrigators are usually not recommended because their use can induce bacteremia.[76] Susceptible patients should be encouraged to maintain the highest level of oral hygiene to control soft tissue inflammation.
3. *Recommended antibiotic prophylactic regimens should be practiced with all high-risk patients during periodontal treatment* (Table 67.3). If any doubt regarding susceptibility exists, the patient's physician should be consulted. In patients who have been receiving continuous oral penicillin for secondary prevention of rheumatic fever, penicillin-resistant α-hemolytic streptococci are occasionally found in the oral cavity. An alternate regimen is recommended instead. If the patient is taking a

TABLE 67.3 Recommended Antibiotic Prophylaxis Regimens for Periodontal / Dental Procedures in Patients at Risk for Infective Endocarditis (Single Dose 30–60 Minutes Prior to Procedure)

Regimen	Antibiotic	Adult Dosage	Child Dosage
Standard oral regimen	Amoxicillin	2.0 g	50 mg/kg
Regimen for patients unable to take oral medications	Ampicillin or Cefazolin or ceftriaxone	2.0 g IM or IV 1.0 g IM or IV	50 mg/kg IM or IV 50 mg/kg IM or IV
Alternate regimen[a] for patients allergic to penicillin or ampicillin (oral)	Cephalexin[b] or Azithromycin or clarithromycin or Doxycycline	2.0 g 500 mg 100 mg	50 mg/kg 15 mg/kg 2.2 mg/kg (<45 kg) 100 mg (>45kg)
Regimen for patients unable to take oral medications and allergic to penicillin or ampicillin	Cefazolin or Ceftriaxone[a]	1.0 g IM or IV	

[a]Clindamycin is no longer recommended for antibiotic prophylaxis due to frequent and severe reactions compared with other antibiotics.[133]

[b]Cephalosporins should not be used in patients with immediate-type hypersensitivity reactions (e.g., urticaria, angioedema, anaphylaxis) to penicillin or ampicillin.

Table updated according to Wilson WR, Gewitz M, Lockhart PB, et al. Prevention of viridans group streptococcal infective endocarditis: a scientific statement from the American Heart Association. *Circulation.* 2021;143(20):e963-e978.[133]

systemic antibiotic, changes in the IE prophylaxis regimen may be indicated. For example, a patient taking a penicillin agent after regenerative therapy can be placed on azithromycin before the next periodontal procedure. Patients with periodontitis-grade C (aggressive periodontitis) often have high levels of *A. actinomycetemcomitans* in the subgingival plaque (biofilm). This organism has been associated with IE and is often resistant to penicillins. In patients with periodontitis grade C (aggressive periodontitis) who warrant antibiotic prophylaxis, Slots and colleagues[106] suggested using tetracycline (250 mg four times daily for 14 days) to eliminate or reduce *A. actinomycetemcomitans*, followed by the conventional prophylaxis protocol at the time of dental treatment.

4. *Periodontal treatment should be designed for susceptible patients to accommodate their degree of periodontal involvement.* The nature of periodontal therapy enhances the problems related to the prophylaxis of subacute IE. Patients are faced with long-term therapy, healing periods that extend beyond a 1-day antibiotic regimen, multiple visits, and procedures that easily elicit gingival bleeding.

The following guidelines can aid in the development of periodontal treatment plans for patients who are highly susceptible to IE:

- Periodontal disease is an infection with potentially wide-ranging systemic effects. For patients at risk for IE, every effort should be made to eliminate this infection. Teeth with severe periodontitis and a poor prognosis may require extraction. Teeth with less severe involvement in a motivated patient should be retained, treated, and monitored closely.
- All periodontal treatment procedures (including probing) require antibiotic prophylaxis; gentle oral hygiene methods are excluded. Pretreatment chlorhexidine rinses are recommended before all procedures, including periodontal probing, because these oral rinses significantly reduce the bacteria on mucosal surfaces.[28]
- To reduce the number of visits required and thereby minimize the risk of developing resistant bacteria, numerous procedures can be accomplished at each appointment, depending on the patient's needs and ability to tolerate dental treatment.[65]
- When possible, allow at least 7 days between appointments (preferably 10 to 14 days). If this is not possible, select an alternative antibiotic regimen for appointments within a 7-day period.
- Evidence does not support or refute a need to place patients at risk for IE on extended antibiotic regimens after treatment.[65] Patients who have had periodontal surgery are not usually placed on antibiotics for the first week of healing unless there are specific indications to do so. If patients are placed on these regimens, the dosages are inadequate to prevent endocarditis during ensuing appointments. The standard prophylactic antibiotic dose is still needed. For example, if a patient was placed on 250 mg of amoxicillin three times a day for 10 days after periodontal surgery and was to return to the office for more treatment on the seventh day, the patient would require a full 2.0-g dose of amoxicillin before that treatment. Alternatively, clindamycin or azithromycin could be used at the second appointment.
- Regular recall appointments, with an emphasis on oral hygiene reinforcement and maintenance of periodontal health, are extremely important for patients susceptible to IE.

There may be instances when health care providers and patients do not agree with the stated guidelines.[132] In these cases, clinicians must be familiar with and understand the guidelines in order to inform patients about risks and benefits of antibiotic prophylaxis. The decision to premedicate is made by the treating clinician in consultation with the patient's physician and based on the specific assessment and needs of the individual patient at the time.

Cerebrovascular Accident

A CVA or stroke is caused by ischemic changes such as a cerebral thrombosis from an embolus, or a hemorrhagic phenomenon. Hypertension and atherosclerosis are predisposing factors for CVA and should alert the clinician to evaluate the patient's medical history carefully for the possibility of early cerebrovascular insufficiency and to be aware of symptoms of the disease. A physician's referral should precede periodontal therapy if the signs and symptoms of early cerebrovascular insufficiency are evident.

To prevent a repeat stroke, active infections should be treated aggressively, because even a minor infection can alter blood coagulation and trigger thrombus formation and ensuing cerebral infarction. The clinician should counsel the patient about maintaining periodontal health and the importance of thorough oral hygiene (biofilm control).[90] Post-stroke weakness of the facial area or paralysis of extremities can make oral hygiene procedures extremely difficult.[75] The clinician may need to modify oral hygiene instruments for ease of use, perhaps in consultation with an occupational therapist. Long-term chlorhexidine rinses greatly aid in biofilm control.

Dental clinicians should treat post-CVA patients with the following guidelines:

1. No periodontal therapy (except for an emergency) should be performed for 6 months after CVA because of the high risk of recurrence during this period.
2. After 6 months, periodontal therapy can be performed during short appointments with an emphasis on minimizing stress. Profound local anesthesia should be obtained, using the minimal effective dose of local anesthetic agents. Concentrations of epinephrine greater than 1:100,000 are contraindicated.
3. Light conscious sedation (i.e., inhalation, oral, or parenteral) can be used for anxious patients. Supplemental oxygen is indicated to maintain thorough cerebral oxygenation.
4. Stroke patients are frequently placed on oral anticoagulants. Previously, it was thought that for procedures entailing significant bleeding, such as periodontal surgery or tooth extraction, the anticoagulant regimen might need adjustment to lower the risk of bleeding. However, evidence regarding the risks of altering anticoagulation therapy suggests that it is safer and more prudent to provide treatment without changing it (see Antiplatelet and Anticoagulant Therapies under Medications below). Any changes in anticoagulant therapy regimens for a stroke patient should only be done in consultation with the patient's physician.
5. Blood pressure should be monitored regularly. Recurrence rates for CVAs are high, as are the rates of associated functional deficits.
6. Dental clinicians are advised to locate and access the nearest stroke center that can screen patients for embolic versus hemorrhagic diagnosis. If screened early and diagnosed with a thromboembolic stroke, treatment with tissue plasminogen activator (TPA) within three hours can be lifesaving and decrease morbidity.

Endocrine Disorders

The endocrine system is comprised of a network of glands that produce and release hormones that regulate and control numerous physiologic functions from energy storage and consumption to tissue repair and maintenance and controlling responses. Alterations or disruptions in the normal functioning of the endocrine system can lead to various diseases and disorders including diabetes mellitus, thyroid or parathyroid disorders, and adrenal insufficiency.

Diabetes

The patient with diabetes requires special precautions before periodontal therapy. Type 1 diabetes was formerly known as insulin-dependent diabetes, and type 2 diabetes was referred to as non–insulin-dependent diabetes.[69] During the past decade, the medical management of diabetes has changed significantly in an effort to minimize the debilitating complications associated with this disease.[1,114]

Blood glucose (i.e., glycemia) levels are more tightly managed through diet, oral agents, and insulin therapy.[66]

If the clinician detects intraoral signs of undiagnosed or poorly controlled diabetes, a thorough history is indicated.[85] The classic signs of diabetes include polydipsia (i.e., excessive thirst), polyuria (i.e., excessive urination), and polyphagia (i.e., excessive hunger, often with unexplained concurrent weight loss). If the patient has any of these signs or symptoms or the clinician suspects diabetes, further investigation with laboratory studies and physician consultation is indicated. Periodontal therapy has limited success in the setting of undiagnosed or poorly controlled diabetes.

If a patient is suspected of having undiagnosed diabetes, the following procedures should be performed:

1. Consult the patient's physician.
2. Analyze laboratory tests (Box 67.3), including fasting blood glucose and casual glucose test results.[6]
3. Rule out acute orofacial infection or severe dental infection; if present, provide emergency care immediately.
4. Establish the best possible oral health through nonsurgical debridement of plaque (biofilm) and calculus. Institute oral hygiene instruction. Limit more advanced care until the diagnosis has been established and good glycemic control obtained.

If a patient is known to have diabetes, it is critical that the level of glycemic control be established before initiating periodontal treatment. The fasting glucose and casual glucose tests provide snapshots of the blood glucose concentration at the time the blood was drawn; these tests reveal nothing about long-term glycemic control. The primary test used to assess glycemic control is the glycated hemoglobin (Hb) assay, also called the HbA1c test (Box 67.4). This assay has been shown by a large international study to provide an accurate measure of the average blood glucose concentrations over the preceding 2 to 3 months.[73] Fig. 67.2 is a simplified graphic representation of the data from that study depicting the average blood glucose concentrations for HbA1c values.

The therapeutic goal for many patients with diabetes is to achieve and maintain an HbA1c below 7%. Patients with well-controlled diabetes (HbA1c < 7%) usually respond to therapy in a manner similar to nondiabetic individuals.[23,113,128] Poorly controlled patients often have a poor response to treatment, with more postoperative complications and less favorable long-term results (see Fig. 25.3 in Chapter 25).[69,113] Improvements in HBA1c values after periodontal therapy may provide an indication of the potential response.

BOX 67.3 Diagnostic Criteria for Diabetes Mellitus

Diabetes mellitus can be diagnosed by any one of the following laboratory methods. Initial results using any method must be confirmed on a subsequent day.

1. Fasting plasma glucose level ≥126 mg/dL (≥7.0 mmol/L). *Fasting* is defined as no caloric intake for at least 8 h. The normal fasting glucose level is 70–100 mg/dL.
2. Two-hour postprandial glucose level ≥200 mg/dL (≥11.1 mmol/L) during an oral glucose tolerance test. The test should be performed using a glucose load containing the equivalent of 75 g anhydrous glucose dissolved in water. The normal 2-hour postprandial glucose level is <140 mg/dL.
3. Glycated hemoglobin (HbA1c) value ≥6.5% (≥48 mmol/L). The test should be performed in a laboratory using a method that is certified by the National Glycohemoglobin Standardization Program (NGSP) and standardized according to the Diabetes Control and Complications Trial (DCCT) assay.[a]
4. Random plasma glucose level ≥200 mg/dL (≥11.1 mmol/L) for a patient with classic symptoms of hyperglycemia or hyperglycemic crisis, which include polyuria, polydipsia, and unexplained weight loss. Blood for casual glucose testing can be drawn without regard to the time since the last meal.

[a] In the absence of unequivocal hyperglycemia, results should be confirmed by repeat testing.
Data from American Diabetes Association. Classification and diagnosis of diabetes. *Diabetes Care.* 2021;44(suppl. 1):S15–S33.

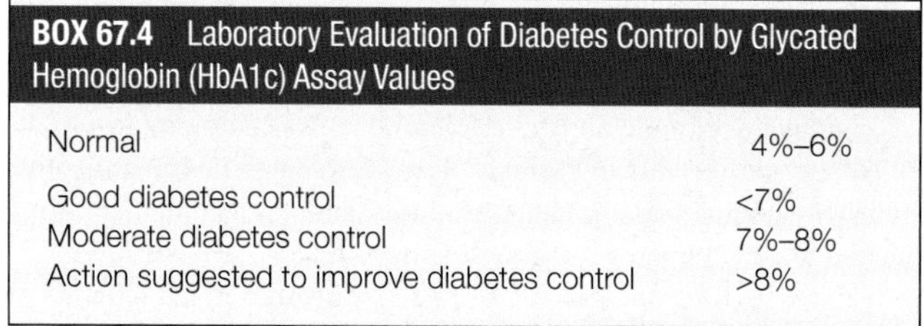

BOX 67.4 Laboratory Evaluation of Diabetes Control by Glycated Hemoglobin (HbA1c) Assay Values

Normal	4%–6%
Good diabetes control	<7%
Moderate diabetes control	7%–8%
Action suggested to improve diabetes control	>8%

Data from American Diabetes Association. Classification and diagnosis of diabetes. *Diabetes Care.* 2021;44(suppl. 1):S15–S33.

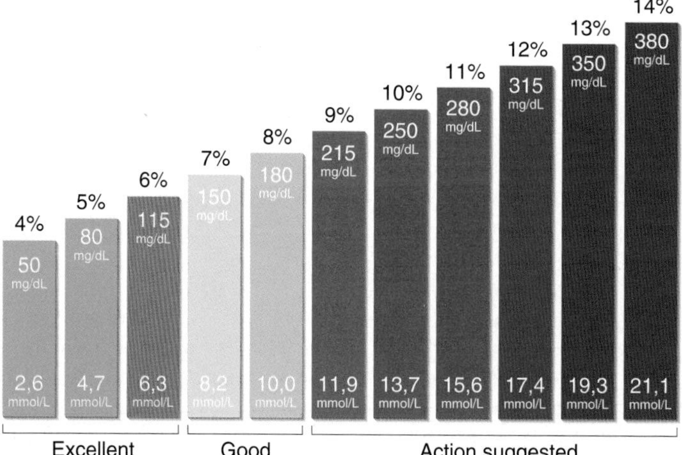

Fig. 67.2 Graphic representation of glycated hemoglobin (HbA1c) values that correspond to estimated average blood glucose levels.

As discussed in Chapters 25 and 26, periodontal infection can worsen glycemic control and should be managed aggressively. Patients with diabetes and periodontitis should receive oral hygiene instructions, mechanical debridement to remove local factors, and regular maintenance. Periodontally hopeless teeth should also be extracted. When possible, HbA1c of less than 8% should be established before elective surgical treatment is performed. Systemic antibiotics are not needed routinely, although evidence indicates that tetracycline antibiotics in combination with scaling and root planing (root debridement) may positively influence glycemic control. If the patient has poor glycemic control and surgery is absolutely needed, prophylactic antibiotics can be given; penicillins are most often used for this purpose. Frequent reevaluation after active therapy is needed to assess treatment response and prevent recurrence of periodontitis.

Almost all patients with diabetes use a glucometer for blood glucose self-monitoring. These devices use capillary blood from a fingerstick to provide blood glucose readings in seconds. Patients with diabetes should be asked whether they have a glucometer and how often they use it. Because these devices provide instantaneous assessment of blood glucose, they are highly beneficial in the dental office environment. The following guidelines should be observed:

1. Patients should be asked to bring their glucometer to the dental office at each appointment.
2. Patients should check their blood glucose before any long procedure to obtain a baseline level. Patients with a blood glucose level at or below the lower end of normal before the procedure may become hypoglycemic intraoperatively. It is advisable to have the patient consume some carbohydrate before starting treatment. For example, if a 2-hour procedure is planned and the pretreatment glucose level is 70 mg/dL (i.e., lower end of normal range), providing 4 ounces of juice preoperatively may help prevent hypoglycemia during treatment. If the pretreatment glucose level is excessively high, the clinician should determine whether the patient's glycemic control has been poor recently. This can be done with thorough patient questioning and by determining the most recent HbA1c values. If glycemic control has been poor over the preceding few months, the procedure may need to be postponed until better glycemic control is established. If glycemic control has been good and the current high glucometer reading is a fairly isolated event, the surgical procedure may proceed.

BOX 67.5 Signs and Symptoms of Hypoglycemia

Shakiness or tremors
Confusion
Agitation and anxiety
Sweating
Tachycardia
Dizziness
Feeling of impending doom
Unconsciousness
Seizures

3. If the procedure lasts several hours, it is often beneficial to check the glucose level during the procedure to ensure that the patient does not become hypoglycemic.
4. After the procedure, the blood glucose can be checked again to assess fluctuations over time.
5. Any time the patient feels the symptoms of hypoglycemia, the blood glucose level should be checked immediately. This may prevent the onset of severe hypoglycemia, a medical emergency.

The most common dental office complication seen in patients with diabetes taking insulin is a symptomatic low blood glucose level (i.e., hypoglycemia) (Box 67.5). Hypoglycemia is also associated with the use of numerous oral agents (Table 67.4). In patients receiving conscious sedation, the warning signs of an impending hypoglycemic episode can be masked, making the patient's glucometer one of the best diagnostic aids. Hypoglycemia does not usually occur until the blood glucose level falls below 60 mg/dL. However, in patients with poor glycemic control who have prolonged hyperglycemia (i.e., high blood glucose levels), a rapid drop in glucose can precipitate signs and symptoms of hypoglycemia at levels well above 60 mg/dL.

As medical management of diabetes has intensified, the incidence of severe hypoglycemia has risen.[115] The clinician should question patients about past episodes of hypoglycemia. Hypoglycemia is more common in patients with better glycemic control. When planning dental treatment, it is best to schedule appointments before or after periods of peak insulin activity. This requires knowledge of the pharmacodynamics of the drugs. Patients taking insulin are at greatest risk, followed by those taking sulfonylurea agents. Oral agents such as metformin, thiazolidinediones, α-glucosidase inhibitors, dipeptidyl peptidase 4 (DPP-4) inhibitors, and sodium-glucose cotransporter-2 (SGLT-2) inhibitors usually do not cause hypoglycemia (see Table 67.4). Likewise, injectable agents known as incretin mimetics (exenatide; liraglutide; albiglutide) generally do not cause hypoglycemia.

Insulins are classified as rapid-acting, short-acting, intermediate-acting, or long-acting agents (Table 67.5). The categories vary in onset, peak, and duration of activity. It is important that the clinician establish exactly which insulin the patient takes, the amount, the number of times per day, and the time of the last dose. Periodontal treatment often can be timed to avoid peak insulin activity. Many patients with diabetes take multiple injections each day, in which case it is difficult, if not impossible, to avoid peak insulin activity. Checking the pretreatment glucose with the patient's glucometer, checking again during a long procedure, and checking again at the end of the procedure provides a better understanding of the patient's insulin pharmacodynamics and can help prevent hypoglycemia.

If hypoglycemia occurs during dental treatment, therapy should be immediately terminated. If a glucometer is available, the blood glucose level should be checked. Treatment guidelines include the following[66]:

1. Provide approximately 15 g of oral carbohydrate to the patient
   - 4 to 6 ounces of juice or soda
   - 3 or 4 teaspoons of table sugar
   - Hard candy with 15 g of sugar
2. If the patient is unable to take food or drink by mouth or if the patient is sedated
   - Give 25 to 30 mL of 50% dextrose intravenously, which provides 12.5 to 15.0 g of dextrose, or
   - Give 1 mg of glucagon intravenously (i.e., glucagon results in rapid release of stored glucose from the liver), or
   - Give 1 mg of glucagon intramuscularly or subcutaneously (if no intravenous access).

Emergencies resulting from hyperglycemia are rare in the dental office. They usually take days to weeks to develop. However, the glucometer may be used to rule out hyperglycemic emergencies such as diabetic ketoacidosis, a life-threatening event.

KEY FACT

The most common dental office complication seen in patients with diabetes who take insulin is a symptomatic low blood glucose level, or hypoglycemia. It does not usually occur until blood glucose level falls below 60 mg/dL. However, in patients with poor glycemic control who have prolonged hyperglycemia, a rapid drop in glucose can precipitate signs and symptoms of hypoglycemia at higher blood glucose levels. Clinicians must recognize the signs of hypoglycemia and be prepared to manage it. Hypoglycemia is more common in individuals with well-controlled glucose levels.

TABLE 67.4 Oral Agents Used for the Management of Diabetes

Agent	Action	Risk of Hypoglycemia[a]
Sulfonylureas (1st gen): Chlorpropae Tolbutamide Tolazamide	Stimulate pancreatic insulin secretion	++
Sulfonylureas (2nd gen): Glyburide Glipizide	Stimulate pancreatic insulin secretion	+++
Sulfonylureas (3rd gen): Glimepiride	Stimulate pancreatic insulin secretion	+
Meglitinides: Repaglinide Nateglinide	Stimulate rapid pancreatic insulin secretion (different mechanism from sulfonylureas)	+
Biguanides: Metformin	Block production of glucose by liver; improve tissue sensitivity to insulin	–
Thiazolidinedio: Rosiglitazone Pioglitazone	Improve tissue sensitivity to insulin	–
α-Glucosidase inhibitors: Acarbose Miglitol	Slow absorption of some carbohydrates from gut, decreasing postprandial peaks in glycemia	–
Dipeptidyl peptidase-4 (DPP-4) inhibitors: Sitagliptin Saxagliptin Alogliptin Linagliptin	Inhibit the enzyme DPP-4; enable the pancreas to produce more insulin but only after food ingestion	–
Sodium-glucose co-transporter 2 (SGLT-2) inhibitors: Canagliflozin Dapagliflozin Empagliflozin	Inhibit reabsorption of glucose in the kidney	–
Combination agents	Combine two different oral agents into single drug	Risk depends on which drugs are combined

[a]Hypoglycemia risk: +++, high; ++, moderate; +, low; –, none.

TABLE 67.5 Types of Insulin

Type	Classification	ACTIVITY		
		Onset	Peak	Duration
Lispro (Humalog), aspart (Novolog), glulisine (Apidra)	Rapid-acting	15 min	30–90 min	<5 h
Regular R or Novolin R, Velosulin (used in insulin pump)	Short-acting	30–60 min	2–3 h 1–2 h	3–6 h 2–3 h
NPH (N), Humulin N, Novolin N	Intermediate-acting	2–4 h	4–12 h	14–18 h
Insulin detemir (Levemir)	Long-acting	1–2 h	Relatively flat (fairly even over 24 h)	Up to 24 h
Glargine (Lantus, Basaglar); Glargine U-300 (Toujeo)	Long-acting	6–8 h	There is no peak	20–24+ h
Degludec (Tresiba U-100 or U-200)	Long-acting	4-6 h	There is no peak	24 h

Because periodontal therapy can render the patient unable to eat for some time, adjustment in insulin or oral agent dosages may be required. It is critical that patients eat a normal meal before dental treatment. Taking insulin without eating is the primary cause of hypoglycemia. If the patient is restricted from eating before treatment (e.g., for conscious sedation), normal insulin doses need to be reduced. As a general guideline, *well-controlled patients with diabetes undergoing routine periodontal treatment may take their normal insulin doses as long as they also eat their normal meal.* If the procedure is going to be particularly long, the insulin dose before treatment may need to be reduced. Likewise, if the patient will have dietary restrictions after treatment, insulin or sulfonylurea dosages may need to be reduced.

Consultation with the patient's physician is prudent and allows both practitioners to review the proposed treatment plan and determine whether modifications are needed. When periodontal surgery is indicated, it is usually best to limit the size of the surgical field so that the patient will be comfortable enough to resume a normal diet immediately.

Hemorrhagic Disorders

Patients with a history of bleeding problems caused by disease or drugs should be managed to minimize the risks of hemorrhage. Identification of these patients through the health history, clinical examination, and clinical laboratory tests is paramount. Health questioning should cover (1) the history of bleeding after previous surgery or trauma, (2) past and current drug history, (3) history of bleeding problems among relatives, and (4) illnesses associated with potential bleeding problems.

Clinical examination can detect jaundice, ecchymosis, spider telangiectasia, hemarthrosis, petechiae, hemorrhagic vesicles, spontaneous gingival bleeding, and gingival enlargement. Laboratory tests include methods to measure the hemostatic, coagulation, or lytic phase of the clotting mechanism, depending on clues regarding which phase is involved (Table 67.6). These tests include bleeding time, tourniquet test, complete blood cell count, prothrombin time (PT), partial thromboplastin time (PTT), and coagulation time. Bleeding disorders are classified as coagulation disorders, thrombocytopenic purpuras, or nonthrombocytopenic purpuras.

Coagulation Disorders

The main inherited coagulation disorders include hemophilia A, hemophilia B, and von Willebrand disease (Table 67.7).[85,95] *Hemophilia A* results in a deficiency of coagulation factor VIII, and the clinical severity of the disorder depends on the level of factor VIII remaining.[77] Patients with severe hemophilia who have less than 1% of normal factor VIII levels can have severe bleeding on the slightest provocation, whereas those with more moderate hemophilia (i.e., 1% to 5% of factor VIII) have less frequent spontaneous hemorrhage but still bleed with minimal trauma.[65] Patients with mild hemophilia (i.e., 6% to 30% of factor VIII) rarely bleed spontaneously but may still hemorrhage after severe trauma or during surgical procedures.

The clinician should consult the patient's physician before dental treatment to determine the risk of bleeding and treatment modifications required. To prevent surgical hemorrhage, a factor VIII level of at least 30% is needed.[65,77] Parenteral 1-deamino-8-D-arginine vasopressin (DDAVP; desmopressin) can be used to raise factor VIII levels twofold to threefold in patients with mild or moderate hemophilia. DDAVP has the significant advantage of avoiding the risk of viral disease transmission from factor VIII infusion and is considered the drug of choice in responsive patients. Most patients with moderate or severe hemophilia require infusion of factor VIII concentrate before surgical procedures. Before 15, the risk of viral disease transmission from these infusions was high. Since then, virally safe, highly purified monoclonal antibody or recombinant deoxyribonucleic acid (DNA) factor VIII products have come into widespread use.

Hemophilia B (i.e., Christmas disease) results in a deficiency of factor IX. The severity of the disorder depends on the relative amount of existing factor IX. Surgical therapy requires a factor IX level of 30% to 50%, which is usually achieved by administration of purified prothrombin complex concentrate or factor IX concentrate.[77]

Von Willebrand disease results from a deficiency of von Willebrand factor, which mediates adhesion of platelets to the injured vessel walls and is required for primary hemostasis. Von Willebrand factor also carries the coagulant portion of factor VIII in the plasma. The disorder has three major subtypes, with a wide range of clinical severity. Many cases of von Willebrand disease go undiagnosed, and bleeding during dental treatment may be the first sign of the underlying disease. More severe forms require preoperative factor VIII concentrate or cryoprecipitate infusion. Patients with milder forms respond favorably to administration of DDAVP before periodontal surgery or tooth extraction.[77,78]

Periodontal treatment can be performed in patients with these coagulation disorders, provided that sufficient precautions are taken. Probing, scaling, and prophylaxis can usually be done without medical modification. More invasive treatment, such as local block anesthesia, root planing (root debridement), or surgery, dictates prior physician consultation.

During treatment, local measures to ensure clot formation and stability are of major importance. Complete wound closure and application of pressure can reduce hemorrhage. Antihemostatic agents, such as oxidized cellulose or purified bovine collagen, can be placed over surgical sites or into extraction sockets. The antifibrinolytic agent *ε-aminocaproic acid* (Amicar), given orally or intravenously, is a potent inhibitor of initial clot dissolution.[50] *Tranexamic acid* is a more potent antifibrinolytic agent than Amicar and can prevent excessive oral hemorrhage after periodontal surgery and tooth extraction.[84] It is available as an oral rinse and may be used alone or in combination with systemic tranexamic acid for several days after surgery.[104]

Not all coagulation disorders are hereditary. Liver disease affects all phases of blood clotting because most coagulation factors are synthesized and removed by the liver. Long-term alcohol abusers or chronic hepatitis patients often demonstrate inadequate coagulation. Coagulation can be impaired by vitamin K deficiency, often caused by malabsorption syndromes, or by prolonged antibiotic administration, which alters the intestinal microflora that produces vitamin K. Dental treatment planning for patients with liver disease should include the following:

1. Physician consultation
2. Laboratory evaluations: PT, bleeding time, platelet count, and PTT (for patients in later stages of liver disease)
3. Conservative, nonsurgical periodontal therapy whenever possible
4. When surgery is required (may require hospitalization)
    - International normalized ratio (INR; PT) in the range of 2.0 to 3.0 is manageable.
    - Platelet count should be more than 80,000/mm^3.

KEY FACT

Periodontal treatment can be performed in patients with coagulation disorders, provided that sufficient precautions are taken. Probing, scaling, and prophylaxis usually can be done without medical modification. However, more invasive treatment, such as local block anesthesia, root planing, or surgery, should be considered only after consultation with their physician.

Leukemia

Altered periodontal treatment for patients with leukemia is based on their enhanced susceptibility to infections, bleeding tendency, and effects of chemotherapy.[65] The treatment plan for leukemia patients is as follows:

1. Refer the patient for medical evaluation and treatment. Close coordination with the physician is required.
2. Before chemotherapy, a complete periodontal treatment plan should be developed with a physician.
    - Monitor hematologic laboratory values daily: bleeding time, coagulation time, PT, and platelet count.

TABLE 67.6 Laboratory Tests for Bleeding Disorders

HEMOSTATIC TESTS			
Vascular	**Platelet**	**Coagulation**	**Lysis**
1. Tourniquet test *N:* 10 petechiae *Abn:* >10 petechiae	1. Platelet count *N:* 150,000–300,000/mm^3 *Abn:* Thrombocytopenia occurs at <100,000/mm^3; clinical bleeding occurs at <80,000/mm^3; spontaneous bleeding occurs at <20,000/mm^3	1. PT measures extrinsic and common pathways: factors I, II, V, VII, and X. *N:* 11–14 s (depending on laboratory) measured against control PT reported as international normalized ratio (INR): *N:* INR = 1.0 *Abn:* INR > 1.5	1. Euglobulin clot lysis time *N:* <90 min *Abn:* >90 min
2. Bleeding time *N:* 1–6 min *Abn:* >6 min	2. Bleeding time 3. Clot retraction 4. Complete blood cell count	2. PTT measures intrinsic and common pathways: factors III, IX, XI, and low levels of factors I, II, V, X, and XII. *N:* 25–40 s (depending on laboratory) measured against control *Abn:* >1.5 times normal 3. Clotting (coagulation) time *N:* 30–40 min *Abn:* >1 h	
Clinical Disease Associations			
Vascular (capillary) wall defect	Thrombocytopenia		Increase in fibrinolytic activity
Rule out:	*Rule out:*	*All three tests:*	
Thrombocytopenia Purpuras Telangiectasia Aspirin or NSAID therapy Leukemia Renal dialysis	Vascular wall defect Acute or chronic leukemia Aplastic anemia Liver disease Renal dialysis	Liver disease Warfarin therapy Aspirin or NSAID therapy Malabsorption syndrome or long-term antibiotic therapy (lack of vitamin K metabolism) PT: factor VII deficiency PTT: hemophilia Renal dialysis	

Abn, Abnormal; *N,* normal; *NSAID,* nonsteroidal antiinflammatory drug; *PT,* prothrombin time; *PTT,* partial thromboplastin time.

TABLE 67.7 Inherited Coagulation Disorders

Type	Prolonged	Normal	Treatment
Hemophilia A	PTT	PT Bleeding time	DDAVP factor VIII concentrate or cryoprecipitate Fresh frozen plasma Fresh whole blood ε-Aminocaproic acid (Amicar) Tranexamic acid
Hemophilia B	PTT	PT Bleeding time	Purified prothrombin complex concentrate Factor IX concentrates Fresh-frozen plasma
Von Willebrand disease	Bleeding time PTT Variable factor VIII deficiency	PT Platelet count	DDAVP factor VIII concentrate or cryoprecipitate

DDAVP, 1-Deamino-8-D-arginine vasopressin (desmopressin); *PT,* prothrombin time; *PTT,* partial thromboplastin time.

- Administer antibiotic coverage before periodontal treatment because infection is a major concern.
- If systemic conditions allow, extract all hopeless, nonmaintainable, or potentially infectious teeth at least 10 days before the initiation of chemotherapy.
- Root debridement (i.e., scaling and root planing) should be performed and thorough oral hygiene instructions given if the patient's condition allows.
- Twice-daily rinsing with 0.12% chlorhexidine gluconate is recommended after oral hygiene procedures.
- Recognize the potential for bleeding caused by thrombocytopenia. Use pressure and topical hemostatic agents as indicated.

3. During the acute phases of leukemia, patients should receive only emergency periodontal care. Any source of potential infection must be eliminated to prevent systemic dissemination. Antibiotic therapy is frequently the treatment of choice, combined with nonsurgical or surgical debridement as indicated.
4. Oral ulcerations and mucositis are treated palliatively with agents such as viscous lidocaine. Systemic antibiotics may be indicated to prevent secondary infection.
5. Oral candidiasis is common in patients with leukemia and can be treated with nystatin suspension (400,000 to 600,000 U/mL four times daily) or clotrimazole vaginal suppositories (10 mg four or five times daily).[67]

6. For patients with chronic leukemia and those in remission, scaling and root planing (root debridement) can be performed without complication, but periodontal surgery should be avoided if possible. Platelet count and bleeding time should be measured on the day of the procedure. If either is low, postpone the appointment and refer the patient to a physician.

Agranulocytosis

Patients with agranulocytosis (i.e., cyclic neutropenia and granulocytopenia) have an increased susceptibility to infection. The total white blood cell count is reduced, and granular leukocytes (i.e., neutrophils, eosinophils, and basophils) are reduced in number or disappear. These disorders are often marked by early, severe periodontal destruction.[126] When possible, periodontal treatment should be done during periods of disease remission. At such times, treatment should be as conservative as possible while reducing potential sources of systemic infection. After physician consultation, severely affected teeth should be extracted. Oral hygiene instruction should include chlorhexidine rinses twice daily. Scaling and root planing (root debridement) should be performed carefully under antibiotic protection.

Medications

Some medications that are prescribed to cure, manage, or prevent diseases may have effects on periodontal tissues, wound healing, or the host immune response that need to be recognized, considered, and possibly modified for treatment. The following medication categories are briefly addressed: bisphosphonates and antiresorptive agents, antiplatelet and anticoagulation therapies, and corticosteroids. Additional information and advice can be found in other sources.

Bisphosphonates and Antiresorptive Agents

Bisphosphonate medications are used to treat metastatic cancer or multiple myeloma via intravenous (IV) administration. They are commonly used to treat osteoporosis via oral and IV administration, albeit with less frequency and lower doses. They act by inhibiting osteoclastic activity, which leads to less bone resorption, remodeling, and turnover.[91] Bisphosphonates are used in cancer treatment to prevent the often-lethal imbalance of osteoclastic activity. In the treatment of osteoporosis, the goal is to harness osteoclastic activity to minimize or prevent bone loss. The major difference between these applications is the potency and route of administration. Potency is influenced by the chemical properties and pharmacokinetics of these agents in bone. Chapter 25 describes the chemical structure, activity, and role of bisphosphonates in the development of bisphosphonate-related osteonecrosis of the jaw (BRONJ). Other non-bisphosphonate antiresorptive agents such as denosumab are also associated with osteonecrosis of the jaw.[74]

Denosumab (Prolia, Xgeva) is an antiresorptive agent used to treat osteoporosis. It is a fully human monoclonal antibody that binds the cytokine RANKL (receptor activator of NFκβ ligand), which is an essential factor that initiates bone turnover. RANKL blocks osteoclast maturation and activity-reducing bone resorption. Thus, denosumab reduces bone resorption.

Although other terms have been suggested and used, the term antiresorptive agent-induced osteonecrosis of the jaw (ARONJ) is currently adopted and is now used to describe the non-healing exposure of bone induced by bisphosphonates or other antiresorptive agents.

KEY FACT

Denosumab (Prolia, Xgeva), a non-bisphosphonate antiresorptive medication used to treat osteoporosis, has also been implicated in osteonecrosis of the jaw.

Romosozumab (Evenity) is an antiresorptive agent used to treat osteoporosis. It is a humanized monoclonal antibody that targets sclerostin, an osteocyte-derived glycoprotein that inhibits the Wnt signaling cascade and activation of osteoblast function, leading to inhibition of bone formation. Thus, romosozumab increases bone formation and reduces bone resorption. Initial animal studies suggest that the osteoporosis dose of romosozumab inhibits bone resorption without inducing ONJ-like lesions.[44]

Clinically, ARONJ manifests as exposed alveolar bone occurring spontaneously or after a dental procedure (see Figs. 25.20 and 25.21 in Chapter 25). Individuals treated with high-potency, nitrogen-containing bisphosphonates, especially those administered intravenously for cancer treatment (e.g., zoledronate), appear to be at greater risk for ARONJ than individuals taking oral bisphosphonates or other antiresorptive agents for prevention and treatment of osteoporosis. In patients treated for cancer, the incidence ranges from 1% to 15%.[52] Estimating the incidence for patients taking oral bisphosphonates for osteoporosis is more difficult but appears to range from 0.001% to 0.01%.[52] Other reports suggest a slightly higher incidence that ranges from 0.004% to 0.11%.[110] Even if this is an underestimation of the actual risk for individuals taking oral bisphosphonates, the incidence appears to be low. The risk for individuals treated with oral bisphosphonates for a period of less than 3 years appears to be minimal or very near zero.[62] Regular use of oral bisphosphonates for a period greater than 3 years suggests a risk profile that increases with time and length of use.[62]

As with many multifactorial diseases and conditions, it is likely that factors in addition to bisphosphonate therapy contribute to the individual risk of ARONJ. Potential comorbidity risk factors include systemic corticosteroid therapy, smoking, alcohol, poor oral hygiene, periodontal disease, chemotherapy, radiotherapy, diabetes, hematologic disease, and the concomitant use of antiresorptive agents with agents that inhibit angiogenesis.[74] Reported treatment-related factors for ARONJ include extractions, root canal treatment, periodontal surgery, and dental implant surgery.[64,74] Periodontal disease and treatment (especially surgery) poses a risk for patients treated with bisphosphonates or other antiresorptive medications. The bacteria-induced inflammatory process of periodontitis that causes bone resorption can lead to bone necrosis. Likewise, periodontal treatment can cause bone necrosis in the setting of bisphosphonates. Caution is warranted for all patients treated with bisphosphonates or other antiresorptive agents.

Health care providers need to evaluate patients carefully, communicate with other medical health care providers, inform patients, and consider treatment options and risks carefully. A careful intraoral examination is prudent for all patients treated with intravenous or oral bisphosphonate therapy (or other antiresorptive agents) to determine whether bone exposure exists and to assess local conditions that may predispose them to ARONJ. A thorough medical history should be reviewed, evaluated, and annotated with details about bisphosphonate or other antiresorptive agent, including medication type, dose, route of administration, and duration. Comorbidities, such as previous and current medications, treatments, and existing disease or pathology, should be considered as well. Radiographs should be carefully evaluated for signs of ARONJ.

Optimal periodontal and oral health should be achieved and maintained for all patients. A thorough inspection of all intraoral tissues should be completed at each periodontal recall maintenance visit. For individuals treated with intravenous bisphosphonates, invasive surgical treatment should be avoided. Risks must be considered before treatment of individuals with a history of taking oral bisphosphonates or antiresorptive agents for longer than 3 years. This area of research will continue to evolve as the pathophysiology becomes better understood. Providers are encouraged to consult other sources for updates on this important topic.

KEY FACT

One or more comorbidity factors along with treatment for osteoporosis with a bisphosphonate medication or other antiresorptive agent contribute to the individual risk of antiresorptive agent-induced osteonecrosis of the jaw (ARONJ). Potential comorbidity risk factors include systemic corticosteroid therapy, smoking, alcohol, poor oral hygiene, periodontal disease, chemotherapy, radiotherapy, diabetes, hematologic disease, and the concomitant use of antiresorptive agents with agents that inhibit angiogenesis.

Antiplatelet and Anticoagulant Therapies

Many patients with a variety of conditions are placed on antiplatelet or anticoagulant medications to prevent thrombosis (i.e., blood clotting) or thromboembolism (Table 67.8). Some patients are treated with a combination of these medications. Patients at risk who may be on antiplatelet or anticoagulant therapy include those with heart valve replacements, heart rhythm disorders, congenital heart defects, or those with a history or risk of myocardial infarction, stroke, or deep vein thrombosis. These patients are frequently placed on oral anticoagulants such as the vitamin K antagonists (VKAs) using coumarin derivatives such as dicumarol and warfarin.[47,61] Over the past decade, there has been increased use of a new class of novel oral anticoagulants (NOACs) or direct oral anticoagulants (DOACs) that have some advantages over VKAs. While antiplatelet and anticoagulant therapies are effective in reducing the risk of thrombosis, they may increase the risk for bleeding complications in patients undergoing surgical procedures.

The traditional approach to managing surgery for patients on antiplatelet or anticoagulant therapy *was* to discontinue therapy about 3 to 5 days (antiplatelet therapy) or 7 to 10 days (anticoagulant therapy) before a planned surgical procedure, in consultation with the patient's physician. However, evidence regarding the care of patients on antiplatelet or anticoagulant therapy suggest that treating them (e.g., with periodontal surgery or extractions) without altering their antiplatelet or anticoagulant medications may be safer and does not lead to greater intraoperative or postoperative bleeding complications.[58] The increased risk of morbidity and mortality for those discontinuing the antiplatelet or anticoagulant therapy may be significant.

Antiplatelet Medications

Many patients are taking oral antiplatelet medications to prevent vascular thrombosis. Aspirin is the most common of these and well known for its antiplatelet activity. It interferes with normal platelet aggregation by irreversibly acetylating cyclooxygenase-1, which inhibits thromboxane-A2 production and reduces platelet aggregation. The effects of aspirin last at least 4 to 7 days. The normal half-life for platelets is 7 to 10 days. Aspirin is typically used in small doses ≤ 325 mg per day, which can increase bleeding time.

Controlled clinical studies have demonstrated that intraoperative bleeding is not likely to be a problem with simple extractions or periodontal surgery if low-dose aspirin antiplatelet therapy is continued.[8,59] In these studies, there were no episodes of uncontrolled bleeding, all bleeding was controlled with local measures, and there were no cases of postoperative bleeding problems.[58] Conversely, the risk of stopping antiplatelet therapy may be serious.

Recent evidence suggests that discontinuing antiplatelet therapy may pose a risk of thrombus formation. In a meta-analysis of 474 studies including 49,590 patients evaluating the thromboembolic risk of discontinuing low-dose aspirin compared to the hemorrhagic risks of continuation for a variety of surgical procedures, including dental, found that discontinuing aspirin therapy resulted in thromboembolic complications, including death.[18] The surgeons who were blinded to the aspirin status were unable to detect a difference in intraoperative bleeding and postoperative bleeding management was identical for both groups. A meta-analysis including 14,981 patients who either continued or discontinued low-dose aspirin in preparation for various surgical procedures revealed that 95 (0.6%) patients who discontinued aspirin experienced an acute vascular event.[18] Fourteen (15.1%) of these were associated with dental surgery. Yet, another review and meta-analysis including 50,279 patients revealed that discontinuing aspirin had a detrimental effect.[60] Thus, it is not advised to discontinue low-dose aspirin therapy prior to oral surgical procedures.

Clopidogrel (Plavix) is an oral antiplatelet medication that reduces platelet aggregation by irreversibly binding and inhibiting adenosine diphosphate (ADP) receptors on platelet membranes. In a prospective study of 192 patients, 5 of 91 patients (5.5%) who had antiplatelet therapy discontinued for surgery experienced an adverse cardiac event.[60] None of the patients who continued antiplatelet therapy experienced an adverse event. The authors suggest that clopidogrel should not be stopped or altered prior to oral surgical procedures.

In a retrospective study of 222 patients receiving one or more extractions (75.7%) or other minor oral surgery (24.3%) with a history of taking antiplatelet medications including aspirin (n = 123; 55.4%), clopidogrel (n = 22; 9.9%), ticagrelor (n = 17; 7.7%), or dual antiplatelet therapy (n = 60; 27%), the overall frequency of bleeding was 4.9% (11 of 222).[31] Postoperative bleeding frequency for aspirin, clopidogrel, ticagrelor, and dual antiplatelet therapy was 3.2%, 4.5%, 5.9%, and 8.3%, respectively, with no statistically significant difference between groups. None of the patients experienced prolonged bleeding. The practical implications of this review, according to published studies and guidelines, is that antiplatelet therapy should not be interrupted for extractions or minor oral surgery.

NSAIDs such as ibuprofen also inhibit platelet function. Because NSAIDs bind reversibly, the effect is transitory, lasting only a short time after the last drug dose. However, due to the antiplatelet effect, these medications should not be prescribed for patients who are receiving antiplatelet or anticoagulation therapy or who have an illness with bleeding tendencies.

Anticoagulant Medications

Oral anticoagulants are prescribed for a variety of conditions to prevent thromboembolic events. The most common oral anticoagulants are the VKAs, such as warfarin, that decrease production of vitamin K–dependent coagulation factors II, VII, IX, and X. The effectiveness of anticoagulation therapy is monitored by a PT laboratory test (PT/INR). The recommended level of therapeutic anticoagulation

TABLE 67.8 Antiplatelet and Anticoagulation Medications

Medication	Class	Mode of Action	Onset / Offset	Reversal
Aspirin	Antiplatelet	Impairs platelet aggregation via inhibition of thromboxane A_2 synthesis. Blocks production of prostaglandins via irreversibly inhibiting cyclooxygenase (COX).	Peak plasma concentration (uncoated 30–40 min; enteric coated 3–4 h)/half-life effect ~7–10 days	None
Clopidogrel (Plavix)	Antiplatelet	Active metabolite irreversibly blocks ADP $P2Y_{12}$ receptor preventing platelet activation	Peak plasma concentration (2 h)/ half-life effect ~7 days	None
Prasugrel (Effient)	Antiplatelet	Active metabolite irreversibly blocks ADP $P2Y_{12}$ receptor preventing platelet activation	Peak plasma concentration (30 min)/half-life effect ~7 days	None
Ticagrelor (Brilinta)	Antiplatelet	Active metabolite reversibly binds to ADP $P2Y_{12}$ receptor preventing platelet activation	Peak plasma concentration (2–3 h)/half-life effect ~12–48 h	PB2452 potential reversal agent under investigation
Dabigatran (Pradaxa)	Direct Oral Anticoagulant	Direct thrombin inhibitor	Peak plasma concentration (0.5–2 h)/~24 h	Idarucizumab (Praxbind)
Apixaban (Eliquis)	Direct Oral Anticoagulant	Activated factor Xa inhibitor	Peak plasma concentration (1–2 h)/~24 h	Andexanet alfa (Andexxa)
Edoxaban (Savaysa)	Direct Oral Anticoagulant	Activated factor Xa inhibitor	Peak plasma concentration (1–2 h)/~24 h	Andexanet alfa (Andexxa)
Rivaroxaban (Xarelto)	Direct Oral Anticoagulant	Activated factor Xa inhibitor	Peak plasma concentration (2–4 h)/~24 h	Andexanet alfa (Andexxa)
Heparin (various)	Anticoagulant	Binds to enzyme inhibitor antithrombin III, which inactivates thrombin, Xa and other proteases	Onset of action (IV immediate; subcutaneous [SQ] 2–4 h)/ duration of action ~2–6 h (IV) ~8–12 h (SQ)	Protamine
Warfarin (Coumadin)	Anticoagulant	Competitively inhibits the vitamin K epoxide reductase complex 1 (VKORC1), which depletes functional vitamin K reserves and reduces synthesis of active clotting factors II, VII, IX, and X	Onset of action (24–72 h)/duration of action ~2–5 days	Oral or IV vitamin K; fresh frozen plasma

for most patients is an INR of 2.0 to 3.0, with prosthetic heart valve patients usually in the range of 2.5 to 3.5.[47]

The traditional recommendations for surgical management of patients taking anticoagulants *was*:

1. Consult the patient's physician to understand medical problem and degree of anticoagulation.
2. Assess the risk of bleeding for the planned procedure and determine an acceptable INR level.
3. The dentist informs physician about anticipated risk of intraoperative and postoperative bleeding.
4. The physician must be consulted about any changes (i.e., discontinuing or reducing) in anticoagulant dosage.
5. The INR was checked on the day of surgery. If the INR was within the acceptable target range, the procedure was done and the anticoagulant resumed immediately after treatment.
6. Meticulous technique and complete wound closure were paramount. Application of cold pressure and other local measures were used to establish hemostasis (e.g., use of oxidized cellulose, microfibrillar collagen, topical thrombin, and tranexamic acid).

Discontinuing anticoagulant therapy before dental surgery *was* common in the past. However, it is no longer recommended because it poses significant risks for the patient.[49,123–125] Evidence related to the risks of altering anticoagulant therapy and the lack of evidence for bleeding complications suggest that treating patients without reducing or discontinuing medications is safe.[58] Specifically, international guidelines, clinical trials, and reviews suggest that dentoalveolar surgical procedures can be safely completed for patients with an INR ≤ 3.5.[58]

Clinical studies of patients on anticoagulant therapy undergoing extractions and other oral surgical procedures have demonstrated minimal bleeding problems when anticoagulant therapy is continued.[16,19,123,124,136] In a review of the literature, Wahl and colleagues[124] reported that only 12 of 950 patients (<1.3%) receiving continuous anticoagulant therapy required more than local measures to control hemorrhage after 2400 minor oral surgical procedures. Most of the 950 patients had anticoagulation levels that were well above currently recommended therapeutic levels. Only three patients (<0.31%) had anticoagulation levels within or below currently recommended therapeutic levels. In contrast, 5 of 526 patients (0.95%) who experienced 575 interruptions of continuous anticoagulant therapy suffered serious embolic complications; 4 patients died.

In a prospective study of 131 patients undergoing 511 extractions, those patients whose oral anticoagulant therapy was reduced 72 hours before surgery to achieve an INR of 1.5 to 2.0 (target INR, 1.8) had postoperative bleeding that warranted subsequent local intervention in 10 of 66 patients (15.1%).[92] Postoperative bleeding occurred in only 6 of 65 patients (9.2%) in the group that continued the regular dosage of oral anticoagulant therapy (mean INR, 2.9).

KEY FACT

Discontinuing anticoagulant therapy before an oral surgical procedure was common in the past. Many clinicians no longer recommend discontinuing anticoagulation for many procedures because it can pose significant risks of thrombus for the patient. Evidence related to the risks of altering anticoagulant therapy and the lack of evidence for bleeding complications in these patients suggest that treating them without discontinuing antiplatelet or anticoagulant medications is safe.

DOACs are medications that inhibit specific activated clotting factors IIa and Xa (Fig. 67.3). They are also known as NOACs or target-specific oral anticoagulants (TSOACs). However, according to the International Society of Thrombosis and Haemostasis, the preferred nomenclature for these medications is DOACs.[12]

This relatively new class of oral anticoagulants includes dabigatran (Pradaxa), rivaroxaban (Xarelto), apixaban (Eliquis), and edoxaban (Savaysa) (see Table 67.8). They act by directly inhibiting an activated clotting factor, either IIa or Xa. Since being approved, physicians are prescribing them more and more as alternatives to the VKA anticoagulant medications. The most significant advantages of these DOACs over VKAs are their predictable pharmacology, limited interaction with other drugs, and rapid onset and offset of activity.[38] The pharmacokinetic and pharmacodynamic properties are more predictable so routine PT testing is not required. Reversal agents are now available for DOACs. Idarucizumab (Praxbind) is the reversal agent for dabigatran (Pradaxa). Andexanet alfa (Andexxa) is the reversal agent for apixaban (Eliquis), edoxaban (Savaysa), and rivaroxaban (Xarelto).

There are a limited number of studies reporting the risks of bleeding associated with continuing DOAC therapy versus the risks of thromboembolic complications associated with discontinuing them. In a prospective clinical comparative study aimed to analyze postoperative bleeding risk in patients continuing their anticoagulation therapy while undergoing dental implant surgery and bone grafting procedures, there were no postoperative bleeding problems reported for patients taking DOACs.[24] A retrospective study including 100 patients (64 with comorbidities; 50% with diabetes) undergoing tooth extraction according to the European Heart Rhythm Association protocol (i.e., continuation of DOAC therapy for up to three extractions at the presumed time of DOAC trough concentration) reported only 4 of 64 patients (6.25%) with bleeding episodes in the comorbidity group (1 moderate episode at one hour after extraction and 3 mild episodes the day after extraction) and no bleeding episodes (0 of 36 patients) in the group without comorbidities.[26] Another retrospective study including 120 patients who received 153 dental procedures while continuing or discontinuing NOACs reported 9 postoperative bleeding episodes in 153 treatments (5.88%). There was no difference in bleeding episodes between groups and all were managed with local measures.[54]

A literature review including 9 studies evaluating bleeding risk in patients undergoing dental implant surgery while taking antiplatelet drugs, oral anticoagulants, or direct oral anticoagulants found that postoperative bleeding occurred in 10 of 456 cases (2.2%).[9] The bleeding incidence for those on antiplatelet therapy was 1 of 253 (0.4%). For those taking oral anticoagulants, the bleeding incidence was 6 of 105 (5.7%). The incidence of postoperative bleeding for patients taking direct oral anticoagulants was 3 of 90 (3.3%). The authors concluded that the evidence supports continuing antiplatelet, oral anticoagulant or direct oral anticoagulant therapy during implant surgery.

These studies suggest that the risk of serious morbidity associated with discontinuing antiplatelet or anticoagulant therapy should be avoided and that the risk of bleeding while maintaining antiplatelet or anticoagulant therapy is minimal.

Patients on anticoagulation therapy should be treated while in the therapeutic range and clinicians must be knowledgeable about and prepared to use local hemostasis procedures. Oral anticoagulant therapy should be continued for periodontal / oral surgical procedures to avoid the risk of thromboembolic complications. It is advisable to request a preoperative PT test to assess the INR level close to the day of surgery (ideally, same day). Clinicians should plan surgical procedures with a minimally invasive approach and attention to local hemostatic measures in these patients to minimize bleeding complications.

Corticosteroids

Approximately 5% of adults in the United States habitually take corticosteroids for the treatment of various conditions, potentially putting them at risk for secondary adrenal insufficiency.[56] Patients who habitually use corticosteroids have an increased likelihood of developing hypertension, osteoporosis, and peptic ulcer disease. Care should be taken to minimize the risk of adverse outcomes in these patients. Blood pressure should be monitored, and medications that may exacerbate peptic ulceration (e.g., aspirin, NSAIDs) should be avoided.

Stressful events, such as trauma, illness, surgery, emotional upset, or athletic events, normally increase circulating endogenous cortisol levels through stimulation of the HPA axis. Pain appears to increase the requirement for cortisol release.[83] There is concern that the normal release of cortisol in response to a stressful event, such as a dental procedure, may be impaired in patients exposed to habitual corticosteroid use. The concern is about whether these patients require perioperative supplementation for dental procedures. Historically, recommendations were based on the type, amount, and duration of corticosteroid use. However, current thinking about the need for perioperative corticosteroid supplementation has been adjusted.

Studies investigating the stress response to minor general and oral surgical procedures concluded that significant increases in cortisol were usually not seen until 1 to 5 hours after surgery and appeared to be associated more with postoperative pain and the loss of local anesthesia than with the preoperative and intraoperative stress of the procedure.[10,100,101] Administration of adequate analgesics in the postoperative period can diminish the release (requirement) of cortisol.[10]

Most individuals with adrenal insufficiency can receive routine dental treatment without the need for supplemental glucocorticosteroids.[17,56] Patients taking corticosteroids usually have enough exogenous and endogenous cortisol to handle routine dental procedures if the usual dose is taken within 2 hours of the planned procedure. For most patients, supplemental corticosteroid administration is not required when uncomplicated minor surgical procedures, including periodontal surgery, are performed with local anesthesia with or without sedation.[56] Topical corticosteroids usually have minimal HPA effect, and steroid supplementation is not required for these patients.

Individuals at risk for adrenal crisis who require supplementation include those undergoing lengthy major surgical procedures, those expected to have significant blood loss, and those who have extremely low adrenal function. Low adrenal function can be identified with an ACTH stimulation test. For these individuals, consultation with the physician and steroid supplementation are indicated.

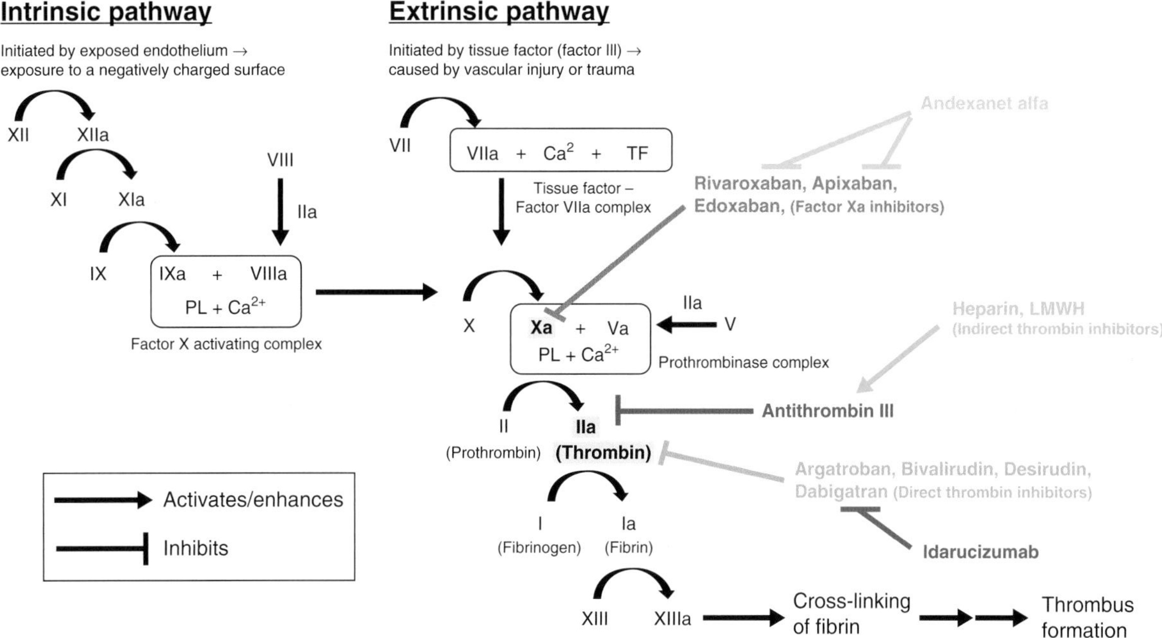

Fig. 67.3 Diagram of the intrinsic and extrinsic coagulation pathways showing factors that are inhibited by various anticoagulation medications.

KEY FACT

Patients taking corticosteroids usually have enough exogenous and endogenous cortisol to handle routine dental procedures if the usual dose is taken within 2 hours of the planned procedure. For most patients, supplemental corticosteroid administration is not required when uncomplicated minor surgical procedures, including periodontal surgery, are performed with local anesthesia with or without sedation.

Cancer Therapies

Many patients are treated for various cancers. These treatments may involve surgery, chemotherapy or radiation as stand-alone therapies or in combination. Cancer therapy can have adverse effects on the patient and may need special consideration or modifications for periodontal treatment. Chemotherapy and radiation therapy are briefly addressed in this section. Additional information and advice can be found in other sources.

Immunosuppression and Chemotherapy

Immunosuppressed patients have an impaired host defense as a result of an underlying immunodeficiency or use of drugs (primarily related to organ transplantation or cancer chemotherapy).[68,97] Because chemotherapy is often cytotoxic to bone marrow, destruction of platelets and red and white blood cells results in thrombocytopenia, anemia, and leukopenia. Immunosuppressed individuals are at greatly increased risk for infection, and even minor periodontal infections can become life-threatening if immunosuppression is severe.[85] Bacterial, viral, and fungal infections can manifest intraorally. Patients undergoing bone marrow transplantation require special attention because they receive extremely high-dose chemotherapy and are particularly susceptible to dissemination of oral infections.

Treatment should be directed toward prevention of oral complications that can be life-threatening. The greatest potential for infection occurs during periods of extreme immunosuppression; treatment should be conservative and palliative. It is always preferable to evaluate the patient before initiation of chemotherapy.[68,97] Teeth with a poor prognosis should be extracted, with thorough debridement of remaining teeth to minimize the microbial load. The clinician must teach and emphasize the importance of good oral hygiene. Antimicrobial rinses, such as chlorhexidine, are recommended, especially for patients with chemotherapy-induced mucositis, to prevent secondary infection.

Chemotherapy is usually performed in cycles, with each cycle lasting several days, followed by intervening periods of myelosuppression and recovery. If periodontal therapy is needed during chemotherapy, it is best done the day *before* chemotherapy is given, when white blood cell counts are relatively high. Coordination with the oncologist is critical. Dental treatment should be done when the white blood cell count is above 2000/mm^3, with an absolute granulocyte count of 1000 to 1500/mm^3.[65]

In consultation with the patient's physician, antibiotic premedication should be considered for any patient who is immunocompromised, including those who are undergoing chemotherapy.

Radiation Therapy

The use of radiotherapy, alone or in conjunction with surgical resection, is common in the treatment of head and neck tumors. The side effects of ionizing radiation include dramatic perioral changes of significant concern to dental health personnel.[46,67,98] The extent and severity of mucositis, dermatitis, xerostomia, dysphagia, gustatory alteration, radiation caries (Fig. 67.4), vascular changes, trismus, temporomandibular joint degeneration, and periodontal changes depend on the type of radiation used, field of irradiation, number of ports, type of tissue in the field, and dosage.

Patients scheduled to receive head and neck radiation therapy require dental consultation *at the earliest possible time* to reduce the morbidity of known perioral side effects.[96] Preirradiation treatment depends on the patient's prognosis, compliance, and residual dentition in addition to the field, ports, dose, and immediacy of radiotherapy. The initial visit should include panoramic and intraoral radiographs, a clinical dental examination, a periodontal evaluation, and a physician consultation. The physician should be asked about the type and amount of radiation to be administered, extent and location of the lesion, nature of surgical procedures already performed

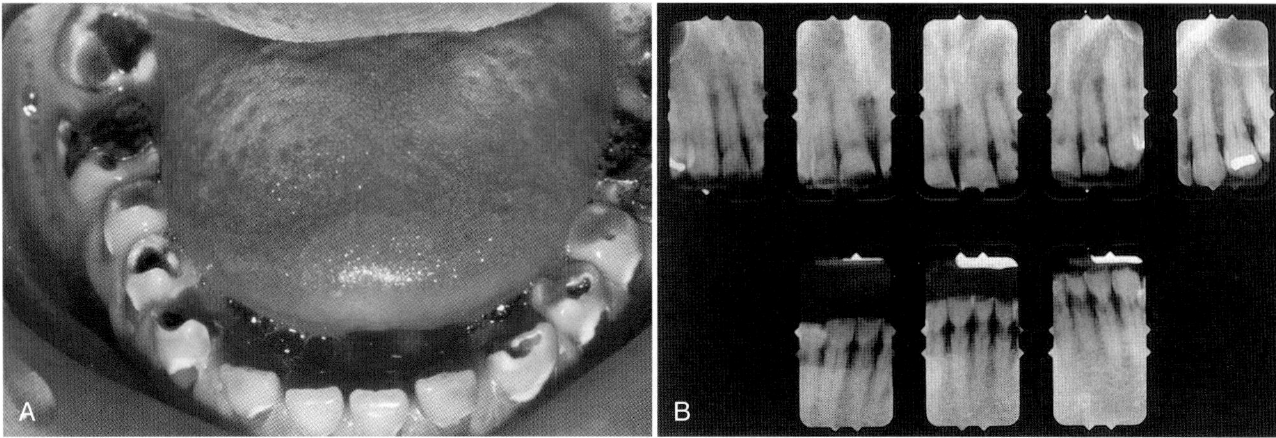

Fig. 67.4 (A) In a clinical view of a patient with radiation caries, notice how the caries primarily affected the smooth tooth surfaces, especially cervical areas and cusp tips. (B) Radiographs of anterior teeth of 52-year-old man with postradiation caries. The patient received a dose of 6000 cGy for radiation treatment of the posterior mandible and base of the tongue for squamous cell carcinoma. Radiation caries developed within 1 year after radiation treatment, affecting the cervical areas and incisal edges of the anterior teeth. (A, Courtesy Dr. Eric Sung, Hospital Dentistry, University of California, Los Angeles.)

or to be performed, number of radiation ports, exact fields to be irradiated, mode of radiation therapy, and patient's prognosis (i.e., likelihood of metastasis). Preirradiation treatment should commence immediately after the physician consultation. The first decision should involve possible extractions because radiation can cause side effects that interfere with healing.

For head and neck squamous cell carcinomas, the radiation dose is usually 5000 to 7000 cGy (1 cGy = 1 rad) delivered in a fractionated method (150 to 200 cGy/day over a 6- to 7-week course).[15,67] This is considered full-course radiation treatment, and the degree of perioral side effects depends on which tissues are irradiated (i.e., radiation fields). If the radiation is administered to the salivary gland tissues, xerostomia will ensue. The parotid is the most radiosensitive of the salivary glands; saliva may become extremely viscous or nonexistent, depending on the dose delivered to the particular gland. Xerostomia causes a decrease in the normal salivary cleansing mechanisms, buffering capacity of saliva, and pH of oral fluids.[67] Oral bacterial populations shift to a preponderance of cariogenic forms (e.g., *Streptococcus mutans, Actinomyces* spp., *Lactobacillus* spp.). Radiation-induced caries may progress rapidly, and they primarily affect smooth tooth surfaces (see Fig. 67.4).

High-dose radiation therapy results in hypovascularity of irradiated tissues, with a reduction in wound-healing capacity.[75,121,122] Most severe among the resulting oral complications is osteoradionecrosis (ORN). Decreased vascularity renders the bone less capable of resolving trauma or infection. These events can cause severe destruction of bone. The risk of ORN continues for the remainder of the patient's life and does not decrease with time.[63]

Periodontal disease can be a precipitating factor in ORN.[20,39] Tooth extraction after radiation treatment involves a high risk of developing ORN, and surgical flap procedures are usually discouraged after radiation therapy. For these reasons, it is important that the clinician address the patient's periodontal disease *before* radiation begins, when possible. Teeth that are nonrestorable or severely periodontally diseased should be extracted, ideally at least 2 weeks before radiation therapy.[67] Extractions should be performed in a manner that allows primary closure. Mucoperiosteal flaps should be gently elevated; teeth should be extracted in segments; alveolectomy should be performed, allowing no rough bony spicules to remain; and primary closure should be provided without tension. It is not necessary to extract teeth that can be retained with conservative restorative, endodontic, or periodontal therapy. However, prudence dictates extraction of questionable teeth because periodontal treatment after irradiation may be limited to nonsurgical forms of therapy. Flap surgery or extraction of teeth after radiation can lead to ORN. Management of ORN is often difficult and costly, involving progressively more aggressive treatment if bone does not respond to conservative therapy. Costly hyperbaric oxygen therapy is frequently required for complete resolution.

During radiation therapy, patients should receive weekly prophylaxis, oral hygiene instruction, and professionally applied fluoride treatments, unless mucositis prevents treatment. Patients should be instructed to brush daily with a 0.4% stannous or 1.0% sodium fluoride gel. Custom gel trays allow optimal fluoride application.[121] All remaining teeth should receive thorough root debridement (i.e., scaling and root planing).

Post-irradiation follow-up consists of palliative treatment provided as needed. Viscous lidocaine can be prescribed for painful mucositis, and salivary substitutes can be given for xerostomia. Daily topical fluoride application and oral hygiene are the best means of preventing radiation caries over time. A long-term, 3-month recall interval is ideal.

Prosthetic Joint Replacement

The main treatment consideration for patients with prosthetic joint replacement *was* the potential need for antibiotic prophylaxis before periodontal therapy. No scientific evidence indicates that prophylactic antibiotics prevent late prosthetic joint infections, which can occur from transient bacteremia induced by dental treatment.[29,65,99] Although dental-induced bacteremia can theoretically cause prosthetic joint infection, scant reports demonstrate dental treatment as a source of joint infection, and none actually documents a cause-and-effect relationship.[23,89,118]

Reports of the American Dental Association (ADA), American Academy of Orthopedic Surgeons (AAOS), American Academy of Oral Medicine (AAOM), and British Society for Antimicrobial Chemotherapy (BSAC) agree that routine antibiotic prophylaxis before dental treatment is not indicated for most patients with prosthetic joint replacement.[3,4,27,35,116]

Between 2009 and 2014, there was controversy and debate among experts, with a complete shift toward recommending prophylactic antibiotics before dental treatment for all patients with prosthetic joint replacement for life. After further review of the evidence and consensus among experts, new recommendations were published that did not recommend prophylactic antibiotics for dental procedures in patients with prosthetic joint replacement to prevent prosthetic joint infection.

Current advice for patients with orthopedic joint replacement stresses the importance of maintaining good dental health and hygiene and seeking prompt attention and treatment for oral infections when they occur. Dental procedures have not been associated with an increased risk of prosthetic joint infection, and the use of prophylactic antibiotics before dental procedures does not reduce the risk of infection.[13,105,135] Given the lack of evidence to support the need for prophylactic antibiotics, the AAOM, ADA, AAOS, and BSAC advise against universal use of antibiotic prophylaxis before dental procedures for the prevention of prosthetic joint infections.

In 2013, the ADA in conjunction with the AAOS published a joint guideline on the prevention of orthopedic implant infections in patients undergoing dental procedures. The publication stated that there was no convincing evidence to support the routine use of prophylactic antibiotics for patients with prosthetic joints.[127] In 2015, the ADA Council on Scientific Affairs published a clinical practice guideline to clearly state the findings of the 2013 ADA/AAOS joint guideline. The clinical practice guideline states that prophylactic antibiotics are *not* recommended before dental procedures for patients with prosthetic joint implants to prevent prosthetic joint infections.[109]

KEY FACT

In 2015, the American Dental Association (ADA) Council on Scientific Affairs published a clinical practice guideline to clearly state the findings published in the 2013 ADA and American Association of Orthopedic Surgeons (AAOS) joint guideline. The clinical practice guideline states that prophylactic antibiotics are not recommended before dental procedures for patients with prosthetic joint implants to prevent prosthetic joint infections. Current advice for patients with orthopedic joint replacement stresses the importance of maintaining good dental health and hygiene and seeking prompt attention and treatment for oral infections when they occur.

Conclusions

Patients with periodontal treatment needs often present with medical diseases or conditions that need to be understood by dentists and dental hygienists. Although some diseases/conditions are mild and may not have an impact on periodontal treatment, others may pose a serious risk of an adverse outcome or complication. Patients also take a variety of medications. It is imperative to review a patient's medical history and to assess the stability of their condition, and the possible need to modify treatment. Whenever a patient's health status is complex, it is prudent to consult with their physician to better understand their condition and to ascertain appropriate modifications for safe periodontal treatment. This chapter reviewed common diseases, conditions, and medications that can have an impact on oral health and patient care.

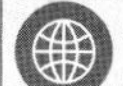

A Case Scenario is found on the companion website eBooks.Health.Elsevier.com.

Suggested Reading

American Association of Orthopaedic Surgeons. *Information Statement: Antibiotic Prophylaxis for Bacteremia in Patients With Joint Replacements*; 2009. http://pacosm.com/wp/wp-content/uploads/2015/08/Antibiotic-Prophylaxis-for-TJA-pts.-AAOS-March-2009.pdf.

American Dental Association: Oral health topics -hypertension. https://www.ada.org/en/member-center/oral-health-topics/hypertension. Last updated July 29, 2020.

American Diabetes Association. 2. Classification and diagnosis of diabetes. *Diabetes Care*. 2021;44(suppl 1):S15–S33.

Centers for Disease Control and Prevention. *Hypertension Cascade: Hypertension Prevalence, Treatment and Control Estimates Among U.S. Adults Aged 18 Years and Older Applying the Criteria from the American College of Cardiology and American Heart Association's 2017 Hypertension Guideline—NHANES 2015–2018*. Atlanta, GA: U.S. Department of Health and Human Services; 2021.

Jeske AH, Suchko GD. Lack of a scientific basis for routine discontinuation of oral anticoagulation therapy before dental treatment. *J Am Dent Assoc*. 2003;134:1492–1497.

Khan AA, Morrison A, Hanley DA, et al. International Task Force on Osteonecrosis of the Jaw. Diagnosis and management of osteonecrosis of the jaw: a systematic review and international consensus. *J Bone Miner Res*. 2015;30(1):3–23.

Lombardi N, Varoni EM, Sorrentino D, Lodi G. International normalized ratio (INR) values in patients receiving oral vitamin K antagonists and undergoing oral surgery: a clinical audit. *Spec Care Dentist*. 2020;40(4):374–381.

Mealey BL. Periodontal implications: medically compromised patients. *Ann Periodontol*. 1996;1:256–321.

Solomon DH, Mercer E, Woo SB, et al. Defining the epidemiology of bisphosphonate-associated osteonecrosis of the jaw: prior work and current challenges. *Osteoporos Int*. 2013;24:237–244.

Whelton PK, Carey RM, Aronow WS, et al. ACC/AHA/AAPA/ABC/ACPM/AGS/APhA/ASH/ASPC/NMA/PCNA Guideline for the Prevention, Detection, Evaluation, and Management of High Blood Pressure in Adults: Executive Summary: A Report of the American College of Cardiology/American Heart Association Task Force on Clinical Practice Guidelines. *Hypertension*. 2018;71(6):1269–1324.

Wilson W, Taubert KA, Gewitz M, et al. Prevention of infective endocarditis: guidelines from the American Heart Association: a guideline from the American Heart Association Rheumatic Fever, Endocarditis and Kawasaki Disease Committee Council on Cardiovascular Disease in the Young, and the Council on Clinical Cardiology Council on Cardiovascular Surgery and Anesthesia, and the Quality of Care and Outcomes Research Interdisciplinary Working Group. *J Am Dent Assoc*. 2008;139(suppl):3S–24S.

Yagiela JA. Adverse drug interactions in dental practice: interactions associated with vasoconstrictors. Part V of a series. *J Am Dent Assoc*. 1999;130:701–709.

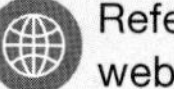

References for this chapter are found on the companion website eBooks.Health.Elsevier.com.

CHAPTER 68

Periodontal Microsurgery

Dennis A. Shanelec† | Leonard S. Tibbetts | Adriana McGregor | J. David Cross*

For online-only content on esthetic periodontal microsurgery and microsurgical knots, please visit the companion website at eBooks.Health.Elsevier.com.

CHAPTER OUTLINE

Microsurgery is surgery performed under a magnification of ×10 or more, which is possible only by using a surgical microscope.[5] The hallmarks of microsurgery are increased visual acuity and improved manual dexterity.[15] When visibility is increased 10-fold, motor movement precision is increased 1 mm to 10 μm.[3] This is the approximate size of an epithelial cell.[12] Large incisions for visibility are therefore unnecessary.

Small surgical instruments are used to advantage in the reduced surgical field (Fig. 68.1). This minimally invasive philosophy results in less injury, diminished morbidity, and rapid healing.[9,12] Sharp microsurgical blades are used to create incisions at a virtually cellular level (Fig. 68.2). These incisions are closed with meticulous apposition to eliminate wound edge gaps and dislocations, allowing healing by primary intention to begin within hours of microsurgical closure. This circumvents the need for an extensive secondary mitotic stage of wound healing to bridge wound gaps and fill surgical voids.

Philosophy of Periodontal Microsurgery

The philosophy of microsurgery embraces three core values. The first is enhanced motor skills for better surgical performance. This is accomplished through improved visual acuity and the use of a precise hand grip to increase accuracy and reduce tremor (Fig. 68.3). The second is minimal tissue trauma, which is accomplished through smaller incisions and reduced surgical fields (Fig. 68.4). The third value is primary passive wound closure.[18] This is accomplished by microsuturing to eliminate gaps and dead spaces at the wound edge (Fig. 68.5).

Advanced periodontics has an increasing need for clinical procedures that require intricate surgical skills. Regenerative procedures, periodontal plastic surgery, and dental implants are a few of the surgical procedures that demand clinical performance that frequently challenge the skills of periodontal surgeons beyond the range of possibility with ordinary vision. Microsurgery establishes a minimally invasive surgical approach to periodontics exemplified by fewer vertical incisions and smaller surgical sites. Every field of microsurgery has recognized the extent to which reduced incision size and less retraction directly correlate with reduced postoperative morbidity and rapid healing[2] (Fig. 68.6).

In addition to the use of magnification and reliance on atraumatic technique, microsurgery requires specially constructed instruments designed specifically to minimize trauma. An important characteristic of microsurgical instruments is their ability to create clean incisions that prepare wounds for healing by primary intention. Microsurgical incisions are established at a 90-degree angle to the surface using ophthalmic microsurgical scalpels (Fig. 68.7).

Microscopy permits easy identification of ragged wound edges for trimming and freshening. For primary wound closure, microsutures in the range of 6-0 to 9-0 are needed to approximate the wound edges accurately (Fig. 68.8). Microsurgical wound apposition minimizes gaps or voids at the wound edges and encourages rapid healing with less postoperative inflammation and less pain. Figs. 68.9 and 68.10 illustrate periodontal surgery cases using microsurgical techniques.

Advantages of Microsurgery

Periodontal microsurgery raises the treatment bar in many ways. Surgical decision-making is enhanced because the quality and

†Deceased.

*Bryan S. Pearson, Scott O. Kissel, Leslie Broline, and Robert Henshaw also contributed to this chapter.

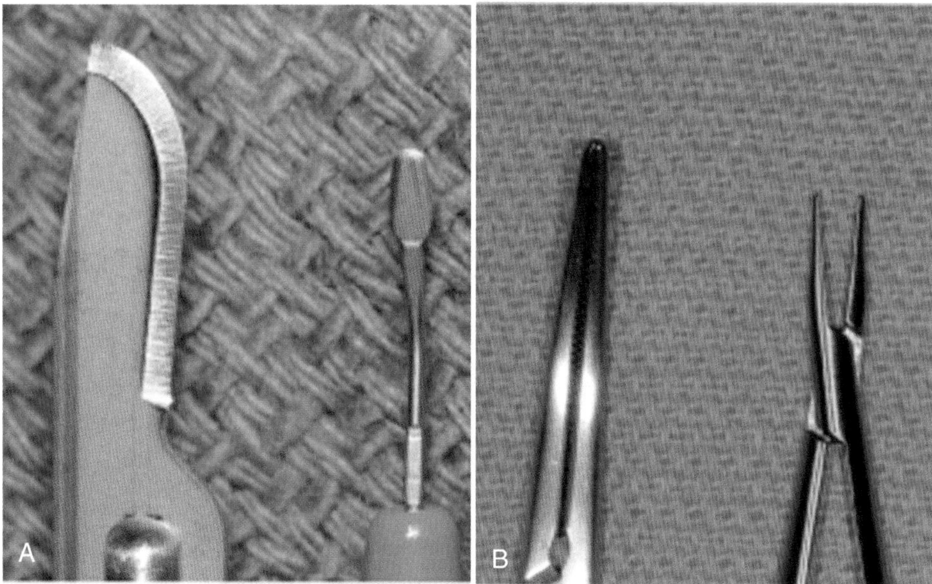

Fig. 68.1 Side-by-side dimensional comparison of commonly used conventional versus microsurgical instruments. (A) A #15 blade versus an ophthalmic blade. (B) Working tip of a conventional needle holder versus a McGregor microsuturing forceps.

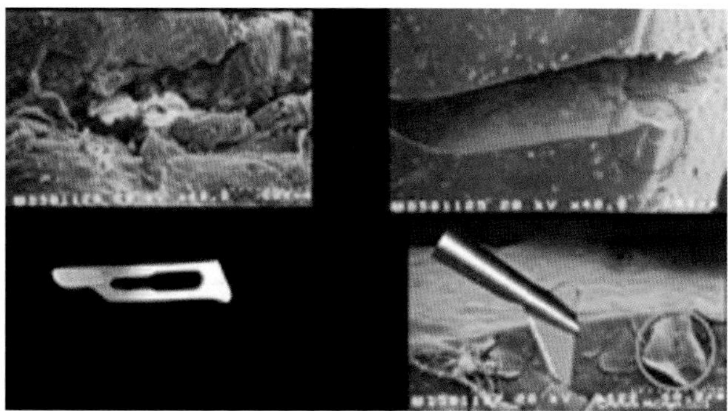

Fig. 68.2 Scanning electron microscopy (SEM) comparison of the incisions made with a #15 blade *(upper left)* and an ophthalmic microsurgical "feather" blade *(upper right and lower right)*. The *red circle* in the upper right image shows the area magnified in the lower right image. The *green circle* shows the disruption of only one epithelial cell. (SEM photographs courtesy Masana Susuki, DDS, Tokyo, Japan.)

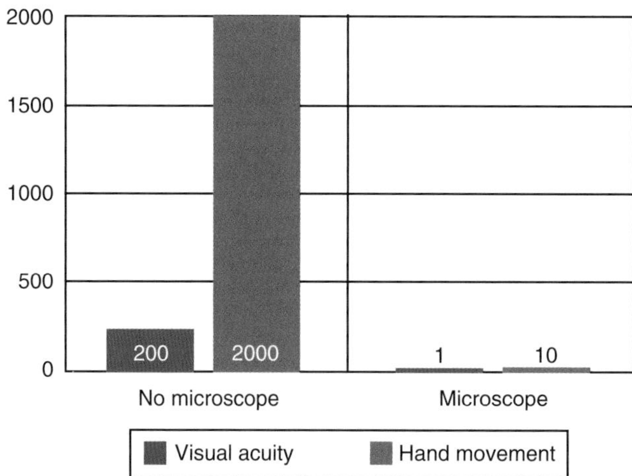

Fig. 68.3 Chart showing the correlation between enhanced visual acuity through magnification and a dramatic reduction in minimal hand movement. (From Shanelec DA. Periodontal microsurgery. *Esthet Restor Dent* 2003;15:402-407.)

quantity of visual data reaching the cerebral cortex are increased by a square of the magnification level. Ergonomic and body posture advantages also occur when using the surgical microscope[1] (Fig. 68.11). Issues such as neuromuscular fatigue and occupational skeletal pathology are reduced. Sitting comfort, good body posture, arm support, and controlled breathing are inherent to proper microscope use. Motor skills are enhanced through instruments designed for a precision grip of the hand. Titanium instruments are used for strength and lightness and are made with round handles to permit precise rotation (Fig. 68.12). This reduces hand fatigue and tremor for precise surgical movement. Ergonomic benefit is a significant aspect of microscope use in periodontics.

An important aspect of periodontal microsurgery is technical improvement in surgical performance. Higher skill levels have been shown in many surgical disciplines and can be fully appreciated when a surgeon tries his or her hand under the microscope. Viewing surgery under the microscope impresses a surgeon with the coarseness of conventional surgical manipulation (Fig. 68.13). What appears to the unaided eye as gentle surgery is revealed under the microscope as gross crushing and tearing of delicate tissues. Periodontics has long advocated atraumatic surgery, but the limits of normal vision have made this goal unattainable.

Proprioceptive guidance is of little value at the microsurgical level. Visual guidance is used for midcourse correction of scalpels and instruments to achieve the finest degrees of skill and dexterity.[4,9] Incisions can be accurately mapped, flaps elevated with minimal damage, and wounds closed accurately without tension (Fig. 68.14). Periodontal microsurgery is a natural progression from conventional surgical principles to a surgical ethic in which the surgical microscope is used for the most accurate and atraumatic handling of tissue (Fig. 68.15).

The resulting appearance of microsurgery is superior to that of conventional surgery. The difference is often startling (Figs. 68.16 to 68.18). As much as judgment and knowledge play a role in surgery, in the end, surgery is a craft. Surgeons appreciate this, especially when microsurgery raises their work to levels of artistic expression. Personal gratification in performing better surgery leads to acceptance of periodontal microsurgery by surgeons motivated to improve the quality of their work.

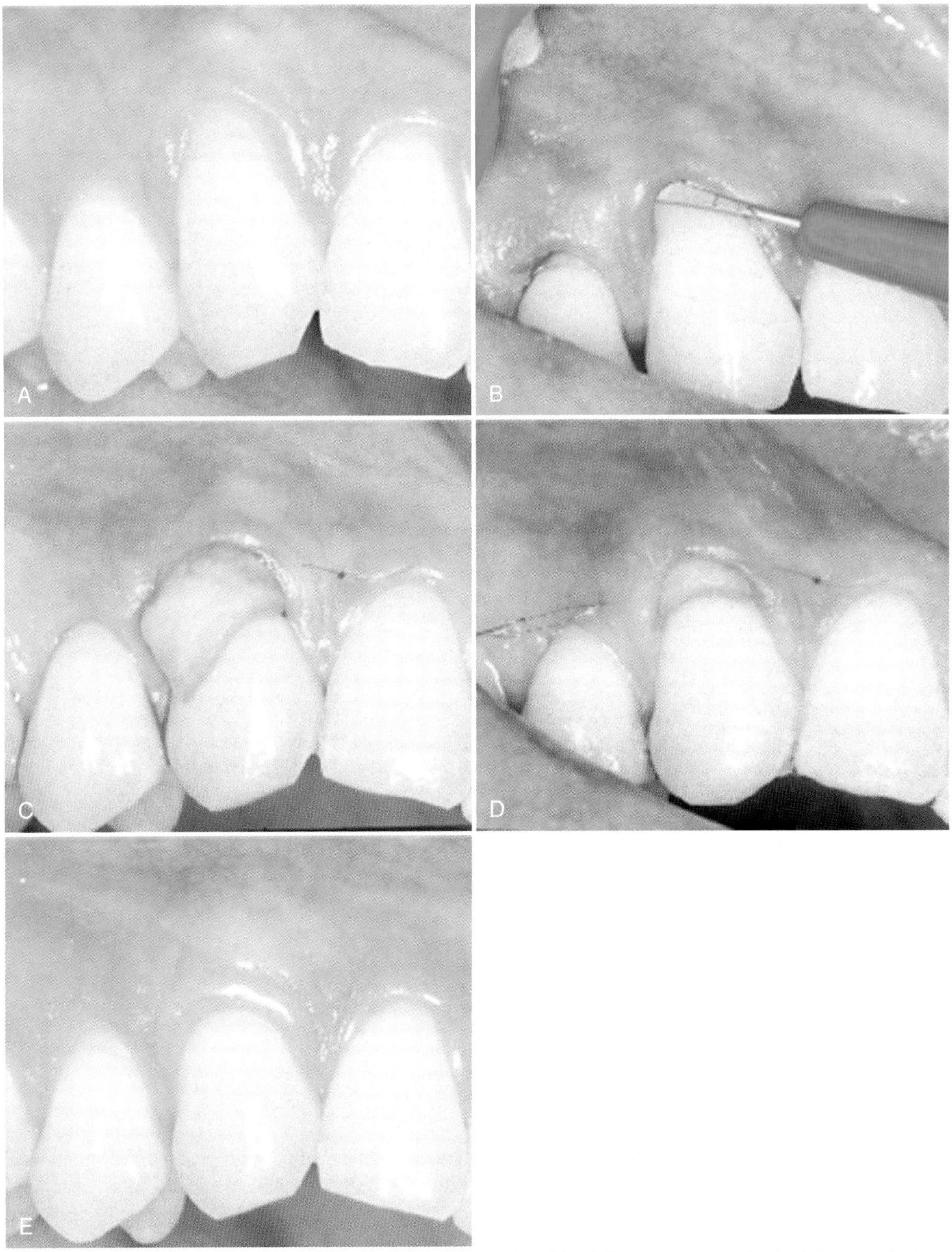

Fig. 68.4 (A–E) For a microsurgical connective tissue graft, minimal tissue trauma during incisions, surgical manipulation, and suturing are accomplished by following microsurgical principles.

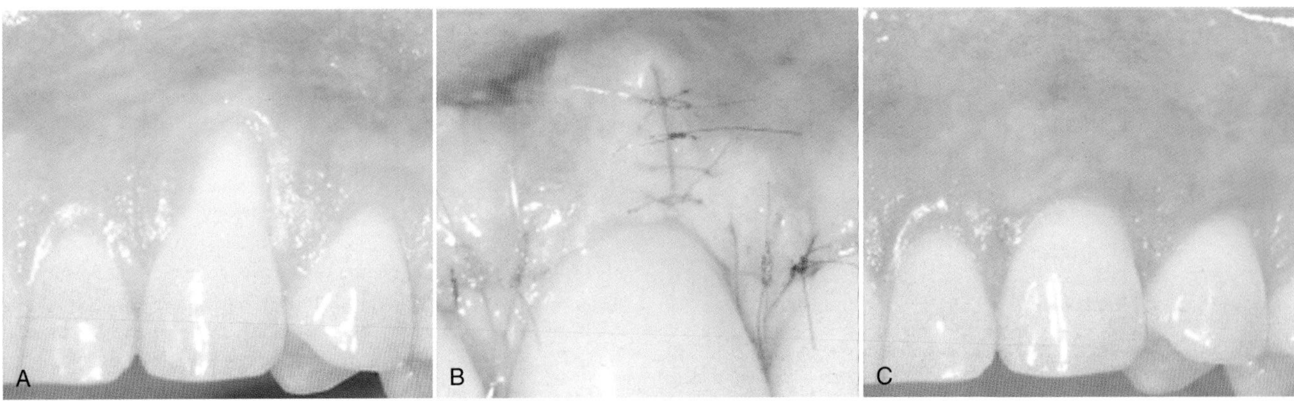

Fig. 68.5 (A–C) Primary wound closure is achieved using microsurgical principles.

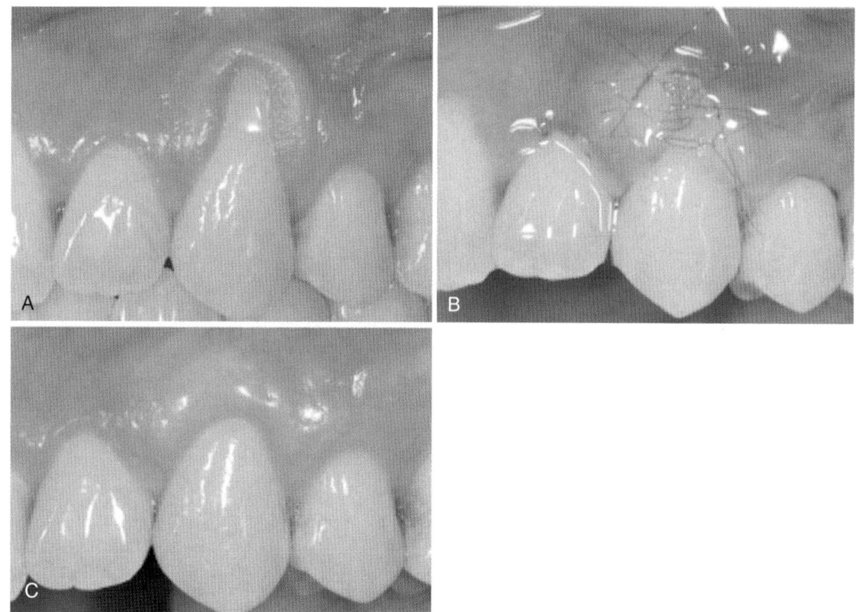

Fig. 68.6 Before (A), during (B), and 8 weeks after (C) healing of a microsurgical connective tissue graft.

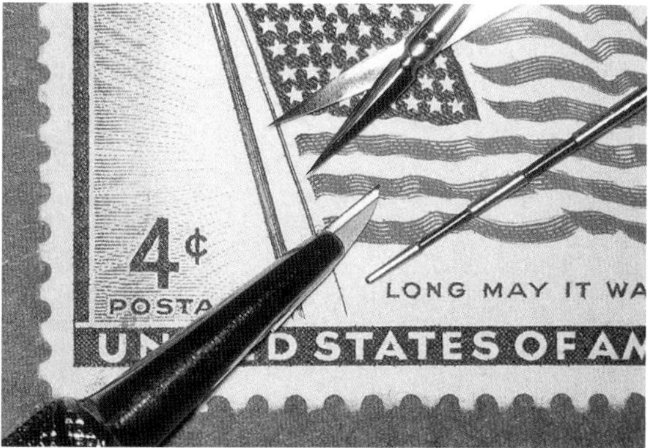

Fig. 68.7 Castroviejo microsurgical scalpel.

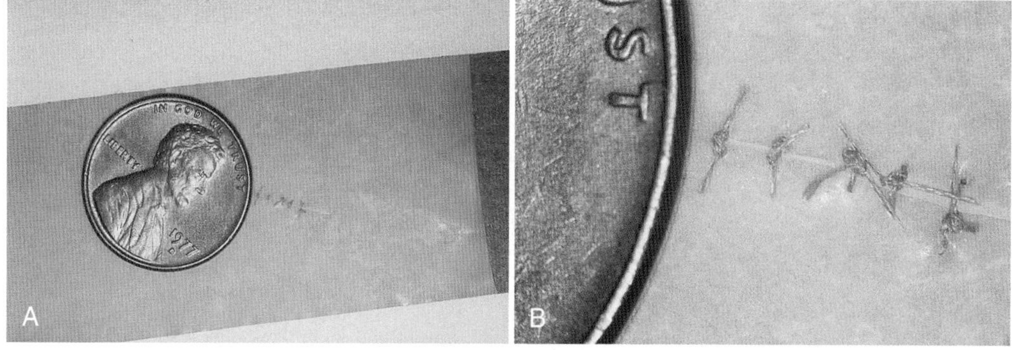

Fig. 68.8 (A and B) Microsurgical suturing.

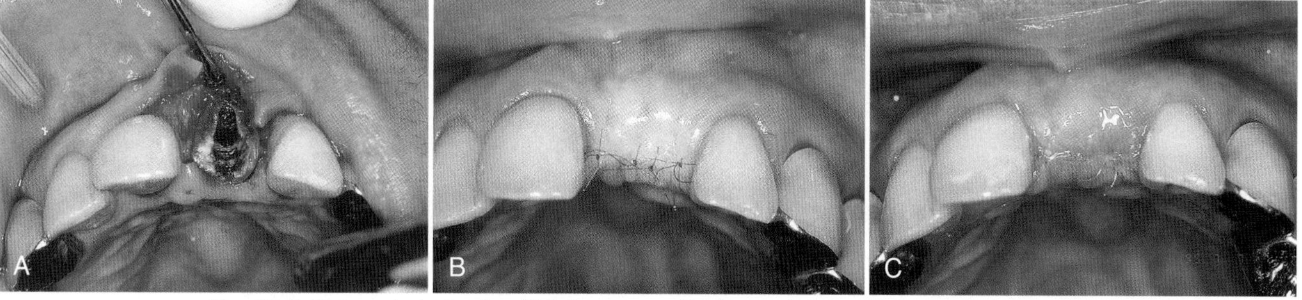

Fig. 68.9 Microsurgical extraction. (A) Before surgery. (B) Microsurgical view. (C) One week after surgery.

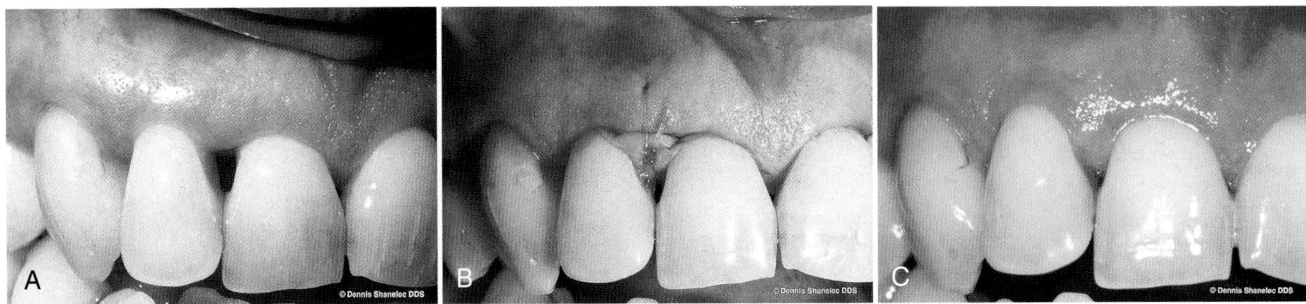

Fig. 68.10 Papilla reconstruction. (A) Before surgery. (B) Microsurgical view. (C) After surgery.

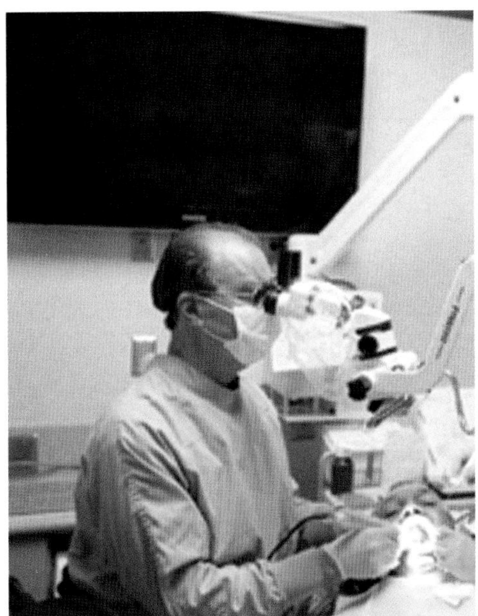

Fig. 68.11 Muscle strain and potential career-ending injuries can be prevented through a more ergonomic position of the surgeon facilitated by the proper use of a microscope.

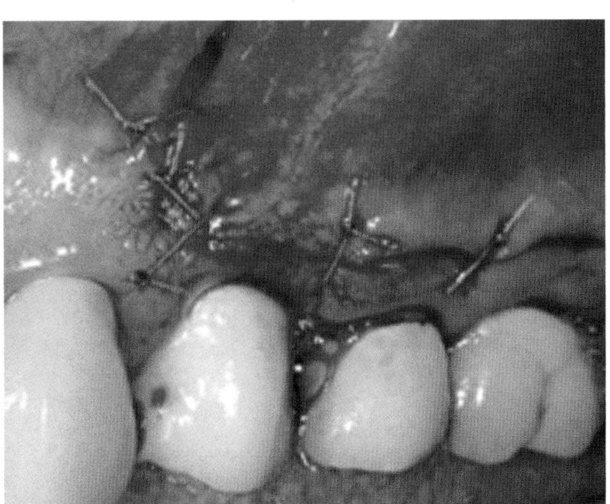

Fig. 68.13 The coarseness of conventional periodontal surgery is readily apparent under microscopic magnification.

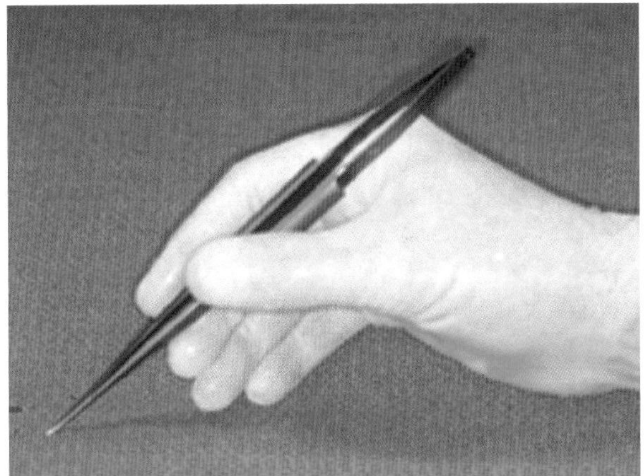

Fig. 68.12 Rounded, titanium microsurgical instruments, ideally 9 mm in diameter, reduce muscle fatigue and facilitate precise, rotational hand movements.

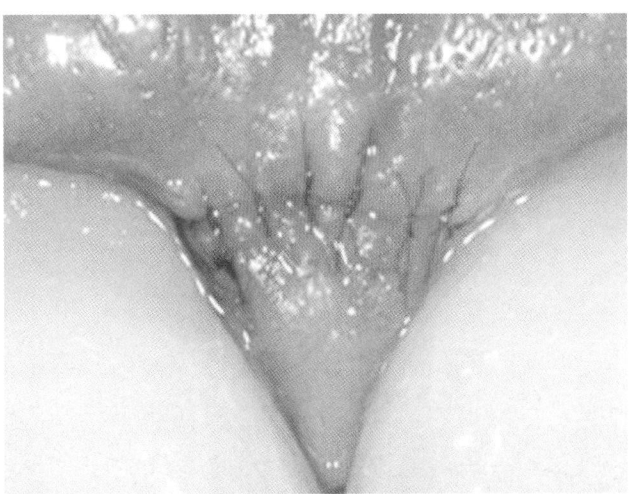

Fig. 68.14 Tension-free wound closure is one of the goals of a microsurgical approach.

Microsurgery offers another advantage in the area of root preparation. The importance of root débridement is recognized universally as an essential component of periodontal therapy.[10,15] Research in clinical dentistry has shown that microscope-enhanced vision more readily accomplishes the established clinical goals of endodontic and restorative dentistry. In periodontics, studies have demonstrated that root débridement performed without magnification was incomplete. When débrided roots were examined with the aid of a microscope, substantial deposits remained. Even in the absence of clinical studies, it may be inferred that microscope-enhanced vision in periodontics permits more definitive root débridement.

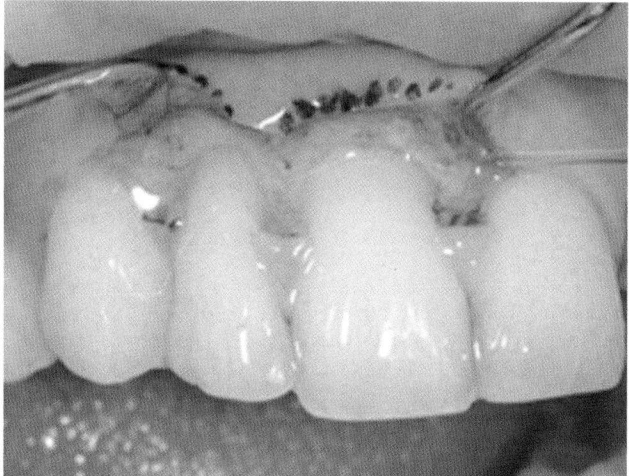

Fig. 68.15 Atraumatic microsurgical tissue manipulation during a microsurgical crown-lengthening procedure.

The primary goals of periodontal surgery include visual access to the root surface for plaque and calculus removal and for removing pathologically altered tooth structures. Magnification greatly improves the surgeon's ability to create a clean, smooth root surface (Fig. 68.19). The root surface represents one opposing edge of the periodontal wound. Root planing is therefore analogous to establishing a clean soft tissue incision. Magnification permits preparation of hard and soft tissue wound surfaces so that they can be joined together according to the accepted microsurgical principle of butt joint wound approximation. This encourages primary wound healing and enhanced periodontal reconstruction. Studies of wound healing show epithelial anastomosis of microsurgically joined surgical wounds in animals within 48 hours.[4,11] With training, the average periodontal microsurgeon can consistently produce better crafted work than the most talented surgeon using conventional methods (Fig. 68.20).

Magnification Systems

Simple and complex magnification systems are available to dentists. They range from simple loupes to prism telescopic loupes and surgical microscopes. Each magnification system has specific advantages and limitations. Although magnification improves the accuracy of clinical and diagnostic skills, it requires an understanding of optical principles that govern all magnification systems. The assumption that "more magnification is better" must always be weighed against the decrease in field of view and depth of focus that can occur as

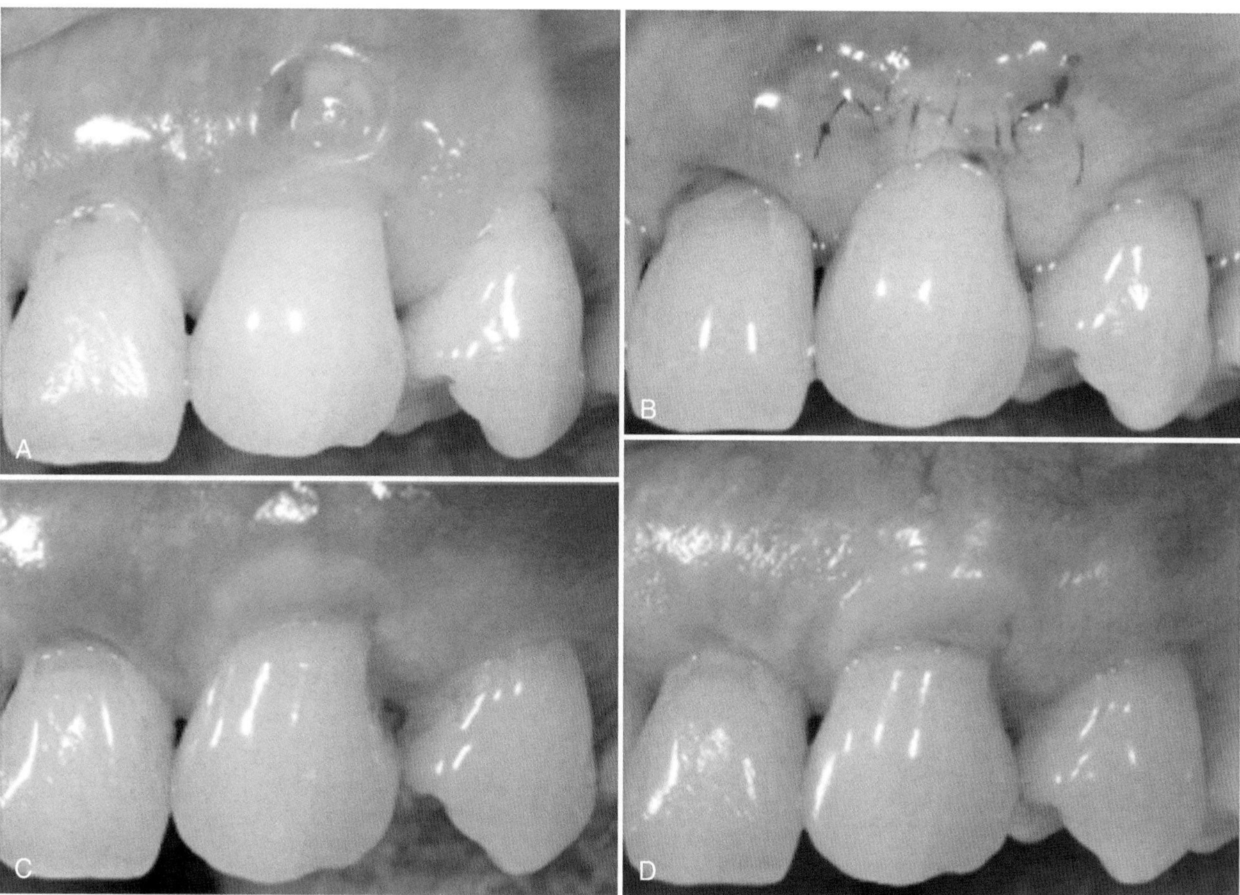

Fig. 68.16 (A) Suppurating gingival fenestration. (B) After careful root planing, a connective tissue graft (CTG) was carefully sutured under the envelope flap. (C) Postoperative healing at 3 weeks. (D) Postoperative follow-up at 1 year.

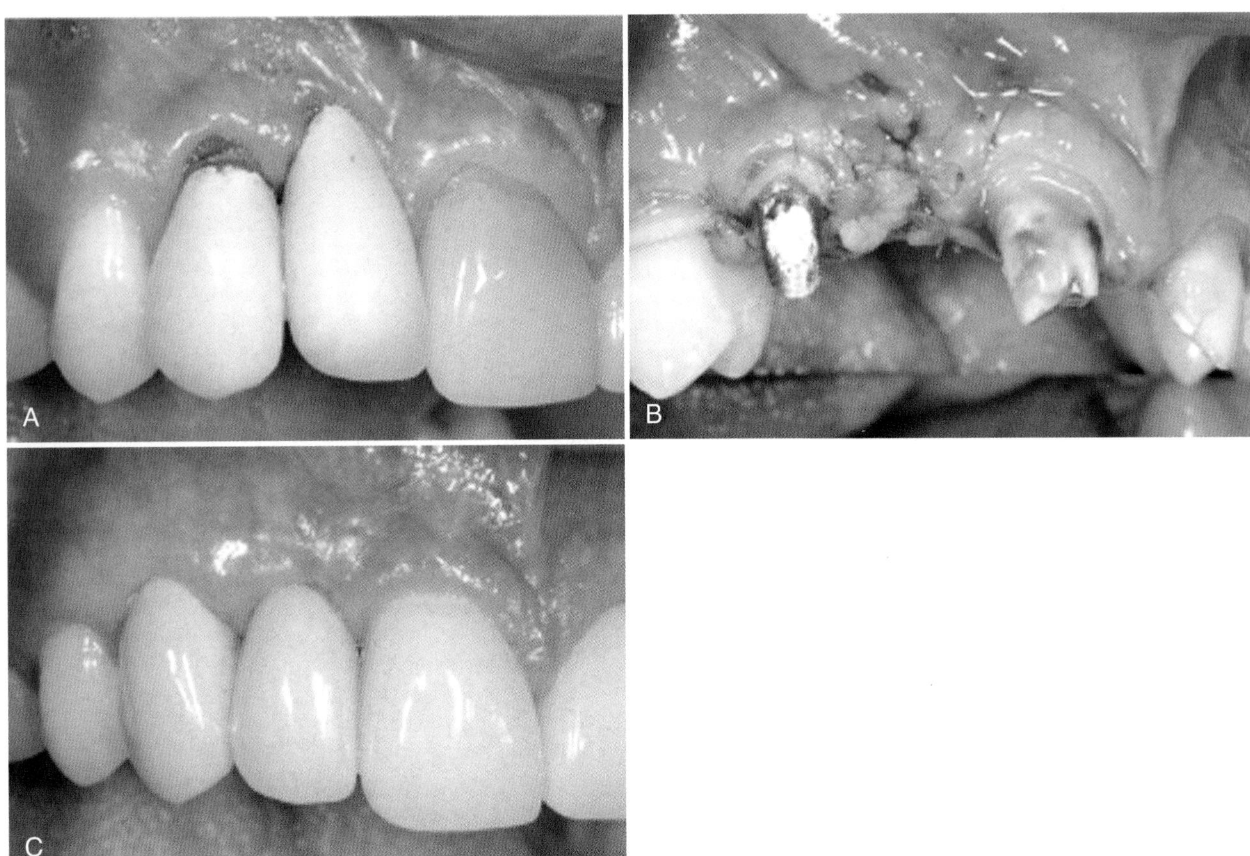

Fig. 68.17 Microsurgical correction of a macrosurgical unsatisfactory outcome. (A) Improper placement caused an unesthetic result. (B) Microsurgical grafting procedure. (C) Final surgical result after fabrication of new crowns.

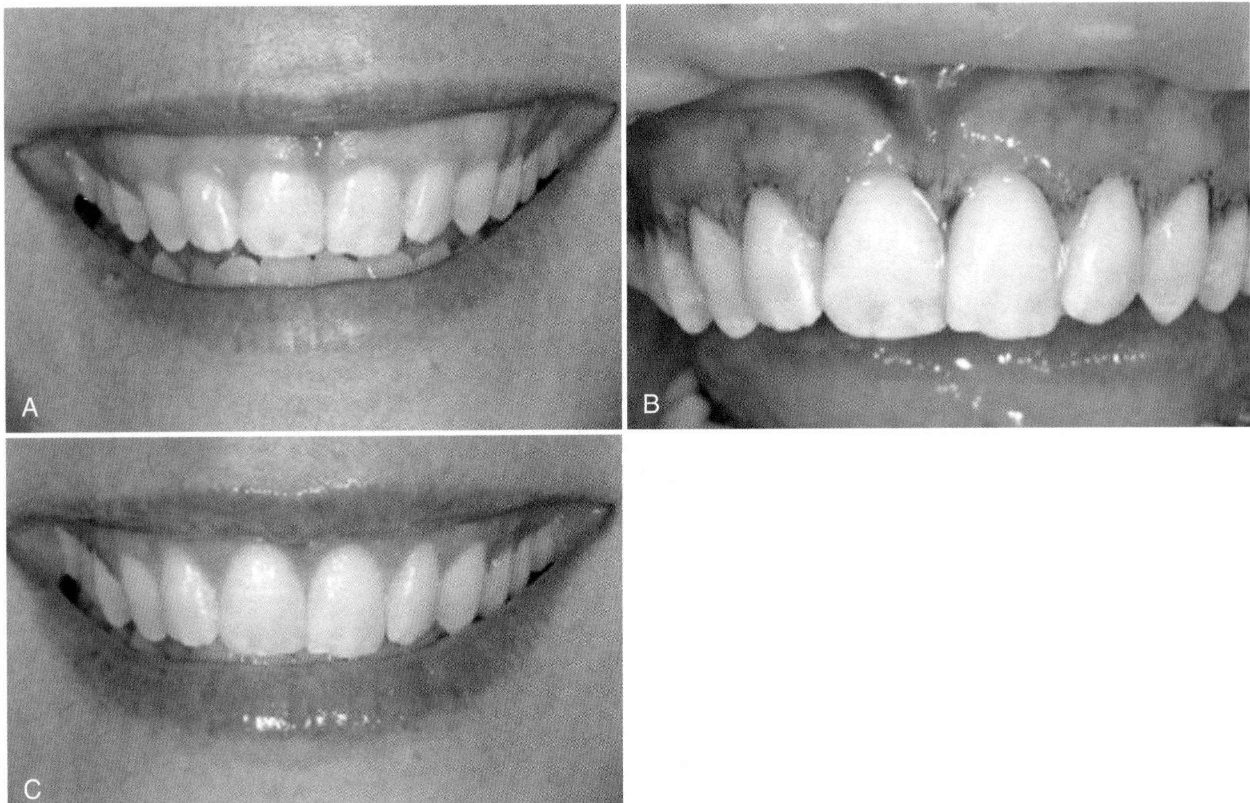

Fig. 68.18 Microsurgical crown-lengthening procedure. (A) Altered passive eruption covering teeth crowns. (B) Immediate microsurgical postoperative result. (C) Postoperative healing at 3 weeks.

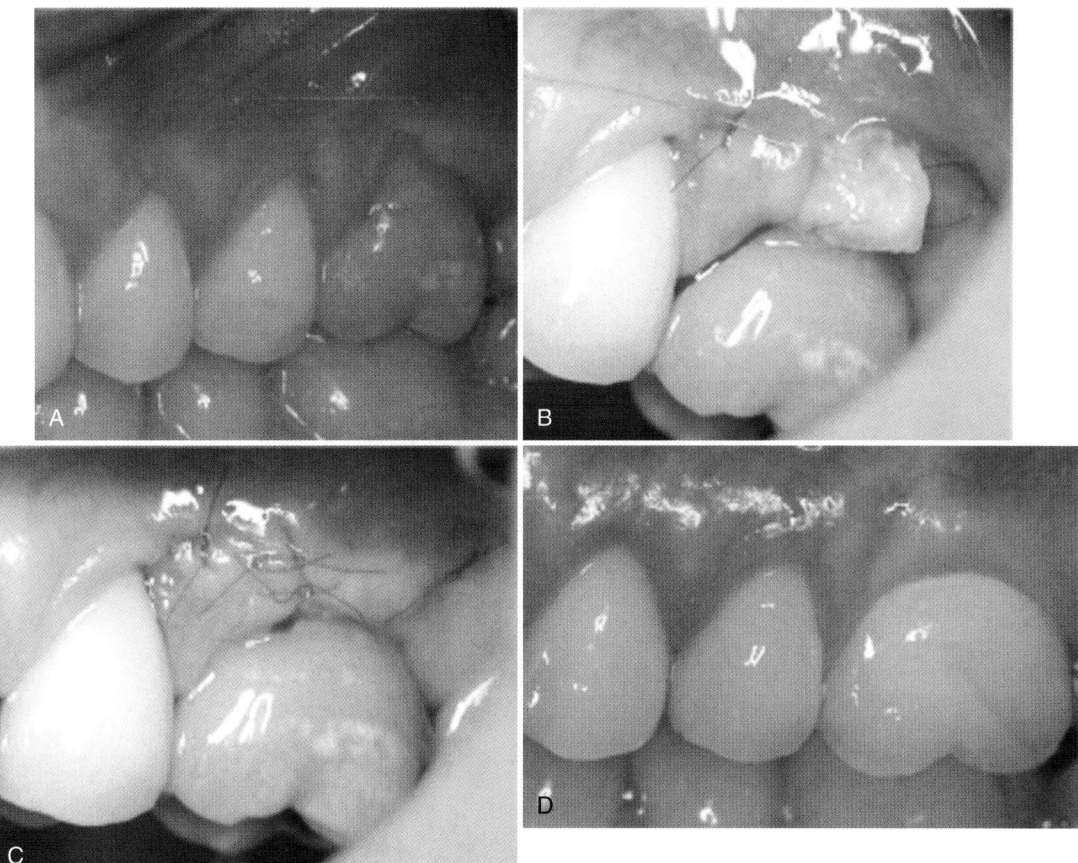

Fig. 68.19 Procedure accessibility is enhanced through microsurgery. (A) Connective tissue graft (CTG) on a maxillary molar. (B) Before surgery. (C) During surgery. (D) Seven weeks postoperatively.

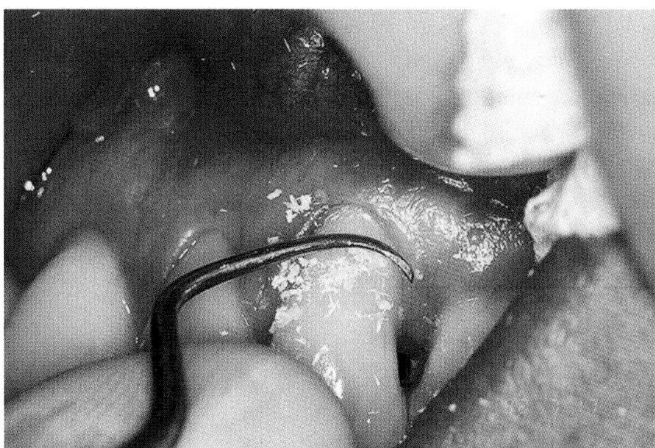

Fig. 68.20 Magnified root planing.

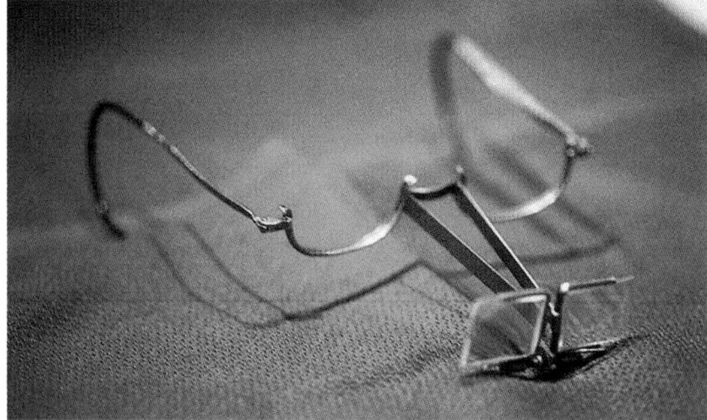

Fig. 68.21 Simple loupes.

magnification increases, which is a problem more common with dental loupes than operating microscopes.

Magnifying Loupes

Dental loupes are the most common system of optical magnification used in periodontics. Loupes are fundamentally dual monocular telescopes with side-by-side lenses that converge to focus on the operative field. The magnified image formed has stereoscopic properties by virtue of their convergence. A convergent lens optical system is called a *Keplerian optical system.*

Although dental loupes are widely used, they have disadvantages compared with the microscope. The clinician's eyes must converge to view the operative field. This can result in eye strain, fatigue, and pathologic vision changes, especially after prolonged use.

Three types of Keplerian loupes are typically used in periodontics: simple or single-element loupes, compound loupes, and prism telescopic loupes. Each type can differ widely in optical sophistication and individual design.

Simple Loupes

Simple loupes consist of a pair of single meniscus lenses (Fig. 68.21). Simple loupes are primitive magnifiers with limited capabilities. Each lens is limited to only two refracting surfaces. Their magnification can increase only by increasing lens diameter and thickness. Size and weight constraints make simple loupes impractical for magnification beyond ×1.5. Another disadvantage of simple loupes is that they are greatly affected by spherical and chromatic aberration. This distorts the image shape and color of objects being viewed.

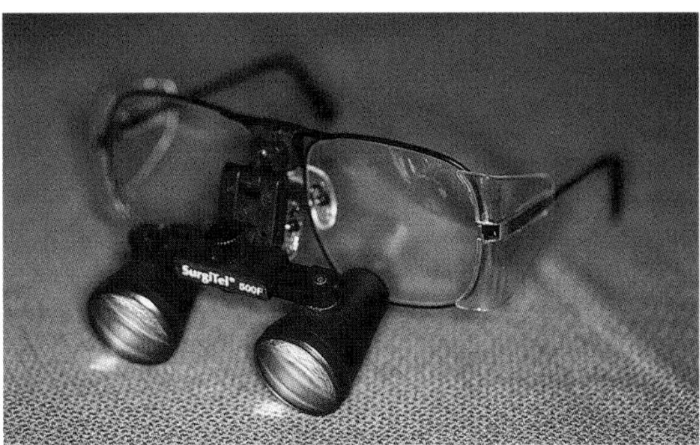

Fig. 68.22 Compound loupes.

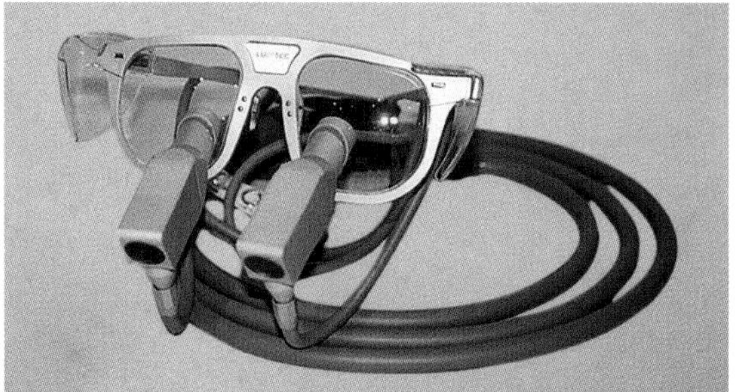

Fig. 68.24 Coaxial light prism loupes.

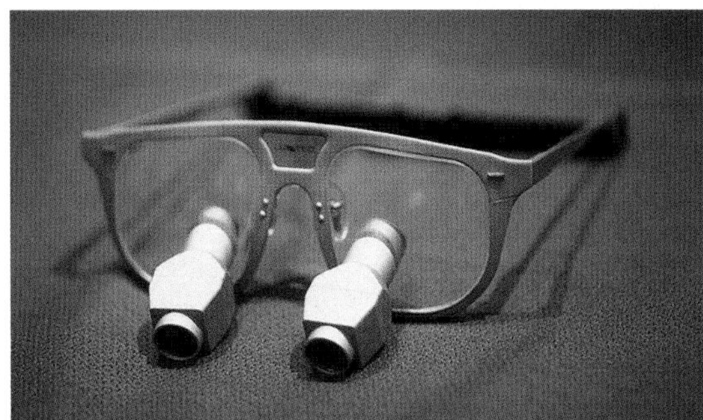

Fig. 68.23 Eyeglass-mounted prism loupes.

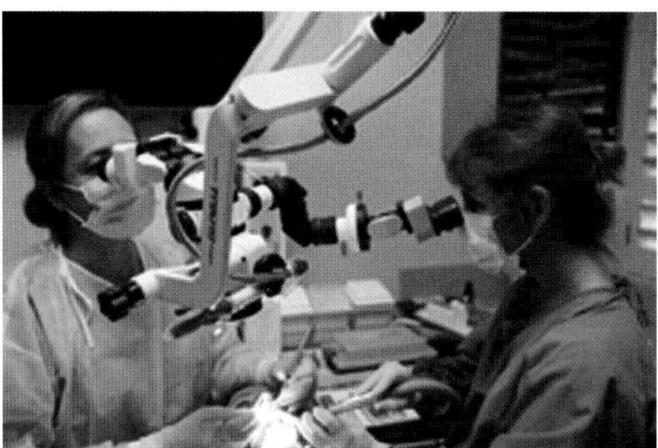

Fig. 68.25 Accessory binocular module allows the assistant to support the operator better during the procedure.

Compound Loupes

Compound loupes use multielement lenses with intervening air spaces to gain additional refracting surfaces (Fig. 68.22). This allows increased magnification with more favorable working distance and depth of field. Magnification of compound loupes can be increased by lengthening the distance between lenses, thereby avoiding excessive size and weight.

In addition to offering improved optical performance, compound lenses can be *achromatic,* which is an optical feature that clinicians should always choose when selecting magnifying loupes. Achromatic lenses consist of two glass lenses joined together with clear resin. The specific density of each lens counteracts the chromatic aberration of its paired lens to produce a color correct image. However, multielement compound loupes become optically inefficient at magnifications above ×3.

Prism Telescopic Loupes

The most advanced loupe optical magnification currently available is the prism telescopic loupe. These loupes use Schmidt or rooftop prisms to lengthen the light path through a series of switchback mirrors between the lenses. This arrangement folds the light so that the barrel of the loupes can be shortened. Prism loupes produce better magnification, wider depths of field, longer working distances, and larger fields of view than other types of loupes. The barrels of prism loupes are short enough to be mounted on eyeglass frames (Fig. 68.23) or headbands. However, the increased weight of prism telescopic loupes with magnification above ×4 makes headband mounting more comfortable and stable than eyeglass frame mounting. Innovations in prism telescopic loupes include coaxial fiberoptic lighting incorporated into the lens elements to improve illumination (Fig. 68.24).

Magnification Range of Surgical Loupes

Dental loupes provide a limited range of magnification (×1.5 to ×6). Loupes delivering magnification of less than ×3 are usually inadequate for the visual acuity necessary for clinical periodontics. Surgical loupes providing magnification of more than ×4 are impractical because of their small field of view, shallow depth of focus, and excessive weight. Excessively heavy loupes can make it difficult to maintain a stable visual field.

For some periodontal procedures, prism telescopic loupes with magnification of ×4 provide an adequate combination of magnification, field of view, and depth of focus. However, the surgical microscope offers much higher magnification and superior optics compared with any of the loupe optical systems mentioned.

The Surgical Microscope

The surgical microscope offers greater versatility than dental loupes by providing a range of magnification with superior optical performance. A surgical microscope can last an entire career, making its long-term expense practical. Proficient use of the microscope requires training and practice. Surgical microscopes designed for dentistry use galilean optics, which have binocular eyepieces joined by offset prisms to establish a parallel optical axis and permit stereoscopic vision without eye convergence or eyestrain. An additional binocular eyepiece can aid the microsurgical assistant (Fig. 68.25).

Surgical microscopes have coated achromatic lenses, high optical resolution, and a rotating magnification element that allows the microsurgeon to change magnification easily to a value appropriate for the surgical task at hand (Fig. 68.26). Because the optical elements of surgical microscopes are more advanced than those in loupes, depth of focus and field of view characteristics are greatly enhanced. Surgical microscopes have objective lenses with various working distances. A useful range in dentistry is 250 to 350 mm.

For practical use, a surgical microscope must have maneuverability and stability. Mountings are available for the ceiling, wall, or floor. Adjustable inclining eyepieces enhance postural flexibility for various procedures (Fig. 68.27). This maneuverability provides visual access to every area of the mouth and is an important factor when choosing to use a surgical microscope.

Illumination of the microsurgical field is also an important consideration. Dentists are accustomed to working with lateral illumination from side-mounted dental lights or headlamps. Fiberoptic coaxial illumination is a major advantage because it focuses light parallel to the microscope's optical axis, which eliminates shadows. Surgeons can visualize the deepest reaches of the oral cavity, including subgingival pockets and angular bony defects. Definitive visualization of root surface to detect deposits and irregularities is possible. Surgeons can view anatomy to make clinical decisions based on accurate assessment of pathology rather than blind educated guesses.

Documentation is important for patient and professional education and for dental-legal reasons. The surgical operating microscope is an ideal platform for documenting periodontal pathology and clinical procedures. Digital images can be captured using a beam splitter and camera attachment. A foot-controlled switch permits a surgeon to record as the procedure unfolds without interrupting surgery. These images represent the surgical field exactly as the surgeon sees it, as opposed to a camera view over the surgeon's shoulder. High-definition video cameras capture still and video images simultaneously to permit documentation of periodontal procedures for educational purposes (Fig. 68.28).

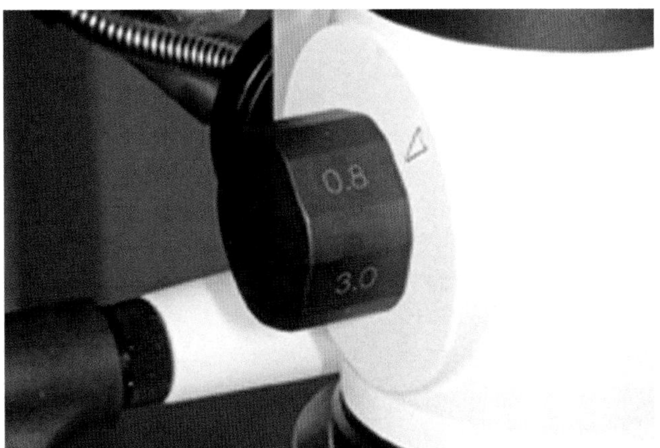

Fig. 68.26 Rotating magnification element with a field of view ranging from the full mouth to approximately 3 cm when using a 250-mm objective lens.

Microsurgical Sutures

To achieve ideal microsurgical wound closure, a surgeon depends on how the incisions were planned and executed, how the surgery was performed, and the suturing technique. Selection of proper suture needles and materials is essential for successful microsurgical wound closure. The choice of suture and needle size is critical for atraumatic tissue passage. Suture material must maintain wound closure until healing is sufficiently advanced to withstand functional stress.

Sutures are classified according to structure as monofilament or braided, according to surface as coated or uncoated, and according to biologic properties as absorbable or nonabsorbable.[2] The suture of choice in microsurgery is a monofilament suture material such as polypropylene or polydioxanone. These materials are bacteriostatic and noninflammatory, hold a knot extremely well, and are easily removed. The purpose of sutures is to provide initial wound support. They are chosen to appropriate wounds based on the fragility of the tissue. The smallest suture capable of supporting the wound

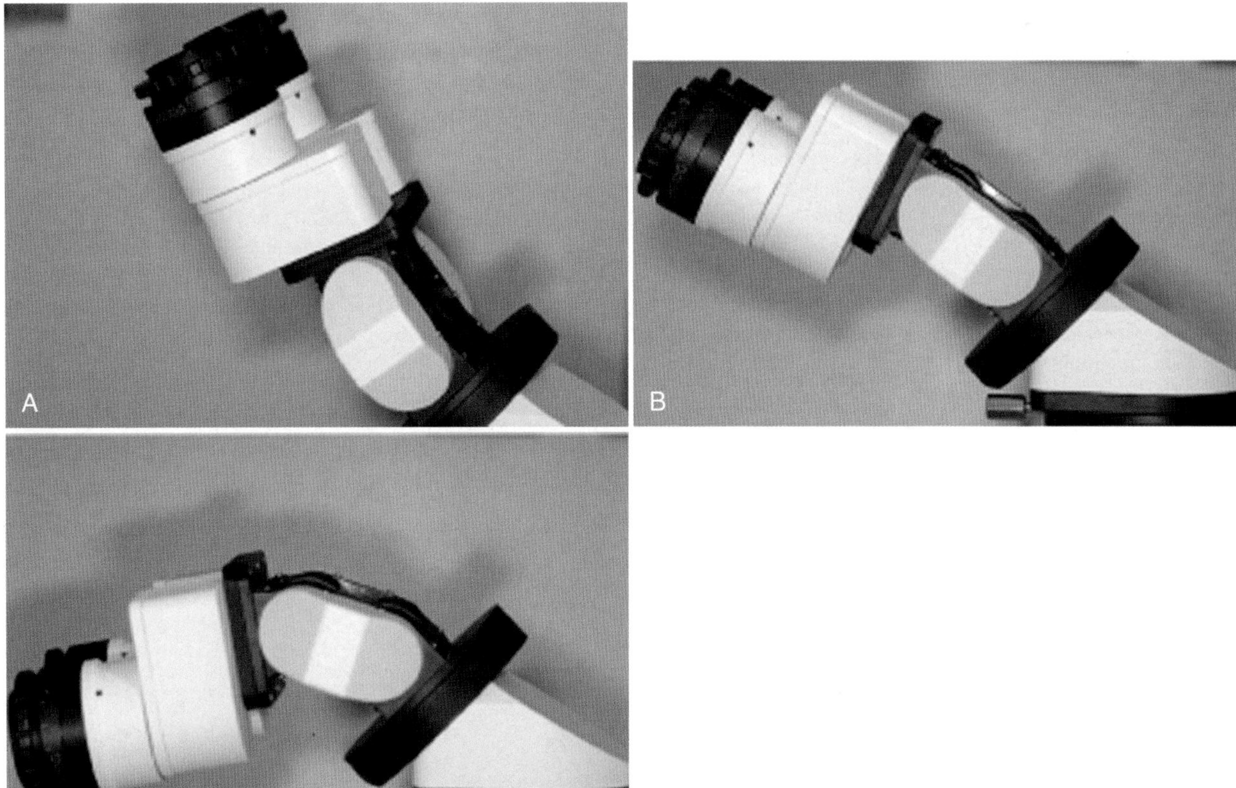

Fig. 68.27 (A–C) The inclinable adjustable eyepieces have a wide range of motion.

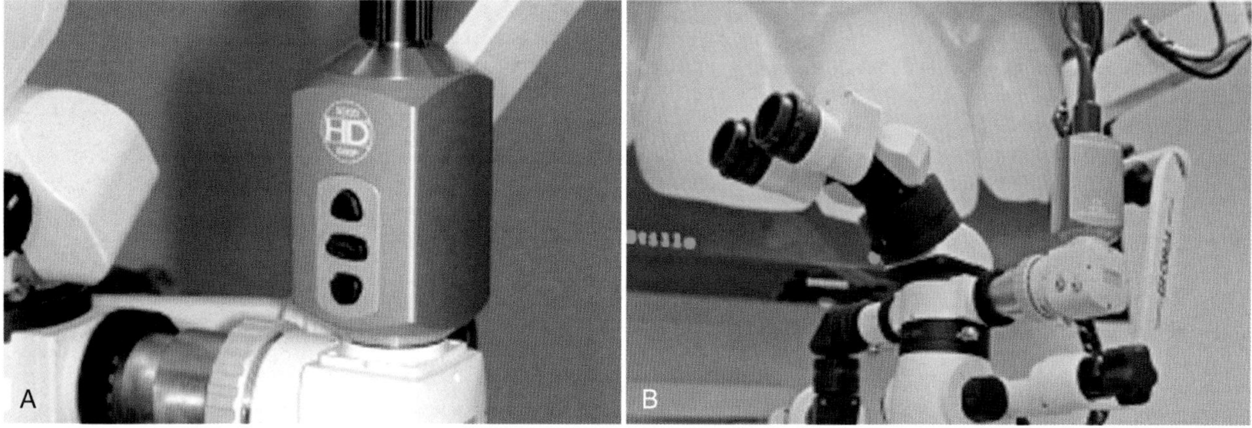

Fig. 68.28 (A) High-definition (HD) video and still capture camera mounts conveniently fit into the microscope and can be viewed in real time on an HD monitor (B). (Courtesy Optronics Microcast HD Studio, Optronics Medical Grade HD Microimaging Systems, Goleta, CA.)

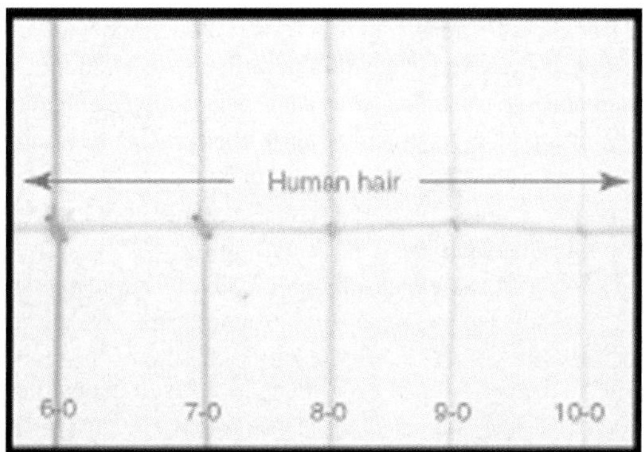

Fig. 68.29 Size comparison of microsutures in relation to the dimension of a human hair.

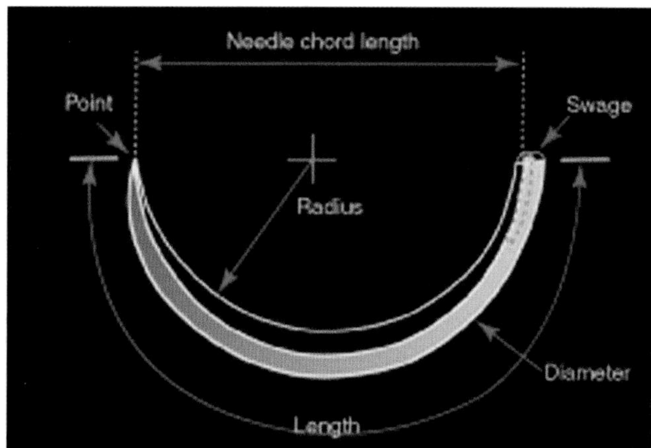

Fig. 68.30 Anatomy of a needle. Microsutures are hand-inserted into the laser-drilled swaged end of the needle, forming a seamless contiguous unit.

produces the least tissue trauma and the least interruption of the blood supply.

In periodontal microsurgery, the suture size ranges from 6-0 (i.e., diameter of a human hair) to 9-0 (Fig. 68.29). The size and shape of the needle used is essential for the atraumatic passage of the suture. The needle diameter is ideally slightly larger than the suture size. Sutures used in microsurgery are swaged, making the needle and the suture continuous[1] (Fig. 68.30). Penetration and passage of the needle depend on the angle of entry of the needle point. Cutting needles pass through gingival tissue easily but can tear tissue. Tapered needles are less traumatic and less likely to tear tissue.

An important component of needle design is the chord distance (see Fig. 68.30). The chord of a needle is the length of a line drawn between the cutting point and the swaged end.[1] The radius of a needle is the arc of its circumference. A half-round needle has an arc of 180 degrees. The chord determines the ease in passing a suture between adjacent teeth. The arc determines the bite size and angle of entry taken by the needle. These needle dimensions are important when selecting sutures for periodontal microsurgery.[4]

Conclusions

As medicine and dentistry continue the pursuit of minimally invasive treatment, periodontal microsurgery and its principles will emerge as the methodology to meet professional and public demand.[13] The microscope provides a tremendous platform from which the microsurgical clinician can gather and observe detailed and precise amounts of information for the diagnosis and treatment of patients with skill and accuracy.[6] Microsurgery leads to improved esthetics, rapid healing, reduced morbidity, and enhanced patient acceptance.[3,11,16]

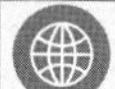 References for this chapter are found on the companion website eBooks.Health.Elsevier.com.

CHAPTER 69

Diagnosis and Management of Periodontal Abscesses

Philip R. Melnick | Henry H. Takei

CHAPTER OUTLINE

The periodontal abscess is a common dental emergency, often resulting in the rapid destruction of periodontal tissues.[3,20,36] It can negatively influence the prognosis of teeth and is a significant cause of tooth loss.[6,15,17,18,22,25,28-32] As a source of infection and inflammation, periodontal abscesses may have serious systemic effects.[16,36] However, with proper treatment followed by consistent supportive therapy, even teeth with significant bone loss may be retained for many years[9] (see Fig. 69.10).

Classification of Abscesses

The periodontal abscess is a localized purulent inflammation of the periodontal tissues.[8,19,26,27]

Periodontal abscesses are primarily classified by *etiology*.[20] *Location, course*[19,33] (acute vs. chronic), and *symptomatology*[23] are considered additional secondary identifiers.[20,33] They may occur at single or multiple sites.[19]

Classification by Etiology

Periodontal abscesses are typically found in patients with untreated, plaque-associated periodontitis, often as acute exacerbations in moderate to deep preexisting periodontal pockets.[6,8,19,26,27,41] (Fig. 69.1). See studies by Herrera, Papapanou, and colleagues.[20,36] Primarily related to extensive calculus deposits or incomplete calculus removal, periodontal abscesses have been linked to several additional clinical situations.[10,11,19,20,22,25,27,39] They have been identified in patients after periodontal surgery,[15] after supportive periodontal therapy (Fig. 69.2),[9,13,28,32] after systemic antibiotic therapy,[44] and as the result of recurrent disease.[19,22,25] Conditions in which periodontal abscesses are not related to periodontitis include tooth perforation or fracture[1,20,39] (Fig. 69.3) and foreign body impaction (e.g., dental floss, toothpick, food particles).[2,20,35] Poorly controlled diabetes mellitus has been considered a predisposing factor for periodontal abscess formation, and is often associated with multiple abscesses[16,20,26,33] (Fig. 69.4).

Identification by Location

Abscesses of the periodontal tissues have also been described by location—gingival abscess, periodontal abscess, and pericoronal abscess.[33] The gingival *abscess* involves the marginal gingival and interdental tissues. The *periodontal abscess* is an infection located contiguous to the periodontal pocket and may result in destruction of the periodontal ligament and alveolar bone. The *pericoronal abscess* is associated with the crown of a partially erupted tooth.[19,26,33]

LEARNING BOX 69.1

Abscesses of the periodontal tissues have also been identified by location—gingival abscess, periodontal abscess, and pericoronal abscess.

LEARNING BOX 69.2

Most periodontal abscesses are a result of the development of large calculus deposits, which impede pocket drainage, or the incomplete removal of subgingival calculus in a periodontal pocket.

Gingival Abscess

The gingival abscess is a localized acute inflammatory lesion that may arise from a variety of sources, including microbial plaque infection, trauma, and foreign body impaction.[26,33] Clinical features include a red, smooth, sometimes painful, often fluctuant swelling (Fig. 69.5).[19] In general, gingival abscesses do not involve clinical attachment loss.

Pericoronal Abscess

The pericoronal abscess results from inflammation of the soft tissue operculum, which covers a partially erupted tooth. This situation is most often observed around the mandibular third molars. As with the gingival abscess, the inflammatory lesion may be caused by the retention of microbial plaque biofilm, food impaction, or trauma.[33]

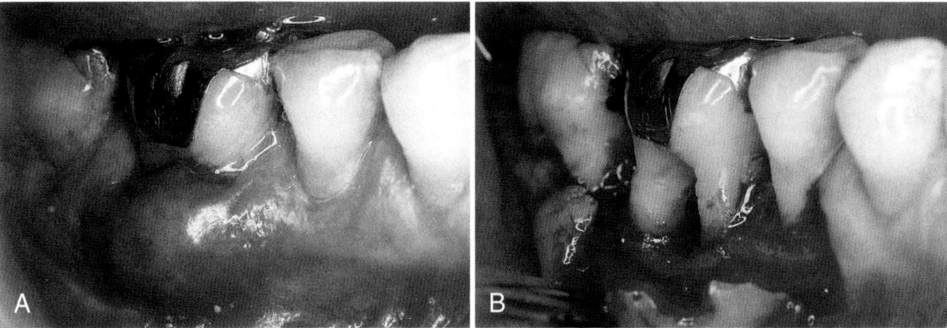

Fig. 69.1 (A) Deep furcation invasions are common locations for the periodontal abscess. (B) Furcation anatomy often prevents the definitive removal of calculus and microbial plaque.

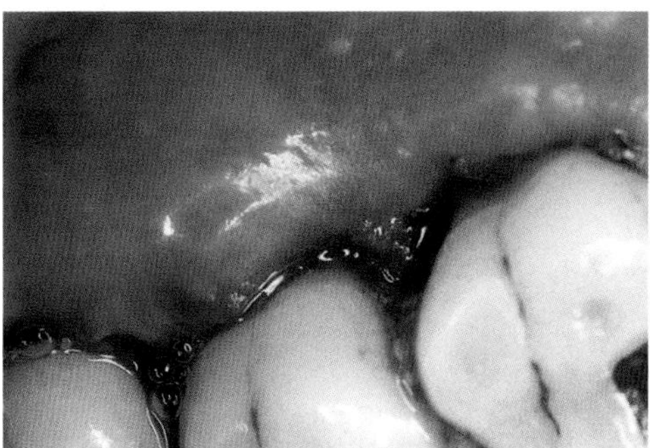

Fig. 69.2 Postprophylaxis periodontal abscess resulting from partial healing of a periodontal pocket over residual calculus.

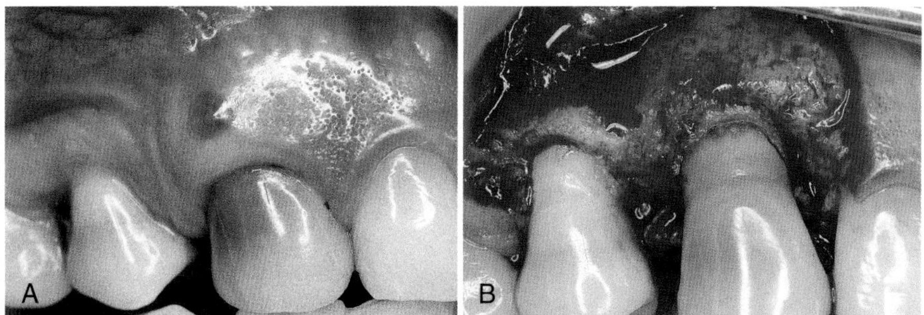

Fig. 69.3 (A) Fistula is observed in attached gingiva of a maxillary right canine. (B) Elevated flap shows the cause to be a root fracture.

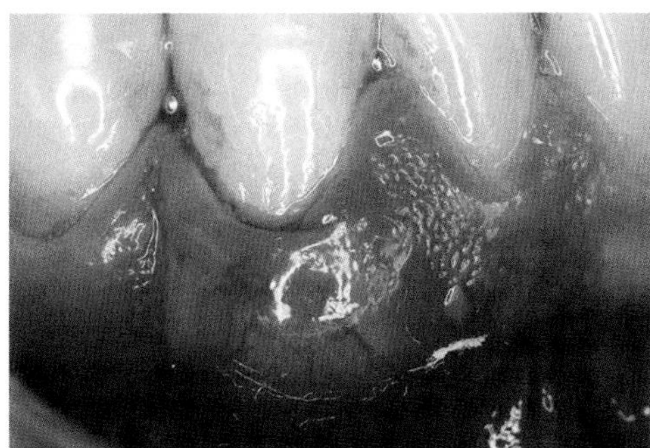

Fig. 69.4 Localized periodontal abscess of a mandibular right canine in a man with poorly controlled type 2 diabetes mellitus. For some patients, periodontal abscess formation may be the first sign of the disease.

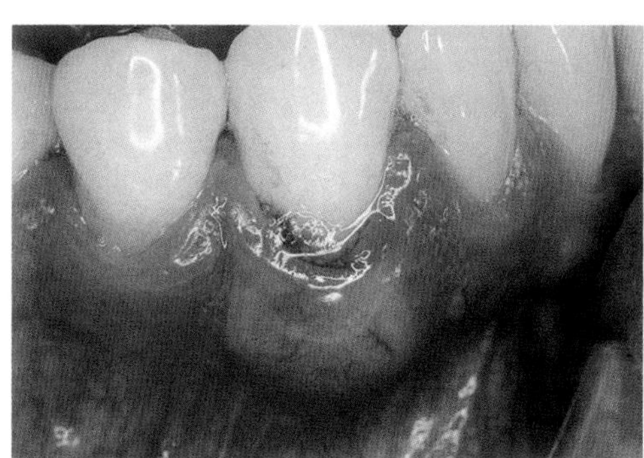

Fig. 69.5 Plaque-associated gingival abscess of a mandibular right canine.

Identification by Course: Onset and Duration

Acute Versus Chronic Abscess

Abscesses have also been described as acute or chronic.[33] Although they are often identified by onset and duration, they can also be distinguished by symptomatology. The *acute abscess* is often an exacerbation of a chronic inflammatory periodontal lesion. Influencing factors include increased numbers and virulence of bacteria combined with lowered tissue resistance and lack of spontaneous drainage.[14,19,41] The drainage may have been prevented by deep, tortuous pocket morphology, debris, or closely adapted pocket epithelium blocking the pocket orifice. Acute abscesses are characterized by painful, red, edematous, smooth, and ovoid swelling of the gingival tissues.[22,25,41] Exudate may be expressed with gentle pressure; the tooth may be percussion sensitive and feel elevated in the socket (Fig. 69.6 and see Fig. 69.9). Fever and regional lymphadenopathy are occasional findings.[33]

The *chronic abscess* develops after the spreading infection has been controlled by spontaneous drainage, host response, or therapy. Once homeostasis between the host and infection has been reached, the patient may have few or no symptoms.[12] However, dull pain may be associated with the clinical findings of a periodontal pocket, inflammation, and a fistulous tract.[33]

Box 69.1 compares the signs and symptoms of acute and chronic abscesses.

As periodontal abscesses usually occur in association with preexisting periodontitis, radiographic evidence of bone loss is not an uncommon finding.

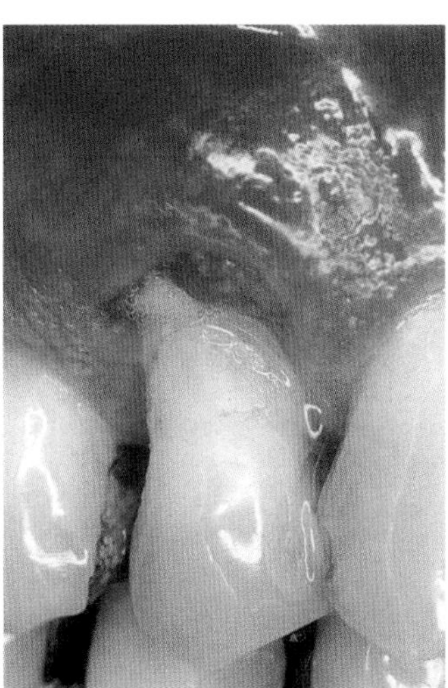

Fig. 69.6 Patient presenting with acute abscess complained of dull pain and a sensation of tooth elevation in the socket. Signs of tissue distention and exudation are evident.

Periodontal Versus Pulpal Abscess

To determine the cause of an abscess and thus establish a proper treatment plan, it is often necessary to perform a differential diagnosis between a periodontal abscess and pulpal abscess[5] (Figs. 69.7 and 69.8). Box 69.2 lists the differential diagnoses comparing the signs and symptoms of the two lesions. Due to the similarity and possible overlap of signs and symptoms, a careful history and examination are essential to reaching a correct diagnosis and treatment. In a small proportion of patients, adjunctive use of cone-beam computed tomography (CBCT) may be useful in situations specifically involving previously root-filled teeth or in periodontally involved maxillary molars.[7,45] However, the inclusion of CBCT should not be used as a substitute for a thorough history and clinical findings and understanding the risks and benefits of radiologic exposure. Selection of the most appropriate imaging protocol for the diagnostic task must be consistent with ALARA principles (***a****s* ***l****ow* ***a****s* ***r****easonably* ***a****chievable*).[40]

Specific Treatment Approaches

Treatment of the periodontal abscess includes two phases—resolving the acute lesion and then managing the resulting chronic condition[19,26,39] (Box 69.3). To ensure proper informed consent, the patient should be advised of the diagnosis, prognosis, treatment options, aftercare, and possible complications. This would include the potential consequences of nontreatment, disease progression, and even tooth loss.[3] Once the condition has been successfully resolved, the need for close monitoring and customized preventive care should be emphasized.[10]

Acute Abscess

The acute abscess is treated to alleviate symptoms, control the spread of infection, and establish drainage.[19,30] Before treatment, the patient's medical history, dental history, and systemic condition are reviewed and evaluated to assist in the diagnosis and determine the possible immediate need for systemic antibiotics[4] (Boxes 69.4 and 69.5). The goal of this phase of treatment is to reduce or eliminate the biofilm and associated mineralized dental deposits within the pocket and initiate the healing process.[10,38]

Drainage Through the Periodontal Pocket

The peripheral area around the abscess is anesthetized with sufficient topical and local anesthetic agents to ensure comfort.

The pocket wall is gently retracted with a periodontal probe or curette in an attempt to initiate drainage through the pocket entrance (Fig. 69.8). Gentle digital pressure and irrigation may be used to express the exudate and drain the pocket (Fig. 69.9). If the lesion is minimal and access is uncomplicated, débridement in the form of scaling and root planing may be undertaken at this appointment. Granulomatous tissue

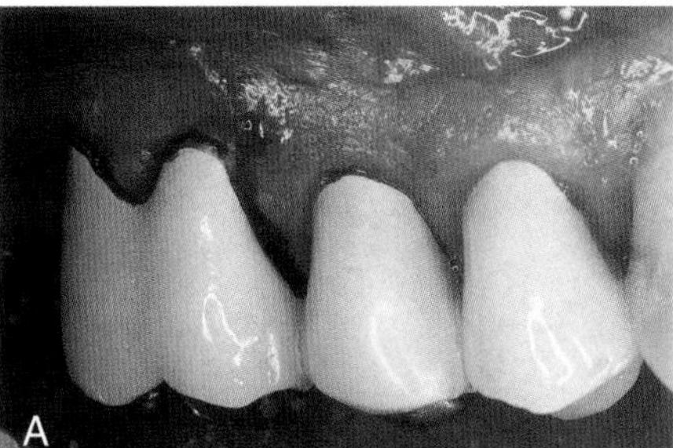
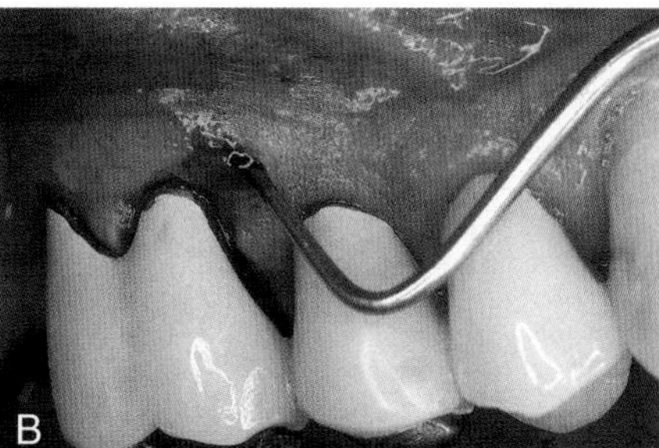
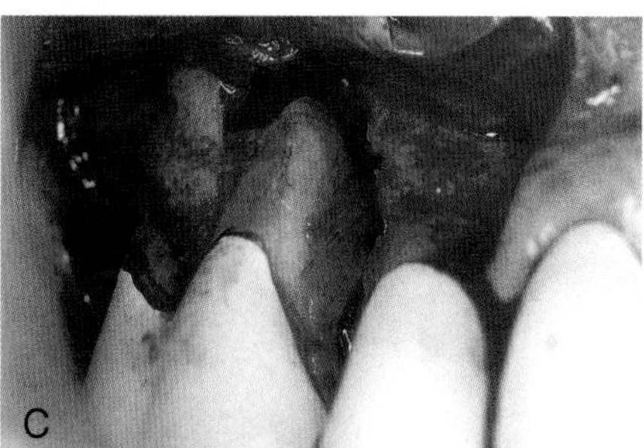

Fig. 69.7 (A) Maxillary right first molar with fistula on the attached gingiva. (B) With local anesthesia, a periodontal probe is introduced through the fistula and angled toward the root end. (C) Surgical flap elevation demonstrates failed endodontic therapy and tooth fracture as causing the fistula.

and tissue tags detached from the internal aspect of the pocket should be removed to forestall postoperative bleeding.

If the lesion is large and drainage cannot be established, root débridement by scaling and root planing or surgical access should be delayed until the major clinical signs have abated.[27,29] In these patients, use of adjunctive systemic antibiotics[17,18,22,25,27] with a short-term, high-dose regimen is recommended[31] (see Box 69.5). Antibiotic therapy alone without subsequent drainage and subgingival scaling is contraindicated[18] because the abscess is likely to re-form because the offending agents, calculus and biofilm, remain in place.[20,33]

Drainage Through an External Incision

To drain the abscess, the lesion is dried and isolated with gauze sponges. A topical anesthetic agent is applied, followed by a local anesthetic agent injected peripherally to the lesion. A vertical incision through the most fluctuant center of the abscess is made with a no. 15 surgical blade. The tissue lateral to the incision can be separated with a curette or periosteal elevator. The fluctuant matter is expressed, and the wound edges are approximated under light digital pressure with a moist gauze pad.

In abscesses manifesting with severe swelling and inflammation, aggressive mechanical instrumentation should be delayed in favor of antibiotic therapy to avoid damage to healthy contiguous periodontal tissues.[39]

Once bleeding and suppuration have ceased, the patient may be dismissed. For patients who do not need systemic antibiotics, posttreatment instructions include frequent rinsing with warm salt water (1 Tbsp per 8-oz glass) and periodic application of chlorhexidine gluconate 0.12% oral rinse, either by rinsing or applying locally with a cotton-tipped applicator. Reduced physical exertion and increased fluid intake are often recommended for patients showing systemic involvement. Analgesics may be prescribed for comfort. By the following day, the signs and symptoms have usually subsided. If the problem continues and the patient is still uncomfortable, the previously recommended regimen is repeated for an additional 24 hours. This often results in satisfactory healing, and the lesion can be treated as a chronic abscess.[41]

BOX 69.1 Signs and Symptoms of Periodontal Abscess

Acute Abscess

- Mild to severe discomfort
- Localized red, ovoid swelling
- Periodontal pocket
- Mobility
- Tooth elevation in socket
- Tenderness to percussion or biting
- Exudation
- Elevated temperature[a]
- Regional lymphadenopathy[a]

Chronic Abscess

- No pain or dull pain
- Localized inflammatory lesion
- Slight tooth elevation
- Intermittent exudation
- Fistulous tract often associated with a deep pocket
- Usually without systemic involvement

[a] May indicate the need for systemic antibiotics.

Data from Dahlén G. Microbiology and treatment of dental abscesses and periodontal-endodontic lesions. *Periodontol 2000* 2002;28:206-239; Meng HX. Periodontal abscess. *Ann Periodontol* 1999;4:79-83; and Sanz M, Herrera D, van Winkelhoff AJ. The periodontal abscess. In Lindhe J, editor: *Clinical periodontology*, Copenhagen, 2003, Munksgaard, pp 260-268.

BOX 69.2 Differential Diagnosis of Periodontal and Pulpal Abscess

Periodontal Abscess

Associated with a preexisting periodontal pocket.
Radiographs show periodontal angular bone loss and furcation radiolucency.
Tests show vital pulp.
Swelling usually includes gingival tissue, with an occasional fistula.
Pain is usually dull and localized.
Sensitivity to percussion may or may not be present.

Pulpal Abscess

The offending tooth may have a large restoration.
The tooth may have no periodontal pocket or, if present, it probes as a narrow defect.
Tests show nonvital pulp.
Swelling is often localized to the apex, with a fistulous tract.
Pain is often severe and difficult to localize.
Sensitivity to percussion is noted.

Modified from Corbet EF: Diagnosis of acute periodontal lesions. *Periodontol 2000* 2004;34:204-216.

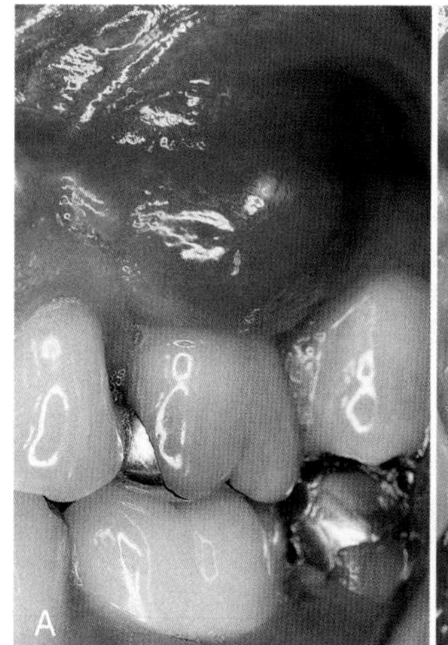

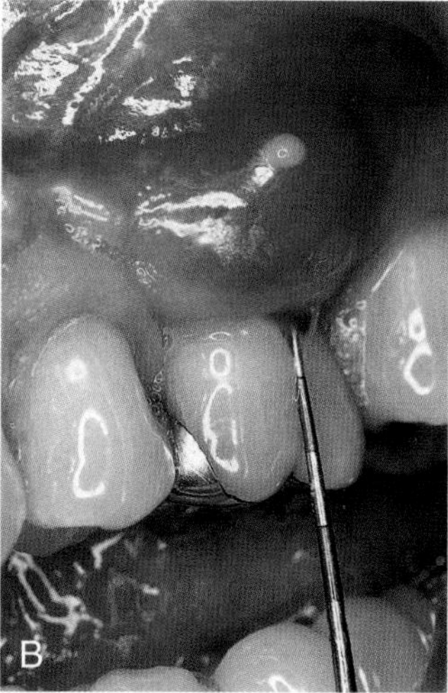

Fig. 69.8 (A) Periodontal abscess of maxillary left first molar. (B) Periodontal probe is used to retract the pocket wall gently.

Chronic Abscess

As with a periodontal pocket, the chronic abscess is usually treated with scaling and root planing and, if indicated, surgical therapy. Surgical treatment is suggested when deep pockets or furcation defects are encountered that are beyond the therapeutic capabilities of nonsurgical instrumentation (see Fig. 69.1). Access to subgingival calculus must be achieved in areas of deep pockets. The patient should be advised of the possible postoperative sequelae usually associated with periodontal nonsurgical and surgical procedures. As with the acute abscess, antibiotic therapy may be indicated.[19,27,34,41]

LEARNING BOX 69.3

Periodontal abscess due to a deep periodontal pocket often requires a surgical flap to access the subgingival calculus. This also allows the clinician to reduce the pocket at the same surgical appointment.

Gingival Abscess

Treatment of the gingival abscess is aimed at reversal of the acute phase and, when applicable, immediate removal of the cause. To ensure comfort, topical or local anesthesia by infiltration is administered. When possible, scaling and root planing are completed to establish drainage and remove microbial deposits. In more acute situations, the fluctuant area is incised with a no. 15 scalpel blade, and exudate may be expressed by gentle digital pressure. Any foreign material (e.g., dental floss, impression material) is removed. The area is irrigated with warm water and covered with moist gauze under light pressure.

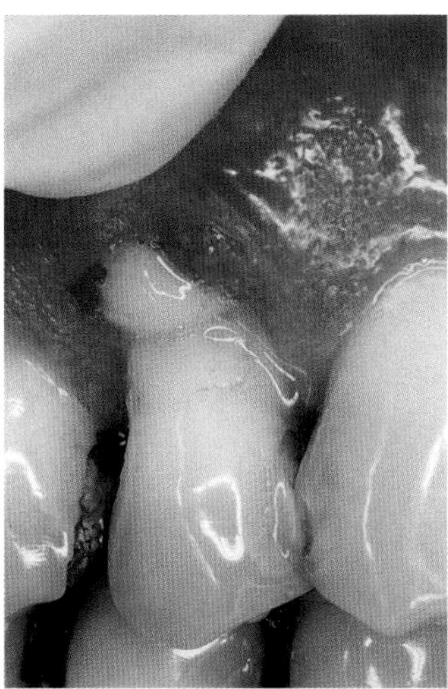

Fig. 69.9 Gentle digital pressure may be sufficient to express purulent discharge.

BOX 69.3 Treatment Options for Periodontal Abscess

1. Drainage through pocket retraction or incision
2. Scaling and root planing
3. Periodontal surgery
4. Systemic antibiotics
5. Tooth removal

Modified from Sanz M, Herrera D, van Winkelhoff AJ: The periodontal abscess. In Lindhe J, editor: *Clinical periodontology,* Copenhagen, 2000, Munksgaard.

BOX 69.4 Indications for Antibiotic Therapy in Patients with Acute Abscess

1. Cellulitis (nonlocalized, spreading infection)
2. Deep inaccessible pocket
3. Fever
4. Regional lymphadenopathy
5. Immunocompromised status

BOX 69.5 Antibiotic Options for Periodontal Infections

Antibiotic of Choice

Amoxicillin, 500 mg

- 1.0-g loading dose, then 500 mg three times a day for 3 days
- Reevaluation after 3 days to determine need for continued or adjusted antibiotic therapy

Penicillin Allergy

Clindamycin

- 600-mg loading dose, then 300 mg four times a day for 3 days

Azithromycin (or Clarithromycin)[a]

- 1.0-g loading dose, then 500 mg four times a day for 3 days

Acute, Severe Lesions: Alternatives

Metronidazole

- 250 mg three times a day for 3 days

Amoxicillin plus Clavulanate (Augmentin)

- 500 mg plus clavulanate 125 ms (Augmentin), 3 times daily for the duration of the acute lesion, usually 23 days

[a]To be used with caution in patients with high baseline cardiovascular risk.

Data from Slots J; Research, Science and Therapy Committee. American Academy of Periodontology: Position paper: systemic antibiotics in periodontics. *J Periodontol* 2004;67:1553-1565; Herrera D, Alonso B, de Arriba L, et al: Acute periodontal lesions. *Periodontol 2000.* 2004;65:149-177.

Once bleeding has stopped, the patient is dismissed with instructions to rinse with warm salt water every 2 hours for the remainder of the day. After 24 hours, the area is reassessed and, if resolution is sufficient, scaling not previously completed is undertaken. If the residual lesion is large or poorly accessible, surgical access may be required.

Pericoronal Abscess

As with other abscesses of the periodontium, treatment of the pericoronal abscess is aimed at management of the acute phase, followed by resolution of the chronic condition. The acute pericoronal abscess is properly anesthetized for comfort, and drainage is established by gently lifting the soft tissue operculum with a curette. If the underlying debris is easily accessible, it may be removed, followed by gentle irrigation with sterile saline. If the patient has regional swelling, lymphadenopathy, or systemic signs, systemic antibiotics may be prescribed.

The patient is dismissed with instructions to rinse with warm salt water every 2 hours, and the area is reassessed after 24 hours. If discomfort was one of the original complaints, appropriate analgesics should be used. Once the acute phase has been controlled, the partially erupted tooth may be definitively treated with either surgical excision of the overlying tissue or removal of the offending tooth.

Microbiology and Antibiotic Therapy

Periodontal abscesses have the clinical and microbiologic characteristics commonly associated with severe forms of periodontitis (stages III and IV; grades B and C). Generally, they have a sizable bacterial mass and a high prevalence of well-recognized putative periodontal pathogens, including *Porphyromonas gingivalis* (50%–100%), *Prevotella intermedia, Prevotella melaninogenica, Fusobacterium nucleatum, Tannerella forsythia, Treponema* spp., *Campylobacter* spp. *Capnocytophaga* spp., *Aggregatibacter actinomycetemcomitans*, and gram-negative enteric rods.[20,23]

Notwithstanding the positive clinical effects of systemic antimicrobials, imprudent use can contribute to the development of drug-resistant species for individual patients and as a global health

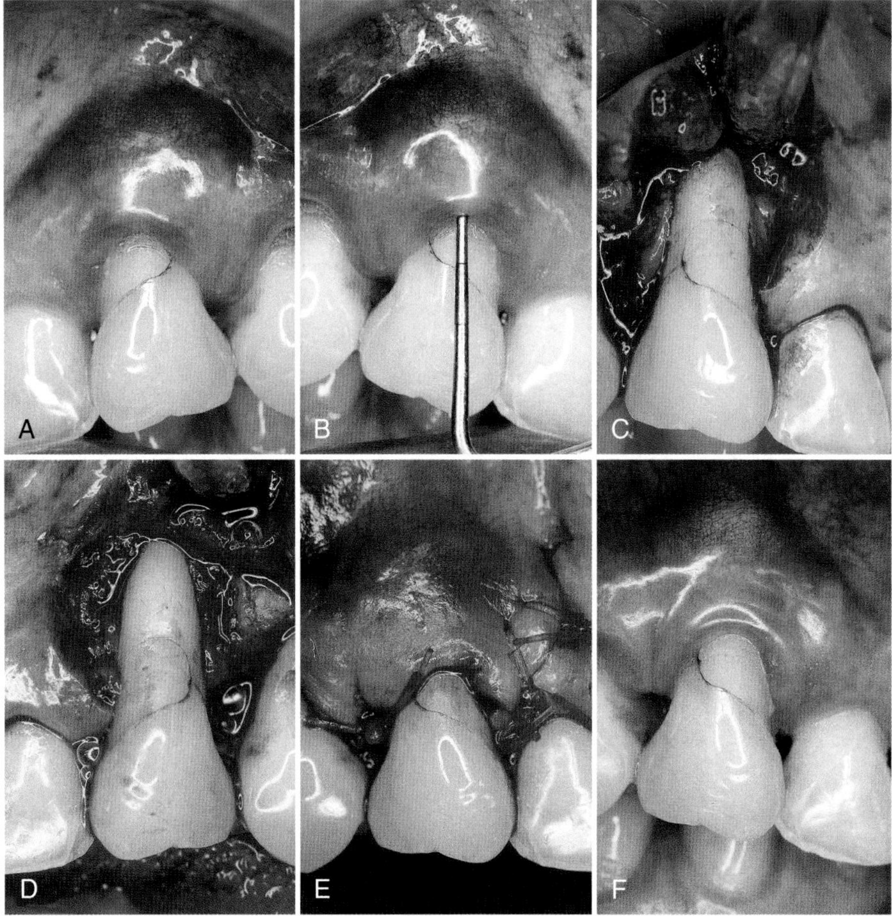

Fig. 69.10 (A) Chronic periodontal abscess of a maxillary right canine. (B) With local anesthesia, a periodontal probe is inserted to determine severity of the lesion. (C) With mesial and distal vertical incisions, a full-thickness flap is elevated, exposing severe bone dehiscence, a subgingival restoration, and root calculus. (D) The root surface has been planed free of calculus, and the restoration has been smoothed. (E) Full-thickness flap has been replaced to its original position and sutured with absorbable sutures. (F) At 3 months, gingival tissues are pink, firm, and well adapted to the tooth, with minimal periodontal probing depth.

BOX 69.6 Periodontal Abscesses Classified According to Etiology

Microbial Plaque–Associated Periodontitis Patients

Preexisting periodontal pocket

- Acute exacerbation of untreated microbial plaque-associated periodontitis
- Periodontitis not responsive to therapy
- During supportive periodontal therapy

After Periodontal Treatment

- Postscaling
- Postsurgery
- Postmedication (systemic antimicrobials)

Nonperiodontitis Patients

- Foreign body impaction
- Factitial habits
- Orthodontic procedures
- Gingival enlargement
- Root fracture
- Root perforation
- External root resorption
- Apical periodontitis

[a]To be used with caution in patients with high baseline cardiovascular risk.
Adapted from Herrera D, Retamal-Valdes B, Alonso B, Feres M. Acute periodontal lesions (periodontal abscesses and necrotizing periodontal diseases) and endo-periodontal lesions. *J Periodontol.* 2018;89(Suppl 1):S85–S102.

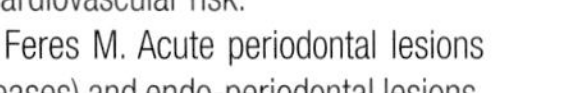

problem. Their use should be restricted as much as possible to patients for whom systemic antimicrobials make a clinically relevant difference, such as severe, diffuse, nondraining lesions, patients showing systemic spread, or those with compromised immune systems.[19,24,42]

The precise effects of the various antibiotics on the different stages and grades of periodontitis, including the periodontal abscess, have yet to be determined. However, several antibiotics and regimens have been identified in the literature as being applicable to the periodontal abscess. Those recommended follow the high-dose, short-course model of use[19,20,24,37,42,46] (Box 69.6).

In general, adjunctive systemic antibiotics should be taken simultaneously with the mechanical removal of supragingival and subgingival deposits and bacterial biofilms.[37] However, if definitive treatment is delayed and antibiotic therapy instituted, follow-up evaluation and therapy should be scheduled for the short term (2–5 days). Failure to do so can have a severe negative effect because a rapid microbiologic rebound may lead to repeated abscess formation and a significantly poorer prognosis.[6,19,21] In fact, a periodontal abscess is the leading cause of tooth loss during supportive periodontal therapy.[6,9]

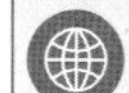
A Case Scenario is found on the companion website eBooks.Health.Elsevier.com.

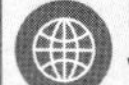
References for this chapter are found on the companion website eBooks.Health.Elsevier.com.

CHAPTER 70

Supportive Periodontal Treatment

Robert L. Merin 

CHAPTER OUTLINE

Preservation of the periodontal health of the treated patient requires a supportive program that is just as important as the therapy used to treat the periodontal disease. After phase I therapy has been completed, patients are placed on a schedule of periodic recall visits for maintenance care to prevent the recurrence of the disease (Figs. 70.1 and 70.2).

LEARNING BOX 70.1

The long-term preservation of the dentition is closely associated with the frequency and quality of recall maintenance.

Transfer of the patient from active treatment status to a maintenance program is a definitive step in total patient care that requires time and effort on the part of the dentist and staff. Patients must understand the purpose of the maintenance program, and the dentist must emphasize that preservation of the teeth depends on maintenance therapy.[6,10,77] Patients who are not maintained in a supervised recall program subsequent to active treatment show obvious signs of recurrent periodontitis (e.g., increased pocket depth, bone loss, or tooth loss).[7,8,10,14,15,21,23,49] The more often patients present for recommended supportive periodontal treatment (SPT), the less likely they are to lose teeth.[23,37,44,49,52,68,73] One study indicated that treated patients who do not return for regular recall have a 5.6 times greater risk for tooth loss than compliant patients.[15]

LEARNING BOX 70.2

Patients who do not return for SPT lose five to six times more teeth than compliant patients.

Cortellini et al, showed that patients with inadequate SPT after successful regenerative therapy have a 50-fold increase in risk of probing attachment loss compared with those who have regular recall visits.[19] Costa et al.[20,24,25] published a group of studies on the benefits of regular compliance with supportive periodontal therapy over a 6-year period. This group found that regular visits during maintenance sustained the reduction in levels of bacteria associated with periodontitis provided by active therapy over a 6-year period.[25] Irregular compliance with SPT led to increased plasma levels of c-reactive protein and higher recurrence of periodontitis.[24] Regular compliers showed improved oral health-related quality of life measures (OHRQL) compared to erratic compliers over a 6-year period.[20]

LEARNING BOX 70.3

Patients who do not have regular SPT have increased plasma levels of c-reactive protein, higher levels of bacteria associated with periodontitis, and more recurrence of periodontitis compared to regular compliers with SPT.

Motivational techniques and reinforcement of the importance of the maintenance phase of treatment should be considered before performing definitive periodontal surgery.[8,77] Studies show that few patients display complete compliance with recommended maintenance schedules (Fig. 70.3A).[1,5,10,43,44,50,51,77,74] Wilson and colleagues[77] presented the results of his efforts to improve patient compliance by simplifying compliance, maintaining records of compliance, informing patients of the consequences of noncompliance, and attempting to identify noncompliers before active periodontal therapy was initiated (see Fig. 70.3B). Because of these efforts the complete compliers improved from 16.4% to 32%. It is important to inform patients that they are to return for periodic recall visits, clearly explain the significance of these visits, and describe what is expected of patients between visits.

The maintenance phase of periodontal treatment starts immediately after the completion of phase I therapy (see Figs. 70.1 and 70.2). While the patient is in the maintenance phase, the necessary surgical and restorative procedures are performed. This ensures that all areas of the mouth retain the degree of health attained after phase I therapy.

Rationale for Supportive Periodontal Treatment

Studies indicate that even with appropriate periodontal therapy, some progression of disease is possible.[22,32,34,46,53,58,60,67,75] One likely explanation for the recurrence of periodontal disease is incomplete subgingival plaque/biofilm and calculus removal.[70,75] If subgingival biofilm is left behind during scaling, it regrows within the pocket. The regrowth of subgingival biofilm is a slow process compared with that of supragingival biofilm. During this period (perhaps months), the subgingival biofilm may not induce inflammatory reactions that can be discerned at the gingival margin. The clinical diagnosis may be further confused by the introduction of

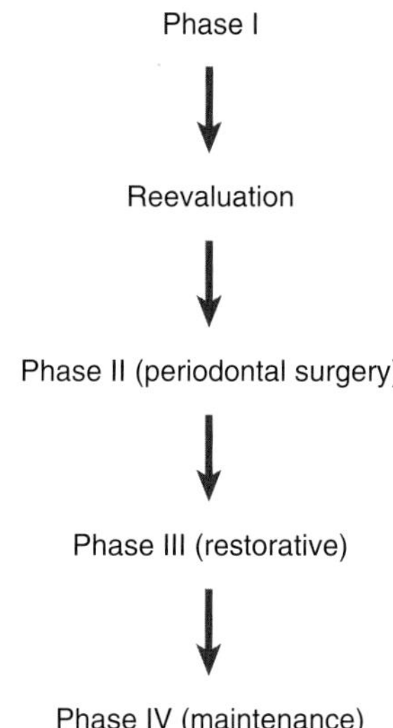

Fig. 70.1 Incorrect sequence of periodontal treatment phases. Maintenance phase should be started immediately after the reevaluation of phase I therapy.

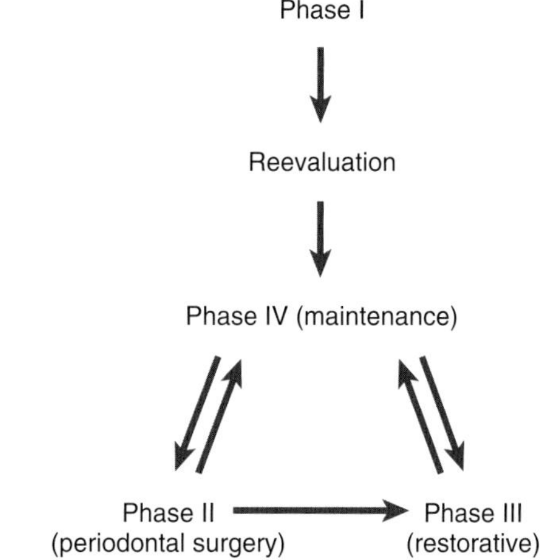

Fig. 70.2 Correct sequence of periodontal treatment phases.

adequate supragingival biofilm control because the inflammatory reactions caused by the biofilm in the soft-tissue wall of the pocket are not likely to manifest clinically as gingival erythema and edema.[26] Thus, inadequate subgingival biofilm control can lead to continued loss of attachment, even without the presence of clinical gingival inflammation. Scaling and root planing are generally not effective at sites with probing depths of 6 mm or greater.[6]

Bacteria are present in the gingival tissues in chronic and aggressive periodontitis cases.[11,17,27,57] Eradication of intragingival microorganisms may be necessary for a stable periodontal result.[27] Scaling, root planing, and even flap surgery may not eliminate intragingival bacteria in some areas.[11] These bacteria may recolonize the pocket and cause recurrent disease.

Bacteria associated with periodontitis can be transmitted between spouses and other family members.[2,69] Patients who appear to be successfully treated can become infected or reinfected with potential pathogens. This is especially likely in patients with remaining pockets.

Another possible explanation for the recurrence of periodontal disease is the microscopic nature of the dentogingival unit healing after periodontal treatment. Histologic studies have indicated that after periodontal procedures, tissues usually heal by the formation of a long junctional epithelium instead of new connective tissue attachment to root surfaces.[13,60,64] It has been speculated that this

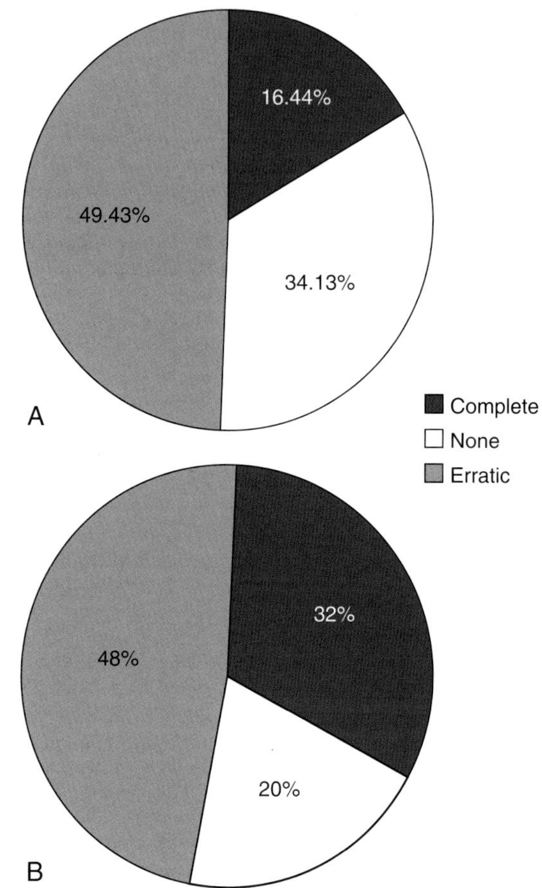

Fig. 70.3 (A) Compliance with maintenance therapy in 961 patients studied for 1 to 8 years. (B) The results of efforts to improve compliance with supportive periodontal treatment. (Modified from Wilson TG Jr, Glover ME, Schoen J, et al. Compliance with maintenance therapy in a private periodontal practice. *J Periodontol.* 1984;55:468.; Adapted from Wilson TG, Hale S, Temple R. The results of efforts to improve compliance with supportive periodontal treatment in a private practice. *J Periodontol.* 1993;64:311.)

type of dentogingival unit may be weaker and that inflammation may rapidly separate the long junctional epithelium from the tooth. Thus treated periodontal patients may be predisposed to recurrent pocket formation if maintenance care is not optimal.

Subgingival scaling alters the microflora of periodontal pockets.[45,56,61] In one study, a single session of scaling and root planing in patients with chronic periodontitis resulted in significant changes in subgingival microflora.[45] Reported alterations included a decrease in the proportion of motile rods for 1 week, a marked elevation in the proportion of coccoid cells for 21 days, and a marked reduction in the proportion of spirochetes for 7 weeks.

Although pocket debridement suppresses components of the subgingival microflora associated with periodontitis, periodontal pathogens may return to baseline levels within days or months.[4,60] The return of pathogens to pretreatment levels generally occurs in approximately 9 to 11 weeks but can vary dramatically among patients.[3]

LEARNING BOX 70.4

Scaling and root planing are generally not effective at sites with probing depths of 6 mm or greater.

Both the mechanical debridement performed by the therapist and the motivational environment provided by the appointment seem to be necessary for good maintenance results. Patients tend to reduce their oral hygiene efforts between appointments.[3,73] Knowing that their hygiene will be evaluated motivates them to perform better oral hygiene in anticipation of the appointment.

In one study, the proportion of spirochetes obtained in baseline samples of subgingival flora was highly correlated with clinical periodontal deterioration over 1 year.[40] However, subsequent reports in the same longitudinal study concluded that the arbitrary assignment of treated periodontitis patients to 3-month maintenance intervals appears to be as effective in preventing recurrences of periodontitis as assignment of recall intervals based on microscopic monitoring of the subgingival flora.[39,40] Microscopic monitoring was found not to be a reliable predictor of future periodontal destruction in patients on 3-month recall programs, presumably because of the alteration of subgingival flora produced by subgingival instrumentation.

In conclusion, there is a sound scientific basis for recall maintenance because subgingival scaling alters the pocket microflora for variable but relatively long periods.

Maintenance Program

Periodic recall visits form the foundation of a meaningful long-term prevention program. The interval between visits is usually set at 3 months but may vary according to the patient's needs.[6,18,28,29,35,36,41,48,55]

Periodontal care at each recall visit comprises three parts (Box 70.1). The first part involves examination and evaluation of the patient's current oral health. The second part includes the necessary maintenance treatment and oral hygiene reinforcement. The third part involves scheduling the patient for the next recall appointment, additional periodontal treatment, or restorative dental procedures. The time required for a recall visit for patients with multiple teeth in both arches is approximately 1 hour.[59]

BOX 70.1 Maintenance Recall Procedures

Part I: Examination
(Approximate time: 14 min)
Patient greeting
Medical history changes
Oral pathologic examination
Oral hygiene status
Gingival changes
Pocket depth changes
Mobility changes
Occlusal changes
Dental caries
Restorative, prosthetic, and implant status

Part II: Treatment
(Approximate time: 36 min)
Oral hygiene reinforcement
Scaling
Polishing
Chemical irrigation or site-specific antimicrobial placement

Part III: Report, Cleanup, and Scheduling
(Approximate time: 10 min)
Write report in chart.
Discuss report with patient.
Clean and disinfect operatory.
Schedule next recall visit.
Schedule further periodontal treatment.
Schedule or refer for restorative or prosthetic treatment.

LEARNING BOX 70.5

There are three parts to an SPT appointment: (1) examination; (2) treatment; and (3) report, cleanup, and scheduling.

Examination and Evaluation

The recall examination is similar to the initial evaluation of the patient (see Chapter 38). However, because the patient is not new to the office, the dentist or hygienist primarily looks for changes that have occurred since the last evaluation. Analysis of the current oral hygiene status of the patient is essential. Updating of changes in the medical history and evaluation of restorations, caries, prostheses, occlusion, tooth mobility, gingival status, and periodontal and peri-implant probing depths are important parts of the recall appointment. The oral mucosa should be carefully inspected for pathologic conditions (Figs. 70.4–70.9).

Radiographic examination must be individualized,[31] depending on the initial severity of the case and the findings during the recall visit (Table 70.1). These are compared with findings on previous radiographs to check the bone height and look for repair of osseous defects, signs of trauma from occlusion, periapical pathologic changes, and caries.

Checking of Plaque/Biofilm Control

To assess the effectiveness of their plaque control, patients should perform their hygiene regimen immediately before the recall appointment. Plaque/biofilm control must be reviewed and corrected until the patient demonstrates the necessary proficiency, even if additional instruction sessions are required. A motivational interviewing technique of teaching may help to produce positive results.[71] Patients instructed in plaque/biofilm control have less biofilm and gingivitis than uninstructed patients,[7,65,66] and because the

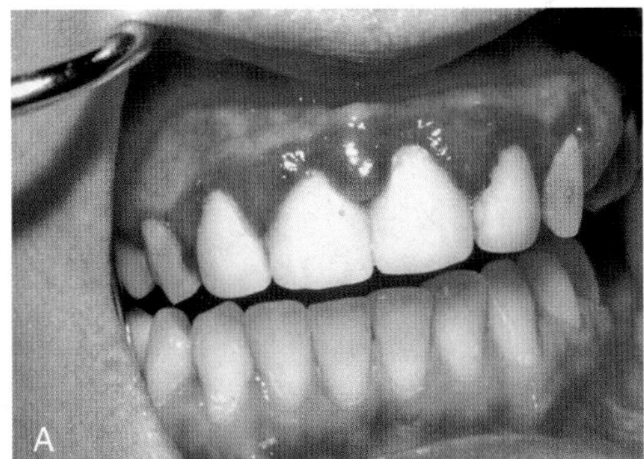

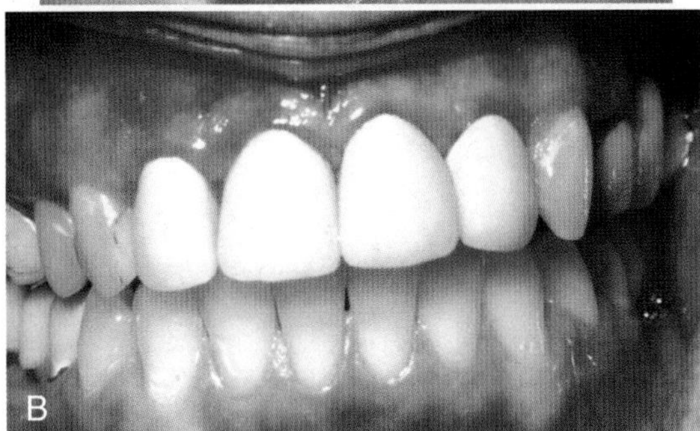

Fig. 70.4 (A) Hyperplastic gingivitis related to crown margins and plaque accumulation in a 27-year-old woman. (B) Four months after treatment, there is significant improvement. However, some inflammation around crown margins still exists, which cannot be resolved without replacing the crowns.

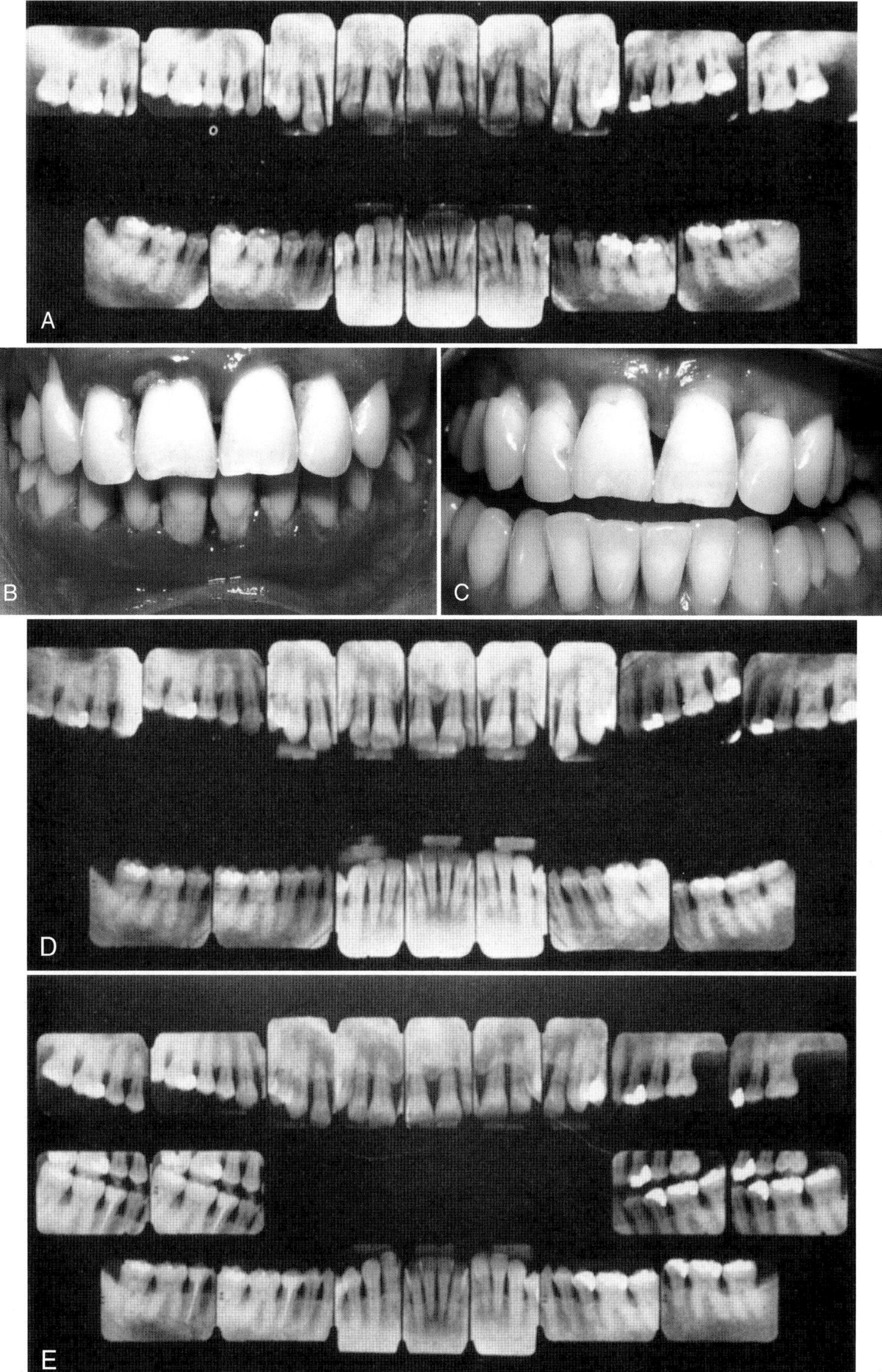

Fig. 70.5 (A) Patient was 38 years old when these original radiographs were taken and was treated with a combination of surgical and nonsurgical therapy. This individual is a classic class C maintenance patient. (B) Pretreatment photograph. Note the inflammation and heavy calculus deposits. (C) Photograph taken 10 years after treatment. (D) Radiographs taken 5 years after treatment. (E) Radiographs taken 10 years after treatment. The radiographic appearance is as good as can be expected in such a severe case. Teeth #15 and #17 were extracted 8 years after treatment.

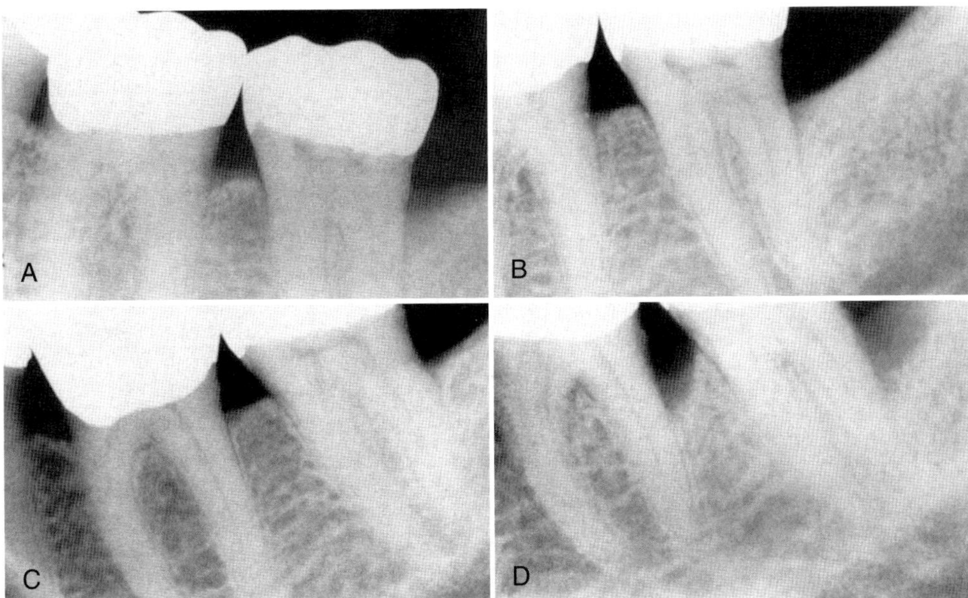

Fig. 70.6 This series of radiographs clearly shows the importance of maintenance therapy. (A) Original radiograph of a 58-year-old male. Note the deep distal bone loss on tooth #18 and the moderate distal lesion of tooth #19. Surgical treatment included osseous grafting. (B) Radiograph 14 months after surgical therapy. The patient had recall maintenance performed every 3 to 4 months. (C) Appearance 3 years after surgery, with regular recalls every 3 to 4 months. (D) Appearance after 2 years without recalls (7 years after surgery). Note the progression of the disease on the distal surfaces of teeth #18 and #19.

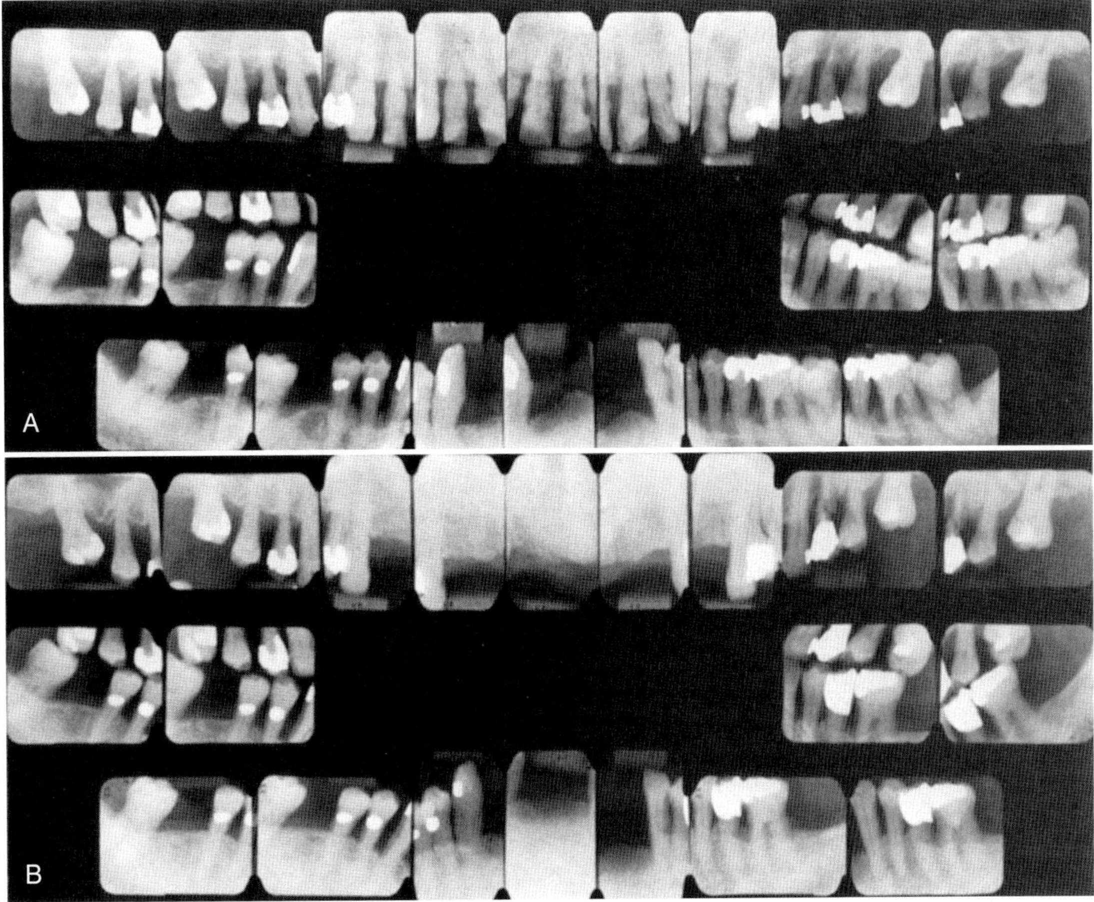

Fig. 70.7 Advanced cases sometimes do better than expected when the patient complies with maintenance therapy. (A) Initial radiographs showing an advanced case. The maxillary arch had extractions and nonsurgical treatment. A plastic partial denture was placed and was expected to grow into a full denture within a few years. The mandibular arch was treated with periodontal surgery, and a permanent, metal and plastic, removable partial denture was placed. (B) Radiographs taken 8 years later. The patient performed good oral hygiene and had 3-month recalls. Teeth #12 and #15 required extraction.

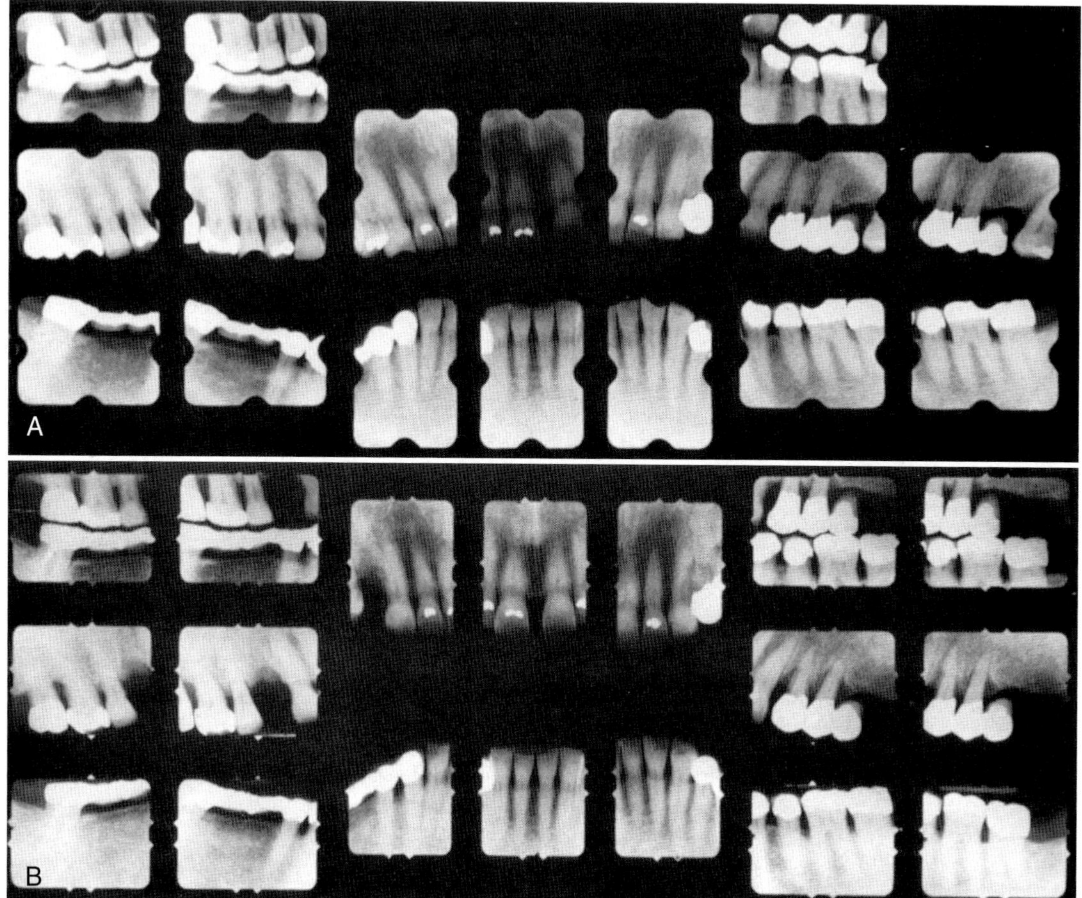

Fig. 70.8 (A) Initial radiographs. The patient was advised to have localized areas of periodontal surgery and periodontal recall every 3 months. However, the patient did not comply and only had dental cleanings once or twice yearly. (B) Radiographs 4 years later. Note the loss of teeth #5 and #15 and the increased bone loss of several premolars and molars.

amount of supragingival plaque/biofilm is less, there is a decrease in the number of subgingival anaerobic organisms.[13,62]

Treatment

Following consultation, examination, and oral hygiene instruction, the required scaling and root planing are performed (see Chapter 51). Care must be taken not to instrument healthy sites with shallow sulci (1- to 3-mm deep) and an absence of gingival inflammation because studies have indicated that repeated subgingival scaling and root planing of sites not periodontally involved result in significant loss of attachment and gingival recession, which will affect esthetics.[38] Irrigation with antimicrobial agents or placement of site-specific antimicrobial devices may be performed in maintenance patients with remaining pockets.[4,33,42]

Recurrence of Periodontal Disease

Occasionally, lesions may recur, which is often due to inadequate plaque/biofilm control on the part of the patient or failure to comply with recommended SPT schedules. It should be understood, however, that it is the responsibility of the dentist to educate and motivate patients to improve their oral hygiene techniques. Surgery should not be undertaken unless the patient participates in disease prevention and demonstrates proficiency in plaque/biofilm control.[8,67,72]

Other causes for recurrence include the following:

1. Inadequate or insufficient treatment that has failed to remove all of the potential factors favoring biofilm accumulation (see Fig. 70.4). Incomplete calculus removal in areas of difficult access is a common source of problems.
2. Inadequate restorations placed after the periodontal treatment was completed.
3. Failure of the patient to return for periodic maintenance care (see Fig. 70.6). This may be a result of the patient's conscious or unconscious decision not to continue treatment or the failure of the dentist and staff to emphasize the need for periodic supportive therapy.
4. Presence of some systemic diseases that may affect host resistance to previously acceptable levels of biofilm.

A failing case can be recognized by the following:

1. Recurring inflammation revealed by gingival changes and bleeding of the sulcus on probing.
2. Increasing depth of sulci, leading to the recurrence of pocket formation.
3. Gradual increases in bone loss, as determined by radiographs.
4. Gradual increases in tooth mobility, as ascertained by clinical examination.

The decision to retreat a periodontal patient should not be made at the preventive maintenance appointment but should be postponed for 1 to 2 weeks.[14] Often, the mouth appears improved at that time because of the resolution of edema and the resulting improved tone of the gingiva. Table 70.2 summarizes the symptoms of the recurrence of periodontal disease and their probable causes.

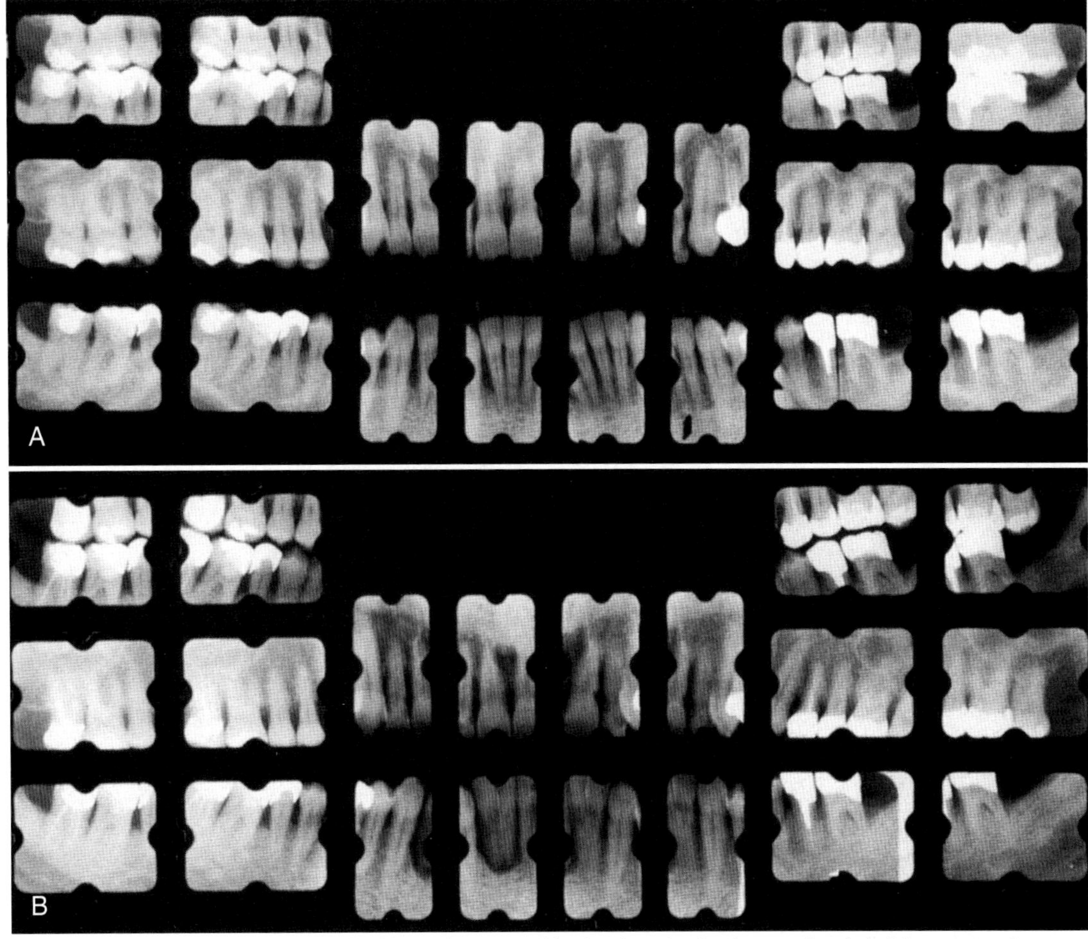

Fig. 70.9 (A) Initial radiographs. The patient was advised to have localized areas of periodontal surgery and periodontal recall every 3 months. However, the patient did not comply and had no treatment other than emergency care and occasional dental cleanings. (B) Radiographs 7 years later. Note the advanced bone loss and caries on many teeth.

TABLE 70.1 Radiographic Examination of Recall Patients for Supportive Periodontal Treatment

Patient Condition/Situation	Type of Examination
Clinical caries or high-risk factors for caries	Posterior bitewing examination at 6- to 18-month intervals
No clinical caries and no high-risk factors for caries	Posterior bitewing examination at 24- to 36-month intervals
Periodontal disease not under good control	Periapical or vertical bitewing radiographs of problem areas every 12–24 months
History of periodontal treatment with disease under good control	Bitewing examination every 24–36 months
Root form dental implants	Periapical or vertical bitewing radiographs after prosthetic placement and at 12 and 24 months, then every 24–36 months unless clinical problems arise
Transfer of periodontal or implant maintenance patients	Full-mouth series if a current set not available; if full-mouth series has been taken within 24 months, radiographs of implants and periodontal problem areas should be taken

Radiographs should be taken when they are likely to affect diagnosis and patient treatment. The recommendations in this table are subject to clinical judgment and may not apply to every patient. Adapted from Guide to Patient Selection and Limiting Radiation Exposure. American Dental Association website. https://www.ada.org/en/member-center/oral-health-topics/x-rays. Accessed September 10, 2021.

Classification of Posttreatment Patients and Risk Assessment

The first year after periodontal therapy is important in terms of indoctrinating the patient in a recall pattern and reinforcing oral hygiene techniques. In addition, it may take several months to evaluate accurately the results of some periodontal surgical procedures. Consequently, some areas may have to be retreated because the results may not be optimal. Furthermore, the first-year patient often has etiologic factors that may have been overlooked and may be amenable to treatment at this early stage. For these reasons, the recall interval for first-year patients should not be longer than 3 months.

Patients who are on a periodontal recall schedule are a varied group. Table 70.3 lists several categories of maintenance patients and a suggested recall interval for each group. Patients can improve

TABLE 70.2 Symptoms and Causes of Recurrence of Disease

Symptom	Possible Causes
Increased mobility	Increased inflammation Poor oral hygiene Subgingival calculus Inadequate restorations Deteriorating or poorly designed prostheses Systemic disease modifying host response to plaque
Recession	Toothbrush abrasion Inadequate keratinized gingiva Frenum pull Orthodontic therapy
Increased mobility with no change in pocket depth and no radiographic change	Occlusal trauma caused by lateral occlusal interference, bruxism, high restoration Poorly designed or worn-out prosthesis Poor crown-to-root ratio
Increased pocket depth with no radiographic change	Poor oral hygiene Infrequent recall visits Subgingival calculus Poorly fitting partial denture Mesial inclination into edentulous space Failure of new attachment surgery Cracked teeth Grooves in teeth New periodontal disease Gingival overgrowth caused by medication
Increased pocket depth with increased radiographic bone loss	Poor oral hygiene Subgingival calculus Infrequent recall visits Inadequate or deteriorating restorations Poorly designed prostheses Inadequate surgery Systemic disease modifying host response to plaque Cracked teeth Grooves in teeth New periodontal disease

or may relapse to a different classification, with a reduction in or exacerbation of periodontal disease. When one dental arch is more involved than the other, the patient's periodontal disease is classified by the arch with the worse condition.

Table 70.3 illustrates a traditional method of assigning the risk of a recurrence of periodontal destruction. A practitioner uses the listed risk factors and his or her own diagnostic and prognostic gestalt to assign a risk category and maintenance schedule. The UK National Institute for Health and Care Excellence (NICE) has developed a checklist form to help dentists assess risk and set patient recall intervals.[18,48] This NICE form with instructions can be accessed at the website for the National Institute for Health and Care Excellence (UK) (www.nice.org.uk). The NICE form can be used for general patients and periodontal patients, and "SCENARIO J" on page 28 of the NICE Guide is an example of the risk assessment summary for a periodontal patient.

Automated factor assessment tools for the prevention of periodontal destruction have been developed.[30,35,36,47] The Periodontal Risk Assessment (PRA) and the Periodontal Risk Calculator (PRC) have the most studies documenting their ability to predict the progression of periodontitis and tooth loss.[35] The PRC is marketed by the PreViser Corporation and offers a web-based system for periodontal risk analysis and prognosis.[30] The PRA is offered free of charge by the Clinical Research Foundation and the University of Bern at http://www.perio-tools.com/PRA/en/index.asp. Patient data are entered into the online form, and the program automatically calculates whether the patient is at low risk, moderate risk, or high risk; an appropriate recall interval is then suggested. Fig. 70.10 is a sample assessment from the PRA website. Because the different assessment tools use different risk factors and algorithms, they will not be in complete agreement.[47,54] In one study, 57 patients were assessed with the PRC and PRA.[47] The PRC classified 14 as low risk, 17 as medium risk, and 26 as high risk, whereas the PRA classified 8 as low risk, 28 as medium risk, and 21 as high risk.[47] In another study, PRC and PRA were in agreement about 60% of the time.[54]

Currently, there is no universally accepted objective method of predicting periodontitis progression, and there has been little research to determine if the risk calculators are more accurate than good clinical judgment.[30] In summary, maintenance care is a critical phase of therapy. The long-term preservation of the dentition is closely associated with the frequency and quality of recall maintenance.

LEARNING BOX 70.6

The therapist should use risk assessment to determine SPT frequency.

Referral of Patients to the Periodontist

A general dentist can properly manage many periodontal patients as a greater number of people retain their teeth throughout their lifetime. Another important fact to consider is that as the proportion of older people in the population increases, more teeth will be at risk for periodontal disease. Numerous studies indicate possible links between periodontal disease and systemic diseases, such as heart disease, stroke, diabetes, and adverse pregnancy outcomes. Therefore the prevalence of patients requiring SPT is likely to increase in the future.

This expected increase in the number of periodontal patients will necessitate a greater understanding of periodontal problems and an increased level of expertise for the solution of such problems on the part of the general practitioner. General dentists must know when co-management with a periodontist is indicated. Specialists are needed to treat difficult periodontal cases, patients with systemic health problems, complicated dental implant patients, and those with a complex prosthetic construction that requires predictable results.

The criteria for cases to be treated in the general dental office and cases to be referred to a specialist vary for different practitioners and patients. The American Academy of Periodontology has issued guidelines to help the general practitioner decide when co-management with a periodontist is indicated.[3] The diagnosis will

TABLE 70.3 Recall Intervals for Various Classes of Recall Patients

Merin Classification	Characteristics	Recall Interval
First year	First-year patient: routine therapy and uneventful healing.	3 months
	First-year patient: difficult case with complicated prosthesis, furcation involvement, poor crown-to-root ratios, or questionable patient cooperation	1–2 months
Class A	Excellent results well maintained for 1 year or longer Patient displays good oral hygiene, minimal calculus, no occlusal problems, no complicated prostheses, no remaining pockets, and no teeth with less than 50% of alveolar bone remaining	6 months to 1 year
Class B	Generally good results maintained reasonably well for 1 year or more, but patient displays some of the following factors: 1. Inconsistent or poor oral hygiene 2. Heavy calculus formation 3. Systemic disease that predisposes to periodontal breakdown 4. Some remaining pockets 5. Occlusal problems 6. Complicated prostheses 7. Ongoing orthodontic therapy 8. Recurrent dental caries 9. Some teeth with less than 50% of alveolar bone support 10. Smoking 11. Positive family history or genetic test 12. More than 20% of pockets bleed on probing	3–4 months (decide on a recall interval based on the number and severity of negative factors)
Class C	Generally poor results after periodontal therapy or several negative factors from the following list: 1. Inconsistent or poor oral hygiene 2. Heavy calculus formation 3. Systemic disease that predisposes to periodontal breakdown 4. Many remaining pockets 5. Occlusal problems 6. Complicated prostheses 7. Recurrent dental caries 8. Periodontal surgery indicated but not performed for medical, psychological, or financial reasons 9. Many teeth with less than 50% of alveolar bone support 10. Condition too far advanced to be improved by periodontal surgery 11. Smoking 12. Positive family history or genetic test	1–3 months (decide on a recall interval based on the number and severity of negative factors; consider retreating some areas or extracting severely involved teeth)

indicate the type of periodontal treatment required. If periodontal destruction necessitates surgery on the distal surfaces of second molars, extensive osseous surgery, or complex regenerative procedures, the patient is usually best treated by a specialist. Patients who require localized nonsurgical therapy or minor flap surgery can usually be managed by the general practitioner. General dentists have a primary responsibility to do what is best in the interest of the patient. According to Christensen, quality dentistry for a complex case requires a team effort partnering with a periodontal specialist to provide optimal care for the patient.[16]

The decision to have the general practitioner treat a patient's periodontal disease should be guided by consideration of the risk that the patient will lose a tooth or teeth due to periodontal involvement or the periodontal disease negatively affecting the patient's systemic health.

The most important factors in the decision to refer a patient to a periodontist are the severity and location of the periodontal disease. Teeth with pockets of 5 mm or more, as measured from the cementoenamel junction, may have a questionable prognosis, as do teeth with furcation invasions even when more than 50% of bone support remains. Therefore, patients with strategically important teeth that have moderate to severe attachment loss or furcation invasions are usually best treated by specialists.

An important question remains: Should the maintenance phase of therapy be performed by the general practitioner or the specialist? This should be determined by the extent and severity of periodontal disease present. Class A recall patients should be maintained by the general dentist, whereas class C patients should be maintained by the specialist (see Table 70.3). Class B patients can alternate recall visits between the general practitioner and the specialist (Fig. 70.11).

Department of Periodontology

Periodontal Risk Assessment

UNIVERSITÄT BERN

Patient Last Name **Perio** First **Patient** Date **Today**

BOP% = 25%

PD≥5mm

Envir.

Tooth loss

Syst./Gen.

BL/Age = 1.05263

Age	38	
Number of teeth and implants	27	(1 - 32)
Number of sites per tooth / implant	○ 2 ○ 4 ● 6	
Number of BOP-pos. sites	40	of 162
Number of sites with PPD≥5mm	4	
Number of missing teeth	1	
% Alveolar bone loss (estimated in % or 10% per 1mm)	40	%
Syst./Gen.	● Yes ○ No	
Envir.	○ Non smoker (NS) ● Former smoker (FS) ○ Occasional smoker (OS) ○ Smoker (S) ○ Heavy smoker (HS)	

Polygon surface: 65.8179

Periodontal Risk: **high**

Suggested Recall interval: **3** Months

Clinical Research Foundation
Periodontal Risk Assessment V3.1
October 30, 2009

design&program
Christoph A. Ramseier
christoph.ramseier@zmk.unibe.ch

Print

Reset

Fig. 70.10 Sample Periodontal Risk Assessment (PRA). (Report completed and downloaded from http://www.perio-tools.com/PRA/en/index.asp.)

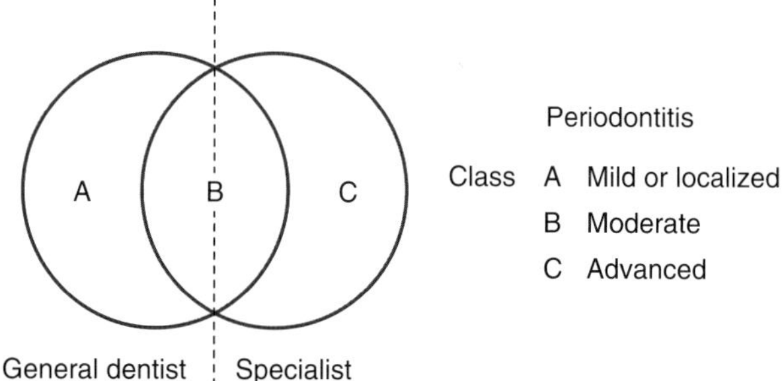

Fig. 70.11 Scheme for determining which practitioner should perform periodontal maintenance in patients with different degrees of periodontitis.

The suggested rule to decide who should maintain the recall therapy is determined by the initial category of the patient's disease and the result of the therapy and the AAP classification of periodontal diseases can be used to help with this.[12] Patients with moderate to severe initial bone loss, advanced grades 2 or 3 furcation invasions, or pockets that could not be completely eradicated are those who should be seen by the periodontist. The specialist and the general dentist must work together, respect the other's knowledge and skills, and decide on a maintenance schedule that is in the best interest of the patient.

LEARNING BOX 70.7

Quality dentistry for a complex case requires a team effort partnering with a periodontal specialist to provide optimal care for the patient.[16]

Tests for Disease Activity

Periodontal patients, even though they have received effective periodontal therapy, are at risk of disease recurrence for the remainder of their lives.[32,33] In addition, pockets in and around the furcation areas are difficult to eliminate even with surgical therapy. These areas with pockets may continue to lose attachment.[4] Comparison of sequential probing measurements gives the most accurate indication of the rate of loss of attachment. A number of other clinical and laboratory variables have been correlated with disease activity.

No accurate method exists to predict disease activity, and clinicians rely on the information obtained from evaluating multiple risk factors.[30,34,39,76] Patients whose disease is clearly refractory are candidates for bacterial culturing and antibiotic therapy in conjunction with additional mechanical therapy.

New methods will undoubtedly be developed in the future to help predict disease activity.[4] The clinician must be able to interpret whether a test may be useful in determining disease activity and future loss of attachment.[9] Tests should be adopted only when they are based on research that includes a critical analysis of the sensitivity, specificity, disease incidence, and predictive value of the proposed test.[30]

Conclusion

The long-term preservation of the dentition is closely associated with the frequency and quality of recall maintenance. The therapist should use risk assessment and educate the patient on the need for periodontal maintenance. Supportive periodontal therapy is a lifetime effort to prevent the disease from recurring. Patients who do not return for supportive periodontal therapy lose more teeth than compliant patients.

Case Scenarios are found on the companion website eBooks.Health.Elsevier.com.

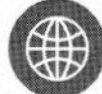
References for this chapter are found on the companion website eBooks.Health.Elsevier.com.

CHAPTER 71

Results of Periodontal Treatment

Robert L. Merin 

CHAPTER OUTLINE

The prevalence of periodontal disease, the resulting high rate of tooth mortality, and the potential for multiple systemic health complications aggravated by chronic periodontitis raise an important question: Is periodontal treatment effective in preventing and controlling the chronic infection and progressive destruction of periodontal disease? Current concepts of evaluating health care require a scientific basis for treatment, referred to as *evidence-based therapy*. Evidence is now overwhelming that periodontal therapy is effective in preventing periodontal disease, slowing the destruction of the periodontium, and reducing tooth loss.

Prevention and Treatment of Gingivitis

LEARNING BOX 71.1

Gingivitis is reversible.

For many years, the belief that good oral hygiene is necessary for the successful prevention and treatment of gingivitis has been widespread among periodontists. In addition, worldwide epidemiologic studies have confirmed a close relationship between the incidence of gingivitis and the lack of oral hygiene.[20,21]

Löe and coworkers[36,67] provided conclusive evidence of the association between oral hygiene and gingivitis. After 9 to 21 days without performing oral hygiene, healthy dental students with previously excellent oral hygiene and healthy gingiva developed heavy accumulations of biofilm and generalized mild gingivitis. When oral hygiene techniques were reinstituted, the biofilm in most areas disappeared in 1 or 2 days, and gingival inflammation in these areas disappeared approximately 1 week after the biofilm was removed. Thus, gingivitis is reversible and can be resolved by daily, effective biofilm removal.

A number of long-term studies have shown that gingival health can be maintained by a combination of effective oral hygiene maintenance and scaling procedures.[1,5,24,28,29,31,38,41,65,66] A 3-year study was conducted on 1248 General Telephone workers in California to determine whether progression of gingival inflammation is reduced in an oral environment in which high levels of hygiene are maintained.[65,66] Experimental and control groups were computer-matched based on periodontal and oral hygiene status, past caries experience, age, and gender. During the study period, several procedures were instituted to ensure that the oral hygiene status of the experimental group was maintained at a high level. Subjects were given a series of frequent oral prophylaxis treatments combined with oral hygiene instruction. Subjects in the control group received no attention from the study team except for annual examinations. They were advised to continue their usual daily practices and accustomed visits for professional care. After 3 years, the increase in biofilm and debris in the control group was four times as great as that in the experimental group. Similarly, gingivitis scores were much higher in control subjects than in the matching experimental group. Therefore, chronic marginal gingivitis can be controlled with good oral hygiene and dental prophylaxis.

LEARNING BOX 71.2

A number of long-term studies have shown that gingival health can be maintained by a combination of effective oral hygiene maintenance and scaling procedures.[1,5,24,28,29,31,38,41,65,66]

Prevention and Treatment of Loss of Attachment

Although periodontal therapy has been used for more than 100 years, it is only since the mid-1970s that studies have been conducted to determine the effect of treatment on reducing the progressive loss of periodontal support for the natural dentition.

Prevention of Loss of Attachment

Löe and coworkers[35,36,54] conducted a longitudinal investigation to study the natural development and progression of periodontal disease. The first study group, established in Oslo, Norway, in 1969, consisted of 565 healthy male nondental students and academicians between 17 and 40 years of age. Oslo was selected mainly because this city had an ongoing preschool, school, and postschool dental program offering systematic preventive, restorative, endodontic, orthodontic, and surgical therapy on an annual recall basis for all children and adolescents, complete with a documented attendance record, for the previous 40 years. Members of the study population had experienced maximum exposure to conventional dental care throughout their lives. A second study group, established in Sri Lanka in 1970, consisted of 480 male tea laborers between 15 and 40 years of age. They were healthy and in excellent physical condition by local standards, and their nutritional condition was clinically fair. The workers had never been exposed to any programs relative to the prevention or treatment of dental diseases. Oral care was unknown, and dental caries was virtually nonexistent.

As the members of the Norwegian group approached 40 years of age, the mean individual loss of attachment was slightly above 1.5 mm; the mean annual rate of attachment loss was 0.08 mm for interproximal surfaces and 0.1 mm for buccal surfaces. As the Sri Lankans approached 40 years of age, the mean individual loss of attachment was 4.5 mm, and the mean annual rate of progression of the lesion was 0.3 mm for interproximal surfaces and 0.2 mm for buccal surfaces. Fig. 71.1 shows a graphic interpretation of the difference between the two groups. This study suggests that without oral care, periodontal lesions progress continually and at a relatively even pace.

Further analysis of the Sri Lankan laborers showed that they were not all losing attachment at the same rate (Figs. 71.2 and 71.3).[36] Virtually all gingival areas showed inflammation, but attachment loss varied tremendously. Based on the interproximal loss of attachment and tooth mortality, three subpopulations were identified as individuals with "rapid progression" (RP) of periodontal disease (8%), individuals with moderate progression (MP) (81%), and individuals who exhibited no progression (NP) of periodontal disease beyond gingivitis (11%). At age 35, the mean loss of attachment in the RP group was 9 mm; in the MP group, 4 mm; and in the NP group, less than 1 mm. At the age of 45 years, the mean loss of attachment in the RP group was 13 mm and in the MP group it was 7 mm. Therefore, under natural conditions and in the absence of therapy, 89% of the Sri Lankan laborers had severe periodontitis that progressed at a much greater rate than that observed in the Norwegian group.

In the previously discussed study of General Telephone workers in California, loss of attachment was measured clinically, and alveolar bone loss was measured radiographically.[65,66] After 3 years, the control group showed loss of attachment at a rate more than three times that of the matching experimental group during the same period (Fig. 71.4). In addition, subjects who received frequent oral prophylaxis and were instructed in good oral hygiene practices showed less bone loss radiographically after 3 years than control subjects. In a systematic review and meta-analysis of the association between oral care habits and periodontitis, Lertpimonchai and associates[30] reviewed 50 publications on this subject and found that poor oral hygiene increases the risk of periodontitis approximately two to five times compared with good oral hygiene. Oral care habits, including regular brushing and dental visits, can decrease the risk of periodontitis and should be promoted as a public health intervention.[22,30,65,66] It is clear that periodontitis with loss of attachment can be reduced by good oral hygiene and frequent dental prophylaxis.

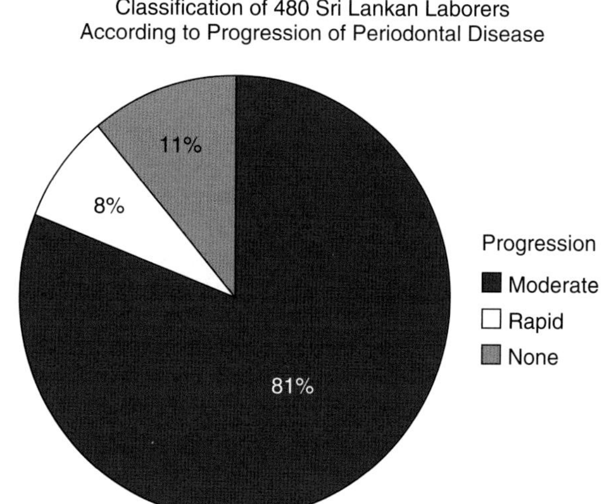

Fig. 71.2 Progression of periodontal disease in an untreated population. (Data from Löe H, Anerud A, Boysen H, et al: Natural history of periodontal disease in man: rapid, moderate and no loss of attachment in Sri Lankan laborers 14 to 31 years of age. *J Clin Periodontol.* 1986;13:431-445.)

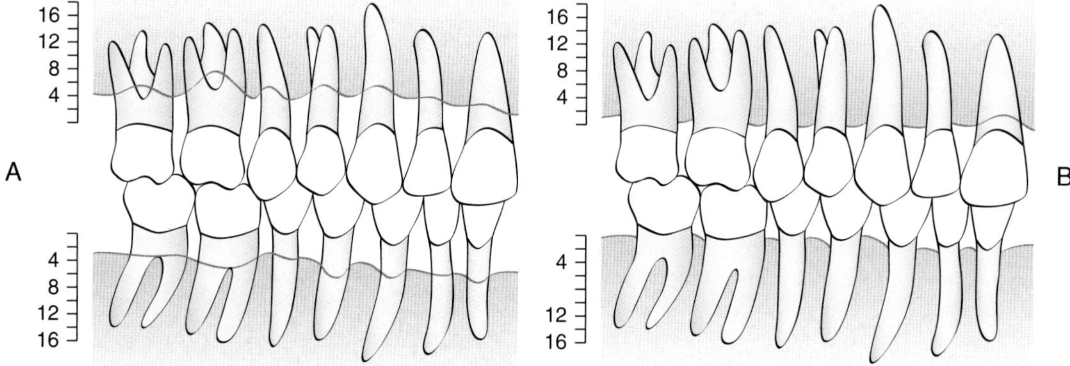

Fig. 71.1 (A) Mean periodontal support of teeth of Sri Lankan tea laborers at approximately 40 years of age. (B) Mean periodontal support of teeth of Norwegian academicians at approximately 40 years of age. (From Löe H, Anerud A, Boysen H, et al: The natural history of periodontal disease in man: the rate of periodontal destruction before 40 years of age. *J Periodontol.* 1978;49:607-620.)

Mean Loss of Attachment at Various Ages (mm)

Age	Progression Group	
	Rapid	Moderate
35	9	4
45	13	7

Fig. 71.3 Loss of attachment in untreated Sri Lankan laborers. (Data from Löe H, Anerud A, Boysen H, et al: Natural history of periodontal disease in man: rapid, moderate and no loss of attachment in Sri Lankan laborers 14 to 46 years of age. *J Clin Periodontol.* 1986;13:431-445.)

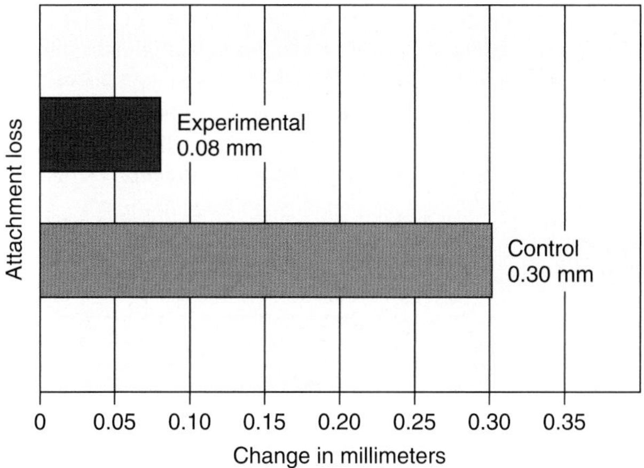

Fig. 71.4 Change in mean attachment level from baseline to third-year examination for experimental and control groups. (From Suomi JD, Greene JC, Vermillion JR, et al: The effect of controlled oral hygiene procedures on the progression of periodontal disease in adults: results after third and final year. *J Periodontol.* 1971;42:152-160.)

Treatment of Loss of Attachment

A longitudinal study of patients with moderate to advanced periodontal disease conducted at the University of Michigan indicated that the progression of periodontal disease can be terminated for 3 years postoperatively, regardless of the modality of treatment.[50-53] With long-term observations, the average loss of attachment was only 0.3 mm over 7 years.[51] These results indicated a more favorable prognosis for treatment of advanced periodontal lesions than previously assumed.

LEARNING BOX 71.3

Patient compliance for regular, thorough biofilm removal by the patient with periodic maintenance therapy can predictably stop ongoing attachment loss.

Another study was conducted in 75 patients with advanced periodontal disease to determine the effect of biofilm control and surgical pocket elimination on the establishment and maintenance of periodontal health.[32] This study indicated that no further alveolar bone loss occurred during the 5-year observation period. The meticulous biofilm control practiced by the patients in this study was considered to be a major factor in the excellent results produced. After 14 years, results for 61 of the initial 75 individuals were reported.[29] Repeated examinations demonstrated that treatment of advanced forms of periodontal disease resulted in clinically healthy periodontal conditions and that this state of health was maintained in most patients and sites during the 14-year period. A more detailed analysis of the data, however, revealed that a small number of sites in a few patients lost a substantial amount of attachment. Approximately 43 surfaces in 15 different patients were exposed to recurrent periodontal disease of significant magnitude. The frequency of sites that lost more than 2 mm of attachment during the 14 years of maintenance was 0.8% to 0.1%/year.

Neither of these studies used a control group because failing to treat advanced periodontal patients cannot be justified for ethical reasons. However, in a study in a private practice, an effort was made to find and evaluate patients with diagnosed moderate to advanced periodontitis who had not followed through with recommended periodontal therapy.[6] Thirty patients ranging in age from 25 to 71 years were evaluated after periods ranging from 18 to 115 months. All untreated patients had progressive increases in pocket depth and radiographic evidence of progressive bone resorption.

In a study of the progression of periodontal disease in the absence of therapy, two different populations were monitored.[34] One group of 64 Swedish adults with mild to moderate periodontal disease and one group of 36 American adults with advanced destructive disease were monitored but not treated for 6 years and 1 year, respectively. During the course of 6 years, 11.6% of all sites in the Swedish population (1.9%/year) showed attachment loss of greater than 2 mm, and the corresponding figure for the American population was 3.2%/year. Thus, the frequency of sites with disease progression was 20 to 30 times higher in untreated groups of patients than in the treated and well-maintained groups described in the preceding discussion.[34] Thus, treatment is effective in reducing loss of attachment.

Tooth Mortality

The ultimate test for the effectiveness of periodontal treatment is whether the loss of teeth can be prevented. Sufficient studies from both private practice and research institutions are now available to document that therapy reduces or prevents loss of teeth.

The combined effect of subgingival scaling every 3 to 6 months and controlled oral hygiene was evaluated over a 5-year period in 1428 factory workers in Oslo.[38] Tooth loss was significantly reduced in all patients. This study showed that frequent subgingival scaling reduces tooth loss, even when oral hygiene is "not good" (Table 71.1).

The previously mentioned longitudinal study conducted at the University of Michigan included 104 patients with a total of 2604 teeth.[50-53] After 1 to 7 years of treatment, 53 teeth were lost for various reasons (Table 71.2). Approximately 32 teeth were lost during the first and second years after the initiation of treatment. The remaining 21 teeth were lost in a random pattern over the next 6 years. Therefore, the loss of teeth caused by advanced periodontal disease after treatment was minimal (1.15%).

Another study was undertaken to test the effect of periodontal therapy in cases of advanced disease.[32,33] The subjects were 75 patients who had lost 50% or more of their periodontal support (Fig. 71.5). Treatment consisted of oral hygiene measures, scaling procedures, extraction of untreatable teeth, periodontal surgery, and prosthetic therapy, if indicated. After completion of periodontal treatment, none of the patients showed further loss of periodontal support for the next 5 years. None of the teeth were extracted in the 5-year posttreatment period. Patients in this study were selected because of their capability to meet the high requirements of biofilm control after repeated instruction in oral hygiene techniques. This does not detract from the validity of the study but tends to indicate the etiologic importance of bacterial biofilm. The results indicate that periodontal surgery coupled with a detailed biofilm control program not only temporarily cures the disease, but also reduces further progression of periodontal breakdown, even in patients with severely reduced periodontal support.

After 14 years, 61 of the original patients were still in the study.[33] Recurrence of destructive periodontal disease in isolated sites of the dentition resulted in loss of a certain number of teeth during the observation period (Fig. 71.6). In the 6 to 10 years after active therapy, one tooth in each of three different patients was lost and, during the final observation period (11 to 14 years), three teeth in one patient, two teeth in each of three patients, and one tooth in each of four patients had to be extracted because of recurrent periodontal disease. In addition, three teeth in each of three different patients and one tooth in each of five patients were extracted because of the development of extensive caries, periapical lesions, or other endodontic complications. Throughout the course of the study, the total loss was 30 teeth (for all reasons) from the total of 1330 teeth. Therefore, the tooth mortality rate was 2.3%.

University-based studies on the treatment of moderate to severe periodontitis have continued to show minimal tooth loss in patients who comply with periodontal maintenance therapy.[13,45]

Several studies in private practice have attempted to measure the frequency of tooth loss after periodontal therapy. In one study, 180 patients who had been treated for chronic destructive periodontal disease were evaluated.[55] The average age of the patients before treatment was 43.7 years. A total of 141 teeth were lost. From the beginning of treatment to the time of the survey, most patients did not lose any teeth (Fig. 71.7). Three of 180 patients (1.7%) lost 35 teeth; approximately 25% of the teeth were lost. Twelve additional patients lost 46 teeth, or 32.6% of the teeth were lost. Many patients in the study had advanced alveolar bone loss, including extensive furcation involvements. However, only a relatively small number (141) of the teeth were lost in the study group of 180 patients

TABLE 71.1 Average Loss of Teeth During a 5-Year Period[a]

	GRADE OF ORAL HYGIENE		
Parameter	**Good**	**Fairly Good**	**Not Good**
Normal loss of teeth[b]	1.1	1.4	1.8
Actual loss of teeth during 5-year period	0.4	0.6	0.9

[a]Compared with normal loss of teeth in 1428 men and women ages 20 through 59 years.
[b]Estimate based on data recorded at initiation of study period.
From Lovdal A, Arno A, Schei O, et al: Combined effect of subgingival scaling and controlled oral hygiene on the incidence of gingivitis. *Acta Odontol Scand.* 1961;19:537-555.

TABLE 71.2 Tooth Mortality After Treatment of Advanced Periodontitis[a]

Teeth Lost[b]	Reason
2	Pulpal disease
3	Accidents
4	Prosthetic considerations
14	Various reasons; for example, one patient wanted a maxillary denture for cosmetic reasons
30	Periodontal
53	All reasons

[a]In 104 patients with 2604 teeth treated over a 10-year period.
[b]Two percent of the teeth were lost during the study period. Note that U.S. health surveys conducted in the 1960s indicated that an average of 4.3 teeth were lost after age 35 in the general population.[9]
Data from Ramfjord SP, Knowles JW, Nissle RR, et al: Longitudinal study of periodontal therapy. *J Periodontol.* 1973;44:66-77.

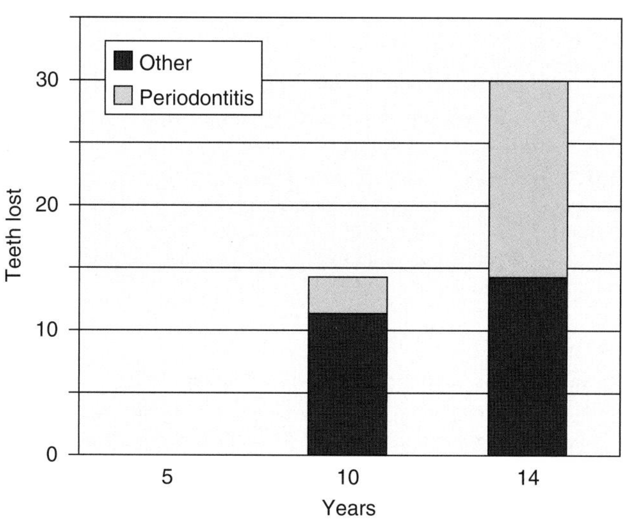

Fig. 71.6 Tooth loss in treated patients with very advanced periodontal disease. (Data from Lindhe J, Nyman S: Long-term maintenance of patients treated for advanced periodontal disease. *J Clin Periodontol.* 1984;11:504-514.)

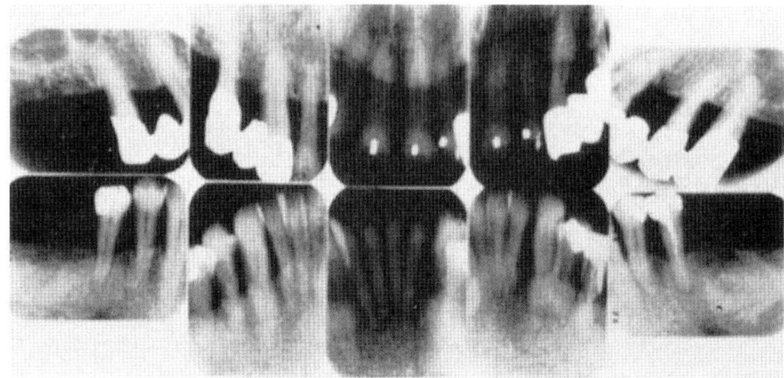

Fig. 71.5 Radiographs taken 5 years after typical periodontal treatment. Note the advanced bone loss, despite the teeth retained in a healthy condition for the duration of the study. (From Lindhe J, Nyman S: The effect of plaque control and surgical pocket elimination on the establishment and maintenance of periodontal health: a longitudinal study of periodontal therapy in cases of advanced disease. *J Clin Periodontol.* 1975;2:67-79.)

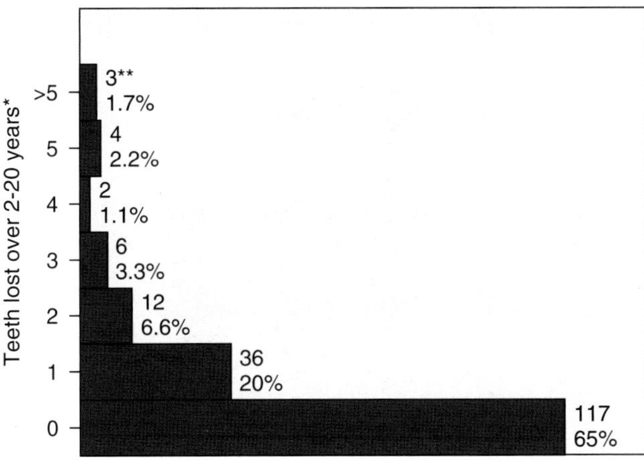

Fig. 71.7 Tooth mortality. Average tooth loss per patient was 0.9/10 years. (Modified from Ross IF, Thompson RH, Galdi M: The results of treatment: a long term study of one hundred and eighty patients. *Parodontologie.* 1971;25:125-134.)

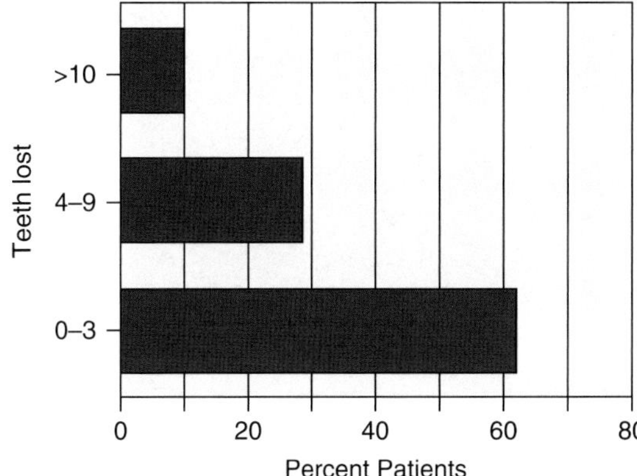

Fig. 71.8 Tooth mortality 15 to 34 years after initiation of therapy (average, 22.2 years). Average tooth loss per patient was 1.6 teeth/10 years. Compare with the same study population in Fig. 71.7. As the treated population ages, the rate of bone loss appears to increase. (Modified from Goldman MJ, Ross IF, Goteiner D: Effect of periodontal therapy on patients maintained for 15 years or longer: a retrospective study. *J Periodontol.* 1986;57:347-353.)

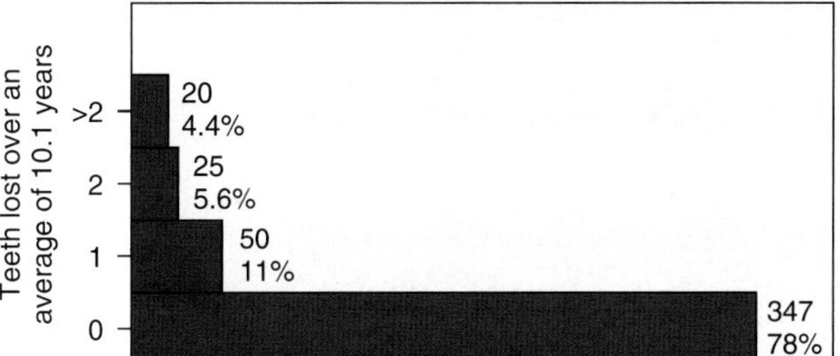

Fig. 71.9 Tooth mortality in 442 periodontal patients treated over 10 years. (Courtesy Dr. R.C. Oliver, Rio Verde, AZ.)

between the beginning of periodontal treatment and the time of the study.

The teeth were lost for several reasons, including periodontal disease, caries, and other nonperiodontal causes. The length of time after treatment varied from 2 to 20 years, with an average of 8.6 years. Of considerable significance is the large number of teeth (81 teeth, or 57.5%) lost by a few patients (15 patients, or 8.4%). Even when this group is considered with the remaining 165 patients, the periodontal care helped retain most teeth because the average loss was slightly less than one tooth (0.9) over the 10 years after treatment.

In a follow-up study, the long-term results of periodontal therapy were evaluated after 15 to 34 years (average, 22.2 years).[18] The average tooth loss at this time was 1.6 teeth/10 years. Patients were classified into three groups according to tooth loss. Approximately 62% had an average tooth loss of 0.45/10 years and were considered "well maintained," 28% lost an average of 2.6 teeth/10 years and were considered "downhill," and 10% lost an average of 6.4 teeth/10 years and were considered "extreme downhill" (Fig. 71.8).

Another study included all patients in a practice who had been treated 5 or more years previously and had received regular preventive periodontal care since that time.[48] The 442 patients had an average of 10.1 years since treatment. Two-thirds of the patients were older than 40 years of age at the time of treatment. These patients had been seen every 4.6 months, on average, for their preventive periodontal care, which consisted of oral hygiene instruction and prophylaxis (Figs. 71.9 and 71.10).

The total tooth loss resulting from periodontal disease was 178 of more than 11,000 teeth available for treatment. More important, 78% of the patients did not lose a single tooth after periodontal therapy, and 11% lost only one tooth. Considering that more than 600 teeth had furcation involvements at the time of the original treatment and that far more than 1000 teeth had less than half the alveolar bone support remaining, there was minimal tooth loss. During the same average 10-year period after periodontal therapy, only 45 teeth were lost through caries or pulpal involvement. Even more surprising are the statistics over an average 10-year period for teeth with a poor prognosis. Only 85 (14%) of a total of 601 teeth with furcation involvement were lost, and 117 (11%) of 1039 teeth with half or less of the bone remaining were lost. Of the 1043 teeth listed as having a "guarded prognosis" by the clinician performing the initial examination, only 126 (12%) were lost over this 10-year period. The average tooth mortality rate was 0.72 tooth lost/patient per 10 years.

In a third study in a private practice, 600 patients were followed for 15 to 53 years after periodontal therapy (Figs. 71.11 and 71.12).[23] The majority (76.5%) had advanced periodontal disease at the start of treatment. There were 15,666 teeth present, for an average of 26 teeth/patient. During the follow-up period (an average of 22 years), a total of 1312 teeth were lost from all causes. Of this number, 1110 were lost for periodontal reasons. The average tooth mortality rate/patient was 2.2 teeth and, when this is converted to a 10-year rate, an average of one tooth was lost/10 years in each patient. During this period of observation, 666 teeth with a questionable prognosis were lost out of a total of 2141. This means that 31% of the teeth with a questionable prognosis were lost over 22 years of treatment. A total of 1464 teeth with furcation involvement were treated, and 31.6% were lost during the period of study. Approximately 83% of the patients lost fewer than three teeth over the 22-year average treatment period and were classified as "well maintained." The remaining 17% of the patients were divided into two groups: downhill (4 to 9 teeth lost) or extreme downhill (10 to 23 teeth lost). Thus, 17% of the patients studied accounted for 69% of teeth lost from periodontal causes. This study also indicated that relatively few teeth are lost after periodontal therapy. In addition,

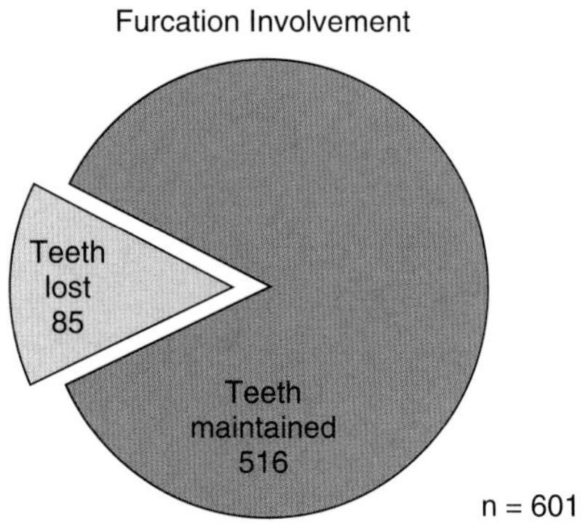

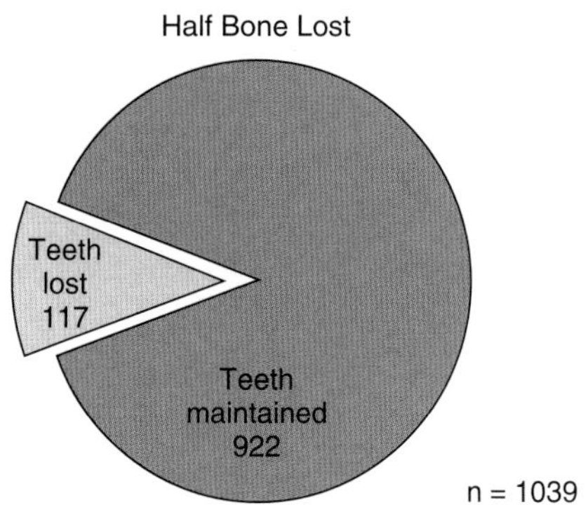

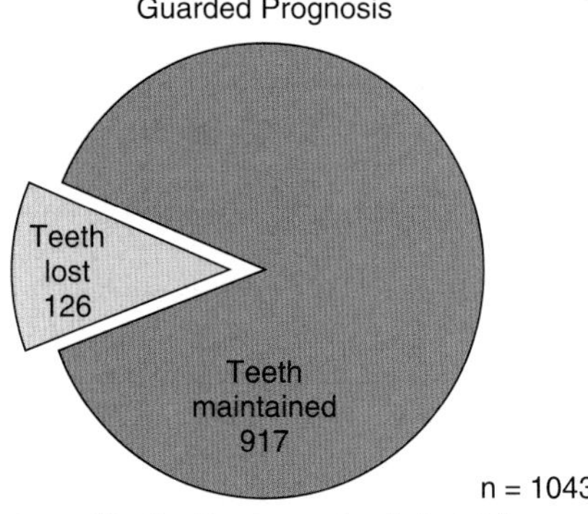

Fig. 71.10 Loss of teeth with advanced periodontal disease over 10 years. (Courtesy Dr. R.C. Oliver, Rio Verde, AZ.)

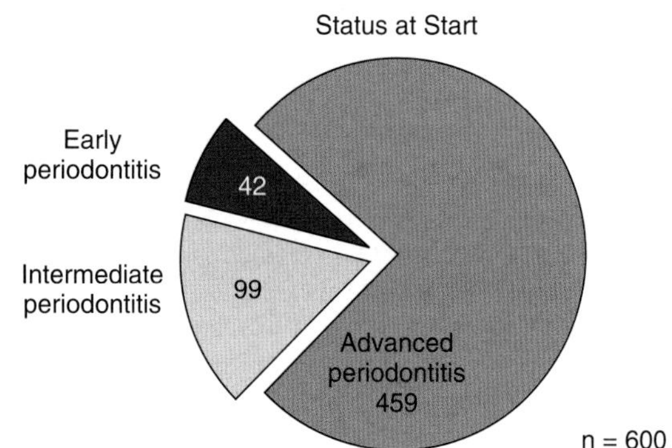

Fig. 71.11 Status at the start of a study of 600 patients. (Data from Hirschfeld L, Wasserman B: A long-term survey of tooth loss in 600 treated periodontal patients. *J Periodontol.* 1978;49:225-237.)

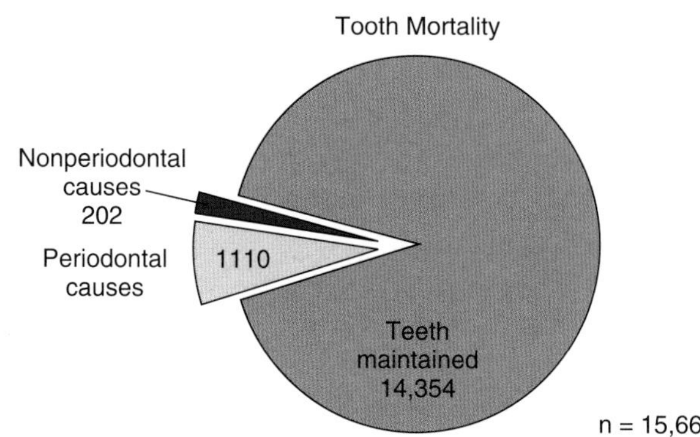

Fig. 71.12 Loss of teeth in 600 patients over 15 to 53 years from nonperiodontal and periodontal causes. (Data from Hirschfeld L, Wasserman B: A long-term survey of tooth loss in 600 treated periodontal patients. *J Periodontol.* 1978;49:225-237.)

few teeth with a guarded prognosis, including those with furcation involvement, are lost, and a small percentage of patients lose most of their teeth.

Clinical studies have also indicated a relatively low rate of tooth loss in patients who are involved in a supportive periodontal maintenance program. One study showed that 0.9% of teeth were lost over 7.8 years, whereas another showed that 1.5% were lost over a 9.8-year period after the initiation of active periodontal treatment.[10,15] Another study showed that questionable teeth in patients with aggressive periodontitis can be maintained for longer than 15 years if the patient is compliant.[70]

A study at the University of Bern looked at the outcome of multirooted teeth treated for longer than 11.5 years.[71] The study found that grade 1 furcation status was not a risk factor for tooth loss compared with no furcation bone loss in patients treated for periodontal disease. Risk factors for the loss of multirooted teeth included furcation involvements grades 2 and 3, smoking, and lack of compliance with regular maintenance therapy (Fig. 71.13).

LEARNING BOX 71.4

Numerous studies indicate the possibility of maintaining teeth in patients with **stage** IV periodontitis if the patient can perform excellent biofilm removal along with regular **supportive periodontal care**.

Three studies have provided insight into tooth mortality in untreated patients. The studies of Löe and colleagues[36,37] in Sri Lankan laborers showed that after age 35, an average of 5 and 16 teeth were lost/10 years in the moderate progression and rapid progression groups, respectively (Fig. 71.14). In a previously discussed study in private practice,[6] an effort was made to find and evaluate patients with diagnosed moderate to advanced periodontitis who did not follow through with recommended periodontal therapy. Patients with untreated periodontal disease were losing teeth at a rate greater than 0.61/year (6.1 teeth/10 years). A total of 83 teeth were lost in 30 patients, but the investigators excluded one patient who had lost 25 teeth. Including this patient would have increased the tooth loss in untreated patients to an even higher rate. In another study, reporting on patients with moderate to advanced periodontitis examined at the Department of Periodontology at the University of Kiel in Germany, Kocher and associates[27] found a marked increase in tooth loss in the untreated patients compared with the treated patients when they were examined after 7 years.

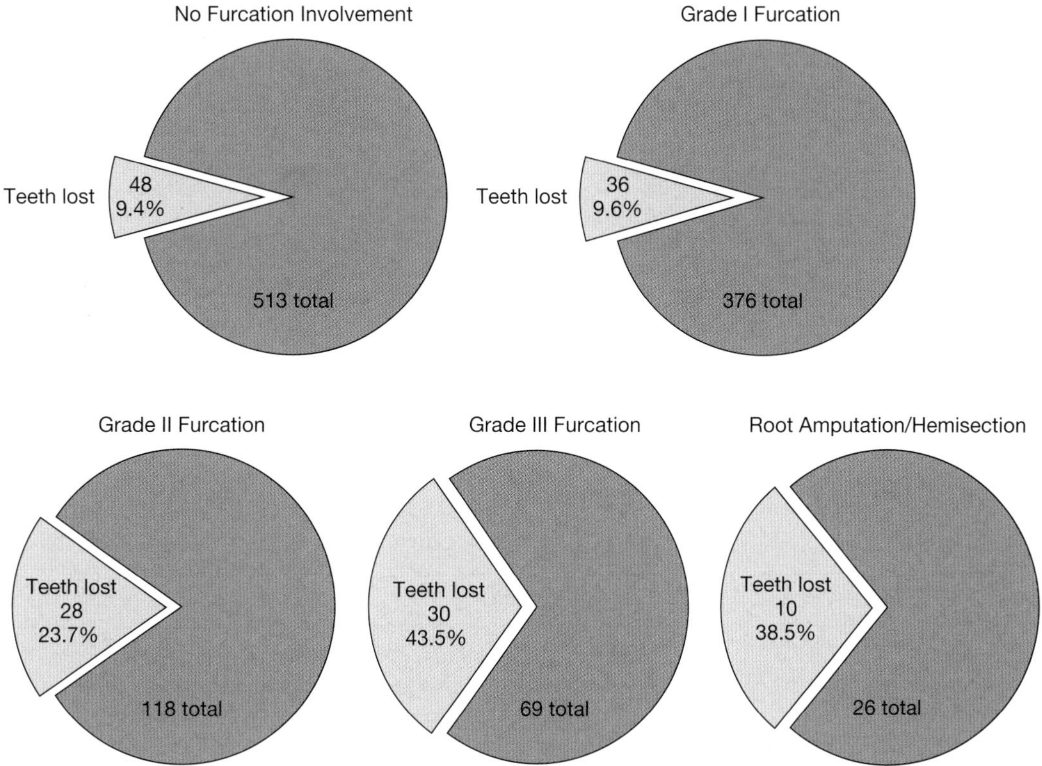

Fig. 71.13 Loss of multirooted teeth during 11.5 years of supportive periodontal therapy. (Data from Salvi GE, Mischler DC, Schmidlin K, et al: Risk factors associated with longevity of multi-rooted teeth: long-term outcomes after active supportive periodontal therapy. *J Clin Periodontol.* 2014;41:701-707.)

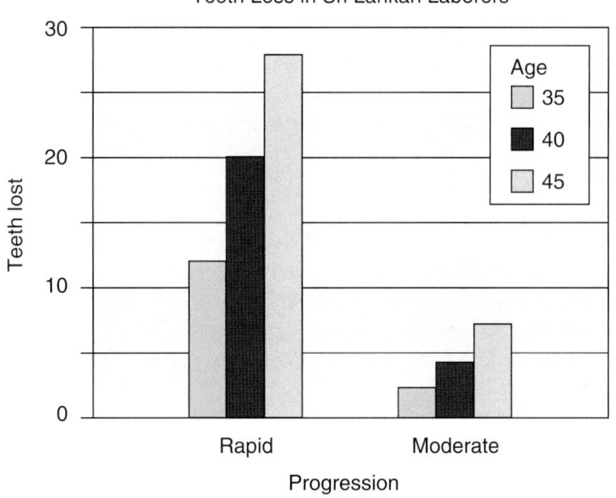

Fig. 71.14 Tooth loss in a population with untreated periodontal disease. (Data from Löe H, Anerud A, Boysen H, et al: Natural history of periodontal disease in man: rapid, moderate and no loss of attachment in Sri Lankan laborers 14 to 46 years of age. *J Clin Periodontol.* 1986;13:431-445.)

When Tables 71.3 and 71.4 are compared, it is obvious that tooth mortality is much higher in untreated groups.

Systematic Reviews and Meta-analyses on the Results of Periodontal Treatment on Clinical Parameters

Smiley and colleagues[60] conducted a review of 72 articles on the results of nonsurgical treatment of chronic periodontitis by means of scaling and root planing, with or without adjuncts. They concluded with a moderate level of certainty that scaling and root planing produced an average improvement in clinical attachment levels of 0.5 mm and that adjunctive therapies could add an additional improvement of 0.2 to 0.6 mm of clinical attachment improvement. This report[60] led to a clinical practice guideline by the same 16 authors,[61] which concluded that scaling and root planing showed a moderate benefit and should be the initial nonsurgical treatment for chronic periodontitis. The evidence for the use of adjunctive therapy with scaling and root planing were rated according to scientific evidence of their effectiveness (Table 71.5).

Zhang and coworkers[75] performed a systematic review and meta-analysis comparing ultrasonic and manual subgingival scaling at different probing pocket depths. Ten randomized controlled trials were included in this review. When initial probing depth was 4 to 6 mm, pocket depth reduction was better with manual subgingival scaling, whereas clinical attachment improvement was the same with ultrasonics. When initial probing depths were greater than 6 mm, pocket depth reduction and clinical attachment level improvements suggested that manual scaling was superior.

Nibali and coworkers[46] presented a review comparing open flap débridement and regenerative surgery for the treatment of intrabony periodontal defects. Seventy-nine randomized clinical trials were included in this review, which found that enamel matrix derivative or resorbable guided tissue regeneration with papilla preservation flaps should be the treatment of choice for deep intrabony defects that have not resolved following nonsurgical therapy. Papillary preservation flaps improve clinical outcomes and should be considered a surgical prerequisite when performing regeneration procedures.[46]

Stavropoulos and colleagues[63] reviewed randomized controlled clinical studies of medium- and long-term clinical benefits of periodontal regenerative and reconstructive procedures in intrabony defects. Thirty studies presenting data 3 to 20 years after treatment with grafting, guided tissue regeneration, and enamel matrix derivatives as monotherapies or combinations, with or without adjunctive

TABLE 71.3 Tooth Mortality in Treated Periodontitis Patients

Study	Average Number of Teeth Lost/10 Years With Periodontal Treatment[a]
Hirschfeld and Wasserman[23]	1.0
Kocher et al.[27]	1.6
McFall[39]	1.4
Oliver[48]	0.7
Ross et al.[55]	0.9
Goldman et al.[18]	1.6
McLeod et al.[41]	1.5
Tsami et al.[68] (nonsmokers)	1.7
Tsami et al.[68] (smokers)	3.7
Ng et al.[45] (compliant with maintenance)	0.8
Ng et al.[45] (noncompliant with maintenance)	2.8
Costa et al.[69] (compliant with maintenance)	1.2
Costa et al.[69] (noncompliant with maintenance)	3.6
Graetz et al.[19] (chronic periodontitis)	1.5

[a]Tooth mortality adjusted to 10 years by chapter author.

TABLE 71.4 Tooth Mortality in Untreated Periodontitis Patients

Study	Average Number of Teeth Lost/10 Years Without Periodontal Treatment[a]
Becker et al[6]	6
Kocher et al[27]	5
Löe et al[36] (moderate progression)	5
Löe et al[36] (rapid progression)	16

[a]Tooth mortality adjusted to 10 years by chapter author.

use of blood-derived growth factor constructs or open flap débridement only. They concluded that periodontal regenerative or reconstructive therapy in intrabony defects results in shallower residual probing depth and larger clinical attachment gain compared with open flap débridement. This produced high rates of tooth survival on a medium- to long-term basis. They also concluded that combination approaches were more efficacious than monotherapy.[63]

LEARNING BOX 71.5

The average pocket reduction with scaling and root planing is 0.5 mm and adjuncts can add 0.2 to 0.6 mm more pocket reduction.

Patient-Reported Outcomes and Oral Health Related Quality of Life

The U.S. Food and Drug Administration (FDA) defines patient-reported outcomes (PROs)[16] as "A measurement based on a report that comes directly from the patient (i.e., study subject) about the status of a patient's health condition without amendment or interpretation of the patient's response by a clinician or anyone else. A PRO can be measured by self-report or by interview provided that the interviewer records only the patient's response.

In treating patients, most of the measures at the clinician's disposal are clinician-centered.[74] Examples of these clinician-centered measurements in periodontics are pocket depth, loss of attachment, and tooth mobility. However, one of the primary goals of health care is to improve how patients feel and function in their daily lives. By including PROs in the design of clinical research and practice, there is a huge potential to improve patient care.[11] High-quality PRO data from trials can improve regulatory and economic analyses and health policy. PRO measurement is a relatively new area of research and international efforts have been made to develop consensus-based, PRO-specific guidelines.[9]

Health-related quality of life (HRQL) is a vital component of PROs. HRQL is multidimensional and is composed of physical functioning, psychological well-being, social and role functioning, and health perceptions. In health research and practice, quality of life is increasingly acknowledged as a valid indicator of service need and intervention outcomes. Box 71.1 is the FDA requirement for claiming a statistical and meaningful improvement in HRQL.

PRO measurements are a partially developed area in clinical dentistry and research, and in the future they have the potential to become the primary or secondary outcome measurements in clinical interventional research.[2,40] Intuitively, one knows that PROs are important in developing the best clinical therapy, but how to incorporate them into periodontal clinical studies and clinical practice are still being refined. As dental patient-reported outcomes gain momentum in dental practice, our understanding of the outcome of dental therapies will be vastly improved.[49]

Oral health related quality of life (OHRQL) is a key component of HRQL because oral health problems can have functional, social, economic, and psychological consequences.[2] In 1994, Slade and Spencer developed the Oral Health Impact Profile (OHIP-49) with forty-eight questions to measure the social impact of oral disorders, and they validated the reliability on a group of 328 patients.[58] In 1997, Slade extracted data from a study of 1217 people aged 60 years and older and found that the OHIP-49 could be reduced to 14 questions (OHIP-14) and have the same reliability, validity, and precision.[59] Although there are several OHRQL measurement tools used in the periodontal literature, OHIP-14 is the one most commonly used.[2-4,49,7,64] Table 71.6 shows the questions in the OHIP-14 so the reader can get an idea of how OHRQL is measured in the most frequently used measurement instrument.

LEARNING BOX 71.6

Subjective outcomes of periodontal therapy, such as quality of life, may be more relevant to patients than clinical changes in probing depths or attachment levels.

Oral Health–Related Quality of Life and Periodontal Diseases

In 2016, Buset and associates[8] carried out a systematic review and asked the question, "Are periodontal diseases really silent?" Among 1134 citations initially, they found 37 articles with clinical periodontal examinations and validated survey instruments. This systematic review investigated the role of periodontal diseases (PDs) in OHRQL and demonstrated that an association between PDs and OHRQL was evident, and the impact was more pronounced with

TABLE 71.5 Clinical Recommendation Statements[a]

Strength Levels	
Strong	Evidence strongly supports providing this intervention
In favor	Evidence favors providing this intervention
Weak	Evidence suggests implementing this intervention only after alternatives have been considered
Expert opinion for	Evidence is lacking; the level of certainty is low. Expert opinion guides this recommendation
Expert opinion against	Evidence is lacking; the level of certainty is low. Expert opinion suggests not implementing this intervention.
Against	Evidence suggests not implementing this intervention
Clinical Recommendation	**Strength**
Scaling and root planing (SRP) (no adjuncts): for patients with chronic periodontitis, clinical should consider SRP as the initial treatment.	In Favor
SRP with systemic subantimicrobial dose doxycycline: for patients with moderate to severe chronic periodontitis, clinicians may consider systemic subantimicrobial dose of doxycycline (20 mg bid) for 3 to 9 months as an adjunct to SRP, with a small net benefit expected.	In Favor
SRP with systemic antimicrobials: for patients with moderate to severe chronic periodontitis, clinicians may consider systemic antimicrobials as an adjunct to SRP, with a small net benefit expected.	Weak
SRP with locally delivered antimicrobials: for patients with moderate to severe chronic periodontitis, clinicians may consider locally delivered chlorhexidine chips as an adjunct to SRP, with a moderate new benefit expected.	Weak
For patients with moderate to severe chronic periodontitis, clinicians may consider locally delivered doxycycline hydrate gel as an adjunct to SRP, but the net benefit is uncertain.	Expert Opinion For
For patients with moderate to severe chronic periodontitis, clinicians may consider locally delivered minocycline microspheres as an adjunct to SRP, but the net benefit is uncertain.	Expert Opinion For
SRP with nonsurgical use of lasers: for patients with moderate to severe chronic periodontitis, clinicians may consider photodynamic therapy (PDT) using diode lasers as an adjunct to SRP, with a moderate net benefit expected.	Weak
For patients with moderate to severe chronic periodontitis, clinicians should be aware that the current evidence shows no net benefit from diode lasers (non-PDT) when used as an adjunct to SRP.	Expert Opinion Against
For patients with moderate to severe chronic periodontitis, clinicians should be aware that the current evidence shows no net benefit from neodymium-yttrium-aluminum-garnet lasers when used as an adjunct to SRP.	Expert Opinion Against
For patients with moderate to severe chronic periodontitis, clinicians should be aware that the current evidence shows no net benefit from erbium lasers when used as an adjunct to SRP.	Expert Opinion Against

[a]From the American Dental Association Council on Scientific Affairs' Nonsurgical Treatment of Chronic Periodontitis Expert Panel.

Adapted from Smiley CJ, Tracy, SL, Abt, E, et al: Evidence-based clinical practice guideline on the nonsurgical treatment of chronic periodontitis by means of scaling and root planing with or without adjuncts. *J Am Dent Assoc.* 2015;146:525-535.

greater severity of PDs. A comprehensive clinical assessment of periodontal parameters using full-mouth periodontal examinations seemed to enhance the detectability of the impairment in OHRQL. The authors concluded that PDs play an important role in the impact of oral health on quality of life and should not be considered silent diseases.

In 2017, Ferreira and colleagues[17] performed a systematic review of the impact of periodontal disease on QL using 34 cross-sectional studies. This review also found that periodontal disease exerts a negative impact on OHRQL, and severe periodontitis has a significantly greater impact than mild to moderate periodontitis. Besides physical pain, the other domains most affected by periodontal disease were functional limitation, psychological discomfort, and physical disability. They concluded that these findings underscore the importance of a periodontal treatment plan based on both the needs diagnosed by the clinician and those perceived by the patient, which allows for the understanding of the clinical consequences that compromise dental function and esthetics.

LEARNING BOX 71.7

Periodontal disease exerts a negative impact on OHRQL, and severe periodontitis has a significantly greater impact than mild to moderate periodontitis.

Impact of Periodontal Status on Oral Health–Related Quality of Life in Patients with Diabetes

In 2015, Irani and coworkers[25] investigated the impact of periodontal status on OHRQL in patients with and without type 2 diabetes.

BOX 71.1 FDA Requirement for Claiming Improvement in Health-Related Quality of Life

HRQL is a multidomain concept that represents the patient's general perception of the effect of illness and treatment on physical, psychological, and social aspects of life. Claiming a statistical and meaningful improvement in HRQL implies the following: (1) that all HRQL domains that are important to interpreting change in how the clinical trial's population feels or functions as a result of the targeted disease and its treatment were measured; (2) that a general improvement was demonstrated; and (3) that no decrement was demonstrated in any domain.

From FDA: Guidance for industry. Patient-reported outcome measures: Use in medical product development to support labeling claims. http://www.fda.gov/Drugs/GuidanceComplianceRegulatoryInformation/Guidances/default.htm.

The OHIP-49 was completed by 61 patients with type 2 diabetes and 74 nondiabetic patients matched for age, gender, and periodontal status. They found that gingivitis and periodontitis are associated with poorer OHRQL in nondiabetic patients with improvements following treatment of periodontitis. No such improvement was observed in patients with diabetes following improved periodontal status.

In 2020, Desai and associates[14] reported on the impact of diabetes and periodontal status on life quality using the Well-being Questionnaire 12 (W-BQ12) and the Audit Diabetes Dependent Quality of Life-19 (ADDQoL-19); 56 type 1 diabetics and 72 type 2 diabetics were matched **for** periodontal status. Analysis of the data revealed that diabetes did have impacts on the OHRQL in both types 1 and 2 diabetics. However, there was no additional impact on OHRQL based on periodontal status. Although the patients with diabetes showed improvements in their clinical condition following treatment, neither of the questionnaires used appeared to be useful in capturing any impact of this improvement in OHRQL. This agrees with the article by Irani and colleagues[25] discussed in the previous paragraph. The lack of improvement in OHRQL may be related to the design of the questionnaires used (OHIP-49, W-BQ12, ADDQoL-19) or to the burden of chronic diabetes minimizing the impact of oral health issues in QL measurements.

LEARNING BOX 71.8

Improved periodontal status does not seem to improve OHRQL measurements in diabetic patients, possibly because the burden of many chronic diabetic problems minimizes the impact of oral health issues.

TABLE 71.6 Questions Used in the Oral Health Impact Profile-14[a]

Dimension: Functional limitation[b]
1. Have you had trouble pronouncing any words because of problems with your teeth mouth or dentures? (0.51)
2. Have you felt that your sense of taste has worsened because of problems with your teeth, mouth, or dentures? (0.49)
Dimension: Physical pain
1. Have you had painful aching in your mouth? (0.34)
2. Have you found it uncomfortable to eat any foods because of problems with your teeth, mouth, or dentures? (0.66)
Dimension: Psychological discomfort
1. Have you been self-conscious because of your teeth, mouth, or dentures? (0.45)
2. Have you felt tense because of problems with your teeth, mouth, or dentures? (0.55)
Dimension: Physical disability
1. Has your diet been unsatisfactory because of problems with your teeth, mouth, or dentures? (0.52)
2. Have you had to interrupt meals because of problems with your teeth, mouth, or dentures? (0.48)
Dimension: Psychological disability
1. Have you found it difficult to relax because of problems with your teeth, mouth, or dentures? (0.60)
2. Have you been a bit embarrassed because of problems with your teeth, mouth, or dentures? (0.40)
Dimension: Social disability
1. Have you been a bit irritable with other people because of problems with your teeth, mouth, or dentures? (0.62)
2. Have you had difficulty doing your usual jobs because of problems with your teeth, mouth, or dentures? (0.38)
Dimension: Handicap
1. Have you felt that life in general was less satisfying because of problems with your teeth, mouth or dentures? (0.59)
2. Have you been totally unable to functions because of problems with your teeth, mouth or dentures? (0.41)

[a]With weights in parentheses.
[b]Responses are made on a five-point scale as follows: 0 = never, 1 = hardly ever, 2 = occasionally, 3 = fairly often, 4 = very often. Within each dimension, responses can be multiplied by weights to give a subscale score
Adapted from Slade GD: Derivation and validation of a short-form oral health impact profile, *Community Dent Oral Epidemiol.* 1997;25:284-290.

The Results of Periodontal Therapy on Oral Health–Related Quality of Life

In 2012, Shanbhag and coworkers[56] performed a systematic review of 11 studies with 639 participants on the impact of periodontal therapy on OHRQL in adults. They found that periodontal therapy improved the OHRQL of adults immediately (1 week) and over the long term (12 months). The domains related to pain as well as functional and emotional aspects benefited from periodontal therapy. The perceived benefit of surgical therapy was relatively less, but overall, they concluded that periodontal therapy is beneficial from a patient-centered perspective.

In 2016, Mendez and associates[42] studied the impact of supragingival and subgingival periodontal treatments on OHRQL; 55 participants with both gingivitis and moderate to severe periodontitis were included. Participants were examined at three time points. Periodontal and OHIP-14 data were collected before treatment, 30 days after the start of supragingival treatment, and 30 days after the end of subgingival scaling and root planing. Overall, the nonsurgical treatment used reduced the negative OHRQL due to periodontal disease, and the supragingival treatment was responsible for the larger proportion of changes in the OHRQL measurements. The supragingival treatment prior to the subgingival interventions is associated with the most significant improvements in OHRQL and gives the opportunity for patients to quickly perceive the benefits of having periodontal therapy.

In 2017, Basher and colleagues[4] studied the impact of nonsurgical periodontal therapy on OHRQL in an obese population in a randomized controlled trial; 66 obese patients with chronic periodontitis were randomly allocated to either the treatment group or control group. The treatment group received oral hygiene instructions and scaling and root planing; the control group only underwent examinations. The OHIP-14 was used in this study. They concluded that periodontal therapy improved the functional and psychological discomfort domains, particularly regarding the items of food impactions and bad breath. However, therapy did not improve most of the domains in the OHIP-14. A major weakness in this study is that they used an inclusion criterion of a BMI of 27.5+, which is not the current definition for obesity. The current Centers for Disease Control and Prevention (CDC) criterion for obesity is 30+.

In 2017, Baiju and coworkers[3] did a systematic review of patient-reported outcome assessment of periodontal therapy; 19 clinical studies with 1345 participants and two systematic reviews were included in this systematic review. Root coverage procedures like connective tissue grafts improved OHRQL of patients with recession, irrespective of the amount of root coverage attained. The results suggested that both surgical and nonsurgical therapy for periodontitis can improve OHRQL of patients. However, the improvement affected by surgical therapy after initial therapy is not significant.

In 2020, Botelho and associates[7] performed a systematic review and meta-analysis on the impact of nonsurgical periodontal treatment on OHRQL; 12 studies were included in the review, which included two randomized clinical trials and ten observational (cohort) studies. Meta-analysis was only possible on seven cohort studies with a total of 519 patients, which used the OHIP-14. They concluded that the use of nonsurgical periodontal treatment procedures improves the OHRQL within 1 month of treatment and this improvement remains stable after 3 months.

In 2021, Khan and colleagues[26] published a systematic review that included 13 studies, including three randomized controlled trials, nine case series, and one quasiexperimental study. Eleven of the 13 reported significant improvement in OHIP-14 scores among participants who had undergone nonsurgical periodontal therapy. Physical disability, psychological discomfort, and functional limitation were the domains that improved significantly in all studies after nonsurgical periodontal therapy. Improvement in OHIP-14 scores was associated with improved clinical periodontal measures. Studies with 12 months of follow-up reported significant reduction in physical pain compared to studies with immediate or short-term follow-up. The study concluded that OHIP-14 was an effective measure in reporting response to change after nonsurgical therapy and that nonsurgical periodontal therapy was significantly associated with improvement in perceived OHRQL.

In 2021, Wong and associates[73] published an umbrella review of systemic reviews on periodontal disease and QL. One of the aims of this umbrella review was to determine the impact of periodontal disease and periodontal therapy (both surgical and nonsurgical) on HRQL and OHRQL. Eight articles met their inclusion criteria. Two systematic reviews investigated the effect of oral health conditions on HRQL, three investigated the effect of periodontal disease on OHRQL, and three evaluated the effect of periodontal therapy on OHRQL. In total, there were 150 studies identified from the eight systematic reviews. The authors concluded that periodontal disease can negatively affect HRQL and OHRQL. Both surgical and nonsurgical therapy can improve OHRQL, although to a different degree as perceived by patients. The impact of surgical therapy may not be as significant when compared to nonsurgical therapy.

PROs are an important part of evaluating periodontal treatment, and periodontal disease has a negative impact on HRQL and OHRQL. Nonsurgical and surgical periodontal therapy can improve OHRQL, with nonsurgical therapy showing a greater improvement in OHRQL than surgical treatment.

Conclusion

The prevalence of periodontal disease and the resulting high rate of tooth mortality have increased the need for effective treatment. Strong evidence now indicates that periodontal disease is associated with numerous health problems, including pregnancy complications, heart disease, stroke, diabetes, and certain cancers.[12,25,43,44,47,57,62,72] Early treatment can prevent periodontal disease, and periodontal treatment can control the progression of advanced disease and greatly reduce tooth mortality. Every dental practitioner should be familiar with the philosophy, recognition, and techniques for periodontal therapy. Failure to diagnose and treat periodontal disease or not to make periodontal treatment available to patients causes unnecessary dental problems and tooth loss, places the patient at risk for other systemic health problems, and reduces patients' quality of life.

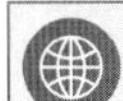
A Case Scenario is found on the companion website eBooks.Health.Elsevier.com.

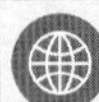
References for this chapter are found on the companion website eBooks.Health.Elsevier.com.

CHAPTER 72

Integrating Implants With Periodontal Therapy

Perry R. Klokkevold

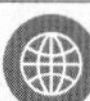 Videos for this chapter can be viewed on the companion website at eBooks.Health.Elsevier.com.

 Animations have been added by the editors as a supplement to the chapter. They are produced by PerioPixel as patient education tools and cover the basic elements in a conceptual manner. They are not intended to be procedural guides for dental professionals.

CHAPTER OUTLINE

Osseointegration

The discovery of osseointegration and the development of endosseous dental implants, by Bränemark and coworkers in the 1960s and 1970s,[8] had a major impact on dentistry (Fig. 72.1). The concept of osseointegration, defined as the intimate contact of vital bone with the implant surface (see Figs. 73.3 and 73.4), and the supporting evidence from clinical studies demonstrating the application and predictability of dental implants was presented to the dental profession at the Toronto Conference in 1982.[41] It marked the beginning of a new era in dentistry that continues today. The original studies and the initial clinical application of osseointegrated dental implants were limited to edentulous patients but were adapted to partially edentulous patients very soon thereafter. The ability to support and/or retain a dental prosthesis (e.g., single crown, fixed partial denture, complete denture) with implant(s) dramatically changed treatment planning and tooth replacement options. In fact, it resulted in a paradigm shift in dentistry from the practice of saving teeth at all costs to one that considered extracting otherwise "maintainable" teeth to improve esthetics, function, and long-term success of implant restorations.[25]

Implant therapy expanded rapidly over the late 1980s through the 1990s and beyond. Initially, there were many challenges adapting the implant system, which was designed for edentulous patients, to the partially edentulous patient, but the number of cases and applications continued to increase and those challenges were addressed. The perceived success and predictability of dental implants made them highly desirable for patients. It seemed to be a panacea for all; patients wanted permanent tooth replacement, clinicians enjoyed increased practice productivity, and implant companies profited from product sales.[40] Along with the lure and profitability of implant therapy came an increased willingness to extract teeth.[15] As a result, more and more teeth were extracted in favor of being replaced with implants.

Advances in Implant Therapy

Many advances in implant therapy over the last several decades have greatly improved our ability to provide esthetic, natural appearing tooth replacement with dental implants. Surgical protocols evolved from placement in completely healed sites only to reconstructing deficient alveolar ridges with augmentation procedures and immediate implant placement in extraction sockets. Restorative protocols advanced from placing restorations only after allowing 4 to 6+ months of healing for osseointegration to earlier loading and/or immediate restoration.

Today, diagnosis and treatment planning for implant sites/cases are greatly facilitated by 3D CBCT imaging, intraoral scanning, and implant planning simulation software. Digital dentistry enhances precision and facilitates the translation of computer-generated plans to the surgical and prosthetic execution of implant therapy—far better than analog methods (see Chapters 84 and 85). Furthermore, in stark contrast to the criteria for surgical placement in healed bone sites only, today's treatment protocols have evolved to include the option of immediate

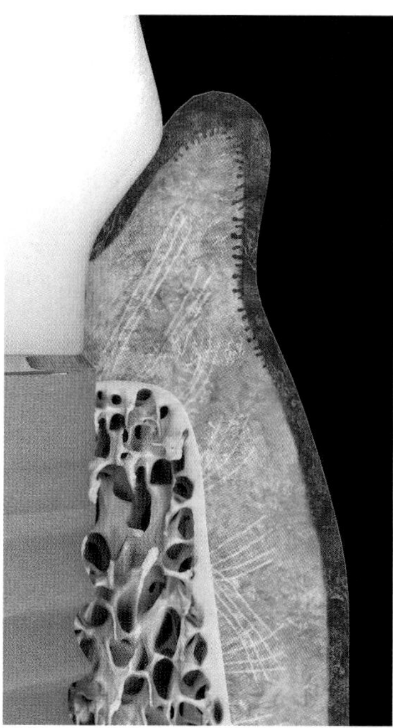

Fig. 72.1 PerioPixel image depicting peri-implant hard and soft tissues. Osseointegration is the intimate contact of vital bone with the implant surface.

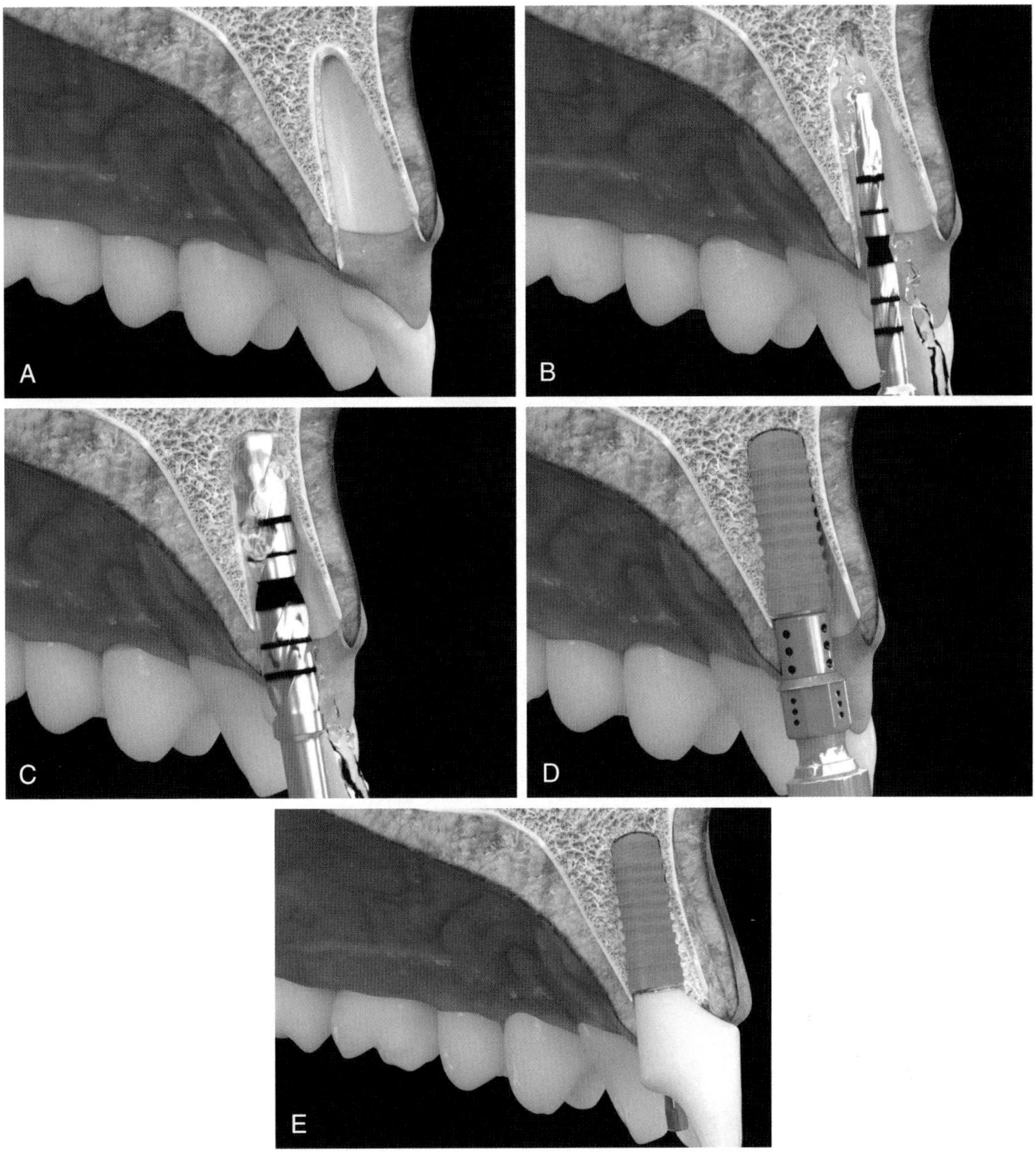

Fig. 72.2 PerioPixel images depicting (A) extraction socket, (B and C) sequential drills preparing implant site osteotomy in the extraction socket, (D) implant placement, and (E) restoration attached to immediate implant.

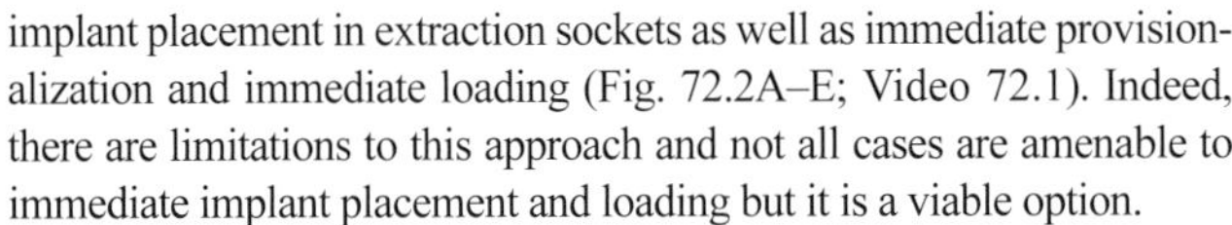

implant placement in extraction sockets as well as immediate provisionalization and immediate loading (Fig. 72.2A–E; Video 72.1). Indeed, there are limitations to this approach and not all cases are amenable to immediate implant placement and loading but it is a viable option.

The overall survival of osseointegrated dental implants has been very good for patients, whether replacing one or several teeth. Regardless of whether patients are missing a single tooth, multiple teeth, or all teeth, their dentition can be functionally and esthetically restored with implant-supported or implant-assisted prostheses that improve patient confidence and quality of life (Fig. 72.3A–G; see Chapters 76, 77, and 88).[34] Unfortunately, the past several decades of clinical experience with implants have also revealed that the incidence of complications is significant.[1,19]

Biological Complications

While implant survival rates are relatively high, implant success is significantly impacted by complications including mechanical, biological, and esthetic (see Chapter 86).[7] In particular, biological complications associated with dental implants are a significant problem, affecting approximately 28% to 56% of patients and 12% to 43% of implant sites.[42]

Similar to periodontitis, peri-implant disease is a host inflammatory response to periodontal pathogens in the bacterial biofilm. Peri-implant mucositis is defined as inflammation of the mucosal tissues surrounding an endosseous implant without the loss of supporting peri-implant bone.[20] The clinical sign of inflammation is bleeding, on probing. Additional signs may include erythema, swelling, and suppuration. Peri-implantitis is defined as a pathologic condition of the peri-implant tissues characterized by inflammation in the surrounding mucosa and progressive loss of supporting bone (Fig. 72.4A).[36] The inflammatory infiltrate is three-fold greater around implants as compared to teeth.[6,16]

Peri-implantitis is a problem that can affect any patient, but patients with a history of periodontitis have a higher incidence of peri-implantitis, especially over longer follow-up periods.[24,26] There is increasing evidence indicating that implants placed in patients with a history of treated periodontitis have a higher incidence of biological complications and lower survival and success as compared to implants placed in patients without a history of periodontitis.[37] There is strong

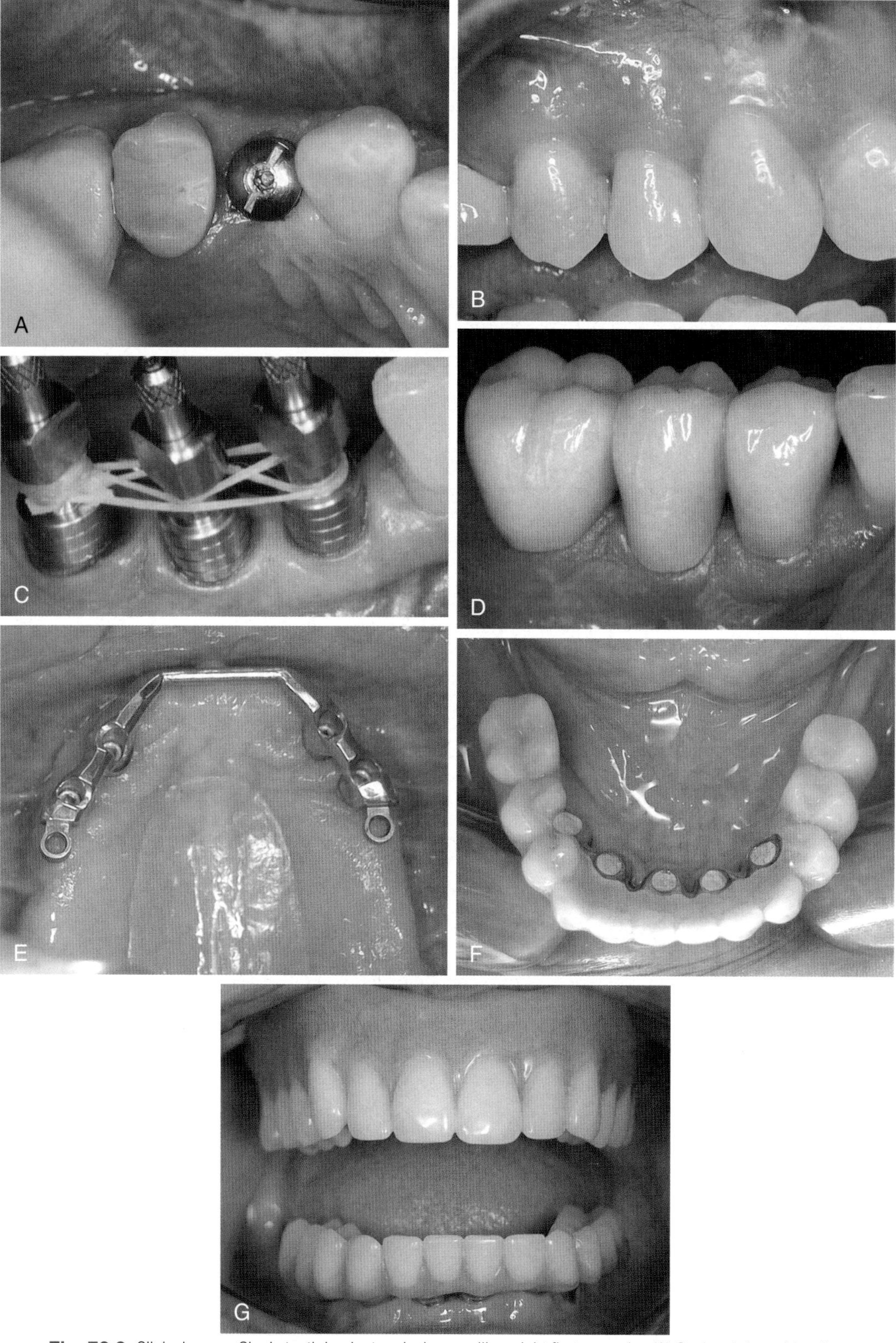

Fig. 72.3 Clinical cases. Single tooth implant replacing maxillary right first premolar. (A) Occlusal view of healing abutment. (B) Buccal view of final implant crown; partially edentulous case with three implants replacing mandibular right posterior teeth. (C) Buccal view of impression copings. (D) Buccal view of final crowns; edentulous case demonstrating an implant-assisted maxillary denture and an implant-supported mandibular hybrid prosthesis. (E) Occlusal view of maxillary implant overdenture bar. (F) Occlusal view of implant-supported hybrid prosthesis. (G) Anterior view of maxillary overdenture and mandibular hybrid prosthesis.

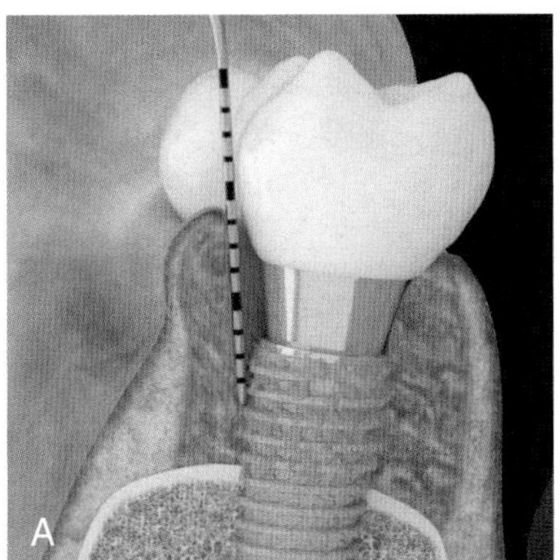

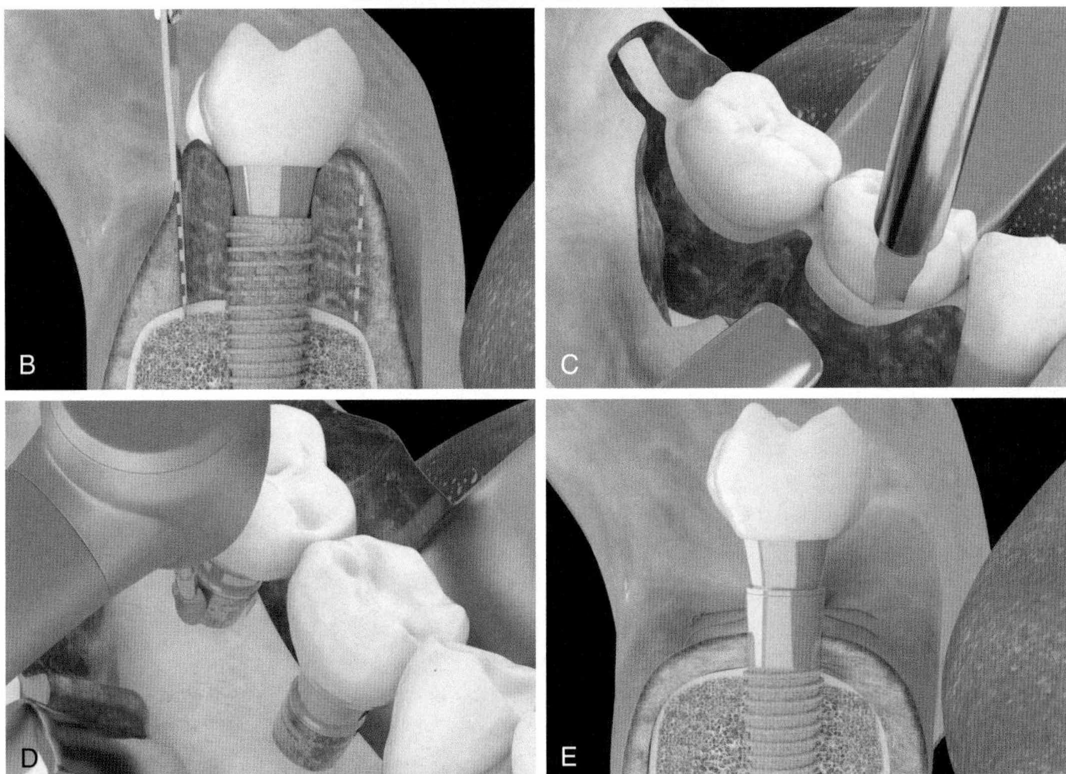

Fig. 72.4 A PerioPixel image depicting resective treatment of peri-implantitis (A) biofilm on implant with inflammatory reaction and inserted probe, (B) outline of proposed incisions, (C) scalloped flap reflected, (D) removing implant threads with rotary instrument, and (E) flaps sutured after resective therapy.

evidence supporting an increased risk of peri-implantitis in patients with a history of periodontitis.[14,33] The incidence of peri-implantitis in patients with a history of periodontitis is 4× higher than the incidence in patients without a history of periodontitis.[10,13]

A recent (2020) study, including 596 patients with implant-supported reconstructions, evaluated the occurrence of mechanical complications, peri-implantitis, and implant loss over a nine-year period. Time of occurrence, potential risk factors, and clustering of complications were evaluated with parametric modeling of survival and hazards.[23] Forty-two percent of patients were affected by mechanical and/or biological complications. Identified risk factors were the extent of therapy and a history of periodontitis. While mechanical complications occurred early (0.7 year) as isolated events, peri-implantitis and implant loss were clustered with other complications. Forty-one percent of subjects with peri-implantitis and 52% of subjects with implant loss presented with other complications. Implant loss peaked early (0.2 year) while peri-implantitis occurred over the entire 9-year follow-up period.

Treatment of Peri-Implantitis

Peri-implantitis is a difficult problem to manage. Treatment is not predictable. The protocols and approach to management frequently follow the principles of therapy and regeneration that have been successful in periodontics. The treatment of peri-implant mucositis is nonsurgical debridement and biofilm control.[5] Adjunctive local delivery agents lack evidence of a beneficial effect.[5] The treatment of peri-implantitis includes open flap surgery, debridement and resection (see Fig. 72.4A–E; Video 72.2), or, when indicated, regenerative procedures with bone grafts and barrier membranes (Fig. 72.5A–H; Video 72.3).[35] Nonsurgical therapy alone is not effective for the management of peri-implantitis. The challenge of treating peri-implantitis is likely related to the unique peri-implant anatomy (i.e., no periodontal ligament, no inserting connective tissue fibers) of surrounding tissues as compared to teeth. The peri-implant mucosal seal is weak. It consists of a long junctional epithelial attachment that is adapted to the implant/abutment/restoration surface and supported by the surrounding tissues, which may be loose, mobile, and not supportive

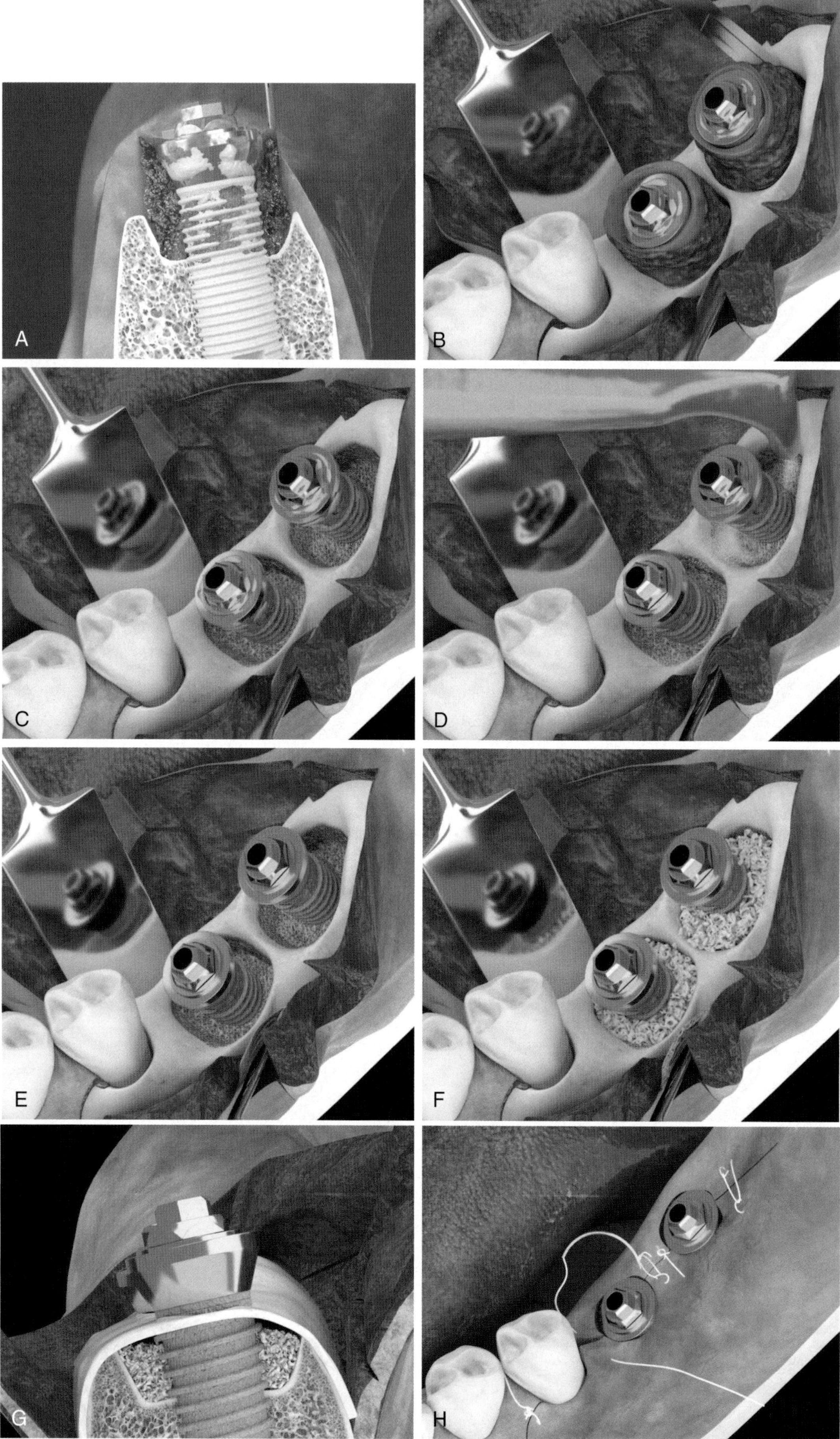

Fig. 72.5 PerioPixel image depicting regenerative treatment of peri-implantitis (A) biofilm on implant with inflammatory reaction and inserted probe, (B) scalloped flap reflected, (C) degranulation of soft tissue from implants and osseous defects, (D) decontamination of implant surfaces, (E) cleaned implant surfaces, (F) application of bone graft material into osseous defect, (G) barrier membrane placed over bone graft, and (H) flaps repositioned and sutured.

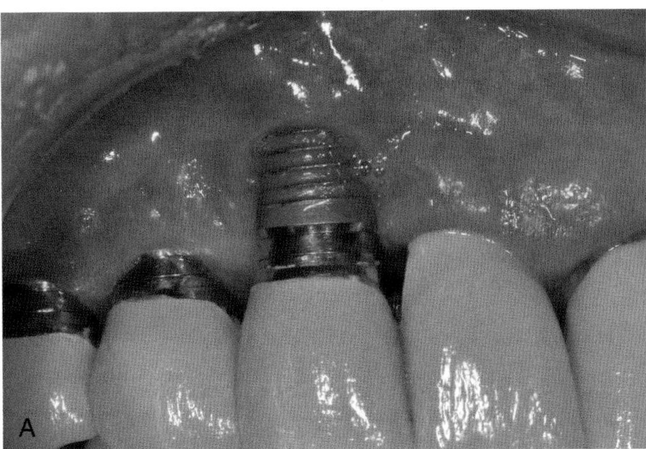
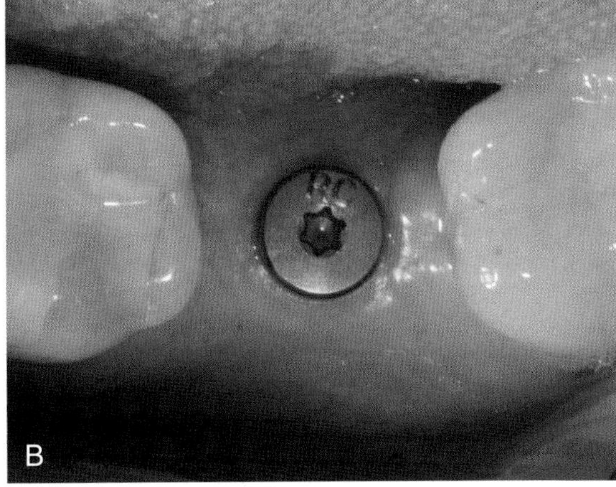

Fig. 72.6 Clinical photos demonstrating (A) maxillary right implant with recession defect surrounded by loose mucosa only, and (B) occlusal view of impalnt healing abutment surrounding by dense keratinized tissue.

(Fig. 72.6A) or dense, firm, and supportive (see Fig. 72.6B) depending on the amount of keratinization and collagen fiber density. An additional factor contributing to the difficulty of peri-implantitis treatment is the inability to effectively clean the implant surface. Macrogeometry threads and microtopography surface characteristics make implant surfaces very challenging to decontaminate.[32,38,39]

Advances in Periodontal Therapy

It is important to remember and recognize that long-term studies have demonstrated the success of periodontal therapy, including periodontal regeneration.[4,21,27] A key element to achieving periodontal treatment success is professional recall maintenance and effective daily biofilm control. Numerous studies, systematic reviews, and meta-analyses have shown that periodontal regeneration is successful.[3,22,28,29] Again, the importance of professional periodontal maintenance and daily biofilm control is critical to success.[12,31]

Integrating implants with periodontal therapy should be recognized as a viable option for the replacement of teeth that are lost, severely compromised, or hopeless. However, it is important to realize and remember that implants should not be considered a solution for "treating" periodontitis.[17]

A recent (2021) retrospective study evaluating the longevity of teeth and implants in a cohort of periodontally compromised patients, treated and maintained in a private periodontal practice, reported the 10-year follow-up results of 58 patients (30 men, 28 women) who received active periodontal therapy and regular periodontal maintenance.[18] Detailed periodontal and peri-implant clinical and radiographic parameters were evaluated along with potential risk factors. The average tooth loss was 0.07 teeth/patient/year (0.04 teeth/patient/year for periodontal reasons), while the average implant loss was 0.4 implants/patient/year, a ten-fold increase. The overall implant loss was 10.08% and the rate of implant failure for biologic reasons was 9.8%. An interesting and compelling finding was that the incidence of implant failure in patients with recurrent periodontitis (defined as PPD ≥ 4 mm with BOP or PPD ≥ 6 without BOP) was 83.3%, while the incidence of implant failure for those with well-maintained periodontitis was only 16.7%. The reported implant survival (90%) was similar to other published long-term reports of implants in treated and maintained periodontitis patients.[24,30]

In a prospective longitudinal study of 73 patients (130 implants), treated surgically for peri-implantitis, assessing the recurrence rate of progressive bone loss, 57 implants (44%) were found to have progressive peri-implant bone loss.[9] Twenty-seven of these implants were lost. Residual deep probing depth (≥6 mm) and reduced marginal bone level at 1 year after surgery were significant risk factors for recurrence/progression of disease, with odds ratio (OR) of 7.4 and 1.4, respectively. Implants with modified surfaces were at higher risk than implants with nonmodified surfaces (OR 5.1).

Conversely, maintenance of the natural dentition with periodontal regeneration has been demonstrated to be highly successful.[2,28,29] In a randomized controlled clinical trial reporting 10-year outcomes, survival analysis and mean cumulative cost of periodontal regeneration versus tooth extraction and implant replacement of periodontally compromised teeth with severe intra-bony defects, Cortellini and coworkers reported 88% survival of teeth and 100% survival of implants with no statistically significant difference.[11] The periodontal attachment gain was 7.3 ± 2.3 mm and residual probing depth was 3.4 ± 0.8 mm. Complication-free survival was similar for teeth and implants in this cohort of severely compromised periodontitis patients. Recurrence analysis showed that costs were significantly higher for implant treatment versus periodontal regeneration over the entire 10-year period.

Conclusions

The integration of dental implants into dentistry/periodontics has revolutionized treatment planning options for all patients who are missing one or more teeth. Implants are a nice option to replace missing or hopeless teeth with implant-supported or implant-assisted prostheses. However, decades of clinical experience with implants have revealed that they are not a panacea for tooth replacement. There are significant biologic complications that are difficult, if not impossible, to resolve. Implants can and do fail! Thus, it is imperative that we diagnose cases accurately and treatment plan well, with an emphasis on preserving the natural dentition when possible. When implants are indicated, it is critical that surgical implant placement and restoration are executed well and that peri-implant maintenance is optimal (i.e., professional care and daily biofilm control). The integration of implants with periodontal therapy has advanced periodontics and facilitated tooth replacement options for patients that were not previously possible.

Suggested Reading

Axelsson P, Nystrom B, Lindhe J. The long-term effect of a plaque control program on tooth mortality, caries and periodontal disease in adults. Results after 30 years of maintenance. *J Clin Periodontol.* 2004;31(9):749–757. https://doi.org/10.1111/j.1600-051X.2004.00563.x.

Berglundh T, Persson L, Klinge B. A systematic review of the incidence of biological and technical complications in implant dentistry reported in prospective longitudinal studies of at least 5 years. *J Clin Periodontol.* 2002;29(suppl 3):197–212; discussion 232-3.https://doi.org/10.1034/j.1600-051x.29.s3.12.x.

Branemark PI, Hansson BO, Adell R, et al. Osseointegrated implants in the treatment of the edentulous jaw. Experience from a 10-year period. *Scand J Plast Reconstr Surg Suppl.* 1977;16:1–132.

Carcuac O, Derks J, Abrahamsson I, Wennstrom JL, Berglundh T. Risk for recurrence of disease following surgical therapy of peri-implantitis-A prospective longitudinal study. *Clin Oral Implants Res.* 2020;31(11):1072–1077. https://doi.org/10.1111/clr.13653.

Cortellini P, Stalpers G, Mollo A, Tonetti MS. Periodontal regeneration versus extraction and dental implant or prosthetic replacement of teeth severely compromised by attachment loss to the apex: A randomized controlled clinical trial reporting 10-year outcomes, survival analysis and mean cumulative cost of recurrence. *J Clin Periodontol.* 2020;47(6):768–776. https://doi.org/10.1111/jcpe.13289.

Costa FO, Takenaka-Martinez S, Cota LO, Ferreira SD, Silva GL, Costa JE. Peri-implant disease in subjects with and without preventive maintenance: a 5-year follow-up. *J Clin Periodontol.* 2012;39(2):173–181. https://doi.org/10.1111/j.1600-051X.2011.01819.x.

Derks J, Tomasi C. Peri-implant health and disease. A systematic review of current epidemiology. *J Clin Periodontol.* 2015;42(suppl 16):S158–S171. https://doi.org/10.1111/jcpe.12334.

Donos N, Laurell L, Mardas N. Hierarchical decisions on teeth vs. implants in the periodontitis-susceptible patient: the modern dilemma. *Periodontol 2000.* 2012;59(1):89–110. https://doi.org/10.1111/j.1600-0757.2011.00433.x.

Greenwell H, Wang HL, Kornman KS, Tonetti MS. Biologically guided implant therapy: A diagnostic and therapeutic strategy of conservation and preservation based on periodontal staging and grading. *J Periodontol.* 2019;90(5):441–444. https://doi.org/10.1002/JPER.18-0495.

Guarnieri R, Di Nardo D, Di Giorgio G, Miccoli G, Testarelli L. Longevity of Teeth and Dental Implants in Patients Treated for Chronic Periodontitis Following Periodontal Maintenance Therapy in a Private Specialist Practice: A Retrospective Study with a 10-Year Follow-up. *Int J Periodontics Restorative Dent.* 2021;41(1):89–98. https://doi.org/10.11607/prd.4674.

Hirschfeld L, Wasserman B. A long-term survey of tooth loss in 600 treated periodontal patients. *J Periodontol.* 1978;49(5):225–237. https://doi.org/10.1902/jop.1978.49.5.225.

Kao RT, Nares S, Reynolds MA. Periodontal regeneration - intrabony defects: a systematic review from the AAP Regeneration Workshop. *J Periodontol.* 2015;86(2 suppl):S77–S104. https://doi.org/10.1902/jop.2015.130685.

Karlsson K, Derks J, Wennstrom JL, Petzold M, Berglundh T. Occurrence and clustering of complications in implant dentistry. *Clin Oral Implants Res.* 2020;31(10):1002–1009. https://doi.org/10.1111/clr.13647.

Karoussis IK, Salvi GE, Heitz-Mayfield LJ, Bragger U, Hammerle CH, Lang NP. Long-term implant prognosis in patients with and without a history of chronic periodontitis: a 10-year prospective cohort study of the ITI Dental Implant System. *Clin Oral Implants Res.* 2003;14(3):329–339. https://doi.org/10.1034/j.1600-0501.000.00934.x.

McFall Jr WT. Tooth loss in 100 treated patients with periodontal disease. A long-term study. *J Periodontol.* 1982;53(9):539–549. https://doi.org/10.1902/jop.1982.53.9.539.

Roccuzzo M, Layton DM, Roccuzzo A, Heitz-Mayfield LJ. Clinical outcomes of peri-implantitis treatment and supportive care: a systematic review. *Clin Oral Implants Res.* 2018;29(suppl 16):331–350. https://doi.org/10.1111/clr.13287.

Roos-Jansaker AM, Lindahl C, Renvert H, Renvert S. Nine- to fourteen-year follow-up of implant treatment. Part I: implant loss and associations to various factors. *J Clin Periodontol.* 2006;33(4):283–289. https://doi.org/10.1111/j.1600-051X.2006.00907.x.

Sousa V, Mardas N, Farias B, et al. A systematic review of implant outcomes in treated periodontitis patients. *Clin Oral Implants Res.* 2016;27(7):787–844. https://doi.org/10.1111/clr.12684.

Wang G, Gao X, Lo EC. Public perceptions of dental implants: a qualitative study. *J Dent.* 2015;43(7):798–805. https://doi.org/10.1016/j.jdent.2015.04.012.

Zarb GA. *Proceedings of the Toronto Conference on Osseointegration in Clinical Dentistry.* St. Louis: Mosby; 1982.

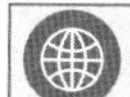
References for this chapter are found on the companion website eBooks.Health.Elsevier.com.

CHAPTER 73

Peri-Implant Anatomy, Biology, and Function

Joseph P. Fiorellini | Keisuke Wada | Hector L. Sarmiento | Perry R. Klokkevold | Kevin W. Luan

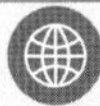

For online-only content on endosseous implants, root form (cylindric) implants, transmandibular implants, subperiosteal implants, and implant surface characteristics (microdesign), go to the companion website at eBooks.Health.Elsevier.com. Some figures may be out of numeric order in this printed chapter.

CHAPTER OUTLINE

The history of modern implant dentistry began with the introduction of titanium implants.[41] In the 1950s, Per-Ingvar Brånemark, a Swedish professor of anatomy, had a serendipitous finding while studying blood circulation in bone that became a historic breakthrough in medicine. He discovered an intimate bone-to-implant apposition with titanium that offered sufficient strength to cope with load transfer. He called the phenomenon *osseointegration* and developed an implant system with a specific protocol to achieve it predictably. The implants were used to anchor prosthetic replacement teeth in the edentulous jaw,[27] and the first patient was successfully treated in 1965.[30,76] Subsequent clinical studies proved that commercially pure (CP) titanium implants, placed with a strict protocol, including an unloaded healing period, could predictably achieve osseointegration and retain a full-arch prosthesis in function with long-term success (15 years).[8]

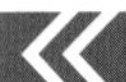

FLASH BACK

The history of modern implant dentistry began with the introduction of titanium implants. In the 1950s, Per-Ingvar Brånemark, a Swedish professor of anatomy, had a serendipitous finding while studying blood circulation in bone that became a historical breakthrough in medicine. He coined the phenomenon *osseointegration* and developed an implant system with a specific protocol to achieve it predictably.

Today, implant designs, surgical placement techniques, healing times, and restorative protocols continue to evolve with the goal of improving outcomes. It is important for clinicians to know peri-implant anatomy, understand the biology, and appreciate the functional capacity of osseointegrated implants. This chapter reviews implant geometry and surface characteristics, as well as the anatomic and biologic relationships of peri-implant tissues.

Implant Geometry (Macrodesign)

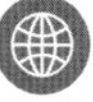

Numerous implant systems with various geometric (macrodesign) designs were developed and used before the current implant systems in use today. Previous implant designs included blade vents (narrow, flat shape; tapped into bony trough prepared with rotary burs),[73] press-fit cylindric (bullet shape; pressed or tapped into prepared hole),[104] subperiosteal (custom-made framework, adapted to the surface of jawbone),[37] and transmandibular (long rods or posts, placed through the anterior mandible).[113] Some of these implant systems were initially stable and appeared to be successful over short-term periods (e.g., 5 years) but failed to remain stable, became symptomatic or loose, and failed over longer periods.[102,125] Lacking predictability, these implant systems are no longer used.

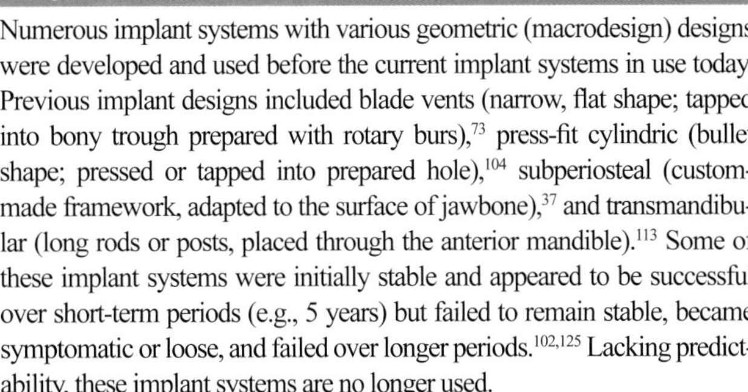

Since the time of the Brånemark studies, millions of patients have been treated worldwide using variations of these techniques with implants of different geometries and surface characteristics. Similar research, including that of André Schroeder in Switzerland in the mid-1970s, contributed to the success of endosseous dental implants. The serendipitous finding of Brånemark was that when a hole is prepared into bone without overheating or otherwise traumatizing the tissues, an inserted biocompatible implantable device would predictably achieve an intimate bone apposition, as long as micromovements at the interface were prevented during the early healing period. The history of the research endeavors in Sweden provides a better understanding of the relevant biologic parameters involved.[76]

The macroscopic configuration of implants has varied widely; the most common types are listed in Box 73.1. Currently, most endosseous implants have a cylindric or tapered, screw-shaped threaded design. The disastrous results with other implant configurations were largely responsible for the evolution toward the current popular designs.[13] See online for a detailed description of the various implant designs, including blades, pins, disks, root form, transmandibular, and subperiosteal implants.

Hard Tissue Interface

The primary goal of implant installation is to achieve and maintain a stable bone to implant connection (i.e., osseointegration).[29,30] Histologically, osseointegration is defined as the direct structural and functional connection between ordered, living bone and the surface of a load-bearing implant without intervening soft tissues (Fig. 73.1).[27,28] Clinically, osseointegration is the asymptomatic rigid fixation of an alloplastic material (implant) in bone with the ability to withstand occlusal forces.[12,127] The hard tissue interface is a fundamental requirement for and an essential component of implant success.

KEY FACT

Histologically, osseointegration is defined as the direct structural and functional connection between ordered, living bone and the surface of a load-bearing implant without intervening soft tissues. Clinically, osseointegration is the rigid fixation of an alloplastic material (implant) in bone with the ability to withstand occlusal forces.

BOX 73.1 Implant Geometry (Macrodesign)

1. Endosseous implants
   - Bladelike
   - Pins
   - Root form, cylindric (hollow and full)
   - Disklike
   - Screw-shaped
   - Tapered and screw-shaped
2. Subperiosteal (custom frame) implants
3. Transmandibular implants

Initial Bone Healing

The osseointegration process observed after implant insertion can be compared with bone fracture healing. Implant site osteotomy preparation (bone wounding) initiates a sequence of events, including an inflammatory reaction, bone resorption, release of growth factors, and chemotactic attraction by osteoprogenitor cells to the site. Differentiation of osteoprogenitor cells into osteoblasts leads to bone formation at the implant surface. Extracellular matrix proteins, such as osteocalcin, modulate apatite crystal growth.[124] Specific conditions, optimal for bone formation, must be maintained at the healing site to achieve osseointegration.

Immobility of the implant relative to the bone must be maintained for bone formation at the surface. A mild inflammatory response enhances bone healing, but moderate inflammation or movement above a certain threshold is detrimental.[6] When micromovements at the interface exceed 150 μm, the movement will impair differentiation of osteoblasts and fibrous scar tissue will form between the bone and implant surface.[94] Therefore it is important to avoid excessive forces, such as occlusal loading, during the early healing period.

Bone tissue damage and debris created by the osteotomy site preparation must be cleared up by osteoclasts for normal bone healing. These multinuclear cells, originating from the blood, can resorb bone at a pace of 50 to 100 μm/day. There is a coupling between bone apposition and bone resorption (Fig. 73.2). Preosteoblasts, derived from primary mesenchymal cells, depend on a favorable oxidation-reduction (redox) potential of the environment. Thus, a proper vascular supply and oxygen tension are needed. If oxygen tension is poor, the primary stem cells may differentiate into fibroblasts, form scar tissue, and lead to implant failure (nonintegration).

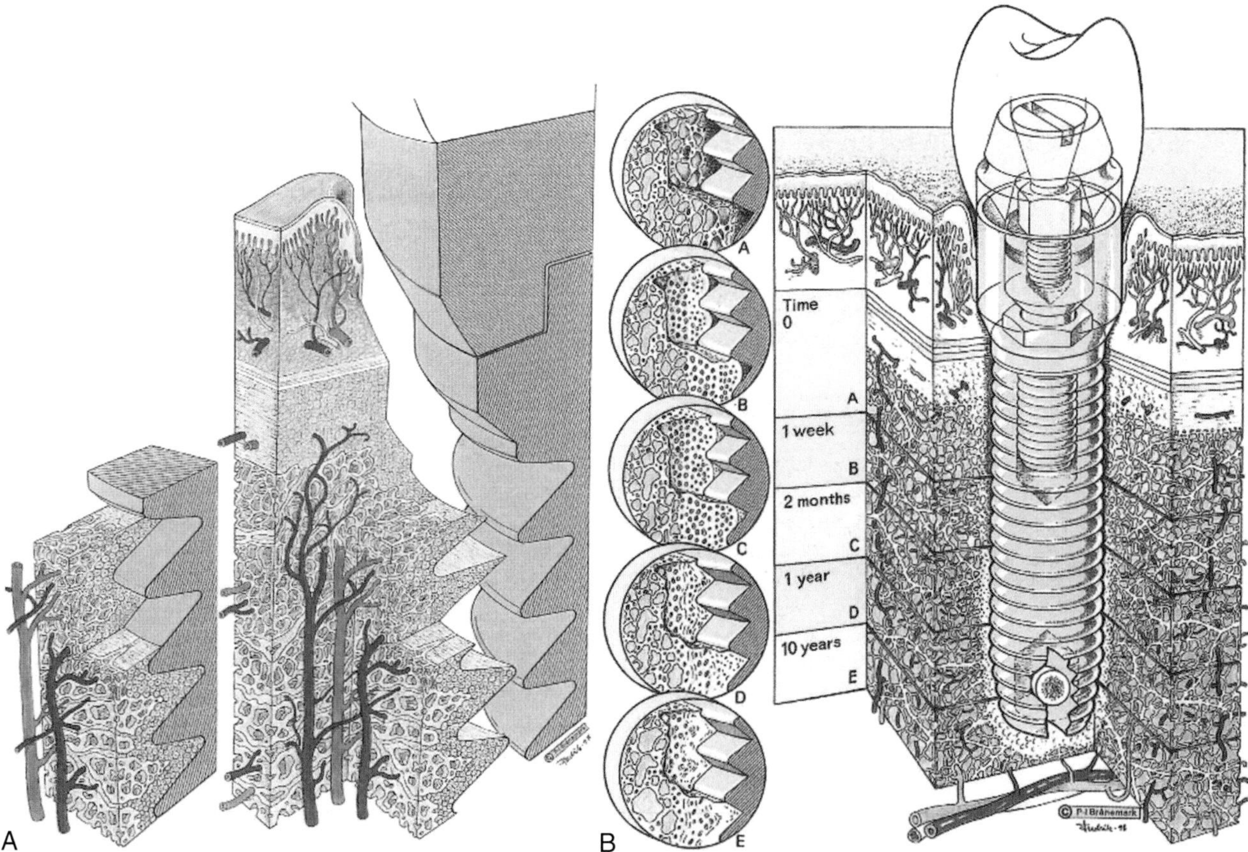

Fig. 73.1 (A) Three-dimensional diagram of the tissue and titanium interrelationship showing an overall view of the intact interfacial zone around the osseointegrated implant. (B) Physiologic evolution of the biology of the interface over time.

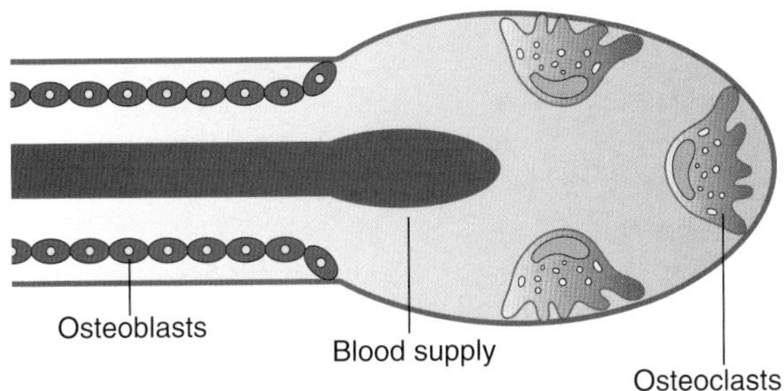

Fig. 73.2 This basic multicellular unit is the basic remodeling process for bone renewal. Osteoclasts are imported by the vascular supply, and the resorption lacunae are soon filled by the lining osteoblasts.

If bone is overheated or crushed during preparation, it will become necrotic and may lead to nonmineralized (soft tissue) scar formation or be sequestered. The critical temperature for bone cells that should not be exceeded is 47°C (116.6°F) at an exposure time of 1 minute.[6] Thus preparation of implant osteotomy sites requires profuse irrigation (cooling) along with gentle, intermittent, moderate-speed drilling using sharp drills. Another complicating factor, well recognized from open wound fractures, is that microbial contamination jeopardizes the normal bone healing. Accordingly, strict aseptic techniques should be maintained.

KEY FACT

Immobility of the implant must be maintained during the early postinsertion healing for bone formation at the surface. Moderate inflammation or movement above a certain threshold is detrimental and may lead to implant failure. If micromovements exceed 150 μm, the movement will impair the differentiation of osteoblasts, and fibrous scar tissue will form between the bone and implant surface.

New bone formation follows a specific sequence of events. Woven bone is quickly formed in the gap between the implant and the bone; it grows fast, up to 100 μm/day, and in all directions. Characterized by a random orientation of its collagen fibrils, high cellularity, and limited degree of mineralization, the biomechanical capacity of woven bone is poor (Fig. 73.3A). Thus, any occlusal load should be well controlled or avoided in the early phase of healing. After several months, woven bone is progressively replaced by lamellar bone with organized, parallel layers of collagen fibrils and dense mineralization. Contrary to the fast-growing woven bone, lamellar bone formation occurs at a slow pace (only a few microns per day). Ultimately, after 18 months of healing, a steady state is reached where lamellar bone is continuously resorbed and replaced (see Fig. 73.3B).[27] At the light microscopic level, an intimate bone to implant contact has been extensively reported (Fig. 73.4).[100] Once the bone to implant interface has reached a steady state, it can maintain itself over decades, as ascertained by human histology from implants retrieved because of hardware fractures.[10]

FLASH BACK

The biomechanical capacity of woven bone is poor. New bone formation adjacent to an implant follows a specific sequence of events, with woven bone forming quickly in the gap; it grows fast (100 μm/day) and in all directions. It is characterized by a random orientation of its collagen fibrils, high cellularity, and a limited degree of mineralization.

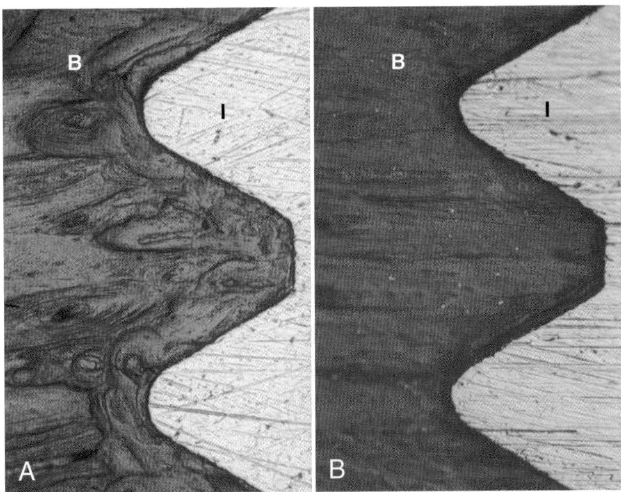

Fig. 73.3 (A) After initial healing, woven bone, as characterized by its irregular pattern, is laid down. (B) After weeks or months, a lamellar bone is laid down progressively, with regular concentric lamellae. *B,* Bone; *I,* implant. (Courtesy Professor T. Albrektsson, Gothenburg, Sweden.)

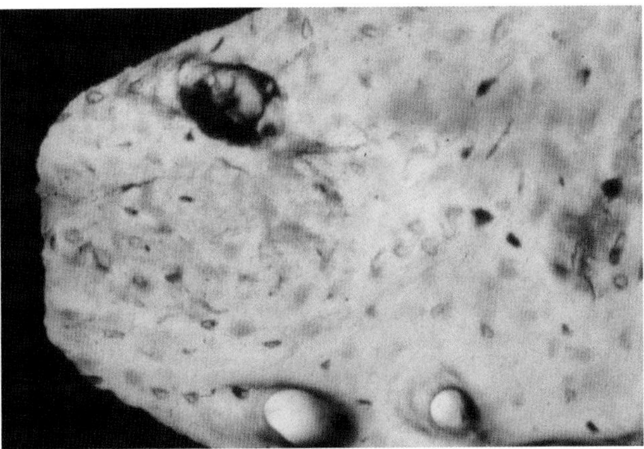

Fig. 73.4 Once a steady state has been achieved at the bone to implant interface, an intimate contact can be observed, with some marrow spaces seen in between at the light microscopic level.

Bone Remodeling and Function

Clinically, both primary and secondary stability of an implant are critical to success. Primary stability, achieved at the time of surgical placement, depends on the implant geometry (macrodesign), as well as the quality and quantity of bone available for implant anchorage at a specific site. Studies using resonance frequency analysis (RFA) have reported decreased implant stability in the early weeks of postinsertion healing.[18,44,58,96] Secondary stability, achieved over time with healing, depends on the implant surface (microdesign), as well as the quality and quantity of adjacent bone, which will determine the percentage of contacts between the implant and bone.[18,50,95,114]

For example, areas such as the anterior mandible have dense cortical bone and provide rigid primary stabilization and good support throughout the healing process. Conversely, areas such as the posterior maxilla have thin cortical bone, and large marrow spaces provide less primary stability. For this reason, the posterior maxilla has been associated with lower success rates compared with other sites with greater bone density and support.[17,63] Interestingly, a new implant with unique knife edge–wide threads (macrodesign) has been shown, in completely healed sites, to maintain stability without the typical drop in the implant stability quotient (ISQ) throughout the early bone remodeling phase.[77]

Once osseointegration is achieved, implants can resist and function under the forces of occlusion for many years. Longitudinal biomechanical assessments seem to indicate that during the first weeks after placement of one-stage implants, decreased rigidity is observed.[47] This may be indicative of bone resorption during the initial phase of healing. Subsequently, rigidity increases and continues to increase for years.[113] Thus, when a prosthesis is installed immediately (in 1 day) or early (in 1 to 2 weeks), care must be taken to control against overload. It is important to recognize that sites with limited primary stability or less bone to implant contact (e.g., posterior maxilla) will likely go through a period of even less bone support in the early stages of bone healing due to the initial phase of bone resorption.

Soft Tissue Interface

Not surprisingly, for two decades, research and clinical interest focused on the bone to implant interface of osseointegrated implants, and the overlying soft tissues were largely ignored. Except for a few descriptive sentences, the classic handbook by Brånemark and colleagues[27] presented no data or information about the soft tissue interface. This may be due in part to the fact that most patients were fully edentulous and the Brånemark system implants had turned (machined) surfaces, which are less likely to be associated with soft tissue inflammatory problems.[5] Today, there is greater interest in and appreciation for peri-implant soft tissues and the soft tissue to implant interface as a function of esthetics and maintenance of a seal or barrier against microbial invasion.

Peri-implant soft tissues are similar in appearance and structure to periodontal soft tissues (see Chapter 4).[5] Clearly, both implants and teeth emerge through the soft tissues on the alveolar ridge. The soft tissues consist of connective tissue covered by epithelium. There is a gingival/mucosal sulcus, a long junctional epithelial attachment, and a zone of connective tissue above the supporting bone (Fig. 73.5). Despite the apparent similarities in soft tissues around teeth and implants, the presence of a periodontal ligament around teeth and not around implants is an important and distinct difference. Whereas natural teeth have a periodontal ligament with connective tissue fibers inserting into the cementum and suspending them in the alveolar bone, osseointegrated implants do not. There are no inserting collagen fibers anywhere along the interface of osseointegrated implants. Bone is in direct contact with the implant surface, without intervening soft tissues.

FLASH BACK

Sharpey's fibers are bundles of collagenous fibers that pass into the outer circumferential lamellae of alveolar bone and the cementum of teeth.

Clinically, the thickness of the peri-implant soft tissues varies from 2 mm to several millimeters (Fig. 73.6). An animal study

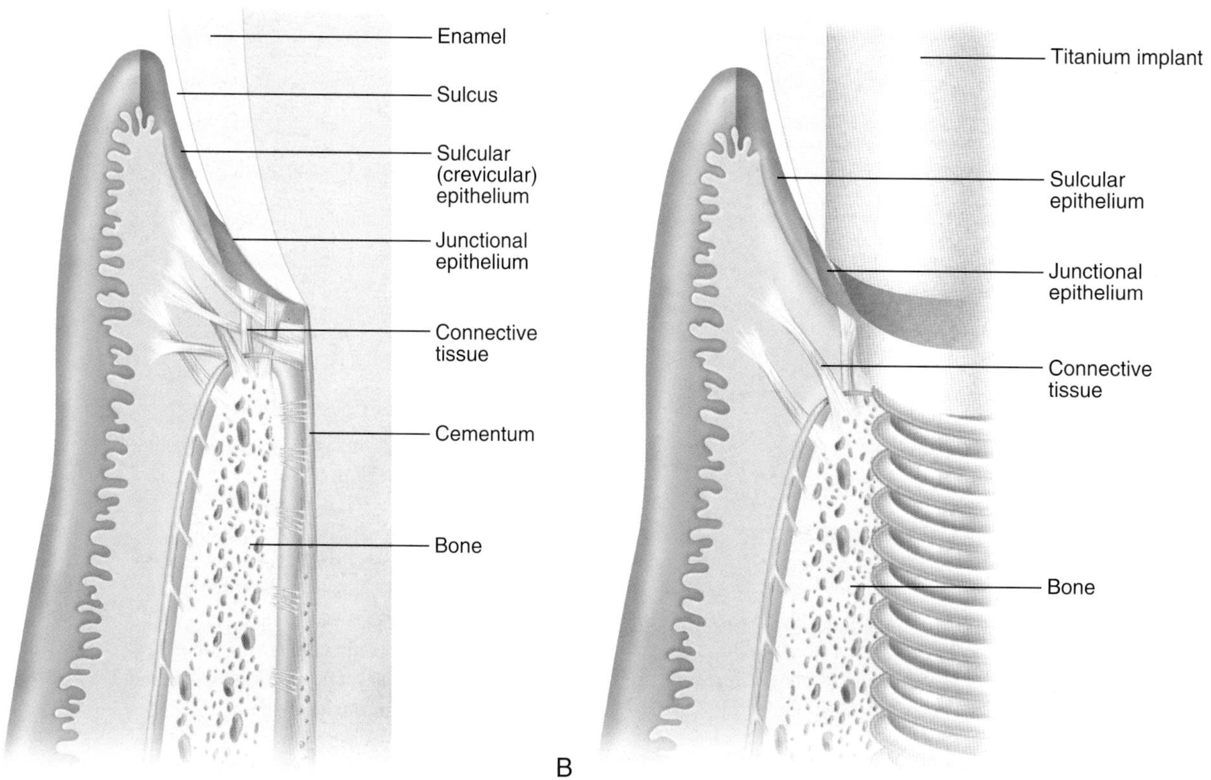

Fig. 73.5 Schematic illustration of hard and soft tissue around a tooth and an implant. (A) Hard and soft tissue anatomy around a natural tooth demonstrates bone support with a periodontal ligament, a connective tissue zone above the crest of bone with connective tissue fibers (Sharpey's) inserting into dentin, a long junctional epithelial attachment, a gingival sulcus lined with sulcular epithelium, and oral gingival epithelium (outer surface of gingiva). (B) Hard and soft tissue anatomy around an implant demonstrates some similarities and some distinct differences. There is supporting bone in direct approximation to the implant surface without any intervening soft tissues (i.e., no periodontal ligament). A connective tissue zone is present above the level of bone, with fibers running parallel to the implant surface and no inserting fibers. There is a long junctional epithelial attachment, a gingival-mucosal sulcus lined with sulcular epithelium, and oral gingival-mucosal epithelium (outer surface of soft tissue).

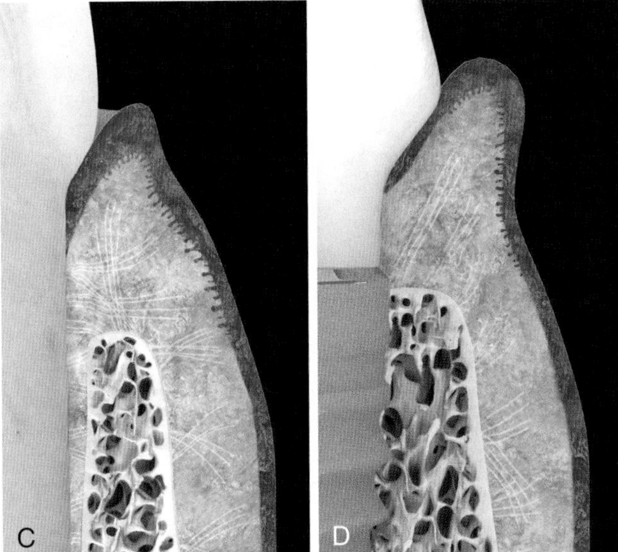

Fig. 73.5 cont'd (C) Hard and soft tissue anatomy around a natural tooth; this demonstrates bone support with a periodontal ligament, a connective tissue zone above the crest of bone with connective tissue fibers (Sharpey's) inserting into dentin, a long junctional epithelial attachment, a gingival sulcus lined with sulcular epithelium, and oral gingival epithelium (outer surface). (D) Hard and soft tissue anatomy around an implant demonstrates some similarities and some distinct differences. There is supporting bone in direct approximation to the implant surface without any intervening soft tissues (i.e., no periodontal ligament). A connective tissue zone is present above the level of bone, with fibers running parallel to the implant surface and no inserting fibers. There is a long junctional epithelial attachment, a gingival/mucosal sulcus lined with sulcular epithelium, and oral gingival/mucosal epithelium (outer surface). (A and B, from Rose LF, Mealey BL: *Periodontics: medicine, surgery, and implants.* St. Louis, 2004, Mosby; C and D, courtesy Periopixel, Madrid, Spain.)

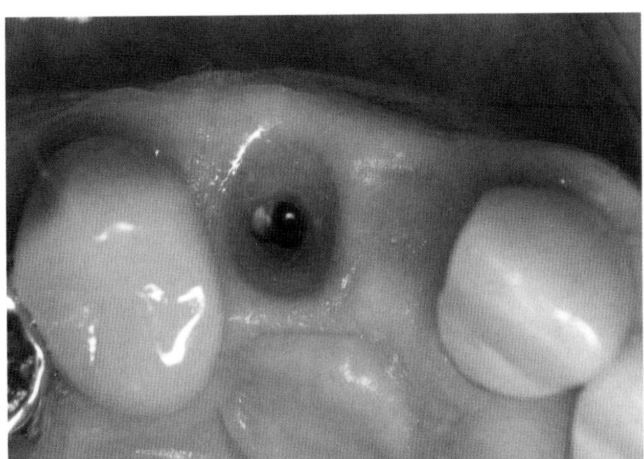

Fig. 73.6 Clinical appearance of normal, healthy peri-implant tissue with implant restoration removed. Soft tissue thickness varies from site to site, depending on the quantity and quality of tissue, as well as the anatomy of the surrounding area (e.g., adjacent to natural teeth with healthy periodontal attachment versus adjacent to a space). Note that the intrasulcular tissue appears more erythematous as the result of the thin, nonkeratinized layer of epithelium overlying the connective tissue.

determined the total height of the peri-implant "biologic width" to be approximately 3 to 4 mm, where about 2 mm is the epithelial attachment and about 1 to 2 mm is the supracrestal connective tissue zone.[19] Consistent with this finding, a human histologic study determined the height of the peri-implant "biologic width," consisting of an epithelial attachment and supracrestal connective tissue, to be about 4 to 4.5 mm[48] (Fig. 73.7).

Epithelium

As in the natural dentition, the oral epithelium around implants is continuous with a sulcular epithelium that lines the inner surface of the gingival sulcus; the apical part of the gingival sulcus is lined

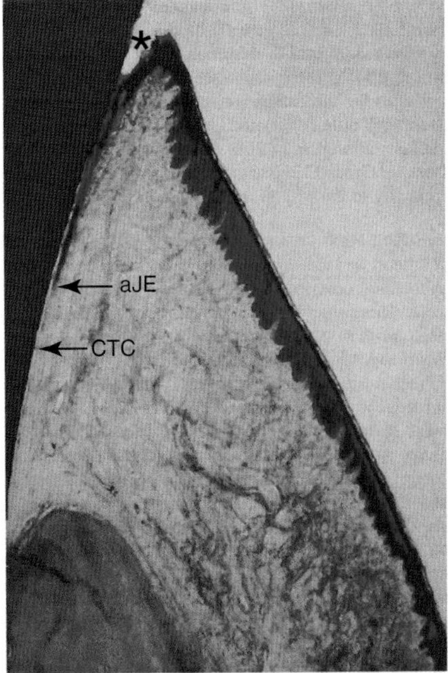

Fig. 73.7 Buccolingual section [basic fuchsin stain; original magnification, ×12.5; one-part sandblasted, large grit, acid-etched implant surface (SLA) implant, 3 months unloaded] showing the gingiva and the most coronal part of alveolar bone. Rete peg formation is only apparent in the area of the keratinized oral gingival epithelium. The oral sulcular epithelium exhibits no keratinization. In the area of the most coronal point of the junctional epithelium (cJE), the soft tissues are slightly torn away (artifact) because of nondecalcified histologic processing. The most apical point of the junctional epithelium is indicated *(aJE)*. No rete peg formation is evident adjacent to the basal cell layer of the junctional epithelium (JE), with all showing healthy and physiologic soft tissue structures. In addition, the area of connective tissue contact *(CTC)* adjacent to the machined titanium surface is marked. A slight round cell infiltrate in the connective tissue indicates a mild inflammation. Note bone remodeling and new bone formation in the crestal bone region indicated by saturated, dark red–stained areas.

with long junctional epithelium.[75] Ultrastructural examination of the long junctional epithelial attachment adjacent to dental implants has demonstrated that epithelial cells attach with a basal lamina and hemidesmosomes[2,4,50,65,116] (Fig. 73.8). Histologic studies indicate that these epithelial structures and the surrounding lamina propria cannot be distinguished from those structures around teeth.[33] In healthy tissues, the dimension of the sulcular epithelium is about 0.5 mm[98] and the dimension of the epithelial attachment is about 2 mm,[19] which is higher than that of the periodontal epithelial attachment.

The apical edge of the epithelial attachment is about 1.5 to 2 mm above the bone margin.[92] In healthy peri-implant tissues, progressive epithelial downgrowth does not occur, indicating that factors other than inserted collagen fiber bundles (i.e., Sharpey's fibers in natural dentition) prevent it.

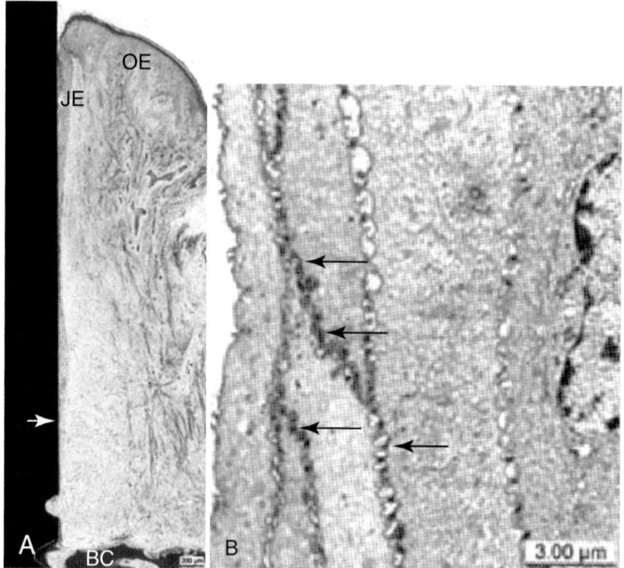

Fig. 73.8 (A) Overview of ground section showing peri-implant tissues covered with keratinizing oral epithelium *(OE)*. Junctional epithelium *(JE)* is interposed between connective tissue and the alveolar bone crest *(BC)*; shown is the apical end of the junctional epithelium *(arrow)* (toluidine blue stain; bar = 200 µm.) (B) Transmission electron microscopic view of sulcular epithelium showing tightly sealed intercellular spaces by numerous spot desmosomes *(arrows)*, contributing to low permeability of this portion of the peri-implant mucosa; bar = 3 µm.

Connective Tissue

Peri-implant connective tissue morphology closely resembles that of natural dentition except that it lacks a periodontal ligament, cementum, and inserting fibers (Fig. 73.9). No significant differences were found at the biochemical level between the peri-implant and periodontal soft tissues,[34] whereas the dimension of the peri-implant connective tissue is 1 to 2 mm, which is higher than that of the average periodontal connective tissue.[19,92]

The zone of supracrestal connective tissue has an important function in the maintenance of a stable soft tissue–implant interface and as a seal or barrier to the "outside" oral environment. The orientation of connective tissue fibers adjacent to an implant differs from that of periodontal connective tissue fibers. In the absence of cementum and inserting connective tissue fibers (i.e., as in a natural tooth), most peri-implant connective tissue fibers run in a direction more or less parallel to the implant surface. Even when the fiber bundles are oriented perpendicularly, which occurs more often in the gingiva than in the mucosa surrounding implants, the bundles are never embedded in the implant surface.

The fiber bundles can also have a cuff-like circular orientation.[20,96] The role of these fibers remains unknown, but it appears that their presence helps create a soft tissue "seal" around the implant. The adaptation of the connective tissue to an implant surface may also be affected by the mobility of the soft tissue around the implant. The connective tissue in direct contact with the implant surface is characterized by an absence of blood vessels and an abundance of fibroblasts interposed between collagen fibers.[72] Several animal and human studies have shown that the alignments of connective fibers

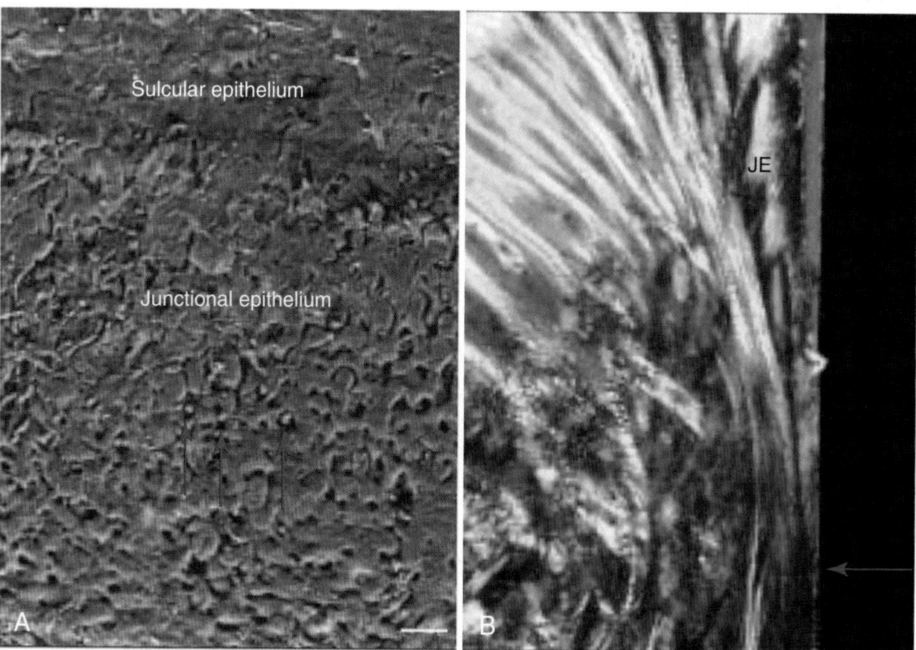

Fig. 73.9 (A) Scanning electron microscope (SEM) image of the junctional epithelium. Note the neutrophils located between the cells *(red arrows)*; bar = 40 µm. (B) Higher magnification of Fig. 73.8 with polarized light showing the apical extent *(red arrow)* of the junctional epithelium *(JE)*. Note the dense collagen fibers running apicocoronal (i.e., parallel to the implant surface).

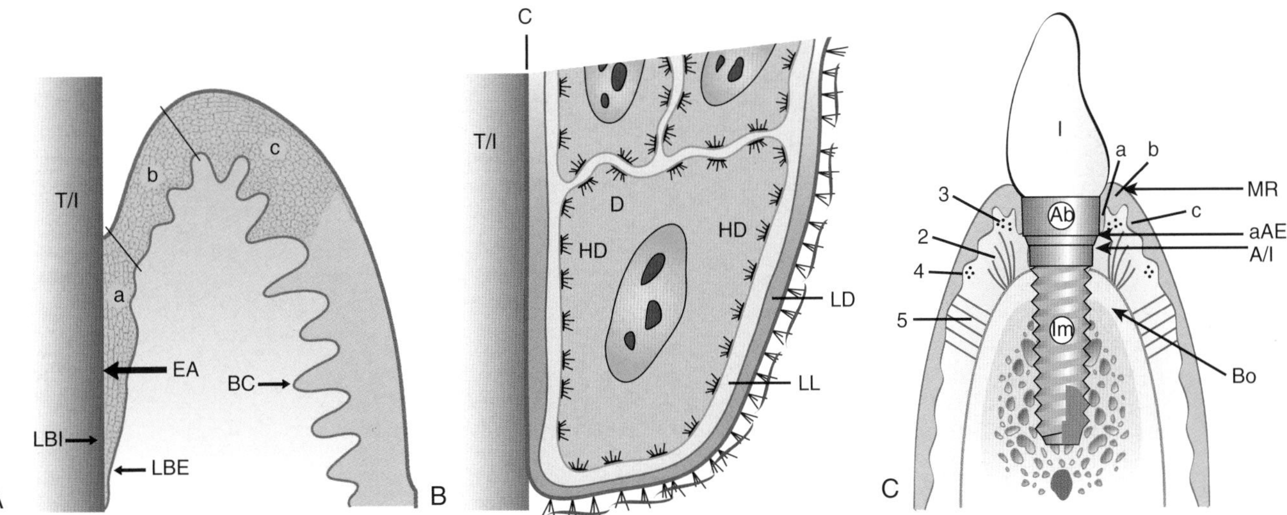

Fig. 73.10 (A) Histologic scheme of epithelial attachment *(EA)* (identical for tooth and implant). *BC,* Basal complex; *LBE,* lamina basalis externa (only location where cell divisions occur); *LBI,* lamina basalis interna; *T/I,* titanium implant; *a,* long junctional epithelial attachment zone; *b,* sulcular epithelial zone; *c,* oral epithelial zone. (B) At the electron microscopic level, basal complex at the epithelial attachment (three most apical cells) and connection with stroma. *C,* Cuticle; *D,* desmosome; *HD,* hemidesmosomes; *LL,* lamina lucida; *LD,* lamina densa.(C) Implant, abutment *(Ab),* and crown within alveolar bone and soft tissues. *aAE,* Apical (point) of attached epithelium; *A/I,* abutment/implant junction; *Bo,* marginal bone level; *Im,* endosseous part of implant; *MR,* margin of gingiva–alveolar mucosa; *1,* implant crown; *2,* vertical alveolar-gingival connective tissue fibers; *3,* circular gingival connective tissue fibers; *4,* circular gingival connective tissue fibers; *5,* periosteal-gingival connective tissue fibers; *a,* junctional epithelium; *b,* sulcular epithelium; *c,* oral epithelium.

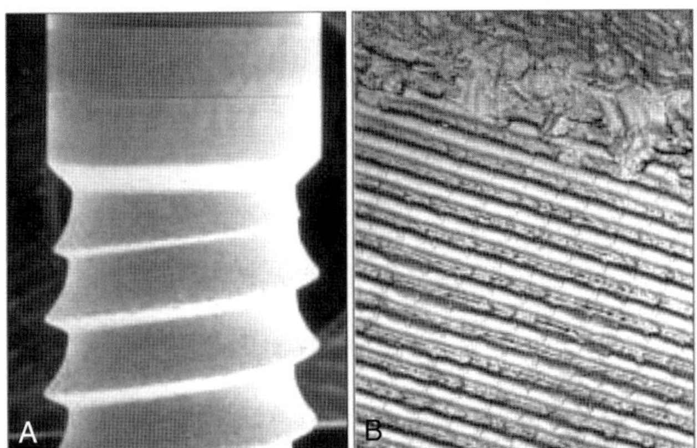

Fig. 73.11 (A) Laser-microtextured surface. (B) Machined collar, original magnification, ×500. (From Botos S, Yousef H, Zweig B, et al: The effects of laser microtexturing of the dental implant collar on crestal bone levels and peri-implant health. *Int J Oral Maxillofac Implants* 2011;26:492-498.)

were circular and horizontal around the implants[1,15,35,49,52,53,101] (Fig. 73.10).

More recent reports have shown histologic evidence of connective tissue attachment perpendicular to the microgrooved implant surface in both animal and human studies.[82-84] These laser-microtextured grooves (Fig. 73.11) have been shown to be able to stop the epithelial downgrowth and establish connective tissue insertion right at the most coronal part of the laser microgrooved area (Fig. 73.12). A prospective controlled clinical study showed that the laser-grooved surface resulted in shallower probing depth and less peri-implant crestal bone loss than that seen around implants with machined collars.[25,89]

This connective tissue interface has been examined by probing attachment level measurements in patients. Probing attachment levels were consistently found coronal to the alveolar crest in patients with peri-implant tissue health, indicating the presence of a zone of direct connective tissue contact to the implant surface. This means that the probing depth measurement performed with a periodontal probe may be about 1.5 mm higher above the bone level in healthy tissues. At inflamed sites, the probe may penetrate to the bone, with the probing depth measurement reflecting the total soft tissue thickness above bone. In cases with inflammatory peri-implant tissue disease, increasing probing depth and reduced attachment levels have been reported.[3,40,90,118]

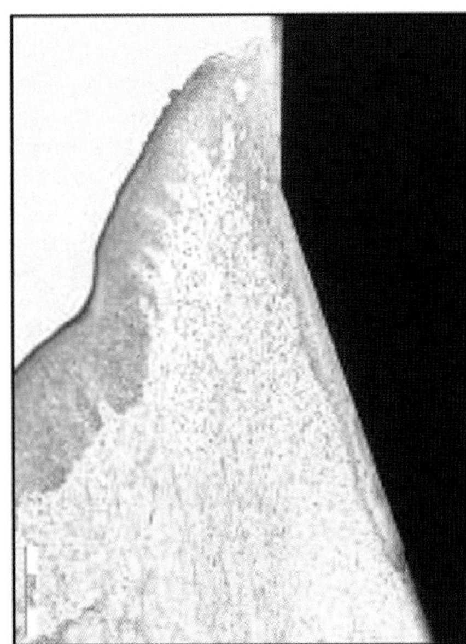

Fig. 73.12 Laser-ablated surface—epithelial downgrowth was stopped right at the coronal-most microgrooved area. Apical to the junctional epithelium, healthy connective tissue fibers attach perpendicularly to the laser-ablated channels. (Courtesy Dr. Myron Nevins.)

Keratinized Tissue

Questions emerged decades ago, as it did for the natural dentition, about the need for keratinized tissue to surround implants. Prospective and cross-sectional studies, evaluating screw-shaped implants with a machined surface, suggest that the presence or absence of keratinized gingiva is not a prerequisite for long-term stability.[103] However, it has been suggested that implants surrounded by mucosa only (i.e., nonkeratinized) are more susceptible to peri-implant problems. An animal study observed that ligature-induced peri-implantitis occurs more frequently when alveolar mucosa surrounds the implant as compared with when keratinized mucosa surrounds the implant.[117]

Keratinized mucosa tends to be more firmly anchored by collagen fibers to the underlying periosteum than nonkeratinized mucosa, which has more elastic fibers and tends to be movable relative to the underlying bone. In clinical studies evaluating intraoral implants, with or without peri-implant keratinized mucosa, no clinically significant difference in implant success was reported.[69,122] However, when there is a lack of keratinized tissue, patients tend to complain about pain and discomfort while performing oral hygiene procedures or other functions in the area. The symptoms are alleviated by increasing the amount of keratinized (firmly bound) tissue around the implant(s) via soft tissue grafting (see online Fig. 65.5, A–L).[9,69,122] Finally, although it may not be comparable to intraoral implants, the mobility of soft tissues surrounding extraoral implants is associated with a higher incidence of implant failure.[9]

Vascular Supply and Inflammation

The vascular supply of the peri-implant gingival or alveolar mucosa may be limited, as compared with periodontal gingiva, due to the lack of a periodontal ligament (Fig. 73.13).[21] This is especially true in the tissue immediately adjacent to the implant surface. However, capillary loops in the connective tissue under the junctional and sulcular epithelium around implants appear to be anatomically similar to those found in the normal periodontium (Fig. 73.14).[115]

Emerging evidence indicates that the peri-implant gingival or alveolar mucosa has the same morphology as the corresponding tissues around teeth. These soft tissues also react the same way to plaque accumulation. Studies investigating the histology (light microscopic and ultrastructural) of healthy and inflamed tissues surrounding implants in humans have indicated that the inflammatory response to plaque is similar to that observed in periodontal tissues.[98] Polymorphonuclear cells and mononuclear cells transmigrate normally through the peri-implant sulcular epithelium (Fig. 73.15).[98]

Clinical Comparison of Teeth and Implants

Although the soft tissue to implant (abutment) interface offers striking similarities with tissue surrounding the natural dentition, some differences should be considered. At the bone level, the lack of a periodontal ligament is the most striking difference. The following discussion elaborates on the clinical perspectives of these similarities and differences.

At the bone level, the absence of the periodontal ligament surrounding an implant has important clinical consequences. This means that no resilient connection exists between implants and supporting bone. Implants cannot intrude or migrate to compensate for the presence of a premature occlusal contact (as teeth can). Implants and the rigidly attached implant restorations do not move. Thus, any occlusal disharmony will have repercussions at either the restoration to implant connection, bone to implant interface, or both.

Proprioception in the natural dentition comes from the periodontal ligament. The absence of a periodontal ligament around implants reduces tactile sensitivity[61] and reflex function.[23] This can become even more challenging when osseointegrated, implant-supported, fixed prostheses are present in both jaws.

The lack of a periodontal ligament and inability of implants to move contraindicates their use in growing individuals. Natural teeth continue to erupt and migrate during growth, whereas implants do not. Implants placed in individuals prior to the completion of growth can lead to occlusal disharmonies with implants.[87] Likewise, it may be problematic to place one or more implants in a location adjacent to teeth that are very mobile from the loss of periodontal support because, as the teeth move in response to or away from the occlusal forces, the implant(s) will bear the entire load.

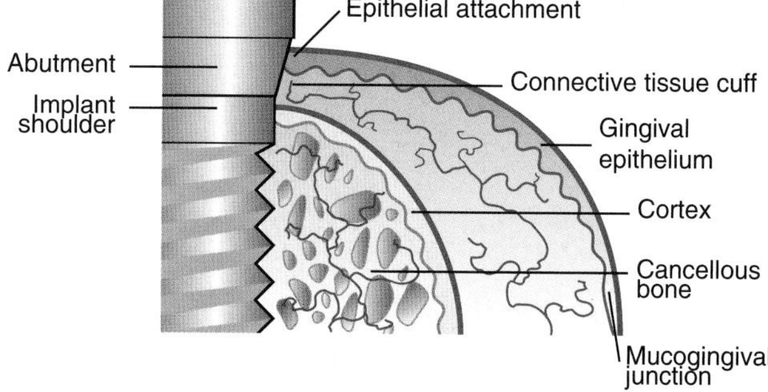

Fig. 73.13 Schematic illustration of the blood supply in the connective tissue cuff surrounding the implant-abutment, which is scarcer than in the gingival complex around teeth because none originates from a periodontal ligament.

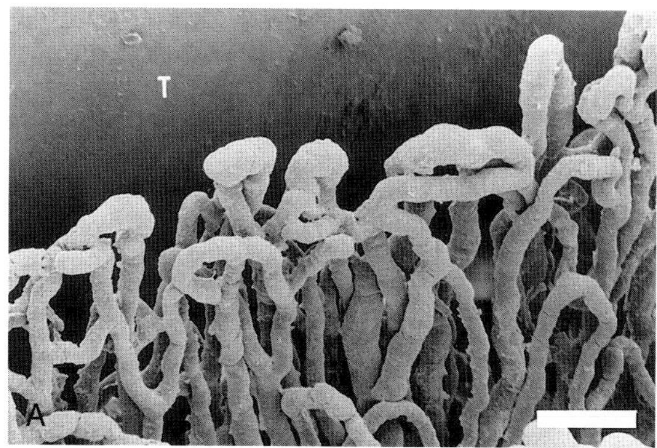

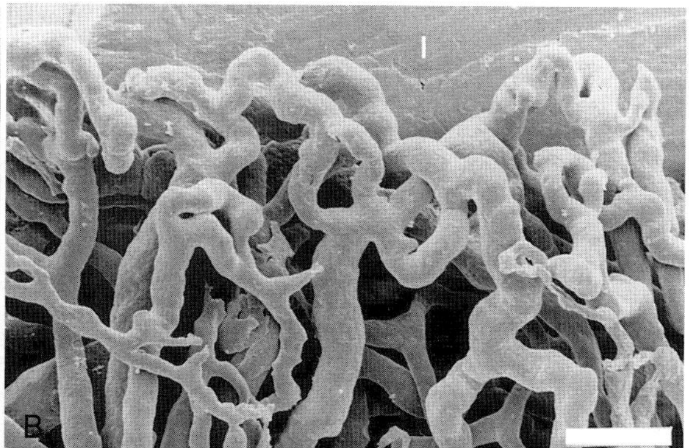

Fig. 73.14 (A) Microvascular topography surrounding a tooth. (B) Microvascular topography surrounding an implant; bar = 5 μm. (Courtesy Dr. N. Selliseth and Dr. K. Selvig, Bergen, Norway.)

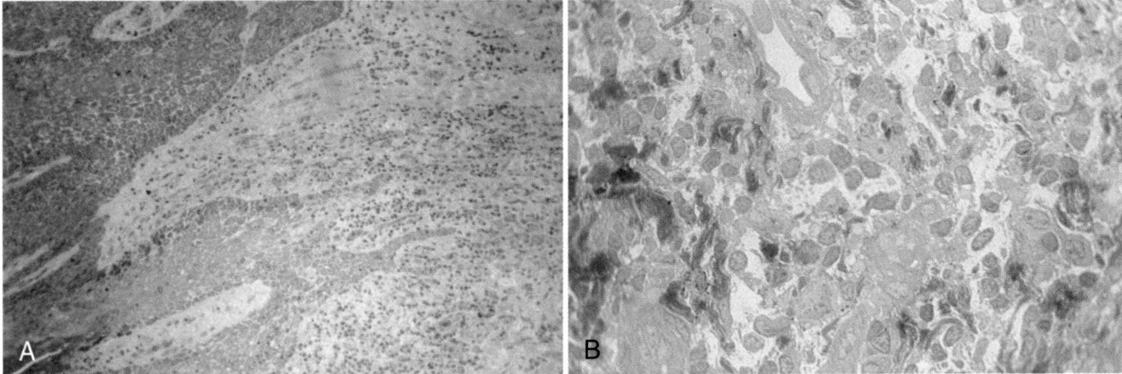

Fig. 73.15 (A) Histologic slide from healthy gingiva surrounding a well-functioning implant in a human patient. No morphologic characteristics differentiate tissue around implant from that around teeth. (B) When gingivitis occurs, a profuse migration of inflammatory cells through the pocket epithelium can be observed. (Courtesy Professor Mariano Sanz, Madrid, Spain.)

Overload, because of improper superstructure design, parafunctional habits, or excessive occlusal load, may cause microstrains and microfractures in the bone, which will lead to bone loss and a fibrous inflammatory tissue at the implant interface.[115]

Conclusions

A thorough understanding of bone biology is essential for clinicians to fully appreciate the phenomenon and limitations of osseointegration. Many factors can interfere with the predictable establishment and maintenance of a long-term rigid connection between the implant surface and the surrounding bone that is able to sustain occlusal loads. The bone to implant interface and its rigidity are a predominant biomechanical aspect of coping with the time and intensity of loading. The quality of the soft tissue to implant interface also plays an important role in the long-term maintenance of stable marginal bone levels around implants. Clinicians must familiarize themselves with the underlying molecular and cellular events to evaluate the future evolution of implant design and implant protocols, including surgical placement, restoration, and maintenance.

A Case Scenario is found on the companion website eBooks.Health.Elsevier.com.

Suggested Readings

Albrektsson T. The host-implant interface: biology. *Int J Prosthodont*. 2003;16(suppl):29–30; discussion 47–51.

Berglundh T, Lindhe J. Dimension of the periimplant mucosa. Biological width revisited. *J Clin Periodontol*. 1996;23:971–973.

Berglundh T, Lindhe J, Ericsson I, et al. The soft tissue barrier at implants and teeth. *Clin Oral Implants Res*. 1991;2:81–90.

Boyan BD, Hummert TW, Dean DD, et al. Role of material surfaces in regulating bone and cartilage cell response. *Biomaterials*. 1996;17:137–146.

Brånemark PI, Zarb G, Albrektsson T. *Tissue-Integrated Prothesis: Osseointegration in Clinical Dentistry*. Chicago: Quintessence; 1987.

Davies JE. Understanding peri-implant endosseous healing. *J Dent Educ*. 2003;67:932–949.

Hermann JS, Buser D, Schenk RK, et al. Biologic width around one- and two-piece titanium implants. *Clin Oral Implants Res*. 2001;12:559–571.

Linkevicius T, Apse P. Biologic width around implants. An evidence-based review. *Stomatologija*. 2008;10:27–35.

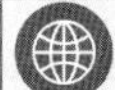
References for this chapter are found on the companion website eBooks.Health.Elsevier.com.

CHAPTER 74

Clinical Evaluation of the Implant Patient

Perry R. Klokkevold | David L. Cochran | Michael Whang

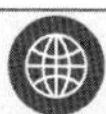 For online-only content on diagnostic study models, please visit the companion website at eBooks.Health.Elsevier.com.

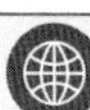 Videos for this chapter can be viewed on the companion website at eBooks.Health.Elsevier.com.

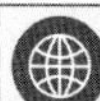 Animations have been added by the editors as a supplement to the chapter. They are produced by PerioPixel as patient education tools and cover the basic elements in a conceptual manner. They are not intended to be procedural guides for dental professionals.

CHAPTER OUTLINE

Over the past several decades, following the landmark research and development of osseointegrated dental implants by Brånemark and colleagues,[15–17] treatment options and treatment planning in dentistry have evolved tremendously. Initially, prosthetic reconstructions with osseointegrated implants were limited to use in the edentulous patient, with many reports documenting excellent long-term success.[1,2,25]

Shortly thereafter, the original implant treatment protocols were adapted for use in partially edentulous patients. There were some transitional challenges associated with the early use of dental implants being adapted to the partially edentulous patient, but ultimately successes were achieved for this population as well. Modifications in implant design, procedural techniques, and treatment planning greatly improved implant therapy for the partially edentulous patient. Currently, the long-term success of dental implants used to replace single and multiple missing teeth in the partially edentulous patient is very good (see Chapter 88).[29,40,42,49,54] The implementation of bone augmentation procedures further increased the option for patients with inadequate bone volume to be successfully restored with implant-retained prostheses.[27,34,55] Virtually any patient with an edentulous space could be a candidate for endosseous implants, and studies suggest that success rates of 90% to 95% can be expected in healthy patients with good bone and normal healing capacity.[24]

The ultimate goal of dental implant therapy is to satisfy the patient's desire to replace one or more missing teeth in an esthetic, secure, functional, and long-lasting manner. To achieve this goal, clinicians must accurately diagnose the dentoalveolar condition, as well as the overall mental and physical well-being of the patient. It is necessary to determine whether implant therapy is possible, practical, and, perhaps most important, whether it is indicated for the particular patient who is seeking implants. Local evaluation of potential jaw sites for implant placement (e.g., measuring available alveolar bone height, width, and spatial relationship) and prosthetic restorability are essential considerations in determining whether an implant(s) is possible. However, making an assessment of the patient and determining whether that patient is a good candidate for implants is an equally important part of the evaluation process. The patient evaluation includes identifying factors that might increase the risk of failure or the possibility of complications, as well as determining whether the patient's expectations are reasonable.

This chapter presents an overview of the clinical aspects of dental implant therapy, including an assessment of possible risk factors and contraindications. It also provides guidelines for the pretreatment evaluation of potential implant patients and the posttreatment evaluation of patients with implants.

Case Types and Indications

Edentulous Patients

The patients who seem to benefit most from dental implants are those with fully edentulous arches. These patients can be effectively restored, both esthetically and functionally, with an implant-assisted removable prosthesis, an implant-supported removable prosthesis, or an implant-supported fixed prosthesis.

The original design for the edentulous arch was a fixed-bone–anchored bridge that used five to six implants in the anterior area of the mandible or the maxilla to support a fixed, hybrid prosthesis. The design is a denture-like complete arch of teeth attached to a substructure (metal framework), which in turn is attached to the implants with cylindrical titanium abutments (Fig. 74.1). The prosthesis is fabricated without flange extensions and does not rely on any soft tissue support. It is entirely implant supported. Usually, the prosthesis includes bilateral distal cantilevers, which extend to replace posterior teeth (back to premolars or first molars).

Another implant-supported design used to restore an edentulous arch is the ceramic-metal fixed bridge (Fig. 74.2). Some patients prefer this design because the ceramic restoration emerges directly from the gingival tissues in a manner that makes its appearance similar to that of natural teeth.

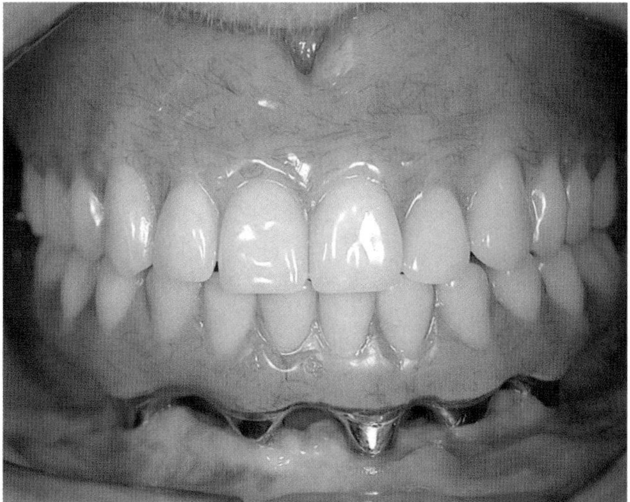

Fig. 74.1 Clinical photograph of patient with a complete maxillary denture opposing a full-arch implant-supported fixed prosthesis in the mandibular arch.

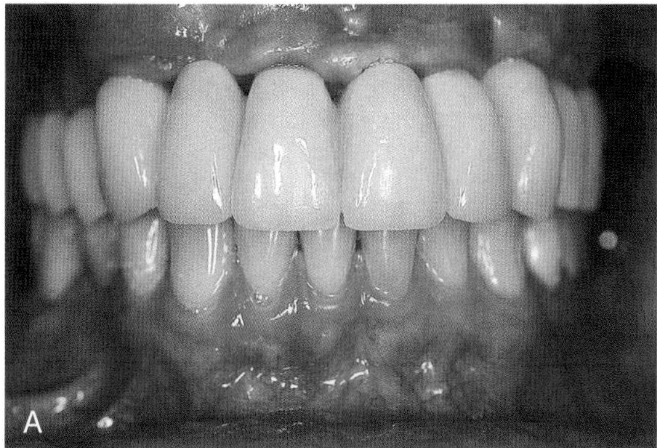

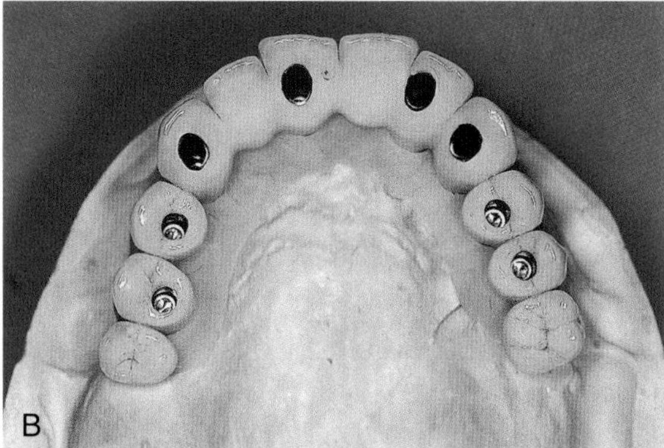

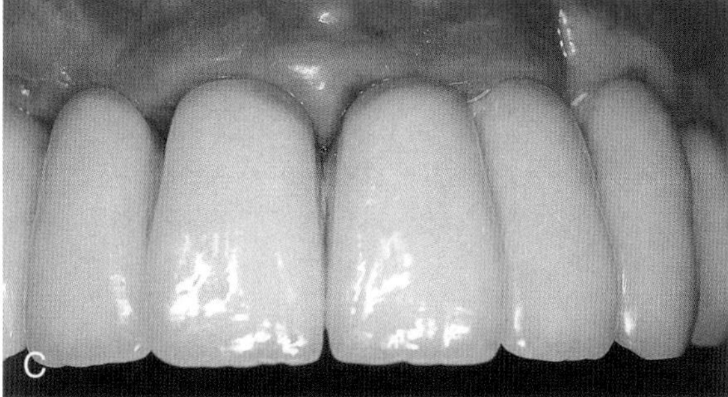

Fig. 74.2 (A) Clinical photograph of acrylic provisional fixed full-arch prosthesis in the maxilla. (B) Clinical photograph of the final ceramometal restoration, anterior view. (C) Occlusal view of final restoration on master cast. *(Courtesy Dr. Russell Nishimura, Westlake Village, California.)*

One limitation of both hybrid and ceramometal implant-supported fixed prostheses is that they provide very little lip support and thus may not be indicated for patients who have lost significant alveolar dimension. This is often more problematic for maxillary reconstructions because lip support is more critical in the upper arch. Furthermore, for some patients, the lack of a complete seal (i.e., spaces under the framework) allows air to escape during speech, thus creating phonetic problems.

Depending on the volume of existing bone, the jaw relationship, the amount of lip support, and phonetics, some patients may not be able to be rehabilitated with an implant-supported fixed prosthesis. For these patients, a removable, complete-denture type of prosthesis is a better choice because it provides a flange extension that can be adjusted and contoured to support the lip, and there are no spaces for unwanted air escape during speech. This type of prosthesis can be retained and stabilized by two or more implants placed in the anterior region of the maxilla or mandible. Methods used to secure the denture to the implants vary from separate attachments on each individual implant to clips or other attachments that connect to a bar, which splints the implants together (Fig. 74.3). It is also possible to design a removable prosthesis to intimately and securely attach to a precision-fit substructure (e.g., milled bar), making it an implant-supported removable prosthesis.

Although the stability of the implant-retained overdenture does not compare with the rigidly attached, implant-supported fixed prosthesis, the increased retention and stability over conventional complete dentures is an important advantage for denture wearers.[57] Additionally, implant-assisted and implant-supported prostheses are thought to lessen the amount of alveolar bone loss associated with long-term use of removable prostheses that bear directly on the alveolar ridges.

Partially Edentulous Patients

Multiple Teeth

Partially edentulous patients with multiple missing teeth represent another viable treatment population for osseointegrated implants, but the remaining natural dentition (occlusal schemes, periodontal health status, spatial relationships, and esthetics) introduces additional challenges for successful rehabilitation.[41] The juxtaposition of implants with natural teeth in the partially edentulous patient presents the clinician with challenges not encountered with implants in the edentulous patient. As a result of distinct differences in the biology and function of implants compared with natural teeth, clinicians must educate themselves and use a prescribed approach to the evaluation and treatment planning of implants for partially edentulous patients (see Chapter 76). In general, endosseous dental implants can support a freestanding fixed partial denture. Adjacent natural teeth are not necessary for support, but their close proximity requires special attention and planning.[11] The major advantage of an implant-supported restoration in the partially edentulous patient is that it replaces missing teeth without invasion or alteration of adjacent teeth. Preparation of natural teeth becomes unnecessary, and larger edentulous spans can be restored with implant-supported fixed bridges.[50] Moreover, patients who previously did not have a fixed option, such as those with Kennedy class I and II partially edentulous situations, can be restored with an implant-supported fixed restoration (Fig. 74.4).

Early attempts to use endosseous implants to replace missing teeth in the partially edentulous patient were a challenge partly because the implants and armamentarium were designed for the edentulous patient and did not have much flexibility for adaptation and use in the partially edentulous patient. Today, clinicians have many choices in terms of implant length, diameter, and abutment connection to choose for the optimal replacement of any missing tooth, large or small (Fig. 74.5).

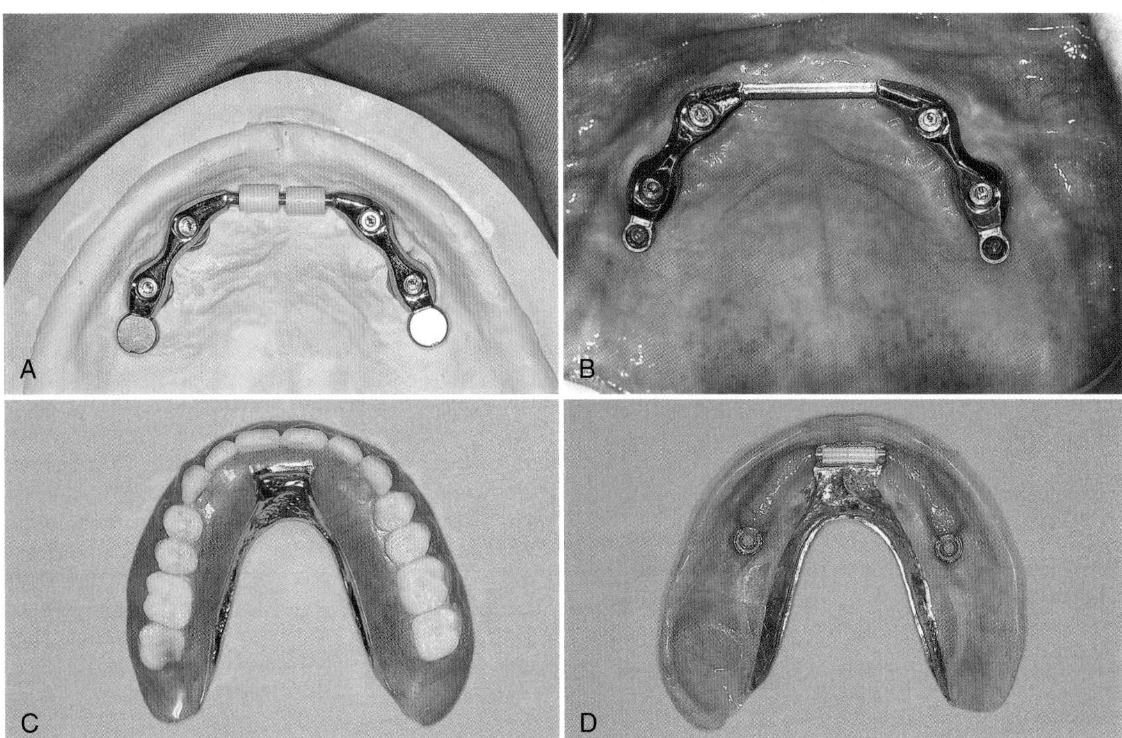

Fig. 74.3 (A) Maxillary overdenture bar attached to four implants with anterior clips and posterior extracoronal resilient attachments (ERAs). (B) Clinical view of maxillary overdenture bar. (C) Palateless maxillary complete overdenture. (D) Tissue surface of the same maxillary implant-assisted overdenture showing clips and ERAs. *(Courtesy Dr. John Beumer, University of California, Los Angeles, Maxillofacial Prosthodontics.)*

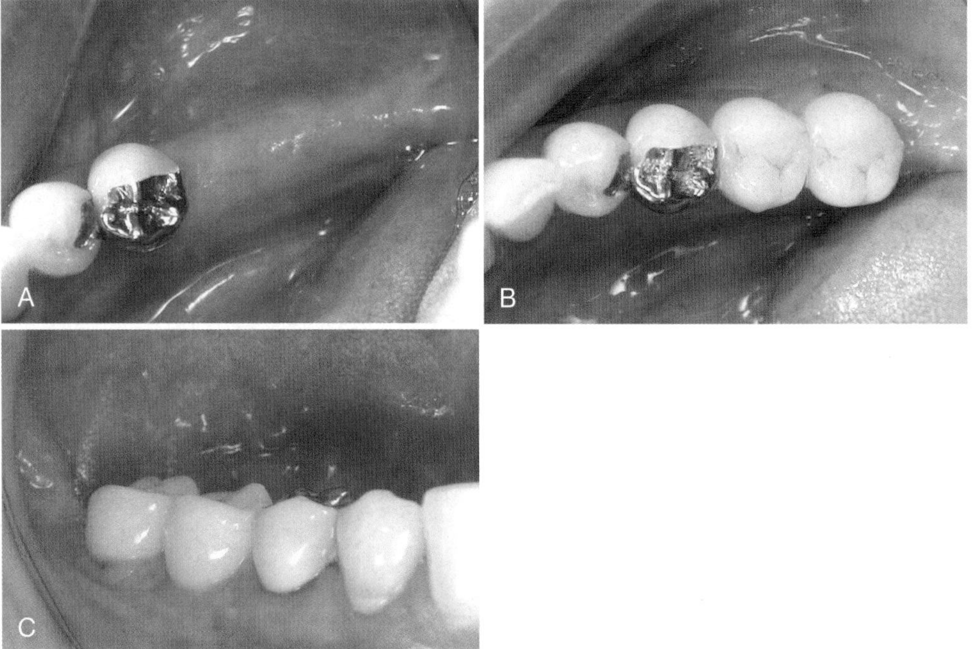

Fig. 74.4 (A) Clinical view of a partially edentulous posterior mandible (Kennedy class II distal extension). (B) Occlusal view of the same patient as in part A restored with an implant-supported fixed restoration replacing teeth #18 and #19. Note that the dimensions of the crowns are smaller than typical mandibular molars (i.e., closer to bicuspid size). (C) Buccal view of the same restorations.

The primary challenge with partially edentulous cases is an underestimation of the importance of treatment planning for implant-retained restorations with an adequate number of implants to withstand occlusal loads. For example, one problem that required correction was the misconception that two implants could be used to support a long-span, multiunit fixed bridge in the posterior area. Multiunit fixed restorations in the posterior jaw are more likely to experience complications or failures (mechanical or biologic) when they are inadequately supported in terms of the number of implants, quality of bone, or strength of the implant material (see Chapter 76).

Fig. 74.5 Diagram representing the use of wide-, narrow-, and standard-diameter implants for molars, mandibular incisors, and other teeth (different-sized implants superimposed over various teeth). (A) Maxillary teeth. (B) Mandibular teeth.

Better treatment planning with the use of an adequate number and size of implants, particularly in areas of poor-quality bone, has solved many of these problems.

FLASH BACK

The Kennedy Classification refers to a system developed by Dr. Edward Kennedy for the classification of an edentulous jaw and partial dentures. It is based on the distribution of edentulous spaces. Kennedy class I is a bilateral free-end posterior edentulous area. Kennedy class II is a unilateral free-end posterior edentulous area. Kennedy class III is a single bounded edentulous area that does not cross the midline (unilateral). Kennedy class IV is a single anterior bounded edentulous area that crosses the midline (bilateral).

Single Tooth

Patients with a missing single tooth (anterior or posterior) represent another type of patient who benefits greatly from the success and predictability of endosseous dental implants (Video 74.1). Replacement of a single missing tooth with an implant-supported crown is a much more conservative approach than preparing two adjacent teeth for the fabrication of a tooth-supported fixed partial denture. It is no longer necessary to "cut" healthy or minimally restored adjacent teeth to replace a missing tooth with a nonremovable prosthetic replacement (Fig. 74.6). Reported success rates for single-tooth implants are excellent.[23]

Replacement of an individual missing posterior tooth with an implant-supported restoration has been successful as well. The greatest challenges to overcome with the single-tooth implant restorations were screw loosening and implant or component fracture. Because of the increased potential to generate forces in the posterior area, the implants, components, and screws often failed. Both of these problems have been addressed with the use of wider-diameter implants and internal fixation of components (Fig. 74.7). Wide-diameter implants often have a wider platform (restorative interface) that resists tipping forces and thus reduces screw loosening. The wide-diameter implant also provides greater strength and resistance to fracture as a result of increased wall thickness (i.e., the thickness of the implant between the inner screw thread and the outer screw thread). Implants with an internal connection are inherently more resistant to screw loosening and thus have an added advantage for single-tooth applications.

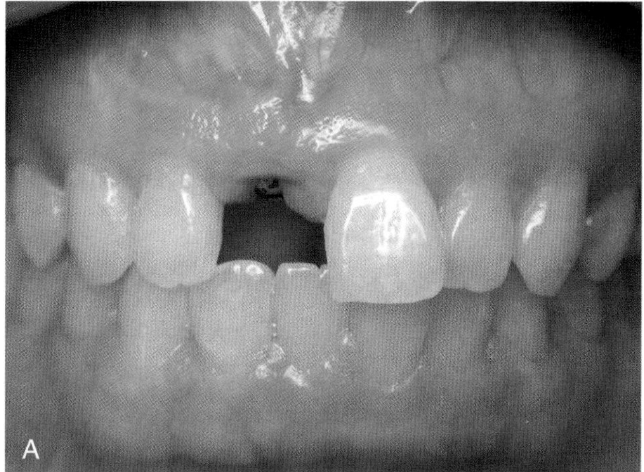

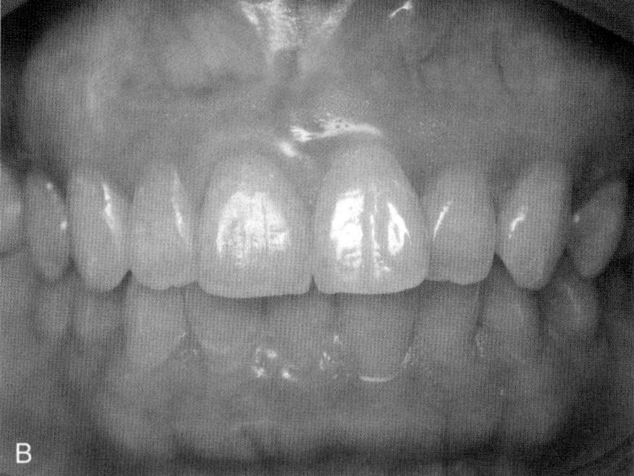

Fig. 74.6 Single-tooth replacement. (A) Implant in place. (B) Metalloceramic crown.

Esthetic Considerations

Anterior single-tooth implants present some of the same challenges as the single posterior tooth supported by an implant, but they also are an esthetic concern for patients. Some cases are more esthetically challenging than others because of the nature of each individual's smile and display of teeth. The prominence and occlusal relationship of existing teeth, the thickness and health of periodontal tissues, and the patient's own psychological perception of esthetics all play a role in the esthetic challenge of the case. Cases with good bone volume, bone height, and tissue thickness can be predictable in terms of achieving satisfactory esthetic results (see Fig. 74.6). However, achieving esthetic results for patients with less-than-ideal tissue qualities poses difficult challenges for the restorative and surgical team.[12] Replacing a single tooth with an implant-supported crown in a patient with a high smile line, compromised or thin periodontium, inadequate hard or soft tissues, and high expectations is probably one of the most difficult challenges in implant dentistry and should not be attempted by novice clinicians.

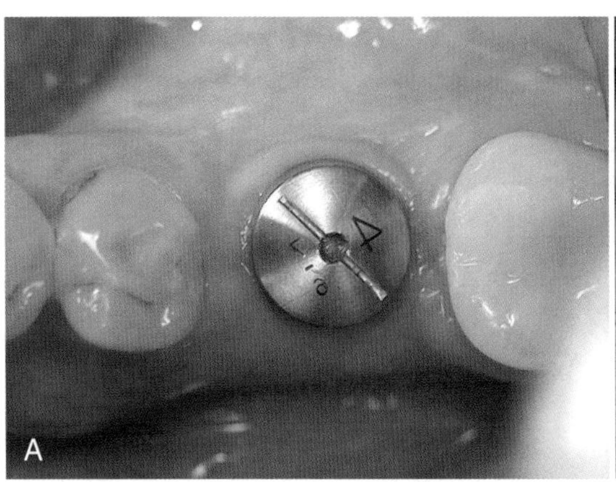

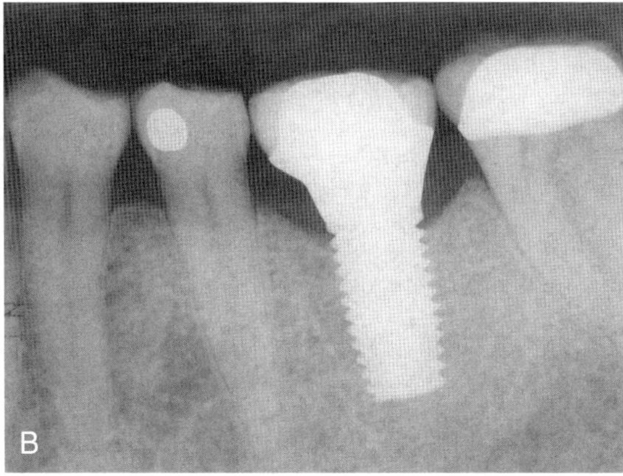

Fig. 74.7 (A) Occlusal view of healing abutment, which is attached to a wide-diameter implant used to replace a single missing molar. (B) Radiograph of the same patient depicted in part A, showing the wide-diameter implant supporting the final restoration (molar replaced with a single-tooth implant-supported crown).

Pretreatment Evaluation

A comprehensive evaluation is indicated for any patient who is being considered for dental implant therapy. The evaluation should assess all aspects of the patient's current health status, including a review the patient's past medical history, medications, and medical treatments. Patients should be questioned about parafunctional habits, such as clenching or grinding teeth, as well as any substance use or abuse, including tobacco, alcohol, and drugs. The assessment should also include an evaluation of the patient's motivations, level of understanding, compliance, and overall behavior. For most patients, this involves simply observing their demeanor and listening to their comments for an impression of their overall sensibility and coherence with other patient norms.

An intraoral and radiographic examination must be done to determine whether it is possible to place implant(s) in the desired location(s). Properly mounted diagnostic study models and intraoral clinical photographs are useful parts of the clinical examination and treatment-planning process to aid in the assessment of spatial and occlusal relationships. Once the data collection is completed, the clinician will be able to determine whether implant therapy is possible, practical, and indicated for the patient.

Conducting an organized, systematic history and examination is essential to obtaining an accurate diagnosis and creating a treatment plan that is appropriate for the patient. Each treatment plan should be comprehensive and provide several treatment options for the patient, including periodontal and restorative therapies. Then, in consultation, the clinician can agree on the final treatment plan with the patient. Information gathered throughout the process will help the clinician's decision-making and determination of whether a patient is a good candidate for dental implants. A thoughtful and well-executed evaluation can also reveal deficiencies and indicate what additional surgical procedures may be necessary to accomplish the desired goals of therapy (e.g., localized ridge augmentation, sinus bone augmentation). Each part of the pretreatment evaluation is briefly discussed here.

KEY FACT

Every treatment plan should be comprehensive. It should provide multiple treatment options, including periodontal and restorative therapies. Then, once presented with good information, the patient can ask questions and make an informed decision about the final treatment plan. Information gathered throughout the process will help the clinician's decision-making and determination of whether a patient is a good candidate for dental implants.

Chief Complaint

What is the problem or concern in the patient's own words? What is the patient's goal of treatment? How realistic are the patient's expectations? The patient's chief concern, desires for treatment, and vision of the successful outcome must be taken into consideration. The patient will measure implant success according to his or her personal criteria. The overall comfort and function of the implant restoration are often the most important factors, but satisfaction with the appearance of the final restoration will also influence the patient's perception of success. Furthermore, patient satisfaction may be influenced simply by the impact that the treatment has on the patient's perceived quality of life. Patients will evaluate for themselves whether the treatment helped them to eat better, look better, or feel better about themselves.

The clinician could consider an implant and the retained prosthesis a success using standard criteria of symptom-free implant function, implant stability, and lack of peri-implant infection or bone loss. At the same time, however, the patient who does not like the esthetic result or does not think the condition has improved could consider the treatment a failure. Therefore it is critical to inquire, as specifically as possible, about the patient's expectations before initiating implant therapy and to appreciate the patient's desires and values. With this goal in mind, it is often helpful and advisable to invite patients to bring their spouses or family members to the consultation and treatment-planning visits to add an independent "trusted" observer to the discussion of treatment options. Ultimately, it is the clinician's responsibility to determine if the patient has realistic expectations for the outcome of therapy and to educate the patient about realistic outcomes for each treatment option.

CLINICAL CORRELATION

It is essential to listen to a patient's chief concerns. The patient will ultimately decide whether the implant is successful based on his or her personal criteria. The overall comfort and function of the implant restoration are often the most important factors, but satisfaction with the appearance will also influence the patient's perception of success. Patient satisfaction will be influenced by the impact of treatment on their perceived quality of life. Patients will evaluate for themselves whether the implant treatment helped them to eat better, look better, or feel better.

Medical History

A thorough medical history is required for any patient in need of dental treatment, regardless of whether implants are part of the plan. This history should be documented in writing by the patient's completion of a standard health history form and verbally through an interview with the treating clinician. The patient's health history should be reviewed for any condition that might put the patient at risk for adverse reactions or complications.

Patients must be in reasonably good health to undergo surgical therapy for the placement of dental implants. Any disorder that may impair the normal wound-healing process, especially as it relates to bone metabolism, should be carefully considered as a possible risk factor or contraindication to implant therapy (discussed later).

A thorough physical examination is warranted if any questions arise about the patient's health status.[15] Appropriate laboratory tests (e.g., coagulation tests for a patient receiving anticoagulant therapy) should be requested to evaluate further any conditions that may affect the patient's ability to undergo the planned surgical and restorative procedures safely and effectively. If any questions remain about the patient's health status, a medical clearance for surgery should be obtained from the patient's treating physician.

Dental History

A review of a patient's past dental experiences can be a valuable part of the overall evaluation. Does the patient report a history of recurrent or frequent abscesses, which may indicate a susceptibility to infections or diabetes? Does the patient have many restorations? How compliant has the patient been with previous dental recommendations? What are the patient's current oral hygiene practices?

The individual's previous experiences with surgery and prosthetics should be discussed. If a patient reports numerous problems and difficulties with past dental care, including a history of dissatisfaction with past treatment, the patient may have similar difficulties with implant therapy. It is essential to identify past problems and to elucidate any contributing factors. The clinician must also assess the patient's dental knowledge and understanding of the proposed treatment, as well as the patient's attitude and motivation toward implants.

Intraoral Examination

The oral examination is performed to assess the current health and condition of existing teeth, as well as to evaluate the condition of the oral hard and soft tissues. It is imperative that no pathologic conditions are present in any of the hard or soft tissues in the maxillofacial region. All oral lesions, especially infections, should be diagnosed and appropriately treated before implant therapy. Additional criteria to consider include the patient's habits, level of oral hygiene, overall dental and periodontal health, occlusion, jaw relationship, temporomandibular joint condition, and ability to open wide.

After a thorough intraoral examination, the clinician can evaluate potential implant sites. All sites should be clinically evaluated to measure the available space in the bone for the placement of implants and in the dental space for prosthetic tooth replacement (Box 74.1). The mesial-distal and buccal-lingual dimensions of edentulous spaces can be approximated with a periodontal probe or other measuring instruments. The orientation or tilt of adjacent teeth and their roots should be noted as well. There may be enough space in the coronal area for the restoration but not enough space in the apical region for the implant if roots are directed into the area of interest (Fig. 74.8). Conversely, there may be adequate space between roots, but the coronal aspects of the teeth may be too close for emergence and restoration of the implant. If either of these conditions is discovered, orthodontic tooth movement may be indicated. Ultimately,

BOX 74.1 How Much Space Is Required for Placement of One or More Implants?[a]

Alveolar Bone

Assuming an implant is 4 mm in diameter and 10 mm long, the minimal width of the jawbone needs to be 6–7 mm, and the minimal height should be 10 mm (minimum of 12 mm in the posterior mandible, where an additional margin of safety is required over the mandibular nerve). This dimension is desired to maintain at least 1–1.5 mm of bone around all surfaces of the implant after preparation and placement.

Interdental Space

Edentulous spaces need to be measured to determine whether enough space exists for the placement and restoration with one or more implant crowns. The minimal space requirements for the placement of one, two, or more implants are illustrated diagrammatically in Fig. 74.9. The minimal mesial-distal space for an implant placed between two teeth is 7 mm. The minimal mesial-distal space required for the placement of two standard-diameter implants (4-mm diameter) between teeth is 14 mm. The required minimal dimensions for wide-diameter or narrow-diameter implants will increase or decrease incrementally according to the size of the implant. For example, the minimal space needed for the placement of an implant 6 mm in diameter is 9 mm (7 + 2 mm). Whenever the available space between teeth is greater than 7 mm and less than 14 mm, only one implant, such as placement of a wide-diameter implant, should be considered. Two narrow-diameter implants could be positioned in a space that is 12 mm. However, the smaller implant may be more vulnerable to implant fracture.

Interocclusal Space

The restoration consists of the abutment, the abutment screw, and the crown (it may also include a screw to secure the crown to the abutment if it is not cemented). This restorative "stack" is the total of all the components used to attach the crown to the implant. The dimensions of the restorative stack vary slightly depending on the type of abutment and the implant-restorative interface (i.e., internal or external connection). The minimum amount of interocclusal space required for the restorative "stack" on an external hex-type implant is 7 mm.

[a]All of the minimal space requirements discussed here are generic averages. The actual space limitations for any particular implant system must be determined according to the manufacturer's specifications.

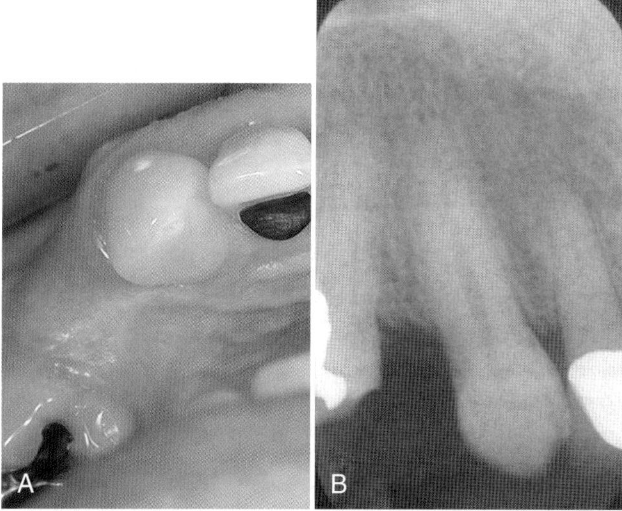

Fig. 74.8 (A) Clinical photograph of maxillary premolar space with apparently adequate space between the remaining teeth for an implant-supported crown. (B) Radiograph clearly shows a lack of space between the roots of the adjacent teeth as a result of convergence into the space (same patient as in part A).

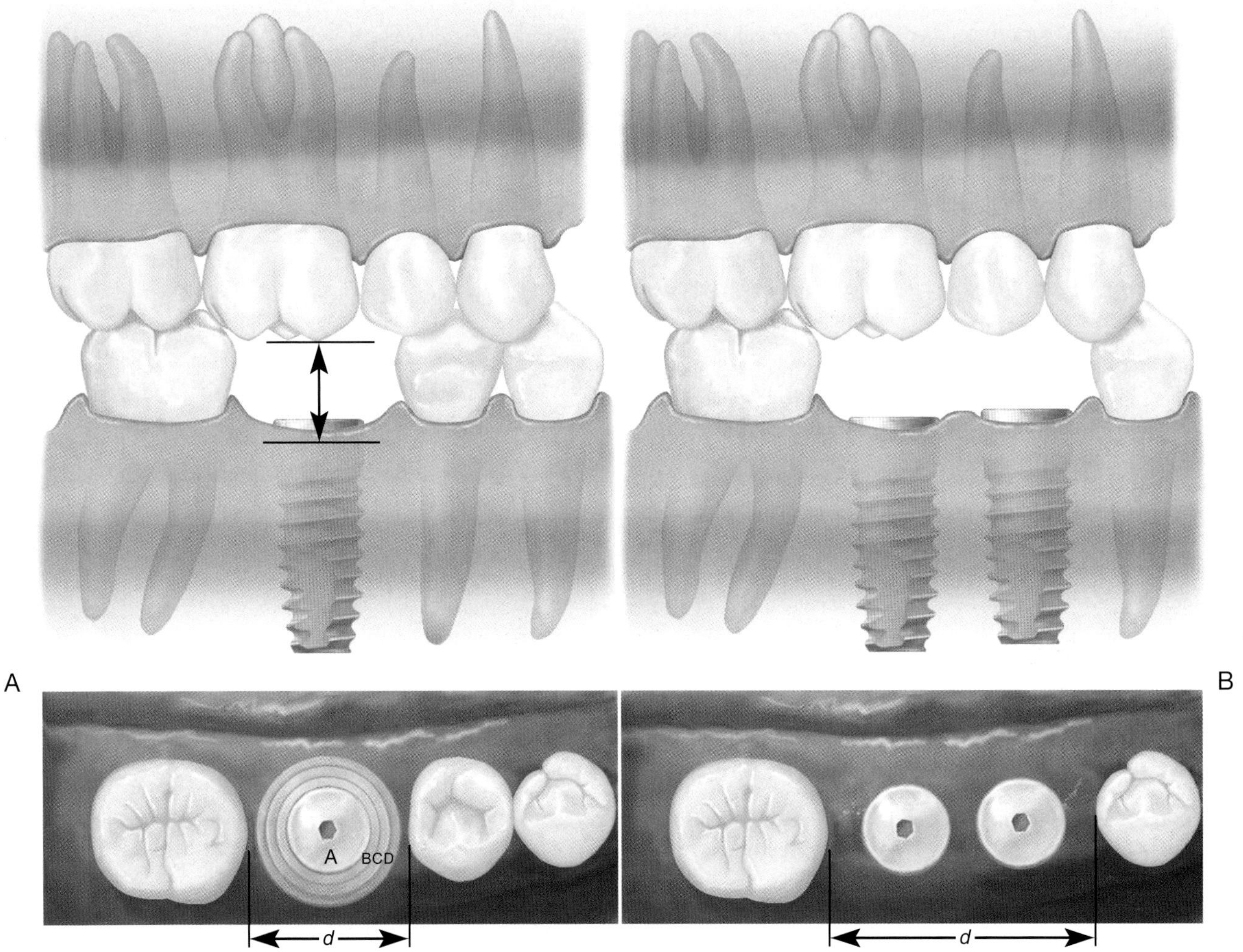

A

B

The minimum mesial-distal space (*d*) required for a:
A. Narrow diameter implant (e.g., 3.25 mm) is 6 mm.
B. Standard diameter implant (e.g., 4.1 mm) is 7 mm.
C. Wide diameter implant (e.g., 5.0 mm) is 8 mm.
D. Wide diameter implant (e.g., 6.0 mm) is 9 mm.

The minimum mesial-distal space (*d*) required for two standard diameter implants is 14 mm wide.

Fig. 74.9 (A) Minimum amount of mesial–distal space *(d)* required for placement of single-tooth implant between natural teeth: *A,* 6 mm for narrow-diameter implant (3.25 mm); *B,* 7 mm for standard-diameter implant (4.1 mm); *C* and *D,* 8 mm and 9 mm, respectively, for wide-diameter implants (5 and 6 mm). (B) Minimum amount of mesial–distal space *(d)* required for placement of two standard-diameter implants (4.1 mm) between natural teeth is 14 mm. This allows approximately 2 mm between teeth/implants and between implant/implant. Minimum amount of space required between implant/restoration interface and opposing occlusal surfaces for restoration of an implant. This dimension will vary depending on implant design and manufacturer component dimensions. The minimal dimension of 7 mm is based on an externally hexed implant and UCLA abutment.

edentulous areas need to be precisely measured using diagnostic study models and imaging techniques to determine whether space is available and whether adequate bone volume exists to replace missing teeth with implants and implant restorations. Fig. 74.9 diagrams the minimal space requirements for standard-, wide-, and narrow-diameter implants placed between natural teeth, and the minimal interocclusal space needed to restore implants.

Diagnostic Study Models

Mounted study models are an excellent means of assessing potential sites for dental implants. Properly articulated models with diagnostic wax-up of the proposed restorations allow the clinician to evaluate the available space and to determine potential limitations of the planned treatment (eFig. 74.1). This is particularly useful when multiple teeth are to be replaced with implants or when a malocclusion is present.

Hard Tissue Evaluation

The amount of available bone is the next criterion to evaluate. Wide variations in jaw anatomy are encountered, and it is therefore important to analyze the anatomy of the dentoalveolar region of interest both clinically and radiographically.

A visual examination can immediately identify deficient areas (Fig. 74.10), whereas other areas that appear to have good ridge width will require further evaluation (Fig. 74.11). Clinical examination of the jawbone consists of palpation to feel for anatomic defects and variations in the jaw anatomy, such as concavities and undercuts. If desired, it is possible with local anesthesia to probe through the soft

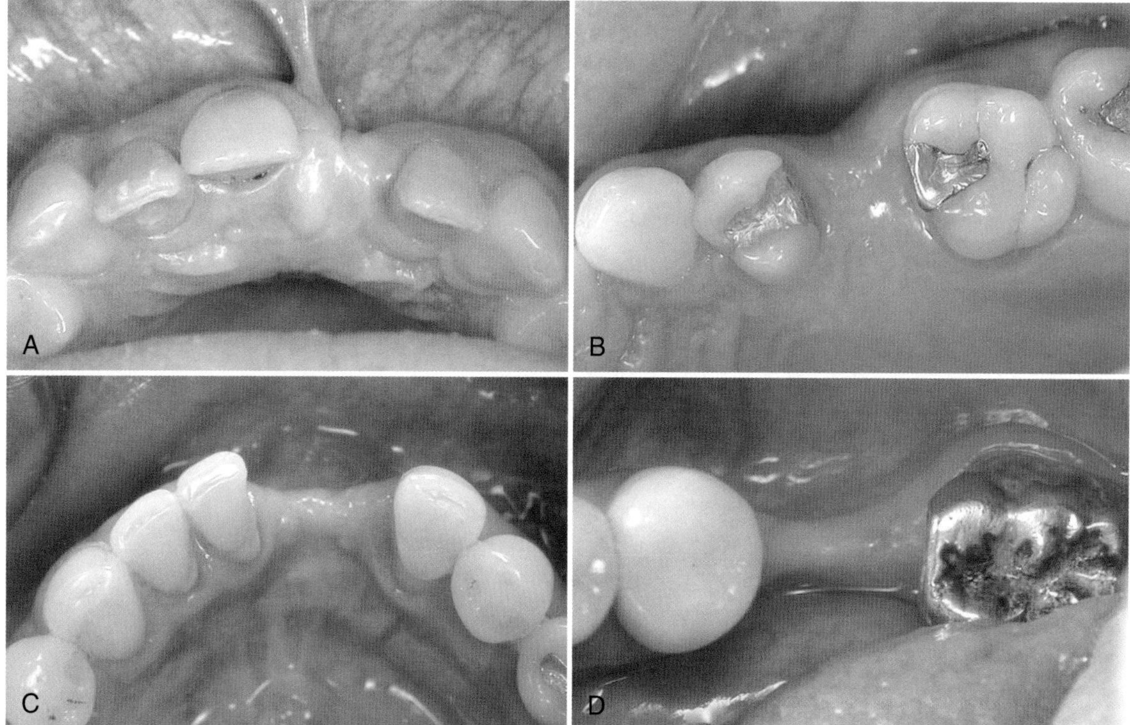

Fig. 74.10 Clinical photographs of edentulous areas with obvious deficient areas of alveolar dimension noted on visual examination: (A) anterior maxilla, (B) posterior maxilla, (C) anterior mandible, and (D) posterior mandible. These clinical images all represent buccal–lingual deficiencies in the alveolar dimensions.

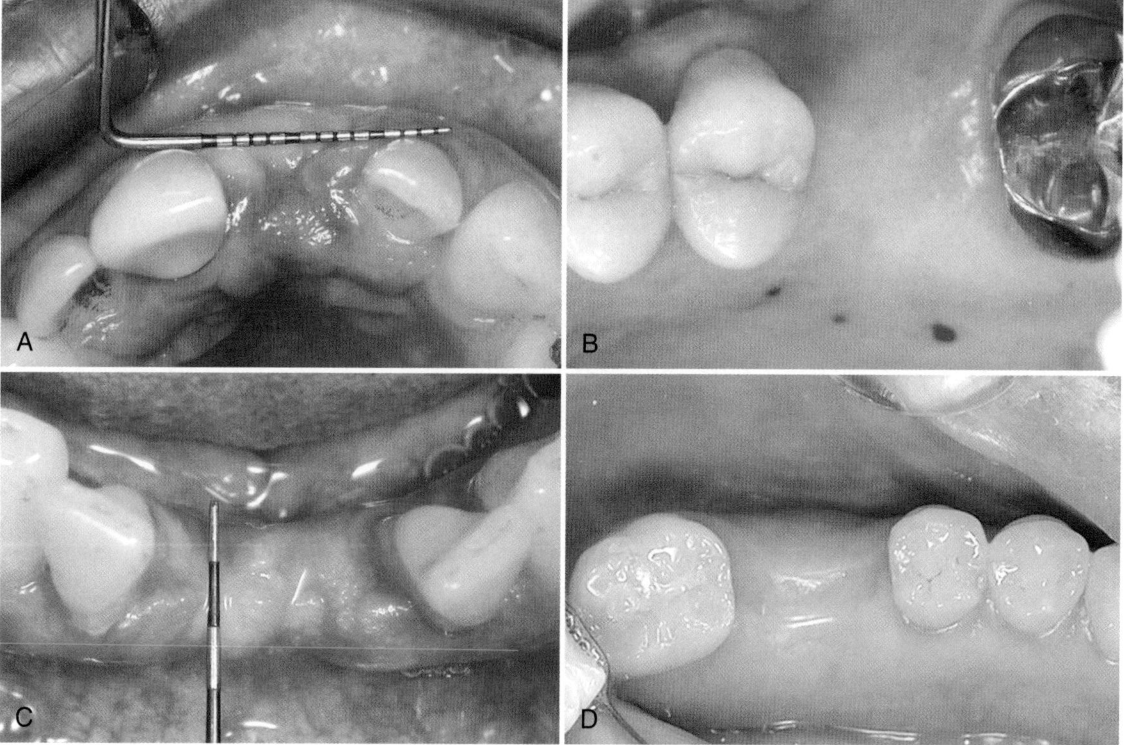

Fig. 74.11 Clinical photographs of edentulous areas with apparent good alveolar dimension noted on visual examination: (A) anterior maxilla, (B) posterior maxilla, (C) anterior mandible, and (D) posterior mandible. It is likely that these sites have adequate bone volume for implant placement. However, it is also possible to find alveolar deficiencies despite the appearance of wide ridges.

tissue (intraoral bone mapping) to assess the thickness of the soft tissues and measure the bone dimensions at the proposed surgical site.

The spatial relationship of the bone must be evaluated in a three-dimensional view because the implant must be placed in the appropriate position relative to the prosthesis. It is possible that an adequate dimension of bone is available in the anticipated implant site (see Box 74.1), but that the bone and thus the implant placement might be located too lingual or too buccal for the desired prosthetic tooth replacement.[30] Bone augmentation procedures may be necessary to facilitate the placement of an implant in an acceptable prosthetic position despite the availability of an adequate quantity of bone (i.e., the bone is in the wrong location). Bone augmentation procedures are discussed in Chapters 79 and 80.

Radiographic Examination

Radiographic assessment of the quantity, quality, and location of available alveolar bone in potential implant sites ultimately determines whether a patient is a candidate for implants and if a particular implant site needs bone augmentation. Appropriate radiographic procedures, including periapical radiographs, panoramic projections, and cross-sectional imaging, can help identify vital structures such as the floor of the nasal cavity, maxillary sinus, mandibular canal, and mental foramen (see Chapter 75). In addition to the absolute dimensional measurement of the alveolar bone, it is important to determine whether the volume of bone radiographically (as well as clinically) is located in a position to allow for the proper position of the implant to facilitate restoration of the tooth/teeth in proper esthetic and functional relationship with the adjacent and opposing dentition. The best way to evaluate the relationship of available bone to the proposed prosthetic tooth replacement is to image the patient with a diagnostically accurate guide using radiopaque markers that are positioned at the proposed prosthetic locations (see Fig. 74.5), ideally with appropriate restorative contours. Alternatively, radiographic images can be merged with digital diagnostic casts using software that allows merging or alignment through a process called registration (see Chapter 84).

KEY FACT

Implant planning should be "prosthetically driven." This can be achieved with a diagnostic wax-up of the proposed prosthesis and radiographic imaging with radiopaque markers, ideally tooth-shaped, that show the desired tooth position(s) relative to the available bone.

Soft Tissue Evaluation

Evaluation of the quality, quantity, and location of soft tissue present in the anticipated implant site helps to anticipate the type of tissue that will surround the implant(s) after treatment is completed (keratinized vs. nonkeratinized mucosa). According to Linkevicius, vertical soft tissue thickness (above the implant platform) should be ≥3 mm to minimize crestal bone loss.[45,51] For some cases, clinical evaluation may reveal a need for soft tissue augmentation (Box 74.2). Areas with minimal or no keratinized mucosa or thin (<3 mm vertical soft tissue) may be augmented with gingival or connective tissue grafts or other techniques (see Chapter 78). Other soft tissue concerns, such as frenum attachments that pull on the gingival margin, should be thoroughly evaluated as well.

BOX 74.2 How Much Keratinized Tissue Is Required for the Health and Maintenance of Implants?

Debate continues about whether it is necessary to have a zone of keratinized tissue surrounding implants. Despite strong opinions and beliefs about the need for keratinized mucosa around implants versus this mucosa being unnecessary, neither argument has been proved.

Some studies have concluded that, in the presence of good oral hygiene, a lack of keratinized tissue does not impair the health or function of implants.[56] Others strongly believe that keratinized mucosa has better functional and esthetic results for implant restorations. Keratinized mucosa is typically thicker and denser than alveolar mucosa (nonkeratinized). It forms a strong seal around the implant with a cuff of circular (parallel) fibers around the implant, abutment, or restoration that is resistant to retracting with mastication forces and oral hygiene procedures. Implants with coated surfaces (i.e., hydroxyapatite [H] or titanium plasma spray [TPS] coating) demonstrate greater peri-implant bone loss and failures in the absence of keratinized mucosa.[13,38]

Risk Factors and Contraindications

Clearly, there are numerous indications for the use of endosseous dental implants to replace missing teeth. Most patients who are missing one or more teeth can benefit from the application of an implant-retained prosthesis provided they meet the requirements for surgical and prosthetic rehabilitation. Edentulous patients who are unable to function with complete dentures and who have adequate bone for the placement of dental implants can be especially good dental implant candidates. More and more partially edentulous patients are also being treated with dental implant restorations. Many patients, whether they are missing one, several, or all of their teeth, can be predictably restored with implant-retained prostheses.

In this era of high implant success and predictability and thus possible complacency, it is imperative for clinicians to recognize risk factors and contraindications to implant therapy so that problems can be minimized and patients can be accurately informed about risks. As such, the clinician must be knowledgeable in this area and inform patients about risk factors and contraindications before initiating treatment. Contraindications for the use of dental implants, although relatively few and often not well defined, do exist. Some conditions are probably best described as "risk factors" rather than "contraindications" to treatment because implants can be successful in almost all patients; implants may be less *predictable* in some situations, and this distinction should be recognized. Ultimately, it is the clinician's responsibility with the patient to make decisions as to when implant therapy is not indicated.

Table 74.1 lists some conditions and factors that are thought to increase the risk for implant failure or otherwise deem the patient a poor candidate for implant therapy. Some of these conditions are briefly discussed here.

Medical and Systemic Health–Related Issues

Although few absolute medical contraindications to implant therapy exist, some relative contraindications are important to consider. The clinician must consider medical and health-related conditions that affect bone metabolism or any aspect of the patient's capacity to heal normally.[10] This category includes conditions such as diabetes, osteoporosis, and immune compromise; medications; and medical treatments such as chemotherapy and irradiation.

Diabetes Mellitus

Diabetes is a metabolic disease that can have significant effects on the patient's ability to heal normally and resist infections. This is particularly true for patients whose diabetes is not well controlled. Patients with poorly controlled diabetes often have impaired wound healing and a predisposition to infections, whereas patients with well-controlled diabetes experience few, if any, problems (see Chapter 25).

TABLE 74.1 Risk Factors and Contraindications for Implant Therapy

	Risk Factor	Contraindication
Medical and Systemic Health–Related Issues		
Diabetes (poorly controlled)	??—Possibly	Relative
Bone metabolic disease (e.g., osteoporosis)	??—Probably	Relative
Radiation therapy (head and neck)	Yes	Relative/absolute
Bisphosphonate therapy (intravenous)	??—Probably	Relative/absolute
Bisphosphonate therapy (oral)	??—Possibly	Relative
Immunosuppressive medication	??—Probably	Relative
Immunocompromising disease (e.g., HIV, AIDS)	??—Possibly	Relative
Psychological and Mental Conditions		
Psychiatric syndromes (e.g., schizophrenia, paranoia)	No	Absolute
Mental instability (e.g., neurotic, hysteric)	No	Absolute
Mentally impaired; uncooperative	No	Absolute
Irrational fears; phobias	No	Absolute
Unrealistic expectations	No	Absolute
Habits and Behavioral Considerations		
Smoking; tobacco use	Yes	Relative
Parafunctional habits	Yes	Relative
Substance abuse (e.g., alcohol, drugs)	??—Possibly	Absolute
Intraoral Examination Findings		
Atrophic maxilla	Yes	Relative
Current infection (e.g., endodontic)	Yes	Relative
Periodontal disease	??—Possibly	Relative

AIDS, Acquired immunodeficiency syndrome; *HIV*, human immunodeficiency virus.

There is concern about the success and predictability of implants in patients with diabetes. Several studies have reported moderate failure rates in patients with diabetes, with implant success ranging from 85.6% to 94.3%.[8,26,36,39] A prospective study demonstrated 2.2% early failures and 7.3% late failures in patients with diabetes.[53] After 5 years, the overall success rate for this group of diabetic patients was 90%.[48] None of these studies was able to correlate gender, age, smoking, diabetes type, or level of diabetic control with implant failure. In a meta-analytical review of implant failures in patients who were not diabetics, the early implant failure rate was 3.2% and the late implant failure rate 5.2%.[22] The finding that patients with diabetes experience slightly more late failures may be related to less tissue integrity caused by reduced tissue turnover and impaired tissue perfusion. These results suggest that diabetes may be a risk factor for implants, particularly for late failures. However, the risk does not appear to be particularly high.

Bone Metabolic Disease

Osteoporosis is a skeletal condition characterized by decreased mineral density. The two main classifications are primary (three types) and secondary (multiple types) osteoporosis. *Primary osteoporosis* has been attributed to menopausal changes (type I), age-related changes (type II), or idiopathic causes (type III). *Secondary osteoporosis* has been attributed to many different diseases and conditions, including diabetes, alcoholism, malnutrition, and smoking.[31]

All the various types of osteoporosis share the same fundamental problem of decreased bone mineral density and the concern that this condition may impair the patient's ability to achieve and maintain implant osseointegration. The premise that implants will not perform as well in a patient with osteoporosis is reasonable given that osseointegration depends on bone formation adjacent to the implant surface and that success rates are highest in dense bone and lowest in poor-quality, loose trabecular bone. However, to date, there is no clear evidence to suggest that implants will not be successful in patients with osteoporosis, so the issue continues to be debated.[9,19] On the positive side, although the evidence is weak, case reports have demonstrated successful implant treatment in patients with osteoporosis.[30] Some investigators advocate the use of longer healing times for osseointegration to occur before loading the implants in patients with osteoporosis.[28] Conversely, in a retrospective analysis of 49 patients who received sinus bone augmentation, individuals (11 patients) with lower bone mass density had significantly lower implant success rates as compared with age- and sex-matched controls.[14] Other parameters evaluated in this study did not demonstrate any significant differences.

Interestingly, there is a trend in aging adults (men older than 50 years and postmenopausal women) for bone mass to decrease progressively through bone demineralization at a rate of 1% to 2% per year and in some individuals as much as 5% to 8% per year throughout their later life.[21,35] If one considers this decline in bone mass with aging along with a continually increasing life expectancy in the population, the number of individuals with osteopenia or osteoporosis will continue to increase, and the concern about this condition's influence on implant success will become increasingly more important for clinicians.

Bisphosphonate Therapy

Some prescribed medications, including steroids and bisphosphonates, may be cause for concern relative to the potential implant patient. A brief statement regarding the risk of bisphosphonate therapy is offered here. Readers are encouraged to review more detailed explanations in Chapters 25 and 67 and to consult online information as well as other resources to get updated information about this important subject as more is learned and recommendations are developed.

Although there is heightened awareness and great concern about risk of bisphosphonate-related osteonecrosis of the jaw (BRONJ), the causal relationship and pathogenesis of the problem have not been fully elucidated. A review of available literature offers information that will guide clinicians in their decision-making, but it is far from definitive. The prevalence and incidence remain uncertain. In general, the risk of BRONJ is between 1 in 10,000 and 1 in 100,000 but may increase to 1 in 300 after an oral surgical procedure. The great majority of BRONJ cases will likely remain in the population of patients who receive intravenous (IV) administration of bisphosphonates. Cofactors, such as smoking, steroid use, anemia, hypoxemia, diabetes, infection, and immune deficiency, have not been firmly established but may be important.[46] Rarely does BRONJ in the oral bisphosphonate patient appear to progress beyond stage 2, and many cases reverse with discontinuation of oral medication. Procedures reported to have contributed to the development of BRONJ include extractions, periodontal surgery, root canal treatment, and dental implant surgery.[47] Dental implant therapy, as well as other surgical procedures, should be avoided in individuals who have been treated with IV bisphosphonate therapy and carefully considered with caution in patients treated with oral bisphosphonate therapy, particularly those with a history of more than 3 years of use.[3] Osteonecrosis of the jaw has been reported following administration of other antiresorptive medications as well. Hence, the newer term, antiresorptive agent-induced osteonecrosis of the jaw, is preferred.

Immune Compromise and Immune Suppression

Corticosteroid therapy, whether used for hormone replacement, cancer treatment, immune suppression, or other chronic conditions, may suppress the immune response, impair wound healing, or compromise the normal adrenal response to stress. See Chapters 25 and 67 for more information on the treatment of patients taking corticosteroids. Individuals undergoing chemotherapy or taking medications that impair healing potential (e.g., steroids) are probably not good candidates for implant therapy because of the effects these agents have on normal healing. This is especially true for cancer chemotherapy. A lowered resistance to infection may also be problematic for these patients. Past history of chemotherapy or immunosuppressive therapy may not be problematic if the patient has recovered from the side effects of treatment.

Patients with an immunocompromising disease, such as human immunodeficiency virus (HIV) infection or acquired immunodeficiency syndrome (AIDS), are not good candidates for implants when their immune system is seriously impaired. Patients with very low or undetectable viral loads and normal (T cell counts) immune function may be candidates for implant therapy (see Chapter 27).

Radiation Therapy

Patients with a history of radiation treatment to the head and neck region may not heal well after surgery. Soft tissue dehiscence may follow surgical manipulation, which may lead to osteoradionecrosis (ORN), a serious condition of nonhealing exposure and infection of bone. This is especially problematic for patients who have received radiation dosages greater than 60 Gy. Surgical procedures, or any procedure that may initiate a wound, are generally avoided in patients with a history of radiation therapy. If deemed necessary, surgical procedures can be done in conjunction with hyperbaric oxygen (HBO) therapy to reduce the risk of ORN.

Several studies have documented poor success rates for implants in patients with a history of radiation therapy.[32,33,44] In a literature review, Sennerby and Roos[52] found irradiation to be associated with high failure rates, as did Esposito and colleagues[24] in their review. Beumer and colleagues[12] reported success rates as low as 60.4% in the irradiated maxilla. Granstrom and colleagues[32] reported a significant improvement in survival rates for implants in patients treated with HBO. However, in a systematic review, Coulthard and colleagues[18] concluded that the evidence is lacking to support the clinical effectiveness of HBO in irradiated patients receiving implants. The application of implants in patients with a history of irradiation, with or without the use of HBO, is not resolved and continues to be debated. Clearly, irradiation is a risk factor for implant success and may be a contraindication.

Psychological and Mental Conditions

In general, any type of psychological abnormality can be considered a contraindication to dental implant treatment because of the patient's uncooperativeness, lack of understanding, or behavioral problems. Physiologically, there is no reason to suspect that implants could not become osseointegrated in these patients. However, the patient's ability to tolerate the number and type of treatment appointments required for implant placement, restoration, and maintenance could be problematic. All psychological conditions have the potential to be absolute contraindications to implant treatment depending on the severity of the condition. The exception might be individuals who demonstrate good cooperative behavior with only mild psychological or mental impairment. The clinician should take great care before accepting a mentally or psychologically impaired individual for treatment with implants.

Habits and Behavioral Considerations

Patients have a variety of habits and behaviors that may increase the risk of failure for dental implants. Smoking, clenching or grinding of teeth, and drug or alcohol abuse are among the most well-known habits that should be identified because of the increased risk for implant failure or complications.

Smoking and Tobacco Use

Moderate to heavy smoking has been documented to result in higher rates of early implant failure and adversely affect the long-term prognosis of dental implant restorations.[6,20,43] This is particularly true for implants placed in poor-quality bone such as the posterior maxilla.[39] The mechanisms of action responsible for higher implant failures associated with smoking are not understood. Plausible explanations include the effect of smoking on white blood cells, vasoconstriction, wound healing, and osteoporosis.[4,37] Smoking is a known risk factor for osteoporosis and thus may adversely affect implant success through its effect on bone metabolism. Smoking cessation may improve the success rate of implants.[5] In a meta-analytical review, Bain and coworkers[7] found that implants with an altered surface microtopography (Biomet 3i, Osseotite; dual acid-etched surface) seemed to significantly lessen the adverse effects of smoking on implant success.

Parafunctional Habits

Parafunctional habits, such as clenching or grinding of teeth (consciously or unconsciously), have been associated with an increased rate of implant failure (e.g., failure to integrate, loss of integration, implant fracture). Repeated lateral forces (i.e., parafunctional habits) applied to implants can be detrimental to the osseointegration process, especially during the early healing period. Patients with known parafunctional habits should be advised of an increased risk of complications or failures as a result of their clenching or grinding. Many consider bruxism to be a contraindication to implant treatment, especially in the case of a short-span, fixed partial denture or a single-tooth implant. If implants are planned for a patient with parafunctional habits, protective measures should be employed, such as creating a narrow occlusal table with flat cusp angles, protected occlusion, and the regular use of occlusal guards.

Substance Abuse

Drug and alcohol abuse should be considered a contraindication for implant therapy for reasons similar to the psychological problems discussed earlier. Patients with drug or alcohol addictions can be irresponsible and noncompliant with treatment recommendations. Depending on the severity and duration of an individual's addiction, some patients may be malnourished or may even have impaired organ function and therefore may not be good surgical candidates because of poor healing capacity. All elective treatments, including implant therapy, should be refused until addictions are treated and controlled.

Posttreatment Evaluation

Periodic posttreatment examination of implants, the retained prosthesis, and the condition of the surrounding peri-implant tissue are important components of successful treatment. Aberrations and complications can often be treated if discovered early, but many problems will go unnoticed by the patient. Thus periodic examination is essential to discovering problems early and to intervening and preventing problems from getting worse. Several parameters are available to evaluate the condition of the prosthesis, the stability of the implants, and the health of surrounding peri-implant tissues after implant integration and prosthetic restoration. Intraoral radiographs should be taken at the time of placement (baseline), at the time of abutment connection (to confirm seating and serve as another baseline), at the time of final restoration delivery (loading), and subsequently to monitor marginal or peri-implant bone changes. Periapical radiographs have excellent resolution and provide adequate details for evaluating bone support around implants if taken at a perpendicular direction.

The long-term success of dental implants is dependent on the health and stability of supporting peri-implant tissues. Good oral hygiene and regular professional care are essential to maintaining peri-implant health, and the importance of good oral hygiene should be stressed as early as possible. Patients should be taught to maintain good oral hygiene. Their performance should be monitored and reinforced at each visit.

See Chapter 87 for a detailed description of important clinical and radiographic monitoring methods as well as oral hygiene and implant maintenance protocols.

Conclusions

Today, clinicians are able to predictably replace missing teeth with endosseous dental implants. Whether missing a single tooth, several teeth, or all teeth, many patients can be candidates for dental implant therapy. It is important for clinicians to recognize factors that influence implant success. In addition to the quantity, quality, and location of available bone, the patient's health, risk factors, and contraindications must be assessed. Patients should be informed about risk factors and provided with treatment options both with and without dental implants. Periodic evaluation, good oral hygiene, and regular maintenance are important aspects of care for the long-term success and the prevention of complications with dental implants.

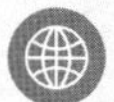
A Case Scenario is found on the companion website eBooks.Health.Elsevier.com.

Suggested Reading

Bain CA. Smoking and implant failure: benefits of a smoking cessation protocol. *Int J Oral Maxillofac Implants*. 1996;11:756–759.

Balshi TJ, Wolfinger GJ. Dental implants in the diabetic patient: a retrospective study. *Implant Dent*. 1999;8:355–359.

Brånemark PI. Osseointegration and its experimental background. *J Prosthet Dent*. 1983;50:399–410.

DeBruyn H, Collaert B. The effect of smoking on early implant failure. *Clin Oral Implants Res*. 1994;5:260.

Fiorellini JP, Nevins ML. Localized ridge augmentation/preservation. A systematic review. *Ann Periodontol*. 2003;8:321–327.

Hammerle CH, Jung RE, Feloutzis A. A systematic review of the survival of implants in bone sites augmented with barrier membranes (guided bone regeneration) in partially edentulous patients. *J Clin Periodontol*. 2002;29(suppl 3):226–231; discussion 232–223.

Klokkevold PR, Han TJ. How do smoking, diabetes, and periodontitis affect outcomes of implant treatment? *Int J Oral Maxillofac Implants*. 2007;22(suppl):173–202.

Linkevicius T, Apse P, Grybauskas S, Puisys A. The influence of soft tissue thickness on crestal bone changes around implants: A 1-year prospective controlled clinical trial. *Int J Oral Maxillofac Implants*. 2009;24: 712–719.

Sennerby L, Roos J. Surgical determinants of clinical success of osseointegrated oral implants: a review of the literature. *Int J Prosthodont*. 1998;11:408–420.

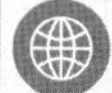
References for this chapter are found on the companion website eBooks.Health.Elsevier.com.

CHAPTER 75

Diagnostic Imaging for the Implant Patient

Mohammed Husain | Sotirios Tetradis | Sanjay M. Mallya | Perry R. Klokkevold

For online-only content on occlusal radiographs and multidetector computed tomography, please visit the companion website at eBooks.Health.Elsevier.com.

CHAPTER OUTLINE

Several radiographic imaging options are available for the diagnosis and treatment planning of patients receiving dental implants.[2,23,24] Options range from standard projections routinely available in the dental office to more complex 3D volumetric radiographic techniques. Standard projections include intraoral (periapical, occlusal) and extraoral (panoramic, lateral cephalometric) radiographs. More complex imaging techniques include cone-beam computed tomography (CBCT) and multidetector computed tomography (MDCT). The CBCT and MDCT image data files can be reformatted and viewed on a personal computer using simulation software, making the diagnosis and treatment-planning process interactive and visually more meaningful. Often, combinations of various modalities are used because no single modality can provide all information pertinent to the radiographic evaluation of the implant patient. Familiarity with the benefits and limitations of various techniques and awareness of the specific clinical questions that need to be answered should guide the decision-making process and selection of radiographic examinations for individual patients.

Multiple factors influence the selection of radiographic technique(s) for a particular case, including cost, availability, radiation exposure, and case type. The decision is a balance between these factors and the desire to minimize risk of complications to the patient. Accurately identifying vital anatomic structures and being able to perform implant placement surgery without injury to these structures are critical to treatment success. Diagnostic imaging must always be interpreted in conjunction with a comprehensive clinical examination.

This chapter discusses common imaging techniques used for evaluation of the implant patient. Indications for each technique are outlined along with the advantages and limitations of each technique.

KEY FACT

Accurate identification of vital anatomic structures is critical to treatment success when performing dental implant surgery. Diagnostic imaging must always be interpreted in conjunction with a clinical examination.

Standard Projections

Standard diagnostic imaging modalities include periapical, panoramic, lateral cephalometric, and occlusal radiographs. Table 75.1 summarizes the advantages and disadvantages of the most widely used modalities.

Periapical Radiographs

Periapical radiographs are often the first imaging modality used to evaluate the implant patient.[25,26] These radiographs provide an overall assessment of the quantity and quality of the edentulous alveolar ridge and the adjacent teeth. They are easy to obtain in the dental office, are relatively inexpensive, and deliver a low radiation dose to the patient (Table 75.2).[12] Dentists are familiar with the depicted anatomy and possible pathology. Among all dental imaging modalities, intraoral radiographs offer the highest detail and *spatial resolution* (Fig. 75.1) and thus are the projection of choice when subtle, localized pathology, such as a retained root tip, needs to be detected and evaluated.

The most significant disadvantage of periapical radiographs is their susceptibility to unpredictable magnification of anatomic structures, which precludes reliable measurements.[21] *Foreshortening* or *elongation* can be minimized by the use of the paralleling technique. However, distortion is particularly accentuated in edentulous areas where missing teeth and resorption of the alveolus necessitate

TABLE 75.1 Advantages and Disadvantages of the Various Radiographic Projections

Modality	Advantages	Disadvantages
Periapical radiography	High resolution and detail, easy acquisition, low radiation exposure, relatively inexpensive	Unpredictable magnification, small imaged area, 2D representation of anatomy
Panoramic radiography	Easy to acquire, images the full dentoalveolar ridge, low radiation dose, relatively inexpensive	Unpredictable magnification, unequal magnification in vertical and horizontal dimensions, 2D representation of anatomy, not detailed
Multidetector computed tomography	3D representation, no magnification, sufficient detail, digital format, images both arches	Requires special equipment, expensive, higher radiation dose, beam hardening artifact
Cone-beam computed tomography	3D representation, no magnification, sufficient detail, digital format, variable FOV, low radiation dose, dental-specific software	Requires special equipment, relatively expensive, beam hardening artifact

2D, Two-dimensional; *3D*, three-dimensional; *FOV*, field of view.

TABLE 75.2 Radiation Dose (Effective Dose in μSv) Received From Common Projections During Evaluation of the Implant Patient

Modality	Effective Dose (μSv)
Full-mouth x-ray (FMX) series	100[a] or 200[b]
Panoramic	20
Limited field-of-view CBCT	50
Medium field-of-view CBCT	100
Large field-of-view CBCT	120
MDCT, maxillofacial	650

[a]Assuming use of PSP or F-speed film and round collimation.
[b]Assuming use of CCD sensors and round collimation.
CBCT, Cone-beam computed tomography; *MDCT*, multidetector computed tomography.
Adapted from Mallya SM. Safety and protection. In: Mallya SM, Lam EW, eds. *White and Pharoah's Oral Radiology: Principles and Interpretation.* 8th ed. St Louis: Elsevier; 2019. Table 3.2: Typical Effective Dose From Radiographic Examinations.

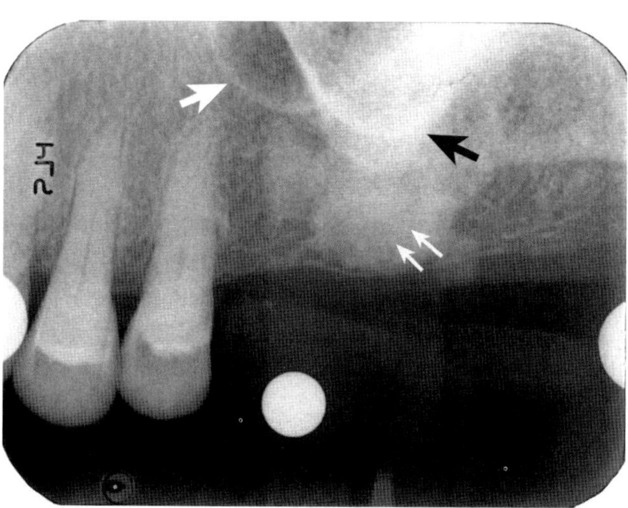

Fig. 75.1 The periapical radiograph offers a high-resolution, detailed image of the edentulous area. Healing of the extraction socket with dense bone (socket sclerosis) can be seen *(small white arrows)*. Some anatomic structures, such as the maxillary sinus *(large white arrow)* and the zygomatic process of the maxilla *(black arrow)*, can also be visualized.

receptor placement at significant angulation in relation to the long axis of the alveolar bone. Additionally, periapical radiographs are two-dimensional representations of three-dimensional objects and do not provide any information of the buccal–lingual dimension of the alveolar ridge. Structures that are distinctly separated in the buccal–lingual dimension appear to be overlapping. Finally, periapical radiographs depict a limited area of the dentoalveolar region. Often, it is not possible to image the entire height of the alveolar ridge, and when a wide span of the ridge needs to be assessed, multiple periapical radiographs are required.

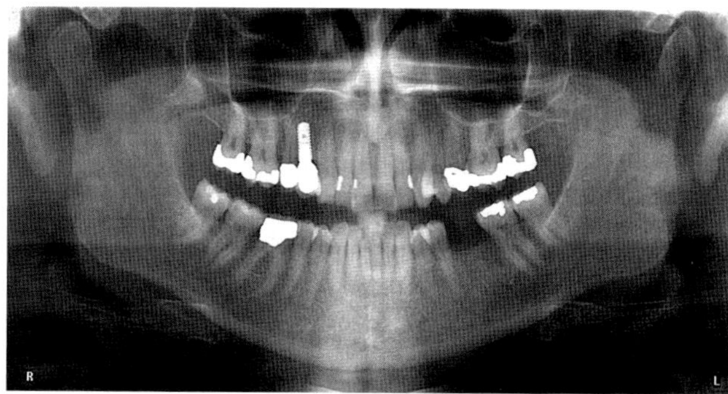

Fig. 75.2 Panoramic radiograph. Both jaws are visualized on the same image. An overall assessment of superoinferior and mesial–distal dimensions of the alveolar ridge can be formulated. Tooth and root positions relative to planned implant sites can be evaluated. Important anatomic structures, such as the maxillary sinus and mandibular canal, can be identified.

Periapical radiographs are useful screening images that offer a detailed view of a small area of the alveolar arch. Limitations that must be considered include the possibility of geometric distortion, superimposition artifact from a two-dimensional representation of anatomic structures, and the possibility of insufficient anatomic coverage of the region of interest.

Panoramic Radiographs

Panoramic radiographs are often used in the evaluation of the implant patient because they offer several advantages over other modalities.[22] Panoramic radiographs[74] provide a broad view of both dental arches at a low radiation dose (see Table 75.2), allowing assessment of longer edentulous spans, the angulation of existing teeth and the occlusal plane, as well as anatomic structures important for implant planning, such as the maxillary sinus, nasal cavity, mental foramen, and mandibular canal (Fig. 75.2). Panoramic units are widely available and easy to operate, and dentists are familiar with the anatomy and pathology depicted by the images. Similar to intraoral projections, panoramic images are two-dimensional and thus do not offer diagnostic information with respect to the buccal–lingual dimension of the alveolar arch.

Panoramic images appear intuitively familiar. However, they combine characteristic physical and radiographic principles that make them distinct from other intraoral and extraoral radiographs. Although outside the scope of this chapter, familiarity with the principles underlying panoramic radiography is central for understanding and thus compensates for the limitations and constraints of the images. The reader is referred to other textbooks for detailed discussions of this topic.[10,14] Briefly, the existence of ghost shadows, unpredictable horizontal and vertical magnification, distortion of structures outside the focal trough, projection geometry generated by the negative vertical angulation of the x-ray beam, and the propensity of patient-positioning errors do not allow consistently detailed and accurate measurements to be generated. As a result, panoramic radiographs do not provide the highly detailed images that are generated by intraoral radiographs.

Measurement distortion is more prevalent and varies across the radiographic image. On average, objects on panoramic radiographs are 15% to 25% magnifications of their actual size.[5] Implant manufacturers often provide transparency sheets with implant size outlines of 25% magnification. However, it is important to appreciate that the 15% to 25% magnification is an estimate. The actual magnification may range from 10% to 30% in different areas within the same image and depends greatly on patient positioning during panoramic radiography. For this reason, precise measurements on panoramic projections are not possible. Nonetheless, panoramic radiographs offer an overall view of the maxilla and mandible that can be used to estimate bone measurements and evaluate the approximate relationships between teeth and other anatomic structures. More precise diagnostic imaging should be used to measure the proximity of critical anatomic structures, such as the maxillary sinus or the mandibular canal, to proposed implant positions.

Panoramic projections provide useful information for the initial assessment of the implant patient. However, due to magnification and distortion errors, panoramic radiographs should not be used for precise measurements of proposed implant sites.

Cross-Sectional Imaging

Cross-sectional diagnostic imaging modalities include CBCT and MDCT. Conventional tomography also provides cross-sectional images with predictable magnification and has been used in the assessment of the implant patient. However, with the introduction and expansion of CBCT imaging, conventional tomography is becoming obsolete and is not described in this chapter.

Cone-Beam Computed Tomography

Cone-beam computed tomography (CBCT) is an imaging modality that offers significant advantages for the evaluation of implant patients.[7,20] CBCT was introduced to dentistry in the late 1990s,[1,17] and since then a multitude of CBCT units have become commercially available for maxillofacial imaging. The x-ray source and the detector are diametrically positioned and make a 180- or 360-degree rotation around the patient's head within the gantry. The x-ray beam is collimated, and the resultant beam is cone or pyramid shaped. Typically, within a single complete rotation, 180 to 500 basis projections of the region of interest are generated and used to reconstruct a digital, three-dimensional map of the face. Once this map is generated, multiplanar reconstructions—axial, coronal, sagittal, or oblique sections of various thicknesses—can be obtained from the data.

KEY FACT

CBCT offers significant advantages for the evaluation of implant patients. The *field of view (FOV)* is an important feature that describes the extent of the imaged volume, from large FOV (greater than 15 cm) to medium FOV (8 to 15 cm) and limited FOV (less than 8 cm). Limited FOV units image a smaller area, deliver less radiation, and produce higher-resolution images.

An important feature of the CBCT units is the ability to modulate the field of view (FOV), which determines the extent of the imaged volume. CBCT units are typically categorized as large FOV (greater than 15 cm), medium FOV (8 to 15 cm), and limited FOV systems (less than 8 cm). Fig. 75.3 schematically depicts the anatomic area covered by large, medium, and limited FOV scans. In general, large FOV units image a more extensive anatomic area, deliver a higher radiation exposure to the patient, and produce lower-resolution images (Fig. 75.4). Conversely, limited FOV units image a smaller area of the face, deliver less radiation, and produce higher-resolution images (Fig. 75.5).

CBCT scans offer several advantages for evaluation of the implant patient compared with two-dimensional (2D) imaging. Most notably, there is a lack of anatomic superimposition, such that cross sections through an edentulous site can be obtained with dimensional accuracy. Reliable measurements of the height and width of the alveolar ridge can be made from these cross sections digitally within the CBCT viewing software utilizing built-in measurement tools.[6,11] Alternatively, relevant cross sections can be printed without magnification, and measurements may be made directly on the printouts with standard rulers (i.e., not magnified). Vertical and horizontal rulers adjacent to each printed cross section allow the clinician to verify dimensional accuracy before making measurements.

Other advantages of CBCT imaging include the ability to easily modulate the FOV for each CBCT scan. This encourages a patient-centric approach in which the imaging protocol is determined by the need to visualize either a single or multiple proposed implant sites. Modulating the FOV to the smallest size for a given diagnostic task is recommended and has the dual benefit of reducing radiation exposure and enhancing *spatial resolution*—defined as the ability to discern small objects that are in close proximity in an image. Being a volumetric imaging modality, CBCT allows the user to visualize and analyze anatomic structures in all three coordinate axes with precision. CBCT-based imaging software is uniquely designed for dental applications and allows for customizable cross sections in any plane—a feature most useful for dentists who routinely evaluate small structures (e.g., teeth, implants, neurovascular canals) not

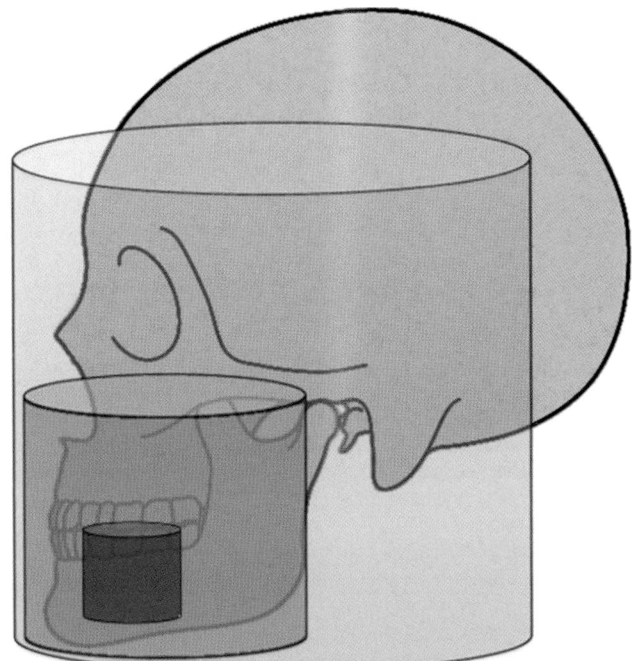

Fig. 75.3 Schematic diagram of the anatomic area imaged with large *(green)*, medium *(blue)*, and limited *(magenta)* field of view cone-beam computed tomography.

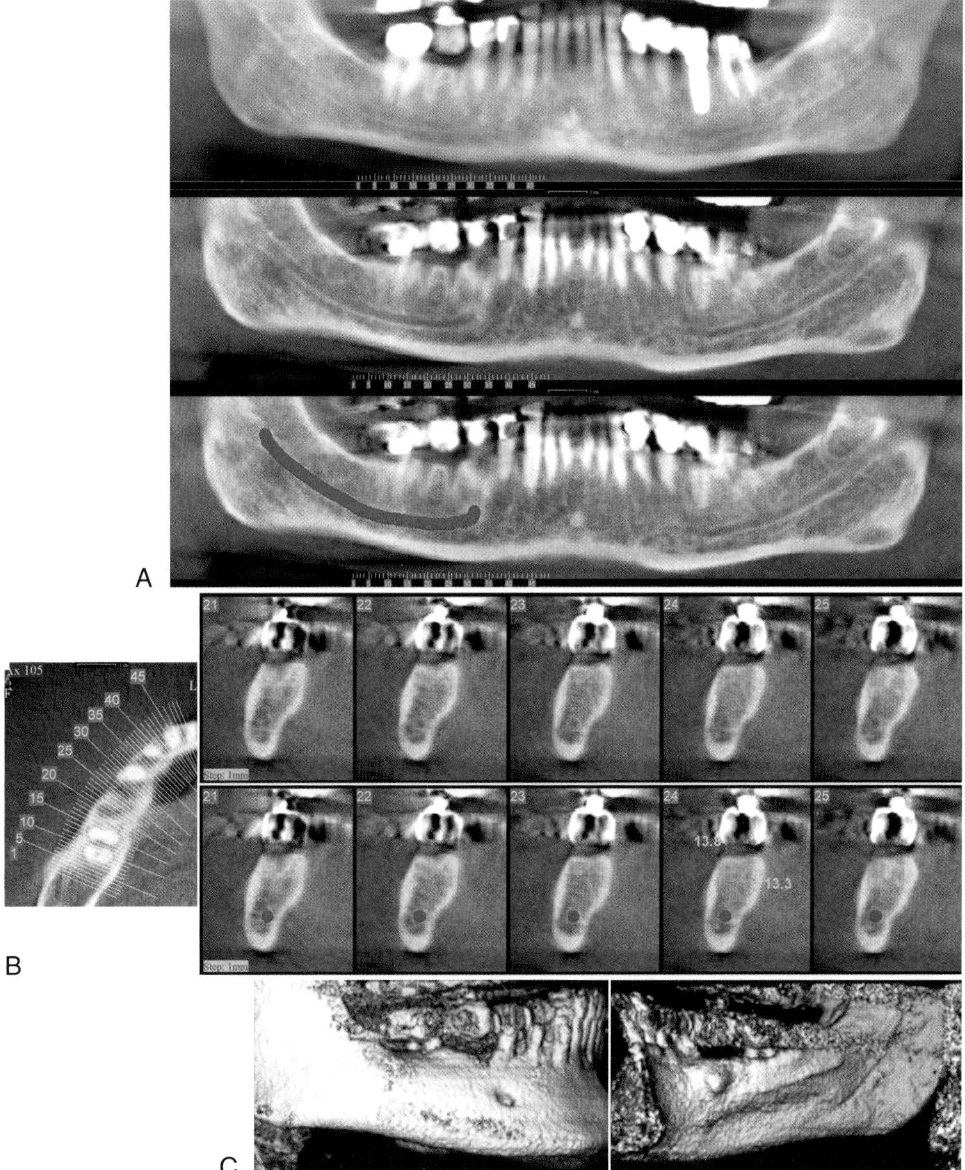

Fig. 75.4 Cone-beam computed tomography images for the evaluation of the edentulous space at the area of missing tooth #30 before implant placement using a large field-of-view unit (NewTom 3G, Verona, Italy, distributed by AFP Imaging, Elmsford, New York). Note the tooth-shaped marker used. (A) A series of "panoramic" reconstructions through the alveolar ridge reveals the relationship of the marker to the adjacent teeth. The top "panoramic" view is 12-mm thick so as to depict most of the extent of the alveolar ridge and adjacent teeth. The middle "panoramic" image is 1-mm thick through the area of the mandibular canal. Note that adjacent teeth are out of the plane of the section and thus not depicted on the image. The bottom "panoramic" view is the same as the middle one, but the position of the mandibular canal has been depicted by the *red line.* (B) Scout axial view and series of cross sections through the area of the marker. The bottom row shows the same axial slices as the top row. However, the position of the *red line* drawn on the panoramic view is also depicted to help localization of the mandibular canal. The height and width of the alveolar ridge have been measured in a selected section. (C) Three-dimensional reconstructions provide an overall impression of the bone contours and shape of the alveolar ridge. Note the small exostosis on the lingual surface of the alveolar ridge.

oriented along any of the standard orthogonal planes (axial, coronal, or sagittal). Like other natively digital imaging modalities, CBCT imaging benefits from the availability of software-based image enhancement and annotation tools and the ability to easily duplicate and store images—all of which facilitate rapid communication between radiologist and surgeon.

In summary, CBCT scanning is a valuable and widely utilized imaging modality for three-dimensional and cross-sectional evaluation of the implant patient. It has similar advantages and disadvantages as CT scanning. The most significant differences are that CBCT imaging offers variable FOVs and substantially reduced radiation exposure to the patient.

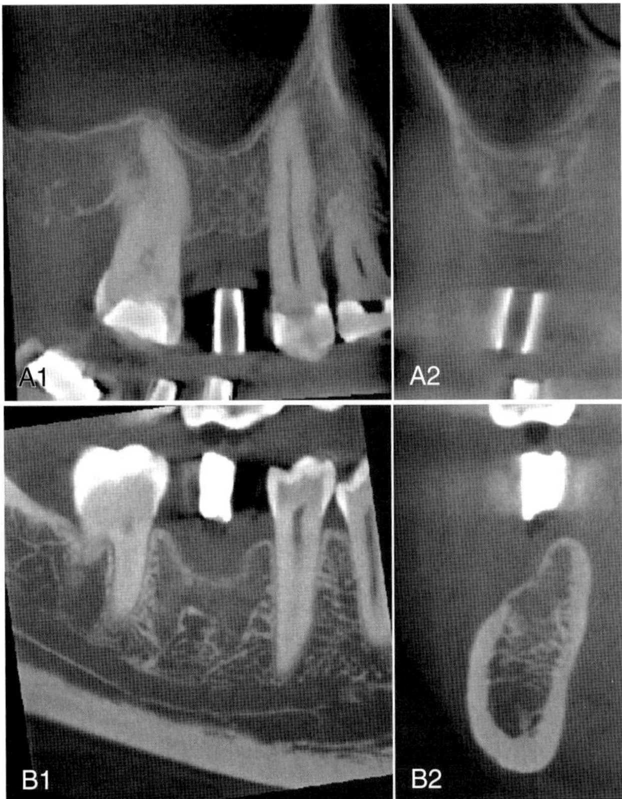

Fig. 75.5 Cone-beam computed tomography images for the evaluation of the edentulous space at the area of missing tooth #4 (A) and missing tooth #30 (B) using a limited field-of-view scan (3D Accuitomo, J. Morita Corporation, Suita City, Osaka, Japan, distributed by J. Morita USA, Inc., Irvine, California). Sagittal and cross-sectional slices are shown. Although the anatomic area imaged is limited, the resolutions of the images are high. (A) Implant site #4 (maxillary right second premolar) in anterior–posterior (A1) and buccolingual (A2) cross-sectional views. (B) Implant site #30 (mandibular right first molar) in anterior–posterior (B1) and buccolingual (B2) cross-sectional views.

Interactive "Simulation" Software Programs

Implant treatment planning can be greatly enhanced by the use of specialized software. In addition to measuring the quantity and quality of bone in potential implant sites, these programs use CT (CBCT or MDCT) scan data to simulate placement of implants and restorations. Using a database of commercially available implant images, the length, width, angulation, and position of implants can be "simulated" in the desired positions and evaluated relative to other structures in three dimensions. In cases of alveolar ridge deficiency or defects, or when sinus bone augmentation is indicated, the additional bone volume needed can be evaluated and quantified. The restoration of the implants can also be simulated and the distribution of mechanical forces onto the implant and adjacent bone predicted.

Software programs specialized in implant treatment planning, such as Simplant Pro (Dentsply, Sweden), coDiagnostiX (DentalWings, Canada), NobelClinician (Nobel Biocare, Switzerland), Implant Studio (3Shape, Denmark), and InVivo (Anatomage, United States) can acquire information directly from CBCT or CT scan data in either *DICOM* or proprietary file formats. The clinician can use the reformatted images on a personal computer in an interactive manner to identify anatomic structures, simulate implant placement positions, and better appreciate relationships between planned implant positions and teeth or anatomic structures (Fig. 75.6). Once implant positions are confirmed, a computer-generated surgical guide is produced to facilitate the surgical placement of implants in the planned positions (Fig. 75.7). See Chapter 84.

Patient Evaluation

Evaluation of the implant patient should be disciplined and objective. Specific questions that can affect implant placement and outcome should be considered and examined carefully and explicitly. The advantages and disadvantages of various radiographic projections should be considered and radiographic modalities chosen based on necessary information for the particular patient. The objectives for any radiographic evaluation, regardless of imaging technique used, should include an evaluation to (1) exclude pathology, (2) identify anatomic structures, and (3) measure the quantity, quality, and location of available bone and its relation to the existing teeth and occlusion as well as the prosthetically planned tooth replacement(s).

CLINICAL CORRELATION

All diagnostic images, regardless of technique, should be evaluated to identify or exclude pathology and to identify normal anatomic structures.

Exclude Pathology

Healthy bone is a prerequisite for successful osseointegration and long-term implant success. The first step in the radiographic evaluation of the implant site is to establish the health of the alveolar bone and other tissues imaged within a particular projection. Local and systemic diseases that affect bone homeostasis can preclude, modify, or alter the placement of implants. Retained root fragments, residual periodontal disease, cysts, and tumors (Fig. 75.8) should be identified and resolved before implant placement. Systemic diseases, such as osteoporosis and hyperparathyroidism, or local bone dysplasias, such as fibrous dysplasia and cemento-osseous dysplasia, alter bone structure and homeostasis and might affect implant osseointegration. Areas of poor bone quality should be identified and, if indicated, adjustments to the treatment plan incorporated. Maxillary sinusitis, polyps, or other sinus pathology should be diagnosed and treated when implants are considered in the posterior maxilla, especially if sinus bone augmentation procedures are planned (Fig. 75.9). See Chapter 80.

Identify Anatomic Structures

Several important anatomic structures are found close to desired areas of implant placement in the maxilla and mandible (Box 75.1). Familiarity with the radiographic appearance of these structures is important during treatment planning and implant placement. Their exact localization is central to prevent unwanted complications and unnecessary morbidity. Important anatomic structures in the maxilla include the floor and anterior wall of the maxillary sinus, incisive canal, floor and lateral wall of the nasal cavity, canalis sinuosus, and canine fossa. Important anatomic structures in the mandible that should be recognized include the mandibular canal, anterior loop of the mandibular canal, mental foramen, anterior extension of the canal, median lingual canal, and submandibular fossa (Fig. 75.10). The existence of anatomic variants, such as incomplete healing of an extraction site, sinus loculation, division of mandibular canal (Fig. 75.11), or absence of a well-defined corticated canal (Fig. 75.12), should also be recognized. See Chapter 59 for important periodontal and implant surgical anatomy.

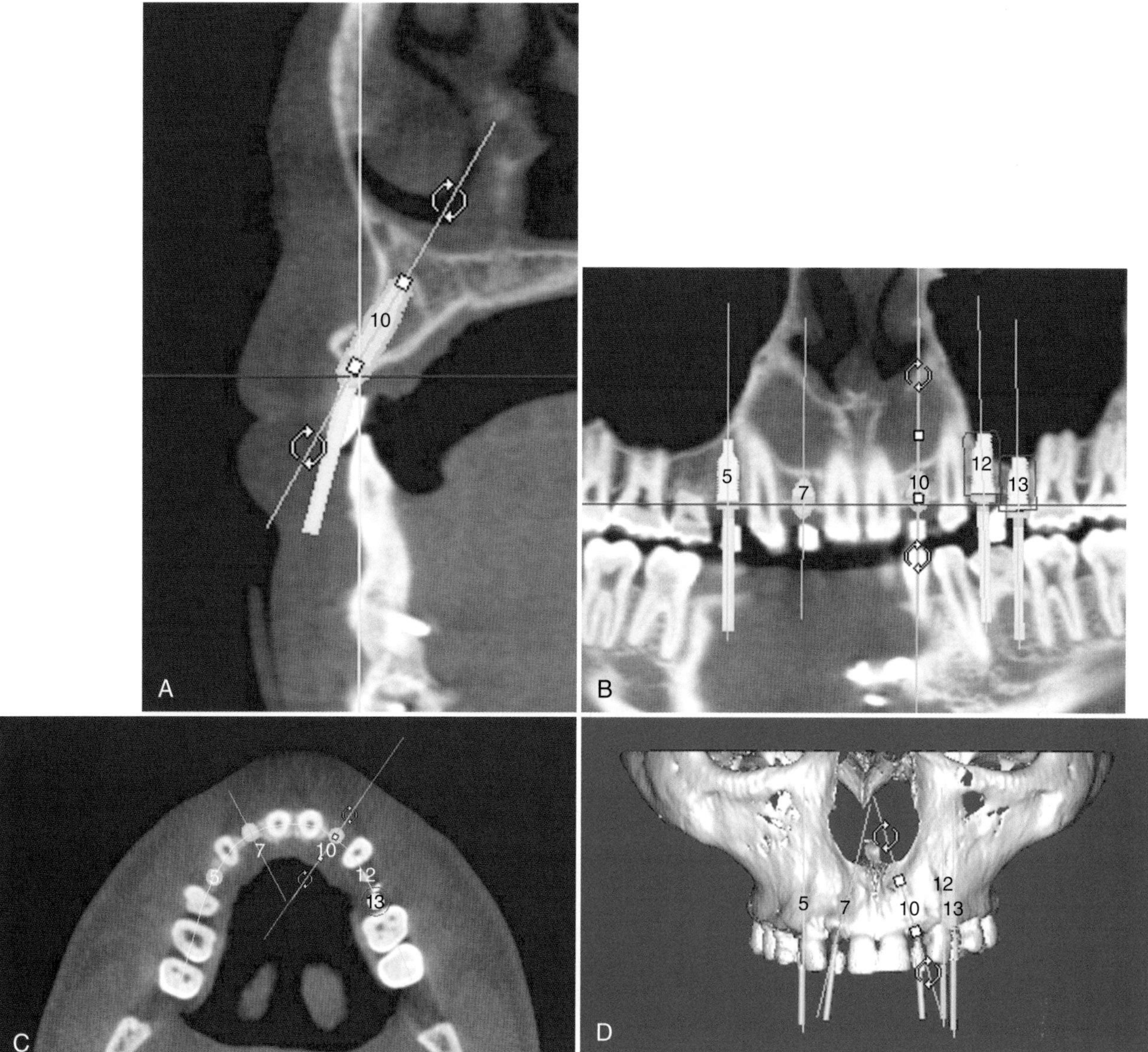

Fig. 75.6 SIM/Plant images. The SIM/Plant software program allows clinicians to measure bone height, width, density, and volume on a personal computer. Scan data are reformatted for interactive evaluation and manipulation. Implant positions can be simulated on the patient's scan data before surgery, allowing the surgeon to anticipate areas of deficiency. (A) Cross-sectional image through simulated implant in anterior maxilla, site #10. (B) Panoramic projection of multiple simulated implant positions, #5, 7, 10, 12, and 13. (C) Axial view of simulated implants. (D) Three-dimensional image of maxilla with simulated implants.

CLINICAL CORRELATION

Several important anatomic structures need to be identified in the jaws prior to implant placement. Violation of structures may cause serious complications and compromise treatment outcomes. Familiarity with the radiographic appearance of vital structures is important, and the existence of anatomic variants should also be recognized.

Assess Bone Quantity, Quality, and Volume

The primary goal of diagnostic imaging for potential implant patients is to evaluate the available bone volume for implant placement in desired anatomic locations. The clinician should verify the presence of adequate height, width, and density of the recipient bone while avoiding damage to critical anatomic structures. Failure to accurately assess the location of important anatomic structures can lead to unnecessary complications. For example, inadvertent penetration and damage to the inferior alveolar nerve can result in serious immediate-term (profuse bleeding), short-term, and long-term (nerve paresthesia/anesthesia) complications. The height and width of the alveolar bone should be accurately assessed. Depending on the imaging technique, diagnostic imaging can estimate or precisely measure the coronal–apical height, the buccal–lingual width, and the mesial–distal spacing available for implants that will be placed in proximity to teeth or relative to other planned implants.

This task can be simple in cases with good bone quality and sufficient bone volume in the desired implant location(s). However, in cases with moderate to severe bone resorption, alveolar defects, or recent extraction sites, obtaining a clear and accurate diagnostic

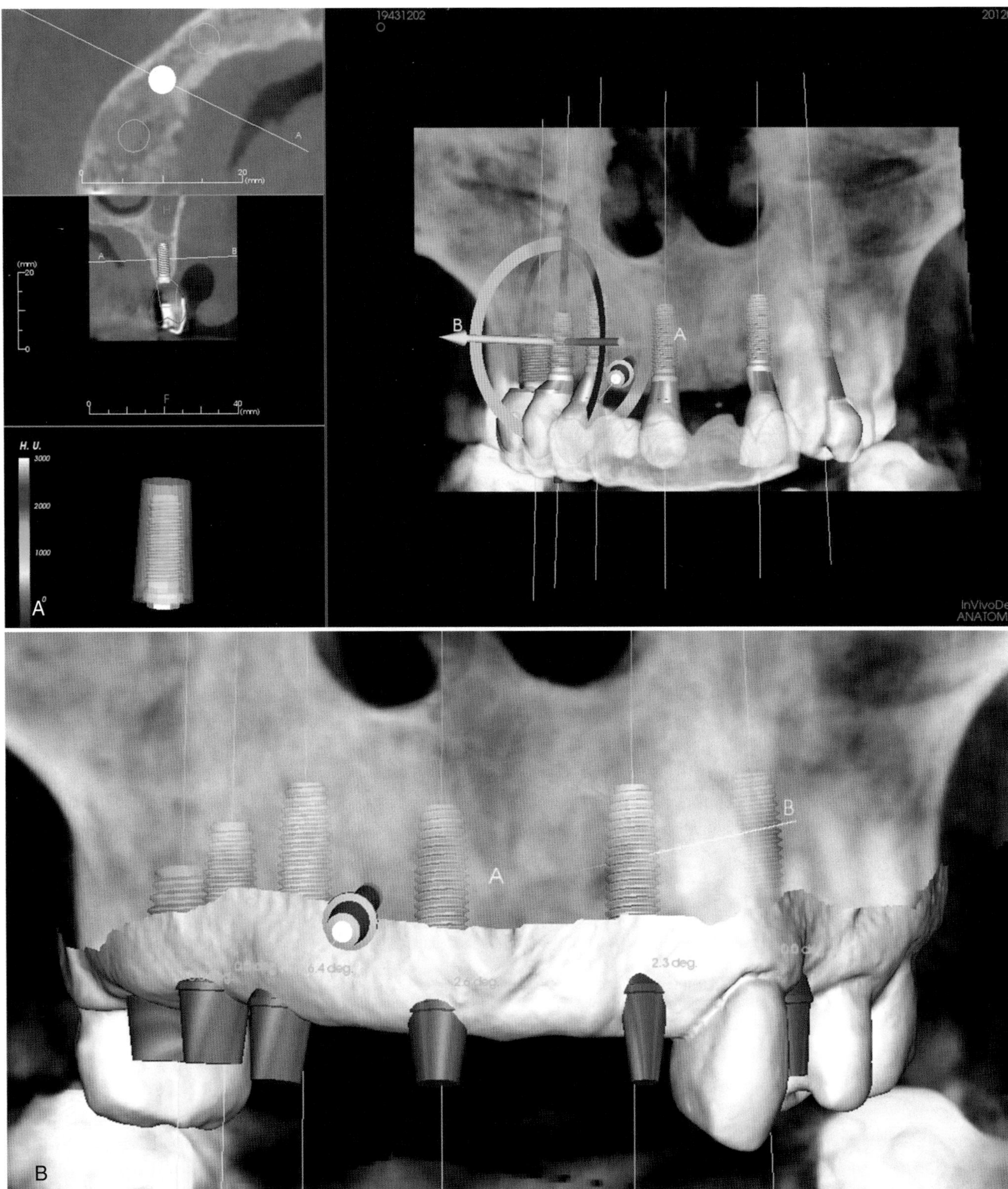

Fig. 75.7 InVivo5 simulation images. The InVivo5 software program allows clinicians to plan implant treatment and simulate virtual implant positions directly from DICOM scan data on a personal computer. (A) Cross-sectional and axial images with three-dimensional simulation of implant positions. (B) Model mockup for computer-generated surgical guide.

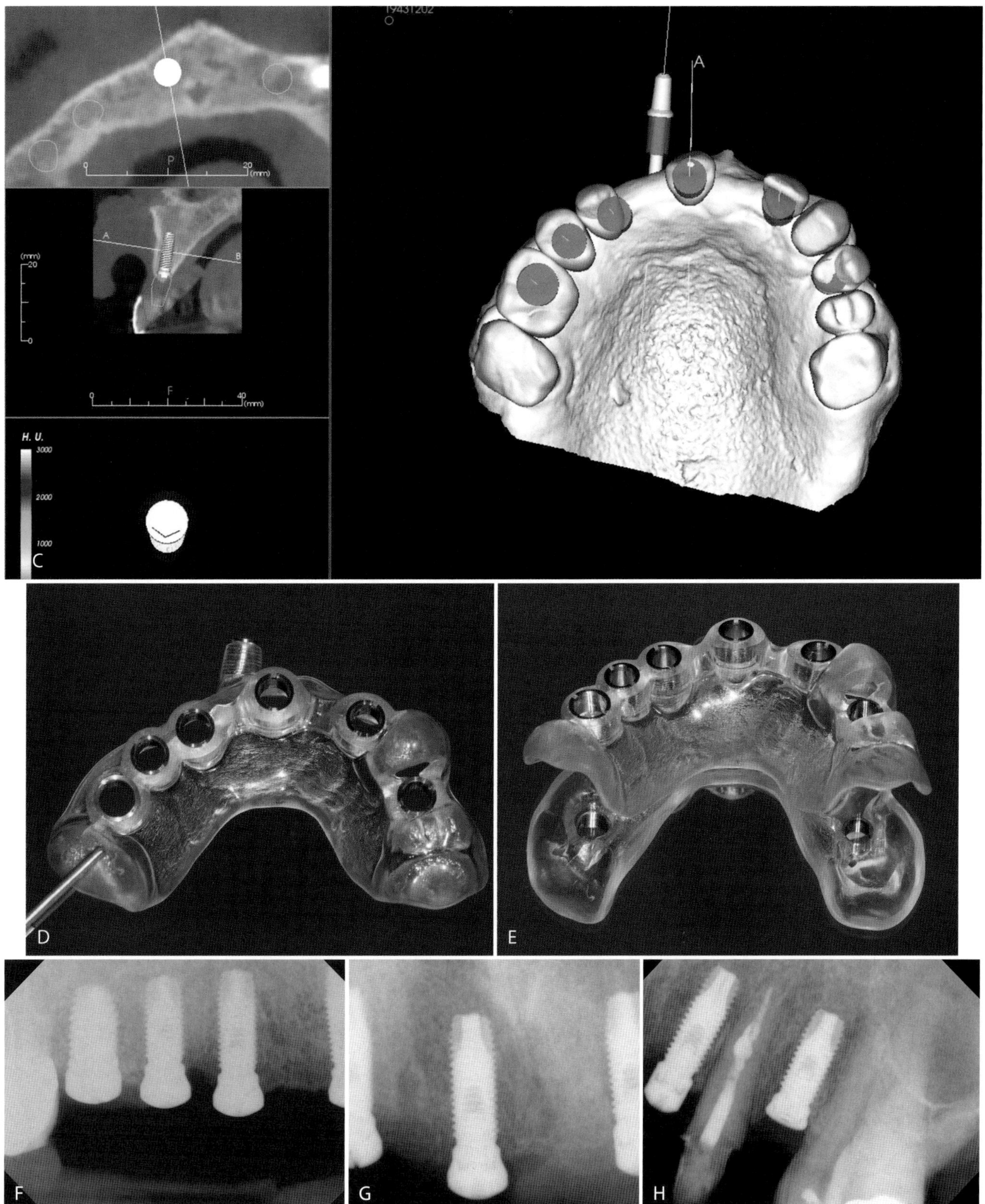

Fig. 75.7 cont'd (C) Cross-sectional and axial images of central incisor simulated implant position and three-dimensional simulation of proposed implant positions from the occlusal view. (D and E) Surgical guide that was created from a simulated plan. (F–H) Periapical radiographs demonstrating the accurate position and alignment of implants that were placed using a computer-generated surgical guide.

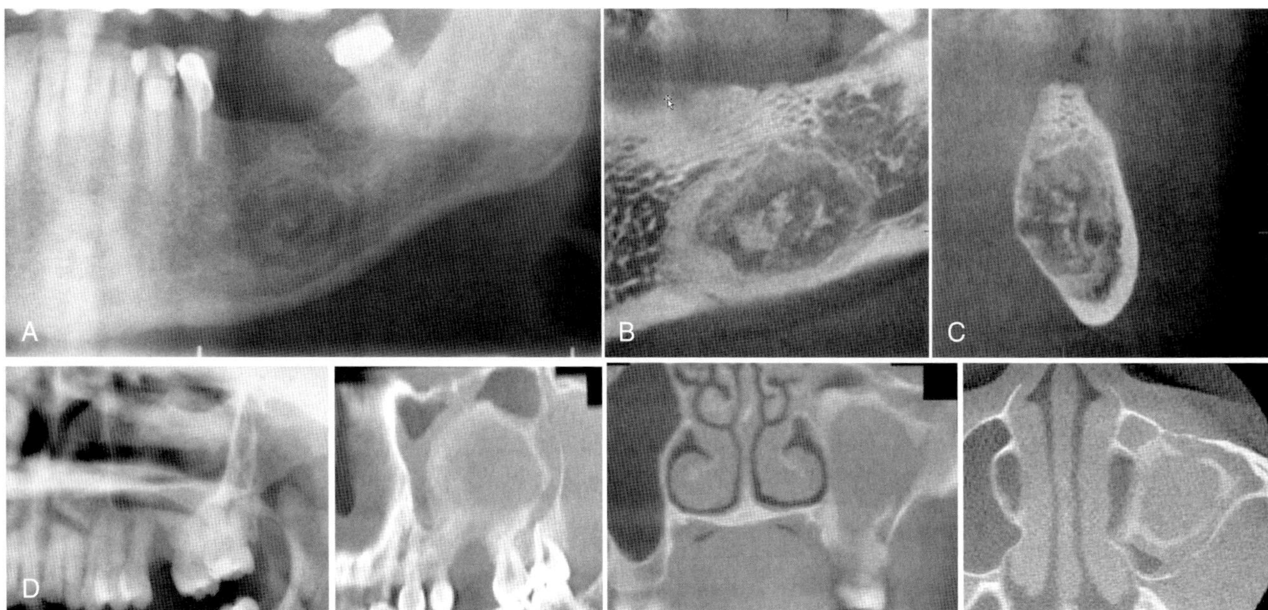

Fig. 75.8 Radiographic examination of a patient with a partially edentulous left posterior mandible. (A) Panoramic radiograph demonstrates an ovoid-shaped, mixed density lesion within the body of the mandible at the area of missing teeth nos. 18–20. (B) Sagittal CBCT image of the area shows the extent of the lesion to the inferior border of the mandible. (C) Cross-sectional view from the same CBCT scan demonstrates lingual cortical expansion and partial encasement of the inferior alveolar canal by the lesion. Biopsy of this incidental finding revealed an ossifying fibroma. (D) Conventional panoramic, reconstructed "panoramic," coronal, and axial sections of the alveolar ridge at the area of the missing first maxillary molar. A large radiolucent lesion at the edentulous alveolar ridge elevates the floor of the maxillary sinus and occupies most of the sinus. Biopsy revealed a keratocystic odontogenic tumor that was an incidental finding in this asymptomatic patient.

image is of critical importance. The diagnostic imaging may reveal inadequate bone volume for the proposed implant(s) and indicate a need for bone augmentation or, depending on the severity of the deficiency, preclude the patient from the possibility of implant therapy. When ridge augmentation is deemed necessary, radiographic evaluation prior to and after surgery informs treatment planning and ensures grafting integrity and quality (Figs. 75.13 and 75.14).

In addition to the amount, the quality of the available bone should also be evaluated. A uniform, continuous cortical outline and a lacy, well-defined trabecular core reflect the normal bone homeostasis necessary for appropriate bone response around the implant. Depending on the timeline of extraction, grafted extraction sockets should be well-condensed along the walls of the extraction sockets and eventually blend in with the adjacent alveolar bone (Fig. 75.15). The presence of thin or discontinuous cortices, sparse trabeculation, large marrow spaces, and altered trabecular architecture should be noted because they might predict poor implant stabilization and less desirable response of the bone. Poor bone quality or poor integration of bone graft may necessitate modifications of the treatment planning, such as waiting longer for healing (osseointegration) to maximize bone-to-implant contact before loading.

Evaluate Relation of Alveolar Ridge With Existing Teeth and Desired Implant Position

Accurate placement (spatial position and angulation relative to adjacent teeth and occlusal plane) will greatly affect the restorative success and long-term prognosis of the implant (see Chapters 74 and 76). A significant variable during the preimplant evaluation is the relation of the desired implant position relative to the existing teeth, alveolar crest, and occlusal plane. Angled or custom abutments can accommodate slight variations in implant position and implant inclination. However, more significant deviations should be avoided.

Prolonged tooth loss is usually associated with atrophy of the alveolar ridge and, in the case of the maxilla, with pneumatization of the sinus floor toward the alveolar crest. Traumatic extractions can compromise the buccal or lingual cortex and alter the shape and buccolingual ridge dimension. Anatomic variants, such as lingual inclination of the alveolus or narrow ridges, should be considered during treatment planning of the implant patient (Fig. 75.16).

An important part of diagnostic imaging must include an evaluation of the available bone relative to the "prosthetically driven" implant position. This aspect of the patient evaluation can be accomplished via analog or digital planning methods. In an analog approach, diagnostic models with wax-up(s) at the sites of planned tooth replacement(s) and a radiographic guide with markers in the desired tooth positions are utilized. Steel balls, brass tubes, gutta-percha, or tooth-shaped, resin-based markers may be used as markers to establish the proposed tooth positions relative to the existing alveolar bone. The radiographic guide is worn during the CBCT or CT imaging examination so that the marker can reveal the location of the planned restoration and thereby direct evaluation of bone height and width to a specific anatomic location (see Figs. 75.5 and 75.17).

In a digital workflow, however, this can be accomplished in different ways, and a radiographic guide may not be necessary. In this approach, a CBCT scan dataset can be registered or aligned with an optical scan (in *STL format*) of the diagnostic cast that includes the diagnostic wax-up at the site of planned restoration. As a result, the datasets are superimposed, thereby facilitating assessment of the alveolar bone at the specific site(s) of the planned restoration (see Chapter 84).

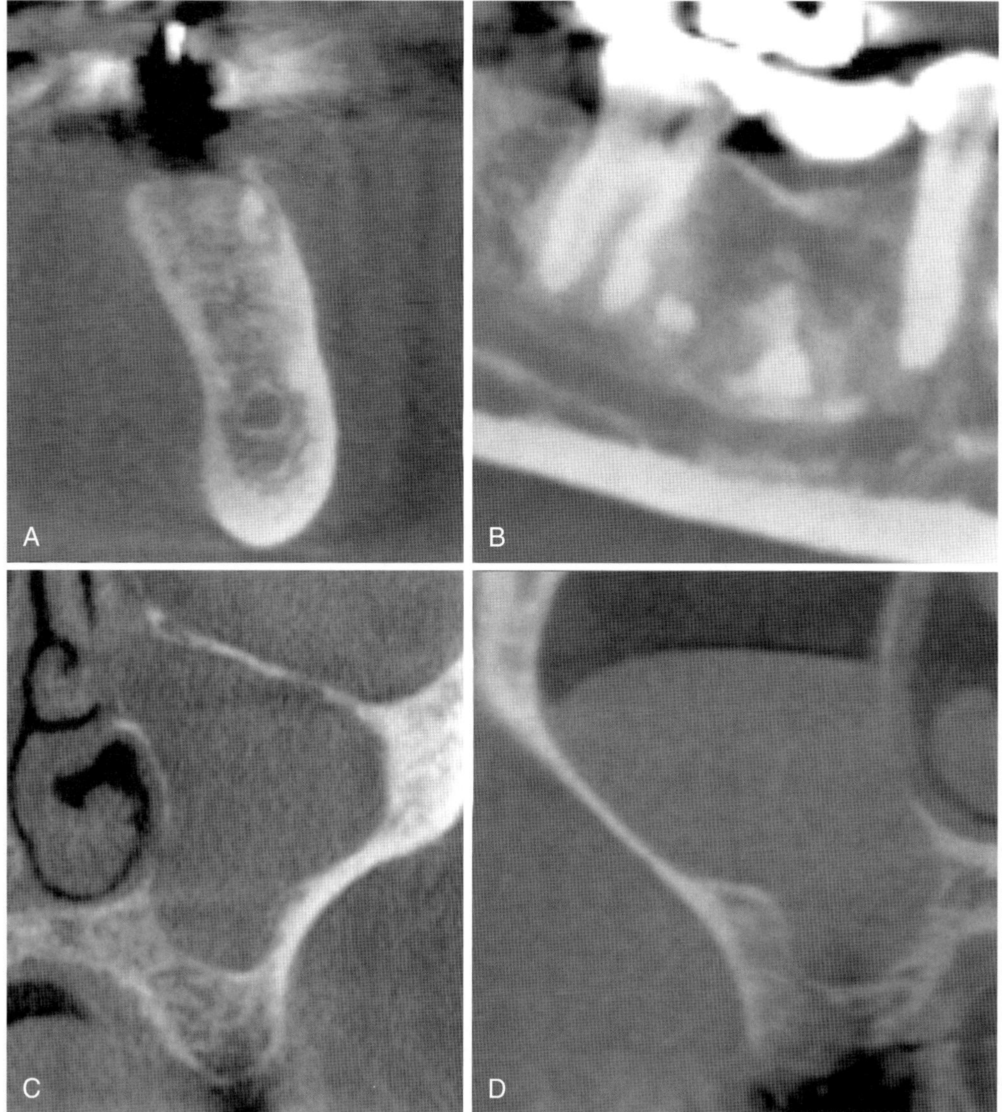

Fig. 75.9 Local abnormalities commonly observed in the vicinity of edentulous sites of the jaws as seen on cone-beam computed tomography. (A) Cross-sectional view demonstrating a small residual root tip near the buccal alveolar crest. (B) Sagittal view showing an amorphous, mixed density lesion consistent with focal cemento-osseous dysplasia near the superior border of the mandibular canal at the site of tooth no. 30. (C) Coronal view reveals complete opacification of the left maxillary sinus consistent with maxillary sinusitis. Note the obstruction of the left ostiomeatal unit. (D) Coronal view of the right maxillary sinus showing a large mucous retention pseudocyst occupying the inferior half of the sinus lumen.

BOX 75.1 Anatomic Structures Pertinent to Treatment Planning of the Implant Patient

Maxilla

Maxillary sinus (floor and anterior wall)
Nasal cavity (floor and lateral wall)
Incisive foramen and canal
Canine fossa
Canalis sinuosus

Mandible

Mandibular canal
Anterior loop of the mandibular canal
Anterior extension of the mandibular canal
Mental foramen
Lingual canal
Submandibular fossa
Retromolar canal
Lingual inclination of the alveolar ridge

KEY FACT

An important part of diagnostic imaging must include an evaluation of the available bone relative to the "prosthetically driven" implant position. This information can be obtained by utilizing a radiographic guide during 3D imaging with radiopaque markers at sites of proposed restoration. Alternatively, if a digital workflow is preferred, one can register the CBCT scan dataset with the digital diagnostic cast, which includes a wax-up at the site of planned prosthesis.

Clinical Selection of Diagnostic Imaging

Radiography is an important diagnostic tool for the evaluation of the implant patient. However, radiographic imaging alone is insufficient. It is important to correlate diagnostic information with a thorough clinical examination. Conversely, a clinical examination is

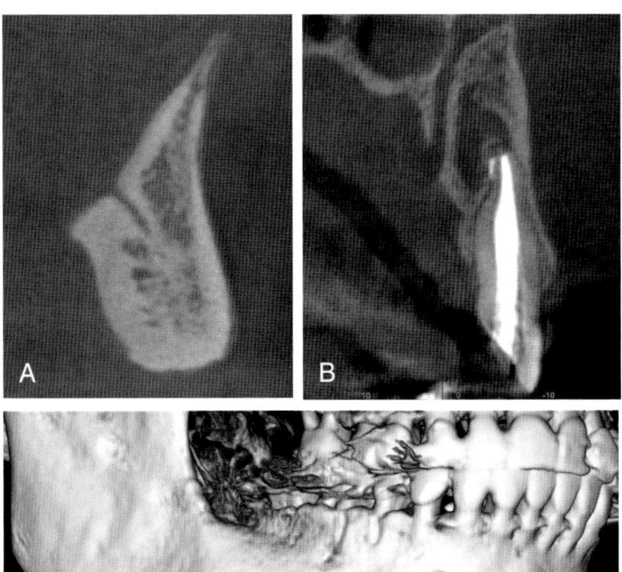

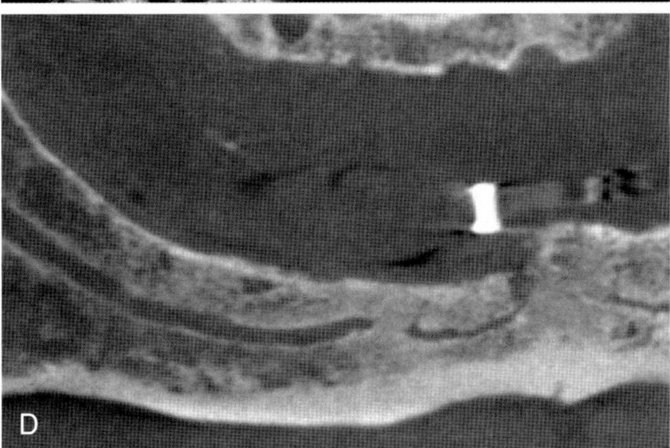

Fig. 75.10 Neurovascular canals of the maxilla and mandible as seen on cone-beam computed tomography. (A) Cross-sectional view through the mandibular midline shows a prominent median lingual canal. Branches of the sublingual artery enter the mandible via this canal. (B) Cross-sectional view through the area of the left maxillary lateral incisor depicts the canalis sinuosus extending from near the floor of the nasal cavity to the palatal cortex. This canal houses nervous structures that innervate the anterior maxilla. (C) 3D volume-rendering view, optimized for bone, demonstrating a double mental foramen, which is an anatomic variation. (D) Panoramic slice view showing a well corticated mandibular canal and prominent anterior extension (incisive branch of the mandibular canal) extending beneath the radiographic marker in the anterior mandible.

insufficient to provide the information needed to plan implant treatment for a patient without some radiographic imaging.

Clinical Examination

Before taking any radiographs, a complete clinical examination of the implant patient is required. This should include the etiology and duration of tooth loss, any history of traumatic extraction, and a review of records and radiographs, if available. A clinical assessment of the edentulous area, covering mucosa, adjacent and opposing teeth, and occlusal plane should be performed. Temporomandibular joint function, mandibular maximal opening, and protrusive and lateral movements should be evaluated.

Screening Radiographs

At this point, an overall assessment of the health of the jaws should be performed. The American Academy of Oral and Maxillofacial Radiology recommends panoramic radiography as the initial evaluation of the dental implant patient, supplemented with periapical radiographs as needed.[23] Periapical radiographs provide a high-resolution image of the alveolus and the surrounding structures, including adjacent teeth. For extended edentulous areas, panoramic radiographs and 3D volumetric imaging techniques can be used to estimate bone height and width. Any pathology of the bone at the prospective implant site as well as of the surrounding structures should be identified and treated as indicated.

KEY FACT

The American Academy of Oral and Maxillofacial Radiology recommends panoramic radiography as the initial evaluation of the dental implant patient, supplemented with periapical radiographs as needed. The organization also recommends that radiographic examination of any potential implant site should include cross-sectional imaging orthogonal to the site of interest.

Fabrication of Radiographic and Surgical Guides

Once the health of the soft and hard tissues is established, casts should be taken (whether analog or digital) and a detailed analysis performed. The clinician should decide on the number of implants and their desired location. If a conventional workflow is followed, a radiographic guide is fabricated with the position of the desired implants indicated by the use of radiopaque objects such as metallic balls, cylinders, or rods; gutta-percha; or composite resin. The design of such a guide greatly enhances the diagnostic information provided by the radiographs because it correlates the radiographic anatomy with the exact position of the proposed implant location. Alternatively, if a digital workflow is preferred, the same information should be sought via co-registration of the CBCT dataset with optical scans of the patient's diagnostic casts (see Chapter 84).

Cross-Sectional Imaging

The American Academy of Oral and Maxillofacial Radiology recommends that radiographic examination of any potential implant site include cross-sectional imaging orthogonal to the site of interest.[23] It further states that CBCT should be considered the imaging modality of choice for preoperative cross-sectional imaging of potential implant sites.[24] The potential morbidity of a compromised anatomic structure and the poor performance and potential failure of a misplaced implant, combined with the relatively wide availability of advanced imaging (CBCT or MDCT), favor the use of cross-sectional imaging in the great majority of implant treatment planning. It is crucial that the cross sections are perpendicular to the curvature of the mandible and parallel to the planned implant. Improper orientation of cross sections can lead to an overestimation of the height and width of the available bone. If the surgeon believes that sections were made at the wrong angulation, new images should be requested.

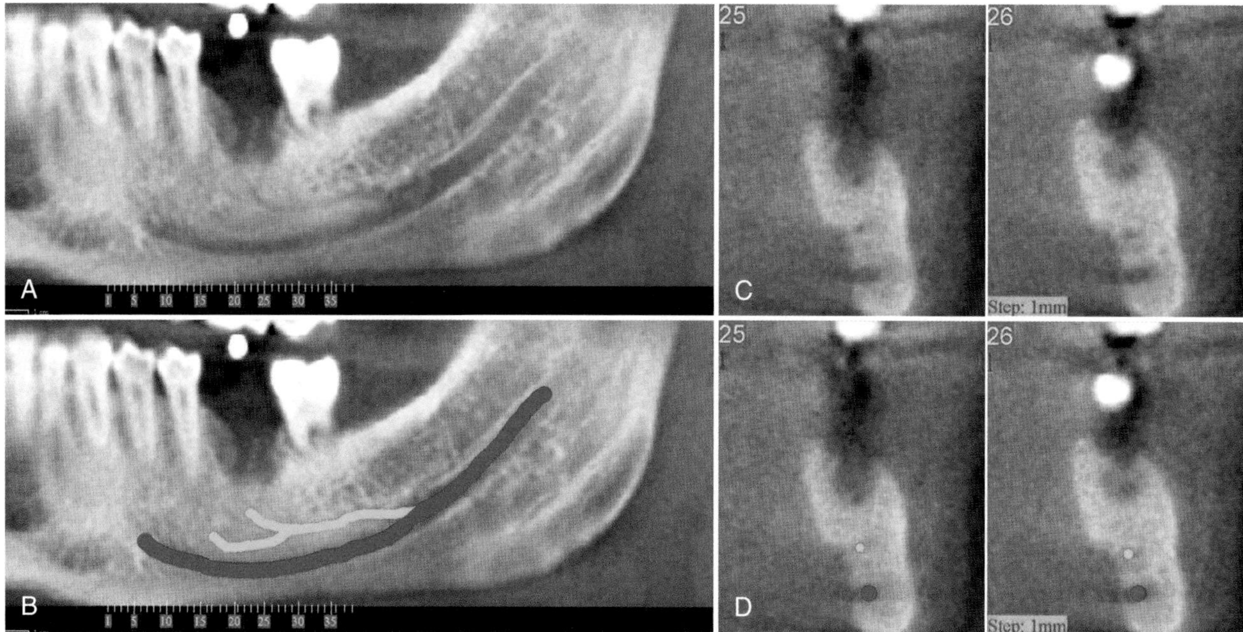

Fig. 75.11 Cone-beam computed tomography examination of the area of missing tooth #19 before implant placement. (A) Panoramic view of the area of interest depicts an accessory mandibular canal. (B) Same panoramic view with the accessory mandibular canal colored blue and the main canal colored red. (C) Cross-sectional views through the area of missing tooth #19. (D) Same cross-sectional images depicting the blue and red markings. Note that the position of the markings coincides with the position of the accessory and main mandibular canals (compare parts C and D).

Intraoperative and Postoperative Radiographic Assessment

Various radiographic modalities can provide valuable information during implant placement. Because of the ease of acquisition and high resolution, periapical radiographs are most commonly used. Intraoperative radiographs can be taken during surgery to evaluate proximity to important anatomic structures. Sequential periapical radiographs guide the clinician to visualize changes in direction and depth of the drilling procedure and parallelism to adjacent teeth and other implants (Fig. 75.18). Digital radiographs are particularly advantageous during an intraoperative assessment of implant placement; images appear on the screen almost instantaneously and can be manipulated to extract the most pertinent diagnostic information (see Chapter 39).

Implant osseointegration and the level of peri-implant alveolar bone are major determinants of implant prognosis. Panoramic and periapical radiographs offer a fast, easy, and low-radiation depiction of the implant and surrounding tissues and aid in the assessment of implant success. To obtain an accurate assessment of peri-implant bone height, the x-ray beam should be directed perpendicular to the implant. In the case of threaded implants, the implant threads should be distinguishable and not overlapping (Fig. 75.19A). Although 2D periapical and panoramic x-rays cannot display buccal–lingual peri-implant bone, the use of CBCT in the regular monitoring of peri-implant bone levels has remained limited due to the presence of *beam hardening artifact* along the implant–bone interface (Fig. 75.20).[18] Advanced defects are often detected on CBCT and may appear with a circumferential pattern of peri-implant bone loss (Fig. 75.21). Nevertheless, due to their higher sensitivity and specificity in detecting peri-implant bone defects, periapical radiographs remain the standard in the routine diagnostics of peri-implant bone sites.[9]

A 1.2-mm marginal bone loss during the first year after implant placement and 0.1 mm per year afterward are expected; however, further bone loss is considered abnormal.[2] Pathologic bone loss could be localized along the full extent of the implant (peri-implant bone loss) or around the crestal part of the implant ("saucerization"), and it could reflect poor osseointegration, peri-implantitis, or unfavorable stress distribution (Fig. 75.19B and C).

In select cases of implant failure (Fig. 75.22) or when poor implant placement (Figs. 75.23 and 75.24) or compromise of vital anatomic structures (Fig. 75.25) is suspected, advanced imaging (CBCT or MDCT) provides a three-dimensional evaluation of the oral structures in relation to the implants. This information can be very important for proper assessment and treatment planning. The treating dentist should recognize relevant signs and symptoms and order appropriate imaging as soon after implant placement as possible. Implant removal, if necessary, would be less complicated before advanced osseointegration.

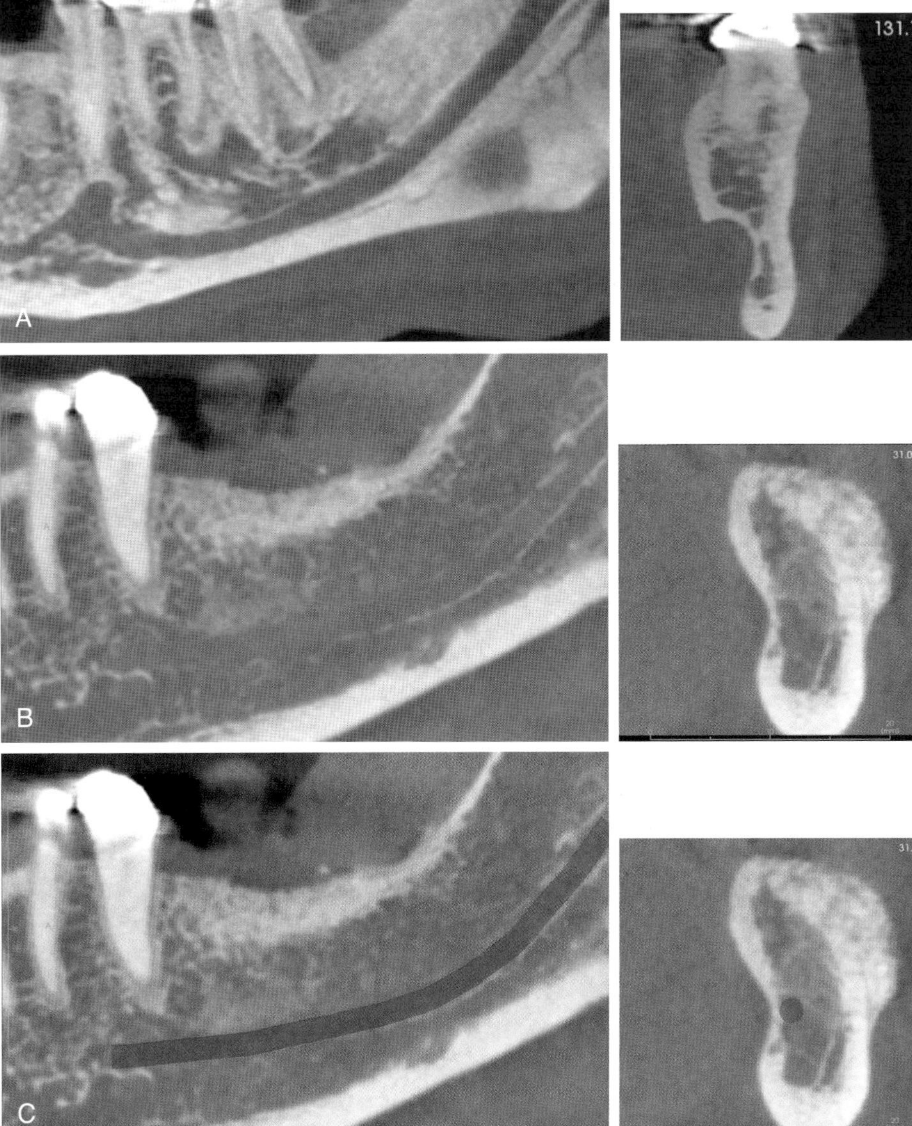

Fig. 75.12 Cone-beam computed tomography images showing normal variations in mandibular canal cortication. (A) Sagittal and cross-sectional views showing an easily identifiable and well corticated mandibular canal. (B) Sagittal and cross-sectional views on a different patient showing an irregular cortication of the mandibular canal with poor visualization of the canal borders in the area of the left first molar. Note the absence of a distinct cortical outline on cross-sectional view. (C) After tracing the mandibular canal on the sagittal view identified by the red line, localization of the canal on the cross-sectional view is attainable. (C) After tracing the mandibular canal on the sagittal view identified by the red line, localization of the canal on the cross-sectional view is attainable.

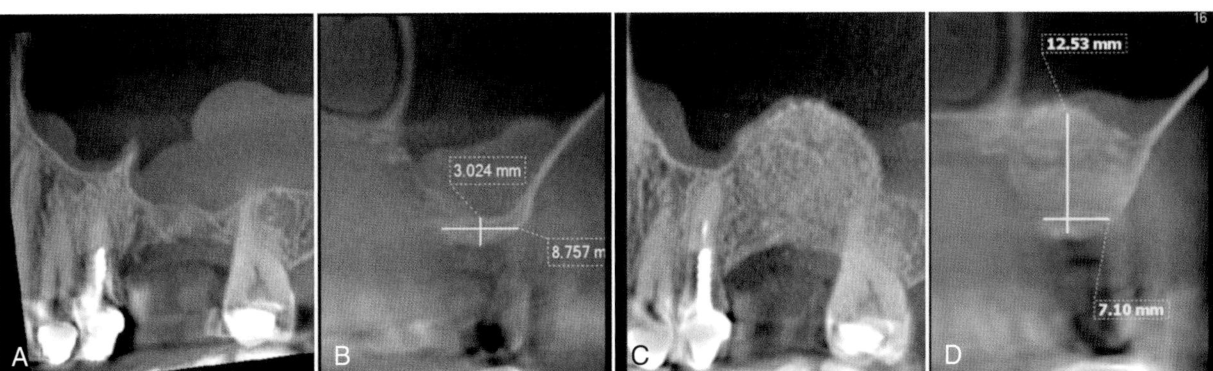

Fig. 75.13 Radiographic evaluation of a patient with missing left maxillary second premolar and first molar. Initial cone-beam computed tomography (CBCT) reveals an atrophic alveolar ridge (A) with inadequate height for implant placement (B). Also note the thickened mucoperiosteum at the floor of the maxillary sinus. CBCT after sinus grafting for ridge augmentation shows the uniformly opaque grafting area blending with alveolar trabeculation and a smooth sinus floor elevation (C), which provides adequate dimensions for implant placement (D).

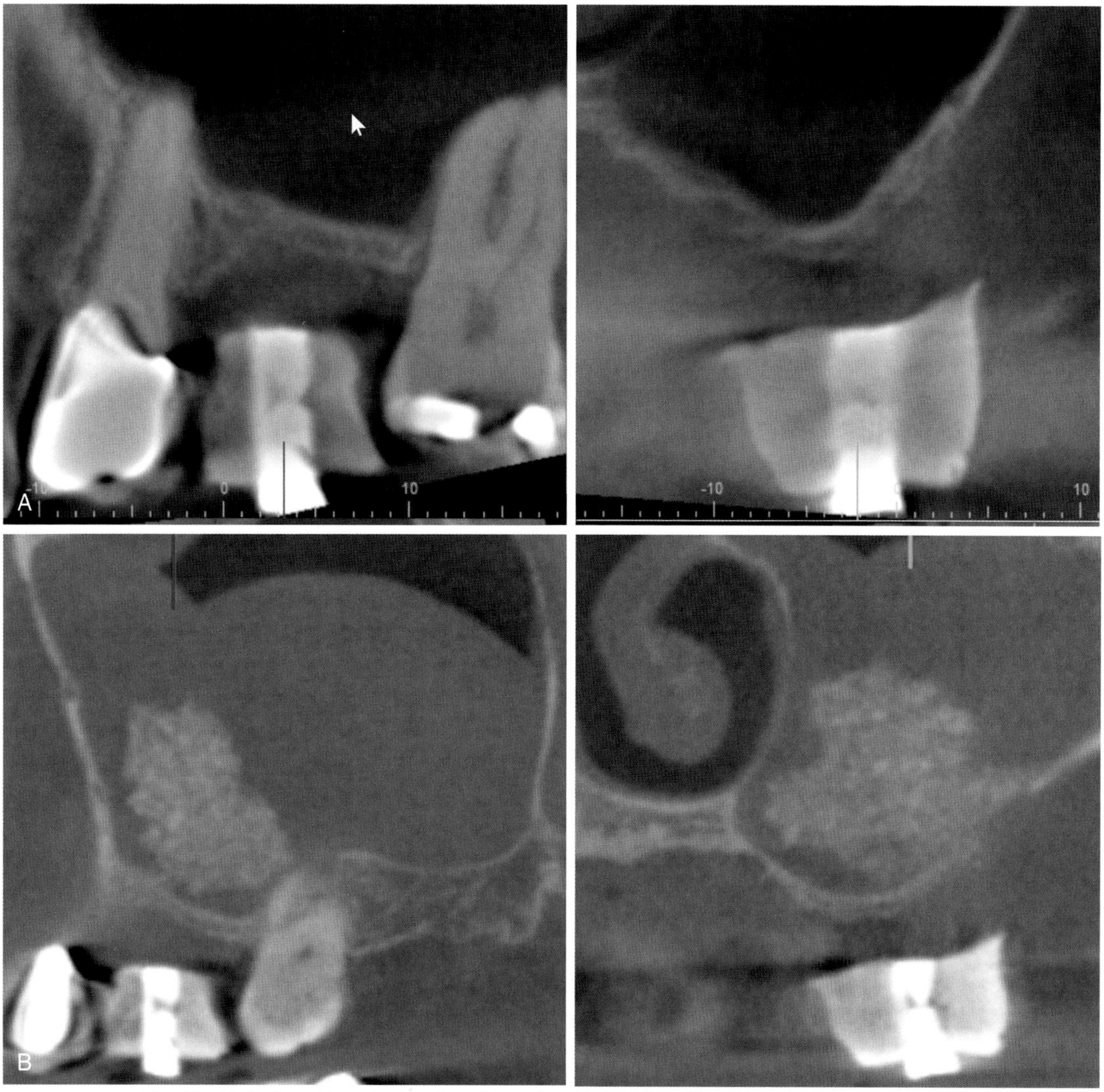

Fig. 75.14 Radiographic evaluation of a patient with a missing left maxillary first molar. (A) Initial cone-beam computed tomography (CBCT) reveals a severely resorbed alveolar ridge with insufficient bone for implant placement. (B) CBCT performed after sinus grafting shows granular, radiopaque material that is largely separated from the underlying alveolar bone in an otherwise mostly opacified left maxillary sinus. These findings are suggestive of maxillary sinusitis and poor osseointegration of graft material.

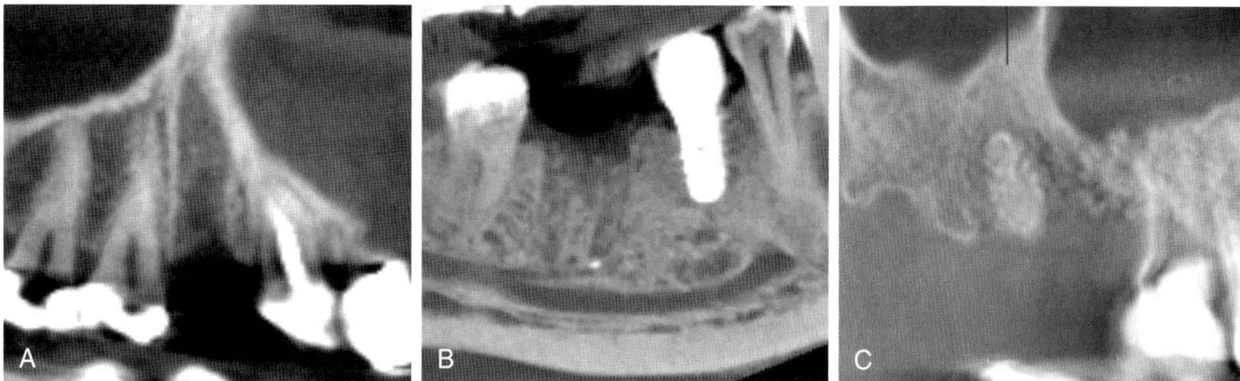

Fig. 75.15 Varied radiographic appearances of grafted extraction sockets on cone-beam computed tomography. Depending on the quantity and type of graft material and the extent of osseous remodeling, radiographic appearances of grafted extraction sockets can vary from relatively radiolucent (A) to mixed density (B) to highly opaque (C).

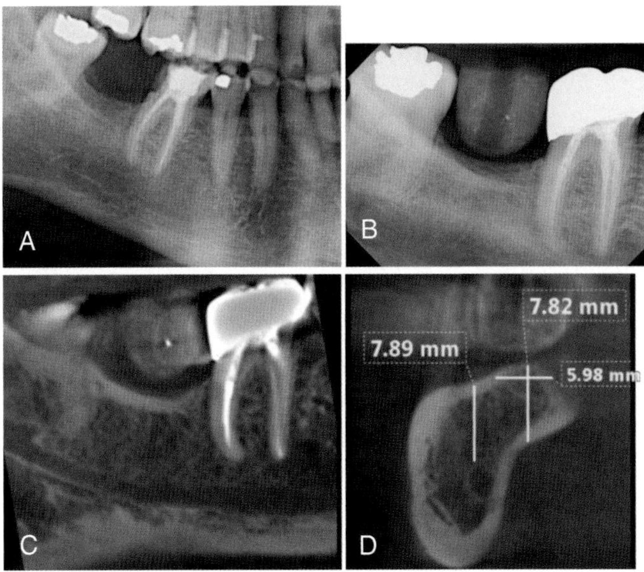

Fig. 75.16 Radiographic evaluation of a patient with an edentulous posterior left mandible before implant placement. Panoramic (A) and periapical (B) radiographs demonstrate sufficient height of the alveolar ridge with little or no resorption. Cone-beam computed tomography sections (C and D) reveal significant lingual inclination of the alveolar ridge with lingual concavity that is not depicted on conventional radiographs.

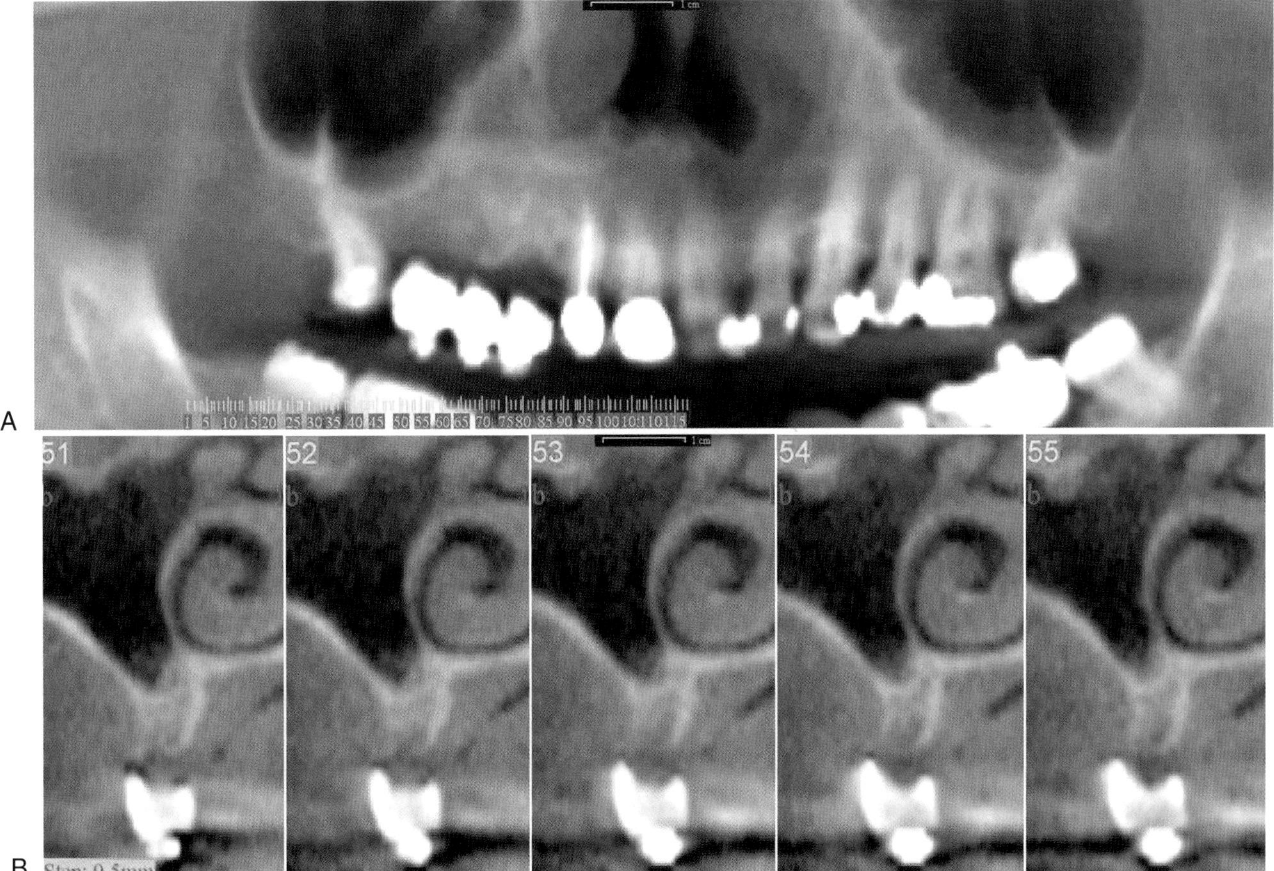

Fig. 75.17 (A) Panoramic view of partially edentulous maxilla with tooth-shaped markers in areas of missing teeth (potential implant sites). (B) Cross-sectional views from a cone-beam computed tomography examination before implant placement in the right maxilla. Appropriately sized and shaped tooth markers placed in the prosthetically desired locations of the planned restorations for the missing teeth help evaluate the existing alveolar ridge relative to the prospective tooth positions and contours.

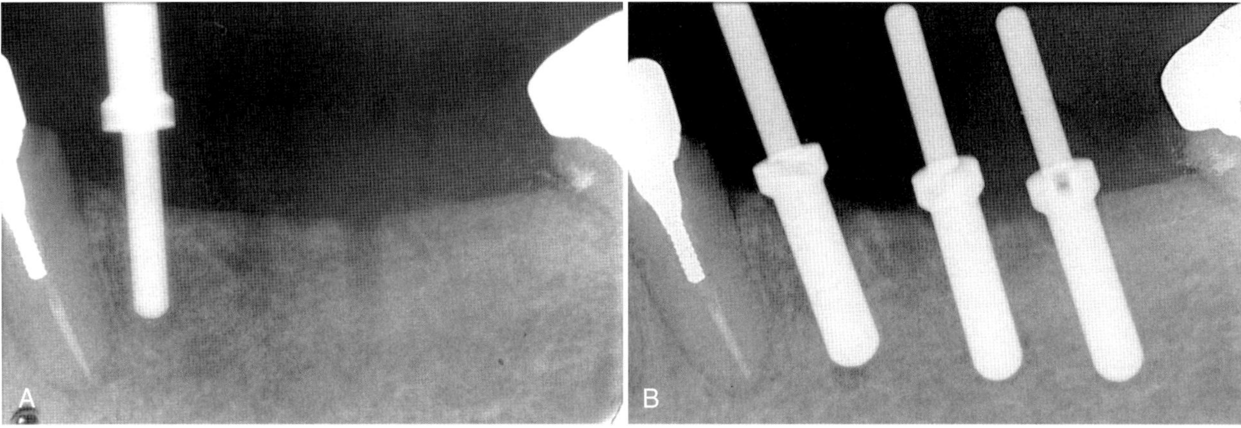

Fig. 75.18 Intraoperative periapical radiographs are valuable in assessing the proximity of adjacent teeth. (A) The 2-mm guide pin is used to determine the direction of the osteotomy site and its proximity to the adjacent root. (B) After angle correction, the osteotomy sites are completed to length with the final drill. Here the 3-mm guide pins confirm the correct angulation and spacing of the final osteotomy site preparation before implant placement.

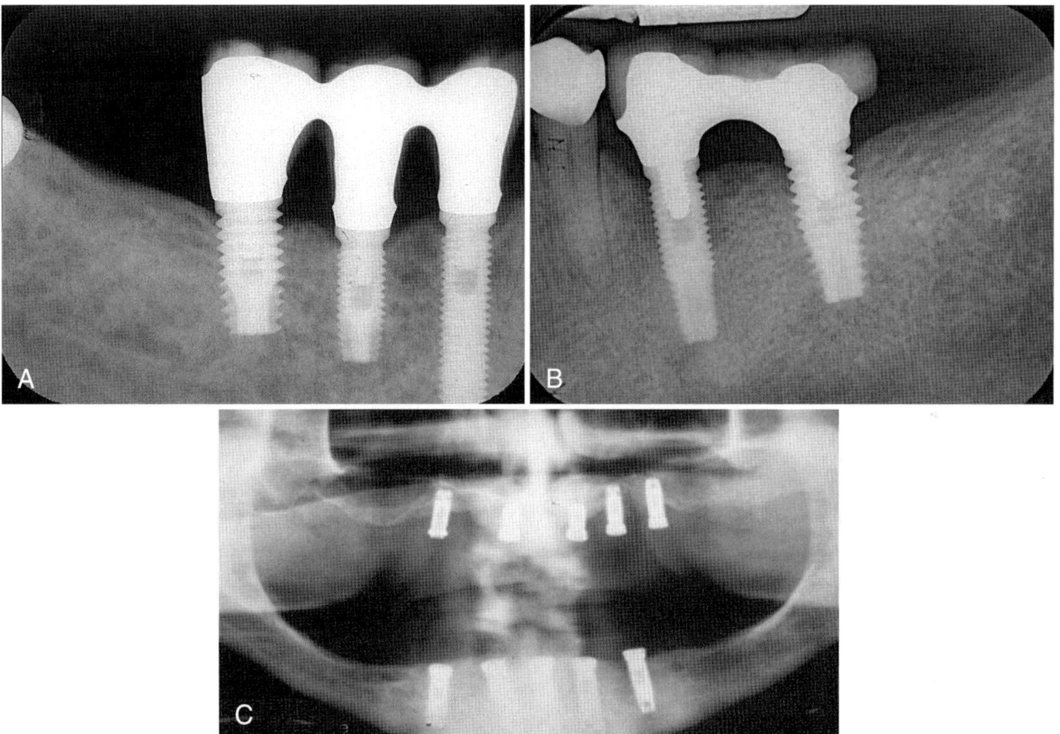

Fig. 75.19 Radiographic follow-up after implant placement in three different patients. (A) Periapical radiograph of three implants in the posterior right mandible. "Normal" bone remodeling around the anterior two implants and slight horizontal bone loss/remodeling around the molar/posterior implant is present. (B) Periapical radiograph of two implants in the left posterior mandible. Severe bone loss (50% of implant length) is seen around the anterior implant, whereas mild bone loss/bone remodeling is observed around the posterior implant. A moderate buccal cantilever in the restoration likely contributed to an adverse occlusal load and the resultant bone loss observed in this case. (C) Panoramic radiograph of maxillary and mandibular implants in an edentulous patient prior to implant loading. The mandibular implants do not show signs of bone loss and appear to be osseointegrated. All maxillary implants show signs of moderate-to-severe peri-implant bone loss, and the success of osseointegration is questionable.

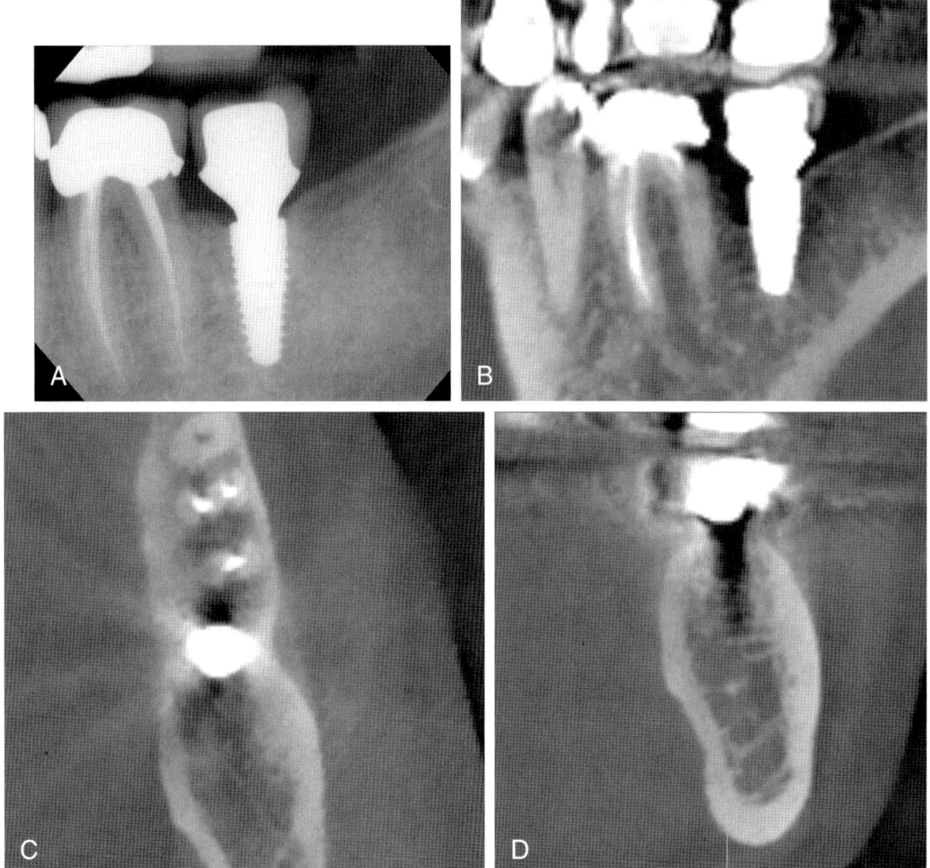

Fig. 75.20 Radiographic follow-up after implant placement. (A) Periapical radiograph shows an implant at the site of the left mandibular second molar with normal bone levels. (B) Sagittal CBCT of the area demonstrates a well-defined radiolucent area along the mesial aspect of the implant fixture to approximately the cervical third consistent with beam hardening artifact. Note that the radiolucent area adjacent to the implant has an airlike radiodensity. (C) Axial view shows alternating radiolucent and radiopaque streaks emanating from the implant fixture. Note that the radiolucent streaks are largely limited to the mesial–distal plane. (D) Cross-sectional slice made mesial to the implant depicts radiolucent artifact in the shape of the implant fixture within the interradicular bone.

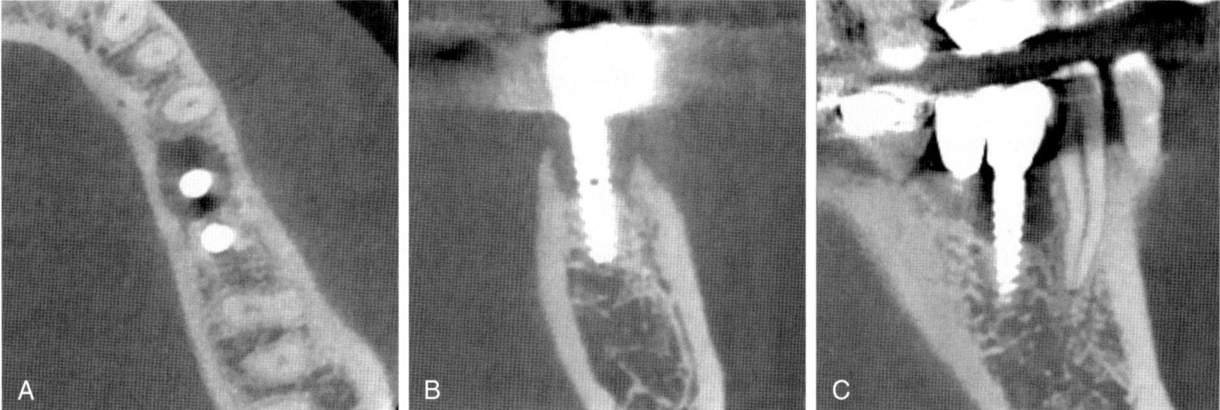

Fig. 75.21 Axial (A), cross-sectional (B), and sagittal (C) CBCT views of a mandibular implant in the left premolar region demonstrating a commonly observed pattern of circumferential peri-implant bone loss. Peri-implant bone loss in this area is advanced and extends to the mid-fixture level.

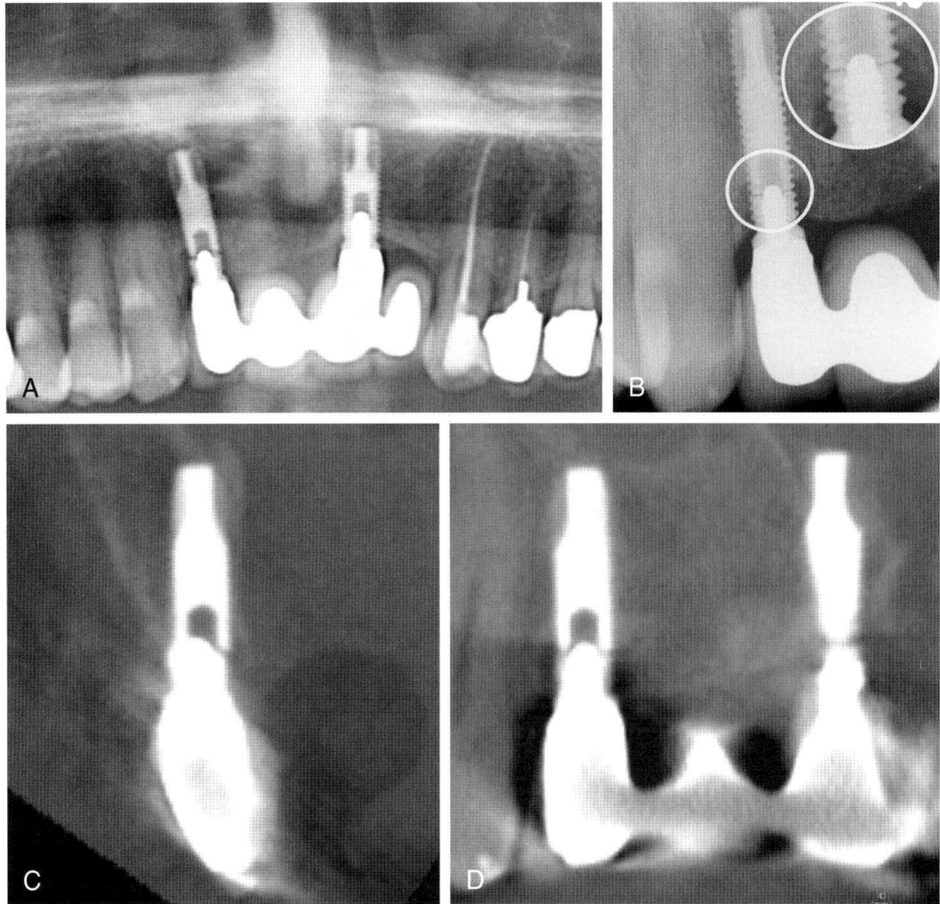

Fig. 75.22 Radiographic follow-up after acute onset of implant mobility. (A) Panoramic radiograph shows fracture of the implant fixture in the cervical third with associated peri-implant bone loss. Slight displacement of the fractured segments can be appreciated. (B) Periapical radiograph also clearly depicts a fracture of the implant fixture, and peri-implant bone loss extending to the fifth thread. (C) Sagittal CBCT view through the implant demonstrates partial fracture of the implant fixture at the buccal aspect. Note the reduced visibility of the fracture line due to beam hardening artifact. (D) Coronal CBCT view of the implant does not obviously display the fracture plane.

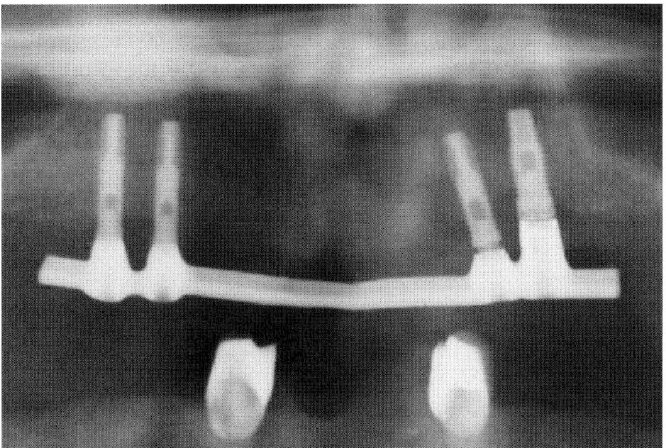

Fig. 75.23 Radiographic follow-up after implant placement. Panoramic radiograph suggests mild-to-moderate bone loss around the neck of all implants. This is especially true for the implants in the left maxilla. These implants appear to be angled, and the distal implant is positioned more apical. The overdenture bar is not completely seated on the left implants. Note that superimposed overlapping anatomic structures in this panoramic radiograph impair the ability to clearly visualize and assess bone loss around implants.

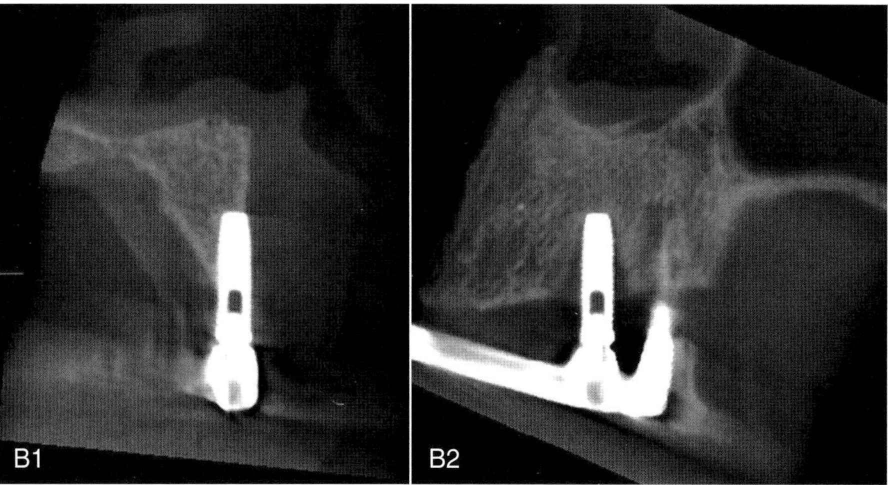

Fig. 75.23 cont'd (B) Cross-sectional (B1) and sagittal cone-beam computed tomography (B2) images of the anterior implant in the left maxilla. Poor implant placement beyond the buccal cortex of the alveolar ridge (cross section) and peri-implant bone loss (sagittal) are revealed.

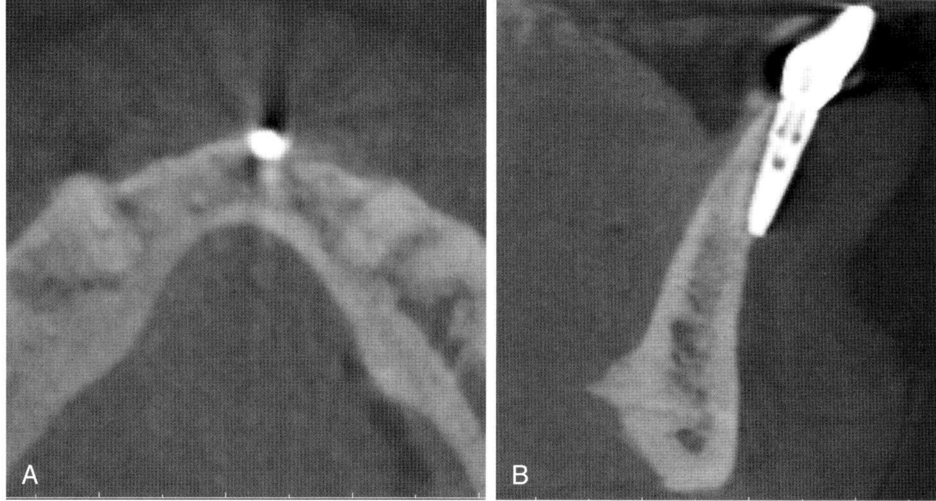

Fig. 75.24 Radiographic follow-up after implant placement. Axial (A) and sagittal (B) cone-beam computed tomography images show poor implant placement beyond the buccal cortex of the alveolar ridge. Note the broad dehiscence of the buccal cortex appreciable on the sagittal view.

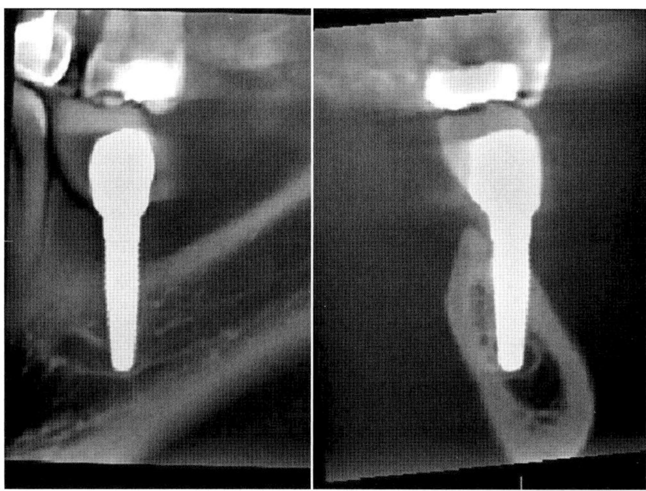

Fig. 75.25 Cone-beam computed tomography sagittal and cross-sectional images clearly demonstrate penetration of the implant into the mandibular canal.

Conclusions

Many radiographic projections are available for the evaluation of implant placement, each with advantages and disadvantages. The clinician must follow sequential steps in patient evaluation, and radiography is an essential diagnostic tool for implant design and successful treatment of the implant patient. Selection of appropriate radiographic modalities will provide the maximum diagnostic information, help avoid unwanted complications, and maximize treatment outcomes while delivering an "as low as reasonably achievable" radiation dose to the patient.[15]

Case Scenarios are found on the companion website eBooks.Health.Elsevier.com.

Suggested Readings

Benson BW, Shetty V. Dental implants. In: White SC, Pharoah MJ, eds. *Oral Radiology: Principles and Interpretation*. 6th ed. St. Louis: Mosby; 2009.

Devlin H, Yuan J. Object position and image magnification in dental panoramic radiography: a theoretical analysis. *Dentomaxillofac Radiol*. 2013;42(1):29951683–29951683.

Fokas G, Vaughn VM, Scarfe WC, Bornstein MM. Accuracy of linear measurements on CBCT images related to presurgical implant treatment planning: a systematic review. *Clin Oral Implants Res*. 2018;29:393–415.

Hatcher DC, Dial C, Mayorga C. Cone beam CT for pre-surgical assessment of implant sites. *J Calif Dent Assoc*. 2003;31:824.

Kühl S, Zürcher S, Zitzmann NU, Filippi A, Payer M, Dagassan–Berndt D. Detection of peri–implant bone defects with different radiographic techniques–a human cadaver study. *Clin Oral Implants Res*. 2016;27(5):529–534.

Langland OE, Langlais RP, Preece JW. *Panoramic and Special Imaging Techniques. Principles of Dental Imaging*. 2nd ed. Baltimore: Lippincott Williams & Wilkins; 2002.

Mallya SM, Lurie AG. Panoramic imaging. In: White SC, Pharoah MJ, eds. *Oral Radiology: Principles And Interpretation*. 7th ed. St. Louis: Mosby; 2013.

Misch CE. *Contemporary Implant Dentistry*. 3rd ed. St. Louis: Mosby Elsevier; 2007.

Rios HF, Borgnakke WS, Benavides E. The use of cone–beam computed tomography in management of patients requiring dental implants: an American Academy of Periodontology best evidence review. *J Periodontol*. 2017;88(10):946–959.

Tyndall DA, Price JB, Tetradis S, et al. Position statement of the American Academy of Oral and Maxillofacial Radiology on selection criteria for the use of radiology in dental implantology with emphasis on cone beam computed tomography. *Oral Surg Oral Med Oral Pathol Oral Radiol*. 2012;113(6):817.

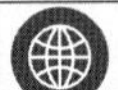

References for this chapter are found on the companion website eBooks.Health.Elsevier.com.

CHAPTER 76

Prosthetic Considerations: Partially Edentulous

Todd R. Schoenbaum | Perry R. Klokkevold

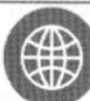
For online-only content on fully edentulous prosthetic considerations, please visit the companion website at eBooks.Health.Elsevier.com.

CHAPTER OUTLINE

Ultimately, successful implant treatment requires a team of clinicians dedicated to excellence in surgical and prosthetic aspects of the process. This chapter reviews the critical aspects of prosthetic implant treatment in partially edentulous patients proven to maximize long-term functional, biologic, and esthetic success.

Implant Considerations

Understanding the Anticipated Load on the System and Its Relation to Implant Diameter

Selecting the appropriate implants for the partially edentulous patient depends in part on the anticipated loads of that particular tooth location. The larger the anticipated loads, the more robust the implant must be to properly support the prosthesis. Notably, for any given implant design, larger-diameter implants result in stronger prostheses.[13] The implant connection design also plays a significant role and will be discussed later. However, the prosthetic advantages of a larger-diameter implant must be balanced with the surgical needs for sufficient (~1.5 mm) surrounding bone. In some locations, this constraint will present itself in the mesiodistal dimension, whereas in others the constraint will come from the buccolingual dimension of the alveolar ridge.

The anticipated load on the implant is affected by its position in the arch. The more posterior the implant is in the arch, the higher the anticipated load. Estimates have been made relating to the ratio of load from anterior to posterior,[41] but such generalizations oversimplify the complexity of the system. Although a tooth located more posteriorly will receive at least twice the load forces (and therefore require a larger implant diameter), there are several other factors that will influence the result. Anterior–posterior position in the arch is part of this consideration, but so are the number and integrity of the other teeth/implants, especially those distal to the proposed implant position. A first molar implant with robust second molar support will receive significantly less force than that same molar with no other molar support.

Often overlooked, the size of the muscles of mastication can provide cursory evidence regarding just how much force a patient is able to produce on his or her dentition. Patients with very large muscles will generate greater forces on their teeth and implants. However, excessive forces do not always show up as attrition. These forces can be delivered in a largely vertical vector with little to no horizontal component. This information should be checked and recorded at the initial patient examination. Patients with a history of cracked or broken teeth and crowns should be expected to place heavier loads on the implants used to replace them.

In the evaluation of the implant patient, special attention should be given to the arch opposing the location of expected implant treatment. If the opposing dentition is a removable appliance (with no plans to change this), then the implant will receive significantly lower forces.[43,48] Conversely, if the opposing dentition is implant-supported fixed restorations, the forces are likely to be quite high. This phenomenon is largely due to the lack of a periodontal ligament (PDL) around the implants. If the implant is opposing a removable appliance, it should be determined if there is any likelihood of converting to a fixed implant-supported prosthesis. If this is the case, then the implant in question should be planned with increased loads in mind.

Occlusal guards have long been employed to protect the dentition and prostheses against excessive forces and destructive wear habits. As implants lack the "cushioning effect" that the PDL provides to natural teeth, the occlusal guard can provide the patient with an added layer of protection against overloading of the implant system. The limiting factor with occlusal guards is patient compliance.

Clinicians looking for a more quantified approach to evaluating the loads placed on teeth and implants might consider digital occlusal analysis systems.

CLINICAL CORRELATION

The anticipated load on the implant is affected by its position in the arch. The more posterior the implant, the higher the anticipated load. Estimates have been made relating to the ratio of load from anterior to posterior, but such generalizations oversimplify the complexity of the system. Although a tooth located more posteriorly will receive at least twice the load forces, there are several other factors that will influence the result. Other important factors to consider are the number of implants, the stability of the surrounding/opposing dentition, and individual mastication forces.

Larger-diameter implants create stronger prosthetics and are less likely to fracture.[13] The use of larger implants becomes more important under the following circumstances: enlarged masseter/temporalis muscles, a history of broken teeth and crowns, distal-most tooth in the arch, opposing other implants, and patients unwilling to wear an occlusal guard. However, the prosthetic advantages of larger platform implants must be balanced with the realities of the surgical site dimensions. In locations with space constraints, other prosthetic modalities may be employed to mitigate the anticipated risks. Innovations in implant connections, manufacturing tolerances, and prosthetic materials have created more and more robust systems that will improve the ability to withstand excessive forces.

Narrow-diameter implants have proven to be a reliable and useful approach to compromised spaces (<7 mm).[65] This constraint can be mesiodistal due to adjacent teeth or implants, or it can be buccolingual due to inadequate volume of the alveolar ridge. Use of such implants is best reserved for sites with low expected loads and constrained spaces, namely the incisors of both jaws.

Number of Implants

Partially edentulous patients with multiple adjacent missing teeth can present some unique challenges. If we use 4 mm as the diameter of a "regular" implant, and the guideline of 1.5 mm of circumferential peri-implant bone, we can quickly estimate the amount of space required for implants by multiplying 7 mm times the number of missing teeth.[121] Or more simply, one tooth requires 7 mm of mesiodistal space, two teeth require 14 mm, three teeth require 21 mm, and so on (Fig. 76.1). This is an oversimplification of the planning process but makes initial estimations of treatment options easier.

Not every missing tooth needs an implant. Two implants with a three-unit fixed dental prosthesis (FDP) have proven to be quite reliable in many situations.[83] Material selection is key; weaker and unproven materials should be used with extreme caution. Gold alloy porcelain-fused-to-metal (PFMs) and zirconia-based FDPs have good (but not perfect) track records. Lithium disilicate materials (and recent derivatives) are not well tested for multiunit FDPs. The use of a pontic between two implants has esthetic advantages in relation to the volume of the peri-implant tissues. This topic will be covered more in depth during the discussion on implants in the esthetic zone.

Cantilevers off one or more implants can be a creative solution to complicated implant treatment planning situations. Such a design is certainly less durable than a non-cantilevered approach, but it does have its place. Cantilever FDPs are best reserved to replace multiple missing incisors (i.e., maxillary central/lateral incisors) in patients with non-excessive occlusal forces.[107] The use of a cantilever pontic should be avoided in most posterior situations, unless

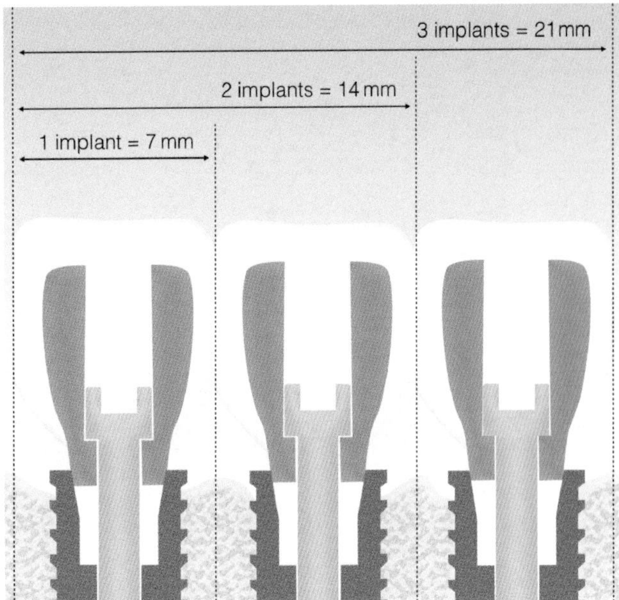

Fig. 76.1 Implants benefit from the presence of 1.5 mm of bone circumferentially. A "normal" diameter implant is ~4 mm. For treatment planning purposes, each implant should have 7 mm of space mesial–distally at the bone crest, two implants would need 14 mm, and so on.

multiple implants are splinted, the length of the cantilever is deemed acceptable, and the opposing dentition/prosthesis reasonable.

Narrow-diameter implants can be implemented in areas with reduced dimensions, but only to a point. Narrower implants are inherently more fragile and more apt to suffer from catastrophic failure. Their minimal dimensions will make more esthetic prosthetic materials (i.e., zirconia abutments) a riskier option. Although manufacturers will continue to produce smaller and smaller implants, their use in patients should be considered cautiously until proven to be successful.

When space constraints push the clinician to select smaller and riskier implants, alternative options should be seriously considered: orthodontics, tooth-borne FDPs (Fig. 76.2), bone augmentation, and additional extractions. Though the last option may sound overly aggressive, it may sometimes be the best choice in scenarios where adequate space cannot be created. This most commonly presents as a single missing mandibular incisor. The two missing incisors can then be replaced with a single implant. In this scenario the implant can be placed centrally between the two missing teeth or off to one side with a larger cantilever (Fig. 76.3). The centrally located implant will reduce the stress due to the decreased length of the cantilever, but the offset implant may allow for the creation of a more natural gingival architecture around the pontic.

Implant-Abutment Connection

Of all the variations in implant designs, perhaps none is as important to prosthetic success as the connection design. The design of an implant abutment junction (IAJ) will influence everything from incidence of screw loosening to maintenance of the hard and soft tissues, to leakage *inside* the implant. The implant(s) should be selected for a particular scenario based on a thorough consideration of the connection that best suits the case. There is no "one size fits all" solution. Certain connections are well suited for fully edentulous patients but are poor choices for a single unit (i.e., older external hex designs), whereas another connection might be well proven in complicated esthetic treatments but perform poorly under heavy loads.

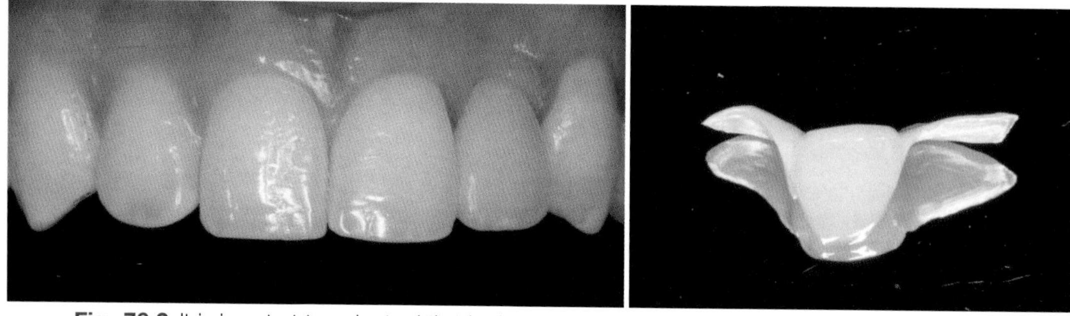

Fig. 76.2 It is important to understand that implants are not the only way to replace missing teeth. In this example a ceramic Maryland bridge is used to replace the upper left lateral incisor.

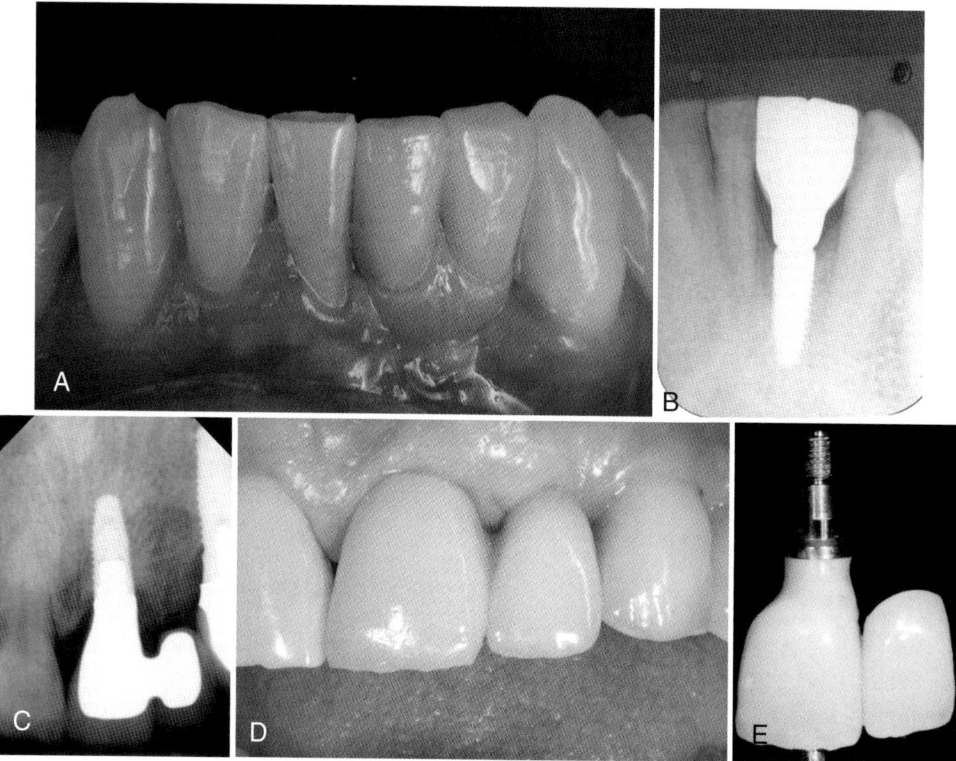

Fig. 76.3 Replacement of two consecutive missing teeth presents a unique challenge. Mesial–distal space requirements often preclude the use of two adjacent implants. The implant can be placed centrally (A and B) or in the position of one of the missing roots (C–E).

Currently available dental implants are classified into three types (Fig. 76.4) based on their abutment connection design: external connection, internal connection, and solid body (the abutment is contiguous with the implant body).

The external connection implant is commonly referred to as an "external hex" implant due to the presence of a raised hexagon connection on most versions of this design. The external connection is one of the older connection designs still in common use today. It offers the advantages of an extremely extensive array of prosthetic products to address even the most complicated of clinical presentations. It is a robust implant and rarely suffers from fracture of the implant body itself. This is a well-tested and widely accepted implant design.[4,5] It is well suited to the restoration of fully edentulous patients desiring a fixed restoration. The wide platform of the implant creates a stable base, whereas the relatively short connection (0.7-mm tall) allows for easy correction of nonparallel implants.

The primary drawback of the external connection implant is screw loosening.[37,38,56,59] The short connection height does little to share the forces between the abutment and the implant body. Even if the hex portion is engaged, there is still very little vertical wall height to transfer the oblique forces of the prosthesis. Inevitably, these forces are transferred largely to the abutment screw, which stretches and deforms under load. Over time this will result in the need to tighten and replace the screws. This problem is significantly reduced with prostheses supported by multiple implants. It is primarily a problem with single tooth replacements on the external connection implant.

KEY FACT

Perhaps the most important implant design factor relative to prosthetic success is the implant-abutment connection design. The design of an implant abutment junction (IAJ) will influence everything from incidence of screw loosening to maintenance of the hard and soft tissues, to leakage inside the implant.

Compared with more modern implant designs, the external connection loses more crestal bone.[6,7,12,19,24,25,40,42,53,93,103,120,122] This is a multifactorial problem, but it is due in large part to the constant opening and closing of the IAJ under load.[50,88,95] This leads to bacterial infiltrate being pumped into and out of the internal aspects of the implant[5,54] and directly into the peri-implant tissues (Fig. 76.5). A move away from the external connection has mitigated (but not eliminated) both screw loosening and excessive crestal bone loss.

The internal connection (in all its variations) has become the implant of choice for most partially edentulous rehabilitations due to improved reliability compared with the external hex design.[44] For most systems, it is a misnomer to call it an "internal hex." The geometry of the connection itself comes in many variations including hexagons, octagons, 12-pointed stars, trilobes, circles with four flat sides, seven-splines, and others. The number of sides to the connection allows the user various positions from which to orient a stock manufacturer abutment. Some manufacturers prescribe which lobe or point of the implant connection should be oriented buccally to address this. Although more sides on the connection allow for more flexibility in positioning a stock abutment, this does increase the difficulty of correctly aligning a custom abutment. There is no overwhelming, independent, peer-reviewed evidence that any one internal connection geometry is superior to all the others.

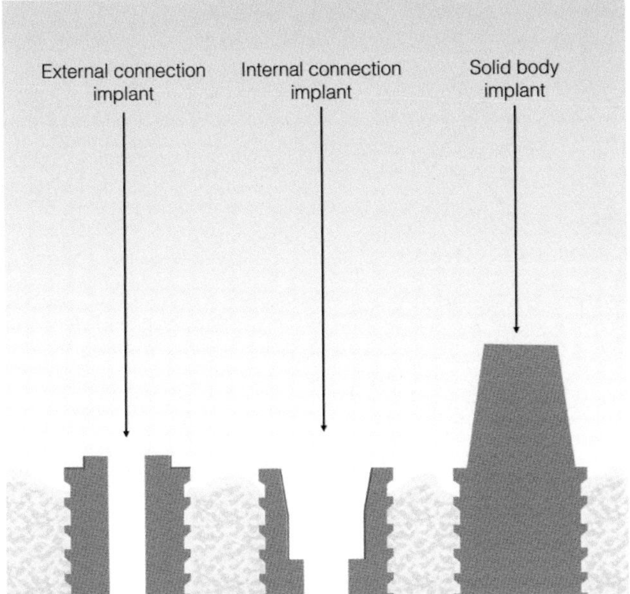

Fig. 76.4 Most currently available implants can be classified as one of three types: external connection, internal connection, or solid body. The external hex connection is primarily indicated for full-arch treatments. The solid body implant must be placed in the ideal position, as there is no way to correct the position with the abutment. The internal connection implant (of which there are many varieties) is indicated for most partially edentulous treatments. Note the abutment engagement areas, as highlighted in *red*.

Many implant systems have begun to incorporate a tapered element into the implant abutment connection. The rationale for incorporating a taper into the connection is to further stabilize the IAJ,[81] thus minimizing leakage, abutment movement, and loosening of screws. This concept comes from the world of machining tools, like lathes and drill presses. For some unknown reason, the dental profession has taken to referring to any tapered connection implant as a "Morse taper," though few implant designs meet the very specific specifications of any Morse taper variation (~3-degree taper inclusive).

Regardless, upon fully torquing the abutment screw, implants with a very narrow taper do create a better seal and will have better long-term stability of the abutment and the screw. Both are advantages in terms of maintenance and persevering the peri-implant tissues at a maximum level. Some tapered connection implant systems even require a special tool to remove the abutments, as after screw removal the components can have such a strong friction fit.

When wide diameter external connection implants were introduced, they remained compatible with the abutments from the narrower implants. Some clinicians and scientists began experimenting with using these narrow abutments on wider implants; they referred to these connections as "platform switched."[68] This term has come to encompass any implant that has an abutment that is narrower than the implant neck (Fig. 76.6). The preponderance of evidence suggests that the platform-switched design maintains bone at a higher level than that of a non-platform-switched design.[6,7,12,19,24,25,40,42,53,93,103,120,122] The reasons for this effect are less leakage at the IAJ (most are tapered connections),[8,35,67,85] less screw loosening,[91,98] less stress on the peri-implant bone,[28,47,78,79] and movement of the non-osseointegrating surface of the abutment away from the bone. The latter concept creates a horizontal space on the implant for supracrestal connective tissue to establish a circumferential peri-implant seal, thereby allowing the bone to maintain its position at a higher level without having to remodel to a lower position.[99,100]

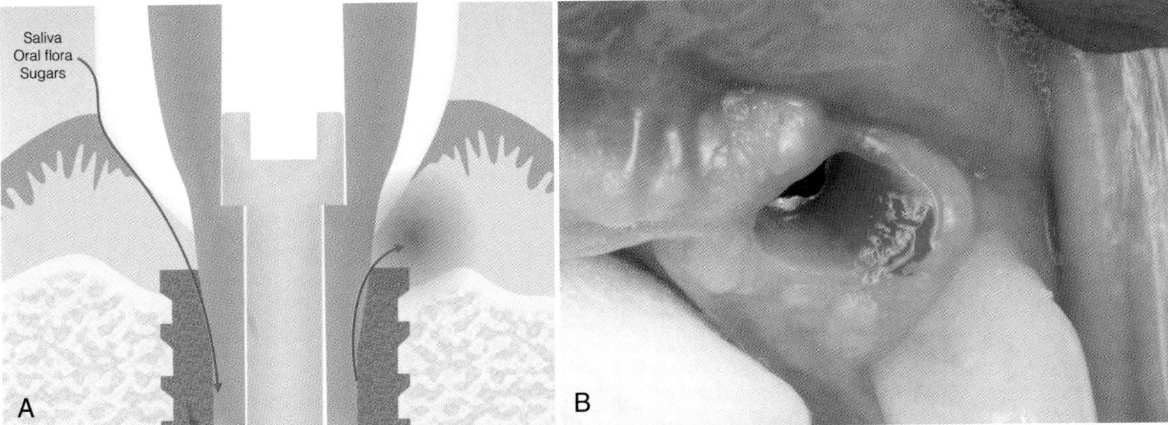

Fig. 76.5 All two-piece implants have hollow internal spaces. Under functional loads, the junction between the implant and the abutment will open slightly and allow saliva, oral flora, and nutrients into the internal aspects of the implant (A). In this oxygen-free environment, anaerobes will proliferate. They will be pumped into the peri-implant tissues and may be partially responsible for typical peri-implant bone loss or inflammation of the peri-implant tissues (B).

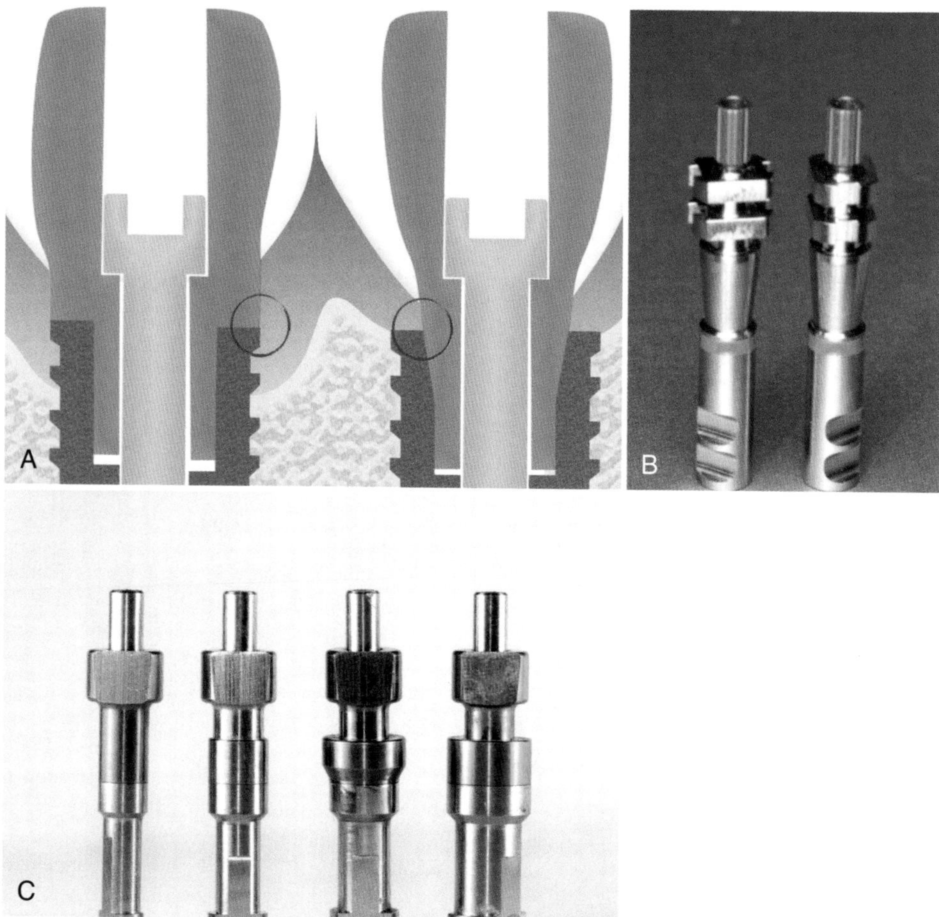

Fig. 76.6 The platform switched implant design (A, *right*) has an abutment that is narrower than the head of the implant (B). The majority of evidence suggests that this design better preserves bone than implants, which use abutments as wide or wider than the head of the implant (C).

The only potential downside to a platform-switched implant system is that the abutment is narrower and therefore more prone to breakage. Data on this concern are sparse, but it stands to reason that for any material (in particular zirconia, but also titanium), the thinner it is, the more easily it will suffer fracture. Many manufacturers have begun to address this problem by offering their zirconia abutments with a titanium insert that interfaces with the implant body (Fig. 76.7). This has the benefit of placing the more fragile zirconia outside the implant and prevents the possibility of the zirconia wearing the implant connection prematurely.

The internal aspect of the implant is hollow to allow for the screw and the abutment connection. However, these spaces inside the implant can serve as a pathogenic reservoir if or when the IAJ leaks.[8,67,85] This internal chamber is anaerobic, body temperature, and when the IAJ leaks, it will become filled with oral bacteria, saliva, and nutrients. The chamber is then fertile breeding ground for anaerobic bacteria and their by-products. Continued movement between the abutment and the implant will pump the bacterial exudate into the fragile peri-implant tissues. It appears that this is one of the primary causes of "normal" bone loss around implants. Excessive amounts of pumping may be culpable in idiopathic incidences of peri-implant mucositis and peri-implantitis. Therefore, clinicians should opt for implants and abutments that have been shown (over extended periods of time) to reduce the micro-gap and leakage. This is best accomplished with a narrow, tapered connection and abutments with titanium interfaces milled by the implant manufacturer. There are additional factors to consider in selecting the appropriate implant for any given scenario, but efforts to minimize the loss of peri-implant tissues is best accomplished with this treatment modality.

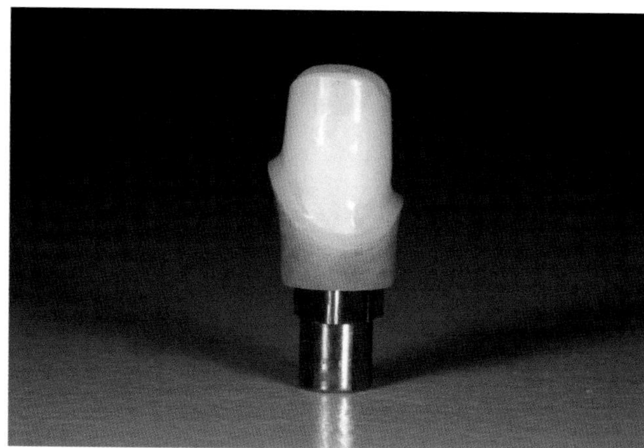

Fig. 76.7 Zirconia abutments are useful to minimize any changes to the color of the peri-implant tissues and allow the use of semitranslucent prosthetic materials. Most manufacturers have developed zirconia abutments, which have a titanium base as shown here. This may make the abutments stronger and will eliminate the failure of the zirconia *inside* the implant body. Such failures are difficult to resolve successfully.

The last type of implant connection to address is the "solid body" implant, or an implant in which the abutment and the implant are one contiguous piece. Such implants have been available for some time but have never gained significant popularity. The challenge with solid

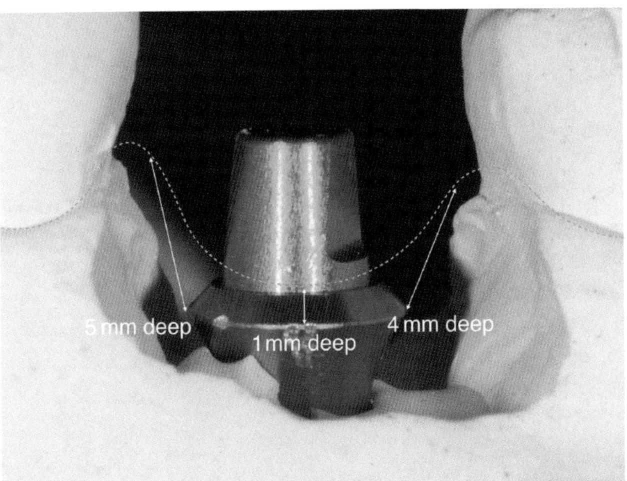

Fig. 76.8 Solid body (and tissue-level) implants present a unique prosthetic challenge due to the margin being on the implant body itself. This often results in mesial and distal margins that are far too deep to reliably remove cement. As such, restorations for tissue-level implants should generally be screw retained. Unfortunately, restorations on solid body implants can only be cemented. Extreme care must be used with solid body implants.

body implants is not surgical, and they may in fact be better for the peri-implant tissues because there is no micro-gap and no leakage. The problem is prosthetic. For these implants, there is no screw-retained option for the prosthesis, and the cement margin is determined at the time of placement. The abutment can be prepped to move the margin apically if absolutely necessary, but there is no reasonable way to move the margin coronally. This presents a serious problem when the gingiva has any significant papilla adjacent to the implant, as the cement margin that is placed perhaps 1 mm subgingival on the facial aspect may now be 3 to 7 mm subgingival at the mesial and distal aspect (Fig. 76.8). With no option for a screw-retained restoration, the restoring clinician is now tasked with fully removing cement far too deep subgingival and will inevitably leave cement behind. This residual cement is likely to induce inflammatory reactions and loss of bone, soft tissue, and perhaps the implant itself.[66,132]

The solid body implant offers no recourse should the abutment break. This is of particular concern as the use of solid body zirconia implants becomes more prevalent. Should the abutment on the solid body implant break, the implant must either be extracted or abandoned. Special care should be taken with solid body implants to avoid over-prepping the abutment area, leading to weakness and increased risk of fracture.

There are a few esoteric implant-abutment connections on the market as well, including press-fit, cemented abutments (where the abutment is cemented *into* the implant), and others. These will not be discussed here due to space constraints and their relative obscurity at the current time.

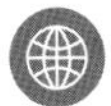

Abutment/Prosthesis Considerations for Single Units

Retention Method for Partially Edentulous Treatment: Cemented Prostheses, Screw-Retained Porcelain-Fused-to-Metal Options, Screw-Retained Full Contour Zirconia, and Hybrid Designs

When treatment planning a partially edentulous case for restoration with an implant, one of the major prosthetic decisions to be made is whether to have a crown that is cemented to an abutment or a crown that is contiguous with the abutment and screwed directly to the implant. For the sake of discussion here, the screw-retained option will be defined as a cast gold alloy abutment with appropriate support of feldspathic porcelain that will be layered directly on it (sometimes referred to as UCLA abutments). More modern variations of the screw-retained crown will be discussed later in this chapter. Many clinicians have developed personal preferences for screw or cement-retained crowns based on their experiences and failures. Much of an individual clinician's anecdotal experience likely has much to do with the skill of his or her technician when considering screw-retained PFMs. Here we will consider the scientific evidence to determine the proven advantages and disadvantages of each type of retention.

TABLE 76.1 Major Versus Minor Complications in Implant Prosthetics

Major Complications	Minor Complications
Implant failure	Screw loosening
Atypical peri-implant bone loss	Chipped porcelain not requiring prosthesis replacement
Persistent inflammation of the soft tissue	Decementation of the prosthesis
Infection of the peri-implant tissues	
Failure of the porcelain requiring replacement of the prosthesis	
Loss of the prosthesis	
Fractured screws or abutments	

For *most* single tooth replacements, either screw or cement-retained crowns have proven to have very high levels of long-term success,[83,101,111,125] provided that the clinician and technician follow critical guidelines. In some clinical scenarios, one type of retention is the overwhelmingly superior choice, but this does not reflect the majority of cases.

It is important to understand the difference between *major* and *minor* complications (Table 76.1). Minor complications are issues that can be resolved with little effort or increased risk, such as loose screws, minor porcelain fracture, and reversible peri-implant mucositis. Major complications are loss of the implant, peri-implantitis, severe bone loss, fractured screws, significant porcelain failure, and loss of the prosthesis.

Screw-retained restorations have a long history of reasonable clinical success. Their introduction in 1988[71] allowed clinicians to create more esthetic restorations than were possible with the available alternatives of the time, and in less vertical space. They can be used in areas with limited interocclusal distances due to their construction design. They can be created with metal occlusal or palatal surfaces for patients with high functional demands. They can have the porcelain carried to within 1 mm of the head of the implant for improved esthetics. The primary disadvantages of the screw-retained restoration are significantly more prosthetic complications[27,33,36,70,83,94,101,131]: porcelain fracture (Fig. 76.9),[62,87,101] screw loosening,[15,33,36,70,83,90,101,130] increased bone loss,[32,49,55,69,87] increased lab costs, and the need for ideal implant angulation. Minor areas of porcelain fracture might be remedied with contouring and polishing. Larger fractures will require replacement of the entire prosthesis, as porcelain should not be repaired after prolonged exposure to the oral environment. A dedicated technician could strip all the porcelain off the metal framework in an attempt to save the costs of a new abutment and alloy, but it may very well be that the reason for the fracture in the first place was a poorly designed framework. As such, it is advisable to fabricate an entirely new prosthesis should the porcelain fail. Screw loosening has been established repeatedly as significantly more common in screw-retained restorations,

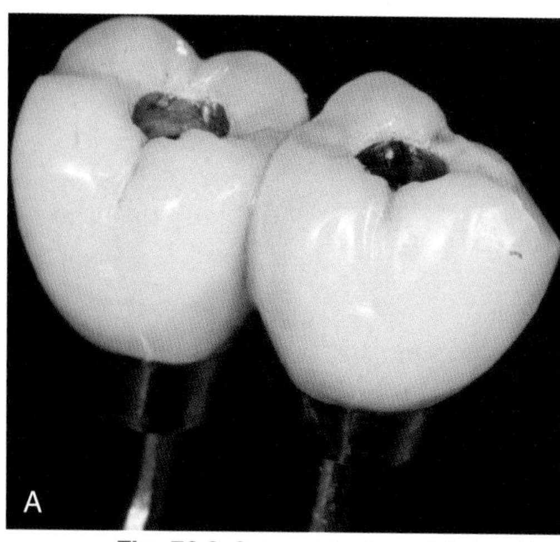

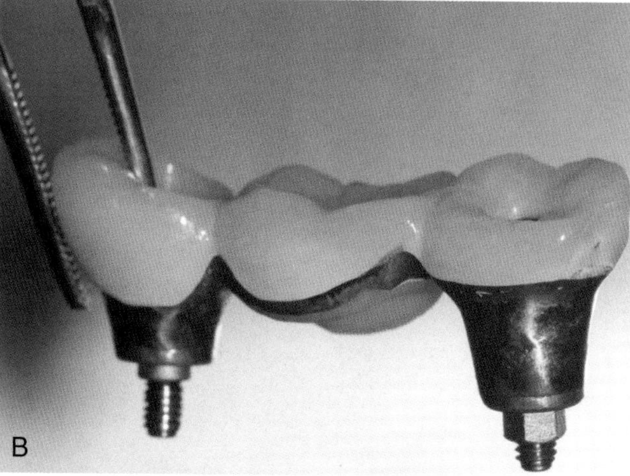

Fig. 76.9 Screw-retained porcelain-fused-to-metal (PFM) restorations have been shown to have significantly more prosthetic complications, most commonly failure of the porcelain and loose abutment screws. Failure of the porcelain is best addressed by replacement. The new prosthesis will need a more robust framework design or alternative materials. (A) Screw-retained PFM crowns with fractured porcelain. (B) Screw-retained PFM bridge being replaced after screws loosened.

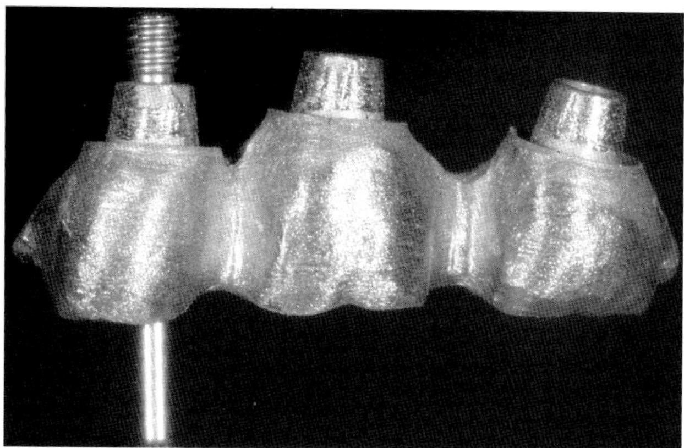

Fig. 76.10 During the fabrication of a screw-retained porcelain-fused-to-metal, the technician must exercise extreme care in creation of the framework so as not to damage the interface area as shown here. The damaged interface will produce a poor-fitting prosthesis leading to increased leakage and screws that loosen more frequently.

although cemented restorations generally use the same screw and torque specifications. The reason for this phenomenon is not exactly known, although it is likely due to poorly casted abutment interfaces, increased preload due to nonpassive frameworks,[82,112,124] the historic use of weaker gold alloy screws, heavy interproximal tooth contact, or damage to the interface during divestment (Fig. 76.10) or finishing. Technicians must exercise care when creating a screw-retained restoration to ensure the integrity of the abutment interface. The UCLA abutment should have a machined interface made by the manufacturer to maximize the integrity of the fit between the abutment and the implant. Because the screw access channel must exit the crown, this option is best reserved for when the implant angulation exits directly through the occlusal surface in posterior regions and through the palatal/lingual surface in the anterior regions.

KEY FACT

For most single tooth implant crowns, both screw and cement-retained methods have proven to be highly successful over the long term provided that the clinician and technician follow critical guidelines. In some clinical scenarios, one type of retention is the overwhelmingly superior choice, but this does not reflect the majority of cases.

The common alternative to the screw-retained crown is the cement-retained crown. This system is made up of an abutment (titanium, gold alloy, or zirconia) that is screwed into the implant and a crown that will be cemented to the abutment. The cement-retained crown allows the restoration of implants that are not placed ideally without having to manage a screw access channel exiting through a crucial esthetic or functional area. This situation is most common in the esthetic zone. When implants are placed angled such that and their line of draw exits through the facial surface of the crown, it becomes esthetically prohibitive to use a "normal" screw-retained crown (Fig. 76.11). There are some workarounds that will be discussed briefly later.

Some clinicians prefer cement-retained restorations because the cementation process is familiar and comfortable. However, the cementation process is not to be taken lightly, as residual cement is one of the major causes (but not the only cause) of peri-implantitis.[1,14,66,132] Cementation details will be discussed later, but note that no attempt should be made to cement an implant crown when margins are more than 1 mm subgingival (Fig. 76.12).[76,77] Cement-retained implant crowns have the main advantage of being far more durable than the screw-retained alternative for any given material, a fact confirmed in multiple reviews.[83,101,111,131,133] Porcelain failure of screw-retained PFM crowns has been reported to be as high as 38%, compared with just 4% for cement-retained PFM crowns at an average of 5 years.[87] For this reason cement-retained implant crowns are indicated in scenarios of higher loads (i.e., molars, patients with enlarged masseters). Should the patient break the cemented crown, retrieval of the remaining abutment is greatly simplified. Drilling through even an intact cemented crown to access the screw channel is a relatively simple matter, akin to routine endodontic access through a crown. Lastly, there is the issue of lab cost. The cemented restorations typically lead to far less expensive lab bills compared with the screw-retained PFM options, though the cost of the latter varies significantly with the market price for gold alloy. The extremely high lab costs of screw retained PFMs may make them financially prohibitive for some clinicians/patients.

One of the reasons cited for selecting a screw-retained restoration is the ease of retrievability. There is a valid concern that should something fail, the cemented crown is slightly more difficult to remove. Although it may seem obvious, removal of the cemented crown is hardly more difficult than for a screw-retained crown (Fig. 76.13).[108] The differences are drilling the access through porcelain

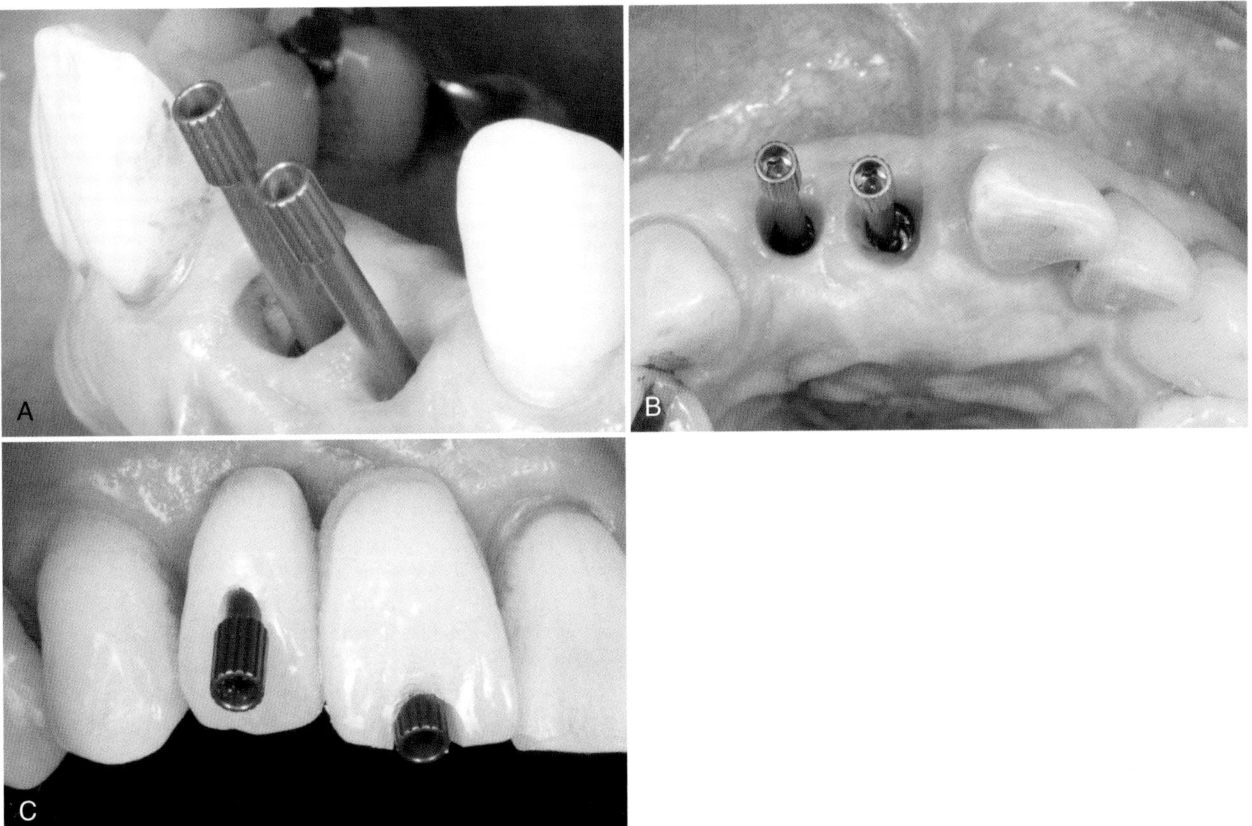

Fig. 76.11 In the esthetic zone, non-grafted alveolar ridges may result in implants angled out to the facial. This results in a relative contraindication to screw retention. With most implant systems, implants angled out through the facial surface will need to be restored with a cement-retained option. Lateral view (A) and occlusal view (B) of maxillary anterior implants with abutment screws showing long-axis projection toward facial surface. (C) Provisional restoration with abutment screws projecting through facial surface.

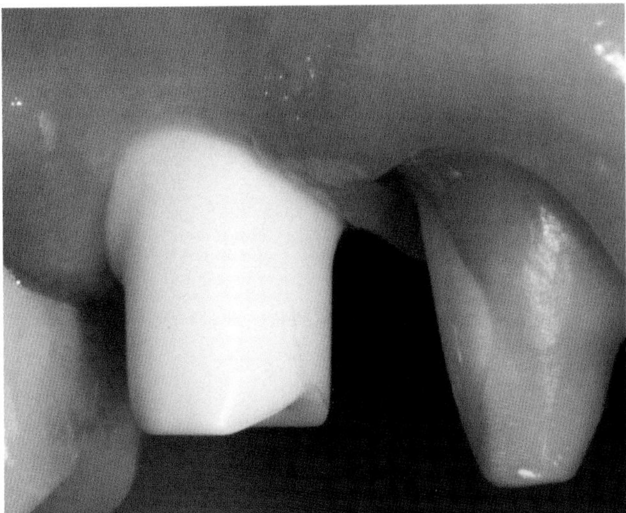

Fig. 76.12 For cemented implant restorations, the abutment must be designed such that the cementation margin is no deeper than 1 mm below the gingival margin. In all but the flattest of ridges, this can only be accomplished with a custom-milled abutment.

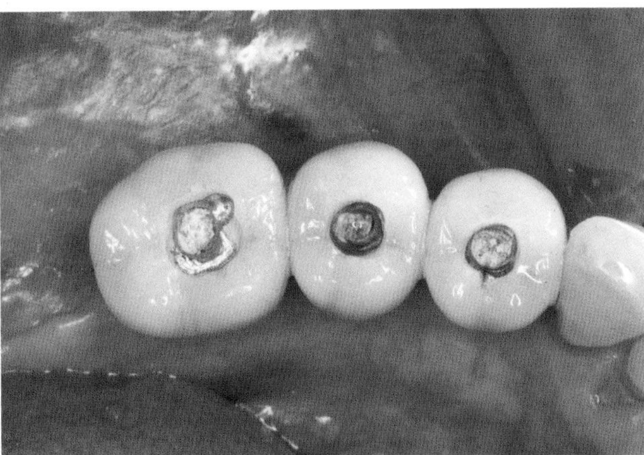

Fig. 76.13 Removal and replacement of failed cement-retained implant crowns are relatively straightforward procedures with most implant designs. The clinician estimates the long access of the implant with radiographs and by palpating the ridge and then simply drills into the screw access through the crown material. The abutments/crowns may still be cemented together and can be removed as one piece.

or metal instead of composite and the location of access may be difficult to discern. Most clinicians are fairly adept at cutting through porcelain, but locating the access channel can be a slight challenge. Most often, the access is fairly easy to locate based off simple radiographs. More sophisticated approaches to recording the location of the access have been proposed, from stents,[51] to guides,[127] to occlusal markings (Fig. 76.14).[104,110] During the era of weaker abutment screws and external connection implants, screw loosening was a common problem. As such, replacement of the screws was a common maintenance requirement, and a screw-retained restoration was ideal. Modern implant connections rarely suffer from loose screws, even for single-unit implants.[83,94]

There are a few other crown retention variations that should be mentioned. One is the hybrid crown (sometimes referred to as a "screwmentable" crown). This system consists of a crown that is cemented to a stock titanium abutment (Fig. 76.15), but the cementation is (usually) performed in the laboratory where excess cement can be easily removed. The screw access is predrilled into the crown.

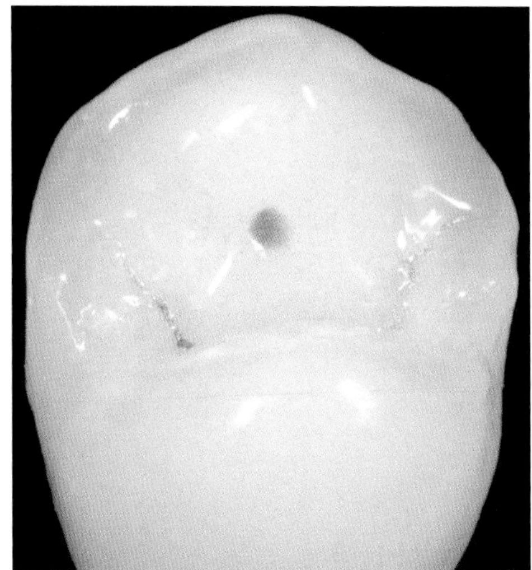

Fig. 76.14 Placement of an occlusal/palatal marker during fabrication of the crown can make finding the screw access more predictable should removal become necessary.

The titanium insert should be used whenever possible, and zirconia extending *into* the implant should be avoided at all costs. This system offers the advantages of minimal risk of retained cement, ease of retrieval, minimal risk of porcelain fracture when stronger ceramics are used, and a lower lab cost than cast gold alloys. Some manufacturers offer this restoration with a screw channel that can be angled up to 25 degrees to allow for screw-retained restorations even when the implant is not in the long access of the crown. This system is relatively new and not fully tested in clinical trials; implement with caution.

Lastly, there is the option of lingual set screws. This system is most commonly employed in the anterior areas of the mouth when the implants are angled too far toward the facial for a traditional screw-retained restoration and the clinician is uncomfortable with a cemented option. The challenges with lingual set screws are increased lab costs, difficulty in locating technicians competent in the technique, leakage between the crown and the abutment, and challenging screw access. In most regions of the world, this is a rarely used treatment option.

Abutment Material Selection

In most bone-level implant designs, the junction between the abutment and the implant is near the crestal bone. In this area the connective tissue and the junctional epithelium may be in intimate contact with the abutment. As such, the abutment material and accuracy of the fit play a critical role in preserving the peri-implant bone and soft tissue. Some abutments better preserve the peri-implant tissues than others. The most relevant options for currently available definitive abutment materials are titanium, titanium with a titanium

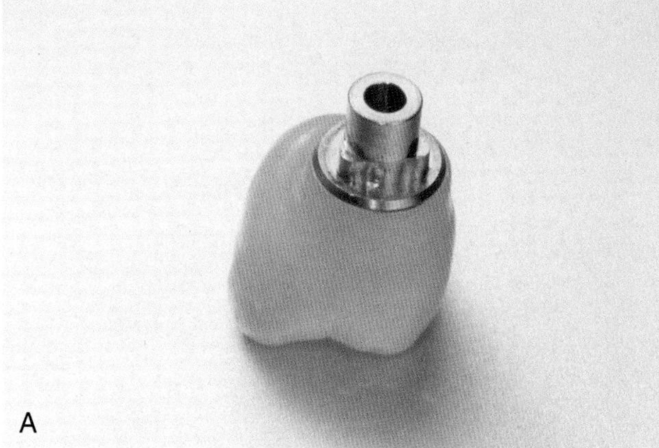

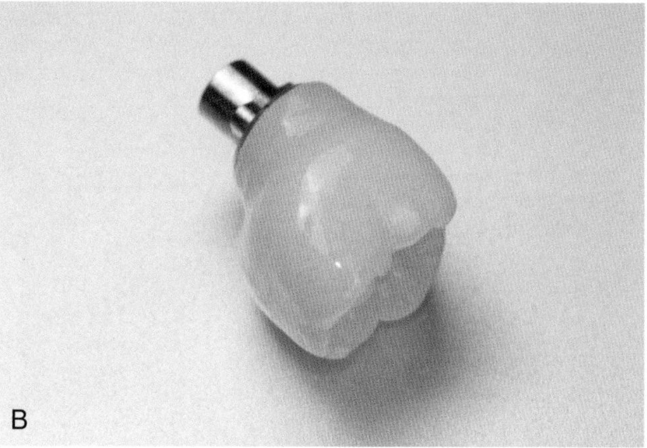

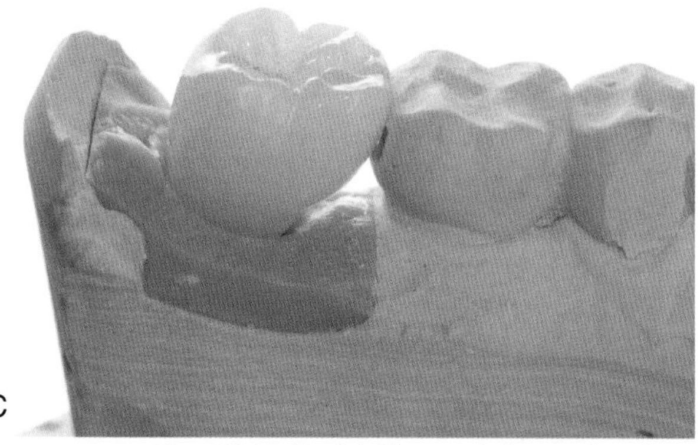

Fig. 76.15 The hybrid crown design consists of a titanium base that is connected to a full contour ceramic (generally zirconia) crown. In the laboratory, the technician follows a specific protocol to cement the titanium base to the ceramic crown. This design produces a screw-retained restoration that should be less prone to the problems of a porcelain-fused-to-metal, although few long-term data are yet available. (A) Abutment view of titanium base crown. (B) Crown view of titanium base crown. (C) Titanium base crown in lab model.

nitride coating, full-contour zirconia, zirconia with a titanium base, and gold alloy (Fig. 76.16). Other less common options include lithium disilicate and chrome-cobalt alloys.

The most rigorous study examining bone and soft tissue reactions to abutment materials found histologic evidence that titanium preserved 1.5 mm more soft tissue and 1 mm more bone compared with the fully cast gold alloy abutment.[2] However, it should be noted that this study was performed in the canine mandible and that when a titanium interface was used in conjunction with a cast gold abutment, there was less bone loss than with the gold alone. It stands to reason that some of the bone and soft tissue loss with gold abutments may have more to do with the less accurate fit of a cast restoration than to the influence of the material itself. More recent clinical studies and reviews have questioned these findings, with gold and titanium showing an equivalent biologic response.[72,123] However, the latter were done with radiographic analysis rather than the histologic measurements of the former. As a whole, the data are not yet conclusive on the biocompatibility of the abutment material and its clinical effects on the tissues. Titanium has been repeatedly shown to perform better on a histologic level than gold alloys, but the difference may be of little clinical significance. What is clear is that the interface between the abutment and the implant must be as accurate as possible. This will ensure minimal leakage, minimal screw loosening, and better maintenance of the peri-implant tissues. Abutments that require casting of the implant interface portion cannot match the fit accuracy of the machined interface.[18]

The strength of the abutment is critical in maintaining long-term success with minimal technical complications. Titanium and gold alloy abutments have a long track record of outstanding strength. Some studies have even shown failure of the implant before failure of the titanium abutment.[117] The primary concern regarding strength is related to zirconia abutments and titanium abutments with thin walls.

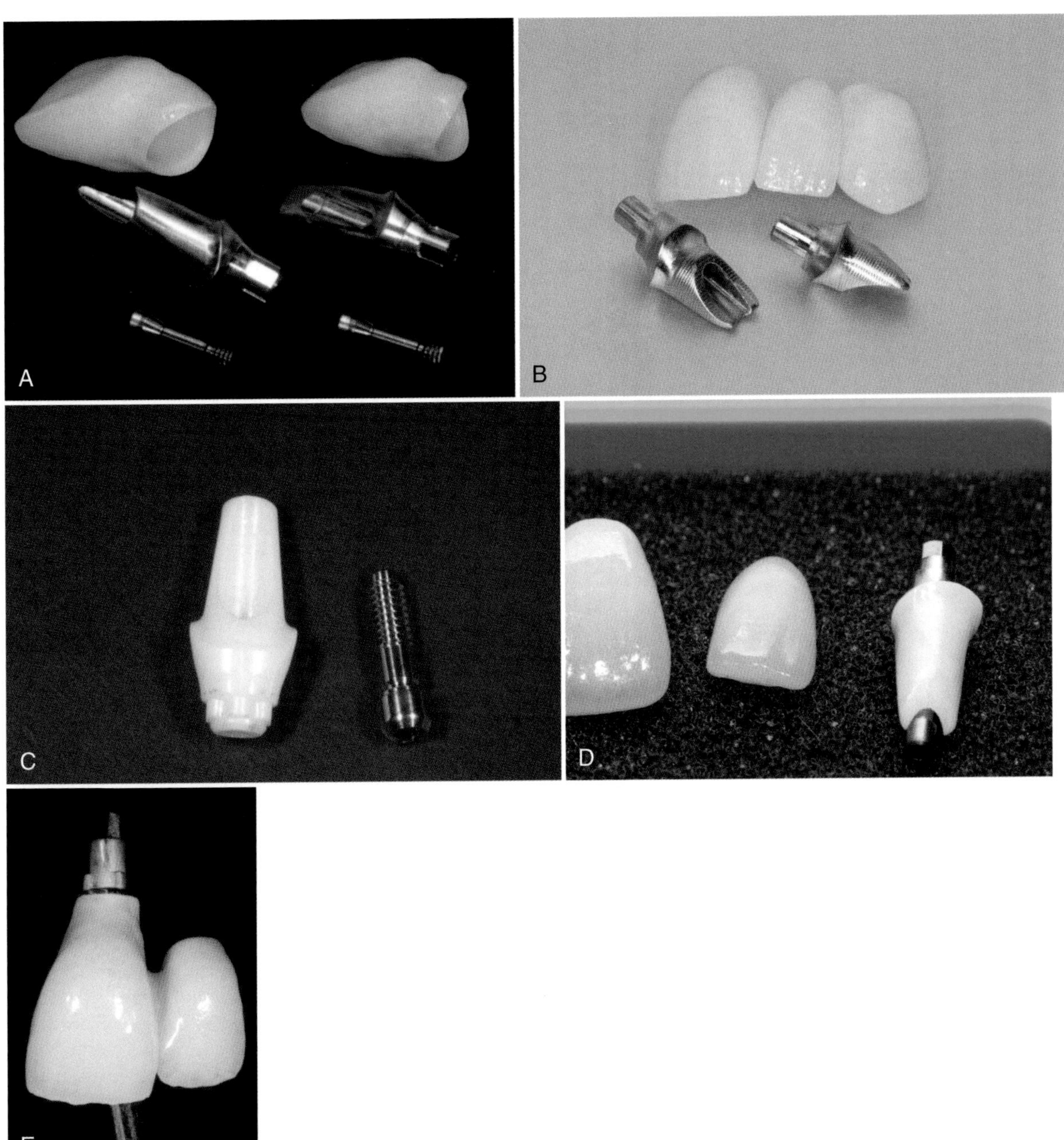

Fig. 76.16 Implant abutments are available in a variety of materials. (A) Titanium. (B) Titanium with a titanium nitride coating. (C) Full-contour zirconia. (D) Zirconia with a titanium base. (E) Gold alloy.

Zirconia abutments can be used with little risk of fracture in many clinical scenarios,[84] but there are a few caveats. The zirconia abutment should have an implant interface component made of titanium (Fig. 76.17).[117] This minimizes the risk of wear to the implant body, and should the zirconia fracture, it is outside the implant where it is much easier to treat. The zirconia abutment should not be used in cases with extreme loads (i.e., molars, patients with enlarged muscles of mastication, long-span FDPs). The zirconia abutments should be made by a reputable manufacturer. Evidence has shown that the manufacturer can have a huge impact on the strength of the material.[63] The abutment walls should be sufficiently thick, no less than 0.7 mm. Every effort should be made to avoid cutting the zirconia after it has been sintered.

Lastly, we must consider the effect of the abutment material on the color of the soft tissue. Gray-colored metallic abutments will darken the tissue more than zirconia abutments, but the effect is not as great as might be expected. Zirconia abutments still cause a significant and perceptible darkening of the soft tissue, confirmed in multiple studies.[16,64,75] Some manufacturers and clinicians have developed techniques to anodize or coat titanium abutments to create gold or pink shades. These may offer some improvement of soft tissue esthetics. The gold-colored abutments (Fig. 76.18) allow predictable use of semi-translucent ceramics with minimal shade change. The thickness of the overlying tissue has been shown to have a greater influence on the perceived color of the gingiva over an implant than the material used. Thick tissues have an almost non-perceptible color shift, whereas with thin tissues the shift is always perceptible, even with zirconia abutments.[58]

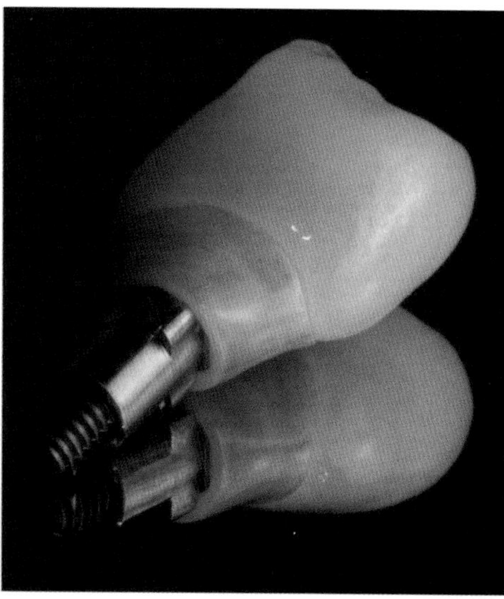

Fig. 76.17 Zirconia implant abutments should be fabricated with a titanium base. This has multiple advantages: increased strength, less complicated failures, and less wear of the internal surface of the implant.

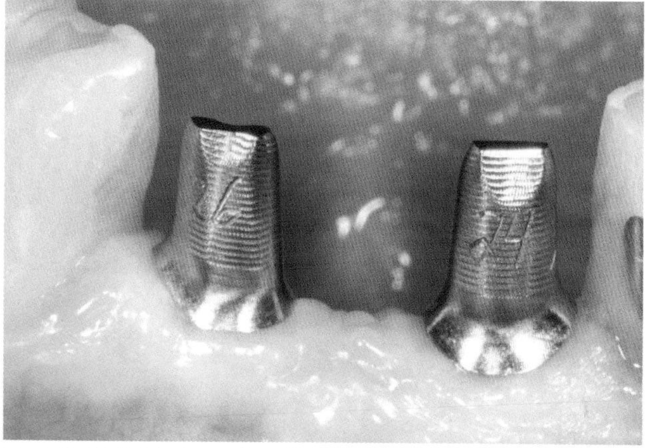

Fig. 76.18 Gold color coating of titanium abutments produces less graying of the soft tissue. This coating is made from titanium nitride or titanium oxide.

KEY FACT

It is clear that the interface between the abutment and the implant must be as accurate as possible. An accurate implant abutment junction fit will ensure minimal leakage, minimal screw loosening, and better maintenance of the peri-implant tissues. Clinicians should understand and appreciate that abutments with casting of the implant interface portion cannot match the fit accuracy of the machined interface.

Abutment Design and Emergence Profile

The design and contours of the abutment play a key role in the shape and dimensions of the peri-implant tissues. If the abutment is overcontoured it will ultimately lead to a loss of bone and soft tissue. This is a common problem when technicians design and shape the abutment without the soft tissue mask on the model. Such overcontoured abutments may require surgery to deliver because the tissue prevents complete seating of the restoration. Alternatively, the restoration can be reshaped to reduce or eliminate impingement on tissues.

The emergence profile of the abutment is the area of the abutment between the head of the implant and the soft tissue margins. More data are showing that undercontouring the emergence profile helps to protect and maintain the peri-implant bone and soft tissue.[99] The "platform switch" style implant helps to create the narrowed abutment design due to the smaller diameter of the connection interface. In most scenarios, the abutment should be designed to emerge from the implant in a narrowed hourglass shape. The narrowed design may allow for increased blood flow around the implant and provide sufficient room for the soft tissues without bone remodeling.[109,121]

Understanding the effects the emergence profile has on the shape and position of the soft tissue is critical for implant treatment in the esthetic zone.[105,114] By selectively over- or undercontouring the emergence zone, the soft tissue can be positioned with a high degree of accuracy.[109,118] More on this technique will be described in the next section with the use of esthetic zone provisional restoration.

For cement restorations, arguably the most critical aspect of the abutment design is the placement of the margins. The peri-implant soft tissue is never perfectly flat, and as such custom abutments are almost universally indicated to avoid deep subgingival margins with the risk of retained cement and the resulting peri-implantitis. The only way for a stock abutment to be used with minimal risk is to select one with completely supragingival margins, but this can be esthetically unacceptable. If a common stock abutment is selected to hide the titanium with a facial margin 1 mm subgingival, in most scenarios the margin at the mesial and distal papilla will be 4 mm or more subgingival. Both in vitro and in vivo studies have shown that for margins beyond 1 mm subgingival, significant amounts of cement will always be left behind.[76,77] No attempt should ever be made to cement restorations on implants with margins more than 1 mm subgingival (Fig. 76.19). A custom abutment can be easily designed to address the natural scalloping of the gingiva. It is fabricated by milling or casting, though casting of custom abutments for cement-retained crowns is no longer the best option due to increased lab costs, increased screw loosening,[15,33,36,70,83,90,101,130] and the less accurate fit at the implant.[18]

CLINICAL CORRELATION

The thickness of the overlying tissue has been shown to have a greater influence on the perceived color of the gingiva over an implant than the abutment/restorative material used. The color shift is almost imperceptible under thick tissues, whereas it is nearly always noticeable when covered by thin tissues, even with zirconia abutments.

Milled custom abutments can be made out of titanium or zirconia. When prescribing these abutments, it is critical to communicate to the technician where the margins should be placed. If left unstated, many technicians will opt to place them deep subgingivally. Several studies[76,77] have clearly shown that cement cannot be predictably removed at depths greater than 1 mm subgingival. If the margins are any deeper than 1 mm, significant amounts of cement will be left behind and will likely start the process of peri-implantitis (Fig. 76.20). It is common for clinicians and technicians to place the margins deeper than 1 mm subgingival in esthetic cases in an attempt to hide the titanium abutment if recession should occur. This strategy is unwise and will inevitably result in retained cement followed by peri-implantitis. The correct approach is to shape the tissue with a provisional, allow it to mature, and place the margin no deeper than 1 mm. The abutment could also be made of zirconia and stained to resemble the root surface. Clinicians should be aware of the significant strength variations in zirconia abutments based on the manufacturer.[63] Zirconia abutments should always have a titanium insert that goes into the implant, rather than full zirconia that goes into the implant.

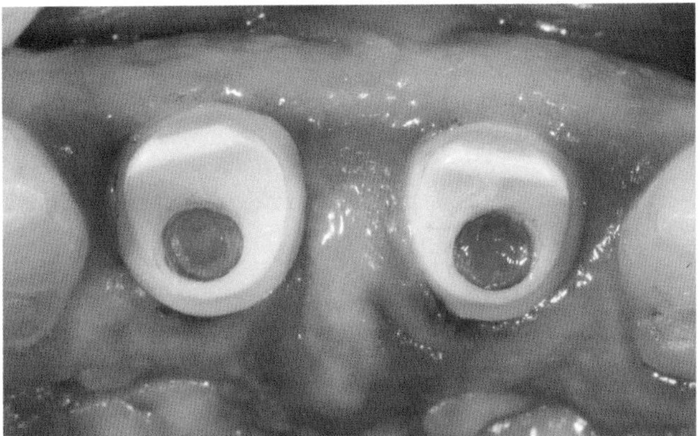

Fig. 76.19 Even in the esthetic zone, the abutment margins should not be placed deeper than 1 mm subgingivally. The margins should be clearly visible circumferentially. This will minimize the risk of cement-induced peri-implantitis.

CLINICAL CORRELATION

No attempt should ever be made to cement restorations on an implant abutment with margins more than 1 mm below the gingival margin. A custom abutment can be easily designed to address the natural scalloping of the gingiva. The probability of leaving (missing) excess cement trapped below the gingival margin is extremely high and problematic. Studies have clearly shown that cement cannot be removed at depths greater than 1 mm subgingival.

Splinting Adjacent Implants

The rationale for splinting adjacent implants (Fig. 76.21) stems from various finite element analysis (FEA)[9,11,129,135] and photo-elastic gel (PEG) experiments.[46] These in vitro studies repeatedly confirm that multiple implants produce less acute forces in the peri-implant bone when splinted compared with multiple individual restorations. However, we do not have a clear notion of how much stress is acceptable for the peri-implant bone and at what threshold we might expect pathologic bone loss. The clinician must consider the length and diameter of the implants as well as the quality and quantity of the bone when determining if multiple implants should be splinted together.

Splinted restorations are advisable when the foundation is compromised (i.e., short or narrow implants, compromised bone).[80,134] This will allow the stronger or better supported implants to "assist" the others. The compromise here is that if the weaker implant fails,

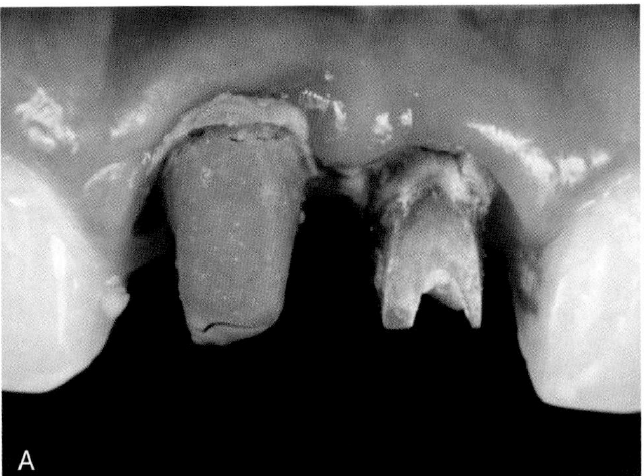

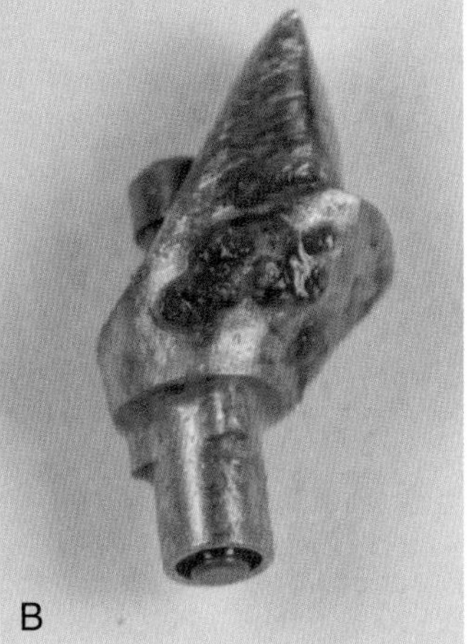

Fig. 76.20 When margins are placed deeper than 1 mm, it is inevitable that cement will be left subgingivally. Regardless of cement type, cement left subgingivally will result in significant loss of bone and soft tissue. Here, a large amount of residual cement has caused catastrophic loss of bone and soft tissue (peri-implantitis). These implants ultimately required extraction and significant reconstruction to treat. (A) Clinical view. (B) Abutment removed.

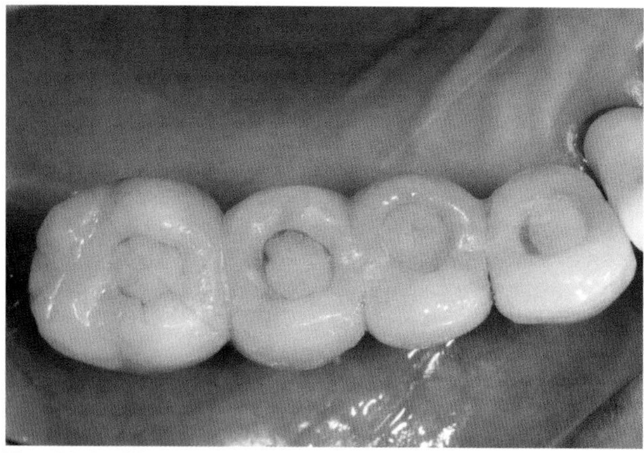

Fig. 76.21 Many in vitro studies have shown that splinting of adjacent implants helps to share occlusal forces between the implants. However, several clinical trials have shown no clinically significant difference in bone levels between splinted and nonsplinted restorations at 3, 5, and 10 years of use.

an entirely new prosthesis may need to be fabricated, usually at a significant expense.

The rationale for splinting adjacent implants involves the intention of "sharing the forces," a concept derived from the in vitro studies of the early 2000s cited earlier. The implication is that clinically we would see fewer implant failures and less bone loss over extended use with splinted restorations. Long-term in vivo randomized controlled trials (RCTs)[29,39,126] have tested this hypothesis in order to quantify the differences in bone loss and implant failure with splinted versus nonsplinted restorations. In the partially edentulous RCT, at 10 years the mean difference in bone loss between splinted and nonsplinted restorations for 132 implants was a mere 0.1 mm.[126] This could hardly be considered clinically significant under most scenarios. In the fully edentulous study with two mandibular implants retaining a full denture, the differences at 3 years were statistically insignificant at most sites and only about 0.5 mm at the most significantly different sites.[39] A prospective split mouth, in vivo trial examining bone levels around splinted and not-splinted restorations showed no significant difference at 36 months.[29] Until better evidence shows otherwise, "sharing forces" in an attempt to reduce bone loss is not a proper consideration for whether or not adjacent implants should be splinted. These data are not necessarily in conflict with the early in vitro experiments; they simply illustrate that higher forces do not necessarily result in more bone loss and that it is difficult to extrapolate data from FEAs and PEGs to clinical realities. Depending on the type of bone and implant, there is likely a threshold below which increased forces will not result in significant bone loss over extended use. Conversely, despite the lack of significance found in these studies, there may be scenarios in which clinical judgment warrants splinting adjacent implants such as multiple implants placed in the posterior maxilla in type IV bone opposing an intact natural dentition or implants.

The downside to splinted restorations is largely related to long-term repair and replacement costs. With patients having implants that must maintain a prosthesis for 30, 40, or 50 years, it is appropriate to consider that the prosthesis will require replacement throughout its life. Most commonly, this is related to porcelain failure on screw-retained PFM FDPs.[87] After a PFM restoration has been in the mouth for any significant period of time, porcelain failure cannot simply be repaired. The restoration must be fully stripped or replaced. Practically speaking, it can be a challenge to find a laboratory willing and able to strip and restack porcelain, and most will opt for complete replacement of the prosthesis. Essentially this has doubled, tripled, or quadrupled the cost of replacement. If an individual unit suffers the same complication, only the unit affected needs to be replaced. Issues related to patient autonomy and desires need to be considered in the replacement of multiple adjacent missing teeth. Some patients may tolerate splinted restorations, whereas others may desire individual units. Oral hygiene techniques and ease of cleansability will vary between restoration types as well.

KEY FACT

Until evidence shows otherwise, "sharing forces" is not a valid reason to splint adjacent implants. These data are not necessarily in conflict with the early in vitro experiments, they simply illustrate that higher forces do not necessarily result in more bone loss and it is difficult to extrapolate data from finite element analysis and photo-elastic gel studies to clinical realities.

Indications for splinting adjacent implants include significant off-axis forces (i.e., canine replacement), multiple adjacent external hex implants, poor bone, and diminutive implants.[45]

Management of Partially Edentulous Implant Treatment in the Esthetic Zone

Treatment of the partially edentulous patient in the esthetic zone is one of the more challenging prosthetic scenarios. The "esthetic zone" is not simply canine to canine in the maxilla. Each patient must be individually evaluated for lip position and movement (Fig. 76.22) to determine the appropriate level of esthetic consideration necessary.

The primary challenge in this treatment is the peri-implant soft tissues.[17] If patients show soft tissue during lip movement, then particular attention should be paid to the creation and preservation of natural appearing gingiva. First, there must be sufficient thickness of the gingiva. Thin tissue biotypes are more prone to recession, peri-implant mucositis, papilla loss, and graying.[60,73,74,96,136] The surgical team may need to employ various techniques prior to, or at the time of, implant placement to increase the tissue thickness.

During the treatment planning phase, the clinical team should consider the shape and position of the soft tissue on all teeth or implants in the area. If any of these positions are planning to be modified, the corresponding implant position may change as well.

Management of potential changes to the tissue color can be challenging, as there is a shift in the gingiva around implants to a gray tone.[16] This can be somewhat managed with the use of UCLA or zirconia abutments, although research has clearly shown that there can still be a perceptible color shift with these more esthetic materials (delta E >3.9).[57] Though zirconia abutments are weaker than titanium, they have shown comparable survival rates for single units in vivo.[137] Some technicians have begun experimenting with the use of fluorescing glazes over the emergence zone of zirconia abutments to decrease the color shift. Some manufacturers and clinicians have coated the titanium abutments with a gold or pink color, again in an attempt to mitigate color changes.[128]

The greatest challenge of implants in the esthetic zone is papilla management. Implants, even with contemporary designs (i.e., platform switch, conical connections), cannot maintain crestal bone height as much as a healthy tooth. The implant is very different than the natural tooth because it does not have PDL (and its blood supply) or supracrestal inserting connective tissue fibers. The clinical appearance (i.e., height and fullness) of the papilla between an implant and a tooth ultimately depends on the periodontal attachment level of the adjacent tooth and not the level of bone adjacent to

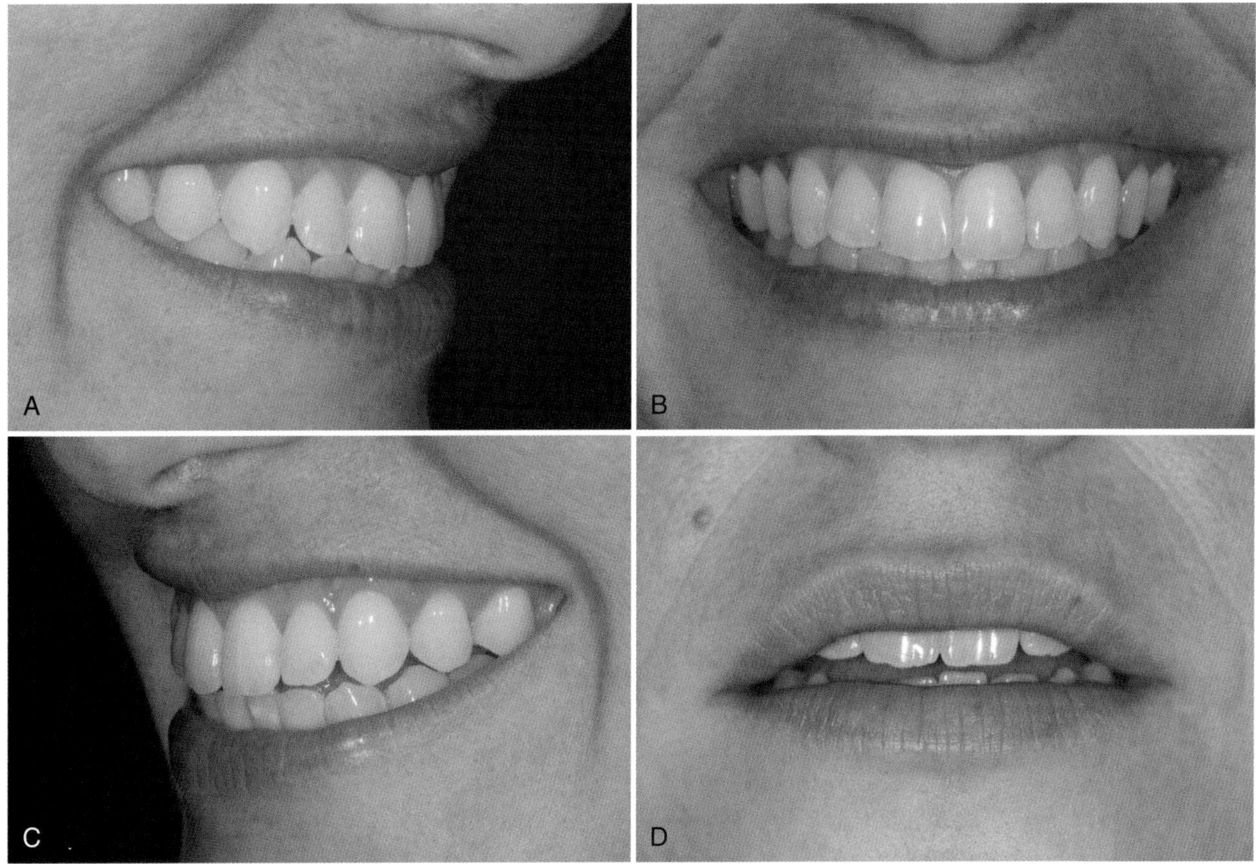

Fig. 76.22 Implant treatment in the esthetic zone is more challenging than in the functional zone. It is important to keep in mind that the esthetic zone differs for each patient. It should be evaluated though a series of basic photos: right, center, and left at maximum smile (A–C), and with lips at rest (D). In this patient the esthetic zone clearly includes the anterior teeth and all premolars.

TABLE 76.2 Anticipated Papilla Height

	Between Natural Teeth	Between Tooth and Implant	Between Adjacent Implants
Average expected papilla height (from crest of bone)	≥5 mm (Tarnow, 1992)[116]	4.2 mm (Kan, 2003)[61]	3.4 mm (Tarnow, 2003)[115]

the implant. Should the papilla fail to meet desires and expectations, the open gingival embrasure is generally best managed through additional surgery or closing the space with restorations.[118] Although there have been good attempts to solve the problem of deficient papilla with pink prosthetics, it is all but impossible to resolve it in a manner that is both esthetically convincing and hygienic in the partially edentulous patient.

Although there will be variations in papilla height adjacent to or between implants, the average papilla height adjacent to a single implant is 4.2 mm.[61] Between adjacent, unrestored natural teeth, the average papilla height is at least 5 mm.[116] Between adjacent (external hex) implants, the average papilla is only 3.4 mm (Table 76.2).[115]

The preceding figures are averages and do not represent the actual value for what is possible for any given patient. The key to predictable, successful treatment in the esthetic zone is the implant-retained provisional restoration. This will allow the clinical team and the patient to truly test the four key criteria of esthetics, phonetics, function, and hygiene. Revisions and alterations are much easier to accomplish with provisionals as compared with the definitive prosthesis.

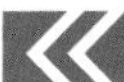

FLASH BACK

The greatest challenge of implants in the esthetic zone is papilla management. Although there have been good attempts to solve the problem of deficient papilla with pink prosthetics, it is all but impossible to resolve it in a manner that is both esthetically convincing and hygienic in the partially edentulous patient.

Tissue Shaping and Management

Following integration of the implant and maturation of the soft tissue, there may be the need to correct slight malpositions of the peri-implant tissues. This can be done through modification of the implant abutment, but it should not be done repeatedly to avoid increased tissue changes that lead to bone loss. Significant deficiencies of tissue may be difficult to correct, whereas others may be able to be addressed with additional surgery.

The emergence profile of the provisional restoration can be added to or contoured back to manipulate the soft tissue position. Applying additional contour will move the gingiva apically, whereas undercontouring will usually allow the tissue to drape more coronally. The abutment can also be modified to apply pressure to the base of the papilla, thus forcing the tip coronally,[118] but this technique should be used with caution around implants due to a diminished blood supply and fragility of the soft tissue.[99] The clinician should minimize the number of reattachments to the head of the implant, as this will weaken the integrity of the tissues and create additional bone loss.[3,100]

Ideally all contours of the soft tissues should be designed in the patient's mouth, and the four keys (esthetics, phonetics, function, and hygiene) should be tested and approved. If done correctly, the transition from the patient to the technician is seamless with the provisional serving as a blueprint for the definitive prosthesis.

Conclusions

Successful implant treatment requires a team of clinicians and technicians dedicated to excellence in surgical and prosthetic aspects. A thorough understanding of the prosthodontic restoration of implants from implant-abutment connections to hard and soft tissue interfaces and compatibility with the implant/abutment/restoration is essential. This chapter reviewed the critical aspects of prosthetic implant treatment proven to maximize long-term functional, biologic, and esthetic success.

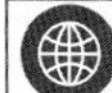
A Case Scenario is found on the companion website eBooks.Health.Elsevier.com.

Suggested Reading

Buser D, Martin W, Belser UC. Optimizing esthetics for implant restorations in the anterior maxilla: anatomic and surgical considerations. *Int J Oral Maxillofac Implants*. 2004;19(suppl):43–61.

Canullo L, Fedele GR, Iannello G, et al. Platform switching and marginal bone-level alterations: the results of a randomized-controlled trial. *Clin Oral Implants Res*. 2010;21(1):115–121.

Clelland N, Chaudhry J, Rashid RG, et al. Split-mouth comparison of splinted and nonsplinted prostheses on short implants: 3-year results. *Int J Oral Maxillofac Implants*. 2016;31(5):1135–1141.

Kan JY, Rungcharassaeng K, Lozada JL, et al. Facial gingival tissue stability following immediate placement and provisionalization of maxillary anterior single implants: a 2-to 8-year follow-up. *Int J Oral Maxillofac Implants*. 2011;26(1):179–187.

Lazzara RJ, Porter SS. Platform switching: a new concept in implant dentistry for controlling postrestorative crestal bone levels. *Int J Perio Rest Dent*. 2006;26:9–17.

Linkevicius T, Vindasiute E, Puisys A, et al. The influence of the cementation margin position on the amount of undetected cement. A prospective clinical study. *Clin Oral Implants Res*. 2013;24(1):71–76.

Millen C, Brägger U, Wittneben JG. Influence of prosthesis type and retention mechanism on complications with fixed implant-supported prostheses: a systematic review applying multivariate analyses. *Int J Oral Maxillofac Implants*. 2015;30(1):110–124.

Sailer I, Mühlemann S, Zwahlen M, et al. Cemented and screw-retained implant reconstructions: a systematic review of the survival and complication rates. *Clin Oral Implants Res*. 2012;23(suppl 6):163–201.

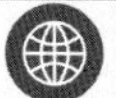
References for this chapter are found on the companion website eBooks.Health.Elsevier.com.

CHAPTER 77

Prosthetic Considerations: Fully Edentulous

Ting-Ling Chang | Evelyn Chung | Perry R. Klokkevold

CHAPTER OUTLINE

Controlled clinical research in implant prosthodontics showed that excellent long-term results can be achieved with appropriate case selection, good occlusal harmony, sufficient oral hygiene, and careful management of patients' soft and hard tissues. With these results, the placement of implants has become one of the most beneficial surgical procedures and treatment modalities. It has also provided a high psychological impact and improvement of quality of life for edentulous patients and the patients transitioning from a hopeless remaining dentition to complete edentulism.

After the first year of implant function, a small loss of marginal bone was noted around most of the implants. However, clinical studies have shown a correlation between insufficient oral hygiene and occlusal overload that can lead to increased bone loss around dental implants. In general, occlusal loading can affect the prognosis of both the implant and implant-supported prosthesis. The occlusal load may exceed the mechanical or biological load-bearing capacity of the osseointegrated oral implant or the prosthesis, causing either a mechanical failure or failure of osseointegration. If this happens, the load can be defined as an overload. The most critical factor to be considered in the prosthodontic planning is to understand the implant load-bearing capacity and to control distribution of the anticipated functional loads to achieve long-term success and avoid overloading.

This chapter describes important biomechanical considerations and prosthodontic guidelines with updates on modern technologies and materials that govern the use of dental implants in edentulous patient applications.

Implant Biomechanics

Knowledge of implant biomechanics is essential if implant-supported prostheses are to be employed predictably. The load-bearing capacity of the implant-supported prosthesis must exceed the loads anticipated during function. If the applied loads exceed the load-bearing capacity of the implants, implant overload may provoke a resorption remodeling response of the bone around the implants.[7,10]

Several factors affect the load-bearing capacity of implants (Fig. 77.1), including implant length, the number of implants used, their arrangement, and their angulation in relation to the plane of occlusion. The quality of the bone-implant interface also greatly influences the load-bearing capacity of the implant-supported prosthesis.

The bone-implant interface is particularly influential. For example, bone anchorage of the implants in the posterior maxilla is poor compared with the anterior mandible. As one progresses posteriorly in the maxilla, the trabecular bone is less dense and the cortical layer is thinner, and, as a result, the bone appositional index in the posterior maxilla may be one-third to one-half of that achieved in the anterior mandible. In addition, pneumatization of the maxillary sinus limits the lengths of implants used, further reducing the load-bearing capacity of implants placed in this region.

The goal of implant biomechanics consideration for the clinician is to form a treatment plan and engineer the design such that the anticipated load is within the load-bearing capacity so that a long-term biomechanics equilibrium is achieved. In clinical situations, the risk of implant overload can be minimized by limiting the width of the occlusal table, flattening the cusp angles, and avoiding excessive cantilevers posterior to the most distal implant.

Edentulous Maxilla

Although a conventional denture may be satisfactory to restore most patients with an edentulous maxilla, an implant-retained prosthesis may be desirable in some situations. When a conventional maxillary denture is only marginally stable, the patient may not be aware of the problem when the conventional mandibular denture is even more unstable. If the edentulous mandible is restored with a stable implant overlay denture, the patient may become aware of the deficiency in the maxillary denture and request the same type of stability for the maxillary prosthesis. Another indication for implants in the maxilla may be to offset the potential destructive effects on the premaxillary area when an edentulous maxilla is opposed by a partially edentulous mandible with natural anterior teeth.

Full-Arch Removable Implant Overlay Prosthesis

Prosthetic options for the patient with an edentulous maxilla include a conventional complete denture, an implant-assisted denture or an implant-supported fixed prosthesis. For many patients, a conventional

Implant biomechanics

Load-bearing capacity	Anticipated load
1. Quality of bone site 2. Quality of bone implant interface 3. Implant microsurfaces Machined vs. rough surfaces 4. Implant Number and arrangement Linear vs. curvilinear Length and diameter Angulation	1. Occlusal factors Cusp angles Width of occlusal table Guidance type Anterior guidance Group function 2. Cantilever forces Connection to natural dentition Size of occlusal table Cantilevered prostheses 3. Parafunctional habits (bruxism) 4. Brachycephalics

Biomechanics equilibrium

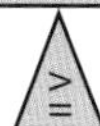

Fig. 77.1 Factors affect the load-bearing capacity and anticipated load of the implant-retained prostheses. Some of the factors are patient-specific and unchangeable by clinicians. Some of the factors are controllable as the implant type/number/arrangement and the prosthetic design. The goal of implant biomechanics consideration for clinician to treatment plan and engineer the design is such that anticipated load is within the load-bearing capacity so that a long-term biomechanics equilibrium is achieved.

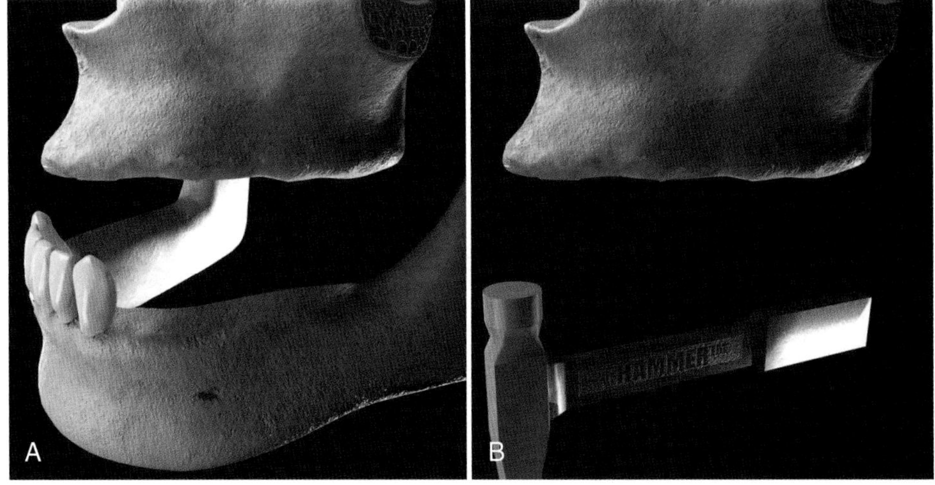

Fig. 77.2 The "hammer and anvil" effect is a useful analogy for the clinician to keep in mind. (A) Model showing mandibular anterior teeth opposing edentulous maxilla without posterior dentition to support vertical dimension of occlusion. (B) Model showing "hammer" opposing edentulous maxilla.

complete denture does not provide the comfort and quality of life that they desire. An implant-assisted or implant-supported prosthesis can provide stability, comfort, and restore confidence to the patient, especially in patients with one or more of the following conditions:

1. *Poor ridge form with a marginally stable conventional maxillary denture.* Two or four implants provide greater stability and security of a maxillary denture in function when the maxillary ridge is severely resorbed and lacks resistance to lateral forces.
2. *Lack of posterior support with an intact mandibular anterior dentition.* Implants in the maxilla can offset the potentially destructive effects on the premaxillary region when a mandible with natural anterior teeth and missing posterior teeth opposes an edentulous maxilla. In this situation, the lack of posterior support leads to a condition often referred to as *combination syndrome,* in which overclosure of the anterior teeth causes a "hammer and anvil" type of destruction of the edentulous anterior maxilla (Fig. 77.2).
3. *Palatal coverage is not tolerated.* Some patients prefer a palateless denture, which may enhance their sensations of taste and texture or may simply provide a psychological advantage. Some patients prefer a palateless denture because the proximity of the denture with the soft palate induces a gag reflex. Patients with large palatal tori (Fig. 77.3) can also benefit from a palateless maxillary denture. A minimum of four implants with adequate anterior–posterior (A–P) spread allows the fabrication of an implant-assisted overdenture without palatal coverage.

The design of a maxillary implant-retained prosthesis is greatly influenced by the anatomy of the maxilla. Most notably, the maxillary sinus limits the height of bone available for implant placement in the posterior region. As a result, implant placement is confined to the anterior region, and the A–P spread that can be achieved is often limited (Fig. 77.4). If the A–P spread is inadequate to provide support, a full-palatal-coverage overlay denture is recommended.

Most patients are best served with an implant-assisted overlay denture.[9] Lower cost, improved hygiene access, and predictable speech articulation are additional benefits that favor the use of an overlay denture in the edentulous maxilla over an implant-supported fixed prosthesis. The four-implant–assisted, palateless overlay denture ideally addresses the needs of most patients (Fig. 77.5). Many patients who are edentulous in the maxilla have lost a significant amount of structure in the premaxillary region resulting in a lack of support for the upper lip. An implant-assisted maxillary overdenture is preferred over an implant-supported fixed prosthesis because the labial flange can provide the needed lip support. The usual resorption pattern of the alveolus places the gingival margin of a fixed restoration either too far superior, too far palatal, or both. Even if the patient has a low enough smile line to hide the appearance of long crowns and deficient soft tissue height, a lack of lip support just beneath the nose can be unsightly with a fixed prosthesis.

Full-Arch Fixed Implant-Supported Prosthesis

For those patients who prefer an implant-supported fixed prosthesis (and do not require additional lip support), six or more implants arranged in an appropriate arc of curvature with at least 2 cm of A–P spread are required (Fig. 77.6). In this situation, the fixed prosthesis can be fabricated with distal extension cantilevers up to half the A–P spread, provided it does not exceed 10 mm.

Modern Manufacturing

Computer-aided manufacturing (CAM) techniques used in early CAM systems for implant-supported frameworks were exclusively subtractive methods, such as milling from a solid block of material.

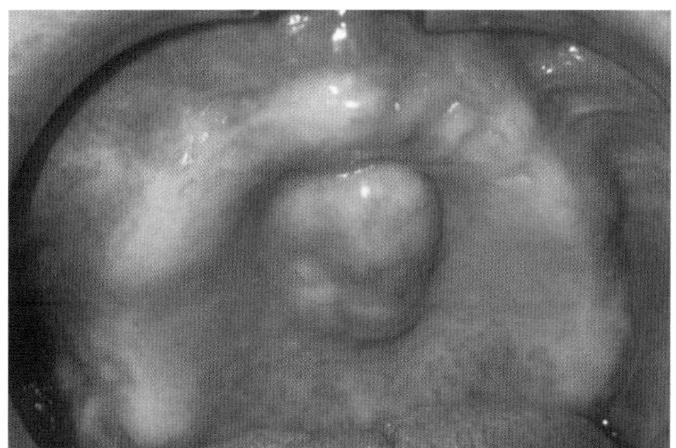

Fig. 77.3 Patients with large palatal tori can also benefit from a palateless maxillary denture.

In recent years, rapid prototyping (RP), a general term used for several additive layer manufacturing techniques, has been refined. The most commonly used are stereolithography (SLA), selective laser melting (SLM), selective laser sintering (SLS), selective deposition modeling, and 3-D printing (3DP). RP allows machines to address every element of a part no matter the complexity of its shape. Both CAD-CAM and RP technologies have provided significant improvement in the cervical adaptation of implant-supported frameworks compared to the conventional analog laboratory procedures, including waxing, investing, and casting. The modern manufacturing technologies also expand the material choices from gold alloys to Titanium, Cobalt-Chrome (Co-Cr), Zirconia, Polymethyl Methacrylate (PMMA) resin, Polyether Ether Ketone (PEEK), and Pekkton. A recent survey study was designed to determine the current prevalence of usage of various treatment modalities and materials for complete-arch fixed implant-supported prostheses in the western United States.[18] The results suggest a plurality (33%) preferred anatomic contour zirconia (with or without layered porcelain) with titanium bases for the maxilla. Laboratory-processed resin with denture teeth over a milled metal bar was preferred (32%) for the mandible.

Edentulous Mandible

Full-Arch Removable Implant Overlay Prosthesis

Similar to the edentulous maxilla, prosthetic options for patients with an edentulous mandible include a conventional complete denture, an implant-assisted denture, or an implant-supported prosthesis. A mandibular complete denture is more problematic for patients than a maxillary complete denture, especially for patients with a severely resorbed (atrophic) mandibular ridge. The lack of stability and retention makes it very challenging for patients to control the denture. In this situation, the addition of implants offers unprecedented control (i.e., stability and retention) for a complete removable prosthesis. The two-implant–assisted overdenture is now the treatment of choice for patients with an atrophic, edentulous mandible.

Implant-assisted overlay dentures are designed so that most of the masticatory load is borne by the primary denture-support areas (i.e., retromolar pad, buccal shelf). A common practice is to place two implants in the anterior mandible with a connecting bar. One

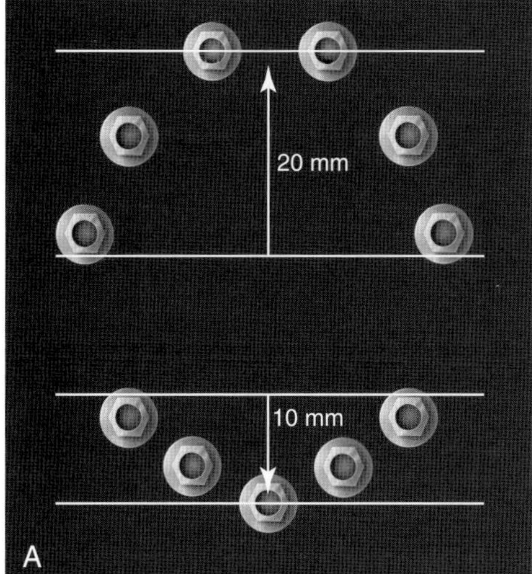

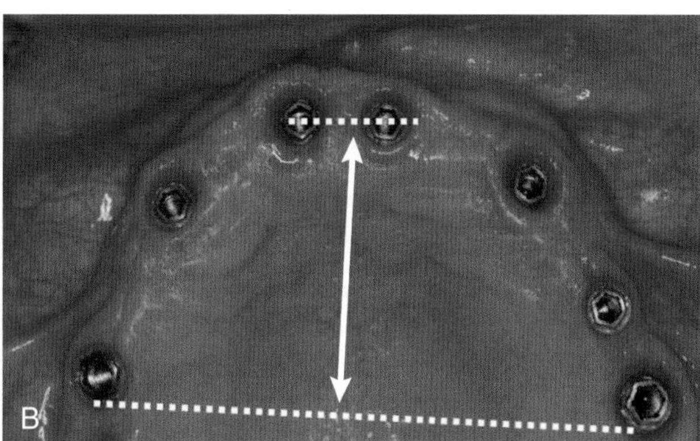

Fig. 77.4 (A) Diagram demonstrating the anterior–posterior (A-P) implant spread. It is defined as the distance from the middle of the most anterior implant to the distal edge of the most posterior implant. (B) Anterior–posterior (A-P) spread of implants is the distance from the center of the most anterior implant(s) to the distal surface of the most posterior implant(s).

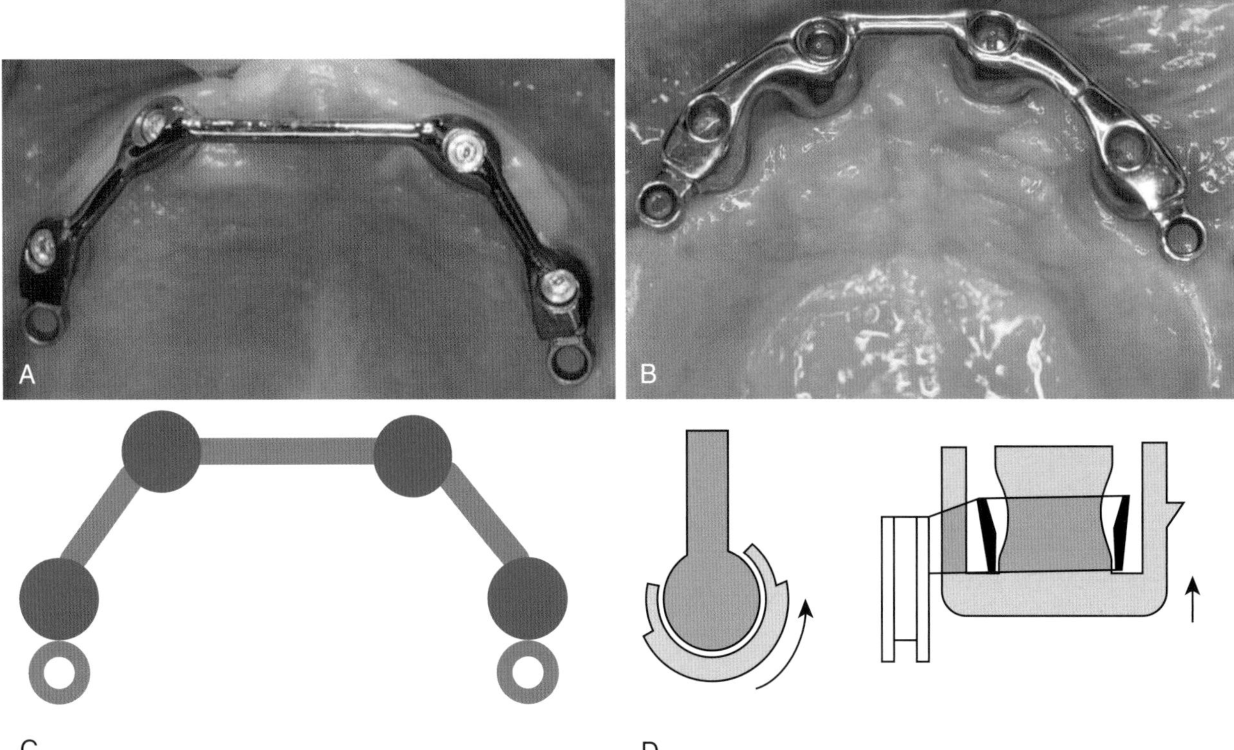

Fig. 77.5 (A) The anterior two implants should be 12 to 20 mm apart. The anterior segment is restored with a Hader bar. If space is adequate, two Hader clips can be employed. (B) The anterior two implants are less than 12 mm apart and the space is only for one Hader clip. (C and D) Extracoronal resilient attachments (ERAs) are positioned adjacent to the distal implants. This attachment permits the overlay prosthesis to be compressed into the mucoperiosteum in the extension areas. As a result, the denture-bearing tissues absorb the posterior occlusal forces.

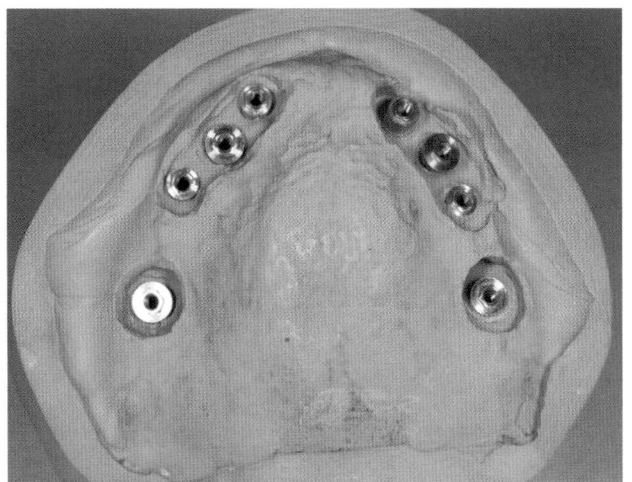

Fig. 77.6 Six or more implants arranged in an appropriate arc of curvature with at least 2 cm of A-P spread are recommended for a maxillary complete-arch fixed implant-supported prosthesis. This case shows favorable biomechanics design with 3 cm of A-P spread and minimum need for distal cantilever due to the molar location of the two posterior implants.

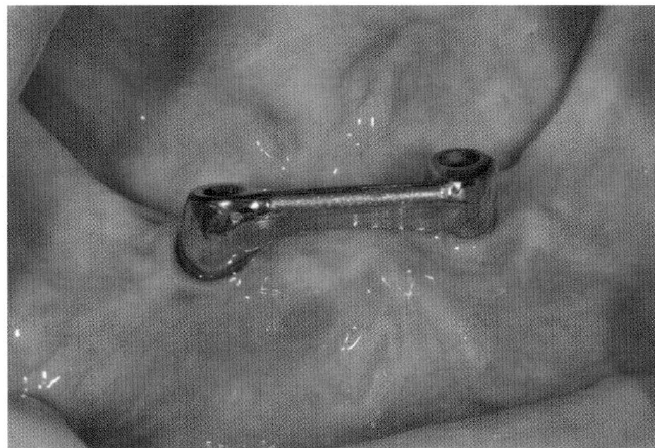

Fig. 77.7 A common practice is to place two implants in the anterior mandible with a connecting bar. It is recommended as a standard of care to restore edentulous mandible. Notice minimum attached keratinized gingiva tissue around the implants. Soft tissue graft is recommended to improve the peri-implant soft tissue quality for this case.

or two clips retain the denture to the bar (Fig. 77.7). When occlusal forces are applied, the denture rotates around the bar (anterior axis of rotation) and depresses slightly in the posterior aspect, directing the forces to the primary denture-bearing areas (Fig. 77.8). The implants provide stability and retention while bearing minimal stress from occlusal loads. Individual attachments secured to each implant offer a simple prosthetic alternative (Fig. 77.9) to the bar and clip design. However, it is more critical for implants with individual attachments to be parallel to one another to facilitate a proper path of insertion and to minimize stress during prosthetic seating and function.

Full-Arch Fixed Implant-Supported Prosthesis

For those patients who prefer an implant-supported fixed prosthesis, four, five, or six implants arranged in an appropriate arc of curvature with at least 1 cm of A–P spread are required (Fig. 77.10). In this situation, the fixed prosthesis can be fabricated with distal extension cantilevers up to twice the A–P spread.

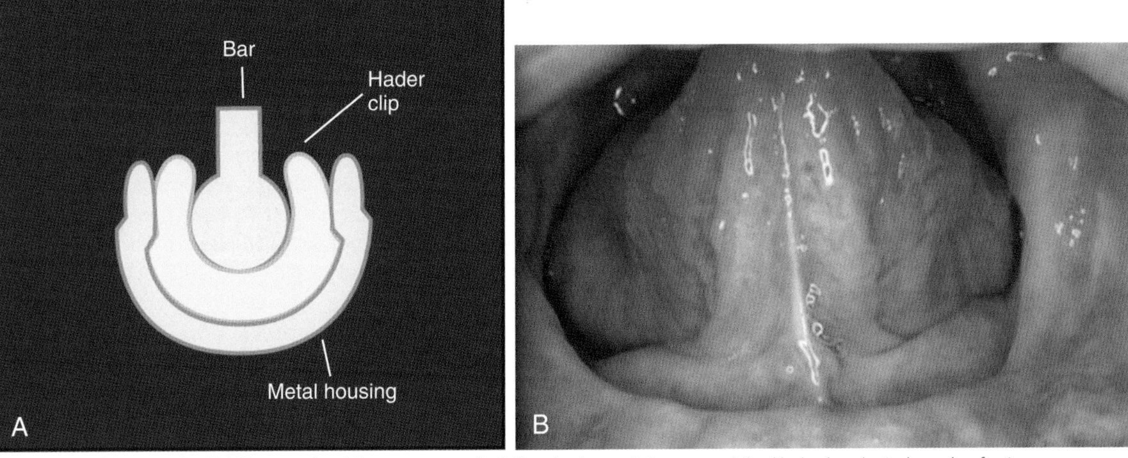

Fig. 77.8 (A) When occlusal forces are applied, the denture rotates around the Hader bar (anterior axis of rotation) and depresses slightly in the posterior aspect, directing the forces to the (B) primary denture-bearing areas (retromolar pad and buccal shelf) of the mandible. These areas are quite resistant to resorption.

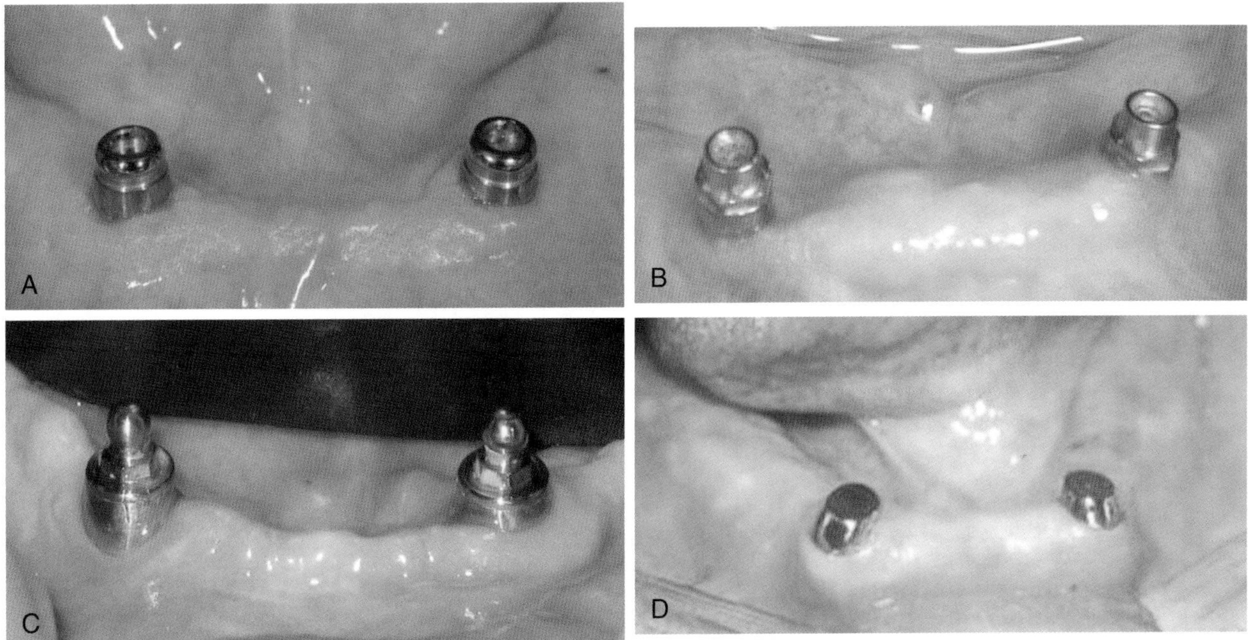

Fig. 77.9 The principal advantages of these individual attachment systems are their simplicity, ease of application, and reduced initial costs. (A) Locator attachment, (B) ERA attachment, (C) O ring attachment, (D) rare-earth magnetic attachment. However, implants need to be reasonably parallel to one another. The overdenture must be properly extended to cover the primary support areas (the retromolar pad and buccal shelf).

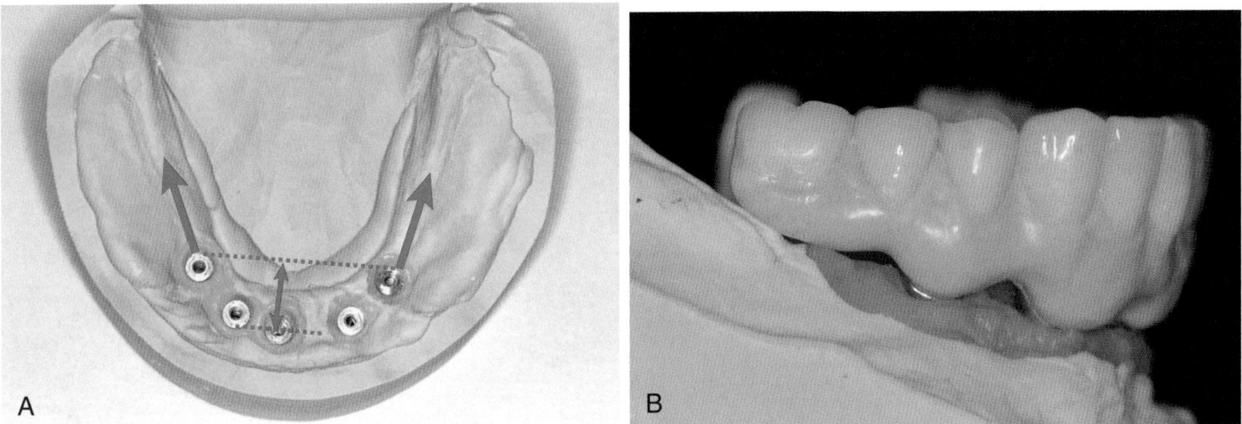

Fig. 77.10 (A) For those patients who prefer an implant-supported fixed prosthesis, four, five, or six implants arranged in an appropriate arc of curvature with at least 1 cm of A-P spread are required. (B) In this situation, the fixed prosthesis can be fabricated with distal extension cantilevers up to twice the A-P spread.

Many patients prefer a fixed option for psychological reasons, but the mastication efficiency provided by a fixed versus removable prosthesis does not appear to be significant.[11] Evidence suggests that such fixed restorations tend to stop resorption of the body of the posterior mandible and in some cases enable regeneration of the bone in this region.[12]

Digital Technology

Digital technology in implant dentistry is rapidly evolving. The digital implant workflow can help clinicians plan more efficiently and execute more accurately. Advances in implant surgical technology include simulation software, static computer-aided design/computer-aided manufacturing (CAD/CAM) surgical guides, and dynamic navigation for dental implant surgery (see Chapter 84). The digitally assisted implant placement offers three major advantages: improved precision in executing the prosthodontically driven guided implant surgery, enhanced predictability in immediate implant placement and provisionalization, and a biological benefit of implant placement prior to significant alveolar bone loss for patients transitioning from failing dentition to edentulism.

Most patients become edentulous due to advanced periodontal disease and/or unrestorable rampant caries. Upon extraction of hopeless teeth, there is often significant horizontal and vertical bone loss. In the past, patients with a terminal stage remaining dentition had to go through a long treatment process from extractions, implant placement, and healing time for osseointegration, to fabrication of the definitive implant prosthesis, which can take several months, and sometimes up to a year for the course of conventional treatment approach. This transition often is long and stressful for patients to endure. Moreover, a fixed implant reconstruction may be considered for a patient who is about to be edentulated and has not experienced significant alveolar bone loss. Digital technology can address these challenges and help this patient group significantly by making the transition much faster and more predictable. Fig. 77.11 highlights digital treatment advantages of transitioning such patients from failing dentition to the immediate implant-supported fixed provisional prostheses. Aires and Berger[2] reported the cumulative survival rates (CSR) were 99.4% at implant level and 96.2% at patient level on a retrospective case series of 228 patients. Distal tilting of implants splinted with a fixed prosthesis does not increase bone stress compared to a vertically placed implant.[19] There is a significant biomechanical advantage to using tilted implants to provide distal abutments for fixed restorations that avoid or reduce distal cantilever extensions.

Contemporary Prosthetic Design and Materials

The use of implant prosthodontics for rehabilitation of the edentulous patient has come a long way during the last 50 years.

Prosthesis design and material selection have been evolving with advances in modern materials and CAD–CAM technology. These advancements broaden the designs and material options for clinicians and offer innovative approaches to optimize the treatment outcomes of restoring edentulism with implants. Fixed implant-supported prostheses for edentulism can be categorized into four general types, including metal-acrylic resin (hybrid) prosthesis, metal ceramic prosthesis, ceramic veneered zirconia prosthesis, and monolithic zirconia prosthesis.

Metal-Acrylic Resin Prosthesis (Hybrid Prosthesis)

The original Branemark prosthetic design with a cast alloy frame veneered with artificial teeth in resin (aka hybrid prosthesis) has demonstrated a high success rate.[3] Prosthesis-related technical complications have been reported for a fixed hybrid prosthesis, including wear and fracture of artificial teeth, as well as discoloration and bacterial contamination of resins.[4,15] They are also susceptible to resin fracture, or resin detachment from the metal substructure, as well as possible metal substructure breakage if poorly designed. However, this design concept remains a vital and cost-effective option. It allows for some flexibility and control over artificial tooth arrangement to achieve optimal esthetics and function irrespective of implant position to some degree. If designed properly, these prostheses allow for easy maintenance and good serviceability at a reasonable cost.

A common finding with use of acrylic resin artificial teeth is wearing of the occlusal surfaces. The rate of wear may be increased with complete arch resin-metal implant-supported prostheses when the maximum occlusal force is twice that of edentulous individuals.[15] The use of zirconia onlays over occlusal surfaces of denture teeth is a viable alternative material for patients with increased tendencies for occlusal wear and may be incorporated to mitigate these complications while offering the advantages of reduced cost, improved esthetics, and superior wear properties.[8]

Metal Ceramic Prosthesis

This prosthetic design offers pleasing esthetics and minimal prosthesis wear. However, material and laboratory costs can be significantly higher. It is more labor intensive and complex to fabricate (Fig. 77.12). Finally, the long-term costs of maintenance of large, fixed metal ceramic prosthesis such as porcelain fracture repair must be kept in mind and needs to be incorporated in the overall cost structure. Long-term clinical studies on the clinical performance and patient satisfaction of this design are lacking in comparison with metal-acrylic resin (hybrid) prostheses.

Ceramic Veneered Zirconia Prosthesis

Digital workflows using all zirconia ceramic materials offer implant patients a metal-free restorative alternative, with potential for enhanced esthetics and time/cost efficiencies, while achieving comparative biocompatibility and mechanical properties. Studies on zirconia-based complete-arch implant-supported prostheses have shown promising short-term clinical outcomes.[13,14] The frequently reported complication of ceramic veneer chipping and the less frequently reported framework failure requires further investigation.

Monolithic Zirconia Prosthesis

In a systematic review of 12 clinical studies in the short-term, zirconia framework, fractures were reported at a low rate of 1.4%, but chipping of the veneered porcelain was 14.7%.[5] The monolithic zirconia design was proposed to address these issues. Using a monolithic zirconia design with a veneered feldspathic gingival region, a cumulative survival rate of 99.3% was documented in a 5-year period.[6] To achieve favorable outcomes when using this design, adherence to clinical procedures and quality control protocols are recommended.[16]

Clinicians should also be mindful that repair is not possible, and adjusting and polishing is difficult for this design. Given the level of evidence and the duration of the studies included, the use of monolithic zirconia prostheses for complete-arch implant supported prostheses warrants additional comprehensive, longer-term investigation.[1]

Conclusions

The importance of biomechanics and the limitations of implant systems were initially underestimated. Over the years, clinical experience and research underscored the importance of biomechanics in the success and predictability of implant-retained prostheses. The rigid nature of implant-retained restorations and the lack of

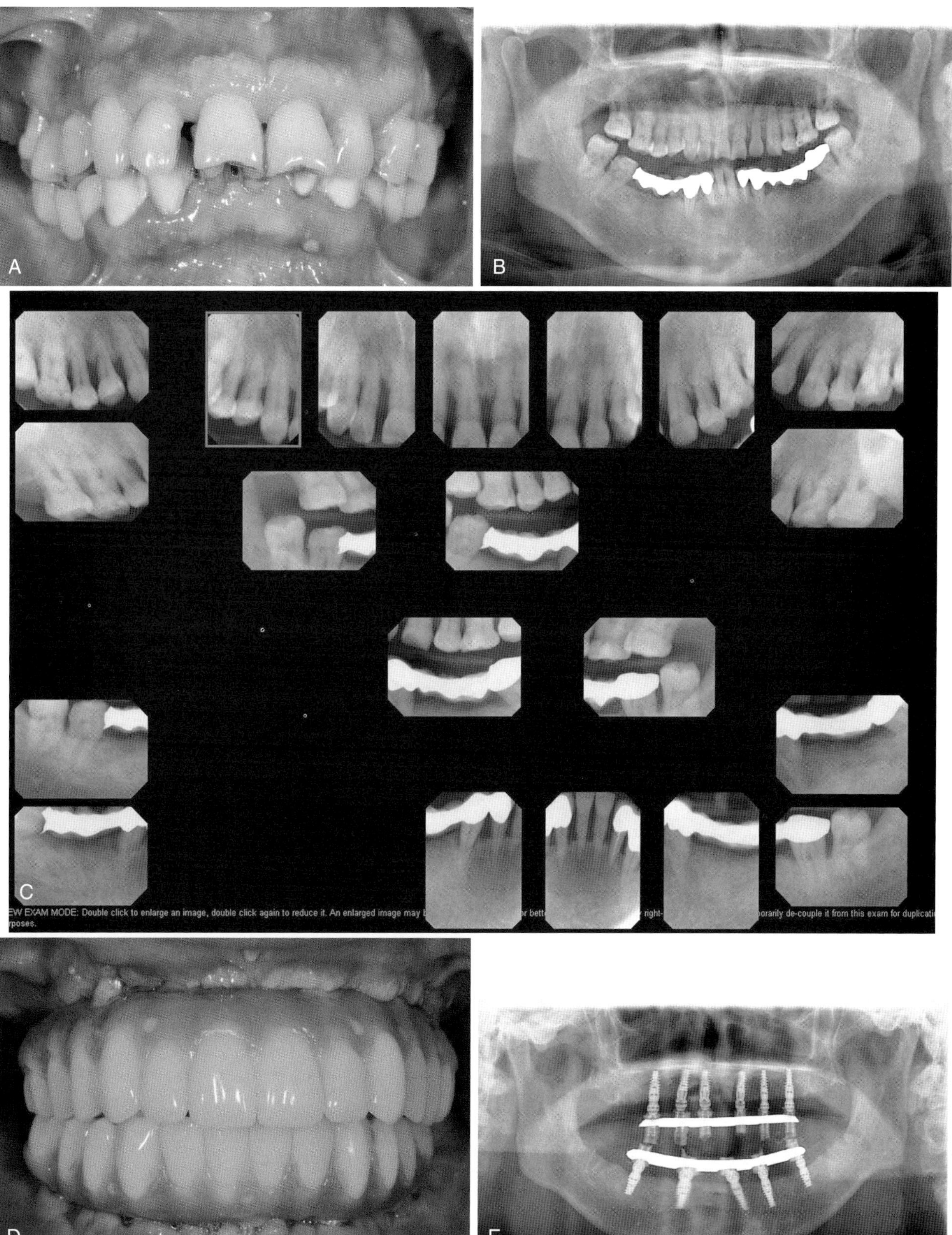

Fig. 77.11 Fifty-one-year-old male patient with failing dentition due to periodontal disease. The transition from failing dentition to extraction, implant placement, and immediate provisionalization was smooth and well-endured by the patient with the help of CAD-CAM technology. (A) to (C) show the pretreatment clinical view, panoramic image, and full mouth radiographs. (D) and (E) represent complete-arch fixed implant-supported provisional prostheses (milled PMMA) and panoramic image 2 months after the extractions and implant placement.

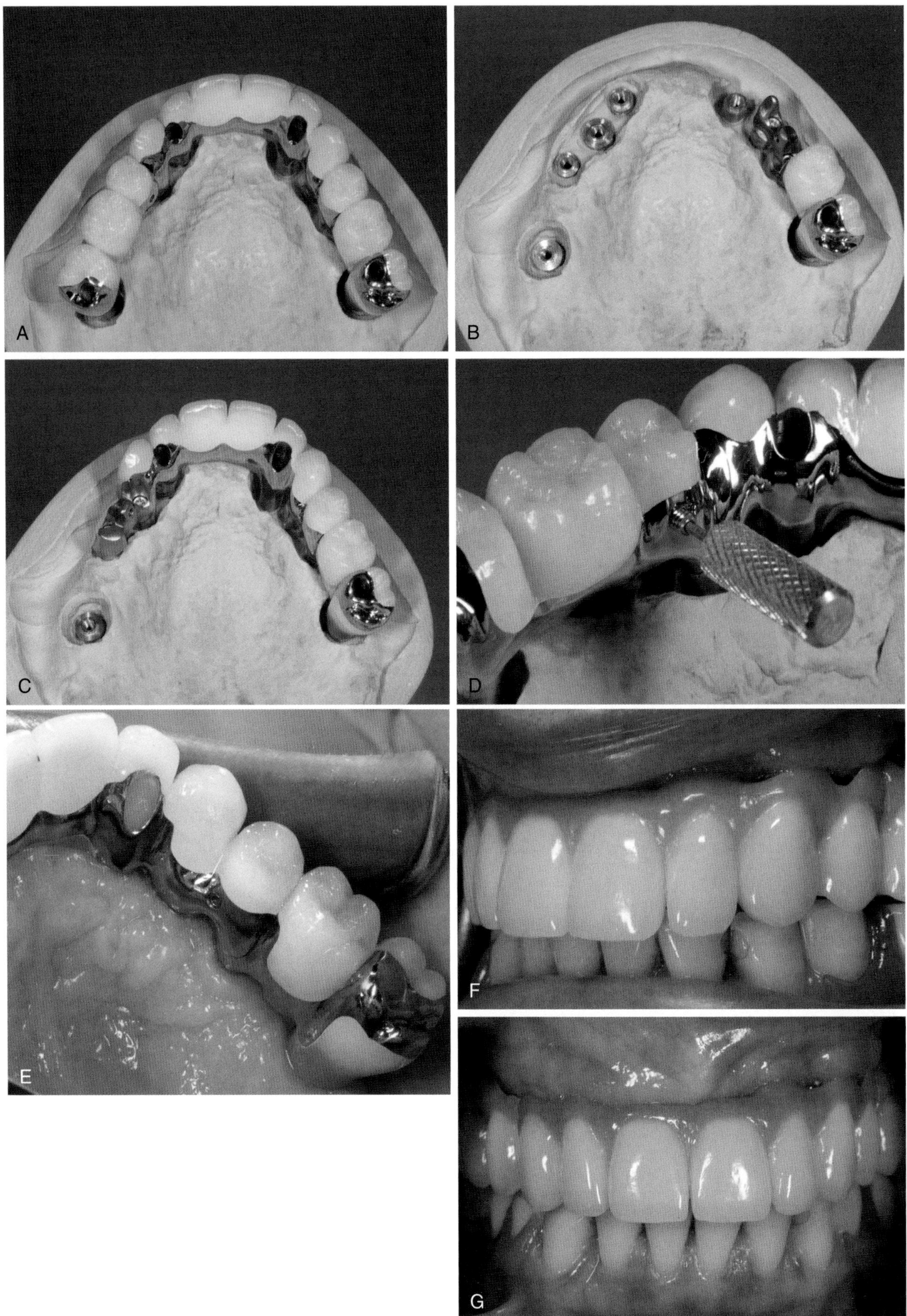

Fig. 77.12 Maxillary complete-arch fixed implant-supported metal-ceramic prosthesis offers superior esthetics. (A-E) show the screw-retained prosthodontic design consists of three segments with lingual-set screws. It is creative design but complex that requires experienced and talented laboratory expertise. (F-G) show tooth colored and pink porcelains are used to optimize esthetic outcomes. The cost of fabrication and maintenance of complete-arch fixed metal ceramic prosthesis must be kept in mind.

forgiveness in these systems demands a revised approach to treatment planning that is now applied. The biomechanics must be factored into the planning at the beginning of any implant treatment to achieve long-term, predictable success. The advances in 3D imaging and CAD–CAM digital technology have had an enormous impact on the contemporary workflow of restoring completely edentulous patients. Digital technologies offer shorter treatment time and a high level of precision compared to the conventional analog workflow. However, clinicians must be mindful that all these evolving technologies, although exciting, are tools and they cannot substitute for proper diagnosis and a thorough knowledge of the sound principles of implant biomechanics and prosthodontic design.

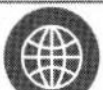
A Case Scenario is found on the companion website eBooks.Health.Elsevier.com.

Suggested Reading

Aires I, Berger J. Planning implant placement on 3d stereolithographic models applied with immediate loading of implant-supported hybrid prostheses after multiple extractions: a case series. *Int J Oral Maxillofac Implants*. 2016;31(1):172–178.

Astrand P, Ahlqvist J, Gunne J, Nilson H. Implant treatment of patients with edentulous jaws: a 20-year follow-up. *Clin Implant Dent Relat Res*. 2008;10(4):207–217.

Attard NJ, Zarb GA. Long-term treatment outcomes in edentulous patients with implant-fixed prostheses: the Toronto study. *Int J Prosthodont*. 2004;17(4):417–424.

Hoshaw S, Brunski J, Cochran C. Mechanical loading of Brånemark implants affects interfacial bone modeling and remodeling. *Int J Oral Maxillofac Implants*. 1994;9:345–360.

Kapur KK. Veterans Administration Cooperative Dental Implant Study–comparisons between fixed partial dentures supported by blade-vent implants and removable partial dentures. Part III: Comparisons of masticatory scores between two treatment modalities. *J Prosthet Dent*. 1991;65:272–283.

Rojas-Vizcaya F. Retrospective 2- to 7-year follow-up study of 20 double full-arch implant-supported monolithic zirconia fixed prostheses: Measurements and Recommendations for optimal design. *J Prosthodont*. 2018;27(6):501–508.

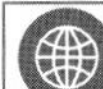
References for this chapter are found on the companion website eBooks.Health.Elsevier.com.

CHAPTER 78

Basic Implant Surgical Procedures[a]

Michael Whang | Perry R. Klokkevold

 Videos for this chapter can be viewed on the companion website at eBooks.Health.Elsevier.com.

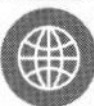 Animations (slide show) from My Dental Hub and and PerioPixel been added by the editors as a supplement to the chapter. They are produced by My Dental Hub and PerioPixel as patient education tools and cover the basic elements in a conceptual manner. They are not intended to be procedural guides for dental professionals.

CHAPTER OUTLINE

The surgical procedures for the placement of nearly all endosseous dental implants currently used are based on the original work of Professor Per-Ingvar Brånemark and colleagues in Sweden in the 1960s and 1970s.[4,5] Their landmark research evaluated the biologic, physiologic, and mechanical aspects of the titanium screw–shaped implant, subsequently known commercially as the Nobelpharma "Brånemark" implant system and currently manufactured by Nobel Biocare. The original Brånemark implant was a parallel-walled, cylindrically shaped, threaded implant with an external hex connection and a machined surface. Since their introduction, many designs of root form implants have been developed, modified, and studied. The same fundamental principles of atraumatic, precise implant site preparation applies to all implant systems. Briefly, this includes a gentle surgical technique and progressive incremental preparation of the bone for a precise fit of the implant at the time of placement.

This chapter outlines the basic surgical procedures for the placement of endosseous dental implants using either a one-stage or two-stage protocol. The principles described here are intentionally generic and meant to serve as guidelines that are applicable to most common implant systems (Videos 78.1 and 78.2). Each implant system is designed with specific armamentarium and recommendations for use (e.g., drilling speeds), and it is advisable to follow the detailed protocols provided by the manufacturer. For the presentation of a dental implant case, see Video 78.3.

General Principles of Implant Surgery

Patient Preparation

Most implant surgical procedures can be done in the office using local anesthesia. Conscious sedation (oral or intravenous) may be indicated (see Chapter 58) for some patients. The risks and benefits of implant surgery specific to the patient's situation and needs should be thoroughly explained prior to surgery. Written informed consent should be obtained for the procedure.

Implant Site Preparation

Some basic principles must be followed to achieve osseointegration with a high degree of predictability[3,4,7] (Box 78.1). The surgical site should be kept aseptic, and the patient should be appropriately prepared and draped for an intraoral surgical procedure. Prerinsing with chlorhexidine gluconate for 1 to 2 minutes immediately before the procedure and removing all supragingival plaque (biofilm) will aid in reducing the bacterial load present around the surgical site. Every effort should be made to maintain a sterile surgical field and avoid contamination of the implant surface. Implant sites should be prepared using gentle, atraumatic surgical techniques with an effort to avoid overheating the bone.

Successful osseointegration occurs predictably for submerged[4] and nonsubmerged[12] dental implants when proven clinical guidelines are followed. Well-controlle[illegible] of patients with good plaque control and appropriate occlus[illegible]ces have demonstrated that root form endosseous dental implants show little change in bone height around the implant over years of function.[1] After initial bone remodeling in the first year (1–1.5 mm of resorption described as "normal remodeling around an externally hexed implant"),[1] the bone level around healthy functioning implants remains stable for many years afterward. The average annual crestal bone loss after the first year in function is expected to be 0.1 mm or less. Hence, implants offer a predictable solution for tooth replacement.

Regardless of the surgical approach, the implant must be placed in healthy bone with good primary stability to achieve osseointegration, and an atraumatic technique must be followed to avoid damage to bone. Drilling of the bone without adequate cooling generates

[a]Editors' note: An animation (slide show) has been added by the editors as a supplement to the chapter. It was produced by My Dental Hub as a patient education tool and covers the basic elements in a conceptual manner. It is not intended to be a procedural guide for dental professionals.

BOX 78.1 Basic Principles of Implant Therapy to Achieve Osseointegration

1. Implants must be sterile and made of a biocompatible material (e.g., titanium).
2. Implant site should be prepared under sterile conditions.
3. Implant site should be prepared with an atraumatic surgical technique that avoids overheating of the bone during preparation of the recipient site.
4. Implants should be placed with good initial stability.
5. Implants should be allowed to heal without loading or micromovement (i.e., undisturbed healing period to allow for osseointegration) for 2 to 4 or 4 to 6 months, depending on the bone density, bone maturation, and implant stability.

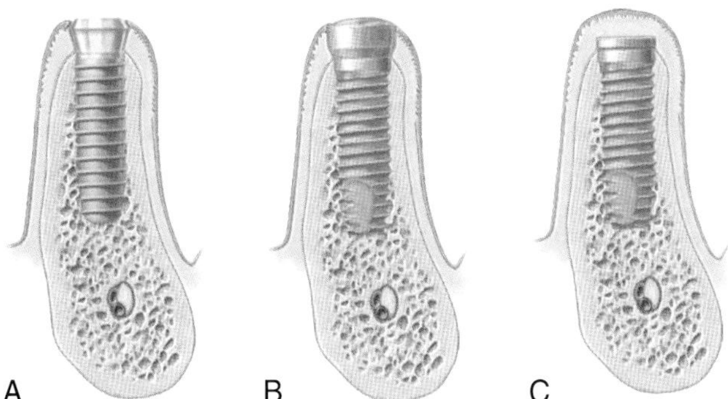

Fig. 78.1 One-stage implant versus two-stage implant surgeries. (A) One-stage surgery with the implant designed so that the coronal portion of the implant extends through the gingiva. (B) One-stage surgery with implant designed to be used for two-stage surgery. A healing abutment is connected to the implant during the first-stage surgery. (C) In the two-stage surgery, the top of the implant is completely submerged under gingiva.

excessive heat, which injures bone and increases the risk of failure.[13] The anatomic features of bone quality (dense compact vs. loose trabecular) at the recipient site influence the interface between bone and implant.[10] Compact bone offers a much greater surface area for bone to implant contact than cancellous bone. Areas of the jaw exhibiting thin layers of cortical bone and large cancellous spaces, such as the posterior maxilla, have lower success rates than areas of dense bone.[10] The best results are achieved when the bone to implant contact is intimate at the time of implant placement.

One-Stage Versus Two-Stage Implant Placement Surgery

Currently, most threaded endosseous implants can be placed using either a one-stage (nonsubmerged) or two-stage (submerged) protocol. In the one-stage approach, the implant or the abutment emerges through the mucoperiosteal gingival tissue at the time of implant placement, whereas in the two-stage approach, the top of the implant and cover screw are completely covered with the flap closure (Fig. 78.1). Implants are allowed to heal, without loading or micromovement, for a period of time to allow for osseointegration. In two-stage implant surgery, the implant must be surgically exposed following a healing period. Some implants, referred to as "tissue level," are specifically designed with the coronal portion of the implant positioned above the crest of bone and extending through the gingival tissues at the time of placement in a one-stage protocol (see Fig. 78.1A). Other implant systems, referred to as "bone level," are designed to be placed at the level of bone and require a healing abutment to be attached to the implant at the time of placement to be used in a one-stage approach[8] (see Fig. 78.1B). Knowledge of the specific characteristics of the implant design must be considered with regard to the depth of implant placement. Polished collars must not be placed subcrestal because bone loss will occur.[9]

A one-stage surgical approach simplifies the procedure because a second-stage exposure surgery is not necessary. The two-stage, submerged approach is advantageous for situations that require simultaneous bone augmentation procedures at the time of implant placement because membranes can be submerged, which will minimize postoperative exposure. Mucogingival tissues can be augmented if desired at the second-stage surgery in a two-stage protocol or as part of the one-stage protocol. Fundamental differences in flap management for these two surgical techniques are described separately.

Two-Stage "Submerged" Implant Placement

In the two-stage implant surgical approach, the first-stage or implant placement surgery ends by suturing the soft tissues together over the implant cover screw so that it remains submerged and isolated from the oral cavity. If the implant fixture is placed more than 1 mm subcrestal, due to lack of restorative space to the opposing occlusion or due to the thin vertical soft tissue thickness (<3 mm), use of a bone profile drill and placement of a short (2-mm) healing abutment is recommended to avoid the difficulty encountered during second-stage surgery with bone covering the cover screw. Placement of a healing abutment with crestal implant placement can also create a "tenting" effect with thin vertical soft tissue thickness that will result in vertical soft tissue gain during healing. This is not recommended in situations with excessively thin soft tissue (<1 mm). Vertical soft tissue thickness can also be gained through augmentation with an autogenous connective tissue graft or soft tissue allograft. In areas with dense cortical bone and good initial implant support, the implants are left to heal undisturbed for a period of 2 to 4 months, whereas in areas of loose trabecular bone, grafted sites, and sites with lesser implant stability, implants may be allowed to heal for periods of 4 to 6 months or more. Longer healing periods are indicated for implants in sites with less bone support. During healing, osteoblasts migrate to the surface and form bone adjacent to the implant (osseointegration).[6] Shorter healing periods are indicated for implants placed in good-quality (dense) bone and for implants with an altered surface microtopography (e.g., acid-etched, blasted, or etched and blasted). Readers are referred to online material and other resources for more information about implant surface microtopography.

In the second-stage (exposure) surgery, the implant is uncovered and a healing abutment is connected to allow emergence of the abutment through the soft tissues. Once healed, the restorative dentist then proceeds with the prosthodontic aspects of the implant therapy (impressions and fabrication of prosthesis).

The following sections describe the steps for osteotomy preparation and first-stage implant placement surgery of the two-stage protocol. Figs. 78.2 and 78.3 illustrate the procedures diagrammatically and Fig. 78.4 depicts the procedures with clinical photographs.

Flap Design, Incisions, and Elevation

Flap management for implant surgery varies slightly, depending on the location and objective of the planned surgery. There are different incision and flap designs, but the most common is the crestal flap design. The incision is made along the crest of the ridge, bisecting the existing zone of keratinized mucosa (see Figs. 78.2A and 78.4B).

A remote incision with a layered suturing technique may be used to minimize the incidence of bone graft exposure when extensive bone augmentation is planned. The crestal incision, however, is preferred in most cases, because closure is easier to manage and typically results in less bleeding, less edema, and faster healing.[11]

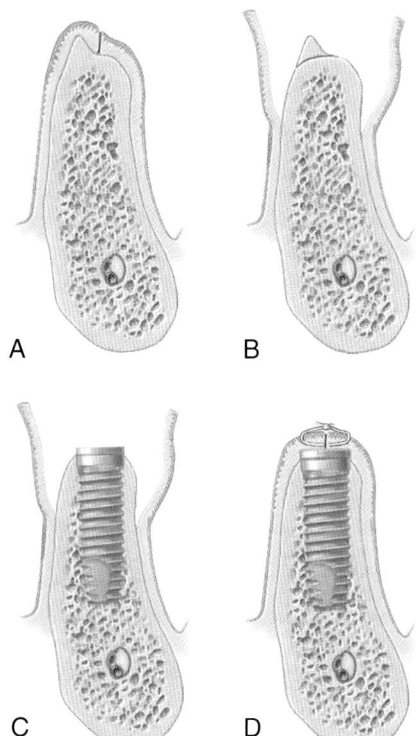

Fig. 78.2 Tissue management for a two-stage implant placement. (A) Crestal incision is made along the crest of the ridge, bisecting the existing zone of keratinized mucosa. (B) Full-thickness flap is raised buccally and lingually to the level of the mucogingival junction. A narrow sharp ridge can be surgically reduced or contoured to provide a reasonably flat bed for the implant. (C) Implant is placed in the prepared osteotomy site. (D) Tissue approximation achieves primary flap closure without tension.

A full-thickness flap is raised (buccal and lingual) up to or slightly beyond the level of the mucogingival junction, exposing the alveolar ridge of the implant surgical sites (see Figs. 78.2B and C). Elevated flaps may be sutured to the buccal mucosa or the opposing teeth to keep the surgical site open during the surgery. The bone at the implant site must be thoroughly débrided of all tissue.

For a "knife edge" alveolar process with sufficient alveolar bone height and distance from vital structures (e.g., inferior alveolar nerve), a large round bur is used to recontour or flatten the bone to provide a wider level surface for the implant site preparation (see Fig. 78.2B). However, if the vertical height of the alveolar bone is limited (e.g., <10 mm), the knife edge alveolar bone height should be preserved. Bone augmentation procedures can be used to increase the ridge width while preserving alveolar bone height (see Chapter 79).

Implant Site Preparation

Once the flaps are reflected and the bone is prepared (i.e., all soft tissue removed and knife edge ridges flattened), the implant osteotomy site can be prepared according to manufacturer recommended protocols. A series of drills are used to prepare the osteotomy site precisely and incrementally for an implant (Fig. 78.5). A surgical guide or stent is inserted, checked for proper positioning, and used throughout the procedure to direct the proper implant placement (see Fig. 78.4E).

Round Bur

A small round bur (or spiral drill) is used to make the initial penetration into bone for the implant site. The surgical guide is removed, and the initial marks are checked for their appropriate buccal-lingual and mesial-distal location, as well as the positions relative to each other and to adjacent teeth (see Fig. 74.9) Slight modifications may be necessary to adjust spatial relationships and avoid minor ridge defects. Any changes should be compared with the prosthetically driven surgical guide positions. Each marked site is then prepared to a depth of 1 to 2 mm with a round drill, breaking through the cortical bone and creating a starting point for the 2-mm twist drill (see Fig. 78.3A).

2-mm Twist Drill

A small twist drill, usually 2 mm in diameter and marked to indicate various lengths (i.e., corresponding to the implant sizes), is used next to establish the depth and align the long axis of the implant recipient site (see Fig. 78.3B). This drill may be externally or internally irrigated. In either case, the twist drill is used at a speed of approximately 800 to 1500 rpm, with copious irrigation to prevent overheating of the bone. Additionally, drills should be intermittently and repeatedly "pumped" or pulled out of the osteotomy site while drilling to expose them to the water coolant and facilitate clearing bone debris from the cutting surfaces. In other words, clinicians should pump the drill (up and down) intermittently and avoid using a constant "push" of the drill in the apical direction only.

When multiple implants are being placed next to one another, a guide pin should be placed in the prepared sites to check alignment, parallelism, and proper prosthetic spacing throughout the preparation process (see Fig. 78.3C). The relationship to neighboring vital structures (e.g., nerve and tooth roots) can be determined by taking a periapical radiograph with a guide pin or radiographic marker in the osteotomy site (see Fig. 75.18). Implants should be positioned with approximately 3 mm between one another to ensure sufficient space for inter-implant bone and soft tissue health and to facilitate oral hygiene procedures. Therefore, the initial marks should be separated by at least 7 mm (center to center) for 4 mm standard-diameter implants. Incrementally more space is needed for wide-diameter implants (see Fig. 74.9).

The 2-mm twist drill is used to establish the final depth of the osteotomy site corresponding to the length of each planned implant. The clinician should also evaluate the bone quality (density) with this drill while preparing the osteotomy to assess the need for modifying subsequent drills used (Box 78.2). If the vertical height of the bone was reduced during the initial ridge preparation, this must be taken into account when preparing the site for a predetermined implant length. For example, if it appears that the implant will be too close to a vital structure, such as the inferior alveolar nerve canal, the depth of the implant osteotomy site and length of the implant may need to be reduced.

The next step is to use a series of drills to incrementally increase the width of the osteotomy site to accommodate the planned implant diameter. The styles, shapes, and final diameter of the drills will differ slightly among different implant systems, but their general purpose is to prepare a recipient site with a precise diameter (and depth) for the selected implant without unduly traumatizing the surrounding bone. It is important to use copious irrigation and a "pumping" action for all drilling.

KEY FACT

A series of drills will be used (speeds determined by manufacturer) sequentially to prepare osteotomy sites. It is essential to prepare sites with copious irrigation to prevent overheating of the bone. Additionally, drills should be intermittently and repeatedly "pumped" or pulled out of the osteotomy site while drilling to expose them to the water coolant and to facilitate clearing bone debris from the cutting surfaces.

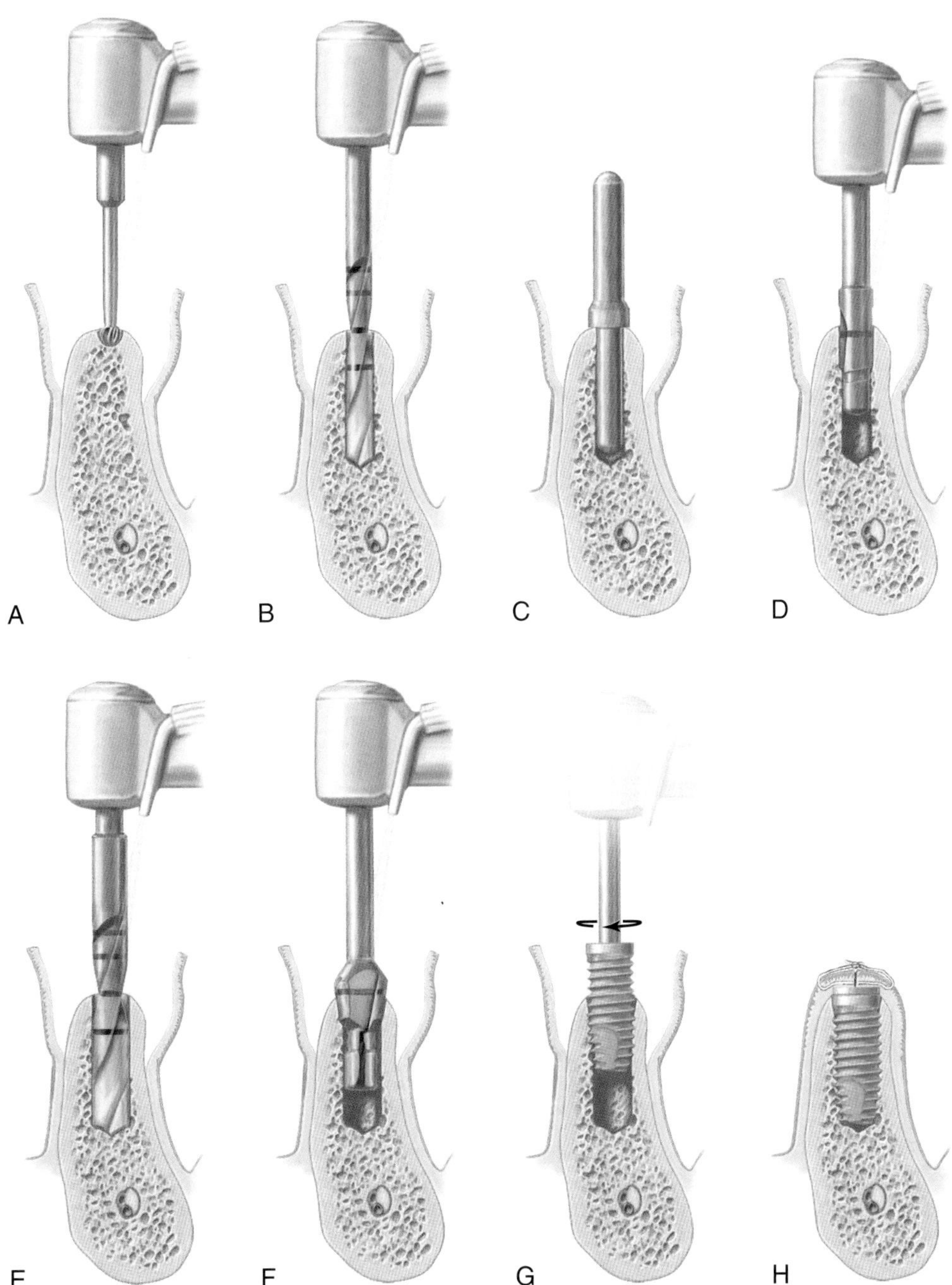

Fig. 78.3 Implant site preparation (osteotomy) for a 4-mm diameter, 10-mm long screw-type, threaded (external hex) implant in a subcrestal position. (A) Initial marking or preparation of the implant site with a round bur. (B) Use of a 2-mm twist drill to establish depth and align the implant. (C) Guide pin is placed in the osteotomy site to confirm position and angulation. (D) Pilot drill is used to increase the diameter of the coronal aspect of the osteotomy site. (E) Final drill used is the 3-mm twist drill to finish preparation of the osteotomy site. (F) Countersink drill is used to widen the entrance of the recipient site and allow for the subcrestal placement of the implant collar and cover screw. Note: An optional tap (not shown) can be used following this step to create screw threads in areas of dense bone. (G) Implant is inserted into the prepared osteotomy site with a handpiece or handheld driver. Note: In systems that use an implant mount, it is removed prior to placement of the cover screw. (H) The cover screw is placed and soft tissues are closed and sutured.

Pilot Drill

Following the 2-mm twist drill, a pilot drill with a noncutting 2-mm–diameter "guide" at the apical end and a cutting 3-mm–diameter (wider) midsection is used to enlarge the osteotomy site at the coronal end, thus facilitating the insertion of the subsequent drill in the sequence (see Fig. 78.3D).

3-mm Twist Drill

The final drill in the osteotomy site preparation for a standard-diameter (4-mm) implant is the 3-mm twist drill. It is the last drill used to widen the site along the entire depth of the osteotomy from the previous diameter (2 mm) to final diameter (3 mm). This final drill in the sequence finishes preparing the osteotomy site and consequently

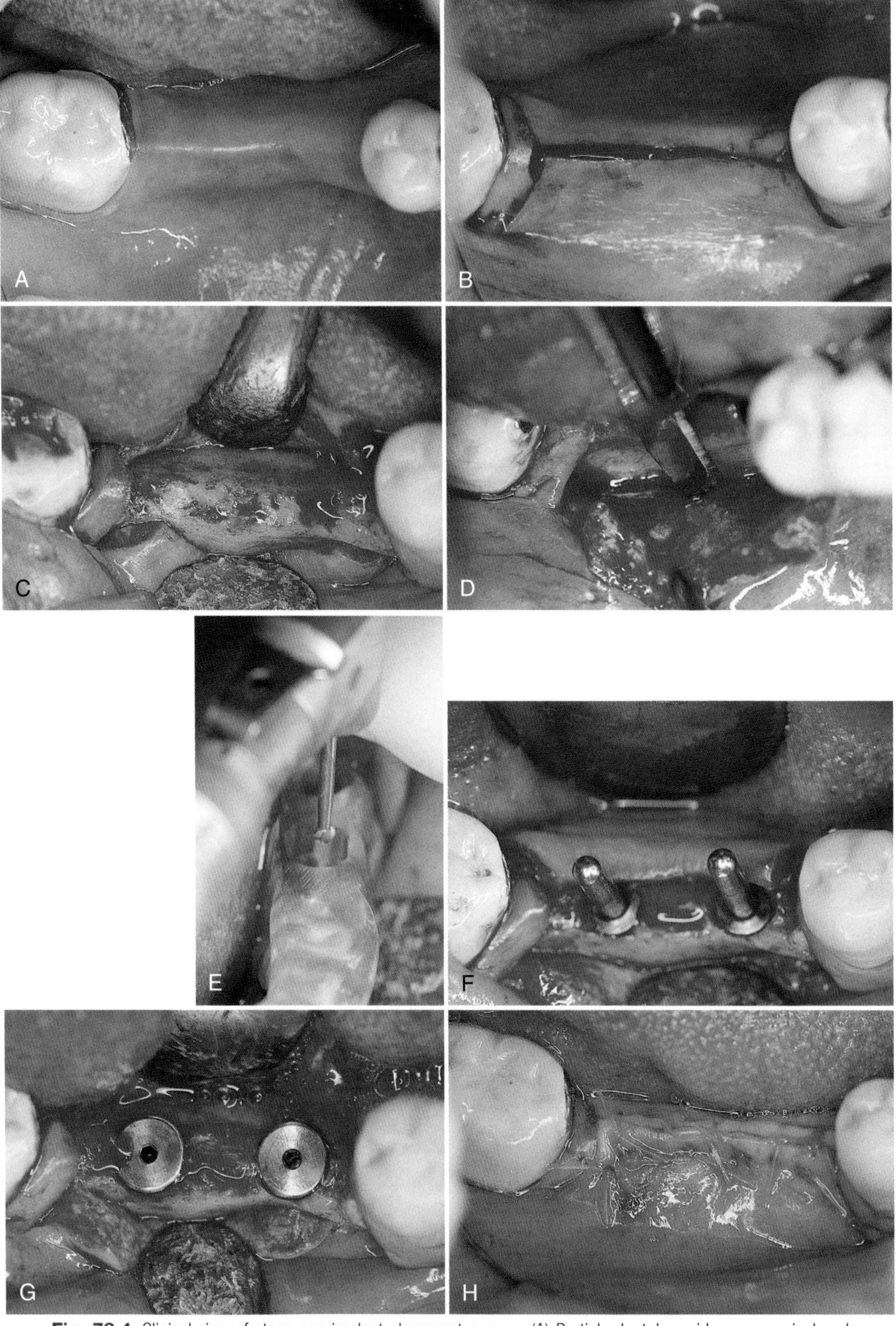

Fig. 78.4 Clinical view of stage-one implant placement surgery. (A) Partial edentulous ridge; presurgical and prosthodontic treatment has been completed. (B) Mesial sulcular and distal vertical incisions are connected by a crestal incision. Notice that bands of gingival collars remain adjacent to the distal molar tooth. (C) Minimal flap reflection is used to expose the alveolar bone. Sometimes a ridge modification is necessary to provide a flap recipient bed. (D) Buccal flap is partially dissected at the apical portion to provide a flap extension. This is a critical step to ensure a tension-free closure of the flap after implant placement. (E) It is important to use the surgical stent to determine the mesial-distal and buccal-lingual dimensions and proper angulation of the implant placement. (F) Frequent use of the guide pins ensures parallelism of the implant placement. (G) After placement of two Nobelpharma implants, the cover screws are placed. The cover screws should be flush with the rest of the ridge to minimize the chance of exposure. This is especially important if the patient will wear a partial denture during the healing phase. (H) Suturing completed. Both regular interrupted and inverted mattress sutures are used intermittently to ensure tension-free, tight closure of the flaps.

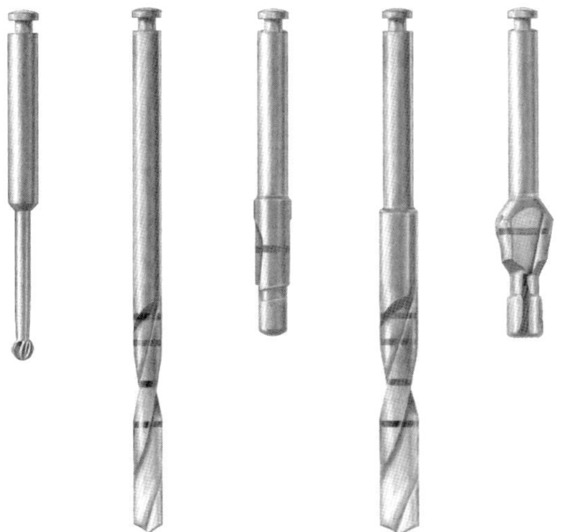

Fig. 78.5 Sequence of drills used for standard-diameter (4-mm) implant site osteotomy preparation: round, 2-mm twist, pilot, 3-mm twist, and countersink. Bone tap (not shown here) is an optional drill that is sometimes used in dense bone before implant placement.

is the step that dictates whether the implant will be stable or not (see Fig. 78.3E). It is critically important that the final diameter drilling be accomplished with a steady hand, without wobbling or changing direction so that the site is not overprepared. Finally, depending on bone density, the diameter of this final drill may be slightly increased or decreased to enhance implant support (see Box 78.2).

Countersink Drill (Optional)

When it is desirable to place the cover screw at or slightly below the crestal bone, countersink drilling is used to shape or flare the crestal aspect of the osteotomy site allowing the coronal flare of the implant head and cover screw to fit within the osteotomy site (see Fig. 78.3F). As with all drills in the sequence, copious irrigation and gentle surgical techniques are used.

Bone Tap (Optional)

As the final step in preparing the osteotomy site in dense cortical bone, a tapping procedure may be necessary (not shown on Fig. 78.3). With self-tapping implants being almost universal, there is less need for a tapping procedure in most sites. However, in dense cortical bone or when placing longer implants into moderately dense bone, it is prudent to tap the bone before implant placement to facilitate implant insertion and to reduce the risk of implant binding (see Fig. 78.3G).

CLINICAL CORRELATION

When faced with a very soft, poor-quality bone (e.g., loose trabecular bone in the posterior maxilla), tapping is not necessary or recommended (see Box 78.2). It is better to allow the threaded implant to "cut" its own path into the osteotomy site.

Bone tapping and implant insertion are both done at very slow speeds (e.g., 20–40 rpm). All other drills in the sequence are used at higher speeds (800–1500 rpm).

It is important to create a recipient site that is accurate in size and angulation. In partially edentulous cases, limited jaw opening or proximity to adjacent teeth may prevent appropriate positioning of the drills in posterior edentulous areas. In fact, implant therapy may be contraindicated in some patients because of a lack of interocclusal clearance, lack of interdental space, or a lack of access for the instrumentation. Therefore, a combination of longer drills and shorter drills, with or without extensions, may be necessary. Anticipating these needs before surgery facilitates the procedure and improves the results.

BOX 78.2 Clinical Advice to Enhance Precision of Final Implant Site Preparation

Clinical Situation 1

If the final drill stops advancing in the apical direction before reaching the desired depth, the added hand pressure necessary to achieve the proper depth can cause wobbling and funneling of the recipient site. This is especially true with "cannon" drills (used for cylindric implants). To minimize this effect, a smaller diameter drill should be used to prepare the site slightly deeper (e.g., ≤0.5 mm). This narrower drill allows the desired depth to be reached without affecting the side walls and facilitates a more precise osteotomy preparation with the final drill. It is also important to use drills that are sharp, especially for dense bone.

Clinical Situation 2

If the final drill is inserted at an inaccurate angle, the result is funneling of the coronal portion of the implant site. To minimize this potential problem, when drilling multiple implant sites, the operator should always keep a direction indicator in an adjacent site. For single-implant sites, the adjacent teeth and surgical guide should serve as direction indicators. When dealing with dense bone, a precise recipient site can be achieved more predictably if there is minimal diameter change from drill to drill. For example, switching from 3 to 5 mm is much less precise than proceeding from 3 to 3.3 mm to 4.2 to 5 mm.

Clinical Situation 3

If the bone is "soft" (e.g., loose trabecular bone), it may be advantageous to underprepare the osteotomy site. A slightly underprepared site can be accomplished by using the final drill to a shallower depth than the previous drill (e.g., half the depth of the osteotomy site). This avoids removing too much bone and increases the implant stability or tightness at the time of placement. Another method to achieve an underprepared site is to use a drill with a slightly smaller diameter as the final drill in the preparation (e.g., a 2.75-mm drill as the final drill rather than a 3-mm or 3.25-mm version as the final drill for a 4-mm implant).

CLINICAL CORRELATION

In areas with loose trabecular bone, such as the posterior maxilla, it may not be necessary to tap the site. If bone is especially loose, it may be beneficial to underprepare the site. For example, the final drill could be omitted to increase the implant stability.

Implant Placement

Implants are inserted with a handpiece rotating at slow speeds (e.g., 25 rpm) or by hand with a wrench. Insertion of the implant must follow the same path or line as the osteotomy site. When multiple implants are being placed, it is helpful to use guide pins in the other sites to have a visual guide for the path of insertion.

Flap Closure and Suturing

Once the implants are inserted and the cover screws secured (see Fig. 78.4G), the surgical sites should be thoroughly irrigated with sterile saline to remove debris and clean the wound. Proper closure of the flap over the implant is essential. One of the most important aspects of flap management is achieving good approximation and primary closure of the tissues in a tension-free manner (see Fig. 78.3H). This is achieved by incising the periosteum (innermost layer of full-thickness flap), which is nonelastic. Once the periosteum is released, the flap becomes very elastic and is able to be stretched over the implant without tension. This is essential when using a healing abutment to "tent" up the soft tissue. One suturing technique that consistently provides the desired result is a combination of alternating horizontal mattress and interrupted sutures (see Fig. 78.4H). Horizontal mattress sutures evert the wound edges and approximate the inner, connective tissue surfaces of the flap to facilitate closure and wound healing. Interrupted sutures help to bring the wound edges together, counterbalancing the eversion caused by the horizontal mattress sutures.

The clinician should choose an appropriate suture for the given patient and procedure. For patient management, it is sometimes simpler to use a resorbable suture that does not require removal during the postoperative visit (e.g., 4-0 chromic gut suture). However, when moderate-to-severe postoperative swelling is anticipated, a nonresorbable suture is recommended to maintain a longer closure period (e.g., 4-0 monofilament suture). These sutures require removal at a postoperative visit.

Postoperative Care

Simple implant surgery in a healthy patient usually does not require therapy. However, antibiotics (e.g., amoxicillin, 500 mg three times a day [tid]) can be prescribed if the surgery is extensive or if the patient is medically compromised. Postoperative swelling is likely after flap surgery. This is particularly true when the periosteum has been incised (released). As a preventive measure, patients should apply cold packs over the first 24 to 48 hours. Chlorhexidine gluconate oral rinses can be prescribed to facilitate plaque control, especially in the days after surgery when oral hygiene is typically poorer. Adequate pain medication should be prescribed (e.g., ibuprofen, 600–800 mg tid).

Patients should be instructed to maintain a relatively soft diet after surgery. Then, as healing progresses, they can gradually return to a normal diet. Patients should also refrain from tobacco and alcohol use after surgery. Provisional restorations, whether fixed or removable, should be checked and adjusted to minimize trauma to the surgical area.

Second-Stage Exposure Surgery

For implants placed using a two-stage "submerged" protocol, a second-stage exposure surgery is necessary. Box 78.3 lists the objectives for second-stage implant exposure surgery. The need for a zone of keratinized tissue surrounding implants is desirable; one long-term study indicated that the presence of keratinized tissue is strongly correlated with soft and hard tissue health.[2]

Simple Circular "Punch" or Crestal Incision

In areas with sufficient zones of keratinized tissue, the gingiva covering the head of the implant can be exposed with a circular or "punch" incision (Fig. 78.6). Alternatively, a crestal incision

BOX 78.3 Objectives of Second-Stage Implant Surgery

1. To expose the submerged implant without damaging the surrounding bone
2. To control the thickness of the soft tissue surrounding the implant
3. To preserve or create attached keratinized tissue around the implant
4. To facilitate oral hygiene
5. To ensure proper abutment seating
6. To preserve soft tissue esthetics

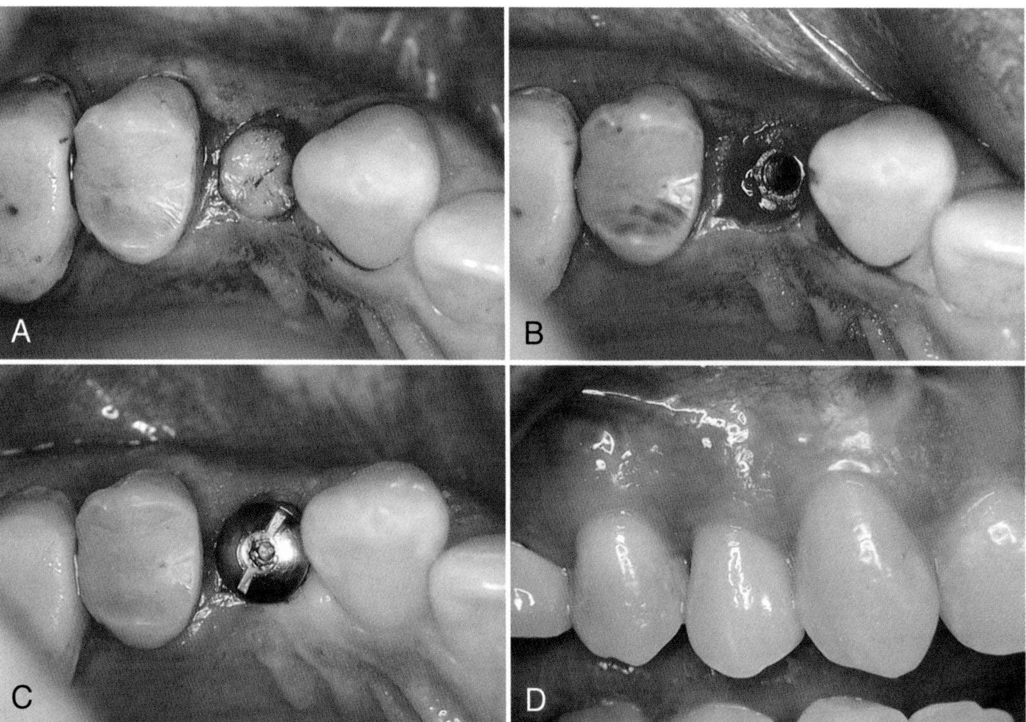

Fig. 78.6 Clinical view of second-stage implant exposure surgery in a case with adequate keratinized tissue. (A) Simple circular "punch" incision used to expose implant when sufficient keratinized tissue is present around the implant. (B) Implant exposed. (C) Healing abutment attached. (D) Final restoration in place, achieving an esthetic result with a good zone of keratinized tissue.

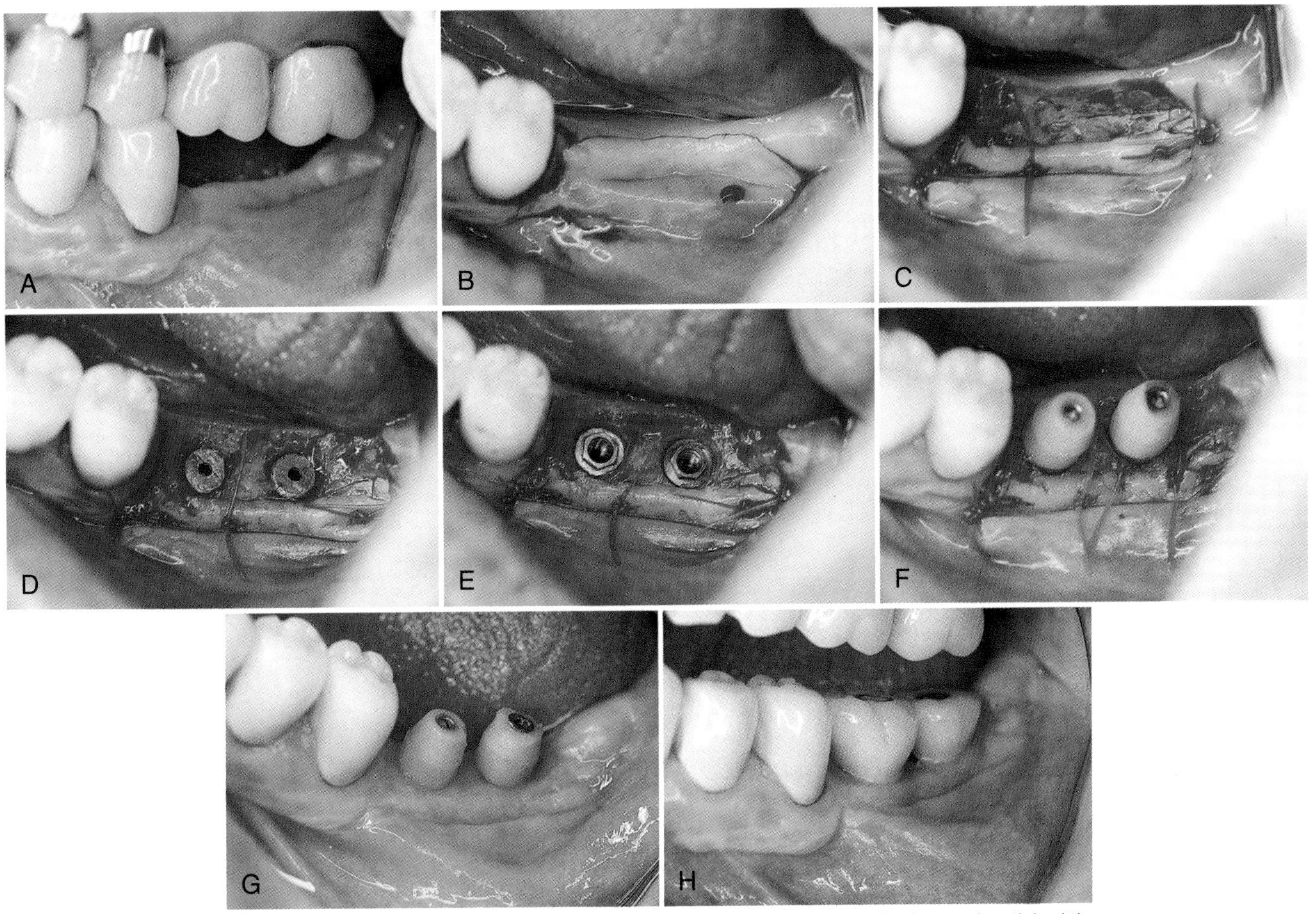

Fig. 78.7 Clinical view of second-stage implant exposure surgery in a case with inadequate keratinized tissue. (A) Two endosseous implants were placed 4 months previously and are ready to be exposed. Note the narrow band of keratinized tissue. (B) Two vertical incisions are connected by a crestal incision. If facial keratinized tissue is insufficient, it is necessary to locate the crestal incision more lingually so that there is at least 2 to 3 mm of keratinized band. (C) Buccal partial-thickness flap is sutured to the periosteum apical to the emerging implants. (D) Gingival tissue coronal to the cover screws is excised using the gingivectomy technique. (E) Cover screws are removed, and heads of the implants are cleared. (F) Abutments are placed. Visual inspection ensures intimate contact between the abutments and implants. (G) Healing at 2 to 3 weeks after second-stage surgery. (H) Four months after the final restoration. Note the healthy band of keratinized attached gingiva around the implants.

through the middle of the keratinized tissue and full-thickness flap reflection can be used to expose implants.

Partial-Thickness Repositioned Flap

If a minimal zone of keratinized tissue exists at the implant site, a partial-thickness flap technique can be used to fulfill the objective of the second-stage surgery (exposing the implant) while increasing the width of keratinized tissue. The initial incision is made within the zone of keratinized tissue so that it becomes the outer edge of the reflected split-thickness flap. Vertical releasing incisions are used on both the mesial and distal ends of the flap (Fig. 78.7A, B). A partial-thickness flap is then raised in so that a nonmobile firm periosteum remains attached to the underlying bone. The flap, containing a narrow band of keratinized tissue, is then repositioned to the facial side of the emerging head of the implant and sutured to the periosteum with a fine needle and resorbable suture, such as a 5-0 gut suture (Fig. 78.8). If the initial amount of keratinized tissue is less than 2 mm, the flap may be started at the labial edge of the keratinized tissue, thus allowing that zone to remain on the lingual aspect of the implant. A partial-thickness flap is apically displaced and sutured to the periosteum without exposing the alveolar bone (see Fig. 78.7C). A free gingival graft may be harvested from the palate and sutured to the periosteum on

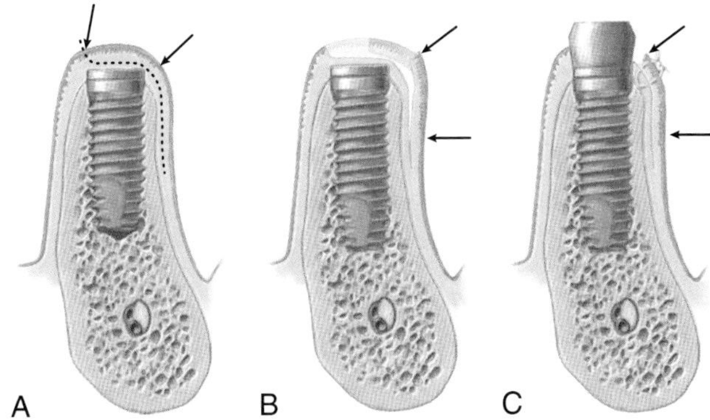

Fig. 78.8 Illustration of the use of a split-thickness flap that is repositioned to the labial surface to preserve and increase the amount of keratinized tissue. (A) Partial-thickness flap is created from the lingual aspect of the crest toward the labial surface to preserve the keratinized tissue on the crest (over the implant). Note: This tissue might be excised in a simple implant exposure. (B) The split-thickness flap is repositioned to the labial surface. (C) The flap is sutured to the periosteum at a more apical position preserving the amount of keratinized tissue *(arrows)*. Finally, the remaining connective tissue over the cover screw (B) is excised with a sharp blade to expose the implant. Care should be taken to avoid removing keratinized tissue from the lingual aspect of the implant.

the labial surface of the implants to increase the zone of keratinized tissue (not shown).

After the flap is repositioned and secured with periosteal sutures, the excess tissue coronal to the cover screw is excised, usually with a surgical blade (see Fig. 78.3B). However, if removal of this tissue would jeopardize the amount of remaining keratinized tissue around the lingual aspect of the implant, a similar partial-thickness flap can be elevated and repositioned on the lingual side as well. Extra care must be taken when creating a split-thickness flap on the lingual surface of mandibular sites because the tissue is often very thin. Alternatively, a full-thickness lingual flap will be safer and will serve a similar purpose of preserving keratinized tissue on the lingual surface of the implant.

A sharp blade is used to eliminate all tissues coronal to the cover screw (see Fig. 78.7D). The cover screw is then removed, the head of the implant is thoroughly cleaned of any soft or hard tissue overgrowth, and the healing abutments or standard abutments are placed on the implant (see Fig. 78.7E and F). The fit of the healing abutments to the implants can often be evaluated visually. However, if it is not possible to visualize the intimate connection between the implant and abutment clearly, an intraoral periapical x-ray film should be taken to confirm complete seating. Bone may need to be removed around the top of the implant to get the abutment to seat properly. Readers are referred to online material for a discussion of bone profiling.

KEY FACT

In sites with limited keratinized tissue, a partial-thickness flap can be used to preserve and reposition the keratinized tissue. A partial-thickness flap is apically displaced and sutured to the periosteum. In cases without keratinized tissue, a free gingival graft may be harvested from the palate and sutured to the periosteum on the labial surface of the implants to increase the zone of keratinized tissue.

Postoperative Care

Once the implant is exposed and soft tissues are sutured, it is important to remind the patient of the need for good oral hygiene around the implant and adjacent teeth. Care should be taken during oral hygiene procedures to avoid dislodging any repositioned or grafted soft tissues. Direct pressure or movement directed toward the soft tissue from a provisional prosthesis can delay healing and should be avoided. Tissues should be monitored regularly, and the provisional prosthesis should be adjusted as needed. Impressions for the final prosthesis fabrication can begin about 2 to 6 weeks after implant exposure surgery, depending on healing and maturation of soft tissues. Fig. 78.7G and H show the postoperative results in a clinical case after 2 to 3 weeks and 4 months, respectively.

One-Stage "Nonsubmerged" Implant Placement

In the one-stage implant surgical approach, a second implant exposure surgery is not needed because the implant is exposed (per gingival) from the time of implant placement (Fig. 78.9). In the standard (classic) implant protocol, the implants are left unloaded and undisturbed for a period similar to that for implants placed in the two-stage approach; that is, in areas with dense cortical bone and good initial implant support, the implants are left to heal undisturbed for a period of 2 to 4 months, whereas in areas of loose trabecular bone, grafted sites, or minimal implant support, they may be allowed to heal for a periods of 4 to 6 months or longer.

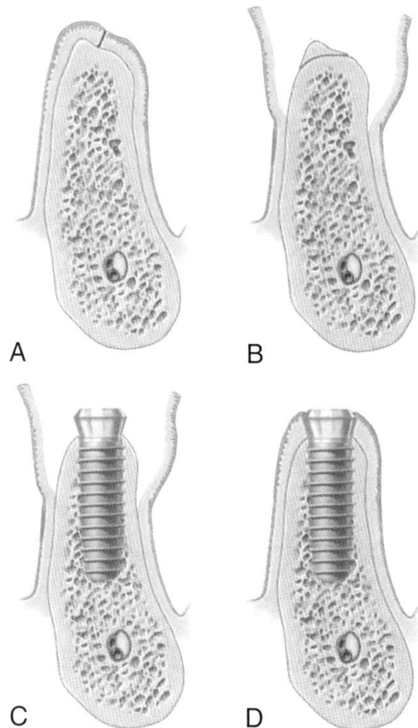

Fig. 78.9 Tissue management for a one-stage implant placement. (A) Crestal incision made along the crest of the ridge, bisecting the existing zone of keratinized mucosa. (B) Full-thickness flap is raised buccally and lingually to the level of the mucogingival junction. A narrow sharp ridge can be surgically reduced or contoured to provide a reasonably flat bed for the implant. (C) Implant is placed in the prepared osteotomy site. (D) Tissues are adapted around the neck of the implant to achieve flap closure, with the implant protruding through the soft tissues.

In the one-stage surgical approach, the implant or healing abutment protrudes approximately 2 to 3 mm from the bone crest, and the flaps are adapted around the implant/abutment. As with the second-stage surgical procedures described, the soft tissues may be thinned, repositioned, or augmented at the implant placement surgery to increase the zone of keratinized tissue surrounding the implant. Vertical soft tissue thickness can be augmented with an autogenous connective tissue graft or soft tissue allograft.

Flap Design, Incisions, and Elevation

The flap design for the one-stage surgical approach is always a crestal incision bisecting the existing keratinized tissue (see Fig. 78.9). Vertical incisions may be needed at one or both ends to facilitate access to the bone or osteotomy site. Tissues can be thinned in posterior areas if excessively thick (>4 mm), but are generally not thinned in anterior esthetic areas. Full-thickness flaps are elevated facially and lingually.

Implant Site Preparation

Implant site preparation for the one-stage approach is identical in principle to the two-stage implant surgical approach. The primary difference is that the coronal aspect of the implant or the healing abutment (two-stage implant) is placed approximately 2 to 3 mm above the bone crest and the soft tissues are approximated around the implant–implant abutment.

Flap Closure and Suturing

The keratinized edges of the flap are sutured with single interrupted sutures around the implant. Depending on the clinician's preference, the wound may be sutured with resorbable or nonresorbable sutures.

When keratinized tissue is abundant, scalloping around the implant provides better flap adaptation.

Postoperative Care

Postoperative care for the one-stage surgical approach is similar to that for the two-stage surgical approach except that the cover screw or healing abutment is exposed to the oral cavity. Patients are advised to avoid chewing in the area of the implant. Prosthetic appliances should not be used if direct chewing forces can be transmitted to the implant, particularly in the early healing period (first 4–8 weeks). When removable prosthetic appliances are used, they should be adequately relieved and a soft tissue liner should be applied.

Conclusions

It is essential to understand and follow basic guidelines to achieve osseointegration predictably. Fundamental protocols must be followed for implant placement (stage one) and implant exposure surgery (stage two). These fundamentals apply to all implant systems.

A Case Scenario is found on the companion website eBooks.Health.Elsevier.com.

Suggested Reading List

Adell R, Lekholm U, Rockler B, et al. A 15-year study of osseointegrated implants in the treatment of the edentulous jaw. *Int J Oral Surg.* 1981;10:387–416.

Brånemark PI, Adell R, Breine U, et al. Intra-osseous anchorage of dental prostheses. I. Experimental studies. *Scand J Plast Reconstr Surg.* 1969;3:81–100.

Brånemark PI, Hansson BO, Adell R, et al. Osseointegrated implants in the treatment of the edentulous jaw. Experience from a 10-year period. *Scand J Plast Reconstr Surg Suppl.* 1977;16:1–132.

Brunski JB. Biomechanics of oral implants: future research directions. *J Dent Educ.* 1988;52:775–787.

Hammerle CH, Bragger U, Burgin W, Lang NP. The effect of subcrestal placement of the polished surface of ITI implants on marginal soft and hard tissues. *Clin Oral Implants Res.* 1996;7:111–119.

Jaffin RA, Berman CL. The excessive loss of Brånemark fixtures in type IV bone: a 5-year analysis. *J Periodontol.* 1991;62:2–4.

Watanabe F, Tawada Y, Komatsu S, et al. Heat distribution in bone during preparation of implant sites: heat analysis by real-time thermography. *Int J Oral Maxillofac Implants.* 1992;7:212–219.

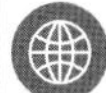
References for this chapter are found on the companion website eBooks.Health.Elsevier.com.

CHAPTER 79

Advanced Implant Surgical Procedures: Horizontal and Vertical Augmentation

Istvan A. Urban | Perry R. Klokkevold | David L. Cochran

For online-only content on staged and delayed implant placement, removal of implants, replacement of failed implants, and growth factors in bone augmentation, please visit the companion website at eBooks.Health.Elsevier.com.

An animation has been added by the editors as a supplement to the chapter. It was produced by PerioPixel as a patient education tool and covers the basic elements in a conceptual manner. It is not intended to be a procedural guide for dental professionals.

CHAPTER OUTLINE

Alveolar Ridge Preservation/Management of Extractions

Because tooth extraction (or loss) often results in alveolar ridge resorption or collapse, preservation of bone volume at the time of extraction is a desirable goal. Most bone loss after extraction occurs in the first 6 to 24 months.[14] Therefore when clinicians are afforded the opportunity to intervene at the time of extraction, preservation of alveolar bone should be initiated. A conservative approach to the management of extraction sites can eliminate or significantly reduce the necessity of advanced bone augmentation procedures.

When extracting a tooth and preparing for implant placement, alveolar bone resorption should be prevented or at least minimized. Experimental animal studies show that the use of a barrier membrane enhances the predictability of bone fill in the extraction site and therefore maintains original bone volume when compared with mucoperiosteal flap coverage alone.[7] Clinical studies also demonstrate the benefits of a regenerative approach to tooth extraction.[45,46,58] These authors found that a non-resorbable barrier membrane results in minimal resorption of alveolar ridge size and shape.

Although earlier studies have proposed the concept of treating extraction sites without flap closure (i.e., an exposed membrane used to cover the graft), more recent studies conclude that complete wound closure over the physical barrier might be associated with greater bone fill.[6,72] The decision about whether to advance a flap to achieve wound closure must be weighed against the soft-tissue changes that will be created (i.e., mucogingival junction discrepancies and esthetic problems) and that may require subsequent surgical correction.

The histologic assessment of allograft healing in extraction sockets has been reported.[2,9,15,28,89,92] In a series of clinical studies, the authors evaluated the quality of bone as well as the dimensions of alveolar ridge preservation with various comparison of allograft properties. Extraction sockets were non-molar sites that were grafted and allowed to heal for a prescribed amount of time. The alveolar dimensions were measured at the time of extraction and again at the time of implant placement. A core biopsy was harvested to assess the percentage of new bone formation, residual bone graft particles, and connective tissue/nonmineralized tissue. In a study[89] evaluating the timing of bone formation in sites grafted with demineralized freeze-dried bone allograft (DFDBA), it was determined that more new bone (47.41% vs. 32.63%) was formed in sites allowed to heal for a long term (18 to 20 weeks) as compared with sites that healed for a short term (8 to 10 weeks), respectively. Another study[2] evaluating new bone formation with mineralized allograft found no greater new bone formation (45% vs. 45.8%) by waiting longer (27 weeks) as compared with the shorter healing period (14 weeks), respectively. When demineralized allograft was compared with mineralized allograft, there was significantly more new bone formation in sites grafted with DFDBA (38.42%) than in sites grafted with freeze-dried bone allograft (FDBA) (24.63%).[92] The DFDBA group also had a significantly lower mean percentage of residual graft particles (8.88% vs. 25.42%). Finally, in another clinical study[28] comparing cortical versus cancellous FDBA, the authors found no difference in the percentage of new bone formation. There was a significantly greater percentage of residual bone graft particles in the cortical FDBA compared with the cancellous FDBA. Except for a great loss of lingual bone crest in the cancellous group of the latter study, none of the other studies found significant differences in clinical measurements between groups.

The timing of implant placement relative to the time of extraction has been widely debated. Depending on the quantity, quality, and support of existing bone, as well as the preferences of the clinician and patient, the placement of implants after tooth extraction can be immediate, delayed, or staged. By definition, *immediate* implant placement occurs at the time of extraction. Delayed implant placement is performed approximately 2 months after extraction to allow for soft-tissue healing. *Staged* implant placement allows for bone healing within the extraction site, which typically requires 4 to 6 months or longer.

Tooth extraction is managed with an atraumatic surgical technique that uses a narrow, flat instrument (e.g., Periotome, Hu-Friedy, Chicago) directed apically into the sulcus to sever the periodontal ligament and slightly expand the adjacent periodontal tissues. The tooth is elevated and removed with forceps using a gentle, rotational movement. Chapter 82 and 83 describe new techniques for atraumatic extraction. Buccolingual forces are avoided to prevent damaging the integrity of the labial bone. No incisions are made, and care is taken to avoid soft-tissue reflection. In this manner, soft tissues maintain their structural anatomy, and the periosteum (blood supply to the bone) remains intact. If the tooth has multiple roots, curved roots, or other anatomic features that make removal difficult, it may be necessary to cut the tooth using a high-speed rotary drill or other cutting device and remove it in smaller pieces. It is important to cut only tooth structure and avoid cutting (overheating) bone when using high-speed rotary drills. The bone within the extraction site is completely debrided of soft tissue with surgical curettes. After debridement, the extraction site is thoroughly irrigated with sterile saline. Finally, the clinician can evaluate the bone level and socket anatomy to determine whether to bone graft the site and when to place the implant (immediate, delayed, or staged placement).

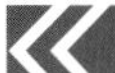

FLASH BACK

The timing of implant placement relative to the time of extraction has been widely debated. Historically, during the early period of osseointegrated implants, immediate or early implant placement was discouraged. Today, these early tenets are being challenged with immediate implant placement and immediate provisionalization.

Delayed Implant Placement

Delayed implant placement shares some advantages of immediate implant placement, including extraction site preservation, and offers additional advantages. Unlike immediate implant placement, which is deficient of soft tissue for coverage, the delayed implant placement technique allows time for soft-tissue healing to close the wound.[40] The delayed placement technique still reduces the length of treatment by a few months because it is not necessary to wait for complete bone healing. Furthermore, because bone formation is active within the first few months after tooth extraction, the delayed technique may facilitate more osteogenesis adjacent to the implant.

The primary advantage of delayed implant placement is that, by allowing for soft-tissue healing and closure of the extraction site, mucogingival flap advancement is not necessary. This alleviates the need for additional surgeries to correct mucogingival discrepancies. Delayed implant placement also allows time for the resolution of infections that may have been present within the extraction site.

As with immediate implant placement, similar limitations of bone support and implant stability exist for delayed placement. The normal osseous healing that occurs within the first 2 months does not significantly affect the anatomy of the alveolar bone. Therefore, limitations in bone support after 2 months of healing are similar to those that exist at the time of extraction.

Staged Implant Placement

Staged implant placement allows adequate time for osseous healing. This may be complete osseous healing of an extraction site without a bone graft (if circumferential bone support is good) or with a bone graft. Staged implant placement, by definition, allows for complete hard- and soft-tissue healing and permits the placement of implants into healed bone sites with adequate coverage by hard and soft tissues.[70] This eliminates the necessity of mucogingival flap advancement, allows for the resolution of preexisting infections, and prevents soft-tissue invasion. Furthermore, by using an extended healing period, the grafted bone also has the opportunity to become vascularized. Bone grafts performed simultaneously with implant placement do not share this advantage. The primary disadvantage of staged implant placement is the length of time required for bone healing.

Delayed Versus Staged Technique

Delayed and staged techniques for implant placement are demonstrated here in one individual using two extraction sites with similar bone morphologies in the anterior maxilla (eFig. 79.1). Both techniques facilitate the esthetic placement of implants into prosthetically driven positions. Delayed and staged approaches maintain alveolar bone volume, reduce the need for advanced bone augmentation, and eliminate the need for subsequent mucogingival surgery. The timing and management of delayed versus staged implant placement are described in the next section.

To decide which implant placement method to use, the quantity and location of bone surrounding the tooth should be assessed. Once the patient has been anesthetized, a periodontal probe can be used to "sound" for the level of bone support through the soft tissue. Using this method, the bone levels surrounding the tooth can be mapped. Bone support that surrounds the extraction site can also be evaluated and confirmed after tooth removal by palpation, probing, and direct (internal) visualization.

If the tooth to be extracted has sufficient bone support on all surfaces, the extraction site can be expected to fill with bone without additional augmentation procedures, except when the labial bone is very thin. A simple extraction followed by a healing period of 4 to 6 months could be sufficient for complete osseous healing. Subsequently, an implant could be placed in the usual manner without the need for bone augmentation. Conversely, if little or no bone exists on the labial surface, it should be anticipated that the site would require bone augmentation to facilitate placement of the implant. In this case, bone grafting at the time of extraction can be used to maintain the alveolar ridge dimensions occupied by the tooth.

Immediate Implant Placement

The primary advantage of immediate implant placement is the reduction of the healing time, which translates to an earlier restorative time (i.e., shorter time to completion for the patient).[51,56,69,91] Because the implant is placed at the time of extraction, the bone-to-implant healing begins immediately with extraction site healing. Another advantage is that the normal bone healing, which generally occurs within the extraction site, takes effect around the implant. This bone-forming activity may enhance the bone-to-implant contact compared with an implant placed in a site with less osteogenic activity.

Possible disadvantages of immediate implant placement include the need for subsequent mucogingival surgeries to correct tissues moved by repositioned flaps and the need for bone grafting to fill extraction site defects around the implant. If inadequate bone exists to stabilize the implant, immediate implant placement is not recommended.

When a two-stage implant is placed at the time of tooth extraction, the mucogingival flap is advanced, with releasing incisions, to cover the implant completely (an exception would be a one-stage implant). It may also be necessary to graft bone into the extraction site in areas that do not contact the implant to avoid soft-tissue invasion around the implant.[69] A 1-year study of 49 immediate extraction site implants treated by a membrane alone demonstrated a 93.6% bone fill. After 1 year (postloading), the implant success rate was 93.9%.[6]

Although some have advocated submerging implants placed in extraction sockets with flap advancement,[40] others have demonstrated success with a nonsubmerged approach. Implants may be placed in extraction sockets along with bone augmentation without flap advancement using a one-stage implant placement approach. Clinical studies evaluating the outcome of bone augmentation around implants placed in extraction sockets reveal good bone fill.[44]

The placement of 21 transmucosal implants in immediate extraction sites treated with a barrier membrane were tested for the implant success rate and the percentage of bone fill. Twenty of the twenty-one transmucosal implants yielded complete bone fill and coverage of the entire plasma-coated implant surface.

A clinical report on the use of resorbable collagen membranes around extraction site implants demonstrated a variable degree of bone fill in nine patients.[60] More clinical review of the use of resorbable membranes for guided bone regeneration (GBR) is required because evidence is insufficient to evaluate the predictability.

In a study of 30 patients, the use of autografts alone in 54 extraction sites was highly effective for simultaneously placed implants completely within the envelope of bone.[4] The study showed that extraction sites, including those with a buccal dehiscence, could be treated with autografts alone. However, because nongrafted sites were not included, the absolute need to graft small defects adjacent to implants was not ascertained by this study. In another study, implants placed in extraction sockets were tested for their potential to regenerate bone with allograft alone, a membrane alone, and a combination treatment.[32] Reentry confirmed 100% thread coverage in all but one implant in the "no-wall" group treated with DFDBA alone. A clinical study of five patients evaluated different treatment modalities for extraction site implants together with bone graft combinations.[72] This small study supported the concept that "non–space-making defects" are best treated with a combination of barrier membrane and an autograft or allograft as compared with treatment with a nonreinforced membrane alone (without a graft).

Immediate placement of an implant into the extraction socket in a one-stage approach along with immediate provisionalization is perhaps the best way to manage the hard and soft tissues following extraction (eFig. 79.2). The immediate placement of a provisional restoration is the best way to support the soft tissues (papilla and marginal gingiva) following tooth extraction.

Horizontal Bone Augmentation

A deficiency in the horizontal dimension of bone may be minimal, such as a dehiscence or fenestration of an implant surface, or it may be more significant, such that the prosthetically positioned implant would have more than one axial surface exposed while having some bone support along the entire vertical length. Dehiscence or fenestration defects can usually be managed simultaneously with implant placement because most of the implant is covered and stabilized by native bone. If the horizontal deficiency is large and the implant placement would result in significant exposure (i.e., implant body is significantly outside the alveolar bone), it may be better to reconstruct the bone first, in a staged approach, with a subsequent surgery for implant placement.

Guided Bone Regeneration

Much of what can be achieved with implant surgery and specifically with bone augmentation procedures is directly related to the fundamental concept of GBR. Historically, augmentation or "regeneration" of alveolar bone that was lost following tooth removal, or from alveolar bone resorption or traumatic injury, presented a significant challenge for clinicians. Allowed to heal without the intervention of regenerative procedures, extraction site defects (especially those lacking a self-supporting bone structure) heal with fibrous connective tissue or scar formation and may not fill completely with bone. The surrounding soft tissues collapse into the bone defect, leaving an alveolar ridge deficiency. Over time, the alveolar ridge continues to resorb, especially when removable prosthetic appliances are used.

Periodontal studies during the last several decades have led to new techniques and a new treatment approach referred to as guided tissue regeneration (GTR). Briefly, this concept is based on the principle that specific cells contribute to the formation of specific tissues.[20,80] Exclusion of the faster-growing epithelium and connective tissue from a periodontal wound for a minimum of 6 to 8 weeks allows the slower-growing tissues to occupy the space adjacent to the tooth. Osteoblasts, cementoblasts, and periodontal ligament cells are then afforded the opportunity to regenerate a new periodontal attachment (defined by new bone and new connective tissue fibers inserted into newly formed cementum) on the previously diseased root surface.

The same basic principle of GTR has been applied to alveolar bone defects to regenerate new bone.[21] Using a canine model, Schenk and colleagues[63] demonstrated with histology that bone regeneration in membrane-protected defects healed in a sequence of steps that simulated bone formation after tooth extraction. They found that after blood clot formation, bone regeneration was initiated by the formation of woven bone initially along new blood vasculature at the periphery of the defect. The new vascular supply emanated from the existing bone bed (recipient site). Cortical perforations surgically created in the recipient site are thought to enhance the blood supply and cellular access to the bone grafted area. The woven bone, which is formed quickly with a disorganized, immature structure, was subsequently replaced by lamellar bone with an organized, mature structure. Over time, bone remodeling continued with new, secondary osteons being formed.

This concept employed the same principles of specific tissue exclusion but was not associated with teeth. Rather, it was space maintenance for bone formation that was being isolated from the surrounding soft tissues. Thus, the term applied to this technique was GBR. Because the objective of GBR is to regenerate a single tissue, namely bone, it is theoretically easier to accomplish than GTR, which strives to regenerate multiple tissues simultaneously in a complex relationship.

Interestingly, long before the current concepts of GBR were introduced, Murray and coworkers[57] demonstrated that when a cavity with a source of osteoblasts and a blood supply was isolated from adjacent soft tissues, it could fill with bone, whereas if the space were not protected, it would fill with fibrous connective tissue. In addition to this observation, they suggested that a bone graft placed in the space might interfere with bone formation because the graft would need to be resorbed before bone could occupy the space.

Bone is a unique tissue that has the capacity to regenerate itself completely. Because of its rigid calcified structure, however, bone has specific requirements that must be respected to achieve regeneration. Because the calcified structure of bone is not conducive to perfusion, new bone formation is critically dependent on establishing an adequate blood supply through the ingrowth of new vasculature while maintaining rigid fixation or stabilization for bone formation. Any movement of the segments of bone relative to one another (even micromotion) during healing results in disruption of the blood supply and a change in the type of tissue formed in the site from mineralized bone to fibrous connective tissue. Table 79.1 lists the biologic requirements for bone regeneration and the associated component of GBR surgical procedures needed to accomplish it.

Barrier Membranes

Barrier membranes are biologically inert materials that protect the blood clot and prevent soft-tissue cells (epithelium and connective tissue) from migrating into the bone defect, allowing osteogenic cells the opportunity to occupy and fill the site with bone. Membranes have been manufactured from biocompatible materials that are either non-resorbable or resorbable. The ideal properties of a barrier membrane are (1) biocompatibility, (2) space maintenance,

TABLE 79.1 Biologic Requirements for Bone Regeneration

Requirement	Surgical Procedure
Blood supply	Cortical perforations
Stabilization	Fixation screws, membrane tacks
Osteoblasts	Autogenous bone (graft or recipient site)
Confined space	Barrier membrane
Space maintenance	Tenting screws, bone graft materials
Wound coverage	Flap management, tension-free suturing

(3) cell occlusive, (4) good handling properties, and (5) either resorbable or ease of removal if non-resorbable. Advantages and disadvantages of the resorbable versus non-resorbable membranes are outlined below.

Non-resorbable Barrier Membranes

Various non-resorbable materials have been used as barrier membranes, including latex and Teflon. Teflon, an expanded polytetrafluoroethylene membrane (ePTFE, Gore-Tex Periodontal and Bone Regenerative Membranes, Gore and Associates, Flagstaff, Arizona), has been used extensively as a barrier membrane in both GTR and GBR procedures. A variety of shapes and sizes have been designed to be custom-fit around teeth and osseous defects. These barrier membranes are non-resorbable and thus require a subsequent surgical procedure to remove them. The advantage of a non-resorbable barrier membrane is its ability to maintain separation of tissues over an extended time period. Unless the barrier is exposed, it can remain in place for several months to years. Typically, non-resorbable GBR membranes are removed after 6 to 12 months. Clinical example of a ridge augmentation using a non-resorbable membrane is demonstrated in Fig. 79.1.

The disadvantage of a non-resorbable barrier membrane is that if it becomes exposed, it will not heal (i.e., wound will remain open) spontaneously and may become progressively more exposed. Exposed membranes become contaminated with oral bacteria, which may lead to infection of the site and result in bone loss. Therefore, exposed membranes must be removed. Contamination or early removal may also result in less bone regeneration.

Space can be maintained under a barrier membrane with bone graft material or tenting screws, thereby facilitating the regeneration of increased bone volume. Titanium-reinforced (TR) membranes are stiffer with space-maintaining capabilities that can regenerate bone without the need for bone grafts or a tenting apparatus.[52,63] Stiffer membranes are able to promote significant amounts of new bone and maintain sufficient space without the addition of supportive devices. Ridge augmentation can be enhanced with a TR membrane in conjunction with implant placement in localized bone defects.[42]

Resorbable Barrier Membranes

The use of resorbable barrier membranes continues to attract widespread interest, primarily because they eliminate the need for an additional surgery to remove them. Copolymers of polylactide and polyglycolide have been used to construct biodegradable membranes. Today, collagen-based resorbable barrier membranes are used extensively. The primary advantage of a resorbable membrane is the elimination of surgical reentry for membrane removal. In the case of a subsequent implant placement procedure (or exposure surgery), this may not be a significant advantage. The other advantage is that resorbable membranes are less likely to become exposed and are less problematic if they do become exposed because they get resorbed and do not usually need to be removed.

A possible disadvantage is that many resorbable membranes degrade before bone formation is completed, and the degradation process may produce varying degrees of inflammation.[95] Developments in resorbable membrane technology include cross-linking of collagen to increase resistance to biodegradation and thus increase longevity of the barrier function.[30] Fortunately, the mild inflammatory reaction caused by bioresorbable membranes does not seem to interfere with osteogenesis. Another disadvantage is that resorbable barrier membranes are quite pliable. The lack of stiffness often results in collapse of the membrane into the defect area.[62] Thus, resorbable membranes are best suited for situations that allow the graft material or hardware (tenting screws, plates) or the adjacent alveolar bone to maintain the desired dimensions.

Human histology has demonstrated that resorbable barrier membranes support the growth of new bone when used in GBR procedures for horizontal, vertical, sinus, and extraction socket def ects.[31,33,53] They have also been shown to reduce bone resorption when used over a monocortical bone block to augment horizontally deficient ridges.[93] Geurs and colleagues[33] demonstrated that a bioabsorbable barrier membrane, used in a GBR procedure along with an allograft, was able to facilitate new bone formation. At present, it can be stated that biodegradable membranes have the potential to facilitate bone formation if they are supported by a bone graft material to resist collapse in small to moderate bone defects.[48,49]

Bone Graft Materials

Unlike other tissues, bone has the unique capacity to completely regenerate itself. The major limiting factors are maintenance of space and structure for bone formation. Bone graft materials have been used to facilitate bone formation within a given space by occupying that space and allowing the subsequent bone ingrowth (and graft replacement) to take place on the structure. The biologic mechanisms that support the use of bone graft materials are osteoconduction, osteoinduction, and osteogenesis.

Osteoconduction is the formation of bone by osteoblasts from the margins of the defect on the bone graft material. Materials that are osteoconductive serve as a scaffold for bone growth. They neither inhibit nor induce bone formation. They simply allow the normal formation of bone by osteoblasts into the grafted defect along the surface of the graft material. Osteoconductive bone graft materials facilitate bone formation by bridging the gap between the existing bone and a distant location that otherwise would not be occupied by bone.

Osteoinduction involves new bone formation through stimulation of osteoprogenitors from the defect (or from the vasculature) to differentiate into osteoblasts and begin forming new bone. This induction of the bone-forming process by cells that would otherwise remain inactive occurs through cell mediators that "turn on" these bone-forming cells. The most widely studied of these mediators is the family of bone morphogenic proteins (BMPs).

Osteogenesis occurs when living osteoblasts are part of the bone graft, as in autogenous bone transplantation. Given an adequate blood supply and cellular viability, these transplanted osteoblasts form new centers of ossification within the graft. Thus, in addition to the bone formation from osteoblasts that already exist in the defect, osteoblasts added as part of the bone graft also form ossification centers and contribute to the total capacity for bone formation.

Numerous bone graft materials have been used to aid in the reconstruction of bone defects. These range from allografts (derived

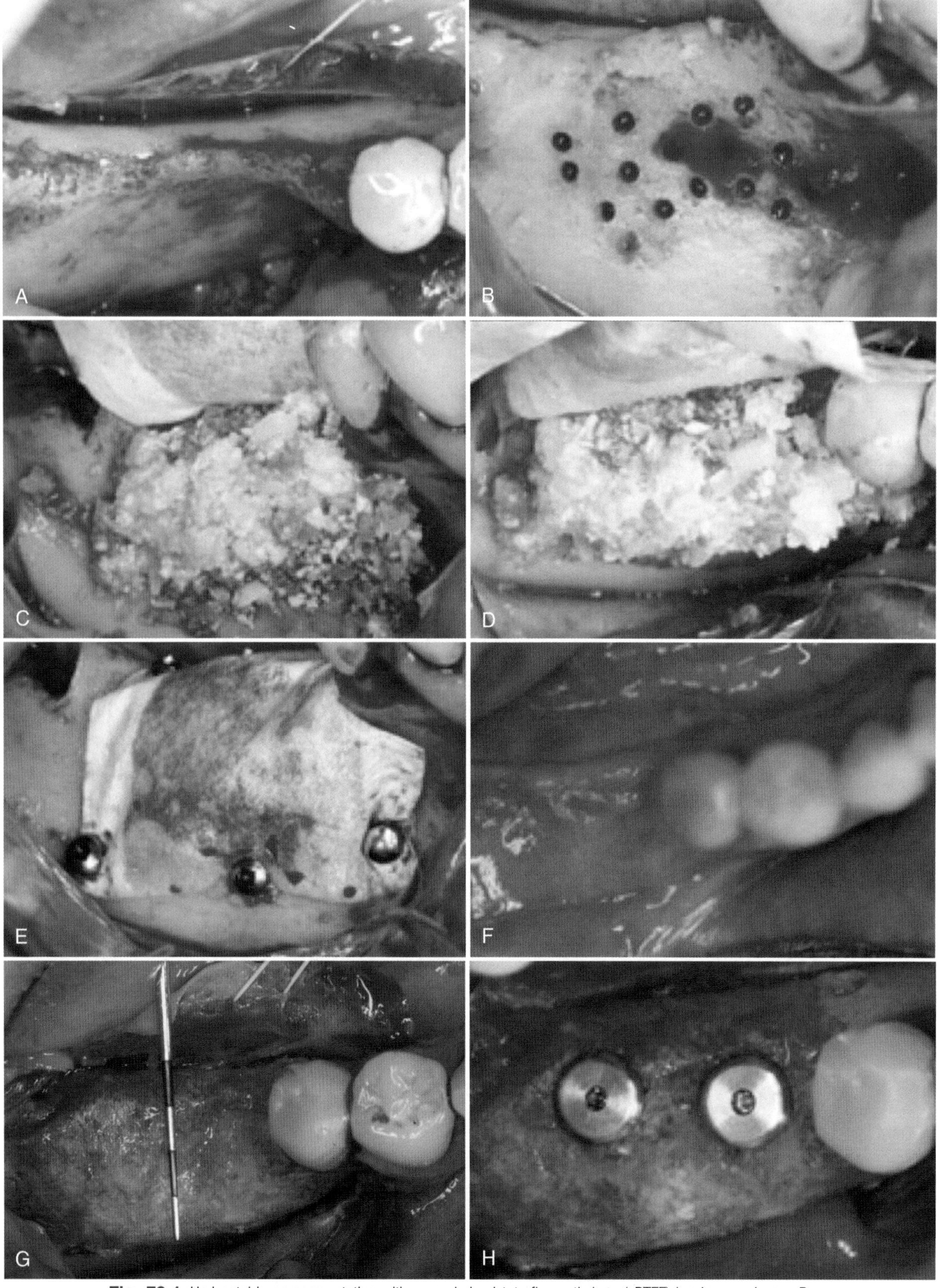

Fig. 79.1 Horizontal bone augmentation with expanded polytetrafluoroethylene (ePTFE) barrier membrane. Bone graft consists of a mixture of autogenous particles harvested from the alveolar ridge and Bio-Oss (Osteohealth Company, Luitpold Pharmaceuticals, Inc., Shirley, New York). (A) Partially edentulous posterior mandible with narrow buccolingual dimensions. (B) Cortical perforations made in buccal bone with small round bur to enhance blood supply to the grafted area. (C) Placement of ePTFE barrier membrane and mixture of autogenous and Bio-Oss particulate bone graft. (D) View of part C from occlusal perspective to visualize horizontal augmentation. (E) Barrier membrane secured to native bone with fixation screws. (F) Clinical photograph of healed site prior to membrane removal. Soft-tissue closure maintained throughout healing without membrane exposure. (G) Clinical photograph of healed ridge after membrane removal. Dimensions of alveolar ridge are significantly wider as demonstrated with periodontal probe. (H) Two standard-diameter implants placed in a "prosthetically driven" ideal position. Notice there are no implant exposures.

TABLE 79.2 Biologic Properties of Various Bone Graft Materials

Source	Osteoconductive	Osteoinductive	Osteogenic
Alloplast	Yes	No	No
Xenograft	Yes	No	No
Allograft	Yes	Yes/no?	No
Autograft	Yes	Yes	Yes

from the same species) to xenografts (derived from a different species) and alloplast or synthetic graft materials. At a minimum, bone graft materials should be osteoconductive. Bone graft materials that are also osteoinductive are believed to be more advantageous than those that are only osteoconductive. Table 79.2 lists the properties of different classes of bone graft materials.

DFDBA is thought to have osteoinductive effects because viable BMPs within the donor tissue matrix are exposed by the decalcification process.[85] In contrast to this view, more recent reports suggest that bone augmentation with DFDBA is not osteoinductive because it does not contain the BMPs necessary to induce bone formation.[5,8] Schwartz and coworkers[65] reported that variations in the amount of bone formation induced by BMPs in DFDBA may be related to the source (i.e., donor tissue) of the bone and the techniques used to process it. In addition to processing variations, it has been demonstrated that young donor bone results in significantly greater quantities of BMPs retained in the bone allograft matrix compared with older donor bone.[66] Therefore, the source of donor bone can greatly influence its osteoinductive capacity.

Bone graft materials help maintain space under a barrier membrane to facilitate the formation of bone within a confined space. Perhaps more importantly, bone graft materials should facilitate neovascularization and the migration of osteoblasts and osteoprogenitors. Because the size of the bone graft particles determines the resultant space available (between particles) for osseous formation, particle size has been carefully selected according to this concept. The typical size of bone graft particles ranges from 100 to 1000 μm, which is conducive to neovascularization and the ingrowth of bone. Bone forms in cones called osteons with a central blood supply. The dimension of these cones (100-μm radius) is determined by the limited distance of nutrient perfusion from the central vasculature supply of the osteon.

Autogenous Bone

Compared with other bone graft materials, autogenous bone is thought to be the best bone graft material because, in addition to being osteoconductive, it is osteoinductive and it also has the potential to be osteogenic. Furthermore, barring contamination, there is no risk of rejection or adverse reaction to the autogenous graft material. Intraoral sources of autogenous bone include edentulous spaces, maxillary tuberosity, mandibular ramus, mandibular symphysis, and extraction sites. Bone harvested from a recent extraction site (e.g., approximately 6 to 12 weeks healing) may have the advantage of increased osteogenic activity compared with other sites, which are more static and undergoing little or no osteogenesis. The maxillary tuberosity provides a more cellular source of autogenous bone compared with other sites. However, the trabecular nature of this site provides a lesser quantity of mineralized matrix, and the resultant total volume of bone available for grafting is often inadequate. For greater amounts of bone, it is more desirable to harvest bone from the mandibular ramus or symphysis. This bone, which is typically more cortical, can be harvested and used as a monocortical block graft (Video 79.1) or it can be ground or shaved into small fragments and used as a particulate graft.

Although the mandibular ramus and symphysis offer good sources of bone for grafting, clinicians are sometimes reluctant to harvest bone from these sites because of an increased risk of morbidity from the surgical procedure. Risks of surgery in the mandibular symphysis region include postoperative bleeding, bruising, wound dehiscence, damage to lower incisors, disfigurement, and injury to nerves. Nerve injury may be the most significant concern because it can be a long-term (possibly permanent), annoying alteration in sensation of the lower lip, chin, anterior teeth, and gingiva for the patient. A more serious risk is the alteration of facial appearance, particularly when the facial muscles are completely elevated from the bone beyond the inferior border of the mandible. A condition referred to as "witch's chin" can occur when the facial muscles and overlying skin of the chin fall, causing a disfiguring sag of facial tissues after surgery.

A retrospective analysis of 48 chin graft–harvesting procedures suggests that maintaining a 5-mm margin of safety between graft harvest sites and vital structures (e.g., lower incisors, the inferior border of the chin, and the mental foramen) will minimize postoperative complications.[36] In the 48 procedures, postoperative sequelae included bruising of the lower face (48/48), bruising of the upper neck (6/48), and paresthesia of the lower lip and incisors (6/48). No patient experienced facial disfigurement or muscle prolapse (chin droop). Three of the six patients with paresthesia experienced transient symptoms and recovered completely within 2 months, whereas symptoms persisted longer than 6 months in the other three patients. Not surprisingly, the larger harvest defects (trephined six-ring sites) resulted in a higher incidence of paresthesia, which was longer lasting than that of the smaller defects (trephined four-ring sites). Harvesting bone in a custom-shaped "block" did not result in paresthesia, presumably because these harvest sites were smaller than the four-ring and six-ring trephine-harvested sites.

Monocortical Block Graft

Horizontal alveolar deficiencies that might be challenging to reconstruct with particulate grafts can easily be reconstructed with a monocortical block bone graft. The technique uses a cortical block of bone harvested from a remote site and used to increase the width of bone. The block graft taken from an intraoral (e.g., mandibular symphysis or ramus) or extraoral (e.g., iliac crest or tibia) site is fixated to the prepared recipient site with screws. The overlying soft tissues can be separated from the bone graft with a barrier membrane or simply covered with the mucoperiosteal flap. Fixation hardware (screws and plates) should be removed after an adequate period of healing (approximately 6 months). The disadvantage of this technique is the biologic limitation of revascularizing large bone blocks. It therefore is crucial to have sufficient osteogenic cells in the residual surface of the surrounding bone and to limit this technique to horizontal augmentation and only minimal vertical defects.

Fig. 79.2 shows the use of a monocortical block graft to reconstruct a horizontal deficiency in the posterior right mandible. The patient presented with a loss of the buccal cortical plate of bone after a traumatic extraction of endodontically treated tooth #29. The surgical extraction also resulted in an iatrogenic cut into the mesial root of tooth #30, rendering the tooth non-restorable. The recommended treatment included extraction of tooth #30, monocortical block graft reconstruction of the buccal defect at site #29, and bone augmentation of the extraction socket #30. The procedure for this case follows.

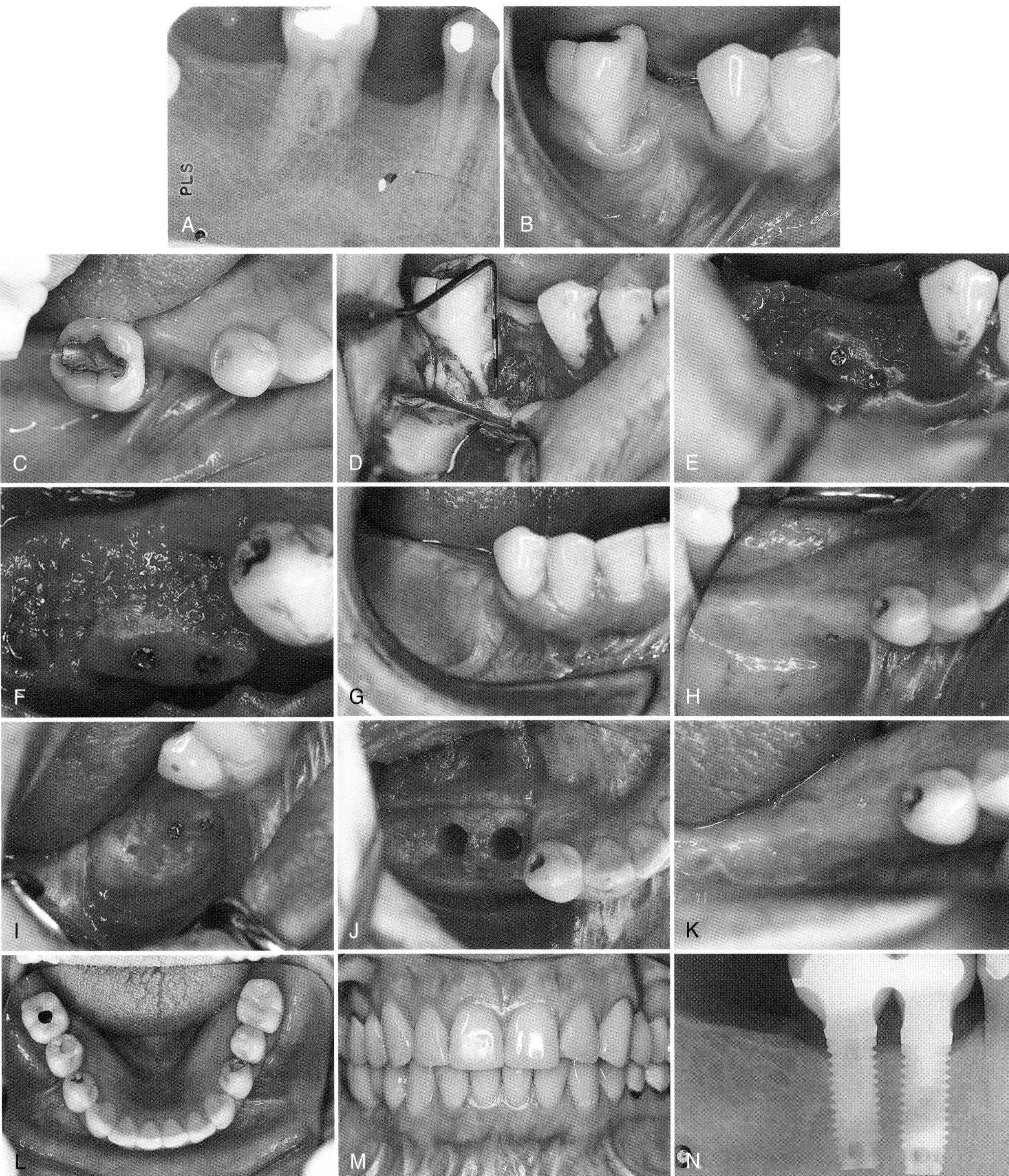

Fig. 79.2 Use of a monocortical block graft to reconstruct a horizontal deficiency in the posterior right mandible. (A) Periapical radiograph shows missing tooth #29 and damaged (i.e., cut) mesial root #30. (B and C) Labial and occlusal views, respectively, of site reveal deficient alveolar ridge on buccal side of #29. (D) Full-thickness flap reflection reveals the extent of missing bone in the buccal aspect of site #29, as well as the periodontal defect and damaged mesial root #30. (E and F) Autogenous monocortical bone block graft secured to native alveolar bone with fixation screws. (G) Good tissue healing after block graft, with evidence of a widened alveolar ridge. (H) After 6 months of healing, posterior fixation screw is observed protruding through the mucosa. (I) Full-thickness flap reveals that bone resorption has resulted in exposure of part of the fixation screw. (J) Osteotomy prepared for wide-diameter implants, taking care to avoid making the labial bone "graft" too thin. (K) Complete closure and good healing of wound after implant placement. (L and M) Clinical photographs of completed restorations. (N) Final radiograph shows good restoration contours on wide-diameter implants.

KEY FACT

Large horizontal alveolar deficiencies can be challenging to reconstruct with particulate grafts. In such a situation, it may be more manageable to use a monocortical block bone graft to reconstruct the area. The technique uses a cortical block of bone harvested from a remote site (e.g., mandibular symphysis or ramus) and fixated to the prepared recipient site with screws.

Procedure

Following local anesthesia, an incision was made in keratinized tissue along the crest and around the molar tooth (#30) with a vertical releasing incision mesial to the first bicuspid (#28). A full-thickness flap was elevated to expose the alveolar bone (see Fig. 79.2.D). All soft tissues were thoroughly removed from the recipient site before bone grafting. After simple forceps delivery of tooth #30, the defect to be grafted was measured to determine the size of block graft to harvest from the mandibular symphysis. Several bleeding points were created using a small round bur.

The autogenous monocortical block graft was harvested from the mandibular symphysis. It was cut to an appropriate size and mortised to intimately fit the recipient defect site. Once properly positioned, the graft was fixated with two fixation screws (Leibinger, Kalamazoo, Michigan) that passed through the graft and into the existing native alveolar bone. A periosteal releasing incision was used to sever the periosteum from anterior to posterior and facilitate coronal advancement of the mucogingival flap.

After 6 months of healing, a full-thickness mucoperiosteal flap was elevated to expose the alveolar bone sites #29 and #30. Mild resorption of the monocortical block graft is evident. Notice that the position of the head of the fixation screws (especially the posterior screw) is more prominent than the grafted bone as a consequence of bone remodeling and resorption (see Fig. 79.2H and I).

The fixation screws are removed, and the sites are prepared in the usual manner for the placement of two-screw type, wide-diameter implants (Implant Innovations, Palm Beach Gardens, Florida). Care is taken to avoid preparing the grafted site too wide or too far to the buccal surface because the grafted bone may be vulnerable to fracture or additional resorption (see Fig. 79.2J).

Anorganic Bovine Bone Mineral

Even though autogenous bone has long been considered the gold standard for bone regeneration procedures, different bone filling materials have also been studied to minimize morbidity associated with the second surgical site to harvest bone.

Anorganic bovine bone mineral (ABBM) is a deproteinized, sterilized, bovine cancellous bone that is osteoconductive and provides a favorable scaffold for bone formation. Newly formed bone incorporates around it and, since it is slowly resorbed, the volume of the graft is very stable. The good osteoconductivity is due to the preserved natural structure. The favorable surface topography allows good contact with the blood clot and the interconnected internal channels facilitate cellular migration and ingrowth of vessels.

Observation of the following basic principles can minimize the risk of postoperative complications and morbidity.

1. Carefully evaluate the harvest site for potential risks. A critical radiographic evaluation before surgery can identify individuals with inferior alveolar nerve branches that extend anterior beyond the mental foramen.
2. Use extreme care in making incisions laterally toward the mental nerve, and dissect the area with blunt instruments to locate the mental foramen.
3. Do not elevate and reflect muscle attachments beyond the inferior border of the mandible.
4. Limit bone cuts to an area at least 5 mm away from the tooth apices, the inferior border of the mandible, and the mental foramen. Do not extend cuts or harvest bone deeper than 6 mm, and do not include both labial and lingual cortical plates.
5. Suture the wound in layers (muscle and overlying mucosa separately) to prevent postoperative wound separation.
6. When harvesting autogenous bone, regardless of site or method used, it is important to use techniques that prevent overheating and maintain viability of the bone cells. Exceeding 47°C (116.6°F) is known to cause bone necrosis.[27] Thus, the use of drills, trephines, or saws to cut bone should always be done with profuse irrigation to keep instruments and bone cooled. Precision of osseous cuts can be facilitated with new technologies such as piezoelectric bone surgery (see Chapter 83).

Flap Management

Soft-tissue management is a critical aspect of bone augmentation procedures. Incisions, reflection, and manipulation should be designed to optimize blood supply and wound closure. The design and management of mucoperiosteal flaps must consider the increased dimensions of the ridge after augmentation as well as esthetics and approximation of the wound margins. The surgical procedure must be executed with the utmost of care to preserve the vascularity of the flap and to minimize tissue injury.[1]

Several flap techniques maintain a "submerged" position of bone grafts and barrier membranes during the entire healing process, including a remote or displaced incision.[13,41] The advantage of a remote incision is that the wound opening is positioned away from the graft. On the other hand, a conventional crestal incision can be used, even in large supracrestal defects, as long as a periosteal releasing incision and coronal advancement of the flap achieve a tension-free closure.[50] Most reports suggest removing sutures approximately 10 to 14 days after surgery.[84] It is also highly advisable to abstain from using removable prosthesis for several weeks (longer is better) after surgery to avoid placing pressure over the wound during the early healing phase.

General concepts for flap management associated with ridge augmentation include the following:

1. It is desirable to make incisions remote relative to the placement of barrier membranes (e.g., vertical releasing incisions at least one tooth away from the site to be grafted). In the anterior maxilla, keeping vertical incisions remote is also an esthetic advantage.
2. Full mucoperiosteal flap elevation at least 5 mm beyond the edge of the bone defect is desirable to expose bone for barrier membrane adaptation.
3. The use of vertical incisions, although often required for surgical access, should be minimized.
4. Use of a periosteal releasing incision to give the flap elasticity and permit tension-free closure with suturing is essential. This permits complete closure without stress on the wound margins.
5. Removable appliances should not be inserted over the wound for 2 to 3 weeks or more to avoid postoperative trauma to the surgical site.
6. Wound closure should incorporate a combination of mattress sutures to approximate connective tissues and interrupted sutures to adapt wound edges.

Although reconstruction of deficient ridges with bone grafts alone (i.e., without barrier membrane) has proved to be effective, variable resorption of the grafted bone has been reported. Preliminary results in a 1- to 3-year study using autografts harvested from the maxillary tuberosity showed an increased ridge width, but resorption of 50% of the graft volume was also noted.[78] Buser and colleagues[13] investigated the lateral ridge augmentation procedure using an autograft from the retromolar or symphysis area covered by a membrane in 40 consecutively treated patients and noted no clinical signs of resorption of the block graft. The researchers emphasized a remote incision technique, perforation of the recipient site bone cortex, stable placement of corticocancellous autografts, precise adaptation and stabilization (with mini-screws) of the polytetrafluoroethylene (ePTFE) membranes, and a tension-free primary soft-tissue closure. After 7 to 13 months, the sites were reopened for membrane removal and implant placement. Of the 40 patients, 38 exhibited excellent ridge augmentation, whereas two sites showed some soft-tissue encapsulation of the grafted bone.

Nevins and Mellonig[59] and Doblin and colleagues[22] reported an increased amount of new bone using FDBAs with membranes, even in the presence of membrane exposure. The biopsies showed viable bone cells and visible osteocytes in lacunae, and a 9-month specimen showed no remaining allograft material.

On the other hand, there are some contradictory results using DFDBA and membrane combinations.[3,7,8] In a human study, seven paired extraction sockets were grafted with either DFDBA or autologous bone. Sites were reentered and biopsied after 3 to 13 months to evaluate bone formation. Histologic specimens revealed non-vital (dead) particles of DFDBA with no evidence of bone formation on the surface and no evidence of osteoclastic resorption. Conversely, the autogenous sites revealed vascular channels with woven and lamellar bone. Some non-vital, cortical bone chips were observed with osteoclastic resorption.

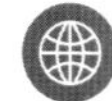

eFig. 79.3 (online) shows an example of the lack of bone formation around DFDBA particles used in a ridge augmentation procedure after more than 20 months of healing under a non-resorbable ePTFE barrier membrane.

Studies investigating GBR to augment the lateral alveolar ridge have shown reproducible results and high implant survival rates long term.[46] Studies have investigated the combination of GBR with simultaneous and subsequent implant placement. The two approaches achieved similar survival rates, indicating they are relatively equivalent.[63] Importantly, implant placement in augmented or pristine bone results in similar implant survival rates, demonstrating the predictability and efficacy of GBR.

Lateral ridge augmentation via GBR with the combination of a resorbable collagen membrane and particulate graft materials is a frequently reported technique in the literature, especially when treating dehiscence defects.[68,86] Application of this technique produces equally high long-term implant survival rates whether used subsequently to or simultaneously with implant placement.[87] Therefore, a simultaneous approach is indicated when small to moderate horizontal deficiency exists, as it reduces the number of surgeries, which lowers morbidity, reduces treatment time, and increases patient comfort.[88] Fig. 79.3 shows a representative case of horizontal ridge augmentation with simultaneous implant placement.

Resorbable membranes have shown better soft tissue compatibility, as compared to non-resorbable membranes.[30,96,97] Reports of clinical and preclinical animal studies have demonstrated that a resorbable membrane in combination with particulated bone or bone substitute can be used for the treatment of knife-edge ridges. Friedmann et al. reported on a clinical study using a slowly resorbing collagen membrane in combination with ABBM for the augmentation of horizontally deficient ridges.[30]

Hämmerle et al. have used ABBM in combination with a collagen membrane, and concluded this was an effective treatment for horizontal ridge augmentation.[34] However, in the reports of GBR using resorbable membranes, the horizontal gain of bone was less than that reported for non-resorbable membranes.[34]

Autogenous monocortical block grafts can be stabilized with screw fixation.

However, the challenge of using GBR is stabilization of the particulated graft. In most cases the necessary bone gain was not achieved and most of the bone growth was achieved apically from the crest. To overcome this difficulty, resorbable membranes were stabilized using multiple tacks. This technique is called the Sausage technique. Fig. 79.4 shows a representative case of a posterior mandibular ridge augmentation using the Sausage technique.

KEY FACT

Dehiscence defects can usually be managed with simultaneous bone grafting during implant placement because most of the implant is covered and stabilized by existing native bone. If the horizontal alveolar deficiency is large such that the implant would be positioned with significant exposure (i.e., more than half of the implant diameter placed outside the alveolar bone), it may be better to reconstruct the bone first, in a staged approach, with a subsequent surgery for implant placement.

Supracrestal/Vertical Bone Augmentation

Supracrestal or vertical bone augmentation presents one of the greatest challenges of bone regeneration in implant dentistry. This is primarily due to difficulty of the surgical procedure and the potential for postoperative complications. Because vertical augmentation can be a challenging procedure with a relatively high rate of complications, it is necessary to justify this particular treatment for each patient. The rate of complications associated with vertical bone augmentation procedures, including membrane exposure or postoperative infection, is reported to range from 2.87% to 17%.[63,75,76,79,82] Alternative treatment options, albeit with limited outcomes, need to be considered. For example, regenerating a vertically deficient ridge may not be necessary if (1) implants can be placed in adjacent sites, (2) short implants can be used, (3) cantilevers or conventional bridges can be used, or (4) in the case of vertical deficiencies in esthetic areas, pink ceramic can be used to create an illusion of "normal" soft tissue anatomy.

Historical attempts to vertically increase alveolar bone height using modalities such as onlay bone grafting have failed. More recent treatment modalities developed for vertical bone growth include vertical GBR and distraction osteogenesis. The techniques and evidence of success are presented.

Guided Bone Regeneration

The surgical technique of GBR for supracrestal regeneration was described in the 1990s.[76] Although available evidence is limited, both animal and human studies demonstrate successful vertical bone augmentation with histologic evidence.[43,76] Some studies have evaluated the effect of space creation by a membrane alone, whereas others have used an autogenous bone graft to maintain space under the membrane. Using TR membranes without bone graft (space filled with blood clot only) in a canine model, Jovanovic and colleagues[43] demonstrated a gain of 1.82 mm of vertical bone height around simultaneously placed implants. In a clinical study, Simion and coworkers[76] treated five patients with

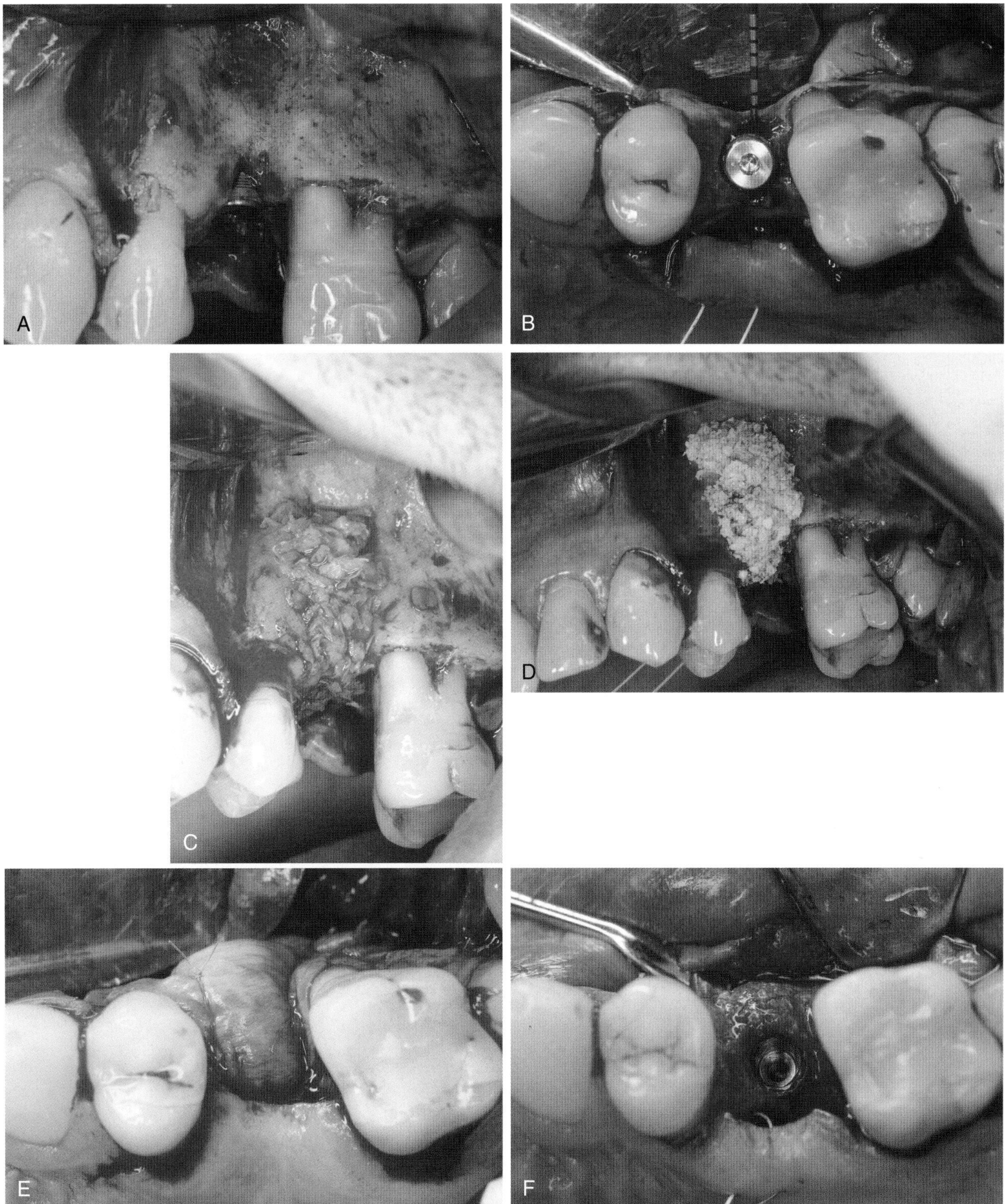

Fig. 79.3 Representative case of horizontal ridge augmentation simultaneously with implant placement. (A and B) Labial and occlusal views of a dehiscence around an implant at the time of implant placement. (C) Labial view of autogenous bone chips placed on the defect as well as the more apical narrow area. (D) Labial view of a xenograft placed as an external layer of the autograft. The rationale was to protect the autograft from resorption as well as to increase the expected bone width. (E) Occlusal view of a native collagen membrane fixated using internal mattress sutures. (F) Occlusal view of the regenerated bone around the implant. Note that a complete regeneration was achieved.

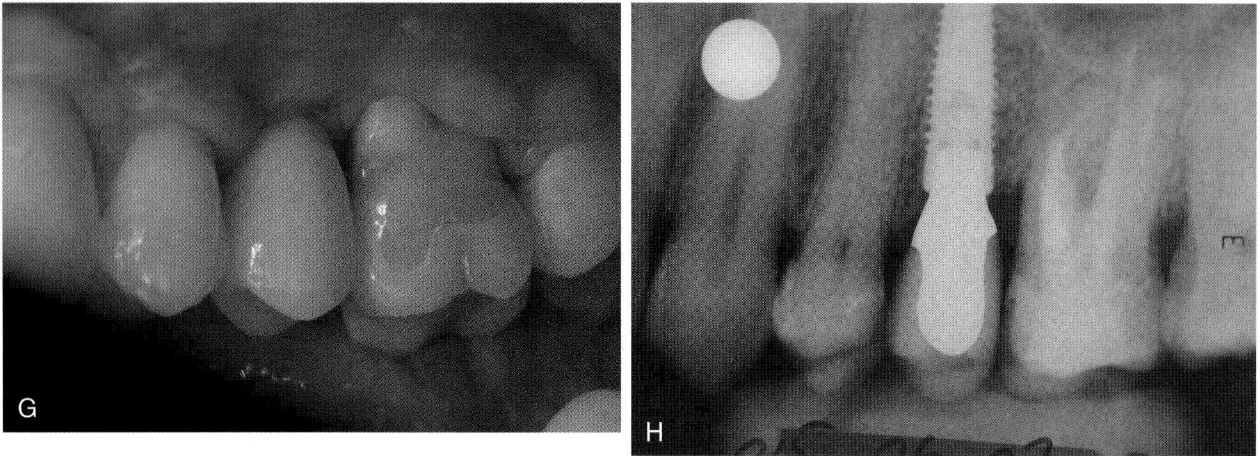

Fig. 79.3, cont'd (G) Labial view of the final restoration in place. (H) Periapical radiograph demonstrates stable crestal bone around the implant.

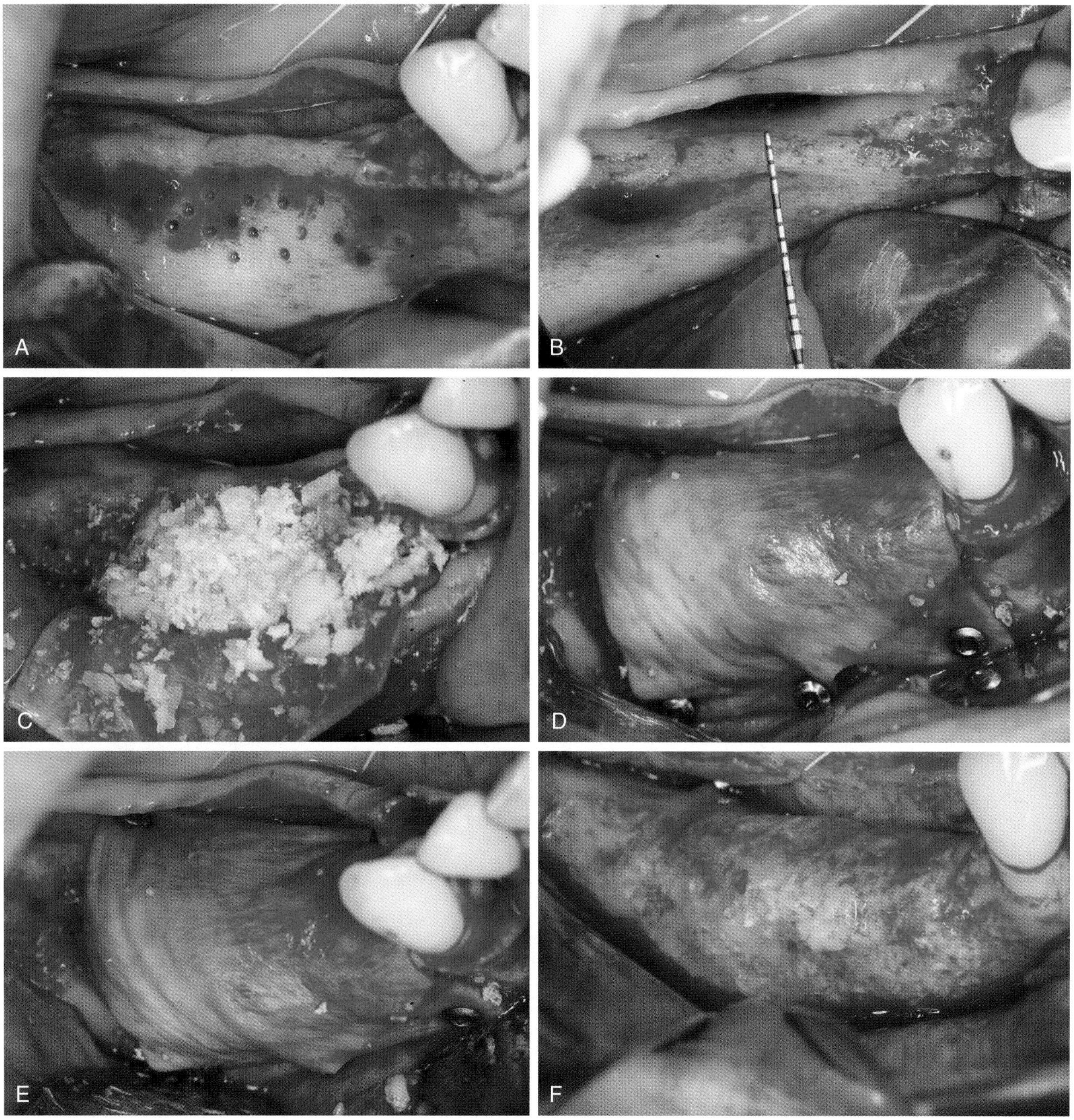

Fig. 79.4 Representative case of a posterior mandibular ridge augmentation using the Sausage technique. (A and B) Labial and occlusal views of a horizontal ridge atrophy in the posterior mandible. Recipient bone bed is prepared with multiple decorticalization holes. (C) Labial view of the membrane stabilized apically and a mixture of autogenous particulated bone and anorganic bovine bone mineral (ABBM) granules is in place. (D and E) Labial and occlusal views of the membrane stabilized further with lingual pins. (F–H) Labial and occlusal views of the regenerated ridge. Note the good incorporation of the ABBM into newly formed bone.

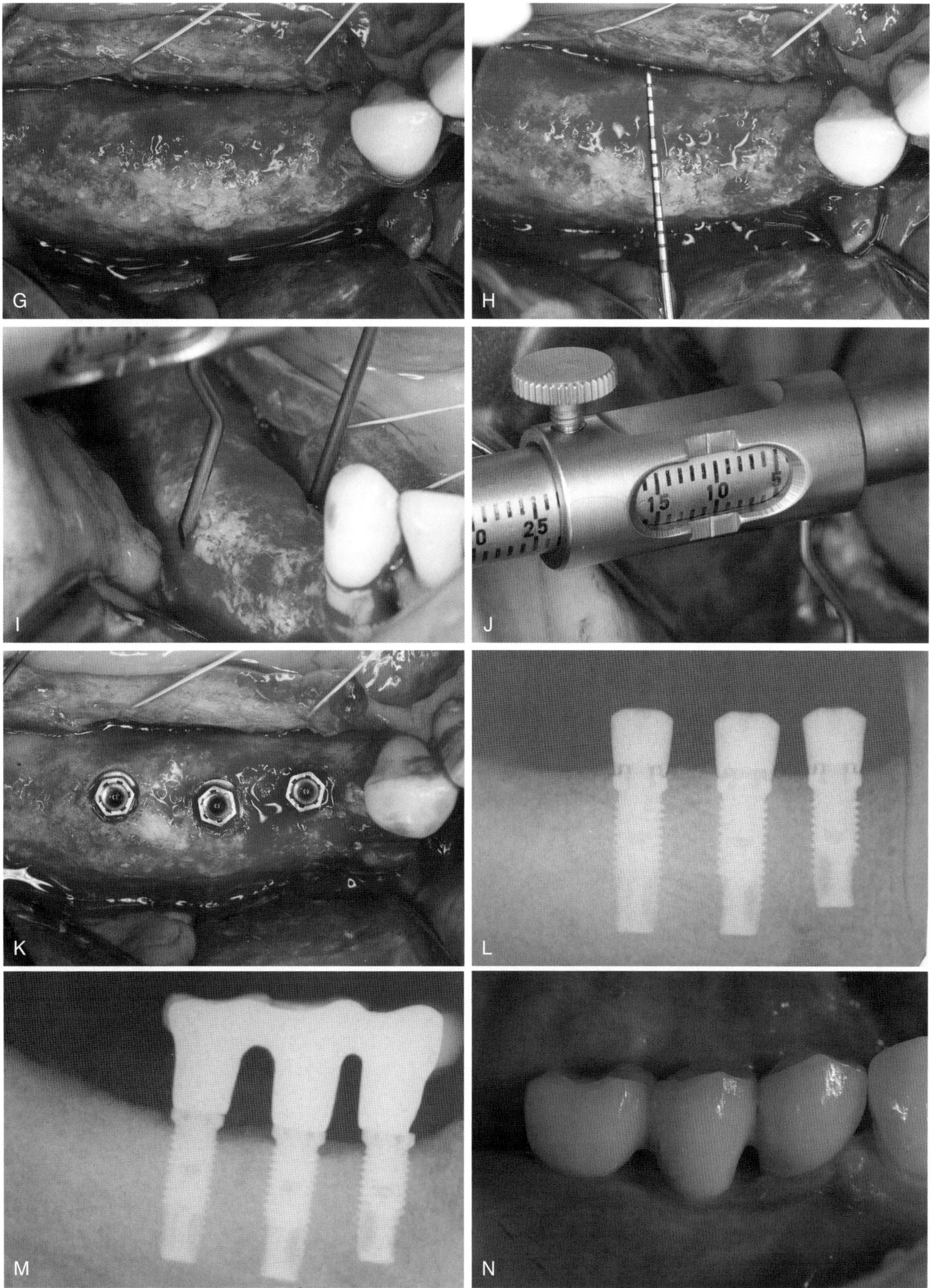

Fig. 79.4 cont'd (I and J) Labial views demonstrating the amount of regenerated bone. (K) Occlusal view of three implants placed into the regenerated bone. (L) Periapical radiograph at the exposure of the implants. (M) Periapical radiograph 5 years after loading demonstrates good crestal bone stability. (N) Final reconstruction in place.

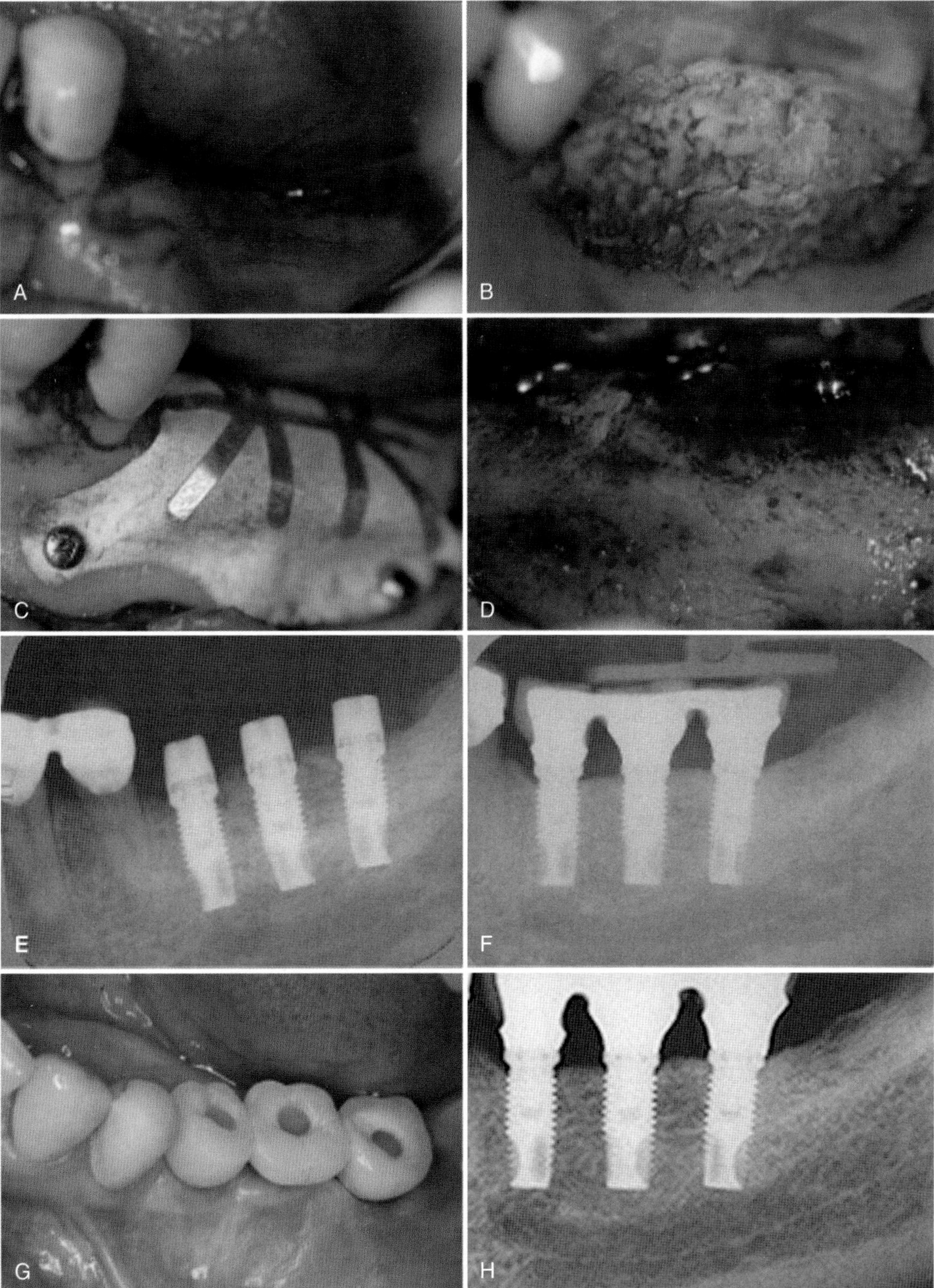

Fig. 79.5 Representative case of a posterior mandibular vertical ridge augmentation. (A) Atrophic posterior mandibular area. (B) Particulated chin bone graft is placed on the ridge. Cortical bone was perforated, and guided tissue regeneration membrane/titanium-reinforced (GTRM-TR) membrane was secured on the lingual side before applying bone graft. (C) GTRM-TR membrane is secured over the graft with titanium pins. (D) Three implants are in place in the newly formed posterior mandibular ridge. Note the well-integrated bone graft. (E) Periapical radiograph at abutment connection. (F) Periapical radiograph at 8-year follow-up with implants in function. (G) Clinical picture demonstrates healthy peri-implant mucosa. (H) Periapical radiograph at 13-year follow-up with implants in function. (A–G from Urban IA, Jovanovic SA, Lozada JL. Vertical ridge augmentation using guided bone regeneration (GBR) in three clinical scenarios prior to implant placement: a retrospective study of 35 patients 12 to 72 months after loading. *Int J Oral Maxillofac Implants.* 2009;24:502–510.)

GBR to gain vertical bone height around 15 implants placed in a supracrestal position with 4 to 7 mm of the implant exposed. Titanium miniscrews were placed distal to the implants in a supracrestal position with 3 to 4 mm exposed. The implants and miniscrews were covered with a TR e-PTFE barrier membrane. Clinical evaluation at implant exposure surgery revealed an average of 3 mm (range from 1 to 4 mm) of vertical bone gain after 9 months. Histomorphometric evaluation of harvested mini-screws showed good bone-to-implant contact (42.5% ± 3.6%) with the regenerated bone. These studies suggest that supracrestal bone formation up to 3 mm is predictable using the GBR technique with a TR barrier membrane–blood clot combination.

Subsequent long-term studies have shown that supracrestal bone formation is more predictable using a bone graft filler material placed under the TR membrane.[75] Therefore, at present, advanced surgical GBR augmentation for vertical bone gain should be achieved with a non-resorbable TR membrane that is supported by a bone graft. Figs. 79.5 and 79.6 show representative cases of horizontal and vertical ridge augmentation using non-resorbable TR membranes supported with bone graft material. The long-term results of vertical GBR after 1 to 5 years of prosthetic loading were examined in a retrospective multicenter study evaluating 123 implants.[75] Three treatment modalities (non-resorbable regenerative membranes in combination with blood clot only, DFDBA, and autogenous bone chips) were studied, and the results from this investigation revealed that vertical bone regeneration greater than 4 mm could only be achieved with the use of autogenous bone chips. These authors reported an overall success rate of 97.5%, leading them to conclude that vertically augmented bone using GBR techniques supports implant placement in a fashion similar to native, non-regenerated bone.

Urban and colleagues[82] used TR membranes with autogenous particulated bone for vertical bone augmentation before implant placement. The study included 35 patients with 36 vertical bone defects. Eighty-two implants were placed in a staged approach, and a resorbable collagen membrane was placed over the newly formed crestal bone during the implant placement surgery to protect the graft from early resorption after removal of the ePTFE membrane. Implants were followed from 1 to 6 years after prosthetic loading. Treatment groups included single and multiple tooth sites, as well as vertical defects in the posterior maxilla. Vertical bone augmentation of the posterior maxillary ridge was done simultaneously with 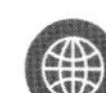 sinus bone augmentation (eFig. 79.4). At membrane removal, the mean vertical bone augmentation was 5.5 mm (±2.29 mm). The mean combined crestal remodeling was 1.01 mm (±0.57 mm) at 12 months, which remained stable through the 6-year follow-up period. There were no statistically significant differences between the treatment groups in mean marginal bone remodeling. The overall implant survival rate was 100% with a cumulative success rate of 94.7%. See Fig. 79.5.

The efficacy of a 1:1 mixture of ABBM and autogenous particulated bone graft using ePTFE membranes was evaluated histologically and histomorphometrically in eight patients (10 ridge defects).[74] After a healing period of 6 to 9 months, a mean vertical gain of 3.15 mm (SD ±1.12 mm) was achieved. A clinical and histologic study evaluating the same graft material and using dense-PTFE membranes in 19 patients achieved an average bone gain of 5.45 mm (SD 1.93). In both studies, histologic evaluation showed that ABBM was surrounded by a dense network of newly formed bone at varying degrees of maturation. See Fig. 79.6.

Simion and coworkers reported the long-term results of machined surface implants placed in vertically augmented bone achieved with GBR. Patients were followed from 13 to 21 years with a mean follow-up of 16 years. The average marginal bone loss from baseline (1-year post-loading) to the final evaluation was 1.06 mm.[73]

There are limited clinical data on the outcomes of simultaneous GBR for horizontal or vertical bone gain for the reconstruction of severely atrophic edentulous maxilla. Urban and colleagues[84] evaluated 16 consecutively treated patients (mean age: 64 years) for vertical and/or horizontal bone augmentation with GBR in combination with bilateral sinus augmentation utilizing a mixture of autologous and anorganic bovine bone. Implant survival, bone gain, intraoperative/postoperative complications, and peri-implant bone loss were calculated up to the last follow-up exam. A total of 122 dental implants were placed into augmented sites and have been followed for up to 15 years (average follow-up of 6.5 years). The vertical bone gain was 5.1 mm; horizontal bone gain was 7 mm. The mean peri-implant bone loss values were consistent within the standards for implant success (1.4 ± 1 mm). At the patient level, only one patient, who had three implants, presented with severe peri-implant bone loss. Fig. 79.7 shows a representative case of GBR for horizontal bone reconstruction of a severely resorbed maxilla with 5-year follow-up.

KEY FACT

Vertical ridge augmentation is one of the most challenging clinical procedures in reconstructing alveolar ridges. Despite the potential for complications with this treatment approach, high success and good long-term implant survival rates have been documented.

Distraction Osteogenesis

Distraction osteogenesis is a surgical technique that has been developed to increase vertical bone height in the deficient jaw site and contrasts with the more conventional method of bone grafting with or without membranes. Under the proper circumstances, most cells in bone can differentiate into osteogenic (or chondrogenic) cells needed for repair. Ilizarov popularized the concept of distraction osteogenesis in the 1980s by developing a protocol for "cutting" long bones and "stretching" them during the healing process.[37–39]

Based on experimental and clinical studies over 35 years, distraction osteogenesis can provide a surgeon with the ability to treat small bones in the hands and feet using external fixation devices. New intraoral devices for vertical bone growth of the alveolar process have been developed and applied in preparation for dental implant placement. One advantage of distraction osteogenesis is the ability to increase bone height in an area using the native autogenous bone without the need for a second surgical site to harvest bone.

A significant disadvantage of distraction osteogenesis for intraoral applications is the unidirectional limitation of current devices. The application of distraction osteogenesis for vertical bone growth has been demonstrated, but the vector or trajectory of the increased bone growth can be challenging to control and there are significant limitations in achieving horizontal bone growth with this method. Secondary bone grafting is frequently needed following vertical distraction osteogenesis, especially for the extremely resorbed (narrow) ridge. Consequently, distraction osteogenesis cannot be expected to solve vertical ridge defects without the use of additional bone augmentation procedures.

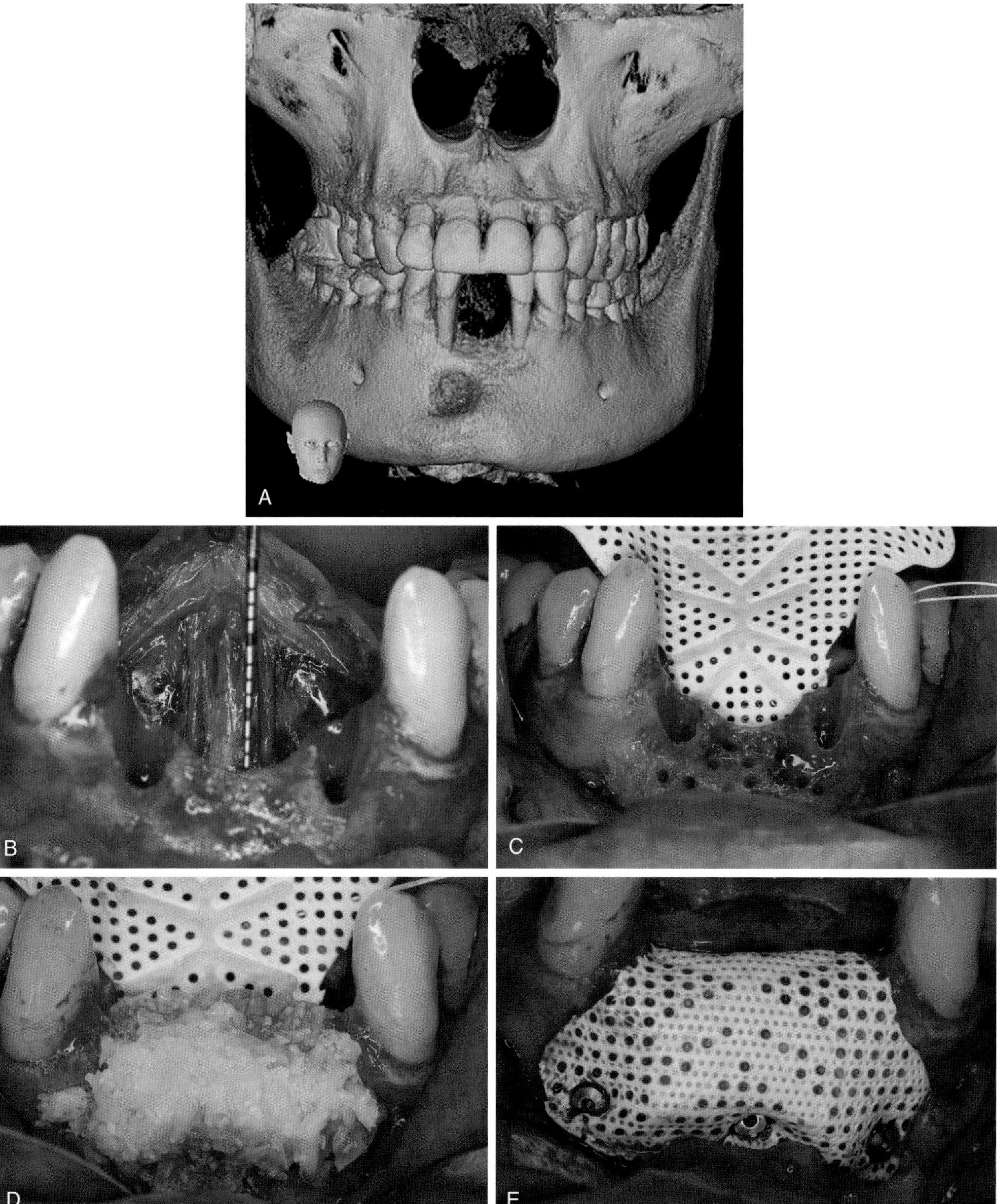

Fig. 79.6 Representative case of an anterior mandibular vertical ridge augmentation. (A) CBCT image demonstrates a vertical defect in the anterior mandible. (B) Labial views of the site after lingual flap advancement. The genioglossus muscle and the two end branches of the arteries are identified during flap elevation. The two lateral incisors with advanced interproximal bone loss were extracted. (C and D) Labial view of the fixated perforated d-PTFE membrane; a 1:1 ratio of autogenous bone and ABBM was utilized. (E) Labial view of the membrane in place.

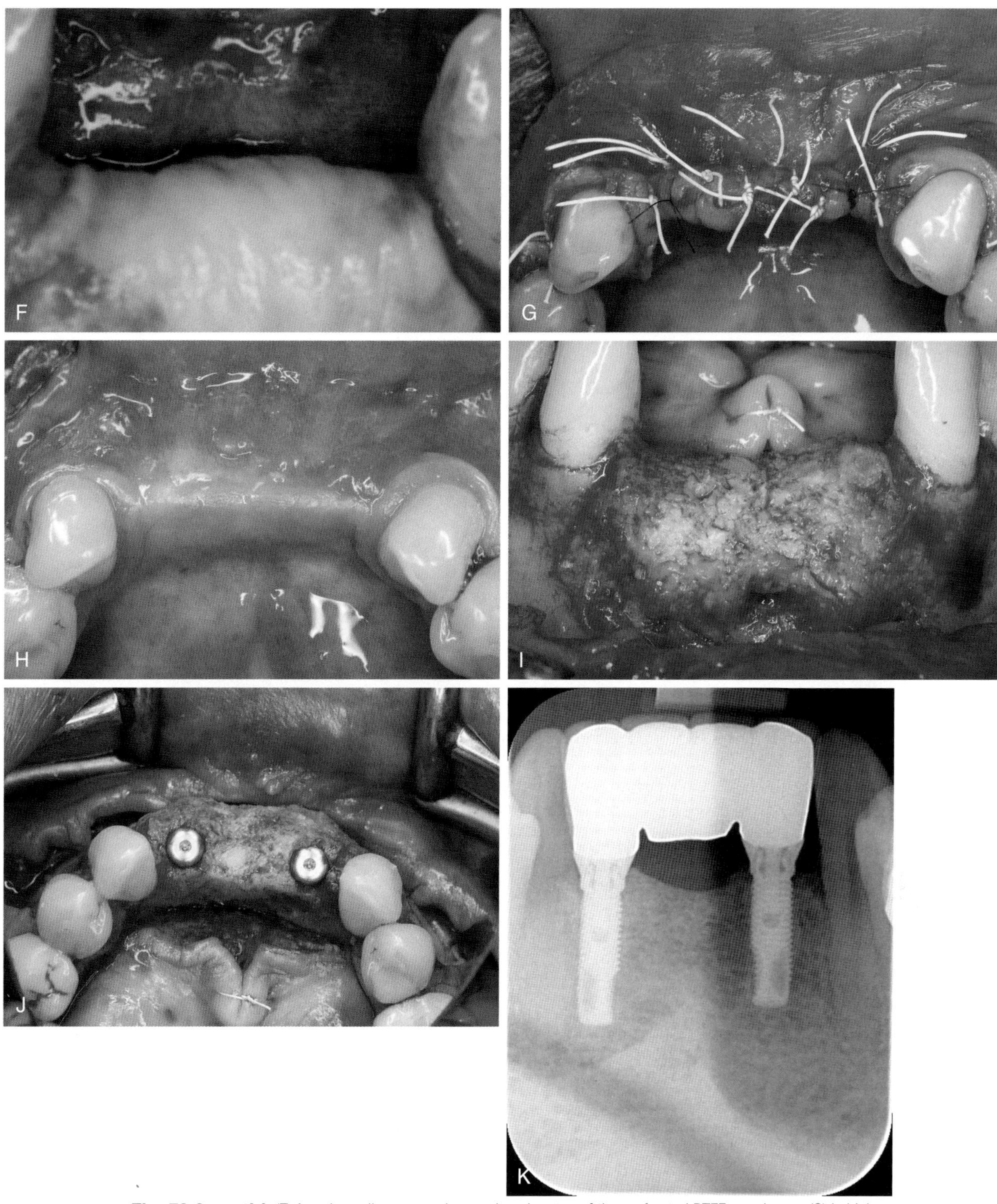

Fig. 79.6 cont'd (F) A native collagen membrane placed on top of the perforated PTFE membrane. (G) Labial view of primary closure at the end of surgery and after 2 weeks. (H) Occlusal view of the site after 9 months of uneventful healing. (I) Labial view of the regenerated vertical bone. (J) Occlusal view of the horizontal bone gain at the site after implant placement. (K) Peri-apical radiograph demonstrates excellent bone level after 2 years of loading.

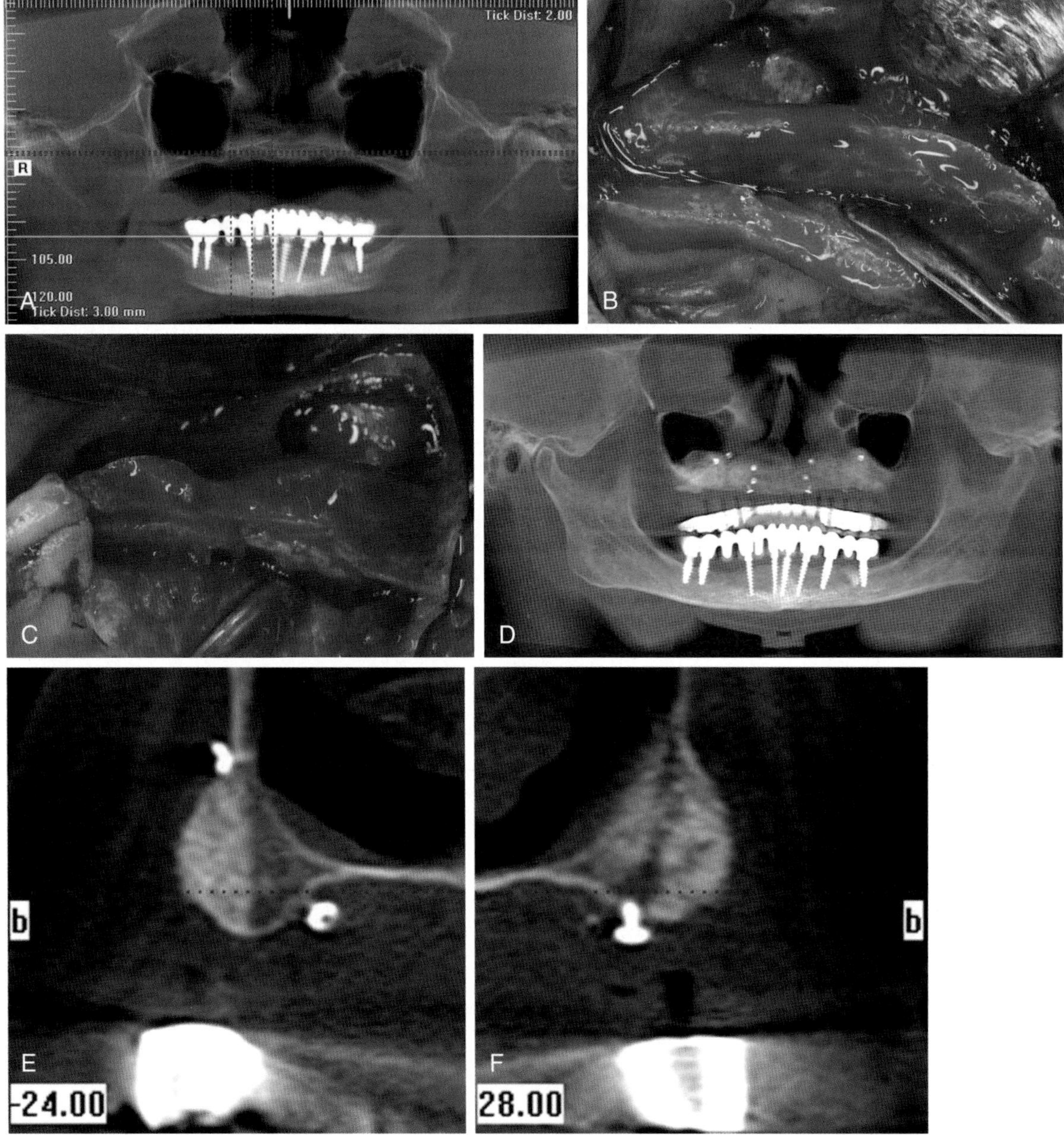

Fig. 79.7 Five-year follow-up of a 60-year-old female after reconstruction of an edentulous and severely resorbed maxilla. (A) Panoramic view of a severely resorbed maxillary case. (B and C) Occlusal views of the ridge atrophies. (D–F) Panoramic and cross-sectional views of the reconstructed ridge.

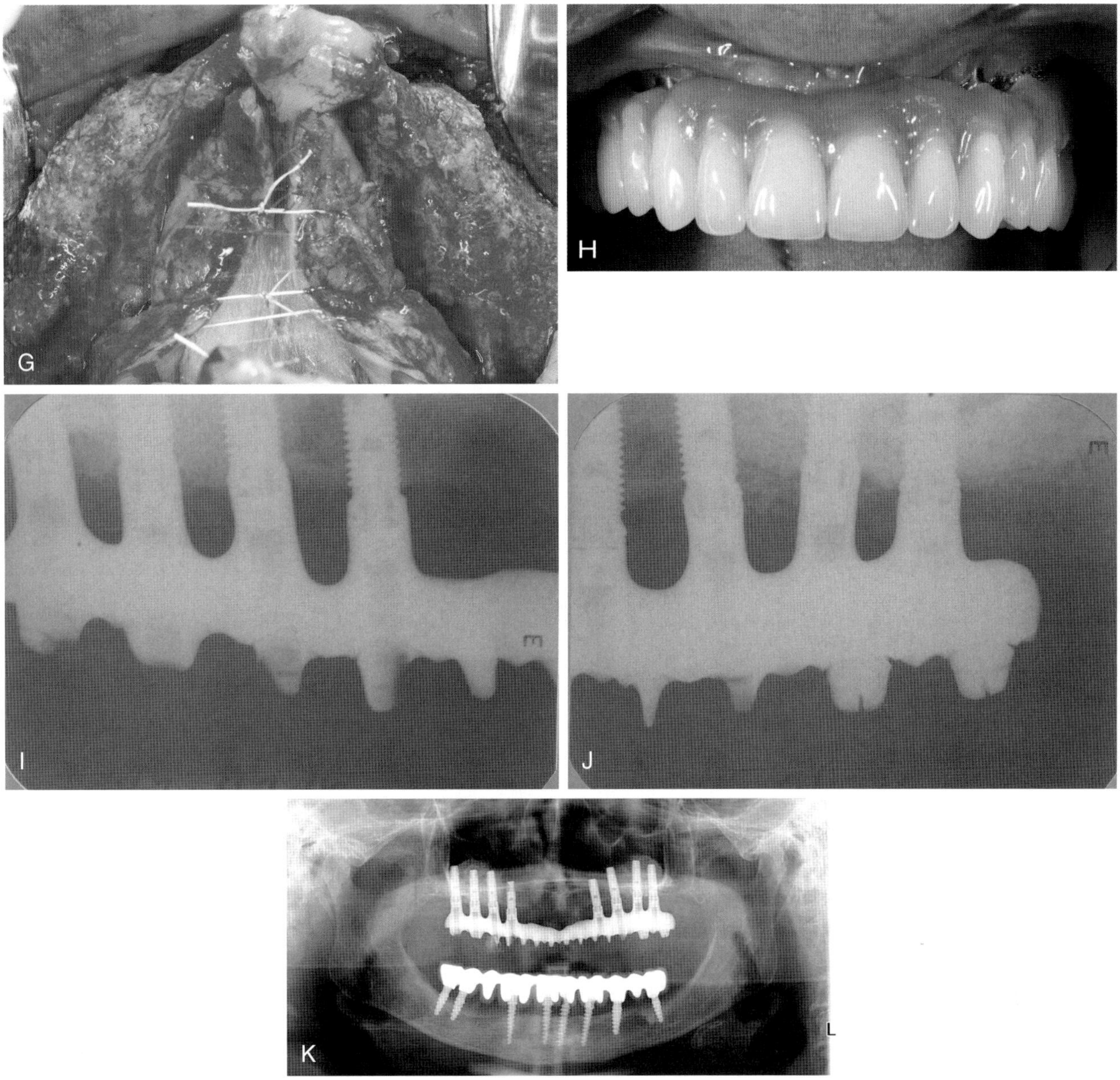

Fig. 79.7 cont'd (G) Occlusal view of the regenerated maxilla. (H) Labial view of the final fixed implant–supported maxillary complete denture (bridge). (I and J) Periapical radiographs after 5 years of loading. (K) Panoramic radiograph of the reconstruction. Note that the lower jaw was reconstructed before the patient sought treatment from the author.

Conclusions

Bone augmentation and advanced implant surgery procedures allow clinicians to reconstruct horizontal and vertical alveolar bone deficiencies and replace missing teeth with endosseous dental implants. Diagnosis, treatment planning, careful execution of the surgical treatment, postoperative follow-up, and appropriate implant loading are all important factors in achieving a predictable outcome and success with these procedures. Reconstruction of vertically deficient ridges remains a significant challenge despite the reported progress and success of new techniques.

A Case Scenario is found on the companion website eBooks.Health.Elsevier.com.

Suggested Reading

Becker W, Becker BE, Caffesse R. A comparison of demineralized freeze-dried bone and autologous bone to induce bone formation in human extraction sockets. *J Periodontol*. 1994;65:1128–1133.

Buser D, Dula K, Hirt HP, et al. Lateral ridge augmentation using autografts and barrier membranes: a clinical study with 40 partially edentulous patients. *J Oral Maxillofac Surg*. 1996;54:420–432; discussion 432–423.

Chan HL, Lin GH, Fu JH, et al. Alterations in bone quality after socket preservation with grafting materials: a systematic review. *Int J Oral Maxillofac Implants*. 2013;28(3):710–720. PMID: 23748301.

Donos N, Mardas N, Chadha V. Clinical outcomes of implants following lateral bone augmentation: systematic assessment of available options (barrier membranes, bone grafts, split osteotomy). *J Clin Periodontol*. 2008;35:173–202.

Fugazzotto PA. GBR using bovine bone matrix and resorbable and non-resorbable membranes. Part 1: histologic results. *Int J Periodontics Restorative Dent*. 2003;23:361–369.

Lazzara RJ. Immediate implant placement into extraction sites: surgical and restorative advantages. *Int J Periodontics Restorative Dent*. 1989;9:332–343.

Nevins M, Mellonig JT. The advantages of localized ridge augmentation prior to implant placement: a staged event. *Int J Periodontics Restorative Dent*. 1994;14:96–111.

Sanz-Sanchez I, Ortiz-Vigon A, Sanz-Martin I, Figuero E, Sanz M. Effectiveness of lateral bone augmentation on the alveolar crest dimension: a systematic review and meta-analysis. *J Dent Res*. 2015;94:S128–S142.

Schenk RK, Buser D, Hardwick WR, et al. Healing pattern of bone regeneration in membrane-protected defects: a histologic study in the canine mandible. *Int J Oral Maxillofac Implants*. 1994;9:13–29.

Tonetti MS, Cortellini P, Lang NP, et al. Clinical outcomes following treatment of human intrabony defects with GTR/bone replacement material or access flap alone. A multicenter randomized controlled clinical trial. *J Clin Periodontol*. 2004;31(9):770–776. https://doi.org/10.1111/j.1600-051X.2004.00562.x. PMID: 15312100.

Urban IA, Jovanovic SA, Lozada JL. Vertical ridge augmentation using guided bone regeneration (GBR) in three clinical scenarios prior to implant placement: a retrospective study of 35 patients 12 to 72 months after loading. *Int J Oral Maxillofac Implants*. 2009;24:502–510.

Urban IA, Monje A, Lozada JL, et al. Long-term evaluation of peri-implant bone level after reconstruction of severely atrophic edentulous maxilla via vertical and horizontal guided bone regeneration in combination with sinus augmentation: a case series with 1 to 15 years of loading. *Clin Implant Dent Relat Res*. 2017;19:46–55.

Urist MR. Bone: formation by autoinduction. *Science*. 1965;150:893–899.

Wang HL, Misch C, Neiva RF. "Sandwich" bone augmentation technique: rationale and report of pilot cases. *Int J Periodontics Restorative Dent*. 2004;24:232–245.

Wessing B, Lettner S, Zechner W. Guided bone regeneration with collagen membranes and particulate graft materials: a systematic review and meta-analysis. *Int J Periodontics Restorative Dent*. 2018;33:87–100.

Whetman J, Mealey BL. Effect of healing time on new bone formation after tooth extraction and ridge preservation with demineralized freeze-dried bone allograft: a randomized controlled clinical trial. *J Periodontol*. 2016;87(9):1022–1029. PMID: 27133791.

Wood RA, Mealey BL. Histologic comparison of healing after tooth extraction with ridge preservation using mineralized versus demineralized freeze-dried bone allograft. *J Periodontol*. 2012;83(3):329–336. PMID: 21749166.

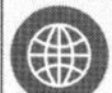

References for this chapter are found on the companion website eBooks.Health.Elsevier.com.

CHAPTER 80

Advanced Implant Surgical Procedures: Maxillary Sinus Augmentation

Perry R. Klokkevold | Istvan A. Urban | Michael Whang

For online-only content on growth factors in bone augmentation, please visit the companion website at eBooks.Health.Elsevier.com.

CHAPTER OUTLINE

The success and predictability of dental implants used to replace missing teeth for any individual patient or in any particular site rely on a multitude of factors, the most important of which is the availability of bone. The loss of teeth, whether caused by disease or trauma, often results in alveolar bone deficiency. The posterior maxilla is particularly susceptible because of a general lack of bone volume and the omnipresent poor bone quality of the area; specifically, posterior maxillary bone often consists of a thin cortical shell and sparse trabecular bone. Thus, edentulous posterior maxillary sites frequently require bone augmentation to increase bone volume for dental implants, and the maxillary sinus is a space that is amenable to grafting.

This chapter reviews advanced surgical procedures used to increase vertical bone height and volume in the maxillary sinus.

Maxillary Sinus Elevation and Bone Augmentation

Rehabilitation of the edentulous posterior maxilla with dental implants often represents a clinical challenge due to insufficient bone volume resulting from *pneumatization* of the maxillary sinus along with a loss of alveolar crestal bone caused by disease or remodeling. Prior to the utilization of bone augmentation procedures, patients with missing teeth and deficient bone in the posterior maxilla could only be rehabilitated with a removable prosthesis, short implants, or a cantilevered restoration (i.e., supported by adjacent teeth). Historically, the failure rate for implants placed in the posterior maxilla was significantly higher than the failure rate for implants placed in other anatomic locations due to inadequate bone volume and density.[10] Procedures such as maxillary sinus elevation and bone augmentation are used to increase vertical bone height in the posterior maxilla for implant placement.

In 1980, Boyne and James[5] first described a procedure to graft the maxillary sinus floor with autogenous marrow and bone to facilitate placement of a blade-type implant. Access to the maxillary sinus was gained through a Caldwell-Luc procedure (i.e., an opening into the maxillary sinus created at the anterior-superior aspect). Since then, several techniques and approaches have been described, including variations on the lateral window osteotomy and a variety of techniques used to lift the sinus floor from a crestal approach.

CLINICAL CORRELATION

The posterior maxilla is a challenging site to rehabilitate with dental implants. Tooth loss in the posterior maxilla, along with the location of the maxillary sinus and poor bone quality, often results in inadequate bone height and volume to place implants. The lack of bone is further exacerbated by the loss of alveolar bone from periodontal disease and tooth loss.

Indications and Contraindications

As with any therapeutic procedure, treatment success depends on a number of factors, including appropriate patient selection, careful evaluation of the anatomy, identification and management of any pathology, sound surgical procedures, and appropriate postsurgical management. The primary indication for maxillary sinus elevation and bone augmentation, specific for the placement of dental implants, is an alveolar bone height in the posterior maxilla that is deficient (e.g., less than 7 or 8 mm of existing vertical bone height). Other factors that must be considered include the health of the patient, the condition of the remaining dentition, and the likelihood of a beneficial outcome. A thorough patient evaluation and the clinician's assessment will ultimately determine whether the procedure is indicated for a particular individual.

Contraindications to maxillary sinus elevation and bone augmentation are like contraindications for other surgical procedures, with added considerations that are specific to the maxillary sinus (Box 80.1). Patients must be in good general health and free of diseases that affect the maxilla or maxillary sinus. Local factors that are considered contraindications to maxillary sinus elevation and bone augmentation include the presence of tumors, obstruction of the ostium, maxillary sinus infection, severe chronic sinusitis, scarring or deformity of the sinus cavity from previous surgery, dental infection, severe allergic rhinitis, or chronic use of topical steroids. Systemic contraindications to treatment include radiation therapy, uncontrolled metabolic disease (e.g., diabetes), excessive tobacco use, drug or alcohol abuse, and psychological or mental impairment.

BOX 80.1 Contraindications for Maxillary Sinus Elevation and Bone Augmentation

Local Factors

Tumors or pathologic growth in the sinus
Maxillary sinus infection
Severe chronic sinusitis
Surgical scar/deformity of sinus cavity
Dental infection involving or in proximity to sinus
Severe allergic rhinitis/sinusitis
Chronic topical steroid use

Systemic Factors

Radiation therapy involving the maxillary sinus
Metabolic disease (e.g., uncontrolled diabetes mellitus)
Excessive tobacco use
Drug/alcohol abuse
Psychologic/mental impairment

Presurgical Evaluation of the Maxillary Sinus

Presurgical evaluation of the maxillary sinus is primarily accomplished using radiographic examination techniques (Fig. 80.1). Several observations about the anatomy can be made with a periapical or panoramic projection, but the internal anatomy is most accurately assessed with a three-dimensional scan, such as computed tomography or cone-beam computed tomography (CBCT) scan. The maxillary sinus should be evaluated for any pathology, masses, or variations in sinus floor anatomy, such as the presence of septa.[32] If three-dimensional scans are available, the lateral wall should also be evaluated for thickness and the presence of medium or large intraosseous vascular channels (see Fig. 59.15). Medium- to large-size vessels occasionally traverse the lateral wall of the maxillary sinus, and identifying them preoperatively helps avoid a bleeding problem during surgery (see Chapters 59 and 75).[18]

Drainage limitations should be evaluated as well. The maxillary sinus drains through the maxillary ostium, which is located at the superior–medial aspect of the maxillary sinus space. The maxillary sinus drains through the ostium, which is about 3 to 6 mm in diameter, into the middle meatus. Patency of the maxillary ostium can be observed in cross-sectional views of a CBCT scan. Fig. 80.2 and Video 80.1.

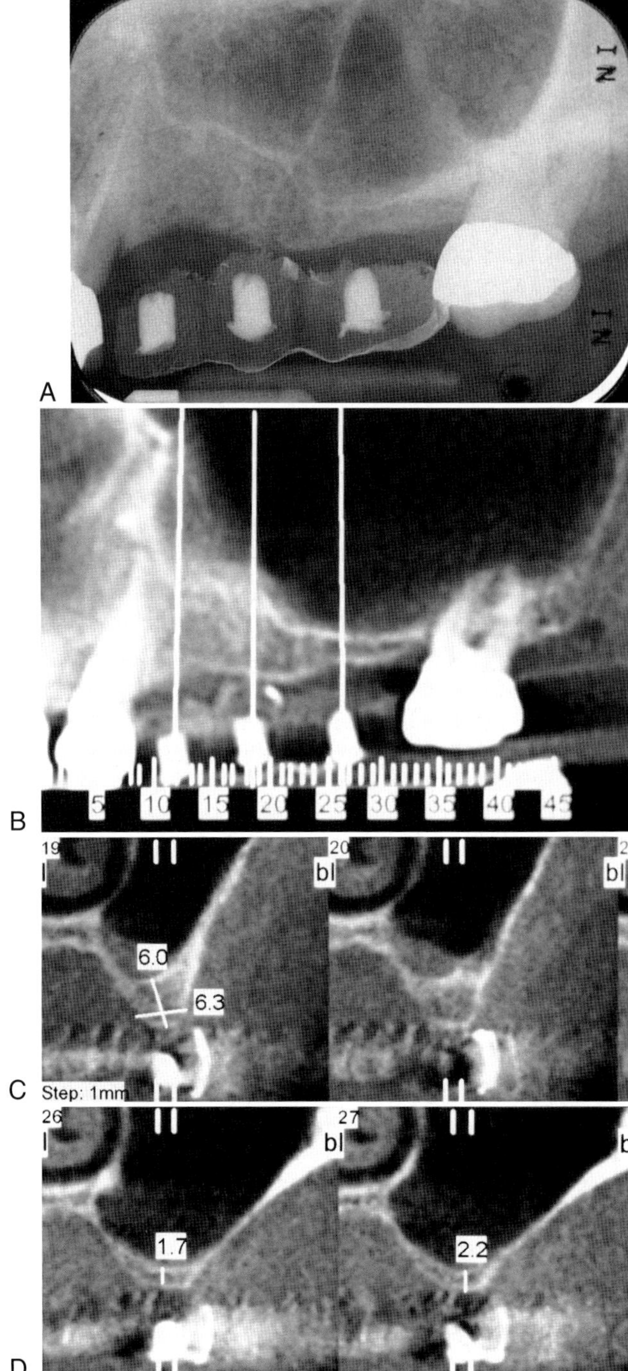

Fig. 80.1 Presurgical evaluation of the maxillary sinus. (A) Periapical radiograph. (B) Panoramic projection from cone-beam scan. Note the presence of maxillary septa in the premolar region. (C) Cross-sectional image in premolar region showing about 6 mm of bone height and the presence of maxillary septa. (D) Cross-sectional image in molar region showing about 2 mm of bone height.

Bone Graft Materials

Autogenous bone is often referred to as the gold standard for bone augmentation because of its osteoconductive, osteoinductive, and osteogenic properties.[1,5,22,23] However, harvesting autogenous bone from intraoral or extraoral locations creates a second surgical site with additional morbidity.

Several clinical studies and reports have attempted to evaluate the effectiveness of the maxillary sinus bone augmentation procedure using a variety of bone-grafting materials, including autogenous bone from the iliac crest or oral cavity and bone substitutes, such as freeze-dried demineralized bone, resorbable and nonresorbable hydroxyapatite, and xenografts. However, only a few studies have critically evaluated the long-term clinical outcome of this procedure, and most have used a small study population. Short- to long-term clinical studies of dental implants placed into grafted sinuses have demonstrated an equivalent or higher survival rate compared with implants placed in native maxillary bone (i.e., without the need of sinus augmentation).[11,28] These results support the clinical predictability of maxillary sinus bone augmentation procedures for the rehabilitation of the edentulous posterior maxilla with implant-supported prostheses (Fig. 80.3).

The 1996 Consensus Conference on Maxillary Sinus Bone Grafting reviewed available data and concluded that many different bone graft materials, including allografts, alloplasts, and xenografts, used alone or in combination with autogenous bone, are effective as bone substitute graft materials for sinus bone augmentation.[11] Recent studies, systematic reviews, and meta-analyses have confirmed the consensus findings that various bone graft materials effectively increase bone height in the maxillary sinus.[15,21] Numerous reports have validated the safety and efficacy of this procedure,[6,8,9,28] and implant success rates are equal to or better than that of implants placed in nongrafted maxillary bone (i.e., areas of the posterior maxilla with adequate height of existing native bone).[28] Thus the evidence supports sinus bone augmentation with various bone graft materials

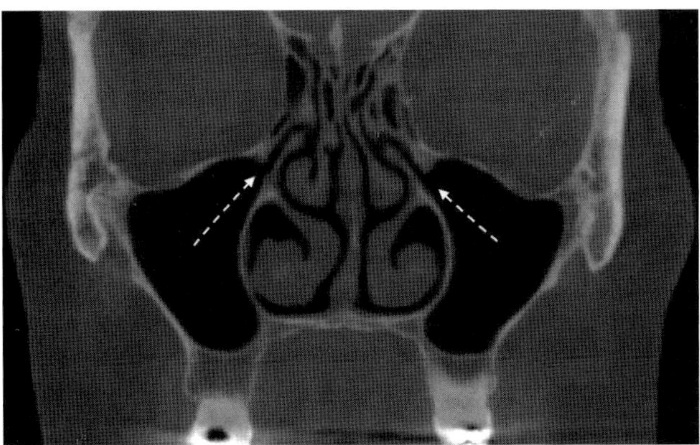

Fig. 80.2 Coronal cone-beam computed tomography cross-sectional image showing maxillary sinus ostium *(arrows)*.

and implant placement as a highly predictable and effective therapeutic modality for the rehabilitation of the posterior maxilla.

The use of bone-substitute graft materials can reduce the morbidity introduced by a second surgical site while maintaining equally good implant success rates.[11] Anorganic bovine bone-derived mineral (ABBM; Bio-Oss, Geistlich Pharma AG, Wolhusen, Switzerland) has been used successfully for sinus augmentation.[31] ABBM has been referred to in the literature as *deproteinized bovine bone mineral, deproteinized anorganic bovine bone,* and *anorganic bovine bone.* This graft material has demonstrated good dimensional stability and high implant survival rates.[8] Overall, ABBM and other bone-substitute graft materials form an osteoconductive scaffold for bone growth but do not have any osteoinductive properties.

A possible exception is demineralized freeze-dried bone allograft (DFDBA). This material has demonstrated osteoinductive potential but has not proved to be particularly advantageous in maxillary sinus

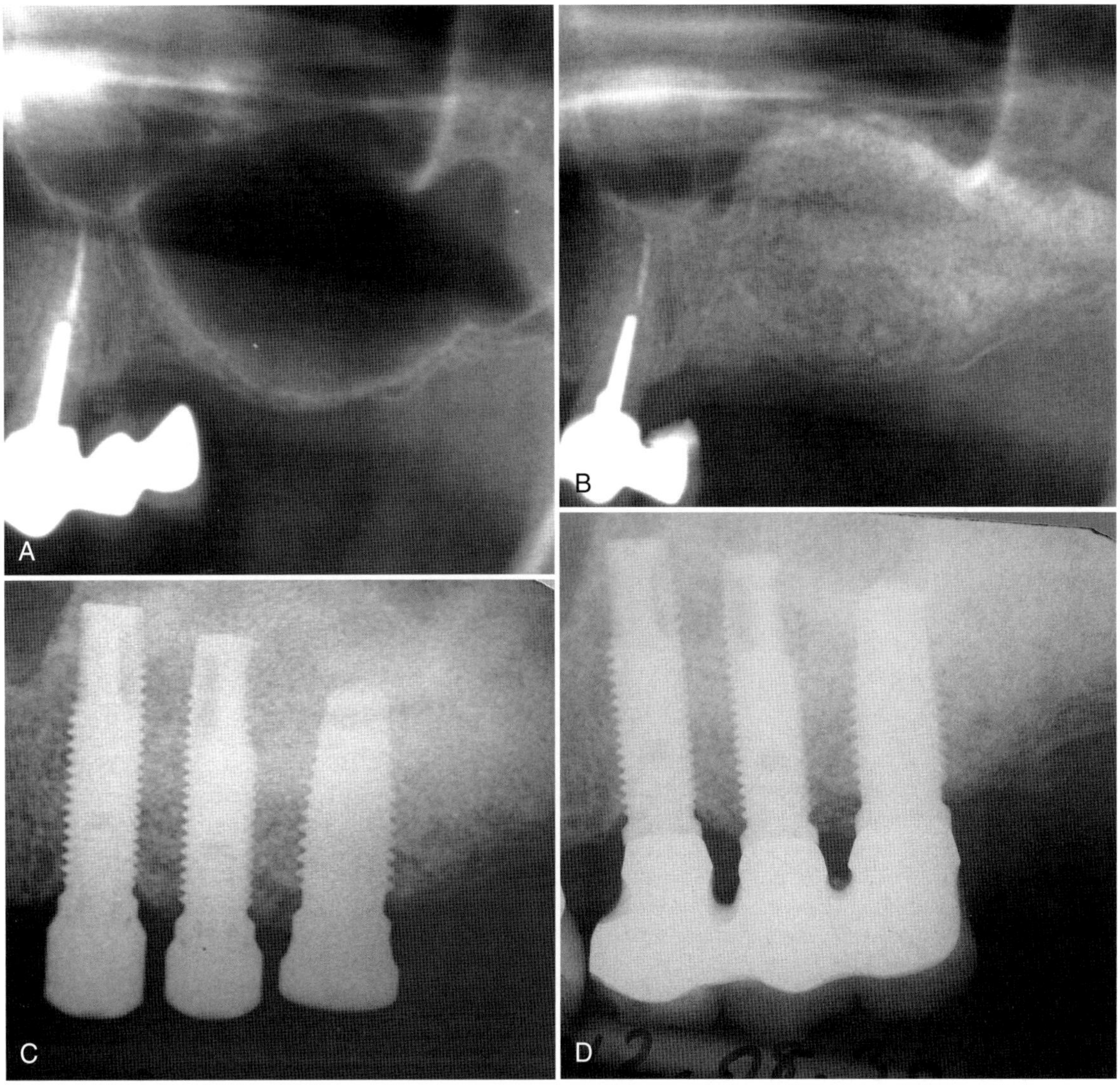

Fig. 80.3 Long-term follow-up of a patient presenting with minimal residual crestal bone height. (A) Preoperative radiograph demonstrates minimal residual crestal bone height. (B) Postoperative radiograph demonstrates sinus graft healing after 6 months. (C) Abutment connection of implants after 6 months of submerged healing. The three distal implants were placed into augmented bone. (D) Periapical radiograph demonstrates stability of crestal bone around implants at 10 years loading. (From Urban IA, Lozada JL. A prospective study of implants placed in augmented sinuses with minimal and moderate residual crestal bone: results after 1 to 5 years. *Int J Oral Maxillofac Implants.* 2010;25:1203–1212.)

bone augmentation.[11,30] In fact, the bone volume gained with DFDBA is less than that achieved with mineralized bone graft materials. The lesser bone volume achieved with DFDBA is due to moderate postoperative shrinkage—presumably because the material is demineralized.

Interestingly, some recent studies and systematic reviews have reported increased bone formation with sinus floor elevation and simultaneous implant placement without the addition of any bone graft materials.[2,16,20,35]

Risks and Complications

The maxillary sinus elevation and bone augmentation procedure is technique sensitive, requiring meticulous surgical skills. Risks and complications of the procedure include tearing or perforation of the Schneiderian membrane, intraoperative and postoperative bleeding, postoperative infection, and loss of bone graft or implants (see Chapter 86).

The reported incidence of perforation or tearing of the Schneiderian membrane varies greatly (up to 60%) and depends largely on the anatomy of the sinus as well as the skill and experience of the operator.[7,13,17,19] The presence of septa in the maxillary sinus increases the likelihood of membrane perforation.[12]

Positioning of the sinus window within 2 to 4 mm from the anterior and inferior borders of the sinus makes it easier to get direct access to the bony walls. This may lessen the amount of membrane perforation during the elevation of the sinus membrane.

Small perforations can often be managed with a resorbable barrier membrane placed over the opening followed by careful packing of the bone graft material. If the perforation or tear is extensive (see eFig. 86.3), it will be necessary to abort the procedure, close the wound, and return later to attempt it again.

Infections have been reported in a small but significant number of cases (up to 10%) after maxillary sinus elevation and bone augmentation procedures.[19,29] Prevention of infection is crucial for bone augmentation procedures. Surgery should always be performed using sterile techniques. Patients should use a presurgical antimicrobial mouthrinse (e.g., chlorhexidine) and take pre- and postoperative antibiotics. The signs and symptoms of sinus graft infection, as well as a detailed protocol for its treatment, was described in a clinical study.[29] The clinical signs include pain, swelling, pus, fistula tracts, and popcorn sign (the exfoliation of graft particles). Sinus graft infections may result in concomitant sinusitis. Consultation with an ear, nose, and throat specialist is strongly recommended in this clinical scenario.

Bleeding is also a risk of this surgical procedure. Opening a window through the lateral wall is accomplished by completely cutting through the bone of the lateral wall up to the Schneiderian membrane. The membrane is highly vascularized and may bleed significantly.[3,18] A more serious bleeding problem can arise if an intraosseous artery is severed in the process. Bone wax and topical hemostatic agents must be available to manage this urgent surgical complication. If a medium-to-large intraosseous vascular channel is identified presurgically via three-dimensional imaging, such as a CBCT scan, the surgical approach can be modified to minimize or avoid the risk of a bleeding complication.

KEY FACT

Maxillary sinus elevation and bone augmentation is a predictable technique to gain vertical bone height in the posterior maxilla. However, despite the high success rates, various intraoperative and postoperative complications have been reported. Patient selection, patient preparation, and precise surgical techniques are the key factors to reduce the incidence of sinus complications.

Surgical Procedures for Maxillary Sinus Elevation

The goal of maxillary sinus elevation and bone augmentation is to lift the Schneiderian membrane from the floor of the sinus, raising it into the sinus cavity to facilitate the generation of bone in the created space. This procedure results in a more superiorly located sinus floor (i.e., elevated membrane) and a newly created space that is filled with autogenous bone and/or a substitute bone graft material to increase the total vertical height of bone in the posterior maxilla for implant placement.

The maxillary sinus bone augmentation procedure was first described in the 1960s by Boyne (unpublished oral presentations to United States [US] Navy Dental postgraduates, 1965–1968) and originally used as a preprosthetic surgical procedure for patients with large tuberosities and pneumatized sinuses.[4] To reduce the size of the tuberosity without creating an oral–antral defect, bone was grafted into the sinus cavity to increase the volume of bone within the maxillary sinus/tuberosity. After a period of healing, the tuberosity was reduced surgically from the alveolar ridge crest. As stated previously, Boyne and James[5] (1980) were the first to describe the use of the maxillary sinus bone-grafting procedure for placement of an implant (blade type) to retain a dental prosthesis. Today, the sinus elevation and bone augmentation procedure has evolved with numerous developments in techniques, especially related to instrumentation for osteotomy access and approach (i.e., lateral vs. crestal).

The variety of techniques used for sinus elevation and bone augmentation is defined by the anatomic location of the osteotomy used to gain access to the maxillary sinus; specifically, four different anatomic locations have been described: (1) the superior lateral wall, or Caldwell-Luc, opening, which is located high on the lateral wall of the maxilla just anterior to the zygomatic arch; (2) the middle lateral wall opening, which is located midway between the alveolar ridge and the zygomatic arch; (3) the inferior lateral wall opening, which is located at the level of the alveolar ridge; and (4) the crestal osteotomy approach, which is an opening through the alveolar bone crest superiorly toward the floor of the sinus. At present, the most common procedure used for sinus elevation and bone augmentation is the lateral wall osteotomy (middle or inferior approach). The crestal approach osteotomy is also common.

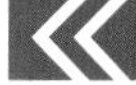

FLASH BACK

Sinus elevation and bone augmentation is a commonly performed procedure to overcome problems associated with the pneumatized sinus and a lack of bone in the posterior maxilla. Several different approaches have been used to access the maxillary sinus for bone augmentation. The lateral window approach currently is the most frequently used technique. The crestal approach is becoming increasingly popular as well.

Lateral Window Technique

The lateral window technique is probably the most effective and efficient way to access the maxillary sinus for bone augmentation. In this procedure, an opening into the maxillary sinus is created in the lateral wall to elevate the Schneiderian membrane and place a bone graft in the space between the membrane and bone, immediately superior to the existing alveolar bone.

Procedure

The lateral wall osteotomy is prepared with a high-speed drill (carbide or diamond), a piezoelectric bone surgery device (see Fig. 80.4 and online video animation), or rotary instruments that were designed to selectively cut bone. All cutting is performed with irrigation. Some clinicians will prepare the lateral window outline only, leaving the

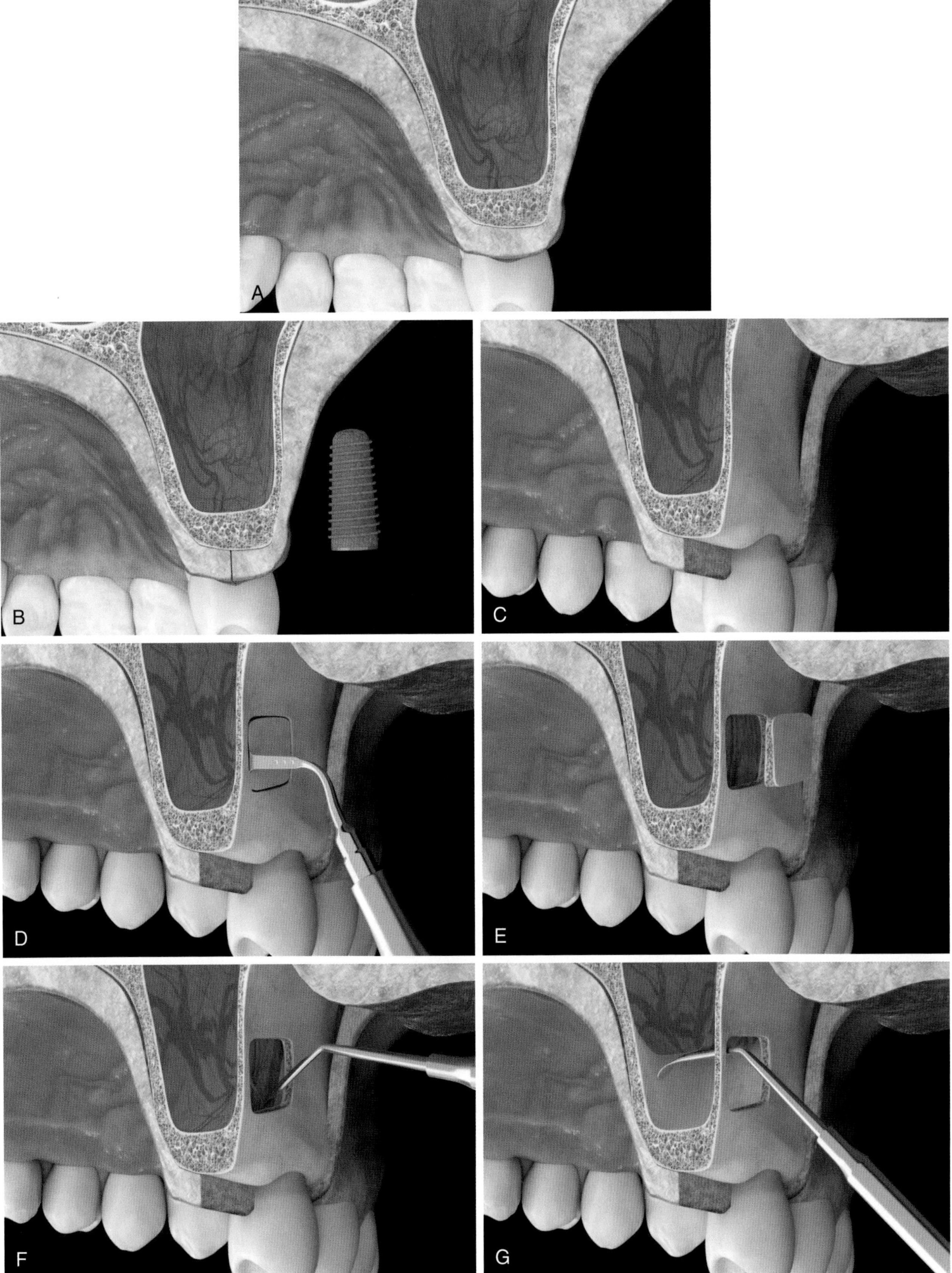

Fig. 80.4 PerioPixel illustrations depicting the steps for maxillary sinus lateral window preparation, Schneiderian membrane elevation, bone augmentation, and implant. (A and B) Notice the lack of vertical bone height in the edentulous posterior maxilla to place a standard size implant. (C) The full-thickness flap is elevated, exposing the lateral wall of the maxillary sinus. (D) The lateral window osteotomy is prepared with a piezosurgery device. (E) The lateral window is removed, leaving Schneiderian membrane intact. (F and G) Sinus elevation instruments are used to gently elevate the membrane from the sinus floor, taking care to keep the instrument on bone at all times.

Continued

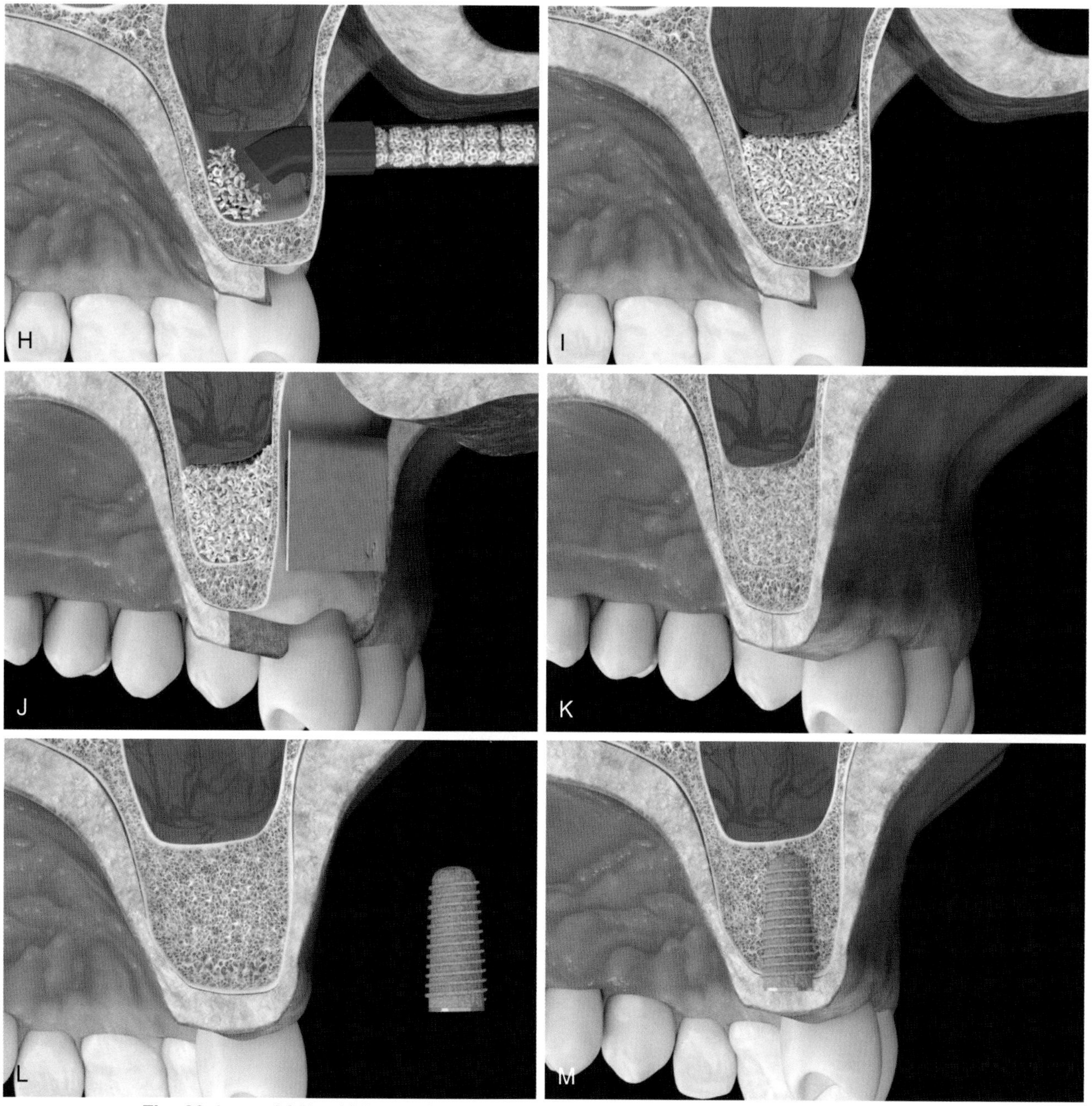

Fig. 80.4 cont'd (H and I) Bone graft material is added to the created space. (J) A resorbable barrier membrane is placed over the lateral window to prevent soft tissue invasion into the grafted maxillary sinus. The flap is sutured and allowed to heal. (K and L) The healed sinus bone augmentation with adequate dimensions for implant placement. (M) Illustration of an implant in the grafted sinus bone.

center bone attached to the membrane as it is elevated and rotated into the sinus, thus becoming the superior wall of the space created for bone grafting (Fig. 80.5A–C) and the new elevated sinus floor. Other clinicians prefer to eliminate the bony window entirely by reducing it or removing it completely (see Fig. 80.5D–F). With the former technique, it is important to create a window that is small enough, relative to the mediolateral width of the maxillary sinus, to allow the window to be pushed completely into the sinus cavity without hitting the medial wall prematurely. If the height of bone from the prepared lateral window cannot be inserted completely, it must be carefully separated from the membrane and removed. The bone removed from the lateral window osteotomy can be harvested, ground, or particulated and incorporated into the bone graft (Video 80.2).

Once the lateral window osteotomy has been created, elevation of the Schneiderian membrane is accomplished with hand instruments that are carefully inserted between the membrane and the bone, along the internal aspect of the bony walls of the sinus (eFig. 80.1). Great care is taken to avoid perforation of the membrane. Small instruments (e.g., a DeMarco curette) are introduced first along the inferior, anterior, posterior, and superior aspects of the prepared window, gradually inserting further along the bone until the membrane begins to separate and lift away from the bone. Subsequently, larger instruments (e.g., a curette or sinus elevators) are gently introduced along the bone to continue lifting the membrane to the desired levels (height, width, and depth). Instruments must always be kept in contact with the bone surface while elevating the Schneiderian membrane, to avoid perforation. An implant surgical guide should be used to estimate the planned anterior–posterior implant positions and to assess the dimensions needed for sinus bone augmentation. Once elevated, the space is filled with

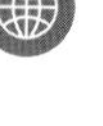

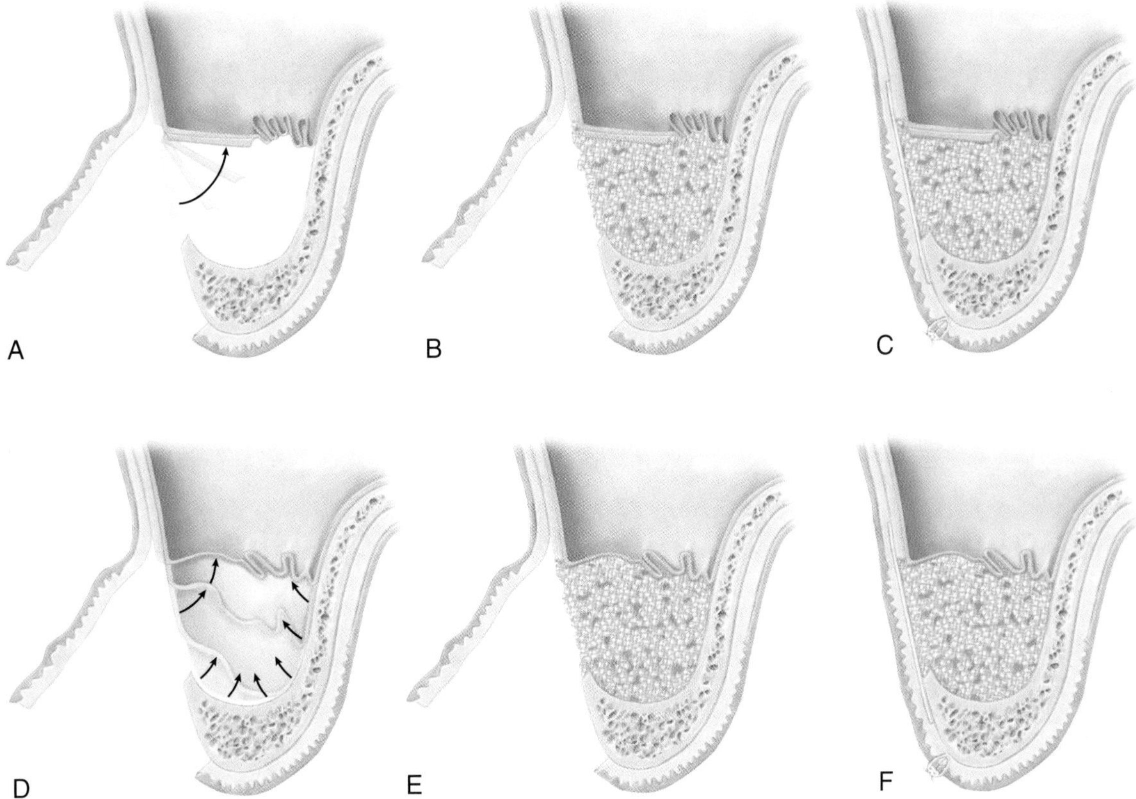

Fig. 80.5 Illustrations showing two techniques for the lateral window procedure to access the maxillary sinus for bone augmentation. The first technique (A–C) preserves the bone of the lateral window, elevating it up into the sinus cavity to create a new sinus floor. The second technique (D–F) completely removes the lateral window as part of the preparation. (A) The lateral window is cut at the periphery of the access window, leaving intact the lateral bony wall in the center of the window. The bony window is then pushed inward to become the new, elevated sinus floor/superior wall of the grafted maxillary sinus space. (B) Bone graft material is packed into the newly created space. (C) A barrier membrane is placed over the lateral window and bone graft material. The full-thickness flap is sutured over the barrier membrane. (D) Lateral window is removed entirely during the preparation of the osteotomy. The Schneiderian membrane is elevated inward and upward to become the superior containment of the grafted maxillary sinus space without a superior bony wall. (E) Bone graft material is packed into the newly created space. (F) A barrier membrane is placed over the lateral window and bone graft material. The full-thickness flap is sutured over the barrier membrane.

bone (autogenous, bone substitute, or a combination). If implants will be simultaneously placed, the implant osteotomy sites should be prepared, and implants placed after the medial, anterior, and posterior aspects of the sinus are filled with bone graft, thereby supporting the schneiderian membrane up and away from the drills and implants. After implant placement, the remaining lateral aspect of the sinus is packed with bone graft. Finally, the lateral window and bone graft are covered with a barrier membrane (e.g., resorbable membrane), and the flap is closed and sutured. Covering the lateral window osteotomy with a barrier membrane has been shown to increase the amount of vital bone and has a positive effect on implant survival.[26,33]

Simultaneous Implant Placement

Simultaneous implant placement is possible with sinus elevation and bone augmentation procedures if the implant can be stabilized in the desired location with the existing native bone (eFig. 80.2).

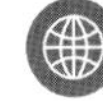

It has been suggested that a minimum of 5 mm of existing native bone in the alveolar crest is required for simultaneous implant placement; however, some clinicians claim that it is possible to place implants simultaneously with as little as 1 mm of remaining bone.[14,34] The most important factor in determining whether implants can be placed at the time of sinus elevation and bone augmentation is the ability to achieve and maintain implant stability in the existing bone regardless of the existing bone's vertical height. Factors that influence implant stability include bone height, bone quality, precision of osteotomy preparation, and the surgeon's skill. If the amount and quality of existing native bone is not sufficient to place and stabilize implants at the time of bone augmentation, then implants should be placed at a subsequent surgery after an appropriate healing period (Fig. 80.6).

Crestal Osteotomy Technique

For cases with a moderate native bone height (e.g., 5 to 7 mm) that require only a small increase in added bone height, a crestal approach to sinus elevation may be desirable. Numerous techniques and procedures have been developed to increase maxillary bone height in the posterior maxilla using a crestal approach, including the use of osteotomes, piezosurgery, osseodensification burs, and more.

The osteotome technique is a procedure that uses osteotomes (eFig. 80.3) to compress bone (internally from the alveolar crest superiorly) against the floor of the sinus, ultimately leading to a controlled "inward fracture" of the sinus floor bone along with the schneiderian membrane, creating a tented space for grafting.

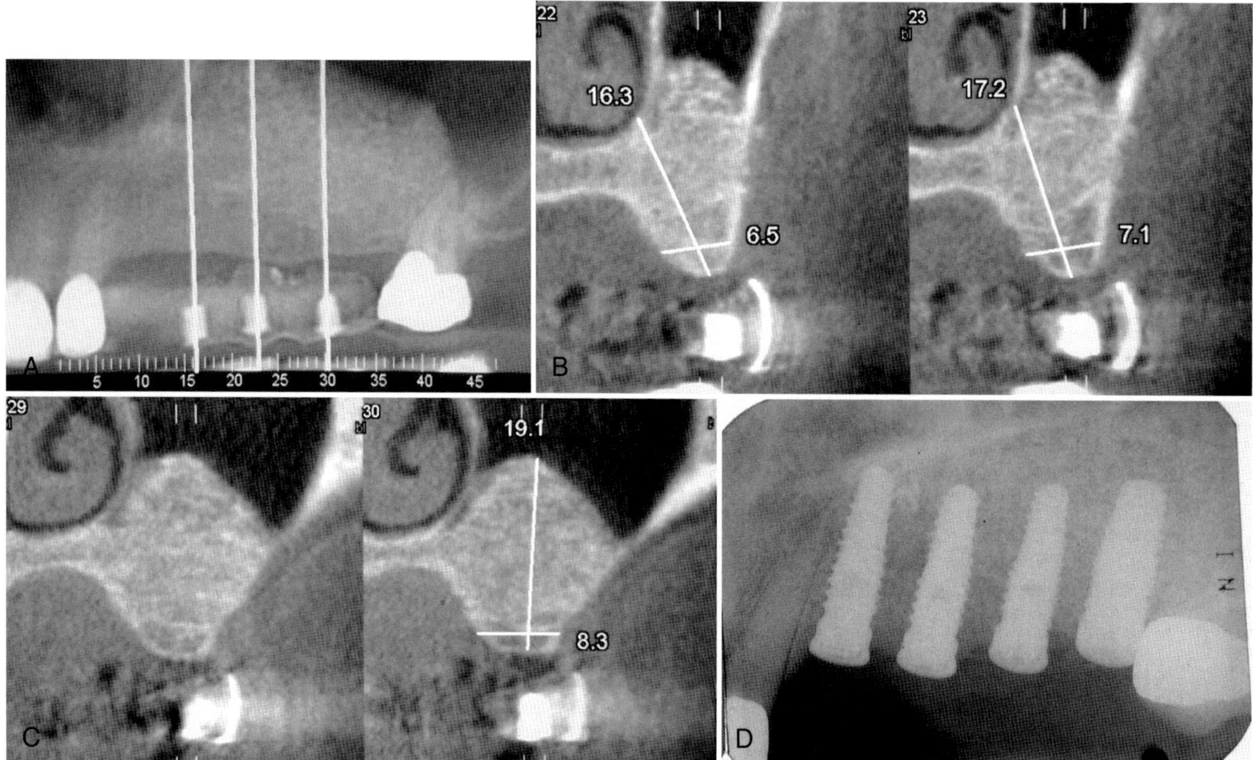

Fig. 80.6 Staged implant placement after sinus elevation and bone augmentation procedure; same patient as in Fig. 80.1. See the preoperative radiograph and preoperative cross-sectional images. (A) Postsurgical panoramic view of bone-augmented maxillary sinus. The maxillary left cuspid has been extracted because of a vertical fracture. (B) Postsurgical cross-sectional image in premolar region demonstrating more than 17-mm vertical bone height. (C) Postsurgical cross-sectional image in molar region demonstrating 19.1-mm vertical bone height. (D) Postsurgical radiograph of implants placed in the previously grafted maxillary sinus (and cuspid site).

The osteotome sinus floor elevation (OSFE) technique was described by Summers.[24,25] It is a conservative approach to sinus elevation, but it is also a "blind" technique because it does not allow the operator to visualize the schneiderian membrane during the procedure. It is a highly technique-sensitive procedure (i.e., the operator must "feel" the bone fracture and the membrane elevation). The increased vertical bone height can only be observed with radiographs that, if successful, will show a raised radio-opaque dome at the treatment site within the sinus cavity. Radiolucent graft materials, such as DFDBA, will not be apparent in the immediate postoperative radiograph.

Procedure

An osteotomy site is prepared with a series of drills (e.g., initial drills used for implant site preparation) to a depth that is approximately 1 to 2 mm from the floor of the maxillary sinus. Osteotomes are used to increase compressive forces gradually against the floor of the sinus by adding small incremental quantities of graft material with osteotome compression until the floor of the sinus fractures inward (Fig. 80.7). The impact force needed to fracture the sinus floor is typically achieved by carefully tapping the osteotome with a mallet using controlled taps. Care must be taken to prevent overinsertion of osteotomes beyond the level of existing sinus floor to avoid instrument perforation through the Schneiderian membrane. After the controlled inward fracture of the maxillary sinus floor, bone graft materials continue to be slowly introduced, through the osteotomy site and gently pushed into the maxillary sinus, which continues to elevate the membrane and thus allows a vertical expansion of the bone height in a localized area of the maxillary sinus. This latter elevation of the membrane is achieved by simply pushing graft material into the tented sinus space with the osteotome alone (i.e., no mallet). Once the sinus membrane is elevated with bone graft material to the desired height, the implant osteotomy can be completed. The final implant osteotomy drill is used to finish preparing the lateral walls to the native bone depth only (i.e., full-depth drilling into the grafted sinus is not necessary), and the implant is inserted. Multiple individual sites can be elevated and prepared simultaneously through separate crestal osteotomy sites.

Published reports of this technique have demonstrated increased bone height from 2 to 7 mm (average, 3.8 mm).[27] Thus, the crestal approach is a useful technique for increasing the vertical height of bone up to approximately 4 mm. If more vertical bone height is needed, or if multiple adjacent sites need sinus bone augmentation, then the lateral wall osteotomy approach may be more advantageous. In addition to the usual precautions and contraindications for sinus elevation and bone augmentation procedures, the osteotome technique may be contraindicated for sinuses that have an acutely sloped floor or septa in the location of the planned osteotomy. An acutely sloped sinus floor will tend to deflect the osteotome in an undesirable direction rather than allowing the osteotome to penetrate the sinus space, and the presence of septa makes it virtually impossible to fracture the sinus floor inward. Box 80.2 provides additional precautions and clinician comments on using the osteotome technique.

Several new instruments and techniques have emerged that improve the ability to create a crestal approach osteotomy while avoiding trauma or injury to the Schneiderian membrane. These instruments and techniques vary from selective rotary drill systems to piezoelectric bone surgery. See Chapter 83 for a description of piezoelectric bone surgery.

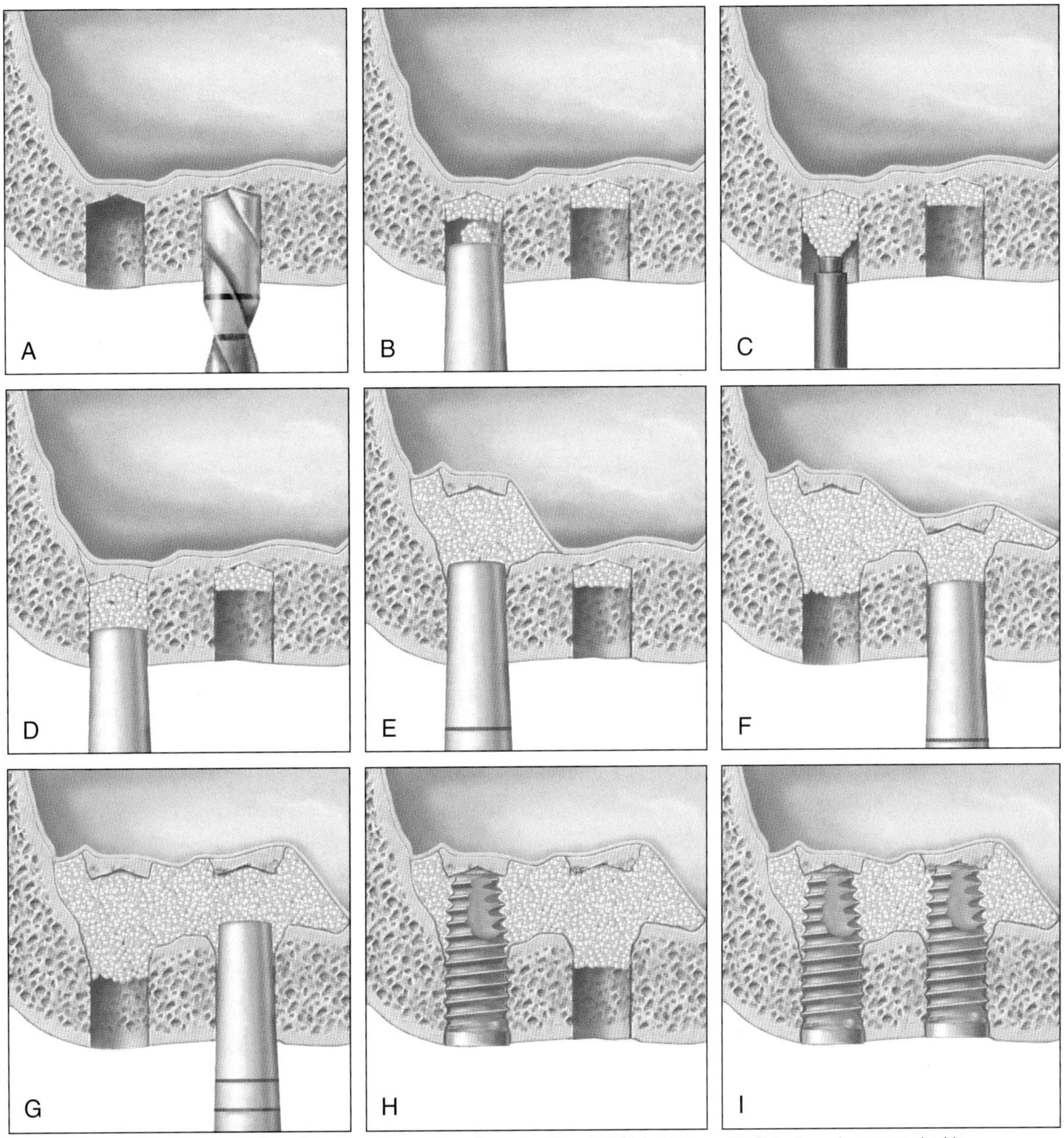

Fig. 80.7 Illustration of the osteotome sinus floor elevation (OSFE) technique. (A) Osteotomy is prepared with drills to a depth that is near the maxillary sinus floor. (B) Graft material is introduced into osteotomy and condensed with osteotome. (C) Additional bone graft material is added to the osteotomy. (D) Bone graft continues to be condensed by osteotomes. (E) This process is continued until floor of sinus is "fractured" up internally and the floor is lifted with the bone graft material. (F) Continuation of process shown in E for second site. (G) Bone graft material continues to be added gradually to both sites with osteotome condensation to elevate the Schneiderian membrane away from the bone (maxillary sinus walls) until sufficient height and volume are created for the placement of implants. (H) The coronal aspect of the osteotomy is carefully prepared for the placement of implants (instrumentation not shown), and the implant is placed. (I) Final view of two implants placed in the grafted maxillary sinus using the OSFE technique.

BOX 80.2 Clinician Comments on Use of the Osteotome Technique

Clinical Perspective 1

The osteotome procedure involves repeated tapping of osteotomes with a mallet to create the necessary pressure to fracture the floor of the maxillary sinus. This tapping can be bothersome to some individuals, especially patients who are not sedated for the procedure. The tapping procedure tends to be more bothersome for patients with dense cortical bone and for those with loose trabecular bone; in fact, a specific postoperative complication, called *benign paroxysmal positional vertigo* (BPPV), has been associated with the osteotome sinus elevation technique. During the osteotomy preparation and sinus floor elevation, the trauma induced by percussion of the osteotome with the surgical hammer, along with hyperextension of the neck during the operation, can displace otoliths in the inner ear and induce BPPV.

Clinical Perspective 2

The osteotome technique requires that the osteotome be properly aligned in the direction of the long axis of the planned implant. Thus, patients must be able to open wide enough to allow a direct insertion of the osteotome into the osteotomy site. Offset osteotomes are available that can facilitate the correct angulation (see eFig. 80.2B, online).

KEY FACT

Published reports of the crestal osteotomy technique have demonstrated increased bone height from 2 to 7 mm (average, 3.8 mm). A significantly higher bone height increase is typically possible with the lateral window approach. When more than 4 mm of bone height increase is desired, the lateral window approach may be advantageous.

Conclusions

Advanced implant surgical procedures such as sinus elevation and bone augmentation allow clinicians to increase bone volume, thus facilitating the replacement of missing teeth with dental implants in the posterior maxilla. This procedure has become widely used and predictable with a variety of approaches. Diagnosis, treatment planning, careful execution of the surgical treatment, postoperative follow-up, and appropriate implant loading are all important factors in achieving a predictable outcome and success with these procedures.

A Case Scenario is found on the companion website eBooks.Health.Elsevier.com.

Suggested Reading

Barone A, Santini S, Sbordone L, et al. A clinical study of the outcomes and complications associated with maxillary sinus augmentation. *Int J Oral Maxillofac Implants*. 2006;21:81–85.

Geurs NC, Wang IC, Shulman LB, et al. Retrospective radiographic analysis of sinus graft and implant placement procedures from the Academy of Osseointegration Consensus Conference on Sinus Grafts. *Int J Periodontics Restorative Dent*. 2001;21:517–523.

Rosano G, Taschieri S, Gaudy JF, et al. Maxillary sinus vascular anatomy and its relation to sinus lift surgery. *Clin Oral Implants Res*. 2011;22: 711–715.

Schwartz-Arad D, Herzberg R, Dolev E. The prevalence of surgical complications of the sinus graft procedure and their impact on implant survival. *J Periodontol*. 2004;75:511–516.

Summers RB. Sinus floor elevation with osteotomes. *J Esthet Dent*. 1998;10:164–171.

Tarnow DP, Wallace SS, Froum SJ, et al. Histologic and clinical comparison of bilateral sinus floor elevations with and without barrier membrane placement in 12 patients: Part 3 of an ongoing prospective study. *Int J Periodontics Restorative Dent*. 2000;20(2):117–125. PMID: 11203554.

Toffler M. Osteotome-mediated sinus floor elevation: a clinical report. *Int J Oral Maxillofac Implants*. 2004;19:266–273.

Urban IA, Lozada JL. A prospective study of implants placed in augmented sinuses with minimal and moderate residual crestal bone: results after 1 to 5 years. *Int J Oral Maxillofac Implants*. 2010;25:1203–1212.

Urban IA, Nagursky H, Church C, et al. Incidence, diagnosis, and treatment of sinus graft infection after sinus floor elevation: a clinical study. *Int J Oral Maxillofac Implants*. 2012;27:449–457.

Valentini P, Abensur DJ. Maxillary sinus grafting with anorganic bovine bone: a clinical report of long-term results. *Int J Oral Maxillofac Implants*. 2003;18:556–560.

Vogiatzi T, Kloukos D, Scarfe WC, Bornstein MM. Incidence of anatomical variations and disease of the maxillary sinuses as identified by cone beam computed tomography: a systematic review. *Int J Oral Maxillofac Implants*. 2014;29(6):1301–1314. https://doi.org/10.11607/jomi.3644. PMID: 25397794.

Wallace SS, Tarnow DP, Froum SJ, et al. Maxillary sinus elevation by lateral window approach: evolution of technology and technique. *J Evid Based Dent Pract*. 2012;12(suppl 3):161–171. PMID: 23040346.

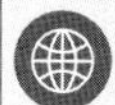
References for this chapter are found on the companion website eBooks.Health.Elsevier.com.

CHAPTER 81

Advanced Surgical Procedures: Simultaneous Implant Placement and Tissue Augmentation in the Esthetic Zone

Thomas J. Han | Kwang-Bum Park | Perry R. Klokkevold

For online-only content on surgical strategy for predictable esthetics, as well as two additional case presentations for the surgical management of difficult cases, please visit the companion website at eBooks.Health.Elsevier.com.

CHAPTER OUTLINE

In recent years, implant dentistry has been increasingly influenced by esthetic considerations. In addition to successful osseointegration, harmonious soft and hard tissues must surround the implant restorations so that they look natural and healthy. A major challenge in implant dentistry is that, in many instances, dental implants need to be placed in an esthetic zone with extensive alveolar bone deficiency from tooth loss, dentoalveolar infection, or other disorders (Fig. 81.1). Gingival morphology follows the shape of the underlying bone, and it is difficult to build esthetically acceptable gingiva in areas with deficient supporting bone. Furthermore, using conventional surgical approaches to accomplish the goal in a patient-friendly manner with minimal trauma and clinical predictability is an extremely demanding task.

Treatment planning in a complex implant case today is often confusing because of the many different surgical and restorative approaches to solve the same problem. Many times these procedures seem to conflict. When considering the surgical placement of implants, clinicians must consider the approach (conventional two-stage approach vs. a one-stage approach) and the timing of implant placement (immediate vs. delayed or staged placement). For bone augmentation procedures, the clinician may choose the more conventional approach of augmenting the ridge first and placing the implant or implants after healing, or the simultaneous implant placement technique with bone augmentation approach in which bone grafting is done at same time as implant placement. All of these approaches can provide a successful outcome if patient selection is appropriate and techniques are performed properly.[7,11,25,35] However, depending on the situation, some of these techniques are more advantageous than others in achieving esthetic results with better predictability and less patient discomfort.

It is easy for a clinician to "dogmatically" choose one approach, usually the one that they feel most comfortable with, and to treat all patients with the same approach. However, with heightened expectations of esthetics pushing the art and science of dentistry, it is essential for clinicians to fully understand all the available options of treatment and to decide appropriately which, where, when, and how to use these options for each patient.

An important clinical development in dental implant surgery is the concept of a "minimally invasive" approach to treatment. Specifically, the drive is toward minimally invasive implant placement. With advances in technologies, materials, and biologic sciences in dentistry, this approach to implant surgery is becoming more popular among clinicians and will most likely dominate the way dental implants will be placed in the near future.

Minimally invasive surgery in implant dentistry implies a surgical approach that minimizes the extent and number of surgical procedures while providing esthetics, predictability, and longevity with minimal surgical morbidity and discomfort to patients. The surgical approach most often required to achieve these goals for anterior implant therapy involves immediate implant placement, a one-stage surgical approach, with or without flap, and simultaneous bone grafting. Furthermore, these surgical techniques need to be guided by a consistent surgical strategy that provides predictable esthetic results in implant dentistry. A minimally invasive approach to implant therapy in posterior sextants where esthetics is not a major concern can be predictably achieved with the use of short, wide implants.[2,18,19,30]

This chapter introduces surgical strategies that enhance the esthetic predictability in implant dentistry. A minimally invasive surgical approach used to manage difficult esthetic and anatomically deficient cases is discussed with examples. The one-stage, immediate implant placement technique, which is the foundation of

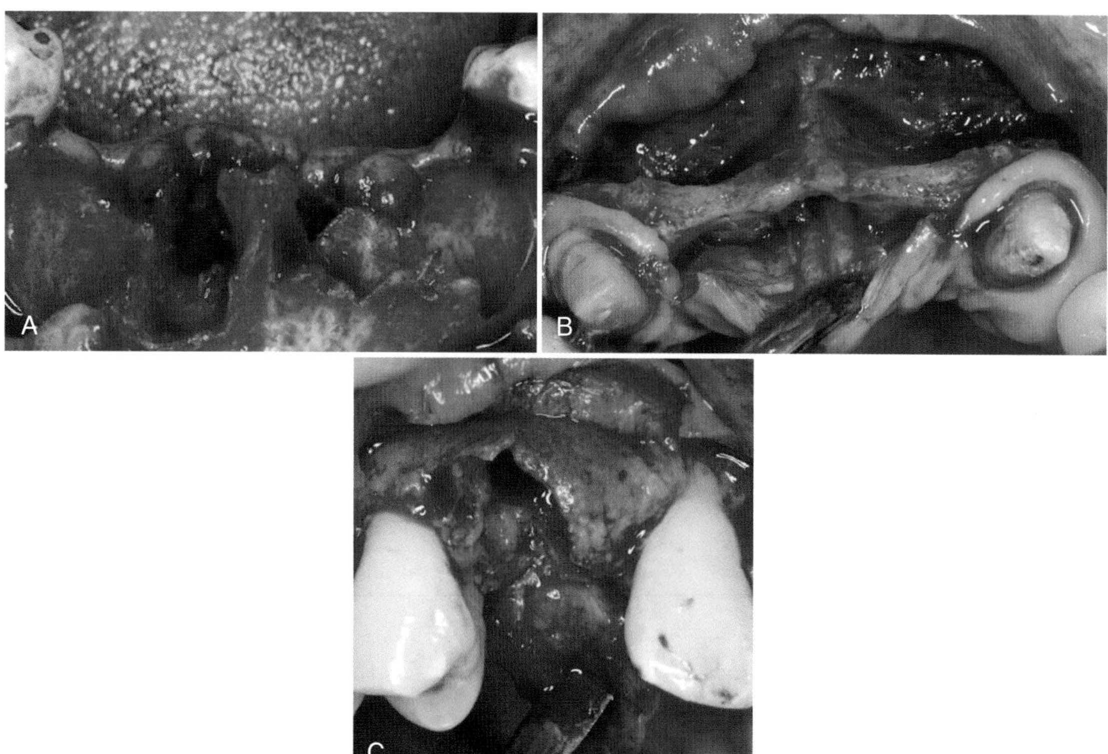

Fig. 81.1 Implant sites in the anterior, esthetic zone with extensive bone loss. (A) Anterior mandibular site showing extensive bone loss following extraction of hopelessly infected mandibular incisors. (B) Extremely narrow (labial-palatal) ridge width in the anterior maxilla that was missing central and lateral incisors for many years. (C) Moderate bone loss associated with the extraction socket of a maxillary cuspid.

a patient-friendly approach to esthetic implant dentistry, is presented in detail. The thought processes involved in case selection, their scientific rationale, and proper techniques of soft and hard tissue management are described with cases.

KEY FACT

Minimally invasive surgery is an approach that minimizes the extent of surgical invasiveness, as well as the number of surgical procedures, while providing esthetics and predictability with minimal surgical morbidity and discomfort to patients. The surgical approach most often required to achieve these goals for anterior implant therapy involves immediate implant placement, a one-stage surgical approach, with or without flap, and simultaneous bone grafting.

Surgical Strategy for Predictable Esthetics

Adherence to the following surgical strategies enhances predictability and outcomes for esthetic dental implant surgical procedures with minimal discomfort to patients (see the online description of the following key points):

1. Determine the level of surgical esthetic goal to be achieved.
2. Visualize the final outcome.
3. Preserve existing tissues important for esthetics.
4. Always overbuild bone and soft tissue in augmentation surgical procedures.

Immediate Implant Placement for Predictability and Esthetics

Immediate implant placement in a one-stage approach in which a healing abutment or provisional restoration is attached to the implant and remains exposed provides more predictable preservation of the interproximal peri-implant gingival tissue with less patient discomfort and treatment time.[24,25] This approach to implant placement is the foundation of a minimally invasive approach to esthetic implant dentistry. However, as with any surgical technique, it takes learning and practice to perform it properly. The criteria and techniques for proper immediate implant placement have previously been established and reported with successful long-term outcomes.[21,35]

One of the more difficult aspects of immediate implant placement is positioning the implant with sufficient primary stability in an extraction socket, often without elevating a flap. The alveolar architecture in relation to the angle of the implant to be inserted, the presence or absence of a bone concavity apical to the extracted tooth, the amount of existing bone apical and palatal to the extraction socket that can provide primary stability for the immediate implant, and the quality of the bone and soft tissues of the ridge should all be thoroughly evaluated clinically and radiographically before surgery.[21,35] While it has been possible for experienced clinicians to successfully place immediate implants without the aid of three-dimensional (3D) scans (e.g., computed tomography [CT] or cone-beam computed tomography [CBCT]), the use of 3D imaging is highly advised because it offers great diagnostic value.

A major disadvantage of placing implants immediately in the changing alveolar bone of an extraction socket is that it may result in progressive recession of the gingival labial margin over the implant restoration.[6,20] Therefore, when placing an immediate implant with a one-stage surgical approach in an esthetic zone, a prudent strategy would be to improve the quality and quantity of labial gingival tissue, which seems to be vital for the stability of the labial gingival margin involving immediate implants.[22,34] One of the most effective ways to keep the implanted socket from collapsing and improve the labial gingival biotype is to simultaneously fill the labial socket void with particulate bone and augment the labial gingival tissue with soft tissue.[3,26,29,33,35] Multiple recent (2020 and 2021) systematic reviews with meta-analyses support the need for soft tissue augmentation to improve and maintain soft tissue esthetics when placing implants immediately in the esthetic zone.[4,5,36,41] One of these (2021)[41] included five randomized controlled trials (RCTs) and three non-randomized controlled studies (NRSs) evaluating the effect of connective tissue graft (CTG) on the vertical mid-facial soft tissue change following immediate implant placement over a period of 12 to 108 months. They reported 0.41 mm ($P < .001$) vertical mid-facial soft tissue stability advantage in favor of soft tissue grafting at the time of implant placement. This is clinically relevant since the risk of a ≥1 mm difference in the mid-facial gingival margin was 12 times greater without soft tissue grafts.

An effective bone and gingival tissue augmentation technique used with flapless, immediate implant placement in a one-stage approach is the bone and crescent-shaped free gingival grafting technique.[21] In this technique, the space between the inner surface of the labial bony wall and the labial surface of the implant is filled with slow-resorbing, mineralized, freeze-dried particulate bone allograft or particulate xenograft to help preserve the horizontal dimension of the ridge (Fig. 81.2A). Then a crescent-shaped soft tissue graft is harvested from the ipsilateral palate (see Fig. 81.2B) and is transplanted into the labial recipient site coronal to the particulate bone graft (see Fig. 81.2C). To provide or maintain the blood supply to the donor tissue, it is important that the outer surface of the crescent graft fits in intimate contact with the bleeding lamina propria of the labial gingiva. Proper suturing ensures good proximity and prevents the graft from being displaced coronally out of the recipient site (see Fig. 81.2D).

The advantages of this approach to gingival augmentation are simplicity and minimal surgical morbidity. In addition to providing a sealed protection for the bone graft, it prevents resorption of the sensitive labial crestal bone. Preparation of the recipient site involves no surgical manipulation other than de-epithelialization, as described. Gingival walls are completely intact with a full blood supply. The donor site wound is small (approximately 3-mm depth × 3-mm height at the widest point) with intact epithelium around the wound, which epithelializes within a week and causes minimal discomfort for the patient. Because each donor tissue graft is small, multiple grafts can be harvested from a single palate so that multiple immediate implants can be augmented at the same time. Furthermore, this gingival augmentation technique frequently improves an unfavorable initial gingival margin because the grafted gingival margin is always coronal to the existing gingival margin. This minimizes a need for other time-consuming techniques, such as orthodontic extrusion or a delayed approach to implant placement when the initial gingival margin is not esthetic or ideal, as recommended by many investigators.[7,37]

The risk-to-benefit ratio of the crescent grafting technique is favorable enough that if the graft does not survive or if more than expected horizontal resorption of the ridge occurs, traditional techniques (e.g., subepithelial connective tissue graft) can be performed to augment the results. This is usually possible without refabrication of the implant restoration because the vertical height of the interdental papilla is sufficiently preserved with immediate implant placement in a one-stage approach.

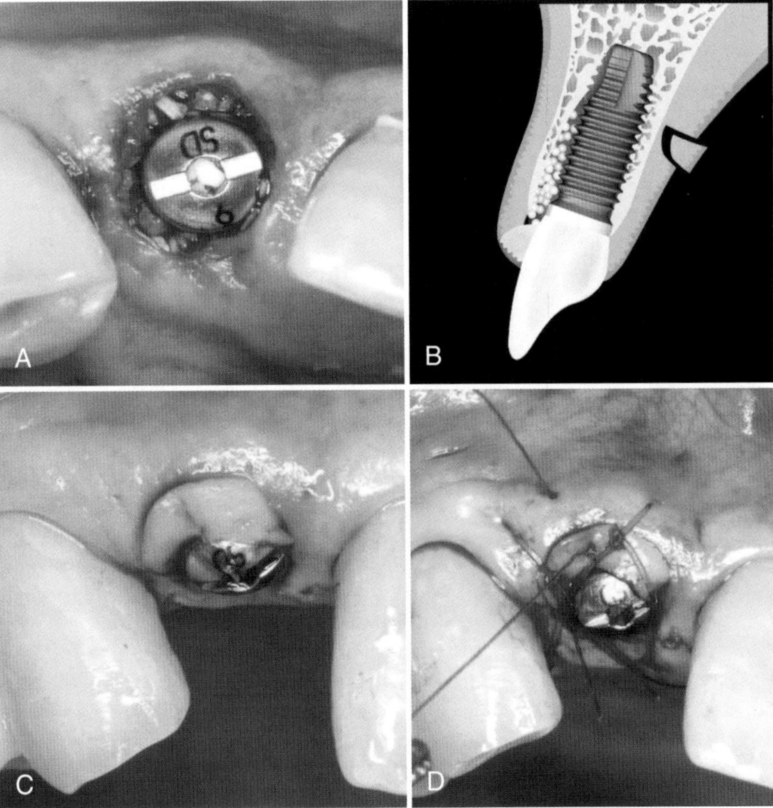

Fig. 81.2 (A) Bone graft material is lightly packed into the extraction socket gap between the labial wall and the implant surface. (B) Diagram of crescent-shaped, free gingival graft tissue being harvested from the palate. (C) Clinical photograph of crescent-shaped, free gingival graft tissue positioned over the bone graft to fit snugly in the gap between the gingival wall and the implant surface. (D) Crescent-shaped, free gingival graft is sutured in place using 5-0 gut sutures. The sutures pass through the gingival graft toward the labial gingival margin and are tied. Then, without cutting the ends, the suture is passed over the graft and tied to the palatal gingival tissue. Three sutures are needed to keep the graft in position.

KEY FACT

An effective bone and gingival tissue augmentation technique used with flapless, immediate implant placement in a one-stage approach is the bone and crescent-shaped free gingival grafting technique. To provide and maintain the blood supply to the donor tissue, it is important that the outer surface of the crescent graft fits in intimate contact with the bleeding lamina propria of the labial gingiva. Proper suturing ensures good proximity and prevents the graft from being displaced coronally. The crescent graft technique enhances gingival thickness following extraction and immediate implant placement.

Surgical Management of Difficult Cases (Minimally Invasive Approach)

The failure to satisfy the esthetic needs of a patient frequently starts with an inadequate examination of the soft and hard tissues surrounding the surgical site and the natural dentition. This can result in an incorrect diagnosis, which leads to an incorrect treatment plan. The wrong treatment plan combined with selection of inappropriate surgical approaches or techniques can result in a disastrous esthetic outcome and unnecessary patient suffering. The first two case presentations describe the examination and thought processes involved in determining the diagnosis and treatment planning of complex anterior cases with extensive alveolar bone loss. The proper application of the surgical strategies and the minimally invasive techniques, as previously described, are illustrated. The final case presentation illustrates the minimally invasive approach to posterior implant therapy with the use of short, wide implants in which esthetics is not the major concern.[2,18,19,30]

Components of Esthetic Examination

The patient's chief complaint, esthetic zone, tooth positions, gingival form, osseous crest position, biotype, tooth shape, horizontal and vertical ridge deficiency, and occlusal status all play important roles in deriving an accurate esthetic treatment plan for the patient. Therefore, developing the necessary skill and knowledge to examine and recognize problems of these components is an essential first step to clinical success.

Case Presentation 1

The first case presented is in a patient with a simultaneous bone and soft tissue augmentation with multiple maxillary anterior immediate implants placed in a one-stage, flapless approach.

Patient Dental History and Chief Complaint

The patient is a 70-year-old woman with severe mobility and discomfort of the maxillary four incisors. Except for a generalized feeling of weakness, she is healthy and does not have any medical contraindications to dental treatment. She presented with a desire to replace her maxillary incisors with dental implants, but she is very concerned about the physical discomfort she may experience from the implant surgery. She does not want to wear a removable prosthesis at all, not even for a short time. She is content with her present dental esthetics.

Examination and Diagnosis

The maxillary incisors exhibit moderate to severe periodontitis with 4- to 7-mm periodontal probing depths. They exhibit severe (2+) mobility with fremitus. The periodontal and restorative prognosis of these teeth is poor. She has an excessive overbite with evidence of moderate mandibular incisor wear, indicating possible parafunctional habits. Her incisors are slightly elongated, but the dentogingival symmetry is acceptable (Fig. 81.3A). The shape of the incisors is slightly triangular with sufficient interdental papilla volume and height. Interproximal gingival tissue is not swollen or edematous. Her gingival biotype appears to be on the thin side with slight marginal inflammation, and the position of the labial gingival margins is already high (i.e., maximal apical position). Any further recession will be unesthetic.

Radiographic evaluation demonstrates moderate to severe vertical and horizontal periodontal bone loss. The osseous crest position in relation to the gingival margins appears too apical to provide adequate gingival support (see Fig. 81.3B). The restorative and periodontal status of the canines is healthy.

Treatment Objectives

Considering her age, reasonable esthetic expectation, concern for surgical morbidity, and a lack of willingness to wear a removable provisional prosthesis, the treatment objective for this patient would be to use a surgical approach that minimizes the extent and number of surgical procedures while providing predictability, longevity, and acceptable esthetics. Recommending orthodontic extrusion or multiple surgical procedures to achieve ideal esthetics on this patient would be considered an excessive treatment plan and would not provide any additional value or benefits for her.

Treatment Options

Considerations for extracting four maxillary incisors include the need to remove sound porcelain-fused-to-metal crowns from the canines to replace them as part of a six-unit fixed prosthesis. This option has a questionable long-term functional and esthetic prognosis. Her dentition exhibits evidence of excessive overbite and parafunctional habit, which may have contributed to the alveolar bone loss of the incisors in the first place. The convex shape of the ridge and the lack of osseous support will most likely result in substantial horizontal and vertical resorption of the edentulous ridge under the pontics of the fixed bridge, even with extraction socket grafting and ovate provisionalization. This will compromise the long-term esthetics.

Even if this patient can tolerate the temporary removable partial denture, which she said she cannot, this option poses a considerable esthetic challenge. The ridge surrounding the extraction sockets will rapidly lose vertical and horizontal dimensions soon after the extractions.[3] The loss of vertical height in the interproximal gingival areas creates an esthetic problem that is very difficult to correct. It often requires multiple surgical procedures that have a high incidence of surgical morbidity and rarely achieve the desired ideal esthetic result. This is especially true in a case such as this in which the patient has extensive periodontal vertical and horizontal bone loss. The anticipated vertical ridge collapse after the extraction is substantial, even with bone grafting of the extraction sockets. More importantly, the need for multiple surgical procedures to achieve "acceptable" esthetic results for this patient may be too traumatic for her.

Extracting four maxillary incisors, immediately placing two implants, and replacing the teeth with a four-unit provisional fixed partial denture supported by two implants is an acceptable but risky treatment option. Immediate provisionalization of the two immediately placed implants, with her occlusion and suspected parafunctional habit, carries the risk of early excessive loading and implant failure. Additionally, it will be challenging to maintain the vertical and horizontal ridge dimensions in the edentulous area under the pontics. Most likely it will require additional soft tissue augmentation procedures to achieve "acceptable" esthetics in the pontic area (i.e., missing central incisor area).

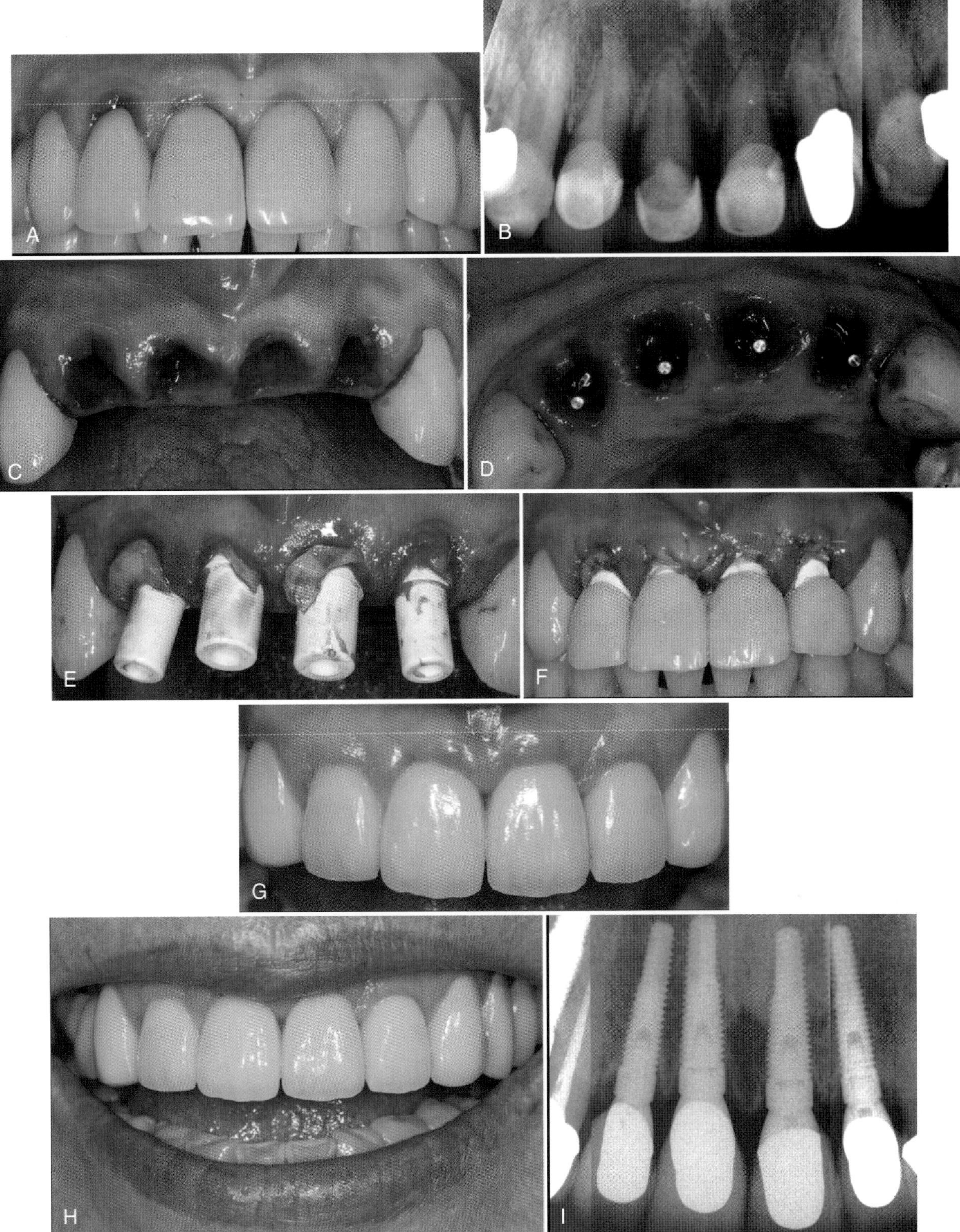

Fig. 81.3 (A) Clinical photograph of periodontally compromised maxillary anterior teeth with long clinical crowns. The presenting esthetic status is not ideal. However, the dentogingival symmetry is fair because the gingival margin is approximately the same for all incisors (cuspid, lateral, and central). (B) Periapical radiographs of the maxillary anterior teeth reveal moderate to severe horizontal periodontal bone loss with vertical intrabony defects. (C) Simple, atraumatic extraction of the maxillary incisors reveals sockets with unsupported interdental tissues. Note the absence of incisions or flap reflection, which has preserved the blood supply and integrity of the interdental soft tissues. (D) Guide pins placed in prepared implant sites reveal good position within the extraction sockets, achieving good primary stability from the palatal aspect of the socket. (E) Implants with temporary abutments and crescent-shaped, free gingival grafts (not yet sutured). (F) Implant provisional abutments are prepared, and provisional restorations are fabricated using conventional methods. (G) One-year post-loading results show nearly complete preservation of the interproximal papilla height and improved labial gingival biotype. Labial gingival margins are substantially coronal in position as compared with the initial levels. (H) The final restorations have a more normal length, offering the patient a much more youthful smile. Preexisting moderate to severe attrition is noted on the incisal edges of the mandibular anterior teeth. (I) Periapical radiographs at 1 year of the implants with final restorations reveal good preservation of interproximal bone height with minimal saucerization. The platform-switched implant restorations likely contribute to the preservation of bone.

CLINICAL CORRELATION

A common cause of esthetic failure is inadequate examination of the soft and hard tissues surrounding the surgical site and the natural dentition. If the examination is incomplete or findings are misinterpreted, an incorrect diagnosis will be made, which in turn will lead to an incorrect treatment plan. The judgment to formulate an appropriate treatment plan depends on making an accurate diagnosis!

Extracting four maxillary incisors, immediately placing four implants in the sockets, and replacing the missing teeth with a four-unit provisional fixed partial denture supported by four implants is another acceptable option. Splinting four provisionals together should provide sufficient resistance and protection to the implants from early excessive loading. Some clinicians do not recommend placing implants next to each other in the lateral and central incisor positions because they are often positioned too close, and it is very difficult to create or maintain an interdental papilla that emulates an interdental papilla between an implant and a tooth or between two natural teeth.[44] However, the more recent use of implants with a platform-switching design may change the spatial requirements for achieving an interdental papilla between implants. The bone between implants appears to be better protected, and as a result the vertical height of the interproximal tissue may be better preserved.[10,28] If procedures are carried out properly, this option can provide a long-term functional and esthetic result with minimal discomfort to the patient.

1. Extract four maxillary incisors and replace them with a conventional (six-unit) fixed prosthesis supported by the canines.
2. Extract four maxillary incisors and wait for healing of the sockets and ridge while temporarily replacing the missing teeth with a removable partial denture. Plan to place two or four implants after 3 to 6 months of healing by using either a one- or two-stage approach.
3. Extract four maxillary incisors, immediately place two implants in the lateral positions, and replace the missing teeth with a four-unit provisional fixed partial denture supported by two implants.
4. Extract four maxillary incisors, immediately place four implants in the sockets, and replace the missing teeth with a four-unit provisional fixed partial denture supported by four implants.

Surgical Strategy for Predictable Esthetics

Because of the patient's age and reasonable expectation, the level of the esthetic goal determined for this patient is not ideal but is acceptable. This level of esthetics can be predictably achieved in a minimally invasive, patient-friendly manner. By mentally visualizing the surgical and prosthetic goal, an acceptable esthetic outcome can be achieved for this patient if the existing heights of the interproximal gingival tissues can be maintained. Additionally, if the existing biotype and the level of the labial gingival margin can be overbuilt with hard and soft tissue augmentation, the final esthetic outcome will be enhanced. If this can be accomplished with simultaneous implant placement, it will minimize the number of surgical procedures required. In this case, especially because the patient appears to have parafunctional habits, it is desirable to place more implants and use them to support the immediate provisionalization.

Considering all of these treatment options, the treatment that is most compatible with this patient's surgical strategy for predictability, acceptable esthetics, and long-term results is treatment option 4—extraction of the incisors followed by immediate placement of four implants with an immediate provisional restoration supported by the implants.

Treatment Plan and Rationale

Four maxillary incisors are to be extracted and four implants placed immediately in a one-stage approach with simultaneous bone and soft tissue grafting. The bone and crescent-shaped free-gingival grafting technique will be used to overbuild labial gingival biotype.[21] A tapered implant with a platform-switching design is to be used. The tapered design has been shown to promote primary stability in sockets, and the platform-switching design better maintains the interimplant bone.[10,28] An immediate provisional restoration without centric contacts will be attached to the implants.

Treatment Sequence

In complex treatments involving dental implants, the treatment plan must be sequenced and coordinated between the restorative dentist and the surgeon before starting the treatment. This is especially true when immediate provisionalization is planned. This will enhance success and help make the treatment more patient friendly.

Surgical Procedure

Once the patient is anesthetized, the incisors are extracted atraumatically, thus ensuring that gingival tissues, especially the interdental papilla, are not damaged (see Fig. 81.3C). The sockets are prepared to receive implants by removing the sulcular epithelium and by completely and thoroughly removing all granulation tissue. Immediately placed implants must have complete primary stability at the time of placement. Proper vertical position, buccolingual position, and mesiodistal position, as well as buccolingual angulation, are all critical factors for a successful outcome. Implants in anterior sockets are prepared and placed toward the palate (see Fig. 81.3D) to ensure sufficient labial bone thickness for labial margin stability.[11] Once the provisional healing abutments are accurately seated (may require bone profiler), the labial void of the sockets is grafted with particulate bone, and a crescent-shaped free gingival tissue graft is harvested and placed over the graft (see Fig. 81.3E) as described previously and in the literature.[21] By using this technique, all four teeth can be augmented in one surgical procedure with minimal discomfort to the patient. Once the soft tissue crescent grafts are secured with sutures, the provisional abutments are prepared for provisional crowns. The provisional crowns (splinted) are fabricated using conventional methods (see Fig. 81.3F). Contours of the provisional crowns may need to be modified as healing and remodeling occurs. Impression taking for the final restoration is relatively easy because the provisional abutments placed at the time of surgery and modified during healing nicely shape the tissues for an optimal prosthetic emergence profile.

Results

The 1-year result shows nearly complete preservation of the interproximal papilla height and an improved labial biotype with labial gingival margins that are substantially coronal to the original gingival margin level (see Fig. 81.3G). The final result consists of crowns with a more normal incisor length and a more youthful smile (see Fig. 81.3H). Some gingival irregularity is noted, and it appears to be a result of the soft tissue grafting. These areas could easily be smoothed with gingivoplasty, but the patient refused. Radiographs reveal preservation of interproximal bone with minimal saucerization around the implants with a platform-switch design (see Fig. 81.3I).

After the surgical strategies described and with the use of minimally invasive surgical techniques, this 70-year-old patient received immediate implant-supported replacement of severely compromised maxillary incisors with an acceptable (or better) esthetic result and minimal treatment discomfort. With one surgery, including the extractions, she was provided with a fixed implant restoration on four implants. In the same surgery, the bone and soft tissue were augmented while preserving the interdental papilla. She experienced very little postoperative pain and was pleased with her new, more youthful-looking smile. The treatment time was only 6 months from extraction to final restoration. She was never without teeth and never wore a removable prosthesis. The improvement of the labial gingival margin was achieved without orthodontic extrusion or multiple surgical procedures.

Conclusions

The clinical science in dentistry has evolved to where placement of dental implants and restoring them require sufficient knowledge in several disciplines of dentistry. In addition to mastering surgical objectives and techniques, periodontists must be able to evaluate and accurately diagnose (and treat or refer) a wide range of related "restorative" issues including but not limited to esthetics, occlusion, temporomandibular joint function, vertical dimension, and dental–skeletal relationships. These "other" aspects of diagnosis are essential for the development of an appropriate treatment plan, which is necessary for a successful outcome in esthetic implant dentistry.

In addition, with heightened expectations of esthetics pushing the art and science of dentistry, it is essential for clinicians to fully understand all the available treatment options and to be able to determine appropriately which option to choose, when to use certain techniques, and how to apply them for each patient's scenario.

The minimally invasive approach and techniques presented in this chapter are not the only ways to manage difficult esthetic cases, and some clinicians may consider them controversial. Certainly, these techniques require learning and practice to make them effective in each clinician's hands. However, they present a sound approach to what is possible in hard and soft tissue management for esthetic implant surgery and provide effective strategies and techniques for solving many difficult esthetic cases in a patient-friendly manner.

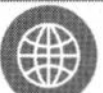
A Case Scenario is found on the companion website eBooks.Health.Elsevier.com.

Suggested Reading

Cappiello M, Luongo R, Di Iorio D, et al. Evaluation of peri-implant bone loss around platform-switched implants. *Int J Periodontics Restorative Dent*. 2008;28:347–355.

Chen ST, Darby IB, Reynolds EC, et al. Immediate implant placement postextraction without flap elevation. *J Periodontol*. 2009;80:163–172.

Grunder U. Stability of the mucosal topography around single-tooth implants and adjacent teeth: 1-year results. *Int J Periodontics Restorative Dent*. 2000;20:11–17.

Han TJ, Jeong CW. Bone and crescent shaped free gingival grafting for anterior immediate implant placement: technique and case report. *J Implant Adv Clin Dent*. 2009;1(5):23–33.

Hermann F, Lerner H, Palti A. Factors influencing the preservation of the periimplant marginal bone. *Implant Dent*. 2007;16:165–175.

Klokkevold PR, Han TJ, Camargo PM. Aesthetic management of extractions for implant site development: delayed versus staged implant placement. *Pract Periodontics Aesthet Dent*. 1999;11:603–610, quiz 612.

Lazzara RJ, Porter SS. Platform switching: a new concept in implant dentistry for controlling postrestorative crestal bone levels. *Int J Periodontics Restorative Dent*. 2006;26:9–17.

Park KB, Han TJ, Kenney EB. Immediate implant placement with immediate provisional crown placement: three case reports. *Pract Periodontics Aesthet Dent*. 2002;14:147–154.

Raghoebar GM, Korfage A, Meijer HJA, Gareb B, Vissink A, Delli K. Linear and profilometric changes of the mucosa following soft tissue augmentation in the zone of aesthetic priority: A systematic review and meta-analysis. *Clin Oral Implants Res*. 2021 Oct;32(Suppl 21):138–156. https://doi.org/10.1111/clr.13759. PMID: 34642988.

Schropp L, Wenzel A, Kostopoulos L, et al. Bone healing and soft tissue contour changes following single-tooth extraction: a clinical and radiographic 12-month prospective study. *Int J Periodontics Restorative Dent*. 2003;23:313–323.

Seyssens L, De Lat L, Cosyn J. Immediate implant placement with or without connective tissue graft: A systematic review and meta-analysis. *J Clin Periodontol*. 2021;48(2):284–301. https://doi.org/10.1111/jcpe.13397. Epub 2020 Nov 20. PMID: 33125754.

Spear FM, Kokich VG, Mathews DP. Interdisciplinary management of anterior dental esthetics. *J Am Dent Assoc*. 2006;137:160–169.

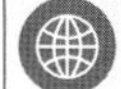
References for this chapter are found on the companion website eBooks.Health.Elsevier.com.

CHAPTER 82

Dental Implant Microsurgery: Immediate Placement

Dennis A. Shanelec† | *Leonard S. Tibbetts*

CHAPTER OUTLINE

The success of dental implants in extraction sites, combined with immediate provisionals for newly placed dental implants, has brought a convergence in restorative and surgical practice for treatment planning dental implants. This convergence reaches its summit in the approach to failing teeth in the maxillary esthetic zone. For anatomic reasons, maxillary anterior teeth are at high risk for traumatic injury (Fig. 82.1).[13,14] Traumatized teeth frequently receive endodontic treatment that may be followed by a horizontal or vertical root fracture.[1,2,15] Dentistry's historical answer to tooth loss has been the fixed bridge. Tooth preparation necessary for a fixed bridge often results in significant reduction of tooth structure.[22] Inherent esthetic limitations of fixed bridges include loss of gingival papillae and resorption of the buccal alveolar plate. For these reasons, dental implants are a preferred choice for tooth replacement in the maxillary esthetic zone.

Implant Microsurgery

Microsurgery is associated with enhanced soft tissue procedures and fine suturing. This procedure is part of the scope of implant microsurgery, but additional benefits include dental implant drilling precision. The ability to discern minute dimensional differences permits implant osteotomy preparations centered exactly between reference points such as adjacent teeth, adjacent implants, or buccal and lingual ridge anatomy. More profoundly, the microscope allows immediate detection of subtle changes in drill position so appropriate feedback corrections can be applied to the handpiece. Enhanced angular perception is also important. The drill's angular position can be oriented relative to small landmarks such as the implant platform surface level or the angle of adjacent implant healing caps, permitting optimal parallel positioning and depth of adjacent implants. The implant drill angle can also be accurately oriented to root surface angulation using just 3 to 4 mm of root anatomy exposed between the cementoenamel junction and the osseous crest. These reference points are simply not visible without a microscope. Detecting subtle angulation reference points and changes in drill position permit feedback correction, which is important for osteotomy preparation in extraction sockets. The microscope-enhanced accuracy of osteotomy microsurgery permits socket implant placement in an ideal position followed by an esthetic implant-supported provisional (Fig. 82.2). As a flapless procedure, this is accomplished with minimal patient morbidity.[22]

KEY FACT

The microscope facilitates the detection of subtle changes in drill position. Enhanced angular perception is possible by focusing on small landmarks such as the implant platform or the healing abutment surface of an adjacent implant. This permits optimal parallel positioning of the drill angle. These reference points are not visible without a microscope. Detection of subtle angulation reference points and changes in drill position permit feedback correction, which is important for osteotomy preparation in extraction sockets.

Microsurgical Tooth Extraction

Tooth extraction has been traumatic for centuries. Conventional tooth extraction may require mucogingival flaps and bone removal, resulting in compromised esthetics. Using a microscope with minimally invasive principles reduces trauma and results in predictable esthetic outcomes.[6] Instrument selection influences the trauma of tooth removal. Periotome luxation or leveraged mechanical extraction using tapped root anchorage systems can carefully separate a tooth from its surrounding ligament and lift it vertically from the socket. This limits injury to papillae and preserves natural gingival anatomy (Fig. 82.3). Subtle nuances in the luxation direction can be microscopically detected for root removal in a proper anatomic path of extraction. Increased visibility under the microscope permits most extractions without mucogingival flaps. Greater visibility also permits atraumatic sectioning of ankylosed roots to leave the alveolar bone and soft tissue uninjured. Apical granulomatous lesions can be completely debrided with full visibility. Such minimally invasive microsurgical techniques translate into reduced patient morbidity with enhanced healing.

Implant Drilling in the Extraction Site

Microsurgical implant drilling in the extraction socket is unique. Under the microscope, a socket appears as large as a room, with its apex and walls clearly visible. A different set of skills is required for socket drilling. For placement of maxillary anterior implants, the most favorable bone lies to the palatal (Fig. 82.4). Drilling therefore must be done at an angle to the palatal socket wall. Twist drills innately track toward the direction of less dense bone and into the open socket. Drilling of sockets under a microscope utilizes visual feedback to constantly redirect the drill to

†Deceased.

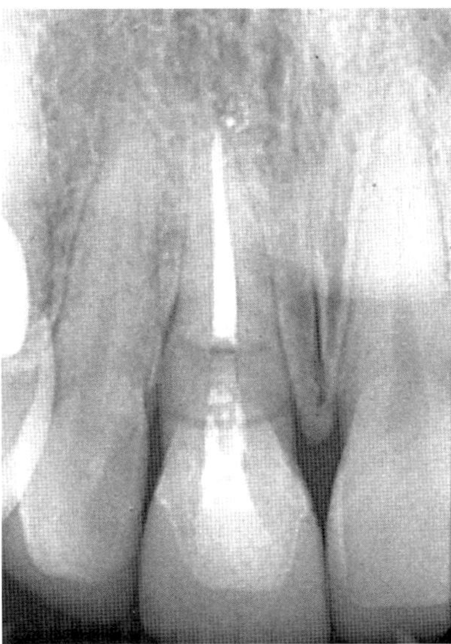

Fig. 82.1 Periapical radiograph of the typical fractured central incisor.

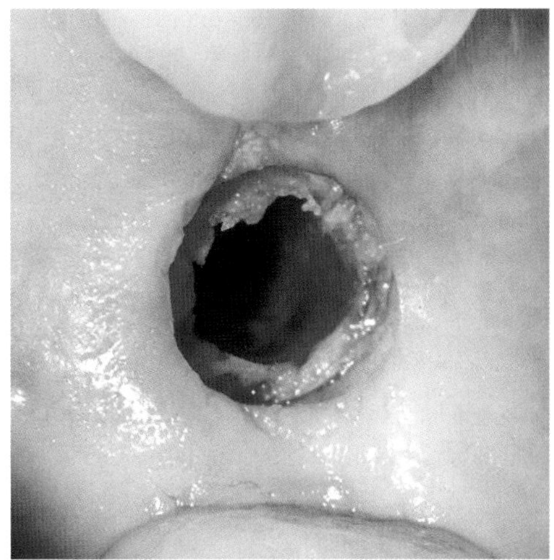

Fig. 82.2 Flapless dental implant microsurgery.

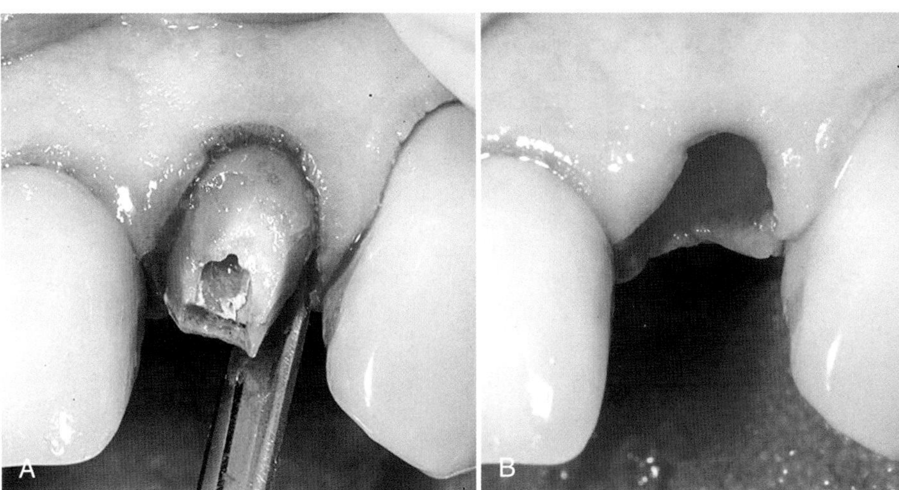

Fig. 82.3 (A) Periotome extraction of lateral incisor. (B) Noninvasive extraction of the lateral incisor. Tissue contours are preserved.

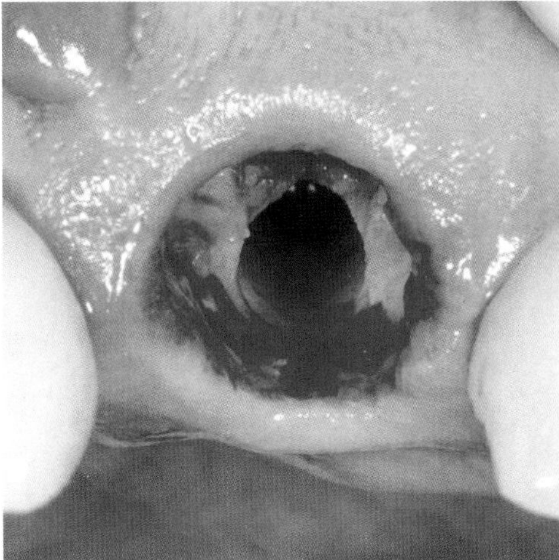

Fig. 82.4 Palatal wall socket osteotomy.

the correct position and angulation. This avoids the common mistake of placing an implant too far toward the buccal. With the magnification and lighting a microscope provides, implants can be placed in the palatal socket wall with good initial stability and ideal esthetic position. Microscope-enhanced dimensional and angular perceptions allow adjustments to correct drilling speed. Too little or too much drill pressure or excessive drill speed causes frictional heat. This adversely affects implant osteointegration. Detecting micromovement of the advancing drill ensures that proper pressure and rotational speed are applied to varying bone densities encountered in the socket. The angular velocity at the cutting edge of a 4-mm drill is several times faster than the velocity at the cutting edge of a 2-mm drill. For this reason, the pressure and rotation of larger diameter drills must be decreased to compensate for their faster cutting speed. Enhanced visual feedback for speed and pressure correction is accomplished through directly viewing the advancing drill under the microscope.

Bone Grafting

The osteotomy in an extraction socket is prepared in the palatal wall. This placement results in a gap between the implant and the buccal socket wall. To avoid displacing a particulate graft, the provisional is finished before a socket bone graft is placed. The socket is filled with xenograft to within a millimeter of its crest. A xenograft is selected to reduce remodeling resorption of the buccal bone.

Filtered bone from the osteotomy preparation is rinsed with a 3% tetracycline solution and then condensed on top of the xenograft. Finally, it is covered with a layer of microfibrillar collagen to contain the graft.

Buccal Gingival Grafting

Recession on the buccal gingival margin around anterior implants placed in extraction sockets has been well documented.[11,17] Multiple factors, such as the periodontal biotype, presence or absence of the buccal cortical plate, surgical trauma, implant position, and the emergence profile of both the provisional and final restorations, are associated with such recession.[9,12,16,18–20] A subepithelial connective tissue graft is harvested from the palate and transferred into a split-thickness envelope incision on the buccal of the implant. A connective tissue graft is done to maintain or augment gingival height and thickness that may have been lost due to injury (Fig. 82.5). Even gingival tissue at a normal height can be expected to recede as much as 1.5 mm unless gingival grafting is performed. Placing a subepithelial connective tissue graft concurrent with implant placement ensures the stability of the postoperative gingival level.[7,21]

Immediate Provisional Fabrication

To preserve natural esthetics and provide support for gingival anatomy, an implant provisional must emerge from the surrounding gingival tissue in exactly the same way as the extracted tooth.[4,23] The surgical microscope gives dentists the visibility necessary to fabricate ideal anatomy for implant provisional crowns. The provisional crown on the implant serves a number of functions, as follows:

1. It provides optimal esthetics and function.
2. It minimizes tissue collapse by supporting the gingival tissue.
3. It obturates the surgical extraction socket to contain particulate and soft tissue grafts.

Creating a provisional implant crown begins before the tooth is removed.[8] A clear silicone impression captures the dentogingival junction and its proximal tooth contours (Fig. 82.6). Tooth color matching is done, and a light-cured flowable composite resin duplicate of the tooth is created using the impression (Fig. 82.7). The duplicate crown is trimmed to the exact location of the dentogingival junction and then hollowed to create a shell crown. It is fitted to a screw-retained titanium provisional abutment that is opaque for a color match (Fig. 82.8). Great attention is paid to the incisal edge position of the shell crown before luting it to the abutment with flowable composite resin. Screw access for removal of the provisional is accomplished by drilling through the incisal one-third of the provisional crown.

The luted abutment and crown are removed and placed on a laboratory handle to facilitate shaping and polishing (Fig. 82.9). Subgingival provisional contours created under the microscope provide tissue support and well-finished margins. Each provisional crown has a uniquely shaped subgingival emergence profile that duplicates the original tooth. Voids and rough edges are eliminated, and the provisional is carefully shaped under the microscope to provide gingival support (Fig. 82.10). Shaping the provisional is accomplished with a 12-fluted finishing bur, glass nail file, and a prophylaxis cup with pumice. Attention to detail is critical. As a final step, the provisional crown is glazed and thoroughly cured.

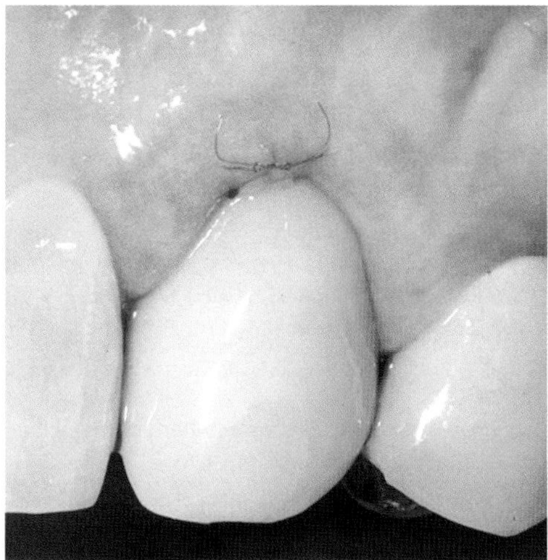

Fig. 82.5 Facial connective tissue graft placed under gingival margin and secured with a fine suture.

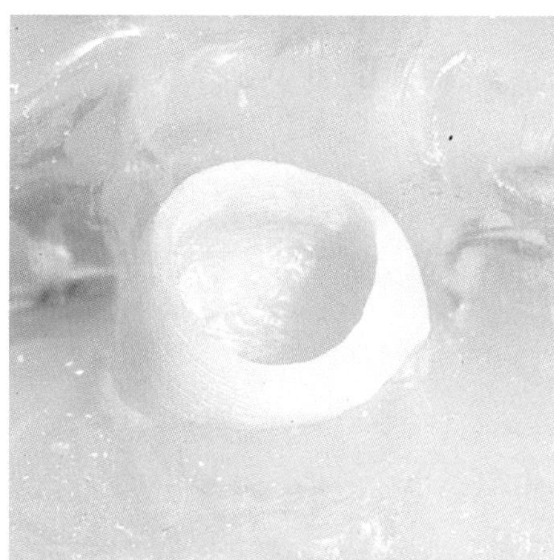

Fig. 82.7 Shell composite crown created from the impression.

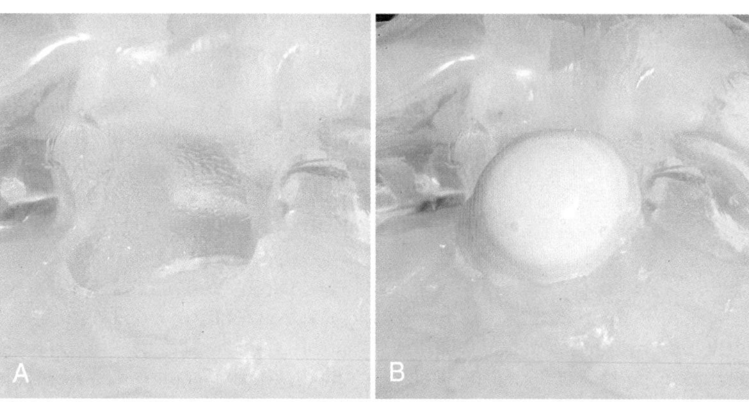

Fig. 82.6 (A) Clear silicone impression of failing tooth crown. (B) Clear silicone impression filled with composite.

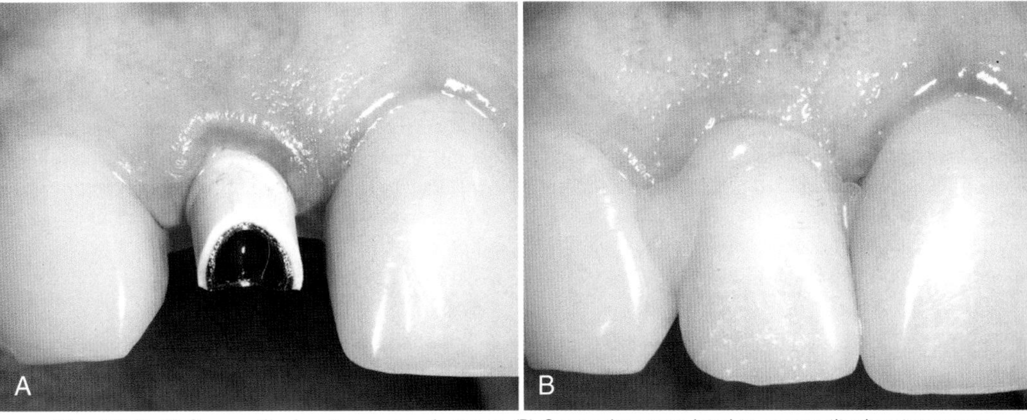

Fig. 82.8 (A) Opaque titanium temporary abutment. (B) Composite crown luted to opaque titanium temporary abutment.

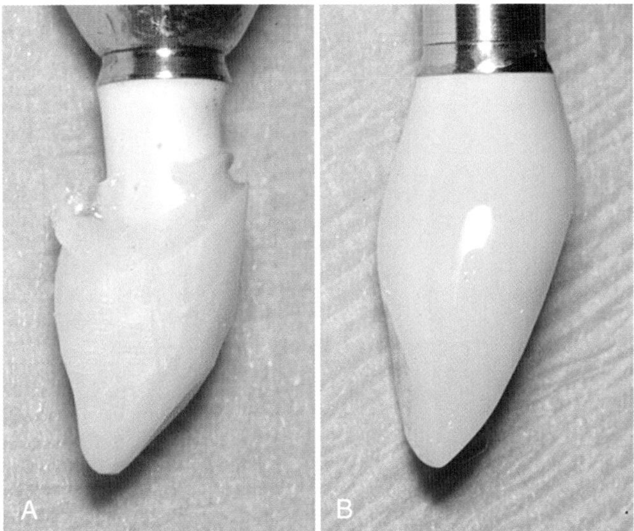

Fig. 82.9 (A) Screw-retained provisional before finishing. (B) Screw-retained provisional after finishing.

Light curing the composite ensures no free monomer is present to irritate soft tissue or bone. The machined titanium provisional abutment ensures good marginal fit and reduces the possibility of loosening.

CLINICAL CORRELATION

An immediate provisional restoration delivered with the immediately placed implant provides optimal esthetics and function, minimizes tissue collapse by supporting the gingival tissue, and helps to obturate the surgical extraction socket to contain particulate and soft tissue grafts.

Immediate Implant Occlusion

Early loading bone trauma is minimized in multiple immediate implant provisional cases by splinting. Early loading bone trauma in single implant cases is reduced by lessening occlusal forces. Symmetric and light mesial and distal proximal contacts are established, and the provisional is taken out of centric and lateral occlusal contact by using 1-mm green occlusal indicator wax. This technique allows patients to leave the dental office with a non-loaded esthetic provisional tooth securely anchored to the implant (Fig. 82.11).

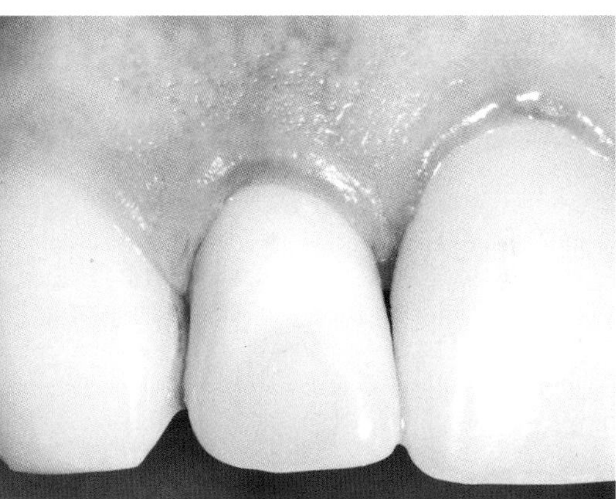

Fig. 82.10 Provisional restoration supporting gingival tissue.

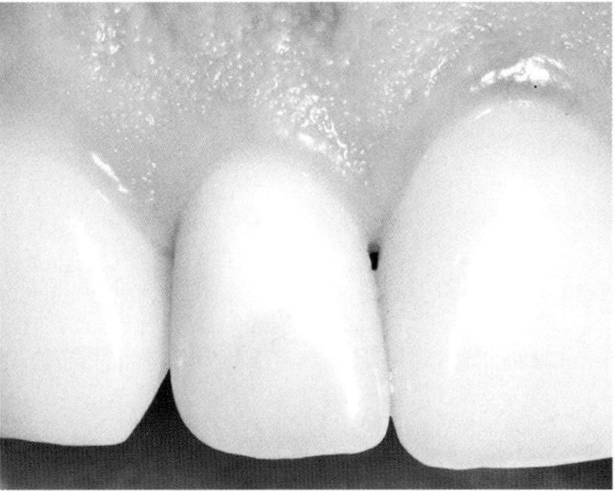

Fig. 82.11 Provisional 1 week after implant microsurgery.

Custom Impression Transfer Coping

A custom impression-transfer coping is necessary to preserve and communicate gingival supporting contours to the ceramicist. The chairside-created provisional anatomy must be precisely reproduced for the dental laboratory via the custom impression-transfer coping.[5,10] To make the custom transfer coping, an impression of the gingival third of the provisional crown is made with an implant analog attached (Fig. 82.12). This registers the implant platform orientation and preserves the provisional anatomy. The crown is removed, and a standard impression coping is attached to the implant analog. Acrylic powder fills the gap between the impression coping and the clear silicone impression. Monomer liquid is then infused into the powder to create a hard acrylic copy of provisional anatomy (Fig. 82.13).[3,5] Using a 25-gauge needle to apply monomer to the powder from the base upward minimizes the inclusion of air bubbles in the custom transfer coping. For orientation, a mark is initially applied to the labial surface of the provisional impression. It is transferred to the custom transfer coping with providing orientation for the restorative dentist during final impressions. This technique allows precise communication from the surgeon to the restorative dentist to the ceramicist of the anatomy required for a final restoration that esthetically supports gingival tissue.

Final Implant Restoration

Final impressions are taken using the custom impression-transfer coping. Computer-assisted scanning and machining create a zirconia abutment and zirconia coping for an all-ceramic crown (Fig. 82.14).

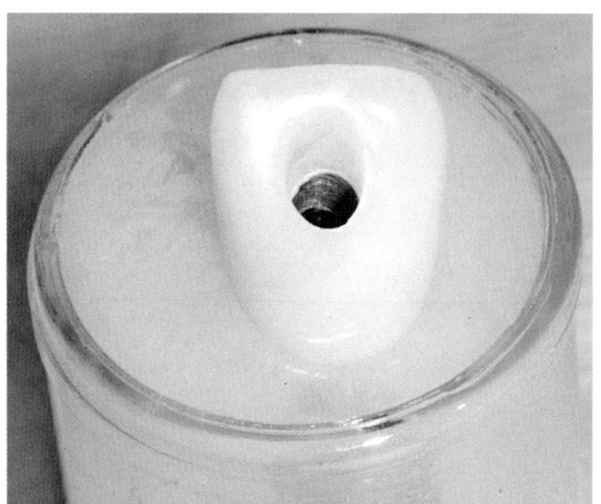

Fig. 82.12 Clear silicon impression of provisional.

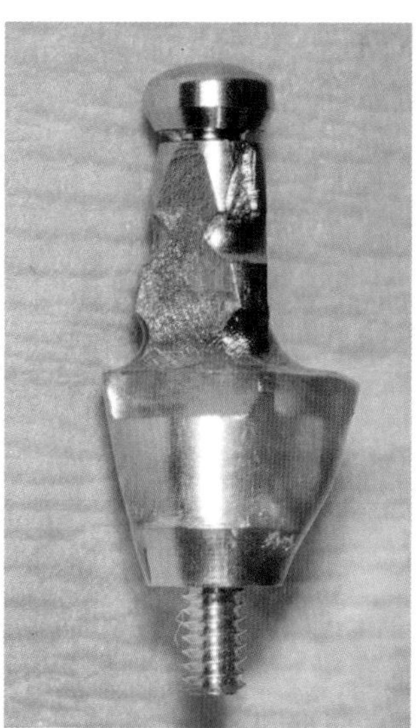

Fig. 82.13 Custom impression-transfer coping reproducing emergence profile.

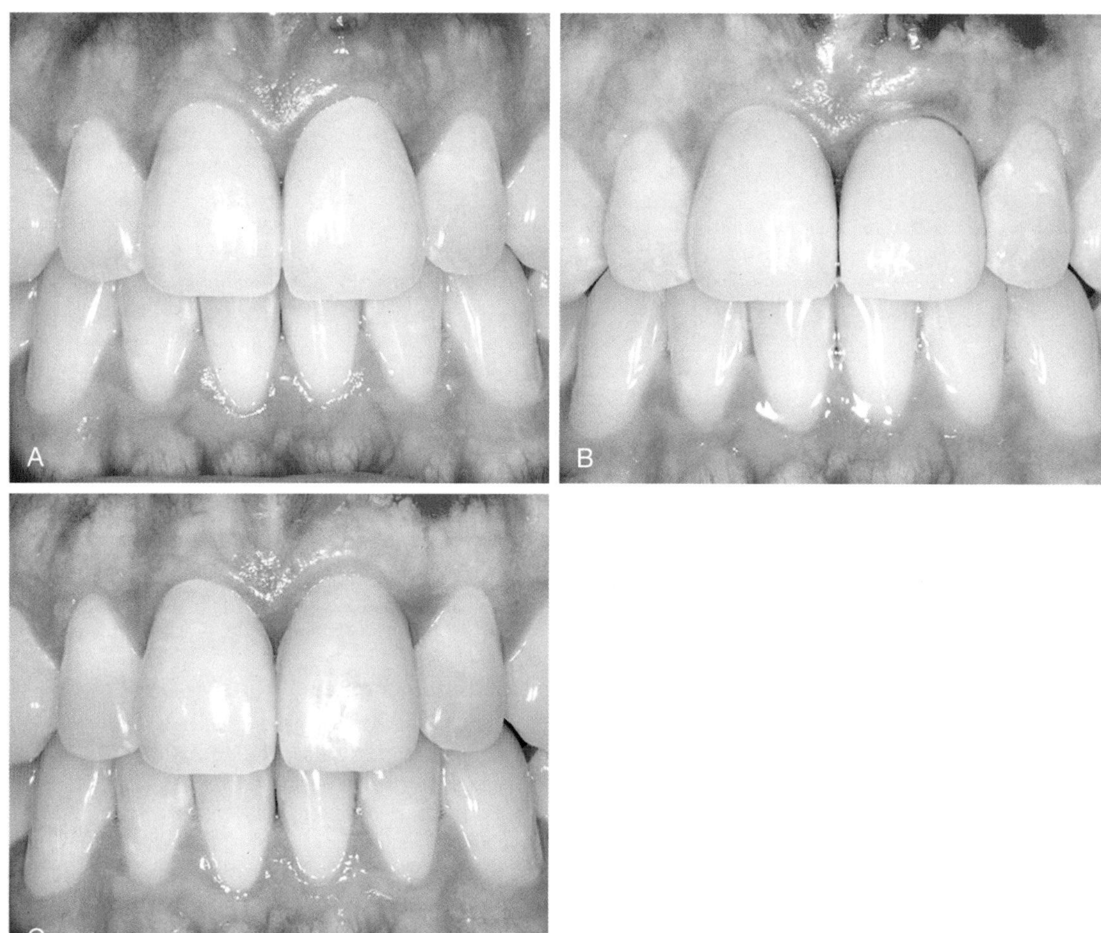

Fig. 82.14 (A) Before microsurgery. (B) Immediately after microsurgery. (C) Provisional 8 weeks after microsurgery.

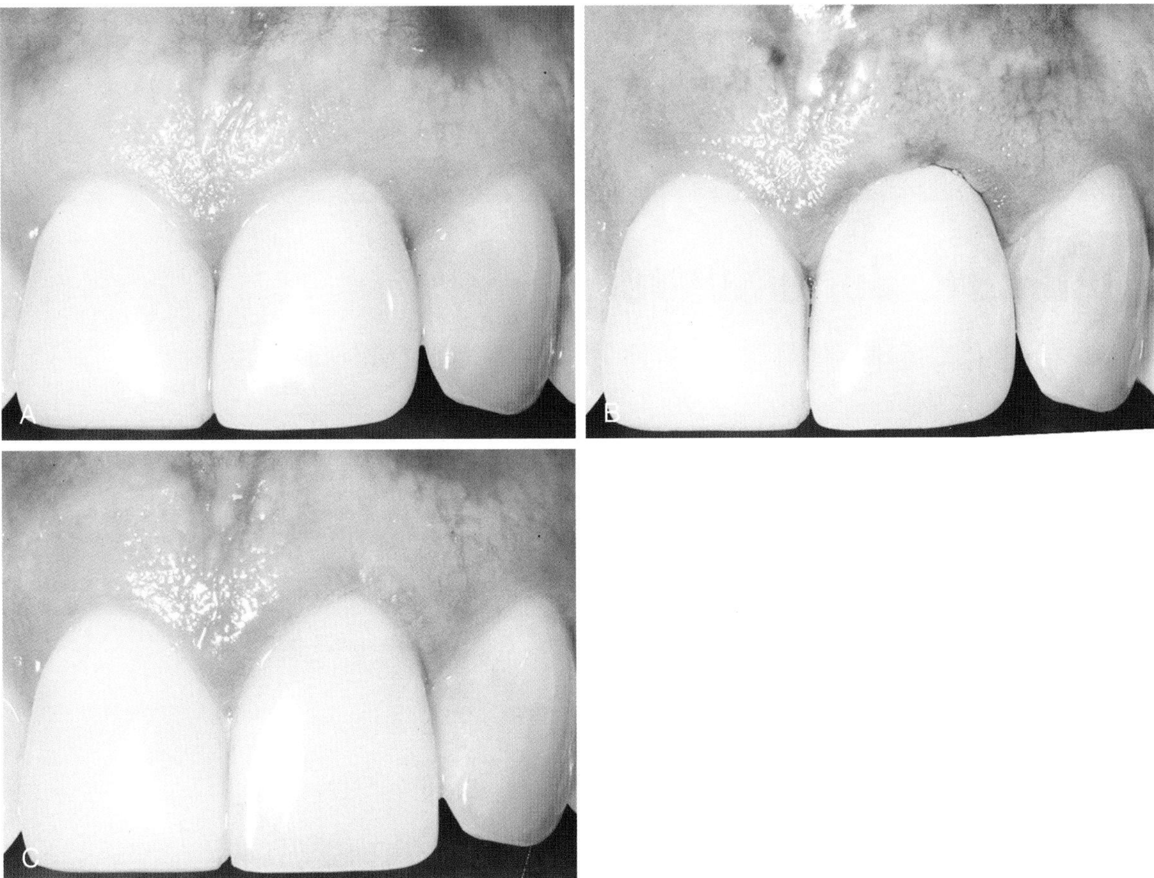

Fig. 82.15 (A) Before microsurgery. (B) Immediately after microsurgery. (C) Final restoration.

Zirconia has the benefit of tissue biocompatibility and light translucency. The sequence described ensures a final implant abutment and crown that exactly matches both the provisional emergence profile and the original tooth shape. Working as a team, the surgeon, restorative dentist, and laboratory technician can create a final restoration in harmony with preserved gingival architecture (Fig. 82.15).

Conclusion

Some of the advantages of microsurgery for extraction and implant placement have been described with an emphasis on tissue management and the ability to enhance visualization of details, which translate into better results. This microsurgery protocol advances dentistry from an era of traumatic tooth extraction to one of seamless, immediate tooth replacement using implant microsurgery.

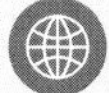
References for this chapter are found on the companion website eBooks.Health.Elsevier.com.

CHAPTER 83

Piezoelectric Bone Surgery

Tomaso Vercellotti | Claudio Stacchi | Perry R. Klokkevold | Giuseppe Vercellotti

For online-only content on advanced clinical applications, including sinus lift, ridge expansion, and bone harvesting, please visit the companion website at eBooks.Health.Elsevier.com.

CHAPTER OUTLINE

Ultrasound has been used for many years in periodontics to remove tartar, debride root surfaces, and degranulate periodontal defects. In recent decades a novel family of ultrasonic-powered devices has been developed that is revolutionizing oral and maxillofacial bone surgery.

This surgical technique, known as piezoelectric bone surgery, was invented by Vercellotti and developed by Mectron Medical Technology (Carasco, Italy). The Piezosurgery device (Fig. 83.1) consists of a piezoelectric ultrasonic transducer powered by an ultrasonic generator capable of driving a range of specially designed cutting inserts.[48,51] The Piezosurgery device employs ultrasonic vibrations to cut mineralized tissues. To this end, a primary frequency at 30 kHz is overmodulated by the superimposition of a sound wave (30 to 60 Hz) to generate a hammering action that effectively cuts bone without harming soft tissues and with minimal heat production. Box 83.1 describes the main cutting properties of Piezosurgery by Mectron, and Box 83.2 describes Piezosurgery inserts. Piezoelectric bone surgery techniques have been developed for clinical applications in dentistry and are becoming state of the art for a variety of procedures.[41,42,47–49,52] Piezosurgery Medical has expanded development of clinical applications to other fields of medicine. The extraordinary cutting properties of piezoelectric bone surgery have been introduced and applied in maxillofacial surgery, facial plastic surgery, otolaryngologic surgery, cranial and spinal neurosurgery, and minute orthopedic surgery.[13–23]

KEY FACT

Ultrasonic scalers use only one frequency and have insufficient power to cut mineralized tissues. In comparison, Mectron surgical devices rely on the juxtaposition of a sound wave (30–60 Hz) to the primary ultrasonic wave (24–36 kHz) to cut bone without overheating. This phenomenon is known as frequency overmodulation.

The most compelling characteristics of piezoelectric bone surgery are low surgical trauma, exceptional control during surgery, and a fast-healing response of tissues. Clinical studies demonstrate that the specificity of operation and the techniques employed with piezoelectric bone surgery make it possible to exploit differences in hard and soft tissue anatomy advantageously.[13,36,38,40] This not only increases treatment effectiveness but also improves postoperative recovery and healing. Experimental studies on animals have shown faster tissue healing when compared with traditional cutting instruments.[13]

KEY FACT

Piezosurgery's cutting action is selective, that is, cutting only mineralized tissues while sparing soft tissues. Selective cutting is made possible by the application of ultrasonic frequencies between 24 and 36 kHz.

Ideally, surgical trauma should be minimized to obtain optimal healing, which depends on gentle management. Surgery, by definition, alters normal physiology by interrupting the vascular supply of tissues. The degree of surgical invasiveness is extremely important for the quality of tissue healing and may affect whether wounds heal by repair or regeneration. Indeed, when surgical trauma is kept to a minimum, it generates enough stimulation to favor healing mechanisms that lead to regeneration, which is actually promoted by ultrasonic frequencies. Conversely, surgical techniques that are more traumatic often lead to greater inflammatory responses with slow healing that may lead to repair and scarring rather than regeneration. For this reason, it is desirable to choose the least traumatic surgical instruments and techniques for any surgical procedure. Piezoelectric bone surgery was conceived and developed precisely to overcome the limits of traditional bone-cutting instruments and to achieve the most effective treatment with the least morbidity.

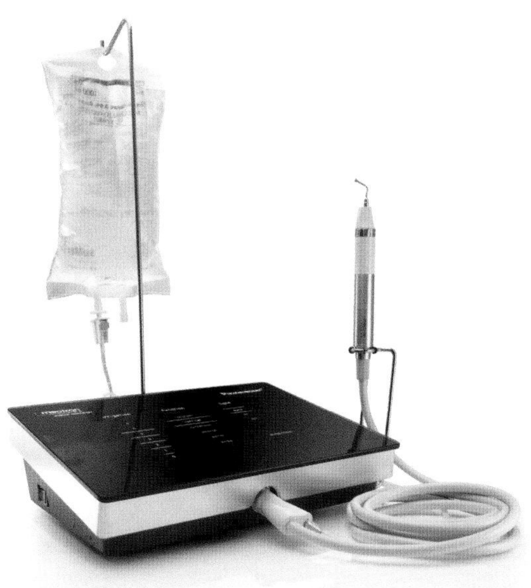

Fig. 83.1 Piezosurgery device by Mectron Medical Technology. (Courtesy Mectron Medical Technology, Carasco, Italy.)

BOX 83.1 Description and Cutting Properties of Piezosurgery by Mectron

Piezosurgery is an electronic device that generates ultrasonic microvibrations at variable frequencies. Its dual-wave technology is unique in the world (US patents 6,695,047 B2, 8,002,783 B2) for the characteristic vibrations generated in parallel and variable frequency modulation for precise cutting of bone with different degrees of density.

The unit has a display that allows the operator to select different operating functions that set the ultrasonic modulated frequency to ideal parameters for cutting bone of different density, shaping, debriding, and smoothing root surfaces (both external [periodontal] and internal [endodontic]) and for separating soft tissues from bone.

Function Settings

Implant

The basic ultrasonic frequency is overmodulated by sound waves that are higher than those for cortical bone, ideally suited for perforating bone for implant site preparation.

Cortical

The basic ultrasonic frequency (30 kHz) is overmodulated by sound waves for cutting and removing small cortical bone fragments.

Cancellous

The basic ultrasonic frequency is overmodulated by sound waves that are slower than those for cortical bone, better for cutting and removing cancellous bone fragments.

Special

The basic ultrasonic frequency operates at a frequency that is most effective when working in proximity with soft tissues.

Perio

The basic ultrasonic frequency, without overmodulation, is set at an ideal power level for scaling, debridement, and root planing.

Endo

The ultrasonic frequency, without overmodulation, is set at an ideal power level for retrocanal and intracanal debridement after root canal treatment.

BOX 83.2 Description of Piezosurgery Inserts

The mechanical action of bone cutting takes place thanks to the linear microvibrations of inserts with a variable range from 20 to 80 μm, depending on the setting selected. Piezosurgery inserts are classified based on their functional and clinical characteristics.

Functional Classification

Sharp: These inserts have sharp ends for osteotomy and osteoplasty. They are made of nitride titanium steel and are gold in color.

Smoothing: These nitride titanium inserts are diamond coated and gold in color. Their different granulometry produces a smoothing action that is generally used to complete the cut near soft tissue.

Blunt: These steel-colored inserts are characterized by rounded ends and are generally used to refine the cut in contact with soft tissue.

The inserts described in the functional classification as sharp, smoothing, and blunt have clinical classification codes that relate to their specific use.

Clinical Classification

OT: The identification code for inserts used to perform osteotomy is *OT* followed by a number.

OP: The identification code for inserts used to perform osteoplasty is *OP* followed by a number.

EX: The identification code for inserts used to perform extraction is *EX* followed by a number.

IM: The identification code for inserts used to perform implant site preparation is *IM* followed by a number.

From a mechanical standpoint, the effect of burs or twist drills on bone is characterized by lamellar fracturing in areas adjacent to the cut surface and the deposition of large bone fragments and debris in the endosteal spaces. This finding is thought to be, at least in part, responsible for the inflammatory process that takes place in immediate postsurgical wound healing and for the delay of osteogenesis observed in these wounds. In contrast, the micromechanical cutting action of piezoelectric bone surgery results in micronization of the cut bone and does not cause lamellar fracturing in adjacent bone; this feature may favor exposure and release of bone morphogenetic proteins (BMPs) and be responsible for the early onset of osteogenesis at these sites (see later). Furthermore, the inflammatory response may be diminished because little or no need exists to remove damaged bone and surgical debris as compared with conventional rotary-drilled sites (Fig. 83.2).

KEY FACT

The most compelling characteristics of piezoelectric bone surgery are low surgical trauma, exceptional precision and control, and fast healing. Clinical studies demonstrate that the specificity of operation and the techniques used with piezoelectric bone surgery make it possible to exploit differences in hard and soft tissue anatomy advantageously.

Clinical Characteristics of Ultrasonic Cutting

The primary clinical characteristics of the Piezosurgery cutting action include microprecision, selective cutting, maximum visibility, and excellent healing.

Microprecision

Piezosurgery cuts mineralized tissues with microprecision and extraordinary surgical control.[28] Piezoelectric osteotomies are

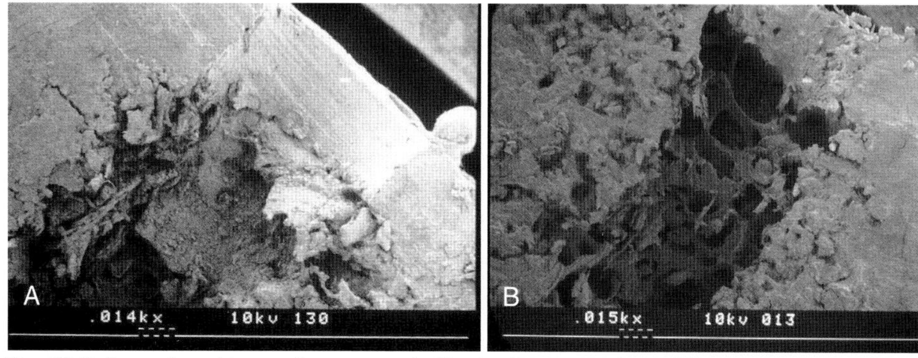

Fig. 83.2 Comparison of bone surfaces prepared with rotary instrumentation and Piezosurgery (Mectron Medical Technology, Carasco, Italy). (A) Rotary technique: in vitro photograph of the implant site following preparation with twist drill of 3.15 mm. The site is ready to receive the implant. Note the compact surface of the cortical bone where no vascular canals are visible. The underlying spongiosa is irregular due to the presence of bone debris in the endosteal spaces. (B) Piezoelectric technique: in vitro image of implant site preparation with 3-mm ultrasonic inserts. The site is ready to receive the implant. Note the cortical bone microporosity where open vascular canals are clearly visible. The underlying spongiosa is intact and free from bone debris. (Courtesy of Dr. Alberto Rebaudi, Genoa, Italy.)

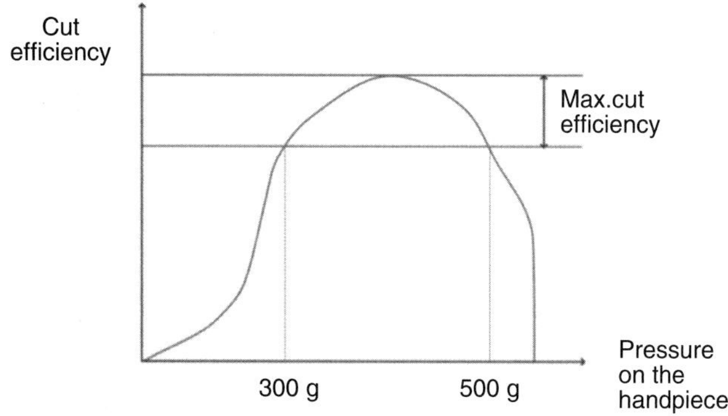

Fig. 83.3 Graph illustrating the relationship between Piezosurgery (Mectron Medical Technology, Carasco, Italy) cutting efficiency and pressure applied on the handpiece. Note that optimal cutting efficiency is found between 300 and 500 g; pressure in excess of 500 g leads to a sudden and complete loss of cutting efficiency. *Max.,* Maximum.

KEY FACT

Heavy pressure or force is not required to operate the piezoelectric bone surgical handpiece. In fact, forceful handling antagonizes the ultrasonic frequency, thus causing a reduction in the cutting efficiency and transforming mechanical energy into thermal energy.

easy to create, but it is important to recognize that the technique and instrument handling are different from the technique using a traditional handpiece with rotary instruments. The Piezosurgery insert is applied to the bone with a relatively light stroke similar to the smooth precision used to draw a picture. Heavy pressure or force is not required and can, in fact, antagonize the ultrasonic frequency, thus reducing efficiency and transforming mechanical energy into thermal energy (Fig. 83.3). The microprecision of this instrument is made possible by the ultrasonic frequency, which produces mechanical microshock waves at a linear range of approximately 80 µm. The extraordinary surgical control that characterizes Piezosurgery is because its microvibrations require only light pressure (approximately 300 g) to be applied to the handpiece. Indeed, the pressure applied by the surgeon to the Piezosurgery handpiece is much lower than the pressure typically applied to a rotary or oscillating type handpiece (approximately 1000 g), which uses mechanical macrovibrations for cutting. This characteristic provides maximum control during surgery and makes this technique unique, especially in areas with delicate anatomy.

Selective Cutting

Piezosurgery's cutting action is selective because it cuts only mineralized tissues, which are characterized by greater mechanical resistance to the action of the ultrasonic microvibrations. Indeed, the linear motion of the vibrations, which is in the order of approximately 80 µm, is absorbed and dispersed by the elastic nature of soft tissues. These microvibrations are physically unable to cut soft tissue, where kinetic energy is easily dissipated and—when in low dosage—stimulates tissue healing by promoting mitotic divisions (see later). Clearly, the most significant demonstrated benefit of Piezosurgery selective cutting is the ability to preserve the integrity of soft tissues, such as the alveolar nerve, the infraorbital nerve, the maxillary sinus membrane, blood vessels, and the dura mater, while effectively cutting the mineralized tissue (bone) in close proximity to these tissues.[11] A study conducted by Schaeren and colleagues[23] revealed that even prolonged contact for up to 5 seconds between Piezosurgery inserts and a peripheral nerve did not dissect the nerve. Combined with maximum operator control, the safety of Piezosurgery's selective cutting dramatically reduces the risk of accidental damage to delicate anatomic structures.

Maximum Visibility

Piezosurgery allows maximum visibility by creating a surgical field that is blood free during cutting because of the cavitation of the cooling irrigation solution. Cavitation is a physical phenomenon that, from a clinical standpoint, happens with the nebulization of the saline solution when it contacts the insert vibrating at ultrasonic frequency. The slight hydropneumatic pressure applied by the nebulized irrigation fluid induces hemostasis in both hard and soft tissues. An important advantage of the cavitation effect is the thorough debridement of the surgical site at the time of the mechanical removal of inflammatory tissue by means of dedicated Piezosurgery inserts. This effect is only temporary, and bleeding resumes shortly after the cutting (and cavitation) action is stopped. Clinically, it is important to ensure proper irrigation and intermittent cutting action to maintain optimal surface microcirculation, especially for long surgical procedures.[54] An added benefit of the temporary hemostasis induced by the cavitation effect is the notably reduced blood loss, especially during longer procedures, which leads to decreased postoperative edema.

KEY FACT

The cavitation effect is a physical phenomenon consisting of the implosion of gaseous bubbles within a fluid. In the context of piezoelectric bone surgery, the cavitation of the irrigation solution creates a microspray that cleans the site of debris and provides temporary hemostasis for maximum visibility of the surgical field.

Excellent Healing

Clinical studies comparing use of piezoelectric bone surgery with traditional rotary instruments for third molar extractions[4,7,10,25] and periodontal surgery[38] have reported better recovery and fewer postoperative symptoms in patients treated with Piezosurgery. Postoperative healing after piezoelectric bone surgery is characterized by minimal swelling and little bleeding, and the rate of postoperative morbidity is lower compared with traditional techniques.[37]

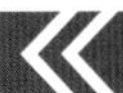

FLASH BACK

Piezosurgery's cutting action is selective because it cuts only mineralized tissues, which are characterized by greater mechanical resistance to the action of the ultrasonic microvibrations.

Improved Hard Tissue Healing

The improved healing response observed at Piezosurgery-treated sites may be explained by the stimulation of healing mechanisms promoted by the device's secondary wave, which operates in the range of 30 to 60 Hz. Indeed, research has shown that the application of low-intensity, high-frequency vibrations in the range of 10 to 50 Hz (i.e., the frequency of postural muscle contractions) to bone tissues mimics mechanical loading and induces the release of several growth factors, including BMPs responsible for osteoblast differentiation and new bone formation.[8,9,34] In an animal study comparing the biomolecular profile of sites prepared with piezoelectric bone surgery or rotary drills, BMP-4 increased earlier at implant sites prepared with piezoelectric bone surgery.[13] As compared with drilled sites, the levels of BMP-4 at Piezosurgery-treated sites were 18.5 times higher at 7 days, 15 times higher at 14 days, and 2 times lower at 56 days. The peak levels of BMP-4 were observed at 14 days for Piezosurgery-treated sites. The level of BMP-4 at drilled sites did not reach the same level of BMP-4 achieved at Piezosurgery-treated sites until day 56. A greater increase in the level of transforming growth factor beta 2 (TGF-β2) was also noted at implant sites prepared with piezoelectric bone surgery techniques. As compared with drilled sites, the levels of TGF-β2 at Piezosurgery-treated sites were 3.5 times higher at 7 days, 19 times higher at 14 days, and diminished below baseline at 56 days. The level of TGF-β2 at drilled sites never exceeded baseline levels.

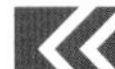

FLASH BACK

BMPs are specialized growth factors that promote new bone formation by inducing mesenchymal stem cells to differentiate into osteoblasts. They are fundamental for proper bone physiologic maintenance and repair.

Proinflammatory cytokine tumor necrosis factor alpha, proinflammatory and bone-resorbing cytokine interleukin-1β (IL-1β), and anti-inflammatory cytokine IL-10 were also measured. In general, the expression of these proinflammatory cytokines was higher in the early experimental phases of drilled sites only, which also showed more inflammatory cells. The piezoelectric bone surgery–treated sites showed a higher expression of the proinflammatory and bone-resorbing cytokine IL-1β at 56 days. This last finding may be indicative of bone remodeling at day 56 in piezoelectric bone surgery–treated sites (IL-1β is involved in osteoclast differentiation). The lower expression of inflammatory factors following the application of Piezosurgery may be explained in terms of reduced trauma to the cut tissues compared with the use of rotatory instruments; this reduced trauma is made possible by the technology's microvibrations and lack of friction overheating.

Improved Soft Tissue Healing

Research on a novel application of Piezosurgery to detach the periosteum from underlying bone tissue investigated the effect of this technology on the integrity and healing of mucoperiosteal flaps.[32] Periosteal activation following surgical intervention is responsible for chondrogenesis, osteogenesis, and angiogenesis, which ultimately promote vascularization and bone remodeling. Periosteal healing response following trauma is directly related to the integrity of the periosteum, which provides nourishment to the underlying bone and is essential in osteoinduction and osteoconduction. To ensure proper healing and clinical success, periosteal integrity should therefore be preserved to the maximum extent possible, especially in patients with compromised health. However, the use of manual instrumentation for periosteal elevation has been shown to damage the cells of the osteogenic layer mechanically. Histologically, the periosteum detached with manual elevators shows visible tears, and individual tissue layers are not clearly visible. In contrast, the use of dedicated Piezosurgery inserts specifically designed for periosteal separation from bone was found to be associated with a clean separation of the tissues, with preservation of the outer fibrous layer and the inner cambium layer. Additionally, fat vacuoles and collagenous connective tissue can also be discerned (Fig. 83.4).[32] At the biomolecular level, expression of collagen (II and IV) and osteocalcin in the 8 days following surgery was significantly greater at Piezosurgery-treated sites, thus indicating a more robust healing response. These findings complement the clinical observation that, following piezoelectric bone surgery procedures, gingival tissues show optimal healing and typically appear light in color.

Clinical Applications

The clinical use of Piezosurgery in osseous surgery advantageously promotes all the benefits of microsurgery, especially when working under optical magnification. Piezosurgery has become an essential instrument in dentistry and in periodontal daily practice to minimize patients' morbidity and increase overall clinical predictability. Piezoelectric bone surgery has many important clinical applications in dentistry. In fact, nearly all techniques previously performed with burs, twist drills, chisels, or oscillating saws have the potential to be performed with piezosurgery. For over 20 consecutive years, one of

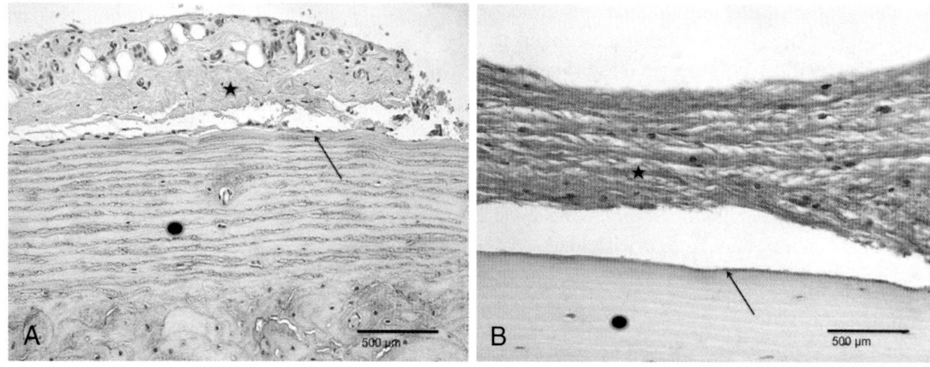

Fig. 83.4 Comparison between periosteal surface elevated with manual instruments and Piezosurgery PR (Mectron Medical Technology, Carasco, Italy) insert tips. (A) Histologic section depicting subperiosteal preparation using manual instrumentation. Note the irregular separation between periosteum *(star)* and bone *(closed circle)* at the boundary between the two layers *(arrow)*. The periosteum shows evidence of mechanical tears. (B) Histologic section showing clear separation between periosteum *(star)* and bone *(closed circle)* at the boundary between the two layers *(arrow)* following preparation with novel piezoelectric inserts. The periosteum is intact and shows no signs of mechanical damage. (Adapted from Stoetzer M, Magel A, Kampmann A, et al. Subperiosteal preparation using a new piezoelectric device: a histological examination. *GMS Interdiscip Plast Reconstr Surg DGPW*. 2014;3:Doc18.)

the authors (T.V.) has used piezosurgery on a daily basis for oral, periodontal, and implant surgical procedures, thus enabling him to develop techniques and protocols for each. Readers are referred to online materials and other publications for detailed descriptions and step-by-step instructions on these Piezosurgery protocols.[53] A brief overview of basic clinical applications using piezoelectric surgery is described here.

Periodontal Surgery

The use of Piezosurgery in periodontal surgery simplifies and improves both soft and hard tissue management (Table 83.1).[43] In osseous resective periodontal surgery, piezoelectric bone surgery represents a notable evolution from the past because it allows the application of concepts of bone microsurgery. In periodontal soft tissue management, after raising the primary flap with a traditional technique, it is easier to detach the secondary flap and remove inflammatory granulation tissue by using a scaler-shaped insert (Piezosurgery insert PS2) (Fig. 83.5A) or an insert in the shape of a rounded scalpel (Piezosurgery insert OP3). Contrary to traditional manual techniques, this phase has little bleeding and better visibility as a result of the cavitation of the saline solution (coolant). Hard tissue management is also improved: with the proper inserts and power mode, the ultrasound device facilitates effective scaling, debridement, and root planing (Fig. 83.5B and C). In particular, debridement with special diamond-coated inserts enables thorough cleaning even for interproximal bone defects, which can therefore be remodeled into even surfaces (Fig. 83.5D). The mechanical action of ultrasonic microvibrations, together with cavitation of the irrigation fluid (pH neutral; isotonic saline solution) eliminates bacteria, toxins, dead cells, and debris, thus creating clean physiology for healing of the wound. Healing is improved by applying ultrasound to produce micropits at the base of the defect to activate cellular response of healing mechanisms. In hard tissue management, the ostectomy maneuver with Piezosurgery is extremely precise and does not pose any risk of damaging the root surface. Typically, to avoid damaging the radicular cementum, conventional ostectomy techniques are incomplete and leave residual "widow's peaks" that require manual removal using hand chisels. When using Piezosurgery for resective procedures, because it is possible to work on the root surface without damaging it, it is possible to perform thorough ostectomies that do not leave behind more than "micro" widow's peaks. These

TABLE 83.1 Piezoelectric Periodontal Surgery Protocol

Management by Tissue Type	Procedure	Inserts Used[a]
Soft Tissue	Soft tissue removal	OP3, PS2, SLC
Hard Tissue		
Bone	Alveolar bone ostectomy	OT13, OT14, OP3, SLC
	Crestal bone osteoplasty	OP3, SLC
	Interproximal osteoplasty	OP4, OP8, OP9
Root	Scaling	PS2
	Debridement	OP5, OP5A
	Planing	PP1

[a]Piezosurgery, Mectron Medical Technology, Carasco, Italy.

minimal formations are easily removed when using the final insert for root planing procedures (Piezosurgery insert PP1). When working on reshaping the crestal bone surface, the osteoplasty maneuver at low irrigation allows for collecting autogenous particulate bone that can be immediately grafted into small bony defects (Fig. 83.5E).The use of this technology not only reduces the invasiveness of traditional surgery by making it faster and by ensuring thorough cleaning of the periodontium, but it also favors tissue healing by using bone removed in the osteoplasty procedure to graft small osseous defects, thus preserving bone architecture.

CLINICAL CORRELATION

The clinical use of Piezosurgery in osseous surgery advantageously promotes all the benefits of microsurgery, especially when working under optical magnification. It simplifies and improves both soft and hard tissue management.

It is our opinion that Piezosurgery in periodontal surgery can redefine the guidelines that mark the border between resective treatment and regenerative treatment. Indeed, the choice between a resective technique and a regenerative technique generally depends on the depth of the bone defect, whether it is more or less than 3.5 mm.

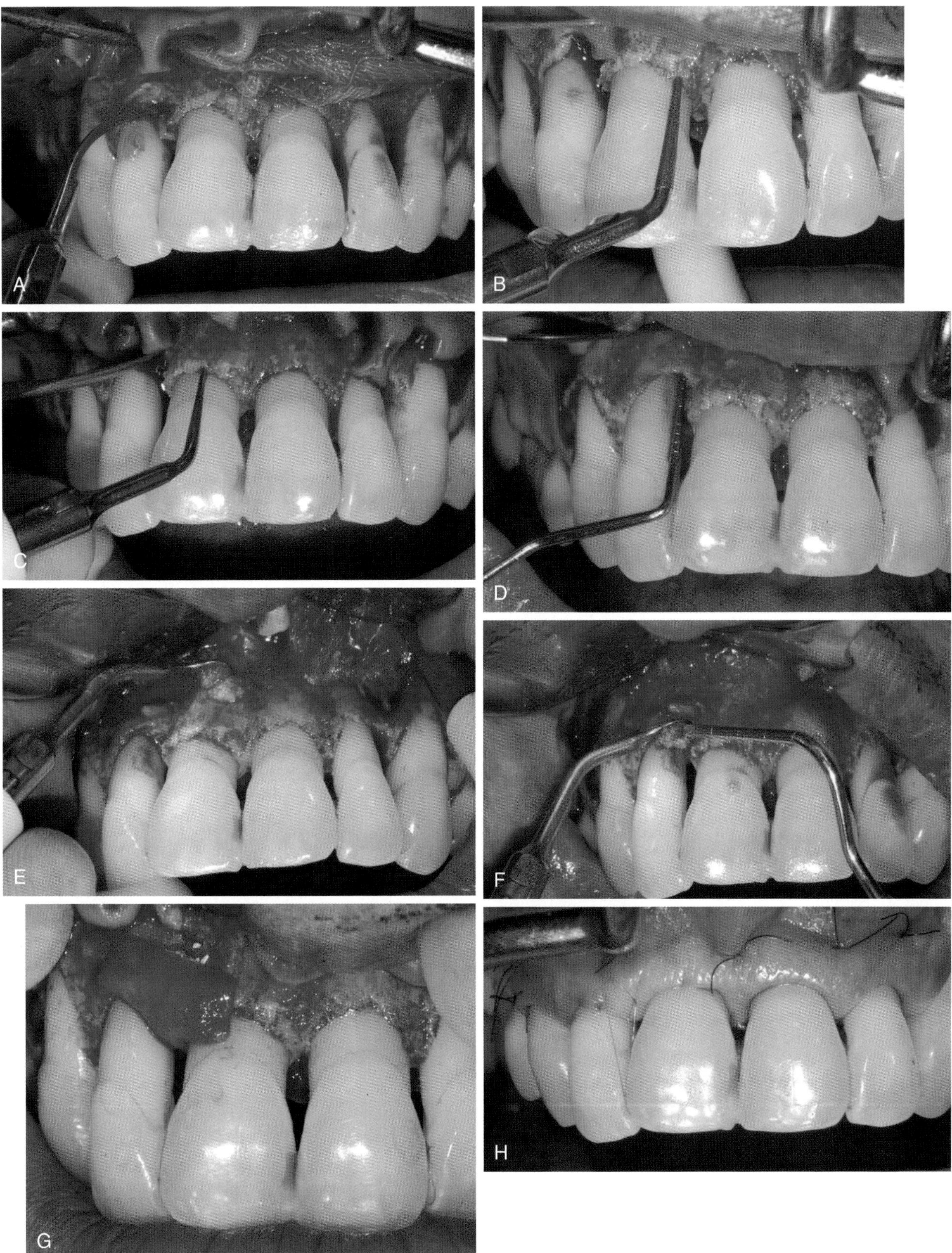

Fig. 83.5 Clinical case demonstrating the use of piezoelectric bone surgery for periodontal surgery. (A) Ultrasonic scaling using Piezosurgery PS2 insert (Mectron Medical Technology, Carasco, Italy). (B) Root surface debridement using Piezosurgery diamond-coated OP5 insert. (C) Ultrasonic root planing using Piezosurgery blunt insert PP1. (D) Interproximal infrabony defect with probe. (E) Autogenous bone chip–harvesting technique using Piezosurgery osteoplasty insert OP3. (F) Autogenous bone-grafting technique. (G) Collagen membrane stabilizing microbone grafting. (H) Flap repositioned and sutured.

Thanks to piezoelectric bone surgery, defects greater than 3.5 mm can now be grafted with particulate bone and covered with resorbable membranes.

The ability to work on the bone defect under magnification (e.g., surgical microscope) makes it possible to exploit the benefits of Piezosurgery microprecision in preparing the recipient site and stabilizing micrografts (Fig. 83.5F–H).

Crown Lengthening

Clinical crown lengthening is the most common periodontal surgical (ostectomy) operation performed in otherwise healthy periodontal conditions. The indication for this procedure is usually associated with a need or desire to expose more tooth structure because of short clinical crowns and/or loss of clinical tooth structure. In general, the goal is to reposition the periodontal bone and soft tissues to a more apical position with appropriate biologic dimensions to avoid periodontal inflammation after tooth restoration.

The clinical crown lengthening technique entails performing a periradicular ostectomy of a few millimeters (1 to 2 mm) combined with an osteoplasty technique to allow for repositioning of the periodontal flap in a more apical position with favorable periodontal tissue architecture. The positive result obtained is that the health of the treated part is preserved even though the normal gingival morphology is altered. Clinical application must include aesthetic assessment, as well as an assessment of the position and health of the adjacent periodontium.

The traditional surgical technique entails raising of a full-thickness flap, ostectomy with manual instruments, osteoplasty with a bur for crest bone architecture recontouring, periradicular bone removal, root planing, and, finally, replacing the flap in an apical position.

The ostectomy is simple to perform using Piezosurgery in direct contact with the root surface because control of the instrument during surgery is precise, even in very difficult proximity cases (Piezosurgery OP3 insert). The root planing phase can be performed very effectively using blunt ultrasonic inserts (Piezosurgery PP1 insert).

Saline solution cavitation reduces bleeding during surgery and facilitates debridement of the surgical area. This effect is likely responsible for the excellent soft tissue healing result, which is always characterized by a light color and the absence of edema.

A histologic animal study conducted at Harvard University in Cambridge, Massachusetts, showed a better healing response for bone and root cementum in teeth that were crown lengthened using Piezosurgery as compared with teeth that were crown lengthened with traditional rotary instruments.[40] Concerning the latter, the tungsten carbide bur was found to be more favorable than the diamond-coated bur for the bone-healing process.

The crown lengthening technique performed with Piezosurgery using appropriate inserts makes it possible to reduce bone effectively while preserving root surface integrity.

Tooth Extraction

Today, tooth extraction is considered the first step in the preparation for implant placement. Maintaining the integrity of the alveolar bone walls is an essential part of this process. Consequently, whether an implant is being placed at the time of extraction or not, the selection of instruments and techniques that minimize trauma to socket walls is critical.

Anatomic differences greatly influence the difficulty of extraction and the challenge of maintaining alveolar bone walls. A newer periodontal classification for dental extractions has been developed (Table 83.2) that makes it easier to choose the best surgical tooth extraction technique for different anatomic situations (Table 83.3).[41] The aim is always to preserve the integrity of the alveolar walls and the morphology of soft tissue. This classification divides anatomy into four types, depending upon the anatomic characteristics of periodontal biotype and anatomy or pathology of the periodontal ligament. Classifying anatomy into type 1, 2, 3, or 4 simplifies the diagnostic process and the subsequent surgical decision. Each type corresponds to a different anatomic issue, which requires a specific extraction technique and determines the most effective surgical instruments.

TABLE 83.2 Periodontal Classification for Dental Extraction

Periodontal Biotype Thickness	Periodontal Ligament	Diagnosis	Anatomic Classification
Normal	Normal	Normal	Type 1
Thin	Normal	Thin	Type 2
Normal	Ankylotic	Ankylotic	Type 3
Thin	Ankylotic	Thin and ankylotic	Type 4

Type 1 anatomy describes a normal periodontal biotype and a normal periodontal ligament (i.e., no pathologic features). This anatomic condition poses little surgical difficulty. A traditional extraction technique using manual instruments is sufficient.

Type 2 anatomy describes a thin periodontal biotype with a normal periodontal ligament. The surgical difficulty for tooth removal is minimal. However, preserving the integrity of the thin alveolar buccal walls makes the extraction more complex. In this situation, the normal displacement operation runs the risk of creating a dehiscence from fracturing the thin buccal cortical plate. To avoid this risk, it is recommended that the surgeon use a root fractioning technique that makes it possible to obtain root mobility inside the alveolus to eliminate the risk of damaging the thin labial and crestal bone.

Type 3 anatomy describes a normal periodontal biotype with an ankylotic periodontal ligament. The surgical difficulty for tooth removal is high because it is not possible to obtain the mobility necessary for displacement. The traditional technique uses a periradicular osteotomy with burs. This is possible without much consequence for mandibular third molars but often results in serious damage to the buccal alveolar walls. The recommended technique creates the space necessary for extraction by operating only on the root surface through a root plasty maneuver. The tooth is removed from the socket by consuming the root surface without touching the alveolar bone. This technique is easy to perform with excellent control using specific Piezosurgery inserts (OP5), used like a bur around the root (eFig. 83.1).

Type 4 anatomy describes a thin periodontal biotype and an ankylotic periodontal ligament, which is a combination of the challenging aspects of type 2 and type 3 anatomy. The surgical difficulty for tooth removal is the highest. In all cases where aesthetics is important, a root-sectioning technique that divides the root into segments with a mesiodistal cut is recommended. This allows the separate pieces (e.g., buccal and palatal) to be removed internal to the socket with minimal force applied just to the mesiodistal socket walls.

To ensure success of the procedure, it is important for the clinician to master the proper technique to perform extractions with Piezosurgery. As in all other procedures, inserts must never be allowed to rest in one single place when the ultrasonic vibration is active. This is particularly important when working in the periodontal ligament space. To avoid pinching of the insert and consequently having the ultrasonic vibration converted into thermal energy, it is important to keep the insert constantly moving.

TABLE 83.3 Root Extraction Surgical Classification by Tomaso Vercellotti

Anatomic Classification	Periodontal Diagnosis	Tissue Damage Risk	Surgery Difficulty	Technique	Maneuver	Surgical Instrument	Piezosurgery[a] Insert
Type 1	Normal	Low	Easy	Standard	Periotomy	Periotome	
					External luxation	Elevator	
					Removal	Forceps	
Type 2	Thin	High	Medium	Advanced	Periotomy	Periotome	
					Root sectioning	Piezosurgery	OT7S-3, EX1-3, OP5
					Internal luxation	Elevator	
					Removal	Forceps	
Type 3	Ankylotic	Low	Complex	Advanced	Periotomy	Periotome	
					Rootplasty	Piezosurgery	OT7S-3, EX1-3, OP5
					External luxation	Elevator	
					Removal	Forceps	
Type 4	Thin and ankylotic	Very high	Severe	Advanced	Periotomy	Periotome	
					Root resection and rootplasty	Piezosurgery	OT7S-3, EX1-3, OP5
					Internal luxation	Elevator	
					Removal	Forceps	

[a]Mectron Medical Technology, Carasco, Italy.

Implant Site Preparation

Special Piezosurgery inserts developed for bone perforation have enabled the development of a newer technique for ultrasonic implant site preparation (UISP). Extensive clinical experience has culminated in the development of a protocol with significant clinical advantages. One article described the protocol in detail and reported the results of a multicenter case series study analyzing 3579 implants with a 1- to 3-year follow-up.[45] The preliminary results indicated that implant site preparation with Piezosurgery is a valid alternative to preparation with conventional rotatory instrumentation, with an overall osseointegration percentage of 97.82% (97.14% maxilla, 98.75% mandible) and an overall implant survival rate of 97.74% (96.99% maxilla, 98.75% mandible). These results are extremely encouraging, especially considering that implant placement was often combined with bone regenerative techniques. Given certain specific advantages of UISP, it is preferable to conventional techniques in the presence of soft bone and limited residual volume, as well as in proximity to delicate anatomic structures such as the inferior alveolar nerve or the Schneiderian membrane.[1]

The first advantage of UISP is related to the cutting characteristics of Piezosurgery, which facilitate differential preparation of the cortical and cancellous bone. A surgical classification system of bone quality at the implant site was developed that simplifies the diagnosis and surgical decision-making process by exploiting differences in bone anatomy (Fig. 83.6). The differential implant site preparation (DISP) technique can be used within the initial osteotomy site to correct the implant axis by selectively directing the cutting action in the desired direction.[48] DISP can also be used in combination with twist drills to facilitate preservation of alveolar crestal bone while achieving maximum primary stability.[55]

The second advantage of UISP is the fast clinical healing of both soft and hard tissue. Animal research demonstrates that new bone formation (neo-osteogenesis) is active at implant sites prepared

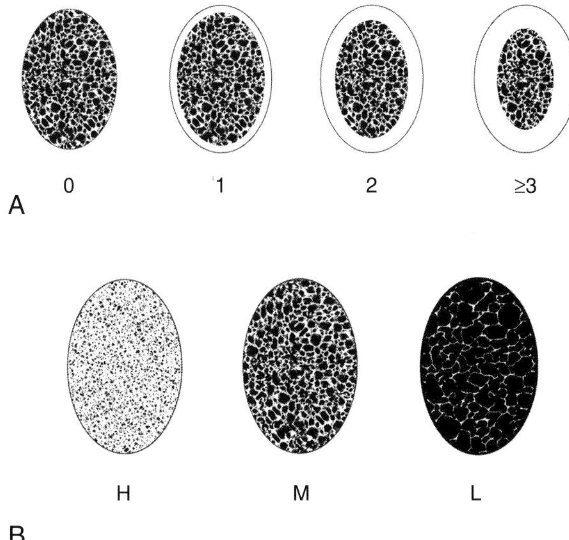

Fig. 83.6 Surgical bone classification by Tomaso and Giuseppe Vercellotti. (A) Cortical crestal thickness in millimeters. (B) Radiographic cancellous bone classification *H*, High; *L*, low; *M*, medium.

with piezoelectric bone surgery earlier than at sites prepared with traditional techniques.[13] A histomorphometric study on mini-pigs showed more bone formation and a greater density of periimplant osteoblasts at implant sites prepared with Piezosurgery as compared with sites prepared with twist drills.[13] Clinically, the minimally invasive nature of the surgery and the stimulation of bone healing translate into better primary stability and likely faster osseointegration compared with conventional instrumentation.[12] In a randomized controlled clinical trial, patients received two identical adjacent implants in the upper premolar area: the test site was prepared with

Piezosurgery, and the control site was prepared using twist drills.[30] Resonance frequency analysis (RFA) measurements were taken by a blinded operator on the day of surgery and at scheduled intervals throughout the first 90 days postoperatively. At the end of this time period, following failure of one implant in the control group, 97.5% of implants were osseointegrated. An initial decrease in mean implant stability quotient (ISQ) values was observed in both groups; however, the decrease in the Piezosurgery group was significantly less than in the control group. The Piezosurgery group also exhibited an earlier stability level reversal, indicating that an overall achievement of better primary stability compared with implants placed with twist drills. These results were subsequently confirmed by numerous clinical trials and a recent meta-analysis with trial sequential analysis, suggesting that piezoelectric implant site preparation improves secondary stability 12 weeks after implant placement when compared with conventional drilling techniques.[3,5,24,27,29]

The surgical technique entails an osteotomy preparation using a series of Piezosurgery inserts. The preparation is initiated with the narrow, pointed IM1 insert (Fig. 83.7A). Parallel pins are used throughout the procedure to check alignment (Fig. 83.7B). The 2-mm–diameter IM2 insert is used to prepare the osteotomy further (Fig. 83.7C). The coronal aspect of the preparation is widened with the pilot 2/3 insert (Fig. 83.7D), and the osteotomy is finished with the IM3 insert (Fig. 83.7E). Final cortical preparation is accomplished with the IM4 insert (Fig. 83.7F). After use of the pilot 3/4 insert (Fig. 83.7G), the implant osteotomy is completed (Fig. 83.7H). If desired, before implant placement, osteoplasty of the crestal bone is possible with the OP3 insert (Fig. 83.7I). Fig. 83.7J shows a final occlusal view of an implant placed in a narrow ridge.

The cutting features of Piezosurgery have also paved the way to new possibilities in the minimally invasive treatment of narrow ridges. The precision of the ultrasonic cut allows for preparation of an implant bed for wedge implants with a rectangular section, specifically designed for ridges with limited horizontal dimension (3.5 to 5 mm), where it would be impossible to insert standard implants without the association of regenerative procedures. Wedge implants (Rex TL 1.8, Rex Implants, Inc., Columbus, OH, USA) are tissue-level implants with a maximum endosseous thickness of 1.8 mm and a diverging transmucosal collar ending in a standard external hex prosthetic connection (Fig. 83.8). A recent multicenter prospective cohort study investigated clinical effectiveness and patient-centered outcomes after implant-supported rehabilitation of narrow ridges with wedge implants,[46] showing promising results after 1 year of functional loading (survival rate 98.3%; mean marginal bone loss 0.60 ± 0.52 mm). Patients reported slight intraoperative discomfort, mild pain on the day of surgery and the first postoperative day, and no pain over the following 5 days, confirming the extremely low invasiveness of this surgical procedure. Even if further investigations are needed to evaluate medium- and long-term clinical outcomes, wedge implants could be considered as an additional resource for the practitioner, allowing implant-supported rehabilitation of selected cases with horizontal ridge deficiencies without the need of advanced regenerative procedures, inevitably associated with higher morbidity, prolonged therapy time, and increased economic costs.

Following a detailed presurgical study of the residual crestal bone characteristics (Fig. 83.9A), confirmed by intraoperatory measurements (Fig. 83.9B), the technique is used for placing wedge-shaped implants entails preparing a pilot osteotomy to determine proper implant axis positioning (Fig. 83.9C), followed by a longitudinal piezoelectric osteotomy (Fig. 83.9D) and bone expansion (Fig. 83.9E and F). The insertion of the implant in the surgical site corrects the horizontal bone defect (Fig. 83.9G and H) without the need for additional augmentation procedures. Implant stability may be assessed through RFA at multiple time points; however, it should be noted that the asymmetrical shape of the Wedge implants implies that different ISQ values should be expected along the mesiodistal (Fig. 83.9I) and buccolingual (Fig. 83.9J) axes, with the latter always exhibiting lower values. Wedge implants' surgical technique, when properly understood, is relatively simple to apply and can provide outstanding clinical outcomes (Fig. 83.9K and L).

Conclusions

Piezoelectric bone surgery is a well-known surgical technique for bone surgery with many clinical applications in dentistry. The extraordinary cutting properties and applications of piezoelectric bone surgery are described in this chapter. The most compelling characteristics of piezoelectric bone surgery are low surgical trauma, exceptional precision, and fast healing response. As a result, Piezosurgery has the ability to increase treatment effectiveness while improving postoperative recovery and healing.

Although a great deal of scientific research focuses on new products for tissue engineering and bone regeneration, the importance of minimal surgical trauma for optimal bone healing and regeneration should not be overlooked. A new appreciation for the effectiveness of Piezosurgery has the potential to redefine the concept of minimally invasive surgery in osteotomy and osteoplasty procedures.

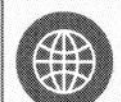
Case Scenarios are found on the companion website eBooks.Health.Elsevier.com.

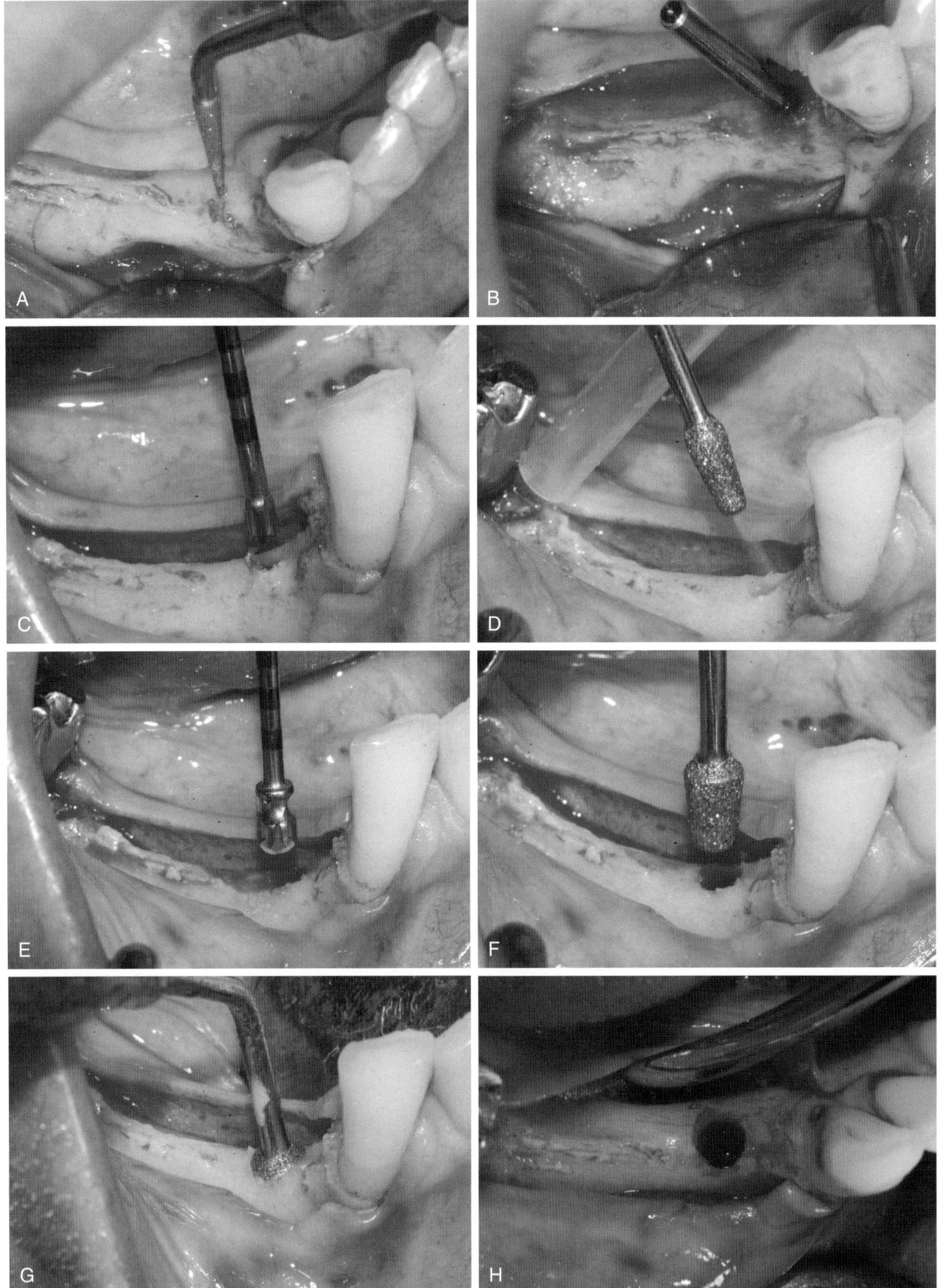

Fig. 83.7 Implant site preparation and placement. (A) Piezosurgery insert (IM1) used to start the implant site preparation (Mectron Medical Technology, Carasco, Italy). (B) Parallel pin in place to check the direction of osteotomy. (C) Piezosurgery 2-mm–diameter insert (IM2) for pilot osteotomy. (D) Piezosurgery insert for cortical preparation (pilot 2/3). (E) Cancellous bone preparation with Piezosurgery insert IM3. (F) Piezosurgery diamond-coated insert (IM4) for final cortical bone preparation. (G) Piezosurgery pilot insert 3/4 in action. (H) Occlusal view of completed implant site preparation.

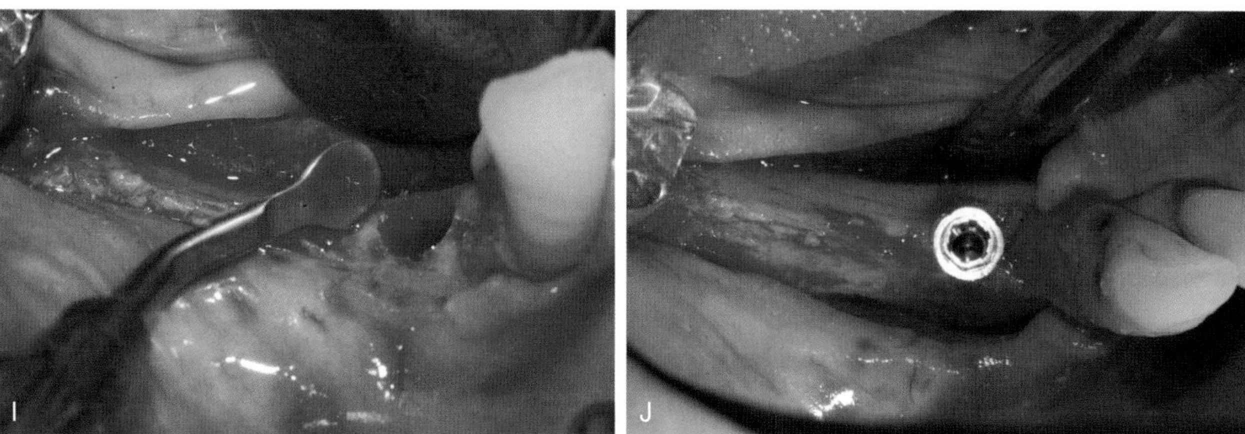

Fig. 83.7 cont'd (I) Osteoplasty of crestal bone in the peri-implant area using Piezosurgery insert OP3. (J) Occlusal view of well-placed implant despite the narrow ridge.

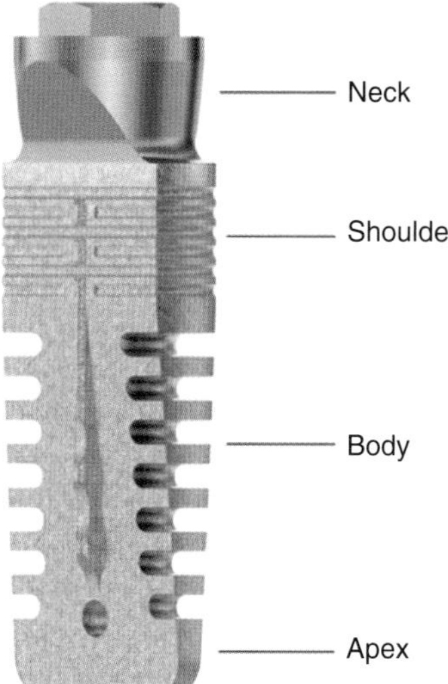

Fig. 83.8 Wedge-shaped implant characterized by rectangular section (Rex Implants, Inc., Columbus, OH).

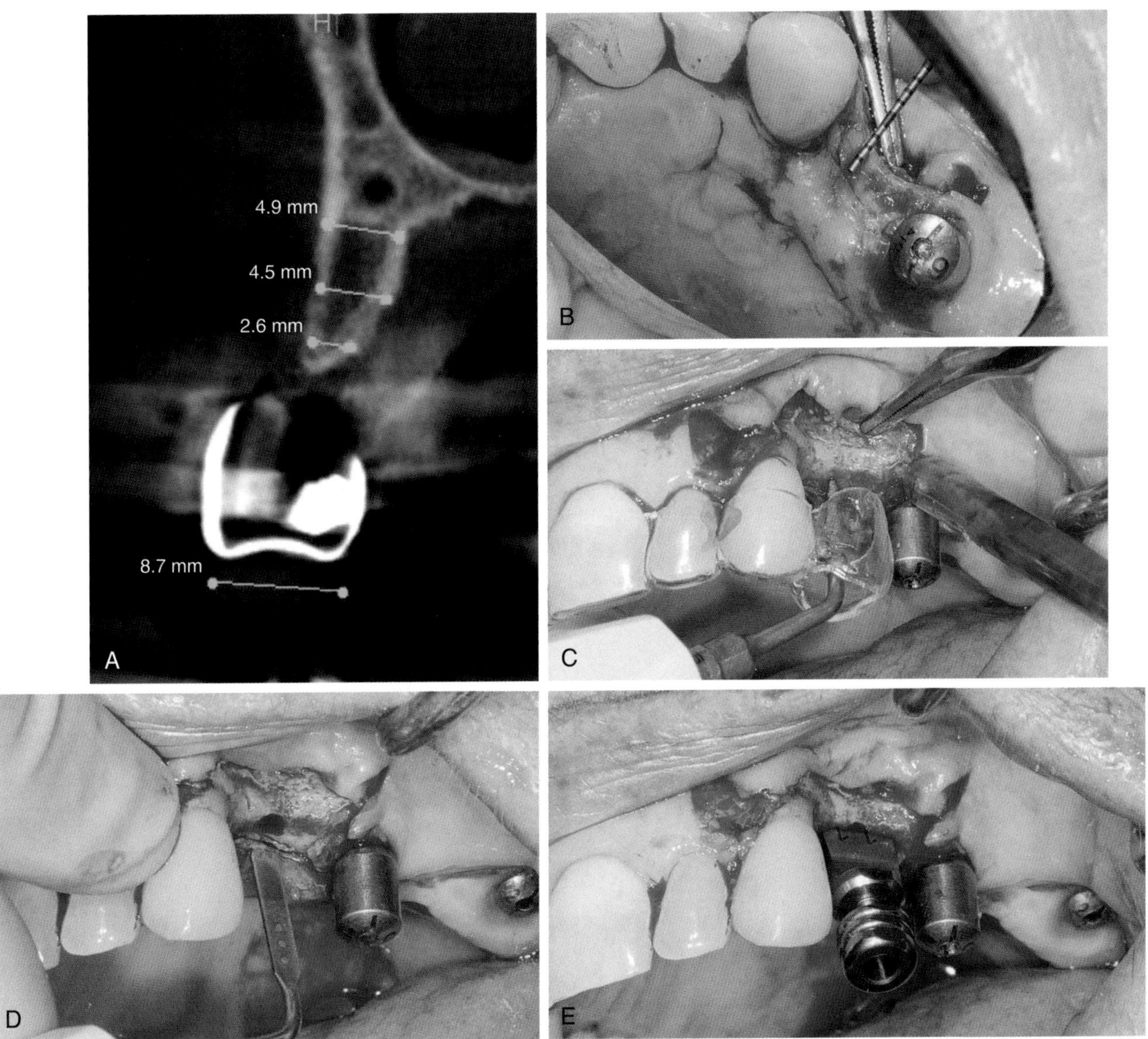

Fig. 83.9 Wedge Implant Placement. (A) CTCB cross-section revealing reduced crestal width. (B) Intra-operatory Crestal Bone Width (approximately 3 mm). (C) Initial pilot osteotomy using conic Piezosurgery insert to establish the mesiodistal and buccolingual implant axis position. (D) Osteotomy using 0.35-mm Piezosurgery insert, which allows removal of minimal bone during the implant site preparation with expansion technique. (E) The expansion of the ridge is performed by inserting two expanders (1.6 mm and 2.0 mm) in a sequence into the horizontal osteotomy.

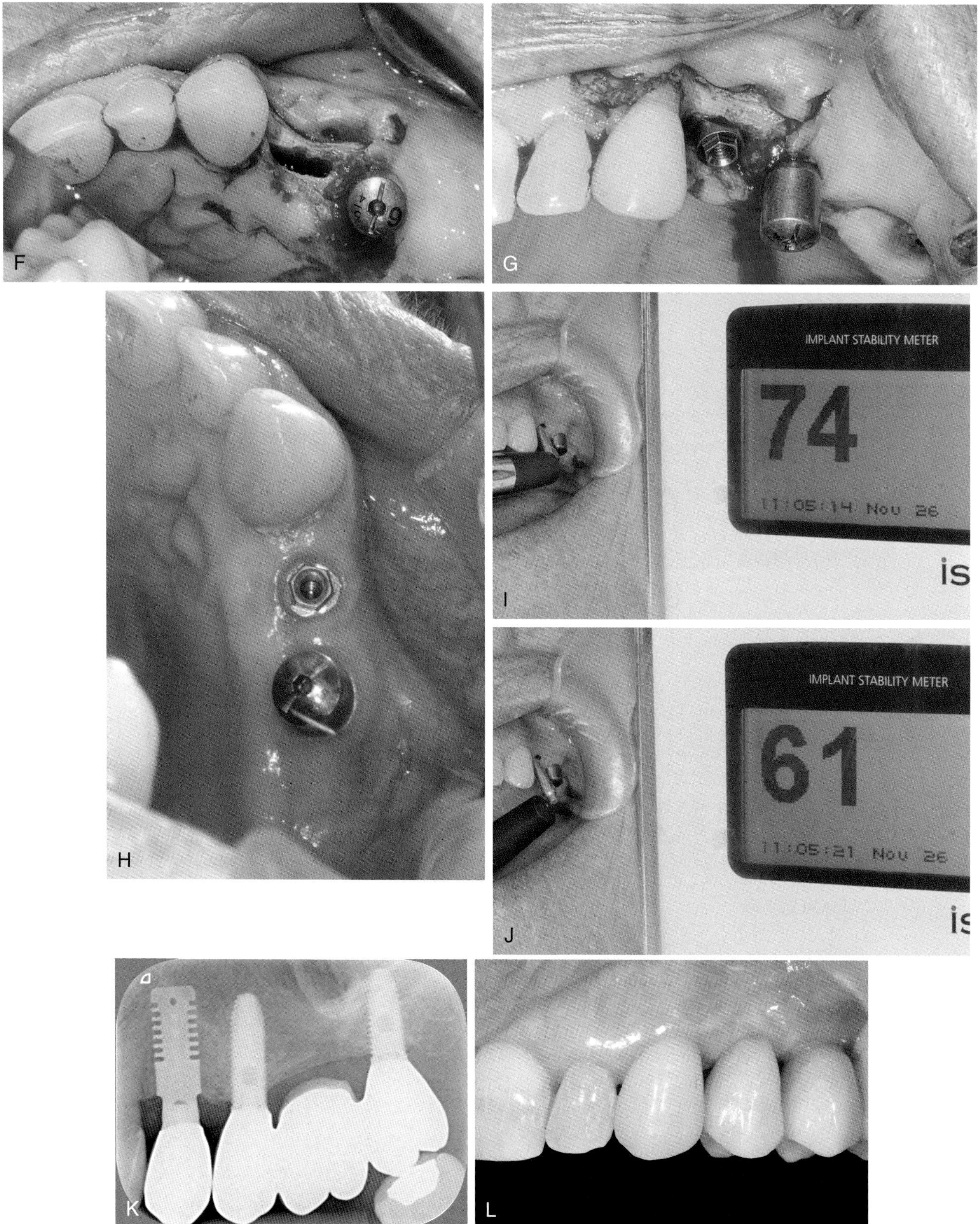

Fig. 83.9 cont'd (F) Correctly prepared site showing the expansion of the implant site and the semicircle pilot osteotomy, necessary to properly position the implant fin. (G) Following implant insertion, the dislocation of the thick bony wall corrected the horizontal bone defect. (H) After soft tissue healing, the correction of the ridge horizontal defect is evident. (I) Mesiodistal implant stability quotient evaluation after 6 months, at time of loading. (J) Buccal-lingual ISQ is always lower compared to the mesiodistal measurement. (K) X-ray after 2 years of loading. (L) Final crown, 2 years of follow-up.

Suggested Readings

Bassi F, Cicciù M, Di Lenarda R, et al. Piezoelectric bone surgery compared with conventional rotary instruments in oral surgery and implantology: Summary and consensus statements of the International Piezoelectric Surgery Academy Consensus Conference 2019. *Int J Oral Implantol (Berl)*. 2020;13(3):235–239. PMID: 32879928.

Canullo L, Peñarrocha D, Peñarrocha M, Rocio AG, Penarrocha-Diago M. Piezoelectric vs. conventional drilling in implant site preparation: pilot controlled randomized clinical trial with crossover design. *Clin Oral Implants Res*. 2014;25(12):1336–1343. https://doi.org/10.1111/clr.12278. Epub 2013 Oct 21. PMID: 24147994.

Cicciù M, Stacchi C, Fiorillo L, et al. Piezoelectric bone surgery for impacted lower third molar extraction compared with conventional rotary instruments: a systematic review, meta-analysis, and trial sequential analysis. *Int J Oral Maxillofac Surg*. 2021;50(1):121–131. https://doi.org/10.1016/j.ijom.2020.03.008. Epub 2020 Apr 11. PMID: 32284166.

Happe A. Use of a piezoelectric surgical device to harvest bone grafts from the mandibular ramus: report of 40 cases. *Int J Periodontics Restorative Dent*. 2007;27:241–249.

Jiang Q, Qiu Y, Yang C, et al. Piezoelectric versus conventional rotary techniques for impacted third molar extraction: a meta-analysis of randomized controlled trials. *Medicine (Baltimore)*. 2015;94(41):e1685.

Peker Tekdal G, Bostanci N, Belibasakis GN, Gürkan A. The effect of piezoelectric surgery implant osteotomy on radiological and molecular parameters of peri-implant crestal bone loss: a randomized, controlled, split-mouth trial. *Clin Oral Implants Res*. 2016;27(5):535–544. https://doi.org/10.1111/clr.12620. Epub 2015 Jun 16. PMID: 26077862.

Preti G, Martinasso G, Peirone B, et al. Cytokines and growth factors involved in the osseointegration of oral titanium implants positioned using piezoelectric bone surgery versus a drill technique: a pilot study in minipigs. *J Periodontol*. 2007;78:716–722.

Schaeren S, Jaquiery C, Heberer M, et al. Assessment of nerve damage using a novel ultrasonic device for bone cutting. *J Oral Maxillofac Surg*. 2008;66:593–596.

Stacchi C, Bassi F, Troiano G, et al. Piezoelectric bone surgery for implant site preparation compared with conventional drilling techniques: A systematic review, meta-analysis and trial sequential analysis. *Int J Oral Implantol (Berl)*. 2020;13(2):141–158. PMID: 32424381.

Stacchi C, Lombardi T, Baldi D, et al. Immediate Loading of Implant-Supported Single Crowns after Conventional and Ultrasonic Implant Site Preparation: A Multicenter Randomized Controlled Clinical Trial. *Biomed Res Int*. 2018;2018:6817154. https://doi.org/10.1155/2018/6817154. PMID: 30186865; PMCID: PMC6112219.

Stacchi C, Vercellotti T, Torelli L, et al. Changes in implant stability using different site preparation techniques: twist drills versus Piezosurgery: a single-blinded, randomized, controlled clinical trial. *Clin Implant Dent Relat Res*. 2011;15:188–197.

Stacchi C, Vercellotti T, Toschetti A, et al. Intraoperative complications during sinus floor elevation using two different ultrasonic approaches: a two-center, randomized, controlled clinical trial. *Clin Implant Dent Relat Res*. 2015;17(suppl 1):e117–e125.

Vercellotti T, Nevins ML, Kim DM, et al. Osseous response following resective therapy with piezosurgery. *Int J Periodontics Restorative Dent*. 2005;25:543–549.

Vercellotti T, Pollack AS. A new bone surgery device: sinus grafting and periodontal surgery. *Compend Contin Educ Dent*. 2006;27:319–325.

Vercellotti T, Stacchi C, Russo C, et al. Ultrasonic implant site preparation using piezosurgery: a multicenter case series study analyzing 3,579 implants with a 1- to 3-year follow-up. *Int J Periodontics Restorative Dent*. 2014;34:11–18.

Vercellotti T, Troiano G, Oreglia F, et al. Wedge-Shaped Implants for Minimally Invasive Treatment of Narrow Ridges: A Multicenter Prospective Cohort Study. *J Clin Med*. 2020;9(10):3301. https://doi.org/10.3390/jcm9103301. PMID: 33066588; PMCID: PMC7602171.

Vercellotti T. *The piezoelectric bone surgery: a new paradigm*. Hanover Park, IL: Quintessence Publishing; 2017.

Wallace SS, Mazor Z, Froum SJ, et al. Schneiderian membrane perforation rate during sinus elevation using piezosurgery: clinical results of 100 consecutive cases. *Int J Periodontics Restorative Dent*. 2007;27:413–419.

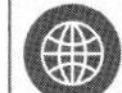
References for this chapter are found on the companion website eBooks.Health.Elsevier.com.

CHAPTER 84

Digitally Assisted Implant Placement Surgery

Denny Chao | Russell J. Crockett | Perry R. Klokkevold

CHAPTER OUTLINE

Introduction

Conventional surgical placement of dental implants involves the elevation of a full-thickness flap to expose the underlying bone. A series of drills with increasingly larger diameters are subsequently employed with copious irrigation to prepare the implant osteotomy site. This is followed by the insertion of the dental implant in the alveolar ridge. The osteotomy and final implant placement must be prosthetically driven to optimize the function and esthetics of the planned dental prosthesis, while avoiding harm to vital structures such as the inferior alveolar nerve, sinus cavities, and adjacent teeth and implants (see Chapter 78).

In conventional presurgical planning, implant positions are determined with a combination of study models, wax-ups of the proposed dental prosthesis, and diagnostic imaging with a laboratory fabricated acrylic resin radiographic guide. This radiographic guide has limited correlation with the underlying bone and needs to be modified (i.e., open access for drills) to be used as a surgical guide following imaging. The transfer of imaging information correlating the prosthetic plan to the alveolar bone via the radiographic/surgical guide is prone to inaccuracies. Furthermore, conventional surgical guides offer minimal guidance. As a result, the final position of the implant is determined by the clinician and how he or she chooses to utilize the surgical guide along with his or her interpretation of the diagnostic information, clinical experience, and surgical skills to replicate the plan.

Digital technology in implant dentistry is rapidly evolving. The digital implant workflow can help clinicians plan more efficiently and execute more accurately. Advances in implant surgical technology include simulation software, static computer-aided design/computer-aided manufacturing (CAD/CAM) surgical guides, and dynamic navigation for dental implant surgery (Table 84.1 and 84.2).

- **Virtual surgical planning or implant simulation software** is used preoperatively to simulate implant placement on a virtual patient. The software allows clinicians to interact with three-dimensional (3D) renderings of the patient created from computed tomography (CT) or cone-beam CT (CBCT) scan data.
- **Static CAD/CAM surgical guides** can be designed from the virtual plan and produced with various technologies including milling and 3D printing. Metal drill sleeves or bushings are manually luted to the guide after production in precise locations designed to receive them. In select manufacturing methods, the drill sleeves can be integrated into the guide and manufactured as a single piece, eliminating the need for inserting metal sleeves. Along with drill handles, keys, or integrated drill stops, the sleeves provide static and physical guidance for the osteotomy drills and implants. The drill handles, keys, or integrated drill stops are system-specific based on the manufacturer.
- **Dynamic navigation** employs real-time tracking and visual guidance to execute the virtual surgical plan. The plan is superimposed onto scan data, registered with the patient via fiducial markers, and observed interactively during live surgery to aid the surgeon in preparing osteotomy sites and placing dental implants.

This chapter provides an overview of the terminology, technical requirements, and limitations of digitally assisted implant placement surgery.

Data and Image Acquisition

The presurgical workup for digitally assisted implant placement begins with the acquisition of diagnostic data. For partially edentulous scenarios, a set of accurate diagnostic casts is needed. This can be accomplished with either conventional impressions or digital impressions via intraoral scanning. If conventional impressions and corresponding diagnostic casts are made, they must be digitized with a desktop or laboratory scanner. These digital scans are commonly exported in the Standard Tessellation Language (STL) format to be utilized for virtual planning and fabrication of tooth-supported surgical guides.

TABLE 84.1 Advantages and Disadvantages of Static CAD/CAM Surgical Guides

Advantages of Static CAD/CAM Surgical Guides
- Implant placement is more accurate compared to the freehand method.
- Flapless surgeries are possible with mucosa-supported surgical guides.
- Less hand-eye coordination is required for implant placement because static surgical guides offer physical guidance.
- A bone-supported alveoloplasty guide can accurately direct the amount of bone removal necessary for the planned prosthesis.
- Static surgical guides can be used to guide the pick-up procedure for an immediately loaded prosthesis.

Disadvantages of Static CAD/CAM Surgical Guides
- Implant placement cannot occur right after imaging because time is required to manufacture the surgical guide.
- It may be difficult to place posterior (second molar) implants and implants in patients with limited mouth opening because the osteotomy drill and handpiece must overcome the height of the surgical sleeve.
- Static surgical guides may not be possible in tight interdental spaces.
- Bone-supported surgical guides are associated with invasive flaps.
- Incorrect guide position that goes unnoticed will result in inaccurate implant placement.
- Cost is associated with guide production (milling, 3D printing, guide sleeve).

CAD/CAM, Computer-aided design/computer-aided manufacturing; *3D,* three-dimensional.

TABLE 84.2 Advantages and Disadvantages of Dynamic Navigation

Advantages of Dynamic Navigation
- Implant placement is more accurate compared to the freehand method.
- Flapless surgeries are possible.
- Implant placement can occur right after imaging.
- It may be less difficult to place posterior (second molar) implants and implants in patients with limited mouth opening.
- Implant placement has the potential to be less invasive because large flaps are not necessary.
- Implant placement in tight interdental spaces is limited only by the diameter of the osteotomy drills.

Disadvantages of Dynamic Navigation
- Hand-eye coordination is needed because dynamic navigation only offers visual guidance.
- Two surgeries are required for completely edentulous patients due to the need to place fiducial markers (bone screws).
- There is no physical guide to guide the pick-up procedure for an immediately loaded prosthesis
- Incorrect patient tracking that goes unnoticed will result in inaccurate implant placement.
- Significant cost may be associated with the dynamic navigation software and hardware.

Conversely, for fully edentulous scenarios, a set of diagnostic casts is not needed for the presurgical workup. Complete dentures or record bases with teeth set in wax are used to convey the necessary information through the dual scan protocol. This protocol involves two CT or CBCT scans: one with patients wearing their dentures with fiducial markers attached and another scan of the denture(s) alone with the fiducial markers still attached. The quality of the complete dentures or record bases with the wax setups are of utmost importance for a successful outcome. If the fit is suboptimal and

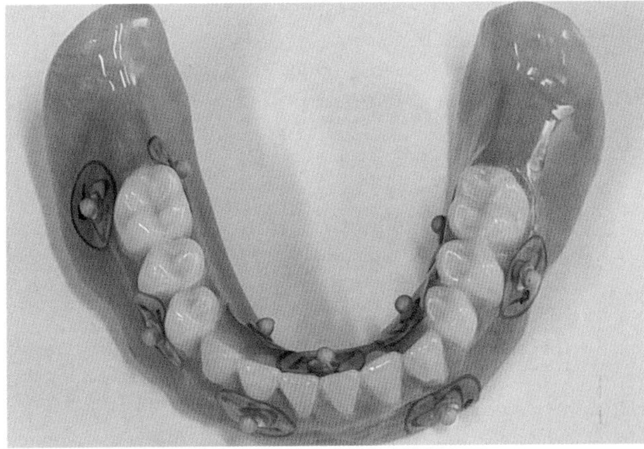

Fig. 84.1 Fiducial markers/stickers are distributed on a mandibular complete denture in preparation for the dual scan protocol.

instability is detected, the denture base must be relined. Likewise, if the occlusal vertical dimension and centric relation are incorrect, they must be addressed at this point in time prior to the dual scan.

Simulation is not possible without the acquisition of CT or CBCT scans. Several factors, such as radiation exposure, limitations in accuracy, and scatter due to the presence of metallic restorations should be considered when utilizing these imaging modalities. Fortunately, the evolution of CBCT imaging technology has made it possible to reduce radiation exposure to near the level of full mouth radiographs while maintaining diagnostic quality for presurgical implant planning (see Table 75.2).[5,7] CBCT scans are obtained in multiple “slices” in Digital Imaging and Communications in Medicine (DICOM) format, which has achieved a near universal level of acceptance among dental simulation software.[12] Clinicians, however, must be cognizant that not all patients should be scanned the same way, and these scans should be prescribed based on how the patient presents at the time dental records are made (see Chapter 75).

- Complete edentulism
  - **With acceptable existing complete dentures:** Due to the lack of intraoral hard structure reference points, the dual scan protocol is recommended.[16,20] Fiducial markers or stickers are attached to the existing prostheses (Fig. 84.1), and the patient is imaged while wearing the dentures. A second scan is acquired of the prostheses extraorally. After completion of the two scans, the fiducial markers are removed, and the unmodified prostheses returned to the patient.
    - **If the existing complete dentures are reinforced with metal,** the prostheses should be duplicated in acrylic resin prior to scanning to avoid metal-induced scatter of the resulting scan data.
  - **Without existing complete dentures or with unacceptable existing complete dentures:** The dual scan protocol is recommended with proper diagnostic setups on well-fitting record bases.
- Partial edentulism
  - **With one to three missing teeth:** CT or CBCT scans can be acquired, as normal, without any appliances.
    - **If numerous metallic restorations are present within the remaining dentition**, a scanning appliance is advised because metal-induced scatter can severely compromise the appearance of the anatomical teeth landmarks (Fig. 84.2).
    - The scanning appliance is made with a full arch impression using the dual scan protocol. Fiducial markers are

attached to the impression tray. The tray with the impression material is then placed intraorally and the patient is scanned with the tray in place prior to removal. Once the patient scan is acquired, the impression tray is removed and scanned extraorally. The resulting scan can be digitally "inverted" to visualize the remaining dentition without scatter (Fig. 84.3).[11]

- **With minimal number of teeth remaining:** Similar to the edentulous scenario, the dual scan protocol is recommended with proper diagnostic setups on well-fitting record bases.

Virtual Surgical Planning Software and Implant Simulation

The DICOM files are imported into a planning software of choice. These programs are categorized as either open or closed architecture. An open architecture software outputs files in the STL format, which can be manipulated across various CAD/CAM programs. A closed architecture software outputs files in proprietary formats, which can only be manipulated by specific proprietary/authorized programs. Generally, open architecture software is preferred for complex cases because the use of multiple programs may be necessary.

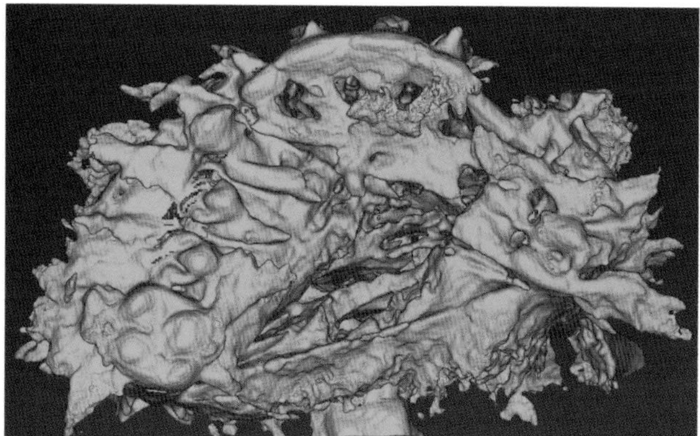

Fig. 84.2 Scatter from metallic restorations can interfere with the 3D reconstruction of the virtual patient. Scatter adjacent to anatomic teeth landmarks can introduce inaccuracies in the registration process.

The virtual patient (i.e., 3D surface models of the patient) is derived from the CBCT dataset using gray value segmentation. Typically, a gray value is assigned to a specific tissue type due to radiation attenuation, which refers to the process by which the number of particles entering a body of matter is reduced by absorption and scattering.[1] Most simulation software has the option to limit the range of gray value displayed on screen, which enables the segmentation of specific tissue types such as soft tissue and bone. Some programs also permit selective editing of segmentations, which allows structures with different densities to be separated (e.g., separating teeth from alveolar bone) (Video 84.1). For complex cases, it is good practice to manually remove any scatter artifacts and to separate structures such as the maxillary teeth, mandibular teeth, maxilla, and mandible into independent objects so they can be turned on and off for planning purposes (Fig. 84.4). Segmentation can be especially useful in the prevention of placing guide fixation pins, which may be required in select scenarios, through the roots of teeth to be extracted.

In most simulation software, certain parameters should be set and modified as necessary to achieve the highest quality output and improve the user interface. One of these parameters is patient data orientation or patient coordinate system. When a CBCT scan is imported into a simulation software, the orientation of the virtual patient is dependent on how the scan was taken. For example, if the patient was off-center or had his or her head rotated or titled during the scan, the virtual patient will be created in a similar manner (i.e., deviated). Prior to implant planning, any deviations in roll, yaw, and pitch should be addressed accordingly (Fig. 84.5).

CLINICAL CORRELATION

Certain parameters, such as patient data orientation, need to be set and modified as necessary to achieve the highest quality output and improve the user interface. The orientation of the virtual patient is dependent on how the CBCT scan was taken. If the patient is scanned off-center or with their head rotated or titled, the virtual patient will be created in a similar deviated manner. Prior to implant planning, deviations in roll, yaw, and pitch need to be adjusted.

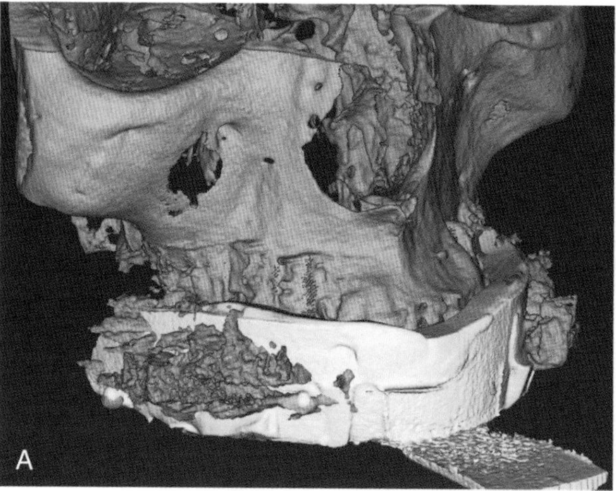

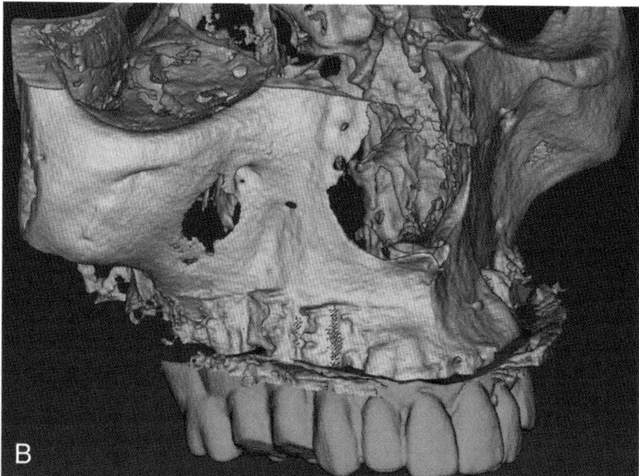

Fig. 84.3 (A and B) Due to the presence of generalized metallic restorations and resulting scatter, the patient is imaged with a scanning appliance via the dual scan protocol. (A) The scanning appliance (impression tray) scan is registered to the patient scan via fiducial markers. (B) The scanning appliance scan is digitally "inverted" to display the anatomical teeth landmarks without scatter.

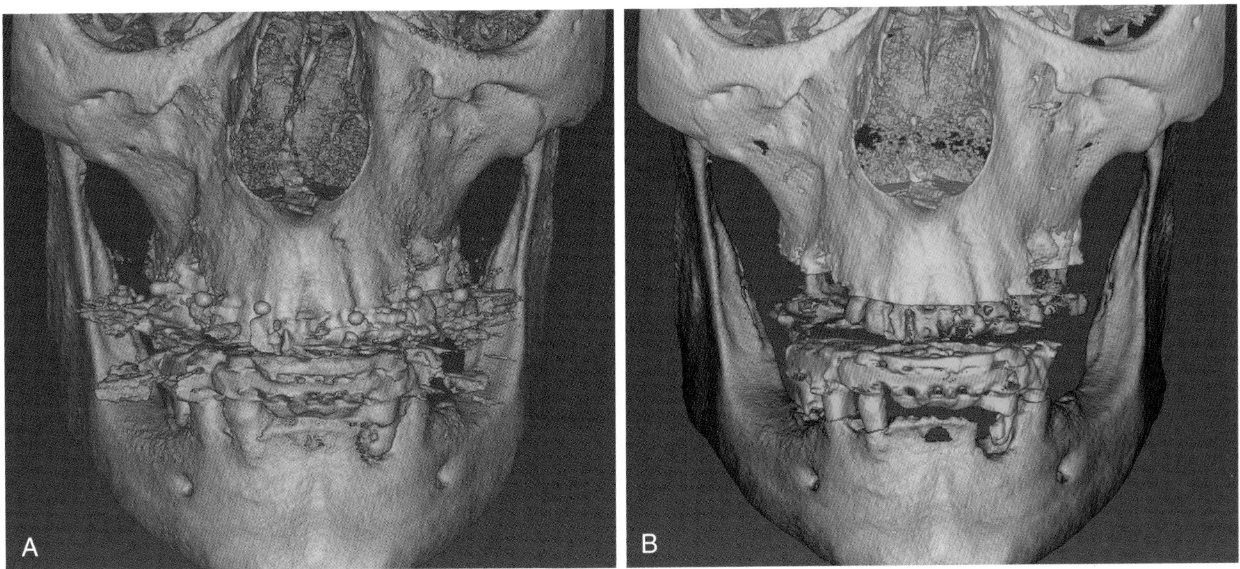

Fig. 84.4 Segmentation of the cone-beam CT (CBCT) scan dataset. (A) The patient is reconstructed from CBCT data. (B) The maxilla *(teal)*, maxillary teeth *(red)*, mandible *(dark gray)*, and mandibular teeth *(green)* are segmented into independent objects for implant planning.

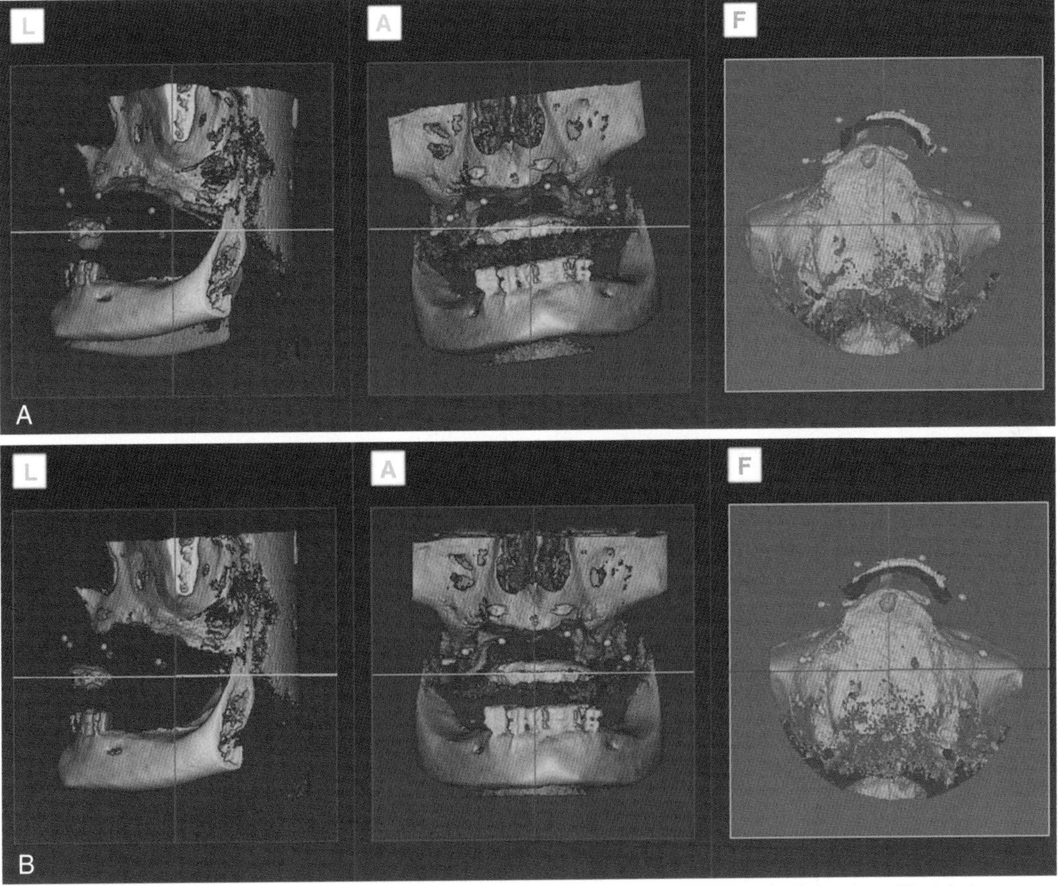

Fig. 84.5 Redefining patient orientation or the patient coordinate system. (A) The patient's head was tilted during the cone-beam CT scan which resulted in a cant in the scan data. (B) Patient orientation is corrected by modifying the roll, yaw, and pitch accordingly.

Another important parameter is the panoramic curve. It is defined by drawing a curve based on the patient's maxilla or mandible in the axial view. The shape, position, and width of the curve determine how the patient's anatomy is visualized in the panoramic and sagittal cross-sectional viewing windows in the user interface. The defined panoramic view is created from the 3D data that falls within the curve. While this is a useful view to visualize the overall plan and structures, it is important to recognize that the panoramic view is prone to distortion and should not be used as the sole view for implant planning. All planned implants must be evaluated in multiple cross-sectional views and in various directions for accurate assessment. Lastly, unlike a conventional panoramic image, the defined panoramic view generated from the panoramic curve will not show anatomic structures that are not within the panoramic curve. Specifically, vital anatomic structures such as the inferior alveolar nerve will only be visible on the defined panoramic view when it is included in the panoramic curve (Fig. 84.6).

Fig. 84.6 Defining the panoramic curve. (A) The panoramic curve is defined incorrectly. The mandible appears to be discontinuous because the curve is positioned lingual to the mandible in the symphysis region. (B) The panoramic curve is defined properly.

The teeth directly segmented from the CBCT dataset are not accurate enough for tooth-supported surgical guide fabrication, especially if metal-induced scatter is present. To circumvent this problem, digital diagnostic casts (with or without analog diagnostic wax-ups) must be imported and aligned prior to the implant planning process. Alignment of the digital diagnostic casts to the CBCT is called registration (Video 84.2).[8,14] Registration is accomplished by selecting common reference points between two datasets. In partially edentulous scenarios, the remaining teeth can be used as common points (Fig. 84.7). If the dual scan protocol is utilized, such as in completely edentulous scenarios, the applied fiducial markers are selected as common points (Fig. 84.8). Once data alignment via common points is achieved, most software programs can refine the alignment through an automated "best-fit" feature (Fig. 84.9). Because the registration between datasets is critical for the accurate transfer of the planned implant position into the surgical guide and in turn, to the intraoral site, the clinician is strongly advised to double-check the registration results. Alignment must be manually corrected if visual deviation is observed (Fig. 84.10).

Following registration of datasets, virtual implant planning can begin. Diagnostic wax-ups remain crucial for the proper positioning of dental implants with the digital workflow. Diagnostic wax-ups can be accomplished manually or digitally. Analog wax-ups must be digitized with diagnostic casts through desktop scanning while digital wax-ups can be directly generated from the simulation software (Fig. 84.11). In cases where the dual scan protocol is utilized, the prosthesis scan itself functions as the diagnostic wax-up. The wax-up of the proposed implant prosthesis must be optimally positioned and take the emergence profile, morphology, occlusal, and proximal contacts into consideration.

Virtual implants from a library or database of manufacturer-defined implants are simulated to the virtual patient's jaw and placed in prosthetically driven positions while avoiding vital anatomic structures. Most implant planning software programs have the ability to apply program or user defined safety checks or boundaries (e.g., 2-mm circumferential zone) around the virtual implants that warn users when implants are positioned too close to vital structures such as neighboring implants, adjacent teeth, sinus cavities, and nerves (Fig. 84.12). The planned implant positions can be viewed and adjusted in two-dimensional (2D)

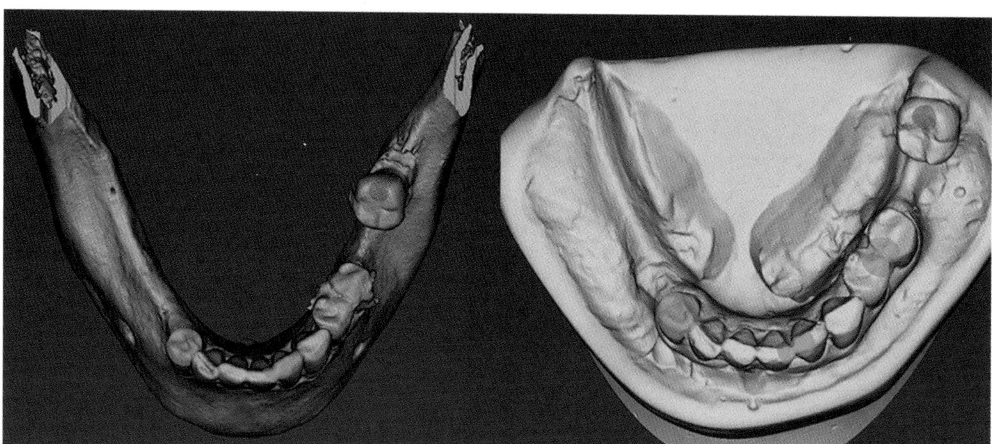

Fig. 84.7 Registration of the cone-beam CT patient dataset with the virtual diagnostic cast in partially edentulous scenarios is accomplished by selecting the remaining dentition as common points.

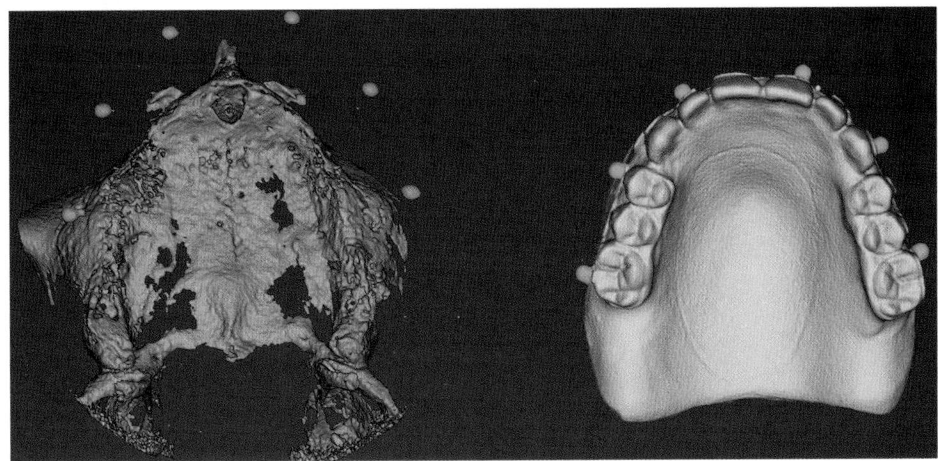

Fig. 84.8 Registration of the cone-beam CT patient dataset with the prosthesis dataset obtained via the dual scan protocol in completely edentulous scenarios is accomplished by selecting fiducial markers as common points.

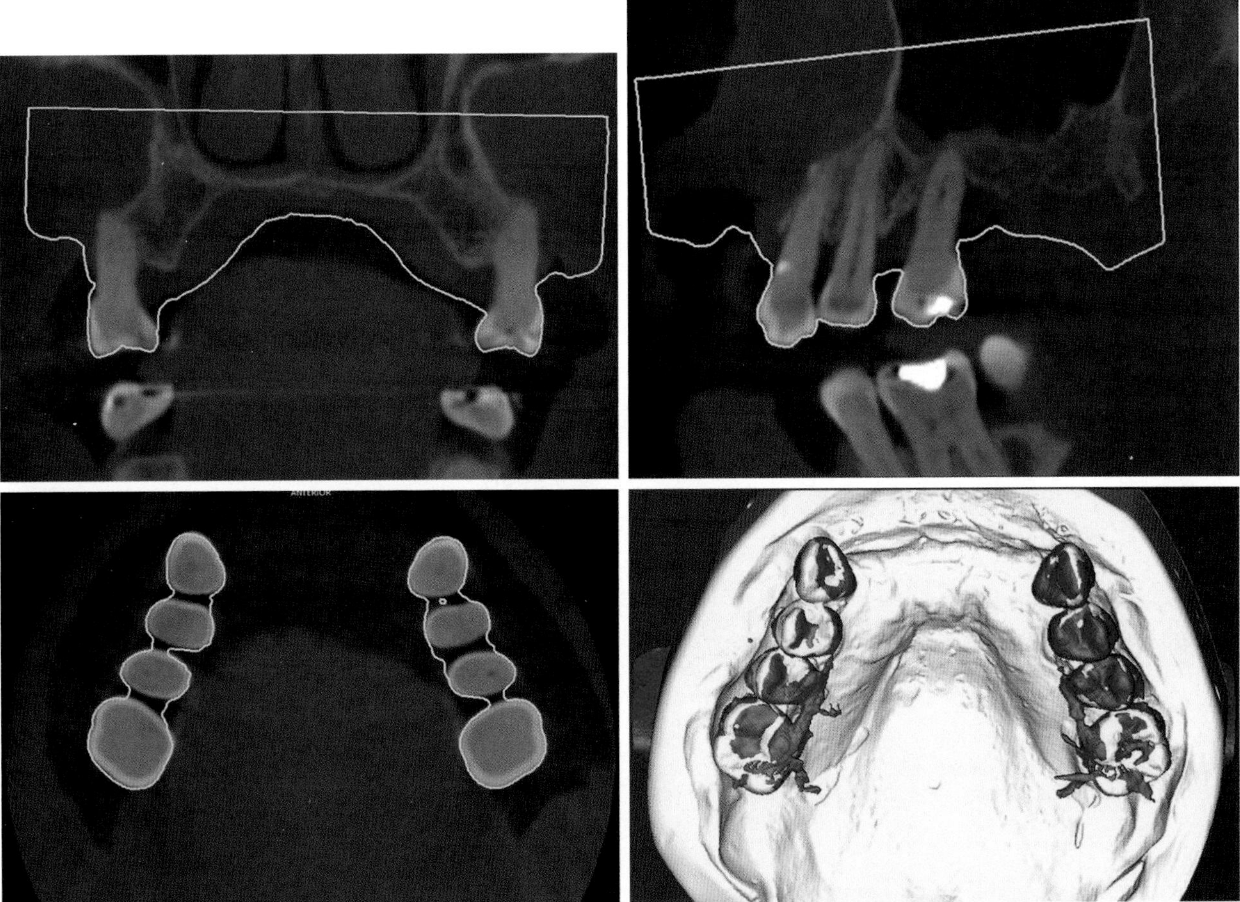

Fig. 84.9 Registration is refined through the software's "best-fit" algorithm. The outline of the virtual diagnostic cast *(yellow)* follows the cone-beam CT scan of the patient closely.

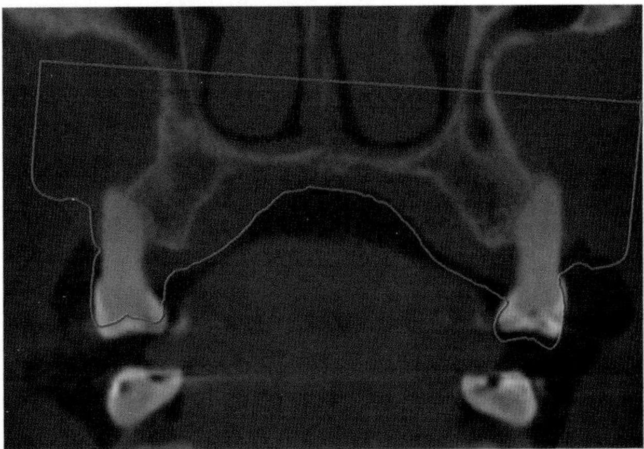

Fig. 84.10 Deviation is observed in the registration process. This must be corrected prior to implant planning and surgical guide design.

cross-sectional images and on the 3D, surface models to ensure these parameters are met.

While prosthetically driven, the proposed implants should be adequately surrounded by bone. If minor bony deficiencies are observed, bone augmentation procedures should be considered. However, if major bony deficiencies not conducive to bone augmentation are observed, the clinician should consider modifying the prosthetic plan. For example, in the event where the long axis of the proposed prosthetically driven implant position deviates significantly from the existing alveolus as viewed in sagittal cross-sections, the clinician may contemplate repositioning the implant within the bone and utilizing angled abutments (Fig. 84.13). Virtual abutments can be generated from a library for planning purposes as well.

In scenarios where no (stable) dentition remains, guide fixation is recommended to maximize guide stability. Fixation is achieved with guide fixation pins. They can be brought in from a library and simulated. Similar to virtual implants, virtual fixation pins should not be placed in close proximity to proposed dental implants, teeth, or vital anatomic structures. The pins should be placed in solid bone for stabilization and should avoid existing teeth and sockets of teeth to be extracted (Fig. 84.14). If the software operator is not the implant surgeon or if the implant surgeon is not present during the implant planning, he or she must review and approve the final implant positions and fixation pins prior to surgical guide design and fabrication.

Static CAD/CAM surgical guides can offer pilot guidance, partial guidance, or full guidance. With pilot and partial guidance, only the pilot drill and/or initial twist drill are guided, and all subsequent osteotomy preparations will be performed without the guide. With full guidance, all drills and implants are utilized through the guide. Drill and implant guidance are provided by

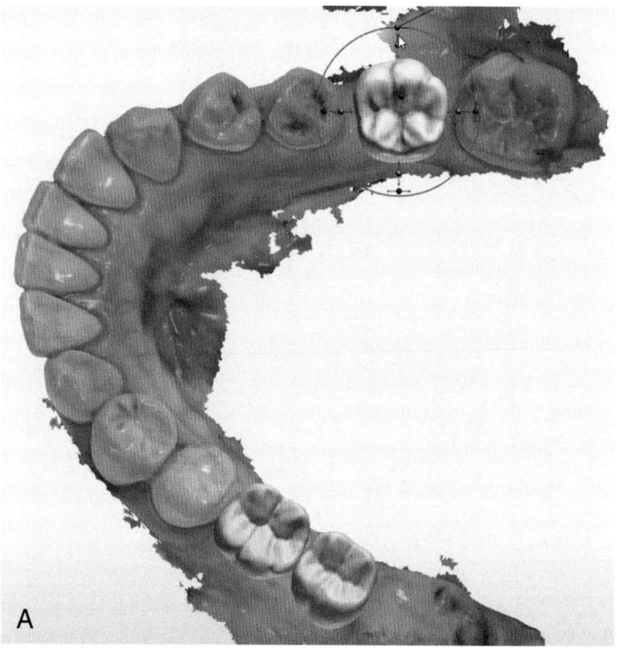

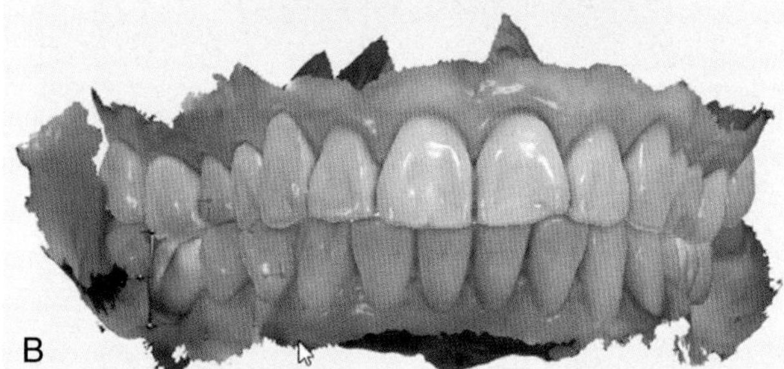

Fig. 84.11 Digital diagnostic wax-ups. (A) The proposed implant restorations are digitally waxed up in the simulation software. (B) The buccal contour and emergence profile of the proposed restorations can be modified from the frontal view.

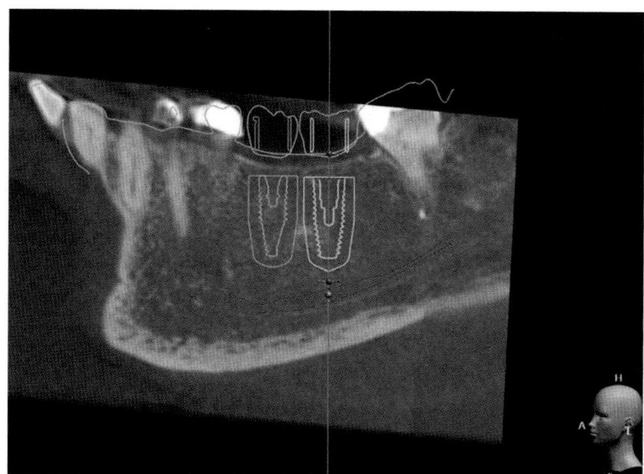

Fig. 84.12 Safety checks or boundaries are available in virtual surgical planning software to prevent potential impingement on vital structures such as adjacent teeth, implants, sinus cavities, and the inferior alveolar nerve.

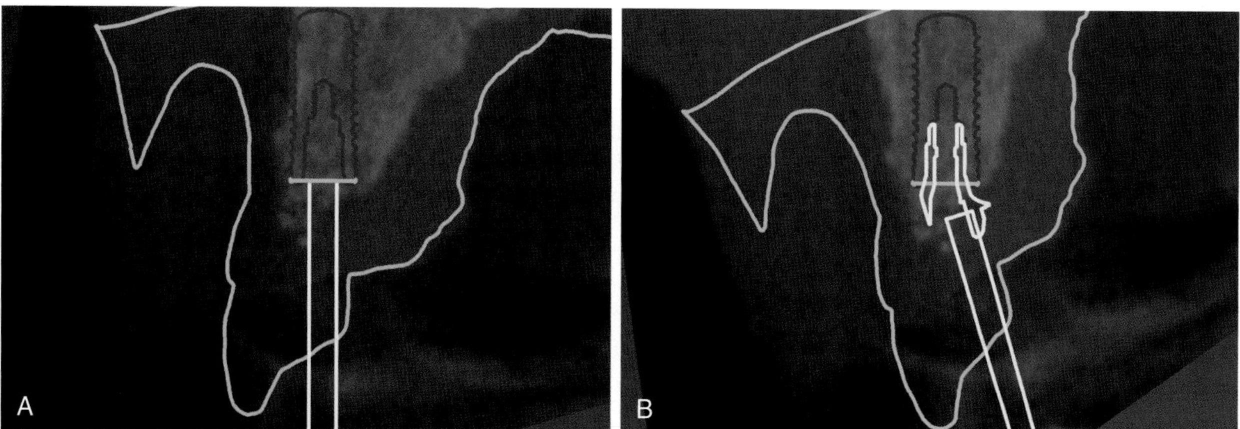

Fig. 84.13 Virtual implant planning. (A) The prosthetically driven position for this proposed implant level restoration is complicated by the lack of buccal bone. (B) The proposed restoration is modified with an angled abutment so the implant can be placed in a more favorable position.

metal drill sleeves, which are brought in from a library for each proposed implant and fixation pin. The sleeves are implant system specific, which means specific sleeves will only work with surgical kits of the corresponding system. While full guidance is preferred, certain situations may necessitate partial guidance. For example, if the interdental space of an edentulous site is too small to accommodate a regular sized metal drill sleeve, a more compact sleeve for partial guidance is indicated (Fig. 84.15).

The buccolingual and mesiodistal position of the metal drill sleeves are based on implant positions and largely fixed. However, the distance from the implant platform to the drill sleeve or the vertical sleeve position (Fig. 84.16) can be modified to create more accessible drilling protocols. Most (but not all) guided systems have several presets available. In general, the vertical sleeve position should be kept to a minimum and as close to the bone (for bone-supported guides) or soft tissue (for mucosa-supported and tooth-supported guides) as possible to maximize access to the surgical site. The consequence of placing drill sleeves too apically, however, is potential interferences with underlying bone or mucosa, which can prevent the complete seating of the guide (Fig. 84.17). In cases where implants are purposely simulated/planned deeper and impediments are inevitable, the underside of the metal sleeves must be manually trimmed prior to surgery, or the interfering bone or soft tissue must be removed during surgery. Following positioning of the drill sleeves, the simulation software will generate a tailored report with drilling protocols specific to the length, diameter, and system of the planned implants (Fig. 84.18).

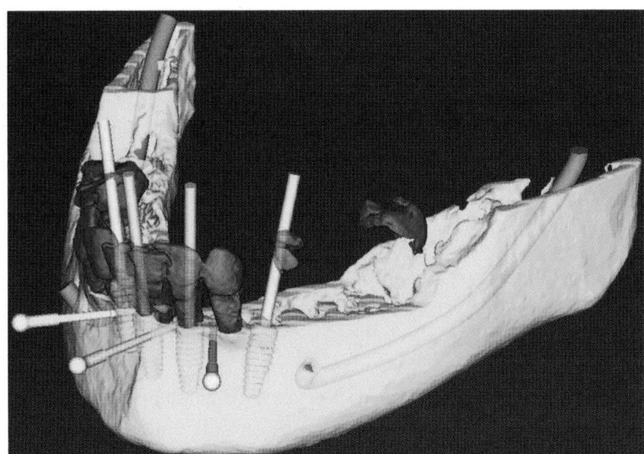

Fig. 84.14 Segmentation of different anatomical structures into independent objects is useful, especially when planning guide fixation pins.

Due to the closed architecture nature of some implant systems, the drilling protocols are only available in the company's own proprietary software. However, some open architecture programs allow the creation of drilling protocols through the custom drill sleeve module. The geometry parameter (diameter and length) and the vertical sleeve position of the third-party drill sleeve(s) to be utilized must be specifically defined for this purpose. If the third-party surgical kit contains osteotomy drills with physical depth stops, the distance from the tip of the drill to the depth stop must be measured so the vertical sleeve position can be defined properly. If the third-party surgical kit does not contain drills with depth stops, the vertical sleeve position can be arbitrarily defined, as long as the drilling depth (or the distance from the apex of the implant to the top of the drill sleeve) does not exceed the length of the longest osteotomy drill in the kit.

Static Computer-Aided Design/Computer-Aided Manufacturing Surgical Guides

Static CAD/CAM implant surgical guides can derive support from several tissue types. In partially edentulous patients, surgical guides are tooth-supported (Fig. 84.19). Hard tissues, such as teeth with normal periodontal support that display minimal mobility and/or compressibility, have been shown to properly support surgical guides for accurate guided implant placement.[17,19] In completely edentulous patients with sufficient bone volume requiring no alveoloplasty or bone reduction, surgical guides can be mucosa-supported (Fig. 84.20). Mucosa-supported surgical guides enable flapless surgery and can reach similar levels of accuracy in guided implant placement compared to tooth-supported surgical guides, provided the soft tissues are minimally compressible.[19,24] In completely edentulous patients with limited restorative space requiring alveoloplasty, surgical guides are bone-supported (Fig. 84.21). While bone is a hard tissue without mobility or compressibility, a systematic review on the accuracy of guided implant placement based on supporting tissue types demonstrated that bone-supported surgical guides are the least accurate.[19,25,22] This inaccuracy could arise from several factors, including the quality of the CBCT scan, the segmentation process, and the guide seating. Complete seating of bone-supported surgical guides requires extensive full thickness flap reflection.

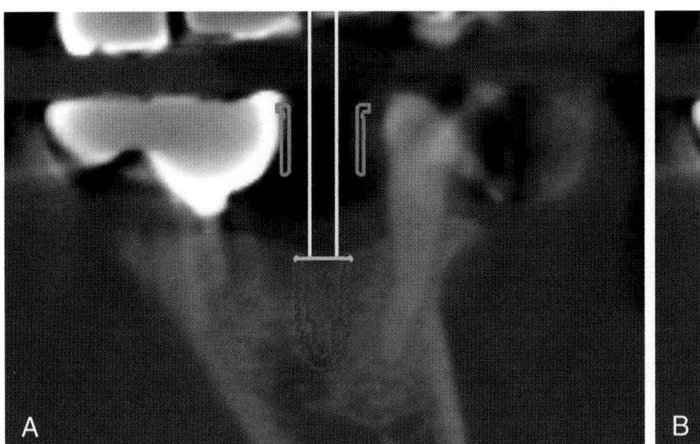

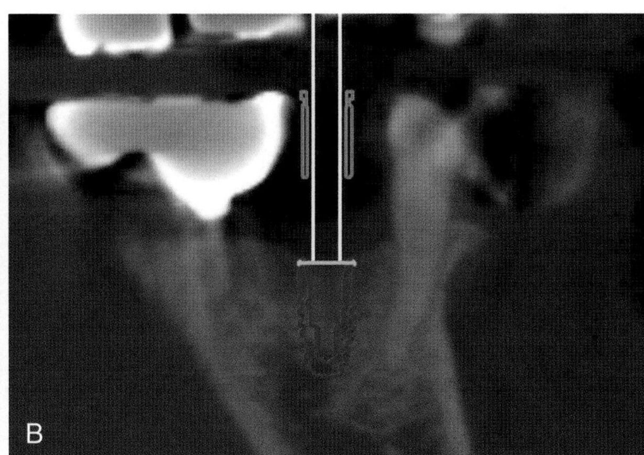

Fig. 84.15 Partially guided surgery due to drill sleeve interference. (A) Full guidance is not possible due to the interference between a standard size metal drill sleeve and an adjacent tooth. (B) Partial guidance is indicated with a narrower metal drill sleeve.

Surgical Guide Design Process

Computer-aided design of static guides starts with defining the insertion direction for the guide. For tooth-supported guides, the insertion direction is defined on the digital diagnostic cast. For mucosa-supported guides or any scenarios where dual scans are involved, the insertion direction is defined from the underside of the dual scanned prosthesis or appliance. And for bone-supported guides, the insertion direction is defined on the bone segmentation of the jaw of interest. Defining the insertion direction ensures that the guide will seat passively because all areas underneath the height of contour, as viewed from the defined insertion direction, are blocked out by the software to prevent the guide from engaging any undercuts (Fig. 84.22).

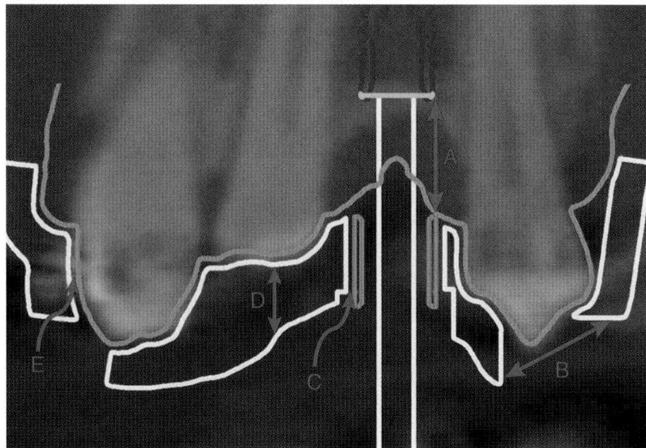

Fig. 84.16 A cross-sectional diagram of a static tooth-supported computer-aided design/computer-aided manufacturing surgical guide. The digital impression of the arch *(orange)* is registered to the cone-beam CT dataset. The surgical guide *(white)* is then designed to be supported by teeth captured in the digital impression. *(A)* Represents the vertical sleeve position. *(B)* Represents an inspection window. *(C)* Represents the sleeve diameter offset. *(D)* Represents the wall thickness. *(E)* represents guide offset.

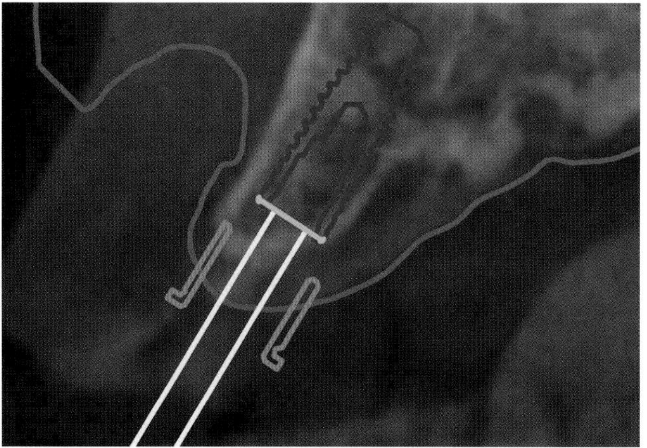

Fig. 84.17 The apical aspect of the drill sleeve intersects with the bony ridge. The surgical guide will not seat fully unless this interference is removed.

LEARNING BOX 84.1

Computer-aided design of static guides starts with defining the insertion direction for the guide. Defining the insertion direction ensures that the guide will seat passively because all areas underneath the height of contour, as viewed from the defined insertion direction, are blocked out by the software to prevent the guide from engaging any undercuts.

Next, contact surfaces or areas used to index and support the guide are highlighted. In tooth-supported scenarios, teeth immediately adjacent to the edentulous span are selected. However, guide stability can be increased by incorporating additional teeth. In mucosa-supported scenarios, the whole intaglio surface of the dual scanned prosthesis is selected and duplicated into the surgical guide. Because the mucosa-supported guide will fit identically to the dual scanned appliance, it is critical that the prosthesis fit optimally (and relined if fit is suboptimal) prior to any imaging. A bone-supported surgical guide is generally indicated when alveoloplasty is needed. Because the ridge crest will be reduced, support and stability of the surgical guide must be derived elsewhere. In these scenarios, the buccal and lingual or palatal slopes of the alveolar bone apical to the level of the alveoloplasty must be selected. The 3D rendering of the surgical guide is then generated by the software through a digital vacuform-like process over the highlighted areas, and the recesses where the metal drill sleeves will occupy are incorporated automatically.

Before finalizing the design, the addition of **inspection windows** is strongly advised. Inspection windows are openings in the surgical guide which allow the operator to verify guide adaptation via visual inspection. These windows are useful regardless of the type of tissue supporting the guide. If a significant amount of space is observed between the surgical guide and the underlying tissues, the guide is likely not seated properly and areas of binding must be adjusted prior to preparing the osteotomies. Inspection windows can be created digitally with a subtraction operation (Fig. 84.23) or manually with a bur following guide production.

Position	Milling cutter	Pilot drill	Guided drill	Guided drill	Guided drill	Profile drill	Tap	Implant	Depth stop
28	ø 3.5 ●	ø 2.2 BLT T1–T3 or dense cortex only = ●	ø 2.8 BLT T1–T4 = ●	ø 3.5 BLT T1–T3 or dense cortex only = ●		ø 4.1 BLT T1–T2 or dense cortex only H4	ø 4.1 BLT T1 H4	021.5310G BLT RC ø 4.1 10 mm SLActive	H4
29	ø 3.5 ●	ø 2.2 BLT T1–T3 or dense cortex only = ●	ø 2.8 BLT T1–T4 = ●	ø 3.5 BLT T1–T3 or dense cortex only = ●		ø 4.1 BLT T1–T2 or dense cortex only H4	ø 4.1 BLT T1 H4	021.5310G BLT RC ø 4.1 10 mm SLActive	H4
30	ø 3.5 ●	ø 2.2 BLT T1–T3 or dense cortex only = ●	ø 2.8 BLT T1–T4 = ●	ø 3.5 BLT T1–T3 or dense cortex only = ●		ø 4.1 BLT T1–T2 or dense cortex only H4	ø 4.1 BLT T1 H4	021.5310G BLT RC ø 4.1 10 mm SLActive	H4

Fig. 84.18 The fully guided drilling protocol is automatically generated by the virtual surgical planning software.

LEARNING BOX 84.2

Inspection windows are openings in the surgical guide which allow the operator to verify guide adaptation via visual inspection. If a significant amount of space is observed between the surgical guide and the underlying tissues, the guide is likely not seated properly and areas of binding must be adjusted prior to preparing the osteotomies.

Prior to manufacturing, several additional parameters which may affect the static surgical guide should be considered and modified as necessary (see Fig. 84.16):

- **Wall thickness** is correlated with the strength of the surgical guide. Overly thin walls are associated with breakages and fractures while excessively thick walls are associated with bulkiness and difficulties in seating due to potential collisions with soft tissues.
  - Depending on the material, this parameter should be kept as low as possible without compromising the rigidity of the guide. For most resin-based materials, wall thickness of 3 to 3.5 mm is appropriate. For metal-based materials, thinner dimensions are possible.
- **Guide offset** is the tolerance between the surgical guide and the tissues that support the guide. Little to no guide offset is associated with binding and incomplete seating while large guide offset is associated with loosely fitting guides. This setting is usually applied to the whole intaglio surface of the surgical guide.
  - Guide offset is a fluid setting based on the accuracy of the manufacturing method. Calibration is recommended to determine the optimal guide offset for a specific method. Guides with different offsets should be manufactured to determine the optimal setting for future guides. This is usually in the range of 0.1 to 0.3 mm.
  - Because bone-supported surgical guides are made directly from the segmentation or 3D reconstruction of the jawbones, the thickness of the CBCT slices may affect the guide offset setting. Thicker slices are associated with a staircase-like appearance (Fig. 84.24) of the reconstructed image and may require additional offset for complete guide seating.
- **Sleeve diameter offset** is the tolerance between the surgical guide and the metal drill sleeve. Like guide offset, calibration is recommended to determine the optimal sleeve diameter offset so metal drill sleeves can fit precisely without additional adjustments. Some software can generate a sleeve calibration matrix which allows the operator to easily identify the best setting.

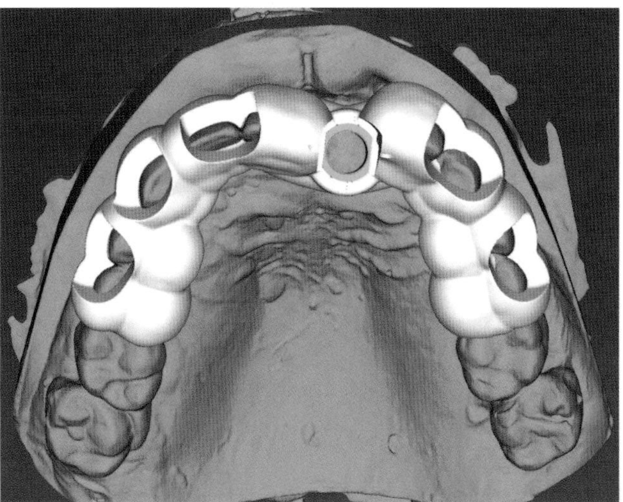

Fig. 84.19 A tooth-supported static computer-aided design/computer-aided manufacturing surgical guide.

Surgical Implant Placement Using Static CAD/CAM Surgical Guide

Surgical implant placement using a static CAD/CAM surgical guide enables clinicians to accurately place implants in the jaw according to the prosthetically driven implant positions as planned in simulation software. As a result, the implant placement surgery is greatly facilitated in terms of reduced time, less need for checking and validating osteotomy position and direction during surgical preparation, and, ultimately, more accurately placed implants. However, the accuracy and surgical expediency is entirely dependent on the care, attention to details, and avoidance of errors during data collection, planning, and processing of surgical guide, as well as the proper positioning of the surgical guide at the time of implant placement surgery. This final step in the process (proper positioning) is the critical key step. Regardless of how precisely the surgical guide was made to capture the planned implant positions, the translation of that information to the patient will only be accurate if the guide fits the patient's jaw and is seated as it was intended.

As described previously, static CAD/CAM implant surgical guides can be used to place implants for the partially edentulous

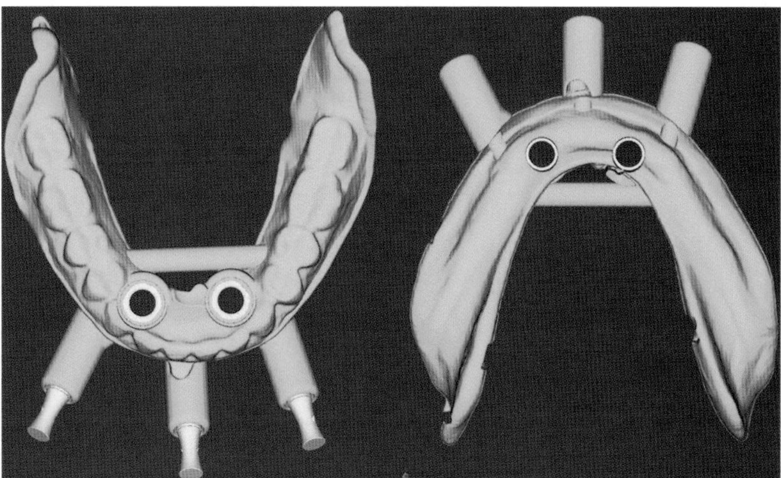

Fig. 84.20 A mucosa-supported static computer-aided design/computer-aided manufacturing surgical guide.

patient/arch with tooth-supported guides or the fully edentulous patient/arch with either a mucosa-supported or a bone-supported guide. In each case, care must be taken to verify the surgical guide is positioned and seated properly and that it is stable and secure for the procedure.

Partially Edentulous Tooth-Supported Surgical Guide

The use of inspection windows in the surgical guide for a partially edentulous arch allows the operator to visualize the intimacy of guide fit and adaptation with the teeth (Fig. 84.25A and B). Depending on the level of guide offset, the operator should be able to see contact or an intimate adaptation between the surgical guide and the supporting teeth through the inspection window. Any moderate-sized spaces or gaps present between the guide and the teeth will indicate the guide is not properly seated. In the case of a guide that does not seat completely, the operator may need to adjust interferences (e.g., excess material on the intaglio surface, sharp angles between teeth and guide surfaces, or sleeve positions that impinge on tissues). If the surgical guide does not fit or adapt completely, it will not reliably guide accurate implant placement.

Once the guide is confirmed to be seated completely, the stability should be assessed. For a surgical guide that is supported by periodontally stable teeth with good cross arch and anterior-posterior distribution, it will be adequately stabilized by the teeth. However, if there are few remaining teeth that are not well distributed (i.e., unilateral), the guide may not be stable. In this case, it will be advantageous to plan the case with fixation pins. If the guide is designed to be both tooth and mucosa-supported, then an occlusal index may be needed to establish the proper position since the mucosa-supported portion will have resilience and movement.

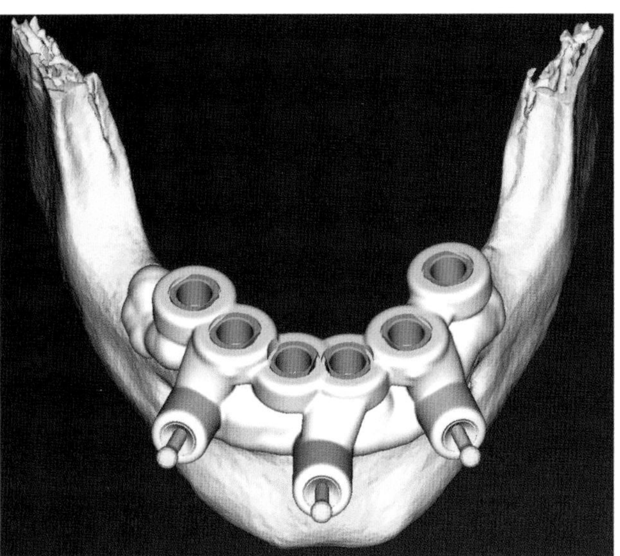

Fig. 84.21 A bone-supported static computer-aided design/computer-aided manufacturing surgical guide.

Fully Edentulous Mucosa-Supported or Bone-Supported Surgical Guide

Similar to their value in the partially edentulous surgical guide, the use of inspection windows in the surgical guide for a fully edentulous arch allows the operator to visualize the intimacy of guide fit and adaptation with the underlying mucosa or bone. The operator should be able to see contact or an intimate approximation between the surgical guide and the mucosal tissue or bone through the inspection windows. Any moderate-sized spaces or gaps present between the guide and the mucosa or bone will indicate the guide is not properly positioned or seated. In the case of a guide that does not seat completely, the operator may need to adjust interferences (e.g., excess material on the intaglio surface, or sleeve positions that impinge on tissues). This is particularly true for bone-supported guides. Incomplete full-thickness flap reflection, inadequate bone exposure, or inaccuracies in the bone/guide modeling may also be reasons for incomplete seating of bone-supported surgical guides on the alveolar bone. If the surgical guide does not fit or adapt completely, it will not reliably guide accurate implant placement.

Once the guide is confirmed to be seated completely, the stability needs to be established. For a fully edentulous surgical guide supported by mucosa or bone, it will be necessary to plan the case using multiple fixation pins. Most fully edentulous surgical guides

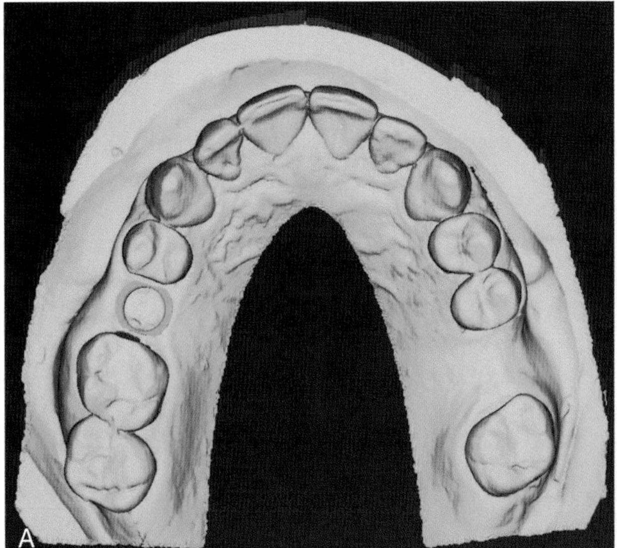

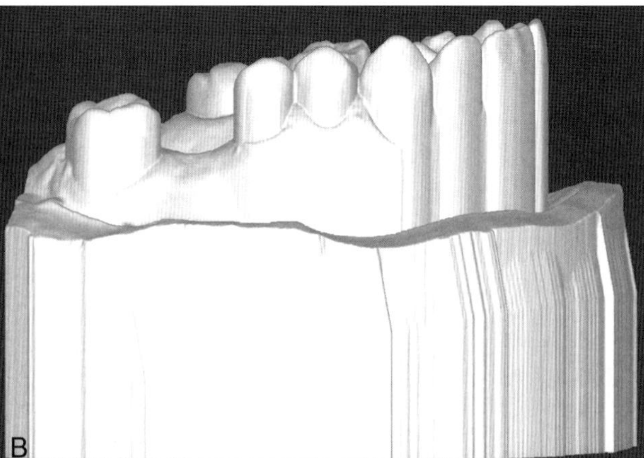

Fig. 84.22 Surgical guide insertion direction. (A) The insertion direction for the surgical guide is generally defined from the occlusal direction. (B) All undercuts beneath the height of contour as viewed from the defined insertion direction are blocked out.

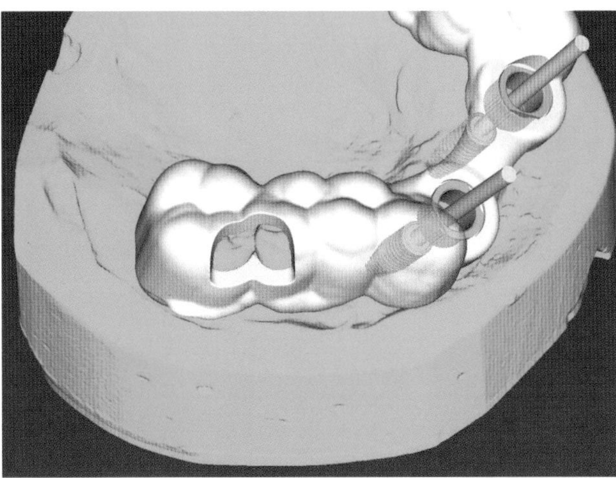

Fig. 84.23 Inspection windows can be created digitally and are essential in confirming that the surgical guide is fully seated.

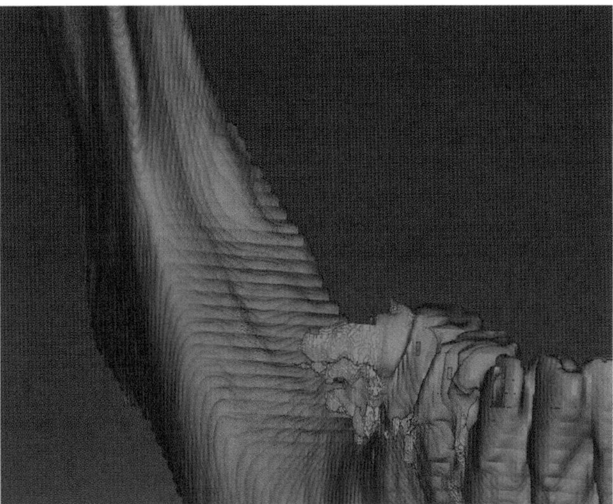

Fig. 84.24 3D reconstructions from thick cone-beam CT slices will have a staircase-like appearance which may necessitate additional guide offset for bone-supported surgical guides.

will require two to three fixation pins to achieve reliable stability. If the guide is mucosa-supported, an occlusal index should be used to establish the proper position since the mucosa-supported portion will have resilience and movement. An occlusal index can be used to position a bone-supported guide as well, but it may not be required since bone is a rigid tissue.

Fixation pins are secured through the guide using a sleeve that has a specific diameter and length for the pins and planned using the implant simulation software. Once the surgical guide is properly positioned, drills are used to prepare fixation pin osteotomies. The fixation pins are then pushed through the sleeve into the bone to stabilize and secure the surgical guide.

Flap Versus Flapless Procedures

The ability to accurately prepare and place implants in planned locations with a static CAD/CAM surgical guide invites the possibility to perform the procedure without soft tissue flap reflection. When implant osteotomies can be prepared and implants can be placed without soft tissue flap reflection, it saves time and decreases surgical morbidity. Both partially edentulous and fully edentulous cases can be successfully executed using a flapless surgical technique with tooth-supported or mucosa-supported guides, respectively. However, there are circumstances that preclude clinicians from preparing and placing implants using flapless surgery, including a lack of bone volume at the implant site(s) and/or a lack of adequate keratinized attached soft tissue at the implant site(s).

If there is a lack of bone volume and a need for bone grafting at the time of implant placement, then a full-thickness flap reflection will be required. This is true regardless of whether the bone deficiency is large or small. Even if the bone deficiency is a minor dehiscence or fenestration, a full-thickness flap reflection should be used because, in addition to the need to graft such defects, if the implant placement is slightly off in the direction of the deficiency, then the deficit of bone surrounding the implant will be significant and the clinician may not recognize the problem without flap reflection. If there is a lack of keratinized attached soft tissue at the implant site such that the soft tissue access incision will be in mobile, unattached mucosa, it is preferable to use a full-thickness flap reflection during implant placement surgery and to manage soft tissue positioning separately. Again, these criteria for adequate bone volume and keratinized attached soft tissue at implant sites apply to both partially edentulous and fully edentulous cases.

The flapless implant placement procedure uses a tissue punch to make a circular incision through the guide at each implant site (see Fig. 84.25B and C). The size of the circular incision is large enough to prepare the osteotomy and place the implant without further soft tissue excision or reflection (see Fig. 84.25D–F). The incised circular soft tissue islands are removed (full thickness) to expose the underlying bone.

Preparing Implant Osteotomy Sites With Static CAD/CAM Surgical Guide

Preparation of implant osteotomy sites are similar regardless of whether the surgical guide is tooth-supported, mucosa-supported, or bone supported. Depending on the implant system, the guide will be designed with drill sleeves that are used with or without drill handles or keys, or the osteotomy drills themselves could have integrated drill stops. Implant osteotomies are prepared with a sequence of increasingly larger diameter drills that are precisely guided in position, direction, and depth by the surgical guide. Some systems will also incorporate timing markers to allow the clinician to specifically align the implant rotation. This may be important for prefabricated prosthesis/crown or to facilitate the use of angled abutments, allowing for predetermined angled abutment selection and positioning. As with all implant site preparations, profuse irrigation should be used to cool drills and flush debris from the osteotomy sites (Video 84.3). It is particularly important when using computer-generated surgical guides because much of the drill is covered by the drill sleeve and guide material.

Depending on bone density, the final steps of the implant osteotomy may be to use bone profilers and taps. Both can be done through the surgical guide using system specific keys or handles. Before implant placement, osteotomy sites should be thoroughly irrigated with sterile saline to flush any residual debris. Implants can be placed through the surgical guide. Some systems will use specific mounts with depth indicators to place implants through the guide sleeve. As mentioned, some systems have timing indicators so implants can be precisely placed in terms of rotation as well as position and depth.

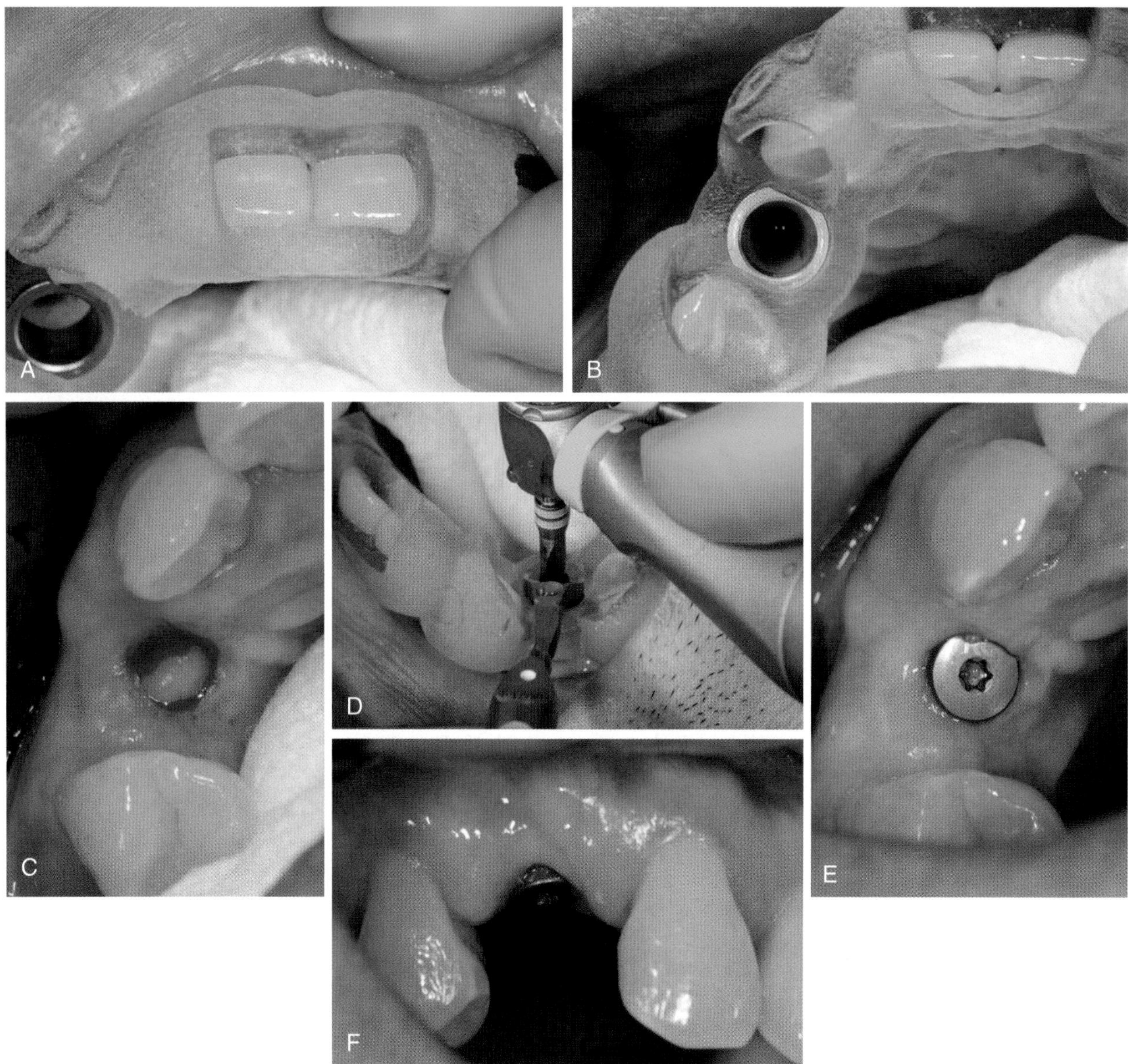

Fig. 84.25 (A–D) Static surgical guide designed for implant placement #6 (maxillary right cuspid) with inspection windows that allow clinician to confirm complete seating of the guide. (A) The intimacy of the surgical guide with the central incisors as observed through the inspection window. (B) Additional inspection windows demonstrate intimate fit of guide with posterior teeth to confirm the guide is properly seated. A tissue punch is used through the guide to remove a circular portion of the gingival tissue to allow implant site osteotomy preparation. (C) Clinical view without guide of tissue incised with circular punch. (D) Preparation of implant site with static surgical guide using handles and following surgical plan. (E) Occlusal and (F) labial clinical views of healing abutment attached to implant immediately after placement with static surgical guide using a flapless approach.

Dynamic Navigation

Dynamically navigated implant placement is a type of computer-assisted surgery that utilizes optical motion tracking. Optical motion tracking systems can be either active or passive. Active system tracker arrays emit infrared light that is tracked by stereo cameras, while passive system tracker arrays use reflective spheres to reflect infrared light emitted from a light source to stereo cameras.[18]

Currently, passive tracking systems are more commonly utilized in dentistry. In passively tracked, dynamically navigated implant surgery, a light source above the surgical field projects infrared light down toward the patient. This light is subsequently reflected off tracking arrays attached to both the patient and the surgical handpiece. The reflected light is detected by stereo cameras so the dynamic navigation program can calculate the real-time position of the patient and the handpiece relative to the surgical plan (Fig. 84.26).[18] Following calculation, a virtual image is displayed on screen that provides the implant surgeon with visual guidance.

The sequence of steps to achieve dynamic navigation includes data and image acquisition, virtual surgical planning, calibration, and, finally, executing the dynamically navigated surgery.

Data and Image Acquisition

The acquisition of quality CT or CBCT scans is a prerequisite for successful dynamic navigation. Because the patient, surgical handpiece, and surgical plan must correlate with each other for implant placement, fiducial markers are necessary during image acquisition and live surgery. Similar to the workflow for static CAD/CAM surgical guides, there are important nuances to consider when scans are taken based on patient presentation.

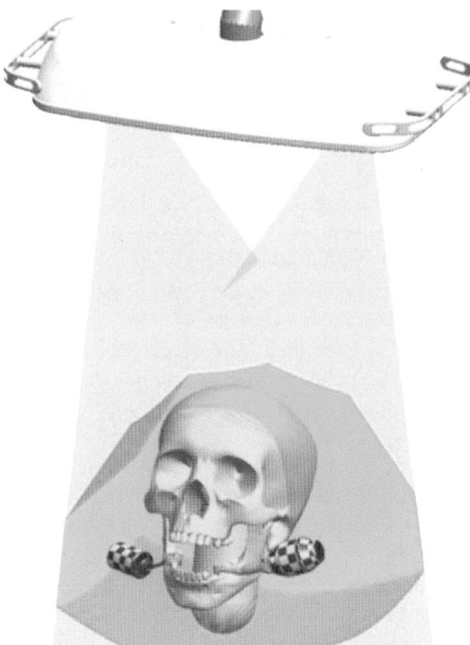

Fig. 84.26 Light is projected inferiorly from a source and reflected off tracking arrays attached to the patient and the surgical instrument. The reflection is captured by stereo cameras above the surgical field so the patient and surgical instrument can be tracked in real-time. (Courtesy X-Nav Technologies, LLC, Lansdale, PA.)

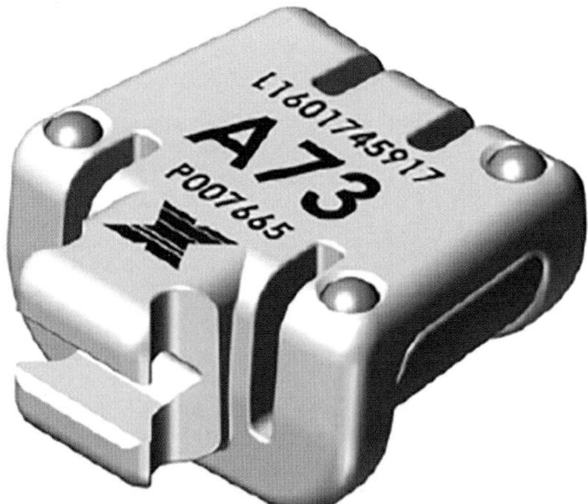

Fig. 84.27 The fiducial clip must be stabilized onto the dentition prior to imaging. The clip is used during registration as the common point between the patient and the cone-beam CT dataset. (Courtesy X-Nav Technologies, LLC, Lansdale, PA.)

- Partial edentulism
  - A clip with fiducial markers or fiducial clip is utilized for imaging (Fig. 84.27). The clip part of the apparatus functions as an impression tray so a sectional impression of the patient's teeth can be made with a thermoplastic material. This fiducial clip must be properly supported and stabilized by the dentition and indexed back into the same location during the CBCT scan and live surgery. If rocking or instability is detected, the thermoplastic material needs to be reheated so the impression can be remade prior to imaging. Teeth that are mobile should not be used to support the clip. The clip should be placed on the arch of interest in a location that will not interfere with surgical instrumentation. Finally, the attachment component on the clip should be facing outward

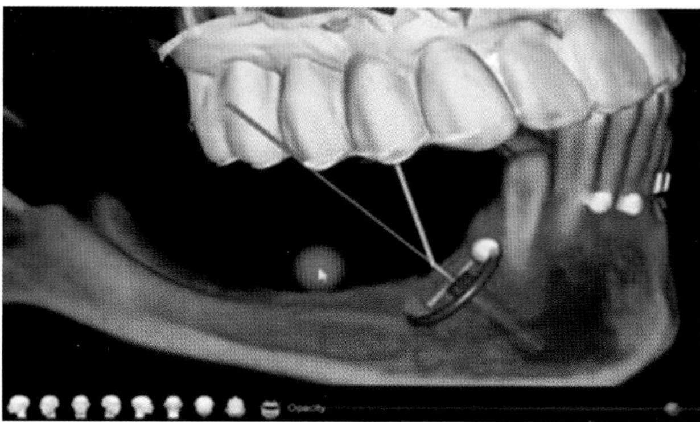

Fig. 84.28 Fiducial screws are fixated into the jawbone of interest prior to imaging. These screws are used during registration as common points between the patient and the cone-beam CT dataset. (Courtesy X-Nav Technologies, LLC, Lansdale, PA.)

(buccal) so an arm with the patient tracker can be attached for the surgery.
  - Although not absolutely required, a set of digital diagnostic casts can be helpful in planning implants in prosthetically driven positions.

> - *New developments* in surface algorithm have made virtual registration possible. With virtual registration, the operator marks three points on the CBCT scan followed by marking the same three points on the live patient (with tracker attached). The surface algorithm is capable of outlining tooth surfaces and register the patient virtually, eliminating the need for fiducial clips during imaging.

- Complete edentulism
  - In edentulous scenarios, fiducial markers come in the form of small bone screws. Four or more screws are placed in the jaw of interest prior to imaging and will not be retrieved until after the implant surgery (Fig. 84.28). They should be well distributed along the arch for optimal triangulation. If alveoloplasty is being considered, the screws must be placed apical to the planned reduction, so they are not accidentally removed when bone is cut. Like the partially edentulous scenario, these fiducial markers need to be rigidly fixed. If movement is detected in a screw, it must be moved to another site. Care should be taken when placing these screws to avoid impingement upon the infraorbital nerve in the maxilla and inferior alveolar nerve in the mandible. Finally, sufficient space is required between the screws for an edentulous fiducial plate to be secured during surgery for the purpose of attaching the patient tracker arm.
  - The dual scan protocol is recommended to aid in planning implants in prosthetically driven positions.

Virtual Surgical Planning

The DICOM files are imported into a planning software specific to the dynamic navigation system of choice. All dynamic navigation planning software is proprietary and must be purchased as a package along with the hardware. All steps involved in the virtual surgical planning process such as segmentation, patient data orientation, panoramic curve, registration of datasets, and implant simulation are identical to the aforementioned steps for static guides.

Simulation of implant positions must be prosthetically driven. The virtual implants should be positioned below the proposed prosthesis and account for proper restorative space and emergence profile mesiodistally as well as buccolingually. As described before, diagnostic wax-ups are crucial for this process. Most dynamic navigation planning software programs can generate individual teeth to be used as wax-ups. Alternatively, analog wax-ups can be performed and converted into the digital realm. For completely edentulous cases, the prosthesis scan obtained from the dual scan protocol is utilized for planning implant positions.

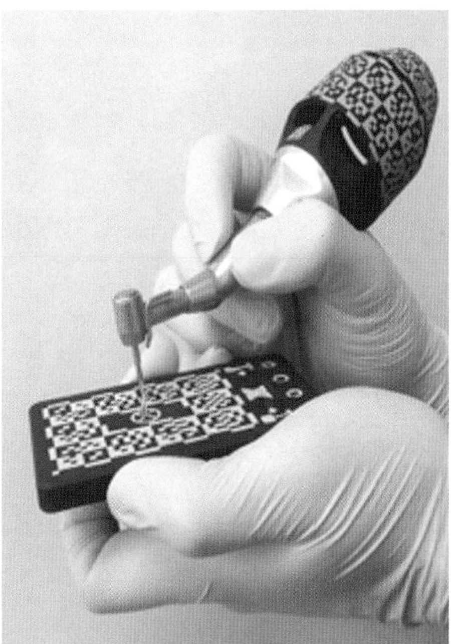

Fig. 84.29 The handpiece is connected to a patterned tracker followed by calibration. Prior to surgical execution, the length of the drill is verified by placing the drill into the calibrated handpiece and positioning the drill at the center of but perpendicular to a calibration plate. (Courtesy X-Nav Technologies, LLC, Lansdale, PA.)

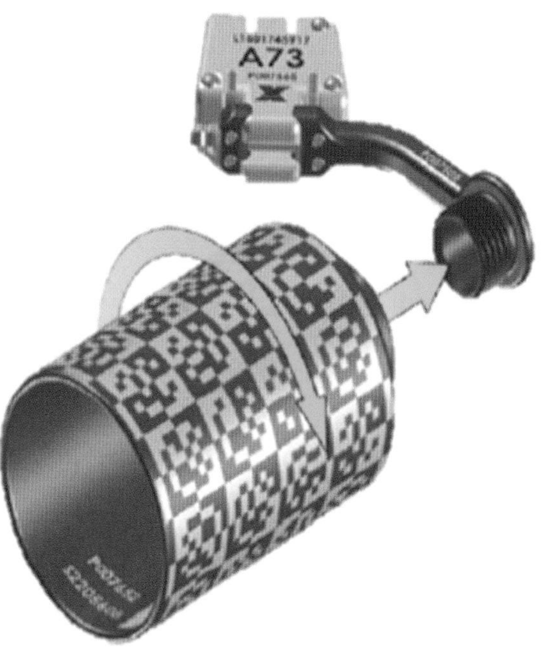

Fig. 84.30 The fiducial clip, patient tracker arm, and tracker are assembled followed by calibration. (Courtesy X-Nav Technologies, LLC, Lansdale, PA.)

Calibration

The surgical instruments (such as the contra-angle handpiece) and the patient must be calibrated prior to live surgery so proper tracking can occur. (Important: Partially edentulous and completely edentulous patients are calibrated differently.)

- Partial edentulism
  - The handpiece is calibrated by attaching a tracker onto the base of the handpiece. This handpiece and tracker assembly is then placed about 60 to 80 cm away from the stereo cameras and rotated slowly so the cameras can read and register the patterns on the tracker (Fig. 84.29).
  - The chuck is calibrated by a chuck plate inserted into the handpiece. The plate is spun slowly underneath the cameras for calibration.
  - The partially edentulous patient is calibrated by attaching a tracker onto a patient tracker arm. The fiducial clip (tailored to the patient's dentition) is then secured to the arm. This assembly is rotated underneath the cameras for calibration (Fig. 84.30).
  - Before surgical execution and between every drill change, drill length must be verified. This is achieved by placing an implant drill into the handpiece and positioning the drill perpendicular at the center of a calibration plate (see Fig. 84.29). If this step fails, the chuck calibration step needs to be performed again.
- Complete edentulism
  - The handpiece, chuck, and drill length are calibrated the same way as described above.

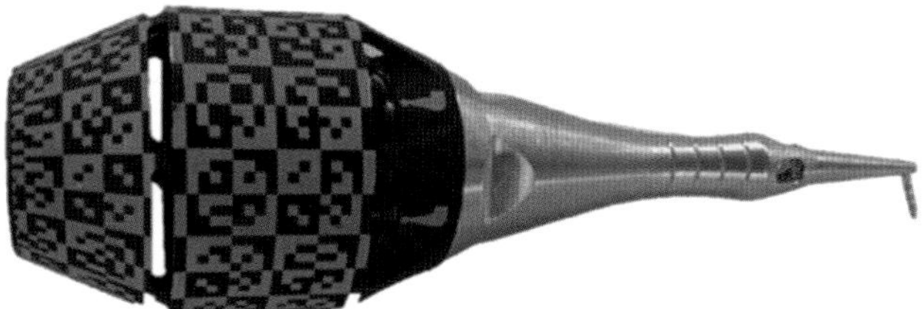

Fig. 84.31 The edentulous patient probe is connected to a patterned tracker and calibrated. (Courtesy X-Nav Technologies, LLC, Lansdale, PA.)

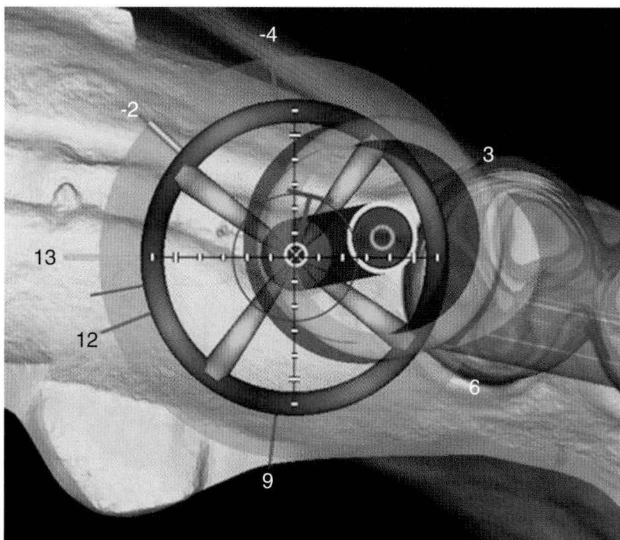

Fig. 84.32 A diagram of the dynamic navigation monitor. The center of the *green X* represents the center of the implant. The *blue dot* represents the drill tip which should be placed at the center of the *green X*. The *green circle* represents the drill angulation which should be superimposed directly over the blue dot prior to drilling. (Courtesy X-Nav Technologies, LLC, Lansdale, PA.)

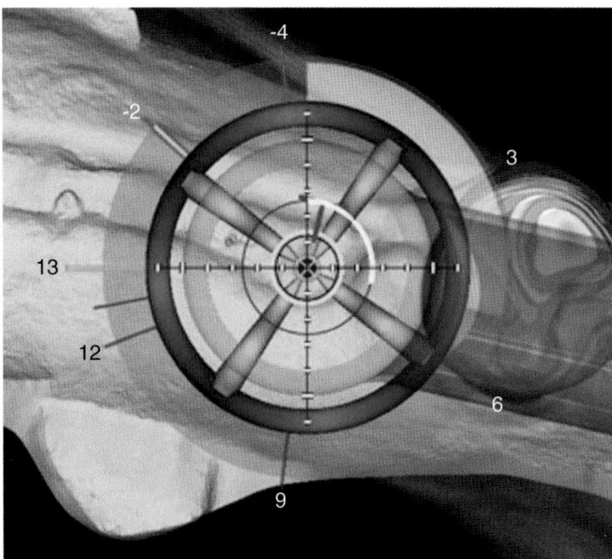

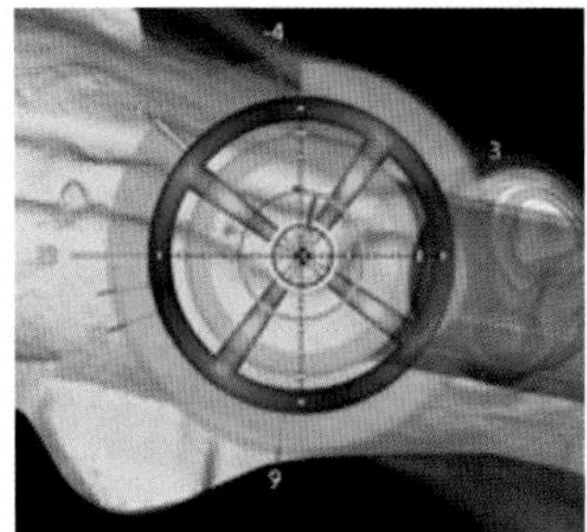

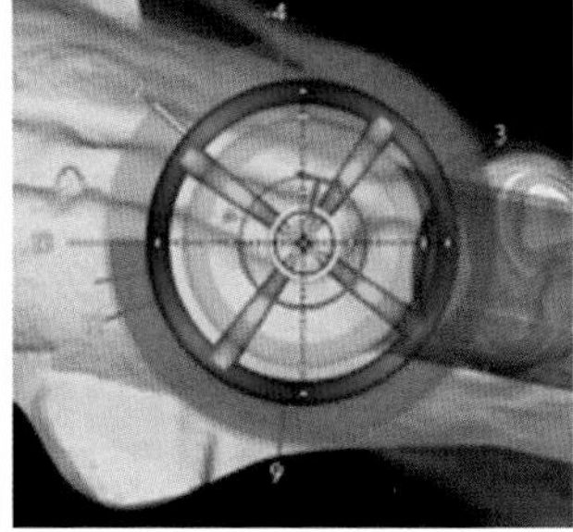

Fig. 84.33 Drilling depth is denoted by an outer ring which can change colors. *Yellow* is a prompt for the operator to start drilling. *Green* denotes the current depth to be 0.5 mm shy of the planned depth while *red* represents that the planned depth has been achieved. (Courtesy X-Nav Technologies, LLC, Lansdale, PA.)

- To calibrate the completely edentulous patient, an edentulous patient probe needs to be calibrated first. This probe is calibrated in a similar manner as the handpiece (Fig. 84.31).
- An edentulous fiducial plate is secured to the jawbone of interest in an area with no fiducial markers or screws (eFig. 84.4). This plate serves as an attachment mechanism for the tracker arm and tracker assembly. The tracker and fiducial screws are then calibrated to the dynamic navigation system via touching the screws with the previously calibrated probe. The fiducial screws register the patient to the virtual surgical plan while the tracker allows the patient to be tracked in real time.

Surgical Implant Placement Using Dynamic Navigation

In dynamic navigation, the surgeon prepares the osteotomies and places the implants by looking at the computer screen. The navigation screen displays the virtual plan with the target implant sites, virtual drills, and indicators specific for drilling angle, drilling depth, and timing of the planned implants (Fig. 84.32).

The tip of the virtual drill is often indicated by a dot on the screen. This dot should be moved to and centered over the target implant site. A circle is usually directly over the dot and signifies drilling angle. The handpiece should be angulated so the dot is centered in the circle prior to drilling. As drilling occurs, depth is commonly displayed by changes in color of the depth indicator. In a popular dynamic navigation system (X-Nav Technologies, Lansdale, PA), the color of the depth indicator changes from yellow to green and green to red, with red denoting that the proper depth has been reached and the surgeon should stop drilling (Fig. 84.33).

During surgery, system checks should be performed frequently to ensure that the dynamic navigation system is tracking correctly. System checks can be accomplished by touching anatomic landmarks with calibrated surgical instruments. The operator can then confirm that the landmark on the screen correlates with what was touched. Optimal landmarks include adjacent teeth or the alveolar ridge near the planned implant site for partially edentulous cases or fiducial markers (screws) for completely edentulous cases.

Conclusions

Digitally assisted implant placement with static CAD/CAM surgical guides has been shown to be more accurate when compared to freehand methods.[9,26,27] Likewise, implant placement via dynamic navigation has displayed comparable results.[2,4] Between static surgical guides and dynamic navigation, however, it is unclear as to which method is superior in terms of accuracy of implant placement.[28] While both methods enable flapless surgeries and are capable of replicating the planned implant position, angulation, and depth, each method has its own set of advantages and disadvantages. At this point in time, the choice between utilizing static guides or dynamic navigation will depend on the operator's personal preference, experience level, and access to required technologies and devices.

Suggested Readings

Kernen F, Kramer J, Wanner L, et al. A review of virtual planning software for guided implant surgery - data import and visualization, drill guide design and manufacturing. *BMC Oral Health*. 2020;20:251.

Raico Gallardo YN, da Silva-Olivio IRT, Mukai E, et al. Accuracy comparison of guided surgery for dental implants according to the tissue of support: a systematic review and meta-analysis. *Clin Oral Implants Res*. 2017;28:602–612.

Tahmaseb A, Wismeijer D, Coucke W, et al. Computer technology applications in surgical implant dentistry: a systematic review. *Int J Oral Maxillofac Implants*. 2014;29:25.

Panchal N, Mahmood L, Retana A, et al. Dynamic navigation for dental implant surgery. *Oral Maxillofac Surg Clin North Am*. 2019;31:539–547.

Varga E, Antal M, Major L, Kiscsatári R, Braunitzer G, Piffkó J. Guidance means accuracy: A randomized clinical trial on freehand versus guided dental implantation. *Clin Oral Impl Res*. 2020;31:417–430.

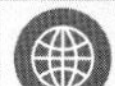
References for this chapter are found on the companion website eBooks.Health.Elsevier.com.

CHAPTER 85

From Implant Placement to Provisional Restoration

Christopher A. Barwacz | Gustavo Avila-Ortiz | Perry R. Klokkevold

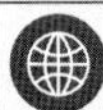 Videos for this chapter can be viewed on the companion website at eBooks.Health.Elsevier.com.

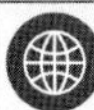 Animations have been added by the editors as a supplement to the chapter. They are produced by PerioPixel as patient education tools and cover the basic elements in a conceptual manner. It is not intended to be procedural guides for dental professionals.

CHAPTER OUTLINE

Introduction

The past decade has seen the maturation and convergence of digital technologies and manufacturing processes in implant dentistry, offering clinicians the ability to optimize both the *surgical* and *prosthetic* phases of tooth replacement therapy with dental implants. On the surgical spectrum, such advancements have enabled more sophisticated and predictable planning of implant placement protocols. On the prosthetic gamut, they have catalyzed the development of patient-specific components that adapt to the patient's individual anatomic and restorative requirements. In recent years, these therapeutic domains, which historically developed in parallel, but in relative isolation from one another, have begun to coalesce, giving rise to robust and streamlined digital workflows not only for implant planning and placement as well as definitive restorations but also for facilitating implant provisionalization. As a result, there is an increasing capacity to effectuate greater customization and personalization of tooth replacement therapy for patients in a more predictable and efficient manner and at earlier stages of therapy.

Regardless of the workflow selected, the end goal of digitally aided implant provisionalization remains the same as in established analog workflows, which includes, but is not limited to:

1. Direction, guidance, and preservation of peri-implant mucosa until maturation;[11]
2. Support for adjunctive soft tissue and bone graft materials;[20,37]
3. Maintenance of coronal form and esthetics post-surgically;
4. Psychosocial support for the patient;[31]
5. Enhanced communication with the laboratory technician.[4]

While implant provisionalization has historically been carried out primarily by restorative clinicians, the lack of adequate curricular time in predoctoral dental education has contributed to preventing the widespread incorporation of such protocols in contemporary general practice.[9] Surgical specialists, such as periodontists and oral surgeons, are increasingly becoming proficient and routinely offer implant provisionalization as part of their surgical regimen to guide and support the peri-implant tissues throughout the healing process, prior to referral to the restorative dentist for fabrication and delivery of the definitive restoration(s). Recent accreditation standards in advanced education programs in periodontics in the United States have reflected such trends. In 2013 the Commission on Dental Accreditation (CODA) instituted Standard 4-10.2.d (Provisionalization of Dental Implants), stating as an intent "*To provide clinical training that incorporates a collaborative team approach to dental implant therapy, enhances soft tissue esthetics and facilitates immediate or early loading protocols. This treatment should be provided in consultation with the individuals who will assume responsibility for completion of the restorative therapy.*" As a result, advanced education programs in periodontics have established formal curricula related to implant provisionalization, with substantial clinical and philosophical consensus within the specialty.[5]

This chapter provides an overview of contemporary digital workflow methodologies predominantly based on computer-guided surgery protocols to facilitate single-tooth implant provisionalization. Digital workflows can support a wide variety of custom healing abutments or full contour provisional restorations. Whether a coronal component is present or absent as part of the provisional prosthesis, the desired endpoint is the same: a peri-implant biologic environment that is free of inflammation, dimensionally stable, and conducive to esthetic contours.

Computer-Guided Implant Placement Surgery: A Foundation for Digitally Aided Provisionalization

The foundation upon which most digitally aided implant provisionalization workflows rest is computer-guided implant surgery. However, non-guided options are also available and will be addressed in this chapter. Historically, analog approaches have been the preeminent methodologies for the manufacturing of transmucosal provisional implant restorations. Such restorations typically consist of prefabricated interim abutments supporting a crown form made of restorative material such as polymethylmethacrylate (PMMA) or bis-acryl composite resin. Implant-supported provisional restorations can be fabricated chairside (direct method) or in a laboratory using a physical model after indexing the implant (indirect method). While such workflows are predictable, they perpetuate a fragmented implant therapy workflow and do not offer the ability to capitalize on the prosthetic benefits that computer-guided surgery offers. Therefore, to better understand the mechanics of digitally aided implant provisionalization, it is first important to understand the fundamentals of computer-guided implant surgery (see Chapter 84). With these concepts in mind, it will be easier to understand the relative advantages and limitations of various digitally aided implant provisionalization workflows and their subsequent definitive prosthetic workflows.

Computer-Guided Implant Placement Workflows

Computer-guided implant placement protocols are supported by several planning software platforms. The adoption of computer-guided implant placement has rapidly expanded within the dental profession in recent years, and its use has demonstrably improved implant planning and placement accuracy when compared with free-hand approaches.[8,30]

KEY FACT

Implant planning software often requires the conversion of DICOM (Digital Imaging and Communications in Medicine) data files (typically displayed with a .dcm file extension) that contain raw radiographic data to a proprietary file format specific to the planning software before a case can be planned. To facilitate guide design and manufacturing, the proprietary conversion file can be merged with either a diagnostic intraoral scan file or a scan of a diagnostic stone model (typically displayed with an .stl file extension).

This is mainly because computer-guided surgery protocols rely on planning that occurs a priori, integrating radiographic and clinical diagnostic records, rather than intra-operatively, when it is significantly more challenging to anticipate and adapt to anatomic, surgical, and prosthetic factors that may influence implant placement decisions.

Surgical guidance can be obtained by two distinct modalities, either *dynamic* or *static* guidance. Both modalities require the patient to undergo a cone-beam computed tomography (CBCT) scan of the involved arch and, as previously mentioned, the use of a proprietary planning software package to virtually plan the implant placement a priori by the interdisciplinary team (Fig. 85.1). The distinction between these two forms of guidance is related to the mode of execution of the surgical intervention.

With dynamic guidance, a physical surgical guide (or stent) is not necessary. Instead, the clinician receives both real-time haptic feedback and, through fiduciary markers in the operative field, visual guidance on the position of the osteotomy drill and the patient's alveolar ridge relative to the a priori surgical plan, as previously designed in the planning software, using imaging tools on a monitor. The clinician can make intraoperative adjustments while performing the osteotomy (e.g., depth and angle) to best match the final implant position in the superimposed virtual plan, as referenced by the planning software.

Comparatively, static guidance depends on the additive (stereolithic) or subtractive (computer-aided machining) manufacturing of a surgical guide from the a priori surgical plan, as dictated via the planning software. Such guides can be supported by various intraoral structures, depending on the clinical scenario, including mucosa, bone, or teeth (Fig. 85.2). Recent evidence has demonstrated that tooth-borne static surgical guides fabricated through computer-aided design and computer-aided manufacturing (CAD/CAM) offer superior accuracy when compared to the mucosa or bone-supported static guides, which may be important when considering subsequent restrictive implant provisionalization protocols.[36,39] Digitally designed and manufactured static surgical guides typically contain embedded metal sleeves that restrict the orientation of the drills during osteotomy preparation (Fig. 85.3). Depending on the level of restriction preferred by the clinician, considering factors such as case complexity, anatomical restrictions, and clinical experience of the operator, guidance may range from pilot-drill guidance, partial guidance, to fully guided surgery (Fig. 85.4).

KEY FACT

Pilot-drill guidance provides restrictions when using the first osteotomy drill, with subsequent steps taking place via mental navigation (i.e., free-handed). Partial guidance provides restriction during several osteotomy enlargement steps but does not provide guidance during placement of the implant fixture. Fully guided (fully restrictive) implant placement facilitates complete restriction of all steps of the osteotomy preparation, as well as the physical placement of the implant body to the correct depth, angle, and rotation.

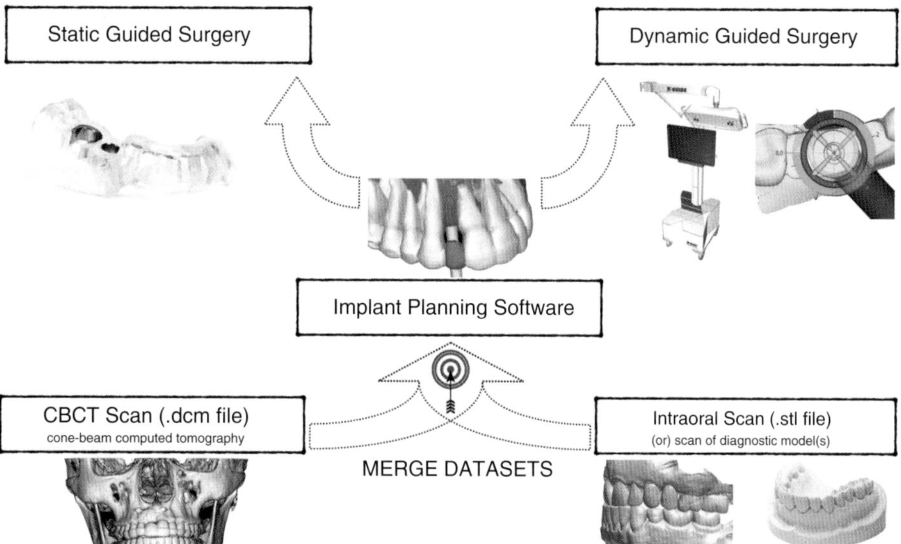

Fig. 85.1 Workflow overview comparing *static* and *dynamic* computer-guided implant placement surgery based on data acquisition.

Studies evaluating comparative accuracy between these different levels of restrictive guidance have demonstrated a significantly better correlation between planned and placed implants in fully guided protocols, as compared with free-handed and pilot guidance, with mixed outcomes on full versus partial guidance.[38,40,44]

When comparing dynamic and static guided implant placement surgery, there are advantages and disadvantages to both modalities. An advantage of dynamic guidance is direct visualization of the surgical field, whereas, with static guidance, the clinician's direct line of view of the osteotomy site is temporarily obscured by the guide. This also applies to the surgical assistant, who can directly apply irrigation to the field in dynamic guidance, while indirect irrigation ports are required in static guidance. Conventional surgical osteotomy drills and kits can be used in dynamic guided surgery, while static guidance necessitates protocol-specific kits and drills, aside from the physical surgical guide, increasing costs and componentry necessary to properly execute the procedure. However, the largest consideration for most clinicians contemplating the incorporation of dynamic guidance in their routine is the cost to purchase and space to store the navigation machinery. This factor tends to compel a larger number of clinicians to choose static guided protocols, as guide fabrication costs are relatively inexpensive, and no additional machinery other than drills and kits is necessary. The comparative accuracy of both dynamic and static guidance has been evaluated in clinical trials that have found equivocal levels of precision.[18,28]

Digital Prosthetic Considerations

Digital technologies have also transformed prosthetic workflows, design (CAD), customization, and manufacturing (CAM) processes. Prior to the adoption of CAD/CAM workflows for fabricating prosthetic components, such as implant abutments, framework

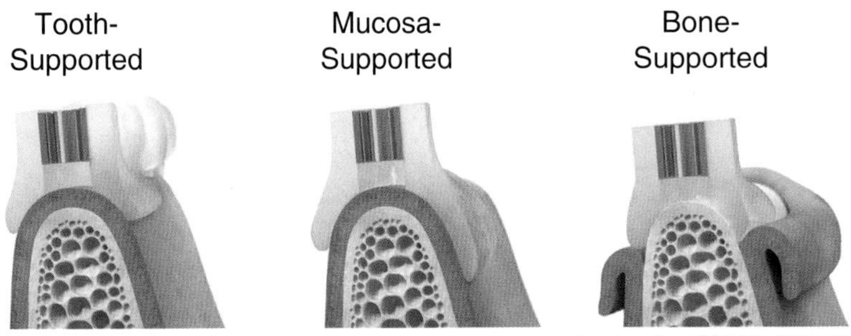

Fig. 85.2 Graphical depiction of retention options for static stereolithic surgical guides, including tooth-supported, mucosa-supported, and bone-supported, depending on the clinical scenario.

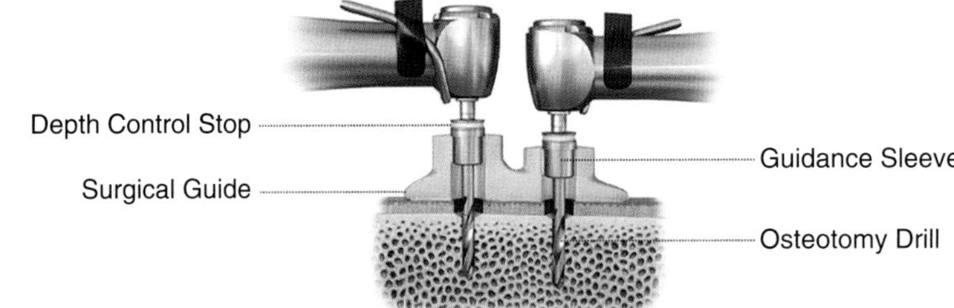

Fig. 85.3 Digital stereolithic surgical guides, manufactured based on computer-guidance software, facilitate osteotomy restriction via the use of specific guidance sleeves and stops, which can either be embedded in the guide, or attached to the osteotomy drill, depending on the manufacturer, and selected protocol.

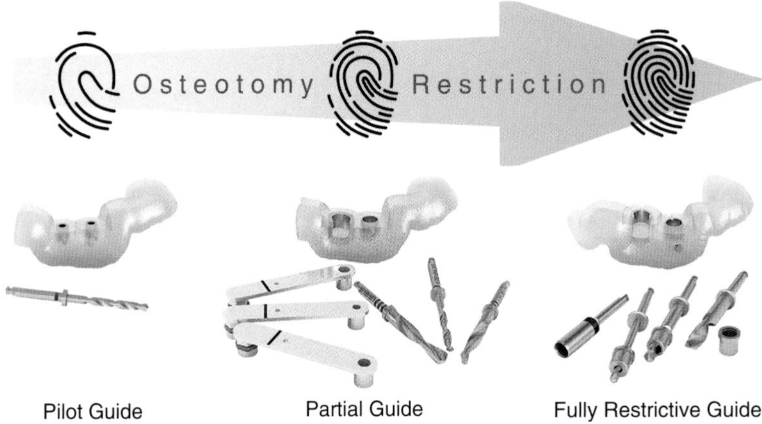

Fig. 85.4 Digitally designed and fabricated surgical guides can vary on the level of surgical restriction, depending on case dynamics, from pilot guidance to full guidance.

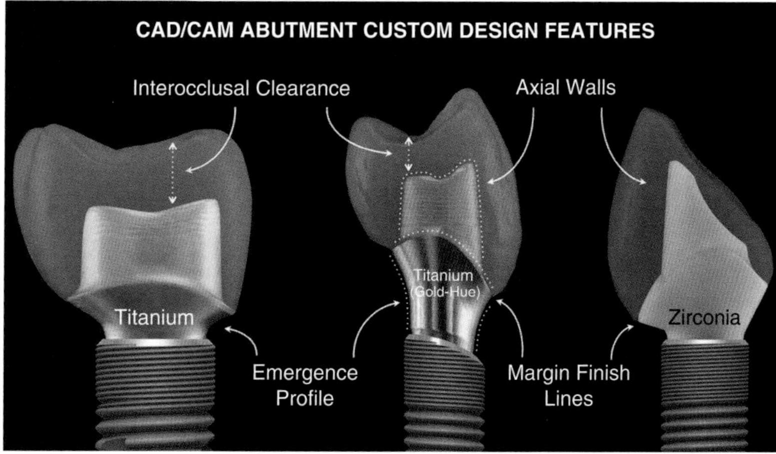

Fig. 85.5 Computer-aided design and computer-aided manufacturing *(CAD/CAM)* prosthetic abutments enable clinicians a full range of parameters for design and fabrication, including biomaterial selection, emergence profile morphology, marginal finish lines, and axial wall taper and interocclusal clearance.

suprastructures, and coronal restorations, most prosthetic components (whether for interim or definitive restorations) were either prefabricated or customized via labor-intensive and often cost-prohibitive methodologies, such as casting with the lost-wax technique.

Abutment Design and Manufacturing

When considering definitive transmucosal abutments, for instance, prefabricated titanium abutments have historically offered clinicians simplicity and cost-effectiveness. However, due to their static emergence design, they are also associated with significant drawbacks when considering clinical situations that exhibit limited restorative space, nonideal implant positioning, and/or compromised soft-tissue esthetics. In contrast, custom abutments designed and fabricated in an analog workflow require castable components that are waxed, invested, and cast by an individual technician, with wide-ranging outcomes. Such castable custom abutments (often referred to as a University of California at Los Angeles [UCLA] abutment) are often associated with compromised biomechanical properties,[19,33] decreased biocompatibility,[2,43] increased cost, and elongated fabrication turnaround time.

KEY FACT

A castable abutment, also known as a **UCLA abutment**, is a prefabricated component, with or without a prefabricated cylinder, used to make a custom abutment for a cement-retained or screw-retained prosthesis. It is created by waxing its plastic burnout pattern and subsequently casting the abutment through a lost-wax technique. The custom-made abutment is then used in the construction of an implant-supported prosthesis. Castable abutments can be made of a variety of materials, including metal alloys such as titanium, gold, or chrome cobalt.[17]

Additionally, analog workflows prevent detailed communication between the clinician and the technician as to the optimal implant abutment prosthetic features, such as emergence profile morphology, interocclusal clearance, and axial wall taper, height, and thickness (Fig. 85.5). Consequently, customization of abutment parameters via digital CAD/CAM workflows has increasingly been adopted as an approach to improve clinical outcomes, while the use of stock abutments has declined.[22]

Further advantages of CAD/CAM custom abutments, when compared with stock abutments, include access to removal of excess cement through prosthetic margin elevation,[21,42,41] conversion of prosthetic screw-channel location and prosthetic fixation method via angulated screw access (ASA) design,[7] optimizing the emergence profile morphology based on implant positioning[10,35] and mucosal phenotype,[24] which allows to predictably support the peri-implant softtissue,[23] and duplication of diagnostic information garnered through implant provisionalization.[15,34] CAD/CAM workflows also make available the opportunity to leverage standardization of manufacturing according to International Organization for Standardization (ISO) 9000 and good manufacturing practices (GMP),[32] CAD-design archiving, and use of abutment design data (via STereoLithography [STL] files) to facilitate expedited design and manufacturing of abutment-supported implant restorations (provisional or definitive) by either the laboratory or clinician.[29] Digital CAD/CAM abutment design technology has also recently been used to design and fabricate custom healing abutments to guide the peri-implant mucosal architecture during non-functional loaded healing, contain bone graft materials, and give the restorative clinician the option to move directly to a properly contoured definitive abutment following osseointegration without the use of an interim coronal restoration (Fig. 85.6).[12,14,16,35] Given the plethora of advantages (e.g., reduced time and cost, design specificity, and flexibility), CAD/CAM abutments have quickly become a standard of care over the past decade, as well as a therapeutic resource to maximize functional and esthetic outcomes for implant-supported restorations.

Digitally Aided Implant Provisionalization: A Union of Workflows

By merging the aforementioned advantages that computer-guided surgery and digital prosthetic design and manufacturing offer into a contiguous workflow, robust opportunities for digitally facilitated implant provisionalization have recently emerged and are likely to continue to evolve in the future across different platforms. The following sections will provide a broad overview of various digitally aided provisionalization workflow options, primarily based on the degree of surgical and prosthetic restriction selected. System- and manufacturer-specific workflow variations need to be considered for the selection of a preferred workflow. Referencing general categories based on the level of restrictive constraints, there are three different workflow domains in digitally aided provisionalization (Fig. 85.7).

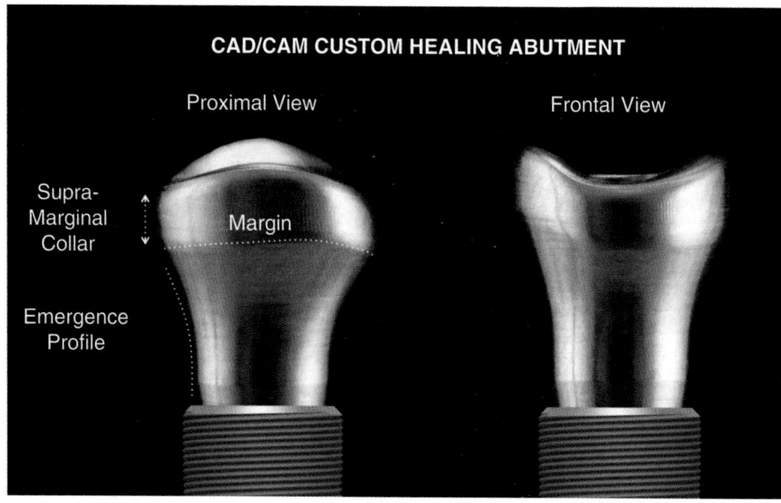

Fig. 85.6 Computer-aided design and computer-aided manufacturing *(CAD/CAM)* custom healing abutments facilitate the development of the peri-implant mucosal architecture and morphology without the need for a coronal component, decreasing chances for occlusal overload in clinical scenarios not suitable for implant provisionalization or in patients that are not compliant with postoperative instructions.

Provisionalization Workflow	Surgical Restriction (Guidance)	Prosthetic Restriction
Non-Restrictive	No Restriction (or) Pilot-Guide	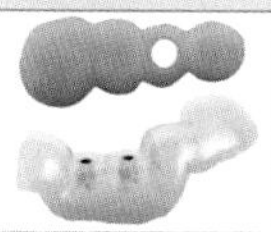 Flexibility to facilitate rotational, apico-coronal, and bodily orientation of interim coronal restoration 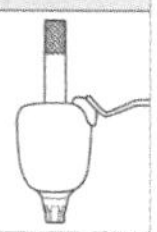
Semi-Restrictive	Partial (or) Full-Guidance	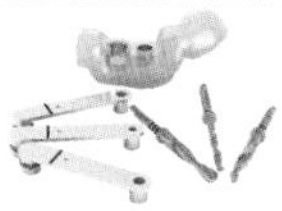 Flexibility to facilitate rotational and apico-coronal, but not bodily orientation of interim coronal restoration 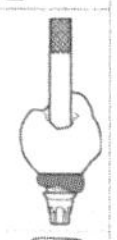
Fully-Restrictive	Full Guidance	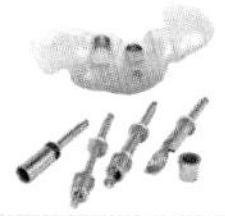 No flexibility for changes in rotation, apico-coronal, or bodily orientation of the interim coronal restoration, components all site-specific 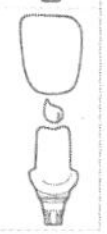

Fig. 85.7 Graphical depiction of the levels of surgical and prosthetic restriction in *digitally aided implant provisionalization.*

Non-Restrictive Digitally Aided Provisionalization

In non-restrictive digitally aided implant provisionalization, both the surgical and prosthetic phases of treatment occur in a non-restrictive workflow. By selecting a non-restrictive workflow, surgical and restorative clinicians prioritize having flexibility in both the osteotomy preparation and implant placement, as well as in interim abutment placement and provisional prosthesis coupling to the interim abutment. Such versatility may be preferable in situations where implants are immediately placed into extraction sockets, and/or the integrity or quality of the residual alveolar bone may be in question, but where either immediate (or) delayed provisionalization may be advantageous. Surgically, such non-restrictive single-tooth implant guides may be designed in various forms and in various digital environments, from laboratory-based design software to chairside intraoral scanners. They can be fabricated by stereolithography using a variety of acrylic and resin materials via 3D printing (additively), or they can be fabricated in subtractive approaches by milling a pre-cured block of resin or acrylic material. Regarding the provisional restorations, such non-restrictive restorations can similarly be fabricated via different digitally aided additive or subtractive approaches, using both lab and clinical-based software platforms and from a variety of acrylic, resin, or resin-ceramic hybrid materials. A pre-fabricated abutment is then coupled to the non-restrictive provisional crown either peri-operatively for immediate provisionalization cases or after osseointegration, and full healing has occurred for delayed provisionalization cases.

Clinical Example

Following several months of healing after a ridge augmentation procedure at site #5, a 57-year-old healthy adult male patient presented for a pre-operative CBCT scan and digital intraoral scan (Fig. 85.8). Per the radiographic assessment, there was sufficient bone volume to facilitate implant placement. A non-restrictive tooth-supported CAD/CAM surgical guide was designed using the intraoral scan captured with a chairside intraoral scanner software (Cerec Omnicam, Dentsply Sirona, York, PA). Attention was given to clearly delineating the desired gingival zenith architecture at the apical aspect of the provisional shell crown and to harmonizing coronal form and occlusion (see Fig. 85.8D). Prior to surgical guide fabrication via a subtractive method using a cross-linked PMMA block (Telio CAD, Ivoclar Vivadent, Schaan, Liechtenstein), it was critical to verify that the planned CAD/CAM surgical guide could be manufactured in its entirety within the dimensions of the block (Fig. 85.9A). After verifying adequate space dimensions, the surgical guide design was sent to

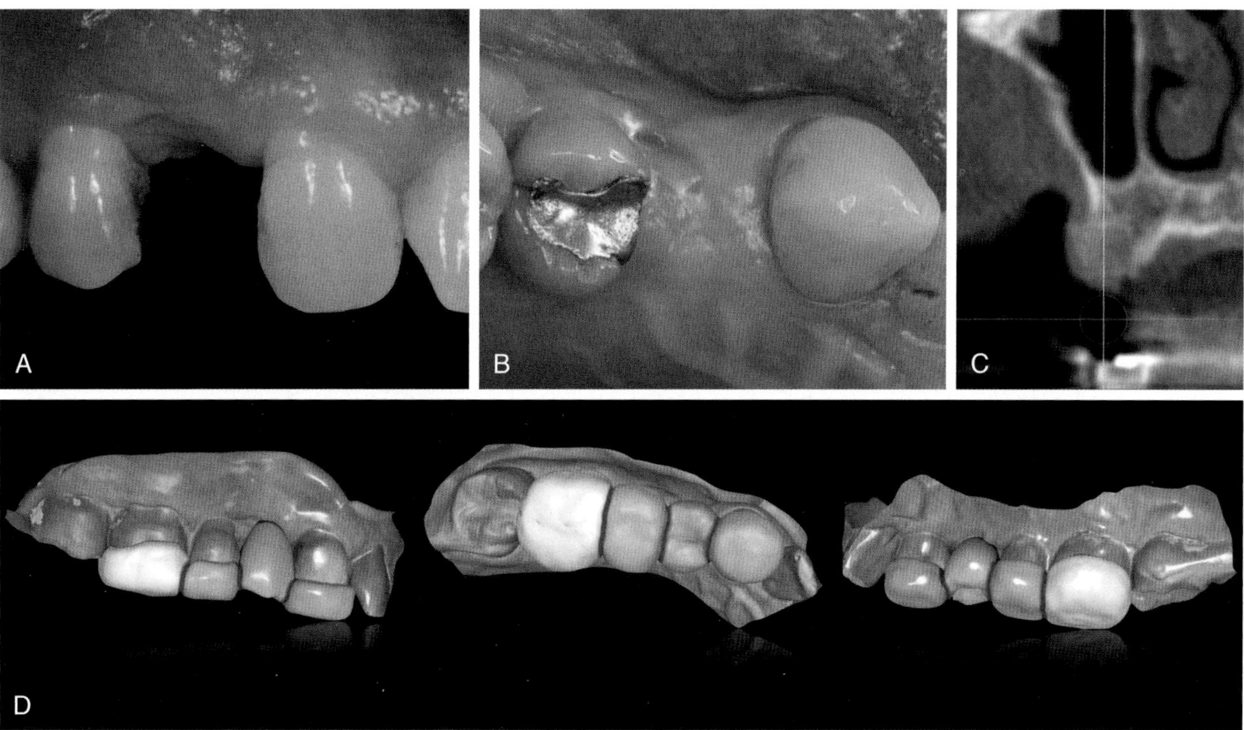

Fig. 85.8 Buccal (A) and occlusal (B) views of site #5 several months after ridge augmentation was performed. A cone-beam computed tomography (CBCT) scan (C) was obtained to verify adequate bone volume, and quality. A non-restrictive static surgical guide (D) was designed from an intraoral scan to communicate the desired coronal form and gingival zenith.

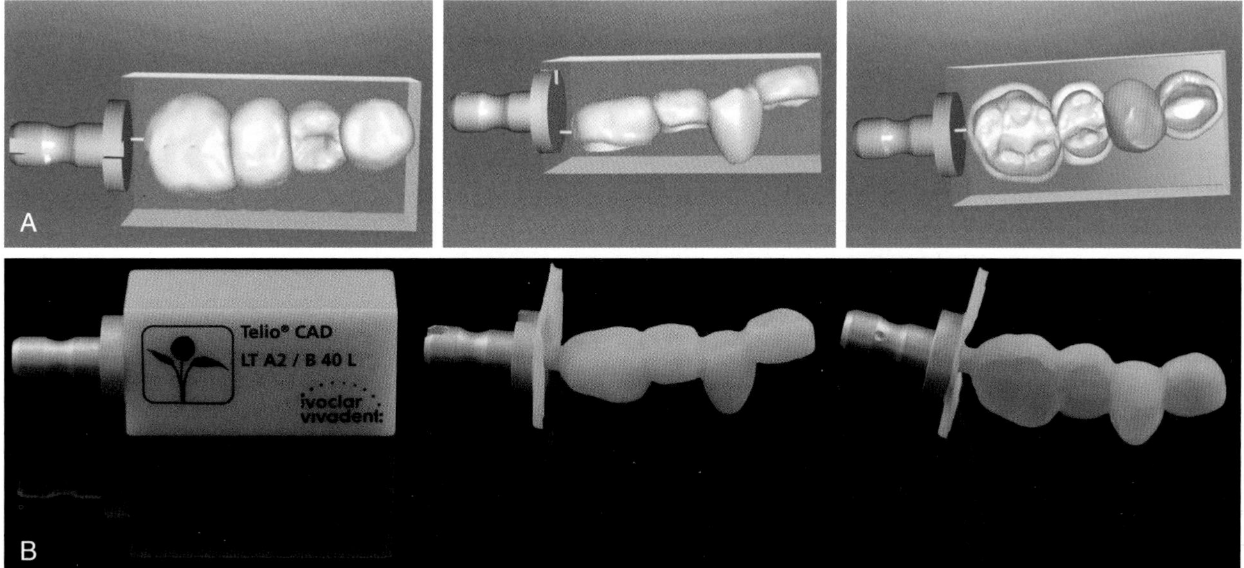

Fig. 85.9 The non-restrictive static surgical guide was previewed in the planning software to verify the dimensions of a cross-linked polymethylmethacrylate (PMMA) block for subtractive manufacturing (A). The surgical guide was milled chairside, requiring removal of the sprue and relief of the intaglio to facilitate non-restrictive guidance at the time of implant placement (B).

a chairside mill (Cerec MC XL, Dentsply Sirona, York, PA) that prepared the tooth-shaded block (see Fig. 85.9B). The surgical guide was utilized at the time of osteotomy preparation in a non-restrictive, prosthetically oriented fashion, delineating the extent of implant bodily (Fig. 85.10A) and depth placement (see Fig. 85.10B). The osteotomy and implant placement orientation were verified radiographically (see Fig. 85.10C and D). Excellent primary stability of the implant (Astra Tech Implant EV Profile 4.2 PS, Dentsply Sirona, York, PA) was obtained, and immediate implant provisionalization ensued. The CAD/CAM surgical guide was converted to a single-tooth implant provisional restoration by prosthetically coupling it via bonding with resin composite to a prefabricated titanium abutment (Temp Abutment Profile EV, Dentsply Sirona, York, PA) (Fig. 85.11A and D).

Proper orientation of the coronal shell within the CAD/CAM surgical guide relative to the interim abutment during pick-up was ensured by visually verifying the full seating of the proximal intaglio

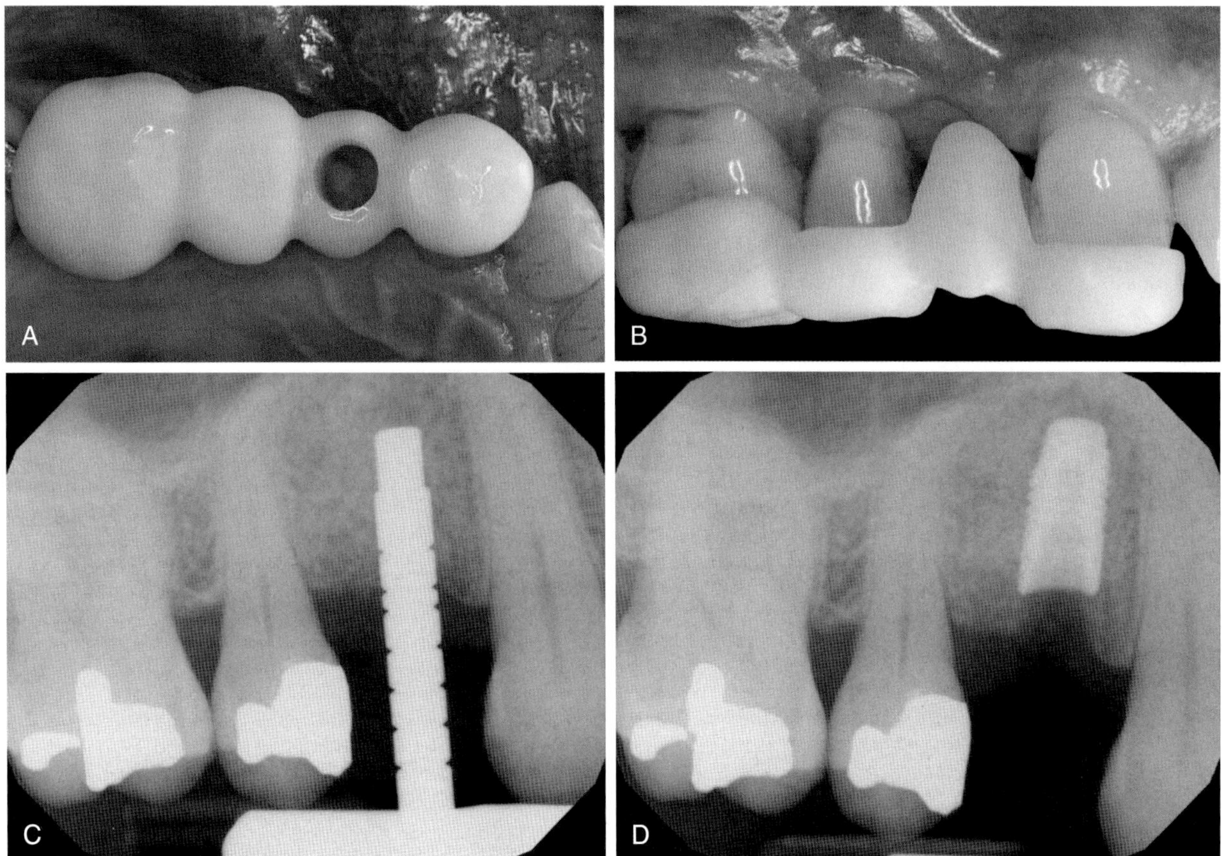

Fig. 85.10 The computer-aided design and computer-aided manufacturing (CAD/CAM) non-restrictive surgical guide facilitated guidance for both lateral and depth orientation of the implant body (A and B), with scout periapical radiographs being used intra-surgically to verify position and depth (C and D).

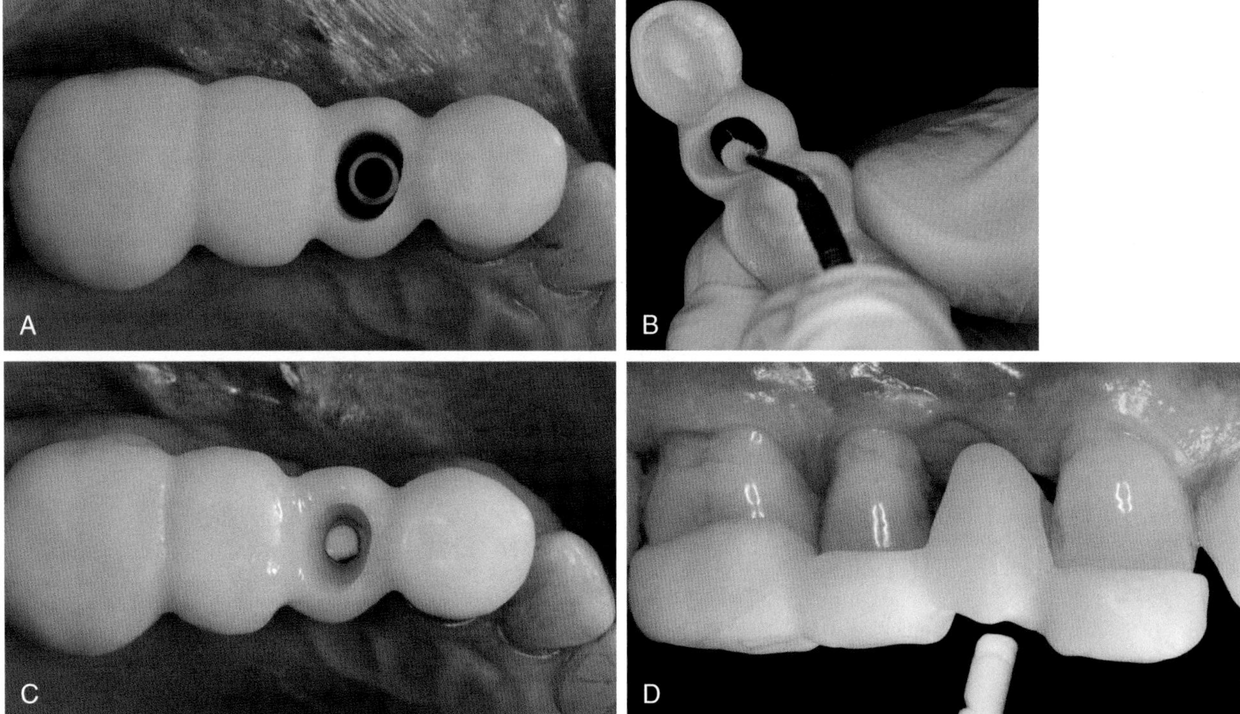

Fig. 85.11 Upon final placement of the implant body, the computer-aided design and computer-aided manufacturing (CAD/CAM) non-restrictive surgical guide were confirmed to have passive seating around a temporary prefabricated titanium abutment (A), and upon blocking of the screw-access, was adhesively coupled to the abutment to facilitate subsequent immediate implant provisionalization (C–D).

surfaces of the guide. Upon coupling the CAD/CAM guide and interim abutment, the proximal supports to the guide were removed by sectioning with a disc (Fig. 85.12A–C). The immediate provisional crown was completed by adding composite resin to the transmucosal aspect of the abutment, which was subsequently polished, and disinfected in an ultrasonic bath. The lack of functional or excursive occlusal contacts was verified, and the provisional restoration was torqued to the manufacturer's recommendation. The screw channel was then sealed with polytetrafluoroethylene (PFTE) tape and resin composite (Fig. 85.13A and B).

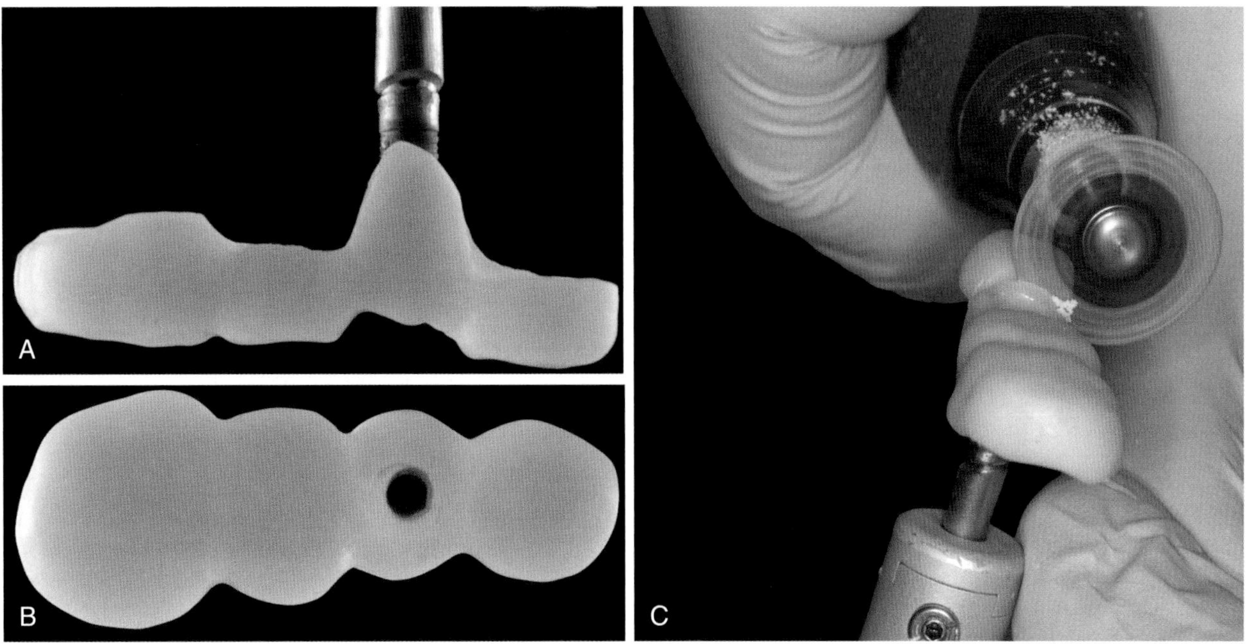

Fig. 85.12 After removal from the oral cavity (A and B), the computer-aided design and computer-aided manufacturing (CAD/CAM) non-restrictive surgical guide were sectioned interproximally to convert the guide into a single-unit immediate implant provisional restoration (C).

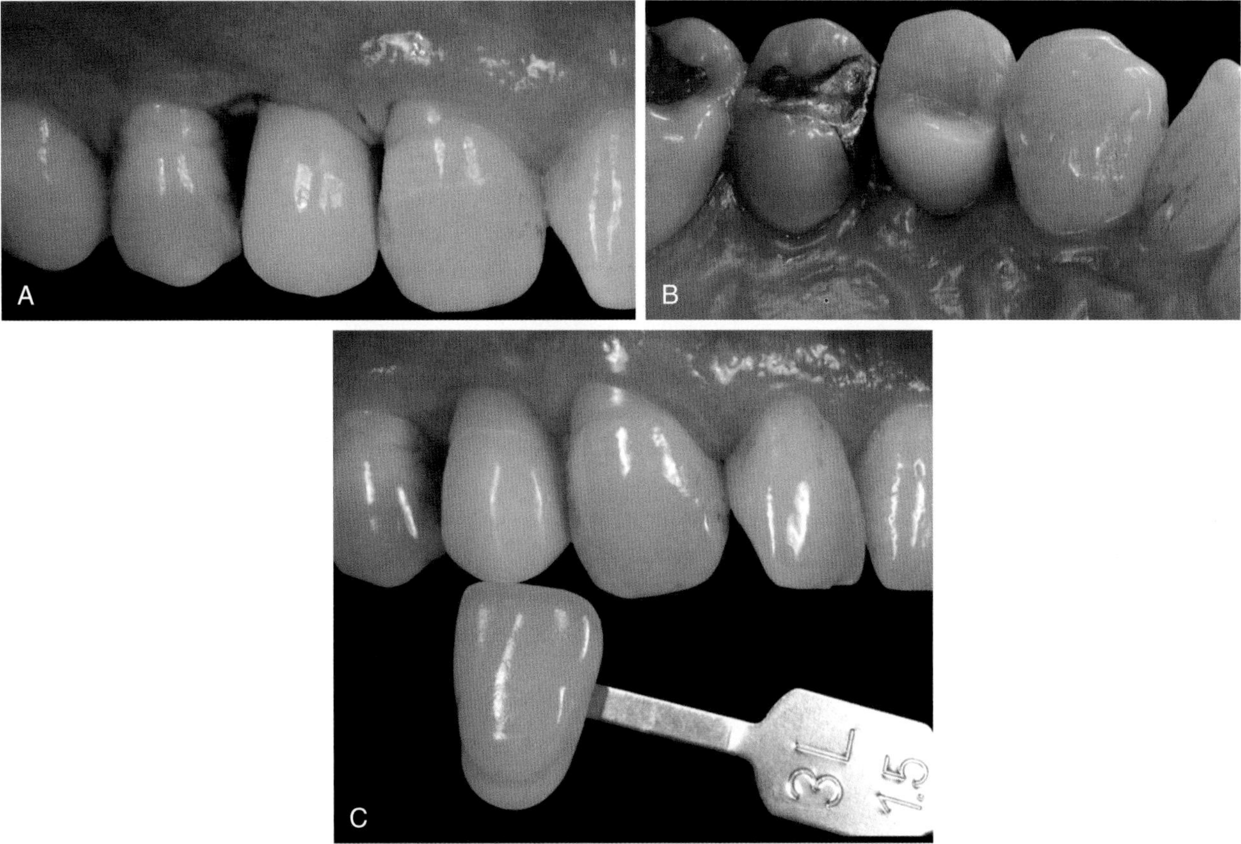

Fig. 85.13 Following completion of the transmucosal emergence profile and verification of proximal and occlusal contacts, the completed immediate provisional restoration was inserted and provisionally torqued to the manufacturer's recommendations and sealed with polytetrafluoroethylene (PTFE) tape and resin composite (A and B). Four months after immediate provisionalization, the health of the peri-implant mucosa and prosthetic stability was verified, and a definitive shade was selected to communicate with the laboratory fabricating the definitive restoration (C).

CLINICAL CORRELATION

Proper disinfection and sealing of implant-supported crowns, whether as a provisional or definitive restoration, helps to minimize bacterial ingress into the implant-abutment interface. It is important to avoid the use of organic compounds, such as cotton pellets, or impression material, as these materials can break down in the presence of moisture or heat and favor bacterial proliferation. PTFE has been demonstrated to be an excellent obturation material, prior to placement of a coronal composite, due to its excellent chemical resistance, satisfactory thermal stability, non-absorbency, ability to be sterilized, resistance to compression, and non-toxicity.[25]

After four months of healing with the provisional crown in place, a ceramic shade was selected and communicated to the laboratory (see Fig. 85.13C). Additionally, an intraoral scan was made with a digital feature locating object (FLO) scan body (Atlantis IO FLO IO-P-06, Dentsply Sirona, York, PA) seated into implant #5 (Fig. 85.14A and B). A definitive CAD/CAM abutment (Atlantis, Dentsply Sirona, York, PA) and a screwmentable high translucent monolithic zirconia crown (ArgenZ Zirconia, Argen, San Diego, CA) were fabricated and verified on a printed model (see Fig. 85.14C and D). Five months after immediate provisionalization, the definitive abutment-crown complex (Fig. 85.15A) was cemented chairside, disinfected, and delivered. Six months after insertion of the definitive restoration, the peri-implant mucosa demonstrated a lack of inflammation and adequate morphology (see Fig. 85.15B and C).

Semi-Restrictive Digitally Aided Provisionalization

Utilizing semi-restrictive digitally aided implant provisionalization protocols offers more guidance as compared with the non-restrictive protocol while still allowing for either the surgeon or restorative clinician, or both, to have control over the implant placement and provisionalization parameters. Semi-restrictive protocols provide opportunities for clinicians to make small adjustments to the osteotomy and implant placement parameters, as well as the orientation and mechanism by which the prosthetic components (abutment and crown) are joined. These protocols may be preferentially indicated in situations where more restrictive implant guidance is necessary (e.g., partial guidance) for anatomic, biologic, or functional reasons but where full guidance may be unnecessary or prohibitive to provisionalization. Conversely, even if full restrictive implant guidance is used, semi-restrictive provisionalization protocols enable greater prosthetic flexibility and can leverage prefabricated prosthetic components, such as stock provisional abutments. Hence, semi-restrictive protocols reduce complexity and cost and offer the clinician carrying out implant provisionalization greater latitude intraoperatively when providing this treatment, as compared to fully restrictive digitally facilitated provisionalization protocols.

Clinical Example

A healthy 46-year-old adult male with a hopeless retained deciduous #H and congenitally missing tooth #11 sought tooth replacement therapy with a dental implant to improve function and esthetics. #H lacked proper occlusal contacts due to incomplete eruption and had become mobile and painful upon function (Fig. 85.16). Due to the extent of apical root resorption associated with #H, as well as a favorable alveolar bone architecture and proximal root orientation, immediate implant placement (IIP) with immediate provisionalization (IP) was planned virtually after obtaining and merging a diagnostic maxillary CBCT scan and intraoral scans of the upper and lower arch. Sufficient alveolar bone height and width were present to facilitate virtual implant placement (Simplant Pro v.18, Dentsply Sirona, York, PA) in a prosthetically oriented position based on a full-contour diagnostic digital design (Fig. 85.17A and B). Festooning of the bucco-coronal aspect of the residual alveolar ridge was planned to facilitate a clinical crown with apico-coronal proportions comparable to those of tooth #6. A virtual preview of the fully restrictive tooth-supported stereolithic surgical guide was

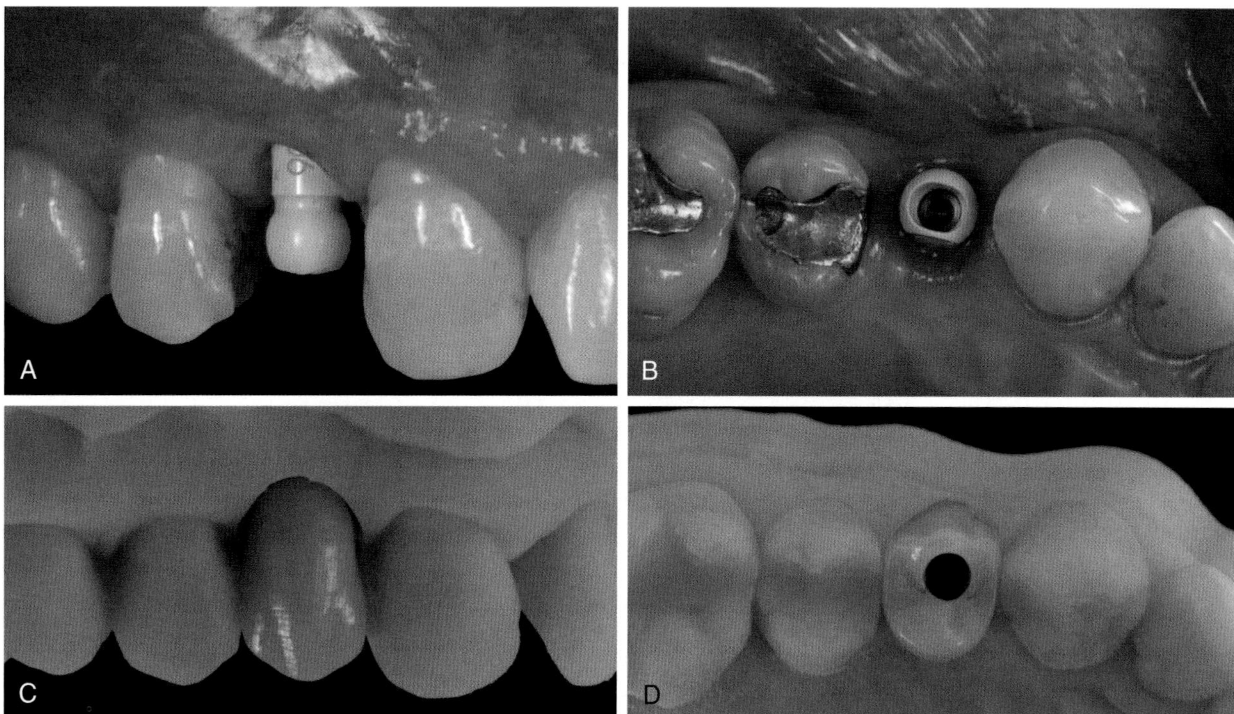

Fig. 85.14 An intraoral scan using an implant digital feature locating object (FLO) scan body was utilized for communicating the final implant position and the architecture of the peri-implant mucosa (A and B). The completed abutment and crown were returned and verified on a master model fabricated by additive manufacturing (C and D).

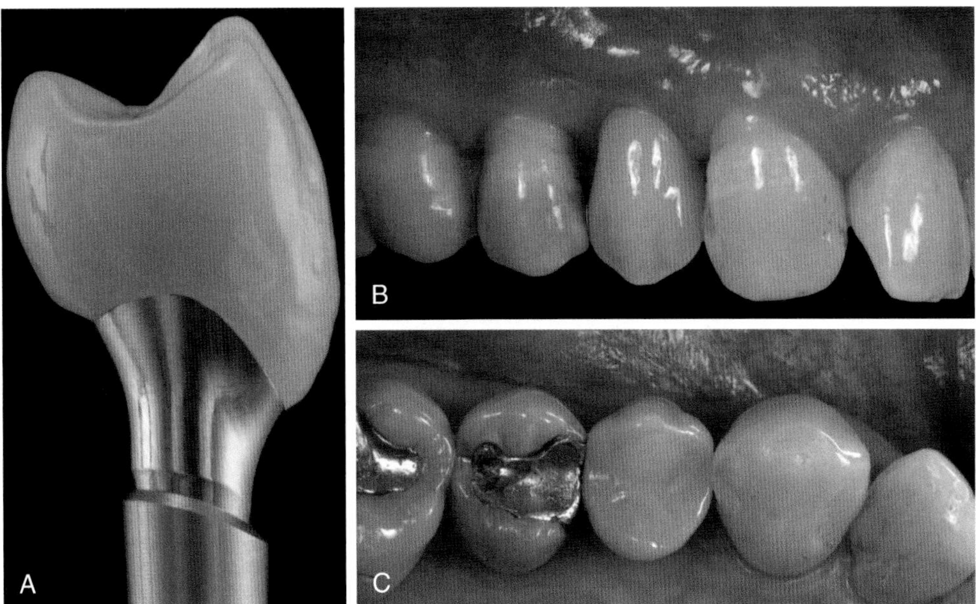

Fig. 85.15 Proper morphological contour and margin placement were required in the design of the definitive computer-aided design and computer-aided manufacturing (CAD/CAM) gold-shaded titanium abutment and zirconia crown (A). Six months after delivery of the definitive restoration, the peri-implant mucosa and functional stability of the prosthesis were verified clinically (B and C).

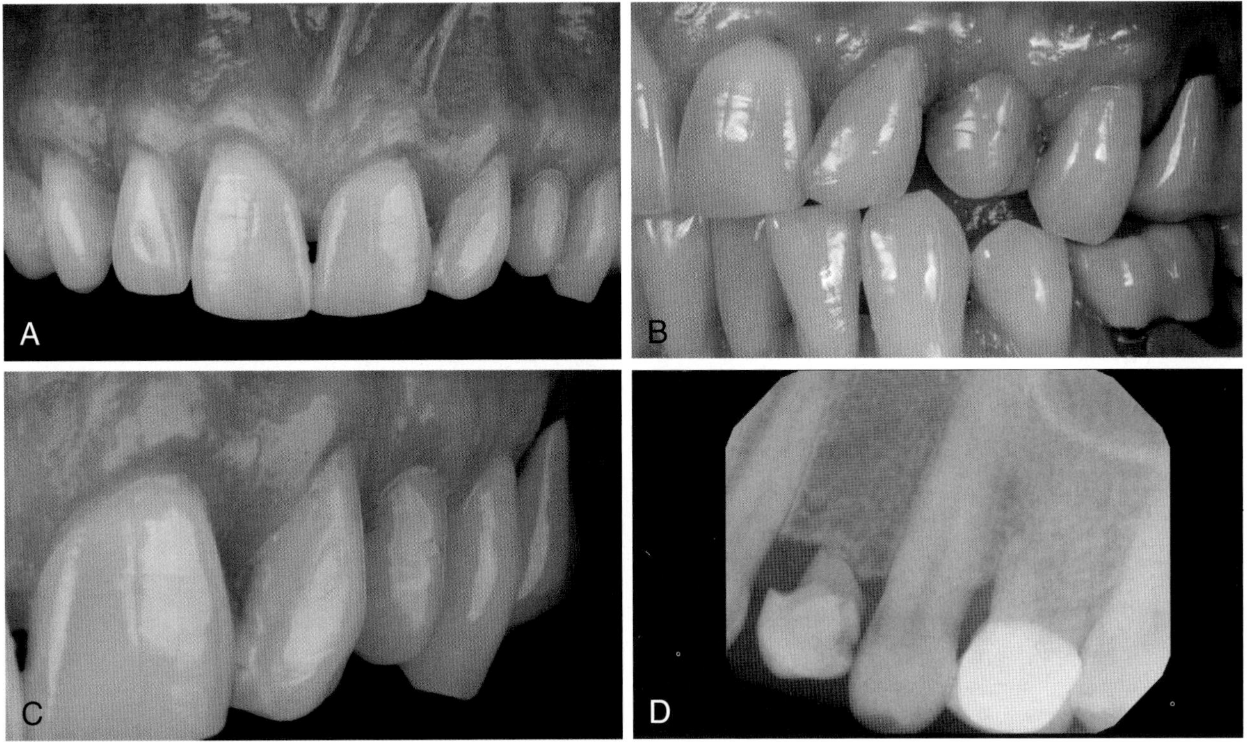

Fig. 85.16 Pre-operative clinical views of a hopeless retained deciduous #H (A–C) and radiographic view demonstrate a hopeless prognosis of #H and a congenitally missing tooth #11 (D).

verified upon finalizing the surgical and prosthetic plan (see Fig. 85.17C and D). Upon fabrication of the stereolithic guide, two STL files were exported from the surgical planning software: one of the diagnostic digital design of the provisional crown #11 and another of the screw-access channel lumen, based on the virtual implant plan (Videos 85.1 and 85.2, respectively). Merging of these two files into a digital design software (3Shape Implant Studio, 3Shape A/S, Copenhagen, Denmark) facilitated the subtractive manufacturing (CAM) of a pre-polymerized PMMA block into a screw-retained immediate provisional restoration. The lumen of the provisional restoration was pre-established based on the STL file of the implant screw-access lumen and therefore required that the implant be placed in the designated position in order to facilitate downstream provisionalization steps. Interproximal seating 'wings' controlled the vertical orientation of the provisional restoration when prosthetically coupling the crown to the interim abutment (Fig. 85.18).

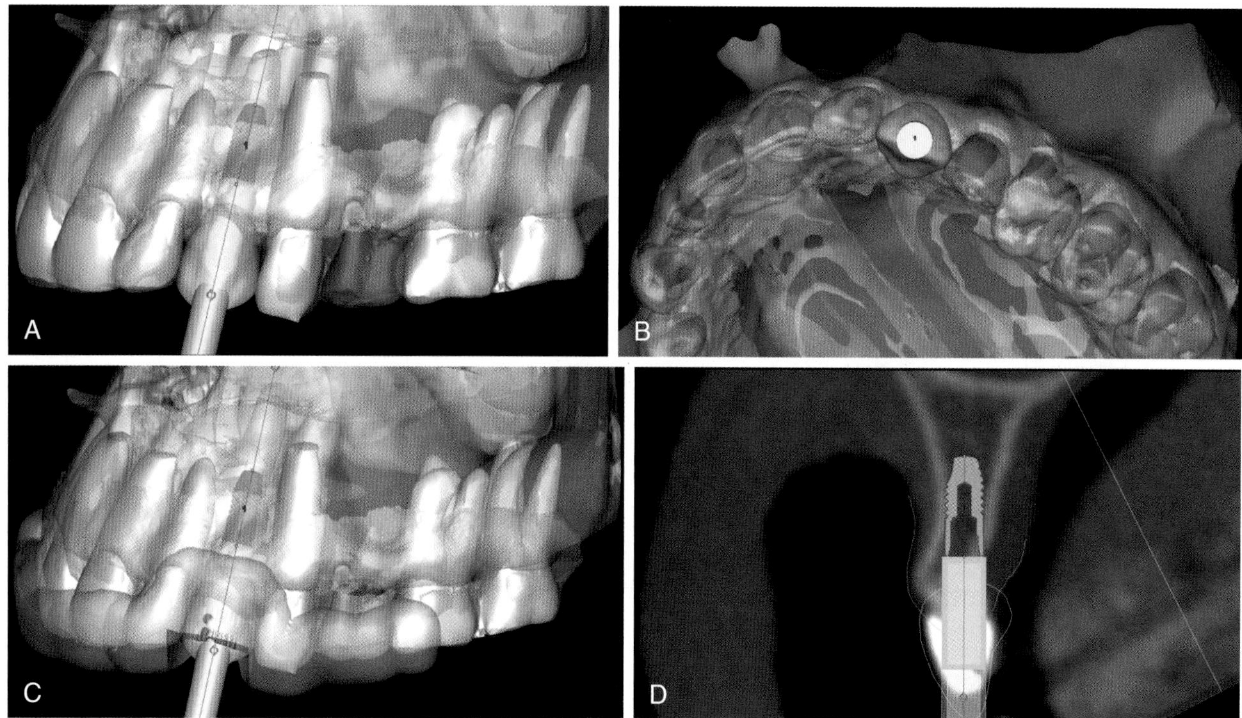

Fig. 85.17 View of merged digital imaging and communications in medicine (DICOM) and STereoLithography (STL) files with a full-contour digital diagnostic wax-up of #11 in digital implant planning software (A and B). A preview of the fully restrictive static stereolithic surgical guide enables communication and planning for adequate surgical guide support and stability (C). A cross-sectional view of the relationship between the planned coronal restoration #11 and the underlying alveolar bone and mucosa to facilitate optimal planning and communication amongst clinical team members (D).

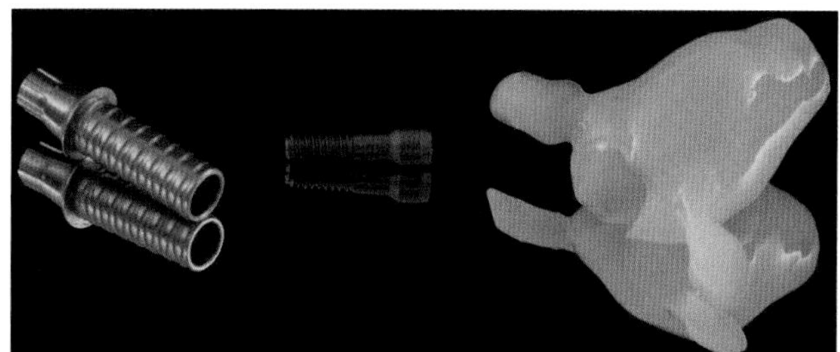

Fig. 85.18 Laboratory view of the components prepared prior to clinical intervention, including the prefabricated titanium temporary abutment *(left)*, the temporary abutment prosthetic screw *(center)*, and the milled semi-restrictive polymethylmethacrylate (PMMA) screw-retained crown *(right)*.

Upon extraction of #H, the adaptation of the stereolithic guide was verified intraorally for passive stability (Fig. 85.19A and D), and the implant osteotomy protocol was followed to completion as dictated by the surgical guide, including the use of a proprietary bone reamer to allow for proper seating of the transmucosal abutment on the implant platform (Fig. 85.20A and B). Sufficient primary stability was achieved to enable immediate implant provisionalization. A prefabricated titanium provisional abutment (Temp Abutment EV, Dentsply Sirona, York, PA) was connected to the implant (see Fig. 85.20C), and the semi-restrictive digitally designed provisional PMMA crown was oriented using the interproximal wings, with lumen passivity noted clinically (see Fig. 85.20D). Flowable resin composite (Flow-It! ALC, Pentron, Orange, CA) was applied after proper priming of both the abutment and intaglio of the PMMA crown to hybridize the components intraorally. The provisional wings were removed, occlusal contacts removed, and the restoration torqued to the manufacturer's recommendation. The screw-access channel was obturated using PTFE tape and resin composite. The flap was approximated with two simple interrupted proximal sutures (4-0 PTFE). Periapical radiographs were made to verify the full seating of the interim abutment into the implant's conical interface (Fig. 85.21). The peri-implant mucosal architecture was monitored from prosthesis insertion (Fig. 85.22A) to four months post-immediate provisionalization (see Fig. 85.22B). Upon verification of adequate peri-implant soft tissue maturation and implant osseointegration, the provisional restoration was disconnected, and an intraoral scan was obtained using a FLO scan body (see Fig. 85.22C and D). The digital design of the final titanium abutment, incorporating angulated screw-access (ASA) to facilitate screw-retention in an optimal position, was finalized (Fig. 85.23A) and subsequently manufactured in gold-shaded titanium nitride with a screwmentable zirconia crown (see Fig. 85.23B). Six months after immediate implant placement and semi-restrictive digitally aided provisionalization, the final CAD/CAM abutment and crown were coupled and definitively delivered (Fig. 85.24A–C). Twelve months after insertion of the final restoration, the peri-implant mucosa was healthy and free of inflammation (Fig. 85.24D).

Fully Restrictive Digitally Aided Provisionalization

With *non-restrictive* and *semi-restrictive* provisionalization workflows, surgical and prosthetic aspects of care can be executed with varying degrees of flexibility, depending on the nature and degree of adjustments that are required. *Fully restrictive* digitally aided implant provisionalization protocols, in contrast, require complete adherence to full guidance during the surgical and prosthetic phases

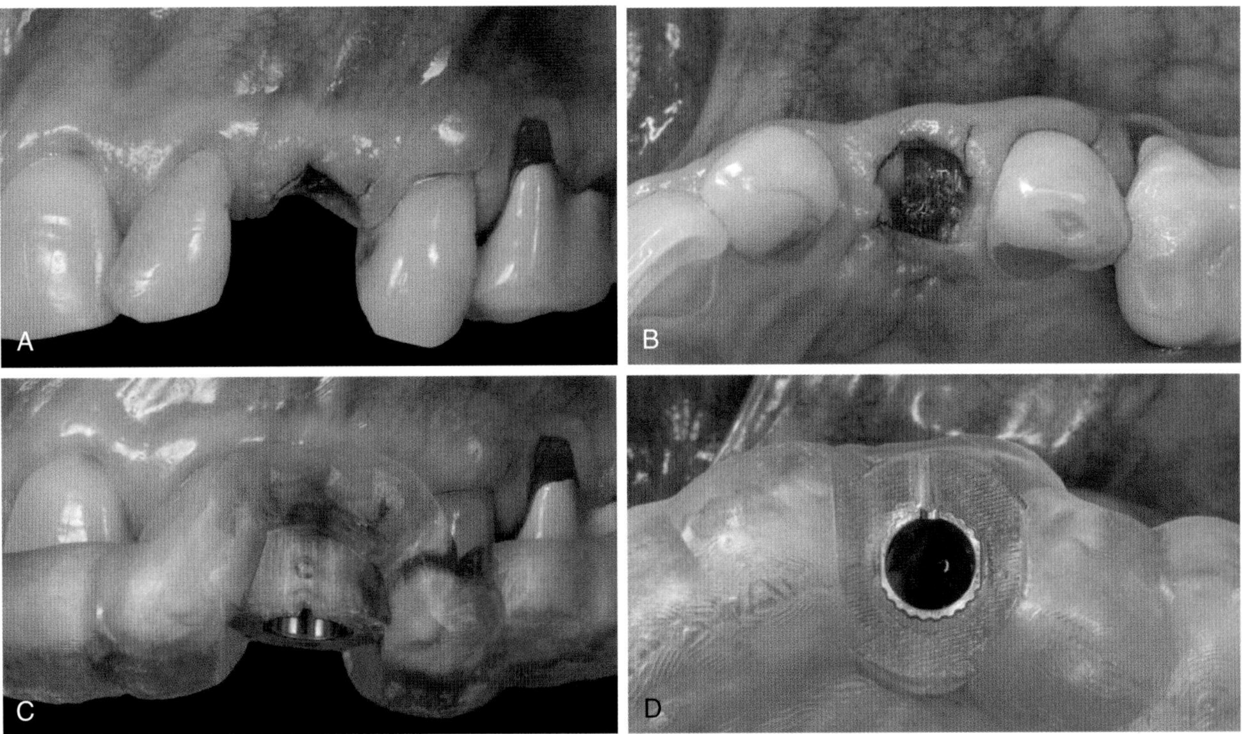

Fig. 85.19 Clinical images of the residual ridge immediately after extraction of #H (A and B). Upon extraction of #H, the static stereolithic surgical could be seated to verify stability and proper guidance (C and D).

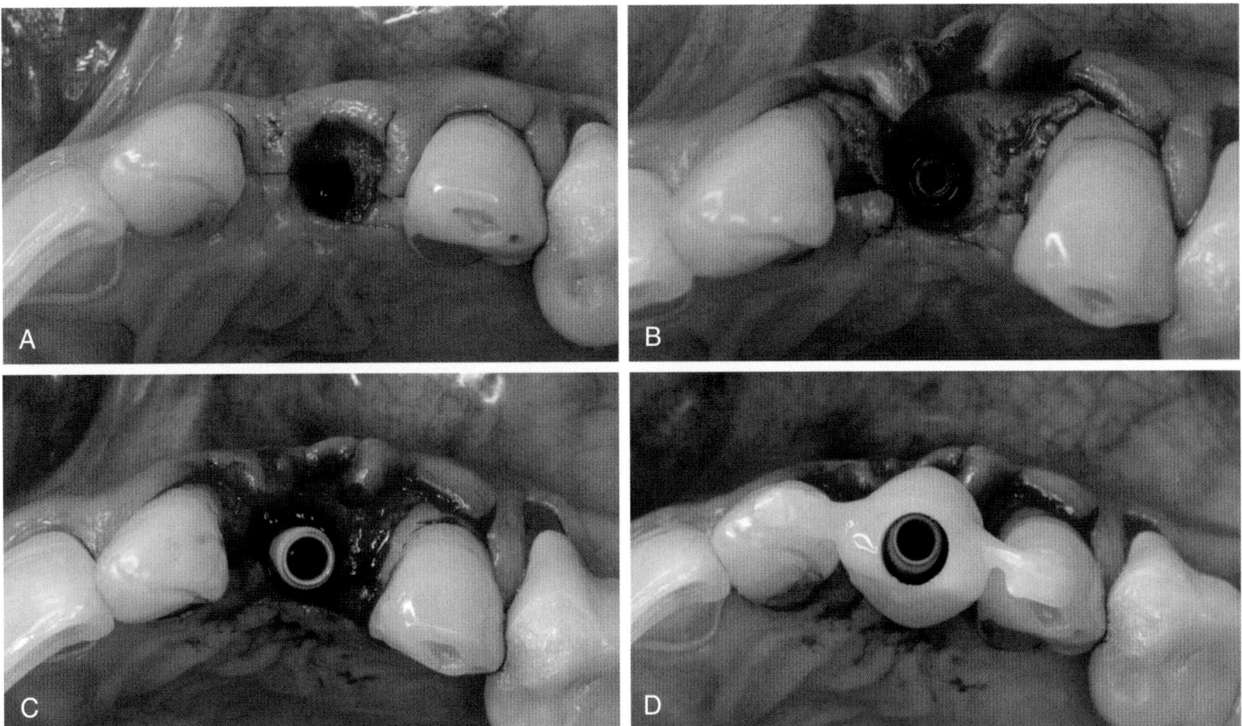

Fig. 85.20 The static fully restrictive stereolithic surgical guide was used for all phases of osteotomy preparation and implant placement (A and B), and upon a temporary prefabricated titanium abutment being secured (C), the semi-restrictive polymethylmethacrylate (PMMA) screw-retained crown was seated to verify passivity to allow for proper positioning and prosthetic coupling (D).

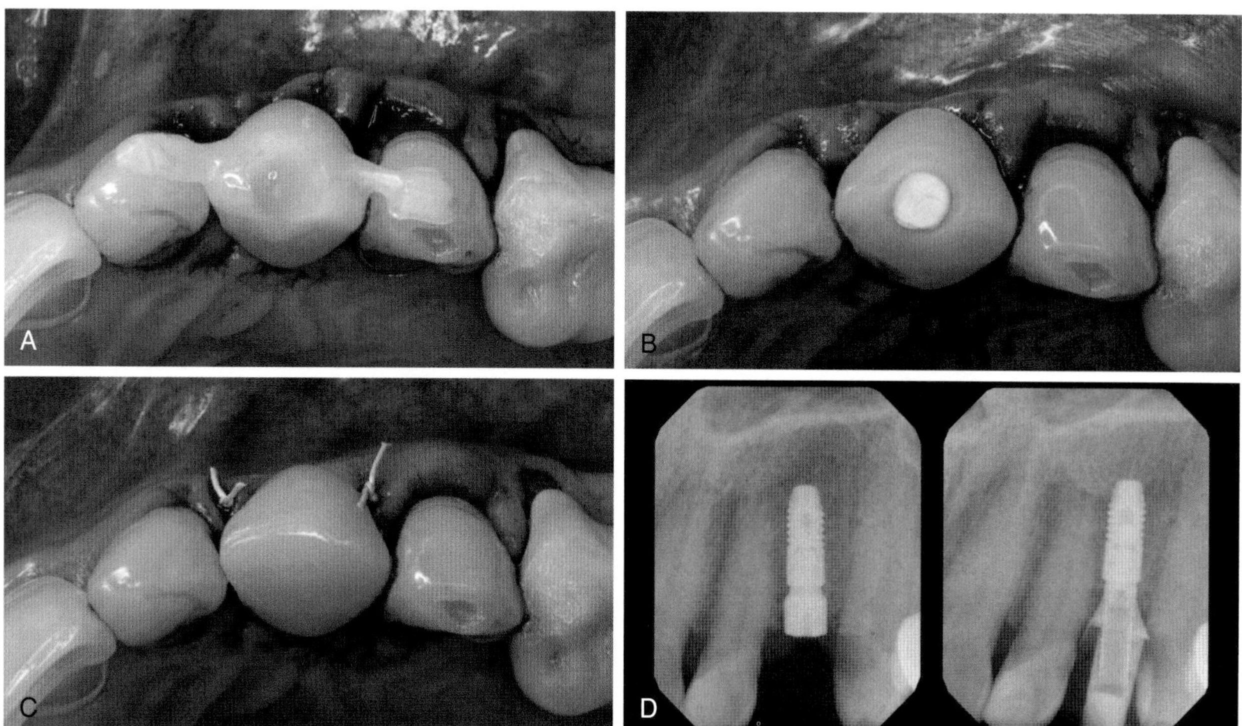

Fig. 85.21 Adhesive resin composite was utilized to prosthetically couple the semi-restrictive polymethylmethacrylate (PMMA) screw-retained crown to the prefabricated titanium abutment after block-out of the screw-access chamber with polytetrafluoroethylene (PTFE) tape (A). Upon light-curing, the chamber was accessed to facilitate the removal of the proximal seating wings and finishing of the transmucosal component with resin composite (B). Upon verification of occlusion and proximal contacts, the provisional restoration was torqued according to the manufacturer's recommendations, and the screw-access channel was obturated with PTFE tape and resin composite (C). Radiographs were made intra-operatively to verify proper implant placement and prosthetic seating of the provisional restorations (D).

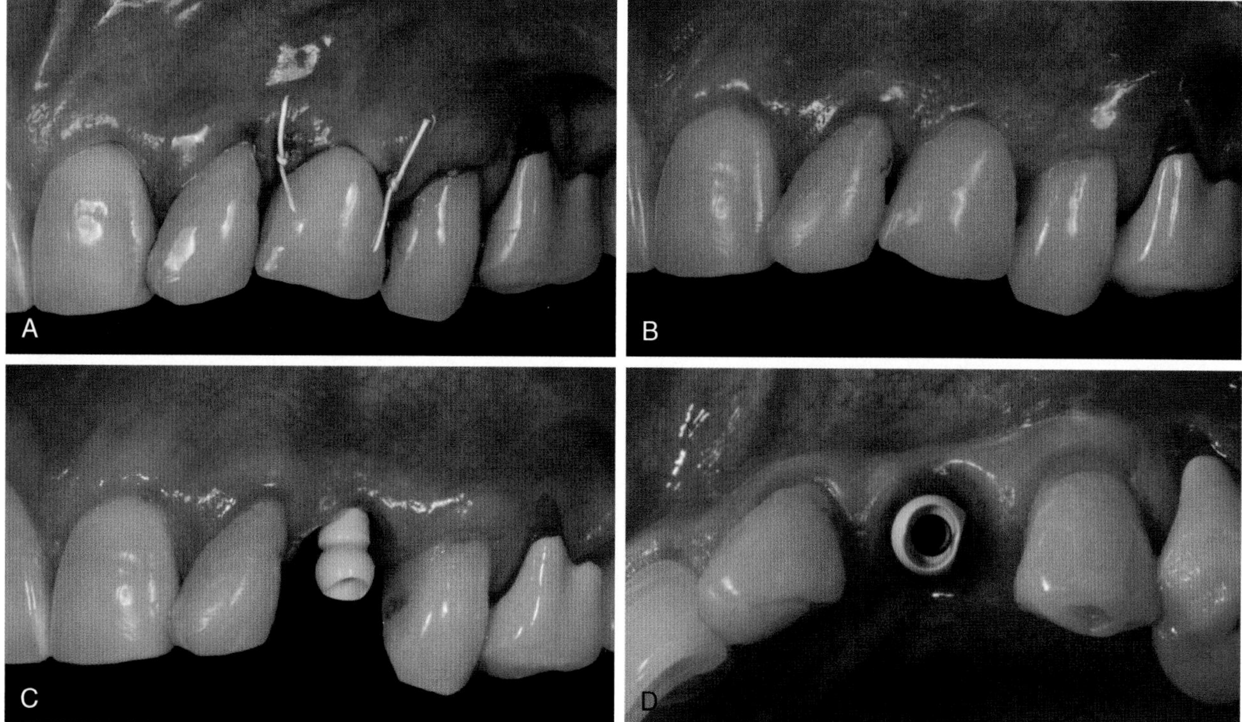

Fig. 85.22 Immediate (A) and four-months (B) postoperative views of the provisional restoration #11. Upon verification of osseointegration and proper peri-implant mucosal architecture, an intraoral scan using an implant digital feature locating object (FLO) scan body was utilized for communicating the implant position and mucosal architecture to the laboratory (C and D).

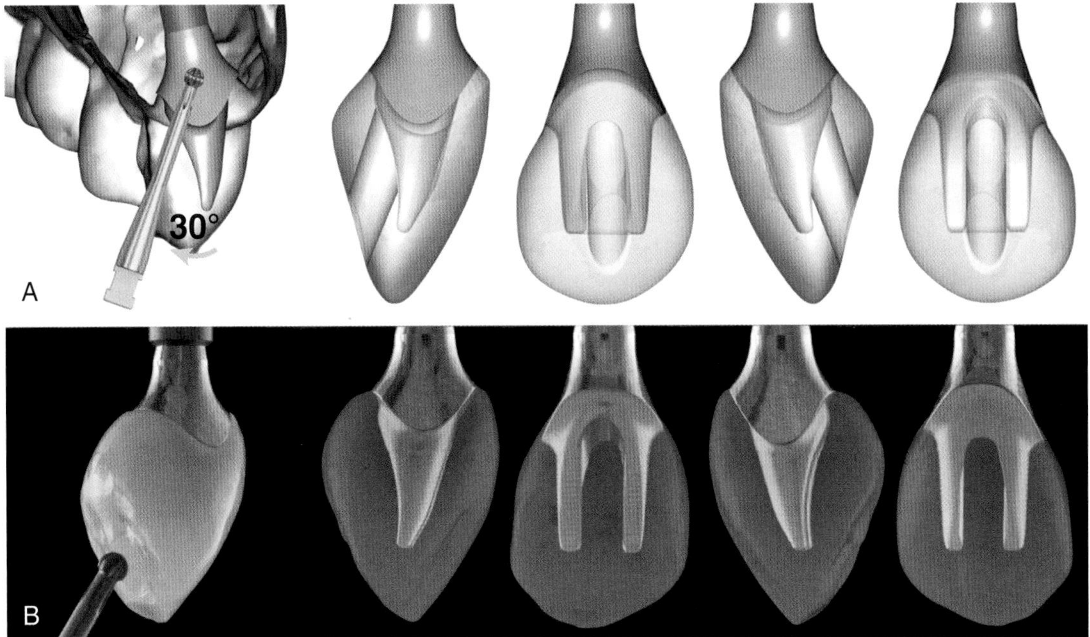

Fig. 85.23 A virtual rendering of the computer-aided design and computer-aided manufacturing (CAD/CAM) gold-shaded custom titanium abutment with angulated screw access (A). A view of the completed restoration demonstrating the use of a hexalobular prosthetic driver to facilitate angulated screw access and a transparent view of the abutment-crown complex to highlight the prosthetic relationship (B).

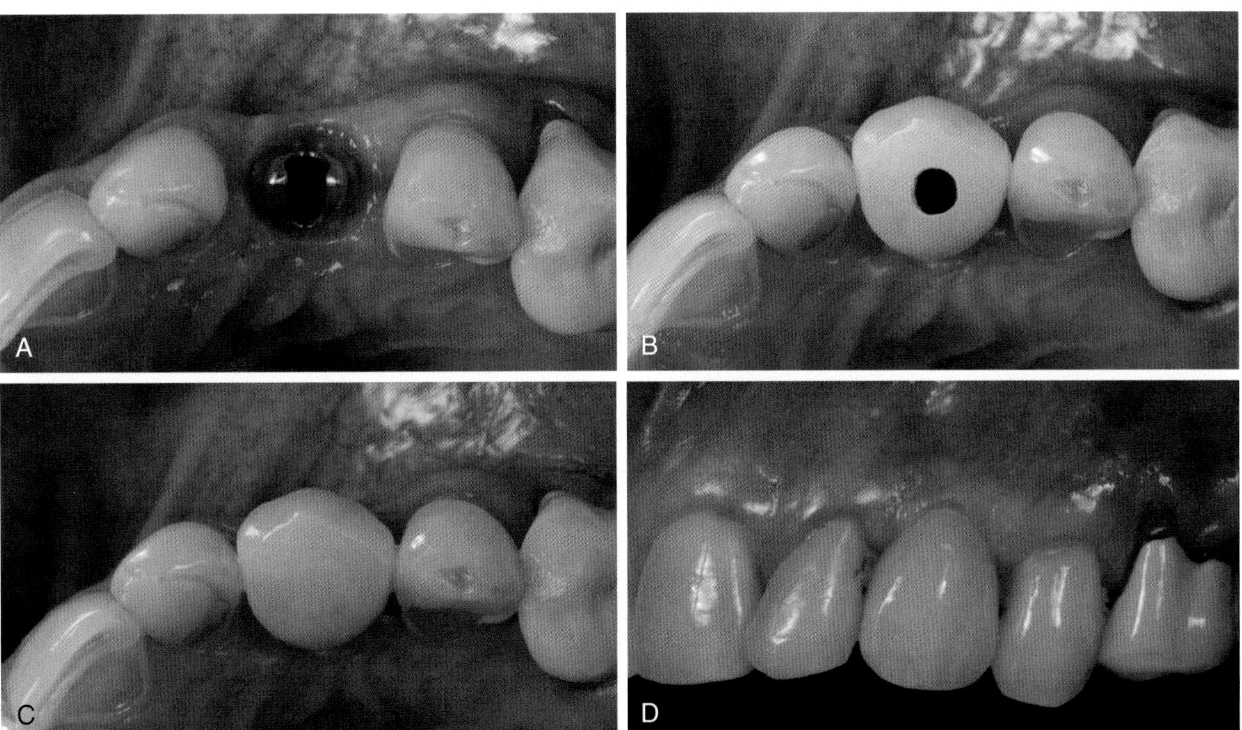

Fig. 85.24 The completed computer-aided design and computer-aided manufacturing (CAD/CAM) gold-shaded custom titanium abutment and screwmentable zirconia crown were seated independently to verify contour, mucosal support, and coronal esthetics prior to coupling (A and B). A view of the coupled abutment-crown complex after sealing the screw-access channel with polytetrafluoroethylene (PTFE) tape and resin composite (C). Clinical view of the restoration #11 12 months after delivery (D).

of treatment, including osteotomy preparation and implant placement and the use of patient and site-specific custom componentry for implant provisionalization. Taken together, this form of provisionalization requires a high degree of coordination during virtual planning of surgery and digital design of the custom prosthetic componentry, as well as between surgical and prosthetic phases during the actual execution of treatment.

The main differentiating factor of fully restrictive digitally aided provisionalization is the use of custom prosthetic componentry, such as custom CAD/CAM abutments and milled or printed provisional crowns. Therefore, this modality requires that implant placement is strictly controlled through the stereolithic guide to constrain implant depth, angulation, and circumferential rotation (sometimes referred to as *timing*) for the site-specific CAD/CAM abutment and provisional crown to fit correctly.[26,6]

Therefore, with regard to workflow considerations, digital planning typically ensues in two phases. First, implant placement planning must be done in planning software that supports fully restrictive implant guidance. After that, a prosthetic design that predicates the design parameters of the abutment and crown on the aspects of implant positioning and depth established previously can occur. Such prosthetic design factors may include abutment material selection, emergence profile morphology, marginal finish line location, axial wall height and clearance, prosthetic crown form and shade, type of prosthetic fixation, and occlusal scheme. Upon completion of design and manufacture of all relevant components, including the stereolithic surgical guide, the CAD/CAM custom abutment, and the provisional crown, they should be sterilized prior to the execution of therapy.

While the most technically and clinically sophisticated of the three forms of digitally aided implant provisionalization reviewed in this chapter, it is important to note that not all cases will be amenable or even fully benefit from *fully restrictive digitally aided provisionalization*. Several factors determine the suitability of such a workflow, including the timing of implant placement (delayed vs. immediate) and the integrity of either the healed ridge or extraction socket, the mucosal phenotype of the implant site, patient compliance, the occlusal status of the patient, and the predictability to accomplish implant placement in the exact a priori planned location to permit implant provisionalization with customized prosthetic components. In clinical scenarios where immediate provisionalization is planned, an additional stipulation must be met: adequate primary stability at the pre-determined position to support immediate provisionalization protocols. Therefore, clinician experience, local factors, and patient compliance are variables that must be carefully considered when selecting the modality of implant provisionalization.

Clinical Example

A healthy 27-year-old female patient with stable occlusion presented with a retained deciduous tooth #K that demonstrated periapical pathosis and discomfort upon function (Fig. 85.25A–D). The patient was interested in tooth replacement therapy with a dental implant, as she had previously undergone implant therapy for the replacement of #T a few years earlier. Diagnostic records, including a mandibular CBCT scan (Video 85.3) and intraoral digital scans of both arches (Video 85.4), were obtained. The CBCT file was segmented to "virtually extract" #K for both guided implant surgery planning (Video 85.5) and for subsequent steps of design and fabrication of a custom abutment and a provisional crown that harmonizes with the proximal surfaces of the adjacent natural teeth. The final implant position was virtually planned in consultation with the treating surgeon (Video 85.6), and a stereolithic surgical guide was designed and fabricated (Simplant Pro v.18, Dentsply Sirona, York, PA) based on this surgical plan.

The guided surgery implant placement parameters were subsequently utilized to digitally design the patient-specific custom prosthetics, including a gold-hue titanium CAD/CAM abutment and a milled provisional screwmentable PMMA crown (Fig. 85.26). While the custom CAD/CAM abutment and crown were required to be "tethered" to the aforementioned implant placement plan, at this

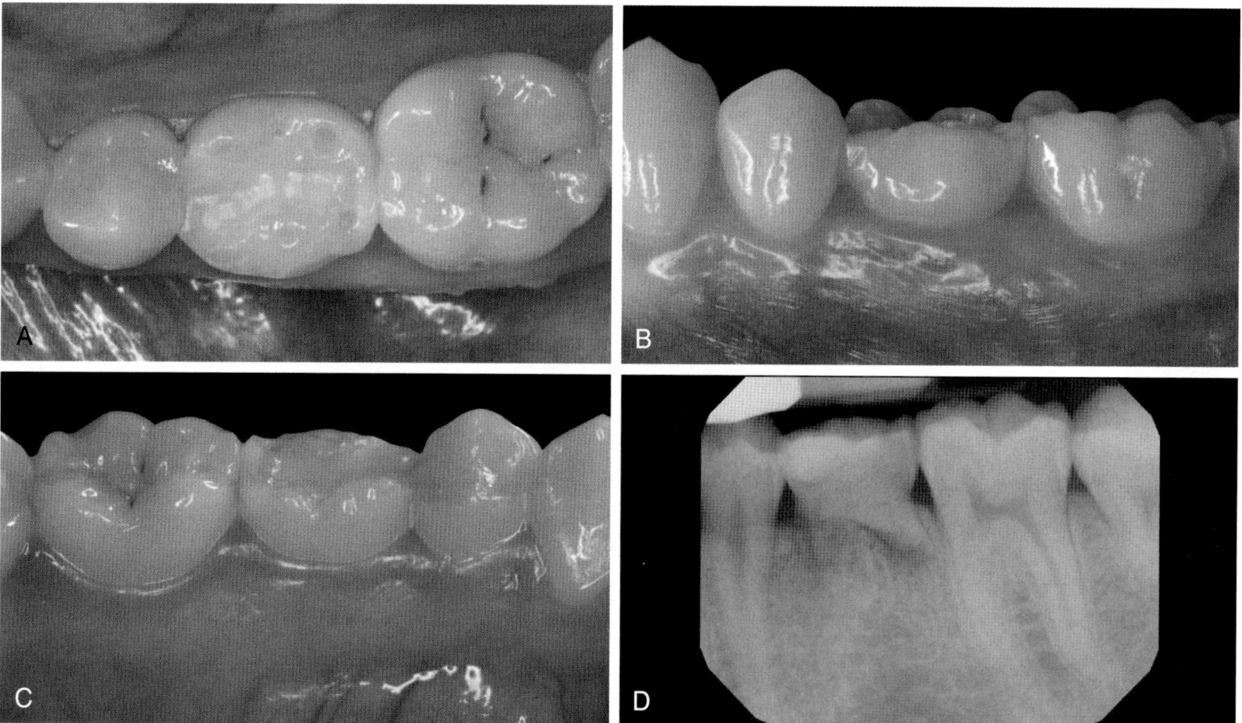

Fig. 85.25 Clinical preoperative views of deciduous tooth #K (A–C) that was deemed hopeless due to apical root resorption and apical pathosis (D).

point, changes to the abutment or provisional crown materials and design could be made, depending on the desired emergence profile, marginal finish line, interocclusal clearance, coronal contours, and screw-access location. Once the appropriate design of the abutment and a provisional crown was verified on the design software (Fig. 85.27A), manufacturing of the components ensued (see Fig. 85.27B). All components were sterilized prior to treatment.

After consent and local anesthesia were obtained, tooth #K was extracted, and the stereolithic, fully restrictive static tooth-supported guide was seated and verified for stability and fit (Fig. 85.28A and B). The implant osteotomy was completed sequentially according to the plan and following the protocol of the implant manufacturer (see Fig. 85.28C andD). After the osteotomy was completed restrictively through the guide, the implant fixture (Astra Tech Implant EV 4.2S, Dentsply Sirona, York, PA) was placed restrictively to proper depth and rotation by adhering to corresponding landmarks on the implant driver carrier and the landed portion of the stereolithic surgical guide platform (Fig. 85.29A and B). Upon verifying that adequate primary stability had been achieved, the CAD/CAM patient-specific abutment was verified to passively engage the implant body without obstruction from the peri-implant bone (see Fig. 85.29C and D). Subsequently, the screwmentable crown was seated on the abutment, and parameters such as marginal adaptation, proximal contact integrity, and occlusion were checked and adjusted where necessary (Fig. 85.30A and B). The abutment-crown complex was cemented with provisional cement (Integrity TempGrip, Dentsply

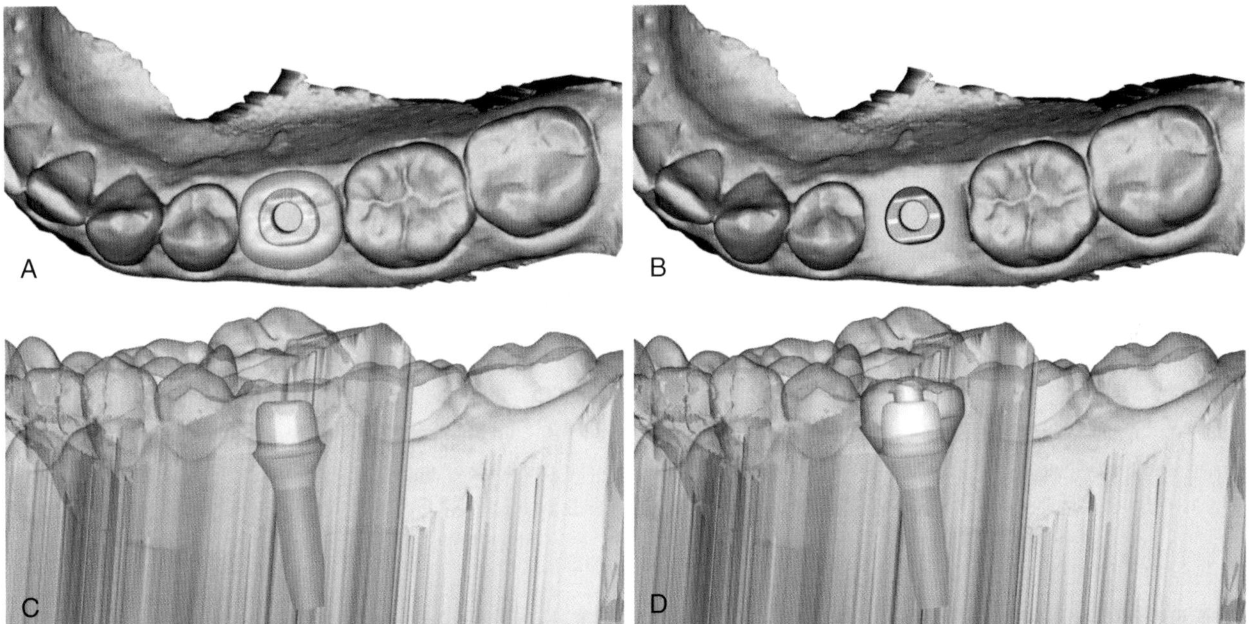

Fig. 85.26 Virtual superimposed occlusal view of the computer-aided design and computer-aided manufacturing (CAD/CAM) gold-shaded custom titanium abutment and screwmentable polymethylmethacrylate (PMMA) crown design (A), and solely the CAD/CAM abutment (B). Virtual buccal views of the same components demonstrate the relationship of the emergence profile, abutment margin design, and screw access channel location in the abutment-crown complex (C and D).

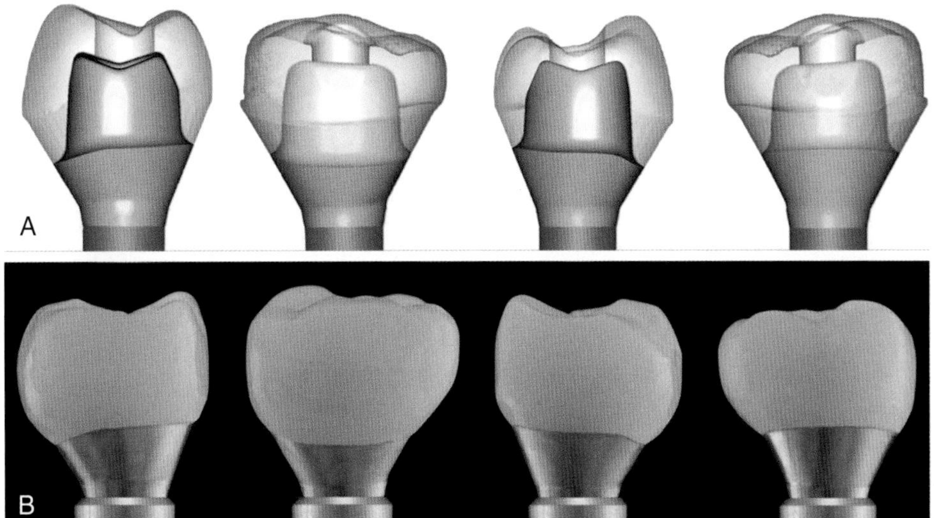

Fig. 85.27 A virtual rendering of the computer-aided design and computer-aided manufacturing (CAD/CAM) gold-shaded custom titanium abutment and overlying custom polymethylmethacrylate (PMMA) provisional crown (A). A view of the completed restoration complex after fabrication (B).

Sirona, York, PA) and cleaned extraorally. Then the peri-implant gap was filled with a particulate bone xenograft (Bio-Oss, Geistlich Pharma, Wolhusen, Switzerland), and the provisional restoration was torqued according to the manufacturer's recommendations. The screw channel was sealed with PTFE tape and resin composite (see Fig. 85.30C and D). Detailed postoperative instructions were provided to the patient regarding dietary and hygiene considerations, as well as potential complications to monitor.

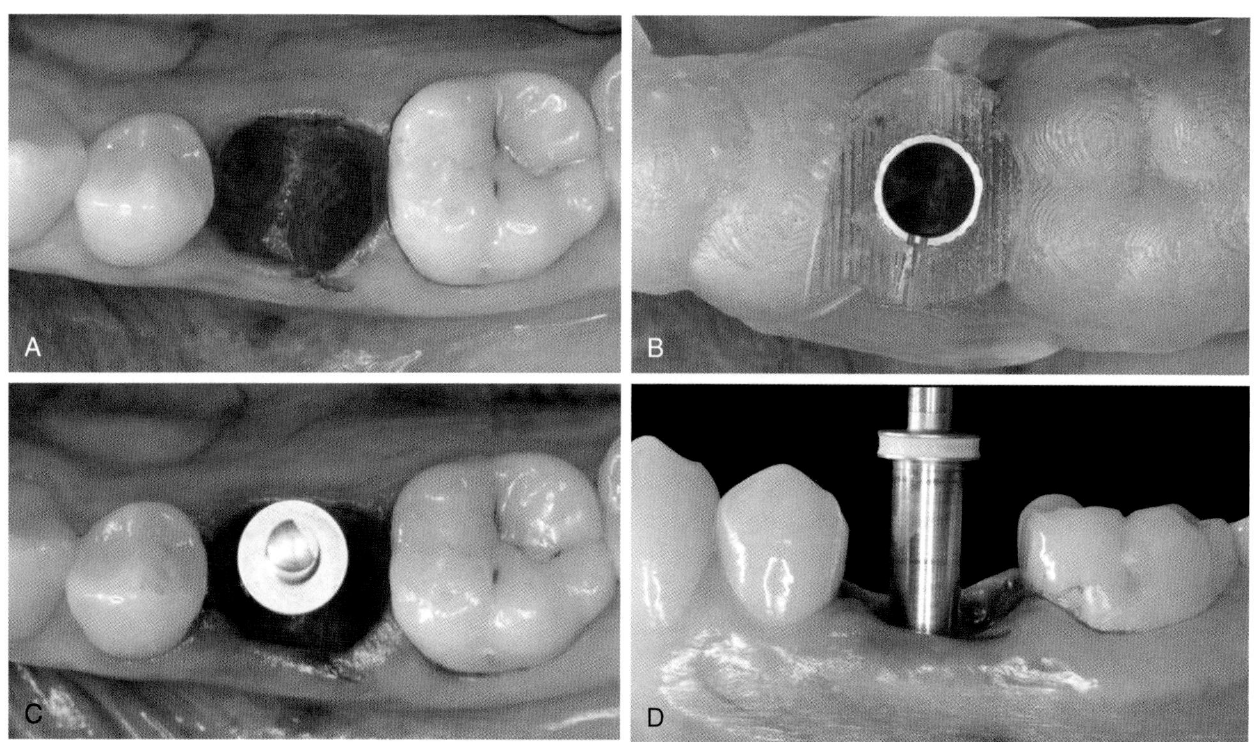

Fig. 85.28 Clinical image of the residual ridge immediately after extraction of #K (A) and subsequent seating of the fully restrictive static stereolithic surgical guide (B). Osteotomy drills correlating with the surgical guidance plan and guide were used to prepare the implant osteotomy (C and D).

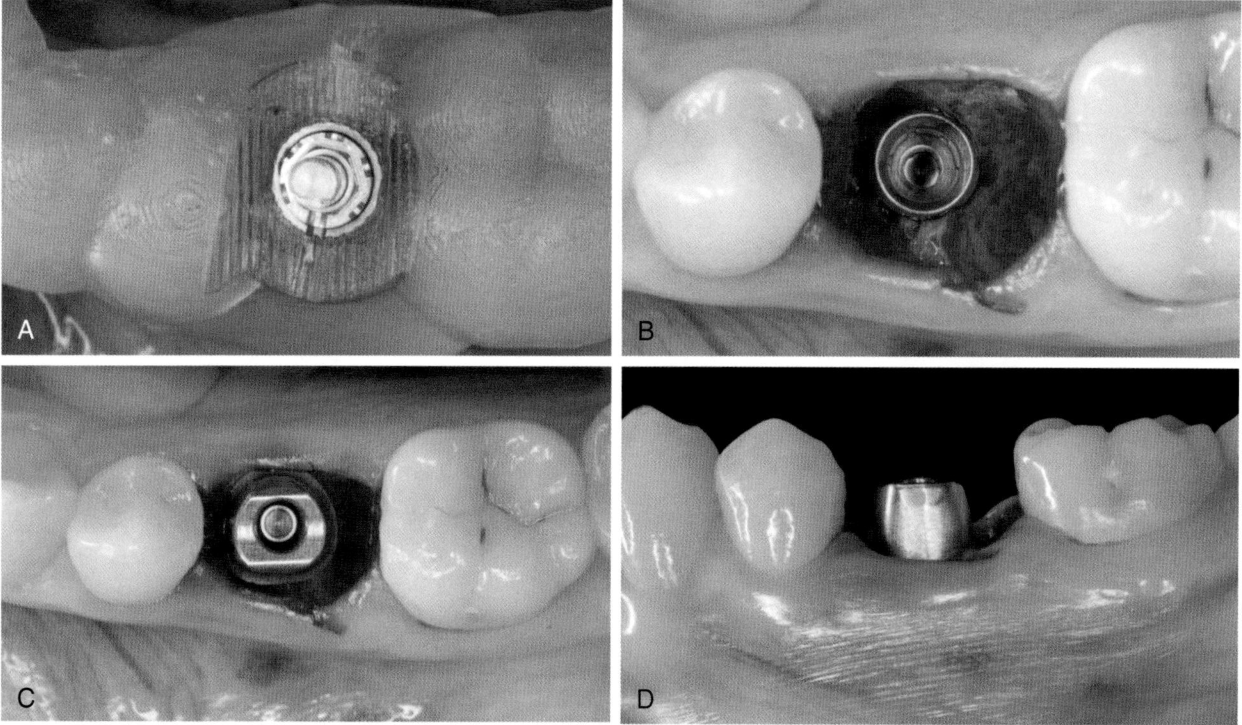

Fig. 85.29 The implant was placed fully restrictively through the stereolithic surgical guide to allow for specific rotational timing of the implant body (A and B). Proper adherence to rotational timing in fully restrictive digitally aided provisionalization is critical to enable proper orientation of the subsequent custom computer-aided design and computer-aided manufacturing (CAD/CAM) abutment (C and D).

Four months after fully restrictive immediate implant placement and immediate implant provisionalization were performed, stability of the peri-implant mucosa and prosthesis was verified clinically (Fig. 85.31). Radiographically, marginal bone levels were stable. A shade was selected, and the same STL file of the CAD/CAM abutment design and adjacent teeth utilized for fabrication of the provisional PMMA crown was again sent to the laboratory, with instructions for fabrication of a monolithic lithium disilicate (e.max, Ivoclar Vivadent)

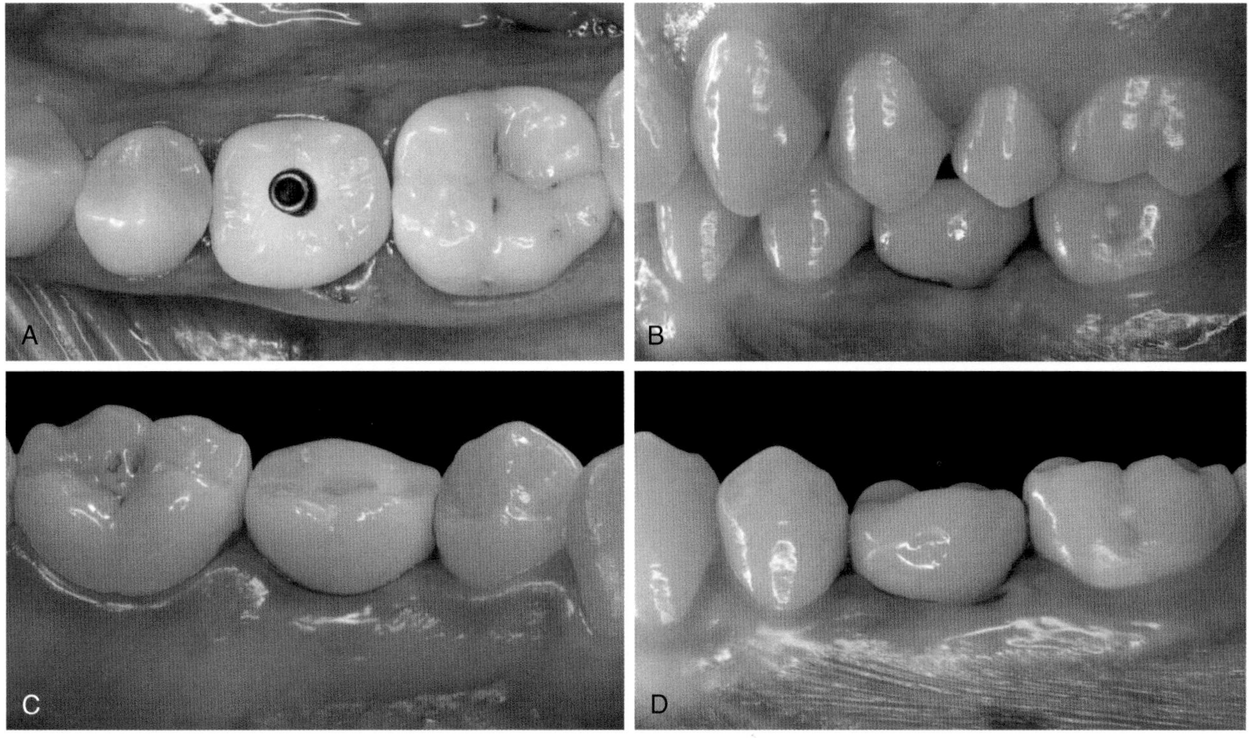

Fig. 85.30 The screwmentable digitally fabricated custom polymethylmethacrylate (PMMA) crown was verified to have proper fit on the computer-aided design and computer-aided manufacturing (CAD/CAM) abutment and subsequently luted with interim cement (A and B). Upon finalizing the prosthesis fit and occlusion, the abutment-crown complex was torqued according to the manufacturer's recommendations and sealed with polytetrafluoroethylene (PTFE) tape and resin composite (C and D).

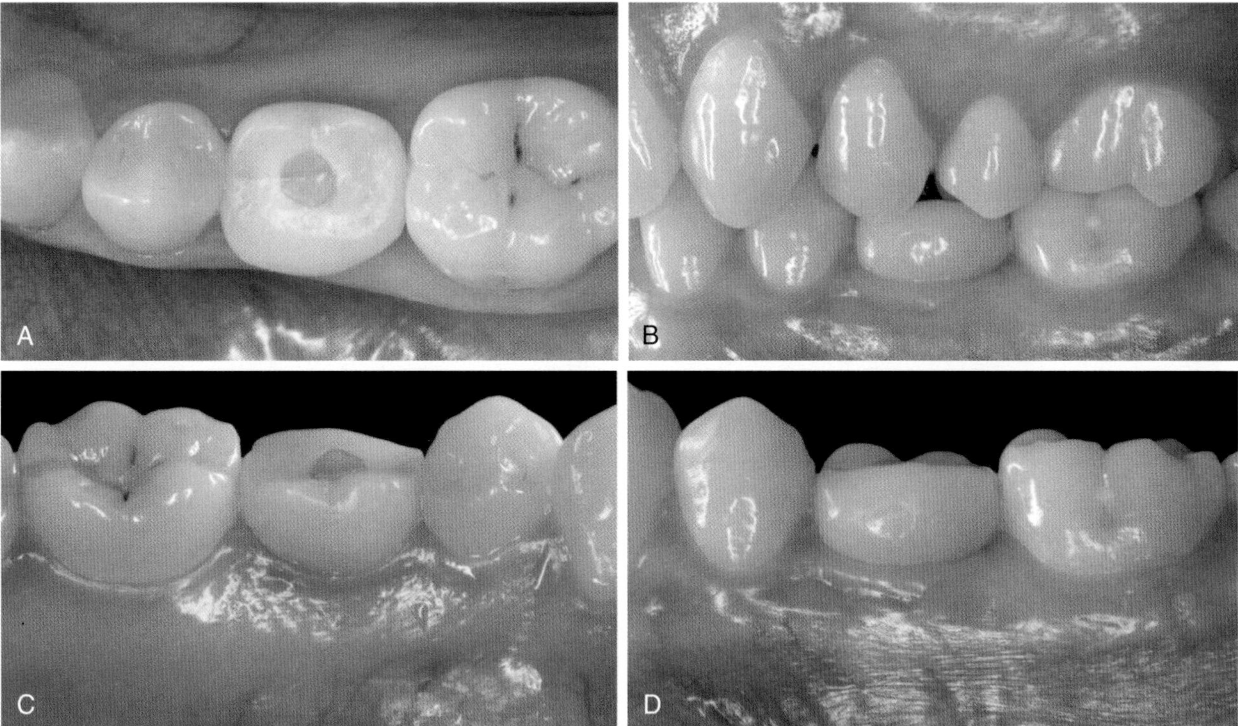

Fig. 85.31 Occlusal (A), functional (B), lingual (C), and buccal (D) views of the provisional restoration at 4-months post-immediate implant placement and immediate provisionalization.

screwmentable crown. As the peri-implant mucosal architecture, coronal form, and esthetics were found to be appropriate with the CAD/CAM abutment and provisional crown, the same STL file could be utilized. This negated the need for a new optical scan of either the implant or the abutment and also prevented an additional disturbance of the implant-abutment interface. A fully digital, model-less workflow was followed for the design and fabrication of the definitive crown (Video 85.7). In the event that either the abutment or crown design was not suitable insitu for the definitive restoration, a new implant or abutment-level scan could be completed to redesign and manufacture the requisite components. Two weeks later, the CAD/CAM abutment and provisional crown were removed, the definitive crown was seated clinically with the abutment, and functional and esthetic parameters were verified. The abutment-crown complex was joined with a definitive self-adhesive resin cement (Rely X Unicem2, 3M, Maplewood, MN), margins cleaned extraorally, and the complex disinfected ultrasonically prior to torquing the restoration to the manufacturer's recommended value and obturating the screw-access channel as previously described (Fig. 85.32A and B). At the one-year recall, stable peri-implant mucosa morphology and negligible levels of inflammation were observed (see Fig. 85.32C and D). A full radiographic sequence of treatment, from implant placement through to one-year recall, is presented (Fig. 85.33), demonstrating adequate marginal bone levels over time.

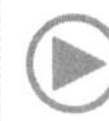

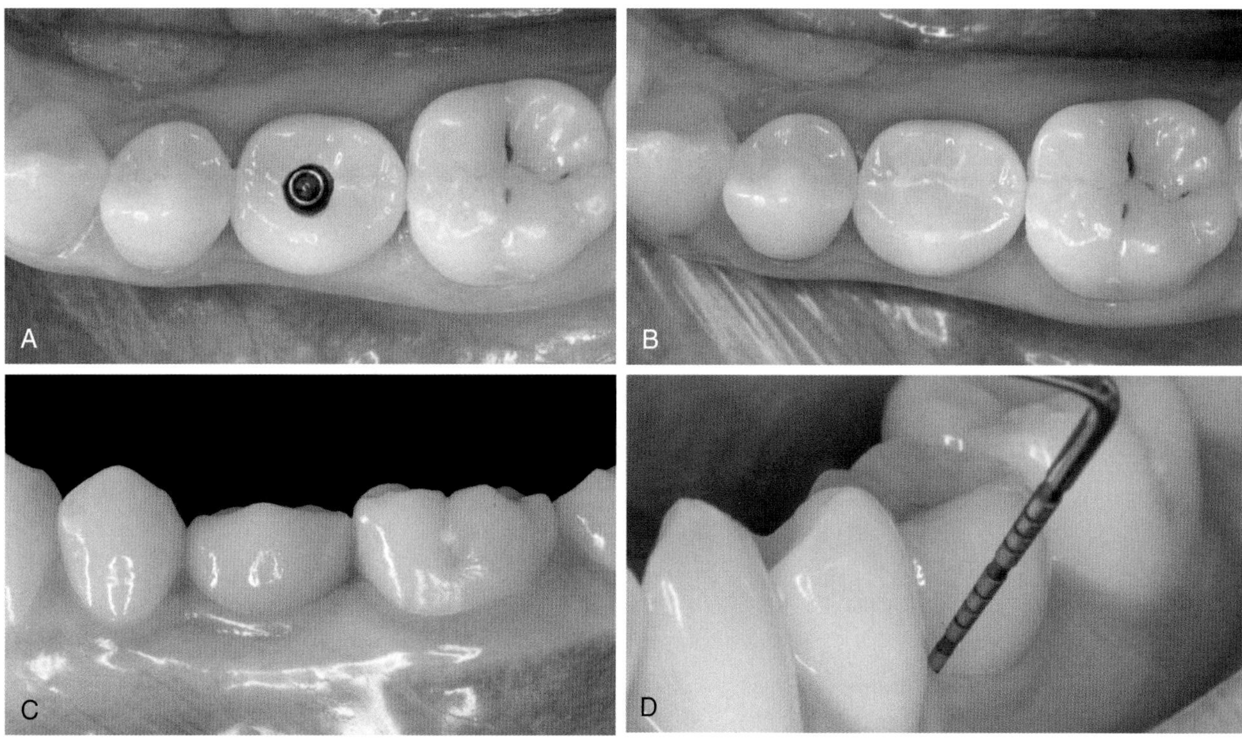

Fig. 85.32 Occlusal view of definitive restoration before (A) and after (B) closure with polytetrafluoroethylene (PTFE) tape and resin composite after verifying fit, occlusion, and contour of the restoration. One year after delivery, the buccal (C) and peri-implant mucosal stability (D) was noted to be free of inflammation and harmonious with the adjacent dentition.

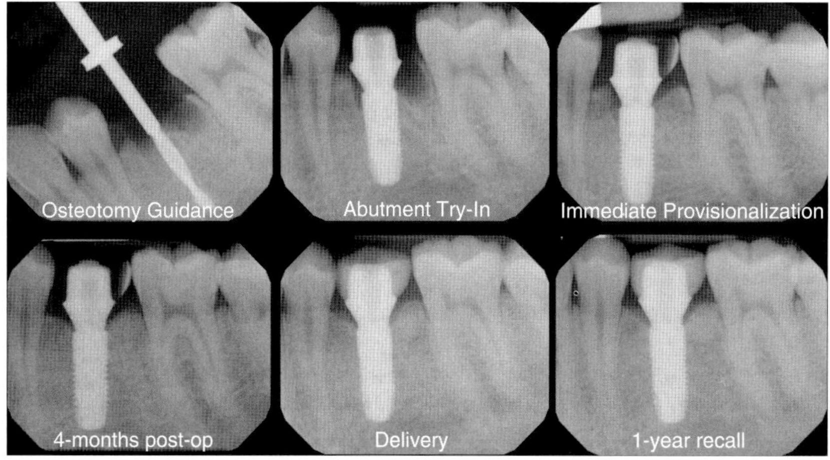

Fig. 85.33 Radiographic sequence of therapy for fully restrictive digitally aided provisionalization, demonstrating stable crestal bone levels at one-year post-provisionalization.

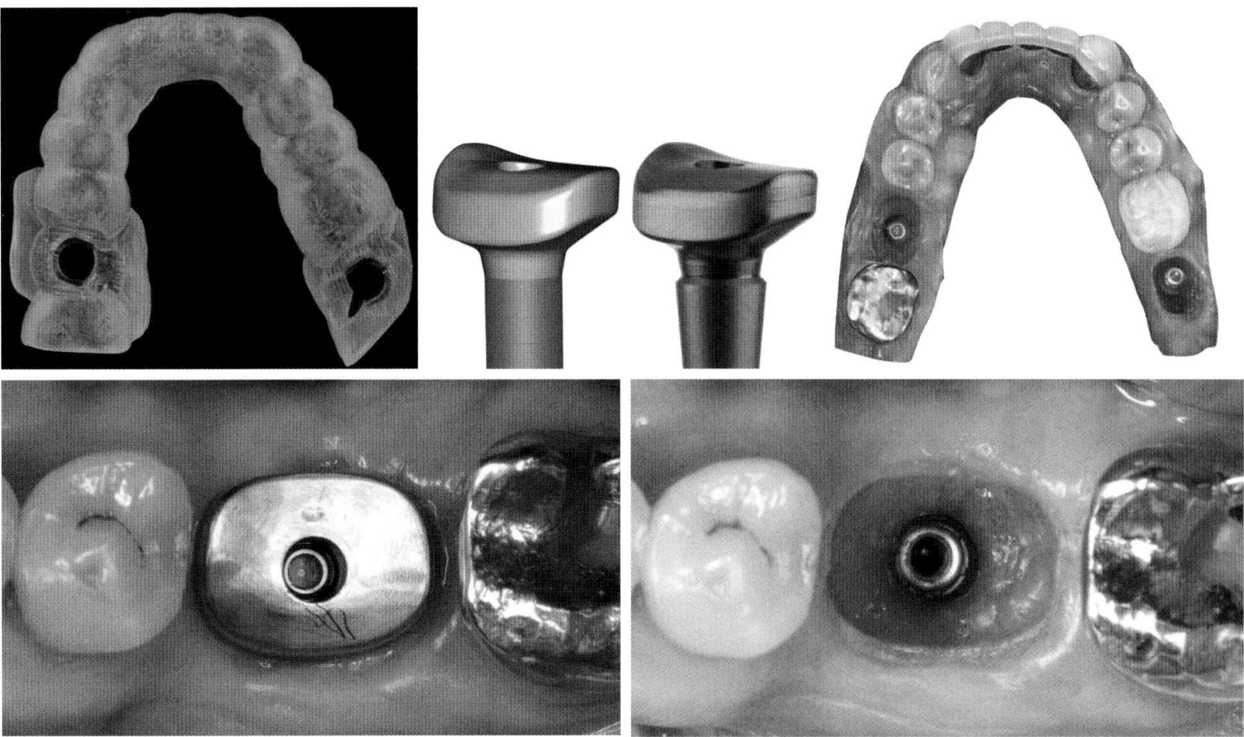

Fig. 85.34 A case-sequence example of the fully restrictive digitally aided custom healing abutment, which lacks a coronal restoration component. Such workflows allow for optimization of implant placement and maturation of the peri-implant mucosa with a custom computer-aided design and computer-aided manufacturing (CAD/CAM) healing abutment, but without the potential risks associated with a full-contour coronal provisional restoration.

Digitally Aided Implant Provisionalization: Alternative Approaches

When clinicians plan implant provisionalization, they may limit their treatment planning process to only consider the replacement of coronal form, function, and esthetics as a means of psychosocial support for the patient. However, an important benefit of implant provisionalization, whether digitally aided or analog, is the optimization of peri-implant soft tissue morphology to improve the design of the definitive restorative components and achieve an optimal esthetic outcome. Such treatment objectives can be achieved with digitally designed and manufactured custom healing abutments in clinical scenarios where conventional, full coronal provisionalization may not be feasible or may jeopardize healing and osseointegration of the implant or where patient compliance may be in doubt. Such workflows enable the achievement of an anatomically correct peri-implant sulcus without many of the potential risk factors at play in the aforementioned digitally facilitated provisionalization scenarios.[1,13,27,43] The design and fabrication methods for such custom CAD/CAM healing abutments vary between manufacturers but will predominantly be based, as summarized previously for digitally aided coronal provisionalization, on some form of computer-guided surgery. In the clinical example (Fig. 85.34), fully restrictive implant placement was planned for implants #19 and 31, and subsequent custom CAD/CAM healing abutments were designed and manufactured based on the desired emergence profile morphology for the future definitive molar-shaped restorations. As seen on the postoperative digital intraoral scan and clinical photograph (see Fig. 85.34), ideal peri-implant mucosal contours can be achieved without the need for a coronal component and can minimize error in the definitive CAD/CAM abutment design, as well as reduce discomfort for the patient during delivery of the final restoration.

Conclusions

Digital approaches and workflows to facilitate implant provisionalization offer the interdisciplinary team flexibility in choosing what level of restriction and customization is appropriate based on their preferences and the presenting clinical scenario(s). As the clinical examples highlight, *digitally aided implant provisionalization* provides the opportunity to customize and accelerate treatment outcomes for patients, providing psychosocial and esthetic benefits while optimizing the peri-implant mucosal architecture. Emerging digital workflows also enable clinicians to provide customized CAD/CAM transmucosal healing abutments that provide some of the benefits of digitally fabricated provisional restorations without the risk of premature loading.

Suggested Reading

Abdel Raheem IM, Hammad IA, Abel Kader SH, Fahmy RA. Fabrication of a CAD-CAM custom healing abutment guided by a conventional dental radiograph for delayed loaded dental implants: a dental technique. *J Prosthet Dent*. 2022;127(1):49–54.

Barwacz CA, Hernandez M. Maximizing esthetics of fixed interim restorations via direct extrinsic characterization. *JCD*. 2013;29:122–131.

Barwacz CA, Summerwill M, Avila-Ortiz G. Leveraging digital workflows for immediate single-tooth replacement therapy: a case report. *Int J Oral Implantol (Berl)*. 2021;14:321–333.

Chen P, Nikoyan L. Guided implant surgery: a technique whose time has come. *Dent Clin North Am*. 2021;65:67–80.

Chu Kan JY, Lee EA, et al. Restorative emergence profile for single-tooth implants in healthy periodontal patients: clinical guidelines and decision-making strategies. *Int J Periodontics Restorative Dent*. 2019;40:19–29.

Hartman MJ. A workflow to design and fabricate a customized healing abutment from a dynamic navigation virtual treatment plan. *Compend Contin Educ Dent*. 2021;42:86–92.

Kaewsiri D, Panmekiate S, Subbalekha K, Mattheos N, Pimkhaokham A.

The accuracy of static vs. dynamic computer-assisted implant surgery in single tooth space: a randomized controlled trial. *Clin Oral Implants Res*. 2019;30:505–514.

Putra RH, Yoda N, Astuti ER, Sasaki K. The accuracy of implant placement with computer-guided surgery in partially edentulous patients and possible influencing factors: a systematic review and meta-analysis. *J Prosthodont Res*. 2021.

Tattan M, Chambrone L, González-Martín O, Avila-Ortiz G. Static computer-aided, partially guided, and free-handed implant placement: a systematic review and meta-analysis of randomized controlled trials. *Clin Oral Implants Res*. 2020;31:889–916.

Van Assche N, Vercruyssen M, Coucke W, Teughels W, Jacobs R, Quirynen M. Accuracy of computer-aided implant placement. *Clin Oral Implants Res*. 2012;23(suppl 6):112–123.

Younes F, Cosyn J, De Bruyckere T, Cleymaet R, Bouckaert E, Eghbali A. A randomized controlled study on the accuracy of free-handed, pilot-drill guided and fully guided implant surgery in partially edentulous patients. *J Clin Periodontol*. 2018;45:721–732.

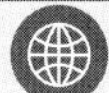

References for this chapter are found on the companion website eBooks.Health.Elsevier.com.

CHAPTER 86

Complications in Dental Implantology

Stuart J. Froum | Perry R. Klokkevold | Sang Choon Cho | Scott H. Froum | Marco Bergamini | Natacha Reis | Adam Barsoum

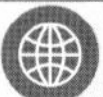
For online-only content on complications related to augmentation procedures and to placement and loading protocols, please visit the companion website at eBooks.Health.Elsevier.com.

CHAPTER OUTLINE

Dental implants, because of documented high long-term success rates have become an often used option for replacement of single or multiple hopeless or missing teeth.[6,162] A systemic review of implants supporting single crowns showed survival rates of 97.2% at 5 years, and 95.2% at 10 years.[140] Two other studies of restorations supported by single or multiple implants documented cumulative implant survival rates of 82.6% up to 15 years and 82.94% up to 16 years, respectively.[8,243]

Despite the long-term predictability and success of dental implants, implant-related complications and failures happen in some cases.[7,43] Complications can be classified as minor, intermediate, major reversible/nonreversible, or major nonreversible. A minor complication (i.e., fractured abutment screw) can be corrected with minimal cost, time, pain, and inconvenience. A major reversible complication (i.e., an implant migrating into the maxillary sinus floor) can be reversed with an increase in cost, time, pain, and inconvenience. A major complication (i.e., damage to the inferior alveolar nerve during implant placement causing neurosensory problems) may or may not be reversed but oftentimes can result in permanent sensory problems for the patients.[94] Complications can be surgical, biologic, mechanical, or esthetic. The most serious complications can result in failure of prostheses, loss of implants, and severe loss of supporting bone and soft tissue.

Surgical complications are those problems or adverse outcomes that result from surgery, including procedures used for implant site development, implant placement, implant exposure, and tissue augmentation. Implant complications commonly arise from placement of an implant in a nonideal position. Malpositioned implants, which usually result from poor preoperative treatment planning or errors in surgical technique, can lead to an array of implant problems ranging in severity from minor to major. Surgical complications include compromised esthetic and prosthetic results, soft tissue and bone dehiscences, impingement on and damage to anatomic structures, and implant failure. Unfortunately, the problems that arise from implant malposition are often not recognized until after osseointegration, when the prosthesis is being fabricated.

Biologic complications involve the hard and soft tissues that support the implant. Peri-implant tissue changes can be limited to inflammation of surrounding soft tissues or be more significant, such as progressive loss of supporting bone. The ultimate biologic complication is implant loss or failure, which can produce soft and hard tissue defects. Loss of implants can be caused by failure to achieve osseointegration in the early stages before restoration or by loss of osseointegration as a result of destruction of supporting bone after the restoration is installed and functioning.

Prosthetic or *mechanical complications* and failures typically occur in the form of material failure, such as abutment and prosthetic screw loosening or fractures. The prosthesis can be rescued from many mechanical problems if they are minor and recognized early. However, some complications, such as implant fractures, are devastating and not salvageable.

Esthetic complications arise when the patient's expectations are not met. Satisfaction with the esthetic outcome of the implant prosthesis varies from patient to patient. The risk of esthetic complications is increased among patients with high esthetic expectations and suboptimal patient-related factors, such as a high smile line, thin gingival tissues, or inadequate bone quantity and quality.

This chapter reviews common implant-related complications. A summary of the literature offers some insight into the prevalence of implant-related complications. Implant failure and surgical complications related to site development and variations in implant placement protocols are discussed.

Definitions of Implant Survival and Success

The criteria used to define and report implant success or failure can vary substantially among publications. Selection of success criteria can be based on the author's preference, study population, or some other study objective. Because the level of success reported in an article is based on the criteria used to define success, recognizing the tremendous variation in the way investigators measure and interpret success is crucial. Sometimes, outcomes are measured by the presence or absence of implants at the time of the last examination, which is a measure only of implant survival and should not be confused with implant success. In contrast to this simplified reporting, some investigators use detailed criteria to measure implant success and failure, with variations of successful outcomes separated and defined by additional criteria. A Consensus Conference proposed a Health Scale for Dental Implants which contains four categories: (1) success (optimum health), (2) satisfactory survival, (3) compromised survival, and (4) failure (clinical or absolute failure) to further make the distinction between implant success and survival.[176]

Implant survival is defined as an implant that remains in place at the time of evaluation, regardless of any untoward signs, symptoms, or history of problems. There is a difference between implants that are functioning under an implant-retained restoration and those that are not connected to a restoration and not providing support or function. These implants are sometimes referred to as sleepers, and they should not be considered successful merely because they remain osseointegrated. Sleeper implants instead should be included in the discussion as surviving but counted as *failures* because they did not fulfill the originally intended treatment objective.

Implant success is defined by the presence of the implant and the criteria evaluating its condition and function at the time of examination. Various criteria for implant success and failure have been published, but not all investigators agree with or use them. In the classic definition, Albrektsson and colleagues[14] defined success as an implant with no pain, no mobility, no radiolucent peri-implant areas, and no more than 0.2 mm of bone loss annually after the first year of loading. Roos-Jansaker and associates[218] added to this by defining a successful implant as one that loses no more than 1 mm of bone during the first year of function.

Sometimes, the criteria are used as proposed, but in other cases, they are used by investigators with modifications and additional criteria. This makes it difficult to compare studies and draw conclusions about any aspect of implant success or failure based on one or a few studies.

Strictly defined, implant success is any implant-retained restoration in which (1) the original treatment plan is performed as intended without complications, (2) all implants that were placed remain stable and functioning without problems, (3) the peri-implant hard and soft tissues are healthy, and (4) the patient and treating clinicians are pleased with the results. When these strict criteria are used, the rate of implant success (i.e., absence of complications) is only about 61% after 5 years for implant-supported fixed partial dentures (FPDs) and 50% after 10 years for combined tooth–implant FPDs.[160]

An additional criterion of implant success that is not typically reported but should be considered is the esthetic success or patient satisfaction with the outcome. Several methods have been proposed to evaluate esthetic results. A restorative index was proposed by Jensen and coworkers[133] to appraise the esthetics of the final restoration. The index uses a scale of 1 to 10, with 1 being an extremely poor result and 10 being a superlative esthetic result. Based on subjective and objective criteria, the index evaluates the size and shape of the implant restoration compared with the equivalent contralateral tooth, how well it blends into the arch, and the papillae, gingival form, color, and other factors considered essential in determining an esthetic result. The pink esthetic score is an index proposed by Furhauser and colleagues[101] that considers seven soft tissue parameters, including evaluation of the color, contour, and texture of the surrounding soft tissues (i.e., papilla and facial mucosa). Each parameter is given a score of 0, 1, or 2, which allows the best score of 14 to determine the highest level of esthetics.

Other indices were proposed for single-tooth implant restorations in the esthetic zone.[33,172] Proposed by Belser and colleagues,[33] one index combines a modified pink esthetic score with a white esthetic score that focuses on the visible part of the implant restoration. Scoring includes five parameters: general tooth form, hue, value, surface texture, and translucency. The maximum white esthetic score is 10. These indices are aimed at quantifying the esthetic result, which can provide an objective method of judging implant esthetic success.

KEY FACT

Implant survival indicates that the implant has become osseointegrated but does not consider associated problems. An implant that is not restored can be included in survival percentages while failing to fulfill its intended purpose. *Implant success* is defined by criteria evaluating the condition and function of the implant. Because different criteria have been used to define implant success, it is difficult to make comparisons between studies and often impossible to make conclusions about implant success or failure based on only one or a few studies.

Types and Prevalence of Implant Complications

The prevalence of implant-related complications has been reported in several reviews. However, a systematic review of the incidence of complications in studies of at least 5 years' duration revealed that biologic complications were considered in only 40% to 60% and technical complications in only 60% to 80% of the studies. The review found that the incidence of technical complications related to implant components and suprastructures was higher for overdentures than for fixed restorations.[35]

In a systematic review of reports on the survival and complication rates of implant-supported FPDs, Lang and associates[160] found that the most common technical complication was fracture of veneers (13.2% after 5 years), followed by loss of the screw access hole restoration (8.2% after 5 years), abutment or occlusal screw loosening (5.8% after 5 years), and abutment or occlusal screw fracture (1.5% after 5 years and 2.5% after 10 years). Fracture of implants occurred infrequently (0.4% after 5 years and 1.8% after 10 years).

A retrospective evaluation of 4937 implants by Eckert and colleagues[74] found that implant fractures occurred more frequently in partially edentulous restorations (1.5%) than in restorations of completely edentulous arches (0.2%), and all observed implant fractures occurred with commercially pure 3.75-mm-diameter threaded implants.

In a literature review that included all types of implant-retained prostheses, Goodacre and colleagues[106] found that the most common

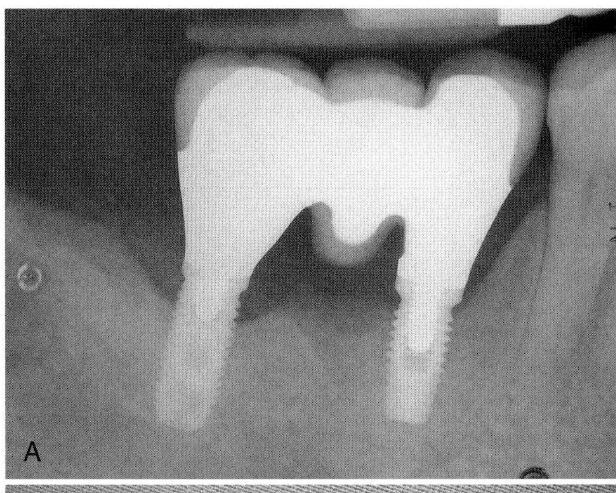

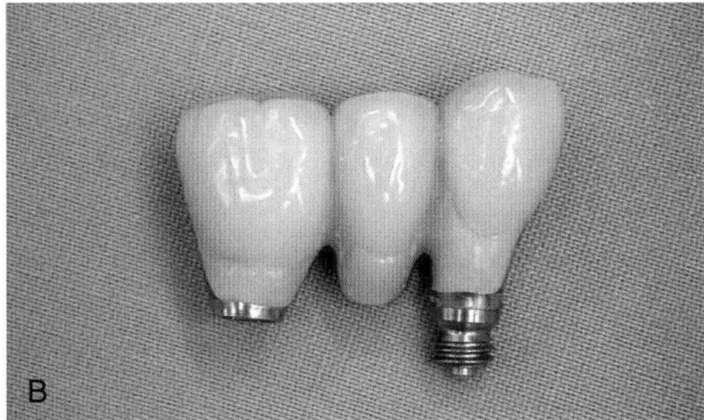

Fig. 86.1 (A) Radiograph of a three-unit, posterior, fixed partial denture supported by two standard-diameter, screw-shaped threaded implants. Notice the long crown height, relatively short implant length, and bone loss around the posterior implant. (B) Photograph of the ultimate implant-supported restoration failure. The anterior implant fractured between the second and third threads, which resulted in loss of the restoration.

technical complications were loosening of the overdenture retentive mechanism (33%), resin veneer fractures with FPDs (22%), overdentures needing to be relined (19%), and overdenture clip or attachment fracture (16%). With the inclusion of edentulous patients having overdentures, their review seemed to indicate a significantly higher percentage of complications than Pjetursson's systematic review[201] of patients with implant-supported FPDs. Goodacre and associates[105] found it impossible to calculate an overall prosthesis complication rate because most studies included in their review did not report several of the complication categories.

The most common complication reported for single crowns was abutment or prosthesis screw loosening. The rate of abutment screw loosening varied dramatically from one study to another, ranging from 2% to 45%.[106] The highest rate of abutment screw loosening was associated with single crowns, followed by overdentures. The rate of prosthesis screw loosening was similar, ranging from 1% to 38% in various studies. A higher frequency was reported for single crowns in the posterior areas (i.e., premolar and molar) than in the anterior region. However, one must note that in the review of Goodacre,[105] 11 of the 13 studies on screw or overdentures loosening used external hex implants.[14,17,19,20,33,45,62,68,69,73,74,87,126] In the same review, the reported failure rate of internal hex implants was 0.9%.[87]

Implant fracture is an uncommon but significant complication. Goodacre and colleagues[105] reported a 1.5% incidence in their literature review. The incidence of implant fracture was higher in FPDs supported by only two implants. Consistent with this finding, Rangert and coworkers[209] reported that most implant fractures occurred in single- and double-implant–supported restorations. They also found that most of these fractures were in posterior partially edentulous segments, in which the generated occlusal forces can be greater than in anterior segments (Fig. 86.1). The data on the percentage of implant fracture is too heterogenous to cite true statistics.[105] Most studies conclude that fracture of implants with greater than 4.0-mm diameter is rare. All other fractures involved 3.75-mm implants of different types (standard, self-tapping, and conical), and different lengths. There were no fractures of 4-mm-diameter implants reported.[209] An article in 2000 concluded that an implant 1 mm wider in diameter will increase surface area by 20% to 30%.[61] In 2007, Albrektsson et al. gathered data for a multicenter study and found 3.5-mm implants had a failure rate of 11.8%, while the 4.3-mm-diameter implants had a failure rate of 2.8%.[12] In 1997, it was concluded that "the increase in diameter decreases the risk of fracture to the power of 4."[177]

In a systematic review of prospective longitudinal studies (i.e., minimum of 5 years' duration) reporting biologic and technical complications associated with implant therapy (i.e., all restoration types included), Berglundh and collegues[35] found that the incidence of technical complications was consistent with Pjetursson's findings, with implant fracture occurring in less than 1% (0.08% to 0.74%) of cases. Consistent with the findings in Goodacre's review, technical complications were higher for implants used in overdenture therapy than implants supporting fixed prostheses.

In Lang and associates' systematic review[160] of survival and complication rates for implant-supported FPDs, biologic complications such as peri-implantitis and soft tissue lesions occurred in 8.6% of patients after 5 years. In a later literature review of the prevalence of peri-implant diseases, Zitzmann and Berglundh[283] reported that although cross-sectional studies were rare, data from the only two studies available showed that peri-implant mucositis occurred in 80% of patients and 50% of implant sites. Peri-implantitis was identified in 28% and 56% or more of patients and in 12% and 43% of implant sites in the two studies that followed patients with functional implants for at least 5 years.

A critical review of the literature by Esposito and associates[85] included 73 publications reporting early and late failures of Brånemark implants; biologically related implant failures were relatively low at 7.7%. Treatments involved all anatomic areas and all types of prosthetic design. The study authors concluded that the predictability of implant treatment was especially good for partially edentulous patients compared with totally edentulous patients; failures in the latter population were twice as high as those in the other group. The incidence of implant failure was three times higher for the edentulous maxilla than for the edentulous mandible, whereas failure rates for the partially edentulous maxilla were similar to those for the partially edentulous mandible.

Risk factors such as smoking, diabetes, and periodontal disease can contribute to implant failure and complications. Several studies with numerous implants and years of follow-up have concluded that smoking is a definite risk factor for implant survival.[22,69,70,77,187] A systematic review of the effect of risk factors on implant outcomes concluded that smoking had an adverse effect on implant survival and success; the effects were more pronounced in areas of loose trabecular bone (i.e., posterior maxilla).[152] The review suggested that type 2 diabetes could have an adverse effect on implant survival rates but did not have enough studies to permit a definitive conclusion.[152] The same review concluded that although patients with a history of treated periodontitis did not show a decrease in implant survival, they did experience more biologic implant complications and lower success rates, especially with longer-term follow-up.[152,219]

Planning to Avoid or Minimize Complications

Prior to placement of implants a thorough dental and medical history should be taken as part of the treatment-planning phase (see Chapter 74). The patient usually presents with a chief complaint of having to replace missing or hopeless teeth. A complete medical history including any current or past systemic diseases the patient has/had and medications the patient is currently taking should be documented. A medical consult, if necessary, with the patient's physician should follow to obtain medical clearance for the surgery planned and whether any of the medications currently being taken (anticoagulants, immunosuppressants, or bone metabolic altering medications such as bisphosphonates) require alteration before implant surgery. If the patient is able to stop any of these medications prior to surgery or if any modification of the duration of the drug therapy is required it should be made by his/her physician. Once medical clearance is obtained a full examination of the mouth, head, and neck, as well as evaluation of any pathology present (i.e., caries, periapical pathology, periodontal conditions, temporomandibular disorder) should be treated prior to implant placement.

Planning for implant placement should begin with taking impressions of both jaws. A radiographic stent should then be made on an ideal wax up on the model of the jaw. The stent should have radiopaque markers (e.g., gutta-percha, composite, or barium sulfate) on the incisal edge, central fossae, and gingival third to allow proper positioning of the implant platform (see Chapter 75). A cone-beam computed tomography (CBCT) scan should be taken while the patient is wearing the stent. A CBCT scan is essential for implant placement, a recent study reported that periapical radiography overestimated and underestimated bone measurements 60% of the time when compared to CBCT when evaluating ridge height in the posterior maxilla with a range of −1.7 mm to +2.1 mm.[143] A virtual implant planning software (e.g., SimPlant) should be used to simulate the exact three-dimensional (3D) position of the implant. A surgical guide should then be fabricated to assist in implant placement during the surgery. With the advent of digital scanners, 3D printers and milling machines, a digital impression can be transferred to the planning software and overlaid on the DICOM file from the CBCT scan to fabricate CBCT-derived surgical guides that assist surgeons in osteotomy preparation and implant placement. The deviation of position of the implant neck was reported in the literature from in vivo and in vitro studies to range from 0.3 to 1.2 mm between the planned and executed position.[36,227,265,266] Therefore, while the use of surgical guides can aid the surgeon during implant placement, surgical experience and expertise is necessary as modification of the planned positions may be needed if the bone quality or quantity differs from what was anticipated from the CBCT scan. As with any surgical procedure informed consent of the possible complications and different outcomes of treatment need to be discussed with the patient and recorded in the form of written consent. A recent study examined claims from 2005 to 2015 and reported 66.3% of claims against dentists were due to unplanned changes to the treatment plan.[4]

Surgical Complications

As with any surgical procedure, implant surgery has risks. Proper precautions must be taken to prevent injuries, including (1) a thorough review of the patient's medical history, (2) a comprehensive clinical and radiographic examination, (3) establishment of a comprehensive interdisciplinary treatment plan, and (4) good surgical techniques.

Intraoperative surgical complications include perilous bleeding/hemorrhage, damage to adjacent structures such as teeth, injury to nerves, displacement into adjacent spaces, swallowing or aspiration, implant malposition, cortical plate perforation, and iatrogenic jaw fracture. Postoperative surgical complications include bleeding/hemorrhage, hematoma, swelling/edema, infection, and emphysema.[16,44] They may be minor, transient, and easily managed or more serious and require postoperative treatment.[94]

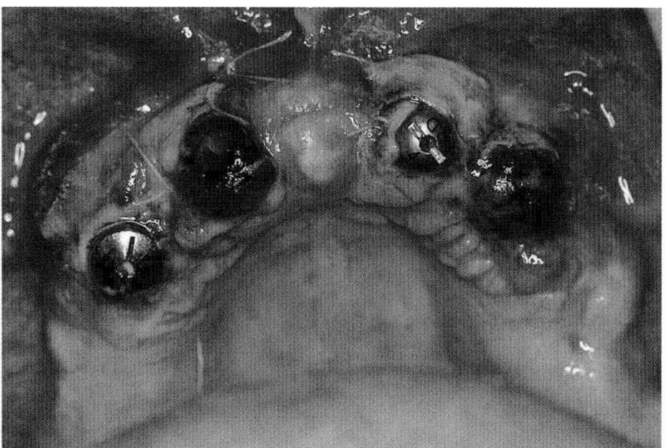

Fig. 86.2 Clinical photograph of postoperative bleeding around healing abutments after second-stage implant exposure surgery.

Hemorrhage and Hematoma

Bleeding during surgery is expected and usually easily controlled. However, if a sizable vessel is incised or otherwise injured during surgery, the hemorrhage can be difficult to control. Smaller vessels naturally constrict or retract to slow the hemorrhage. If bleeding continues, it may be necessary to apply pressure or suture the hemorrhaging vessel. Cauterizing the hemorrhaging vessel also may be warranted. This can be especially difficult if there is a vascular injury to an artery that is inaccessible, such as in the floor of the mouth or posterior maxilla. Serious bleeding from an inaccessible vessel can be life-threatening, not by exsanguination but rather as a result of airway obstruction. This is most problematic when the point of bleeding is inaccessible and internal (i.e., in connective tissues and soft tissue spaces).

Postoperative bleeding is an equally important problem to manage (Fig. 86.2). Patients should be given postoperative instructions on normal expectations for bleeding and how to prevent and manage minor bleeding. Historically, standard practice is that they should be advised, with their physician's approval, to discontinue or reduce medications that increase bleeding tendency 3 to 10 days before surgery. However, recent evidence suggests that this may not be necessary and may increase the risk of hematologic or cardiovascular problems[134,135,187,221] (see Chapter 67). Moreover, it is important to understand that there are other risk factors that could affect intraoperative and/or postoperative bleeding, such as taking dietary supplements (garlic, vitamin E, magnesium, selenium, coenzyme Q10, glucosamine, vitamin A complex, fish oil, *Ginkgo biloba*, ginseng, and ginger) due to their interfering in the coagulation process.[111]

Dental health care providers should consult with medical health care providers regarding the best management for each patient. Dental health care providers and patients should always include the treating medical practitioner in management decisions if postoperative bleeding is excessive or persistent.

Submucosal or subdermal hemorrhage into the connective tissues and soft tissue spaces can result in hematoma formation. Postoperative bruising is a typical example of minor submucosal or subdermal bleeding into the connective tissues (Fig. 86.3). Bruising and small hematomas typically resolve without special treatment or consequence. However, larger hematomas or those that occur in

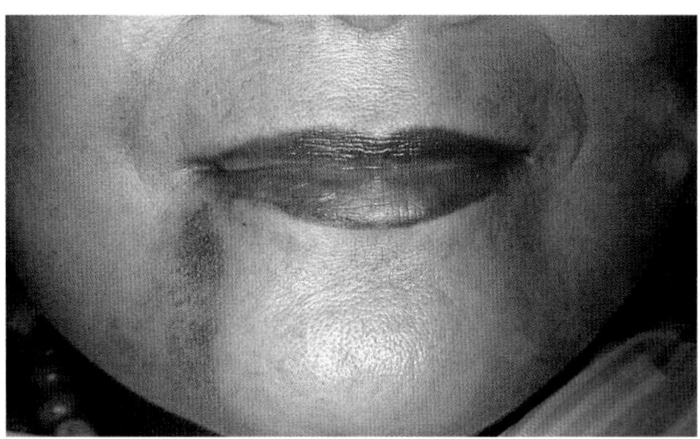

Fig. 86.3 Clinical photograph of postoperative (extraoral) bruising indicative of subdermal bleeding into connective tissue spaces. This is a normal expectation that resolves in 7 to 14 days.

medically compromised individuals are susceptible to infection as a result of the noncirculating blood that sits in the space. It is prudent to prescribe antibiotics for patients who develop a noticeably large hematoma. Referral to the appropriate medical physician may be warranted for nonresolving hematomas.[126]

Although the incidence of a life-threatening hemorrhage[261] from implant surgery is extremely low, the seriousness of the problem warrants the attention of everyone who participates in this type of surgery. Potentially fatal complications have been reported for implant surgical procedures in the mandible, especially the anterior region.[29,64,66,90,127,191,193,253] Massive internal bleeding in the highly vascular region of the floor of the mouth can result from instrumentation or implants that perforate the lingual cortical plate and sever or injure the arteries running along the lingual surface. Depending on the severity and location of the injury, bleeding may become apparent immediately or only after some delay. In either case, the progressively increasing hematoma dissects and expands to displace the tongue and soft tissues of the floor of the mouth, ultimately leading to upper airway obstruction.

Emergency treatment includes airway management (primary importance) and surgical intervention to isolate and stop the bleeding. Clinicians must be aware of this risk and be prepared to act quickly. It is important to recognize that bleeding, although considered a complication at the time of surgery, can become a serious complication in the hours and days after surgery.[66]

CLINICAL CORRELATION

Although the incidence of a life-threatening hemorrhage from implant surgery is extremely low, it is a serious problem that can occur. Implant surgical procedures in the anterior mandible have been associated with potentially fatal complications. Massive internal bleeding in the floor of the mouth from inadvertent injury to lingual arteries can cause an expanding hematoma that displaces the tongue and soft tissues, obstructing the upper airway. Emergency treatment includes airway management and surgical intervention to isolate and stop the bleeding. Clinicians must be aware of this risk and be prepared to act quickly.

Damage to Adjacent Structures

When performing implant surgery adjacent to teeth or implants, there is always a risk of injuring these by drilling through the tooth/implant, by placing the implant in direct contact with the tooth/implant, or even indirectly by overheating the bone. If this occurs, these adjacent teeth/implants may be damaged and require further treatment. In case of direct contact between tooth and implant, the implant should be immediately removed to avoid further complications. To prevent these complications, preoperative treatment planning should be performed, a CBCT scan used, and intraoperative surgical guides, made from an ideal wax-up or laboratory (if guided surgery is planned) should be used. In addition, when performing implant surgery in the posterior mandible injury can occur to the sublingual salivary gland by penetration of the drill or implant. This can result in a ranula formation. This complication can be avoided by preoperative treatment planning including analysis of CBCT scans and use of surgical guides intraoperatively.[44,56,178]

Displacement Into Adjacent Spaces

During implant surgery, there is a risk of migration of implants into adjacent spaces such as sinuses, nasal floor, anterior cranial fossa, and mandibular medullary space (Figs. 86.4A–C and 86.5). In this situation, implant removal from the space should be immediately performed, but if not possible the patient should be referred to an oral maxillofacial or head and neck surgeon.[44,95]

Swallowing or Aspiration

Intraoperatively, swallowing or aspiration of foreign objects can occur during implant surgery. In case of aspiration, the foreign object will be located in the respiratory tract and if it is blocking the airway the patient will start coughing, choking, wheezing, or develop hoarseness, with dyspnea and cyanosis. This can result in a life-threatening situation, or if the foreign body remains in the lungs can cause a future infection. In case of ingestion, the foreign object will be located in the digestive tract and usually patients are asymptomatic. It can become a life-threatening situation if the foreign object is not removed, causing inflammation, obstruction, perforation, and/or infection in the gastrointestinal tract. In both cases, after the occurrence, the patient should be sent to the hospital for chest and abdominal radiographs. The best way to prevent this occurrence is to use gauze as a throat pack and attach dental floss (whenever possible) to small instruments and have a clear and illuminated surgical area.[57,95,108,178]

Neurosensory Disturbances

One of the more problematic surgical complications is neuropathic injuries. Neurosensory alterations caused by damage to a nerve may be temporary or permanent. Neuropathy can be caused by a drilling injury (i.e., cut, tear, or puncture of the nerve), by implant compression, or damage to the nerve including transection of the nerve during incision or suturing[141] (see Fig. 75.25; and Figs. 86.6 and 86.7). According to the literature, implant-related surgeries are the second most common cause of neurosensory alterations after impacted third molar removal.[124,163] Nerve injury causes neuroma formation, and different patterns of clinical neuropathy may occur including hypoesthesia, anesthesia, dysesthesia, and neuralgia. *Hypoesthesia* is a neuropathy defined by impaired sensory function that is sometimes associated with phantom pain. *Anesthesia* consists of an absence of sensation for the affected subject. *Dysesthesia* is a neuropathy defined by pain with minimal or no sensory impairment.[110] Neuralgia is defined as a spontaneous or evoked abnormal paroxysmal pain. Some of these neuropathies resolve, whereas others persist. The recovery depends upon the degree of injury and upon the time of diagnosis.[200,237] For several reasons, it is likely that neurosensory disturbances occur more frequently after implant surgery than is reported in the literature. First, many of the changes are transient in nature, and most patients recover completely or at least recover to a level that is below a threshold of annoyance or daily perception. Second, wide variation exists in the postoperative evaluation of patients by clinicians. Some clinicians do not assess

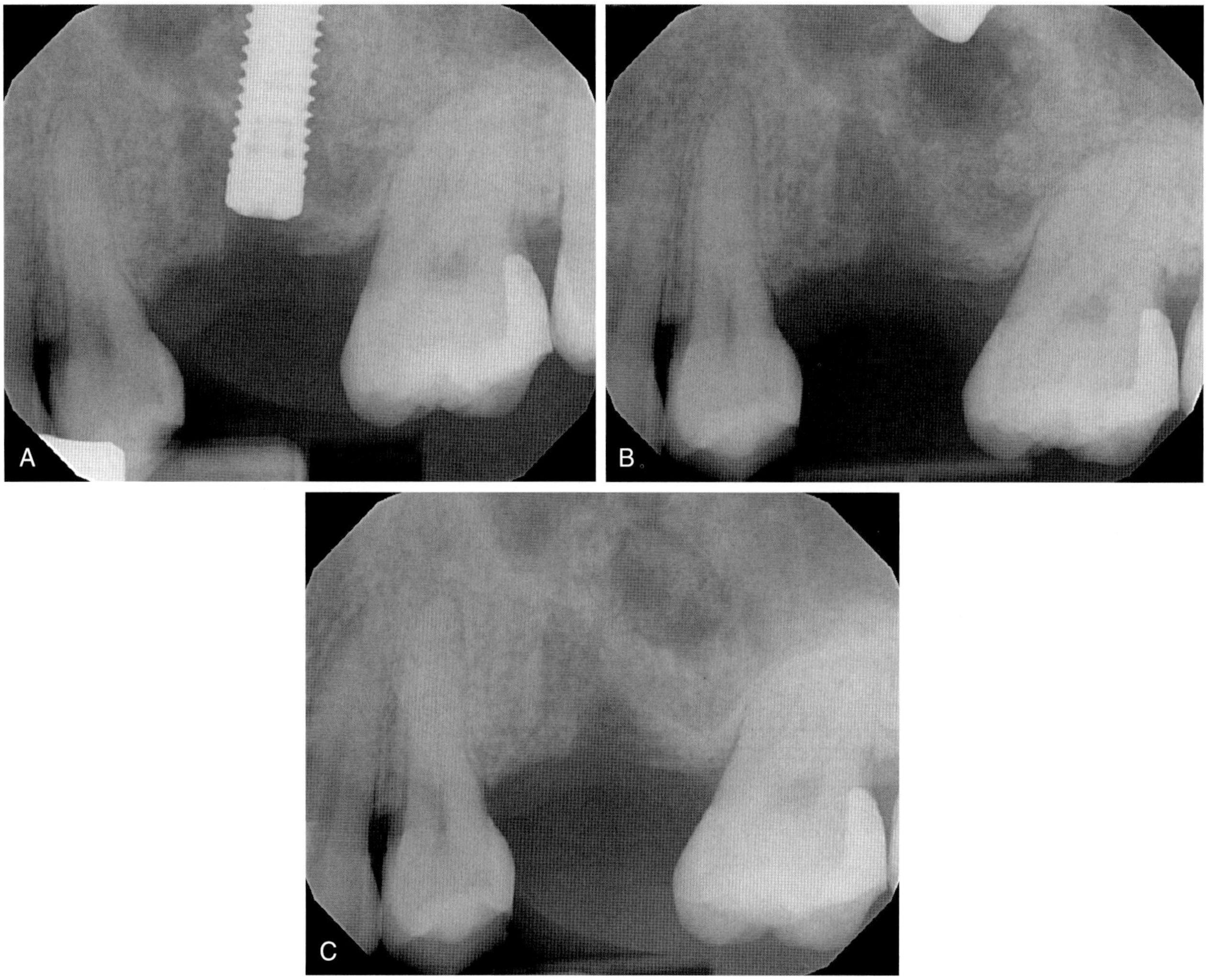

Fig. 86.4 (A) Sinus augmentation with simultaneous implant placement. (B) Implant displaced into the maxillary sinus. (C) Implant was removed from the maxillary sinus through the lateral window.

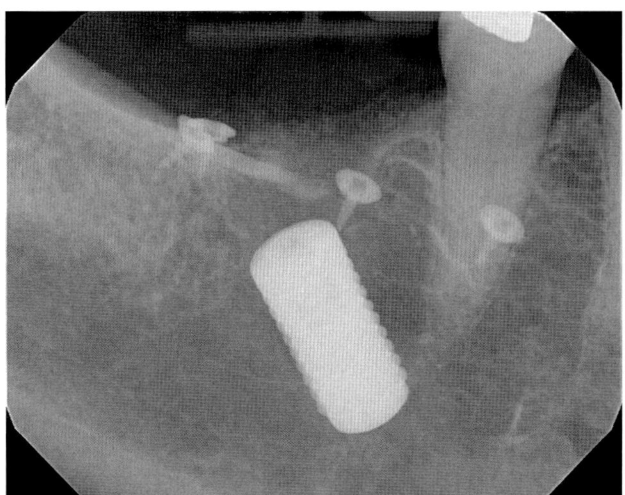

Fig. 86.5 After implant placement and guided bone regeneration, implant was displaced into the mandibular medullary bone.

or inquire about postsurgical neurosensory disturbances, allowing this complication to go unnoticed. Likewise, some patients expect altered sensation as part of surgery and may never acknowledge or comment on its presence, especially if the disturbance is minor. It is therefore likely that minor neuropathies exist but go unrecognized and unreported.[2,119,267]

According to a systematic review of inferior alveolar nerve injuries after implant placement, the importance of early diagnosis and treatment is considered essential for preventing long-term, permanent neurologic problems.[9] If a diagnosis is established and treatment is rendered within the first 36 hours, a high percentage of successful outcomes can be achieved. An estimated 25% of patients with iatrogenic paresthesia suffer permanent effects.[148]

Neurosensory disturbances reported in the literature are most significant when they are more serious and occur more frequently, such as those associated with lateral transposition of the mandibular nerve.[131,144,268] This relatively uncommon procedure is used to reposition the nerve and allow longer implants to be placed in the atrophic posterior mandible. Lateral nerve transposition procedures are associated with an almost 100% incidence of neurosensory dysfunction immediately after surgery. According to some studies, more than 90% of the nerve injuries have transient change in sensation and increased possibility of recovery.[3] Nevertheless, some other reports mentioned that more than 50% (range, 30% to 80%) of these neurosensory changes are permanent.[144] Different treatment modalities for neurosensory disturbances are reported in the literature. The treatment depends upon injury type, injury timing, type of neurosensory disturbances, and intraoperative findings.[141] Some authors report that pharmacologic therapy might be beneficial in minimizing neuropathy with nonsteroidal antiinflammatory drugs (NSAIDs) or adrenocorticosteroids.[117,142,157] In addition, several researchers and clinicians evidenced positive outcomes of early implant removal (i.e., within the first 24 to 36 hours after implant placement).[148,149] The results showed that the removal of the endosseous implants may lead to a physiologic return of sensation. Hence, if neurologic disturbances occur, early removal of the implant is always the suggested treatment of choice.

Implant Malposition

Many of the complications that arise during implant surgery can be attributed to the dental implant being placed in an undesired or unintended position. Malpositioning of dental implants is usually the result of poor treatment planning before surgery, lack of surgical skill, and/or lack of execution between the surgical and restorative phases of implant dentistry. Optimal implant esthetics and the avoidance of positional complications can be achieved by placing the implant in a prosthetically driven manner.[173,194] The ideal placement of an implant should be placed with reference to the three dimensions dictated by the position and emergence profile of the final restoration, not by the availability of bone.[86]

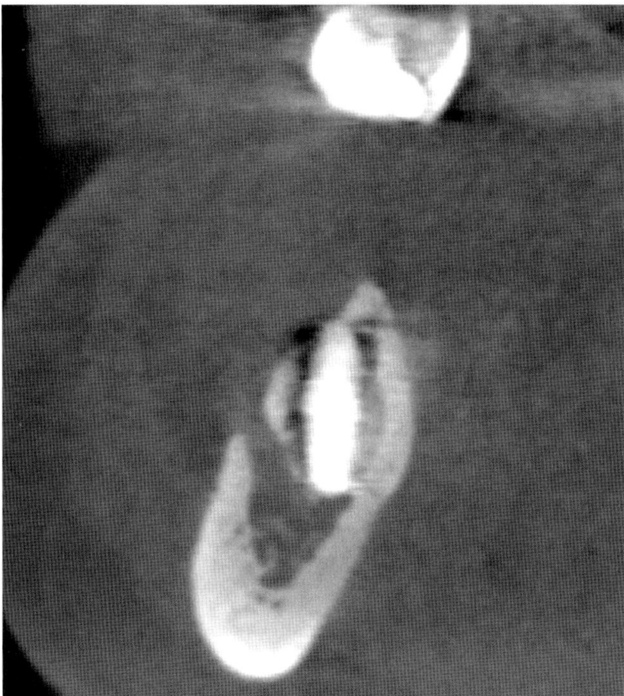

Fig. 86.6 Cone-beam computed tomography cross-sectional image of an incorrect implant placement encroaching on the inferior alveolar nerve canal near the mental foramen.

Angulation is another important determinant of implant position that affects outcome esthetics. The ideal implant position entails an accurate preparation, insertion, and placement into the alveolus in a proper 3D geometry according to apicocoronal, mesiodistal, and buccolingual parameters and implant angulation relative to the final prosthetic restoration and gingival margins[153,222] (see Chapter 78).

Apicocoronally, the implant should be placed so the platform is about 3 to 4 mm apical to the zenith of the gingival margin of the anticipated restoration.[42] If the platform is placed at or above the level of the gingival margin, the metal collar or implant exposure can occur, yielding an unesthetic result (Fig. 86.8). If the implant has a roughened surface or the exposed metal collar is damaged, this may act as a nidus for biofilm deposition leading to inflammation of the proximal tissues. If the implant platform is placed too far apically, a long transmucosal abutment will be necessary to restore the implant. This can lead to a deep pocket and difficult hygiene access for the patient and clinician. This deep pocket can also result in cement retention during implant insertion if the case is going to have a cementable restoration.[189]

The implant should be placed at a distance of 1.5 to 2 mm from an adjacent natural tooth and 2 to 3 mm from an adjacent implant to maintain an adequate biologic dimension of width.[113] Similar to natural teeth, violation of biologic width around an implant can lead to bone loss.[123] In addition, dental implants that are placed too close to each other (Fig. 86.9) or to natural teeth can be difficult to restore (Figs. 86.10 and 86.11). Restoring implants placed in close proximity to adjacent teeth or implants may require modification of proximal crowns, impression copings, and impression-taking techniques.[239]

Embrasure form can be compromised leading to the inability to perform adequate hygiene and can invariably lead to chronic inflammation and peri-implantitis.[78,260] Conversely, an implant placed at an excessive distance from an adjacent tooth or implant may require prosthetic compensation in the form of mesial or distal cantilevers which can predispose the implant to biologic (i.e., bone loss) and mechanical (i.e., screw loosening,[106] screw fracture,[257] and implant fracture[209]) complications and difficulties with hygiene.[260]

Ideally, an implant should be placed buccolingually so there is at least 2 mm of bone circumferentially around it.[246] Implant exposure

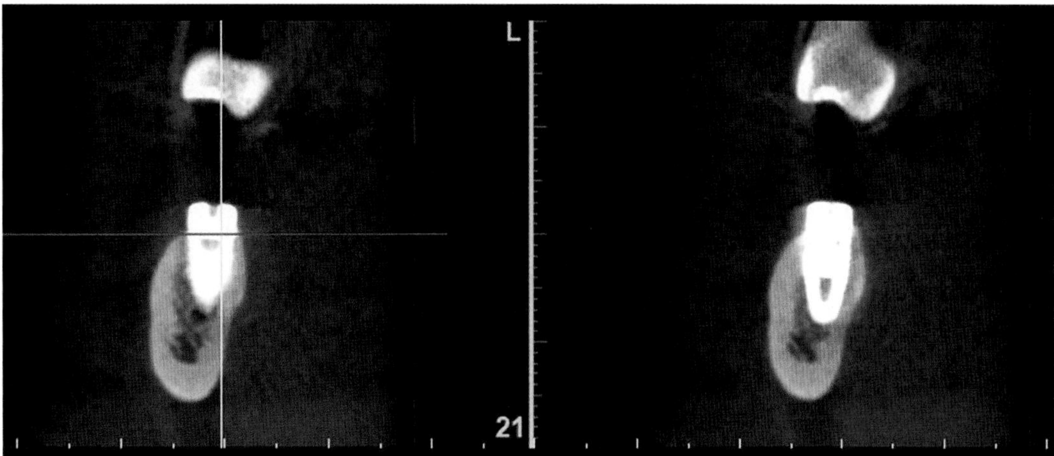

Fig. 86.7 Cone-beam computed tomography cross-sectional images of an implant placement violating the inferior alveolar nerve canal space.

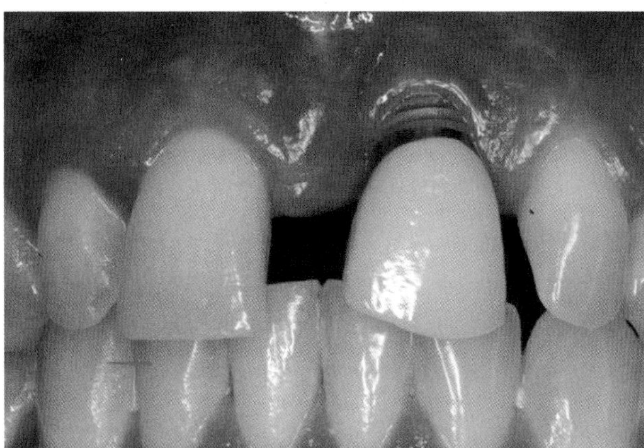

Fig. 86.8 Clinical photograph of gingival recession and implant exposure around a maxillary anterior implant (left central incisor) that was placed too coronal relative to the desired gingival margin resulting in exposure of the crown margin, the implant collar, and several threads of the implant.

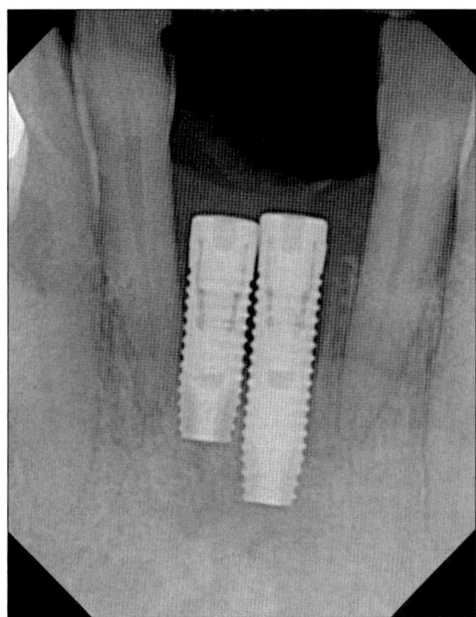

Fig. 86.9 Radiograph of two mandibular anterior implants placed too close together (i.e., no proximal space), resulting in implants that are impossible to restore.

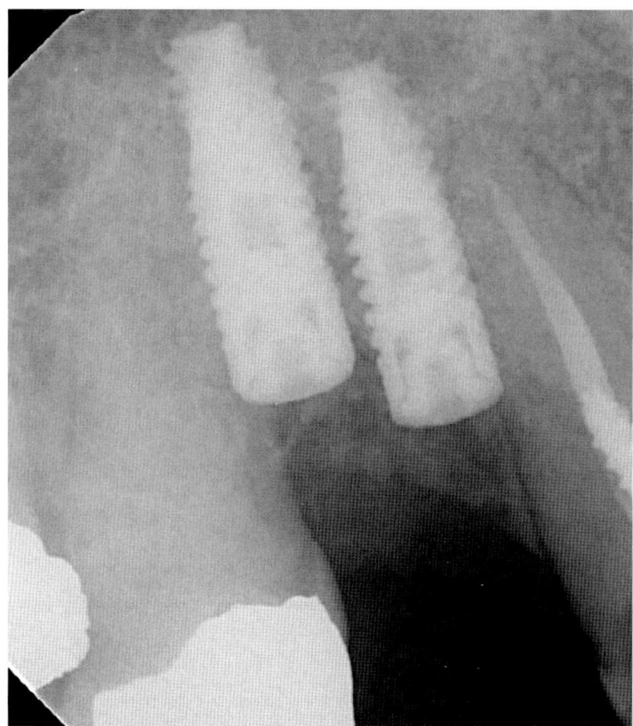

Fig. 86.10 Two implants were placed in the space of one not respecting the three-dimensional rule of implant placement.

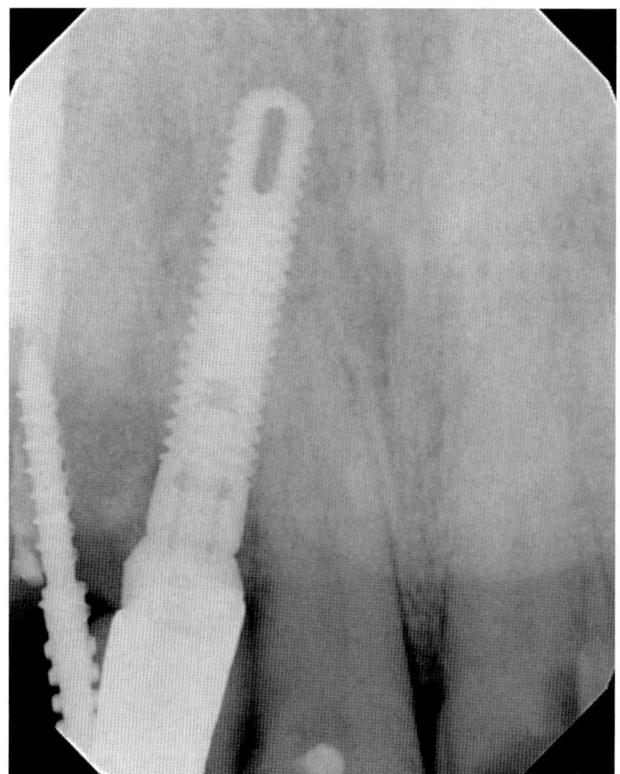

Fig. 86.11 Implant placement with wrong angulation and too close to the root of adjacent tooth.

through the lingual or buccal cortex can predispose an individual to abscess and suppuration.[53] Implants that are placed too palatally or lingually require prosthetic compensation in the form of a buccal ridge lap, which may be difficult for the patient to clean and can lead to tissue inflammation.[32]

To obtain ideal esthetics, to avoid potential esthetic complications, and to correct bodily placement of the dental implant, it must be correctly angulated on insertion. Insertion angulation is dependent upon whether the restoration will be screw-retained or cemented. In most anterior cases, it is desirable to have the long axis of the implant directed so it is emerging toward the cingulum in cases where the prosthesis will be screw-retained. In cementable cases, the long axis of the implant should be directed anywhere from the restorative cingulum to the incisal edge. In the posterior region, the implant axis should be directed toward the central fossa or the stamp cusp of the opposing tooth. Implants that are placed with mild to moderate misangulations can often be corrected prosthetically with implant abutments. Minor misangulations (i.e., 15 to 20 degrees) can be corrected with prefabricated or customized angled abutments; moderate misangulations (i.e., 20 to 35 degrees) can usually be managed with customized UCLA-type abutments or intermediate abutments; and extreme errors in implant angulations

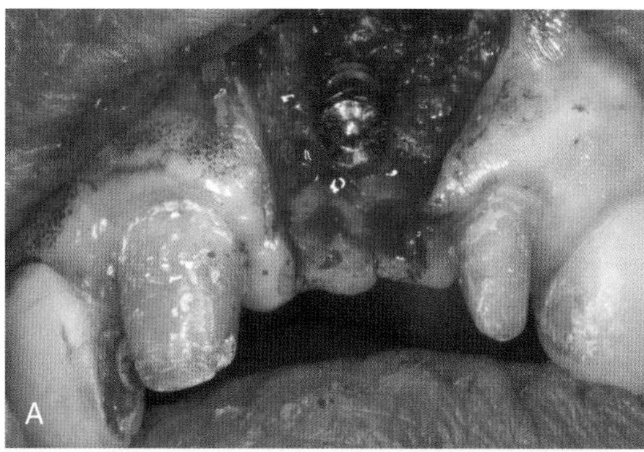

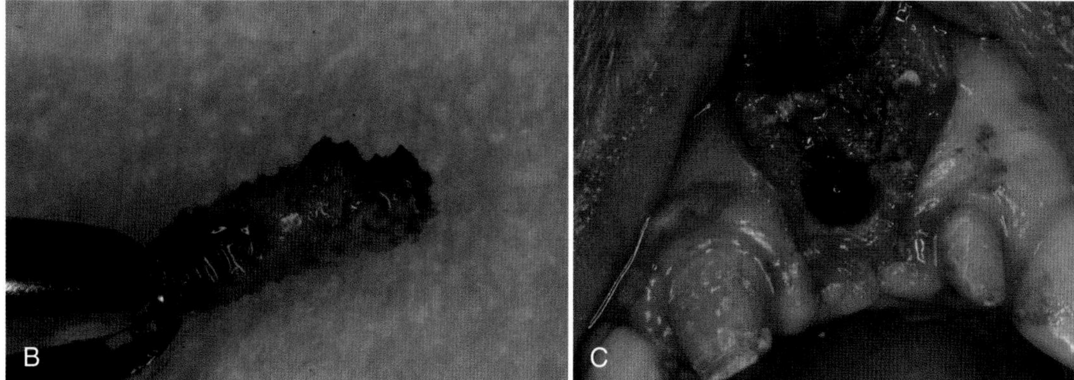

Fig. 86.12 Clinical photograph of a maxillary anterior implant (i.e., left central incisor) placed with an extreme facial angulation, resulting in an implant that emerges through the gingiva at a level that is more apical than the adjacent natural tooth gingival margins. (A) Surgical exposure of the malpositioned implant. (B) Surgically removed implant. (C) Alveolar defect resulting from surgical removal of the malpositioned implant.

(>35 degrees) may make an implant unrestorable and require it to be left submerged (i.e., a sleeper) or be removed (Fig. 86.12).

The ultimate complication of malpositioning is implant or instrument invasion into vital structures. The most common violation of neighboring anatomy is placement of the dental implant into the adjacent tooth root. Surgical procedures used to prepare osteotomy sites and place implants adjacent to teeth can injure them by directly cutting into the tooth structure or by damaging nearby supporting tissues and nerves. Instrumentation (e.g., drills) directed at or near the adjacent tooth can injure the periodontal ligament, tooth structure, and nerve of the tooth. Depending on the extent of the injury, the tooth can require endodontic therapy or extraction.

On insertion, dental implants follow the trajectory of the osteotomy prepared by the drill. Care must be taken when preparing the osteotomy to stay true to the planned path of insertion. Lateral correction of an improperly prepared osteotomy can be accomplished with the use of a Lindemann side-cutting bur.[109]

Radiographs taken periodically during implant surgery with a guide pin in the osteotomy site can greatly reduce the potential for damaging adjacent teeth (see Fig. 75.18). Radiographic analysis before implant surgery should include detection of curved, convergent, or dilacerated root structures of adjacent teeth that can limit implant placement.

Particular care must be taken when placing implants in the mandible so as to not encroach on the inferior alveolar canal or the mental foramen (see Chapter 59). Encroachment on the mandibular canal or mental foramen during osteotomy or implant placement by direct contact or mechanical compression of bone can injure nerves and blood vessels. Paresthesia, hypoesthesia, hyperesthesia, dysesthesia, or anesthesia of the lower lip, skin, mucosa, and teeth can result, as can arterial or venous bleeding.[107] The reported incidence of sensory disturbances after mandibular implant placement is 0% to 40%.[27,148]

In the maxilla, care must be taken to avoid dental implant perforation into the maxillary sinus or nasal cavity. Displacement of the entire dental implant into the maxillary sinus cavity may require a Caldwell-Luc procedure for retrieval. See online material for complications related to sinus bone augmentation.

The risks of surgery always exist, but the complications can be minimized by an understanding of the causes and with proper diagnosis and treatment planning. Three-dimensional imaging (i.e., computed tomography [CT] and cone-beam CT [CBCT]) provides the surgeon with useful preoperative information for diagnosis and treatment planning (see Chapter 75). Careful surgical exposure for direct visualization and identification of the mental nerve are indicated. The surgeon should establish a *zone of safety* and keep instrumentation and implants a safe margin (≥2 mm) away from the nerve.[107]

KEY FACT

Malpositioned implants can be avoided by proper planning, good communication, and meticulous surgical skills. Radiographs taken periodically during implant surgery with guide pins in the osteotomy site can greatly reduce damage to adjacent teeth. Radiographic analysis before implant surgery should include detection of curved, convergent, or dilacerated root structures of adjacent teeth that can limit implant placement.

Cortical Plate Perforation

Perforation of the buccal or lingual cortical plate is a complication that can occur during implant surgery causing possible further problems (bleeding, hematoma, swelling, injury of other anatomical structures). It is easily avoided by adequate treatment planning and the use of surgical guides.[56,178]

Latrogenic Jaw Fracture

In rare instances (incidence is approximately 0.2%), fracture of the jaw during or after implant surgery can occur, especially in the mandible, when the alveolar ridge is severely atrophic, and the bone quality is poor. This complication can lead to osteomyelitis, paresthesia, malunion, nonunion, and functional and nutritional disorders. The treatment should be immediate to relieve patients' signs and symptoms and to restore function. Patients should be referred immediately to the hospital and the appropriate treatment should be performed under general anesthesia in the emergency room by an oral and maxillofacial surgery (OMFS) or head and neck surgeon. The prevention of this event consists of careful treatment planning and execution. Evaluation of the quantity and quality of bone in the potential implant site should be done with CBCTs prior to implant placement.[44,178,108,195]

Swelling/Edema

This is a common complication related to the extent of the surgical trauma and the duration of the surgical procedure. It is caused by accumulation of plasma in the interstitial spaces. The swelling usually starts in a few hours after the surgery, increases until 48 hours after, and reaches a peak at 72 hours. It then usually starts decreasing. To minimize this occurrence, ice packs should immediately be applied after surgery and NSAIDs may be prescribed. However, use of corticosteroids is most effective to reduce swelling and edema. To prevent this complication, surgical procedures should be performed in a reasonable time, and surgical trauma should be minimized. Planning for surgery and estimating the time preoperatively should be performed for each surgical procedure.[16,195]

Infection

Postoperative infection can occur after implant placement due to bacterial contamination. The signs and symptoms of a postoperative infection are swelling/edema, exudate/pus or fistula, pain, redness, and sometimes fever. To prevent contamination, the working area and the instruments should be sterile, the environment should be clean and aseptic protocols should be used. Antibiotics are widely prescribed for implant surgery; however, the timing of administration is still controversial. Antibacterial prescription mouthwash used before and after implant surgery are recommended. Infection can be treated with continued administration of antibiotics and in some cases changing the type of antibiotic. In cases of abscess formation, incision and drainage is the treatment of choice.[108,167,40,225]

Emphysema

This occurs due to an increase of pressure causing air entering in the tissues under the skin and mucosa, which can enter the fascial spaces. This is a rare complication in implant surgery, but it can occur when high-speed instruments, such as high-speed handpieces or air-powder abrasives, are used during open flap surgery. Usually the patient will present with a unilateral swelling in the face that can extend to the neck. When the skin in the area is palpated, it will often produce a crackling sound. Treatment includes massage and compression of the area with ice packs together with analgesics, antibiotics, and observation. To avoid this complication, high-speed instruments should be used carefully when flaps are reflected, and flaps should be held against the bone to close any spaces when these instruments are used. In addition, patients should be told not to blow their nose for several days after the surgical procedure.[16,108]

Biologic Complications

Biologic complications involve pathologies surrounding peri-implant hard and soft tissues. Frequently, soft tissue problems are an inflammatory response to bacterial accumulation on or around implants. In addition, bacteria can accumulate at the junction of an ill-fitting implant–abutment or abutment–crown connection. Literature suggested that some of the highly textured, macroscopically rough implant surfaces (e.g., titanium plasma-sprayed [TPS] or hydroxyapatite [HA] coating) may be prone to accumulation of bacteria on the implant surface.[133]

Inflammation and Proliferation

Because inflammation of the peri-implant soft tissues is similar to the inflammatory response in gingival and other periodontal tissues, the clinical appearance is similar. Inflamed peri-implant tissues demonstrate the same erythema, edema, and swelling around teeth.[19,206] Occasionally, the reaction of peri-implant soft tissues to bacterial accumulation due to its different attachment may be profound and unusual, with dramatic inflammatory proliferation (Fig. 86.13).[220] This type of lesion is somewhat characteristic around implants and indicates bacteria contaminating the implant surface due to a loose-fitting implant-to-abutment connection or trapped excess cement that remains buried within the soft tissue space (i.e., peri-implant pocket).[34]

The precipitating local factor ultimately becomes infected with bacterial pathogens, leading to mucosal hypertrophy or proliferation and possible abscess formation (Fig. 86.14). Correction of the precipitating factors (e.g., loose connection, loose abutments, or retained cement) may effectively resolve the lesion.[192,264] Another type of lesion resulting from a loose abutment connection or abutment, is a fistula (Fig. 86.15) which if treated properly can result in resolution of the complication (Figs. 86.16 and 86.17).[254]

Dehiscence and Recession

Dehiscence and recession of the peri-implant soft tissues occur when support for the tissues is lacking or has been lost. Recession is a common finding that may result in an esthetic complication and failure of the restoration. This problem should be identified after implant placement, and proper correction be carried out prior to the installation of the final prosthesis, especially when the soft tissues' thickness is limited and not well supported (Fig. 86.18).[11] Improper implant positioning also predisposes peri-implant tissues to recession. Placement or angulation of the implant too far buccally causes the buccal plate to resorb, resulting in greater recession (Fig. 86.19).[245,217]

Another factor that plays an important role in the esthetic outcome and the longevity of the restoration is the thickness of the buccal plate of bone. Spray and colleagues[246] recommended a buccal bone thickness of 2 mm or greater to support the buccal soft tissue. If it is insufficient, preoperative or simultaneous site development using guided bone regeneration (GBR) is indicated.[217] Recession is a problem that is particularly disconcerting in anterior esthetic areas. Patients with a high smile line or high esthetic demands consider recession a failure (Fig. 86.20).

The anatomy and soft tissue support around implants differ from those around teeth. Periodontal tissues have the advantage of soft tissue support supplied by circumferential and transseptal connective tissue fibers that insert into the cementum at a level that is more coronal than the supporting bone. In the absence of inflammation, these fibers support periodontal soft tissues far above the level of crestal bone. As a result, gingival margins and interdental papillae are supported and maintained higher around teeth than around implants, even when the periodontal tissues are very thin.

Peri-implant soft tissues, however, depend entirely on the surrounding bone for support. Soft tissue thickness accounts for some soft tissue height, but there are no supracrestal inserting connective tissue fibers to aid the soft tissue support around an implant. The soft tissue height around implants is typically limited to about 3 or 4 mm, and peri-implant bone loss often leads to recession.[259] Excessive forces are distributed differently to the peri-implant tissue when compared to the natural dentition and may play a role in bone resorption. According to some authors, connecting multiple implants with a splinted restoration may be beneficial in preserving hard and soft tissues and reducing technical complications.[210]

FLASH BACK

The peri-implant soft tissue seal is weaker than the periodontal soft tissue seal. The soft tissue seal around implants depends on tissue thickness and a long junctional epithelial attachment with hemidesmosomes. It is inferior to the periodontal attachment around natural teeth because it lacks the inserting connective tissue fibers (i.e., Sharpey fibers) of the periodontium. Periodontal papillae and gingival margins are also supported at a higher supracrestal level compared with peri-implant soft tissues. Periodontal soft tissues are supported by circumferential and transseptal connective tissue fibers that insert into the cementum at a level that is more coronal than the supporting bone.

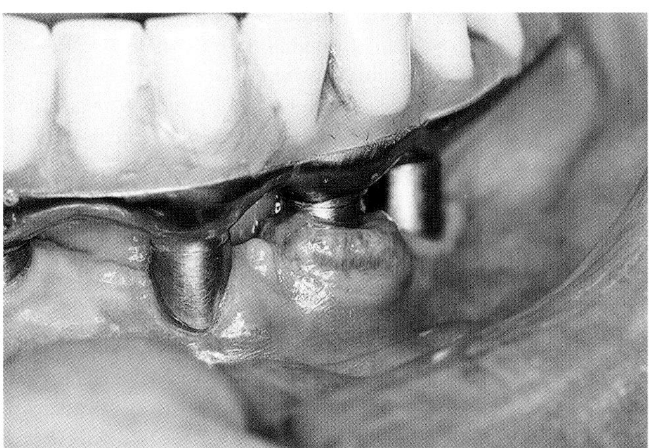

Fig. 86.13 Inflammatory proliferation caused by a loose-fitting connection between the abutment and the implant. (Courtesy Dr. John Beumer, UCLA Maxillofacial Prosthetics, Los Angeles, CA.)

Peri-Implantitis and Bone Loss

Peri-implant mucositis is a term used to describe a reversible inflammatory reaction in the mucosa adjacent to an implant without evidence of bone loss.[13] The reported prevalence of this disease (bleeding on probing and no bone loss) was reported to be about 79% of subjects and 50% of the implants.[219] A cause-and-effect relationship between bacterial plaque and the developing mucositis was established for all implants when patients discontinued all oral hygiene for a period of 3 weeks.[203] In a study by Salvi, subjects were asked to refrain from oral hygiene practice in the mandible for a period of 21 days during which bacterial deposits were allowed to accumulate on all surfaces. Following this period, all subjects resumed their optimal mechanical plaque control practices to reach preexperimental levels of oral cleanliness and gingival/mucosal health.[224] Peri-implant soft tissue developed a stronger inflammatory response to experimental plaque accretions when compared to their gingival counterparts. Experimental gingivitis and peri-implant mucositis were

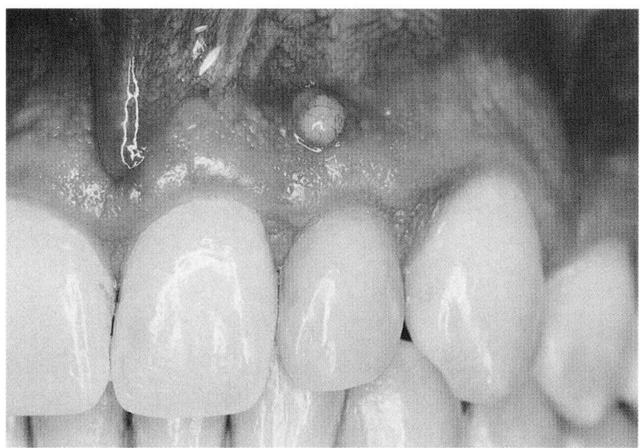

Fig. 86.15 Fistula caused by a loose implant–abutment connection (i.e., maxillary left lateral incisor).

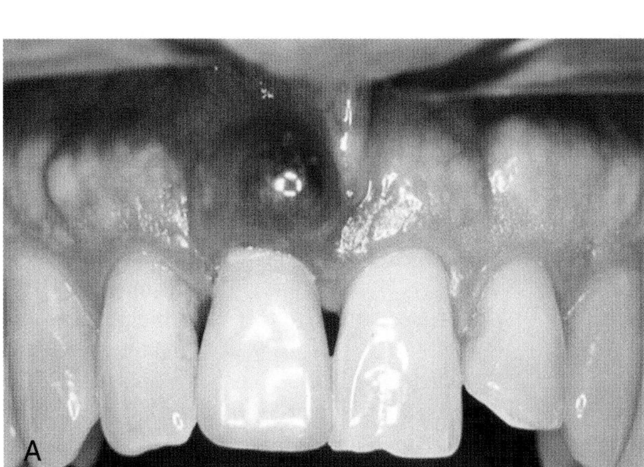

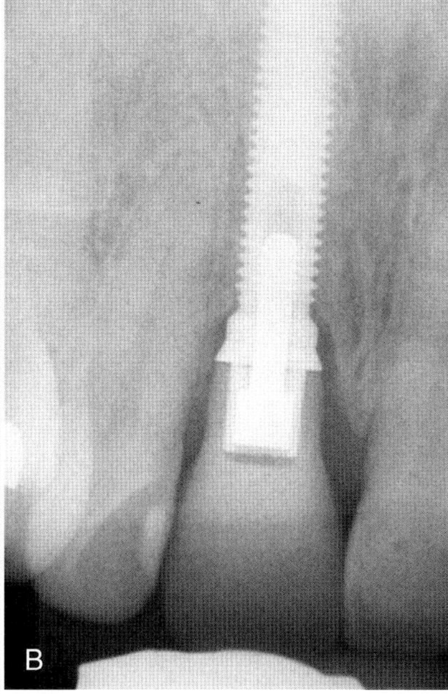

Fig. 86.14 (A) Clinical photograph of an abscess caused by excess cement trapped within the soft tissues. (B) Radiograph of an implant with a cemented crown (same patient as in A). Notice the subgingival depth of the crown–abutment (cement line) junction, which is below the level of the adjacent interproximal bone and therefore impossible to adequately access with an explorer to remove the excess cement. (Courtesy Dr. John Beumer, UCLA Maxillofacial Prosthetics, Los Angeles, CA.)

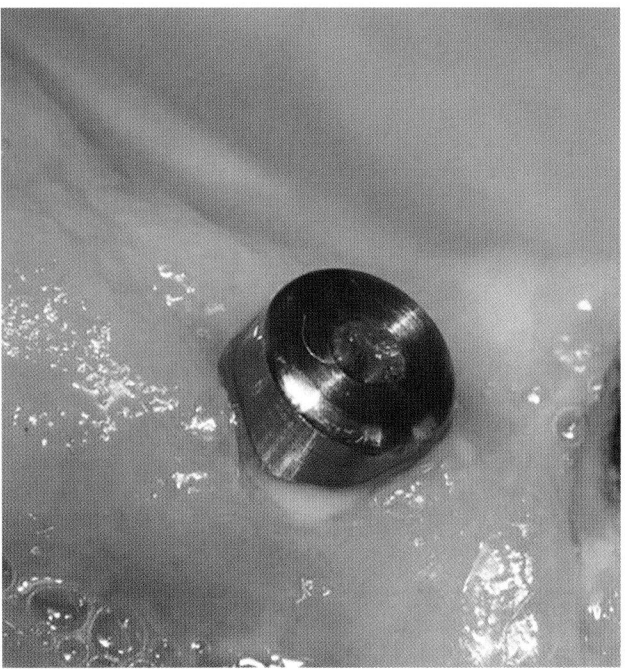

Fig. 86.16 Improper seating of healing abutment leading to purulence.

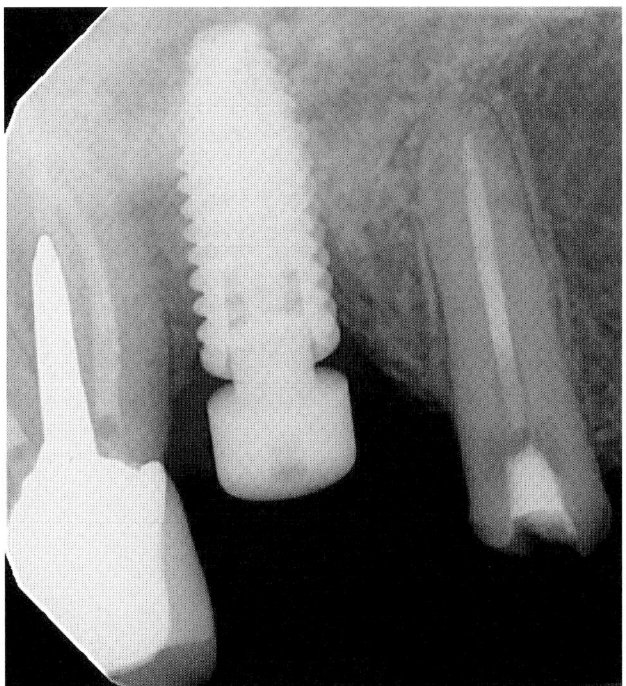

Fig. 86.17 Periapical radiograph of improper or incomplete seating of healing abutment.

reversible at the biomarker level, but 3 weeks of resumed biofilm control did not yield preexperimental levels of gingival and peri-implant mucosal health. In a randomized controlled clinical trial on antiinfective treatment of peri-implant mucositis, investigators found that this treatment and oral hygiene were effective in reducing peri-implant mucositis, but did not always result in complete resolution of inflammation.[121] This is why a review of the management of peri-implant mucositis and peri-implantitis defined the former as an inflammatory lesion limited to the surrounding mucosa of an implant.[88] This is also why a recent review of the treatment of peri-implant mucositis, after evaluating the results of various methods of treatment, urged the removal of the word "reversible" from the definition since complete elimination of the inflammation was not achieved in any study.[96] *Peri-implantitis* is an inflammatory process that affects the tissues around an osseointegrated implant and results in the loss of supporting bone[181] (Fig. 86.21). The reported prevalence of peri-implantitis varies from less than 7% to 37% of implants.[151] The variation can be attributed to differences in studied populations, length of follow-up time, implant variables, and the criteria used to define peri-implantitis.[154,219] Two systematic reviews concluded that peri-implantitis affected 10% of implants and 20% of patients during the 5 to 10 years after placement.[19,183]

A classification for early, moderate, and advanced peri-implantitis based on the degree of bone loss was proposed to improve communication when describing prevalence and treatment.[98] Soft tissue measurements using manual or automated probes have been suggested to diagnose a compromised implant site.[99] Although some reports state that probing is contraindicated, careful monitoring of probing depth over time seems useful in detecting changes of the peri-implant tissue.[63,208,249,250] Standardized radiographic techniques, with or without computerized analysis, have been useful in evaluating peri-implant bone levels.[7,37,43,138,208] Periodic evaluation of tissue appearance, probing depth changes, and radiographic assessment are the best means of detecting changes in bone support.

Clinicians should monitor the surrounding tissues for signs of peri-implant disease by observing changes in probing depth and radiographic evidence of bone destruction, suppuration, calculus buildup, swelling, color changes, and bleeding.[182,190] Peri-implantitis can be perpetuated by bacterial infection that has contaminated a rough (e.g., TPS- or HA-coated) implant surface and by excessive biomechanical forces.[277,278] The classic trough-type defect is typically associated with peri-implantitis (Fig. 86.22). In cases with severely reduced bone support extending into the apical half of the implant (Fig. 86.23) and definitely in cases demonstrating implant mobility, implant removal should be considered.[14,188]

The number and distribution of implants as well as the occlusal relationships influence the biomechanical forces applied to implants.[207,213] A review by Lindhe and Meyle from the Consensus Report of the Sixth European Workshop on Periodontology concluded that risk indicators for peri-implantitis included (1) poor oral hygiene, (2) a history of periodontitis, (3) diabetes, (4) cigarette smoking, (5) alcohol consumption, and (6) implant surface.[166] Risk factors 1 to 4 have been recognized and reported in the literature.[152] The report suggests that although data for risk factors 5 and 6 are limited, they appear to be relevant to peri-implantitis.[166] One study found little evidence to support smoking as a risk factor for peri-implantitis.[235] Another proposed risk factor involves individual genetic polymorphisms.[48,159] More research is needed to study the relation of this risk factor to the development of peri-implantitis. Another risk factor involves a deficiency of keratinized mucosa (KM) around the implant. In a systematic review and meta-analysis of the effect of KM on peri-implant health, it was concluded that "Based on current available evidence, a lack of adequate KM around endosseous dental implants is associated with more plaque accumulation, tissue inflammation, mucosal recession and attachment loss".[164]

Other risk factors, including excess and retained cement, have been implicated in peri-implantitis. One article said that excess

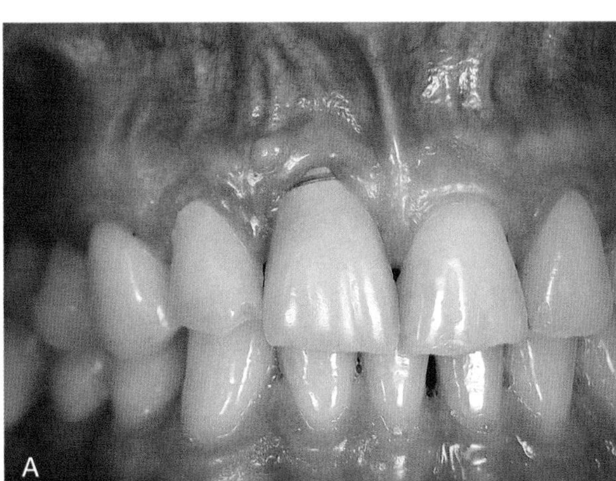

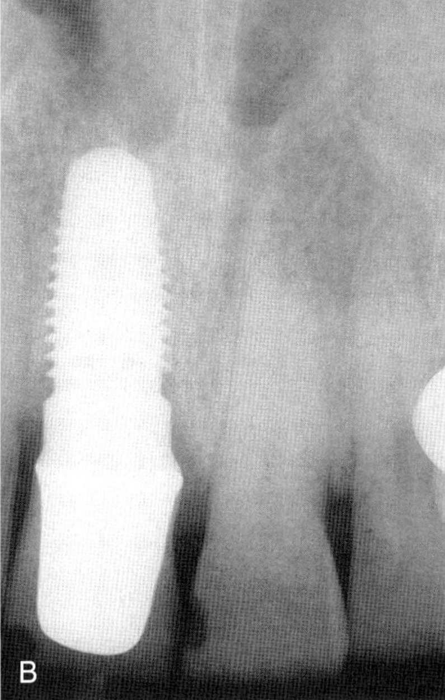

Fig. 86.18 (A) Clinical photograph of a single-tooth implant crown (maxillary right central) with moderate recession that occurred 1 year after the final restoration. In this case, recession most likely occurred because the labial bone around this wide-diameter implant was very thin or nonexistent. (B) Radiograph of a wide-diameter (6-mm) implant supporting a maxillary central incisor crown (same patient as in A).

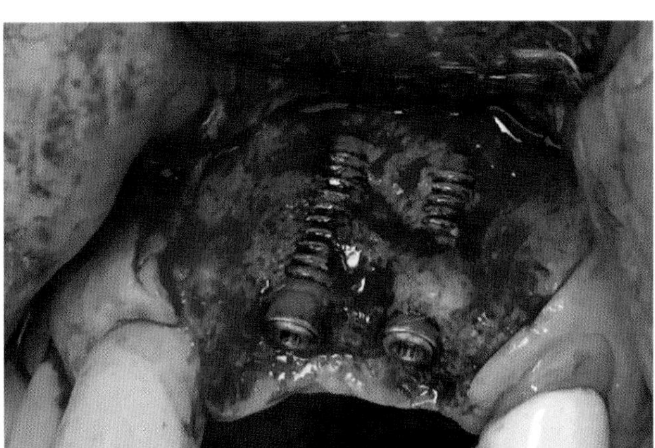

Fig. 86.19 Dehiscence of the implant.

dental cement was associated with signs of peri-implant disease in 81% of cases evaluated using a dental endoscope.[274] The radiopacity of some commonly used cements affects their detectability.[169] This emphasizes the importance of proper cementation, use of screw-retained rather than cemented restorations when possible, and careful clinical examination after final crown cementation on implants.

Other proposed peri-implantitis predisposing factors include the presence of aggressive bacteria, excessive mechanical stress, and corrosion. Each was documented as a factor that could act synergistically with biofilm or existing peri-implantitis to worsen the condition.[186]

The type of implant surface has been proposed as a risk factor for peri-implantitis. A systemic review of the literature on peri-implantitis and implants body roughness concluded that peri-implantitis is clearly linked with surface roughness and the higher the surface roughness, the higher the mean peri-implantitis rate.[137]

However, another systematic review comparing peri-implantitis in implants with tapered and rough surfaces concluded that rough implant surfaces do not seem to increase the incidence of peri-implants in comparison to tapered implant surfaces.[228] Certainly, more controlled studies are needed to determine the effect of implant surface roughness on the prevalence of peri-implantitis.

Another potential risk factor is titanium particles in the peri-implant mucosa. These particles were looked at in a systematic review of the literature. A search of 141 articles (26 included in the review) found titanium (Ti) particles in the soft tissue and hard tissue (bone crest and bone marrow) around dental implants. Moreover, peri-implantitis sites presented a higher number of particles compared to healthy implants. Various mechanisms were described as cause of Ti release including friction during implant insertion, corrosion of the implant surface, friction at the implant abutment interface, implantoplasty as part of the treatment of peri-implantitis, and several methods used for implant surface detoxification.[251]

A recent commentary was published that discussed metallosis, the process of particles and ions of titanium released into the surrounding tissues by the action of biofilm and/or mechanical forces which, as the author states, can be responsible for bone loss around some dental implants.[275] These particles of Ti have been found in greater numbers in submucosal plaque around implants associates with peri-implantitis compared to healthy sites.[92] A critical review regarding Ti particles concluded that there is a relationship between titanium particles and implant complications but at present, there is not enough evidence to prove a unidirectional causal relationship.[185]

Multiple systematic reviews and long-term clinical trials concluded that no predicable method of treatment for peri-implantitis could be recommended.[49,55,79,83,120,155,192,212,215,219] However, a clinical study of 170 consecutively treated implants with peri-implantitis using a regenerative protocol reported a more than 98% success rate.[97]

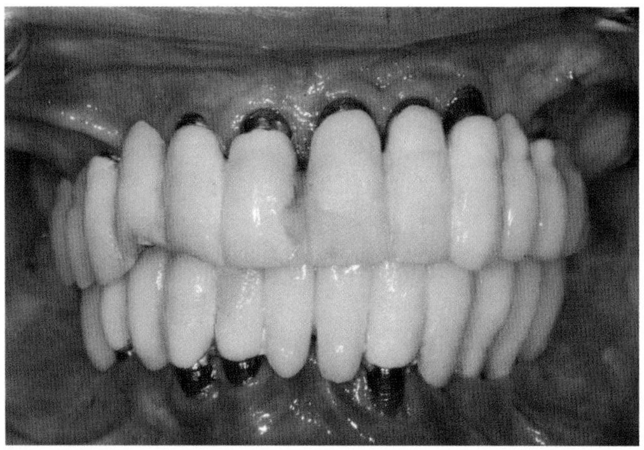

Fig. 86.20 Poor esthetics resulting from gingival recession and exposure of the crown margins, implant collars, and threads of several maxillary and mandibular implants supporting full-arch, fixed partial dentures. Notice the thin labial tissues and erythema, especially around the mandibular implant sites.

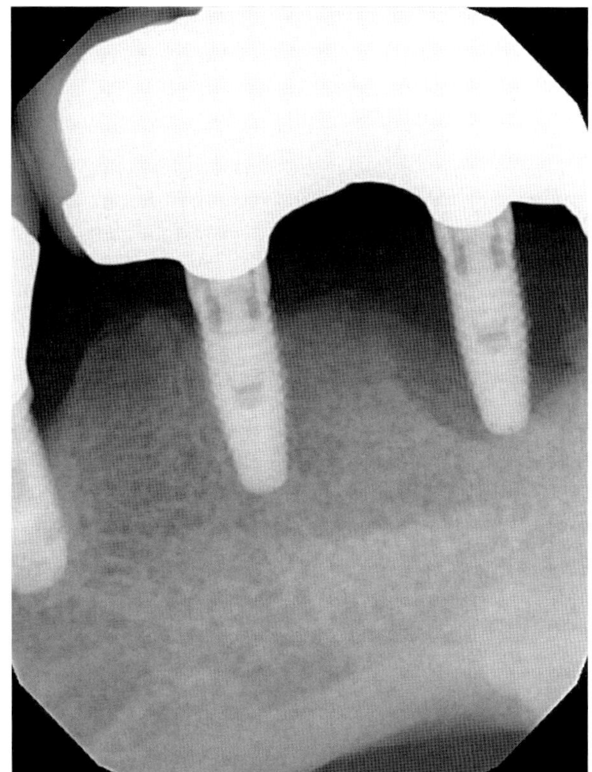

Fig. 86.21 Periapical radiograph showing bone loss around implant in the anterior mandible.

Implant Loss or Failure

Implant loss or failure is considered relative to the time of placement or restoration. Early implant failures occur before implant restoration. Late implant failures occur after the implant has been restored. When an implant fails before restoration, it probably did not achieve osseointegration, or the integration was weak or jeopardized by infection, movement, or impaired wound healing (Fig. 86.24). Late implant failures occur after prosthesis installation for a variety of reasons, including infection and implant overload (Fig. 86.25). In a review of the literature to evaluate biologic causes for implant failure, Esposito and colleagues[84] found that infections,

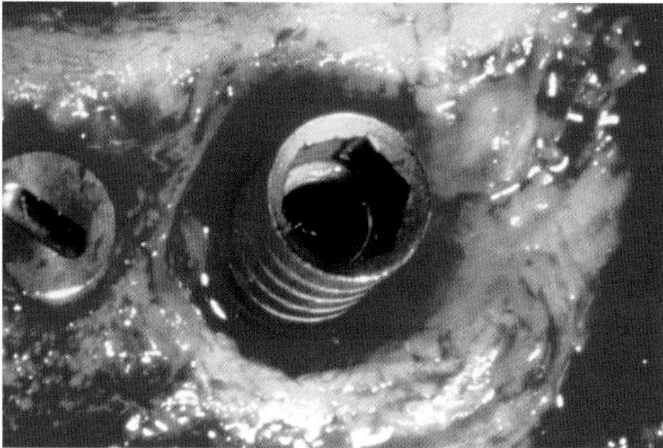

Fig. 86.22 Moderately advanced bone loss around an implant with the typical circumferential trough type of bony defect. (From Garg AK. *Implant Dentistry: A Practical Approach*. 2nd ed. St. Louis: Mosby; 2010.)

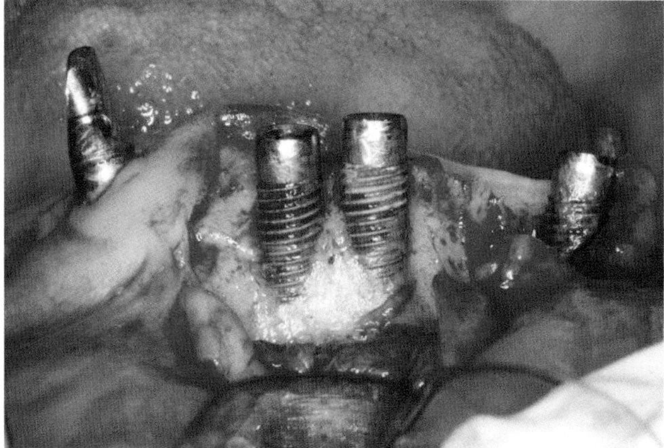

Fig. 86.23 Severe horizontal and vertical bone loss around several mandibular implants.

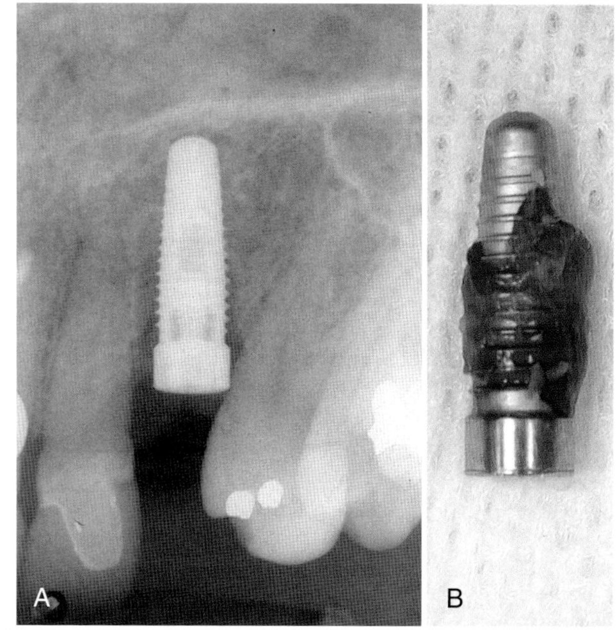

Fig. 86.24 (A) Radiograph of an early failed implant caused by lack of osseointegration. In addition to the crestal bone loss, notice the radiolucency along the sides of the implant. (B) Photograph of the failed (nonintegrated) implant (shown in A) that was easily removed along with surrounding connective tissue.

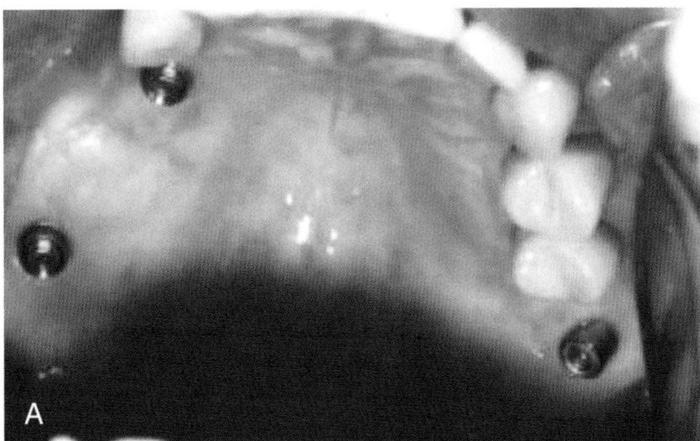

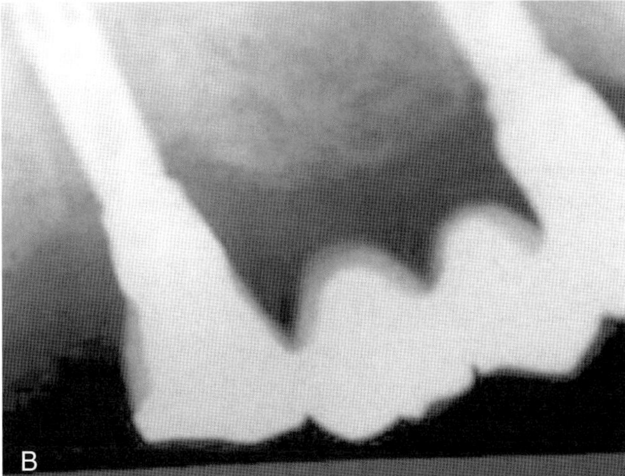

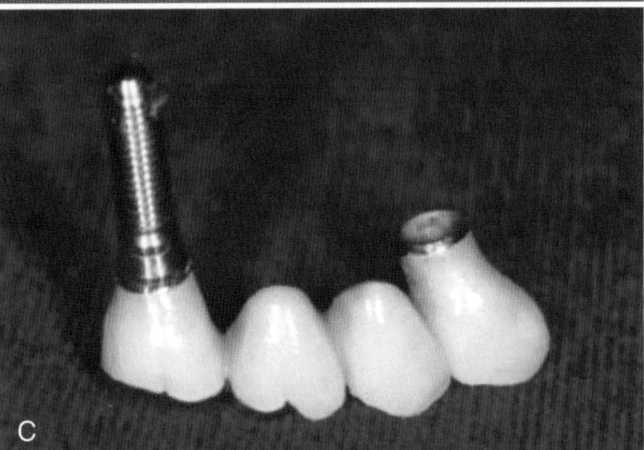

Fig. 86.25 A four-unit fixed partial denture in the posterior maxilla was supported by only two implants. (A) Clinical photograph of implant abutments in the posterior maxilla. (B) Radiograph taken 30 months after restoration. Notice the bone loss around the distal implant. (C) Failed distal implant attached to a failed prosthesis. The biologic failure of one (posterior) implant resulted in a long-span cantilever extension from the other (anterior) implant that ultimately led to its mechanical failure (i.e., abutment screw fracture). (Courtesy Dr. John Beumer, UCLA Maxillofacial Prosthetics, Los Angeles, CA.)

impaired healing, and overload were the most important contributing factors. Two systematic reviews of the literature concluded that a single dose of preoperative antibiotic therapy could decrease the failure rate of dental implants.[81,236]

Failure of oral implants have been attributed to several factors including a low insertion torque on immediately placed or early loaded implants, inexperienced surgeons, implants inserted in the maxilla and posterior regions of the jaws, implants placed in heavy smokers, implant placed in poor-quality (i.e., type III and type IV) bone, lack of initial stability, and prosthetic rehabilitation with implant-supported overdentures.[54]

Retrograde peri-implantitis (RPI) has emerged as a distinct entity that originates at the apex of the involved implant. It was first defined as zed osteomyelitis, believed to arise secondary to endodontic pathosis in adjacent teeth.[252] The definition has since been changed to any clinically symptomatic periapical lesion at a dental implant.[204] Some research groups have proposed that RPI results from either residual or active bacterial infection from a previous endodontic therapy.[226,280] Others have suggested that a history of apical surgeries is the main predisposing factor for RPI and bacterial contamination of the implant body remains a possibility after apical surgery.[85,21]

A recent study including 502 teeth that had apicoectomy and were replaced with implants found a cumulative survival rate of 92%.[223] There was an increased trend for RPI cases (35.7%) with persistent apical periodontitis but was not statistically significant. The authors concluded that implants placed in sites with previous apical surgery are not at an increased risk of implant failure or RPI.[223]

The risk of implant failure varies among patients, but patterns of loss tend to cluster. A second attempt at dental implant placement should be approached cautiously if placing the implant in the same site as the one that previously failed. It is often challenging to achieve adequate diameter, length, and stability of replacement implants due to the residual defect created by removal of the failed implant. In 2007, Grossmann and Levin reported an overall survival rate of 71% for dental implants that were placed in sites of previously failed single implants. In that study, all of the original implants failed during the early healing phase (mean of 2.3 to 3.2 months after placement).[112] In 2008, Machtei and colleagues[169] reported an overall survival rate of 83.5% for the second attempt at dental implants. They concluded that replacing failed implants resulted in a lower survival rate compared with that for implants placed in pristine sites. This could not be associated with conventional implant- or patient-related factors. They suggested that a site-specific negative effect might be associated with this phenomenon.[169]

In 2011, Machtei and coworkers reported a lower survival rate (60%) for third reimplanted sites.[168] This outcome represents a further diminished prognosis compared with implants in original sites or after a second attempt.[62] Replacement of a failed implant poses a challenge in achieving osseointegration in a healed bone site and can reduce the implant survival rate.[168]

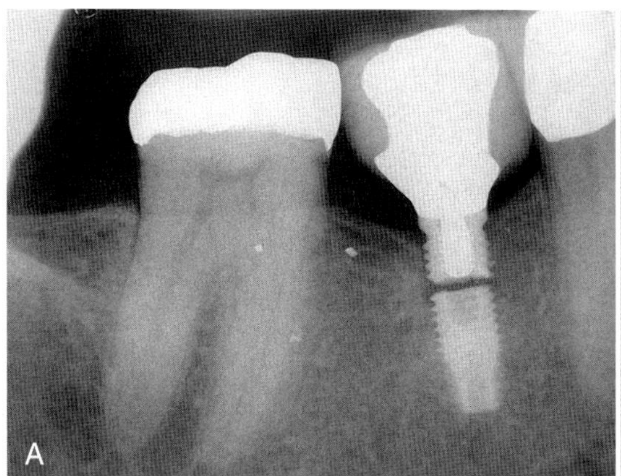

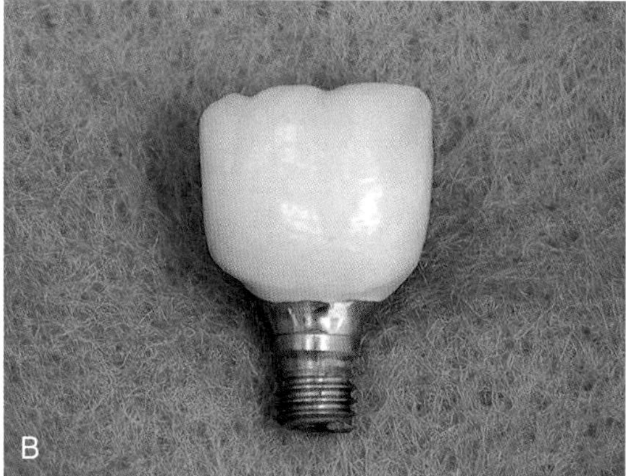

Fig. 86.26 (A) Radiograph of a fractured standard-diameter implant used to support a molar-sized single crown in the posterior mandible. (B) Crown and coronal portion of the implant (same as shown in A) that fractured between the third and fourth threads.

Prosthetic or Mechanical Complications

Prosthetic or mechanical complications occur when the strength of materials is no longer able to resist the forces that are being applied. As materials fatigue, they begin to stretch and bend. Ultimately, depending on the applied forces, they will fracture. Material failures lead to prosthetic complications such as loose, broken, and failed restorations.

Screw Loosening and Fracture

Screw loosening has occurred frequently in screw-retained FPDs. Screw-retained single crowns attached to externally hexed implants (i.e., those with narrow- or standard-diameter restorative interface connection surfaces) are particularly prone to this type of mechanical complication. Screw loosening has been reported for 6% to 49% of cases at the first annual checkup.[129,184]

Screw loosening causes many complications that may contribute to crestal bone loss, screw fracture, implant fracture, or implant failure.

Abutment or prosthesis screw loosening is often corrected by retightening the screws, but if screws continue to be stretched over time, they become fatigued and eventually fracture. This problem is evident in the patient with a loose single crown. In the patient with a prosthesis retained by multiple implants, the ability to detect a loose screw is greatly diminished, and the problem may go unnoticed until additional screws stretch, fatigue, and fracture. In either case, the biomechanical support (and resistance) for the restoration must be evaluated and, if possible, changed to prevent recurrence of the problem.

The ideal torque force (preload) applied to an abutment screw varies by manufacturer and may range from 10 to 35 N-cm. This preload is determined by many variables, including the screw material, screw head design, abutment material, and abutment surface characteristics. Preventative techniques for screw loosening include lightly finger tighten the abutment screw with an implant driver to around 10 N-cm followed by maximal finger tightening to 20 N-cm. Use an implant torque driver to tighten the abutment screw to the manufacturer's specifications. After 5 to 10 minutes, the screw should be retorqued to the manufacturer's specifications, as this will regain preload lost due to settling.[276]

Implant Fracture

The ultimate mechanical failure is implant fracture because it results in loss of the implant and possibly of the prosthesis. (Figs. 86.26–86.28). Removal of a fractured implant creates a large osseous defect. Factors such as fatigue of implant materials (Fig. 86.29) and weakness in prosthetic design or dimension are the usual causes of implant fractures.[7,25] Balshi[25] listed three categories

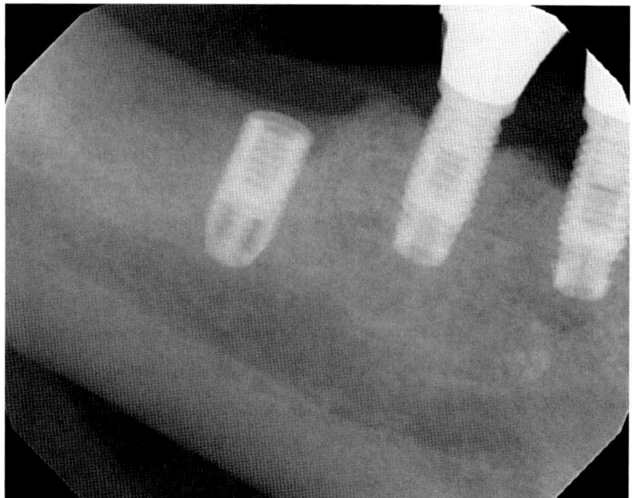

Fig. 86.27 Implant fractured on site #30 in closure with the inferior alveolar canal.

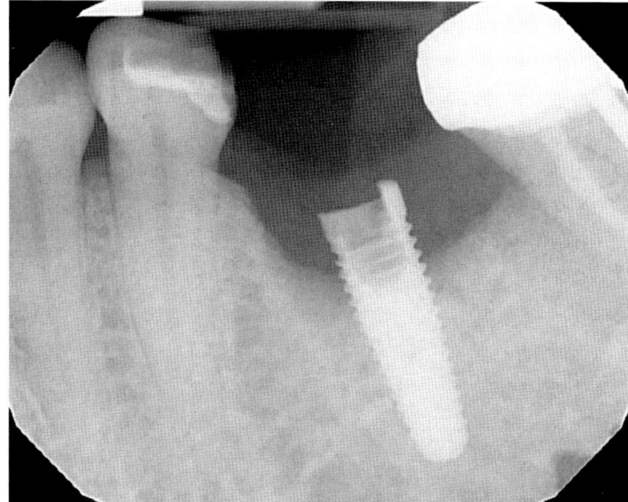

Fig. 86.28 Implant fractured on site #19 with bone loss.

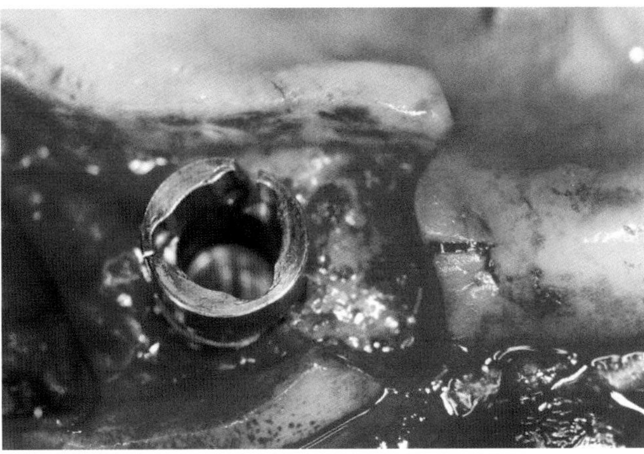

Fig. 86.29 The implant fractured at the internal connection collar. Fracture was caused by rotational forces applied to the implant at the time of placement into dense bone and was likely the result of combined material weakness and density of the prepared site.

of causes that may explain implant fractures: (1) design and material, (2) nonpassive fit of the prosthetic framework, and (3) physiologic or biomechanical overload. Patients with bruxism seem to be at higher risk for these events and therefore need to be screened, informed, and treated accordingly.[24,25] These patients should be fitted with occlusal guards in conjunction with placement of the final prostheses.

Multiple methods have been suggested for the removal of fractured implants including reverse torquing the implant with and implant insertion driver, trephination, and implant retrieval kits.[100]

Conclusions

Although implants offer a highly predictable treatment option for the replacement of single and multiple missing teeth, surgical, biologic, mechanical, prosthetic, and esthetic complications can occur. Careful diagnosis and treatment planning with the use of diagnostic imaging, surgical guides, meticulous techniques, and adherence to proven principles can prevent many of the problems discussed in this chapter.

A thorough understanding of anatomy, biology, and wound healing can reduce the incidence of complications. There is no substitute for good training, knowledge, and clinical experience. The clinician who places or restores implants must be well prepared to diagnose, prevent, and manage complications.

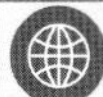

A Case Scenario is found on the companion website eBooks.Health.Elsevier.com.

Suggested Reading

Adler L, Buhlin K, Jansson L. Survival and complications: A 9- to 15-year retrospective follow-up of dental implant therapy. *J Oral Rehabil.* 2020;47:67–77.

Berglundh T, Persson L, Klinge B. A systematic review of the incidence of biological and technical complications in implant dentistry reported in prospective longitudinal studies of at least 5 years, *J Clin Periodontol* 2002; 29(suppl 3):197–212, discussion 232–233.

Clarkson E, Jung E, Lin S. How to avoid life threatening complications associated with implant surgery. *Dent Clin N Am.* 2021;65:33–41.

Cooper LF, De Kok IJ, Thalji G, Bryington MS. Prosthodontic management of implant therapy esthetic complications. *Dent Clin N Am.* 2019;63:199–216.

Draenert FG, Kämmerer PW, Berthold M, et al. Complications with allogeneic, cancellous bone blocks in vertical alveolar ridge augmentation: prospective clinical case study and review of the literature. *Oral Surg Oral Med Oral Pathol Oral Radiol.* 2016;122:e31–e43.

Figuero E, Graziani F, Sanz I, Herrera D, Sanz M. Management of peri-implant mucositis and peri-implantitis. *Periodontology 2000.* 2014;66:255–273.

Froum SJ. The team approach to managing dental implant complications: The periodontist's point of view. *Compendium.* 2013;34:4–11.

Froum SJ, Froum SH, Rosen PS. A regenerative approach to the successful treatment of peri-implantitis: a consecutive series of 170 implants in 100 patients with 2- to 10-year follow-up. *Int J Periodontics Restorative Dent.* 2015;35:857–863.

Froum SJ, Rosen PS. A proposed classification for peri-implantitis. *Int J Periodontics Restorative Dent.* 2012;32:533–540.

Goodacre CJ, Bernal G, Rungcharassaeng K, et al. Clinical complications with implants and implant prostheses. *J Prosthet Dent.* 2003;90:121–132.

Greenstein G, Cavallaro J, Romanos G, Tarnow D. Clinical recommendations for avoiding and managing surgical complications associated with implant dentistry: a review. *J Periodontol.* 2008;79:1317–1329.

Heitz-Mayfield LJ, Needleman I, Salvi GE, et al. Consensus statements and clinical recommendations for prevention and management of biologic and technical implant complications. *Int J Oral Maxillofac Implants.* 2014;29(suppl):346–350.

Jung RE, Zembic A, Pjetursson BE, Zwahlen M, Thoma DS. Systematic review of the survival rate and the incidence of biological, technical and aesthetic complications of single crowns on implants reported in longitudinal studies with a mean follow-up of 5 years. *Clin Oral Implant Res.* 2012;23(suppl 6):2–21.

Lang NP, Pjetursson BE, Tan K, et al. A systematic review of the survival and complication rates of fixed partial dentures (FPDs) after an observation period of at least 5 years. II. Combined tooth–implant-supported FPDs. *Clin Oral Implants Res.* 2004;15:643–653.

Misch K, Wang H-L. Implant surgery complications: Etiology and treatment. *Implant Dentistry.* 2008;17(2):159–167.

Roos-Jansaker AM, Lindahl C, Renvert H, et al. Nine- to fourteen-year follow-up of implant treatment. Part II: presence of peri-implant lesions. *J Clin Periodontol.* 2006;33:290–295.

Rosen P, Clem D, Cochran D, et al. Peri-implant mucositis and peri-implantitis: a current understanding of their diagnoses and clinical implications. *J Periodontol.* 2013;84(4):436–443.

Wadhwani C, Rapoport D, La Rosa S, et al. Radiographic detection and characteristic patterns of residual excess cement associated with cement-retained implant restorations: a clinical report. *J Prosthet Dent.* 2012;107:151–157.

Wallace SS, Mazor Z, Froum SJ, et al. Schneiderian membrane perforation rate during sinus elevation using piezosurgery: clinical results of 100 consecutive cases. *Int J Periodontics Restorative Dent.* 2007;27:413–419.

Wang I-C, Barootchi S, Tavelli L, Wang H-L. The peri-implant phenotype and implant esthetic complications. Contemporary overview. *J Esthet Restor Dent.* 2021;33:212–223.

Zembic A, Kim S, Zwahlen M, Kelly JR. Systematic review of the survival rate and incidence of biologic, technical, and esthetic complications of single implant abutments supporting fixed prostheses. *Int J Oral Maxillofac Implants.* 2014;29(suppl):99–116.

Zijderveld SA, van den Bergh JP, Schulten EA, et al. Anatomical and surgical findings and complications in 100 consecutive maxillary sinus floor elevation procedures. *J Oral Maxillofac Surg.* 2008;66:1426–1438.

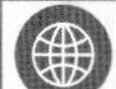

References for this chapter are found on the companion website eBooks.Health.Elsevier.com.

CHAPTER 87

Supportive Implant Treatment

Jonathan H. Do | Perry R. Klokkevold

CHAPTER OUTLINE

Dental implant therapy does not end with the final prosthetic restoration of the implant. Predictability and long-term success of a dental implant and its restoration require sound treatment planning, precise surgical and restorative execution, and impeccable long-term maintenance, which depend on daily patient compliance with home care as well as periodic re-evaluation and professional, supportive implant treatment.

Peri-implant maintenance begins as the implant becomes exposed to the oral cavity and continues at regular intervals during the life of the implant. The recall interval is determined by the patient's oral hygiene and susceptibility to biofilm-induced inflammatory diseases. For the first year after treatment, recall maintenance visits should be scheduled at 3-month intervals and then adjusted to suit the patient's needs. Patients who have good oral hygiene, minimal deposits, and disease resistance require infrequent professional hygiene maintenance, whereas those who have poor oral hygiene, heavy deposits, and disease susceptibility require more frequent follow-up care.

Rationale for Supportive Implant Treatment

Although dental implants are not vulnerable to dental caries, they are susceptible to mechanical complications and peri-implant, biofilm-induced inflammatory tissue changes. A 10-year retrospective study[49] of 397 fixed-implant reconstructions in 300 patients observed a mechanical complication rate of 24.7%. The most frequent complication was ceramic chipping (20.31%), followed by occlusal screw loosening (2.57%) and loss of retention (2.06%). Although relatively infrequent, occlusal screw loosening can result in a subgingival gap at the implant–abutment junction that retains plaque and stimulates an inflammatory reaction in soft and hard tissues.

Biologically, biofilm accumulation due to inadequate or no access to oral hygiene can result in peri-implant mucositis and peri-implantitis. Peri-implant mucositis is characterized by inflammation confined to the soft tissue and is reported to affect up to 80% of patients with dental implants.[24] Peri-implantitis is characterized by peri-implant inflammation with progressive crestal bone loss beyond the initial remodeling. The prevalence of peri-implantitis among patients is 11.2% to 53%.[28,38–41] Poor oral hygiene, residual cement, current or history of periodontitis, cigarette smoking, and diabetes mellitus are risk factors for peri-implant diseases.[1,10]

The relationship between peri-implant mucositis and peri-implantitis is similar to that between gingivitis and periodontitis. Although peri-implant mucositis does not necessarily progress to peri-implantitis, it is likely the precursor to peri-implantitis.[1] The inflammatory response in peri-implant disease appears to be similar to that in periodontal disease.[42] However, the severity and rate of disease progression appear to be more pronounced around implants.[9] This may be caused by the absence of a self-limiting process, which is observed in periodontitis, around implants that separates the inflammatory cell infiltrate from the bone.[6] Experimental models demonstrated that peri-implant mucositis was reversible at the biomarker level (i.e., matrix metalloproteinase 8 [MMP-8] and interleukin-1β [IL-1β]).[42]

A review of the literature[37] reported that peri-implant mucositis could be effectively treated with nonsurgical mechanical therapies, but these modalities tended to be ineffective against peri-implantitis. Results of surgical treatment for peri-implantitis are not predictable. Prevention, early detection, and early treatment of peri-implant diseases are therefore crucial. Periodic and well-regimented supportive implant treatment is essential to the long-term success of dental implant therapy.

KEY FACT

Implants are susceptible to mechanical complications and biofilm-induced inflammatory diseases, such as peri-implant mucositis and peri-implantitis.

Examination of Implants

The supportive implant treatment appointment should include an inquiry about new concerns, problems, or pain; review of changes

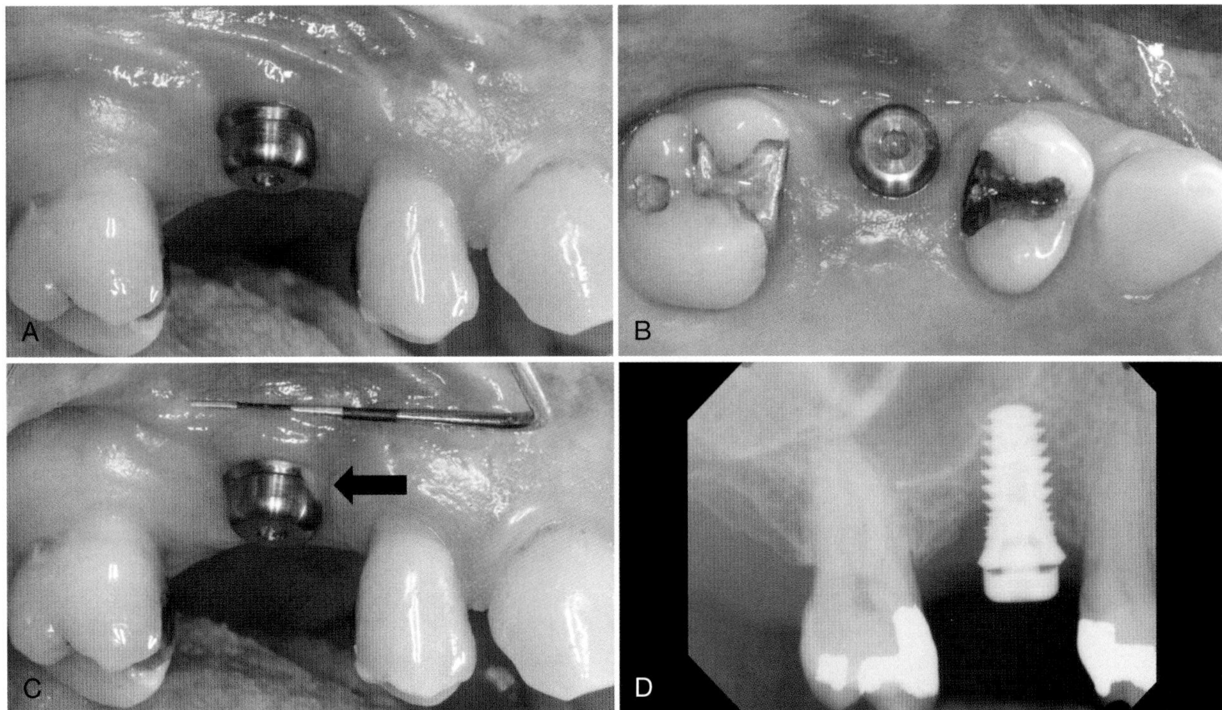

Fig. 87.1 Peri-implantitis. (A and B) Minimal biofilm accumulation is seen. The peri-implant mucosa exhibits minimal erythema and edema. Notice the buccal placement of the implant in B. (C) Manipulation of tissue indicates a lack of buccal keratinized attached gingiva and exudation from the peri-implant sulcus *(arrow)*. (D) The periapical radiograph shows peri-implant bone loss to the apex of the implant.

in the patient's systemic and oral health status; evaluation and reinforcement of oral hygiene; examination and evaluation of soft and hard tissue health; evaluation of implants and the associated implant restorations' stability and integrity; and professional, supportive treatment. Assessment should determine the appropriate recall interval and plan for the next visit.

Examination begins with visual inspection for biofilm and calculus accumulation; signs of inflammation and swelling; peri-implant soft tissue quality, color, consistency, and contour; and aberrations in the implant prosthesis. Peri-implant soft tissue can be digitally palpated to detect edema, tenderness, exudation, or suppuration. Peri-implant probing can be done to assess the condition and level of soft and hard tissues surrounding implants. Radiographic images can be obtained to help verify the level of the peri-implant crestal bone. Determination of implant stability or mobility and percussion testing can help verify implant osseointegration (Fig. 87.1).

CLINICAL CORRELATION

Implant examination includes evaluation of biofilm control, visual and tactile assessment of peri-implant tissue for inflammatory changes and changes in probing depths, and radiographic examination of the mesial and distal bone level.

Peri-Implant Probing

Probing of implants can be done with light force (i.e., 0.25 N) using a traditional steel probe without adverse effects on the peri-implant mucosa.[16] Implant probing should be recorded at the time of final restoration as the baseline measurement and done at least annually thereafter.[24]

Clinicians should use caution when evaluating peri-implant probing because these measures cannot be interpreted the same as probing depths around teeth. Although periodontal probing around natural teeth is useful for assessing the health of periodontal tissues, the sulcus or pocket depth, and the level of attachment, probing around implants may not provide comparable results.[7] Due to distinct differences in the tissues that surround and support teeth compared with those that surround and support implants, the probe inserts and penetrates differently. Around teeth, the periodontal probe is resisted by the health of the periodontal tissues and importantly, by the insertion of supracrestal connective tissue fibers into the cementum of the root surface. These fibers, unique to teeth, are the primary source of resistance to the probe.[3] There is no equivalent fiber attachment around implants. Connective tissue fibers around implants usually run parallel to the implant or restorative surface and do not have perpendicular or inserting fibers (see Chapter 73). The primary source of resistance to the probe depends on the conditions around the implant.[13,23] At noninflamed sites, the most coronal aspect of connective tissue adhesion to the implant resists the probe. At inflamed sites, the probe tip consistently penetrates farther into the connective tissue until less inflamed connective tissue is encountered, which is often close to or at the level of bone.

The value of peri-implant probing is different from periodontal probing and offers comparatively limited information. Probing around implants can measure the level of the mucosal margin relative to a fixed position on the implant or restoration and can also measure the depth of tissue around the implant. The peri-implant probing depth is often a measure of the thickness of the surrounding connective tissues and correlates most consistently with the level of the surrounding bone. However, peri-implant probing is affected by several conditions, including the size of the probe, the force and direction of insertion, the health and resistance of peri-implant tissues, the level of bone support, and the features of the implant, abutment, and prosthesis design (Fig. 87.2A and B).

A comparison[46] of probing pocket depth of implants with peri-implantitis before and after the removal of the prosthetic restorations reported similar probing depths in only 37% of sites. In 39%

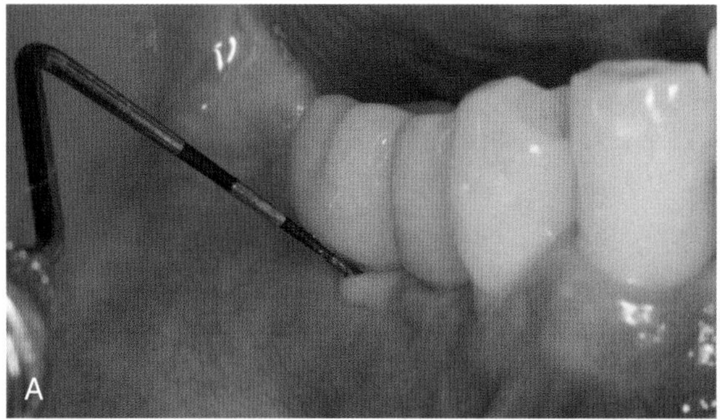

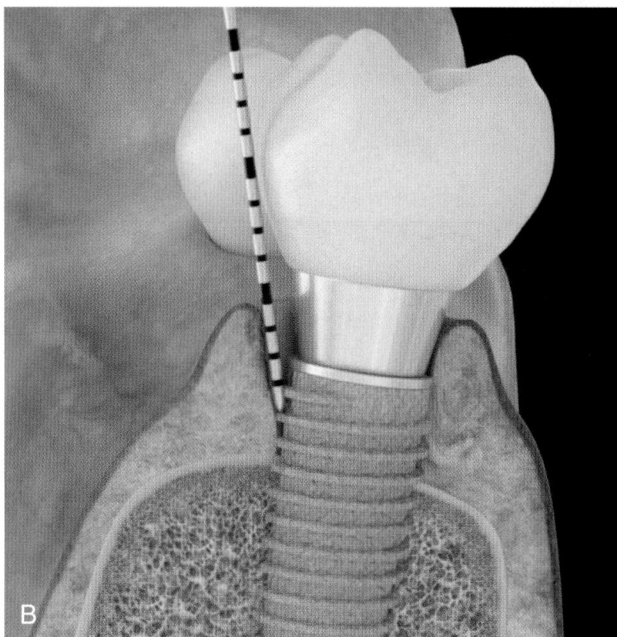

Fig. 87.2 (A) Buccal probing of the implant is impeded by implant restoration. (B) PerioPixel illustration of problem depicted in (A). Buccal probing of the implant is impeded by the implant restoration. In this case, the probe contacts the thread on the implant and cannot accurately assess the peri-implant probing depth.

of sites, the difference was ±1 mm; in 15% of sites, it was ±2 mm; and in 9% of sites, it was ±3 mm. Probing measurements can be an accurate measure of soft tissue thickness around an implant (i.e., peri-implant soft tissue above the bone level), but in many cases or sites, the inability to properly angle and direct the probe along the implant can lead to inaccurate assessment of soft tissue thickness. In these situations, the clinician must appreciate the limitations and know that other clinical parameters and radiographs are required to help evaluate the peri-implant's condition.

Probing around implants is likely to vary more than around teeth. Studies have shown that a change in probing force around implants results in more dramatic changes than a similar change in probing force around teeth.[30] The probing depth around implants presumed to be healthy (and without bleeding) has been documented as about 3 mm around all surfaces.[2,8] The absence of bleeding upon probing teeth has been established as an indicator of health and predictor of periodontal stability.[20] Studies comparing bleeding on probing around teeth and implants in the same patient have reported that bleeding around implants occurs more frequently.

Bleeding on probing at implant sites can indicate inflammation in the peri-implant mucosa. However, the ability to use bleeding on probing as an indicator for assessing diseased or healthy sites around implants has not been established. Due to the potential for false-positive bleeding (i.e., provoked bleeding) with probing, the use of marginal bleeding, which is a more sensitive indicator of inflammation and is less likely to elicit false-positive bleeding, has been proposed to assess peri-implant inflammation.[51] Marginal bleeding can be evaluated by running a probe circumferentially along the coronal portion in the implant sulcus. Overall, the value of peri-implant probing is in monitoring changes in the probing pocket depth over time rather than the initial value because some implants are placed apically for esthetics.[1]

CLINICAL CORRELATION

Probing of implants can be accomplished with a traditional steel probe. It is valuable for detecting tactilely inflammatory changes in the tissue, such as loss of tissue to resistance to probe penetration, sponginess of peri-implant mucosa, and bleeding on probing, and for monitoring changes in probing depth over time.

Microbial Testing

Studies in animals and humans have demonstrated the development of peri-implant mucosal inflammation in response to the accumulation of bacterial plaque (biofilm).[5,34,42,52] Microbiologic studies suggest that greater probing depths (i.e., pockets) around implants harbor higher levels of pathogenic microorganisms.[31,36,44] Studies have also documented similarities in the microbial composition of plaque (biofilm) in healthy periodontal sites compared with healthy peri-implant sites.[32] Evidence indicates that the microbiota of diseased periodontal pockets harbor the same pathogenic microorganisms as those observed in inflamed peri-implant sites (i.e., peri-implantitis).[32,44] However, there is no evidence to prove that periodontal pathogens cause peri-implant disease, and the pathogenesis of inflammatory disease around implants has not been defined.[11]

One report[1] accepted the idea that peri-implant disease, like periodontal disease, occurs primarily because of an overwhelming bacterial insult and subsequent host response. Human biopsies indicate that peri-implantitis and periodontitis exhibit similar histologic features, including an inflammatory cell infiltrate in the connective tissue dominated by B lymphocytes and plasma cells and by upregulation of inflammatory biomarkers. No evidence indicates that laboratory tests for the identification of suspected periodontal pathogens are of use in the evaluation of implants.[15] The usefulness of microbial testing may be limited to the evaluation of peri-implant sites that are showing signs of infection and bone loss, allowing the clinician to prescribe appropriate antibiotics.

Stability Measures

The assessment of implant stability or mobility is an important measure for determining whether osseointegration is being maintained. Important as it is, however, this measure has extremely low sensitivity but high specificity. An implant can exhibit significant bone loss and remain stable; the stability measure, in this case, has a low sensitivity for the detection of bone loss. Conversely, if implant mobility is detected, it is likely that the implant is not surrounded by bone; mobility is highly specific for the detection of implant failure or lack of osseointegration. Mobility demands differentiation of loss of implant osseointegration from a loose implant restoration.

There is great interest in evaluating the stability of bone-to-implant contact in a noninvasive manner. Two noninvasive techniques for evaluating implant stability are impact resistance (e.g., Periotest) and resonance frequency analysis (RFA). Originally designed to evaluate tooth mobility quantitatively, the Periotest

(Gulden, Bensheim, Germany) is a noninvasive electronic device that provides an objective measurement of the reaction of the periodontium to a defined impact load applied to the tooth crown. The Periotest value depends to some extent on tooth mobility but mainly on the dampening characteristics of the periodontium. Despite dependence on the periodontium, the Periotest has been used to evaluate implant stability. However, unlike teeth, the movement of implants and surrounding bone is minuscule, and Periotest values, therefore, fall within a much smaller range compared with those for teeth. Detection of horizontal mobility may be a significant advantage of the Periotest because it is much more sensitive to horizontal movement than similar detection by other means, such as manual assessment.[15]

Another noninvasive method used to measure the stability of implants is RFA,[29] which uses a transducer attached to the implant or abutment. A steady-state signal is applied to the implant through the transducer, and the response is measured. The RFA value is a function of the stiffness of the implant in the surrounding tissues. The stiffness is influenced by the implant, the interface between the implant, the bone, soft tissues, and the surrounding bone itself. The height of the implant or abutment above the bone influences the RFA value. Unlike the Periotest, the RFA does not depend on movement in only one direction. The absolute RFA values vary from one implant design to another and from one site to another, but there is high consistency for any one implant or location.

The value of RFA is most appreciated with repeated measures of the same implant over time because it is very sensitive to changes in the bone-implant interface. Small changes in tissue support can be detected using this method. An increase in RFA value indicates increased implant stability, whereas a decrease indicates loss of stability. However, this is a relative measure, and it has not been determined whether RFA is capable of detecting impending failure before the implant fails.

Much interest and research have focused on the use of noninvasive methods to evaluate implant stability. Mobility remains the cardinal sign of implant failure, and detecting mobility is therefore an important parameter.

Implant Percussion

Tapping an implant's healing abutment or restoration with an instrument produces a sound that can help determine its osseointegration. A solid resonating sound and the absence of pain usually indicate osseointegration. A dull sound can indicate that the implant is fibrous encapsulated; radiographic and other clinical findings are needed for diagnosis. Video 87.1 demonstrates percussion testing, which distinguishes between an osseointegrated implant and a failed implant.

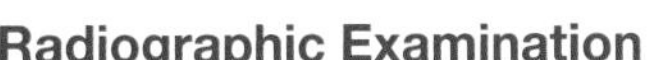

Radiographic Examination

Perpendicular intraoral periapical radiographs should be taken at implant placement, at abutment connection, and at final restoration for baseline documentation of bone levels and annually[12] thereafter to monitor marginal or peri-implant bone changes. In the setting of peri-implant inflammation, a periapical radiograph is indicated for peri-implant bone evaluation and disease diagnosis. Periapical radiographs have excellent resolution and, when taken perpendicular to an implant, can provide valuable details of the implant-abutment junction, mesial and distal crestal bone level relative to the implant platform, and bone-to-implant interface along the length of the implant (Fig. 87.3). Periapical radiographs are difficult to standardize and great variation is inherent in the acquisition process, but they are relatively simple, inexpensive, and readily available in the dental office. It is diagnostically important to obtain images that clearly show implant threads (i.e., not blurred by non-perpendicular angulation) and the restorative implant-abutment connection.

The objective of the radiographic examination is to measure the height of bone adjacent to the implant, evaluate the quality and proximity of bone along the length of the implant, and detect peri-implant radiolucencies. Although the predictive value of assessing implant stability with radiographs is low, films do offer a reasonable method to measure changes in bone levels.[46] The predictive value of detecting implant failure or loss of stability is good when radiolucent lesions are discovered with periapical radiographs. Identification of unstable implants is reliable when radiographs are obtained as part of an annual examination and when examining patients on a routine long-term basis.[19]

The radiographic examination remains one of the primary tools for the detection of failed or failing implants in routine clinical evaluations, although it is not as accurate as mobility tests. In one study designed to evaluate the accuracy and precision of radiographic diagnosis of mobility, the probability of predicting implant mobility in a population with a low prevalence of implant failures was low.[47] Other studies, however, have demonstrated a much higher predictive value for radiographic diagnosis of implant mobility.[18,19] Investigators concluded that the most important factors for making an accurate radiographic diagnosis are the quality of the radiograph and the experience of the clinician.[19,47]

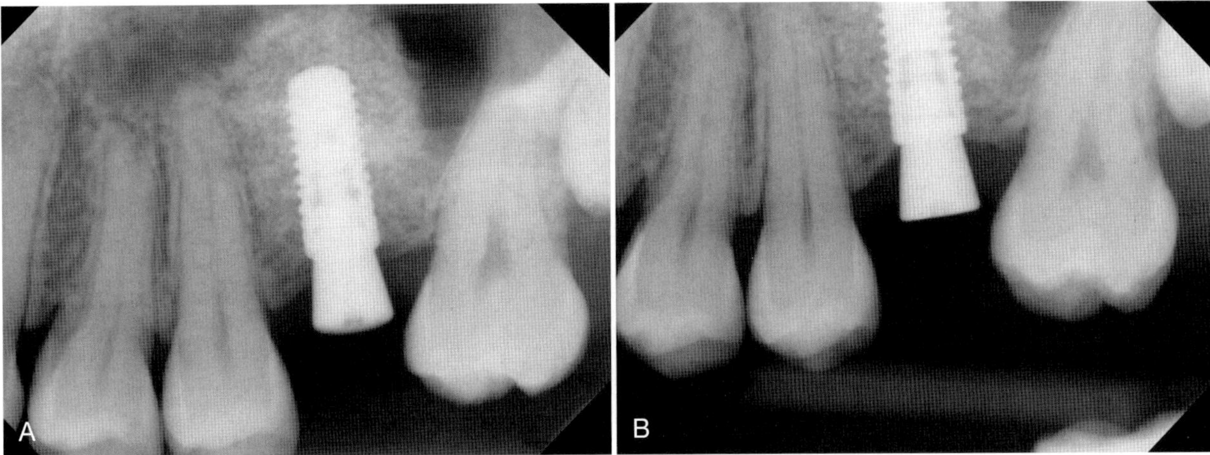

Fig. 87.3 (A) A periapical radiograph captures the whole implant. (B) A second perpendicular periapical radiograph is necessary to assess the crestal bone level. Platform switching is seen at the implant–abutment junction.

FLASH BACK

Intraoral periapical radiographs of implants must be taken with the x-ray beam perpendicular to the implant fixture to enable clear visualization of implant threads and the mesial and distal crestal bone levels.

Assessment of Peri-Implant Health

Evaluation of Biofilm Control

Impeccable biofilm control is crucial to peri-implant tissue health. Poor biofilm control is associated with peri-implant disease (odds ratio =14.3).[24] It is advantageous to evaluate biofilm control before tissue manipulation. The amount and location of biofilm and calculus accumulation should be assessed visually. Poor control is typically associated with biofilm and calculus retention and with erythematous and edematous gingival tissue. When biofilm control is inadequate, the patient should be asked to demonstrate his or her oral hygiene routine in front of a mirror so that the clinician can evaluate the patient's technique. If the patient fails to remove biofilm in any area, the patient's attention should be directed to the location of the biofilm. An instrument can be used to remove the biofilm, with the patient paying attention so that he or she can see its color and consistency. At this time, oral hygiene instruction should be demonstrated and reinforced.

Evaluation of Peri-Implant Health and Disease

Peri-implant mucosal health is characterized by pink, firm, and well-adapted gingival tissue. Peri-implant disease is associated with clinical erythema, edema, and loss of tissue tightness around the implant. Peri-implant mucosa can be nonkeratinized and unattached (see Fig. 87.1C) or keratinized and attached (Fig. 87.4C). In the setting of keratinized, attached mucosa, a gingival seal or gingival cuff is established around the implant.[4] The gingival cuff can protect the underlying bone and reduce subgingival plaque formation. Due to the mobile nature of oral mucosa, the protective function of nonkeratinized, unattached peri-implant mucosa may not be as effective. However, the presence of keratinized, attached gingiva, which can facilitate oral hygiene, is not a requisite for peri-implant health if the biofilm is well controlled.[45,50] Nonetheless, sites deficient in keratinized, attached tissue typically exhibit vertical or horizontal ridge deficiencies, shallow vestibular depths, and long or bulky restorations. All these factors can impede oral hygiene access and contribute to biofilm accumulation and peri-implant inflammation.

KEY FACT

Peri-implant health is characterized by pink, firm, and well-adapted peri-implant mucosa. Peri-implant disease is associated with erythema, edema, and loss of tissue tightness around the implant.

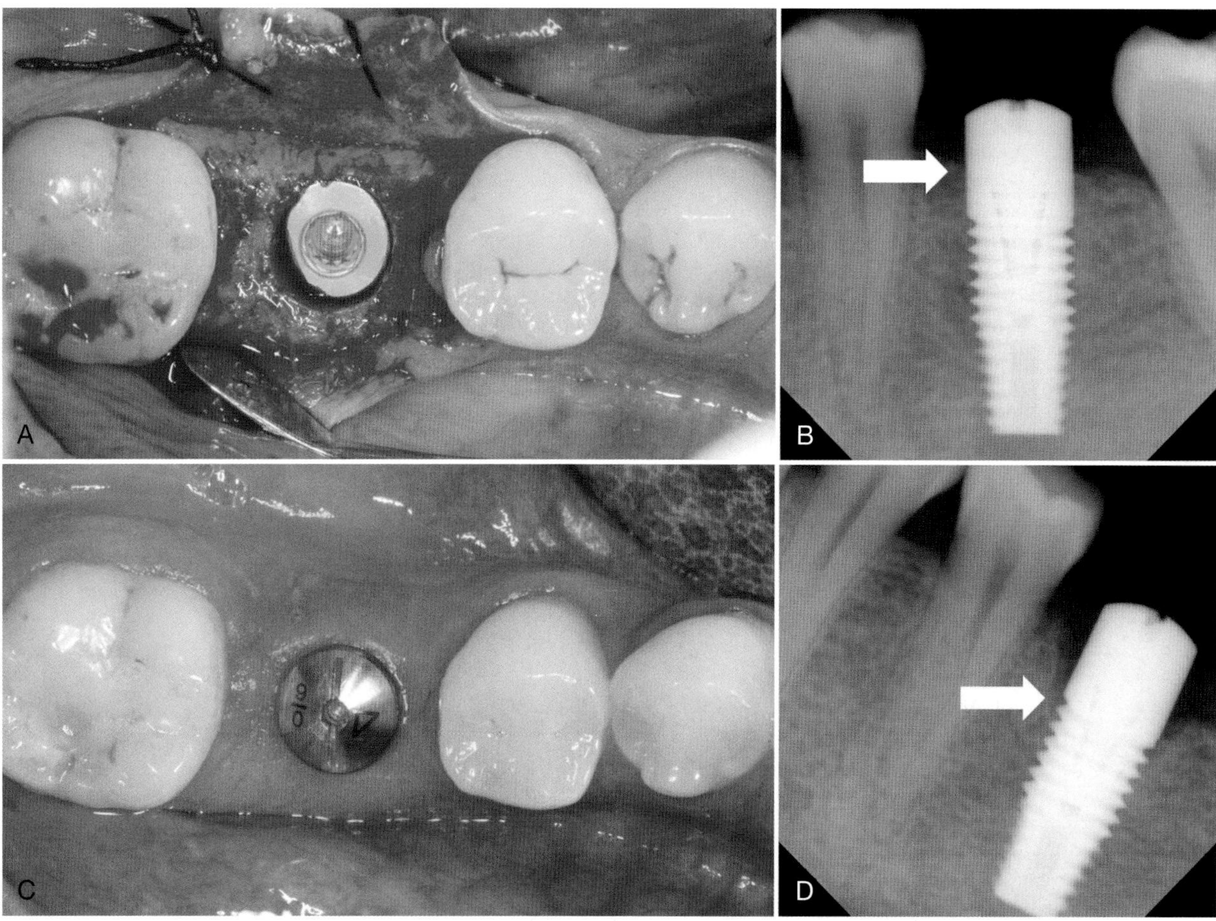

Fig. 87.4 (A) Subcrestal placement of an implant with adequate buccal and lingual bone thickness. (B) Periapical radiograph at the time of implant placement. (C) Implant at the 5-month osseointegration check exhibits adequate peri-implant keratinized attached tissue. (D) It also shows crestal bone remodeling to the first thread. *Arrows* indicate the mesial crestal bone level.

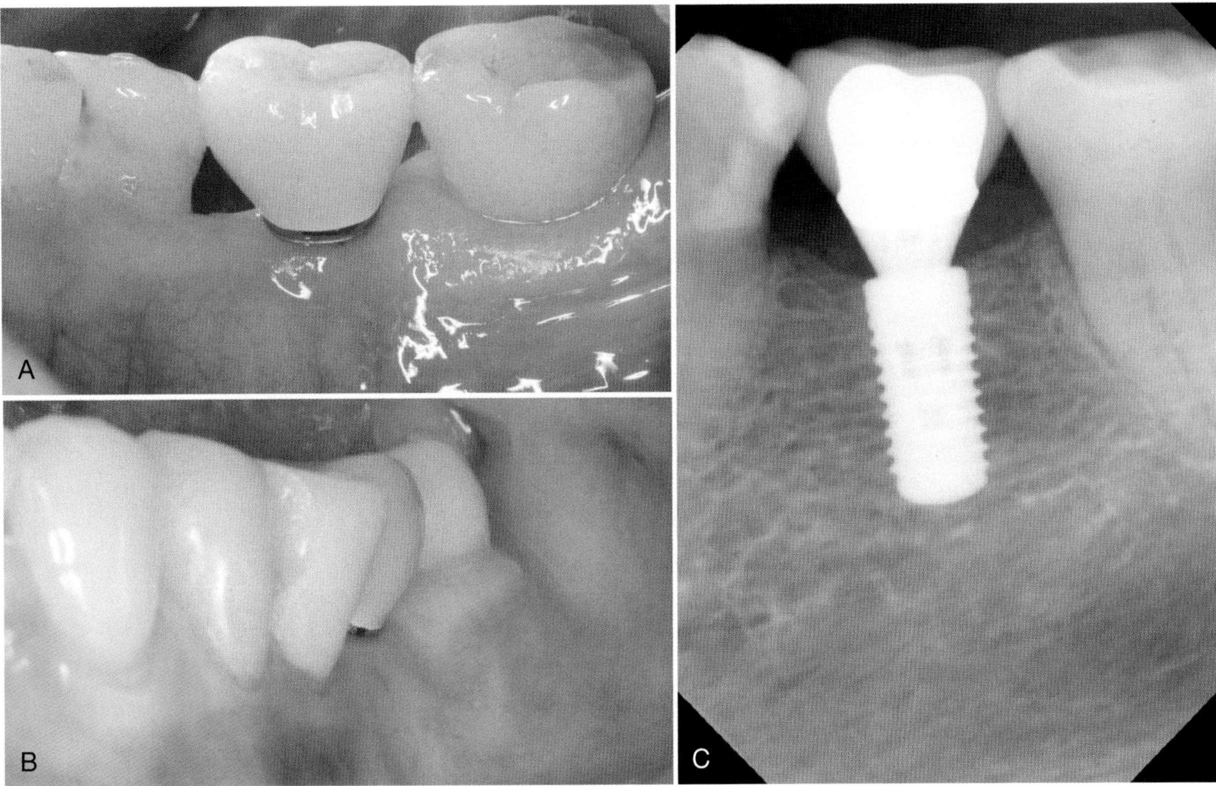

Fig. 87.5 Restoration is designed with adequate hygiene access. (A) Lingual view. (B) Mesial view of the buccal contour. (C) The periapical radiograph shows a gradual transition from the implant fixture to the restoration. Platform switching is seen at the implant–abutment junction.

In cases of inflammation, the peri-implant tissue must be palpated for tenderness and suppuration, the implant must be probed, and periapical radiographs must be obtained and compared with baseline images to determine peri-implant bone loss. Suppuration often indicates peri-implantitis.[24] Radiographic crestal bone loss beyond the implant baseline level at the time of final prosthesis delivery in conjunction with bleeding on probing is characteristic of peri-implantitis.[21] Due to potential measurement errors, a threshold of detectable bone loss of 1.0 to 1.5 mm is recommended for the diagnosis of peri-implantitis.[43] In the absence of a baseline radiograph, a vertical distance of 2 mm from the expected marginal bone level after the initial crestal bone remodeling is recommended as the threshold for diagnosing peri-implantitis.[43]

The amount of initial marginal bone remodeling depends on the design of the implant–abutment junction. Platform-switched implants (Fig. 87.5C; see Fig. 87.3), in which the abutment is internally offset relative to the implant fixture at the implant–abutment junction, may exhibit less crestal bone remodeling than non–platform-switched implants (see Fig. 87.4), in which the abutment is flush or even with the implant fixture at the implant–abutment junction. Bone level stability may also be influenced by soft tissue thickness or lack thereof. According to Linkevicius, vertical soft tissue thickness (above the implant platform) should be ≥3 mm to minimize crestal bone loss.[25,26]

Evaluation of Implant Osseointegration

Implant osseointegration must be determined before the fabrication and delivery of the final implant prosthesis. Implant osseointegration can be definitively determined only histologically, which requires the implant and the surrounding bone to be removed. A combination of radiographic and clinical parameters is used to assess implant osseointegration or to rule out lack of osseointegration. They include the absence of peri-implant inflammation and pain in response to palpation and percussion, a solid resonating sound in reaction to percussion, complete radiographic bone-to-implant contact along the implant surface (i.e., absence of radiolucencies along the bone-implant interface), and implant stability.

Evaluation of Implant Restorations

Implant superstructures, frameworks, and restorations should be fabricated to accommodate and facilitate oral hygiene (e.g., embrasure spaces made to allow passage of a proxy brush) (see Fig. 87.4). Occlusal schemes of implant restorations should provide adequate posterior support, maximize axial loading, and minimize incline contacts, nonaxial loading, and interferences in excursive movements.

During delivery, radiographs perpendicular to the implant should be obtained for baseline documentation and to verify the complete seating of the restorations. After delivery, cement-retained implant restorations should be thoroughly evaluated for residual excess cement, which must be removed. During follow-up visits, implant restorations should be carefully examined for heavy contacts, fractures, loose screws, and in removable prostheses, worn-out retentive components (i.e., Hader clips and locator attachment inserts). Occlusion should be adjusted accordingly to prevent implant overload and fractures of implant parts. Loose abutment and set screws must be evaluated, possibly replaced, and properly torqued down. Worn-out retentive components must be replaced periodically to ensure proper retention, stability, and function of the removable prosthesis. Occlusal wear of teeth and fit of tissue-borne surfaces of an implant prosthesis should be assessed and corrected as indicated. In patients with oral parafunction and heavy occlusal forces, occlusal guards are recommended to protect implants and restorations.

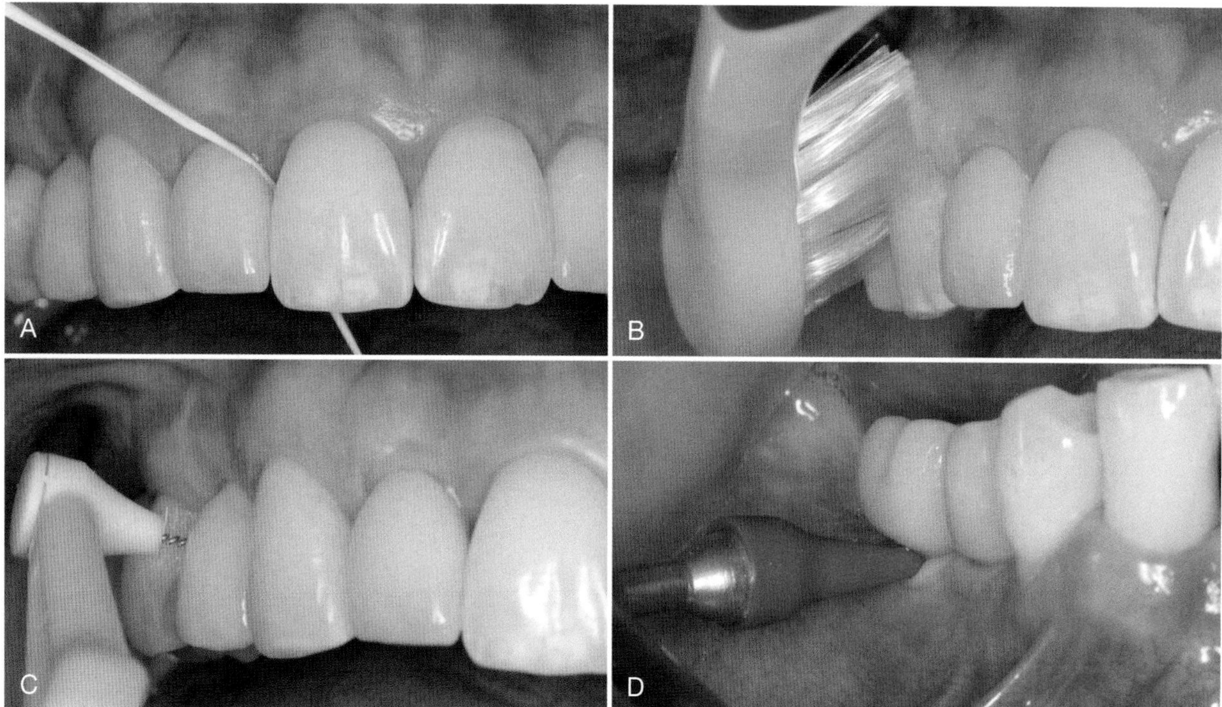

Fig. 87.6 Methods for patient oral hygiene are shown. (A) Flossing. (B) Bass method of brushing with an extra-soft toothbrush. (C) Interproximal brushing. (D) Removal of biofilm with a rubber tip. Hygiene methods remove biofilm along the gingival margin.

Implant Maintenance

Methods for Patient Oral Hygiene

The importance of good oral hygiene should be stressed even before implants are placed, and peri-implant oral hygiene for biofilm control should begin as early as possible after the implant is exposed to the oral cavity. A cotton tip, cotton gauze, or soft toothbrush can be used to gently remove biofilm from healing abutments or provisional restorations during the early postoperative phase of healing. Before implant osseointegration, the use of powered toothbrushes should be avoided.

After implant osseointegration has been achieved and verified, brushing with dentifrice can help remove deposits and increase the smoothness of exposed implant and restoration surfaces.[33] Other dental hygiene aids, such as dental floss, rubber tips, and interdental brushes, can be employed (Fig. 87.6). Oral hygiene should emphasize the removal of biofilm and deposits along the gingival margin. Evidence for the use of a powered oral irrigator around implants is limited. One study reported that subgingival irrigation of 0.06% chlorhexidine gluconate with a Waterpik device (Water Pik, Inc., Fort Collins, CO) was more effective at reducing biofilm and gingival inflammation and produced fewer stains than rinsing with 0.12% chlorhexidine gluconate once daily.[17]

Methods for Professional Recall Maintenance

Professional maintenance consists of the removal of dental biofilm and calculus from implant components exposed to the oral environment.[27] Like root surfaces, the transmucosal surfaces of implants should be smooth to minimize plaque accumulation and to facilitate oral hygiene practices.[22] At sites with excellent biofilm control and peri-implant health, the need for professional instrumentation is minimal, and instrumentation should be limited to prevent iatrogenic damage to implant components that can contribute to plaque and calculus accumulation. In the setting of biofilm, calculus, and tenacious deposits, care should be taken to minimize damage to transmucosal implant surfaces. However, priority should be placed on the complete removal of implant surface deposits.

All metal instruments, including metal curettes, scalers, and ultrasonic scalers, increase the surface roughness of polished titanium.[27] The use of plastic, Teflon-coated, and carbon and gold-coated curettes and nonmetal ultrasonic tips have been advocated to protect the titanium implant surface and the titanium abutment from contamination by other metals and to reduce the likelihood of scratching the surface. Unfortunately, the large size and flexibility of nonmetal curettes may not allow effective biofilm and calculus removal,[35] and Teflon- and gold-coated curettes cannot be sharpened.

Most implant prostheses are made with gold alloys or ceramic materials, which are usually identical to the materials used in restorations for natural dentition. The location of the connection between the restorative material and the implant is typically below the mucosa and often near the crest of bone; most calculus removal is done above this level. The fear of contaminating the titanium implant is, therefore, unwarranted. Gold alloy or ceramic surfaces can be debrided with most scalers and curettes (e.g., plastic, gold-coated, stainless steel) without damaging the surface. Rubber cups and polishing paste can be used to remove biofilm and to enhance the smoothness of machined and polished surfaces. Magnetostrictive and piezoelectric ultrasonic instruments with metal tips (e.g., Cavitron) should be used with caution because of irregularities that can easily be created in the surface.

Treatment of Peri-Implant Diseases

The goals of treatment are the elimination of all peri-implant infectious and inflammatory processes, prevention of disease progression, and preservation and restoration of function and esthetics. Treatment begins with patient education about the causes, pathogenesis, and prevention of peri-implant diseases, along with oral hygiene instruction. Although bacteria are the main etiologic factor, systemic (e.g., smoking, poorly controlled diabetes) and local factors (e.g., residual excess cement, poorly designed restorations that inhibit hygiene access) should also be identified and modified.

Peri-Implant Mucositis

Peri-implant mucositis can be effectively treated with nonsurgical mechanical therapy.[35] Treatment requires complete removal of supramucosal and submucosal biofilm, calculus, and deposits using curettes, ultrasonic scalers, and polishing cups with prophy paste. Antimicrobials (e.g., chlorhexidine irrigation and mouthrinse) can be used with mechanical debridement to enhance treatment outcomes.[35]

Peri-Implantitis

The treatment of peri-implantitis includes nonsurgical and surgical interventions, which can be combined with the adjunctive use of antimicrobials. Nonsurgical interventions include antimicrobial rinse and irrigation, local antibiotics, ultrasonic debridement, mechanical debridement with air-abrasive devices, and laser therapy. Surgical treatment includes full-thickness flap elevation for access, followed by degranulation, surface debridement by laser or mechanical instruments, surface decontamination with laser or antimicrobials, and bone augmentation. The data from two systematic reviews[14,48] are insufficient to suggest which intervention for peri-implantitis is most effective or to allow specific recommendations for the use of locally or systematically administered antibiotics.

Implant surface decontamination or disinfection remains challenging, especially for implants with roughened surfaces. For some treatment modalities, recurrence of peri-implantitis appears to be high (up to 100%) after 1 or more years of treatment, and retreatment may be necessary. Surgical access appears to be necessary to arrest peri-implant bone loss. Surgical treatment can result in gingival recession and compromised esthetics. At sites with high esthetic demands, definitive treatment of peri-implantitis can include the removal of the implant, grafting of the site, and placement of another implant.

Treatment of peri-implant mucositis is effective, whereas treatment of peri-implantitis is unpredictable. Prevention, early detection, and treatment of peri-implant inflammatory diseases are essential for successful outcomes.

Referral of Patients to the Periodontist

The previously described guidelines allow many implants to be maintained quite well by primary dental care providers (i.e., general dentists). Referral to a periodontist should be considered if peri-implantitis or peri-implant mucositis is diagnosed and cannot be resolved with improved oral hygiene and professional maintenance care. Early referral is advantageous for stopping progression and limiting the extent of bone loss.

Conclusions

Dental implants are not vulnerable to caries, but they are susceptible to mechanical and inflammatory-related biologic complications. Long-term success of dental implants requires sound treatment planning, precise surgical and restorative execution, and impeccable long-term maintenance. This chapter described the evaluation and maintenance of dental implants.

Video 87.1

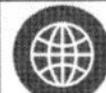
A Case Scenario is found on the companion website eBooks.Health.Elsevier.com.

Suggested Readings

Berglundh T, Lindhe J, Ericsson I, et al. The soft tissue barrier at implants and teeth. *Clin Oral Implants Res*. 1991;2:81–90.

Berglundh T, Zitzmann NU, Donati M. Are peri-implantitis lesions different from periodontitis lesions? *J Clin Periodontol*. 2011;38(suppl 11):188–202.

Carcuac O, Abrahamsson I, Albouy JP, Linder E, Larsson L, Berglundh T. Experimental periodontitis and peri-implantitis in dogs. *Clin Oral Implants Res*. 2013;24(4):363–371. https://doi.org/10.1111/clr.12067. Epub 2012 Nov 26. PMID: 23176551.

Cooper L, Moriarty J. Prosthodontic and periodontal considerations for implant-supported dental restorations. *Curr Opin Periodontol*. 1997;4:119–126.

De Bruyn H, Vandeweghe S, Ruyffelaert C, et al. Radiographic evaluation of modern oral implants with emphasis on crestal bone level and relevance to peri-implant health. *Periodontol 2000*. 2013;62:256–270.

Lang NP, Nyman SR. Supportive maintenance care for patients with implants and advanced restorative therapy. *Periodontol 2000*. 1994;4:119–126.

Linkevicius T, Apse P, Grybauskas S, Puisys A. The influence of soft tissue thickness on crestal bone changes around implants: a 1-year prospective controlled clinical trial. *Int J Oral Maxillofac Implants*. 2009;24:712–719.

Linkevicius T, Puisys A, Steigmann M, Vindasiute E, Linkeviciene L. Influence of vertical soft tissue thickness on crestal bone changes around implants with platform switching: a comparative clinical study. *Clin Implant Dent Relat Res*. 2015;17(6):1228–1236. https://doi.org/10.1111/cid.12222. Epub 2014 Mar 28. PMID: 24673875.

Louropoulou A, Slot DE, Van der Weijden FA. Titanium surface alterations following the use of different mechanical instruments: a systematic review. *Clin Oral Implants Res*. 2012;23:643–658.

Mombelli A. Microbiology and antimicrobial therapy of peri-implantitis. *Periodontol 2000*. 2002;28:177–189.

Park JB, Kim N, Ko Y. Effects of ultrasonic scaler tips and toothbrush on titanium disc surfaces evaluated with confocal microscopy. *J Craniofac Surg*. 2012;23:1552–1558.

Renvert S, Roos-Jansåker AM, Claffey N. Non-surgical treatment of peri-implant mucositis and peri-implantitis: a literature review. *J Clin Periodontol*. 2008;35(suppl):305–315.

Roos-Jansåker AM, Lindahl C, Renvert H, et al. Nine- to fourteen-year follow-up of implant treatment. Part II: presence of peri-implant lesions. *J Clin Periodontol*. 2006;33:290–295.

Serino G, Turri A, Lang NP. Probing at implants with peri-implantitis and its relation to clinical peri-implant bone loss. *Clin Oral Implants Res*. 2013;24:91–95.

Zeza B, Pilloni A. Peri-implant mucositis treatments in humans: a systematic review. *Ann Stomatol (Roma)*. 2012;3:83–89.

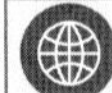
References for this chapter are found on the companion website eBooks.Health.Elsevier.com.

CHAPTER 88

Results of Implant Treatment

Perry R. Klokkevold

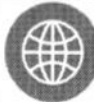
An animation has been added by the editors as a supplement to the chapter. It was produced by PerioPixel as a patient education tool and covers the basic elements in a conceptual manner. It is not intended to be a procedural guide for dental professionals.

CHAPTER OUTLINE

The landmark Göteborg study and the replica study at the University of Toronto supported expectations for the success and predictability of root form dental implants. The study, conducted over a 15-year period at the University of Göteborg, Sweden, by Bränemark and coworkers, began in 1965 and concluded in 1980. The results, which were reported in several articles, defined the concept of osseointegration, described protocols for success, and shared clinical experiences.

The most significant article from the study, published in 1981, was on osseointegrated implants in the treatment of the edentulous jaw.[2] The Göteborg study included 2768 root form implants placed into 410 edentulous jaws in 371 consecutive patients. The data were usually reported in subsets according to the three study phases—initial, developmental, and routine. Cases treated in the routine period with standardized procedures and an observation time of 5 to 9 years were thought to reflect the potential of the method and were the basis of data reported in that historic publication. The subset consisted of 895 implants placed in 130 jaws. The implant survival rate was 81% in the maxilla and 91% in the mandible. The prosthesis survival (i.e., continuous stability) rate was 89% in the maxilla and 100% in the mandible.

The replica study, which was conducted at the University of Toronto, demonstrated that comparable results could be predictably achieved using the same implant design and treatment protocols.[5,85-87] Together, these studies demonstrated that an implant survival of 81% or more and prosthesis survival of 89% or more could be expected in the edentulous patient.

In the decades since the landmark discovery of osseointegration and the documentation of its clinical effectiveness, clinicians have had tremendous success in replacing missing teeth with endosseous root form dental implants in both partially edentulous and edentulous patients.[1,51] In 2017, Buser and colleagues published a comprehensive report detailing the successes, current trends, and pending questions following 50 years of modern implant dentistry.[12] Despite the high level of success and long-term predictability, a 100% success rate cannot be achieved.

Complications and implant failures do occur.[2,13] Some implants fail to achieve osseointegration, some achieve osseointegration but lose bone progressively over time, leading to failure, and other implants rapidly lose bone and fail in a short time. Some implants achieve and maintain osseointegration but fail because they do not meet the esthetic expectations of the patient or clinician.

The reporting of implant success varies widely in the literature, which makes defining an absolute implant success rate impractical. This chapter considers implant treatment results in light of the factors that influence implant survival and success. The intent is to outline important aspects that need to be considered in evaluating implant outcomes and offer guidelines for understanding published results.

Defining Implant Outcomes

Implant outcomes are reported in a variety of ways in the literature. Various levels of implant success and failure are described in case reports, case series, retrospective studies, controlled studies, and prospective studies. The type of study and method of reporting are decided by the authors and are often influenced by the data collected and the study objectives. Each type of study or report has recognized limitations but, because of the tremendous variation that exists in how individual investigators measure, interpret, and report implant outcomes, differences in the results from one study to another may not be obvious.

Some implant outcomes are reported as the presence or absence of the implant at the time of the last examination, regardless of whether the implant was functional, suffered from bone loss, or had other problems. This type of assessment is a measure of implant *survival* and should not be confused with implant *success*. In contrast to such an overly simplified assessment, some investigators report implant outcomes using specific criteria to determine implant success.

Implant success is defined by specific criteria used to evaluate the condition and function of the implant. Criteria for implant success have been proposed in the literature but have not been used consistently. The problem is that a universally accepted and agreed on definition of implant success has not been established. In the classic definition, Albrektsson and colleagues[3] defined success as an implant with no pain, no mobility, no radiolucent peri-implant areas, and less than 0.2 mm of bone loss annually after the first year of loading.[3] Bone loss in the first year was recognized but was not defined or quantified as part of the success criteria until later, in a separate definition by Roos and associates.[66]

The challenge in comparing reported data between studies is that investigators use different criteria for success. As a result, it is difficult or impossible to make comparisons between studies, and drawing conclusions about implant success or failure from data reported in different studies is tenuous at best.

Success rates are dramatically affected by variations in the criteria used to define them. In strict terms, if implant success is considered to be an outcome without adverse effects or problems, the treatment would be performed as planned, implants would remain stable and function without problems, peri-implant tissues would be stable and healthy, and the patient and treating clinician would be pleased with the outcome (Fig. 88.1). Use of strict criteria would produce implant success rates lower than those determined using less stringent criteria.

Table 88.1 illustrates the powerful effect that small changes in success criteria have on reported success rates. The data

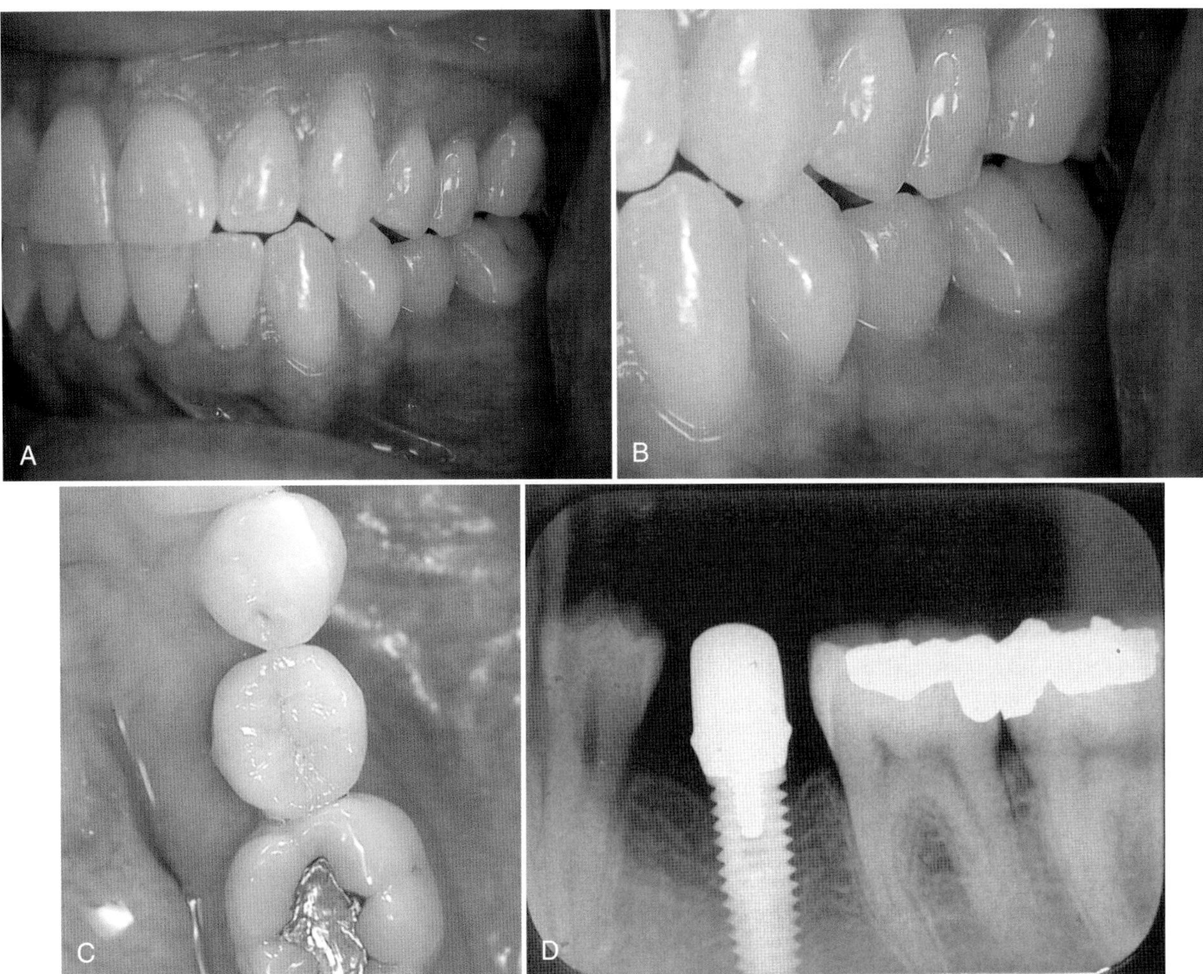

Fig. 88.1 Clinical implant success was demonstrated when a single implant was placed in the mandible to replace the lower second premolar (as planned). The implant osseointegrated, and function was successfully restored. The patient and clinicians were pleased with the outcome. (A) Photograph of the dentition in occlusion (from the left side). (B) Close-up photograph of the dentition in occlusion. The mandibular second premolar is an implant-supported crown. (C) Occlusal view of an implant-supported crown in the second premolar position. Replacement of the mandibular second premolar with an implant is a conservative treatment, obviating the need to prepare adjacent teeth. (D) Periapical radiograph of the posterior mandibular teeth and implant in the second premolar position. Bone support is good, and bone loss is minimal and consistent with expectations for this implant design.

TABLE 88.1 Effect of Slight Modifications of Implant Success Criteria on Successful Outcomes[a]

Group	PPD ≤ 5 mm, no BOP, BL < 0.2 mm/yr (%)	PPD ≤ 6 mm, no BOP, BL < 0.2 mm/yr (%)	PPD ≤5 mm, no BOP (%)	PPD ≤ 6 mm, no BOP (%)	Implant Survival (%)
Group A	52.4	62	71.4	81	90.5
Group B	79.1	81.3	94.5	96.7	96.5

[a]The initial success criteria at 10 years were set as a PPD ≤ 5 mm, no BOP, and BL < 0.2 mm annually. The implant success rates for group A (patients with a history of periodontitis) and group B (patients with periodontal health) using these initial criteria are listed in the first column. Notice how dramatically the success rates change when the criteria used to define success are modified to include PPD ≤ 6 mm (second column). The next two columns show the success rates for each group using PPD ≤ 5 mm and PPD ≤ 6 mm when the criteria are modified to omit bone loss as a determinant. The last column shows the implant survival rate for each group, which demonstrates that the survival rate is different than the success rate.

BL, Bone loss; *BOP,* bleeding on probing; *PPD,* probing pocket depth.

Data from Karoussis IK, Salvi GE, Heitz-Mayfield LJ, et al: Long-term implant prognosis in patients with and without a history of chronic periodontitis: a 10-year prospective cohort study of the ITI Dental Implant System. *Clin Oral Implant Res.* 2003;14:329-339.

demonstrate that changing the criteria of success to include a probing pocket depth (PPD) of 5 mm or less to 6 mm or less changed the implant success rates from 52.4% to 62% and from 79.1% to 81.3% for patients with and without a history of periodontitis, respectively.[45] This also shows that implant survival is quite different from implant success.

KEY FACT

Implant success is defined by specific criteria used to evaluate the condition and function of the implant. Criteria for implant success have been proposed in the literature but have not been used consistently across different studies. The problem is that depending on the criteria used, the rates of reported implant success can vary substantially from one study to another.

Implant survival is defined as an implant that remains in place at the time of evaluation, regardless of untoward signs and symptoms or a history of problems. Extant implants that are healthy and functioning under an implant-retained restoration are different from those that are suffering from peri-implant bone loss or those that are not connected to a restoration and are not functioning (Fig. 88.2), but these operational differences do not affect calculations of implant survival. Implants that are osseointegrated but not functional are referred to as sleepers and should not be considered successful merely because they are present and osseointegrated.

Implant survival and implant success are different outcome measures. Consider the dramatic difference between survival and success rates for implants reported in a systematic review that included 21 studies of implants supporting fixed partial dentures.[63] The 5-year implant survival rate was 95.4%, whereas the overall 5-year success rate (individual implant success rates were not calculated), defined as free of complications, was only 61.3%.[63]

In a 10-year retrospective study of 397 fixed implant reconstructions in 300 patients, the observed mechanical complication rate was 24.7%.[83] The most frequent complication was ceramic chipping (20.31%), followed by occlusal screw loosening (2.57%) and loss of retention (2.06%).[83] Although relatively uncommon, occlusal screw loosening can result in a subgingival gap at the implant-abutment junction that retains plaque (biofilm) and stimulates an

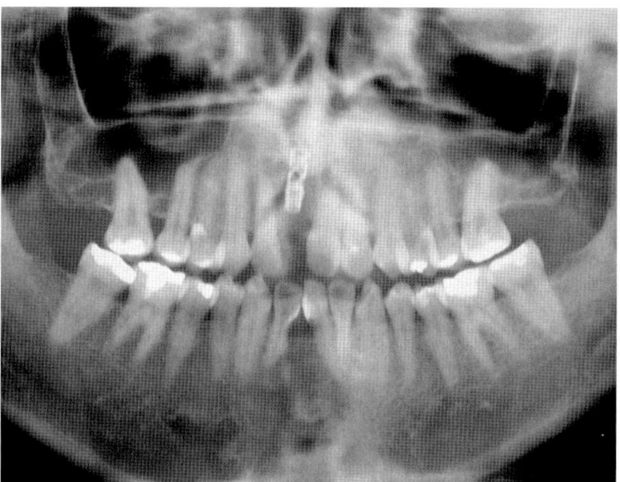

Fig. 88.2 Panoramic radiograph shows an implant placed in the position of a missing maxillary right central incisor. The implant appears to be placed in a nonrestorable position. It is osseointegrated and could technically be counted as a surviving implant, but it must be considered a failure because it does not meet the intended goal and function has not been restored.

inflammatory reaction in the soft and hard tissues, leading to bone loss around the implant. Although surviving, these implants would fail to meet optimal success criteria.

Defining implant results in absolute terms is difficult and confusing. Implant survival, which typically is reported in studies, can overestimate good implant outcomes. Implant success, which is reported less often, could offer a better measure if specific success criteria were universally defined, accepted, and used. However, implant success is difficult or impossible to compare across studies because of differences in evaluation criteria used by investigators. Implant success in a single study or series of studies using the same success criteria is meaningful only in the context of that study or series.

Currently, the usefulness of implant success rates from different studies is limited. Implant survival is important but is only an indicator of surviving implants and does not reveal whether they are functioning or had problems associated with them over time. The incidence of peri-implant problems is more significant than once thought. A systematic review of the literature evaluating the prevalence of peri-implant disease reported that peri-implant mucositis and peri-implantitis occurred in 19% to 65% and 1% to 47% of cases, respectively.[24]

Factors That Influence Implant Outcomes

Many issues influence implant outcomes, including available bone, implant design, placement and loading protocols, and host-related factors.

Anatomic Location

Osseointegration depends on the availability of an adequate quantity and quality of bone at the implant site. Areas with abundant bone volume in the desired location are better than those with deficient bone volume. Areas with good bone density provide more predictable outcomes than those with poor bone density.

The bone classification system described by Lekholm and Zarb[52] defines bone with different levels of support for implants and the likely impact on survival and success. The quality of bone support is greatly influenced by the anatomic location, and implant outcomes are sometimes categorized according to location. Extreme examples are the anterior mandible and posterior maxilla. The anterior mandible typically consists of dense cortical bone, which offers great support and high bone to implant contact, whereas the posterior maxilla is often limited in volume because of alveolar resorption and sinus pneumatization; it typically consists of a loose trabecular structure and a thin cortical bone shell.

Implants placed in the posterior maxilla are less well supported compared with implants placed in the anterior mandible. Jaffin and Berman[38] demonstrated the significance of bone quality on implant survival in a report of 1054 Bränemark implants. Of these implants, 90% were placed in type I, II, or III bone, with a failure rate of only 3%. Of the 10% that were placed in type IV bone, 35% failed.[38] Excluding those placed in the mandible, 23 (44%) of 52 implants placed in type IV bone in the maxilla failed, for a dismal survival rate of 56%. The study authors concluded that bone quality was the single greatest determinant of implant loss.

Anatomic location has a significant effect on implant outcome, particularly for the posterior maxilla. The implants used in the study by Jaffin and Berman[38] had machined surfaces, and current implants with altered microtopography are thought to perform better in the posterior maxilla due to increased bone to implant contact. When all 1054 implants, placed in all types of bone, are considered together, the combined implant survival rate (93.9%) in the study is within or slightly higher than the reported range in the Göteborg study (done with similar implants).

Implant Design

Implant design influences outcome. Hundreds of companies manufacture and market dental implants worldwide, and the number continues to grow. Implant dimensions, geometries, and surface characteristics vary tremendously and continue to evolve as innovation and research findings pave the way for changes that are thought to improve outcomes. Very few implant designs have been studied. They instead rely on being clinically similar to researched and approved designs without additional studies or documentation to support their effectiveness. In most cases, it is impossible to appreciate the effect of a particular implant design feature on outcomes. Nonetheless, novel implant designs are being used, and outcomes are being reported from studies that evaluated other aspects of treatment that are not specific to the design, which makes comparisons and assessments more confusing and unreliable.

The studies that have documented the success of dental implants based on design characteristics have shaped current standards for selection and use. For example, many clinicians adhere to the premise that longer implants, threaded implants, and rough-surfaced implants are better than shorter, unthreaded, and smooth designs. As changes in design and use have evolved over time, some beliefs have been disproved, such as the successful application of short implants.[61,64] Continued advances and research will undoubtedly refute other firmly held beliefs.

Clinicians would like to know whether one implant design performs better than the rest, but it is almost impossible to determine which design characteristics are important because there are many variables to consider and implants are successful most of the time. Given the generally high rate of success, it appears that subtle differences in implant design are probably not significant for most patients and situations.[26,30] However, in patients with inadequate sites, risk factors, or challenging circumstances, certain implant designs may perform better than others. An example is the effect of implant surface characteristics. Implants with altered surface microtopography (e.g., acid-etched or blasted) enhance the bone to implant interface[47,48] and can improve outcomes, especially in compromised sites.[76,77] Lower success rates have been associated with smooth-surfaced (i.e., machined) implants.[39,65,69]

Implant length is another consideration. Many studies have supported the principle that longer is better for implant success,[70,71] but later studies have challenged this.[33] Another important feature is the macrothread design of implants. Clinical research[55] evaluating the stability (assessed by resonance frequency analysis) of a novel implant designed with a wide thread depth and increased pitch found that it did not cause the typical decrease in stability in the early postoperative healing period. This finding may have an impact on early and immediate loading protocols.

KEY FACT

Many features influence outcomes, including available bone, implant design, placement and loading protocols, and host-related factors. Defining implant results in absolute terms can be difficult and confusing.

Placement and Loading Protocols

The traditional placement protocol required a healed edentulous ridge into which implants were placed and allowed to osseointegrate for a period without occlusal loading (see Chapter 78). The nonloading period after implant placement was empirically determined to be 3 to 4 months in the mandible and 6 months in the maxilla.[10] A strongly held belief was that early loading would lead to higher failure rates.[11] However, several studies have challenged this belief.

In contrast to the early standards, some current protocols advocate dramatically different approaches, including implant placement immediately after tooth extraction and implant occlusal loading immediately or shortly after placement. Each of these approaches has distinct advantages, but they are accompanied by challenges that have the potential to affect outcomes adversely.

Immediate Implant Placement

The immediate implant placement protocol describes the procedure in which an implant is placed in an extraction socket after tooth removal and socket débridement. This procedure, described by Schulte and colleagues[73] in 1978 and by Lazzara in 1989,[50] has been reported with survival rates equivalent to those of implants placed into healed ridges.[15,54] The advantages of immediate placement include decreased surgery, cost, and healing time.[74] Immediate implant placement introduces an additional risk of complications, including poor implant position, compromised esthetic outcome, and implant failure (see Chapter 86). Despite the increased risk, a high long-term (1- to 16-year) survival rate of 96% has been reported for implants immediately placed into extraction sockets.[80] A recent (2019) systematic review and meta-analysis of the literature, including eight clinical trials that met inclusion criteria, concluded that immediate implants placed into infected sites presented a statistically significant higher risk of implant failure (almost three times higher) when compared to immediate implants placed in noninfected sites.[23]

Immediate Occlusal Loading

Brånemark established the concept of the osseointegrated dental implant as a predictable treatment modality for the edentulous patient on the empirically based requirement that the implant remain submerged and unloaded for a healing period of 3 to 6 months.[10] This original protocol, requiring the implant to remain stress-free, was based on the concern that premature loading would cause micromotion of the dental implant, leading to fibrous encapsulation and implant failure. However, studies have shown this assumption to be incorrect, demonstrating that immediately loaded implants can achieve success rates (>90%) similar to those for conventionally loaded dental implants.[16,20,31,35,43] The long-term predictability of immediately loaded implants requires strict surgical and prosthodontic protocols.[7]

Bone Augmentation

A common problem encountered in implant dentistry is insufficient bone quantity to allow implant placement. Deficiencies in alveolar bone result from developmental defects, periodontal disease, tooth loss, or trauma.[6,14,72] For most cases with alveolar ridge resorption, bone regenerative procedures are required to correct the defects before or simultaneously with implant placement (see Chapters 79 and 80). The question is whether implants placed in sites that are reconstructed with bone augmentation procedures can achieve the same survival and success rates as implants placed in native bone sites.

The results of implants and bone augmentation procedures reported in the literature have been assessed by expert clinicians in several workshops.[17,32,36,37] One systematic review of the literature—2003 Workshop on Contemporary Science in Clinical Periodontics—including 13 studies (guided bone regeneration) with 1741 patients and 5 studies (distraction osteogenesis) with 92 patients, found that survival rates of dental implants in augmented bone achieved a high level of predictability that was similar to that for implants placed in natural (nongrafted) bone.[32]

Another systematic review of the literature, 2008 Consensus Report of the Sixth European Workshop on Periodontology,[78] pointed out that bone augmentation procedures can fail and that implants placed in these areas do not enjoy the high long-term survival rates of dental implants placed in pristine sites.[78] The 2003 systematic review did not include an assessment of whether bone augmentation procedures failed; it intentionally focused on implants placed in sites that were successfully treated with bone augmentation. More research is needed to determine the long-term performance of dental implants placed in augmented bone and the clinical benefits of bone augmentation with respect to alternative treatments (e.g., use of short implants).

Risk Factors

Most patients enjoy similar rates of survival and success with dental implants. Only a few patients experience implant failure.

In addition to the factors previously discussed, host-related factors can adversely affect healing, osseointegration, and maintenance of dental implants. Smoking, diabetes, and periodontitis have been identified as risk factors that can adversely affect implant outcomes. In a systematic review of the literature, Klokkevold and Han[46] evaluated the influence of smoking, diabetes, and periodontal disease on outcomes and found that smoking has an adverse effect on implant survival and success, with the effects being more pronounced in areas of loose trabecular bone (e.g., posterior maxilla).

The review also suggested that type 2 diabetes had an adverse effect on implant survival rates, but the limited number of included studies did not permit a definitive conclusion.[46] The review did conclude that although patients with a history of treated periodontitis did not show a decrease in implant survival, they did experience more complications and lower success rates, especially when the implants were followed over longer periods (10+ years).[46] A recent systematic review and meta-analysis, including 10 published studies evaluating the association between diabetes and dental implant complications, confirms this earlier finding—that patients with diabetes have more implant complications, including marginal bone loss, probing depth, and bleeding around dental implants.[42] A further subgroup analysis of this report suggested that as level of glycated hemoglobin (HbA1c) increases, peri-implant bleeding increases.

Smoking

Above all other risk factors, smoking has a significant negative impact on implant survival and success. In a study of 2194 implants, Bain and Moy reported a significantly greater rate of failure among smokers (11.28%) than nonsmokers (4.76%).[7a] De Bruyn and Colleart reported an early failure rate of 9% among smokers compared with 1% among nonsmokers.[19] Two studies, one of 10 years' duration[27] and the other with a follow-up assessment of 6 months to 21 years,[59] concluded that smoking was a definite risk factor for implant survival.[21,22] Peri-implant bone loss appears to be more significant in smokers with a history of periodontal disease, based on a 9-year follow-up study.[79]

Diabetes

The role of diabetes mellitus as a risk factor for implant outcomes is less clear. Although a metabolic disease such as diabetes was expected to have an adverse effect on bone healing[81] and tissue support for implants, the research has not definitively determined that diabetes has a negative impact on implant survival or success.[4]

Moy and coworkers[59] reported a significantly lower success rate (68.7%) for patients with diabetes compared with the success rate (85.1%) for the entire study population (1140 patients with 4680 implants); individual implant survival and success rates were not reported. However, the low success rate (i.e., high failure rate) may be an overestimate of the actual implant failure rate for patients with diabetes because it counts the number of patients with failures regardless of how many implants they had; implants successfully inserted and maintained in these patients were not counted. There were 48 patients with diabetes in the study, 4.2% of the 1140 total. Of these, 15 patients experienced implant failures.

Conversely, in a systematic review of the literature (33 studies), Javed and Romanos found that patients with good metabolic control (i.e., HbA1c levels in the normal range) achieve success rates with osseointegrated implants that are similar to those for patients without diabetes.[40] Dowell and coworkers[25] also noted similar success for implants placed in patients with controlled diabetes. As stated above, patients with poorly controlled diabetes appear to have higher complications with implant treatment.[42]

Periodontitis

A limited number of studies have assessed the prognosis of implant treatment in patients with a history of periodontitis.[44] Most of these studies suggest that implants are equally successful in patients with a history of chronic periodontitis (periodontitis, grade B). Short-term studies demonstrate 90–100% implant survival in patients with a history of periodontitis, grade B (chronic).[56,58] Long-term studies report 90% to 97% implant survival rates for patients with a history of periodontitis, grade B (chronic).[45,53,67,82] Short-term implant survival rates for patients treated for aggressive periodontitis (periodontitis, grade C) are 95% to 100%.[56,57] One long-term study reported an 88.8% implant survival rate over 5 years for patients treated for periodontitis, grade C (aggressive).[58]

Implant survival in patients with a history of periodontitis appears to be highly predictable. However, the lack of long-term studies to support implant survival in patients treated for periodontitis, grade C (aggressive) leaves the prognosis for these patients open to question.[44]

Long-term studies evaluating implant treatment in periodontally compromised patients suggest that they may experience more peri-implant problems.[45] When these patients are followed for extended periods, there appear to be more complications (e.g., peri-implantitis) associated with implants than in periodontally healthy patients. In a 10-year prospective study of patients with and without a history of chronic periodontitis, the rate of biologic complications (e.g., peri-implantitis) was higher for those with a history of periodontitis, grade B (28.6%), than those with periodontal health (5.8%).[45] This controlled study by Karoussis and coworkers[45] found a statistically significant difference in mean peri-implant bone loss between patients with a history of periodontitis, grade B, and patients who were periodontally healthy.

Peri-implant problems may be attributed to a continuous increase in the percentage of implants exhibiting probing pocket depths of 4 mm or deeper over time.[28] A systematic review of implant outcomes in patients treated for periodontitis concluded that these individuals had a greater incidence of biologic complications and lower success and survival rates compared with periodontally healthy subjects.[75]

KEY FACT

Smoking, diabetes, and periodontitis are risk factors that can adversely affect implant outcomes.

Esthetic Results and Patient Satisfaction

The ultimate goal of treatment is to achieve natural-appearing, optimally functioning, implant-supported tooth replacements. Proper

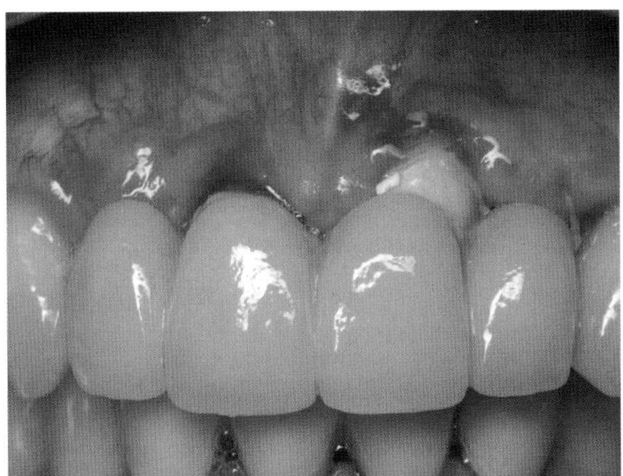

Fig. 88.3 Clinical photograph shows a maxillary anterior fixed restoration supported by two malpositioned implants in the central incisor positions. The patient was dissatisfied with the esthetic outcome. The left implant was positioned between the central and lateral incisor and angled toward the facial surface at a level above the gingival margin. A tooth-colored material was used to mask the exposed framework in the gingival area.

tooth dimensions and contours and ideal soft tissue support are key factors for successful esthetic outcomes.[49] If crown form, dimension, and shape and gingival harmony around the implants are not ideal, the patient may consider the implant restoration unacceptable because the result does not represent a natural dental profile (Fig. 88.3). For some patients, such as those with severe alveolar deficiency, an ideal esthetic outcome may be impossible because reconstructive surgical procedures are complex, require extensive time, and remain unpredictable. For others, a less than ideal esthetic outcome may be acceptable (see Chapter 81).

Esthetic problems and patient dissatisfaction occur when results are inferior to what was expected. Satisfaction with the esthetic outcome of the implant prosthesis varies from patient to patient, depending on a number of factors. The risk for esthetic failure is increased for patients with high esthetic expectations. The risk is also higher when patients present with patient-related risk factors such as a high smile line, thin periodontal soft tissues, and compromised bone support. Two systematic reviews reported that the patient's perceptions and desires greatly influence and determine how well the implant outcome is accepted.[18,60]

Although infrequently reported, esthetic success and patient satisfaction need to be included when considering the results of implant therapy. Although patient-reported esthetic outcome measures are becoming increasingly more important and studied, there is a lack of standardized methods to collect and report them.[84] Despite several proposed methods for evaluating esthetic results, reports of esthetic parameters in the scientific literature are scarce.[9,84] A restorative index appraises the white esthetics of the final restoration,[41] a soft tissue or pink esthetic score considers soft tissue parameters,[34] and an esthetic index uses a combination of pink and white esthetic scores, focusing on the visible part of the implant restoration.[8] These indices quantify the esthetic result, providing an objective method of judging esthetic success.

In a survey of patient satisfaction, more than 90% of patients were completely satisfied in terms of function and esthetics.[62] A questionnaire was given to 104 patients 5 to 15 years (mean, 10.2 years) after implant placement to assess subjective perceptions of treatment. Of these patients, 48% were treated with single implant crowns and 52% were treated with fixed partial dentures. The survival rate for all implants was 93%. Most patients had favorable responses to the questions regarding function, esthetics, hygiene, and cost. Table 88.2 lists the percentage of patients responding as highly satisfied or satisfied for each category. Comparing chewing comfort for teeth or implants, 72.1% perceived no difference, 17.3% felt more secure chewing on teeth, and 7.7% felt more secure chewing on implants. A systematic review and meta-analysis focused on the esthetics of implant and tooth-supported fixed dental prostheses (FDPs) concluded that patient satisfaction was high for implant-supported FDPs and surrounding mucosa.[84]

TABLE 88.2 Patient Satisfaction with Implant Treatment

Implant Experience	Highly Satisfied or Satisfied (%)[a]
Function or chewing	97
Phonetics	96
Esthetics	97
Oral hygiene ease	93
Complete fulfillment	92
Would do treatment again	94
Would recommend to friend or relative	89
Reasonable or justified cost	87

[a]Percentage of patients subjectively responding with *highly satisfied* or *satisfied* to survey questions about their implant experience. More than 90% responded favorably and thought implant treatment was a positive experience.

Data from Pjetursson BE, Karoussis I, Burgin W, et al: Patients' satisfaction following implant therapy. A 10-year prospective cohort study. *Clin Oral Implants Res.* 2005;16:185-193.

In another survey, patient satisfaction with implant-supported prostheses in totally edentulous jaws was evaluated.[68] Experience with an implant-supported prosthesis was assessed over a period of 10 years, and 97% of the 135 patients reported overall satisfaction with treatment. Chewing satisfaction was reported as good or very good by all but one patient (99.3% positive response rate). Improved lifestyle and greater self-confidence in public were reported by 75% and 82% of patients, respectively.

A systematic review of the literature, which included all randomized controlled trials published in English or French up to April 2007 comparing conventional mandibular dentures and implant overdentures in adult edentulous patients, identified eight publications for meta-analysis.[29] The study reported that patients were more satisfied with implant overdentures than with conventional mandibular dentures. However, there was a lack of evidence to show a patient's perception of the impact of mandibular implant overdentures on general health.

CLINICAL CORRELATION

Esthetic problems and dissatisfaction occur when results do not match a patient's expectations. Satisfaction with the esthetic outcome of an implant prosthesis varies among patients. The risk of failure is greater among those with high esthetic demands and risk factors such as a high smile line, thin periodontal soft tissues, or compromised bone support.

Conclusions

The use of dental implants to replace missing teeth is highly predictable, advantageous, and beneficial for patients. Because of variations in implant designs, study protocols, and populations studied, results are difficult to compare and an absolute definition of implant success remains elusive. The results of implant treatment are reported using a wide range of criteria from being present (i.e., survival) to being functional without complications (i.e., success). Patient-reported outcomes (PROs) are becoming increasingly more important, yet a reliable protocol for collecting and reporting them is limited.

It is challenging to compare the results of studies because the number of variables continues to change. Clinical research suggests that certain risk factors can decrease success rates for some patients. Understanding what is being reported in the literature helps patients and clinicians appreciate implant treatment results.

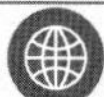
A Case Scenario is found on the companion website eBooks.Health.Elsevier.com

Suggested Readings

Albrektsson T, Zarb G, Worthington P, et al. The long-term efficacy of currently used dental implants: a review and proposed criteria of success. *Int J Oral Maxillofac Implants*. 1986;1:11–25.

Buser D, Sennerby L, De Bruyn H. Modern implant dentistry based on osseointegration: 50 years of progress, current trends and open questions. *Periodontol 2000*. 2017;73(1):7–21.

Cosyn J, Thoma DS, Hämmerle CH, et al. Esthetic assessments in implant dentistry: objective and subjective criteria for clinicians and patients. *Periodontol 2000*. 2017;73:193–202.

DeLuca S, Habsha E, Zarb GA. The effect of smoking on osseointegrated dental implants. Part I: implant survival. *Int J Prosthodont*. 2006;19:491–498.

DeLuca S, Zarb G. The effect of smoking on osseointegrated dental implants. Part II: peri-implant bone loss. *Int J Prosthodont*. 2006;19:560–566.

de Oliveira-Neto OB, Lemos CA, Barbosa FT, et al. Immediate dental implants placed into infected sites present a higher risk of failure than immediate dental implants placed into non-infected sites: systematic review and meta-analysis. *Med Oral Patol Oral Cir Bucal*. 2019;24(4):e518–e528.

Derks J, Tomasi C. Peri-implant health and disease. A systematic review of current epidemiology [review]. *J Clin Periodontol*. 2015;42(suppl 16):S158–S171.

Fugazzotto PA, Beagle JR, Ganeles J, et al. Success and failure rates of 9 mm or shorter implants in the replacement of missing maxillary molars when restored with individual crowns: preliminary results 0 to 84 months in function. A retrospective study. *J Periodontol*. 2004;75:327–332.

Jaffin RA, Berman CL. The excessive loss of Brånemark fixtures in type IV bone: a 5-year analysis. *J Periodontol*. 1991;62:2–4.

Javed F, Romanos GE. Impact of diabetes mellitus and glycemic control on the osseointegration of dental implants: a systematic literature review. *J Periodontol*. 2009;80:1719–1730.

Jiang X, Zhu Y, Liu Z, et al. Association between diabetes and dental implant complications: a systematic review and meta-analysis. *Acta Odontol Scand*. 2021;79(1):9–18.

Karoussis IK, Kotsovilis S, Fourmousis I. A comprehensive and critical review of dental implant prognosis in periodontally compromised partially edentulous patients. *Clin Oral Implants Res*. 2007;18:669–679.

Klokkevold PR, Han TJ. How do smoking, diabetes, and periodontitis affect outcomes of implant treatment? *Int J Oral Maxillofac Implants*. 2007;22(suppl):173–202.

McCullough JJ, Klokkevold PR. The effect of implant macro-thread design on implant stability in the early post-operative period: a randomized, controlled pilot study. *Clin Oral Implants Res*. 2017;28:1218–1226.

Mengel R, Flores-de-Jacoby L. Implants in patients treated for generalized aggressive and chronic periodontitis: a 3-year prospective longitudinal study. *J Periodontol*. 2005;76:534–543.

Papaspyridakos P, De Souza A, Vazouras K, et al. Survival rates of short dental implants (≤6 mm) compared with implants longer than 6 mm in posterior jaw areas: a meta-analysis. *Clin Oral Implants Res*. 2018;29(suppl 16):8–20.

Pjetursson BE, Tan K, Lang NP, et al. A systematic review of the survival and complication rates of fixed partial dentures (FPDs) after an observation period of at least 5 years. *Clin Oral Implants Res*. 2004;15:625–642.

Ravidà A, Galli M, Bianchi M, et al. Clinical outcomes of short implants (≤ 6 mm) placed between two adjacent teeth/implants or in the most distal position: a systematic review and meta-analysis. *Int J Oral Implantol (Berl)*. 2021;14(3):241–257.

Vervaeke S, Collaert B, Cosyn J, De Bruyn H. A 9-year prospective case series using multivariate analyses to identify predictors of early and late peri-implant bone loss. *Clin Implant Dent Relat Res*. 2016;18(1):30–39.

Wittneben JG, Wismeijer D, Brägger U, et al. Patient-reported outcome measures focusing on aesthetics of implant- and tooth-supported fixed dental prostheses: a systematic review and meta-analysis. *Clin Oral Implants Res*. 2018;29(suppl 16):224–240.

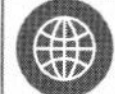
References for this chapter are found on the companion website eBooks.Health.Elsevier.com.

INDEX

Note: Page numbers followed by "*f*" refer to illustrations; page numbers followed by "*t*" refer to tables; page numbers followed by "*b*" refer to boxes.

G

Q

R